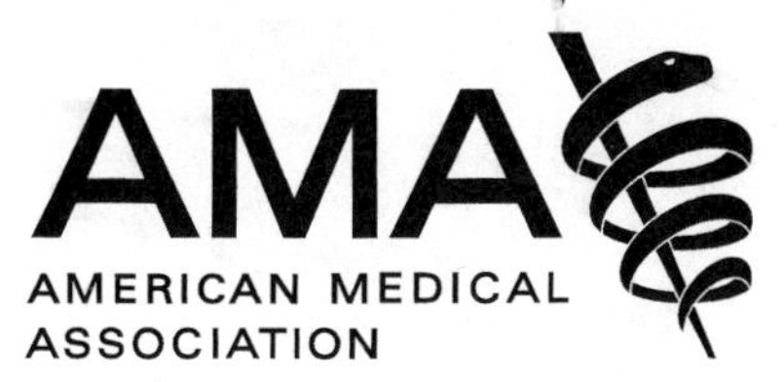

cpt® CODING ESSENTIALS

Urology and Nephrology | 2022

CPT® Coding Essentials Urology and Nephrology 2022

Fee schedules, relative value units, conversion factors and/or related components are not assigned by the AMA, are not part of CPT, and the AMA is not recommending their use. Neither DecisionHealth nor the AMA directly or indirectly practices medicine or dispenses medical services. The AMA and DecisionHealth assume no liability for data contained or not contained herein. The AMA and DecisionHealth disclaim responsibility for any consequences or liability attributable to or related to any use, nonuse or interpretation of information contained in this product.

This publication does not replace the AMA's Current Procedural Terminology codebook or other appropriate coding authority. The coding information in this publication should be used only as a guide.

Disclaimer

This publication is sold with the understanding that neither DecisionHealth nor the American Medical Association is engaged in rendering legal, medical, accounting, or other professional services in specific situations. Although prepared for professionals, this publication should not be used as a substitute for professional services in specific situations. If legal or medical advice is required, the services of a professional should be sought.

Printed in the United States of America

ISBN: 978-1-64016-146-7
OP260022

Additional copies of this book or other AMA products may be ordered by calling 612-435-6065 or visiting the AMA Store at amastore.com. Refer to product number OP260022.

AMA publication and product updates, errata, and addendum can be found at *amaproductupdates.org.*

Published by DecisionHealth, an HCPro brand
100 Winners Circle, Suite 300
Brentwood, TN 37027
www.codingbooks.com

Contents

Codes List

The CPT surgery and ancillary codes and code ranges that appear in this book are listed below.

Surgery Codes

10004
10005-10008
10009-10012
10021
10030
10180
11004-11006
11420-11426
11620-11626
12001-12007
12020-12021
12041-12047
13131-13133
13160
17270-17276
35800-35860
36000
36011-36012
36245-36248
36251-36252
36253-36254
36415-36416
36593
36600
36800-36815
36818-36820
36821
36825-36830
36831
36832-36833
36835
36838
36860-36861
36901-36903
36904-36906
36907-36908
36909
37788
37790
38500-38505
38531
38562-38564
38570
38760-38765
38770
38780
44660-44661
49000-49002
49010
49020
49060
49082-49083
49084
49180
49185
49320
49321
49324-49325
49327
49400
49402
49405-49407
49411-49412
49418
49419
49421-49422
49423-49424
49435
49436
50010
50020
50040
50045
50060-50065
50070-50075
50080-50081
50100
50120-50135
50200-50205
50220-50225
50230
50234-50236
50240
50250
50280
50290
50300
50320
50323-50325
50327-50328
50329
50340
50360-50365
50370
50380
50382-50384
50385-50386
50387
50389
50390
50391
50396
50400-50405
50430-50431
50432-50433
50434-50435
50436-50437
50500
50520
50525-50526
50540
50541-50542
50543
50544
50545
50546
50547
50548
50551-50553
50555-50557
50561
50562
50570-50572
50574
50575
50576
50580
50590
50592
50593
50600
50605
50606
50610-50630
50650
50660
50684
50686
50688
50690
50693
50694-50695
50700
50705
50706
50715
50722-50725
50727-50728
50740-50750
50760-50770
50780-50785
50800
50810
50815-50820
50825
50830
50840
50845
50860
50900
50920-50930
50940
50945
50947-50948
50951-50953
50955-50961
50970-50972
50974-50980
51020-51030
51040
51045

51050
51060
51065
51080
51100-51102
51500
51520-51530
51535
51550-51565
51570-51575
51580-51585
51590-51595
51596
51597
51600
51605
51610
51700
51701
51702-51703
51705-51710
51715
51720
51725
51726-51729
51736-51741
51784-51785
51792
51797
51798
51800-51820
51840-51841
51860-51865
51880
51900
51920-51925
51940
51960
51980
51990
52000
52001
52005-52007
52010
52204
52214
52224-52240
52250
52260-52265
52270-52276
52277
52281
52282
52283
52285
52287
52290
52300-52301
52305
52310-52315
52317-52318
52320-52325
52327
52330
52332
52334
52341-52343
52344-52346
52351
52352-52353
52354-52355
52356
52400
52402
52441-52442
52450
52500
52601
52630
52640
52647
52648
52649
52700
53000-53010
53020-53025
53040
53060
53080-53085
53200
53210
53215
53220
53230
53235
53240
53250
53260
53265
53270
53275
53400-53405
53410
53415
53420-53425
53430
53431
53440
53442
53444
53445
53446-53448
53449
53450
53451-53454
53460
53500
53502
53505-53510
53515
53520
53600-53601
53605
53620-53621
53660-53665
53850
53852
53854
53855
53860
54000-54001
54015
54050-54065
54100-54105
54110-54112
54115
54120
54125
54130-54135
54150
54160-54161
54162
54163
54164
54200-54205
54220
54230
54231
54235
54240
54250
54300
54304
54308-54316
54318
54322-54326
54328
54332
54336
54340-54348
54352
54360
54380-54390
54400-54401
54405
54406
54408
54410-54411
54415
54416-54417
54420-54430
54435
54437
54438
54440
54450
54500-54505
54512
54520
54522
54530-54535
54550-54560
54600-54620
54640
54650
54660
54670
54680
54690
54692
54700
54800
54830
54840
54860-54861
54865
54900-54901
55000
55040-55041
55060
55100
55110
55120
55150
55175-55180
55200
55250
55300
55400
55500
55520
55530-55535

55540
55550
55600-55605
55650
55680
55700-55705
55706
55720-55725
55801
55810-55815
55821
55831
55840-55845
55860-55865
55866
55870
55873
55874
55875
55876
55880
55920
57220
57230
57240
57284
57285
57287
57288
57289
57423
60540-60545
60650
64566
64581

Ancillary Codes

72191
72192-72194
72195-72197
74018-74022
74150-74170
74174
74175
74176-74178
74181-74183
74190
74400
74410
74415
74420
74425
74430
74440
74445
74450
74455
74470
74485
75831
75833
75984
75989
76000
76700-76705
76770-76775
76776
76870
76872-76873
76940
76942
77002
77012
77013
77021
77022
78700-78701
78707-78709
78725
78730
78740
78761
80047-80048
80050
80051
80053
80069
80169
80197
80200
80408
80416
80417
81000-81003
81005
81007
81015
81020
81050
81224
81225
81226
81227
81250
81539
81541
81542
81551
82009-82010
82040
82042
82043-82044
82108
82127-82131
82136-82139
82140
82163
82340
82355-82360
82365-82370
82379
82435
82436
82441
82507
82565-82575
82610
82615
82642
82947-82948
82950
82951-82952
83735
84066
84100-84105
84119-84120
84132
84133
84134
84152-84154
84155
84156
84160
84165
84166
84206
84244
84295-84302
84402-84403
84410
84520
84525-84545
84550
84560
84578-84583
84588
85004
85007-85008
85009
85013-85014
85018
85025-85027
85032
85041
85048
85049
85060
86294
86328
86386
86609
86631-86632
86694-86696
86769
86780
87086
87088
87110
87164-87166
87270
87273-87274
87285
87320
87389-87391
87490-87492
87500
87528-87530
87534-87536
87537-87539
87563
87590-87592
87623-87625
87635
87850
87901
87905
88104-88106
88120-88121
88160-88162
88172-88173
88177
88302-88309
88311
89260-89261
89264
89310-89320
89321
89322
89331
90935-90937
90940
90945-90947

90951-90953
90954-90956
90957-90959
90960-90962
90963-90965
90966
90967-90970
90989-90993
90997
93975-93976
93980-93981
93985-93986
93990
96360-96361
96365-96368
96372
96373
96374-96376
97802
97803-97804
98960-98962
98966-98968
98970-98972
99000-99001
99058-99060
99151-99153
99155-99157
0421T
0443T
0487T
0499T
0582T
0587T-0588T
0589T-0590T
0596T-0597T
0602T-0603T
0619T
0655T
0672T

Introduction

Unlike other specialty coding books on the market, CPT® *Coding Essentials for Urology and Nephrology 2022* combines urology- and nephrology-specific procedural coding and reimbursement information with verbatim guidelines and parenthetical information from the Current Procedural Terminology (CPT®) codebook. In addition, *CPT® Coding Essentials for Urology and Nephrology 2022* enhances that CPT-specific information by displaying pertinent diagnostic codes, procedural descriptions, illustrations, relative value units (RVUs), and more on the same page as the CPT code being explained. This one book provides urology and nephrology coding and billing knowledge that otherwise might take years of experience or multiple resources to accumulate. It sets a foundation for urology and nephrology coders and subspecialty coding experts that facilitates correct code assignment.

This book includes reporting rules for CPT code submission as written and enforced by the Centers for Medicare & Medicaid Services (CMS). *CPT® Coding Essentials for Urology and Nephrology 2022* is not intended to equip coders with information to make medical decisions or to determine diagnoses or treatments; rather, it is intended to aid correct code selection that is supported by physician or other qualified health care professional (QHP) documentation. This reference work does not replace the need for a CPT codebook.

IMPORTANT: The RVU file that contains the modifier values for new CPT codes was not released as the *2022 CPT Coding Essentials* specialty books went to press. Once the data are available, the file will be posted at www.amaproductupdates.com.

The pending RVU modifier data affect the following new 2022 codes: 33267-33268, 33269, 33370, 33509, 33894-33895, 33897, 43497, 53451-53454, 63052-63053, 64628-64629, 66989, 66991, 68841

About the *CPT® Coding Essentials* Editorial Team and Content Selection

The *CPT® Coding Essentials* series is developed by a team of veteran clinical technical editors and certified medical coders. When developing the content of this book, the team members consider all annual new, revised, and deleted medical codes. They adhere to authoritative medical research; medical policies; and official guidelines, conventions, and rules to determine the final content presented within this book. In addition, the team monitors utilization and denial trends when selecting the codes highlighted in *CPT® Coding Essentials for Urology and Nephrology 2022.*

The main section of *CPT® Coding Essentials for Urology and Nephrology 2022* is titled "CPT® Procedural Coding." This section is organized for ease of use and simple lookup by displaying CPT codes in numeric order. Each code-detail page of this section presents a single code or multiple codes representing a code family concept.

The procedures featured are those commonly performed by a urologist or nephrologist but more difficult to understand or miscoded in claims reporting. This book does not provide a comprehensive list of all services performed in the specialty, nor all sites within the cardiovascular body system. Similarly, the CPT to ICD-10-CM crosswalks are intended to illustrate those conditions that would most commonly present relative to the procedure and the specialist. The crosswalks are not designed to be an exhaustive list of all possible conditions for each procedure, nor medical necessity reasons for coverage.

The "CPT® Procedural Coding" section is complemented by other sections that review urology and nephrology terminology and anatomy, ICD-10-CM conventions and coding, ICD-10-CM documentation tips, and the ICD-10-PCS procedure coding and format. The appendices contain data from the CMS National Correct Coding Initiative, multiple ICD-10-CM compliant urology and nephrology conditions documentation checklists, and the evaluation and management (E/M) documentation guidelines.

Sections Contained Within This Book

What follows is a section-by-section explanation of *CPT® Coding Essentials for Urology and Nephrology 2022.*

Terminology, Abbreviations, and Basic Anatomy

This section provides a quick reference tool for coders who may come across unfamiliar terminology in medical record documentation. This review of basic terminology displays lists of alphabetized Greek and Latin root words, prefixes, and suffixes associated with urology and nephrology.

The combination of root words with prefixes and suffixes is the basis of medical terminology and enables readers to deduce the meaning of new words by understanding the components. For example, *neuro* is a root word for *nerve,* and *–algia* is a suffix for *pain*; thus, *neuralgia* describes nerve pain.

Also included in this section are a glossary of urology and nephrology-specific terms and a list of acronyms and abbreviations. Keep in mind that these glossary definitions are specific to urology and nephrology. The same word may have a different meaning in a different specialty. In some cases, a parenthetical phrase after the term may provide the reader with a common acronym or synonym for that term. Pay particular attention to the use of capitalization in the abbreviation and acronym list, as the same letters sometimes have varied meaning in clinical nomenclature, depending on capitalization.

Introduction to ICD-10-CM and ICD-10-PCS

For coders who want a review, *CPT® Coding Essentials for Urology and Nephrology 2022* recaps the development of the ICD-10-CM and ICD-10-PCS code sets and outlines important concepts pertaining to both.

Lists of common ICD-10-CM diagnoses and conditions from the for each selected CPT code or code range may be found within the "CPT® Procedural Coding" section.

The ICD-10-CM content provided within this book complements your use of the ICD-10-CM 2022 codebook. This section provides a chapter-by-chapter overview of ICD-10-CM that includes common new diagnoses and their codes, as well as identification of new or substantially changed chapter-specific guidelines for 2022.

ICD-10-PCS is not used for reporting physician services; however, an understanding of ICD-10-PCS is essential to physician practices because physician inpatient surgical documentation is used by hospitals for the abstraction of ICD-10-PCS codes for hospital billing. An overview of this structure is reviewed in this section.

ICD-10-CM Anatomy and Physiology

Advanced understanding of the urinary system is essential to accurate coding for urology and nephrology. A detailed study of the anatomy and physiology gives beginner or intermediate coders the information boost they may need to abstract the medical record accurately.

The anatomy and physiology explanations are accompanied by labeled and detailed illustrations for urology and nephrology, beginning at the cellular level and extending to the functions and interactions of the various body parts and tissues. This section also includes discussion of common disorders affecting the urinary system, their pathophysiology, as well as coding exercises to assess mastery of the coding topic.

ICD-10-CM Documentation

Accurate, complete coding of diseases, disorders, injuries, conditions, and even signs and symptoms using ICD-10-CM codes requires extensive patient encounter documentation. This section highlights commonly encountered conditions that require a high level of specificity in documentation and reporting.

The documentation information is presented in an easy-to-understand bulleted format that enables the physician, other QHP, and/or coder to identify quickly the specificity of documentation required for accurate ICD-10-CM code abstraction. This section also includes coding exercises to assess mastery of the documentation topic.

CPT® Procedural Coding

"CPT® Procedural Coding" is the main section of this book and displays pertinent coding and reimbursement data for each targeted CPT code or code family on code-detail pages. The following is presented within each surgical code detail page:

- CPT code and verbatim description with icons (when required)
- Parentheticals (when they exist)
- Official CPT coding guidelines
- Plain English descriptions
- Illustrations
- ICD-10-CM diagnostic codes
- AMA *CPT® Assistant* newsletter references
- CMS Pub 100 references
- CMS relative value units
- CMS global periods
- CMS modifier edits

Category III codes and codes from diagnostic (ancillary) sections will contain a truncated version of the code-detail page content, as diagnostic tests are too broad for all data elements contained in the surgical code-detail pages.

CPT Coding Guidelines

The guidelines and parenthetical instructions included in the CPT codebook provide coders with insight into how the CPT Editorial Panel and CPT Advisory Committee intend the codes to be used. This information is critical to correct code selection, and until now, has been unavailable in books other than official AMA CPT codebooks.

Section guidelines for the pertinent sections of the CPT code set (Surgery, Radiology, Pathology, and Medicine) appear before the code-detail pages associated with the respective CPT section. Guidelines that appear elsewhere within a CPT code set section are displayed on the code-detail pages, whenever appropriate. The reproduction of coding guidelines and parenthetical information in *CPT® Coding Essentials for Urology and Nephrology 2022* is verbatim from the AMA CPT codebook.

CPT Codes and Descriptions

CPT codes are listed in numerical order and include anesthesia, surgery, radiology, pathology and laboratory, medicine, and Category III codes pertinent to urology and nephrology.

The CPT code set has been developed as stand-alone descriptions of medical services. However, not all descriptions of CPT codes are presented in their complete form within the code set. In some cases, one or more abbreviated code descriptions (known as *child codes*) appear indented and without an initial capital letter. Such codes refer back to a common portion of the preceding code description (known as a *parent code*) that includes a semi-colon (;) and includes all of the text prior to the semi-colon. An example of this parent–child code system is as follows:

55810 Prostatectomy, perineal radical;

55812 with lymph node biopsy(s) (limited pelvic lymphadenectomy)

55815 with bilateral pelvic lymphadenectomy, including external iliac, hypogastric and obturator nodes

The full descriptions for indented codes 55812 and 55815 are:

55812 Prostatectomy, perineal radical; with lymph node biopsy(s) (limited pelvic lymphadenectomy)

55815 Prostatectomy, perineal radical; with bilateral pelvic lymphadenectomy, including external iliac, hypogastric and obturator nodes

When a group of similar codes is found on a code-detail page in *CPT® Essentials*, a full description of each code will be displayed.

Icons

Icons on the code-detail page may affect ICD or CPT codes. The male (♂) and female (♀) edit icons are applied to ICD codes. New or revised CPT codes are identified with a bullet (●) or triangle (▲), respectively. The plus sign (✚) identifies add-on codes. Add-on codes may never be reported alone, but are always reported in addition to the main procedure, and should never be reported with modifier 51, *Multiple Procedures*.

A bullet with the numeral 7 within it (❼) is displayed next to ICD-10-CM codes that require a seventh character. Consult the ICD-10-CM codebook for appropriate seventh characters.

The bolt symbol (⚡) identifies CPT codes for vaccines pending FDA approval.

The star symbol (★) identifies CPT codes that may be used to report telemedicine services when appended by modifier 95.

The right/left arrows symbol (⇄) identifies where the full range of lateral codes would be appropriate. To conserve space in the *CPT® Coding Essentials* series, we have chosen to use this icon to denote laterality.

The cell phone icon (▯) denotes the *CPT® QuickRef*, a mobile app created by the AMA and available from the App Store and Google Play. The icon indicates that additional dynamic information can be accessed within the app (in-app purchases required).

Parenthetical Information

The CPT code set sometimes provides guidance in the form of a parenthetical note. For example:

> (For injection procedure for urethrocystography, see 51600-51610)

Code-detail pages include parenthetical instructions specific to both the code and the section within which the code is placed within the CPT code set. Not all codes and/or sections have associated parenthetical notes.

CPT® Assistant References

CPT® Assistant is a monthly newsletter published by the AMA to provide supplemental guidance to the CPT codebook. If a CPT code is the subject of discussion in a past issue of *CPT® Assistant*, the volume and page numbers are noted beneath the code to direct readers to the relevant newsletter archives to keep abreast of compliant coding rules.

Plain English Description

A simple description of what is included in the service represented by each CPT code is provided as a guide for coders to select the correct CPT code while reading the medical record. Not all approaches or methodologies are described in the Plain English Description; rather, the most common approaches or methodologies are provided. In some cases, the description provides an overview to more than one code, as some code-detail pages have multiple codes listed.

Illustrations

Streamlined line drawings demonstrate the anatomical site of the procedure, illustrating the basics of the procedure to assist in code selection. In some cases, not all codes on code-detail pages and not all approaches or methodologies are captured in the single illustration.

Diagnostic Code Crosswalk

ICD-10-CM codes commonly associated with the service represented on the code-detail pages are listed with their official code descriptions. These crosswalk codes were selected by trained coding professionals based on their knowledge and experience. The most common and medically related ICD-10-CM codes appropriate to the procedure or services represented on the code-detail pages are provided within space constraints. The intent is not to provide a list of codes that are deemed medically necessary or relate to payment policies.

When a seventh character is required for a code, a bullet with the numeral 7 within it (❼) alerts the coder. Sometimes, a seventh character is appended to a code with only three, four, or five characters. In those cases, "X" placeholders should be appended to the codes so that only the seventh character must be added. For example, the following ICD-10-CM diagnosis code:

T83.84	Pain from genitourinary prosthetic devices, implants and grafts requires a seventh character; therefore, it is displayed with six characters in this manner:
❼T83.84X	Pain from genitourinary prosthetic devices, implants and grafts

Within ICD-10-CM, many diagnoses have different codes based on laterality (for example, right kidney, left kidney, bilateral kidneys). Due to space constraints, not every laterality code is listed. Rather, a representative code is listed along with an icon indicating that other laterality code versions are available.

The provided crosswalks are not meant to replace your ICD-10-CM codebook. Please consult your manual for all seventh characters needed to complete listed codes and additional laterality choices, as well as ICD-10-CM coding conventions essential to proper use.

Pub 100

CMS Pub 100 (Publication 100-04; "Medicare Claims Processing Manual") is an online resource of federal coding regulations that often relate to CPT coding. If a CPT code or its associated procedure is the topic of discussion in a CMS Pub 100 entry, the Pub 100 reference is noted so that coders may access it at www.cms.gov/Regulations-and-Guidance/Guidance/Manuals/Internet-Only-Manuals-IOMs.

Payment Grids

Information in the payment grids that appear on code-detail pages comes from CMS. These grids identify the relative value of providing a specific professional service in relation to the value of other services, the number of postoperative follow-up days associated with each CPT code, and other reimbursement edits. All data displayed in the payment grids are relevant to physicians participating in Medicare.

Global Period

During the follow-up, or global surgery period, any routine care associated with the original service is bundled into the original service. This means that, for example, an E/M visit to check the surgical wound would not be billable if it occurs during the global surgery period.

Possible global periods under Medicare are 0, 10, and 90 days. "XXX" indicates that the global period concept does not apply to the service.

Relative Value Units (RVUs)

RVU data show the breakout of work, practice expense (PE), and malpractice expense (MP) associated with a code, and provide a breakout for the service depending on whether it was performed in the physician's office or in a facility not belonging to the physician. Understandably, the physician payment for a surgical procedure is reduced if a procedure is hosted by a facility, as the facility would expect payment to cover its share of costs. A physician who performs the surgery in his or her own office is not subject to the same cost-sharing. This cost difference is shown in the PE column.

The payment information provided is sometimes used to set rates or anticipate payments. Payment information may be affected by modifiers appended to the CPT code.

Modifiers

Sometimes, modifiers developed by the AMA and CMS may be appended to CPT codes to indicate that the services represented by the codes have been altered in some way. For example, modifier 26 reports the professional component (PC) of a service that has both a professional and a technical component (TC). A patient who undergoes an ultrasound might have a technician perform the ultrasound itself, while the physician interprets the ultrasound results to determine a diagnosis. The technician's service would be reported with the same ultrasound CPT code as the physician, but the physician would use modifier 26 to indicate the PC only, and the technician would report modifier TC, which is a Healthcare Common Procedure Coding System (HCPCS; pronounced as "hick-picks") Level II modifier identifying the service as the technical portion only. If the physician performs the ultrasound and interprets the results, no modifier is required.

When such circumstances affect the code, users may find the payment information provided for the full code, the professional services–only code, and the technical component–only code.

Many modifiers affect payment for services or with whom payment is shared when multiple providers or procedures are involved in a single surgical encounter. CMS provides definitions for the payments, based on the number listed in the modifier's field.

Modifier 50 (Bilateral Procedure)

This modifier indicates which payment-adjustment rule for bilateral procedures applies to the service.

0 150% payment adjustment for bilateral procedures does not apply. If a procedure is reported with modifier 50 or with modifiers RT and LT, Medicare bases payment for the two sides on the lower of (a) the total actual charge for both sides or (b) 100% of the fee-schedule amount for a single code. For example, the fee-schedule amount for code XXXXX is $125. The physician reports code XXXXX-LT with an actual charge of $100 and XXXXX-RT with an actual charge of $100.

Payment would be based on the fee-schedule amount ($125) because it is lower than the total actual charges for the left and right sides ($200). The bilateral adjustment is inappropriate for codes in this category (a) due to physiology or anatomy or (b) because the code descriptor specifically states that it is a unilateral procedure and there is an existing code for the bilateral procedure.

1 150% payment adjustment for bilateral procedures applies. If a code is billed with the bilateral modifier or is reported twice on the same day by any other means (such as with RT and LT modifiers or with a "2" in the units field), payment is based for these codes when reported as bilateral procedures on the lower of (a) the total actual charge for both sides or (b) 150% of the fee-schedule amount for a single code. If a code is reported as a bilateral procedure and is reported with other procedure codes on the same day, the bilateral adjustment is applied before any applicable multiple procedure rules are applied.

2 150% payment adjustment for bilateral procedure does not apply. RVUs are already based on the procedure being performed as a bilateral procedure. If a procedure is reported with modifier 50, or is reported twice on the same day by any other means (such as with RT and LT modifiers with a "2" in the units field), payment is based for both sides on the lower of (a) the total actual charges by the physician for both sides or (b) 100% of the fee-schedule amount for a single code. For example, the fee-schedule amount for code YYYYY is $125. The physician reports code YYYYY-LT with an actual charge of $100 and YYYYY-RT with an actual charge of $100.

Payment would be based on the fee-schedule amount ($125) because it is lower than the total actual charges for the left and right sides ($200). The RVUs are based on a bilateral procedure because (a) the code descriptor specifically states that the procedure is bilateral, (b) the code descriptor states that the procedure may be performed either unilaterally or bilaterally, or (c) the procedure is usually performed as a bilateral procedure.

3 The usual payment adjustment for bilateral procedures does not apply. If a procedure is reported with modifier 50, or is reported for both sides on the same day by any other means (such as with RT and LT modifiers or with a "2" in the units field), Medicare bases payment for each side or organ or site of a paired organ on the lower of (a) the actual charge for each side or (b) 100% of the fee-schedule amount for each side. If a procedure is reported as a bilateral procedure and with other procedure codes on the same day, the fee-schedule amount for a bilateral procedure is determined before any applicable multiple procedure rules are applied. Services in this category are generally radiology procedures or other diagnostic tests that are not subject to the special payment rules for other bilateral procedures.

9 Concept does not apply.

Modifier 51 (Multiple Procedures)

This modifier indicates which payment-adjustment rule for multiple procedures applies to the service.

0 No payment-adjustment rules for multiple procedures apply. If the procedure is reported on the same day as another procedure, payment is based on the lower of (a) the actual charge or (b) the fee-schedule amount for the procedure.

1 This indicator is only applied to codes with a procedure status of "D." If a procedure is reported on the same day as another procedure with an indicator of "1," "2," or "3," Medicare ranks the procedures by the fee-schedule amount, and the appropriate reduction to this code is applied (100%, 50%, 25%, 25%, 25%, and by report). Carriers and Medicare Administrative Contractors (MACs) base payment on the lower of (a) the actual charge or (b) the fee-schedule amount reduced by the appropriate percentage.

2 Standard payment-adjustment rules for multiple procedures apply. If the procedure is reported on the same day as another procedure with an indicator of "1," "2," or "3," carriers and MACs rank the procedures by the fee-schedule amount and apply the appropriate reduction to this code (100%, 50%, 50%, 50%, 50%, and by report). MACs base payment on the lower of: (a) the actual charge, or (b) the fee-schedule amount reduced by the appropriate percentage.

3 Special rules for multiple endoscopic procedures apply if a procedure is billed with another endoscopy in the same family (ie, another endoscopy that has the same base procedure). The base procedure for each code with this indicator is identified in field 31G of Form CMS-1500 or its electronic equivalent claim. The multiple endoscopy rules apply to a family before ranking the family with other procedures performed on the same day (for example, if multiple endoscopies in the same family are reported on the same day as endoscopies in another family or on the same day as a non-endoscopic procedure). If an endoscopic procedure is reported with only its base procedure, the base procedure is not separately paid. Payment for the base procedure is included in the payment for the other endoscopy.

4 Diagnostic imaging services are subject to multiple procedure payment reduction (MPPR) methodology. Technical component (TC) of diagnostic imaging services is subject to a 50% reduction of the second and subsequent imaging services furnished by the same physician (or by multiple physicians in the same group practice using the same group national provider identifier [NPI]) to the same beneficiary on the same day, effective for services July 1, 2010, and after. Physician component (PC) of diagnostic imaging services are subject to a 25% payment reduction of the second and subsequent imaging services effective January 1, 2012.

5 Selected therapy services are subject to MPPR methodology. Therapy services are subject to 20% of the PE component for certain therapy services furnished in office or other non-institutional settings, and a 25% reduction of the PE component for certain therapy services furnished in institutional settings. Therapy services are subject to 50% reduction of the PE component for certain therapy services furnished in both institutional and non-institutional settings.

6 Diagnostic urology/nephrology services are subject to the MPPR methodology. Full payment is made for the TC service with the highest payment under the Medicare physician fee schedule (MPFS). Payment is made at 75% for subsequent TC services furnished by the same physician (or by multiple physicians in the same group practice using the same group NPI) to the same beneficiary on the same day.

7 Diagnostic urology/nephrology services are subject to the MPPR methodology. Full payment is made for the TC service with the highest payment under the MPFS. Payment is made at 80% for subsequent TC services furnished by the same physician (or by multiple physicians in the same group practice using the same group NPI) to the same beneficiary on the same day.

9 Concept does not apply.

Modifier 62 (Two Surgeons)

This modifier indicates services for which two surgeons, each in a different specialty, may be paid.

0 Co-surgeons not permitted for this procedure.

1 Co-surgeons could be paid. Supporting documentation is required to establish medical necessity of two surgeons for the procedure.

2 Co-surgeons permitted. No documentation is required if two specialty requirements are met.

9 Concept does not apply.

Modifier 66 (Surgical Team)

This modifier indicator services for which a surgical team may be paid.

0 Team surgeons not permitted for this procedure.

1 Team surgeons could be paid. Supporting documentation is required to establish medical necessity of a team; paid by report.

2 Team surgeons permitted; paid by report.

9 Concept does not apply.

Modifier 80 (Assistant Surgeon)

This modifier indicates services for which an assistant at surgery is never paid.

0 Payment restriction for assistants at surgery applies to this procedure unless supporting documentation is submitted to establish medical necessity.

1 Statutory payment restriction for assistants at surgery applies to this procedure. Assistants at surgery may not be paid.

2 Payment restriction for assistants at surgery does not apply to this procedure. Assistants at surgery may be paid.

9 Concept does not apply.

Because many of the services represented by CPT codes in the Radiology, Pathology, and Medicine sections of the CPT code set are diagnostic in nature, crosswalks to the ICD-10-CM code set are too numerous to list. Instead, a narrative description of the service is followed by RVU, modifier, and global information. The official CPT parenthetical information associated with the CPT code is included as well.

The following page presents a guide to the information contained within a code-detail page.

HCPCS Level II Codes

The HCPCS Level II code set is a collection of codes that are used to report health care procedures, supplies, and services. HCPCS Level I codes are CPT codes, developed and copyrighted by the AMA. HCPCS Level II codes include alphanumeric codes developed by CMS to report services, procedures, and supplies that are not reported with CPT codes. These codes include; ambulance services; durable medical equipment; prosthetics, orthotics, and supplies (DMEPOS); drugs; and quality-measure reporting. HCPCS Level II codes also include two-character modifiers

Master code or code family for this code-detail page. All information on this page links to or crosswalks to this code(s).

Citations for *CPT® Assistant* are provided so coders know when to seek further information from this authoritative reference.

Simple line illustrations bring clarity and understanding to complex procedures.

Plain English Descriptions of the procedure or service explain what the master code represents, enabling the coder to verify code selections against the medical record.

Parenthetical instructions that are part of the official CPT codebook give crucial direction to prevent coding errors.

Official CPT code description(s) for the master code(s) enable coders to double-check their code selections.

Common diagnoses associated with the procedure are linked to the ICD-10-CM code set. Icons identify when a seventh character is required, and Xs have been added to codes as placeholders to prevent errors when assigning the seventh character. Diagnoses that are limited to one sex are noted with an icon. Diagnoses that apply to multiple sides/regions of the body are noted with an icon.

RVUs are national Medicare relative value units, or a breakdown of the costs of medical care based on CPT code. Physician work, practice expense, malpractice expense, and total expense differ for facility and nonfacility, so both are listed. RVUs may be used to predict or set fees for physician payment. RVUs shown are for physicians participating in the Medicare program.

From the CMS database, key CPT code modifiers affecting relative values when they indicate multiple procedures or multiple providers, as in co-surgery, team surgery, or assistant surgery are listed here.

The Medicare global period indicates the number of postoperative days during which any routine care associated with the original service is bundled into the original service. Possible global periods are 0, 10, and 90 days.

® Coc ...ology & N...

...l Coding

50323-50325

50323 Backbench standard preparation of cadaver donor renal allograft prior to transplantation, including dissection and removal of perinephric fat, diaphragmatic and retroperitoneal attachments, excision of adrenal gland, and preparation of ureter(s), renal vein(s), and renal artery(s), ligating branches, as necessary

(Do not report 50323 in conjunction with 60540, 60545)

50325 Backbench standard preparation of living donor renal allograft (open or laparoscopic) prior to transplantation, including dissection and removal of perinephric fat and preparation of ureter(s), renal vein(s), and renal artery(s), ligating branches, as necessary

...IA Coding Guideline

...nal Transplantation Procedures

...nal autotransplantation includes reimplantation ...the autograft as the primary procedure, along ...h secondary extra-corporeal procedure(s) (eg, partial nephrectomy, nephrolithotomy) reported with modifier 51 (see 50380 and applicable secondary procedure(s)).

Renal allotransplantation involves three distinct components of physician work:

1. Cadaver donor nephrectomy, unilateral or bilateral, which includes harvesting the graft(s) and cold preservation of the graft(s) (perfusing with cold preservation solution and cold maintenance) (use 50300). Living donor nephrectomy, which includes harvesting the graft, cold preservation of the graft (perfusing with cold preservation solution and cold maintenance), and care of the donor (see 50320, 50547).

2. Backbench work:

Standard preparation of a cadaver donor renal allograft prior to transplantation including dissection and removal of perinephric fat, diaphragmatic and retroperitoneal attachments; excision of adrenal gland; and preparation of ureter(s), renal vein(s), and renal artery(s), ligating branches, as necessary (use 50323).

Standard preparation of a living donor renal allograft (open or laparoscopic) prior to transplantation including dissection and removal of perinephric fat and preparation of ureter(s), renal vein(s), and renal artery(s), ligating branches, as necessary (use 50325).

Additional reconstruction of a cadaver or living donor renal allograft prior to transplantation may include venous, arterial, and/or ureteral anastomosis(es) necessary for implantation (see 50327-50329).

includes transplantation of the allograft (with or without recipient nephrectomy) and care of the recipient (see 50360, 50365).

AMA Coding Notes

Renal Transplantation Procedures

(For dialysis, see 90935-90999)

(For laparoscopic donor nephrectomy, use 50547)

(For laparoscopic drainage of lymphocele to peritoneal cavity, use 49323)

Surgical Procedures on the Urinary System

(For provision of chemotherapeutic agents, report both the specific service in addition to code(s) for the specific substance(s) or drug(s) provided)

AMA *CPT Assistant* ◻

50323: Apr 05: 10-11

Plain English Description

Standard backbench (backtable) preparation of a kidney harvested from a cadaver or living donor is performed prior to transplant. The kidney is unpackaged and transferred to a backtable basin and placed in iced Ringers lactate solution. Cultures are taken of the preservation fluid and sent to the laboratory. Fat and surrounding tissue is dissected off the external surface of the kidney. The adrenal gland is excised. The kidney is inspected and all open ends of small blood vessels are suture ligated to prevent post transplant bleeding. Lymphatic vessels are also suture ligated to prevent post transplant lymphocele formation. Large blood vessels are then addressed. The gonadal, adrenal, and any lumbar vein branches are divided and ligated. The renal vein is trimmed. If any reconstruction of the renal vein is required it is reported separately. The renal arteries are evaluated. Some donors have only a single renal artery and others have multiple renal arteries. The renal arteries are trimmed and branches ligated as needed. If any reconstruction is required on the renal arteries, it is reported separately. The ureter is then prepared leaving as much surrounding tissue as possible undisturbed to prevent damage to the vascular structures. The renal vessels are then flushed with Ringers lactate to identify any vascular defects or leaks that may require additional preparation or repair. Report 50323 for backbench preparation on a cadaver donor kidney and 50325 for backbench preparation on a living donor kidney.

...ndard pr... ...renal allo... transplantatic...

For 50323, a donor kidney is prep... cadaver or living donor. Report 5... tissue and fat from the kidney...

ICD-10-CM Diagnostic ...

Z52.4 Kidney don...

CCI Edits

Refer to Appendix A for CCI e...

Pub 100

50323: Pub 100-04, 3, 90.1...

50325: Pub 100-04, 3, 90.1-90.6

Facility RVUs ◻

Code	Work
50323	0.00
50325	0.00

Non-facility RVU...

Code	Work			
50323	0.00			
50325	0.00	0.00	0.00	0.00

Modifiers (PAR) ◻

Code	Mod 50	Mod 51	Mod 62	Mod 66	Mod 80
50323	0	2	1	0	2
50325	0	2	1	0	2

Global Period

Code	Days
50323	XXX
50325	XXX

● New ▲ Revised ✚ Add On ⊘Modifier 51 Exempt ★Telemedicine ◻ CPT QuickRef ⁄FDA Pending ⇄ Laterality ❼ Seventh Character ♂Male ♀Female

226

used to identify anatomic sites, describe the provider of care or supplies, or describe specific clinical findings.

Modifiers

HCPCS Level II and CPT modifiers appropriate to urology/nephrology coding are included in this chapter. A modifier provides the means to report or indicate that a service reported with a CPT or HCPCS Level II code has been altered by some specific circumstance but unchanged in its definition or code. The service may have been greater, or lesser, or may have been performed by multiple physicians who will share in reimbursement for the service. Modifiers also enable health care professionals to effectively respond to payment policy requirements established by other entities, and often affect reimbursement.

Modifiers may be part of the CPT code set or part of the HCPCS Level II code set. Both types are included in this chapter. CMS rules specific to the assignment of modifiers are presented in numeric (CPT modifiers) or alphanumeric order (HCPCS Level II modifiers).

Appendices

What follows is an explanation the appendices contained within *CPT® Coding Essentials for Urology and Nephrology 2022.*

Appendix A: National Correct Coding Initiative Edits

The National Correct Coding Initiative (CCI) was developed by CMS to restrict the reporting of inappropriate code combinations and reduce inappropriate payments to providers. The CCI edits essentially identify when a lesser code should be bundled into the parent code and not separately reported, and when two codes are mutually exclusive. In either case, only one of the codes is eligible for reimbursement. In other cases, it is only appropriate to report both codes concurrently if modifier 59 is appended to identify that one of the codes reported is a distinct procedural service.

Each of the CCI edits presented in this appendix includes a superscript that identifies how the edit should be applied. With a superscript of 0 (12001^{0}), the two codes may never be reported together. With a superscript of 1 (12001^{1}), a modifier may be applied and both codes reported, if appropriate. A superscript of 9 (12001^{9}) indicates that the modifier issue is not applicable to this code pairing, and the two codes should not be reported together. Remember, the modifier can only be used when the paired codes represent distinct procedural services. The modifier would be appended to the lesser of the two codes, as defined by their RVUs.

The CCI edits for each of the CPT codes found in this guide are included in this appendix, listed in numeric order for simple lookup. CCI edits are updated quarterly. Those listed in this guide are effective January 1, 2022, through March 31, 2022. Future quarterly CCI edits can be found at www.cms.gov/Medicare/Coding/NationalCorrectCodInitEd/Version_Update_Changes.

Appendix B: Clinical Documentation Checklist

One of the greatest challenges of ICD-10-CM coding is ensuring that the clinical documentation from providers is sufficient.

The Clinical Documentation Checklists were developed to be used as a communication tool between coder and physician, or as a document that can be reproduced as a template for documentation by the physician. Essentially, the checklist identifies those documentation required for complete and accurate code selection. For example, in ICD-10-CM, secondary diabetes is divided into diabetes due to underlying condition (E08) and diabetes induced by drugs or chemicals (E09). Furthermore, another category, other specified diabetes mellitus (E13), has been added. This category is selected for patients who have postsurgical or postpancreatectomy diabetes, or when the cause of secondary diabetes is not documented. Type 1 is reported with E10 codes, and type 2 with E11 codes.

Appendix C: Documentation Guidelines for Evaluation and Management (E/M) Services

As the author and owner of E/M codes found in the CPT code set, the AMA has developed detailed guidelines on how to determine which code is appropriate to report, based on the medical record for the encounter. These guidelines look at the quality and quantity of the data in the record:

- History
- Examination
- Medical decision making
- Counseling
- Coordination of care
- Nature of the presenting problem
- Length of the visit

In 1995, CMS published its own documentation guidelines (DGs). Recognizing that the 1995 DGs did not appropriately reflect the work performed in some specialties, CMS published a second set of DGs in 1997. Both sets are still in use. The 1995 DGs are appropriate for multisystem examinations (eg, internal medicine physician). The 1997 DGs are appropriate for in-depth, single-system examinations (eg, retinal specialist).

For Medicare and Medicaid, either the 1995 or 1997 DGs is to be followed, depending on the preference of the provider or coder. The CPT guidelines, while largely incorporated into the 1995 and 1997 DGs, still have unique features accepted by some private payers. Unabridged copies of all three sets of DGs are presented in Appendix C.

Terminology, Abbreviations, and Basic Anatomy

The Terminology, Abbreviations, and Basic Anatomy chapter can be used as a reference tool if there is confusion when reading medical record documentation or when a more extensive understanding of medical terminology is needed. The following chapter includes terms, abbreviations, symbols, prefixes, suffixes, and anatomical illustrations that will help clarify some of the more difficult issues, and give a firmer understanding of information that is in medical record documentation.

Medical Terminology

Majority of medical terms are composed of Greek and Latin word parts and can be broken down into different elements. One element is the root word. The root word is the foundation of the medical term and contains the fundamental meaning. All medical terms have one or more roots.

Examples:

hydr = water

lith = stone

path = disease

Combining forms (or vowel, usually "o") links the root word to the suffix or to another root word. This combining vowel does not have a meaning on its own; it only joins one part of a word to another.

Prefixes and suffixes are two of the other elements used in medical terminology and consist of one or more syllables placed before or after root words to show various kinds of relationships. Prefixes come before the root word and suffixes come after the root word and consist of one or more letters grouped together. They are never used independently; however, they can modify the meaning of the other word parts.

Examples:

Prefixes:

micro = small

peri = surrounding

Suffixes:

algia = pain

an = pertaining to

The following are lists of prefixes and suffixes typically seen in urology:

Root Words/Combining Forms

abdomin/o	abdomen
acr/o	extremities, top, extreme point
aden/o	gland
adip/o	fat
andr/o	male
ankyl/o	stiff, bent, crooked
anter/o	front
arthr/o	joint
ather/o	yellowish, fatty plaque
aut/o	self
axill/o	armpit
balan/o	glans penis
bi/o	life
blast/o	developing cell
brachi/o	arm
bronch/o	bronchial tubes
carcin/o	cancer
cardi/o	heart
cele	prolapse
cheil/o	lip
chol/o	gall, bile
cholangi/o	bile duct
chondr/o	cartilage
cis/o	to cut
colp/o	vagina
coron/o	heart
cost/o	ribs
cry/o	cold
cutane/o	skin
cyan/o	blue
cyst/o	urinary bladder
cyt/o	cell
derm/o	skin
dermat/o	skin
dipl/o	double, two
dips/o	thirst
dist/o	distant, far
ech/o	sound
encephal/o	brain
enter/o	intestine
erythr/o	red
erythem/o	red
eti/o	cause of disease
gastr/o	stomach
gluc/o	sugar
glyc/o	sugar

gon/o	seed
gravid/o	pregnancy
gynec/o	female, woman
hemat/o	blood
hepat/o	liver
hidr/o	sweat
hist/o	tissue
home/o	sameness
inguin/o	groin
isch/o	to hold back
kal/o	potassium
labi/o	lip
lapar/o	abdomen, abdominal
lei/o	smooth
leuk/o	white
lith/o	stone
melan/o	black
ment/o	mind
metr/o	uterus
morph/o	shape, form
my/o	muscle
myc/o	fungus
natr/o	sodium
necr/o	death
nephr/o	kidney
neur/o	nerve
noct/o	night
olig/o	few, scanty
omphal/o	naval, umbilicus
onc/o	tumor
oophor/o	ovary
or/o	mouth
orch/o	testis
orchi/o	testis
orchid/o	testis
orth/o	straight
ov/o	egg
ovul/o	egg
pachy/o	thick
path/o	disease
phag/o	to eat, swallow
phleb/o	vein
phot/o	light
phren/o	diaphragm
plas/o	formation, development
pneumon/o	lungs
proct/o	rectum and anus
pulmon/o	lungs
psych/o	mind
py/o	pus
quadr/o	four
ren/o	kidney
rhiz/o	nerve root
salping/o	fallopian tubes
sial/o	salivary gland
sarc/o	flesh
sect/o	to cut
spir/o	breathing
squam/o	scale-like
staphyl/o	clusters
steat/o	fat
strept/o	twisted chains
terat/o	monster
thec/o	sheath
thorac/o	chest
thromb/o	clot
vas/o	vessel
ven/o	vein
viscer/o	internal organs
xanth/o	yellow
xer/o	dry

Prefixes

a(d)-	towards
a(n)-	without
ab-	from
ab(s)-	away from
ad-	towards
allo-	other, another
ambi-	both
amphi-	on both sides, around
ana-	up to, back, again, movement from
aniso-	different, unequal
ante-	before, forwards
anti-	against, opposite
ap-, apo-	from, back, again
bi(s)-	twice, double
bio-	life
brachy-	short
cata-	down
circum-	around
con-	together
contra-	against
cyte-	cell
de-	from, away from, down from
deca-	ten
di(s)-	two
dia-	through, complete
di(a)s	separation
diplo-	double
dolicho-	long
dur-	hard, firm
dys-	bad, abnormal

e-, ec-, ek-	out, from out of
ecto-	outside, external
em-	in
en-	into
endo-	into
ent-	within
epi-	on, up, against, high
eso-	will carry
eu-	well, abundant, prosperous
eury-	broad, wide
ex-, exo-	out, from out of
extra-	outside, beyond, in addition
haplo-	single
hapto-	bind to
hemi-	half
hept-	seven
hetero-	different
hex-	six
homo-	same
hyper-	above, excessive
hypo-	below, deficient
im-, in-	not
in-	into, to
infra-	below, underneath
inter-	among, between
intra-	within, inside, during
intro-	inward, during
iso-	equal, same
juxta-	adjacent to
kata-	down, down from
macro-	large
magno-	large
medi-	middle
mega-	large
megalo-	very large
meso-	middle
meta-	beyond, between
micro-	small
neo-	new
non-	not
ob-	before, against
octa-	eight
octo-	eight
oligo-	few
pachy-	thick
pan-	all
para-	beside, to the side of, wrong
pent-	five
per-	by, through, throughout
peri-	around, round-about
pleo-	more than usual
poly	many
post-	behind, after
pre-	before, in front, very
pros-	besides
prox-	besides
pseudo-	false, fake
quar(r)-	four
re, red-	back, again
retro-	backwards, behind
semi-	half
sex-	six
sept-	seven
sub-	under, beneath
super-	above, in addition, over
supra-	above, on the upper side
syn-	together, with
sys-	together, with
tetra-	four
thio-	sulfur
trans-	across, beyond
tri-	three
uni-	one
ultra-	beyond, besides, over

Suffixes

-ase	enzyme
-ate	do
-cide	killer
-c(o)ele	cavity, hollow
-ectomy	removal of, cut out
-form	shaped like
-ia	pathological condition
-iasis	infestation, pathological state
-ile	little version
-illa	little version
-illus	little version
-in	stuff
-ism	condition indicated by root/prefix
-itis	inflammation
-ity	makes a noun of quality
-ium	structure; tissue
-ize	do
-logy	study of, reasoning about
-megaly	large
-noid	mind, spirit
-oid	resembling, image of
-ogen	precursor
-ol(e)	alcohol
-ole	little version
-oma	tumor (usually)
-osis	full of
-ostomy	artificial opening

-pathy	disease of, suffering
-penia	lack
-pexy	fix in place
-plasty	re-shaping
-philia	affection for
-rhage	burst out
-rhea	discharge, flowing out
-rhexis	shredding
-sis	state of; condition
-tomy	cut; incise
-ule	little version
-um	thing (makes a noun, typically concrete)

Urology Terms

The following definitions are medical terms commonly seen while coding/billing for Urology/Nephrology:

Absorbent products – Pads and garments, disposable or reusable, worn to absorb leaked urine. Absorbent products include shields, undergarment pads, combination pad-pant systems, diaper-like garments, and bed pads.

Acinar – Cluster of cells that resembles a berry.

Acute – Acute often means urgent. An acute disease happens suddenly. It lasts a short time. Acute is the opposite of chronic, or long lasting.

Agenesis – Failure to develop during gestation.

Albuminuria – More than normal amounts of a protein called albumin in the urine. Albuminuria may be a sign of kidney disease.

Anemia – A condition in which the blood is deficient in red blood cells, in hemoglobin, or in total volume.

Antidiuretic – A natural body chemical that slows down the production of urine. Some children who wet their beds regularly may lack normal amounts of antidiuretic hormone.

Anuria – A condition in which the body stops making urine.

Areflexic – Diminished or absent reflex. A bladder that fails to react or has diminished reactions is areflexic. Also called flaccid.

Artificial Urinary Sphincter (AUS) – Complicated cases of urinary incontinence require implantation of a device known as an artificial urinary sphincter. People who might benefit from this treatment include those who are incontinent after surgery for prostate cancer or stress incontinence, trauma victims, and people with congenital defects in the urinary system. The artificial sphincter has three components, including a pump, balloon reservoir, and a cuff that encircles the urethra and prevents urine from leaking out. The cuff is connected to the pump, which is surgically implanted in the scrotum (in men) or labia (in women). The pump can be activated (usually by squeezing or pressing a button) to deflate the cuff and permit the bladder to empty. After a brief interval, the cuff refills itself and the urethra is again closed.

Atonic – Same as areflexic. Also, a bladder that shows no "tone" or muscle strength; flaccid.

Atrophy – Usually attributed to muscle, it is a shrinking in size, usually following a period of disuse or immobility.

Autonomous – Acting independently. Used to describe a bladder that acts on its own, with no control by the patient.

Balanoposthitis – Inflammation of the glans and foreskin in an uncircumcised male.

Balloon dilation – Treatment for benign prostatic hyperplasia or prostate enlargement. A tiny balloon is inflated inside the urethra to make it wider so urine can flow more freely from the bladder.

Benign Prostatic Hyperplasia (BPH) – Normal, benign enlargement of the prostate that occurs as a natural process of aging in men.

Benign tumor – A tumor that is not cancerous.

Bilateral – A term describing a condition that affects both sides of the body or two paired organs, such as kidneys.

Biofeedback – The use of instrumentation to bring covert physiological processes to the conscious awareness of the individual, usually by visual or auditory signals.

Biopsy – A procedure in which a tiny piece of a body part, such as the kidney or bladder, is removed for examination under a microscope.

Bladder – A hollow muscular balloon shaped organ that stores urine until it is excreted from the body.

Bladder neck – The area of the bladder where the bladder muscle converges to form the urethra.

Bladder training – A behavioral technique that teaches the patient to resist or inhibit the urge to urinate, and to urinate according to a schedule rather than urinating at the urge.

Blood Urea Nitrogen (BUN) – A waste product in the blood that comes from the breakdown of food protein. The kidneys filter blood to remove urea. As kidney function decreases, the BUN level increases.

Calcium – A mineral that the body needs for strong bones and teeth. Calcium may form stones in the kidney.

Catheter – A tube passed through the body for draining fluids or injecting them into body cavities. It may be made of elastic, elastic web, rubber, glass, metal, or plastic.

Catheterization – Insertion of a slender tube through the urethra or through the anterior abdominal wall into the bladder, urinary reservoir, or urinary conduit to allow urine drainage.

Chancre – A hard, syphilitic primary ulcer, the first sign of syphilis, appearing approximately 2 to 3 weeks after infection. The ulcer begins as a painless lesion or papule that ulcerates. Occurs generally singly, but sometimes may be multiple.

Chemolysis – Certain types of kidney stones can be dissolved with the application of chemicals. Uric acid stones, for example, can be dissolved with a solution of sodium bicarbonate in saline.

Cystine stones may be treated successfully with a combination of acetylcysteine and sodium bicarbonate in saline. Struvite and carbon apatite stones can be treated with an acidic solution of hemiacidrin. The procedure involves infusing the chemical solution into the affected area by means of a ureteral catheter in a series of treatments over time until the stone is dissolved. The patient's urine must be cultured regularly throughout the course of treatment to guard against urinary infection and prevent the buildup of excessive chemical levels, particularly magnesium, which can cause other health problems.

Chordee – Condition in which the head of the penis curves either up or down.

Chronic – Lasting a long time. Chronic diseases develop slowly. Chronic renal failure may develop over many years and lead to end-stage renal disease.

Chronic Prostatitis – Inflammation of the prostate gland, developing slowly and lasting a long time.

Collagen – The major protein found in tissues, cartilage, and bones. Collagen injections are used to treat stress urinary incontinence.

Continence – The successful storage of urine.

Contraction – The shortening of the bladder muscle causing the bladder to get smaller and force urine out.

Corpora cavernosa – Two chambers in the penis which run the length of the organ and are filled with spongy tissue. Blood flows in and fills the open spaces in the spongy tissue to create an erection.

Creatinine – A waste product that is filtered from the blood by the kidneys and expelled in urine.

Cryotherapy – During an operation probes are placed in the prostate. The probes are then frozen which kills the prostatic cells.

Cyst – A lump filled with either fluid or soft material, occurring in any organ or tissue; may occur for a number of reasons but is usually harmless unless its presence disrupts organ or tissue function; prefix for bladder.

Cystectomy – Surgical removal of the bladder.

Cystine Stone – A rare form of kidney stone consisting of the amino acid cystine.

Cystinuria – A condition in which urine contains high levels of the amino acid cystine. If cystine does not dissolve in the urine, it can build up to form kidney stones.

Cystica, Cystitis – Inflammation of the bladder, causing pain and a burning feeling in the pelvis or urethra.

Cystocele – Fallen bladder. When the bladder falls or sags from its normal position down to the pelvic floor, it can cause either urinary leakage or urinary retention.

Cystometrogram – A line graph that records urinary bladder pressure at various volumes.

Cystometry – Measurement of the bladder. Bladder pressure is measured as the bladder is filled. A volume versus pressure graph is produced called a cystometrogram.

Cystoscope – An optical instrument which is inserted in the urinary bladder through the urethra. Besides the optical port there is an additional port in the instrument for insertion of various instruments for biopsy, treatment of some bladder tumors, stone removal, and removal of the prostate (prostatectomy).

Cystoscopy – A flexible scope is inserted into the urethra and then into the bladder to determine abnormalities in the bladder and lower urinary tract.

Denervation – Resection (cutting) or removal of the nerves to a certain organ or part of the body.

Detrusor – The smooth muscle that forms the bladder.

Detrusor pressure – The pressure in the bladder caused exclusively by the contraction of the detrusor muscle.

Diabetes Insipidus – A disease of the pituitary gland or kidney. The signs of diabetes insipidus are a need to drink and urinate often, and a feeling of weakness. However, blood sugar levels are normal. (*See also* nephrogenic diabetes insipidus.)

Diabetes Mellitus – A condition characterized by high blood sugar resulting from the body's inability to use sugar (glucose) as it should. In type 1 diabetes, the pancreas is not able to make enough insulin; in type 2 diabetes, the body is resistant to using available insulin.

Dilate – To open or stretch a tubular organ (such as the urethra) beyond its normal dimensions.

Distend – To stretch outward. For example, when the bladder is filled, it is distended.

Diuretic – A drug that increases the amount of water in the urine, removing excess water from the body; used in treating high blood pressure and fluid retention

Dysplasia – Difficult or painful coitus

Dyspareunia – Difficult or painful coitus.

Dysuria – Difficult or painful urination.

Ecchymosis – Bruising.

Ejaculation – Ejection of semen during male orgasm.

Ejaculation, retrograde – The discharge of semen into the bladder rather than through the urethra and out of the body.

Electrical stimulation – Provides a situation whereby there is an electrical generation of action potentials, giving rise to therapeutically significant physiological responses, e.g. increased muscle strength, stimulated lymph and blood flow, analgesia, kinesthetic awareness, and autonomic nervous system responses.

Electrohydraulic lithotripsy (EHL) – This technique uses a special probe to break up small stones with shock waves generated by electricity. Through a flexible ureteroscope, the physician positions the tip of the probe 1 mm from the stone. Then, by means of a foot switch, the physician projects electrically generated hydraulic shock waves through an irrigating fluid at the stone until it is broken into small fragments. These can be passed by the patient or removed through the previously described extraction methods. EHL has some limitations: it requires general anesthesia, and is generally not used in close proximity to the kidney itself, as the shock waves can cause tissue damage. Fragments produced by the hydraulic shock also tend to scatter widely, making retrieval or extraction more difficult.

Electromyography – The measurement of relative nerve activity by electronically measuring and amplifying nerve signals.

Endoscope – An optical instrument which allows a deep look inside the body. Specialized endoscopes are named depending where they are intended to look. Examples of some specialized endoscopes are: cystoscope, nephroscope, ureteroscope, bronchoscope, laryngoscope, otoscope, arthroscope, laparoscope, and gastrointestinal endoscopes. They can be rigid or flexible.

Enterocele – Herniation of small bowel into vagina.

Enuresis – Urinary incontinence not caused by a physical disorder.

Epispadias – Rare malformation of the penis in which the urethral ends in an opening on the upper aspect (dorsum) of the penis, or in which the urethra is too short in females.

Erectile dysfunction (impotence) – Persistent inability to obtain and maintain an erection sufficient for sexual intercourse.

Erection – Enlargement and hardening of the penis caused by increased blood flow into the penis and decreased blood flow out of it as a result of sexual excitement.

Estrogen – Hormones responsible for the development of female sex characteristics; produced by the ovary.

Exstrophy – Congenital malformation in which the bladder is flat and exposed.

External beam radiation therapy – A 25-28 treatment protocol that utilizes external beam radiation. Approximately 6800-7400 rads of radiation energy is delivered to the prostate. There can be some radiation effect on surrounding tissues.

Extracorporeal shock wave lithotripsy (ESWL) – Extracorporeal shock wave lithotripsy uses highly focused impulses projected from outside the body to pulverize kidney stones.

Fluoroscopy – A method of using x-ray to produce real-time video images. After the x-rays pass through the patient, instead of using film, they are captured by a device called image intensifier and converted into light. The light is captured by a TV camera and displayed on a CRT monitor.

Foley Catheter – A tube that is inserted through the urethra to the bladder to drain urine.

Fulguration – Destruction of small growth or areas of tissues using diathermy.

Genitals – Sex organs, including the penis and testicles in men and the vagina and vulva in women.

Hematuria – Blood in urine. Microhematuria—visible only under microscope. Gross hematuria—visible with naked eye. Painless hematuria—number of causes including cancer.

Hormonal therapy – Involves the use of anti-androgens. An androgen is a male hormone needed for the production of testosterone. By depriving the cancer cells of the testosterone they need for growth, tumors regress in size and cellular activity. Side effects include gynecomastia, the enlargement of breast tissue, hot flashes, and loss of libido. Some long-term hormonal therapy is associated with the loss of muscle mass, osteoporosis, and malaise.

Hormone – A natural chemical produced in one part of the body and released into the blood to trigger or regulate particular functions of the body. Antidiuretic hormone tells the kidneys to slow down urine production.

Hydrocele – A painless swelling of the scrotum, caused by a collection of fluid around the testicle; commonly occurs in middle-aged men.

Hydronephrosis – Dilatation, distension, enlargement of the collecting system in the kidney. Hydronephrosis is usually caused by ureteral obstruction, most commonly by ureteral stones. Other causes are: a) ureteral strictures, b) ureteral tumor, c) compression from outside of the ureter, d) congenital ureteral narrowing, e) high bladder pressure transmitted to the kidney, f) abnormal flow of urine from bladder back to the kidney during voiding (vesico-ureteral reflux).

Hydrotherapy – Rehabilitation exercises performed in an appropriately designed pool.

Hydroureter – Dilatation, distension of the ureter, commonly because of obstruction.

Hypercalciuria – Abnormally large amounts of calcium in the urine.

Hyperemia – Increased blood flow to tissue

Hyperoxaluria – Unusually large amounts of oxalate in the urine, leading to kidney stones.

Hyperplasia – Excessive growth of normal cells of an organ.

Hyperreflexic – Refers to the bladder that contracts too soon or too much.

Hypertonic – Similar to hyperreflexic. A bladder with unusually high pressure or one that contracts too soon.

Hypertrophy – An increase in the size of tissue.

Hypomobility – A decrease in the normal range of joint movement. Often characterized by the loss of accessory movements.

Hyporeflexic – Underactive or weakened muscle reflexes.

Hypospadias – A birth defect in which the opening of the urethra, called the urinary meatus, is on the underside of the penis instead of at the tip.

Hypotonic – A lack of muscle strength and tone.

Hypoxia – Depletion of oxygen to tissues. Often caused by a cessation of blood flow and hence oxygen carrying cells.

Impotence – The inability to get or maintain an erection of the penis for sexual activity. Also called erectile dysfunction.

Incomplete voiding – The failure of the lower urinary tract to expel all the urine in the bladder (a 20-50 cc residual normally remains).

Incontinence – Loss of bladder or bowel control; the accidental loss of urine or feces.

Infertility – Inability to achieve a pregnancy.

Inhibit – Refers to conscious effort that keeps the bladder from contracting. Conscious inhibition of the detrusor reflex.

Insemination – The placement of semen into a woman's uterus, cervix, or vagina.

Integrated EMG – A technique of averaging the signals received from electromyography in order to be able to graph the information with standard recording devices. This is as opposed to direct EMG, which shows individual nerve impulses. The individual pulses happen too fast to record on paper with most devices.

Interstim continence control therapy – A therapy used in treating urge incontinence. A device, about the size of a pacemaker, is implanted into the sacral nerves of the lower spine, where it delivers electrical impulses that help regulate bladder function.

Interstitial cystitis (IC) – A disorder that causes the bladder wall to become swollen and irritated, leading to scarring and stiffening of the bladder, decreased bladder capacity, and, in rare cases, ulcers in the bladder lining. IC is also known as painful bladder syndrome.

Interstitial laser – A laser probe is placed within prostatic tissue. Laser energy is then used to destroy prostatic tissue which makes urination easier.

Intra-abdominal pressure – Pressure in the abdomen that in turn applies pressure to the bladder.

Intravenous pyelogram – An x-ray of the urinary tract. A dye is injected to make urine visible on the x-ray and show any blockage in the urinary tract.

Intrinsic – Pertaining exclusively to a part. Intrinsic bladder pressure is pressure created only by the bladder, not for example, abdominal pressure.

Intrinsic sphincter deficiency (ISD) – Weakening of the urethra sphincter muscles. As a result of this weakening the sphincter does not function normally regardless of the position of the bladder neck or urethra. This condition is a common cause of stress urinary incontinence.

Irritable bladder – Involuntary contractions of muscles in the bladder, which can cause lack of control of urination.

Kegel exercises – Tightening and relaxing the muscles that hold urine in the bladder and hold the bladder in its proper position.

Kidney stone – A stone that develops from crystals that form in urine and build up on the inner surfaces of the kidney, in the renal pelvis, or in the ureters.

Kidneys – The two bean-shaped organs that filter wastes from the blood. The kidneys are located near the middle of the back. They send urine to the bladder through tubes called ureters.

KUB – A radiograph of the abdomen and pelvis (short for kidney, ureter and bladder)

Laparoscopy – Surgery using a laparoscope to visualize internal organ through a small incision. Generally less invasive than traditional surgeries requiring a shorter recovery period.

Laser therapy – Use of low powered lasers, for treatment of pain, swelling, inflammation and promotion of healing.

Lithotripsy – A method of breaking up kidney stones using shock waves or other means.

Magnetic Resonance Imaging (MRI) – A method for producing sectional images of the inside of the body with a strong magnet and radio waves.

Menopause – The period that marks the permanent cessation of menstrual activity, usually occurring between the ages of 40 and 58.

Metastasis – The spreading of a cancerous tumor to another part of the body.

Microwave – A catheter is placed within the bladder and positioned within the prostate, then the antenna emits microwaves. This procedure increases the passageway allowing for easier urination.

Mixed incontinence – Having both stress and urge incontinence.

Nephrectomy – Removal of an entire kidney.

Nephrogenic diabetes insipidus – Constant thirst and frequent urination because the kidney tubules cannot respond to antidiuretic hormone and therefore pass too much water.

Nephrolithiasis – Kidney stones.

Nephrologist – An internal medicine specialist in medical diseases involving kidneys, kidney failure, kidney dialysis, and kidney transplantation.

Nephroscope – An optical instrument which is inserted in the collecting system of the kidney via the ureter or a cutaneous tract, for the purpose of examining the inside of the kidney or treatment of kidney stones, strictures, and some kidney tumors.

Nephrotic syndrome – A collection of symptoms that indicate kidney damage. Symptoms include high levels of protein in the urine, lack of protein in the blood, and high blood cholesterol.

Neurogenic bladder – Loss of bladder control caused by damage to the nerves controlling the bladder.

Nuclear scan – A test of the structure, blood flow, and function of the kidneys. The doctor injects a mildly radioactive solution into an arm vein and uses x-rays to monitor its progress through the kidneys.

Obstruct – Refers to something blocking the urethra and restricting or preventing urine outflow.

Open nephrolithotomy – Deep anesthesia is required, after which the surgeon makes a large (10-20 centimeter) incision in the patient's back or abdomen, depending upon where the stone is located. Either the ureter or the kidney is opened and the stone extracted.

Orchiectomy – The surgical removal of one or both of the testicles.

Orchitis – Inflammation of a testicle.

Outlet – Refers to the bladder neck, urethra, and sphincter as a combined mechanism.

Overactive bladder – A condition in which the patient experiences two or all three of the following conditions:

- urinary urgency
- urge incontinence
- urinary frequency—defined for this condition as urination more than seven times a day or more than twice at night.

Overflow incontinence – A type of incontinence brought about because of incomplete emptying and a large amount of urine always being present in the bladder.

Oxalate – A chemical that combines with calcium in urine to form the most common type of kidney stone (calcium oxalate stone).

Pelvic floor muscles – Muscles that support the bladder.

Pelvis – The bowl-shaped bone that supports the spine and holds up the digestive, urinary, and reproductive organs. The legs connect to the body at the pelvis.

Penis – The male organ used for urination and sex.

Percutaneous nephrolithotomy – A method for removing kidney stones through keyhole surgery.

Perineal prostatectomy – A perineal incision is utilized to remove the prostate. The advantages are less blood loss, easier visualization of the bladder/urethral anastomosis, and decreased recovery time because the incision does not involve muscle or any other vital tissue.

Periurethral bulking injections – A surgical procedure in which injected implants are used to "bulk up" the area around the neck of the bladder allowing it to resist increases in abdominal pressure which can push down on the bladder and cause leakage.

Pessary – A specially designed object worn in the vagina to hold the bladder in its correct position and prevent leakage of urine. Pessaries come in many shapes and sizes.

Peyronie's disease – A plaque (hardened area) that forms on the penis, preventing that area from stretching. During erection, the penis bends in the direction of the plaque, or the plaque may lead to indentation and shortening of the penis.

Phimosis – Tightened foreskin which cannot be pulled back.

Post-void residual (PVR) volume – A diagnostic test which measures how much urine remains in the bladder after urination. Specific measurement of PVR volume can be accomplished by catheterization, pelvic ultrasound, radiography, or radioisotope studies.

Prepuce – Foreskin.

Priapism – Prolonged erection usually without arousal.

Prostaglandin – Any of various oxygenated unsaturated cyclic fatty acids of animals that have a variety of hormone-like actions (as in controlling blood pressure or smooth muscle contraction).

Prostate – A walnut-shaped gland that surrounds the urethra at the neck of the bladder found in men. The prostate supplies fluid that goes into semen.

Prostate cancer – Uncontrolled growth of abnormal, malignant cells in the prostate.

Prostatectomy – Surgical removal of the prostate.

Prostate-specific antigen (PSA) – A protein made only by the prostate gland. High levels of PSA in the blood may be a sign of prostate cancer.

Prostatic stent – Inserted through a cystoscope, it is a wire device that expands after placement thus pushing prostate tissue away from passageway allowing for easier urination.

Prostatitis – Inflammation of the prostate gland. Chronic prostatitis means the prostate gets inflamed over and over again. The most common form of prostatitis is not associated with any known infecting organism.

Prostatron – Also called TUMT or transurethral microwave thermotherapy. A catheter is placed within the bladder and positioned within the prostate, then the antenna emits microwaves. This procedure increases the passageway allowing for easier urination.

Proteinuria – The presence of protein in the urine, indicating that the kidneys may not be working properly.

Pubovaginal sling – A surgical procedure in which a man-made or cadaveric piece of material is placed under the bladder neck to support and immobilize. This technique improves sphincter function and decreases bladder neck movement, improving continence.

Pyelonephritis – Acute bacterial infection of the kidney. Symptoms are flank pain, fever, shaking chills, sometimes foul-smelling urine, urgency, frequency, and general malaise. Tenderness is elicited on gently tapping over the kidney with a fist (percussion). Urinalysis will discover white blood cells (pyuria) and bacteria (bacteriuria). There is an increase in circulating white cells in the blood (leucocytosis). Therapy involves appropriate antibiotics under physician's supervision.

Pyuria – The presence of pus in the urine; usually an indication of kidney or urinary tract infection.

Radical retropubic prostatectomy – Removal of prostate through an abdominal incision. The prostate is completely removed. The advantage is that the lymph nodes can be sampled at the time of the operation and the nerve-sparing procedure is easier to do via this operation.

Radiopaque – That which is white on radiograph. Most stones are radiopaque. Those that are not are called radiolucent.

Rectocele – A herniation of the rectum into the vagina.

Residual – The urine remaining in the bladder just after urination.

Retention – The symptom of retaining too much urine in the bladder. Incomplete voiding or complete inability to void.

Sensation – The feeling of the bladder filling.

Sexually transmitted disease (STD) – Infections that are most commonly spread through sexual intercourse or genital contact.

Sling procedures – Surgical methods for treating urinary incontinence involving the placement of a sling, made either of tissue obtained from the person undergoing the sling procedure or a synthetic material. The sling is anchored to retropubic and/or abdominal structures.

Sphincter – A round muscle that opens and closes to let fluid or other matter pass into or out of an organ. Sphincter muscles keep the bladder closed until it is time to urinate.

Stent – Ureteral stent is a catheter or a plastic tube, 1-3 mm in diameter, which is inserted in the ureter between the bladder and the kidney. Its function is to bypass a ureteral obstruction caused by a stone, stricture, tumor or outside compression upon the ureter. It is usually inserted from below by a urologist using a cystoscope (retrograde stent placement). If a nephrostomy is in place it can also be inserted from above (antegrade stent placement).

Stress test – A diagnostic test that requires patients to lift something or perform an exercise to determines if there is urine loss when stress is placed on bladder muscles.

Stress urinary incontinence – Leakage of urine caused by actions—such as coughing, laughing, sneezing, running, or lifting—that place pressure on the bladder from inside the body. Stress urinary incontinence can result from either a fallen bladder or weak sphincter muscles.

Stricture – The reduced diameter of a tubular passage or orifice, such as the urethra, restricting or blocking flow through it.

Struvite stone – A type of kidney stone caused by infection.

Subtracted pressure – Pressure created only by the detrusor muscle. Abdominal pressure is electronically subtracted from total bladder pressure to get this value.

Suprapubic/retropubic prostatectomy – The removal of obstructing prostatic tissue through a suprapubic incision (a cut below the belly button). Suprapubic prostatectomy requires incising the bladder to remove the obstructing tissue while a retropubic approach involves incising the prostatic capsule to remove the obstructing tissue.

Testosterone – The sex hormone that stimulates development of male sex characteristics and bone and muscle growth; produced by the testicles and in small amounts by the ovaries.

Transient urinary incontinence – Temporary episodes of urinary incontinence that is gone when the cause of the episode is identified and treated, such as a bladder infection.

Transurethral – Through the urethra. Several transurethral procedures are treatments for BPH:

- TUIP (transurethral incision of the prostate): widens the urethra by making a few small cuts in the bladder neck, where the urethra joins the bladder, and in the prostate gland itself.
- TUMT (transurethral microwave thermotherapy): destroys excess prostate tissue interfering with the exit of urine from the body by using a probe in the urethra to deliver microwaves.
- TUNA (transurethral needle ablation): destroys excess prostate tissue with electromagnetically generated heat by using a needle-like device in the urethra.
- TURP (transurethral resection of the prostate): removes the excess prostate tissue by using an instrument with an electrical loop.

Transurethral Needle Ablation (TUNA) – The instrument is placed into prostate tissue through a cystoscope. The tissue between the needles is destroyed via thermal energy.

Transurethral Resection of the Prostate (TURP) – A surgical telescope is used through the urethra to core out the inside of the prostate, creating a larger channel and making the passage of urine easier.

Trigone – A sensitive area in the bladder, defined as the area bounded by the two ureteral orifices and the bladder neck.

Ultrasonic lithotripsy – Use of an optical scope and electronic probe inserted into the ureter under epidural (spinal) anesthesia, to locate a stone. High-frequency ultrasound waves then are directed at the stone to break it up gradually. The fragments can either be passed naturally by the patient or removed by grasping forceps, basket extraction or suction through the scope instrument. The instrument is not flexible, however, so ultrasonic lithotripsy typically can be employed only when a straight path directly from outside the body to the stone is possible.

Ultrasound – A technique that bounces painless sound waves off organs to create an image of their structure.

Underactive bladder – A condition characterized by a bladder contraction of inadequate magnitude and/or duration to effect bladder emptying in a normal timespan. This condition can be caused by drugs, fecal impaction, and neurologic conditions such as diabetic neuropathy or low spinal cord injury or as a result of radical pelvic surgery. It also can result from a weakening of the detrusor muscle from vitamin B12 deficiency or idiopathic causes. Bladder underactivity may cause overdistension of the bladder, resulting in overflow incontinence (*See* overflow incontinence).

Urea – A waste product found in the blood and caused by the breakdown of protein in the liver. Urea is normally removed from the blood by the kidneys and then excreted in the urine.

Urea breath test – Test used to detect Helicobacter pylori infection. The test measures breath samples for urease, an enzyme H. Pylori produces.

Ureter – The tube that drains urine from the kidney to the bladder.

Ureteroscopy – A flexible, fiberoptic instrument resembling a long, thin telescope is inserted through the urethra and bladder up to the ureter to visualize the tube. Often used for retrieval of kidney stones.

Urethra – The tube that carries urine from the bladder to the outside of the body.

Urethral obstruction – A blockage in the urethra. A kidney stone is the most common cause.

Urethral pressure profile – A test that measures pressures along the length of the urethra.

Urethral pressure static – Refers to measurement of pressure at a single point in the urethra.

Urethritis – Inflammation of the urethra.

Urge – The feeling of the need to urinate.

Urge incontinence – The inability to hold urine.

Urgency – The symptom of sudden onset of a strong urge to urinate.

Uric acid stone – A kidney stone that may result from animal protein in the diet.

Urinalysis – A test of a urine sample that can reveal many problems of the urinary system and other body systems. The sample may be observed for physical characteristics, chemistry, the presence of drugs or germs, or other signs of disease.

Urinary frequency – Urination eight or more times a day.

Urinary incontinence (UI) – Involuntary loss of urine sufficient to be a problem. There are several types of UI, but all are characterized by an inability to restrain voiding.

Urinary retention – The inability to empty the bladder.

Urinary tract – The system that takes wastes from the blood and carries them out of the body in the form of urine. The urinary tract includes the kidneys, ureters, bladder, and urethra.

Urinary tract infections (UTI) – UTIs are caused by bacteria that invade the urinary system and multiply, leading to an infection.

Urinary urgency – Inability to delay urination.

Urinate –To release urine from the bladder.

Urine – Liquid waste product filtered from the blood by the kidneys, stored in the bladder, and expelled from the body through the urethra by the act of voiding or urinating.

Urodynamic tests – Measures of the bladder's ability to hold and release urine.

Uroflow test – Measurement of the rate at which urine flows out of the body. A lower than normal rate can indicate obstruction.

Urolithiasis –Stones in the urinary system.

Urologist – A surgeon specializing in diseases involving the urinary systems of both sexes and the reproductive organs of men. Four to six years of specialized training after the medical school.

Uroradiologist – A radiologist specializing in diagnosis of genitourinary tract.

Urostomy – An opening through the skin to the urinary tract to allow urine to drain when normal voiding is not possible.

Vagina – The tube in a woman's body that runs beside the urethra and connects the womb (uterus) to the outside of the body. Sometimes called the birth canal.

Valsalva – Bearing down to apply pressure to the bladder.

Vaportrode – A type of cautery electrode that vaporizes prostatic tissue. This creates a larger prostatic channel which makes urination easier.

Vasoepididymostomy – A microsurgical procedure that uses a microscopic camera and very small operative tools to correct obstructions in the genital tract. The procedure requires removal of the blockage in the epididymis (the coiled tube that extends the length of each testis and connects with a larger duct - the vas deferens) and re-attachment of the epididymis to the vas deferens.

Vasovasostomy – Vasovasostomy is a vasectomy reversal, the re-connection of the severed ends of the vas deferens restoring the flow of sperm through the vas deferens.

Vesica sling procedure – A surgical sling procedure used to stabilize the bladder neck and provide support for the urethra using autologous or synthetic sling material. This procedure treats both hypermobility and ISD.

Vesicoureteral reflux – An abnormal condition in which urine backs up into the ureters and occasionally into the kidneys, raising the risk of infection.

Abbreviations/Acronyms

The following abbreviations and acronyms are commonly seen in documentation for Urology/Nephrology:

A	without, lack of
A & P	anterior and posterior; auscultation and percussion
Ab	antibody
Ab	away from
abd	abdomen
ABG	arterial blood gases
ABP	arterial blood pressure
Ac	before meals
ACT	anticoagulant therapy; active motion
ACTH	adrenocorticotropic hormone
Ad	to, toward, near to
Ad lib	as desired
ADH	antidiuretic hormone
AFB	acid-fast bacilli
AIDS	acquired immune deficiency syndrome
ALP	alkaline phosphatase
ALT	alanine transaminase, alanine aminotransferase

AMA	against medical advice
AMB	ambulatory
Ambi	both
Amphi	about, on both sides, both
Ana	up, back, again, excessive
Ant	before, forward
Anti	against, opposed to, reversed
AO	angle of; aorta
AP	apical pulse
Apo	from, away from
APSGN	acute poststreptococcal glomerulonephritis
ARF	acute renal failure
AST	aspartate aminotransferase
ATN	acute tubular necrosis
BBS	bilateral breath sounds
BE	barium enema
BG	blood glucose
Bi	twice, double
BID	twice a day
bilat	bilateral
BM	bowel movement or breast milk
BMR	basal metabolic rate
BP	blood pressure
BPH	benign prostatic hypertrophy
BRM	biologic response modifiers
BRP	bathroom privileges
BS	bowel sounds
BSA	body surface area
BT	bowel tones
BUN	blood urea nitrogen
bx	biopsy
C	Celsius (centigrade)
c	with
C & S	culture and sensitivity
c/o	complaint of
Ca	calcium, cancer, carcinoma
CA	cardiac arrest
CAPD	continuous ambulatory peritoneal dialysis
CAT	computerized tomography scan
Cata	down, according to, complete
CBC	complete blood count
CBD	common bile duct
CBI	continuous bladder irrigation
CBR	complete bed rest
CC	chief complaint
CCK	cholecystokinin
CCPD	continuous cyclic peritoneal dialysis
CFT	complement-fixation test
CHF	congestive heart failure
CI	cardiac insufficiency
CIN	cervical intraepithelial neoplasm
Circum	around, about
CMS	circulation, motion, sensation

CO	cardiac output
CO2	carbon dioxide
Com	with, together
Con	with, together
Contra	against, opposite
COPD	chronic obstructive pulmonary disease
CRF	chronic renal failure
CRRT	continuous renal replacement therapy
CRT	capillary refill time
CSF	cerebrospinal fluid, colony stimulating factors
CT	chest tube, computed tomography
CVP	central venous pressure
CX	circumflex
Cx'd	cancelled
CXR	chest x-ray
D5LR	dextrose 5% with lactated ringers
D5W	dextrose 5% in water
DAT	diet as tolerated
DBP	diastolic blood pressure
DC (dc)	discontinue
DCCT	Diabetes Control and Complication Trials
De	away from
DEX (DXT)	blood sugar
Di	twice, double
Dia	through, apart, across, completely
DIC	disseminated intravascular coagulation
Dis	reversal, apart from, separation
DKA	diabetic ketoacidosis
DM	diabetes mellitus
DNA	deoxyribonucleic acid
DNR	do not resuscitate
Dx	diagnosis
Dys	bad, difficult, disordered
E, ex	out, away from
EBV	Epstein-Barr Virus
Ec	out from
ECF	extracellular fluid, extended care facility
ECG (EKG)	electrocardiogram/electrocardiograph
Ecto	on outer side
EHL	electrohydraulic lithotripsy
Endo	within
Epi	upon, on
ESRD	end stage renal disease
ESWL	extracorporeal shock wave lithotripsy
Exo	outside, on outer side, outer layer
Extra	outside
F & R	force and rhythm
FA	fatty acid
FBS	fasting blood sugar
FD	fatal dose, focal distance
FDA	Food & Drug Administration
FUO	fever of unknown origin
FVD	fluid volume deficit

GB	gallbladder
GFR	glomerular filtration rate
GGT	gamma-glutamyl transferase
GI	gastrointestinal
GOT	glutamic oxalic transaminase
GU	genitourinary
GVHD	graft-versus-host-disease
h/o	history of
Hb	hemoglobin
hCG	human chorionic gonadotropin
HCO3	bicarbonate
HCT	hematocrit
HD	heart disease, hemodialysis
HDL	high density lipoprotein
HEENT	head, eye, ear, nose and throat
Hemi	half
Hgb	hemoglobin
HIV	human immunodeficiency virus
HPI	history of present illness
HRT	hormone replacement therapy
HS	hour of sleep
HTN (BP)	hypertension
Hx	history
Hyper	over, above, excessive
Hypo	under, below, deficient
I & O	intake and output
IBC	iron binding capacity
IBD	inflammatory bowel disease
IBS	irritable bowel syndrome
IBW	ideal body weight
ICF	intermediate care facility
ICS	intercostal space
ICU	intensive care unit
IDDM	insulin dependent diabetes mellitus
IH	infectious hepatitis
IHR	intrinsic heart rate
IIP	implantable insulin pump
IM	intramuscular
im, in	in, into
Imp	impression
Infra	below
INR	international normalization ratio
Inter	between
Intra	within
Intro	into, within
IPD	intermittent peritoneal dialysis
ISD	intrinsic sphincter deficiency
ITP	immune thrombocytopenic purpura
IV	intravenous
IVP	intravenous pyelography
JAMA	Journal of the American Medical Association
K	potassium
KCl	potassium chloride

KI	potassium iodide
KUB	kidney, ureter, bladder
KVO	keep vein open
LB	large bowel
LDL	low density lipoprotein
LE	lupus erythematosus
LFTs	liver function tests
LLQ	left lower quadrant
LMP	last menstrual period
LP	lumbar puncture
LUQ	left upper quadrant
Lytes	electrolytes
MAP	mean arterial pressure
MAR	medication administration record
MDI	multiple daily vitamin
Meta	beyond, after, change
MLC	midline catheter
MM	mucous membrane
MoAbs	monoclonal antibodies
MRDD	mental retarded/developmentally disabled
MRI	magnetic resonance imaging
MS	multiple sclerosis, morphine sulfate
Na	sodium
NaCl	sodium chloride
NAD	no apparent distress
NED	no evidence of disease
Neg	negative
NIDDM	noninsulin dependent diabetes mellitus
NKA	no known allergies
NKDA	non-ketotic diabetic acidosis
NKMA	no known medication allergies
noc	night
NPD	nightly peritoneal dialysis
NPO	nothing by mouth
NS	normal saline
NS (NIS)	normal saline
NSAID	nonsteroidal anti-inflammatory drug
NSR	normal sinus rhythm
NTD	neural tube defect
NV	nausea & vomiting
NYD	not yet diagnosed
O_2	oxygen
OOB	out of bed
Opistho	behind, backward
p	after
P	pulse
PABA	para-aminobenzoic acid
Para	beside, beyond, near to
PCA	patient controlled analgesia, posterior communicating artery
PCN	penicillin, primary care nurse
PCV	packed cell volume
PD	peritoneal dialysis
PDA	patent ductus arteriosus

PDR	physician's desk reference
PE	physical examination
PEG	percutaneous endoscopic gastrostomy
PEJ	percutaneous endoscopic jejunostomy
Peri	around
PERL	pupils equal, react to light
Permeate	pass through
PERRLA	pupils equal, round, react to light, accommodation
PET	positron emission tomography
PG	prostaglandin
PH	past history
PI	present illness
PICC	peripherally inserted central venous catheter
PID	pelvic inflammatory disease
PMH	past medical history
PMI	point of maximal impulse
PNH	paroxysmal nocturnal hemoglobinuria
PO	by mouth
post	after, behind
post op	post-operative
PRBC	packed red blood cells
pre	before, in front of
pre op	pre-operative
prep	preparation
PRN	as needed
Pro	before, in front of
PS	pyloric stenosis
PSA	prostate specific antigen
PT	prothrombin time
PTT	partial thromboplastin time
px	pneumothorax
Q	every
Q2H	every 2 hours
QD	everyday
QH	every hour
QID	four times a day
qns	quantity not sufficient
QOD	every other day
Qs	quantity sufficient, quantity required
R	respirations
RAI	radioactive iodine
RAIU	radioactive iodine uptake
RBC	red blood cells
RDW	red cell distribution width
Re	back, again, contrary
REEDA	redness, edema, ecchymosis, drainage, approximation
Retro	backward, located behind
RLQ	right lower quadrant
RM	respiratory movement
RO	rule out
ROS	review of systems
RT or R	right
RUQ	right upper quadrant

Rx	prescription, pharmacy
S (s)	without
S/S	signs & symptoms
SAST	serum aspartate aminotransferase
Semi	half
SGPT	serum glutamic-pyruvic transaminase
SLE	systemic lupus erythematosus
SNF	skilled nursing facility
SOB	shortness of breath
SOBOE	shortness of breath on exertion
SOP	standard operating procedure
SR	sinus rhythm
SS	social services
STAT	immediately
STD	sexually transmitted disease
STH	somatotropic hormone
sub	under
SUI	stress urinary incontinence
super	above, upper, excessive
supra	above, upper, excessive
SVR	systemic vascular resistance
Sx	symptoms
sym	together, with
T	temperature
T3	triiodothyronine
T4	thyroxine
TBSA	total body surface area
TCDB	turn, cough, deep breathe
TED (hose)	thrombo-embolism deterrent
TIA	transient ischemic attack
TIBC	total iron binding capacity
TID	three times a day
TIL	tumor infiltrating lymphocytes
TNF	tumor necrosis factor
TNM	tumor, node, metastases
TNTC	too numerous to mention
TPN	total parenteral nutrition
TPR	temperature, pulse, respiration
Trans	across, through, beyond
TUMT	transurethral microwave thermotherapy
TUNA	transurethral needle ablation
TUPR	trans-urethral prostatic resection
TUR (or TURP)	trans-urethral resection of the prostate
TWB	touch weight bear
TWE	tap water enema
Tx	treatment, traction
UA	urinalysis
UBW	usual body weight
UGA	under general anesthesia
UGI	upper gastrointestinal
UI	urinary incontinence
Ultra	beyond, in excess

up ad lib	up as desired
UPJ	ureteropelvic junction
US	ultrasonic, ultrasound
UTI	urinary tract infection
UVJ	ureterovesical junction
VBP	venous blood pressure
VC	ventricular contraction
VENT	ventral
VF/Vfib	ventricular fibrillation
VLDL	very low density lipoprotein
VMA	vanillylmandelic acid
VP	venous pressure, venipuncture
VS	vital signs
VW	vessel wall
WBC	white blood cell
WD	well developed
WHO	World Health Organization
WN	well nourished
WNL	within normal limits
X	times

Anatomy

Anatomy is the science of the structure of the body. This section will address systemic, regional, and clinical anatomy as it applies to coding in the Urology/Nephrology setting. Anatomical terms have distinct meanings and are a major part of medical terminology.

Anatomical Positions

Often in medical records, anatomical positional terms are used to identify specific areas of body parts and body positions. The following list is commonly used terms that may be found in medical documentation:

- Superior = Nearer to head
- Inferior (caudal) = Nearer to feet
- Anterior (ventral) = Nearer to front
- Proximal = Nearer to trunk or point of origin (e.g., of a limb)
- Distal = Farther from trunk or point of origin (e.g., of a limb)
- Superficial = Nearer to or on surface
- Deep = Farther from surface
- Posterior (dorsal) = Nearer to back
- Medial = Nearer to median plane
- Lateral = Farther from median plane

Anatomical Planes

Anatomical descriptions are based on four anatomical planes that pass through the body in the anatomical position:

- Median plane (midsagittal plane) is the vertical plane passing longitudinally through the body, dividing it into right and left halves
- Paramedian (parasagittal) plane is a sagittal plane that divides the body into unequal right and left regions.
- Coronal (frontal) planes are vertical planes passing through the body at right angles to the median plane, dividing it into anterior (front) and posterior (back) portions
- Horizontal planes are transverse planes passing through the body at right angles to the median and coronal planes; a horizontal plane divides the body into superior (upper) and inferior (lower) parts (it is helpful to give a reference point such as a horizontal plane through the umbilicus).

Anatomical Planes

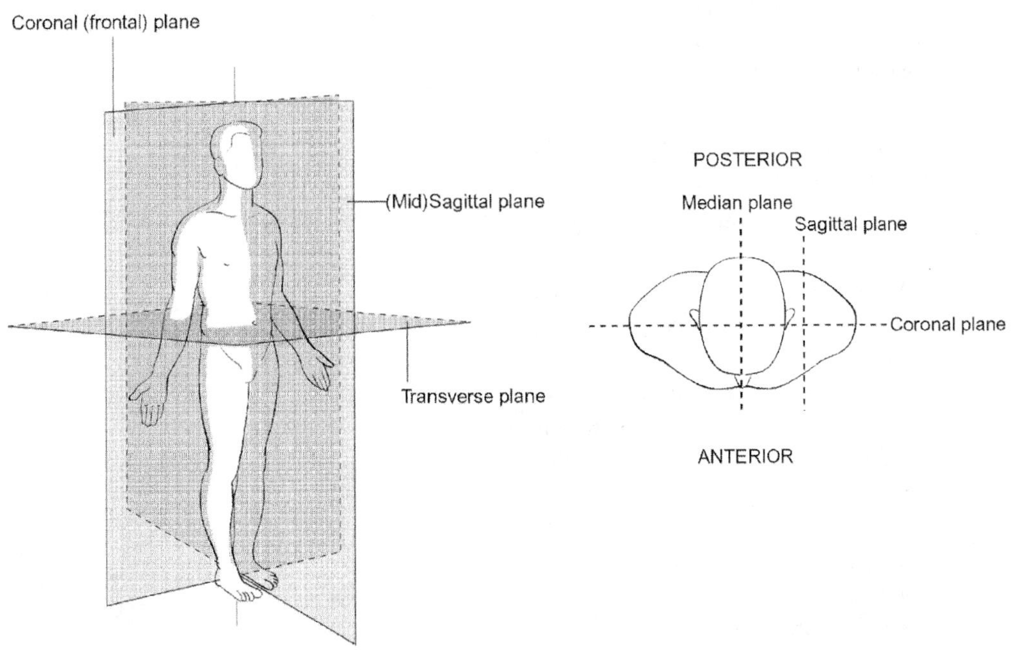

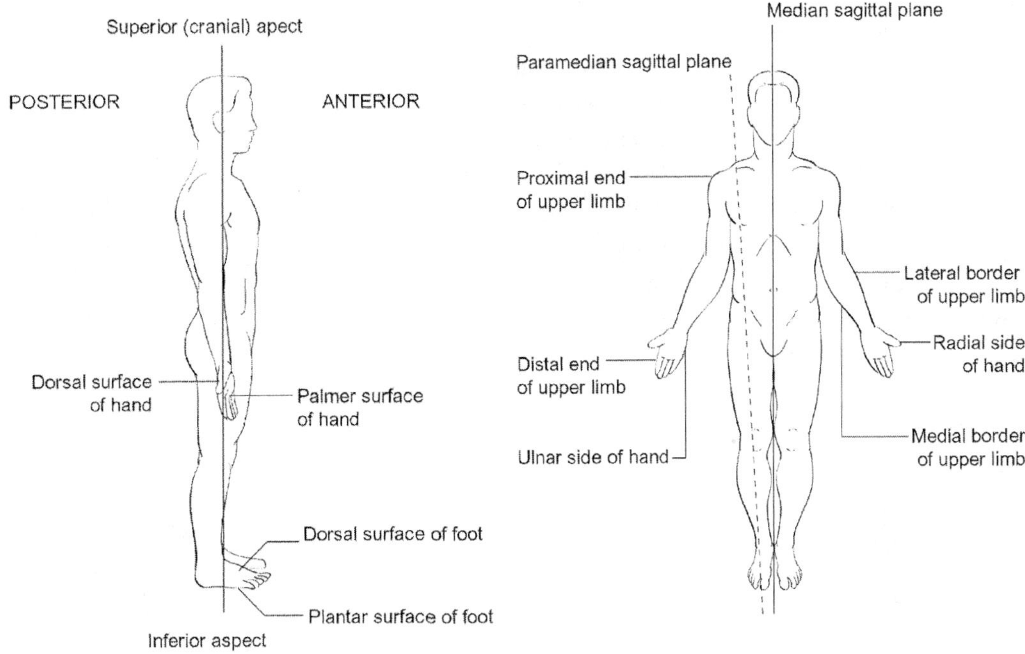

Anatomical Movement Terms

Various terms are used to describe movements of the body. Movements take place at joints where two or more bones or cartilages articulate with one another. They are described as pairs of opposites.

Flexion	Bending of a part or decreasing the angle between body parts.
Extension	Straightening a part or increasing the angle between body parts.
Abduction	Moving away from the median plane of the body in the coronal plane.
Adduction	Moving toward the median plane of the body in the coronal plane. In the digits (fingers and toes), abduction means spreading them, and adduction refers to drawing them together.
Rotation	Moving a part of the body around its long axis. Medial rotation turns the anterior surface medially and lateral rotation turns this surface laterally.
Circumduction	The circular movement of the limbs, or parts of them, combining in sequence the movements of flexion, extension, abduction, and adduction.
Pronation	A medial rotation of the forearm and hand so that the palm faces posteriorly.
Supination	A lateral rotation of the forearm and hand so that the palm faces anteriorly, as in the anatomical position.
Eversion	Turning sole of foot outward.
Inversion	Turning sole of foot inward.
Protrusion (protraction)	To move the jaw anteriorly.
Retrusion (retraction)	To move the jaw posteriorly.

Urology/Nephrology Anatomy

The illustrations on the following pages detail anatomical images which relate to Urology/Nephrology:

Male Figure
(Anterior View)

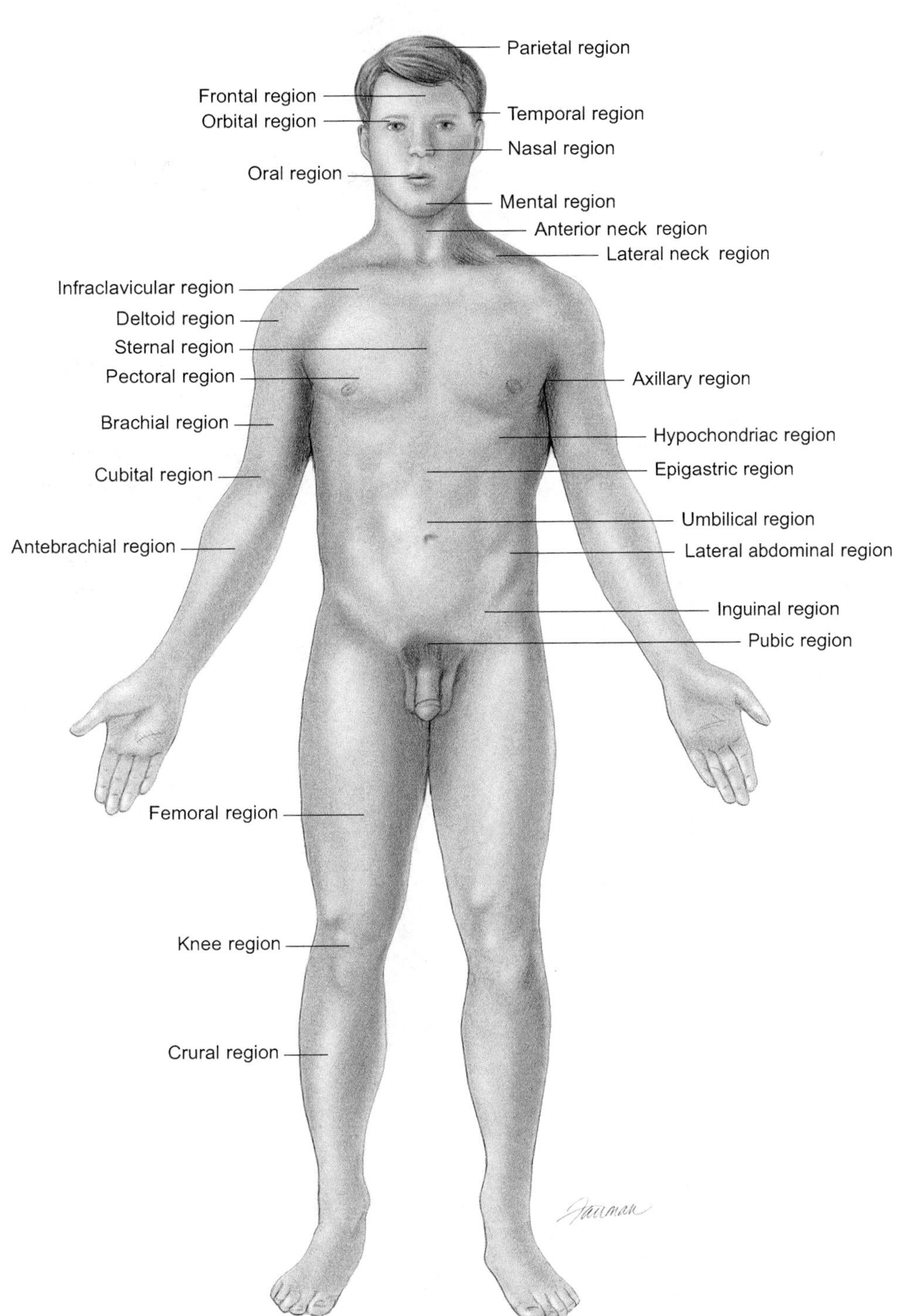

Female Figure
(Anterior View)

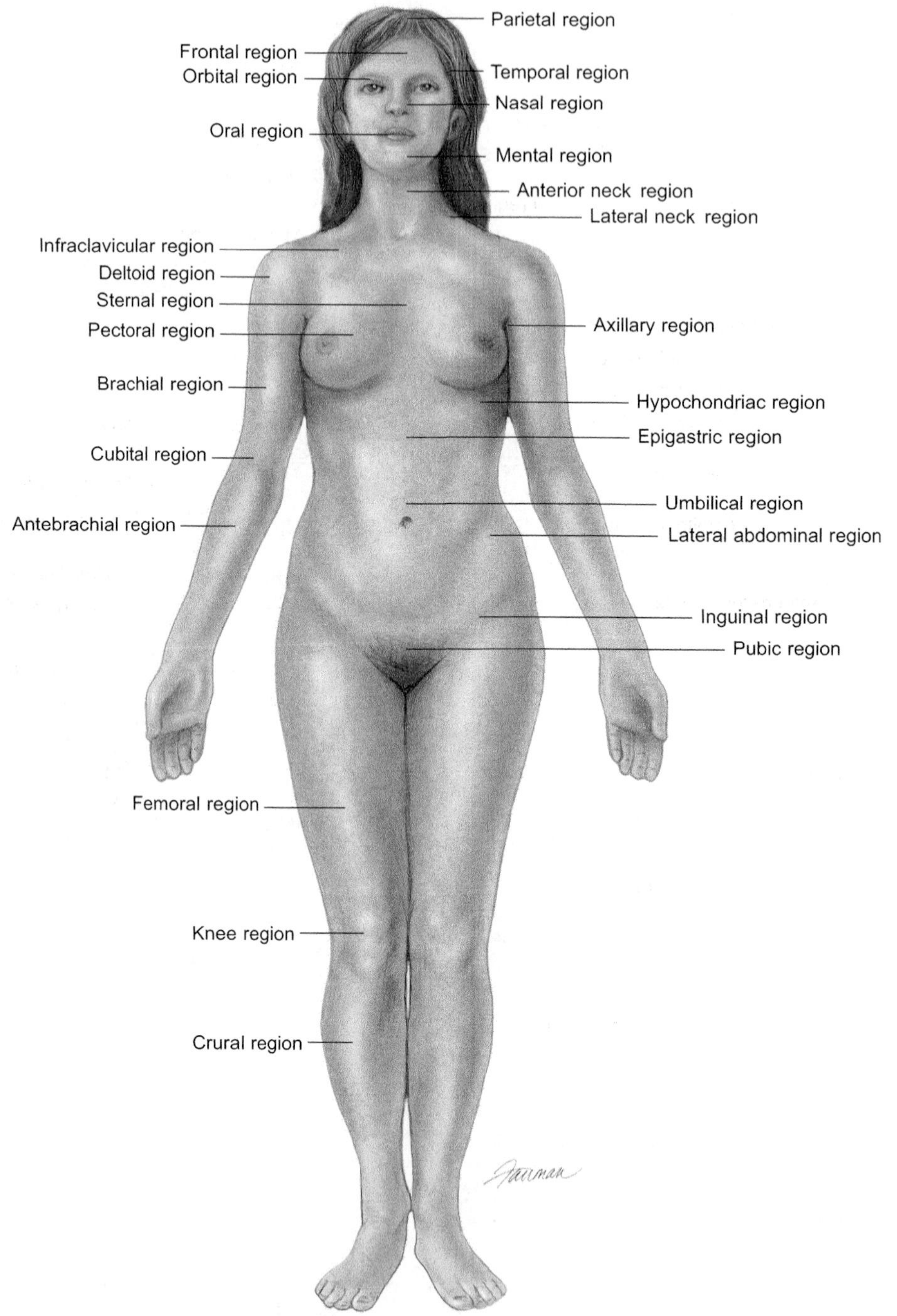
Parietal region
Frontal region
Orbital region
Temporal region
Nasal region
Oral region
Mental region
Anterior neck region
Lateral neck region
Infraclavicular region
Deltoid region
Sternal region
Pectoral region
Axillary region
Brachial region
Hypochondriac region
Epigastric region
Cubital region
Umbilical region
Antebrachial region
Lateral abdominal region
Inguinal region
Pubic region
Femoral region
Knee region
Crural region

Vascular System

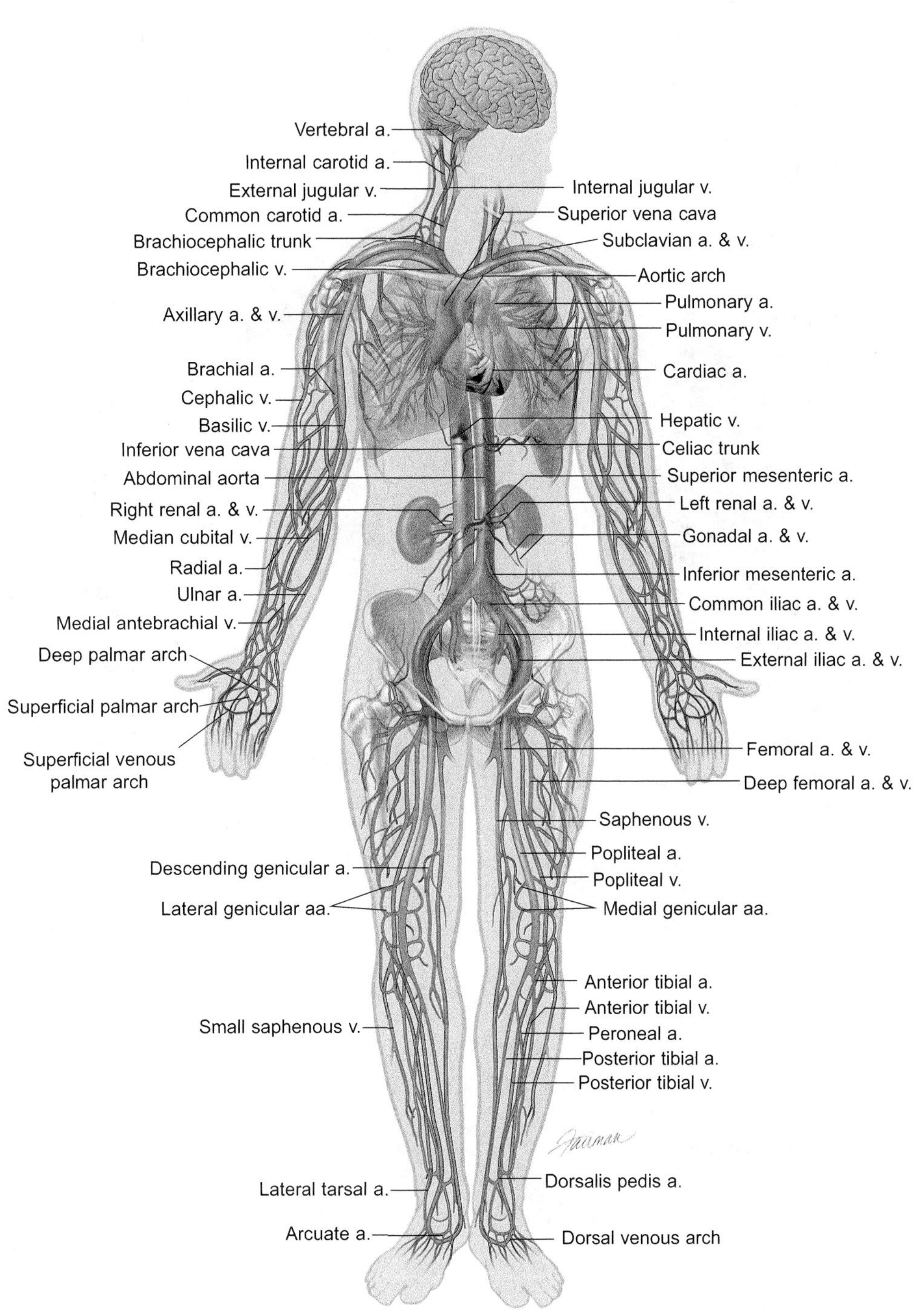
Vertebral a.
Internal carotid a.
External jugular v.
Common carotid a.
Brachiocephalic trunk
Brachiocephalic v.
Axillary a. & v.
Brachial a.
Cephalic v.
Basilic v.
Inferior vena cava
Abdominal aorta
Right renal a. & v.
Median cubital v.
Radial a.
Ulnar a.
Medial antebrachial v.
Deep palmar arch
Superficial palmar arch
Superficial venous palmar arch
Descending genicular a.
Lateral genicular aa.
Small saphenous v.
Lateral tarsal a.
Arcuate a.
Internal jugular v.
Superior vena cava
Subclavian a. & v.
Aortic arch
Pulmonary a.
Pulmonary v.
Cardiac a.
Hepatic v.
Celiac trunk
Superior mesenteric a.
Left renal a. & v.
Gonadal a. & v.
Inferior mesenteric a.
Common iliac a. & v.
Internal iliac a. & v.
External iliac a. & v.
Femoral a. & v.
Deep femoral a. & v.
Saphenous v.
Popliteal a.
Popliteal v.
Medial genicular aa.
Anterior tibial a.
Anterior tibial v.
Peroneal a.
Posterior tibial a.
Posterior tibial v.
Fairman
Dorsalis pedis a.
Dorsal venous arch

Urinary System

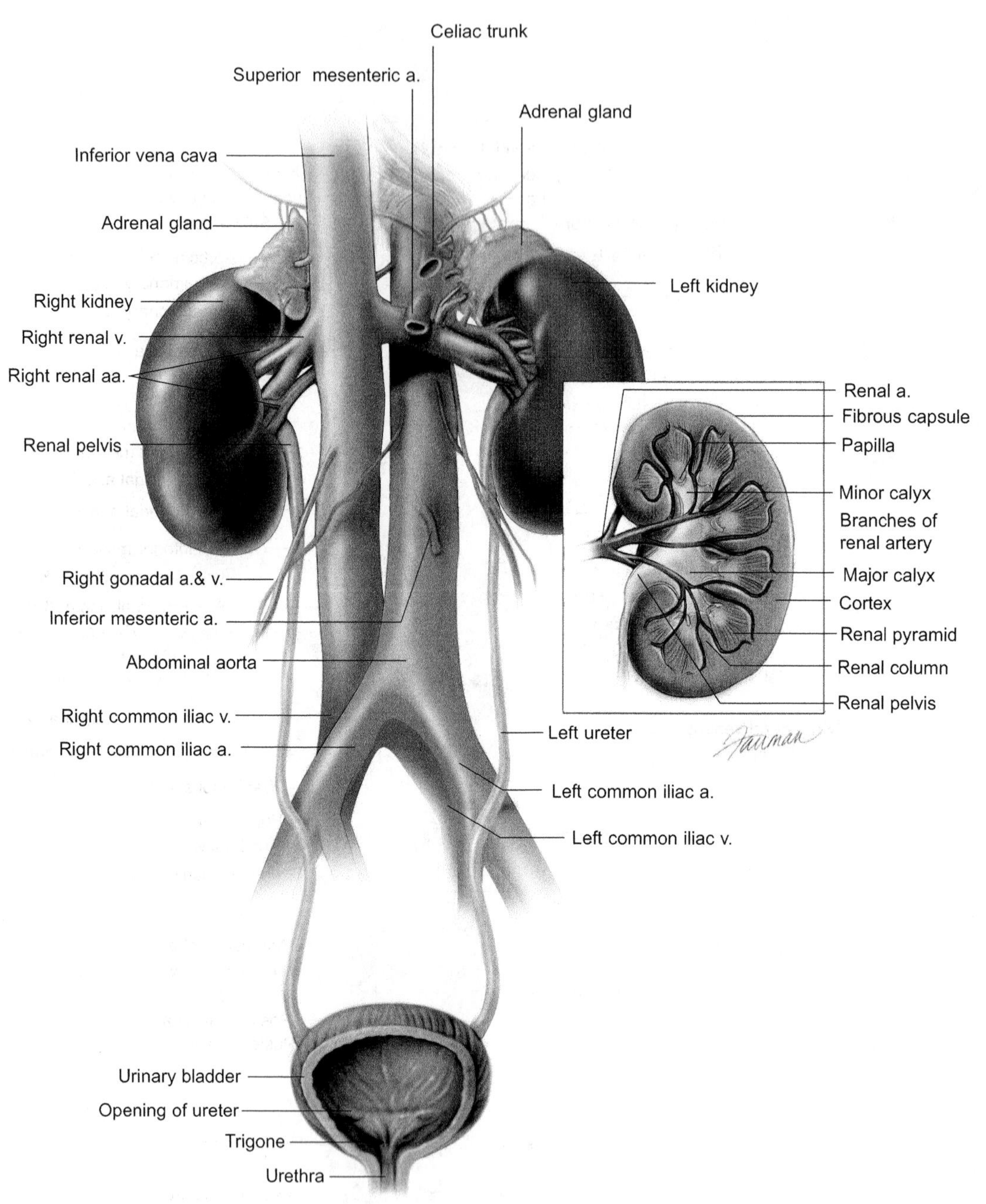
Celiac trunk
Superior mesenteric a.
Adrenal gland
Inferior vena cava
Adrenal gland
Left kidney
Right kidney
Right renal v.
Right renal aa.
Renal pelvis
Renal a.
Fibrous capsule
Papilla
Minor calyx
Branches of renal artery
Major calyx
Cortex
Renal pyramid
Renal column
Renal pelvis
Right gonadal a.& v.
Inferior mesenteric a.
Abdominal aorta
Right common iliac v.
Right common iliac a.
Left ureter
Left common iliac a.
Left common iliac v.
Urinary bladder
Opening of ureter
Trigone
Urethra

Male Genital System

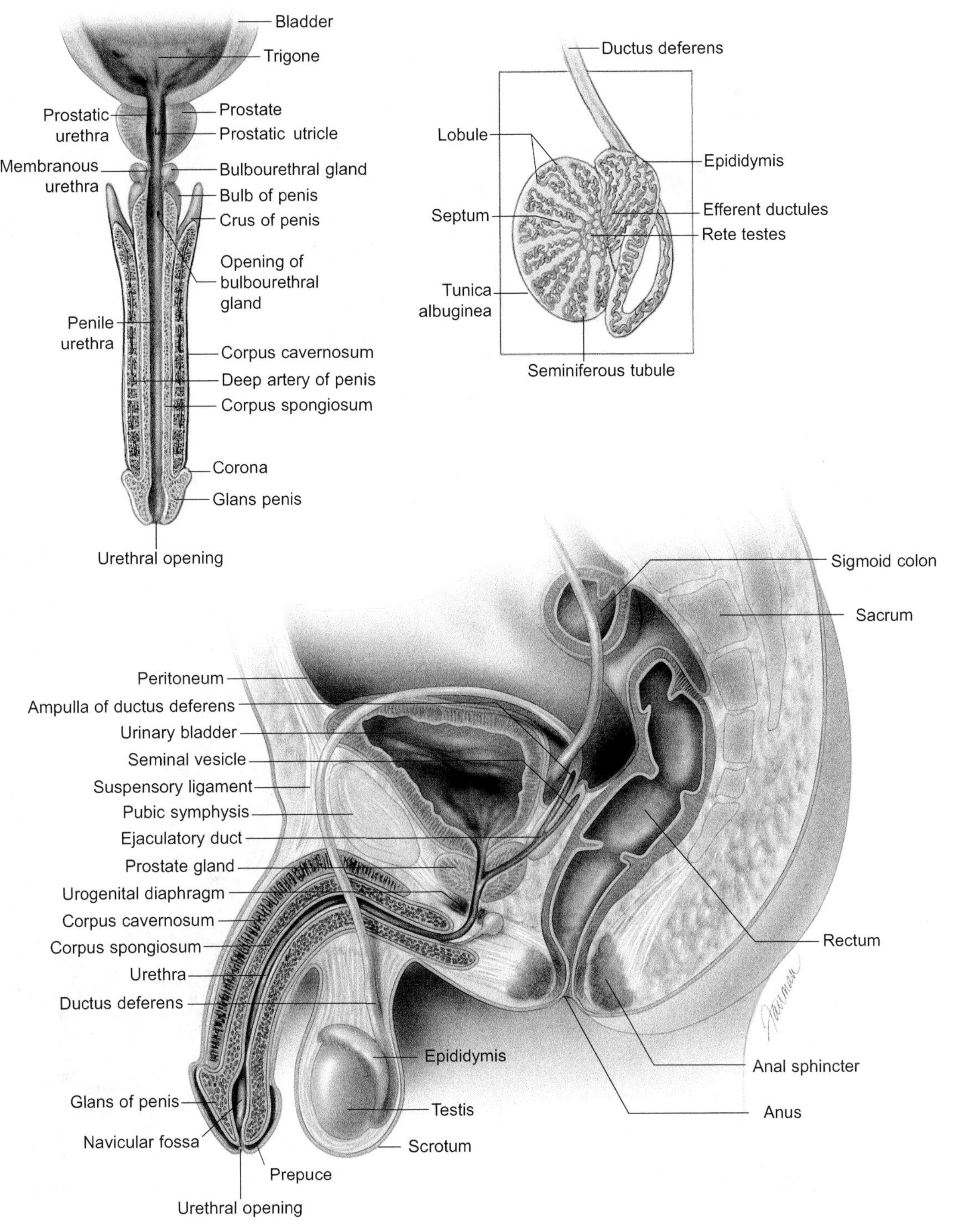

Female Genital System

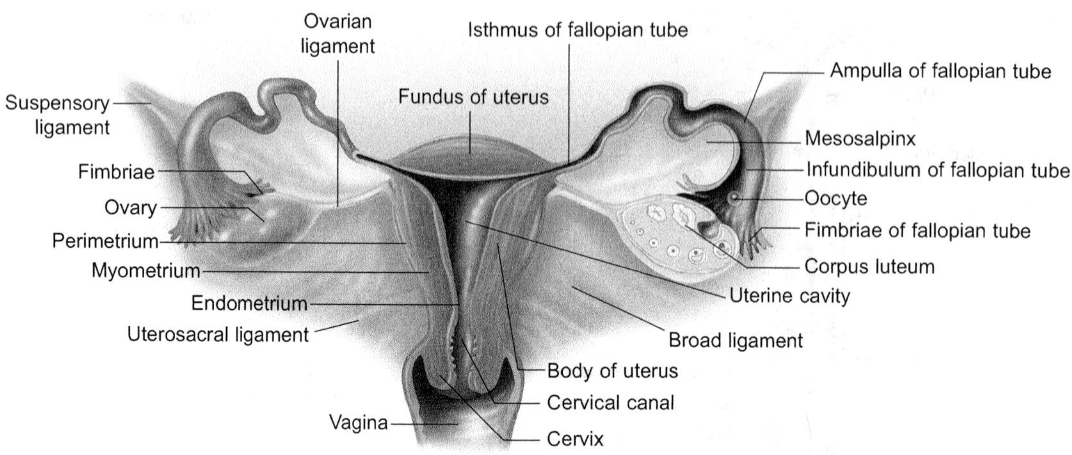

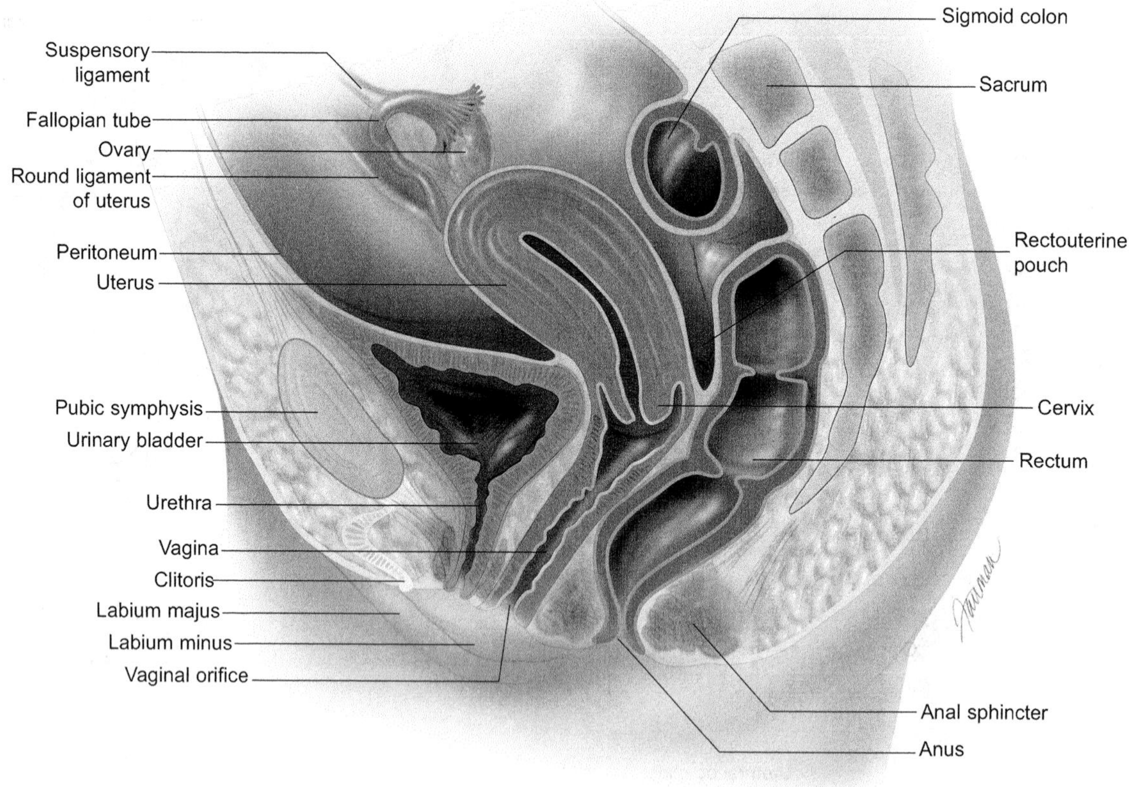

Introduction to ICD-10-CM and ICD-10-PCS Coding

ICD-10

The International Classification of Diseases (ICD) is designed to promote international comparability in the collection, processing, classification, and presentation of mortality statistics. This includes providing a format for reporting causes of death on the death certificate. The reported conditions are translated into medical codes through use of the classification structure and the selection and modification rules contained in the applicable revision of the ICD, published by the World Health Organization (WHO). These coding rules improve the usefulness of mortality statistics by giving preference to certain categories, consolidating conditions, and systematically selecting a single cause of death from a reported sequence of conditions.

ICD-10 is used to code and classify mortality data from death certificates, having replaced ICD-9 for this purpose as of January 1, 1999. The ICD-10 is copyrighted by the WHO, which owns and publishes the classification. WHO has authorized the development of an adaptation of ICD-10 for use in the United States for U.S. government purposes.

Development of ICD-10-CM

The National Center for Health Statistics (NCHS) is the Federal agency responsible for use of the *International Statistical Classification of Diseases and Related Health Problems,* 10th revision (ICD-10) in the United States. The NCHS has developed ICD-10-CM, a clinical modification of the classification for morbidity purposes. As agreed, all modifications must conform to WHO conventions for the ICD. ICD-10-CM was developed following a thorough evaluation by a Technical Advisory Panel and extensive additional consultation with physicians, clinical coders, and others, including public comment, to assure clinical accuracy and utility.

On August 22, 2008, the Department of Health and Human Services (DHHS) published a proposed rule to adopt ICD-10-CM (and ICD-10-PCS) to replace ICD-9-CM in HIPAA transactions. On January 16, 2009, the final rule on adoption of ICD-10-CM and ICD-10-PCS was published. The final initial implementation date was October 1, 2015.

The ICD-10-CM Coordination and Maintenance Committee

Annual modifications are made through the ICD-10-CM Coordination and Maintenance Committee. The Committee is made up of representatives from two Federal Government agencies, the National Center for Health Statistics (NCHS) and the Centers for Medicare and Medicaid Services (CMS). The Committee holds meetings twice a year which are open to the public. Modification proposals submitted to the Committee for consideration are presented at the meetings for public discussion. Approved modification proposals are incorporated into the official government version and become effective for use October 1.

ICD-10-CM Official Guidelines for Coding and Reporting

The structure and format of the Guidelines for Coding and Reporting are as follows:

- Section I. Conventions, general coding guidelines and chapter-specific guidelines
- Section II. Selection of principal diagnosis
- Section III. Reporting additional diagnoses
- Section IV. Diagnostic coding and reporting guidelines for outpatient services
- Appendix I. Present on admission reporting guidelines

Section I – Conventions, General Coding Guidelines and Chapter-Specific Guidelines

Section I of the Guidelines is divided into three general areas:

A. Conventions of the ICD-10-CM
B. General Coding Guidelines
C. Chapter-Specific Coding Guidelines

Conventions

The conventions for the ICD-10-CM are the general rules for its use independent of the guidelines. These conventions are incorporated within the Alphabetic Index and the Tabular List as instructional notes, which take precedence over general guidelines.

The Alphabetic Index and Tabular List

The ICD-10-CM is divided into the Alphabetic Index of terms and their corresponding code, and the Tabular List, a chronological list of codes divided into chapters based on body system or condition. The Alphabetic Index contains the Index of Diseases and Injury, the Index of External Causes of Injury, the Table of Neoplasms, and the Table of Drugs and Chemicals.

Format and Structure

The ICD-10-CM Tabular List contains categories, subcategories, and codes made up of characters that are either a letter or a number. All categories are 3 characters. A three-character category with no further subdivision is equivalent to a code. Subcategories are either 4 or 5 characters. Valid codes may consist of 3, 4, 5, 6 or 7 characters. Each level of subdivision after a category is a subcategory. The final level of subdivision is the valid code. Codes that have applicable 7th characters are still referred to as codes, not subcategories. A code that requires an applicable 7th character is considered invalid without the 7th character.

When locating a code in ICD-10-CM, it is important to note that the 7th characters do not appear in the Alphabetic Index. The Tabular List must be checked to determine whether a 7th character should be assigned, and if so, which one to select.

7th Characters

Certain categories have applicable 7th characters. The meanings of the 7th character are dependent on the chapters, and in some cases the categories, in which they are used. The applicable 7th characters and their definitions are found under each category or subcategory to which they apply in the Tabular List. When 7th character designations are listed under a category or subcategory, the 7th character is required for all codes in that category or subcategory. Failing to assign a 7th character results in an invalid diagnosis code that will not be recognized by payers. Because the 7th character must always be in the 7th place in the data field, codes that are not 6 characters in length require the use of the placeholder 'X' to fill the empty characters. There are a number of chapters that make use of 7th characters including:

- Chapter 7 – Diseases of the Eye and Adnexa (H00-H59). The 7th character is used for glaucoma codes to designate the stage of the glaucoma.
- Chapter 13 – Diseases of the Musculoskeletal System and Connective Tissue (M00-M99). A 7th character is required for chronic gout codes to identify the condition as with or without tophus. The 7th character is also used for stress fractures and pathological fractures due to osteoporosis, neoplastic or other disease to identify the episode of care (initial, subsequent, sequela). For subsequent encounters the 7th character also provides information on healing (routine, delayed, with nonunion, with malunion).
- Chapter 15 – Pregnancy, Childbirth, and the Puerperium (O00-O9A). The 7th character identifies the fetus for those conditions that may affect one or more fetuses in a multiple gestation pregnancy. The 7th character identifies the specific fetus as fetus 1, fetus 2, fetus 3, and so on – NOT the number of fetuses.
- Chapter 18 – Symptoms, Signs and Abnormal Clinical/ Laboratory Findings, NOS (R00-R99). There are subcategories for coma that identify elements from the coma scale and the 7th character provides information on when the coma scale assessment was performed.
- Chapter 19 – Injury, Poisoning and Certain Other Consequences of External Causes (S00-T88). The 7th character is used to identify the episode of care (initial, subsequent, sequela). For fractures it identifies the episode of care, the status of the fracture as open or closed, and fracture healing for subsequent encounters as routine, delayed, nonunion, or malunion.
- Chapter 20 – External Causes of Morbidity (V01-Y99). The 7th character is used to identify the episode of care (initial, subsequent, sequela).

Examples of codes with applicable 7th characters:

- M48.46XA Fatigue fracture of vertebra, lumbar region, initial encounter for fracture
- M80.051D Age-related osteoporosis with current pathological fracture, right femur, subsequent encounter for fracture with routine healing
- O33.4XX0 Maternal care for disproportion of mixed maternal and fetal origin, fetus not applicable or unspecified. Note: 7th character 0 is used for single gestation
- O36.5932 Maternal care for other known or suspected poor fetal growth, third trimester, fetus 2
- S52.121A Displaced fracture of head of right radius, initial encounter for closed fracture
- T88.2XXS Shock due to anesthesia, sequela
- W11.XXXA Fall on and from ladder, initial encounter

Note the use of the placeholder 'X' for those codes that are less than 6 characters in the examples above.

Excludes Notes

There are two types of excludes notes in ICD-10-CM which are designated as Excludes1 and Excludes2. The definitions of the two types differ, but both types indicate that the excluded codes are independent of each other. A type 1 Excludes note, identified in the Tabular as ***Excludes1***, is a pure excludes. It means that the condition referenced is "NOT CODED HERE." For an Excludes1 the two codes are never reported together because the two conditions cannot occur together, such as a congenital and acquired form of the same condition. An exception to the Excludes1 definition is the circumstance when the two conditions are unrelated to each other. If it is not clear whether the two conditions involving an Excludes1 note are related or not, query the provider. For example, code F45.8, Other somatoform disorders, has an Excludes1 note for "sleep related teeth grinding (G47.63)," because "teeth grinding" is an inclusion term under F45.8. Only one of these two codes should be assigned for teeth grinding. However psychogenic dysmenorrhea is also an inclusion term under F45.8, and a patient could have both this condition and sleep related teeth grinding. In this case, the two conditions are clearly unrelated to each other, and so it would be appropriate to report F45.8 and G47.63 together.

A type 2 Excludes note, identified in the Tabular as ***Excludes2***, indicates that the excluded condition is "NOT INCLUDED HERE." This means that the excluded condition is not part of the condition represented by the code, but the patient may have both conditions at the same time and the two codes may be reported together when the patient has both conditions.

General Coding Guidelines

Locating a Code in the ICD-10-CM

To select a code in the classification that corresponds to a diagnosis or reason for visit documented in a medical record, first locate the term in the Alphabetic Index, and then verify the code in the Tabular List. Read and be guided by instructional notations that appear in both the Alphabetic Index and the Tabular List.

It is essential to use both the Alphabetic Index and Tabular List when locating and assigning a code. The Alphabetic Index does not always provide the full code. Selection of the full code, including laterality and any applicable 7th character can only be done in the Tabular List. A dash (-) at the end of an Alphabetic Index entry indicates that additional characters are required. Even if a dash is not included at the Alphabetic Index entry, it is necessary to refer to the Tabular List to verify that no 7th character is required.

Each unique ICD-10-CM diagnosis code may be reported only once for an encounter. This applies to bilateral conditions when there are no distinct codes identifying laterality or two different conditions classified to the same ICD-10-CM diagnosis code.

Laterality

Some ICD-10-CM codes indicate laterality, specifying whether the condition occurs on the left, right or is bilateral. If no bilateral code is provided and the condition is bilateral, assign separate codes for both the left and right side. When laterality is not documented by the provider, code assignment for the affected side may be based on documentation from other clinicians. If there is conflicting documentation regarding the affected side, the patient's attending provider should be queried for clarification. Codes for "unspecified" side should rarely be used, such as when the documentation in the record is insufficient to determine the affected side and it is not possible to obtain clarification.

Documentation by Clinicians Other than the Patient's Provider

The assignment of a diagnosis code is based on the provider's (i.e., physician or other qualified healthcare practitioner legally accountable for establishing the patient's diagnosis) documentation that the condition exists. The few exceptions include codes for body mass index, pressure ulcer stage, depth of non-pressure ulcers, coma scale, NIH stroke scale, laterality, blood alcohol level, and social determinants of health. This information may be documented by "clinicians" other than the patient's provider, such as healthcare professionals who are permitted, based on regulatory or accreditation requirements, to document in the medical record. The provider's statement that the patient has a particular condition is sufficient. Code assignment is not based on clinical criteria used by the provider to establish the diagnosis.

ICD-10-CM Coding for Urology/Nephrology

Diseases of the genitourinary system and related symptoms are coded in ICD-10-CM Chapter 14. The table below shows examples of genitourinary conditions and their corresponding ICD-10-CM codes:

Condition	ICD-10-CM
Coital incontinence	N39.491
Continuous leakage	N39.45
Incontinence without sensory awareness	N39.42
Mixed incontinence	N39.46
Nocturnal enuresis	N39.44
Other specified urinary incontinence	N39.498
Overflow incontinence	N39.490
Postural (urinary) incontinence	N39.492
Post-void dribbling	N39.43
Stress incontinence	N39.3
Urge incontinence	N39.41

Chapter-Specific Coding Guidelines

The information that follows provides an overview of each chapter and highlights some of the more significant aspects of the guidelines. Using this overview is a good starting point for learning about ICD-10-CM; however, this resource must be combined with more intensive training using the Official Guidelines for Coding and Reporting and the current code set in order to attain the proficiency needed to accurately assign ICD-10-CM codes accurately to the highest level of specificity.

Chapter 1 – Certain Infectious and Parasitic Diseases (A00-B99)

Infectious and parasitic diseases are those that are generally recognized as communicable or transmissible. Examples of diseases in Chapter 1 include: human immunodeficiency virus, scarlet fever, sepsis due to infectious organisms, meningococcal infection, and genitourinary tract infections. It should be noted that not all infectious and parasitic diseases are found in Chapter 1. Localized infections are found in the body system chapters. Examples of localized infections found in other chapters include strep throat, pneumonia, influenza, and otitis media.

Chapter Guidelines

Guidelines in Chapter 1 relate to coding of infections that are classified in chapters other than Chapter 1 and for infections resistant to antibiotics. Note that only severe sepsis and septic shock require additional codes from Chapter 18 – Symptoms, Signs, and Abnormal Clinical Findings NOS. Exceptions include sepsis complicating pregnancy, childbirth and the puerperium and congenital/newborn sepsis which are found in Chapters 15 and 16 respectively. In order to report sepsis, severe sepsis, and septic shock accurately, both the guidelines and coding instructions in the Tabular List must be followed.

Some infections are classified in chapters based on the body system that is affected rather than in Chapter 1. For infections that are classified in other chapters that do not identify the infectious organism, it is necessary to assign an additional code from the following categories in Chapter 1:

- B95 Streptococcus, Staphylococcus, and Enterococcus as the cause of diseases classified elsewhere
- B96 Other bacterial agents as the cause of diseases classified elsewhere
- B97 Viral agents as the cause of diseases classified elsewhere

Codes for infections classified to other chapters that require an additional code from Chapter 1 are easily identified by the instructional note, "Use additional code (B95-B97) to identify infectious agent."

In addition to the extensive guidelines related to MRSA infections, there are also guidelines for reporting bacterial infections that are resistant to current antibiotics. An additional code from category Z16 is required for all bacterial infections documented as antibiotic resistant for which the infection code does not also capture the drug resistance.

Chapter 2 – Neoplasms (C00-D49)

Codes for all neoplasms are located in Chapter 2. Neoplasms are classified primarily by site and then by behavior (benign, carcinoma in-situ, malignant, uncertain behavior, and unspecified). In some cases, the morphology (histologic type) is also included in the code descriptor. Many neoplasm codes have more specific site designations and laterality (right, left) is a component of codes for paired organs and the extremities. In addition, there are more malignant neoplasm codes that capture morphology.

Chapter Guidelines

Careful review of the guidelines related to neoplasms, conditions associated with malignancy, and adverse effects of treatment for malignancies is required. The guidelines provide instructions for coding primary malignancies that are contiguous sites versus primary malignancies of two sites where two codes are required. Another coding challenge related to neoplasms is determining when the code for personal history should be used rather than the malignant neoplasm code. For blood cancers, this is further complicated because it is necessary to determine whether the code for "in remission" or "personal history" should be assigned.

Primary malignancies that overlap two or more sites that are next to each other (contiguous) are classified to subcategory/code .8 except in instances where there is a combination code that is specifically indexed elsewhere. When there are two primary sites that are not contiguous, a code is assigned for each specific site. For example, a large (primary) malignant mass in the right breast (female) that extends from the upper outer quadrant to the lower outer quadrant would be reported with code C50.811 Malignant neoplasm of overlapping sites of right female breast. However, if there are two distinct lesions in the right breast (female), a 0.5 cm lesion in the upper outer quadrant and a noncontiguous 1 cm lesion in the lower outer quadrant, two codes would be required, C50.411 for the 0.5 cm lesion in the upper outer quadrant and C50.511 for the 1 cm lesion in the lower outer quadrant.

Malignant neoplasms of ectopic tissue are coded to the site of origin. For example, ectopic pancreatic malignancy involving the stomach is assigned code C25.9 Malignant neoplasm of pancreas, unspecified.

There are guidelines for anemia associated with malignancy and for anemia associated with treatment. When an admission or encounter is for the management of anemia associated with a malignant neoplasm, the code for the malignancy is sequenced first followed by the appropriate anemia code, such as D63.0 Anemia in neoplastic disease. For anemia associated with chemotherapy or immunotherapy, when the treatment is for the anemia only, the anemia code is sequenced first followed by the appropriate code for the neoplasm and code T45.1X5- Adverse effect of antineoplastic and immunosuppressive drugs. For anemia associated with an adverse effect of radiotherapy, the anemia should be sequenced first, followed by the code for the neoplasm and code Y84.2 Radiological procedure and radiotherapy as the cause of abnormal reaction in the patient.

Code C80.0 Disseminated malignant neoplasm, unspecified is reported only when the patient has advanced metastatic disease with no known primary or secondary sites specified. It should not be used in place of assigning codes for the primary site and all known secondary sites. Cancer unspecified is reported with code C80.1 Malignant (primary) neoplasm, unspecified. This code should be used only when no determination can be made as to the primary site of the malignancy. This code would rarely be used in the inpatient setting.

The guidelines provide detailed information on sequencing of neoplasm codes for various scenarios, such as sequencing for an encounter for a malignant neoplasm during pregnancy. Be sure to review the Official Guidelines for Coding and Reporting for this chapter before assigning a code.

Coding for a current malignancy versus a personal history of malignancy is dependent on two factors. First, it must be determined whether the malignancy has been excised or eradicated. Next, it must be determined whether any additional treatment is being directed to the site of the primary malignancy.

Primary malignancy excised/or eradicated?	Still receiving treatment directed at primary site?	Code Assignment
No	Yes	Use the malignant neoplasm code
Yes	Yes	Use the malignant neoplasm code
Yes	No	Use a code from category Z85 Personal history of primary or secondary malignant neoplasm

There are also guidelines related to coding for leukemia in remission versus coding for personal history of leukemia. These guidelines also apply to multiple myeloma and malignant plasma cell neoplasms. Categories with codes for "in remission" include:

- C90 Multiple myeloma and malignant plasma cell neoplasms
- C91 Lymphoid leukemia
- C92 Myeloid leukemia
- C93 Monocytic leukemia
- C94 Other leukemias of specified cell type

Coding for these neoplasms requires first determining, based on the documentation, whether or not the patient is in remission. If the documentation is unclear as to whether the patient has achieved remission, the physician should be queried.

Coding is further complicated because it must also be determined whether a patient who has achieved and maintained remission is now "cured," in which case the applicable code for personal history of leukemia or personal history of other malignant neoplasms of lymphoid, hematopoietic and related tissues should be assigned. If the documentation is not clear, the physician should be queried. Categories that report a history of these neoplasms include:

- Z85.6 Personal history of leukemia
- Z85.79 Personal history of other malignant neoplasms of lymphoid, hematopoietic and related tissues

Multiple myeloma, malignant plasma cell neoplasm, leukemia eradicated?	Still receiving treatment for the neoplasm?	Documentation that patient is currently in remission or has maintained remission and is now "cured"?	Code Assignment
No	Yes	No	Use the malignant neoplasm code with fifth character '0' for not having achieved remission or fifth character '2' for in relapse
Yes	No	In remission	Use the malignant neoplasm code with fifth character '1' for in remission
Yes	No	Maintained remission/cured	Use a code from category Z85 Personal history of primary or secondary malignant neoplasm

Chapter 3 – Diseases of the Blood and Blood-Forming Organs and Certain Disorders Involving the Immune Mechanism (D50-D89)

Diseases of the blood and blood-forming organs include disorders involving the bone marrow, lymphatic tissue, platelets, and coagulation factors. Certain disorders involving the immune mechanism such as immunodeficiency disorders (except HIV/AIDS) are also classified to Chapter 3.

Chapter Guidelines

There are no chapter-specific guidelines for Chapter 3. However, Chapter 2 guidelines should be reviewed for anemia associated with a malignancy or with treatment of a malignancy.

Chapter 4 – Endocrine, Nutritional, and Metabolic Diseases (E00-E89)

Chapter 4 covers diseases and conditions of the endocrine glands which include the pituitary, thyroid, parathyroids, adrenals, pancreas, ovaries/testes, pineal gland, and thymus; malnutrition and other nutritional deficiencies; overweight and obesity; and metabolic disorders such as lactose intolerance, hyperlipidemia, dehydration, and electrolyte imbalances. One of the most frequently treated conditions, diabetes mellitus, is found in this chapter.

Diabetes Mellitus

Diabetes mellitus, one of the most common diseases treated by physicians, is classified in Chapter 4 and, since complications of diabetes can affect one or more body systems, all physician specialties must be familiar with diabetes coding. Two significant concepts to note in diabetes coding include 1) the code categories, and 2) most codes are combination codes that capture the type of diabetes, the body system affected as well as the specific manifestations/complications. However, some categories include instructional notes to assign additional codes from other chapters for added specificity. Diabetes mellitus code categories include:

- E08 Diabetes mellitus due to an underlying condition. Examples of underlying conditions include:
  - Congenital rubella
  - Cushing's syndrome
  - Cystic fibrosis
  - Malignant neoplasm
  - Malnutrition
  - Pancreatitis and other diseases of the pancreas
- E09 Drug or chemical induced diabetes mellitus
- E10 Type 1 diabetes mellitus
- E11 Type 2 diabetes mellitus
- E13 Other specified diabetes mellitus. This category includes diabetes mellitus:
  - Due to genetic defects of beta-cell function
  - Due to genetic defects in insulin action
  - Postpancreatectomy
  - Postprocedural
  - Secondary diabetes not elsewhere classified

Combination codes capture information about the body system affected and specific complications/manifestations affecting that body system. Specific information regarding some types of complications may be captured in a single code:

- Ketoacidosis which is further differentiated as with or without coma
- Kidney complications with specific codes for diabetic nephropathy, diabetic chronic kidney disease, and other diabetic kidney complications
- Ophthalmic complications with specific codes for diabetic retinopathy including severity (nonproliferative - mild, moderate, severe; proliferative; unspecified) and whether there is any associated macular edema or retinal detachment; diabetic cataract; and other ophthalmic complications
- Diabetic neurological complications with specific codes for amyotrophy, autonomic (poly)neuropathy, mononeuropathy, polyneuropathy, other specified neurological complication
- Diabetic circulatory complications with specific codes for peripheral angiopathy differentiated as with gangrene or without gangrene
- Diabetic arthropathy with specific codes for neuropathic arthropathy and other arthropathy
- Diabetic skin complication with specific codes for dermatitis, foot ulcer, other skin ulcer, and other skin complication

- Diabetic oral complications with specific codes for periodontal disease and other oral complications
- Hypoglycemia which is further differentiated as with or without coma

"Uncontrolled" and "not stated as uncontrolled" are not components of the diabetes codes. 'Uncontrolled' diabetes may mean either with hyperglycemia or hypoglycemia per the Alphabetic Index. Terms such as 'poorly controlled', 'out of control', or 'inadequately controlled' default to the specified type of diabetes with hyperglycemia. Therefore, diabetes with hyperglycemia should be based only on the documentation to avoid reporting cases of uncontrolled diabetes meant with hypoglycemia incorrectly.

Chapter Guidelines

All chapter-specific guidelines for Chapter 4 relate to coding diabetes mellitus. Some of the guidelines are discussed below.

Diabetics may have no complications, a single complication or multiple complications related to their diabetes. For diabetics with multiple complications it is necessary to report as many codes within a particular category (E08-E13) as are necessary to describe all the complications of the diabetes mellitus. Sequencing is based on the reason for the encounter. In addition, as many codes from each subcategory as are necessary to completely identify all of the associated conditions that the patient has should be assigned. For example, if an ophthalmologist is evaluating a patient with type 1 diabetes who has mild nonproliferative diabetic retinopathy without macular edema and diabetic cataracts, two codes from the subcategory for type 1 diabetes with ophthalmic complications must be assigned, code E10.329 for mild nonproliferative retinopathy without macular edema and code E10.36 to capture the diabetic cataracts.

The physician should always be queried when the type of diabetes is not documented. However, the guidelines do provide instructions for reporting diabetes when the type is not documented. Guidelines state that when the type of diabetes mellitus is not documented in the medical record the default is E11 Type 2 diabetes mellitus. In addition, when the type of diabetes is not documented but there is documentation of long-term insulin or hypoglycemic drug use, a code from category E11 Type 2 diabetes mellitus is assigned along with code Z79.4 Long-term (current) use of insulin or Z79.84, Long term (current) use of oral hypoglycemic drugs.

If both oral hypoglycemic medication and insulin use is documented, assign code Z79.4 Long term (current) use of insulin and code Z79.84 Long term (current) use of oral hypoglycemic drugs.

If the patient is treated with both insulin and an injectable non-insulin antidiabetic drug, assign code Z79.4 Long term (current) use of insulin and code Z79.899 Other long term (current) drug therapy.

If the patient is treated with both oral hypoglycemic drugs and an injectable non-insulin antidiabetic drug, assign codes Z79.84 Long term (current) use of oral hypoglycemic drugs and Z79.899 Other long term (current) drug therapy.

Diabetes mellitus in pregnancy and gestational diabetes are reported with codes from Chapter 15 Pregnancy, Childbirth, and the Puerperium as the first listed diagnosis. For pre-existing diabetes mellitus, an additional code from Chapter 4 is reported to identify the specific type and any systemic complications or manifestations.

Complications of insulin pump malfunction may involve either overdosing or underdosing of insulin. Underdosing of insulin or other medications is captured by the addition of a column and codes in the Table of Drugs and Chemicals specifically for underdosing. Underdosing of insulin due to insulin pump failure requires a minimum of three codes. The principal or first-listed diagnosis code is the code for the mechanical complication which is found in subcategory T85.6-. Fifth, sixth and seventh characters are required to capture the specific type of mechanical breakdown or failure (fifth character), the type of device which in this case is an insulin pump (sixth character '4'), and the episode of care (seventh character). The second code T38.3X6- captures underdosing of insulin and oral hypoglycemic [antidiabetic] drugs. A seventh character is required to capture the episode of care. Then additional codes are assigned to identify the type of diabetes mellitus and any associated complications due to the underdosing.

Secondary diabetes mellitus is always caused by another condition or event. Categories for secondary diabetes mellitus include: E08 Diabetes mellitus due to underlying condition, E09 Drug and chemical induced diabetes mellitus, and E13 Other specified diabetes mellitus. For patients with secondary diabetes who routinely use insulin or hypoglycemic drugs, code Z79.4 Long-term (current) use of insulin or Z79.84, Long term (current) use of oral hypoglycemic drugs should be reported. Code Z79.4 is not reported for temporary use of insulin to bring a patient's blood sugar under control during an encounter. Coding and sequencing for secondary diabetes requires review of the guidelines as well as the instructions found in the tabular. For example, a diagnosis of diabetes due to partial pancreatectomy with postpancreatectomy hypoinsulinemia requires three codes. Code E89.1 Postprocedural hypoinsulinemia is the principal or first-listed diagnosis followed by a code or codes from category E13 that identifies the type of diabetes as "other specified" and the complications or manifestations, and lastly code Z90.411 is reported for the acquired partial absence of the pancreas.

Chapter 5 – Mental and Behavioral Disorders (F01-F99)

Mental disorders are alterations in thinking, mood, or behavior associated with distress and impaired functioning. Many mental disorders are organic in origin, where disease or injury causes the mental or behavioral condition. Examples of conditions classified in Chapter 5 include: schizophrenia, mood (affective) disorders such as major depression, anxiety and other nonpsychotic mental disorders, personality disorders, and intellectual disabilities.

Chapter Guidelines

Detailed guidelines are provided for coding certain conditions classified in Chapter 5, including pain disorders with related psychological factors, and mental and behavioral disorders due to psychoactive substance use, abuse, and dependence.

Pain related to psychological disorders may be due exclusively to the psychological disorder, or may be due to another cause that is exacerbated by the psychological factors. Documentation of any psychological component associated with acute or chronic pain is essential for correct code assignment. Pain exclusively related to psychological factors is reported with code F45.41, which is the only code that is assigned. Acute or chronic pain disorders with related psychological factors are reported with code F45.42 Pain disorder with related psychological factors and a second code from category G89 Pain not elsewhere classified for documented acute or chronic pain disorder.

Mental and behavioral disorders due to psychoactive substance use are reported with codes in categories F10-F19. Both the guidelines and tabular instructions must be followed to code mental and behavioral disorders due to psychoactive substance use correctly. As with all other diagnoses, the codes for psychoactive substance use correctly, abuse, and dependence may only be assigned based on provider documentation and only if the condition meets the definition of a reportable diagnosis. In addition, psychoactive substance use codes are reported only when the condition is associated with a mental or behavioral disorder and a relationship between the substance use and the mental or behavioral disorder is documented by the physician.

The codes for mental and behavioral disorders caused by psychoactive substance use are specific as to substance; selecting the correct code requires an understanding of the differences between use, abuse, and dependence. Physicians may use the terms use, abuse and/or dependence interchangeably; however only one code should be reported for each behavioral disorder documented when the documentation refers to use, abuse and dependence of a specific substance. When these terms are used together or interchangeably in the documentation the guidelines are as follows:

- If both use and abuse are documented, assign only the code for abuse
- If both use and dependence are documented, assign only the code for dependence
- If use, abuse and dependence are all documented, assign only the code for dependence
- If both abuse and dependence are documented, assign only the code for dependence

Coding guidelines also provide instruction on correct reporting of psychoactive substance dependence described as "in remission." Selection of "in remission" codes in categories F10-F19 requires the physician's clinical judgment. Codes for "in remission" are assigned only with supporting provider documentation. If the documentation is not clear, the physician should be queried.

Chapter 6 – Diseases of Nervous System (G00-G99)

Diseases of the Nervous System include disorders of the brain and spinal cord (the central nervous system) such as cerebral degeneration or Parkinson's disease, and diseases of the peripheral nervous system, such as polyneuropathy, myasthenia gravis, and muscular dystrophy. Codes for some of the more commonly treated pain diagnoses are also found in Chapter 6 including: migraine and other headache syndromes (categories G43-G44); causalgia (complex regional pain syndrome II) (CRPS II) (G56.4-, G57.7-); complex regional pain syndrome I (CRPS I) (G90.5-); neuralgia and other nerve, nerve root and plexus disorders (categories G50-G59); and pain, not elsewhere classified (category G89).

Chapter Guidelines

Chapter-specific coding guidelines for the nervous system and sense organs cover dominant/nondominant side for hemiplegia and monoplegia, and pain conditions reported with code G89 Pain not elsewhere classified.

Codes for hemiplegia and hemiparesis (category G81) and monoplegia of the lower limb (G83.1-), upper limb (G83.2-), and unspecified limb (G83.3-) are specific to the side affected and whether that side is dominant or non-dominant. Conditions in these categories/subcategories are classified as:

- Unspecified side
- Right dominant side
- Left dominant side
- Right non-dominant side
- Left non-dominant side

When documentation does not specify the condition as affecting the dominant or non-dominant side the guidelines provide specific instructions on how dominant and non-dominant should be determined. For ambidextrous patients, the default is dominant. If the left side is affected, the default is non-dominant. If the right side is affected, the default is dominant.

There are extensive guidelines for reporting pain codes in category G89, including sequencing rules and when to report a code from category G89 as an additional code. It should be noted that pain not specified as acute or chronic, post-thoracotomy, postprocedural, or neoplasm-related is not reported with a code from category G89. Codes from category G89 are also not assigned when the underlying or definitive diagnosis is known, unless the reason for the encounter is pain management rather than management of the underlying condition. For example, when a patient experiencing acute pain due to vertebral fracture is admitted for spinal fusion to treat the vertebral fracture, the code for the vertebral fracture is assigned as the principal diagnosis, but no pain code is assigned. When pain control or pain management is the reason for the admission/encounter, a code from category G89 is assigned and in this case the G89 code is listed as the principal or first-listed diagnosis. For example, when a patient with nerve impingement and severe back pain is seen for a spinal canal steroid injection, the appropriate pain code is assigned as the principal or first-listed diagnosis. However, when an admission or encounter is for treatment of the underlying condition and a neurostimulator is also inserted for pain control during the same episode of care, the underlying condition is reported as the principal diagnosis and a code from category G89 is reported as a secondary diagnosis. Pain codes from category G89 may be used in conjunction with site-specific pain codes that identify the site of pain (including codes from chapter 18) when the code provides additional diagnostic information such as describing whether the pain is acute or chronic. In addition to the general guidelines for assignment of codes in category G89, there are also specific guidelines for postoperative pain, chronic pain, neoplasm related pain and chronic pain syndrome.

Postoperative pain may be acute or chronic. There are four codes for postoperative pain: G89.12 Acute post-thoracotomy pain, G89.18 Other acute post-procedural pain, G89.22 Chronic post-thoracotomy pain, and G89.28 Other chronic post-procedural pain. Coding of postoperative pain is driven by the provider's documentation. One important thing to remember is that routine or expected postoperative pain occurring immediately after surgery is not coded. When the provider's documentation does support reporting a code for post-thoracotomy or other postoperative pain, but the pain is not specified as acute or chronic, the code for the acute form is the default. Only postoperative pain that is not associated with a specific postoperative complication is assigned a postoperative pain code in category G89. Postoperative pain associated with a specific postoperative complication such as painful wire sutures is coded to Chapter 19, Injury, Poisoning, and Certain Other Consequences of External Causes with an additional code from category G89 to identify acute or chronic pain.

Chronic pain is reported with codes in subcategory G89.2- and includes: G89.21 Chronic pain due to trauma, G89.22 Chronic post-thoracotomy pain, G89.28 Other chronic post-procedural pain, and G89.29 Other chronic pain. There is no time frame defining when pain becomes chronic pain. The provider's documentation directs the use of these codes. It is important to note that central pain syndrome (G89.0) and chronic pain syndrome (G89.4) are not the same as "chronic pain," so these codes should only be used when the provider has specifically documented these conditions.

Code G89.3 is assigned when the patient's pain is documented as being related to, associated with, or due to cancer, primary or secondary malignancy, or tumor. Code G89.3 is assigned regardless of whether the pain is documented as acute or chronic. Sequencing of code G89.3 is dependent on the reason for the admission/encounter. When the reason for the admission/encounter is documented as pain control/pain management, code G89.3 is assigned as the principal or first-listed code with the underlying neoplasm reported as an additional diagnosis. When the admission/encounter is for management of the neoplasm and the pain associated with the neoplasm is also documented, the neoplasm code is assigned as the principal or first-listed diagnosis and code G89.3 may be assigned as an additional diagnosis. It is not necessary to assign an additional code for the site of the pain.

Chapter 7 – Diseases of Eye and Adnexa (H00-H59)

Chapter 7 classifies diseases of the eye and the adnexa. The adnexa includes structures surrounding the eye, such as the tear (lacrimal) ducts and glands, the extraocular muscles, and the eyelids. Coding diseases of the eye and adnexa can be difficult due to the complex anatomic structures of the ocular system. Laterality is required for most eye conditions. For conditions affecting the eyelid, there are also specific codes for the upper and lower eyelids.

Not all eye conditions are found in Chapter 7. For example, some diseases that are coded to other chapters have associated eye manifestations, such as eye disorders associated with infectious diseases (Chapter 1) and diabetes (Chapter 4). There are also combination codes for conditions and common symptoms or manifestations. Most notable are combination codes for diabetes mellitus with eye conditions (E08.3-, E09.3-, E10.3-, E11.3-, E13.3-). Because the diabetes code captures the manifestation, these conditions do not require additional manifestation codes from Chapter 7.

Chapter Guidelines

All guidelines for Chapter 7 relate to assignment of codes for glaucoma. Glaucoma codes (category H40) are specific to type and, in most cases, laterality (right, left, bilateral) is a component of the code. For some types of glaucoma, the glaucoma stage is also a component of the code. Glaucoma stage is reported using a 7th character extension as follows:

- 0 – Stage unspecified
- 1 – Mild stage
- 2 – Moderate stage
- 3 – Severe stage
- 4 – Indeterminate stage

Indeterminate stage glaucoma identified by the 7th character 4 is assigned only when the stage of the glaucoma cannot be clinically determined. If the glaucoma stage is not documented, 7th character 0, stage unspecified, must be assigned.

Because laterality is a component of most glaucoma codes, it is possible to identify the specific stage for each eye when the type of glaucoma is the same, but the stages are different. When the patient has bilateral glaucoma that is the same type and same stage in both eyes, and there is a bilateral code, a single code is reported with the seventh character for the stage. When laterality is not a component of the code (H40.10-, H40.20-) and the patient has the same stage of glaucoma bilaterally, only one code for the type of glaucoma with the appropriate 7th character for stage is assigned. When the patient has bilateral glaucoma but different types or different stages in each eye and the classification distinguishes laterality, two codes are assigned to identify appropriate type and stage for each eye rather than the code for bilateral glaucoma. When there is not a code that distinguishes laterality (H40.10-, H40.20-) two codes are also reported, one for each type of glaucoma with the appropriate seventh character for stage. Should the glaucoma stage evolve during an admission, the code for the highest stage documented is assigned.

Chapter 8 – Diseases of the Ear and Mastoid Process (H60-H95)

Chapter 8 classifies diseases and conditions of the ear and mastoid process by site, starting with diseases of the external ear, followed by diseases of the middle ear and mastoid, then diseases of the inner ear. Several diseases with associated ear manifestations are classified in other chapters, such as otitis media in influenza (J09.X9, J10.83, J11.83), measles (B05.3), scarlet fever (A38.0), and tuberculosis (A18.6).

Chapter Guidelines

Currently, there are no chapter-specific guidelines for diseases of the ear and mastoid process.

Chapter 9 – Diseases of the Circulatory System (I00-I99)

This chapter conditions affecting the heart muscle and coronary arteries, diseases of the pulmonary artery and conditions affecting the pulmonary circulation, inflammatory disease processes such as pericarditis, valve disorders, arrhythmias and other conditions affecting the conductive system of the heart, heart failure, cerebrovascular diseases, and diseases of the peripheral vascular system.

Hypertension

Essential hypertension is reported with code I10 Essential hypertension and is not designated as benign, malignant or unspecified. The classification presumes a causal relationship between hypertension and heart involvement and between hypertension and kidney involvement, as the two conditions are linked by the term "with" in the Alphabetic Index.

For hypertension and conditions not specifically linked by relational terms such as "with," "associated with" or "due to" in the classification, provider documentation must link the conditions in order to code them as related. These conditions should be coded as related even in the absence of provider documentation explicitly linking them, unless the documentation clearly states the conditions are unrelated.

There are categories for hypertensive heart disease (I11), hypertensive chronic kidney disease (I12), hypertensive heart and chronic kidney disease (I13), and secondary hypertension (I15).

Myocardial Infarction

The period of time for initial treatment of acute myocardial infarction (AMI) is 4 weeks. Codes for the initial treatment should be used only for an AMI that is equal to or less than 4 weeks old (category I21). If care related to the AMI is required beyond 4 weeks, an aftercare code is reported. Codes for subsequent episode of care for AMI (category I22) are used only when the patient suffers a new AMI during the initial 4-week treatment period of a previous AMI. In addition, codes for initial treatment of acute type 1 ST elevation myocardial infarction (STEMI) are more specific to site requiring identification of the affected coronary artery. Type 1 anterior wall AMI is classified as involving the left main coronary artery (I21.01), left anterior descending artery (I21.02), and other coronary artery of anterior wall (I21.09). A type 1 AMI of the inferior wall is classified as involving the right coronary artery (I21.11) or other coronary artery of the inferior wall (I21.19). Codes for other specified sites for type 1 STEM include an AMI involving the left circumflex coronary artery (I21.21) or other specified site (I21.29). There is also a code for an initial type 1 STEMI of an unspecified site (I21.3). Type 1 NSTEMI (I21.4) is not specific to site. A subsequent type 1 STEMI within 4 weeks of the first AMI is classified as involving the anterior wall (I22.0), inferior wall (I22.1), or other sites (I22.8). There is also a code for a subsequent STEMI of an unspecified site (I22.9). No site designation is required for a subsequent type 1 NSTEMI (I22.2).

ICD-10-CM provides codes for different types of myocardial infarction. Type 1 myocardial infarctions are assigned to codes I21.1-I21.4. Type 2 myocardial infarction, and myocardial infarction due to demand ischemia or secondary to ischemic balance, is assigned to code I21.A1, Myocardial infarction type 2 with a code for the underlying cause. Assign code I21.A1 when a type 2 AMI code is described as NSTEMI or STEMI. Acute myocardial infarctions type 3, 4a, 4b, 4c, and 5 are assigned to code I21.A9, Other myocardial infarction type. If the type of AMI is not documented, code I21.9 Acute myocardial infarction, unspecified would be assigned.

Coronary Atherosclerosis

Codes for coronary atherosclerosis (I25.1-, I25.7-, I25.81-) continue to be classified by vessel type, but codes also capture the presence or absence of angina pectoris. When angina is present the codes capture the type of angina (unstable, with documented spasm, other forms of angina, unspecified angina).

Nontraumatic Subarachnoid/Intracerebral Hemorrhage

These codes are specific to site. For nontraumatic subarachnoid hemorrhage (category I60), the specific artery must be identified, and laterality is also a component of the code. For example, code I60.11 reports nontraumatic subarachnoid hemorrhage from right middle cerebral hemorrhage. Nontraumatic intracerebral hemorrhage (category I61) is specific to site as well with the following site designations: subcortical hemisphere, cortical hemisphere, brain stem, cerebellum, intraventricular, multiple localized, other specified, and unspecified site.

Cerebral Infarction

Codes for cerebral infarction (category I63) are specific to type (thrombotic, embolic, unspecified occlusion or stenosis), site, and laterality. The site designations require identification of the specific precerebral or cerebral artery.

Chapter Guidelines

Guidelines for coding diseases of the circulatory system cover five conditions which include hypertension, acute myocardial infarction, atherosclerotic coronary artery disease and angina, intraoperative and postprocedural cerebrovascular accident, and sequelae of cerebrovascular disease.

As was stated earlier, hypertension is not classified as benign, malignant, or unspecified. Hypertension without associated heart or kidney disease is reported with the code I10 Essential hypertension.

There are combination codes for atherosclerotic coronary artery disease with angina pectoris. Documentation of the two conditions are reported with codes from subcategories I25.11- Atherosclerotic heart disease of native coronary artery with angina pectoris, and I25.7- Atherosclerosis of coronary artery bypass grafts and coronary artery of transplanted heart with angina pectoris. It is not necessary to assign a separate code for angina pectoris when both conditions are documented because the combination code captures both conditions. A causal relationship between the atherosclerosis and angina is assumed unless documentation specifically indicates that the angina is due to a condition other than atherosclerosis.

Intraoperative and postprocedural complications and disorders of the circulatory system are found in category I97. Codes from category I97 for intraoperative or postprocedural cerebrovascular accident are found in subcategory I97.8-. Guidelines state that a cause and effect relationship between a cerebrovascular accident (CVA) and a procedure cannot be assumed. The physician must document that a cause and effect relationship exists. Documentation must clearly identify the condition as an intraoperative or postoperative event. The condition must also be clearly documented as an infarction or hemorrhage. Intraoperative and postoperative cerebrovascular infarction (I97.81-, I97.82-) are classified in the circulatory system chapter while intraoperative and postoperative cerebrovascular hemorrhage (G97.3-, G97.5-) are classified in the nervous system chapter.

Category I69 Sequelae of cerebrovascular disease is used to report conditions classifiable to categories I60-I67 as the causes of late effects, specifically neurological deficits, which are classified elsewhere. Sequelae/late effects are conditions that persist after the initial onset of the conditions classifiable to categories I60-I67. The neurologic deficits may be present at the onset of the cerebrovascular disease or may arise at any time after the onset. If the patient has a current CVA and deficits from an old CVA, codes from category I69 and categories I60-I67 may be reported together. For a cerebral infarction without residual neurological deficits, code Z86.73 Personal history of transient ischemic attack (TIA) is reported instead of a code from category I69 to identify the history of the cerebrovascular disease.

Acute myocardial infarction (AMI) is reported with codes that identify type 1 AMI as ST elevation myocardial infarction (STEMI) and non ST elevation myocardial infarction (NSTEMI). Initial acute type 1 myocardial infarction is assigned a code from category I21 for STEMI/NSTEMI not documented as subsequent or not occurring within 28 days of a previous myocardial infarction. All encounters for care of the AMI during the first four weeks (equal to or less than 4 full weeks/28 days), are assigned a code from category I21. Encounters related to the myocardial infarction after 4 full weeks of care are reported with the appropriate aftercare code. Old or healed myocardial infarctions are assigned code I25.2 Old myocardial infarction.

Code I21.9 Acute myocardial infarction, unspecified is the default for unspecified acute myocardial infarction or unspecified type. If only type 1 STEMI or transmural MI without the site is documented, assign code I21.3 ST elevation (STEMI) myocardial infarction of un-specified site.

Subsequent type 1 or unspecified AMI occurring within 28 days of a previous AMI is assigned a code from category I22 for a new STEMI/NSTEMI documented as occurring within 4 weeks (28 days) of a previous myocardial infarction. The subsequent AMI may involve the same site as the initial AMI or a different site. Codes in category I22 are never reported alone. A code from category I21 must be reported in conjunction with the code from I22. Codes from categories I21 and I22 are sequenced based on the circumstances of the encounter.

Do not assign code I22 for subsequent myocardial infarctions other than type 1 or unspecified. For subsequent type 2 AMI assign only code I21.A1. For subsequent type 4 or type 5 AMI, assign only code I21.A9.

Chapter 10 – Diseases of the Respiratory System (J00-J99)

Diseases of the respiratory system include conditions affecting the nose and sinuses, throat, tonsils, larynx and trachea, bronchi, and lungs. Chapter 10 is organized by the general type of disease or condition and by site with diseases affecting primarily the upper respiratory system or the lower respiratory system in separate sections.

Chapter Guidelines

The respiratory system guidelines cover chronic obstructive pulmonary disease (COPD) and asthma, acute respiratory failure, influenza due to avian influenza virus, and ventilator associated pneumonia.

Codes for COPD in category J44 differentiate between uncomplicated cases and those with an acute exacerbation. For coding purposes an acute exacerbation is defined as a worsening or decompensation of a chronic condition. An acute exacerbation is not the same as an infection superimposed on a chronic condition, though an exacerbation may be triggered by an infection.

Guidelines for reporting acute respiratory failure (J96.0-) and acute and chronic respiratory failure (J96.2-) relate to sequencing of these codes. Depending on the documentation these codes may be either the principal or first-listed diagnosis or a secondary diagnosis. Careful review of the provider documentation and a clear understanding of the guidelines including the definition of principal diagnosis are required to sequence these codes correctly.

There are three code categories for reporting influenza which are as follows: J09 Influenza due to certain identified influenza viruses, J10 Influenza due to other identified influenza virus, and J11 Influenza due to unidentified influenza virus. All codes in category J09 report influenza due to identified novel influenza A virus with various complications or manifestations such as pneumonia, other respiratory conditions, gastrointestinal manifestations or other manifestations. Identified novel influenza A viruses include avian (bird) influenza, influenza A/H5N1, influenza of other animal origin (not bird or swine), and swine influenza. Codes from category J09 are reported only for confirmed cases of avian influenza and the other specific types of influenza identified in the code description. This is an exception to the inpatient guideline related to uncertain diagnoses. Confirmation does not require a positive laboratory finding. Documentation by the provider that the patient has avian influenza or influenza due other identified novel influenza A virus is sufficient to report a code from category J09. Documentation of "suspected," "possible," or "probable" avian influenza or other novel influenza A virus is reported with a code from category J10.

Ventilator associated pneumonia (VAP) is listed in category J95 Intraoperative and postprocedural complications and disorders of respiratory system not elsewhere classified, and is reported with code J95.851. As with all procedural and postprocedural complications, the provider must document the relationship between the conditions, in this case VAP, and the procedure. An additional code should be assigned to identify the organism. Codes for pneumonia classified in categories J12-J18 are not assigned additionally for VAP. However, when a patient is admitted with a different type of pneumonia and subsequently develops VAP, the appropriate code from J12-J18 is reported as the principal diagnosis and code J95.851 is reported as an additional diagnosis

Chapter 11 – Diseases of the Digestive System (K00-K95)

Diseases of the digestive system include conditions affecting the esophagus, stomach, small and large intestines, liver, and gallbladder. Some of the most frequently diagnosed digestive system diseases and conditions, such as cholecystitis and cholelithiasis, have specific elements incorporated into the codes. For example, cholecystitis is classified as acute, chronic, or acute and chronic regardless of whether the cholecystitis occurs alone or with cholelithiasis. Combination codes for cholelithiasis with cholecystitis identify the site of the calculus as being in the gallbladder and/or bile duct and the specific type of cholecystitis. Combination codes also report cholelithiasis of the bile duct with cholangitis. There are other digestive system conditions that require an acute or chronic designation as well as more combination codes that capture diseases of the gallbladder and associated complications.

Chapter Guidelines

Currently there are no guidelines for the digestive system.

Chapter 12 – Diseases of the Skin and Subcutaneous Tissue (L00-L99)

Diseases of the skin and subcutaneous tissue include diseases affecting the epidermis, dermis and hypodermis, subcutaneous tissue, nails, sebaceous glands, sweat glands, and hair and hair follicles. Common conditions of the skin and subcutaneous tissue include boils, cellulitis, abscess, pressure ulcers, lymphadenitis, and pilonidal cysts.

Chapter Guidelines

All guidelines related to coding of diseases of the skin and subcutaneous tissue relate to pressure ulcers and non-pressure chronic ulcers. Codes from category L89 Pressure ulcer are combination codes that identify the site of the pressure ulcer as well as the stage of the ulcer. For patients with multiple pressure ulcers, multiple codes should be assigned to capture all pressure ulcer sites.

Pressure ulcer stages are based on severity. Severity is designated as:

- Stage 1 – Pressure ulcer skin changes limited to persistent focal edema
- Stage 2 – Pressure ulcer with abrasion, blister, partial thickness skin loss involving epidermis and/or dermis
- Stage 3 – Pressure ulcer with full thickness skin loss involving damage or necrosis of subcutaneous tissue
- Stage 4 – Pressure ulcer with necrosis of soft tissues through to underlying muscle, tendon, or bone
- Unstageable – Pressure ulcer stage cannot be clinically determined
- Unspecified – Pressure ulcer stage is not documented

Assignment of the pressure ulcer stage code should be guided by clinical documentation of the stage or documentation of the terms found in the Alphabetic Index. For clinical terms describing the stage that are not found in the Alphabetic Index and when there is no documentation of the stage, the provider should be queried. Assignment of the code for unstageable pressure ulcer (L89.--0) should be based on the clinical documentation. These codes are used for pressure ulcers whose stage cannot be clinically determined (e.g., the ulcer is covered by eschar or has been treated with a skin or muscle graft) and pressure ulcers that are documented as deep tissue injury, but not documented as due to trauma. Unstageable pressure ulcers should not be confused with the codes for unspecified stage (L89.--9). When there is no documentation regarding the stage of the pressure ulcer, the appropriate code for unspecified stage (L89.--9) is assigned.

The depth of non-pressure chronic ulcers and the stage of pressure ulcers may be coded from documentation provided by a clinician other than the patient's provider, such as a wound care nurse. The actual diagnosis must be made by the patient's provider. Code assignment for the specific type and site of the ulcer must be based on information in the provider's documentation.

Patients admitted with pressure ulcers documented as healing should be assigned the appropriate pressure ulcer stage code based on the documentation in the medical record. If the documentation does not provide information about the stage of the healing pressure ulcer, a code for unspecified stage is assigned. If the documentation is unclear as to whether the patient has a current (new) pressure ulcer or if the patient is being treated for a healing pressure ulcer, query the provider. No code is assigned if the documentation states that the pressure ulcer is completely healed.

If a patient is admitted with a pressure ulcer at one stage and it progresses to a higher stage, two separate codes should be assigned: one code for the site and stage of the ulcer on admission and a second code for the same ulcer site and the highest stage reported during the stay. For ulcers that were present on admission but healed at the time of discharge, assign the code for the site and stage of the pressure ulcer at the time of admission.

Non-pressure ulcers described as healing should be assigned the appropriate non-pressure ulcer code based on the documentation in the medical record. If the documentation does not provide information about the severity of the healing non-pressure ulcer, assign the appropriate code for unspecified severity. For ulcers that were present on admission but healed at the time of discharge, assign the code for the site and severity of the non-pressure ulcer at the time of admission.

If the patient is admitted with a non-pressure ulcer at one severity level and it progresses to a higher severity level, two separate codes should be assigned: one code for the site and severity level of the ulcer on admission and a second code for the same ulcer site and the highest severity level reported during the stay.

Chapter 13 – Diseases of the Musculoskeletal System and Connective Tissue (M00-M99)

Coding of musculoskeletal system and connective tissue conditions requires both precise site specificity and laterality. For example, conditions affecting the cervical spine require identification of the site as occipito-atlanto-axial, mid-cervical or cervicothoracic. Laterality is also included for most musculoskeletal and connective tissue conditions affecting the extremities. For some conditions only right and left are provided, but for other conditions that frequently affect both sides, codes for bilateral are also listed. For example, osteoarthritis of the hips has designations for bilateral primary osteoarthritis (M16.0), bilateral osteoarthritis resulting from hip dysplasia (M16.2), bilateral post-traumatic osteoarthritis (M16.4), and other bilateral secondary osteoarthritis of the hip (M16.6). In addition, there are 7th characters for some code categories.

7th Characters

In Chapter 13, 7th characters are required for chronic gout to identify the presence or absence of tophus (tophi). Tophi are solid deposits of monosodium urate (MSU) crystals that form in the joints, cartilage, bones, and elsewhere in the body. Chronic gout is reported with codes in category M1A. The required 7th characters identify chronic gout as without tophus (0) or with tophus (1).

Fatigue and compression fractures of the vertebra, stress fractures, and pathological fractures due to osteoporosis, neoplastic or other disease also require 7th characters to identify the episode of care. For fatigue fractures of the vertebra (M48.4-) and collapsed vertebra (M48.5-) the 7th character designates episode of care as: initial encounter for fracture (A), subsequent encounter for fracture with routine healing (D), subsequent encounter for fracture with delayed healing (G), and sequela (S). For age-related osteoporosis with current pathological fracture (M80.0-), other osteoporosis with current pathological fracture (M80.1-), stress fracture (M84.3-), pathological fracture not elsewhere classified (M84.4-), pathological fracture in neoplastic disease (M84.5-), and pathological fracture in other disease (M84.6-), 7th character designations include those listed for fatigue and compression fractures of the vertebra, and also include two additional 7th characters for subsequent encounter with nonunion (K) or malunion (P). The table below explains and defines the 7th characters used for fractures classified in Chapter 13.

Character	Definition	Explanation
A	Initial encounter for fracture	Use 'A' for as long as the patient is receiving active treatment for the pathologic fracture. Examples of active treatment are: surgical treatment, emergency department encounter, evaluation and treatment by a new physician
D	Subsequent encounter with routine fracture healing	For encounters after the patient has completed active treatment and when the fracture is healing normally
G	Subsequent encounter for fracture with delayed healing	For encounters when the physician has documented that healing is delayed or is not occurring as rapidly as normally expected
K	Subsequent encounter for fracture with nonunion	For encounters when the physician has documented that there is nonunion of the fracture or that the fracture has failed to heal. This is a serious fracture complication that requires additional intervention and treatment by the physician
P	Subsequent encounter for fracture with malunion	For encounters when the physician has documented that the fracture has healed in an abnormal or nonanatomic position. This is a serious fracture complication that requires additional intervention and treatment by the physician
S	Sequela	Use for complications or conditions that arise as a direct result of the pathological fracture, such as a leg length discrepancy following pathological fracture of the femur. The specific type of sequela is sequenced first followed by the pathological fracture code.

Chapter Guidelines

Chapter specific guidelines are provided for musculoskeletal system and connective tissue coding related to the following: site and laterality, acute traumatic versus chronic or recurrent musculoskeletal conditions, osteoporosis, and pathological fractures. Guidelines related to coding of pathological fractures relate to the use of 7th characters which are discussed above.

Most codes in Chapter 13 have site and laterality designations. Site represents either the bone, joint or muscle involved. For some conditions where more than one bone, joint, or muscle is commonly involved, such as osteoarthritis, there is a "multiple sites" code available. For categories where no multiple site code is provided and more than one bone, joint or muscle is involved, it is necessary to report multiple codes to indicate the different sites involved. Because some conditions involving the bones occur at the upper and/or lower ends at the joint, it is sometimes difficult to determine whether the code for the bone or joint should be reported. The guidelines indicate that when a condition involves the upper or lower ends of the bones, the site code assigned should be designated as the bone, not the joint.

Many musculoskeletal conditions are a result of a previous injury or trauma to a site, or are recurrent conditions. Musculoskeletal conditions are classified either in Chapter 13, Diseases of the Musculoskeletal System and Connective tissue or in Chapter 19, Injury, Poisoning, and Certain Other Consequences of External Causes. The table below identifies where various conditions/injuries are classified.

Condition	Chapter
Healed injury	Chapter 13
Recurrent bone, joint, or muscle condition	Chapter 13
Chronic or other recurrent conditions	Chapter 13
Current acute injury	Chapter 19

Osteoporosis is a systemic condition, meaning that all bones of the musculoskeletal system are affected. Therefore, site is not a component of the codes under category M81 Osteoporosis without current pathological fracture. The site codes under M80 Osteoporosis with current pathological fracture identify the site of the fracture not the osteoporosis. A code from category M80, not a traumatic fracture code, should be used for any patient with known osteoporosis who suffers a fracture, even if the patient had a minor fall or trauma, if that fall or trauma would not usually break a normal, healthy bone. For a patient with a history of osteoporosis fractures, status code Z87.31, Personal history of osteoporosis fracture should follow the code from category M81.

Chapter 14 – Diseases of the Genitourinary System (N00-N99)

The Genitourinary System includes the organs and anatomical structures involved with reproduction and urinary excretion in both males and females. Female genitourinary disorders include pelvic inflammatory diseases, vaginitis, salpingitis and oophoritis. Common male genitourinary disorders include prostatitis, benign prostatic hyperplasia, premature ejaculation and erectile dysfunction.

Chapter Guidelines

All coding guidelines relate to coding of chronic kidney disease. The guidelines cover stages of chronic kidney disease (CKD), CKD and kidney transplant status, and CKD with other conditions.

Chapter 15 – Pregnancy, Childbirth and the Puerperium (O00-O9A)

The majority of codes for complications that occur during pregnancy require identification of the trimester.

Trimester

The trimester is captured by the fourth, fifth or sixth character. The fourth, fifth or sixth character also captures the episode of care for complications that can occur at any point in the pregnancy, during childbirth or postpartum, such as eclampsia (O15). Some complications of pregnancy that typically occur or are treated only in a single trimester such as ectopic pregnancy (O00) do not identify the trimester. In addition, complications that occur only during childbirth or the puerperium contain that information in the code description, such as obstructed labor due to generally contracted pelvis (O65.1) or puerperal sepsis (O85).

7th Character

A 7th character identifying the fetus is required for certain categories. Some complications of pregnancy and childbirth occur more frequently in multiple gestation pregnancies. These complications may affect one or more fetuses and require a 7th character to identify the fetus or fetuses affected by the complication. The following categories/subcategories require identification of the fetus:

- O31 Complications specific to multiple gestation
- O32 Maternal care for malpresentation of fetus
- O33.3 Maternal care for disproportion due to outlet contraction of pelvis
- O33.4 Maternal care for disproportion of mixed maternal and fetal origin
- O33.5 Maternal care for disproportion due to unusually large fetus
- O33.6 Maternal care for disproportion due to hydrocephalic fetus
- O35 Maternal care for known or suspected fetal abnormality and damage
- O36 Maternal care for other fetal problems
- O40 Polyhydramnios
- O41 Other disorders of amniotic fluid and membranes
- O60.1 Preterm labor with preterm delivery
- O60.2 Term delivery with preterm labor
- O64 Obstructed labor due to malposition and malpresentation of fetus
- O69 Labor and delivery complicated by umbilical cord complications

The 7th character identifies the fetus to which the complication code applies. For a single gestation, when the documentation is insufficient, or when it is clinically impossible to identify the fetus, the 7th character '0' for not applicable/unspecified is assigned. For multiple gestations, each fetus should be identified with a number as fetus 1, fetus 2, fetus 3, etc. The fetus or fetuses affected by the condition should then be clearly identified using the number assigned to the fetus. For example, a triplet gestation in the third trimester with fetus 1 having no complications, fetus 2 in a separate amniotic sac having polyhydramnios, and fetus 3 having hydrocephalus with maternal pelvic disproportion would require reporting of the complications as follows: Fetus 1 – No codes; Fetus 2 – O40.3XX2, Polyhydramnios, third trimester, fetus 2; Fetus 3 – O33.6XX3, Maternal care for disproportion due to hydrocephalic fetus, fetus 3. An additional code identifying the triplet pregnancy would also be reported. Applicable 7th characters are:

- 0 – not applicable or unspecified
- 1 – fetus 1
- 2 – fetus 2
- 3 – fetus 3
- 4 – fetus 4
- 5 – fetus 5
- 9 – other fetus

Chapter Guidelines

Chapter 15 guidelines include information covering general rules and sequencing of codes and coding rules for specific conditions. Only guidelines related to trimester, pre-existing conditions versus conditions due to pregnancy, and gestational diabetes are discussed here. Consult the Official Guidelines for Coding and Reporting for the complete Chapter 15 guidelines.

Most codes for conditions and complications of pregnancy have a final character indicating the trimester. Assignment of the final character for trimester is based on the provider's documentation which may identify the trimester or the number of weeks of gestation for the current encounter. Trimesters are calculated using the first day of the last menstrual period and are as follows:

- First trimester – less than 14 weeks 0 days
- Second trimester – 14 weeks 0 days to less than 28 weeks 0 days
- Third trimester – 28 weeks 0 days to delivery

There are codes for unspecified trimester; however, these codes should be used only when the documentation is insufficient to determine the trimester and it is not possible to obtain clarification from the provider. If a delivery occurs during the admission and there is an "in childbirth" option for the complication, the code for "in childbirth" is assigned.

When an obstetric patient is admitted and delivers during that admission, the condition that prompted the admission should be sequenced as the principal diagnosis. If multiple conditions prompted the admission, sequence the one most related to the delivery as the principal diagnosis. A code for any complication of the delivery should be assigned as an additional diagnosis.

For inpatient services, when an inpatient admission encompasses more than one trimester, the code is assigned based on when the condition developed not when the discharge occurred. For example, if the condition developed during the second trimester and the patient was discharged during the third trimester, the code for the second trimester is assigned. If the condition being treated developed prior to the current admission/encounter or was a pre-existing condition, the trimester character at the time of the admission/encounter is used.

Certain categories in Chapter 15 distinguish between conditions that existed prior to pregnancy (pre-existing) and those that are a direct result of the pregnancy. Two examples are hypertension (O10, O11, O13) and diabetes mellitus (O24). The physician must provide clear documentation as to whether the condition existed prior to pregnancy or whether it developed during the pregnancy or as a result of the pregnancy. Categories that do not distinguish between pre-existing conditions and pregnancy related conditions may be used for either. If a puerperal complication develops during the delivery encounter and a specific code for the puerperal complication exists, the code for the puerperal complication may be reported with codes related to complications of pregnancy and childbirth.

Gestational diabetes can occur during the second and third trimesters in women without a pre-pregnancy diagnosis of diabetes mellitus. Gestational diabetes may cause complications similar to those in patients with pre-existing diabetes mellitus. Gestational diabetes is classified in category O24 along with pre-existing diabetes mellitus. Subcategory O24.4- Gestational diabetes mellitus, cannot be used with any other codes in category O24. Codes in subcategory O24.4- are combination codes that identify the condition as well as how it is being controlled. In order to assign the most specific code, the provider must document whether the gestational diabetes is being controlled by diet or insulin. If documentation indicates the gestational diabetes is being controlled with both diet and insulin, only the code for insulin-controlled is assigned. Code Z79.4 for long-term insulin use is not reported with codes in subcategory O24.4-. Codes for gestational diabetes are not used to report an abnormal glucose tolerance test which is reported with code O99.81 Abnormal glucose complicating pregnancy, childbirth, and the puerperium.

Chapter 16 – Newborn (Perinatal) Guidelines (P00-P96)

Perinatal conditions have their origin in the period beginning before birth and extending through the first 28 days after birth. Codes from this chapter are used only on the newborn medical record, never on the maternal medical record. These conditions must originate during this period but for some conditions morbidity may not be manifested or diagnosed until later. As long as the documentation supports the origin of the condition during the perinatal period, codes for perinatal conditions may be reported. Examples of conditions included in this chapter are maternal conditions that have affected or are suspected to have affected the fetus or newborn, prematurity, light for dates, birth injuries, and other conditions originating in the perinatal period and affecting specific body systems.

Chapter Guidelines

The principal diagnosis for the birth record is always a code from Chapter 21, category Z38 Liveborn according to place of birth and type of delivery. Additional diagnoses are assigned for all clinically significant conditions identified on the newborn examination. Other guidelines relate to prematurity, fetal growth retardation, low birth weight and immaturity status.

In determining prematurity, different providers may utilize different criteria. A code for prematurity should not be assigned unless specifically documented by the physician. Two code categories are provided for reporting prematurity and fetal growth retardation, P05 Disorders of newborn related to slow fetal growth and fetal malnutrition and P07 Disorders of newborn related to short gestation and low birth weight, not elsewhere classified. Assignment of codes in categories P05 and P07 should be based on the recorded birth weight and estimated gestational age.

To identify those instances when a healthy newborn is evaluated for a suspected condition that is determined after study not to be present, assign a code from category Z05, Observation and evaluation of newborns and infants for suspected conditions ruled out. Do not use a code from category Z05 when the patient has identified signs or symptoms of a suspected problem; in such cases code the sign or symptom. A code from category Z05 may also be assigned as a principal or first-listed code for readmissions or encounters when the code from category Z38 code no longer applies. Codes from category Z05 are for use only for healthy newborns and infants for which no condition after study is found to be present. On a birth record, a code from category Z05 is to be used as a secondary code after the code from category Z38, Liveborn infants according to place of birth and type of delivery.

Chapter 17 – Congenital Malformations, Deformations, and Chromosomal Abnormalities (Q00-Q99)

Congenital anomalies are conditions that are present at birth. Congenital anomalies include both congenital malformations, such as spina bifida, atrial and ventricular septal heart defects, undescended testes, and chromosomal abnormalities such as trisomy 21 also known as Down's syndrome. Chapter 17 is organized with congenital anomalies, malformations, or deformations grouped together by body system followed by other congenital conditions such as syndromes that affect multiple systems with the last block of codes being chromosomal abnormalities.

Codes for congenital malformations, deformations and chromosomal abnormalities require specificity. For example, codes for encephalocele (category Q01) are specific to site and must be documented as frontal, nasofrontal, occipital, or of other specific sites. Cleft lip and cleft palate (categories Q35-Q37) require documentation of the condition as complete or incomplete but do require more specific documentation of the site of the opening in the palate as the hard or soft palate and the location of the cleft lip as unilateral, in the median, or bilateral.

Chapter Guidelines

When a malformation, deformation, or chromosomal abnormality is documented, the appropriate code from categories Q00-Q99 is assigned. A malformation, deformation, or chromosomal abnormality may be the principal or first-listed diagnosis or it may be a secondary diagnosis. For the birth admission the principal diagnosis is always a code from category Z38 and any congenital anomalies documented in the birth record are reported additionally. In some instances there may not be a specific diagnosis code for the malformation, deformation, or chromosomal abnormality. In this case the code for other specified is used and additional codes are assigned for any manifestations that are present. However, when there is a specific code available to report the congenital anomaly, manifestations that are an inherent component of the anomaly should not be coded separately. Additional codes may be reported for manifestations that are not an inherent component of the anomaly. Although present at birth the congenital malformation, deformation, or chromosomal abnormality may not be diagnosed until later in life and it is appropriate to assign a code from Chapter 17 when the physician documentation supports a diagnosis of a congenital anomaly. If the congenital malformation or deformity has been corrected, a personal history code should be used to identify the history of the malformation or deformity.

Chapter 18 – Symptoms, Signs, and Abnormal Clinical and Laboratory Findings, Not Elsewhere Classified (R00-R99)

Codes for symptoms, signs, abnormal results of laboratory or other investigative procedures, and ill-defined conditions without a diagnosis classified elsewhere are classified in Chapter 18. There are 7 code blocks that identify symptoms and signs for specific body systems followed by a code block for general symptoms and signs. The last 5 code blocks report abnormal findings for laboratory tests, imaging and function studies, and tumor markers. Examples of signs and symptoms related to specific body systems include: shortness of breath (R06.02), epigastric pain (R10.13), cyanosis (R23.0), ataxia (R27.0), and dysuria (R30.0). Examples of general signs and symptoms include: fever (R50.9), chronic fatigue (R53.82), abnormal weight loss (R63.4), systemic inflammatory response syndrome (SIRS) of non-infectious origin (R65.1-), and severe sepsis (R65.2-). Examples of abnormal findings include: red blood cell abnormalities (R71.-), proteinuria (R80-), abnormal cytological findings in specimens from cervix uteri (R87.61-), and inconclusive mammogram (R92.2).

Combination Codes

A number of codes identify both the definitive diagnosis and common symptoms of that diagnosis. When using these combination codes, an additional code should not be assigned for the symptom. For example, R18.8 Other ascites is not reported with the combination code K70.31 Alcoholic cirrhosis of the liver with ascites because code K70.31 identifies both the definitive diagnosis (alcoholic cirrhosis) and a common symptom of the condition (ascites).

Coma Scale

One significant ICD-10-CM coding concept relates the coma scale codes (R40.2-). Coma scale codes can be used by trauma registries in conjunction with traumatic brain injury codes, acute cerebrovascular disease, and sequela of cerebrovascular disease codes or to assess the status of the central nervous system. These codes can also be used for other non-trauma conditions, such as monitoring patients in the intensive care unit regardless of medical condition. The coma scale codes are sequenced after the diagnosis code(s).

The coma scale consists of three elements, eye opening (R40.21-), verbal response (R40.22-), and motor response (R40.23-) and a code from each subcategory must be assigned to complete the coma scale. If all three elements are documented, codes for the individual scores should be assigned. In addition, a 7th character indicates when the scale was recorded and the 7th character should match for all three codes. The 7th characters identify the time/place as follows:

- 0 – Unspecified time
- 1 – In the field (EMT/ambulance)
- 2 – At arrival in emergency department
- 3 – At hospital admission
- 4 – 24 hours or more after hospital admission

If all three elements are not known but the total Glasgow coma scale is documented, the code for the total Glasgow coma score is assigned. The Glasgow score is classified as follows:

- Glasgow score 13-15
- Glasgow score 9-12
- Glasgow score 3-8
- Other coma without documented Glasgow coma scale score or with partial score reported

Chapter Guidelines

There are a number of general guidelines for the use of symptom codes and combination codes that include symptoms as well as some specific guidelines related to repeated falls, the coma scale (discussed above), and systemic inflammatory response syndrome (SIRS) due to non-infectious process. There are also some guidelines referencing signs and symptoms in Section II Selection of Principal Diagnosis. For example, the first guideline related to the use of symptom codes indicates that these codes are acceptable for reporting purposes when a related definitive diagnosis has not been established (confirmed) by the provider. It may also be appropriate to report a sign or symptom code with a definitive diagnosis. However, this is dependent upon whether or not the symptom is routinely associated with the definitive diagnosis/disease process. When the sign or symptom is not routinely associated with the definitive diagnosis, the codes for signs and symptoms may be reported additionally. The definitive diagnosis should be sequenced before the symptom code. When the sign or symptom is routinely associated with the disease process, the sign or symptom code is not reported additionally unless instructions in the Tabular indicate otherwise.

There is a code for repeated falls (R29.6) and another code for history of falling (Z91.81). The code for repeated falls is assigned when a patient has recently fallen and the reason for the fall is being investigated. The code for history of falling is assigned when a patient has fallen in the past and is at risk for future falls. Both codes may be assigned when the patient has had a recent fall that is being investigated and also has a history of falling.

Guidelines related to SIRS due to a non-infectious process (R65.1-) relate to sequencing of codes. Also discussed is the need to verify whether any documented acute organ dysfunction is associated with the SIRS or due to the underlying condition that caused the SIRS or another related condition as this affects code assignment.

Chapter 19 – Injury, Poisoning, and Certain Other Consequences of External Causes (S00-T88)

Codes for injury, poisoning and certain other consequences of external causes are found in Chapter 19. One of the important characteristics to note is that injuries are organized first by body site and then by type of injury. Another is that laterality is included in the code descriptor. The vast majority of injuries to paired organs and the extremities identify the injury as the right or left. In addition, most injuries are specific to site. For example, codes for an open wound of the thorax (category S21), are specific to the right back wall, left back wall, right front wall or left front wall. For open wounds of the abdominal wall (S31.1-, S31.6-), the site must be identified as right upper quadrant, left upper quadrant, epigastric region, right lower quadrant, or left lower quadrant. Also, the vast majority of codes require a 7th character to identify episode of care. Episode of care designations have been discussed previously and many of the same designations are used in Chapter 13. However, there are some additional 7th characters for episode of care that are used only in this chapter for fractures of the long bones. Additionally, the codes for poisoning, adverse effects and toxic effects are combination codes that capture both the drug and the external cause. The Table of Drugs and Chemicals includes an underdosing column.

Application of 7th Characters

Most categories in the injury and poisoning chapter require assignment of a 7th character to identify the episode of care. For most categories there are three (3) 7th character values to select from: 'A' for initial encounter; 'B' for subsequent encounter and 'S' for sequela. Categories for fractures are an exception with fractures having 6 to 16 7th character values in order to capture additional information about the fracture including, whether the fracture is open or closed and whether the healing phase is routine or complicated by delayed healing, nonunion, or malunion. Detailed guidelines are provided related to selection of the 7th character value. Related guidelines and some examples of encounters representative of the three episodes of care 7th character values found in the majority of categories are as follows:

A Initial encounter. Initial encounter is defined as the period when the patient is receiving active treatment for the injury, poisoning, or other consequences of an external cause. An 'A' may be assigned on more than one claim. For example, if a patient is seen in the emergency department (ED) for a head injury that is first evaluated by the ED physician who requests a CT scan that is read by a radiologist and a consultation by a neurologist, the 7th character 'A' is used by all three physicians and also reported on the ED claim. If the patient required admission to an acute care hospital, the 7th character 'A' would be reported for the entire acute care hospital stay because the 7th character extension 'A' is used for the entire period that the patient receives active treatment for the injury.

D Subsequent encounter. This is an encounter after the patient has completed the active phase of treatment and is receiving routine care for the injury or poisoning during the period of healing or recovery. Unlike aftercare following medical or surgical services for other conditions which are reported with codes from Chapter 21, Factors Influencing Health Status and Contact with Health Services (Z00-Z99), aftercare for injuries and poisonings is captured by the 7th character D. For example, a patient with an ankle sprain may return to the office to have joint stability re-evaluated to ensure that the injury is healing properly. In this case, the 7th character 'D' would be assigned.

S Sequela. The 7th character extension 'S' is assigned for complications or conditions that arise as a direct result of an injury. An example of a sequela is a scar resulting from a burn.

Fracture Coding

Two things of note related to fracture coding include the 7th character extensions which differ from the 7th character extensions for other injuries, and the incorporation of information from certain fracture classification systems in the code descriptors. In fact, for open fractures of the long bones, correct assignment of the 7th character requires an understanding of the Gustilo classification system. For most fractures the 7th character extensions are the same as those detailed in Chapter 13 for pathological fractures. The designations are again summarized here and are as follows:

7th Character	Description
A	Initial encounter for closed fracture
B	Initial encounter for open fracture type
D	Subsequent encounter for fracture with routine healing
G	Subsequent encounter for fracture with delayed healing
K	Subsequent encounter for fracture with nonunion
P	Subsequent encounter for fracture with malunion
S	Sequela

For fractures of the shafts of the long bones, the 7th characters further describe the fracture as open or closed. When documentation does not indicate whether the fracture is open or closed, the default is closed. For open fractures, the 7th character also captures the severity of the injury using the Gustilo classification. The Gustilo classification applies to open fractures of the long bones including the humerus, radius, ulna, femur, tibia, and fibula. The Gustilo open fracture classification groups open fractures into three main categories designated as Type I, Type II and Type III with Type III injuries being further divided into Type IIIA, Type IIIB, and Type IIIC subcategories. The categories are defined by characteristics that include the mechanism of injury, extent of soft tissue damage, and degree of bone injury or involvement. The table below identifies key features of Gustilo fracture types. When the Gustilo classification type is not specified for an open fracture, the 7th character for open fracture type I or II should be assigned.

Type	Wound/ Contamination	Soft Tissue Damage	Type of Injury	Most Common Fracture Type(s)
Gustilo Type I	< 1 cm/ Wound bed clean	Minimal	Low-energy	Simple transverse, short oblique, minimally comminuted
Gustilo Type II	> 1 cm/ Minimal or no contamination	Moderate	Low-energy	Simple transverse, short oblique, minimally comminuted
Gustilo Type III	> 1 cm/ Contaminated wound	Extensive Type IIIA – • Adequate soft tissue coverage open wound • No flap coverage required Type IIIB • Extensive soft tissue loss • Flap coverage required Type IIIC • Major arterial injury • Extensive repair • May require vascular surgeon for limb salvage	High-energy	Unstable fracture with multiple bone fragments including the following: • Open segmental fracture regardless of wound size • Gun-shot wounds with bone involvement • Open fractures with any type of neurovascular involvement • Severely contaminated open fractures • Traumatic amputations • Open fractures with delayed treatment (over 8 hours)

The applicable 7th character extensions for fractures of the shafts of the long bones are as follows:

7th Character	Description
A	Initial encounter for closed fracture
B	Initial encounter for open fracture type I or II
C	Initial encounter for open fracture type IIIA, IIIB, or IIIC
D	Subsequent encounter for closed fracture with routine healing
E	Subsequent encounter for open fracture type I or II with routine healing
F	Subsequent encounter for open fracture type IIIA, IIIB, or IIIC with routine healing
G	Subsequent encounter for closed fracture with delayed healing
H	Subsequent encounter for open fracture type I or II with delayed healing
J	Subsequent encounter for open fracture type IIIA, IIIB, or IIIC with delayed healing
K	Subsequent encounter for closed fracture with nonunion
M	Subsequent encounter for open fracture type I or II with nonunion
N	Subsequent encounter for open fracture type IIIA, IIIB, or IIIC with nonunion
P	Subsequent encounter for closed fracture with malunion
Q	Subsequent encounter for open fracture type I or II with malunion
R	Subsequent encounter for open fracture type IIIA, IIIB, or IIIC with malunion
S	Sequela

Chapter Guidelines

There are detailed guidelines for reporting of injury, poisoning and certain other consequences of external causes. The following topics are covered in the chapter-specific guidelines: application of 7th characters; coding of injuries, traumatic fractures, burns and corrosions; adverse effects, poisoning, underdosing and toxic effects; adult and child abuse, neglect and other maltreatment; and complications of care.

The principles for coding traumatic fractures are the same as coding of other injuries. Applicable 7th characters for fractures have already been discussed. Two additional guidelines of note provide default codes when certain information is not provided. A fracture not indicated as open or closed is coded as closed. A fracture not indicated as displaced or nondisplaced is coded as displaced.

Burns are classified first as corrosion or thermal burns and then by depth and extent. Corrosions are burns due to chemicals. Thermal burns are burns that come from a heat source but exclude sunburns. Examples of heat sources include: fire, hot appliance, electricity, and radiation.

The guidelines are the same for both corrosions and thermal burns with one exception: corrosions require identification of the chemical substance. The chemical substance that caused the corrosion is the first-listed diagnosis and is found in the Table of Drugs and Chemicals. Codes for drugs and chemicals are combination codes that identify the substance and the external cause or intent, so an external cause of injury code is not required. However, external cause codes should be assigned for the place of occurrence, activity, and external cause status when this information is available. The correct code for an accidental corrosion is found in the column for poisoning, accidental (unintentional).

Codes for adverse effects, poisoning, underdosing and toxic effects are combination codes that include both the substance taken and the intent. If the intent of the poisoning is unknown or unspecified, code the intent as accidental intent. The undetermined intent is only for use if the documentation in the record specifies that the intent cannot be determined. No additional external cause code is reported with these codes. Underdosing is defined as taking less of a medication than is prescribed by the provider or the manufacturer's instructions. Underdosing codes are never assigned as the principal or first-listed code. The code for the relapse or exacerbation of the medical condition for which the drug was prescribed is listed as the principal or first-listed code and the underdosing code is listed secondarily. An additional code from subcategories Z91.12- or Z91.13-, Z91.14- should also be assigned to identify the intent of the noncompliance if known. For example, code Z91.120 would be assigned for intentional underdosing due to financial hardship.

Complications of surgical and medical care not elsewhere classified are reported with codes from categories T80-T88. However, intraoperative and post-procedural complications are reported with codes from the body system chapters. For example, ventilator associated pneumonia is considered a procedural or post-procedural complication and is reported with code J95.851 Ventilator associated pneumonia from Chapter 10 – Diseases of the Respiratory System. Complication of care code assignment is based on the provider's documentation of the relationship between the condition and the care or procedure. Not all conditions that occur following medical or surgical treatment are classified as complications. Only conditions for which the provider has documented a cause-and-effect relationship between the care and the complication should be classified as complications of care. If the documentation is unclear, query the provider. Some complications of care codes include the external cause in the code. These codes include the nature of the complication as well as the type of procedure that caused the complication. An additional external cause code indicating the type of procedure is not necessary for these codes.

Pain due to medical devices, implants, or grafts requires two codes, one from the T-codes to identify the device causing the pain, such as T84.84- Pain due to internal orthopedic prosthetic devices, implants, and grafts and one from category G89 to identify acute or chronic pain due to presence of the device, implant, or graft.

Transplant complications are reported with codes from category T86. These codes should be used for both complications and rejection of transplanted organs. A transplant complication code is assigned only when the complication affects the function of the transplanted organ. Two codes are required to describe a transplant complication, one from category T86 and a secondary code that identifies the specific complication. Patients who have undergone a kidney transplant may have some form of chronic kidney disease (CKD) because the transplant may not fully restore kidney function. CKD is not considered to be a transplant complication unless the provider documents a transplant complication such as transplant failure or rejection. If the documentation is unclear, the provider should be queried. Other complications (other than CKD) that affect function of the kidney are assigned a code from subcategory T86.1- Complications of transplanted kidney and a secondary code that identifies the complication.

Chapter 20 – External Causes of Morbidity (V00-Y99)

Codes for external causes of morbidity are found in Chapter 20. External cause codes classify environmental events and other circumstances as the cause of injury and other adverse effects.

Codes in this chapter are always reported as a secondary code with the nature of the condition or injury reported as the first-listed diagnosis. Codes for external causes of morbidity relate to all aspects of external cause coding including: cause, intent, place of occurrence, and activity at the time of the injury or other health condition.

External cause codes are most frequently reported with codes in Chapter 19, Injury, Poisoning and Certain Other Consequences of External Causes (S00-T88). There are conditions in other chapters that may also be due to an external cause. For example, when a condition, such as a myocardial infarction, is specifically stated as due to or precipitated by strenuous activity, such as shoveling snow, then external cause codes should be reported to identify the activity, place and external cause status. As was discussed previously, separate reporting of external cause codes is not necessary for poisoning, adverse effects, or underdosing of drugs and other substances (T36-T50), or for toxic effect of nonmedicinal substances (T51-T65), since the external cause is captured in a combination code from Chapter 19.

External Cause Coding and Third Party Payer Requirements

While not all third party payers require reporting of external cause codes, they are a valuable source of information to public health departments and other state agencies regarding the causes of death, injury, poisoning and adverse effects. In fact, more than half of all states have mandated that hospitals collect external cause data using statewide hospital discharge data systems. Another third of all states routinely collect external cause data even though it is not mandated. There are also 15 states that have mandated statewide hospital emergency department data systems requiring collection of external cause data.

These codes provide a framework for systematically collecting patient health-related information on the external cause of death, injury, poisoning and adverse effects. These codes define the manner of the death or injury, the mechanism, the place of occurrence of the event, the activity, and the status of the person at the time death or injury occurred. Manner refers to whether the cause of death or injury was unintentional/accidental, self-inflicted, assault, or undetermined. Mechanism describes how the injury occurred such as a motor vehicle accident, fall, contact with a sharp object or power tool, or being caught between moving objects. Place identifies where the injury occurred, such as a personal residence, playground, street, or place of employment. Activity indicates the activity of the person at the time the injury occurred such as swimming, running, bathing, or cooking. External cause status is used to indicate the status of the person at the time death or injury occurred such as work done for pay, military activity, or volunteer activity.

7th Characters

Most external cause codes require a 7th character to identify the episode of care. The 7th characters used in Chapter 20 are A, D and S. These external cause codes have the same definitions as they do for most injury codes found in Chapter 19. Initial encounter is defined as the period when the patient is receiving active treatment for the injury, poisoning, or other consequences of an external cause and is reported with 7th character 'A'. Subsequent encounters are identified with 7th character 'D'. This is an encounter after the active phase of treatment and when the patient is receiving routine care for the injury or poisoning during the period of healing or recovery. Sequela is identified by 7th character 'S' which is assigned for complications or conditions that arise as a direct result of an injury.

Chapter Guidelines

As with other chapter guidelines, the guidelines for Chapter 20 External Causes of Morbidity are provided so that there is standardization in the assignment of these codes. External cause codes are always secondary codes, and these codes can be used in any health care setting. An overview of the guidelines is provided here. For the complete guidelines related to external causes, the Official Guidelines for the Code Set should be consulted.

The general external cause coding guidelines relate to all external cause codes including those that describe the cause, the intent, the place of occurrence, the activity of the patient, and the patient's status at the time of the injury. External cause codes may be used with any code in ranges A00.0-T88.9 or Z00-Z99 when the health condition is due to an external cause. The most common health conditions related to external causes are those for injuries in categories S00-T88. It is appropriate to assign external cause codes to infections and diseases in categories A00-R99 and Z00-Z99 that are the result of an external cause, such as a heart attack resulting from strenuous activity.

External cause codes are assigned for the entire length of treatment for the condition resulting from the external cause. The appropriate 7th character must be assigned to identify the encounter as the initial encounter, subsequent encounter, or sequela. For conditions due to an external cause, the full range of external cause codes are used to completely describe the cause, intent, place of occurrence, activity of patient at time of event, and patient's status. No external cause code is required if the external cause and intent are captured by a code from another chapter. For example, codes for poisoning, adverse effect and underdosing of drugs, medicaments, and biological substances in categories T36-T50 and toxic effects of substances chiefly nonmedicinal as to source in categories T51-T65 capture both the external cause and the intent.

When applicable, place of occurrence (Y92), activity (Y93), and external cause status (Y99) codes are sequenced after the main external cause codes. Regardless of the number of external cause codes assigned, there is generally only one place of occurrence code, one activity code, and one external cause status code assigned. However, if a new injury should occur during hospitalization, it is allowable in such rare instances to assign an additional place of occurrence code. Codes from these categories are only assigned at the initial encounter for treatment so these codes do not make use of 7th characters. If the place, activity, or external cause status is not documented, no code is assigned. These codes do not apply to poisonings, adverse effects, misadventures, or sequela.

If the intent (accident, self-harm, assault) of the cause of an injury or other condition is unknown or unspecified, code the intent as accidental. All transport accident categories assume accidental intent. A code for undetermined intent is assigned only when the documentation in the medical record specifies that the intent cannot be determined.

The external cause of sequelae are reported using the code for the external cause with the 7th character extension 'S' for sequela. An external cause code is assigned for any condition described as a late effect or sequela resulting from a previous injury.

Chapter 21 – Factors Influencing Health Status and Contact with Health Services (Z00-Z99)

The codes for factors influencing health and contact with health services represent reasons for encounters. These codes are located in Chapter 21 and the initial alpha character is Z so they are referred to as Z-codes. While code descriptions in Chapter 21, such as Z00.110 Health examination of newborn under 8 days old may appear to be a description of a service or procedure, codes in this chapter are not procedure codes. These codes represent the reason for the encounter, service, or visit. The procedure must be reported with the appropriate procedure code.

Chapter Guidelines

There are extensive chapter-specific coding guidelines for factors influencing health status and contact with health services. The guidelines identify broad categories of Z-codes, such as status Z-codes and history Z-codes. Each of these broad categories contains categories and subcategories of Z-codes for similar types of patient visits/encounters with similar reporting rules. Z-codes may be used in any health care setting and most Z-codes may be either a principal/first-listed or secondary code depending on the circumstances of the encounter. However, certain Z-codes, such as Z02 Encounter for administrative examination, may only be used as a first-listed or principal diagnosis. An overview of the guidelines for the broad categories of Z-codes is provided here. Consult the Official Guidelines for the complete guidelines for Chapter 21.

Contact/Exposure – There are two categories of contact/exposure codes which may be reported as either a first-listed or secondary diagnosis although they are more commonly reported as a secondary diagnosis. Category Z20 indicates contact with, and suspected exposure to communicable diseases. These codes are reported for patients who do not show signs or symptoms of a disease but are suspected to have been exposed to it either by a close personal contact with an infected individual or by currently being in or having been in an area where the disease is epidemic. Category Z77 indicates contact with or suspected exposure to substances that are known to be hazardous to health. Code Z77.22 Exposure to tobacco smoke (second hand smoke) is included in this category.

Inoculations and Vaccinations – Inoculations and vaccinations may also be either the first-listed or a secondary diagnosis. There is a single code Z23 Encounter for immunization for reporting inoculations and vaccinations. A procedure code is required to capture the administration of the immunization of vaccination and to identify the specific immunization/vaccination provided.

Status – Status codes indicate that a patient is either a carrier of a disease or has the sequelae or residual of a past disease or condition. Codes for the presence of prosthetic or mechanical devices resulting from past treatment are categorized as status codes. Status codes should not be confused with history codes which indicate that a patient no longer has the condition. Status codes are not used with diagnosis codes that provide the same information as the status code. For example, code Z94.1 Heart transplant status should not be used with a code from subcategory T86.2- Complications of heart transplant because codes in subcategory T86.2- already identify the patient as a heart transplant recipient.

History (of) – There are two types of history Z-codes, personal and family. Personal history codes explain a patient's past medical condition that no longer exists and is not receiving any treatment, but that has the potential for recurrence, and therefore may require continued monitoring. Family history codes are for use when a patient has a family member who has had a particular disease that causes the patient to be at higher risk of also contracting the disease.

Screening – Screening is testing for disease or disease precursors in seemingly well individuals so that early detection and treatment can be provided for those who test positive for the disease (e.g. screening mammogram). The testing of a person to rule out or confirm a suspected diagnosis because the patient has some sign or symptom is a diagnostic examination not a screening and a sign or symptoms code is used to explain the reason for the visit.

Observation – There are three observation categories (Z03-Z05) for use in very limited circumstances when a person is being observed for a suspected condition that has been ruled out. The observation codes are to be used as principal diagnosis only. The only exception to this is when the principal diagnosis is required to be a code from category Z38, Liveborn infants according to place of birth and type of delivery. Then a code from category Z05, Encounter for observation and evaluation of newborn for suspected diseases and conditions ruled out, is sequenced after the Z38 code. Additional codes may be used in addition to the observation code, but only if they are unrelated to the suspected condition being observed.

Aftercare – Aftercare visit codes cover situations when the initial treatment of a disease has been performed and the patient requires continued care during the healing or recovery phase, or for the long-term consequences of the disease. Aftercare for injuries is not reported with Z-codes. The injury code is reported with the appropriate 7th character for subsequent care. Aftercare Z-codes/categories include Z42-Z49 and Z51. Z51 includes other after-care and medical care.

Follow-up – The follow-up Z-codes are used to explain continuing surveillance following completed treatment of a disease, condition, or injury. They imply that the condition has been fully treated and no longer exists. Do not confuse follow-up codes with aftercare codes or injury codes with 7th character 'S'. Follow-up Z-codes/categories include: Z08-Z09 and Z39.

Donor – Codes in category Z52 Donors of organs and tissues are used for living individuals who are donating blood or other body tissue. These codes are only for individuals donating for other individuals, not for self-donations. The only exception to this rule is blood donation. There are codes for autologous blood donation in subcategory Z52.01-. Codes in category Z52 are not used to identify cadaveric donations.

Counseling – Counseling Z-codes are used when a patient or family member receives assistance in the aftermath of an illness or injury or when support is required in coping with family or social problems. They are not used in conjunction with a diagnosis code when the counseling component of care is considered integral to standard treatment. Counseling Z-codes/categories include: Z30.0-, Z31.5, Z31.6-, Z32.2-Z32.3, Z69-Z71, and Z76.81.

Encounters for Obstetrical and Reproductive Services – Routine prenatal visits and postpartum care are reported with Z-codes. Codes in category Z34 Encounter for supervision of normal pregnancy are always the first-listed diagnosis and are not to be used with any other code from the OB chapter. Codes in category Z3A Weeks of gestation may be assigned to provide additional information about the pregnancy. Codes in category Z37 Outcome of delivery should be included on all maternal delivery records. Outcome of delivery codes are always secondary codes and are never used on the newborn record. Examples of other conditions reported with Z-codes include family planning, and procreative management and counseling. Codes in category Z3A, Weeks of gestation, may be assigned to provide additional information about the pregnancy. Category Z3A codes should not be assigned for pregnancies with abortive outcomes (categories O00-O08), elective termination of pregnancy (code Z33.32), nor for postpartum conditions, as category Z3A is not applicable to these conditions. The date of the admission should be used to determine weeks of gestation for inpatient admissions that encompass more than one gestational week.

Newborns and Infants – There are a limited number of Z-codes for newborns and infants. Category Z38 Liveborn infants according to place of birth and type of delivery is always the principle diagnosis on the birth record. Subcategory Z00.11- Newborn health examination reports routine examination of the newborn. A 6th character is required that identifies the age of the newborn as under 8 days old (0) or 8-28 days old (1).

Routine and Administrative Examinations – An example of a routine examination is a general check-up. An example of an examination for administrative purposes is a pre-employment physical. These Z-codes are not to be used if the examination is for diagnosis of a suspected condition or for treatment purposes. In such cases the diagnosis code is used. During a routine exam, should a diagnosis or condition be discovered, it should be coded as an additional code. Some of the codes for routine health examinations distinguish between "with" and "without" abnormal findings. An examination with abnormal findings refers to a condition/diagnosis that is newly identified or a change in severity of a chronic condition (such as uncontrolled hypertension, or an acute exacerbation of chronic obstructive pulmonary disease) during a routine physical examination. Code assignment depends on the information that is known at the time the encounter is being coded. For example, if no abnormal findings were found during the examination, but the encounter is being coded before the test results are back, it is acceptable to assign the code for "without abnormal findings" diagnosis. When assigning a code for "with abnormal findings," additional codes should be assigned to identify the specific abnormal findings. Z-codes/categories for routine and administrative examinations include: Z00-Z02 (except Z02.9)and Z32.0-.

Miscellaneous Z-Codes – The miscellaneous Z-codes capture a number of other health care encounters that do not fall into one of the other categories. Certain of these codes identify the reason for the encounter; others are for use as additional codes that provide useful information on circumstances that may affect a patient's care and treatment. Miscellaneous Z-codes/categories are as follows: Z28 (except Z28.3), Z29, Z40-Z41 (except Z41.9) Z53, Z55-Z60, Z62-Z65, Z72-Z75 (except Z74.01 and only when the documentation specifies that the patient has an associated problem), Z76.0, Z76.3, Z76.5, Z91.1-, Z91.83, and Z91.84-, and Z91.89.

Chapter 22 – Codes for Special Purposes (U00-U85)

This chapter is for the provisional assignment of new diseases of uncertain etiology or emergency use. Specifically, codes U00-U49 are to be used by WHO for the provisional assignment of new diseases of uncertain etiology or emergency use. Included in Chapter 22 are three codes:

- U07.0 Vaping-related disorder

- U07.1 COVID-19
- U09.9 COVID-19

U07.0 Vaping Related Disorder

The purpose of U07.0 is for coding encounters related to E-cigarette, or vaping, product use. This code has been implemented in response to the recent occurrences of vaping-related disorders. E-cigarettes work by heating a liquid in a pod or cartridge into an aerosol that is inhaled. Base ingredients, such as glycerol (vegetable glycerin) and propylene glycol create the vapor when heated. Other additives like nicotine, artificial flavorings, THC (tetrahydrocannabinol) or CBD (cannabinoid) oil, and vitamin E acetate are combined with the base liquid.

E-cigarette or vaping product use associated lung injury (EVALI) is the name given by the CDC to the dangerous lung disease linked to vaping. Symptoms include cough, shortness of breath, acute respiratory distress, chest pain, fever, stomach pain, diarrhea, nausea, vomiting, and weight loss. Damaging lung effects can be so severe as to stop the lungs from functioning.

Coding Guidance for U07.0

For patients documented with E-cigarette or vaping product use associated lung injury (EVALI), or acute lung injury, without further documentation identifying a specific condition [e.g., pneumonitis, bronchitis], assign only code U07.0. Per tabular instructions, when assigning U07.0, use additional code(s) to identify manifestations, such as:

- abdominal pain (R10.84)
- acute respiratory distress syndrome (J80)
- diarrhea (R19.7)
- drug-induced interstitial lung disorder (J70.4)
- lipoid pneumonia (J69.1)
- weight loss (R63.4)

Lung-related Complications – For patients presenting with lung conditions related to vaping, assign code U07.0 as the principal diagnosis. Assign additional codes for other specified respiratory manifestations, such as:

- J68.0 Bronchitis and pneumonitis due to chemicals, gases, fumes and vapors
- J69.1 Pneumonitis due to inhalation of oils and essences
- J80 Acute respiratory distress syndrome
- J82.8- Pulmonary eosinophilia, not elsewhere classified
- J84.114 Acute interstitial pneumonitis
- J96.0- Acute respiratory failure

Associated respiratory signs and symptoms due to vaping, such as cough, shortness of breath, etc., are not coded separately, when a definitive diagnosis has been established. However, it would be appropriate to code separately any gastrointestinal symptoms, such as diarrhea and abdominal pain.

Poisoning and Toxicity – Acute nicotine exposure can be toxic. Children and adults have been poisoned by swallowing, breathing, or even absorbing e-cigarette liquid through their skin or eyes. For these patients, assign code T65.291- Toxic effect of other nicotine and tobacco, accidental (unintentional). For a patient with acute tetrahydrocannabinol (THC) toxicity, assign code T40.711 Poisoning by cannabis, accidental (unintentional) or code T40.721 Poisoning by synthetic cannabinoids, accidental (unintentional).

Substance Use, Abuse, and Dependence – For patients with documented substance use, abuse, or dependence, additional codes identifying the substance(s) used should be assigned. When the provider documentation refers to use, abuse, and dependence of the same substance (e.g. nicotine, cannabis, etc.) together or interchangeably, only one code should be assigned to identify the pattern of use based on coding guidelines:

- If both use and abuse are documented, assign only the code for abuse
- If both abuse and dependence are documented, assign only the code for dependence
- If use, abuse and dependence are all documented, assign only the code for dependence
- If both use and dependence are documented, assign only the code for dependence

Assign as many codes as appropriate to identify each substance documented. Examples:

- F12.--- Cannabis related disorders
- F17.--- Nicotine related disorders

For vaping of nicotine with dependence, assign code F17.29- Nicotine dependence, other tobacco products since electronic nicotine delivery systems (ENDS) are non-combustible tobacco products.

U07.1 COVID-19

The purpose of U07.1 is for coding encounters related to infections due to SARS-CoV-2, the newly discovered strain of coronavirus emerging in December of 2019 causing the disease responsible for the recent pandemic. The disease it causes is named "coronavirus disease 2019", abbreviated as COVID-19. The disease causes respiratory illness with flu-like symptoms that range from mild to severe illness and death. Severe cases require hospitalization and ventilator assistance. Most patients will recover with supportive care.

Symptoms may appear 2-14 days after exposure and include cough, fever, shortness of breath, or difficulty breathing in serious cases. Older persons and those with an existing medical condition such as heart or lung disease, cancer, or diabetes are at greater risk for developing more serious illness. Emergency warning signs for COVID-19 infection that require immediate medical attention include trouble breathing; continual pain or pressure in the chest; a newly altered mental state such as confusion or the inability to be aroused; and a bluish tint to the lips or face.

Coding Guidance for U07.1

Code only a confirmed diagnosis of the 2019 novel coronavirus disease (COVID-19) as documented by the provider or documentation of a positive COVID-19 test result. For a confirmed diagnosis, assign code U07.1 COVID-19. This is an exception to the hospital inpatient guideline Section II, H. In this context, "confirmation" does not require documentation of a positive test result for COVID-19; the provider's documentation that the individual has COVID-19 is sufficient. If the provider documents "suspected," "possible," "probable," or "inconclusive" COVID-19, do not assign code U07.1. Instead, code the signs and symptoms reported.

Acute Respiratory Illnesses Due to COVID-19 – When the reason for the encounter/admission is a respiratory manifestation of COVID-19, assign U07.1 as the principal or first-listed diagnosis and assign code(s) for the respiratory manifestation(s) as additional diagnoses. The following conditions are examples of common respiratory manifestations of COVID-19:

- Pneumonia: Assign codes U07.1 COVID-19 and J12.82 Pneumonia due to coronavirus disease 2019.
- Acute bronchitis: Assign codes U07.1 and J20.8 Acute bronchitis due to other specified organisms. Note: Bronchitis not otherwise specified (NOS) due to COVID-19 should be coded using code U07.1 and J40 Bronchitis, not specified as acute or chronic.
- Lower respiratory infection: If the COVID-19 is documented as being associated with a lower respiratory infection, not otherwise specified (NOS), or an acute respiratory infection, NOS, assign codes U07.1 and J22 Unspecified acute lower respiratory infection. If the COVID-19 is documented as being associated with a respiratory infection, NOS, assign codes U07.1 and J98.8 Other specified respiratory disorders.
- Acute respiratory distress syndrome (ARDS) due to COVID 19: Assign codes U07.1 and J80 Acute respiratory distress syndrome.
- Acute respiratory failure due to COVID 19: Assign codes U07.1 and J96.0- Acute respiratory failure.

Note: When the reason for the encounter/admission is a non-respiratory manifestation (e.g., viral enteritis) of COVID-19, assign code U07.1 COVID-19 as the principal diagnosis and assign the appropriate code(s) for the non-respiratory manifestation(s) as additional diagnoses.

When COVID-19 meets the definition of principal diagnosis, code U07.1 COVID-19, should be sequenced first, followed by the appropriate codes for associated manifestations, except when another guideline requires that certain codes be sequenced first, such as for obstetric, sepsis, or transplant complications. (*See Section I.C.1.d. Sepsis, Severe Sepsis, and Septic Shock for a COVID-19 infection that progresses to sepsis. See Section I.C.19.g.3.a. Transplant complications other than kidney for a COVID-19 infection in a lung transplant patient.*)

Pregnancy, Childbirth, and Puerperium – When COVID-19 is the reason for the admission or encounter, assign code O98.5- Other viral diseases complicating pregnancy, childbirth and the puerperium, as the principal diagnosis, and code U07.1 COVID-19 along with the appropriate code(s) for any associated manifestation(s) as additional diagnoses. Codes from Chapter 15 always take sequencing priority. (*See Section I.C.15.s. for COVID-19 infection in pregnancy, childbirth, and the puerperium.*)

Newborns – For a newborn that tests positive for COVID-19, assign code U07.1 COVID-19, and the appropriate codes for any associated manifestation(s) in neonates/newborns in the absence of documentation indicating a specific type of transmission. For a newborn that tests positive for COVID-19 and the provider documents the condition was contracted in utero or during the birth process, assign codes P35.8 Other congenital viral diseases, and U07.1 COVID-19. When coding the birth episode in a newborn record, the appropriate code from category Z38 Liveborn infants according to place of birth and type of delivery, should be assigned as the principal diagnosis. (*See Section I.C.16.h. for COVID-19 infection in newborn.*)

Exposure – For asymptomatic individuals with actual or suspected exposure to COVID-19, assign code Z20.822 Contact with and (suspected) exposure to COVID-19. For symptomatic individuals with actual or suspected exposure to COVID-19 and the infection has been ruled out, or test results are inconclusive or unknown, assign code Z20.822 Contact with and (suspected) exposure to COVID-19. (*See Section I.C.21.c.1, Contact/Exposure, for additional guidance regarding the use of category Z20 codes.*)

Screening – During the COVID-19 pandemic, a screening code is generally not appropriate. For encounters for COVID-19 testing, including preoperative testing, code as exposure to COVID-19.

Note: Coding guidance will be updated as new information concerning the pandemic status becomes available.

Signs and Symptoms without Definifitive Diagnosis – For patients who have any signs/symptoms associated with COVID-19, but a definitive diagnosis has not be confirmed, assign the appropriate codes for each of the presenting signs and symptoms, such as:

- R05.1 Acute cough or R05.9 Cough, unspecified
- R06.02 Shortness of breath
- R50.9 Fever, unspecified

If a patient with signs/symptoms associated with COVID-19 also has an actual or suspected contact with or exposure to COVID-19, assign Z20.822.

Asymptomatic Individuals Testing Positive – For patients who are asymptomatic and test positive for COVID-19, assign U07.1. Although the individual is asymptomatic, the person has tested positive and is considered to have the COVID-19 infection.

Personal History – For patients with a history of COVID-19, assign code Z86.16 Personal history of COVID-19.

Follow-Up Visits – For individuals who previously had COVID-19, without residual symptom(s) or condition(s) and are being seen for a follow-up evaluation, when COVID-19 test results are negative, assign codes Z09 Encounter for follow-up examination after completed treatment for conditions other than malignant neoplasm and Z86.16 Personal history of COVID-19.

Encounter for Antibody Testing – For antibody testing that is not being performed to confirm a current COVID-19 infection, nor as a follow-up test after resolution of a previous COVID-19 infection, assign code Z01.84 Encounter for antibody response examination.

Multisystem Inflammatory Syndrome – For individuals with multisystem inflammatory syndrome (MIS) and COVID-19, assign code U07.1 COVID-19 as the principal diagnosis and code M35.81 Multisystem inflammatory syndrome, as an additional diagnosis.

If an individual with a history of COVID-19 develops MIS, assign codes M35.81 Multisystem inflammatory syndrome and U09.9 Post COVID-19 condition, unspecified.

Assign additional code(s) for an associated complications of MIS.

Post COVID-19 Condition – For sequela of a COVID-19 infection, or associated symptoms/conditions that develop following a previous COVID-19 infection, assign a code(s) for the specific symptoms/ conditions related to the previous COVID-19 infection, if known, and code U09.9 Post COVID-19 condition, unspecified. Do not use code U09.9 for manifestations of an active (current) COVID-19 infection.

If a patient has a condition(s) associated with a previous COVID-19 infection and develops a new active (current) COVID-19 infection, code U09.9 may be assigned together with code U07.1 to identify that the patient also has a condition(s) associated with a previous COVID-19 infection. Code(s) for the specific condition(s) associated with the previous COVID-19 infection and code(s) for manifestation(s) of the new active (current) COVID-19 infection should also be assigned.

Introduction to ICD-10-PCS

ICD-10-PCS is a procedure coding system used to report inpatient procedures beginning October 1, 2015. As inpatient procedures associated with changing technology and medical advances are developed, the structure of ICD-10-PCS allows them to be easily incorporated as unique codes. This is possible because during the development phase, four attributes were identified as key components for the structure of the coding system – completeness, expandability, multiaxial, and standardized terminology. These components are defined as follows:

Completeness

Completeness refers to the ability to assign a unique code for all substantially different procedures, including unique codes for procedures that can be performed using different approaches.

Expandability

Expandability means the ability to add new unique codes to the coding system in the section and body system where they should reside.

Multiaxial

Multiaxial signifies the ability to assign codes using independent characters around each individual axis or component of the procedure. For example, if a new surgical approach is used for one of the root operations on a specific body part, a value for the new surgical approach can be added to the approach character without a need to add or change other code characters.

Standardized Terminology

ICD-10-PCS includes definitions of the terminology used. While the meaning of specific words varies in common usage, ICD-10-PCS does not include multiple meanings for the same term, and each term is assigned a specific meaning. For example, the term "excision" is defined in most medical dictionaries as surgical removal of part or all of a structure or organ. However, in ICD-10-PCS excision is defined as "cutting out or off, without replacement, a portion of a body part." If all of a body part is surgically removed without replacement, the procedure is defined as 'resection' in ICD-10-PCS.

General Development Principles

In the development of ICD-10-PCS, several general principles were followed:

Diagnostic Information is Not Included in Procedure Description

When procedures are performed for specific diseases or disorders, the disease or disorder is not contained in the procedure code. There are no codes for procedures exclusive to aneurysms, cleft lip, strictures, neoplasms, hernias, etc. The diagnosis codes, not the procedure codes, specify the disease or disorder.

Limited Use of Not Elsewhere Classified (NEC) Option

Because all significant components of a procedure are specified, there is generally no need for an NEC code option. However, limited NEC options are incorporated into ICD-10-PCS where necessary. For example, new devices are frequently developed, and therefore it is necessary to provide an "Other Device" option for use until the new device can be explicitly added to the coding system.

Level of Specificity

All procedures currently performed can be specified in ICD-10-PCS. The frequency with which a procedure is performed was not a consideration in the development of the system. Rather, a unique code is available for variations of a procedure that can be performed.

ICD-10-PCS Structure

ICD-10-PCS has a seven-character alphanumeric code structure. Each character contains up to 34 possible values. Each value represents a specific option for the general character definition (e.g., stomach is one of the values for the body part character). The ten digits 0-9 and the 24 letters A-H, J-N and P-Z may be used in each character. The letters O and I are not used in order to avoid confusion with the digits 0 and 1.

Procedures are divided into sections that identify the general type of procedure (e.g., medical and surgical, obstetrics, imaging). The first character of the procedure code always specifies the section. The sections are shown in Table 1.

Table 1: ICD-10-PCS Sections

0	Medical and Surgical
1	Obstetrics
2	Placement
3	Administration
4	Measurement and Monitoring
5	Extracorporeal or Systemic Assistance and Performance
6	Extracorporeal or Systemic Therapies

7	Osteopathic
8	Other Procedures
9	Chiropractic
B	Imaging
C	Nuclear Medicine
D	Radiation Therapy
F	Physical Rehabilitation and Diagnostic Audiology
G	Mental Health
H	Substance Abuse Treatment
X	New Technology

The second through seventh characters mean the same thing within each section, but may mean different things in other sections. In all sections, the third character specifies the general type of procedure performed, or root operation (e.g., resection, transfusion, fluoroscopy), while the other characters give additional information such as the body part and approach. In ICD-10-PCS, the term "procedure" refers to the complete specification of the seven characters.

ICD-10-PCS Format

The ICD-10-PCS is made up of three separate parts:

- Tables
- Index

The Index allows codes to be located by an alphabetic lookup. The index entry refers to a specific location in the Tables. The Tables must be used in order to construct a complete and valid code.

Tables in ICD-10-PCS

Each page in the Tables is composed of rows that specify the valid combinations of code values. ***Table 2*** is an excerpt from the ICD-10-PCS tables. In the system, the upper portion of each table specifies the values for the first three characters of the codes in that table. In the administration section, the first three characters are the section, the body system and the root operation.

In ICD-10-PCS, the values 3E0 specify the section Administration (3), the body system Physiological Systems/Anatomical Region (E), and the root operation Introduction (0). As shown in Table 2, the root operation (i.e., introduction) is accompanied by its definition. The lower portion of the table specifies all the valid combinations of the remaining characters four through seven. The four columns in the table specify the last four characters. In the administration section they are labeled Body System, Approach, Substance and Qualifier, respectively. Each row in the table specifies the valid combination of values for characters four through seven. The Tables contain only those combinations of values that result in a valid procedure code.

ICD-10-PCS for Urology and Nephrology

Urinary, Female Reproductive, and Male Reproductive system procedures are reported with codes from Medical and Surgical sections 0T1-0VW.

Table 2: Excerpt from the ICD-10-PCS tables

3 Administration E Physiological Systems/Anatomical Regions 0 Introduction: Putting in or on a therapeutic, diagnostic, nutritional, physiological, or prophylactic substance except blood or blood products			
Character 4	**Character 5**	**Character 6**	**Character 7**
T Peripheral Nerves and Plexi X Cranial Nerves	3 Percutaneous	3 Anti-inflammatory B Anesthetic Agent T Destructive Agent	Z No Qualifier

There are 6 code options for the table above:

3E0T33Z	Introduction (injection) anti-inflammatory peripheral nerves and plexi
3E0T3BZ	Introduction (injection) anesthetic agent peripheral nerves and plexi
3E0T3TZ	Introduction (injection) destructive agent peripheral nerves and plexi
3E0X33Z	Introduction (injection) anti-inflammatory peripheral cranial nerves
3E0X3BZ	Introduction (injection) anesthetic agent peripheral nerves and plexi
3E0X3TZ	Introduction (injection) destructive agent cranial nerves

ICD-10-CM Anatomy and Physiology

Genitourinary System

Chapter Objectives

After studying this chapter, you should be able to:

- Define the following:
  - Urinary System
    - » Kidneys
    - » Urinary Bladder
    - » Ureter
    - » Urethra
  - Male Genital System
    - » Testes
    - » Excretory Ducts
      - Epididymis
      - Vas Deferens
      - Ejaculatory Ducts
    - » Seminourethral glands
    - » Prostate
    - » Bulbourethral glands
    - » Penis
  - Female Genital System
    - » Ovaries
    - » Fallopian Tubes
    - » Uterus
    - » Vagina
    - » External Genitalia
    - » Breasts
    - » Pregnancy, Childbirth, and the Puerperium
- Identify infectious diseases of the urinary and reproductive systems
- Identify neoplasms of the urinary and reproductive systems
- Identify other diseases and conditions of the genitourinary system
- Define congenital anomalies
- Identify pregnancy disorders and pregnancy-related disorders
- Assign ICD-10-CM codes for a variety of diseases, injuries, and other conditions affecting the genitourinary system

Overview

The genitourinary system contains the reproductive organs and the urinary system organs. These are grouped together because of their close proximity to one another, shared origin, and the use of common pathways for both the reproductive and urinary systems. It is also called the urogenital system and urogenital tract.

Urinary System

The urinary system contains organs, tubes, muscles, and nerves that work together to create, store, and eliminate urine. The urinary system includes:

- Two kidneys
- Two ureters
- Urinary bladder
- Two sphincter muscles
- Urethra

Waste products that are left behind after the body has taken what it needs from food and fluids are eliminated through the urinary system. It works with other organs that excrete waste—the skin (sweat), lungs (exhalation), and intestines (solid waste)—to keep chemicals and water balanced in the body. The urinary system removes urea, a waste product, from the blood. Urea is produced by the breakdown of protein in food and carried in the bloodstream to the kidneys. The urinary system also maintains the proper fluid volume by regulating the amount of water, which is excreted in urine. Other functions are to regulate the concentrations of various electrolytes in bodily fluids and to maintain normal pH of the blood.

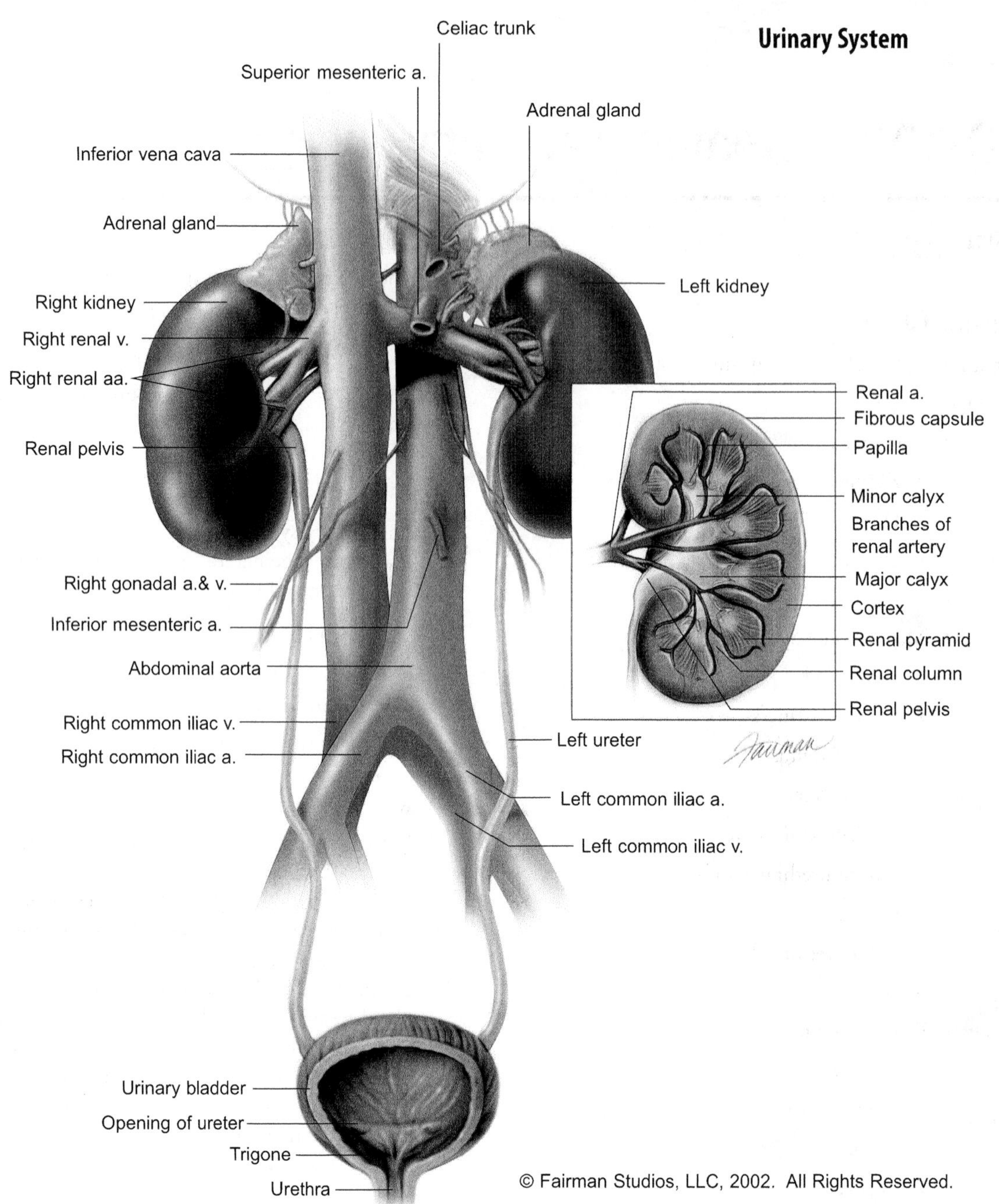

Kidneys

Kidney Structure

The kidneys are paired retroperitoneal organs that are the approximate size of a fist. They are situated near the posterior wall of the abdomen on each side of the vertebral column, around the twelfth rib.

There are two surfaces of the kidney, the concave and the convex. The concave surface, the renal hilum, is the where the renal artery enters the kidney, and the renal vein and ureter leave. The renal capsule is the tough, fibrous tissue surrounding the kidney and covered by a thick layer of perinephric fat and the renal fascia, known as Gerota's fascia. The capsule provides protection from trauma. The anterior border of these tissues is the peritoneum, and the posterior border is the transversalis fascia.

The parenchyma is the functional part of the kidney and is divided into two major parts: the superficial renal cortex and the deep renal medulla. The renal cortex is the smooth outer portion of the kidney that lies between the capsule and the medulla. The medulla is the innermost part, divided into 10 to 18 cone-shaped pyramids. The base of each pyramid lies at the corticomedullary border and the apex of each pyramid points inward to the minor calyx. The pyramids are composed of nephrons and collecting ducts. Located between the renal pyramids are columns extending down from the cortex.

The nephrons are the basic functional units of the kidney. The first part of the filtering process of a nephron is the renal corpuscle, located in the cortex, and made up of two structures—a glomerulus and Bowman's capsule. Glomeruli are small tufts of capillaries at the beginning of the nephron. Bowman's capsule is a walled, cup-shaped structure surrounding the glomerulus of each nephron that filters waste, excess salts, and water from the blood. The glomerular filtrate passes through a renal tubule before becoming urine. Water and salts are reabsorbed back into the blood along the length of the long, convoluted tubules. The interstitium is the functional space in the kidney that absorbs the fluid recovered from urine. It is rich in blood vessels and lies beneath the glomeruli.

The medullary ray is the collection of renal tubules that eventually drain urine into a single collecting duct. The papilla (tip) of each pyramid empties urine into a minor calyx, and then empties into the major calyces, which empty into the renal pelvis and then into the ureter.

Kidney Function

The kidneys are regulatory organs, which maintain the volume and composition of body fluid by blood filtration and selective reabsorption or secretion of filtered solutes. The kidneys remove urea through filtering units called nephrons. Each of these nephrons contains a ball formed of small blood capillaries (glomerulus) and a small tube, which is the renal tubule. Urea, along with water and other waste substances, forms the urine as it passes through the nephrons and down the renal tubules of the kidney.

The main roles of the kidneys are:

- **Regulation of ionic plasma composition** – Plasma composition is regulated by the concentration of ions such as sodium, potassium, calcium, magnesium, chloride, bicarbonate, and phosphates.
- **Regulation of plasma volume** – Plasma volume is controlled by how much water is excreted which has a direct effect on the total blood volume, and is an element in determining blood pressure.
- **Regulation of plasma osmolarity** – Osmolarity in plasma is sensitive to hydration status changes during rehydration and dehydration. The kidneys regulate this because they have direct control over how many ions are contained in the plasma and how much water is excreted.
- **Regulation of pH** (plasma hydrogen ion concentration) – Working together with the lungs and respiration, the kidneys play a part in maintaining bodily pH by controlling the amount of bicarbonate ions held in the blood and excreting hydrogen.
- **Removal of metabolic waste from plasma** – The kidneys excrete toxic nitrogenous waste. The liver produces ammonia as it breaks down amino acids produced by digesting proteins and combines the toxic ammonia molecule with carbon dioxide, which creates urea (a less-toxic nitrogenous compound). The urea is released into the bloodstream. The kidneys filter it and remove it in the urine.
- **Secretion of hormones**
  - Renin – an enzyme released by the kidneys that leads to the secretion of aldosterone from the adrenal cortex. The aldosterone promotes the kidneys' reabsorption of sodium ions.
  - Erythropoietin – a hormone produced by the kidneys that promotes the formation of red blood cells in the bone marrow. The kidneys secrete erythropoietin when the blood is lacking the capacity to carry oxygen.

Kidney Blood Supply

The kidney's blood supply is from the aorta through the renal arteries, which branch directly from the abdominal aorta. Each renal artery branches into segmental arteries, dividing further into interlobar arteries, which penetrate the renal capsule and extend though the renal columns between the renal pyramids. The blood supply then goes to the arcuate arteries that run through the boundary of the cortex and medulla. Each of the arcuate arteries supplies several interlobular arteries, which feed into the afferent arterioles that supply the glomeruli.

After filtration of the blood occurs, the blood moves through a small network of venules that converge into interlobar veins. The interlobar veins provide blood to the arcuate veins then back to the interlobar veins, which join to form the renal vein, exiting the kidney.

Ureters

The ureters are two thin tubes that connect the kidneys to the urinary bladder and are about 8-10 inches (20 to 25 cm) long. Muscles located in the ureter constantly tighten and relax to force urine downward toward the bladder and away from the kidney. Small amounts of urine are emptied into the bladder from the ureters about every 10 to 15 seconds.

The ureters begin on the medial aspect of each kidney and descend downward towards the bladder on the front of the psoas major muscle. They then run posteroinferiorly on the lateral walls of the pelvis and curve anteromedially to enter the bladder through the back, at the vesicoureteric junction, running within the wall of the bladder. The pelviureteric junction is where the ureters cross the pelvic brim near the bifurcation of the iliac arteries. Valves in the ureters (ureterovesical valves) prevent the backflow of urine. In the female, the ureters pass through the mesometrium (mesentery of the uterus) on the way to the bladder.

The ureteric lumen is lined with transitional epithelium, which contains layers of smooth muscle. The epithelial cells of the ureter are in many layers (stratified) and round but become flat when stretched.

The ureter contains a thin layer beneath the transitional epithelium called the lamina propria made up of loose connective tissue. Together with the transitional epithelium, it makes up the mucosa, which secretes a substance that protects the inner walls. The lamina propria contains capillaries, the central lymph vessel, and lymphoid tissue. It also consists of glands with ducts opening on the mucosal epithelium that secrete mucus and serous secretions.

In the ureteral wall, there are two spiral layers of smooth muscle: inner loose spiral (longitudinal), and outer tight spiral (circular). The distal third layer of the ureter contains another layer of outer longitudinal muscle.

Urinary Bladder

The bladder is a hollow muscular organ located in the pelvis and held in place by ligaments attached to other organs and the pelvic bones. It stores urine until it is emptied through excretion. It increases in size into a round shape when it is full and gets smaller when empty. If the urinary system is healthy, the bladder can hold up to 16 ounces (2 cups) of urine comfortably for two to five hours.

In males, the base of the bladder lies between the rectum and the pubic symphysis. It is superior to the prostate and separated from the rectum by the rectovesical excavation. In females, the bladder is situated inferior to the uterus and anterior to the vagina. It is separated from the uterus by the vesicouterine excavation.

Similar to the ureters, the innermost portion of the urinary bladder is the mucosa. It is composed of transitional epithelium, which has domed-shaped cells on the apical surface and connective tissue. The epithelial layer does not contain blood vessels or lymphatics. The epithelium lies upon the lamina propria which is composed of areolar connective tissue and consists of blood vessels, nerves, and in some areas, glands.

The detrusor muscle is another layer in the wall of the bladder and is made of smooth muscle fibers arranged in spiral, longitudinal, and circular bundles. When the bladder is stretched because of urine, this signals the parasympathetic nervous system to contract the muscle and expel urine. Continence during sleep results from the unconscious inhibition of detrusor muscle contraction. Support of the bladder neck and urethra entails the interconnection of three structures:

1. **Arcus tendineus fasciae pelvis** – Called the tendinous arch or white line of the pelvic fascia, this is a thickened, condensed band of the endopelvic fascia that extends from the body of the pubic bone and attaches to the ischial spine, and provides support to the bladder by resisting caudal movement of the anterior vaginal wall and urethra in upright posture.
2. **Levator ani muscle** – This is a broad, thin muscle formed by three muscle components: the puborectalis, the pubococcygeus muscle, and the iliococcygeus, attached to either side of the lower pelvis and uniting to make up the main part of the pelvic diaphragm (pelvic floor). It functions to support all the viscera in the pelvic cavity and raise the bladder.
3. **Endopelvic fascia** – A group of connective tissues, also known as the vesical layer that is attached to the diaphragmatic part of the pelvic fascia along the tendinous arch. It forms the anterior and lateral ligaments of the bladder.

Urethral Sphincter Muscles

Two sphincter muscles facilitate urine being expelled from the bladder:

1. **Internal sphincter muscle of urethra** – This muscle is located at the inferior end of the bladder and the urethra's proximal end where it connects to the bladder. The internal sphincter muscle is a continuation of the detrusor muscle. Because it is made up of smooth muscle, it is under involuntary or autonomic control. This is the main muscle for retention of urine in the bladder.
2. **External sphincter muscle** – This muscle is located at the inferior end of the bladder in females; in males, it is inferior to the prostate, at the level of the membranous urethra. It is the secondary sphincter to control the flow of urine through the urethra. This muscle is made up of skeletal muscle and is under voluntary control of the pudendal nerve (somatic nerve), which acts to constrict the urethra.

These muscles are used to control micturition (flow of urine) from the urinary bladder. Both muscles are required to control the exit of urine from the bladder. They envelop the urethra and when they are contracted, the urethra is sealed shut.

Bladder Nerves

Both spinal and peripheral nerves affect the bladder. The two nerves that have the most impact on bladder function are sacral nerves – the pudendal nerve and the pelvic splanchnic nerve. Through signals and reflexes, the nerves and bladder coordinate with the pelvic floor muscles and external urinary sphincters. This coordination keeps the sphincters closed except during urination. The nerves sense the pressure in the bladder and impulses are sent to the brain. The brain then sends signals back through the nerves to keep the external sphincter closed, called the guarding reflex. When urination is to occur, the nerves send signals to the bladder to empty.

Urethra

The urethra is the last part of the urinary system through which urine is passed for elimination. The anatomy for the urethra is different in women and men:

In women, it is around 1 to 1 ½ inches (3 to 4 cm) long and lies directly behind the symphysis pubis, anterior to the vagina. The external urethral orifice is the most contracted portion of the urethra that is situated directly in front of the vaginal opening and behind the glans clitoridis. It is a vertical slit and sits between the two labia.

The lining of the urethra is a membrane with numerous mucous glands and follicles (urethral glands) situated in the submucosal tissue. There are three layers of the membrane, also referred to as 'coats':

- **Muscular coat** – This is a portion of the bladder that extends the entire length of the urethra and consists of circular fibers.
- **Erectile tissue** – This thin, spongy layer contains a plexus of large veins and is intermixed with bundles of muscular fibers. It lies immediately beneath the mucous coat.

- **Mucous coat.** – Pale in color, this is a continuous part of the vulva and the bladder. It is lined with stratified squamous epithelium, which becomes transitional near the bladder.

In men, the urethra is about 7 to 8 inches (17.5 to 20 cm) long and begins at the bladder at the internal urethral orifice. It is divided into three portions:

- **Prostatic** – This section has the most ability to dilate due to its wideness. It runs vertically through the prostate from its base to its apex. It is spindle-shaped, being wider in the middle and narrowest where it joins the membranous portion.
- **Membranous** – This is the shortest portion of the urethra; it extends downward and forward, with a slight anterior concavity. It is located behind the pubic symphysis and surrounded by the fibers of the sphincter urethrae membranacea.
- **Cavernous** – This is the longest portion of the urethra and is a part of the corpus cavernosum urethrae. It is approximately 6 inches (15 cm) long and narrow, extending from the end of the membranous portion of the urethra and joining with the glans penis to form the fossa navicularis urethrae.

The urethra is composed of a mucous membrane, which derives its support from the submucosal tissue that connects it with the structures through which is passes.

- **Mucous coat** – Part of the mucous membrane that is included in the bladder, ureters, kidneys, and the integument covering the glans penis. It is also included in the gland ducts that open into the urethra, bulbo-urethral glands, prostate, ductus deferens, and vesiculae seminales, through the ejaculatory ducts.
- **Submucous tissue** – This tissue consists of muscular fibers arranged in a circular direction, which separates the mucous membrane and this tissue from the tissue of the corpus cavernosum urethrae. It also has a layer of vascular erectile tissue.

In men, the urethra also serves as a passageway for semen. The urethra passes through the prostate gland where it connects with the ejaculatory duct and then passes through the penis to the meatus, or opening, at the tip of the glans penis.

Male Genital System

The male genital system consists of external and internal organs involved in sexual reproduction, located in the lower trunk area. The external organ is the penis and the internal organs include the testes (gonads), epididymis, vas deferens, and ejaculatory duct, with the associated glands, which include the prostate and seminal bulbo-urethral glands. These assist in producing semen and sperm, which are used to fertilize an ovum for sexual reproduction.

Penis

The penis is one of the main male reproductive organs. The root (radix) is attached to the trunk and consists of the median urethral bulb in the middle of two diverging crura on either side and lies within the superficial perineal pouch. The body of the penis has two surfaces:

1. Dorsal – posterosuperior in the erect penis
2. Ventral (urethral) – facing downwards and backwards in the flaccid penis. This has a visible median raphe running between the lateral halves of the penis.

The penis is made up of three columns of tissue:

1. **Two corpora cavernosa** – These lie next to each other on the dorsal side of the shaft of the penis, running from the pubic bones to the head of the penis, where the corpora cavernosa join. These are made up of erectile tissue, which contain the majority of blood in the penis during erection. This tissue is expandable and sponge-like and contains irregular blood-filled spaces lined by endothelium and separated by connective tissue septa.
2. **One corpus spongiosum** – This lies between the two corpora cavernosa on the ventral side of the penile shaft. The corpus spongiosum is large and bulbous-shaped at the end with the opening known as the meatus at the tip of the glans penis. This supports the prepuce, or foreskin, a loose fold of skin which can be retracted to expose the glans. On the underside of the penis is the frenum, or frenulum, where the foreskin attaches. The urethra is a passageway for both urine and the ejaculation of semen through the meatus.

During certain situations, nitric oxide is released prior to relaxation of muscles in the corpora cavernosa and corpus spongiosum. The spongy tissue fills with blood to cause an erection. A function of the corpus spongiosum is to prevent urethral compression during erection.

Testes

The testes are components of both the reproductive system and the endocrine system. The main functions of the testes are:

- Production and storage of sperm (reproduction). The production of spermatozoa is best at a temperature slightly less than core body temperature.
- Production of male sex hormones (e.g., testosterone – endocrine)

Both of these functions are controlled by gonadotropic hormones, luteinizing hormone (LH) and follicle-stimulating hormone (FSH), which are produced by the anterior pituitary gland.

In healthy males, there are two testes, which are located behind the penis in a pouch of skin called the scrotum.

There are three layers of tissue in the testes:

1. **Tunica vaginalis** – The serous outer membrane enveloping the testes in a double layer, except where the spermatic cord and epididymis adhere. The tunica vaginalis is a remnant derived from the saccus vaginalis of the peritoneum.
2. **Tunica albuginea** – A layer of tough connective tissue that covers the testes, composed of white fibrous tissue interlaced in various directions. It is covered by the tunica vaginalis, except at the points of attachment of the epididymis, and along the posterior border, where the spermatic vessels enter.

3. **Tunica vasculosa** – A vascular layer of tissue located on the inner surface of the tunica albuginea and in the septa in the interior of the gland that consists of a plexus of blood vessels held together by areolar tissue.

Seminiferous Tubules

Located in the testicles, the seminiferous tubules are the structures where meiosis takes place — the formation of gametes (spermatozoa). The epithelium of the tubule is consistent with Sertoli cells, which are tall, columnar-type cells that line the tubule. In between the Sertoli cells are spermatogenic cells, which eventually become sperm cells through the process of meiosis. There are two types of tubules:

1. **Convoluted** – Placed toward the lateral side of the testicle
2. **Straight** – Sitting medially to form ducts that exit the testes

Developing sperm travel from the seminiferous tubules to the rete testis, a network of delicate tubules located in the hilum of the testes (mediastinum testis), which then carry the sperm from the seminiferous tubules to the efferent ducts, and finally through the epididymis.

Leydig Cells

In between the tubules are Leydig cells (interstitial cells), which produce and secrete testosterone and other androgens that are key for sexual development and puberty and the development of secondary sex characteristics (e.g., facial hair, libido), as well as supporting spermatogenesis and erectile function.

Epididymis

The epididymis is where newly created sperm cells mature through spermatogenesis. Spermatogenesis is the process by which the spermatogonia, an intermediary male gametogonium, a type of germ cell, develop into mature sperm. This starts at puberty and typically continues until death. The sperm then move into the vas deferens.

Vas deferens

The vas deferens, also called the ductus deferens, transport sperm from the left and right epididymis to the ejaculatory ducts for expulsion out the urethra via ejaculation by the action of muscular contractions. These two ducts are about 10 to 12 inches long (25 to 30 cm), about 3-5 mm in diameter and surrounded by smooth muscle. The vas deferens are part of the spermatic cords.

The smooth muscle in the wall of the vas deferens contracts during ejaculation, propelling the sperm forward. The sperm are transferred from the vas deferens into the urethra, collecting secretions from the male accessory sex glands (e.g., seminal vesicles, prostate gland) which form semen.

Spermatic Cord

The spermatic cord is a cord-like structure formed by the vas deferens and surrounding tissue that goes through the deep inguinal ring and fascial coverings down to each testicle. Its purpose is to suspend the testes in the scrotum and to house structures running to and from the testes.

The spermatic cord is covered in three layers of tissue:

- **External spermatic fascia** – An extension of the innominate fascia that overlies the aponeurosis of the external oblique muscle. It is a thin membrane that progresses downward around the surface of the spermatic cord and testis. It is separated from the dartos tunic (layer of smooth muscular tissue that assists in regulating the temperature of the testicles) by loose areolar tissue.
- **Cremasteric muscle** – Formed by a continuation of the internal oblique muscle and fascia. When this muscle contracts, the cord is shortened and the testicle is moved closer up toward the body where there is more warmth to maintain optimal testicular temperature. If cooling is necessary, the muscle relaxes and the testicle is lowered away from the warm body where it is able to cool, known as the cremasteric reflex.
- **Internal spermatic fascia** – This thin layer of tissue is a continuation of the transversalis fascia that supports the spermatic cord.

Prostate

The prostate is a tubuloalveolar exocrine gland that assists in making and storing seminal fluid, the medium which helps sperm to move. It is about 1 to 1.25 inches (2.5 to 3 cm) long and located under the urinary bladder and in front of the rectum. The prostate surrounds part of the urethra and is sheathed in the muscles of the pelvic floor, which assist in contraction during the ejaculatory process. The ducts in the prostate are lined with transitional epithelium.

The prostate stores and secretes an alkaline, prostatic fluid which is milky white. This fluid composes part of semen, along with spermatozoa and seminal vesicle fluid. The alkalinity of semen, derived from seminal vesicle secretions, helps neutralize the acidity of the vaginal tract, which prolongs the life of the sperm. The prostatic fluid is expelled in the first part of ejaculation along with most of the spermatozoa. The few spermatozoa expelled with seminal vesicular fluid have better motility, longer survival, and better protection of genetic material.

The prostate also controls the flow of urine during ejaculation. A complex system of valves sends semen into the urethra during the ejaculatory process and the sphincter seals the bladder, preventing urine entry into the urethra.

Bulbourethral Glands

The bulbourethral glands (Cowper's gland) are two exocrine glands located posterior and lateral to the membranous portion of the urethra, at the base of the penis. They lie between two layers of the fascia of the urogenital diaphragm, deep in the perineal pouch, and are enclosed by transverse fibers of the sphincter urethrae membranacea muscle.

The glands are compound tubulo-alveolar, and are composed of several lobules held together by a fibrous covering. Each of the lobules are made up of acini, lined by columnar epithelial cells, which open up into a duct that joins with the ducts of other lobules to form a single excretory duct. It is approximately 1¾ to 2 inches (2.0 to 2.5 cm) long. The glands diminish in size as a person ages.

During sexual arousal, each of the bulbourethral glands produces a clear, viscous fluid (pre-ejaculate). This fluid assists in lubricating the urethra for spermatozoa to pass through, neutralizing the traces of acidic urine in the urethra and helps in flushing out any residual urine or other foreign matter. It also produces a small amount of the prostate-specific antigen (PSA).

Female Genital System

The female genital system contains organs and other body parts necessary for reproduction. It carries out several functions, which include production of ova or oocytes (egg cells), transporting ova/oocytes to the site of fertilization, conception, or fertilization of the ova/oocytes by male sperm, and implantation of the fertilized egg into the uterine wall, leading to pregnancy.

If fertilization of the ova/oocyte does not take place, then menstruation (monthly shedding of the uterine lining) occurs. The female genital system also produces female sex hormones that maintain the reproductive cycle.

Hymen

Located at the beginning of the reproductive tract, the hymen lies just inside the opening of the vagina. This is a mucous membrane that encircles or covers the opening like a tight ring. It assists in protecting the genital tract, but is not a necessary component for health. It is typically broken during the first attempt at sexual intercourse, or it may be soft and pliable and tearing does not occur. It may also be torn during exercise or insertion of a tampon or diaphragm. Tearing may or may not cause bleeding.

External Genitalia

The external genital organs, called the pudendum, function to enable sperm to enter the body and protect the internal reproductive organs from infectious organisms.

Labia

The labia have multiple anatomical parts with different functions:

Labia majora – The outer paired lips of the pudendum that enclose and protect the other external reproductive tissues. They are large and fleshy and comparable to the scrotum in males. The labia majora consist of sweat and oil-secreting glands, and after puberty, are covered with hair.

Labia minora – The inner paired lips of the pudendum that protect the vaginal opening and prevent infectious and other foreign organisms from entering. They are smaller and lie just inside the labia majora surrounding the openings to the vagina and the urethra.

Bartholin's gland – These glands produce a mucous-filled secretion that assists in sexual intercourse. They are located beside the vaginal opening.

Clitoris – The small female sex organ of arousal, very sensitive to stimulation and able to become erect. It is covered by a fold of skin (prepuce), similar to the foreskin on the penis.

Uterus and Cervix

The uterus is a thick-walled, muscular, pear-shaped organ located in the middle of the pelvis, behind the bladder and in front of the rectum. It consists of the cervix, which opens into the vagina, and the corpus (main body), which is connected to the fallopian tubes and the dome-shaped top of the fundus. The uterus is anchored by several ligaments, such as the round, cardinal, broad, and uterosacral ligaments.

There are three layers of tissue in the wall of the uterus. The inner layer is the endometrium, the middle layer is the myometrium, and the outer is the perimetrium.

Endometrium – The inner layer of the uterus that has a main role in the conception and menstruation cycle. During conception, the glands and the blood vessels increase in size and number. The vascular spaces become interconnected by fusion to form the placenta. Before menstruation, the endometrium grows to a thick, blood vessel rich layer of glandular tissue.

Myometrium – Made up of muscle tissue, this middle layer of the uterus stretches during pregnancy as the smooth muscle cells expand in size and number. It also contracts during labor to expel the fetus. After delivery, it contracts to expel the placenta and reduce blood loss. After pregnancy, it assists in returning the uterus to its pre-pregnancy size.

Perimetrium – The outer, serosal layer of the uterus composed of a smooth, thin layer of cells that secrete serous fluid. This serous fluid lubricates to reduce friction from muscle movement.

The lining of the uterus grows and thickens each month to prepare for fertilization of the ova (egg), progressing to pregnancy. If fertilization of the egg does not happen, menstruation occurs, and the thick, blood vessel-rich, glandular lining flows out through the vagina.

The main purpose of the uterus is to house the fetus after fertilization. It also provides structural integrity and support to other organs, such as the bladder, bowel, and pelvic bones. The uterus helps separate and keep the bladder in its natural position above the pubic bone and the bowel in place behind the uterus.

Another purpose of the uterus is in sexual response. It directs blood flow to the pelvis, external genitalia (e.g., labia, clitoris), and the ovaries and is essential for orgasm.

In reproduction, the uterus accepts a fertilized ovum, which passes from the fallopian tube. It then becomes implanted into the endometrium and derives nourishment from blood vessels specifically for this purpose. Eventually, the fertilized ovum becomes an embryo, attaches to the wall of the uterus, a placenta develops, and a fetus develops until childbirth.

Uterine Corpus

The body of the uterus can stretch to accommodate a growing fetus because it is highly muscular. Its muscular walls contract during labor to push the baby out through the cervix and vagina. During the reproductive years, the corpus uteri is twice as long as the cervix, but after menopause, the reverse is true.

A woman's reproductive cycle typically lasts 28 days. During this time, the endometrium lining the corpus thickens. If pregnancy does not take place, a majority of the endometrium is shed and bleeding occurs, resulting in a menstrual period.

Cervix

The lower part of the uterus, the cervix protrudes into the upper end of the vagina. It is lined with a smooth, mucous membrane and is usually a narrow channel. The cervix is a passageway for sperm to enter the internal reproductive tract, but also one for menstrual blood to exit. During labor, the channel widens to allow the fetus to pass into the birth canal. It is also a barrier against bacteria, except during sexual intercourse when bacteria can potentially enter the uterus, causing sexually transmitted disease.

The cervical channel is lined with glands that secrete mucus. This mucus is thick and impenetrable to sperm until just before ovulation—the release of an ova/oocyte. At ovulation, the consistency of the mucus changes to allow sperm to get through and fertilize the ova/oocyte. The typical time the mucus-secreting gland can store sperm is up to 5 days. These sperm can later move up through the corpus uteri and into the fallopian tube to fertilize an ova. Most pregnancies occur from intercourse that happens during the 3 days before ovulation, but to a lesser extent, up to 6 days before ovulation or 3 days after ovulation.

Vagina

The vagina is a muscular, elastic, tubular organ about 4 to 5 inches (10 to 12 ½ cm) long in an adult female. It connects the external genital organs to the uterus and is the main female reproductive organ of sexual intercourse. It is also part of the passageway for sperm to reach the ova/oocyte for fertilization, as well as the passage for shedding of menstrual blood and transporting a fetus to the external environment.

There is typically no space inside the vagina unless stretched (e.g., childbirth, intercourse). The lower third is surrounded by elastic muscle that controls the diameter of its opening and contracts rhythmically and involuntarily during orgasm.

The lining of the vagina is a mucous membrane that is kept moist by fluid seeping from cells on its surface and by secretions from glands in the cervix in the lower part of the uterus. Normally, a small amount of clear or milky white secretions will discharge. During the reproductive years, the lining has folds and wrinkles. The lining is smooth prior to puberty and after menopause.

Ovaries

There are two ovaries that sit on each side of the pelvis, at the ends of the uterine tubes. They are normally about the size of a walnut. They are attached to the uterus by ligaments and contain follicles, or fluid-filled cavities within their walls. Each of these follicles contains one developing egg cells. One egg (ovum) is typically released every 28 days and travels down the fallopian tube, where it may become fertilized.

Fallopian Tubes

There are two fallopian tubes, also called salpinges, that extend from the upper edges on either side of the uterus toward the ovaries. They are 2 to 3 inches (5 to 7 cm) long. They do not connect directly to the ovaries, but instead, each of the tubes flares into a funnel shape with fimbriae, or finger-like extensions, at the ovaries.

When an egg is released from an ovary, the fimbriae guide the egg into the fallopian tube opening. The fallopian tubes are lined with cilia, tiny hair-like projections which, together with the muscles in the tube wall, propel an egg downward through the tube toward the uterus. The egg is typically fertilized within the fallopian tube. There are different parts of the fallopian tube:

Infundibulum – The funnel-shaped end of the fallopian tube with the fimbriae and closest to the ovary.

Ampullary region – The major portion of the lateral tube.

Isthmus – The narrower portion of the tube that connects to the uterus and the interstitial portion that traverses the uterine musculature.

Tubal ostium – The proximal or distal opening of the fallopian tube. The distal ostium is the opening in the infundibulum to the abdominal cavity, though which an oocyte enters the tube at ovulation. The proximal ostium is located within the uterus at the uterotubal junction.

Fallopian Tube Cells

Within the simple columnar epithelium of the fallopian tubes, there are two types of cells:

Ciliated cells – Found throughout the tubes, but most numerous in the infundibulum and ampulla, the cilia of these cells help propel the egg through the tube. The hormone estrogen increases the production of cilia on these cells.

Peg cells – Interspersed between the ciliated cells, the peg cells consist of apical granules and produce tubular fluid. This fluid contains nutrients for spermatozoa, oocytes, and zygotes. The hormone progesterone increases the number of peg cells and estrogen increases their secretory activity.

Breasts

Located in the upper ventral region, the breasts are modified sudoriferous (sweat) glands that contain mammary glands to produce milk. It is mainly the larger of the mammary glands distributed throughout the breast that produce milk.

On each breast there is one nipple surrounded by the areola. The areola can vary in color from pink to dark brown and contains many sebaceous glands. The mammary glands are drained of milk through the nipple by lactiferous ducts, where each of the ducts has its own opening. The milk is located in the back of the breast. When suckling occurs on the breast, the smooth muscles of the glands push more milk forward to the ducts.

The breast also consists of connective tissue (i.e., collagen and elastin), adipose tissue (fat), and Cooper's ligaments. The breast sits over the pectoralis major muscle and usually extends from the level of the 2nd rib to the 6th rib. The superior lateral quadrant of the breast extends diagonally upwards towards the tail of Spence. Mammary tissue extends from the clavicle above to the seventh or eighth rib below, and from the midline to the edge of the Latissimus dorsi posteriorly.

The nipples have a large concentration of blood vessels. Blood supply to the breasts comes from the internal thoracic (internal mammary), lateral thoracic, thoracoacromial, and posterior intercostal arteries. Drainage is from the axillary, internal thoracic, and intercostal veins.

The nipples also contain a large amount of nerves. The breasts are innervated by the anterior and lateral cutaneous branches of the fourth through sixth intercostal nerves. In conjunction with the blood vessels, the nipples can become erect in response to sexual stimuli, cold, and touch because of the nerves and blood supply.

Some lymph nodes travel from the breast to the ipsilateral axillary lymph nodes and the remaining travel to the parasternal nodes and to other breast or abdominal lymph nodes. The axillary nodes include the pectoral, subscapular, and humeral groups of lymph nodes. These drain to the central axillary lymph nodes and then to the apical axillary lymph nodes.

Breasts develop as a result of changing sex hormones (e.g., estrogen) during puberty. Changes to breasts also occur during pregnancy when they become larger and firmer, due to hypertrophy of the mammary gland because of prolactin hormone. The size of the nipples may increase and the pigmentation typically becomes darker. The menstrual cycle may also cause breast and nipple changes.

Genitourinary Coding Guidelines

Diseases of the Genitourinary System are contained in Chapter 14 in ICD-10-CM.

ICD-10-CM – Chapter 14: Diseases of Genitourinary System (N00-N99)

1. Chronic kidney disease

   a. Stages of chronic kidney disease (CKD)

   The ICD-10-CM classifies CKD based on severity. The severity of CKD is designated by stages 1-5. Stage 2, code N18.2, equates to mild CKD; stage 3, code N18.3, equates to moderate CKD; and stage 4, code N18.4, equates to severe CKD. Code N18.6, End stage renal disease (ESRD), is assigned when the provider has documented end-stage-renal disease (ESRD).

   If both a stage of CKD and ESRD are documented, assign code N18.6 only.

   b. Chronic kidney disease and kidney transplant status

   Patients who have undergone kidney transplant may still have some form of chronic kidney disease (CKD) because the kidney transplant may not fully restore kidney function. Therefore, the presence of CKD alone does not constitute a transplant complication. Assign the appropriate N18 code for the patient's stage of CKD and code Z94.0, Kidney transplant status. If a transplant complication such as failure or rejection or other transplant complication is documented, see section I.C.19.g for information on coding complications of a kidney transplant. If the documentation is unclear as to whether the patient has a complication of the transplant, query the provider.

   c. Chronic kidney disease with other conditions

   Patients with CKD may also suffer from other serious conditions, most commonly diabetes mellitus and hypertension. The sequencing of the CKD code in relationship to codes for other contributing conditions is based on the conventions in the Tabular List.

   See I.C.9. Hypertensive chronic kidney disease.

   See I.C.19. Chronic kidney disease and kidney transplant complications.

Documentation Elements of Genitourinary System

Some key documentation elements for genitourinary system coding include the following:

- Instead of using a separate code to report hematuria in conjunction with cystitis or prostatitis, a combination code is used to capture the specific type of cystitis or prostatitis and the hematuria.
- Post-traumatic and post-infective urethral stricture codes are specific to gender. In males, documentation must identify of site of the stricture as meatal, bulbous, membranous, or anterior. In females, post-traumatic urethral stricture requires documentation as to whether the stricture was due to childbirth or another cause.
- Spermatocele needs to be documented as single or multiple.
- Inflammation of the testes or epididymis is specific to site and must be designated as epididymitis only, orchitis only, or epididymo-orchitis.
- Azoospermia and oligospermia conditions related to infertility in males require documentation as organic or due to drug therapy, radiation, infection, obstruction of efferent ducts, systemic disease, or of other extratesticular cause.
- Priapism requires documentation of the cause as due to trauma, disease classified elsewhere, drug-induced, or other specified cause.
- Inflammation of the ovaries or fallopian tubes are specific to site and must be designated as oophoritis only, salpingitis only, or salpingitis with oophoritis.
- Inflammation of the vagina or vulva must be specified as acute, or subacute and chronic and must be designated as vulvitis alone, vaginitis alone, or as vulvovaginitis.

- Additional codes have been added to the subcategory for other female genital prolapse to allow identification of the type of prolapse as:
  - Perineocele
  - Incompetence or weakening of pubocervical tissue
  - Incompetence or weakening of rectovaginal tissue
  - Pelvic muscle wasting
  - Cervical stump prolapse
  - Other specified genital prolapse
- Fistulas of the female genital tract require designation as vesicovaginal, other urinary-genital fistula, vaginal to small intestine, vaginal to large intestine, other intestinal-genital tract fistula, genital tract to skin, or female genital tract to other specified site.
- Laterality must be documented as right, left, or bilateral for most diseases and conditions involving paired organs located in this section.

Section 1 – Infectious Diseases of the Urinary and Reproductive Systems

Infections of the genitourinary tract can be divided into those with a sexual mode of transmission and other types of infections. In addition, there are infections with a sexual mode of transmission that affect other organ systems or are systemic in nature. Lastly, there are maternal infections that affect the fetus during pregnancy.

Genitourinary Sexually Transmitted Diseases

Genitourinary infections with a predominantly sexual mode of transmission include: chlamydia, gonorrhea, herpes simplex, human papilloma virus (HPV), syphilis, and trichomoniasis.

Chlamydia

Chlamydia is a bacterial infection caused by *Chlamydia trachomatis* and is the most common sexually transmitted disease (STD). In men, chlamydia produces the following symptoms: burning on urination, discharge from the penis or rectum, testicular tenderness or pain, or rectal pain. However, up to 25% of men report no symptoms. In women, symptoms include: burning on urination, painful sexual intercourse, rectal pain or discharge, pelvic pain, liver inflammation, and vaginal discharge. However, only about 30% of women report any symptoms indicative of infection. Untreated chlamydia in women can cause pelvic inflammatory disease (PID) and fallopian tube scarring leading to infertility and ectopic pregnancy. Men rarely suffer reproductive damage from chlamydia.

Gonorrhea

Gonorrhea is a bacterial infection caused by *Neisseria gonorrhea* and is also a common STD. In men, symptoms include: burning and pain on urination, urinary urgency or frequency, purulent discharge from the urethra, red or swollen urethral meatus, and tender or swollen testicles. In women, symptoms may be mild or nonspecific and may be mistaken for other conditions. Symptoms in women include: vaginal discharge, burning and pain on urination, urinary frequency, painful sexual intercourse, pelvic or abdominal pain, and fever. Another presenting symptom in both men and women who practice oral sex is sore throat. Untreated gonorrhea can lead to infertility or to a systemic infection called disseminated gonococcemia. Disseminated gonococcemia can affect the joints and heart valves. In women, *N. gonorrhea* can infect the uterus, fallopian tubes, and ovaries and is one of the primary causes of PID.

Herpes Simplex

There are two types of herpes simplex virus (HSV). Type 1 (HSV-1) typically causes oral herpes, also referred to as cold sores, but can also cause genital infections. Type 2 (HSV-2) typically causes genital herpes. Genital herpes affects the skin and mucous membrane of the genitals. During the initial infection the patient may experience generalized symptoms including: decreased appetite, fever, malaise, and body aches. In addition to the generalized symptoms, small, painful blisters filled with clear or straw-colored fluid appear at the site of the infection which may be the genitalia or mouth. Before the blisters appear, the skin may tingle, burn or itch. The blisters eventually break causing shallow ulcers that heal slowly over a 7-14 day period. After the initial infection, a second outbreak may occur weeks or months later. It is usually less severe and shorter than the first. Outbreaks can continue to occur at intervals throughout the rest of the patient's life.

Human Papilloma Virus

HPV is actually a group of more than 100 viruses. Some strains cause STDs such as genital warts. Certain high-risk strains have been shown to cause cervical cancer.

Syphilis

Treponema pallidum is the causative agent of syphilis. Infection with *T. pallidum* produces symptoms that are divided into stages. During the primary stage of syphilis, a sore called a chancre appears at the site where the syphilis bacterium entered the body. The chancre resolves without treatment in 3-6 weeks but the patient remains infected. Untreated primary stage syphilis progresses to second stage syphilis which is characterized by a skin rash and mucous membrane lesions. The most common site of the rash is the palms of the hands and soles of the feet. Other symptoms of second stage syphilis include fever, swollen lymph nodes, sore throat, hair loss, headaches, weight loss, muscle aches, and fatigue. Symptoms of second stage syphilis also resolve spontaneously but the patient remains infected. The patient then enters the late or latent stage which may not produce symptoms for 10-20 years following infection. Central and peripheral nervous system symptoms appear during late stage syphilis and include difficulty coordinating muscle movements, paralysis, numbness, gradual blindness and dementia. Late stage syphilis also damages other internal organs including the eyes, heart, blood vessels, liver, bones, and joints.

Trichomoniasis

Trichomoniasis is an STD caused by the parasite *Trichomonas vaginalis.* In men, the infection may not cause any symptoms and typically resolves on its own. Some men do report burning on urination or ejaculation, urethral itching or slight urethral discharge. Rarely, some men will develop prostatitis or epididymitis from the infection. In women, symptoms include vaginal itching, vaginal discharge, vaginal odor, itching of inner thighs and discomfort with intercourse.

Other Genitourinary Tract Infections

Other infections of the genitourinary tract may be generally described as urinary tract infections (UTIs) and or they may be described by the site of the infection such as urethritis, cystitis, pyelonephritis, epididymitis, prostatitis, or pelvic inflammatory disease (PID). These terms may refer to inflammation that is due to infection or inflammation due to other causes. When the inflammation is due to an infection the inflammation is typically identified using a code from the genitourinary system chapter and a code from the chapter for certain infectious and parasitic diseases to identify the infectious organism. However, there are some exceptions to this rule.

Urinary Tract Infection (UTI)

Urine is usually sterile. It is usually free of bacteria, viruses and fungi, but does contain fluids, salts and waste products. An infection can occur when tiny organisms, such as *Escherichia coli* (*E. coli*) (bacteria from the digestive tract), cling to the opening of the urethra and begin to multiply. The bacteria first travel to the urethra and multiply, causing an infection.

Women are more prone to UTIs than males because females have a shorter urethra, and the urethra is closer to the anus. Although, as males age, UTIs in men become equal in proportion as in women, mostly due to the prostate enlarging. As the prostate grows, it obstructs the urethra, leading to increased difficulty in urination. Because there is less urine flushing the urethra, there is a higher incidence of *E. coli* colonization.

UTI is also more common in young women who are sexually active. Other causes are urinary catheters, with *Staphylococcus epidermidis* the most common organism; spermicide use; and a familial predisposition for UTIs. Other risk factors include diabetes, sickle-cell diseases, and anatomical malformations of the urinary tract.

Urethritis

Urethritis is an inflammation that is limited to the urethra. There are two primary types of urethritis-gonococcal urethritis and non-gonococcal urethritis (NGU). NGU, also called non-specific urethritis, has both infectious and non-infectious causes. Infectious causes include adenovirus, *E. coli*, *C. trachomatis*, and *T. vaginalis*. Symptoms of NGU include white cloudy discharge and pain on urination. In addition, men may experience penile irritation or itchiness.

Urethritis that is inadequately treated or not treated can eventually cause a stricture of the urethra that may increase the risk that infections will develop in the future. An abscess is another complication that can occur due to an accumulation of the pus around the urethra, which can produce outpouchings in the urethral wall called diverticula. If the abscess perforates the skin, the vagina or rectum, a fistula may form.

Cystitis

Cystitis is an inflammation of the urinary bladder that more often affects women due to a shorter urethra and closer proximity of the urethra to the anus. Sexual intercourse may increase the risk of cystitis because organisms can be introduced into the bladder through the urethra during sexual activity. Infectious organisms are normally removed through urination, but if they multiply faster than they can be removed, an infection may result.

There are several different types of cystitis, but only two are commonly associated with infection, traumatic cystitis and bacterial cystitis. Traumatic cystitis is the most common type of cystitis in women. It is caused by bruising of the bladder usually due to sexual intercourse. This is often followed by bacterial infection. Bacterial cystitis is caused by bacteria being transferred from the anus through the urethra into the bladder. The bacteria most often associated with cystitis are *E. coli* and *Staphylococcus saprophyticus*.

The risks of developing cystitis include obstruction of the bladder or urethra, catheterization or other insertion of instruments into the urinary tract, pregnancy, diabetes, and a history of nephropathy. Other risks include benign prostatic hypertrophy (BPH), prostatitis, urethral strictures, lack of adequate fluids, bowel incontinence, and immobility.

Pyelonephritis

Pyelonephritis is an inflammation of the kidney, more specifically the renal parenchyma, which is the functional tissue of the kidney, calyces and renal pelvis. Inflammation is most often due to an infection of the kidney that typically originates as a lower urinary tract infection, such as cystitis or prostatitis. It may be acute or chronic in form.

Acute pyelonephritis is an inflammation of the renal pelvis and the kidney that is exudative and purulent (containing pus). There may also be interstitial abscesses of the renal parenchyma containing neutrophils, fibrin, cell debris and central germ colonies. Renal tubules are typically damaged by the exudates and may contain neutrophil casts.

In **chronic pyelonephritis**, there is hemorrhage and suppuration (pus) in the renal pelvis through to the renal cortex. This may result in fibrosis (formation of excess connective tissue) in the kidney.

Some of the more common occurrences of pyelonephritis are due to certain types of bacteria, such as *E. coli, Enterococcus faecalis*, and *Pseudomonas aeruginosa*

In some cases, pyelonephritis can lead to sepsis.

Epididymitis

Epididymitis, inflammation of the epididymis, is most often caused by infection or a sexually transmitted disease, such as *C. trachomatis* or *E. coli*. It may also follow a viral illness, be associated with urinary tract anomaly, or be caused by sterile reflux of urine through the ejaculatory ducts.

Epididymitis causes scrotal pain and swelling, and in severe cases may spread to the adjacent testicle, causing fever and abscess. If left untreated, scar tissue can be produced, that can block the sperm from leaving the testicle and may result in infertility.

Pelvic Inflammatory Disease (Disorder) (PID)

Pelvic inflammatory disease is inflammation of the uterus, fallopian tubes, and/or ovaries that eventually progresses to form scars with adhesions to tissues and organs that are in close proximity and may lead to other types of infections. Although most pelvic inflammatory diseases are bacterial infections, they may also be caused by viruses, fungi, and/or parasites. Organisms that are considered normal vaginal flora can be involved and individual cases can be due to a single or multiple organisms. PID is classified by the affected organ(s), the stage of the infection and the organism.

The main cause of pelvic inflammatory disease is transmission of the infecting organism during sexual intercourse. Other modes of transmission include through the lymph nodes, postabortal (miscarriage or abortion), postpartum or because of an intrauterine contraceptive device (IUD).

Many patients are unaware they have PID. If left untreated, it can lead to infertility; in fact, PID is the leading cause of infertility in women.

Other Sexually Transmitted Diseases

Other infections with a sexual mode of transmission affect other organ system or are systemic in nature. The two described here include human immunodeficiency virus (HIV) and hepatitis B virus (HBV).

Human Immunodeficiency Virus

HIV is an STD but can also be transmitted from unscreened blood, shared needles, and from mother to child in utero or by breast feeding. There are two HIV serotypes, HIV-1 and HIV-2, but both types cause similar disease processes. Shortly after infection approximately 50% of those who are infected develop flu-like symptoms including fever, muscle aches, joint pain, sore throat, and enlarged lymph nodes. After the primary phase of infection, individuals with HIV go through an asymptomatic (symptom free) period. During the asymptomatic phase, HIV attacks the immune system by destroying CD4 T-cells, which are a type of white blood cell. This hampers the body's ability to fight infection. Some HIV infected individuals show evidence of immune system compromise within a year of infection. However, for the majority of individuals with HIV, immune system compromise may not be evident for 8-10 years or even longer. Symptomatic HIV infected individuals usually progress from having early symptoms and then go on to develop acquired immunodeficiency syndrome (AIDS), which is the final stage of an HIV infection. AIDS is defined as a CD4 T-cell count below 200 cells/mm^3. For coding purposes, individuals are considered to have AIDS if their physician uses the term AIDS to describe the illness or if the patient is being treated for an HIV-related illness or is described as having any conditions resulting from the HIV positive status.

Hepatitis B

HBV is spread through direct contact with blood, semen, vaginal secretions, or other body fluids. HBV causes inflammation of the liver and is discussed in more detail in the gastrointestinal system. It is mentioned here only because one primary form of transmission is unprotected sex with an HBV infected partner.

Maternal Infection Affecting the Fetus

There are a number of infections that can cause adverse outcomes for the fetus, particularly when the maternal infection occurs during the first trimester of pregnancy. Some of the more common maternal infections known to affect the fetus include: toxoplasmosis, rubella, cytomegalovirus. Two other viruses that can affect the fetus, HSV and HIV, have already been discussed.

Toxoplasmosis

Toxoplasmosis is caused by the parasite Toxoplasma gondii. If a woman contracts toxoplasma during pregnancy, the fetus can become infected. The fetus can also become infected during labor and delivery. Infection of the fetus is referred to as congenital toxoplasmosis. Toxoplasmosis often produces minimal symptoms in the mother and the mother may not know that she has contracted the parasite. However, infection particularly during early pregnancy can cause serious problems for the fetus including: preterm birth and damage to the fetus' eyes, nervous system, skin, and ears. To prevent infection pregnant women are typically instructed to avoid undercooked meats, use good hand washing technique after handling raw meat, and avoid contact with cat feces, litter boxes and dog feces.

Rubella

When a pregnant woman is infected with rubella during the first trimester of pregnancy the fetus can suffer a number of conditions directly related to the infection. Complications of congenital rubella include: cataracts, glaucoma, retinitis, patent ductus arteriosus, pulmonary artery stenosis, mental retardation, motor retardation, encephalitis, meningitis, and deafness. The incidence of congenital rubella has decreased significantly since the introduction of the rubella vaccine. Women of childbearing age who have not had rubella should have the vaccine prior to becoming pregnant.

Cytomegalovirus

Cytomegalovirus (CMV) is a member of the herpes virus family. Between 50 and 85% of people over age 40 have had a CMV infection. CMV is typically a mild infection in healthy individuals and typically only causes concern in high-risk groups which includes pregnant women due to the effects of the virus on the fetus. Infants who are infected before birth may show no symptoms at birth, but some infants will develop problems over time including hearing, vision, neurological, and developmental problems.

Section 1 Coding Practice

Condition	ICD-10-CM
Urinary tract infection, due to E. coli	N39.0, B96.20
Acute gonococcal urethritis	A54.01
Chronic pyelonephritis with associated vesicoureteral reflux	N11.0
Epididymitis, due to Chlamydia	A56.19
Pelvic inflammatory disease	N73.9
Congenital cytomegalovirus	P35.1
HIV positive status, asymptomatic	Z21
Encounter for treatment of severe oral and esophageal candidiasis due to AIDS (HIV-1)	B37.81, B37.0, B20

Section 1 Questions

Would chronic gonococcal urethritis be reported with the same code?

Is code A56.19 specific for chlamydial epididymitis?

Is code N73.9 reported for PID complicating pregnancy?

What other term(s) is used to describe congenital cytomegalovirus?

Why isn't asymptomatic HIV-1 positive status reported with the same code as AIDS?

Is symptomatic HIV-2 infection reported with the same code as HIV-1 infection?

See end of chapter for Coding Practice answers.

Section 2 – Neoplasms of the Urinary and Reproductive Systems

Neoplasms of the urinary and reproductive system may be benign, pre-malignant, carcinoma in situ, malignant, or of uncertain behavior. There are a number of different types of benign neoplasms that affect the urinary tract and reproductive system, such as simple renal cysts, bladder polyps, and uterine fibroids. Premalignant lesions or tissues are those that are in a transitional state between normal tissue and carcinoma in situ. Examples include villous or dysplastic bladder polyps, atypical hyperplasia of the urothelium, and mild to moderate dysplasia of the uterine cervix, vagina or vulva.

Carcinoma in situ, also sometimes referred to as severe dysplasia, is a common type of neoplasm of the female reproductive tract and is most commonly found in the uterine cervix, vagina, and vulva using routine screening procedures such as a PAP smear. Most people are familiar with the most common types of malignancies of the male and female reproductive organs with common sites being the prostate, testicles, breast and uterus. Urinary tract malignancies are less common than reproductive system malignancies but kidney, bladder, and other urinary tract cancers are still fairly common. The more common types of urinary and reproductive system neoplasms are discussed here.

Renal Cyst

Renal cysts are typically classified as simple or complex. Simple cysts are benign lesions consisting of spherical spaces within the kidney filled with either clear or yellow liquid or blood. The lining of simple cysts is thin with no irregularities. Complex cysts are those that are irregular in shape and contain irregularities inside the cyst itself such as septations, calcifications, and/or a blood supply that can be seen on enhanced radiological studies. Complex renal cysts may be benign, pre-malignant, or malignant.

Renal Cell Carcinoma

Renal cell carcinoma originates in the renal tubules and is the most common type of kidney cancer in adults, occurring most often in men aged 50-70. The cancer may be found in only one kidney but is often bilateral. It is an aggressive cancer that metastasizes to the lungs and other organs. At the time of diagnosis one-third of all patients have metastatic disease.

Wilms Tumor

Wilms tumor, also known as nephroblastoma, is the most common type of renal malignancy in children. These types of tumors can become quite large without metastasizing, although they can metastasize to the lungs, liver, bone, and brain. Wilms tumor that has not spread to other organs has a 90% cure rate when treated with surgery alone or a combination of surgery, chemotherapy, and radiation therapy.

Transitional Cell Carcinoma

The renal pelvis, ureters, and bladder are lined with transitional cells. These specialized cells are able to stretch and change shape. Transitional cell carcinoma is type of malignant neoplasm that originates in these cells. This is the most common type of bladder cancer.

Other Bladder Malignancies

Other types of bladder cancer include squamous cell carcinoma (thin, flat cells in the bladder) and adenocarcinoma (cells that make and release mucus and other fluids). The cells that form squamous cell carcinoma and adenocarcinoma develop in the inner lining of the bladder as a result of chronic irritation and inflammation.

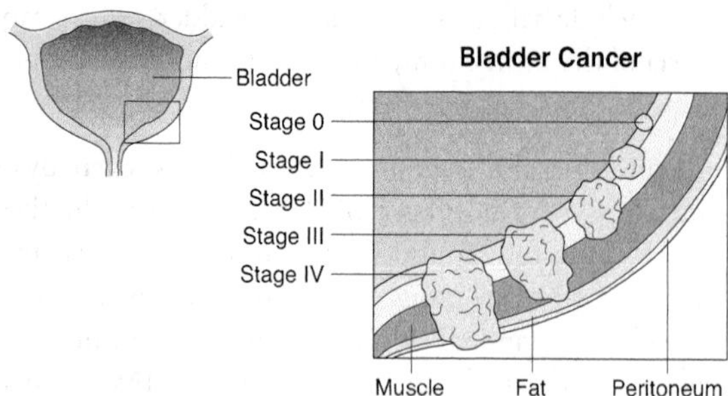

Bladder Polyps

Bladder polyps are outpouchings or growths the bladder lining. There are three common types, hamartomatous, adenomatous, and villous or dysplastic polyps. Hamartomatous and adenomatous bladder polyps are benign lesions that do not require removal unless they are very large or are causing symptoms. Villous or dysplastic polyps are classified as premalignant lesions and typically require removal.

Prostate Malignancy

Prostate cancer forms in the prostate gland in males. There are several types of cells in the prostate, but most of these cancers begin in the gland cells and are adenocarcinomas. Prostate cancer starts with very small changes in the size and shape of the prostate gland cells, known as prostatic intraepithelial neoplasia (PIN). This type of cancer grows slowly, and in autopsies of older men (80+) 8 out of 10 men who have died from other conditions or diseases, show they did have prostate cancer, but it did not cause problems in their lifetime.

Signs of prostate cancer may be pain, difficulty in and painful urination, nocturia, urinary retention, hematuria, erectile dysfunction and/or problems during sexual intercourse (e.g., painful ejaculation).

Risk factors include:

- Age – 60+
- Genetics – Family history of prostate cancer
- Diet – High fat intake, lack of vegetables
- Lifestyle
- Medications
- Increased testosterone levels
- Cadmium exposure

Testicular Malignancy

Cancer of the testes occurs when abnormal cells in the testicles divide and grow uncontrollably. It can develop in one of both testicles. Signs of this cancer include a lump, irregularity or enlargement in either testicle, a pulling sensation or unusual heaviness in the scrotum, a dull ache in the groin or lower abdomen, and pain or discomfort in a testicle or the scrotum, which may come and go.

Risk factors include:

- Age – Usually occurs between the ages of 15 to 40 years
- Family history
- Race – Caucasian men have five times the risk of African-American men and more than double than that of Asian men.
- Pre-existing condition – Undescended testicle(s) (cryptorchidism) – Testicles that do not descend from the abdomen are a major risk factor.

Breast Malignancy

Breast cancer originates in the breast tissue, with the most common forms occurring in the milk duct inner lining (ductal carcinoma) and the lobules that supply the ducts with milk (lobular carcinoma).

Some types of breast cancers require estrogen and progesterone to grow because they have receptors for those hormones, such as estrogen receptor positive cancer (ER positive cancer). Certain drugs can stop the production of those hormones and prevent the spread of the cancer. Those without hormone receptors or which have become metastatic may have genetic characteristics. Women with human epidermal growth factor receptor 2 (HER2) positive breast cancer are higher risk. HER2 is a gene that assists in cell growth, division and repair. Cancer cells can copy the genes and multiply quickly, causing the cancer to be more aggressive.

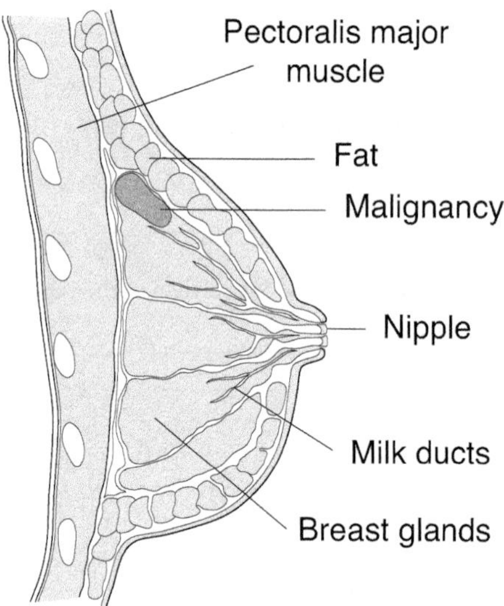

Risk factors include:

- Advanced age
- Genes – Breast cancer susceptibility type 1 (BRCA1) and breast cancer susceptibility type 2 (BRCA2) mutated genes
- Obesity
- Hormone replacement therapy (HRT)
- Nulligravida (no children)
- Dense breasts

Malignant Neoplasms of Uterus and Uterine Cervix

Endometrial carcinoma is the most common type of uterine cancer. This type of cancer begins in the endometrium which is the tissue that lines the uterus. It occurs most frequently in women over age 40 and symptoms include abnormal uterine bleeding, abdominal pain or cramping, and thin clear vaginal discharge after menopause. Endometrial cancer is usually diagnosed at an early stage before it has metastasized to organs outside the uterus. It is most commonly treated with hysterectomy alone, but radiation and/or chemotherapy may also be used if the cancer has spread to the lymph nodes or other abdominal organs.

Cervical cancer originates in the cells on the surface of the cervix. The two types of cells on the surface of the cervix are squamous and columnar cells. Most cervical cancers originate in the squamous cells and almost all squamous cell carcinoma is caused by certain strains of the human papilloma virus (HPV), a common virus spread by sexual intercourse. Other strains of HPV cause genital warts. Squamous cell carcinoma of the cervix is typically very slow growing and starts with pre-malignant cell changes called cervical dysplasia. Cervical dysplasia, also referred to as cervical intraepithelial neoplasia (CIN), can be detected by a PAP smear and is grouped into three categories as follows:

1. CIN I – Mild cervical dysplasia. Only the lower one-third of cells in the top (upper) layer of the cervix is abnormal.
2. CIN II – Moderate to marked cervical dysplasia. Up to two-thirds of the cells in the upper layer of the cervix are abnormal.
3. CIN III – Severe dysplasia to carcinoma in situ. Precancerous cells are present in the entire upper layer of the cervix.

Treatment of CIN depends on the degree of dysplasia and may include cryosurgery, electrocauterization, laser vaporization, LEEP procedure, or cone biopsy/excision of abnormal tissue.

Uterine Fibroids

Common benign tumors, or fibroids, grow in the muscle of the uterus. Fibroids are also called leiomyomas, fibromyomas, or myomas; they are not associated with uterine cancer and almost never develop into a malignancy. They occur mostly in women in their forties, and many women have multiple fibroids, but fibroids typically do not develop into cancer. When menopause is reached, fibroids are likely to become smaller and sometimes disappear.

Fibroids can cause bleeding, vaginal discharge, and frequent urination. They may also cause heavy bleeding or may press on surrounding organs causing pain.

There are three types of fibroids:

1. **Submucous** – This type is located just under the endometrium (uterine mucosa) and may be on a pedicle (long, thin stalk) or sessile (broad-based).
2. **Intramural** – This type is located predominantly within the myometrium and may distort the uterine cavity when it grows. They can also cause an irregular shape of the external uterus.
3. **Subserosal** – Located just under the uterine serosa this type can form into a pedicle that remains attached to the uterine wall but can protrude into the uterus, and eventually, enter into the vagina. This type may also be sessile.

Submucous leiomyoma of uterus

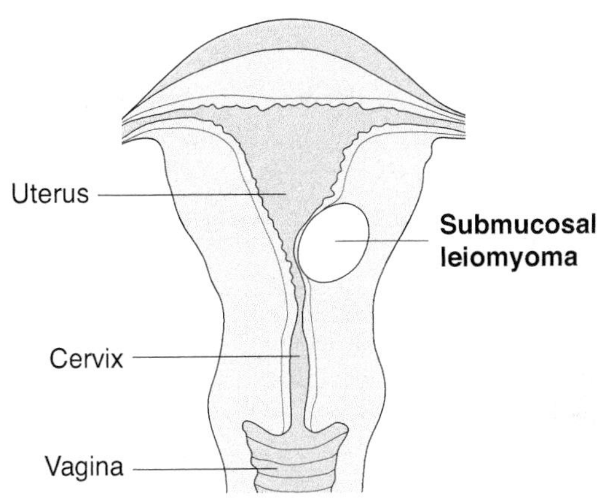

ICD-10-CM Anatomy & Physiology

Section 2 Coding Practice

Condition	ICD-10-CM
Bladder cancer of the trigone	C67.0
Prostate cancer	C61
Right testicular cancer	C62.91
A 52-year-old woman with infiltrating ductal carcinoma, center section of right breast	C50.111
Interstitial leiomyoma of the uterus	D25.1

Section 2 Questions

Since there is no excludes note under C67 indicating that carcinoma in situ is not reported under C67, would it be correct to report carcinoma in situ of the bladder trigone with code C67.0?

Is malignant neoplasm of the prostatic utricle reported with the same code as malignant neoplasm of the prostate? What is the prostatic utricle?

Code C62.91 reports malignant neoplasm of right testis, unspecified. What additional information is required to report a more specific code?

Does the type of breast cancer make a difference in code selection?

How is it determined that interstitial leiomyoma should be reported with code D25.1 for intramural leiomyoma?

See end of chapter for Coding Practice answers.

Section 3 – Other Diseases and Conditions of the Genitourinary System

Diseases of the genitourinary system are divided into four broad categories in ICD-10-CM. Diseases of the urinary system are listed first including: kidneys, ureters, bladder, and urethra. Diseases of the male genital organs are listed second. The third broad category is disorders of the breast. While disorders of the breast are typically associated with females, male conditions such as gynecomastia are also listed in this category. The last broad category is diseases of the female genital tract.

Diseases of the Urinary System

Diseases of the kidney are divided into conditions affecting the glomeruli called glomerular diseases, diseases that affect the renal tubules and the interstitial spaces between the tubules, and acute kidney failure and chronic kidney disease. Some of the more common diseases of the bladder and urethra include: interstitial and irradiation cystitis, bladder diverticulum, overactive bladder, and urethral stricture.

Glomerular Diseases

Glomerular diseases fall into two broad categories, glomerulonephritis which is an inflammatory process affecting the glomeruli, and glomerulosclerosis which refers to hardening or scarring of the tiny blood vessels that make up the glomeruli. These conditions may be acute, chronic, or congenital. Other terms used to describe diseases of the glomeruli include: nephritic syndrome and nephropathy.

Glomerular diseases damage the glomeruli. This damage can cause protein and red blood cells to leak into the urine and interfere with the clearance of waste products by the kidney, so they begin to build up in the blood. When protein leaks into the urine in excessive amounts it can cause their levels in the bloodstream to fall. Loss of blood proteins like albumin can cause excessive amounts of fluid to accumulate in body tissues resulting in edema. In the blood stream, albumin acts like a sponge, drawing excess fluid from the body into the bloodstream. The kidneys then remove the excess fluid from the bloodstream and it is excreted as urine. However, when albumin leaks into the urine, the blood loses its capacity to absorb extra fluid from the body.

Signs and symptoms of glomerular disease include:

- Proteinuria (large amounts of protein in the urine)
- Hematuria (blood in the urine)
- Reduced glomerular filtration rate which results in inefficient filtering of wastes from the blood
- Hypoproteinemia (low blood protein)
- Edema

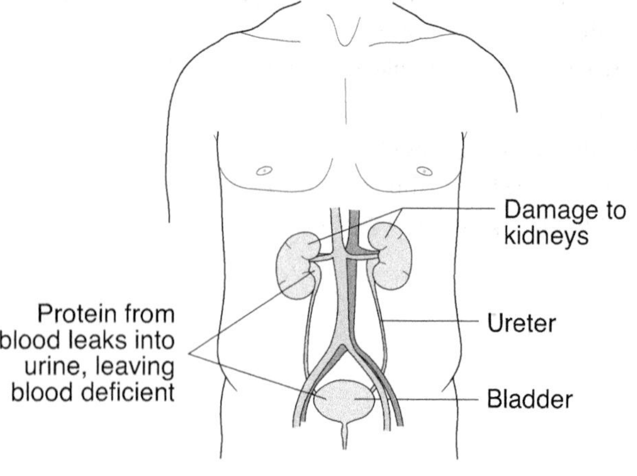

Renal Tubulo-Interstitial Diseases

Renal tubulo-interstitial diseases, also referred to as pyelitis, pyelonephritis, infectious interstitial nephritis, or tubular necrosis, are due to inflammatory processes that damage the renal tubules and interstitium, which in turn causes impaired renal function. These conditions may be acute or chronic and they may be primary diseases or secondary to another disease process. Acute conditions are most often associated with drug reactions or infection. Chronic conditions may be due to genetic or metabolic disorders, obstructive disorders such as ureteral strictures, renal or ureteral calculus, vesicoureteral reflux, drugs or environmental toxins such as heavy metals, or other underlying diseases.

Vesicoureteral Reflux

Vesicoureteral reflux (VUR) is when the flow of urine has reversed, causing the urine to travel from the bladder back up into the ureters or kidneys. Normal flow of the urine occurs when the ureters enter the urinary bladder and run submucously for a distance. This, along with the ureters' muscular attachments assists in securing and supporting them. These features together produce a valve-like effect that occludes the ureteric opening during the storage of urine, as well as urine elimination. In VUR, this mechanism fails, with the urine flowing backwards (retrograde).

Primary Vesicoureteral Reflux – If the submucosal length of the ureter relative to its diameter is insufficient, it causes valvular inadequacies. This is caused by a congenital anatomical deformity or lack of longitudinal muscle of the intravesical ureter, resulting in an anomaly of the ureterovesical junction (UVJ).

Secondary Vesicoureteral Reflux – The valvular mechanism begins normally, but an obstruction can cause raised vesicular pressures, deforming the UVJ. Also, there are functional reasons that cause secondary UVR, like bladder instability, neurogenic bladder, and non-neurogenic bladder.

Acute Kidney Failure

Acute kidney failure is the sudden loss of kidney function. Acute renal failure has many causes. Some causes include: burns, traumatic injuries, infection, autoimmune disorders, serious illness, septic shock, surgery, complications of pregnancy, clotting disorders, and urinary tract obstruction. In acute renal failure the goal is to treat the disease or condition that has caused the failure and restore kidney function.

Chronic Kidney Disease (CKD)

Chronic kidney disease is the loss of kidney function over a period of time (months or years). Usually this is caused by another disease, such as high blood pressure, diabetes, and or glomerulonephritis. Patients with these conditions are typically screened to prevent any further kidney damage. Kidney failure may lead to other complications, such as cardiovascular disease or anemia.

There are five stages of kidney disease:

1. Stage 1 – mildest form, with slightly diminished kidney function. Kidney damage with normal or high GFR*
2. Stage II – Kidney damage and mild decrease in GFR*
3. Stage III – Moderate decrease in GFR*
4. Stage IV – Severe decrease in GFR*
5. Stage V – Established kidney failure. Previously termed chronic kidney failure (CKF), or chronic renal failure (CRF)

Note: *Stage 5 chronic kidney disease that requires dialysis to sustain the life of the patient is reported as N18.6 End stage renal disease.*

*GFR level, or glomerular filtration rate, is a measure of how well the kidneys are cleaning waste product out of the blood.

Urolithiasis

Urolithiasis is a general term that refers to the presence of calculi or stones in the urinary tract.

Nephrolithiasis, also known as kidney stones, result from renal calculi in the kidney. Ureterolithiasis is the condition of having calculi in the ureter and ureterolithiasis is the condition of having calculi in the urethra. The stones are solid concretions (crystal aggregations) formed from dissolved urinary materials. There are several types, with type being based on the type of crystals of which they are made. The most common are calcium oxalate, then calcium phosphate, but a few stones are struvite, produced by urea-splitting bacteria from previous UTIs, and other metabolic abnormalities may produce uric acid or cystine stones.

These stones typically leave the body by passage through the urinary stream. If stones grow to a significant size before passage, they may obstruct the urinary tract at some point. The result of the obstruction causes dilation or stretching of the ureter and renal pelvis, and muscle spasms of the ureter to try and move the stone, which causes severe pain (renal colic) and nausea and vomiting. Blood in the urine (hematuria) may appear due to the damage to the lining of the urinary tract.

Calculus in urethra

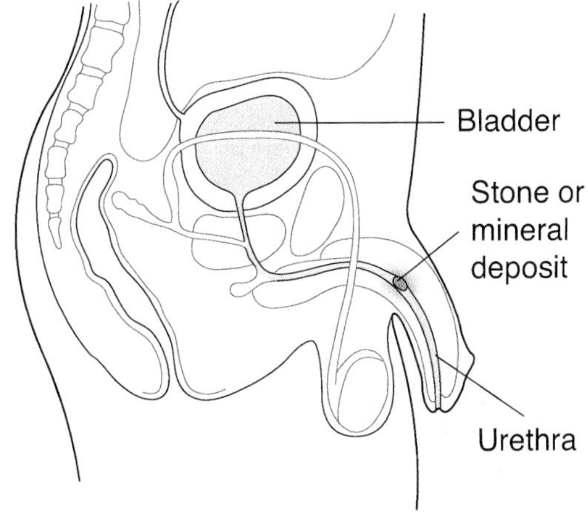

Gout

The kidneys excrete nitrogenous waste. As the liver breaks down amino acids, it also releases ammonia. The liver then combines the ammonia with carbon dioxide, creating urea, which is a less toxic form of nitrogenous waste than ammonia and the primary end product of metabolism. Some ammonia, creatinine, and uric acid are also excreted. The creatinine comes from the metabolic breakdown of creatine phosphate (high-energy phosphate in the muscles). Uric acid comes from the breakdown of nucleotides. It is insoluble and too much uric acid in the blood can build up and form crystals that can collect in the joints, tendons, and/or surrounding tissues, causing gout.

Gout presents as an acute and very painful attack of inflammatory arthritis, where the joint is red, tender, and swollen. It typically affects the first metatarsophalangeal joint at the base of the toe, because of the foot's lower temperature.

Patients who suffer from hyperuricemia (abnormally high uric acid level in the blood) can also form tophi (uric acid crystal deposits) in the tissues. The tophi deposits are hard and typically not as painful, although extensive tophi can invade bone with arthritis due to bone erosion.

Chronic gout can lead to decreased kidney function due to blockage of the kidney-filtering tubules with uric acid crystals and the formation of kidney stones.

Note: *Although gout can be directly related to kidney function and disease, both acute gout (M10) and chronic gout (M1A) are reported with codes from Chapter 13 Diseases of the Musculoskeletal System and Connective Tissue.*

Interstitial and Irradiation Cystitis

Cystitis caused by bacterial infection was discussed in the infection section of this chapter. However, there are other types of cystitis. Interstitial cystitis is a chronic inflammation of the tissues of the bladder wall of unknown cause. Irradiation cystitis is a type of radiation injury to the bladder that is a complication of treatment of malignancies of the pelvic organs including the uterus, ovary, vagina/vulva, prostate, bladder, colon, and rectum. Inflammation may be acute or chronic and may be complicated by hematuria.

Bladder diverticulum

A bladder diverticulum is a herniation of the bladder mucosa through the bladder wall musculature. Diverticula vary in size with some attaining a size larger than the bladder. The mouths of diverticula may be wide or narrow and depend on the size of the defect in the musculature. Narrow mouthed diverticula can cause additional complications if urine in the diverticula does not empty completely on urination (voiding). Complications include calculus formation and epithelial dysplasia.

Overactive bladder

Overactive bladder describes a condition in which there is sudden involuntary contraction of the bladder wall musculature. This causes an immediate need to urinate (void) even though the bladder may only contain a small amount of urine.

Urethral Stricture

Urethral stricture is an abnormal narrowing of urethra that may be acquired or congenital. Acquired strictures are most often caused by scar tissue following surgery, disease, or injury. Strictures are more common in men than women.

Section 3 Coding Practice

Condition	ICD-10-CM
Chronic hypertensive kidney disease, stage 3	I12.9, N18.3
Renal calculi	N20.0
Secondary vesicoureteral reflux, left ureter, with reflux nephropathy	N13.721
Renal calculus due to chronic gout of multiple sites	M1A.09, N22
Chronic interstitial cystitis with hematuria	N30.11

Section 3 Questions

Why is the hypertensive kidney disease reported as the first listed diagnosis and the chronic kidney disease as the second diagnosis?

What other terms are synonymous with renal calculus?

Is documentation of vesicoureteral reflux as primary or secondary or as right or left ureter (laterality) required for assignment of the most specific code?

Why is the code for gout reported first when it is associated with a renal calculus?

What type of code is N39.0? What type of information would be required to select a more specific code?

See end of chapter for Coding Practice answers.

Section 4 – Diseases of Male Genital Organs

Diseases and disorders of the male genital organs can be divided into several broad categories which include diseases of the prostate, diseases of the spermatic cord, testes, and tunica vaginalis, infertility, diseases of the prepuce and penis, erectile dysfunction and other sexual dysfunction, and other disorders of the male genital system. Some of the more common conditions include:

- Enlarged prostate
- Inflammatory diseases of the prostate
- Prostatic intraepithelial neoplasia
- Hydrocele and spermatocele
- Testicular torsion
- Male Infertility
- Phimosis and paraphimosis

Enlarged Prostate

An enlarged prostate, also referred to as benign prostatic hypertrophy (BPH,) is a non-malignant, non-neoplastic enlargement of the prostate. Prostate enlargement occurs over many years as a result of exposure to male hormones, particularly testosterone. Because prostate enlargement occurs over a long period of time, BPH is primarily a disease of older men. Most men are not aware that they have BPH until the prostate has enlarged to the point that it impinges on the urethra causing difficulty with urination. When enlargement of the prostate begins to affect the ability to pass urine it is referred to as BPH with lower urinary tract symptoms (LUTS). Lower urinary tract symptoms may include incomplete bladder emptying, nocturia, straining, urinary frequency, urinary hesitancy, incontinence, urinary obstruction, urinary retention, urgency, or weak urinary stream.

Prostatitis

Prostatitis is an inflammation of the prostate. The condition may be acute or chronic. The most common and well understood cause of both acute and chronic prostatitis is bacterial infection. Bacterial infection is believed to occur when urine leaks into the prostate through the urethra. For some types of chronic prostatitis with pelvic pain, no single factor has been identified as the causative factor. Possible causes of chronic prostatitis with chronic pelvic pain may be due to one or more of the following: an immune or nervous system disorder, infection, pressure on the prostate from diseased tissue, traumatic injury, or psychological stress.

Prostatic Intraepithelial Neoplasia

Prostatic intraepithelial neoplasia (PIN) is a condition in which there is abnormal tissue development. The abnormal tissue is composed of abnormal prostatic epithelial cells that divide more rapidly than normal epithelium. Even though these abnormal prostatic epithelial cells are not cancerous, PIN is considered to be a precursor to prostate cancer. PIN is classified by grade as high, medium or low. Low grade PIN is considered less likely to become cancerous than medium or high grade PIN.

Hydrocele and Spermatocele

A **hydrocele** is a collection of serous fluid in the tunica vaginalis of the scrotum or in a pocket along the spermatic cord or the canal of Nuck. Hydroceles may occur alone or in conjunction with an inguinal hernia. Hydroceles may be communicating or non-communicating. A communicating hydrocele is patent, which means that the processus vaginalis has failed to close during prenatal development. Failure of this thin membrane to close allows fluids from the abdominal (peritoneal) cavity to accumulate in the tunica vaginalis or along the spermatic cord or canal of Nuck. Non-communicating hydroceles are not patent so there is no communication with the peritoneal cavity. A **spermatocele** is a cyst of the epididymis that contains sperm.

Spermatocele

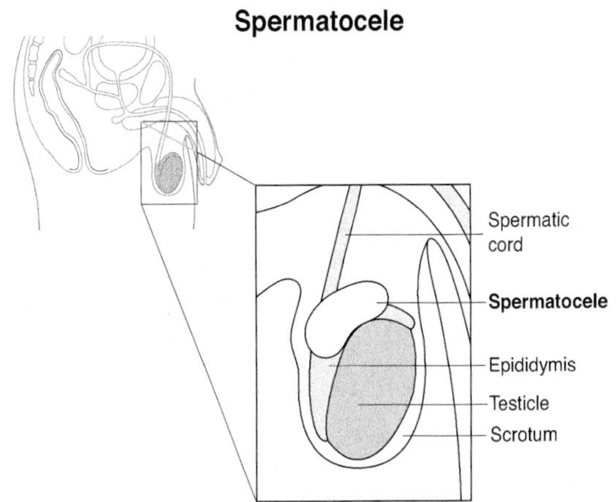

Testicular Torsion

The testicles are secured at one end by the spermatic cord within the scrotum. At times, this cord gets twisted, cutting off the testicle's blood supply. Most often occurring in men 12 to 18, it can be a result from an injury to the testicles or from strenuous activity. It can also occur randomly, for no apparent reason and is considered an emergent condition. If the blood supply to the testicle is cut off for a long period of time, it can become permanently damaged and may require removal.

Symptoms of testicular torsion include sudden and severe pain in the genital area, enlargement of the affected testicle, tenderness and swelling.

Male Infertility

The causes of male infertility can be divided into two broad categories, infertility caused by an endocrine disorder and infertility due to other causes. Male infertility due to an endocrine disorder, such as hypogonadism, is reported with codes from the endocrine system. Other causes of male infertility are reported with codes from the genitourinary system. Some causes of infertility include:

- Impaired production or function of sperm
  - Azoospermia
  - Oligospermia
  - Impaired motility
- Other medical causes
  - Varicocele
  - Undescended testicles
  - Infection
  - Retrograde ejaculation
  - Antisperm antibodies
  - Use of certain medications
  - Certain systemic diseases
- Endocrine/hormone causes
  - Hypogonadism

Azoospermia and Oligospermia

Azoospermia refers to the absence of living spermatozoa in semen. Oligospermia refers to a subnormal number of spermatozoa in semen. Azoospermia and oligospermia may be of testicular origin which is referred to as organic.

Impaired Motility

Spermatozoa must be able to move rapidly toward the egg for fertilization to occur. Any abnormalities in morphology (shape and structure) may affect motility and/or the ability to penetrate the egg may be impaired.

Medical Causes of Infertility

A few of the medical causes of infertility are listed above. Some of these causes have been discussed previously in this chapter or in chapters for other body systems. Others are self-explanatory. The two conditions not discussed previously include retrograde ejaculation and anti-sperm antibodies. Retrograde ejaculation refers to semen entering the bladder during orgasm instead being propelled through the urethra and out the external urethral orifice. Anti-sperm antibodies are antibodies in the male that attack and kill or damage the sperm.

Hypogonadism

Hypogonadism occurs when the testicles do not produce enough testosterone. Other diseases may cause this condition, such as Klinefelter's syndrome, undescended testicles, hemochromatosis, testicular trauma, normal aging, pituitary disorders and medications.

It is divided into two types:

Primary – Occurs when there is a problem within the testicle itself.

Secondary – Occurs when there is a problem with the pituitary gland, which sends messages to the testicles to produce testosterone.

Hypogonadism can happen during fetal development, at puberty, or in adult males. When it occurs in adult males, it may cause the following issues:

- Decrease in body hair growth
- Decrease in size and firmness of the testicles
- Decrease in muscle mass
- Increase in body fat
- Infertility
- Erectile dysfunction
- Decreased sex drive
- Gynecomastia (enlarged breast tissue)

Phimosis and Paraphimosis

The prepuce, more commonly referred to as the foreskin, is a free fold of skin that covers the glans penis in the uncircumcised male. The glans penis is the cone-shaped expansion of the corpus spongiosum that forms the head of the penis. Phimosis is the inability to retract the foreskin behind the glans penis in adult males. The condition may be physiologic or pathologic. Physiologic phimosis is present in infants and children and is not a cause for concern. Pathologic phimosis is due to scarring and adhesions that prevent retraction of the foreskin and is typically treated by circumcision in adult males. Paraphimosis, also referred to as capistration, is a rare condition in which the foreskin when retracted cannot be returned to its original position covering the glans penis. In the retracted position, the foreskin can become edematous and restrict blood supply to the glans penis. Treatment of paraphimosis requires prompt medical intervention.

Section 4 Coding Practice

Condition	ICD-10-CM
Testicular torsion	N44.00
BPH with urinary frequency, urinary retention, and urinary obstruction	N40.1, N13.8, R35.0, R33.8
Prostatic dysplasia presenting as ASAP suspicious for malignancy	N42.32
Single spermatocele	N43.41
A 28-year-old male with history of Hodgkin lymphoma presents with infertility. Patient has been cancer free for 5+ years. Complete absence of sperm is due to ABVD chemotherapy regimen for Hodgkin disease. ABVD regimen includes use of Adriamycin, Bleomycin, Vinblastine, Dacarbazine	N46.021, T45.1X5S, Z85.71
Primary hypogonadism in male	E29.1

Section 4 Questions

Why isn't testicular torsion reported with a code for an injury from Chapter 19?

Why is the BPH reported with a code for BPH with LUTS when the diagnosis does not specifically state that the patient has LUTS?

What does ASAP stand for regarding dysplasia of the prostate? If the patient was diagnosed with prostatic intraepithelial neoplasia (PIN) III would the condition still be reported with a code from N42.3-?

Why is it necessary to identify the drugs that caused the infertility? Why is only a single code reported for the four drugs that caused the infertility? Why is 7th character 'S' used?

Why is hypogonadism reported with a code from the endocrine chapter?

See end of chapter for Coding Practice answers.

Section 5 – Disorders of the Breasts

While disorders of the breasts are most often associated with women, men can develop many of the same disorders as women. Common disorders of the breast include: cysts, fibrocystic breast disease, fibroadenosis, gynecomastia, and hypertrophy, breast lump or mass, and complications associated with breast augmentation and breast reconstruction.

Fibrocystic Breast Disease

Fibrocystic breast disease, also referred to as cystic breast, mammary dysplasia, diffuse cystic mastopathy, or chronic cystic mastitis, is a very common condition in which there are benign tissue changes in the breast. The cause is not completely understood, but the tissue changes are believed to be associated with hormone production as the condition typically completely resolves at menopause.

Fibroadenosis

Fibroadenosis refers to tissue changes in the breast usually occurring after ovulation during the second half of the menstrual cycle. In fibroadenosis, the breasts become lumpy or nodular and painful to touch. The condition is temporary, usually resolving with the onset of menstruation. Fibroadenosis should not be confused with the term fibroadenoma. Fibroadenomas are benign neoplasms of the breast and are reported with a code from the neoplasm chapter.

Gynecomastia

Gynecomastia is the excessive development of breast tissue in males usually caused by ductal proliferation and periductal edema. The condition is considered to be secondary to increased estrogen levels. During puberty many males develop transient gynecomastia due to normal hormonal changes. While the condition does not pose a medical risk, the psychological effects of the development of significant amounts of breast tissue may warrant surgical intervention or treatment with hormones or other drugs.

Complications of Breast Augmentation and Reconstruction

One of the most common complications of breast augmentation is capsular contracture. It is caused by the development of scar tissue that hardens around the implant. Capsular contracture is more likely to occur following other complications associated with breast augmentation, such as infection, hematoma, or seroma.

Other complications of breast augmentation include: asymmetry, implant displacement, implant leak or rupture, keloid formation, rippling, skin irregularities, swelling and inflammation.

The two most common complications of breast reconstruction following mastectomy are deformity and disproportion. Deformity refers to irregularities in the breast contour, misshapen breasts, or excess tissue in the reconstructed breast. Disproportion refers to asymmetry between the native and reconstructed breast.

Section 5 Coding Practice

Condition	ICD-10-CM
Lump in auxiliary tail of the right breast	N63.31
Gynecomastia	N62
Bilateral fibrocystic disease of the breasts	N60.11, N60.12
Ptosis of native breast in relation to reconstructed breast	N65.1
Status post bilateral breast augmentation. Initial consultation (new physician) for evaluation of left breast capsular contraction	T85.44XA

Section 5 Questions

A breast lump or nodule is reported with an unspecified code. What additional information is required to report a more specific code for a mass in the breast?

Should code N62 Hypertrophy of breast, which is used to report gynecomastia, be used only for males?

Why are two codes required to report bilateral fibrocystic breast disease?

How is the coding of capsular contraction following breast augmentation classified?

See end of chapter for Coding Practice answers.

Section 6 – Diseases of Female Pelvic Organs and Genital Tract

Diseases and disorders and female genital tract are generally divided for coding purposes into two broad categories, inflammatory diseases and noninflammatory disorders. Some of the more common conditions include:

- Endometriosis
- Genital prolapse
- Cervical dysplasia
- Endometrial hyperplasia
- Abnormal uterine and vaginal bleeding
- Female infertility

Endometriosis

Endometriosis is a condition in which endometrial tissue normally confined to the inner layer of the uterus begins to grow outside the uterus. Common sites of endometriosis include the pelvic peritoneum, fallopian tubes, ovaries, bowel, rectum, and bladder. The condition is typically diagnosed between ages

25-35 when symptoms become more severe, but onset of the condition is believed to occur when regular menstruation begins. The condition is more common in women who have never been pregnant. Symptoms may include painful menstruation, abnormal bleeding, pain during intercourse, pain with bowel movements, and pain in the pelvis or lower back, although some women with severe endometriosis have no symptoms. Women with endometriosis are at risk for loss of fertility.

Endometriosis of ovary

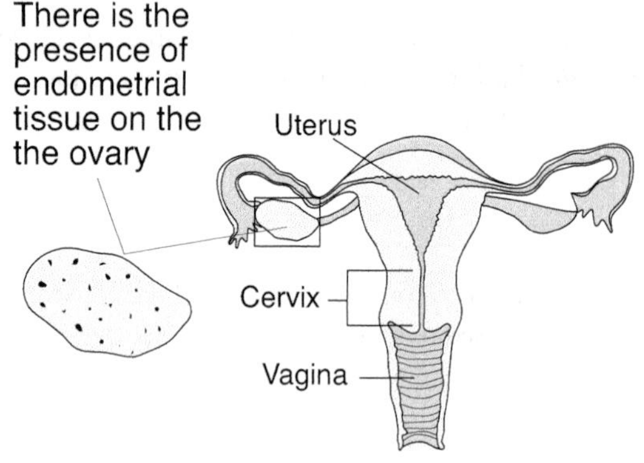

Genital Prolapse

Female genital prolapse is a general term used to describe slippage of the pelvic organs, including the uterus, bladder, intestine or rectum, from their normal anatomical position where they then protrude into the vagina or press against the wall of the vagina. This is due to weakening or damage of the ligaments, muscles, connective tissue, and fascia that make up the pelvic floor. Prolapse of bladder is referred to as a cystocele. An enterocele is prolapse of the intestine. A rectocele is prolapse of the rectum. A perineocele is prolapse of the perineum.

Endometrial Hyperplasia

Endometrial hyperplasia is an abnormal thickening of the lining of the uterus typically caused by an elevated level of estrogen in conjunction with a deficiency of progesterone. Endometrial hyperplasia is sometimes a precursor to uterine cancer.

Endometrial hyperplasia

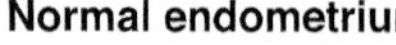

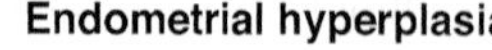

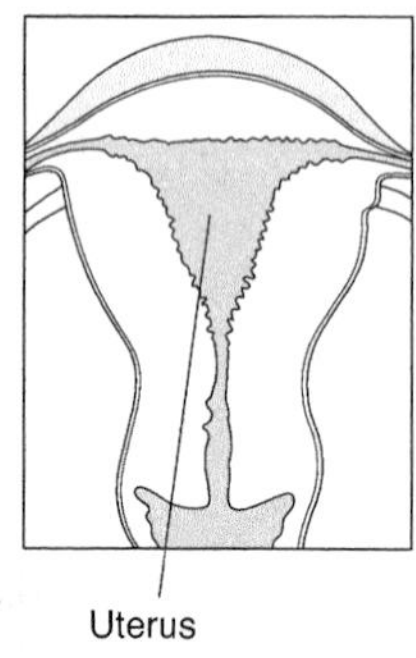

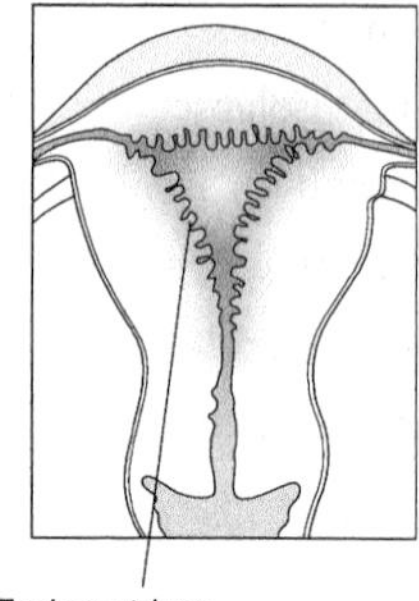

As menopause nears, a woman produces lower amounts of estrogen and progesterone. After menopause, when a menstruation has stopped, very little of these hormones are produced. The lining of the uterus may thicken due to proliferation of the cells of the endometrium if there is estrogen without enough progesterone, it may lead to endometrial hyperplasia. The following are different types of endometrial hyperplasia:

Simple – There are irregular and systemic expansion of glands without changes in the appearance of individual gland cells.

Complex – Crowding and budding of glands without changes in the appearance of individual gland cells.

Atypical – May be simple or complex, but there are atypical changes in the gland cells, which include cell stratification, tufting, loss of nuclear polarity, enlarged nuclei and an increase in mitotic activity. The changes are similar to what is seen in cancer cells and may eventually lead to uterine cancer.

Female Infertility

Female infertility like male infertility is divided into two broad categories, infertility caused by an endocrine disorder and infertility from other causes. Infertility caused by endocrine disorders is reported with codes from the endocrine chapter. Other causes include failure to ovulate (anovulation), tubal anomalies, occlusion or stenosis, uterine anomaly, and failure of implantation of a fertilized egg. Two other conditions that are not classified under female infertility include cervical incompetence which is considered to be a disorder of the cervix and habitual abortion which is not a type of infertility because the patient does become pregnant but is unable to carry the products of conception (embryo or fetus) to term.

Menopause

Menopause is the cessation of menstruation for a period of one year where the ovaries stop releasing eggs for fertilization. The ovaries begin to decline in hormone production, typically starting in the mid-30's. Usually beginning in the late forties, the process accelerates and hormone levels (estrogen and progesterone) fluctuate more, causing irregular menstrual cycles and episodes of heavy bleeding. As menopause approaches, the menstrual cycle may become shorter or longer. These changes may continue over a 2 to 8 year period before menstruation ceases completely. At menopause, estrogen production does not completely stop. The ovaries significantly decrease their output but may still produce a small amount.

Surgical menopause occurs when the ovaries are removed, typically during a hysterectomy.

Perimenopause is the time two to eight years (including one year after the last menstrual period) prior to menopause. Estrogen levels begin to rise and fall unevenly and menstrual cycles occur without ovulation. There are also irregular menstrual periods that usually start occurring in the 40's, but some women experience symptoms as early as the mid-30's. Symptoms include hot flashes, night flashes, mood swings, vaginal dryness, fluctuations in libido (sexual desire), forgetfulness, trouble sleeping, and fatigue.

Section 6 Coding Practice

Condition	ICD-10-CM
Endometriosis of the uterus	N80.0
Atypical endometrial hyperplasia	N85.02
Menopause with sleeplessness and irritability	N95.1, G47.01, R45.4

Section 6 Questions

Does the site of the endometriosis make a difference in code selection?

Is atypical endometrial hyperplasia identified with its own code, or included with endometrial intraepithelial neoplasia [EIN]?

What coding instruction is present related to coding for symptomatic menopause?

See end of chapter for Coding Practice answers.

Section 7 – Signs and Symptoms

Urinary Incontinence

During urination the muscles in the wall of the bladder contract forcing urine from the bladder into the urethra. The muscles in the sphincter surrounding the urethra relax, allowing the urine to exit the body. If the bladder muscles suddenly contract or the sphincter muscles are not strong enough to hold the urine, incontinence occurs. Also, urine may leak with less force than usual if the muscles are damaged.

Urinary incontinence affects women more than men because of the structure of the female urinary tract, pregnancy and childbirth, and menopause. Although, other factors may cause incontinence, such as birth defects, neurological injury, stroke, multiple sclerosis and physical issues associated with aging.

In many cases, multiple types of incontinence (mixed incontinence) occur at the same time.

Stress Incontinence

This type of incontinence is due to some sort of physical activity, such as coughing, sneezing, laughing, or exercise. Any physical changes because of pregnancy, childbirth, and menopause can cause stress incontinence. Pelvic floor muscles, the vagina and ligaments that support the bladder can be weakened from those physical changes. The bladder can drop lower toward the vagina, preventing the muscles from squeezing tightly enough to keep the urethra closed. During the week prior to menstruation, lower estrogen levels may lead to lower muscular pressure around the urethra, increasing leakage.

Stress incontinence, female

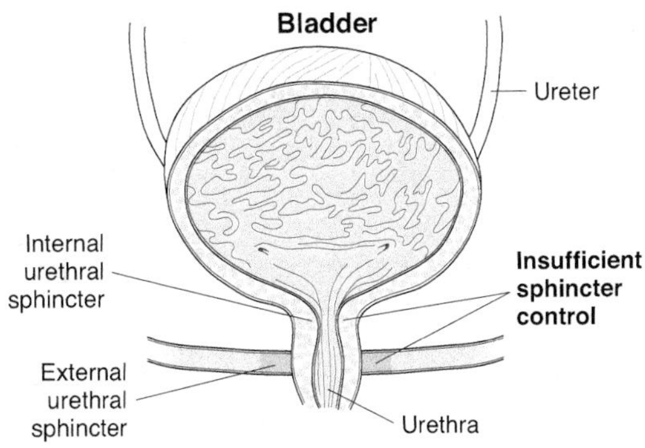

Urge Incontinence

In urge incontinence, there is a loss of urine after suddenly needing to urinate. This is typically caused by inappropriate bladder contractions or abnormal nerve signals causing bladder spasms. This can happen nocturnally, after drinking a small amount of fluid. It may occur with the sound or touch of running water. There are some fluids and medications (e.g., diuretics) that can exacerbate urge incontinence.

Functional Incontinence

Functional incontinence is associated with physical and medical conditions that interfere with the ability to urinate on demand.

Overflow Incontinence

If the bladder does not empty properly, urine may overflow. This may be caused by weak bladder muscles, a blocked urethra, urinary calculi, or nerve damage from diabetes or another disease.

Transient Incontinence

Transient incontinence occurs when urine leaks due to a temporary cause, such as an infection, new medication, restricted mobility, and colds.

Coital Incontinence

Coital incontinence is the spontaneous leakage of urine during sexual activity. This is a disorder of the pelvic floor muscles. A high percentage of women with overactive bladder experience coital incontinence. Postmenopausal women are at greatest risk. This often points to stress incontinence as well.

Postural (Urinary) Incontinence

Postural incontinence is the involuntary escape of urine associated with changing body position, such as standing up or rising from a lying down position. The change in the tilt of the pelvis changes the bony structure support and the amount of pressure applied to the pelvic floor muscles and can allow for pelvic contents to shift, resulting in involuntary urine leakage.

Section 7 Coding Practice

Condition	ICD-10-CM
Stress incontinence of 38-year-old woman	N39.3
Overactive bladder with urge incontinence	N32.81, N39.41
Mixed incontinence	N39.46
Overflow incontinence	N39.490
Coital incontinence with overactive bladder	N39.491, N32.81

Section 7 Questions

Does gender make a difference in ICD-10-CM code selection?

Urge incontinence may be a symptom of overactive bladder and general coding guidelines indicate that symptoms of an established condition are not reported additionally. Why is urge incontinence reported with overactive bladder?

See end of chapter for Coding Practice answers.

Section 8 – Congenital Anomalies

Hypospadias

Hypospadias is a congenital anomaly in the urethra of a male in which the urinary meatus is abnormally placed. Instead of the opening at the tip of the glans of the penis, it will be anywhere along the ventral aspect (underside) of the shaft, to the junction of the penis and scrotum or perineum. Hypospadias is commonly associated with chordee and possibly undescended testes.

There are different degrees of hypospadias:

1. **First degree** – The opening is somewhere on the glans penis, but not in the normal area where it is typically located.
2. **Second degree** – The opening is on the shaft of the penis.
3. **Third degree** – The opening is on the perineum.

Chordee

Chordee is a condition in which the head of the penis is curved downwards or upwards. This occurs when the connective tissue between the urethral opening and the glans and/or the urethra is shorter than normal.

Undescended Testicles

Undescended testes are also called cryptorchidism. This is a congenital condition in which one or both testicles do not descend from the abdomen to their proper position within the scrotum as they should before birth. Undescended testicles may be found in the abdomen, the inguinal canal, or high within the scrotum along the normal descent pathway, or in an ectopic position such as the perineum.

Klinefelter's Syndrome

Klinefelter's syndrome involves abnormal sex chromosomes. In males, there is one X chromosome and one Y chromosome. The Y chromosome contains genetic material with the codes that determine the male gender, related masculine characteristics, and other male developmental features. In this syndrome, there is the presence of an extra X chromosome, meaning these individuals have 47 chromosomes instead of 46, which causes abnormal development of the testicles.

Section 8 Coding Practice

Condition	ICD-10-CM
Hypospadias	Q54.9
Two-year-old with chordee	Q54.4
Bilateral undescended testicles	Q53.20
Klinefelter's syndrome	Q98.4

Section 8 Questions

Does laterality make a difference in code selection when coding undescended testicles?

What other information is required to avoid reporting an unspecified code for unilateral or bilateral undescended testes?

See end of chapter for Coding Practice answers.

Section 9 – Injuries of the Genitourinary Tract

Contusions and lacerations are the most common types of injuries to genitourinary tract organs. Lacerations may result from closed injuries or penetrating open wounds. The external genitalia are also subject to crushing and traumatic amputation injuries. Another cause of injury particularly to the ureters is accidental puncture or laceration during a surgical procedure.

Renal Trauma

Contusion or laceration of the kidney due to blunt or penetrating trauma is the most common type of urinary tract injury. Motor vehicle accidents are the most common cause of renal trauma. Falls from a height and assault are also associated with renal trauma but are less common. Injuries to the kidneys are categorized as minor, moderate or major depending on the extent of the injury which is determined by the size of the contusion or the length of the laceration.

Testicular Trauma

The testicles are located in the scrotum, which is on the external portion of the body and can be easily subjected to outside trauma because of a lack protection from muscles or bones. This makes it easier for them to be struck, hit, or crushed, especially during contact sports. Injury to the testes can cause severe pain, bruising and/or swelling.

Intraoperative Injury of Genitourinary Tract

The ureters are particularly vulnerable to intraoperative injury due to their proximity to the intestines and female reproductive organs. Iatrogenic ureteral injury is most often associated with gynecologic procedures on the uterus, fallopian tubes and ovaries. After gynecological procedures, injury during colorectal procedures and procedures on the abdominal vasculature are the next most frequent causes.

Section 9 Coding Practice

Condition	ICD-10-CM
A 3 cm left kidney contusion sustained in fall from ladder at work on a new home construction site	S37.022A, W11.XXXA, Y92.61, Y93.H3, Y99.0
ED evaluation of 19-year-old male involved in fight with knife wound penetrating the retroperitoneum, with 2 cm laceration of the right kidney.	S37.051A, S36.893A, S31.031A, X99.1XXA
Right testicle crushed by falling bookcase, initial visit	S38.02XA, W20.8XXA
Accidental laceration of left ureter during abdominal adhesiolysis of left fallopian tube and ovary	N99.71

Section 9 Questions

How are contusions of the kidney classified?

Why aren't codes for the site and activity reported for the knife wound to the kidney?

Does laterality affect code selection for testicular injuries?

How is accidental laceration or puncture coded?

See end of chapter for Coding Practice answers.

Quiz — Genitourinary System

1. Which of the following is NOT a function of the kidneys?
   a. Regulation of ionic plasma composition.
   b. Regulation of plasma volume.
   c. Regulation of urinary output.
   d. Regulation of pH.
2. Support of the bladder and urethra entails:
   a. Two fascia, one muscle
   b. Three fascia, one muscle
   c. Two muscles, two fascia
   d. Two muscles, one fascia
3. The main function of the testes is:
   a. To contract during ejaculation, propelling the sperm forward
   b. Produce and store sperm
   c. Transport sperm from the epididymis to the urethra and out of the urethral orifice through ejaculation
   d. Control the flow of urine during ejaculation
4. What are the two types of cells located in the fallopian tubes?
   a. Tubal ostium cells and ciliated cells
   b. Peg cells and ampullary cells
   c. Ciliated cells and peg cells
   d. Ampullary cells and infundibulum cells
5. Which of the following is not a form of cystitis?
   a. Nocturnal
   b. Traumatic
   c. Interstitial
   d. Eosinophilic
6. How many stages are there in chronic kidney disease?
   a. 4
   b. 3
   c. 5
   d. 2
7. Which of the following describes an intramural fibroid?
   a. Grows under the endometrium
   b. Located predominately in the myometrium
   c. Located in the uterine serosa
   d. Forms into a pedicle

8. Which of the following is not a form of urinary incontinence?
   a. Overflow
   b. Transitional
   c. Functional
   d. Urge
9. Undescended testicle is also called:
   a. Chordee
   b. Hypospadias
   c. Klinefelter's
   d. Cryptorchidism

See next page for answers.

Quiz Answers—Genitourinary System

1. Which of the following is NOT a function of the kidneys?

   c. Regulation of urinary output.

2. Support of the bladder and urethra entails:

   a. Two fascia, one muscle

3. The main function of the testes is:

   b. Produce and store sperm

4. What are the two types of cells located in the fallopian tubes?

   c. Ciliated cells and peg cells.

5. Which of the following is not a form of cystitis?

   a. Nocturnal

6. How many stages are there in chronic kidney disease?

   c. 5

7. Which of the follow describes an intramural fibroid?

   b. Located predominately in the myometrium

8. Which of the following is not a form of urinary incontinence?

   b. Transitional

9. Undescended testicle is also called:

   d. Cryptorchidism

Coding Practice Answers

Answers to the coding practices throughout this chapter are provided in this section.

Section 1 Coding Practice

Question: Would chronic gonococcal urethritis be reported with the same code?

Answer: Yes. In ICD-10-CM, the same code (A54.01) is used for both acute and chronic gonococcal urethritis.

Question: Is code A56.19 specific for chlamydial epididymitis?

Answer: No. Code A56.19 is reported for chlamydial infections of specified sites in the genitourinary tract that do not have a more specific code provided. For example, A56.19 is also used to report chlamydial infection of the testes (orchitis).

Question: Is code N73.9 reported for PID complicating pregnancy?

Answer: No. A code from Chapter 15 Pregnancy, Childbirth and the Puerperium is reported instead. Category O23.- is used for an identified genitourinary tract infection complicating pregnancy, or code O99.89 for unspecified pelvic inflammatory disease complicating pregnancy.

Question: What other term(s) is used to describe congenital cytomegalovirus?

Answer: Congenital cytomegalic inclusion disease.

Question: Why isn't asymptomatic HIV-1 positive status reported with the same code as AIDS?

Answer: ICD-10-CM Official Coding Guidelines state that the code for AIDS is only reported when documentation states that the patient has AIDS, when the patient is admitted for an HIV-related illness or disease, or has any conditions resulting from HIV positive status.

Question: Is symptomatic HIV-2 infection reported with the same code as HIV-1 infection?

Answer: No. HIV-2 as the cause of disease classified elsewhere is reported with code B97.35.

Section 2 Coding Practice

Question: Since there is no excludes note under C67 indicating that carcinoma in situ is not reported under C67, would it be correct to report carcinoma in situ of the bladder trigone with code C67.0?

Answer: No. The Neoplasm Table indicates that the correct code for carcinoma in situ of the bladder trigone is D09.0.

Question: Is malignant neoplasm of the prostatic utricle reported with the same code as malignant neoplasm of the prostate? What is the prostatic utricle?

Answer: No. Malignant neoplasm of the prostatic utricle is reported with code C68.0 Malignant neoplasm of urethra. The prostatic utricle is a small pouch in the prostate that opens on the seminal colliculus, which is a portion of the urethral crest.

Question: Code C62.91 reports malignant neoplasm of right testis, unspecified. What additional information is required to report a more specific code?

Answer: Documentation would need to specify whether the right testis was undescended or descended.

Question: Does the type of breast cancer make a difference in code selection?

Answer: Yes. For example, noninfiltrating intraductal carcinoma of the right breast is reported with code D05.11 Carcinoma in situ of the right breast.

Question: How is it determined that interstitial leiomyoma should be reported with code D25.1 for intramural leiomyoma?

Answer: Interstitial leiomyoma is listed under D25.1 in the Tabular List as an inclusion term for intramural leiomyoma.

Section 3 Coding Practice

Question: Why is the hypertensive kidney disease reported as the first listed diagnosis and the chronic kidney disease as the second diagnosis?

Answer: There is a code first note under N18 indicating that the hypertensive chronic kidney disease is to be listed first.

Question: What other terms are synonymous with renal calculus?

Answer: Nephrolithiasis, renal stone, staghorn calculus, kidney stone.

Question: Is documentation of vesicoureteral reflux as primary or secondary or as right or left ureter required for assignment of the most specific code?

Answer: No. In order to select the most specific code, documentation needs to indicate whether the vesicoureteral reflux occurs with or without reflux nephropathy and if reflux nephropathy is present, whether it is with or without hydroureter. The specific side affected is not reported, only whether it affects one side alone, or both. Primary vs secondary is not an axis of classification.

Question: Why is the code for gout reported first when it is associated with a renal calculus?

Answer: Gout is the underlying disease and per coding guidelines, the underlying disease is the first listed diagnosis.

Question: What type of code is N39.0? What type of information would be required to select a more specific code?

Answer: Code N39.0 is nonspecific. The site of the urinary tract infection such as the bladder (cystitis) or urethra (urethritis) is required to select a more specific code.

Section 4 Coding Practice

Question: Why isn't testicular torsion reported with a code for an injury from Chapter 19?

Answer: Torsion of the testis typically occurs spontaneously and not from an injury. However, if the testicular torsion was caused by an injury, refer to Chapter 19, categories S30-S39.

Question: Why is the BPH reported with a code for BPH with LUTS when the diagnosis does not specifically state that the patient has LUTS?

Answer: Even though LUTS is not specifically stated in the diagnosis, the patient does have lower urinary tract symptoms which include urinary obstruction, urinary urgency, and urinary retention.

Question: What does ASAP stand for regarding dysplasia of the prostate? If the patient was diagnosed with prostatic intraepithelial neoplasia (PIN) III would the condition still be reported with a code from N42.3-?

Answer: ASAP stands for atypical small acinar proliferation of prostate. This pre-cancerous lesion is often suspicious for malignancy with a highly predictive outcome of subsequent prostatic adenocarcinoma. No. A code from N42.3- would not be used. PIN III, which may also be referred to as severe prostatic dysplasia, is reported with D07.5 for carcinoma in situ of the prostate.

Question: Why is it necessary to identify the drugs that caused the infertility? Why is only a single code reported for the four drugs that caused the infertility? Why is 7th character 'S' used?

Answer: Identification of the drugs is required because there is a coding instruction to code the cause of the infertility in addition to the infertility. T45.1X5S is only reported once because all four drugs are in the same drug class. The 7th character 'S' is used because the infertility is a sequela of the chemotherapy.

Question: Why is hypogonadism reported with a code from the endocrine chapter?

Answer: Hypogonadism is an endocrine disorder; male infertility caused by endocrine disorders are reported with codes from the endocrine chapter.

Section 5 Coding Practice

Question: A breast lump or nodule is reported with an unspecified code. What additional information is required to report a more specific code for a mass in the breast?

Answer: Documentation would need to indicate laterality and location of the mass such as in the auxiliary tail, subareolar area, or specific quadrant.

Question: Should code N62 Hypertrophy of breast, which is used to report gynecomastia, be used only for males?

Answer: No. Macromastia, which is the term to indicate extremely enlarged female breasts, is also reported with code N62.

Question: Why are two codes required to report bilateral fibrocystic breast disease?

Answer: Since there is no code for bilateral fibrocystic breast disease, the codes for right and left breast are reported.

Question: How is the coding of capsular contraction following breast augmentation classified?

Answer: It is listed in Chapter 19 Injury, Poisoning and Certain Other Consequences of External Causes under mechanical complication of breast prosthesis and implant, and is not reported within Chapter 15.

Section 6 Coding Practice

Question: Does the site of the endometriosis make a difference in code selection?

Answer: Yes. There are various codes for different sites located under category N80.

Question: Is atypical endometrial hyperplasia identified with its own code, or included with endometrial intraepithelial neoplasia [EIN]?

Answer: Both EIN and atypical endometrial hyperplasia are reported with code N85.02.

Question: What coding instruction is present related to coding for symptomatic menopause?

Answer: There is an instruction to use additional codes for associated symptoms.

Section 7 Coding Practice

Question: Does gender make a difference in ICD-10-CM code selection?

Answer: For some codes, yes, gender does make a difference, but not for others. For example, the stress incontinence code, N39.3, can be used for both females and males, but code N35.112 Postinfective bulbous urethral stricture, not elsewhere classified is male-specific and N35.12 Postinfective urethral stricture, not elsewhere classified, female, is female-specific.

Question: Urge incontinence may be a symptom of overactive bladder and generally coding guidelines indicate that symptoms of an established condition are not reported additionally. Why is urge incontinence reported with overactive bladder?

Answer: There is a 'code also' instruction under subcategory N39.4 that states that any associated overactive bladder is also coded.

Section 8 Coding Practice

Question: Does laterality make a difference in code selection when coding undescended testicles?

Answer: ICD-10-CM does not distinguish between right or left, but it does indicate whether the condition is unilateral or bilateral.

Question: What additional information is required to avoid reporting an unspecified code for unilateral or bilateral undescended testes?

Answer: The location of the undescended testicle(s) within the abdomen, inguinal canal, or high within the scrotum is required to assign a specified code for unilateral or bilateral undescended testes.

Section 9 Coding Practice

Question: How are contusions of the kidney classified?

Answer: Kidney contusions must be identified as minor or major. A minor contusion is one less than 2 cm. A major contusion is greater than 2 cm. Any open wound is reported with an additional code from S31.-.

Question: Why aren't codes for the site and activity reported for the knife wound injury?

Answer: Even though there are codes for unspecified site and activity, the coding guidelines state that the unspecified codes should not be reported if the site and activity are not included in the documentation.

Question: Does laterality affect code selection for testicular injuries?

Answer: No.

Question: How is accidental laceration or puncture coded?

Answer: Accidental laceration or puncture is coded as body system specific. The codes are listed in each body system's chapter under Intraoperative and Postprocedural Complications and Disorders.

ICD-10-CM Documentation

Genitourinary System

Introduction

Codes for genitourinary diseases are found in Chapter 14 in ICD-10-CM. The genitourinary system (or the urogenital system) includes the organs and anatomical structures involved with reproduction and urinary excretion in both males and females. Female genitourinary disorders include pelvic inflammatory diseases, vaginitis, salpingitis, and oophoritis. Common male genitourinary disorders include prostatitis, benign prostatic hyperplasia, urogenital cancers, premature ejaculation, and erectile dysfunction.

The code blocks for Diseases of the Genitourinary System chapter are displayed in the table below.

ICD-10-CM Blocks	
N00-N08	Glomerular Diseases
N10-N16	Renal Tubulo-Interstitial Diseases
N17-N19	Acute Kidney Failure and Chronic Kidney Disease
N20-N23	Urolithiasis
N25-N29	Other Disorders of Kidney and Ureter
N30-N39	Other Diseases of the Urinary System
N40-N53	Diseases of Male Genital Organs
N60-N65	Disorders of Breast
N70-N77	Inflammatory Diseases of Female Pelvic Organs
N80-N98	Noninflammatory Disorders of Female Genital Tract
N99	Intraoperative and Postprocedural Complications and Disorders of Genitourinary System, Not Elsewhere Classified

ICD-10-CM incorporates similar codes into related categories. For example, for urolithiasis the different sites where a calculus occurs are classified together in a code block created to group into one location all calculus-related codes for all sites. There is also a category that classifies all intraoperative and postprocedural complications of treatment for genitourinary disorders (N99) together, as well as a code block entitled Renal Tubulo-Interstitial Diseases (N10-N16) that classifies all types of pyelonephritis. For some conditions, terminology has been updated with changes made to several block and category titles to reflect the currently accepted diagnostic terminology.

In Chapter 14, diseases of the genitourinary system in both males and females are organized by site and then by specific disease or condition. Genitourinary disorders in diseases classified elsewhere are located in a separate category at the end of each code block. For example, category N08 Glomerular disorders in diseases classified elsewhere identifies glomerulonephritis, nephritis, and nephropathy in diseases classified elsewhere. In addition, certain genitourinary diseases are classified by etiology (e.g., due to transmissible infections) rather than by site in Chapter 14.

Exclusions

Neoplastic diseases, certain infectious and parasitic diseases, and conditions complicating pregnancy, childbirth, and the puerperium are examples of conditions classified in other chapters. Reviewing all of the chapter level exclusions provides information on conditions classified in other chapters.

At the chapter level, there are no Excludes1 notes; however there are several Excludes2 notes for Chapter 14 directing the coder to report these conditions, when they are present, with codes from another chapter.

ICD-10-CM Excludes1	ICD-10-CM Excludes2
None	Certain conditions originating in the perinatal period (P04-P96) Certain infectious and parasitic diseases (A00-B99) Complications of pregnancy, childbirth, and the puerperium (O00-O9A) Congenital malformations, deformations, and chromosomal abnormalities (Q00-Q99) Endocrine, nutritional, and metabolic diseases (E00-E88) Injury, poisoning, and certain other consequences of external causes (S00-T88) Neoplasms (C00-D49) Symptoms, signs, and abnormal clinical and laboratory findings, not elsewhere classified (R00-R94)

Reclassification of Codes

Nongonococcal urethritis is not classified as an infectious and parasitic disease in Chapter 1, but as nonspecific urethritis, code N34.1, in Chapter 14. Incontinence is considered a disease rather than a symptom, so the codes for incontinence are listed in the genitourinary diseases chapter.

Revised Terminology

The clinical terminology used to describe genitourinary disorders in ICD-10-CM has been updated from that which was traditionally used for classification to reflect advances in medical diagnostics and treatment for conditions such as male erectile dysfunction. For example, instead of reporting impotence of organic origin, ICD-10-CM provides codes that identify the various causes of erectile dysfunction as seen in the table below.

ICD-10-CM	
N52.01	Erectile dysfunction due to arterial insufficiency
N52.02	Corporo-venous occlusive erectile dysfunction
N52.03	Combined arterial insufficiency and corporo-venous occlusive erectile dysfunction
N52.1	Erectile dysfunction due to diseases classified elsewhere (Code first underlying disease)
N52.2	Drug-induced erectile dysfunction
N52.31	Erectile dysfunction following radical prostatectomy
N52.32	Erectile dysfunction following radical cystectomy
N52.33	Erectile dysfunction following urethral surgery
N52.34	Erectile dysfunction following simple prostatectomy
N52.35	Erectile dysfunction following radiation therapy
N52.36	Erectile dysfunction following interstitial seed therapy
N52.37	Erectile dysfunction following prostate ablative therapy
N52.39	Other and unspecified postprocedural erectile dysfunction
N52.8	Other male erectile dysfunction
N52.9	Male erectile dysfunction, unspecified

Chapter Guidelines

Coding guidelines include the coding conventions, the general coding guidelines, and the chapter-specific coding guidelines. Coding and sequencing guidelines for genitourinary diseases and complications due to the treatment of genitourinary diseases are incorporated into the Alphabetic Index and the Tabular List. To assign the most specific code possible, pay close attention to the coding and sequencing instructions in the Tabular List and Alphabetic Index, particularly the Excludes1 and Excludes2 notes. Detailed guidelines are provided for chronic kidney disease (CKD), which is classified based on stage of severity, described in the following table.

ICD-10-CM	
CKD Severity Stages	CKD, Stage 1 (N18.1) CKD, Stage 2 (N18.2) equates to mild CKD CKD, Stage 3 (N18.3) equates to moderate CKD CKD, Stage 4 (N18.4) equates to severe CKD CKD, Stage 5 (N18.5) excludes CKD requiring chronic dialysis CKD, Stage 5 (N18.6) includes CKD requiring chronic dialysis (ESRD)

Coding and sequencing guidelines for chronic kidney disease in patients who have undergone a kidney transplant state:

- A kidney transplant status patient may still have some form of chronic kidney disease because the transplanted kidney may not fully restore kidney function
- The presence of CKD alone does not constitute a transplant complication
- Assign the appropriate N18 code for the patient's stage of CKD and code Z94.0 Kidney transplant status
- If a transplant complication such as failure or rejection or other transplant complication is documented, see Section1.C.19.g for information on coding complications of a kidney transplant
- If the documentation is unclear as to whether the patient has a complication of the transplant, query the provider

Section I.C.19.g of the ICD-10-CM guidelines provides guidance on coding kidney transplant complications:

- Assign code T86.1- for documented complications of a kidney transplant (e.g., transplant failure or rejection or other transplant complication). Code T86.1- should not be assigned for post kidney transplant patients who have chronic kidney disease (CKD) unless a transplant complication such as transplant failure or rejection is documented. The provider should be queried if the documentation is unclear as to whether the patient has a complication of the transplant
- Conditions that affect the function of the transplanted kidney, other than CKD, should be assigned a code from subcategory T86.1 Complications of transplanted organ, kidney along with a secondary code that identifies the complication

Patients with CKD may also suffer from other serious conditions, most commonly diabetes mellitus and hypertension. The guidelines for coding patients with CKD and other serious conditions, indicate that the sequencing of the CKD code in relationship to codes for other contributing conditions is based on the conventions in the Tabular List.

General Documentation Requirements

Documentation requirements depend on the particular genitourinary disease or disorder. Some of the general documentation requirements are discussed here, but greater detail for some of the more common genitourinary system diseases will be provided in the next section.

In general, basic medical record documentation requirements include the severity or status of the disease (e.g., acute or chronic), as well as the site, etiology, and any secondary disease process. Physician documentation of the significance of any findings or confirmation of any diagnosis found in laboratory or other diagnostic test reports is necessary for code assignment.

ICD-10-CM requires specificity regarding the type and cause of the genitourinary disorder which must be documented in the medical record. Provider documentation should clearly specify any cause-and-effect relationship between medical treatment and a genitourinary disorder such as post-catheterization urethral stricture, or prolapse of vaginal vault after hysterectomy. Documentation in the medical record should specify whether a complication occurred intraoperatively or postoperatively, such as intraoperative versus postoperative hemorrhage.

Many codes also require documentation of the site, including laterality (right, left, bilateral) for paired organs and the extremities, such as in the example below.

ICD-10-CM Code(s)	
N60.01	Solitary cyst of right breast
N60.02	Solitary cyst of left breast
N60.09	Solitary cyst of unspecified breast

Chapter-Specific Documentation Requirements

In this section, categories, subcategories, and subclassifications for some of the more frequently reported genitourinary diseases are reviewed. Valid codes are listed and documentation requirements are identified. The focus is on conditions with additional pieces of specific clinical documentation required in order to select the correct diagnostic code(s). Although not all codes with significant documentation requirements are discussed, this section will provide a representative sample of the type of additional documentation needed for genitourinary diseases. The section is organized alphabetically by the topic.

Cystitis

Cystitis, or inflammation of the bladder, is most often caused by a bacterial infection of the urinary tract. Cystitis may also result from a reaction to certain drugs, radiation therapy, irritants such as long-term use of a catheter, or as a complication of another illness. Documentation in the medical record needs to specify the type and cause of the cystitis and identify any infectious agent or organism, such as *E. coli*. Proper coding also requires documentation of cystitis as with or without hematuria.

Cystitis caused by certain specific infectious organisms are coded differently within the infectious disease chapter and are not included in the genitourinary chapter, so careful review of the documentation is needed to identify certain conditions such as candidal cystitis, chlamydial cystitis, diphtheritic cystitis, gonococcal cystitis, monilial cystitis, trichomonal cystitis, and tuberculous cystitis. Prostatocystitis is coded to N41.3 and not in category N30.

Coding and Documentation Requirements

Identify the type of cystitis:

- Acute
  - With hematuria
  - Without hematuria
- Chronic
  - Interstitial
    - With hematuria
    - Without hematuria
  - Other chronic
    - With hematuria
    - Without hematuria
- Irradiation
  - With hematuria
  - Without hematuria
- Trigonitis
  - With hematuria
  - Without hematuria
- Other specified type
  - With hematuria
  - Without hematuria
- Unspecified
  - With hematuria
  - Without hematuria

Use additional code to identify any infectious agent.

Note: Some types of cystitis are classified in Chapter 1 Infectious and Parasitic diseases. See Alphabetic Index when causative organism is documented to determine whether a code from category N30 should be assigned.

ICD-10-CM Code/Documentation	
N30.00	Acute cystitis without hematuria
N30.01	Acute cystitis with hematuria
N30.10	Interstitial cystitis (chronic) without hematuria
N30.11	Interstitial cystitis (chronic) with hematuria
N30.20	Other chronic cystitis without hematuria
N30.21	Other chronic cystitis with hematuria
N30.30	Trigonitis without hematuria
N30.31	Trigonitis with hematuria
N30.40	Irradiation cystitis without hematuria
N30.41	Irradiation cystitis with hematuria
N30.80	Other cystitis without hematuria
N30.81	Other cystitis with hematuria
N30.90	Cystitis, unspecified without hematuria
N30.91	Cystitis, unspecified with hematuria

Documentation and Coding Example

Twenty-nine-year-old Caucasian female is referred to Urology Clinic by her GYN for c/o ongoing urinary frequency, urgency, and pain. She was initially seen 3 months ago by her Internist for acute onset of symptoms and was prescribed Macrodantin for a UTI. Her symptoms improved but did not clear completely and she began to have pain with intercourse. She saw her GYN who diagnosed a yeast infection and prescribed Monistat®. When her symptoms did not improve her GYN suggested she see a urologist. On examination, this is an anxious appearing, well-dressed woman who looks younger than her stated age. Voided UA was positive for blood, negative for protein, WBCs. Physical exam is unremarkable and informed consent obtained for cystoscopy. Patient positioned comfortably in dorsal lithotomy and cystoscope inserted without difficulty through the urethral meatus into the bladder. A patchy area of nonkeratinizing squamous metaplasia is easily identified at the trigone of the bladder by its glistening, fluffy white appearance. A biopsy is taken since patient does have hematuria. Remainder of the exam is unremarkable. Patient tolerated the procedure well and was interviewed after she had rested and gotten dressed. Advised patient she has **acute urethrotrigonitis** and biopsy should confirm that. Most appropriate treatment is Doxycycline 100 mg BID x 2 weeks for both she and her partner followed by Doxycycline 100 mg daily for 2 weeks for her. They should use a condom during intercourse for one month or abstain from intercourse altogether.

Diagnosis: **Hematuria due to acute urethrotrigonitis**

Diagnosis Code(s)

N30.31 Trigonitis with hematuria

Coding Note(s)

Urethrotrigonitis is listed as an included condition under the code for trigonitis, which includes both the acute and chronic forms of the disease. When coding cases of cystitis, an additional code is assigned for the infectious agent when it is identified in the medical record documentation.

Hydronephrosis

Hydronephrosis is a condition in which the kidney's urine collecting system becomes dilated, usually due to an underlying illness or medical condition. In hydronephrosis, distention of the kidney with urine is caused by the backward pressure placed on the kidney when the flow of urine is obstructed. Obstruction or blockage is the most frequent cause of hydronephrosis, but the condition may also be congenital or occur as a response to pregnancy, or it may be caused by trauma, neoplastic disease, calculi, inflammatory processes, or surgical procedures. Documentation of the etiology is essential for code assignment.

Careful review of the medical record documentation is necessary to assign the correct code. For example, calculus of the kidney and ureter without hydronephrosis must be distinguished from cases with hydronephrosis. Other examples include congenital obstructive defects of the renal pelvis and ureter, and obstructive pyelonephritis. All of these conditions are coded differently.

Obstruction can occur anywhere from the urethral meatus to the calyceal infundibula and the physiological effects depend on the level of the obstruction, the extent of involvement, the patient's age at onset, and whether it is acute or chronic. Medical record documentation identifying the location of the obstruction is needed for code assignment. Hydronephrosis can also be unilateral involving just one kidney or bilateral involving both, although specific code selection does not require laterality.

Clinically, the term hydronephrosis describes dilation and swelling of the kidney, while the term hydroureter describes swelling of the ureter. These conditions, along with congenital hydronephrosis, are coded differently and therefore need to be clearly differentiated in the documentation.

Acquired hydronephrosis is a combination code that identifies the underlying medical condition causing the obstruction of urine and the resulting distension of the kidney.

Coding and Documentation Requirements

For acquired hydronephrosis, identify type of obstruction present:

- With infection
- With renal and ureteral calculous obstruction
- With ureteral stricture
- With ureteropelvic junction obstruction
- Other hydronephrosis

ICD-10-CM Code/Documentation	
N13.0	Hydronephrosis with ureteropelvic junction obstruction
N13.1	Hydronephrosis with ureteral stricture, not elsewhere classified
N13.2	Hydronephrosis with renal and ureteral calculous obstruction
N13.30	Unspecified hydronephrosis
N13.39	Other hydronephrosis
N13.4	Hydroureter
N13.6	Pyonephrosis

Note: Pyonephrosis reports hydronephrosis/hydroureter with infection.

Documentation and Coding Example

Twenty-four-year-old male patient presents to ED with c/o worsening left flank pain with nausea and vomiting for the past 2 hours. PMH is significant for kidney stone at age 20 that resolved without intervention. Patient states he is a professional backup dancer for a well-known recording artist who performed locally this evening. On examination, this is a well-developed, well-nourished Black male who looks exhausted from recent physical exertion. Temp 99, Pulse 70, Resp 14, BP 102/66, O2 sat 99%. PERRL, neck supple. HR regular, breath sounds clear and equal. CVA tenderness present on left side with fullness detected in the kidney area. Abdomen soft with decreased bowel sounds. Liver and spleen not palpated. IV started in right forearm infusing LR. UA obtained and blood drawn for CBC, comprehensive metabolic panel. Medicated with MS and Phenergan with patient reporting decreased pain and nausea. Urology consult obtained and Spiral CT ordered. Patient is comfortable while waiting for CT scanner to be available.

Urology Note: Patient was examined after CT scan. He is resting comfortably after repeat IV morphine sulfate. Spiral CT shows a **stone in the left ureter with subsequent hydronephrosis of the left kidney**. Movement of the stone is noted from the time lapse of the scan with the **stone now mid-way between the kidney and bladder**. It should clear the ureter and enter the bladder in a few hours. Labs are unremarkable other than UA showing a slightly elevated pH and microscopic hematuria. Patient admitted to medical floor for continued IV hydration and pain management. Strain all urine and send all solid material to lab for analysis.

Diagnosis: **Unilateral hydronephrosis secondary to mid ureteral calculus**

Diagnosis Code(s)

N13.2 Hydronephrosis with renal and ureteral calculous obstruction

Coding Note(s)

A combination code reports both the hydronephrosis and the obstruction due to the ureteral calculus.

Male Infertility

Male infertility is defined as an inability to achieve pregnancy in a fertile female after one year of unprotected intercourse. The scope of male infertility is widespread. An estimated 15% of couples are considered infertile, with approximately 30%-40% due to male factors alone, and 20% due to a combination of female and male factors. The quality and the quantity of sperm greatly influence reproductive outcomes. Male infertility may be due to low or absent sperm production, immobile sperm, or blockages in the delivery of sperm. Other factors that can play a role in causing male infertility include illnesses, injuries, and chronic health problems.

Azoospermia describes a complete absence of sperm in the ejaculate, while hypospermatogenesis is abnormally decreased spermatozoa production. Because germ cells are precursors to spermatozoa, germ cell aplasia is often the cause of non-obstructive azoospermia.

Coding and Documentation Requirements

Identify the specific type and cause of infertility:

- Azoospermia
  - Due to extratesticular cause
    - » Drug therapy
    - » Infection
    - » Obstruction of efferent ducts
    - » Other extratesticular causes
    - » Radiation
    - » Systemic disease
  - Organic
- Oligospermia
  - Due to extratesticular cause
    - » Drug therapy
    - » Infection
    - » Obstruction of efferent ducts
    - » Other extratesticular causes
    - » Radiation
    - » Systemic disease
  - Organic
- Other male infertility
- Unspecified male infertility

For azoospermia and oligospermia due to extratesticular causes, code also associated cause.

ICD-10-CM Code/Documentation	
N46.01	Organic azoospermia
N46.8	Other male infertility
N46.9	Male infertility, unspecified
N46.11	Organic oligospermia
N46.021	Azoospermia due to drug therapy
N46.022	Azoospermia due to infection
N46.023	Azoospermia due to obstruction of efferent ducts
N46.024	Azoospermia due to radiation
N46.025	Azoospermia due to systemic disease
N46.029	Azoospermia due to other extratesticular causes
N46.121	Oligospermia due to drug therapy
N46.122	Oligospermia due to infection
N46.123	Oligospermia due to obstruction of efferent ducts
N46.124	Oligospermia due to radiation
N46.125	Oligospermia due to systemic disease
N46.129	Oligospermia due to other extratesticular causes

Documentation and Coding Example

Fifty-two-year-old Caucasian male is referred to PMD for comprehensive physical as part of an infertility work up. Patient was able to father 3 healthy children with his first wife but his new wife has been unable to get pregnant despite unprotected intercourse x 8 months. His wife's work up has been benign thus far. Patient comes reluctantly to the appointment because he has an extremely busy work schedule. He travels in the continental US frequently and goes to Europe and/or Asia at least once a month. Accessibility is not a problem as his wife travels with him, nor does performance appear to be an issue. He states that he is able to maintain an erection, penetrate, and ejaculate. A recent semen analysis showed a very low sperm count but the sperm present in the ejaculate were healthy and motile.

Temp 97.6, Pulse 80, Resp 12, BP 142/90, Ht. 72 inches, Wt. 184 lbs. His Blackberry and phone vibrate every few minutes and although he does not answer them, he is clearly distracted by the interruptions and is anxious to get the exam over with. He had a company nurse draw blood and he provided a urine sample prior to this visit so lab results are available. His only medication is occasional OTC Tagamet and Tums for heartburn. On examination, this is a well-developed, well-nourished man who looks younger than his stated age. PERRL, neck supple without lymphadenopathy. Nares patent, mucous membranes moist and pink. Cranial nerves grossly intact. Pulses and reflexes normal in extremities. Heart rate regular without bruit, rub, murmur. Breath sounds clear, equal bilaterally. Abdomen soft, bowel sounds present. Liver palpated at 3 cm below RCM, spleen at 1 cm below LCM. No evidence of hernia, testicles smooth.

Penis is circumcised without urethral drainage. Rectal exam shows good sphincter tone with a smooth, normal size prostate gland.

Patient allowed to dress and labs are reviewed with him seated in the consultation room. Of significance his FBGL is 125 and HgbA1C is 7.1. TSH is 5.8. Lipid and triglyceride levels are in high normal range but liver and renal function tests are mildly elevated. Patient admits to **smoking 2-3 cigarettes daily, cigars 1-2 x week**. His alcohol consumption includes 2-4 oz. of Scotch and 2-3 glasses of wine per day.

Impression: **Low sperm count due to underlying hypothyroid and insulin resistant diabetes Type II**.

Plan: Patient is given samples and a prescription for Synthroid 0.05 mg to take daily in the AM at least 30 minutes before breakfast. He is given samples and a prescription for Metformin 500 to be taken 2 x day with meals. He is advised to stop smoking, cut down on his alcohol consumption, and avoid taking Tagamet as all 3 of these can decrease sperm count. He is to repeat labs in 1 month and call at his convenience to discuss results. This note is electronically sent to his wife's infertility doctor. Further arrangements should be made with them for semen analysis.

Diagnosis: **Hypospermatogenesis due to systemic disease**.

Diagnosis Code(s)

N46.125 Oligospermia due to systemic disease

E11.69 Type 2 diabetes with other specified complication

E03.9 Hypothyroidism unspecified

Z72.0 Tobacco use

Coding Note(s)

There is a specific code for infertility due to systemic disease; in this case, hypospermatogenesis, or oligospermia. Code(s) that specifically identify the systemic disease(s) present are coded additionally. The low sperm count is attributed to both hypothyroidism and type 2 diabetes. The type of hypothyroidism is not specified, and since there is no diabetes combination code specifically for reporting that occurring with infertility as a complication, the code for type 2 diabetes with other specific complication is assigned.

Redundant Prepuce and Phimosis

Phimosis is the inability of the prepuce or foreskin to be retracted behind the glans penis in uncircumcised males. This tightening of the foreskin may close the opening of the penis. Circumcision is the most common treatment to correct phimosis. In paraphimosis, the foreskin is retracted behind the crown of the penis which may cause entrapment of the penis, impairing blood flow.

Phimosis can be congenital or it may be due to infection. The symptoms of phimosis and paraphimosis are similar to other medical disorders, so clear documentation of the patient's condition is necessary. When the cause of the phimosis or paraphimosis is infection, the medical record documentation should also identify the infectious agent.

When balanitis (inflammation of the glans) and posthitis (inflammation of the foreskin) occur together, it is called balanoposthitis. Correct coding requires documentation clearly describing the patient's condition. Balanoposthitis is classified as a disorder of the prepuce and is reported within category N47 Disorders of prepuce, which provides specific codes for adherent prepuce of newborn, phimosis, paraphimosis, deficient foreskin, benign cyst, adhesions, and balanoposthitis. There is an additional code for other inflammatory disease of the prepuce and another code for other disorders (noninflammatory) of the prepuce.

Coding and Documentation Requirements

Identify type of prepuce disorder:

- Adherent prepuce, newborn
- Adhesions of prepuce and glans penis
- Balanoposthitis
- Benign cyst of prepuce
- Deficient foreskin
- Paraphimosis
- Phimosis
- Other disorders of prepuce
- Other inflammatory disease of prepuce

Use additional code as needed to identify any infectious agent.

ICD-10-CM Code/Documentation	
N47.0	Adherent prepuce, newborn
N47.1	Phimosis
N47.2	Paraphimosis
N47.3	Deficient foreskin
N47.4	Benign cyst of prepuce
N47.5	Adhesions of prepuce and glans penis
N47.6	Balanoposthitis
N47.7	Other inflammatory diseases of prepuce
N47.8	Other disorders of prepuce

Documentation and Coding Example

Patient is an 18-month-old Hispanic male brought to ED by his grandmother and older sister. Parents are out of the country. Child is crying and appears uncomfortable. Through an interpreter, sister states her little brother woke this morning fussy and when she removed his diaper she saw that the tip of his penis was swollen. Child is seen immediately by the pediatric resident. On examination, the glans penis is red and swollen with an edematous, proximally retracted foreskin forming a circumferential constricting band. The penile shaft is soft and there is no evidence of necrosis in the glans or the shaft. EMLA cream is applied liberally to the penis, patient placed on monitors, and medicated with Demerol IM. Manual compression of the glans penis and foreskin x 10 minutes allows the foreskin to be easily reduced over the glans using gentle pressure. Patient monitored following procedure and discharged home in good condition. Family is given instructions for care/cleaning of uncircumcised penis and will follow up in Urology Clinic in one week.

Diagnosis: **Paraphimosis**.

Diagnosis Code(s)

N47.2 Paraphimosis

Spermatocele

A spermatocele is a cyst on the epididymis usually filled with fluid and dead sperm cells. These spermatic cysts may occur alone or as multiple cysts. ICD-10-CM provides specific codes for spermatocele of the epididymis to identify the occurrence as single, multiple, or unspecified.

Coding and Documentation Requirements

Identify the occurrence of spermatocele:

- Multiple
- Single
- Unspecified

ICD-10-CM Code/Documentation	
N43.40	Spermatocele of epididymis, unspecified
N43.41	Spermatocele of epididymis, single
N43.42	Spermatocele of epididymis, multiple

Documentation and Coding Example

Twenty-three-year-old male presents to urologist concerned about a painless lump he discovered in his scrotum when he did a testicular self-exam. He has practiced TSE since the age of 17 when his brother-in-law was diagnosed with testicular cancer. Patient is a graduate student in International Relations and an elite cyclist on his college team. On examination, this is a muscular, but thin young man. He is very intense, extremely articulate, and able to provide a detailed health history on both himself and his family. On examination, the abdomen is very firm and muscular. He denies pain with palpation. There is no evidence of hernia in the inguinal area. Penis is circumcised, no urethral drainage. Scrotum has normal rugae. Left testicle is smooth and slightly higher than the right. The right testicle is also smooth with a soft, spherical, well circumscribed fullness in the epididymis at the superior aspect of the testicle. The area is positive to trans-illumination. Testicular ultrasound confirms that this is a **single spermatocele** located at the head of the epididymis on the right testicle. Patient is reassured that this is a benign cystic type of lesion and no treatment is necessary at this time. He should continue to do TSE and return if he has pain or the lump becomes larger.

Diagnosis: **Solitary spermatocele of epididymis**

Diagnosis Code(s)

N43.41 Spermatocele of epididymis, single

Urethral Stricture

Urethral strictures result from various causes and present a range of manifestations. Causes of urethral stricture include trauma, an adverse effect or complication from medical treatment, inflammatory or infectious processes, and malignancy. Urethral strictures may also be congenital.

Most urethral strictures are the result of trauma to the perineum, such as traumatic catheter placement or removal or a chronic indwelling Foley catheter. Postprocedural urethral stricture is classified at the end of the code block with other intraoperative and postprocedural complications and disorders of the genitourinary system.

Codes for urethral stricture capture the cause (postinfective, post-traumatic, postprocedural, other specified), gender, and for males the site of the stricture as the meatus, bulbous urethra, membranous urethra, anterior urethra, or unspecified site. For postinfective stricture, there are more specific codes for postinfective stricture due to the following organisms: schistosomiasis (B65.-, N29), gonorrhea (A54.01), syphilis (A52.76).

Coding and Documentation Requirements

Identify the cause of urethral stricture:

- Postinfective, NEC
- Postprocedural
- Post-traumatic
- Other specified cause
- Unspecified cause

Identify gender:

- Male
- Female

For male with postinfective, postprocedural, and post-traumatic stricture, identify site:

- Anterior urethra
- Bulbous urethra
- Meatus
- Membranous urethra
- Unspecified

For female with post-traumatic stricture, identify cause:

- Due to childbirth
- Other specified trauma

ICD-10-CM Code/Documentation	
N35.010	Post-traumatic urethral stricture, male, meatal
N35.011	Post-traumatic bulbous urethral stricture
N35.012	Post-traumatic membranous urethral stricture
N35.013	Post-traumatic anterior urethral stricture
N35.014	Post-traumatic urethral stricture, male, unspecified
N35.021	Urethral stricture due to childbirth
N35.028	Other post-traumatic urethral stricture, female
N35.111	Postinfective urethral stricture, not elsewhere classified, male, meatal
N35.112	Postinfective bulbous urethral stricture, not elsewhere classified, male
N35.113	Postinfective membranous urethral stricture, not elsewhere classified, male
N35.114	Postinfective anterior urethral stricture, not elsewhere classified, male
N35.119	Postinfective urethral stricture, not elsewhere classified, male, unspecified
N35.12	Postinfective urethral stricture, not elsewhere classified, female
N99.110	Postprocedural urethral stricture, male, meatal
N99.111	Postprocedural bulbous urethral stricture, male

ICD-10-CM Code/Documentation	
N99.112	Postprocedural membranous urethral stricture, male
N99.113	Postprocedural anterior bulbous urethral stricture
N99.114	Postprocedural urethral stricture, male, unspecified, male
N99.115	Postprocedural fossa navicularis urethral stricture
N99.12	Postprocedural urethral stricture, female
N37	Urethral disorders in diseases classified elsewhere
N35.8	Other urethral stricture
N35.9	Urethral stricture, unspecified

Documentation and Coding Example

Patient is a thirty-four-year-old Hispanic female who presents for a second urethral dilatation. This healthy woman delivered her first child vaginally six months ago. The infant was over 10 lbs. with fetal distress which necessitated an emergency delivery using forceps. Patient sustained deep lacerations to the vagina, one of which extended close to the urethra. She was subsequently unable to void post-delivery and was straight cathed once and finally had a Foley placed for 24 hours. She mentioned to her OB at her postpartum checkup that she was having pain and urgency with voiding. Exam showed excellent healing of the vaginal mucosa without evidence of fistula and urine culture was negative. She was referred to urology where cystoscopic exam revealed **1 cm long urethral stricture, most likely due to catheterization following delivery**. The stricture was dilated using serial sounds and patient's urinary symptoms resolved. In the past 3 weeks, she has again noticed urinary urgency and frequency. She came into the office and was seen by the PA who found a PVR of 220 cc and sent a cathed urine specimen to the lab for culture which was negative at 72 hours. Procedure Note: Patient is prepped and draped in lithotomy position. The cystoscope inserted without difficulty through the urethral meatus and almost immediately encountered a **urethral stricture which is the same size as previously mentioned**. Cystoscope advanced into the bladder which appears normal and the scope removed. The urethra is dilated with serial sounds and cystoscope inserted again to visualize the urethra. Excellent dilatation achieved. Patient tolerated procedure well.

Diagnosis: **Urethral stricture, post-catheterization**

Diagnosis Code(s)

N99.12 Postprocedural urethral stricture, female

Coding Note(s)

Coding post-operative or postprocedural urethral stricture to the highest level of specificity available requires identification of the patient's gender. In a male, the anatomical position of the urethral stricture is also required. In females, the cause is reported as post-traumatic due to childbirth or other trauma, postinfective, and postprocedural. Postprocedural stricture has an inclusion term that specifies postcatheterization urethral stricture.

Vesicoureteral Reflux

Vesicoureteral reflux is the abnormal flow of urine back up the ureters and is usually diagnosed in infants and children. Vesicoureteral reflux can be unilateral or bilateral and documentation of laterality is necessary for the most accurate code assignment. Vesicoureteral reflux can damage the kidneys. When this occurs, it is referred to as reflux nephropathy. Coding requires documentation indicating the presence or absence of damage to the kidneys caused by the reflux of urine. Codes for vesicoureteral reflux also capture the presence or absence of hydroureter. Vesicoureteral reflux with reflux nephropathy is not the same as reflux associated pyelonephritis and the two conditions are coded differently, so the two conditions must be clearly differentiated in the documentation.

Coding and Documentation Requirements

Identify the type/presentation of vesicoureteral reflux:

- With reflux nephropathy
  - With hydroureter
    - Bilateral
    - Unilateral
    - Unspecified
  - Without hydroureter
    - Bilateral
    - Unilateral
    - Unspecified
- Without reflux nephropathy
- Unspecified

ICD-10-CM Code/Documentation	
N13.70	Vesicoureteral reflux
N13.71	Vesicoureteral-reflux without reflux nephropathy
N13.721	Vesicoureteral-reflux with reflux nephropathy without hydroureter, unilateral
N13.722	Vesicoureteral-reflux with reflux nephropathy without hydroureter, bilateral
N13.729	Vesicoureteral-reflux with reflux nephropathy without hydroureter, unspecified
N13.731	Vesicoureteral-reflux with reflux nephropathy with hydroureter, unilateral
N13.732	Vesicoureteral-reflux with reflux nephropathy with hydroureter, bilateral
N13.739	Vesicoureteral-reflux with reflux nephropathy with hydroureter, unspecified

Documentation and Coding Example

Ten-year-old Caucasian female presents to Urology Clinic for annual exam. The patient is well known to our practice having been followed since the age of five when she presented with a UTI and subsequent work up revealed **vesicoureteral reflux with reflux nephropathy and hydroureter**. She had an ultrasound prior to this appointment that shows her condition to be stable, unchanged. Physical exam is unremarkable. Labs are significant for mildly elevated BUN and creatinine. Urine culture showed no growth of bacteria. She will continue to take daily Macrodantin and bring in a monthly clean catch voided urine for culture. RTC in 1 year, sooner if problems arise.

Diagnosis: **Vesicoureteral reflux with reflux nephropathy and hydroureter.**

Diagnosis Code(s)

N13.739 Vesicoureteral-reflux with reflux nephropathy with hydroureter, unspecified

Coding Note(s)

An unspecified code is assigned because the medical record documentation does not specify whether the patient's condition was affecting only one kidney or both.

Summary

Maintaining best practices in documentation of genitourinary disorders requires detailed information on the diagnosis and treatment of these conditions. Coders will find that some aspects of coding are streamlined thanks to an increased number of combination codes that identify both the (type of) disorder and its manifestation or status. For example, cystitis is a combination code which bases the code selection on the type of cystitis and whether the patient has hematuria or not. The urinary section includes subchapters that classify each code into a code family, making it easier for coders to select the correct code. Many conditions affecting bilateral organs require code assignment that includes the side affected, such as torsion, prolapse, hernia, and testicular pain; or whether the condition affects only one side or both sides, such as vesicoureteral reflux.

The clinical terminology used to describe genitourinary disorders has been updated from that used previously in order to include advances in medical diagnosis and treatment for conditions. An example of this is erectile dysfunction following radiation therapy, interstitial seed therapy, or prostate ablative therapy. This, in turn, requires an understanding of specific coding terms as well as detailed documentation of the patient's condition.

Resources

A documentation checklist is available in Appendix B for the following condition:

- Undescended/Retractile Testes

Genitourinary System Quiz

1. What information is NOT required to code vesicoureteral reflux to the highest level of specificity?
   a. Documentation of the presence/absence of reflux nephropathy
   b. Documentation of unilateral vesicoureteral reflux as left or right
   c. Documentation of with or without hydroureter
   d. Documentation of laterality as unilateral or bilateral

2. Where is postprocedural urethral stricture classified?
   a. In the code block for urethral disorders in Chapter 14
   b. In a separate code block for intraoperative and postprocedural complications at the end of Chapter 14
   c. In Chapter 21 Factors Influencing Health Status and Contact with Health Services
   d. With infectious and parasitic diseases in Chapter 1

3. Which of the following statements is true regarding coding hydronephrosis and ureteral calculus? a. Dual coding is required to report hydronephrosis and ureteral calculus
   b. A combination code reports hydronephrosis with ureteral calculus
   c. A combination code reports hydronephrosis with ureteral calculus and the side affected
   d. Dual coding is required to report hydronephrosis by laterality and ureteral calculus by laterality

4. How is endometriosis classified?
   a. By site
   b. By etiology
   c. By site and laterality
   d. By both site and etiology

5. Coding post-traumatic urethral stricture to the highest level of specificity available requires identification of ____________________.
   a. The patient's gender
   b. The underlying cause
   c. The manifestation
   d. All of the above

6. When coding dysmenorrhea, what distinction is made for proper code selection?
   a. Site
   b. Etiology
   c. Type as primary or secondary
   d. With or without endometriosis

7. How is Chronic Kidney Disease (CKD) coded?
   a. Based on stage of severity
   b. Based on type
   c. Based on etiology
   d. Based on duration of the patient's chronic condition

8. The physician documents the patient's diagnosis as "subacute vaginitis." How is this coded?
   a. With the code for acute and subacute vaginitis
   b. With the code for chronic vaginitis
   c. With the code for subacute and chronic vaginitis
   d. With the code for unspecified vaginitis

9. According to the coding and sequencing guidelines for chronic kidney disease in a kidney transplant patient, which of the following is true?
   a. A kidney transplant status patient may still have some form of chronic kidney disease
   b. The presence of CKD alone does not constitute a transplant complication
   c. If the documentation does not clarify whether the CKD constitutes a transplant complication, the provider should be queried
   d. All of the above

10. What is the correct coding and sequencing for a patient diagnosed with hematuria and cystitis?
   a. A code for the type of cystitis is listed first, followed by a code for the hematuria
   b. A code for the hematuria is listed first, followed by the code for cystitis
   c. A combination code is assigned that includes the type of cystitis with hematuria
   d. A code for the underlying infection is listed first, followed by a code for the cystitis, and a code for the hematuria

See next page for answers and rationales.

Genitourinary System Answers and Rationales

1. What information is NOT required to code vesicoureteral reflux to the highest level of specificity?

   b. Documentation of unilateral vesicoureteral reflux as left or right

   Rationale: While laterality is an element of coding vesicoureteral reflux, the codes only differentiate the condition as unilateral or bilateral. Unilateral vesicoureteral reflux does not need to be specified as right or left to assign the most specific code. Documentation of the presence or absence of reflux nephropathy and the presence or absence of hydroureter is needed to assign the most specific code.

2. Where is postprocedural urethral stricture classified?

   b. In a separate code block for intraoperative and postprocedural complications at the end of Chapter 14

   Rationale: ICD-10-CM has a separate code block at the end of Chapter 14 (N99) where all intraoperative and postprocedural complications from treatment of genitourinary disorders are classified.

3. Which of the following statements is true regarding coding hydronephrosis and ureteral calculus?

   b. A combination code reports hydronephrosis with ureteral calculus

   Rationale: Codes in category N13 Obstructive and reflux uropathy are combination codes which report hydronephrosis with ureteral stricture, with infection, and with renal and ureteral calculous obstruction. Separate codes are not required and laterality is not an axis of classification.

4. How is endometriosis classified?

   a. By site

   Rationale: Codes in category N80 Endometriosis specify endometriosis of the uterus, ovary, fallopian tube, pelvic peritoneum, rectovaginal septum and vagina, intestine, cutaneous scar, and other sites. Etiology and laterality are not components of coding endometriosis.

5. Coding post-traumatic urethral stricture to the highest level of specificity available requires identification of ________________.

   a. The patient's gender

   Rationale: Identification of the patient's gender is required for code assignment because category N35.0 Post-traumatic urethral stricture includes subcategories of codes specifically for male types of post-traumatic urethral stricture and female causes of post-traumatic urethral stricture.

6. When coding dysmenorrhea, what distinction is made for proper code selection?

   c. Type as primary or secondary

   Rationale: Codes for dysmenorrhea (N94) specify primary type versus secondary type dysmenorrhea.

7. How is Chronic Kidney Disease (CKD) coded?

   a. Based on stage of severity

   Rationale: Chronic kidney disease is specified as stage 1-5.

8. The physician documents the patient's diagnosis as "subacute vaginitis." How is this coded?

   c. With the code for subacute and chronic vaginitis

   Rationale: Codes in category N76 Other inflammation of vagina and vulva specify cases of vaginitis as either acute (which is the default for unspecified cases), or as subacute and chronic together.

9. According to the coding and sequencing guidelines for chronic kidney disease in a kidney transplant patient, which of the following is true?

   d. All of the above

   Rationale: According to the ICD-10-CM Official Guidelines for Coding and Reporting Section I.C.14: patients who have undergone kidney transplant may still have some form of chronic kidney disease (CKD) because the kidney transplant may not fully restore kidney function. Therefore, the presence of CKD alone does not constitute a transplant complication. The guidelines further state that if the documentation is unclear as to whether the patient has a complication of the transplant, query the provider.

10. What is the correct coding and sequencing for a patient diagnosed with hematuria and cystitis?

    c. A combination code is assigned that includes the type of cystitis with hematuria

    Rationale: In the Tabular List, codes in category N30 for cystitis specify the type of cystitis as with or without hematuria in one combination code, so multiple codes are not needed.

CPT® Procedural Coding

Introduction

Current Procedural Terminology (CPT®) codes are published by the American Medical Association (AMA). The purpose of this coding system is to provide a uniform language for reporting services provided to patients.

A CPT Category I code is a five-digit numeric code used to describe medical, surgical, radiological, laboratory, anesthesiology, and evaluation and management (E/M) services performed by physicians, and other health care providers or entities. There are over 8,000 CPT codes ranging from 00100 through 99607. Beginning in 2002, the AMA added Category III (emerging technology) codes. In 2004, the AMA introduced Category II (supplemental tracking) codes. Both Category II and III codes are five-digit alphanumeric codes.

The entire family of procedure codes acceptable to Medicare is referred to as HCPCS, which is an acronym for:

H Healthcare

C Common

P Procedure

C Coding

S System

This family is comprised of two distinct parts or levels: Level I and Level II.

HCPCS Level I Codes (CPT)

HCPCS Level I codes consist of the five-digit codes listed in the *CPT®* codebook published by the American Medical Association. These are the most frequently used codes to report services and procedures, since the codebook mainly consists of physician procedures. The codes are updated annually, and the new codes for the upcoming year are available at the end of the preceding year for use on January 1.

HCPCS Level II Codes

HCPCS Level II codes consist of five-digit alphanumeric codes using letters A-V, and were developed specifically by the Centers for Medicare & Medicaid Services (CMS) to report services and supplies not found in Level I. HCPCS Level II is a standardized coding system that is used primarily to identify products; supplies; drugs and biologicals; durable medical equipment, prosthetics, orthotics, and supplies (DMEPOS); quality reporting measures; some physician and non-physician provider services; and other services, such as ambulance services. HCPCS Level II codes are recognized by Medicare and many other third-party payers.

The CPT Codebook

This coding reference book, which is updated annually, is organized into nine sections, sixteen appendices, and an alphabetic index. There are specific guidelines listed in the CPT codebook at the beginning of each section. These guidelines indicate interpretations and appropriate reporting of codes contained in that particular section. The guidelines should be reviewed prior to using any code in that section. The sections include:

- **Introduction and Illustrated Anatomical and Procedural Review** — Contains basic instructions for using the CPT codebook and reviews basic medical terminology and anatomy with additional information, references, and illustrations.
- **Evaluation and Management** — Provides the codes and guidelines for reporting patient evaluation and management services, most of which are face-to-face with the provider and based on established or new patient status. The codes are broadly grouped into place of service, such as office, hospital, outpatient or ambulatory surgical center, emergency department, or nursing home or other residential facility and/or type of service, such as observation, consultations, critical care, newborn care, and preventive care.
- **Anesthesia** — Provides guidelines, codes, and modifiers for reporting services involving the administration of anesthesia for different types of procedures and on various locations of the body.
- **Surgery** — Identifies surgical procedures performed across all specialties and body systems. The procedure normally includes the necessary, related services in the surgical package without being stated as part of the code description.
- **Radiology** — Lists codes for diagnostic imaging, ultrasound, radiological guidance, radiation oncology, and nuclear medicine. Procedures in this section include X-ray, fluoroscopy, computed tomography, magnetic resonance imaging, angiography, lymphangiography, mammography, radiological supervision and interpretation for therapeutic transcatheter procedures, bone studies, radiation treatment and planning for cancer, brachytherapy, and radiopharmaceutical procedures.
- **Pathology and Laboratory** — Contains codes for reporting procedures and services processed in a laboratory facility. Tests include organ or disease panels, drug assays, urinalysis, chemistry profiles, microorganism identification, immunoassays, pathological examination of surgical samples, and reproductive-related procedures.
- **Medicine** — Identifies procedures that usually do not require operating room services. The medicine codes provided in this section cover a wide spectrum of specialties and include

both diagnostic and therapeutic procedures. This section includes procedures, such as neuromuscular testing, cardiac catheterization, acupuncture, dialysis, chemotherapy, vaccine administration, and psychiatric services.

- **Category II Codes** — Lists, supplemental, optional tracking codes composed of four digits and the letter F. These codes are intended to reduce the need for record abstraction and chart review and facilitate data collection by those seeking to measure quality of patient care.
- **Category III Codes** — Provides temporary codes composed of four digits and the letter T, established for reporting and tracking data for emerging technology, services, and procedures. When a Category III code is available, it must be used rather than reporting an unlisted code. These codes may or may not be assigned a Category I code at a future date.

The appendices include:

- **Appendix A – Modifiers** — Lists all the applicable modifiers for the CPT codes to identify when a service or procedure was altered by a specific circumstance or to provide additional information about the procedure performed. This includes anesthesia physical status modifiers, CPT Level I modifiers approved for ambulatory surgical centers and hospital outpatient departments, Category II modifiers, and Level II National HCPCS modifiers.
- **Appendix B – Summary of Additions, Deletions, and Revisions** — Shows the current year's changes that were made to the codes.
- **Appendix C – Clinical Examples** — Gives real-life clinical scenarios and examples of patient evaluation and management encounters to help medical offices in reporting services provided to the patient.
- **Appendix D – Summary of CPT Add-on Codes** — Lists in numerical sequence all the codes designated in CPT as add-on codes. The add-on codes are only to be assigned in addition to the principal procedure and never stand alone. Add-on codes are also not subject to modifier 51 rules. These codes are additionally identified with a ✚ symbol.
- **Appendix E – Summary of CPT Codes Exempt from Modifier 51** — Lists in numerical sequence all the CPT codes designated as exempt from the use of modifier 51 that have not been identified as add-on procedures or services. These codes are additionally identified with a ⊘ symbol.
- **Appendix F – Summary of CPT Codes Exempt from Modifier 63** — Lists in numerical sequence all the CPT codes designated as exempt from the use of modifier 63. These codes are additionally identified with a parenthetical instruction.
- **Appendix G – Summary of CPT Codes That Include Moderate (Conscious) Sedation** — Summary of CPT codes that include moderate (conscious) sedation (formerly Appendix G) has been removed from the CPT code set. The codes that were previously included were revised to remove the moderate (conscious) sedation symbol.
- **Appendix H – Alphabetical Clinical Topics Listing** — The Alphabetical Clinical Topics Listing (formerly Appendix H) has been removed from the CPT codebook. Since performance measures are subject to change each year, the alphabetic index to performance measures is now maintained on the AMA website at www.ama-assn.org/go/cpt. The online version will continue to provide measures in table format listed alphabetically by the disease or condition and crosswalked to the Category II codes used to report the quality measure.
- **Appendix I – Genetic Testing Code Modifiers** — The list of Genetic Testing Code Modifiers (formerly Appendix I) has been removed from the CPT code set. The addition of hundreds of molecular pathology codes resulted in the deletion of the stacking codes to which these modifiers applied. For the most current updates for molecular pathology coding in the CPT code set, see the AMA CPT website at www.ama-assn.org/go/cpt.
- **Appendix J – Electrodiagnostic Medicine Listing of Sensory, Motor, and Mixed Nerves** — Assigns each sensory, motor, and mixed nerve with its proper nerve conduction study code in order to improve accurate reporting of codes 95907-99913.
- **Appendix K – Product Pending FDA Approval** — Identifies vaccines that have already been assigned Category I codes that are still awaiting FDA approval. These are identified with the symbol ⚡.
- **Appendix L – Vascular Families** — Outlines the tree of vascular families and identifies first-, second-, and third-order branches, assuming the beginning point is the aorta, vena cava, pulmonary artery, or portal vein.
- **Appendix M – Renumbered CPT Codes – Citations Crosswalk** — This listing identifies codes that were deleted and renumbered from 2007 to 2009 and their crosswalk to current year code(s).
- **Appendix N – Summary of Resequenced CPT Codes** — This list identifies codes that do not appear in numeric sequence. Instead of deleting and renumbering existing codes that need to be moved, the existing codes are now being moved to the correct location without being renumbered. Resequenced codes are relocated to appear with codes for the appropriate code concept. The CPT codebook lists the code in numeric sequence without the code description. Instead, a parenthetical note is listed referencing the range of codes in which the resequenced code appears. The resequenced code is identified with a # symbol, and the full code description is listed for the resequenced code.
- **Appendix O – Multianalyte Assays with Algorithmic Analyses** — This list identifies codes for Multianalyte Assays with Algorithmic Analyses (MAAA) procedures that use utilize multiple results derived from various types of assays (e.g., molecular pathology assays, non-nucleic acid based assays) that are typically unique to a single clinical laboratory or manufacturer.

- **Appendix P – CPT Codes That May Be Used For Synchronous Telemedicine Services** — This appendix first appeared in 2017 to lists codes that may be used for reporting real-time telemedicine services when appended by modifier 95. These procedures include interactive electronic communication using audio-visual telecommunications equipment. These are identified with the ★ symbol.
- **Appendix Q – Severe Acute Respiratory Syndrome Coronavirus 2 (SARS-CoV-2) (coronavirus disease [COVID-19]) Vaccines** — This appendix is new to the CPT 2022 code set. The table in Appendix Q links the COVID-19 vaccine product codes (91300, 91301, 91302, 91303, 91304) to their associated immunization administration codes (0001A, 0002A, 0011A, 0012A, 0021A, 0022A, 0031A, 0041A, 0042A), manufacturer name, vaccine name(s), 10- and 11-digit National Drug Code (NDC) Labeler Product ID, and interval between doses. These codes are also located in the **Medicine** section of the CPT code set.
- **Appendix R – Digital Medicine—Services Taxonomy** — This appendix is new to the CPT 2022 code set. Appendix R is a listing of digital medicine services described in the CPT code set. The digital medicine–services taxonomy table in this appendix classifies CPT codes that are related to digital medicine services into discrete categories of clinician-to-patient services (eg, visit), clinician-to-clinician services (eg, consultation), patient-monitoring services, and digital diagnostic services.

Locating a CPT Code

Once familiar with the CPT codebook, identifying appropriate codes becomes less of a task. The numbers at the top of each page are for easy reference and give the range of codes located on that particular page.

Most sections list the sequence of codes in the following order:

- Top to bottom of body (head to toe)
- Central to peripheral in some subsections (i.e., cardiovascular and nervous system codes)
- Outside to inside of body (incision/excision)

There are two ways to locate a code in the CPT codebook:

- By anatomical site (numerically)
- The Index (alphabetically)

A code can be located simply by knowing the site or body system. For example, if a patient had an EKG performed in the emergency department, the user should try to locate a code through the Index. Alternatively, the coder could rationalize that a medicine service was performed to monitor the patient's heart, which is part of the cardiovascular system. Since those medicine codes are found in the 93000 series of codes, the coder could then look in this section of the CPT codebook to locate the appropriate code.

The Index is organized by main terms, shown in bold typeface. There are four primary classes of main entries:

- Procedure or service – e.g., Cardiac Catheterization, Angioplasty
- Organ or other anatomic site – e.g., Heart, Chest, Abdomen
- Condition – e.g., Angina, Myocardial Infarction
- Synonyms, eponyms, and abbreviations – e.g., EKG, EMG, DXA

The main term is divided into specific sub-terms that help in selecting the appropriate code.

Whenever more than one code applies to a given index entry, a code range is listed. If two or more nonsequential codes apply, they will be separated by a comma. For example:

> **Electrocardiography**
>
> Evaluation ... 0178T-0180T, 93000, 93010, 93660

If more than one sequential code applies, they will be separated by a hyphen. For example:

> **Office and/or Other Outpatient Services**
>
> Established patient ... 99211-99215

A cross-reference provides instructions to the user on where to look when entries are listed under another heading.

> **See** directs the user to refer to the term listed. This is used primarily for synonyms, eponyms, and abbreviations, such as:
>
> **Ear Canal**
> *See* Auditory Canal

The alphabetic index is not a substitute for the main text of CPT. The user must always refer to the main text to ensure that the code selection is accurate and not assign any codes from the Index entry alone.

CPT Symbols

In addition to understanding the layout of CPT and knowing how to reference the book, the user must also understand symbols and their meanings.

● Indicates a new code has been added to the edition the coder is referencing. For example:

● 65874 **Percutaneous transluminal mechanical thrombectomy and/or infusion for thrombolysis, dialysis circuit, any method, including all imaging and radiological supervision and interpretation, diagnostic angiography, fluoroscopic guidance, catheter placement(s), and intraprocedural pharmacological thrombolytic injection(s)**

▲ Indicates the code number is the same, but the definition or description has changed since the last edition

▲ 36908 **Transcatheter placement of intravascular stent(s), central dialysis segment, performed through dialysis circuit, including all imaging and radiological supervision and interpretation required to perform the stenting, and all angioplasty in the central dialysis segment (List separately in addition to code for primary procedure**

; Indicates a selection of suffixes that append to the main portion (prefix) of the code. For example:

96374 **Therapeutic, prophylactic, or diagnostic injection (specify substance or drug); subcutaneous or intramuscular**

96375 Therapeutic, prophylactic, or diagnostic injection (specify substance or drug); intra-arterial

96376 Therapeutic, prophylactic, or diagnostic injection (specify substance or drug); intravenous push, single or initial substance/drug

⊘ Identifies codes that are exempt from the use of modifier 51 but have not been designated as add-on procedures/services.

⊘ 31500 Intubation, endotracheal, emergency procedure

Note: For more information on modifier 51, see the Modifier chapter.

★ Identifies telemedicine codes.

★ 90832 Psychotherapy, 30 minutes with patient

⚡ Identifies codes that have been created for vaccines that are pending FDA approval (at the time of the publication of that year's CPT codebook).

⚡ 90739 Hepatitis B vaccine (HepB), adult dosage, 2 dose schedule, for intramuscular use

Add-on Codes

Add-on procedures or services are ones that are performed in addition to the primary procedure/service. In the CPT codebook, a ✚ indicates a CPT add-on code.

99291 Critical care, evaluation and management of the critically ill or critically injured patient; first 30-74 minutes

✚ 99292 each additional 30 minutes (List separately in addition to code for primary service)

The add-on procedure is performed on the same day by the same provider that performed the primary procedure/service. These codes should never be reported alone and should not be reported with modifier 51.

Modifiers

Modifiers consist of two numeric or alphanumeric digits appended to a code to indicate when a service or procedure that still fits the code description was altered by a specific circumstance or when additional information about the procedure performed needs to be provided.

Unlisted Procedure or Service

The procedure performed may not always be found with a designated code assignment in the CPT codebook. Unlisted procedure codes are provided in every section to be used in these cases. An accompanying operative report or other visit documentation is required when reporting unlisted codes in order for the payer to identify what the procedure entailed and determine its eligibility for reimbursement. An unlisted procedure code should not be used when a Category III code best describes the procedure performed.

Surgical Package

The concept of a global fee for surgical procedures is a long-established concept under which a single fee is billed that pays for all necessary services normally furnished by the surgeon before, during, and after the procedure. Since the fee schedule is based on uniform national relative values, it is necessary to have a uniform national definition of global surgery to assure that equivalent payment is made for the same amount of work and resources.

The following items are included in the global package reimbursement:

- Local anesthesia, digital block, or topical anesthesia
- After the decision for surgery is made, one E/M service one day before or the day of surgery
- Postoperative care that occurs directly after the procedure
- Examining the patient in the recovery area
- Any postoperative care occurring during the designated postoperative period

To assist in this uniform implementation, the CPT Editorial Panel created five modifiers (24, 25, 59, 78, and 79) to identify a service or procedure furnished during a global period that is not a part of the global surgery fee, such as a service unrelated to the condition requiring surgery or for treating the underlying condition and not for normal recovery from the surgery. Use of these modifiers allows such services to be reported in addition to the global fee.

Category II Codes

The Category II section of CPT contains a set of supplemental tracking codes that can be used for performance measurement. This section of codes was implemented in 2004 to facilitate data collection about the quality of care rendered for specific conditions. These codes report certain services and test results that support nationally established performance measures with evidence of contributing to increased quality patient care. It is not required for providers to report these codes; the use of these codes is optional.

Category II codes consist of five-digit alphanumeric codes that end in an F, and the following categories are included in this code set:

- Composite Codes
- Patient Management
- Patient History
- Physical Examination
- Diagnostic/Screening Processes or Results
- Therapeutic, Preventive, or Other Interventions
- Follow-up or Other Outcomes
- Patient Safety
- Structural Measures
- Nonmeasure Code Listings

Category III Codes

Category III codes are temporary codes that identify emerging technologies, services, and procedures and allow for data collection to determine clinical efficacy, utilization, and outcomes. They are alphanumeric codes that consist of four numbers, followed by the letter T.

A Category III code should be reported instead of an unlisted code whenever it accurately describes the procedure that was performed. These temporary codes may or may not be assigned a Category I CPT code in the future.

2022 Urology/Nephrology CPT Codes and Crosswalks

The 2022 Urology/Nephrology CPT codes and crosswalks begin following the Surgery Guidelines section. Each code includes official CPT descriptions, official CPT Guidelines, Plain English Descriptions (PED), ICD-10-CM crosswalks, and Medicare-related information including: RVUs, Modifiers, and CCI edits (also known as NCCI).

Note: This Urology/Nephrology coding book is not intended to replace the AMA's CPT codebook. Use this book in conjunction with the official AMA 2022 CPT codebook.

Surgery Guidelines

Guidelines to direct general reporting of services are presented in the **Introduction**. Some of the commonalities are repeated here for the convenience of those referring to this section on **Surgery**. Other definitions and items unique to Surgery are also listed.

Services

Services rendered in the office, home, or hospital, consultations, and other medical services are listed in the **Evaluation and Management Services** section (99202-99499) beginning on page 19.* "Special Services, Procedures, and Reports" (99000-99082) are listed in the **Medicine** section.

CPT Surgical Package Definition

By their very nature, the services to any patient are variable. The CPT codes that represent a readily identifiable surgical procedure thereby include, on a procedure-by-procedure basis, a variety of services. In defining the specific services "included" in a given CPT surgical code, the following services related to the surgery when furnished by the physician or other qualified health care professional who performs the surgery are included in addition to the operation per se:

- Evaluation and Management (E/M) service(s) subsequent to the decision for surgery on the day before and/or day of surgery (including history and physical)
- Local infiltration, metacarpal/metatarsal/digital block or topical anesthesia
- Immediate postoperative care, including dictating operative notes, talking with the family and other physicians or other qualified health care professionals
- Writing orders
- Evaluating the patient in the postanesthesia recovery area
- Typical postoperative follow-up care

Follow-Up Care for Diagnostic Procedures

Follow-up care for diagnostic procedures (eg, endoscopy, arthroscopy, injection procedures for radiography) includes only that care related to recovery from the diagnostic procedure itself. Care of the condition for which the diagnostic procedure was performed or of other concomitant conditions is not included and may be listed separately.

Follow-Up Care for Therapeutic Surgical Procedures

Follow-up care for therapeutic surgical procedures includes only that care which is usually a part of the surgical service. Complications, exacerbations, recurrence, or the presence of other diseases or injuries requiring additional services should be separately reported.

Supplied Materials

Supplies and materials (eg, sterile trays/drugs), over and above those usually included with the procedure(s) rendered are reported separately. List drugs, trays, supplies, and materials provided. Identify as 99070 or specific supply code.

Reporting More Than One Procedure/Service

When more than one procedure/service is performed on the same date, same session or during a post-operative period (subject to the "surgical package" concept), several CPT modifiers may apply (see Appendix A* for definition).

Separate Procedure

Some of the procedures or services listed in the CPT codebook that are commonly carried out as an integral component of a total service or procedure have been identified by the inclusion of the term "separate procedure." The codes designated as "separate procedure" should not be reported in addition to the code for the total procedure or service of which it is considered an integral component.

However, when a procedure or service that is designated as a "separate procedure" is carried out independently or considered to be unrelated or distinct from other procedures/services provided at that time, it may be reported by itself, or in addition to other procedures/services by appending modifier 59 to the specific "separate procedure" code to indicate that the procedure is not considered to be a component of another procedure, but is a distinct, independent procedure. This may represent a different session, different procedure or surgery, different site or organ system, separate incision/excision, separate lesion, or separate injury (or area of injury in extensive injuries).

 * Pages in this section refer to the AMA *CPT® 2022 Professional Edition.*

Unlisted Service or Procedure

A service or procedure may be provided that is not listed in this edition of the CPT codebook. When reporting such a service, the appropriate "Unlisted Procedure" code may be used to indicate the service, identifying it by "Special Report" as discussed in the section below. The "Unlisted Procedures" and accompanying codes for **Surgery** are as follows:

15999 Unlisted procedure, excision pressure ulcer

17999 Unlisted procedure, skin, mucous membrane and subcutaneous tissue

19499 Unlisted procedure, breast

20999 Unlisted procedure, musculoskeletal system, general

21089 Unlisted maxillofacial prosthetic procedure

21299 Unlisted craniofacial and maxillofacial procedure

21499 Unlisted musculoskeletal procedure, head

21899 Unlisted procedure, neck or thorax

22899 Unlisted procedure, spine

22999 Unlisted procedure, abdomen, musculoskeletal system

23929 Unlisted procedure, shoulder

24999 Unlisted procedure, humerus or elbow

25999 Unlisted procedure, forearm or wrist

26989 Unlisted procedure, hands or fingers

27299 Unlisted procedure, pelvis or hip joint

27599 Unlisted procedure, femur or knee

27899 Unlisted procedure, leg or ankle

28899 Unlisted procedure, foot or toes

29799 Unlisted procedure, casting or strapping

29999 Unlisted procedure, arthroscopy

30999 Unlisted procedure, nose

31299 Unlisted procedure, accessory sinuses

31599 Unlisted procedure, larynx

31899 Unlisted procedure, trachea, bronchi

32999 Unlisted procedure, lungs and pleura

33999 Unlisted procedure, cardiac surgery

36299 Unlisted procedure, vascular injection

37501 Unlisted vascular endoscopy procedure

37799 Unlisted procedure, vascular surgery

38129 Unlisted laparoscopy procedure, spleen

38589 Unlisted laparoscopy procedure, lymphatic system

38999 Unlisted procedure, hemic or lymphatic system

39499 Unlisted procedure, mediastinum

39599 Unlisted procedure, diaphragm

40799 Unlisted procedure, lips

40899 Unlisted procedure, vestibule of mouth

41599 Unlisted procedure, tongue, floor of mouth

41899 Unlisted procedure, dentoalveolar structures

42299 Unlisted procedure, palate, uvula

42699 Unlisted procedure, salivary glands or ducts

42999 Unlisted procedure, pharynx, adenoids, or tonsils

43289 Unlisted laparoscopy procedure, esophagus

43499 Unlisted procedure, esophagus

43659 Unlisted laparoscopy procedure, stomach

43999 Unlisted procedure, stomach

44238 Unlisted laparoscopy procedure, intestine (except rectum)

44799 Unlisted procedure, small intestine

44899 Unlisted procedure, Meckel's diverticulum and the mesentery

44979 Unlisted laparoscopy procedure, appendix

45399 Unlisted procedure, colon

45499 Unlisted laparoscopy procedure, rectum

45999 Unlisted procedure, rectum

46999 Unlisted procedure, anus

47379 Unlisted laparoscopic procedure, liver

47399 Unlisted procedure, liver

47579 Unlisted laparoscopy procedure, biliary tract

47999 Unlisted procedure, biliary tract

48999 Unlisted procedure, pancreas

49329 Unlisted laparoscopy procedure, abdomen, peritoneum and omentum

49659 Unlisted laparoscopy procedure, hernioplasty, herniorrhaphy, herniotomy

49999 Unlisted procedure, abdomen, peritoneum and omentum

50549 Unlisted laparoscopy procedure, renal

50949 Unlisted laparoscopy procedure, ureter

51999 Unlisted laparoscopy procedure, bladder

53899 Unlisted procedure, urinary system

54699 Unlisted laparoscopy procedure, testis

55559 Unlisted laparoscopy procedure, spermatic cord

55899 Unlisted procedure, male genital system

58578 Unlisted laparoscopy procedure, uterus

58579 Unlisted hysteroscopy procedure, uterus

58679 Unlisted laparoscopy procedure, oviduct, ovary

58999 Unlisted procedure, female genital system (nonobstetrical)

* Pages in this section refer to the AMA *CPT® 2022 Professional Edition.*

59897 Unlisted fetal invasive procedure, including ultrasound guidance, when performed

59898 Unlisted laparoscopy procedure, maternity care and delivery

59899 Unlisted procedure, maternity care and delivery

60659 Unlisted laparoscopy procedure, endocrine system

60699 Unlisted procedure, endocrine system

64999 Unlisted procedure, nervous system

66999 Unlisted procedure, anterior segment of eye

67299 Unlisted procedure, posterior segment

67399 Unlisted procedure, extraocular muscle

67599 Unlisted procedure, orbit

67999 Unlisted procedure, eyelids

68399 Unlisted procedure, conjunctiva

68899 Unlisted procedure, lacrimal system

69399 Unlisted procedure, external ear

69799 Unlisted procedure, middle ear

69949 Unlisted procedure, inner ear

69979 Unlisted procedure, temporal bone, middle fossa approach

Special Report

A service that is rarely provided, unusual, variable, or new may require a special report. Pertinent information should include an adequate definition or description of the nature, extent, and need for the procedure, and the time, effort, and equipment necessary to provide the service.

Imaging Guidance

When imaging guidance or imaging supervision and interpretation is included in a surgical procedure, guidelines for image documentation and report, included in the guidelines for Radiology (Including Nuclear Medicine and Diagnostic Ultrasound), will apply. Imaging guidance should not be reported for use of a nonimaging-guided tracking or localizing system (eg, radar signals, electromagnetic signals). Imaging guidance should only be reported when an imaging modality (eg, radiography, fluoroscopy, ultrasonography, magnetic resonance imaging, computed tomography, or nuclear medicine) is used and is appropriately documented.

Surgical Destruction

Surgical destruction is a part of a surgical procedure and different methods of destruction are not ordinarily listed separately unless the technique substantially alters the standard management of a problem or condition. Exceptions under special circumstances are provided for by separate code numbers.

▶Foreign Body/Implant Definition◀

▶An object intentionally placed by a physician or other qualified health care professional for any purpose (eg, diagnostic or therapeutic) is considered an implant. An object that is unintentionally placed (eg, trauma or ingestion) is considered a foreign body. If an implant (or part thereof) has moved from its original position or is structurally broken and no longer serves its intended purpose or presents a hazard to the patient, it qualifies as a foreign body for coding purposes, unless CPT coding instructions direct otherwise or a specific CPT code exists to describe the removal of that broken/moved implant.◀

Surgical Procedures on the Cardiovascular System

Selective vascular catheterizations should be coded to include introduction and all lesser order selective catheterizations used in the approach (eg, the description for a selective right middle cerebral artery catheterization includes the introduction and placement catheterization of the right common and internal carotid arteries).

Additional second and/or third order arterial catheterizations within the same family of arteries supplied by a single first order artery should be expressed by 36218 or 36248. Additional first order or higher catheterizations in vascular families supplied by a first order vessel different from a previously selected and coded family should be separately coded using the conventions described above.

The Central Venous Access Procedures Table

	Non-tunneled	Tunneled Without Port or Pump (w/out port or pump)	Central Tunneled	Tunneled With Port (w/port)	Tunneled With Pump (w/pump)	Peripheral	<5 years	≥5 years	Any Age
Insertion									
Catheter (without imaging guidance)	36555						36555		
	36556							36556	
		36557	36557				36557		
		36558	36558					36558	
	36568 (w/o port or pump)					36568 (w/o port or pump)	36568 (w/o port or pump)		
	36569 (w/o port or pump)					36569 (w/o port or pump)		36569 (w/o port or pump)	
Catheter (with bundled imaging guidance)						36572 (w/o port or pump)	36572 (w/o port or pump)		
						36573 (w/o port or pump)		36573 (w/o port or pump)	
Device			36560	36560			36560		
			36561	36561				36561	
			36563		36563				36563
		36565	36565						36565
			36566	36566					
	36570 (w/port)			36570 (w/port)		36570 (w/port)	36570 (w/port)		
	36571 (w/port)			36571 (w/port)		36571 (w/port)		36571 (w/port)	
Repair									
Catheter	36575 (w/o port or pump)	36575 (w/o port or pump)	36575 (w/o port or pump)			36575 (w/o port or pump)			36575
Device	36576 (w/port or pump)					36576 (w/port or pump)			36576

 * Pages in this section refer to the AMA *CPT® 2022 Professional Edition.*

	Non-tunneled	Tunneled Without Port or Pump (w/out port or pump)	Central Tunneled	Tunneled With Port (w/port)	Tunneled With Pump (w/pump)	Peripheral	<5 years	≥5 years	Any Age
Partial Replacement - Central Venous Access Device (Catheter only)									
			36578	36578	36578	36578			36578
Complete Replacement - Central Venous Access Device (Through Same Venous Access Site)									
Catheter (without imaging guidance)	36580 (w/o port or pump)								36580
		36581	36581						36581
Catheter (with bundled imaging guidance)	36584 (w/o port or pump)					36584 (w/o port or pump)			36584 (w/o port or pump)
Device			36582	36582					36582
			36583		36583				36583
				36585 (w/port)		36585 (w/port)			36585
Removal									
Catheter		36589							36589
Device			36590	36590	36590	36590			36590
Removal of Obstructive Material from Device									
	36595 (pericatheter)	36595 (pericatheter)	36595 (pericatheter)	36595 (pericatheter)	36595 (pericatheter)	36595 (pericatheter)			36595 (pericatheter)
	36596 (intraluminal)	36596 (intraluminal)	36596 (intraluminal)	36596 (intraluminal)	36596 (intraluminal)	36596 (intraluminal)			36596 (intraluminal)
Repositioning of Catheter									
	36597	36597	36597	36597	36597	36597	36597	36597	36597

 * Pages in this section refer to the AMA *CPT® 2022 Professional Edition.*

10004

✚ **10004 Fine needle aspiration biopsy, without imaging guidance; each additional lesion (List separately in addition to code for primary procedure)**

(Use 10004 in conjunction with 10021)

(Do not report 10004, 10021 in conjunction with 10005, 10006, 10007, 10008, 10009, 10010, 10011, 10012 for the same lesion)

(For evaluation of fine needle aspirate, see 88172, 88173, 88177)

AMA Coding Guideline

Fine Needle Aspiration Biopsy Procedures

A fine needle aspiration (FNA) biopsy is performed when material is aspirated with a fine needle and the cells are examined cytologically. A core needle biopsy is typically performed with a larger bore needle to obtain a core sample of tissue for histopathologic evaluation. FNA biopsy procedures are performed with or without imaging guidance. Imaging guidance codes (eg, 76942, 77002, 77012, 77021) may not be reported separately with 10004, 10005, 10006, 10007, 10008, 10009, 10010, 10011, 10012, 10021. Codes 10004, 10005, 10006, 10007, 10008, 10009, 10010, 10011, 10012, 10021 are reported once per lesion sampled in a single session. When more than one FNA biopsy is performed on separate lesions at the same session, same day, same imaging modality, use the appropriate imaging modality add-on code for the second and subsequent lesion(s). When more than one FNA biopsy is performed on separate lesions, same session, same day, using different imaging modalities, report the corresponding primary code with modifier 59 for each additional imaging modality and corresponding add-on codes for subsequent lesions sampled. This instruction applies regardless of whether the lesions are ipsilateral or contralateral to each other, and/or whether they are in the same or different organs/structures. When FNA biopsy and core needle biopsy both are performed on the same lesion, same session, same day using the same type of imaging guidance, do not separately report the imaging guidance for the core needle biopsy. When FNA biopsy is performed on one lesion and core needle biopsy is performed on a separate lesion, same session, same day using the same type of imaging guidance, both the core needle biopsy and the imaging guidance for the core needle biopsy may be reported separately with modifier 59. When FNA biopsy is performed on one lesion and core needle biopsy is performed on a separate lesion, same session, same day using different types of imaging guidance, both the core needle biopsy and the imaging guidance for the core needle biopsy may be reported with modifier 59.

AMA *CPT® Assistant* ▢

10004: Feb 19: 8, Apr 19: 4

Plain English Description

A fine gauge needle (22- or 25-gauge) and syringe are used to sample fluid from a lump, lesion, or cyst or to remove clusters of cells from a solid mass. The fine needle aspiration (FNA) biopsy site is cleansed and the physician locates the lump by palpation and guides the needle into the target site. After the needle is placed into the mass, a vacuum is created and multiple in-and-out needle motions are performed. Several needle insertions are usually required to ensure that an adequate tissue sample is taken. The samples are then prepared by smear onto a microscope slide and allowed to air dry, then fixed by spraying or immersion in a liquid. The fixed smears are stained and examined by a pathologist under the microscope. FNA does not require stitches and is usually performed on an outpatient basis. A small bandage is placed over the site after the procedure. Many patients resume a normal routine the same day. Report code 10021 for the first lesion biopsied by FNA with no imaging guidance and 10004 for each additional lesion.

ICD-10-CM Diagnostic Codes

See Primary Procedure code for crosswalks.

CCI Edits

Refer to Appendix A for CCI edits.

Facility RVUs ▢

Code	Work	PE Facility	MP	Total Facility
10004	0.80	0.35	0.11	1.26

Non-facility RVUs ▢

Code	Work	PE Non-Facility	MP	Total Non-Facility
10004	0.80	0.60	0.11	1.51

Modifiers (PAR) ▢

Code	Mod 50	Mod 51	Mod 62	Mod 66	Mod 80
10004	0	0	0	0	0

Global Period

Code	Days
10004	ZZZ

10005-10008

10005 Fine needle aspiration biopsy, including ultrasound guidance; first lesion

+ 10006 Fine needle aspiration biopsy, including ultrasound guidance; each additional lesion (List separately in addition to code for primary procedure)

(Use 10006 in conjunction with 10005)

(Do not report 10005, 10006 in conjunction with 76942)

(For evaluation of fine needle aspirate, see 88172, 88173, 88177)

10007 Fine needle aspiration biopsy, including fluoroscopic guidance; first lesion

+ 10008 Fine needle aspiration biopsy, including fluoroscopic guidance; each additional lesion (List separately in addition to code for primary procedure)

(Use 10008 in conjunction with 10007)

(Do not report 10007, 10008 in conjunction with 77002)

(For evaluation of fine needle aspirate, see 88172, 88173, 88177)

AMA Coding Guideline

Fine Needle Aspiration Biopsy Procedures

A fine needle aspiration (FNA) biopsy is performed when material is aspirated with a fine needle and the cells are examined cytologically. A core needle biopsy is typically performed with a larger bore needle to obtain a core sample of tissue for histopathologic evaluation. FNA biopsy procedures are performed with or without imaging guidance. Imaging guidance codes (eg, 76942, 77002, 77012, 77021) may not be reported separately with 10004, 10005, 10006, 10007, 10008, 10009, 10010, 10011, 10012, 10021. Codes 10004, 10005, 10006, 10007, 10008, 10009, 10010, 10011, 10012, 10021 are reported once per lesion sampled in a single session. When more than one FNA biopsy is performed on separate lesions at the same session, same day, same imaging modality, use the appropriate imaging modality add-on code for the second and subsequent lesion(s). When more than one FNA biopsy is performed on separate lesions, same session, same day, using different imaging modalities, report the corresponding primary code with modifier 59 for each additional imaging modality and corresponding add-on codes for subsequent lesions sampled. This instruction applies regardless of whether the lesions are ipsilateral or contralateral to each other, and/or whether they are in the same or different organs/structures. When FNA biopsy and core needle biopsy both are performed on the same lesion, same session, same day using the same type of imaging guidance, do not separately report the imaging guidance for the core needle biopsy. When FNA biopsy is performed on one lesion and core needle biopsy is performed on a separate lesion, same session, same day using the same type of imaging guidance, both the core needle biopsy and the imaging guidance for the core needle biopsy may be reported separately with modifier 59. When FNA biopsy is performed on one lesion and core needle biopsy is performed on a separate lesion, same session, same day using different types of imaging guidance, both the core needle biopsy and the imaging guidance for the core needle biopsy may be reported with modifier 59.

AMA *CPT® Assistant*

10005: Feb 19: 8, Apr 19: 4, May 19: 10
10006: Feb 19: 8, Apr 19: 4
10007: Feb 19: 8, Apr 19: 4
10008: Feb 19: 8, Apr 19: 4

Plain English Description

A fine gauge needle (22- or 25-gauge) and syringe are used to sample fluid from a cyst or remove clusters of cells from a solid mass. The fine needle aspiration (FNA) biopsy site is cleansed and the physician locates the lump by palpation. If the lump is non-palpable, imaging guidance is used to assist the FNA biopsy procedure. For more easily localized masses, fluoroscopic guidance or ultrasound guidance may be used. After the needle is placed into the mass, a vacuum is created and multiple in-and-out needle motions are performed pulling back on the syringe. Several needle insertions are usually required to ensure that an adequate tissue sample is taken. The samples are then prepared by smear onto a microscope slide and allowed to air dry, then fixed by spraying or immersion in a liquid. The fixed smears are stained and examined under the microscope by a pathologist. FNA does not require stitches and is usually performed on an outpatient basis. A small bandage is placed over the site after the procedure. Many patients resume a normal routine the same day. Report code 10005 for the first lesion biopsied by FNA with ultrasound guidance and 10006 for each additional lesion. Code 10007 for the first lesion biopsied by FNA with fluoroscopic guidance and 10008 for each additional lesion.

Fine needle aspiration biopsy, including ultrasound guidance; first lesion (10005); each additional lesion (10006); including fluoroscopic guidance; first lesion (10007); each additional lesion (10008)

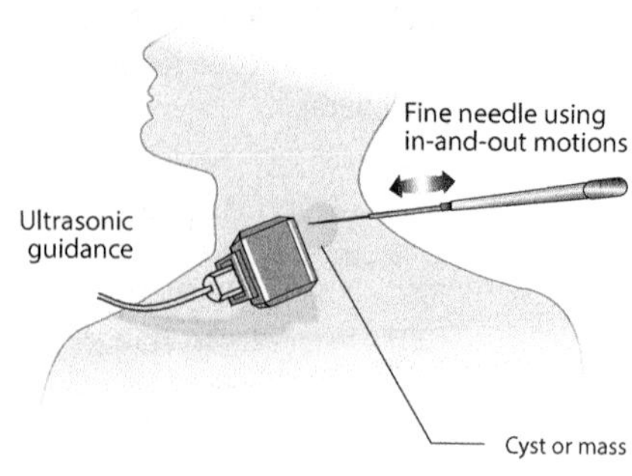

ICD-10-CM Diagnostic Codes

	C61	Malignant neoplasm of prostate ♂
⇄	C62.01	Malignant neoplasm of undescended right testis ♂
⇄	C62.02	Malignant neoplasm of undescended left testis ♂
⇄	C62.11	Malignant neoplasm of descended right testis ♂
⇄	C62.12	Malignant neoplasm of descended left testis ♂
⇄	C63.0	Malignant neoplasm of epididymis
⇄	C63.1	Malignant neoplasm of spermatic cord
	C63.2	Malignant neoplasm of scrotum ♂
	C63.7	Malignant neoplasm of other specified male genital organs ♂
⇄	C64	Malignant neoplasm of kidney, except renal pelvis
⇄	C65	Malignant neoplasm of renal pelvis
⇄	C66	Malignant neoplasm of ureter
	C67.0	Malignant neoplasm of trigone of bladder
	C67.1	Malignant neoplasm of dome of bladder
	C67.2	Malignant neoplasm of lateral wall of bladder
	C67.3	Malignant neoplasm of anterior wall of bladder
	C67.4	Malignant neoplasm of posterior wall of bladder
	C67.5	Malignant neoplasm of bladder neck
	C67.6	Malignant neoplasm of ureteric orifice
	C67.7	Malignant neoplasm of urachus
	C68.0	Malignant neoplasm of urethra
	C68.1	Malignant neoplasm of paraurethral glands
	C77.2	Secondary and unspecified malignant neoplasm of intra-abdominal lymph nodes
	C77.4	Secondary and unspecified malignant neoplasm of inguinal and lower limb lymph nodes
	C77.5	Secondary and unspecified malignant neoplasm of intrapelvic lymph nodes

⇄ C79.0 Secondary malignant neoplasm of kidney and renal pelvis
C79.82 Secondary malignant neoplasm of genital organs
C7B.04 Secondary carcinoid tumors of peritoneum
D29.0 Benign neoplasm of penis ♂
D29.1 Benign neoplasm of prostate ♂
⇄ D29.2 Benign neoplasm of testis
⇄ D29.3 Benign neoplasm of epididymis
D29.4 Benign neoplasm of scrotum ♂
D29.8 Benign neoplasm of other specified male genital organs ♂
⇄ D30.0 Benign neoplasm of kidney
⇄ D30.1 Benign neoplasm of renal pelvis
⇄ D30.2 Benign neoplasm of ureter
D30.3 Benign neoplasm of bladder
D30.4 Benign neoplasm of urethra
D30.8 Benign neoplasm of other specified urinary organs
D40.0 Neoplasm of uncertain behavior of prostate ♂
⇄ D40.1 Neoplasm of uncertain behavior of testis
D40.8 Neoplasm of uncertain behavior of other specified male genital organs ♂
⇄ D41.0 Neoplasm of uncertain behavior of kidney
⇄ D41.1 Neoplasm of uncertain behavior of renal pelvis
⇄ D41.2 Neoplasm of uncertain behavior of ureter
D41.3 Neoplasm of uncertain behavior of urethra
D41.4 Neoplasm of uncertain behavior of bladder
E27.8 Other specified disorders of adrenal gland
E29.0 Testicular hyperfunction ♂
N00.0 Acute nephritic syndrome with minor glomerular abnormality
N00.1 Acute nephritic syndrome with focal and segmental glomerular lesions
N00.2 Acute nephritic syndrome with diffuse membranous glomerulonephritis
N00.3 Acute nephritic syndrome with diffuse mesangial proliferative glomerulonephritis
N00.4 Acute nephritic syndrome with diffuse endocapillary proliferative glomerulonephritis
N00.5 Acute nephritic syndrome with diffuse mesangiocapillary glomerulonephritis
N00.6 Acute nephritic syndrome with dense deposit disease
N00.7 Acute nephritic syndrome with diffuse crescentic glomerulonephritis
N00.8 Acute nephritic syndrome with other morphologic changes
N00.9 Acute nephritic syndrome with unspecified morphologic changes
N00.A Acute nephritic syndrome with C3 glomerulonephritis
N01.0 Rapidly progressive nephritic syndrome with minor glomerular abnormality
N01.1 Rapidly progressive nephritic syndrome with focal and segmental glomerular lesions
N01.2 Rapidly progressive nephritic syndrome with diffuse membranous glomerulonephritis
N01.3 Rapidly progressive nephritic syndrome with diffuse mesangial proliferative glomerulonephritis
N01.4 Rapidly progressive nephritic syndrome with diffuse endocapillary proliferative glomerulonephritis
N01.5 Rapidly progressive nephritic syndrome with diffuse mesangiocapillary glomerulonephritis
N01.6 Rapidly progressive nephritic syndrome with dense deposit disease
N01.7 Rapidly progressive nephritic syndrome with diffuse crescentic glomerulonephritis
N01.8 Rapidly progressive nephritic syndrome with other morphologic changes
N01.A Rapidly progressive nephritic syndrome with C3 glomerulonephritis
N02.0 Recurrent and persistent hematuria with minor glomerular abnormality
N02.1 Recurrent and persistent hematuria with focal and segmental glomerular lesions
N02.2 Recurrent and persistent hematuria with diffuse membranous glomerulonephritis
N02.3 Recurrent and persistent hematuria with diffuse mesangial proliferative glomerulonephritis
N02.4 Recurrent and persistent hematuria with diffuse endocapillary proliferative glomerulonephritis
N02.5 Recurrent and persistent hematuria with diffuse mesangiocapillary glomerulonephritis
N02.6 Recurrent and persistent hematuria with dense deposit disease
N02.7 Recurrent and persistent hematuria with diffuse crescentic glomerulonephritis
N02.8 Recurrent and persistent hematuria with other morphologic changes
N02.A Recurrent and persistent hematuria with C3 glomerulonephritis
N03.0 Chronic nephritic syndrome with minor glomerular abnormality
N03.1 Chronic nephritic syndrome with focal and segmental glomerular lesions
N03.8 Chronic nephritic syndrome with other morphologic changes
N03.A Chronic nephritic syndrome with C3 glomerulonephritis
N04.0 Nephrotic syndrome with minor glomerular abnormality
N04.1 Nephrotic syndrome with focal and segmental glomerular lesions
N04.8 Nephrotic syndrome with other morphologic changes
N04.A Nephrotic syndrome with C3 glomerulonephritis
N28.89 Other specified disorders of kidney and ureter
N36.8 Other specified disorders of urethra
N40.0 Benign prostatic hyperplasia without lower urinary tract symptoms ♂
N40.1 Benign prostatic hyperplasia with lower urinary tract symptoms ♂
N40.2 Nodular prostate without lower urinary tract symptoms ♂
N40.3 Nodular prostate with lower urinary tract symptoms ♂
N42.83 Cyst of prostate ♂
Q55.69 Other congenital malformation of penis ♂
Q61.00 Congenital renal cyst, unspecified
Q61.01 Congenital single renal cyst
Q64.79 Other congenital malformations of bladder and urethra
R19.09 Other intra-abdominal and pelvic swelling, mass and lump
R22.2 Localized swelling, mass and lump, trunk

CCI Edits

Refer to Appendix A for CCI edits.

Facility RVUs

Code	Work	PE Facility	MP	Total Facility
10005	1.46	0.54	0.17	2.17
10006	1.00	0.38	0.10	1.48
10007	1.81	0.66	0.20	2.67
10008	1.18	0.39	0.11	1.68

Non-facility RVUs

Code	Work	PE Non-Facility	MP	Total Non-Facility
10005	1.46	2.48	0.17	4.11
10006	1.00	0.68	0.10	1.78
10007	1.81	7.01	0.20	9.02
10008	1.18	3.63	0.11	4.92

Modifiers (PAR)

Code	Mod 50	Mod 51	Mod 62	Mod 66	Mod 80
10005	0	2	0	0	0
10006	0	0	0	0	0
10007	0	2	0	0	0
10008	0	0	0	0	0

Global Period

Code	Days
10005	XXX
10006	ZZZ
10007	XXX
10008	ZZZ

10009-10012

10009 Fine needle aspiration biopsy, including CT guidance; first lesion

✚ **10010 Fine needle aspiration biopsy, including CT guidance; each additional lesion (List separately in addition to code for primary procedure)**

(Use 10010 in conjunction with 10009)

(Do not report 10009, 10010 in conjunction with 77012)

(For evaluation of fine needle aspirate, see 88172, 88173, 88177)

10011 Fine needle aspiration biopsy, including MR guidance; first lesion

✚ **10012 Fine needle aspiration biopsy, including MR guidance; each additional lesion (List separately in addition to code for primary procedure)**

(Use 10012 in conjunction with 10011)

(Do not report 10011, 10012 in conjunction with 77021)

(For evaluation of fine needle aspirate, see 88172, 88173, 88177)

(For percutaneous needle biopsy other than fine needle aspiration, see 19081-19086 for breast, 20206 for muscle, 32400 for pleura, 32408 for lung or mediastinum, 42400 for salivary gland, 47000 for liver, 48102 for pancreas, 49180 for abdominal or retroperitoneal mass, 50200 for kidney, 54500 for testis, 54800 for epididymis, 60100 for thyroid, 62267 for nucleus pulposus, intervertebral disc, or paravertebral tissue, 62269 for spinal cord)

(For percutaneous image-guided fluid collection drainage by catheter of soft tissue [eg, extremity, abdominal wall, neck], use 10030)

AMA Coding Guideline

Fine Needle Aspiration Biopsy Procedures

A fine needle aspiration (FNA) biopsy is performed when material is aspirated with a fine needle and the cells are examined cytologically. A core needle biopsy is typically performed with a larger bore needle to obtain a core sample of tissue for histopathologic evaluation. FNA biopsy procedures are performed with or without imaging guidance. Imaging guidance codes (eg, 76942, 77002, 77012, 77021) may not be reported separately with 10004, 10005, 10006, 10007, 10008, 10009, 10010, 10011, 10012, 10021. Codes 10004, 10005, 10006, 10007, 10008, 10009, 10010, 10011, 10012, 10021 are reported once per lesion sampled in a single session. When more than one FNA biopsy is performed on separate lesions at the same session, same day, same imaging modality, use the appropriate imaging modality add-on code for the second and subsequent lesion(s). When more than one FNA biopsy is performed on separate lesions, same session, same day, using different imaging modalities, report the corresponding primary code with modifier 59 for each additional imaging modality and corresponding add-on codes for subsequent lesions sampled. This instruction applies regardless of whether the lesions are ipsilateral or contralateral to each other, and/or whether they are in the same or different organs/structures. When FNA biopsy and core needle biopsy both are performed on the same lesion, same session, same day using the same type of imaging guidance, do not separately report the imaging guidance for the core needle biopsy. When FNA biopsy is performed on one lesion and core needle biopsy is performed on a separate lesion, same session, same day using the same type of imaging guidance, both the core needle biopsy and the imaging guidance for the core needle biopsy may be reported separately with modifier 59. When FNA biopsy is performed on one lesion and core needle biopsy is performed on a separate lesion, same session, same day using different types of imaging guidance, both the core needle biopsy and the imaging guidance for the core needle biopsy may be reported with modifier 59.

AMA *CPT® Assistant* ▯

10009: Feb 19: 8, Apr 19: 4
10010: Feb 19: 8, Apr 19: 4
10011: Feb 19: 8, Apr 19: 4
10012: Feb 19: 8, Apr 19: 4

Plain English Description

A fine needle aspiration (FNA) biopsy is performed to obtain a sample of fluid from a cyst or remove clusters of cells from a solid mass using CT or MRI for visual guidance of the FNA biopsy procedure. FNA biopsy is used when open biopsy would be potentially dangerous for disrupting surgical planes or causing tumor seeding, such as in previously surgically treated or irradiated lesions. CT and MRI guidance are employed for lesions that are not easily localized or are inaccessible by routine methods, such as abdominal or thoracic lesions or masses within the lungs, pancreas, liver, or kidneys, or deep-seated nodules within the neck. In the case of CT guidance, a radiopaque marker is placed over the lesion site and the patient is scanned in small increments until the best location for the biopsy is obtained. Intravenous (IV) sedation may be administered in some cases. The site is prepared with local anesthesia and antiseptic solution. A coaxial biopsy guide needle is inserted and a second scan is obtained with the needle in place to confirm its placement. A biopsy gun with a long internal needle is then attached to the guide needle in position and activated to plunge into the mass and aspirate sample cells or fluid as many times as necessary. The specimens are then prepared by smear onto a microscope slide and allowed to air dry, then fixed and stained. The slides are examined microscopically immediately in order to ascertain if the specimens obtained are adequate or more samples need to be obtained. Report code 10009 for the first lesion biopsied by FNA with CT guidance and 10010 for each additional lesion. Report 10011 for the first lesion biopsied by FNA with MRI guidance and 10012 for each additional lesion.

Fine needle aspiration biopsy, including CT guidance; first lesion (10009); each additional lesion (10010); including MR guidance; first lesion (10011); each additional lesion (10012)

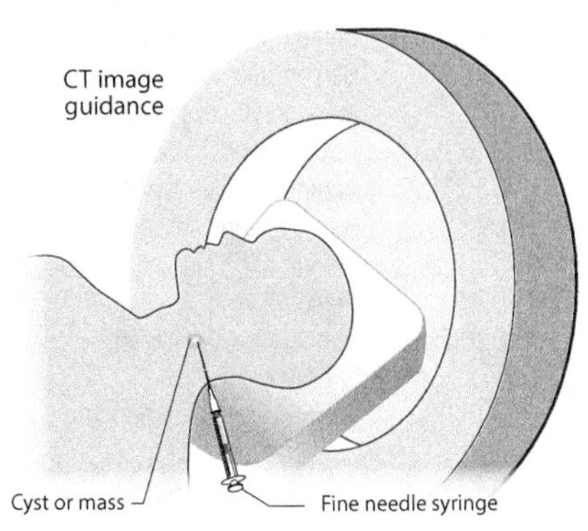

ICD-10-CM Diagnostic Codes

	C61	Malignant neoplasm of prostate ♂
⇄	C62.01	Malignant neoplasm of undescended right testis ♂
⇄	C62.02	Malignant neoplasm of undescended left testis ♂
⇄	C62.11	Malignant neoplasm of descended right testis ♂
⇄	C62.12	Malignant neoplasm of descended left testis ♂
⇄	C63.0	Malignant neoplasm of epididymis
⇄	C63.1	Malignant neoplasm of spermatic cord
	C63.7	Malignant neoplasm of other specified male genital organs ♂
⇄	C64	Malignant neoplasm of kidney, except renal pelvis
⇄	C65	Malignant neoplasm of renal pelvis
⇄	C66	Malignant neoplasm of ureter
	C67.0	Malignant neoplasm of trigone of bladder
	C67.1	Malignant neoplasm of dome of bladder
	C67.2	Malignant neoplasm of lateral wall of bladder
	C67.3	Malignant neoplasm of anterior wall of bladder
	C67.4	Malignant neoplasm of posterior wall of bladder
	C67.5	Malignant neoplasm of bladder neck
	C67.6	Malignant neoplasm of ureteric orifice
	C67.7	Malignant neoplasm of urachus
	C68.0	Malignant neoplasm of urethra

C77.2 Secondary and unspecified malignant neoplasm of intra-abdominal lymph nodes
C77.4 Secondary and unspecified malignant neoplasm of inguinal and lower limb lymph nodes
C77.5 Secondary and unspecified malignant neoplasm of intrapelvic lymph nodes
⇄ C79.0 Secondary malignant neoplasm of kidney and renal pelvis
C79.82 Secondary malignant neoplasm of genital organs
C7B.04 Secondary carcinoid tumors of peritoneum
D29.1 Benign neoplasm of prostate ♂
⇄ D29.2 Benign neoplasm of testis
⇄ D29.3 Benign neoplasm of epididymis
D29.8 Benign neoplasm of other specified male genital organs ♂
⇄ D30.0 Benign neoplasm of kidney
⇄ D30.1 Benign neoplasm of renal pelvis
⇄ D30.2 Benign neoplasm of ureter
D30.3 Benign neoplasm of bladder
D30.4 Benign neoplasm of urethra
D30.8 Benign neoplasm of other specified urinary organs
D40.0 Neoplasm of uncertain behavior of prostate ♂
⇄ D40.1 Neoplasm of uncertain behavior of testis
D40.8 Neoplasm of uncertain behavior of other specified male genital organs ♂
⇄ D41.0 Neoplasm of uncertain behavior of kidney
⇄ D41.1 Neoplasm of uncertain behavior of renal pelvis
⇄ D41.2 Neoplasm of uncertain behavior of ureter
D41.3 Neoplasm of uncertain behavior of urethra
D41.4 Neoplasm of uncertain behavior of bladder
E27.8 Other specified disorders of adrenal gland
E29.0 Testicular hyperfunction ♂
N00.0 Acute nephritic syndrome with minor glomerular abnormality
N00.1 Acute nephritic syndrome with focal and segmental glomerular lesions
N00.2 Acute nephritic syndrome with diffuse membranous glomerulonephritis
N00.3 Acute nephritic syndrome with diffuse mesangial proliferative glomerulonephritis
N00.4 Acute nephritic syndrome with diffuse endocapillary proliferative glomerulonephritis
N00.5 Acute nephritic syndrome with diffuse mesangiocapillary glomerulonephritis
N00.6 Acute nephritic syndrome with dense deposit disease
N00.7 Acute nephritic syndrome with diffuse crescentic glomerulonephritis
N00.8 Acute nephritic syndrome with other morphologic changes
N00.A Acute nephritic syndrome with C3 glomerulonephritis
N01.0 Rapidly progressive nephritic syndrome with minor glomerular abnormality
N01.1 Rapidly progressive nephritic syndrome with focal and segmental glomerular lesions
N01.2 Rapidly progressive nephritic syndrome with diffuse membranous glomerulonephritis
N01.3 Rapidly progressive nephritic syndrome with diffuse mesangial proliferative glomerulonephritis
N01.4 Rapidly progressive nephritic syndrome with diffuse endocapillary proliferative glomerulonephritis
N01.5 Rapidly progressive nephritic syndrome with diffuse mesangiocapillary glomerulonephritis
N01.6 Rapidly progressive nephritic syndrome with dense deposit disease
N01.7 Rapidly progressive nephritic syndrome with diffuse crescentic glomerulonephritis
N01.8 Rapidly progressive nephritic syndrome with other morphologic changes
N01.A Rapidly progressive nephritic syndrome with C3 glomerulonephritis
N02.0 Recurrent and persistent hematuria with minor glomerular abnormality
N02.1 Recurrent and persistent hematuria with focal and segmental glomerular lesions
N02.2 Recurrent and persistent hematuria with diffuse membranous glomerulonephritis
N02.3 Recurrent and persistent hematuria with diffuse mesangial proliferative glomerulonephritis
N02.4 Recurrent and persistent hematuria with diffuse endocapillary proliferative glomerulonephritis
N02.5 Recurrent and persistent hematuria with diffuse mesangiocapillary glomerulonephritis
N02.6 Recurrent and persistent hematuria with dense deposit disease
N02.7 Recurrent and persistent hematuria with diffuse crescentic glomerulonephritis
N02.8 Recurrent and persistent hematuria with other morphologic changes
N02.A Recurrent and persistent hematuria with C3 glomerulonephritis
N03.0 Chronic nephritic syndrome with minor glomerular abnormality
N03.1 Chronic nephritic syndrome with focal and segmental glomerular lesions
N03.8 Chronic nephritic syndrome with other morphologic changes
N03.A Chronic nephritic syndrome with C3 glomerulonephritis
N04.0 Nephrotic syndrome with minor glomerular abnormality
N04.1 Nephrotic syndrome with focal and segmental glomerular lesions
N04.8 Nephrotic syndrome with other morphologic changes
N04.A Nephrotic syndrome with C3 glomerulonephritis
N28.89 Other specified disorders of kidney and ureter
N36.8 Other specified disorders of urethra
N40.0 Benign prostatic hyperplasia without lower urinary tract symptoms ♂
N40.1 Benign prostatic hyperplasia with lower urinary tract symptoms ♂
N40.2 Nodular prostate without lower urinary tract symptoms ♂
N40.3 Nodular prostate with lower urinary tract symptoms ♂
N42.83 Cyst of prostate ♂
Q55.69 Other congenital malformation of penis ♂
Q61.00 Congenital renal cyst, unspecified
Q61.01 Congenital single renal cyst
Q64.79 Other congenital malformations of bladder and urethra
R19.09 Other intra-abdominal and pelvic swelling, mass and lump
R22.2 Localized swelling, mass and lump, trunk

CCI Edits

Refer to Appendix A for CCI edits.

Facility RVUs

Code	Work	PE Facility	MP	Total Facility
10009	2.26	0.77	0.22	3.25
10010	1.65	0.54	0.14	2.33
10011	0.00	0.00	0.00	0.00
10012	0.00	0.00	0.00	0.00

Non-facility RVUs

Code	Work	PE Non-Facility	MP	Total Non-Facility
10009	2.26	11.09	0.22	13.57
10010	1.65	6.17	0.14	7.96
10011	0.00	0.00	0.00	0.00
10012	0.00	0.00	0.00	0.00

Modifiers (PAR)

Code	Mod 50	Mod 51	Mod 62	Mod 66	Mod 80
10009	0	2	0	0	0
10010	0	0	0	0	0
10011	0	2	0	0	0
10012	0	0	0	0	0

Global Period

Code	Days
10009	XXX
10010	ZZZ
10011	XXX
10012	ZZZ

10021

10021 Fine needle aspiration biopsy, without imaging guidance; first lesion

AMA Coding Guideline

Fine Needle Aspiration Biopsy Procedures

A fine needle aspiration (FNA) biopsy is performed when material is aspirated with a fine needle and the cells are examined cytologically. A core needle biopsy is typically performed with a larger bore needle to obtain a core sample of tissue for histopathologic evaluation. FNA biopsy procedures are performed with or without imaging guidance. Imaging guidance codes (eg, 76942, 77002, 77012, 77021) may not be reported separately with 10004, 10005, 10006, 10007, 10008, 10009, 10010, 10011, 10012, 10021. Codes 10004, 10005, 10006, 10007, 10008, 10009, 10010, 10011, 10012, 10021 are reported once per lesion sampled in a single session. When more than one FNA biopsy is performed on separate lesions at the same session, same day, same imaging modality, use the appropriate imaging modality add-on code for the second and subsequent lesion(s). When more than one FNA biopsy is performed on separate lesions, same session, same day, using different imaging modalities, report the corresponding primary code with modifier 59 for each additional imaging modality and corresponding add-on codes for subsequent lesions sampled. This instruction applies regardless of whether the lesions are ipsilateral or contralateral to each other, and/or whether they are in the same or different organs/structures. When FNA biopsy and core needle biopsy both are performed on the same lesion, same session, same day using the same type of imaging guidance, do not separately report the imaging guidance for the core needle biopsy. When FNA biopsy is performed on one lesion and core needle biopsy is performed on a separate lesion, same session, same day using the same type of imaging guidance, both the core needle biopsy and the imaging guidance for the core needle biopsy may be reported separately with modifier 59. When FNA biopsy is performed on one lesion and core needle biopsy is performed on a separate lesion, same session, same day using different types of imaging guidance, both the core needle biopsy and the imaging guidance for the core needle biopsy may be reported with modifier 59.

AMA *CPT® Assistant* ▢

10021: Aug 02: 10, Mar 05: 11, Apr 19: 4, May 19: 10

Plain English Description

A fine gauge needle (22- or 25-gauge) and syringe are used to sample fluid from a lump, lesion, or cyst or to remove clusters of cells from a solid mass. The fine needle aspiration (FNA) biopsy site is cleansed and the physician locates the lump by palpation and guides the needle into the target site. After the needle is placed into the mass, a vacuum is created and multiple in-and-out needle motions are performed. Several needle insertions are usually required to ensure that an adequate tissue sample is taken. The samples are then prepared by smear onto a microscope slide and allowed to air dry, then fixed by spraying or immersion in a liquid. The fixed smears are stained and examined under the microscope by a pathologist. FNA does not require stitches and is usually performed on an outpatient basis. A small bandage is placed over the site after the procedure. Many patients resume a normal routine the same day. Report code 10021 for the first lesion biopsied by FNA with no imaging guidance and 10004 for each additional lesion.

Fine needle aspiration

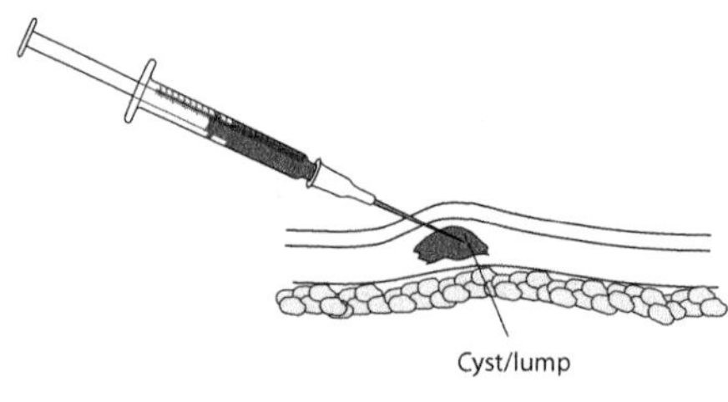

A tissue sample is taken for analysis. No image guidance is used.

ICD-10-CM Diagnostic Codes

⇄	C62.11	Malignant neoplasm of descended right testis ♂
⇄	C62.12	Malignant neoplasm of descended left testis ♂
	C63.2	Malignant neoplasm of scrotum ♂
	C63.7	Malignant neoplasm of other specified male genital organs ♂
	C79.82	Secondary malignant neoplasm of genital organs
	D07.69	Carcinoma in situ of other male genital organs ♂
	D29.0	Benign neoplasm of penis ♂
⇄	D29.21	Benign neoplasm of right testis ♂
⇄	D29.22	Benign neoplasm of left testis ♂
	D29.4	Benign neoplasm of scrotum ♂
	D29.8	Benign neoplasm of other specified male genital organs ♂
⇄	D40.11	Neoplasm of uncertain behavior of right testis ♂
⇄	D40.12	Neoplasm of uncertain behavior of left testis ♂
	D40.8	Neoplasm of uncertain behavior of other specified male genital organs ♂
	E29.0	Testicular hyperfunction ♂
	N43.0	Encysted hydrocele ♂
	N43.1	Infected hydrocele ♂
	N43.2	Other hydrocele ♂
	N43.3	Hydrocele, unspecified ♂
	N44.1	Cyst of tunica albuginea testis ♂
	N44.2	Benign cyst of testis ♂
	N44.8	Other noninflammatory disorders of the testis ♂
	N45.2	Orchitis ♂
	N45.4	Abscess of epididymis or testis ♂
⇄	R19.03	Right lower quadrant abdominal swelling, mass and lump
⇄	R19.04	Left lower quadrant abdominal swelling, mass and lump
	R19.05	Periumbilic swelling, mass or lump
	R22.2	Localized swelling, mass and lump, trunk

CCI Edits

Refer to Appendix A for CCI edits.

Facility RVUs ▢

Code	Work	PE Facility	MP	Total Facility
10021	1.03	0.45	0.12	1.60

Non-facility RVUs ▢

Code	Work	PE Non-Facility	MP	Total Non-Facility
10021	1.03	1.87	0.12	3.02

Modifiers (PAR) ▢

Code	Mod 50	Mod 51	Mod 62	Mod 66	Mod 80
10021	0	2	0	0	0

Global Period

Code	Days
10021	XXX

10030

10030 Image-guided fluid collection drainage by catheter (eg, abscess, hematoma, seroma, lymphocele, cyst), soft tissue (eg, extremity, abdominal wall, neck), percutaneous

(Report 10030 for each individual collection drained with a separate catheter)

(Do not report 10030 in conjunction with 75989, 76942, 77002, 77003, 77012, 77021)

(For image-guided fluid collection drainage, percutaneous or transvaginal/transrectal of visceral, peritoneal, or retroperitoneal collections, see 49405-49407)

AMA *CPT® Assistant* ☐

10030: May 14: 3, 9, Aug 17: 9

Plain English Description

A soft tissue fluid collection such as an abscess, hematoma, seroma, lymphocele, or cyst is drained by percutaneous technique. Using fluoroscopy, ultrasound, or CT guidance, the fluid collection in the soft tissue is identified. The skin and soft tissue over the fluid collection are punctured and a catheter is placed. The fluid is drained. The soft tissue cavity may be flushed with sterile saline or antibiotic solution to clear all pus, blood, and other fluid from the site. The catheter may be secured to the skin and is left to provide continuous drainage as needed before being removed.

ICD-10-CM Diagnostic Codes

	L02.211	Cutaneous abscess of abdominal wall
	L02.214	Cutaneous abscess of groin
	L02.215	Cutaneous abscess of perineum
	L04.1	Acute lymphadenitis of trunk
	L05.01	Pilonidal cyst with abscess
	L05.02	Pilonidal sinus with abscess
	L05.91	Pilonidal cyst without abscess
	L72.0	Epidermal cyst
	L72.3	Sebaceous cyst
	L76.32	Postprocedural hematoma of skin and subcutaneous tissue following other procedure
	L76.34	Postprocedural seroma of skin and subcutaneous tissue following other procedure
	M72.8	Other fibroblastic disorders
	M79.81	Nontraumatic hematoma of soft tissue
❼	T79.2	Traumatic secondary and recurrent hemorrhage and seroma
❼	T81.41	Infection following a procedure, superficial incisional surgical site
❼	T81.42	Infection following a procedure, deep incisional surgical site
❼	T81.43	Infection following a procedure, organ and space surgical site

ICD-10-CM Coding Notes

For codes requiring a 7th character extension, refer to your ICD-10-CM book. Review the character descriptions and coding guidelines for proper selection. For some procedures, only certain characters will apply.

CCI Edits

Refer to Appendix A for CCI edits.

Facility RVUs ☐

Code	Work	PE Facility	MP	Total Facility
10030	2.75	0.94	0.25	3.94

Non-facility RVUs ☐

Code	Work	PE Non-Facility	MP	Total Non-Facility
10030	2.75	16.91	0.25	19.91

Modifiers (PAR) ☐

Code	Mod 50	Mod 51	Mod 62	Mod 66	Mod 80
10030	9	2	0	0	0

Global Period

Code	Days
10030	000

10180

10180 Incision and drainage, complex, postoperative wound infection

(For secondary closure of surgical wound, see 12020, 12021, 13160)

AMA Coding Notes

Incision and Drainage Procedures on the Skin, Subcutaneous and Accessory Structures

(For excision, see 11400, et seq)

AMA *CPT® Assistant*

10180: Nov 14: 5

Plain English Description

Incision and drainage are performed when infection occurs after an operation and the wound must be drained. The physician prepares the area by removing any sutures or staples or by creating additional incisions. Any necrotic (dead) tissue is removed after the wound has been drained. The wound is irrigated with saline and may be resutured or packed with gauze to allow additional drainage. Suction or latex drains may be used if the physician closes the wound. If the wound is left open, it may require future closure.

Incision and drainage, complex, postoperative wound infection

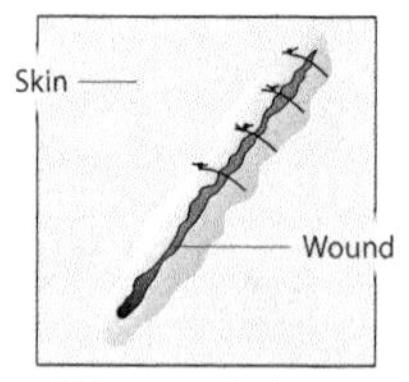

Sutures or staples are removed and wound is drained

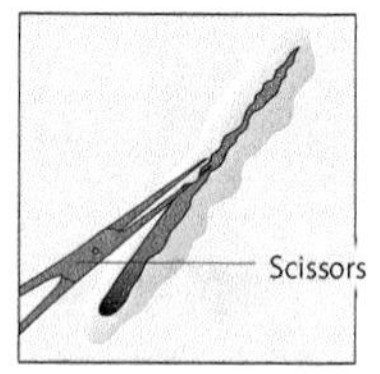

Any necrotic tissue is removed

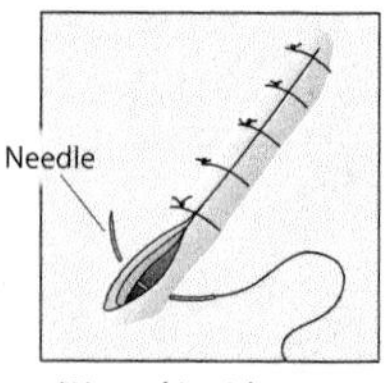

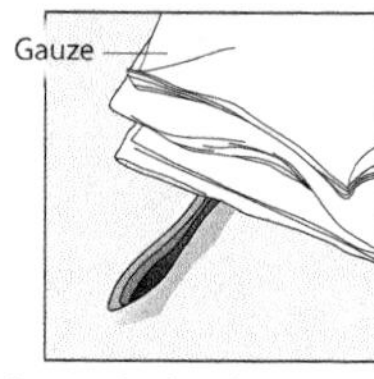

Wound is either resutured or packed with gauze.

ICD-10-CM Diagnostic Codes

	A48.52	Wound botulism
	K68.11	Postprocedural retroperitoneal abscess
	N99.511	Cystostomy infection
	N99.521	Infection of incontinent external stoma of urinary tract
	N99.531	Infection of continent stoma of urinary tract
➐	T81.41	Infection following a procedure, superficial incisional surgical site
➐	T81.42	Infection following a procedure, deep incisional surgical site
➐	T81.43	Infection following a procedure, organ and space surgical site
➐	T81.49	Infection following a procedure, other surgical site
➐	T83.510	Infection and inflammatory reaction due to cystostomy catheter
➐	T83.511	Infection and inflammatory reaction due to indwelling urethral catheter
➐	T83.512	Infection and inflammatory reaction due to nephrostomy catheter
➐	T83.518	Infection and inflammatory reaction due to other urinary catheter
➐	T83.591	Infection and inflammatory reaction due to implanted urinary sphincter
➐	T83.592	Infection and inflammatory reaction due to indwelling ureteral stent
➐	T83.593	Infection and inflammatory reaction due to other urinary stents
➐	T83.598	Infection and inflammatory reaction due to other prosthetic device, implant and graft in urinary system
➐	T83.61	Infection and inflammatory reaction due to implanted penile prosthesis
➐	T83.62	Infection and inflammatory reaction due to implanted testicular prosthesis
➐	T83.69	Infection and inflammatory reaction due to other prosthetic device, implant and graft in genital tract

ICD-10-CM Coding Notes

For codes requiring a 7th character extension, refer to your ICD-10-CM book. Review the character descriptions and coding guidelines for proper selection. For some procedures, only certain characters will apply.

CCI Edits

Refer to Appendix A for CCI edits.

Facility RVUs

Code	Work	PE Facility	MP	Total Facility
10180	2.30	2.46	0.50	5.26

Non-facility RVUs

Code	Work	PE Non-Facility	MP	Total Non-Facility
10180	2.30	5.08	0.50	7.88

Modifiers (PAR)

Code	Mod 50	Mod 51	Mod 62	Mod 66	Mod 80
10180	0	2	0	0	1

Global Period

Code	Days
10180	010

11004-11006

11004 Debridement of skin, subcutaneous tissue, muscle and fascia for necrotizing soft tissue infection; external genitalia and perineum

11005 Debridement of skin, subcutaneous tissue, muscle and fascia for necrotizing soft tissue infection; abdominal wall, with or without fascial closure

11006 Debridement of skin, subcutaneous tissue, muscle and fascia for necrotizing soft tissue infection; external genitalia, perineum and abdominal wall, with or without fascial closure

(If orchiectomy is performed, use 54520)

(If testicular transplantation is performed, use 54680)

AMA Coding Guideline

Debridement Procedures on the Skin

Wound debridements (11042-11047) are reported by depth of tissue that is removed and by surface area of the wound. These services may be reported for injuries, infections, wounds and chronic ulcers. When performing debridement of a single wound, report depth using the deepest level of tissue removed. In multiple wounds, sum the surface area of those wounds that are at the same depth, but do not combine sums from different depths. For example: When bone is debrided from a 4 sq cm heel ulcer and from a 10 sq cm ischial ulcer, report the work with a single code, 11044. When subcutaneous tissue is debrided from a 16 sq cm dehisced abdominal wound and a 10 sq cm thigh wound, report the work with 11042 for the first 20 sq cm and 11045 for the second 6 sq cm. If all four wounds were debrided on the same day, use modifier 59 with either 11042, or 11044 as appropriate.

AMA Coding Notes

Debridement Procedures on the Skin

(For dermabrasions, see 15780-15783)

(For nail debridement, see 11720-11721)

(For burn(s), see 16000-16035)

(For pressure ulcers, see 15920-15999)

AMA *CPT® Assistant* ☐

11004: Jan 12: 6, Oct 12: 3, Oct 13: 15, Feb 18: 10, Nov 19: 14

11005: Jan 12: 6, Oct 12: 3, Oct 13: 15, Feb 18: 10, Nov 19: 14

11006: Jan 12: 6, Oct 12: 3, Oct 13: 15, Nov 19: 14

Plain English Description

Skin, subcutaneous tissue, muscle, and fascia of the external genitalia and perineum are debrided due to necrotizing soft tissue infection (NSTI) in 11004. NSTI of the perineum is also referred to as Fournier's gangrene. The skin is incised. The area of NSTI is explored to determine the extent of tissue involvement. All apparent necrotic tissue is aggressively debrided, extending beyond the skin to subcutaneous tissues, fascia, and muscle, until the presence of arterial bleeding is noted and viable tissue is identified. All nonviable skin is resected, taking care to preserve as much viable skin and subcutaneous tissue as possible. Cultures are taken and sent to the lab for identification of infectious organisms and sensitivity testing. Use 11005 for debridement of skin, subcutaneous tissue, muscle, and fascia for NSTI of the abdominal wall, with or without closure of the fascia, and 11006 for NSTI debridement of the external genitalia, perineum, and the abdominal wall, with or without closure of the fascia.

Debridement of necrotic soft tissue

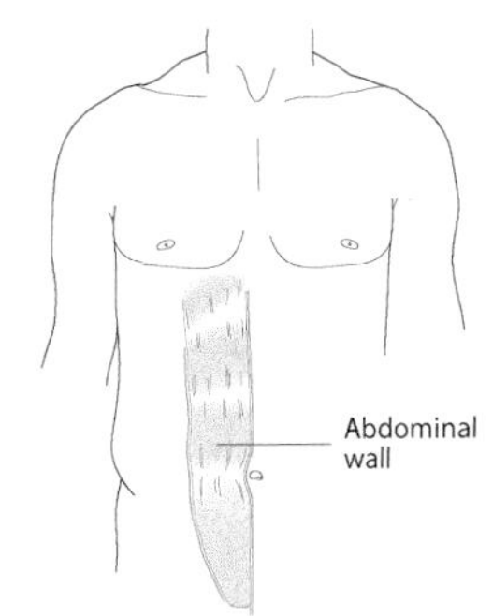

Skin, subcutaneous tissue, muscle, and fascia of the external genitalia, perineum, and/or abdominal wall are debrided due to necrotizing soft tissue infection.

ICD-10-CM Diagnostic Codes

	A48.52	Wound botulism
	A49.01	Methicillin susceptible Staphylococcus aureus infection, unspecified site
	A49.02	Methicillin resistant Staphylococcus aureus infection, unspecified site
	B95.0	Streptococcus, group A, as the cause of diseases classified elsewhere
	B95.1	Streptococcus, group B, as the cause of diseases classified elsewhere
	B95.2	Enterococcus as the cause of diseases classified elsewhere
	B95.3	Streptococcus pneumoniae as the cause of diseases classified elsewhere
	B95.4	Other streptococcus as the cause of diseases classified elsewhere
	B95.61	Methicillin susceptible Staphylococcus aureus infection as the cause of diseases classified elsewhere
	B95.62	Methicillin resistant Staphylococcus aureus infection as the cause of diseases classified elsewhere
	B95.7	Other staphylococcus as the cause of diseases classified elsewhere
	B96.1	Klebsiella pneumoniae [K. pneumoniae] as the cause of diseases classified elsewhere
	B96.21	Shiga toxin-producing Escherichia coli [E. coli] [STEC] 0157 as the cause of diseases classified elsewhere
	B96.22	Other specified Shiga toxin-producing Escherichia coli [E. coli] [STEC] as the cause of diseases classified elsewhere
	B96.23	Unspecified Shiga toxin-producing Escherichia coli [E. coli] [STEC] as the cause of diseases classified elsewhere
	B96.5	Pseudomonas (aeruginosa) (mallei) (pseudomallei) as the cause of diseases classified elsewhere
	B96.6	Bacteroides fragilis [B. fragilis] as the cause of diseases classified elsewhere
	B96.7	Clostridium perfringens [C. perfringens] as the cause of diseases classified elsewhere
	B96.82	Vibrio vulnificus as the cause of diseases classified elsewhere
	I96	Gangrene, not elsewhere classified
	K61.0	Anal abscess
	K61.1	Rectal abscess
	L03.311	Cellulitis of abdominal wall
	L03.315	Cellulitis of perineum
	L88	Pyoderma gangrenosum
	L98.0	Pyogenic granuloma
	M72.6	Necrotizing fasciitis
	M72.8	Other fibroblastic disorders
	M79.A3	Nontraumatic compartment syndrome of abdomen
	M79.A9	Nontraumatic compartment syndrome of other sites
	N49.3	Fournier gangrene ♂
❼⇄	S31.103	Unspecified open wound of abdominal wall, right lower quadrant without penetration into peritoneal cavity
❼⇄	S31.104	Unspecified open wound of abdominal wall, left lower quadrant without penetration into peritoneal cavity
❼	S31.30	Unspecified open wound of scrotum and testes
❼	T81.41	Infection following a procedure, superficial incisional surgical site
❼	T81.42	Infection following a procedure, deep incisional surgical site
❼	T83.510	Infection and inflammatory reaction due to cystostomy catheter
❼	T83.511	Infection and inflammatory reaction due to indwelling urethral catheter
❼	T83.61	Infection and inflammatory reaction due to implanted penile prosthesis
❼	T83.62	Infection and inflammatory reaction due to implanted testicular prosthesis
❼	T83.69	Infection and inflammatory reaction due to other prosthetic device, implant and graft in genital tract

ICD-10-CM Coding Notes

For codes requiring a 7th character extension, refer to your ICD-10-CM book. Review the character descriptions and coding guidelines for proper selection. For some procedures, only certain characters will apply.

CCI Edits

Refer to Appendix A for CCI edits.

Facility RVUs ▯

Code	Work	PE Facility	MP	Total Facility
11004	10.80	3.95	2.04	16.79
11005	14.24	5.37	3.33	22.94
11006	13.10	4.87	2.73	20.70

Non-facility RVUs ▯

Code	Work	PE Non-Facility	MP	Total Non-Facility
11004	10.80	3.95	2.04	16.79
11005	14.24	5.37	3.33	22.94
11006	13.10	4.87	2.73	20.70

Modifiers (PAR) ▯

Code	Mod 50	Mod 51	Mod 62	Mod 66	Mod 80
11004	0	2	0	0	1
11005	0	0	0	0	0
11006	0	2	0	0	1

Global Period

Code	Days
11004	000
11005	000
11006	000

11420-11426

11420 Excision, benign lesion including margins, except skin tag (unless listed elsewhere), scalp, neck, hands, feet, genitalia; excised diameter 0.5 cm or less

11421 Excision, benign lesion including margins, except skin tag (unless listed elsewhere), scalp, neck, hands, feet, genitalia; excised diameter 0.6 to 1.0 cm

11422 Excision, benign lesion including margins, except skin tag (unless listed elsewhere), scalp, neck, hands, feet, genitalia; excised diameter 1.1 to 2.0 cm

11423 Excision, benign lesion including margins, except skin tag (unless listed elsewhere), scalp, neck, hands, feet, genitalia; excised diameter 2.1 to 3.0 cm

11424 Excision, benign lesion including margins, except skin tag (unless listed elsewhere), scalp, neck, hands, feet, genitalia; excised diameter 3.1 to 4.0 cm

11426 Excision, benign lesion including margins, except skin tag (unless listed elsewhere), scalp, neck, hands, feet, genitalia; excised diameter over 4.0 cm

(For unusual or complicated excision, add modifier 22)

AMA Coding Guideline

Excision-Benign Lesions Procedures on the Skin

Excision (including simple closure) of benign lesions of skin (eg, neoplasm, cicatricial, fibrous, inflammatory, congenital, cystic lesions), includes local anesthesia. See appropriate size and area below. For shave removal, see 11300 et seq, and for electrosurgical and other methods see 17000 et seq.

Excision is defined as full-thickness (through the dermis) removal of a lesion, including margins, and includes simple (non-layered) closure when performed. Report separately each benign lesion excised. Code selection is determined by measuring the greatest clinical diameter of the apparent lesion plus that margin required for complete excision (lesion diameter plus the most narrow margins required equals the excised diameter). The margins refer to the most narrow margin required to adequately excise the lesion, based on individual judgment. The measurement of lesion plus margin is made prior to excision. The excised diameter is the same whether the surgical defect is repaired in a linear fashion, or reconstructed (eg, with a skin graft).

The closure of defects created by incision, excision, or trauma may require intermediate or complex closure. Repair by intermediate or complex closure should be reported separately. For excision of benign lesions requiring more than simple closure, ie, requiring intermediate or complex closure, report 11400-11446 in addition to appropriate intermediate (12031-12057) or complex closure (13100-13153) codes. For reconstructive closure, see 15002-15261, 15570-15770. For excision performed in conjunction with adjacent tissue transfer, report only the adjacent tissue transfer code (14000-14302). Excision of lesion (11400-11446) is not separately reportable with adjacent tissue transfer.

AMA Coding Notes

Excision-Benign Lesions Procedures on the Skin

(For destruction [eg, laser surgery, electrosurgery, cryosurgery, chemosurgery, surgical curette] of benign lesions other than skin tags or cutaneous vascular proliferative lesions, see 17110, 17111; premalignant lesions, see 17000, 17003, 17004; cutaneous vascular proliferative lesions, see 17106, 17107, 17108; malignant lesions, see 17260-17286)

(For excision of cicatricial lesion[s] [eg, full thickness excision, through the dermis], see 11400-11446)

(For incisional removal of burn scar, see 16035, 16036)

(For fractional ablative laser fenestration for functional improvement of traumatic or burn scars, see 0479T, 0480T)

AMA *CPT® Assistant* ▢

11420: Summer 92: 22, Fall 95: 3, Jul 08: 5, Jul 10: 10, May 12: 13, Jan 13: 15, Mar 14: 4, 12, Apr 16: 3, Feb 18: 10, Sep 18: 7, Nov 19: 3

11421: Summer 92: 22, Fall 95: 3, May 96: 11, Jul 10: 10, May 12: 13, Jan 13: 15, Mar 14: 4, 12, Apr 16: 3, Feb 18: 10, Sep 18: 7, Nov 19: 3

11422: Summer 92: 22, Fall 95: 3, May 96: 11, Aug 00: 5, Jul 10: 10, Mar 12: 4, May 12: 13, Jan 13: 15, Mar 14: 4, 12, Apr 16: 3, Feb 18: 10, Sep 18: 7, Nov 19: 3

11423: Summer 92: 22, Fall 95: 3, May 96: 11, Jul 10: 10, May 12: 13, Jan 13: 15, Mar 14: 4, 12, Apr 16: 3, Feb 18: 10, Sep 18: 7, Nov 19: 3

11424: Summer 92: 22, Fall 95: 3, May 96: 11, Jul 10: 10, May 12: 13, Jan 13: 15, Mar 14: 4, 12, Apr 16: 3, Feb 18: 10, Sep 18: 7, Nov 19: 3

11426: Summer 92: 22, Fall 95: 3, May 96: 11, Jul 10: 10, May 12: 13, Jan 13: 15, Mar 14: 4, 12, Apr 16: 3, Feb 18: 10, Sep 18: 7, Nov 19: 3

Plain English Description

A benign lesion other than a skin tag of the scalp, neck, hands, feet, or genitalia is excised along with a margin of normal tissue. Commonly excised benign lesions include: lipomas, dermatofibromas, pyogenic granulomas, epidermoid cysts, and benign nevi. The area is cleansed and a local anesthetic injected. A narrow margin of healthy tissue is identified and a full-thickness incision is made through the dermis. The incision is carried around the lesion and the entire lesion is excised. The lesion is sent to the laboratory for separately reportable histologic evaluation. Bleeding is controlled by electrocautery or chemical cautery. The wound may be closed using simple single-layer suture technique. Separately reportable intermediate (layer) closure, complex repair, skin graft, or pedicle flap may also be used to close the surgical wound. Use 11420 for excision diameter 0.5 cm or less; 11421 for excision diameter 0.6-1.0 cm; 11422 for excision diameter of 1.1-2.0 cm; 11423 for excision diameter of 2.1-3.0 cm; 11424 for excision diameter of 3.1-4.0; and 11426 for excision diameter of over 4.0 cm.

Excision, benign lesion

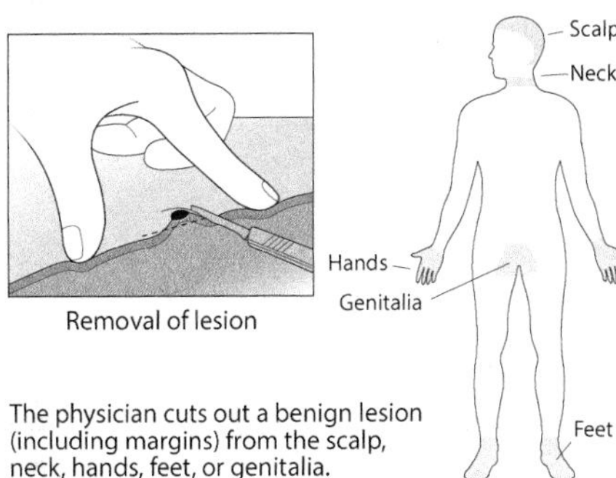

The physician cuts out a benign lesion (including margins) from the scalp, neck, hands, feet, or genitalia.

ICD-10-CM Diagnostic Codes

A54.89	Other gonococcal infections
A63.0	Anogenital (venereal) warts
B07.8	Other viral warts
B08.1	Molluscum contagiosum
D17.1	Benign lipomatous neoplasm of skin and subcutaneous tissue of trunk
D17.39	Benign lipomatous neoplasm of skin and subcutaneous tissue of other sites
D18.01	Hemangioma of skin and subcutaneous tissue
D22.5	Melanocytic nevi of trunk
D23.5	Other benign neoplasm of skin of trunk
D29.0	Benign neoplasm of penis ♂
D29.4	Benign neoplasm of scrotum ♂
L57.5	Actinic granuloma
L72.11	Pilar cyst
L72.12	Trichodermal cyst
L72.3	Sebaceous cyst
L72.8	Other follicular cysts of the skin and subcutaneous tissue
L82.1	Other seborrheic keratosis
L90.5	Scar conditions and fibrosis of skin
L91.0	Hypertrophic scar
L92.3	Foreign body granuloma of the skin and subcutaneous tissue
L92.8	Other granulomatous disorders of the skin and subcutaneous tissue
L98.0	Pyogenic granuloma
L98.8	Other specified disorders of the skin and subcutaneous tissue
P83.81	Umbilical granuloma

CCI Edits

Refer to Appendix A for CCI edits.

Facility RVUs

Code	Work	PE Facility	MP	Total Facility
11420	1.03	1.28	0.10	2.41
11421	1.47	1.56	0.17	3.20
11422	1.68	2.08	0.21	3.97
11423	2.06	2.23	0.27	4.56
11424	2.48	2.38	0.35	5.21
11426	4.09	3.26	0.65	8.00

Non-facility RVUs

Code	Work	PE Non-Facility	MP	Total Non-Facility
11420	1.03	2.68	0.10	3.81
11421	1.47	3.13	0.17	4.77
11422	1.68	3.46	0.21	5.35
11423	2.06	3.77	0.27	6.10
11424	2.48	4.16	0.35	6.99
11426	4.09	5.18	0.65	9.92

Modifiers (PAR)

Code	Mod 50	Mod 51	Mod 62	Mod 66	Mod 80
11420	0	2	0	0	1
11421	0	2	0	0	1
11422	0	2	0	0	1
11423	0	2	0	0	1
11424	0	2	0	0	1
11426	0	2	0	0	1

Global Period

Code	Days
11420	010
11421	010
11422	010
11423	010
11424	010
11426	010

11620-11626

11620 Excision, malignant lesion including margins, scalp, neck, hands, feet, genitalia; excised diameter 0.5 cm or less

11621 Excision, malignant lesion including margins, scalp, neck, hands, feet, genitalia; excised diameter 0.6 to 1.0 cm

11622 Excision, malignant lesion including margins, scalp, neck, hands, feet, genitalia; excised diameter 1.1 to 2.0 cm

11623 Excision, malignant lesion including margins, scalp, neck, hands, feet, genitalia; excised diameter 2.1 to 3.0 cm

11624 Excision, malignant lesion including margins, scalp, neck, hands, feet, genitalia; excised diameter 3.1 to 4.0 cm

11626 Excision, malignant lesion including margins, scalp, neck, hands, feet, genitalia; excised diameter over 4.0 cm

AMA Coding Guideline

Excision-Malignant Lesions Procedures on the Skin

Excision (including simple closure) of malignant lesions of skin (eg, basal cell carcinoma, squamous cell carcinoma, melanoma) includes local anesthesia. (See appropriate size and body area below.) For destruction of malignant lesions of skin, see destruction codes 17260-17286.

Excision is defined as full-thickness (through the dermis) removal of a lesion including margins, and includes simple (non-layered) closure when performed. Report separately each malignant lesion excised. Code selection is determined by measuring the greatest clinical diameter of the apparent lesion plus that margin required for complete excision (lesion diameter plus the most narrow margins required equals the excised diameter). The margins refer to the most narrow margin required to adequately excise the lesion, based on the physician's judgment. The measurement of lesion plus margin is made prior to excision. The excised diameter is the same whether the surgical defect is repaired in a linear fashion, or reconstructed (eg, with a skin graft).

The closure of defects created by incision, excision, or trauma may require intermediate or complex closure. Repair by intermediate or complex closure should be reported separately. For excision of malignant lesions requiring more than simple closure, ie, requiring intermediate or complex closure, report 11600-11646 in addition to appropriate intermediate (12031-12057) or complex closure (13100-13153) codes. For reconstructive closure, see 15002-15261, 15570-15770. For excision performed in conjunction with adjacent tissue transfer, report only the adjacent tissue transfer code (14000-14302). Excision of lesion (11600-11646) is not separately reportable with adjacent tissue transfer.

When frozen section pathology shows the margins of excision were not adequate, an additional excision may be necessary for complete tumor removal. Use only one code to report the additional excision and re-excision(s) based on the final widest excised diameter required for complete tumor removal at the same operative session. To report a re-excision procedure performed to widen margins at a subsequent operative session, see codes 11600-11646, as appropriate. Append modifier 58 if the re-excision procedure is performed during the postoperative period of the primary excision procedure.

AMA *CPT® Assistant* ▯

11620: Fall 95: 3, Nov 02: 5, Oct 04: 4, Feb 08: 8, Feb 10: 3, May 12: 13, Jul 12: 12, Mar 14: 4, 12, Sep 18: 7, Nov 19: 3

11621: Fall 95: 3, May 96: 11, Nov 02: 5, Feb 08: 8, Feb 10: 3, May 12: 13, Mar 14: 4, 12, Sep 18: 7, Nov 19: 3

11622: Fall 95: 3, May 96: 11, Nov 02: 5, Feb 08: 8, Feb 10: 3, May 12: 13, Mar 14: 4, 12, Sep 18: 7, Nov 19: 3

11623: Fall 95: 3, May 96: 11, Nov 02: 5, Feb 08: 8, Feb 10: 3, May 12: 13, Mar 14: 4, 12, Sep 18: 7, Nov 19: 3

11624: Fall 95: 3, May 96: 11, Nov 02: 5, Feb 08: 8, Feb 10: 3, May 12: 13, Mar 14: 4, 12, Sep 18: 7, Nov 19: 3

11626: Fall 95: 3, May 96: 11, Nov 02: 5, Feb 08: 8, Feb 10: 3, May 12: 13, Mar 14: 4, 12, Sep 18: 7, Nov 19: 3

Plain English Description

A malignant lesion of the scalp, neck, hands, feet, or genitalia is excised along with a margin of normal tissue. Commonly excised malignant lesions include: basal cell carcinoma, squamous cell carcinoma, verrucous carcinoma, and melanoma. The area is cleansed and a local anesthetic injected. A margin of healthy tissue is identified and a full-thickness incision is made through the dermis. The incision is carried around the lesion and the entire lesion is excised. Separately reportable frozen section may be performed at the time of the excision to ensure that an adequate margin has been excised. If malignant tissue is identified at the margin, additional tissue is excised until all margins are clean. The lesion is sent to the laboratory for separately reportable histologic evaluation. Bleeding is controlled by electrocautery or chemical cautery. The wound may be closed using simple single-layer suture technique. Separately reportable intermediate (layer) closure, complex repair, skin graft, or pedicle flap may also be used to close the surgical wound. Use 11620 for excision diameter 0.5 cm or less; 11621 for excision diameter 0.6-1.0 cm; 11622 for excision diameter of 1.1-2.0 cm; 11623 for excision diameter of 2.1-3.0 cm; 11624 for excision diameter of 3.1-4.0; and 11626 for excision diameter of over 4.0 cm.

Excision, malignant lesion
(scalp, neck, hands, feet, genitalia)

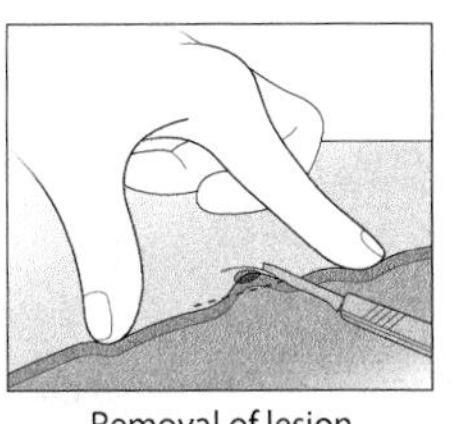

Removal of lesion

0.5 cm or less (11620);
0.6 cm to 1.0 cm (11621);
1.1 cm to 2.0 cm (11622);
2.1 cm to 3.0 cm (11623);
3.1 cm to 4.0 cm (11624);
larger than 4.0 cm (11626)

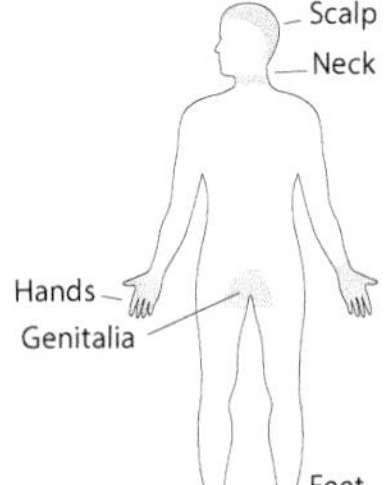

Location of lesion

A malignant lesion is cut out (including margins).

ICD-10-CM Diagnostic Codes

C60.0	Malignant neoplasm of prepuce ♂
C60.1	Malignant neoplasm of glans penis ♂
C60.2	Malignant neoplasm of body of penis ♂
C60.8	Malignant neoplasm of overlapping sites of penis ♂
C63.2	Malignant neoplasm of scrotum ♂
C79.2	Secondary malignant neoplasm of skin
C79.82	Secondary malignant neoplasm of genital organs
D03.59	Melanoma in situ of other part of trunk
D03.8	Melanoma in situ of other sites
D07.4	Carcinoma in situ of penis ♂
D07.61	Carcinoma in situ of scrotum ♂

CCI Edits

Refer to Appendix A for CCI edits.

Facility RVUs

Code	Work	PE Facility	MP	Total Facility
11620	1.64	1.75	0.21	3.60
11621	2.08	2.03	0.25	4.36
11622	2.41	2.25	0.27	4.93
11623	3.11	2.61	0.39	6.11
11624	3.62	2.84	0.50	6.96
11626	4.61	3.22	0.76	8.59

Non-facility RVUs

Code	Work	PE Non-Facility	MP	Total Non-Facility
11620	1.64	4.08	0.21	5.93
11621	2.08	4.50	0.25	6.83
11622	2.41	4.82	0.27	7.50
11623	3.11	5.29	0.39	8.79
11624	3.62	5.89	0.50	10.01
11626	4.61	6.73	0.76	12.10

Modifiers (PAR)

Code	Mod 50	Mod 51	Mod 62	Mod 66	Mod 80
11620	0	2	0	0	1
11621	0	2	0	0	1
11622	0	2	0	0	1
11623	0	2	0	0	1
11624	0	2	0	0	1
11626	0	2	0	0	1

Global Period

Code	Days
11620	010
11621	010
11622	010
11623	010
11624	010
11626	010

12001-12007

12001 Simple repair of superficial wounds of scalp, neck, axillae, external genitalia, trunk and/or extremities (including hands and feet); 2.5 cm or less

12002 Simple repair of superficial wounds of scalp, neck, axillae, external genitalia, trunk and/or extremities (including hands and feet); 2.6 cm to 7.5 cm

12004 Simple repair of superficial wounds of scalp, neck, axillae, external genitalia, trunk and/or extremities (including hands and feet); 7.6 cm to 12.5 cm

12005 Simple repair of superficial wounds of scalp, neck, axillae, external genitalia, trunk and/or extremities (including hands and feet); 12.6 cm to 20.0 cm

12006 Simple repair of superficial wounds of scalp, neck, axillae, external genitalia, trunk and/or extremities (including hands and feet); 20.1 cm to 30.0 cm

12007 Simple repair of superficial wounds of scalp, neck, axillae, external genitalia, trunk and/or extremities (including hands and feet); over 30.0 cm

AMA Coding Guideline

Repair-Simple Procedures on the Integumentary System

Sum of lengths of repairs for each group of anatomic sites.

Surgical Repair (Closure) Procedures on the Integumentary System

Use the codes in this section to designate wound closure utilizing sutures, staples, or tissue adhesives (eg, 2-cyanoacrylate), either singly or in combination with each other, or in combination with adhesive strips. Chemical cauterization, electrocauterization, or wound closure utilizing adhesive strips as the sole repair material are included in the appropriate E/M code.

Definitions

The repair of wounds may be classified as Simple, Intermediate, or Complex.

Simple repair is used when the wound is superficial (eg, involving primarily epidermis or dermis, or subcutaneous tissues without significant involvement of deeper structures) and requires simple one-layer closure. Hemostasis and local or topical anesthesia, when performed, are not reported separately.

Intermediate repair includes the repair of wounds that, in addition to the above, require layered closure of one or more of the deeper layers of subcutaneous tissue and superficial (non-muscle) fascia, in addition to the skin (epidermal and dermal) closure. It includes limited undermining (defined as a distance less than the maximum width of the defect, measured perpendicular to the closure line, along at least one entire edge of the defect). Single-layer closure of heavily contaminated wounds that have required extensive cleaning or removal of particulate matter also constitutes intermediate repair.

Complex repair includes the repair of wounds that, in addition to the requirements for intermediate repair, require at least one of the following: exposure of bone, cartilage, tendon, or named neurovascular structure; debridement of wound edges (eg, traumatic lacerations or avulsions); extensive undermining (defined as a distance greater than or equal to the maximum width of the defect, measured perpendicular to the closure line along at least one entire edge of the defect); involvement of free margins of helical rim, vermilion border, or nostril rim; placement of retention sutures. Necessary preparation includes creation of a limited defect for repairs or the debridement of complicated lacerations or avulsions. Complex repair does not include excision of benign (11400-11446) or malignant (11600-11646) lesions, excisional preparation of a wound bed (15002-15005) or debridement of an open fracture or open dislocation.

Instructions for listing services at time of wound repair:

1. The repaired wound(s) should be measured and recorded in centimeters, whether curved, angular, or stellate.

2. When multiple wounds are repaired, add together the lengths of those in the same classification (see above) and from all anatomic sites that are grouped together into the same code descriptor. For example, add together the lengths of intermediate repairs to the trunk and extremities. Do not add lengths of repairs from different groupings of anatomic sites (eg, face and extremities). Also, do not add together lengths of different classifications (eg, intermediate and complex repairs).

When more than one classification of wounds is repaired, list the more complicated as the primary procedure and the less complicated as the secondary procedure, using modifier 59.

3. Decontamination and/or debridement: Debridement is considered a separate procedure only when gross contamination requires prolonged cleansing, when appreciable amounts of devitalized or contaminated tissue are removed, or when debridement is carried out separately without immediate primary closure.

4. Involvement of nerves, blood vessels and tendons: Report under appropriate system (Nervous, Cardiovascular, Musculoskeletal) for repair of these structures. The repair of these associated wounds is included in the primary procedure unless it qualifies as a complex repair, in which case modifier 59 applies.

Simple ligation of vessels in an open wound is considered as part of any wound closure.

Simple "exploration" of nerves, blood vessels or tendons exposed in an open wound is also considered part of the essential treatment of the wound and is not a separate procedure unless appreciable dissection is required. If the wound requires enlargement, extension of dissection (to determine penetration), debridement, removal of foreign body(s), ligation or coagulation of minor subcutaneous and/or muscular blood vessel(s) of the subcutaneous tissue, muscle fascia, and/or muscle, not requiring thoracotomy or laparotomy, use codes 20100-20103, as appropriate.

AMA Coding Notes

Surgical Repair (Closure) Procedures on the Integumentary System

(For extensive debridement of soft tissue and/or bone, not associated with open fracture(s) and/ or dislocation(s) resulting from penetrating and/or blunt trauma, see 11042-11047.)

(For extensive debridement of subcutaneous tissue, muscle fascia, muscle, and/or bone associated with open fracture(s) and/or dislocation(s), see 11010-11012.)

AMA *CPT® Assistant*

12001: Jun 96: 7, Feb 98: 11, Jan 00: 11, Feb 00: 10, Apr 00: 8, Jul 00: 10, Jan 02: 10, Feb 07: 10, Feb 08: 8, Mar 12: 5, Dec 17: 15, Sep 18: 7

12002: Feb 00: 10, Jan 02: 10, Feb 08: 8, Oct 14: 14, Sep 18: 7

12004: Feb 00: 10, Jan 02: 10, Feb 08: 8, Sep 18: 7

12005: Feb 00: 10, Jan 02: 10, Feb 08: 8, Sep 18: 7

12006: Feb 98: 11, Feb 00: 10, Jan 02: 10, Feb 08: 8, Sep 18: 7

12007: Feb 00: 10, Jan 02: 10, Feb 08: 8, Sep 18: 7

Plain English Description

Simple repair of superficial wounds of the scalp, neck, axillae, external genitalia, trunk, and/or extremities is performed. The wound is cleansed and a local anesthetic is administered. The wound is inspected and determined to be superficial involving only the epidermis, dermis, or subcutaneous tissue without involvement of deeper tissues and without heavy contamination. A simple, one-layer closure using sutures, staples, or tissue adhesive is performed. Alternatively, chemical cautery or electrocautery may be used to treat the wound without closure. Use 12001 for simple repair of a wound 2.5 cm or less, 12002 for a wound 2.6 to 7.5 cm, 12004 for a wound 7.6 to 12.5 cm, 12005 for a wound 12.6 to 20.0 cm, 12006 for a wound 20.1 to 30.0 cm, or 12007 for a wound over 30.0 cm.

Simple repair of superficial wounds

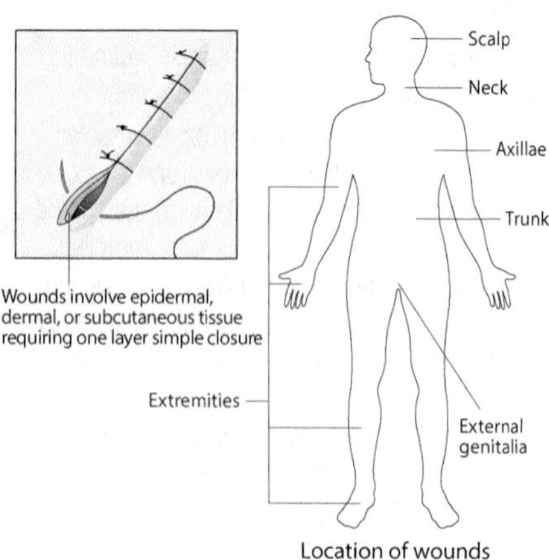

Location of wounds

ICD-10-CM Diagnostic Codes

- ❼ S31.000 Unspecified open wound of lower back and pelvis without penetration into retroperitoneum
- ❼ S31.010 Laceration without foreign body of lower back and pelvis without penetration into retroperitoneum
- ❼ S31.030 Puncture wound without foreign body of lower back and pelvis without penetration into retroperitoneum
- ❼ S31.050 Open bite of lower back and pelvis without penetration into retroperitoneum
- ❼⇄ S31.103 Unspecified open wound of abdominal wall, right lower quadrant without penetration into peritoneal cavity
- ❼⇄ S31.104 Unspecified open wound of abdominal wall, left lower quadrant without penetration into peritoneal cavity
- ❼⇄ S31.113 Laceration without foreign body of abdominal wall, right lower quadrant without penetration into peritoneal cavity
- ❼⇄ S31.114 Laceration without foreign body of abdominal wall, left lower quadrant without penetration into peritoneal cavity
- ❼⇄ S31.133 Puncture wound of abdominal wall without foreign body, right lower quadrant without penetration into peritoneal cavity
- ❼⇄ S31.134 Puncture wound of abdominal wall without foreign body, left lower quadrant without penetration into peritoneal cavity
- ❼⇄ S31.153 Open bite of abdominal wall, right lower quadrant without penetration into peritoneal cavity
- ❼⇄ S31.154 Open bite of abdominal wall, left lower quadrant without penetration into peritoneal cavity
- ❼ S31.20 Unspecified open wound of penis
- ❼ S31.21 Laceration without foreign body of penis
- ❼ S31.23 Puncture wound without foreign body of penis
- ❼ S31.25 Open bite of penis
- ❼ S31.30 Unspecified open wound of scrotum and testes
- ❼ S31.31 Laceration without foreign body of scrotum and testes
- ❼ S31.33 Puncture wound without foreign body of scrotum and testes
- ❼ S31.35 Open bite of scrotum and testes

ICD-10-CM Coding Notes

For codes requiring a 7th character extension, refer to your ICD-10-CM book. Review the character descriptions and coding guidelines for proper selection. For some procedures, only certain characters will apply.

CCI Edits

Refer to Appendix A for CCI edits.

Facility RVUs ▯

Code	Work	PE Facility	MP	Total Facility
12001	0.84	0.32	0.17	1.33
12002	1.14	0.38	0.22	1.74
12004	1.44	0.44	0.27	2.15
12005	1.97	0.45	0.39	2.81
12006	2.39	0.59	0.47	3.45
12007	2.90	0.84	0.56	4.30

Non-facility RVUs ▯

Code	Work	PE Non-Facility	MP	Total Non-Facility
12001	0.84	1.79	0.17	2.80
12002	1.14	2.01	0.22	3.37
12004	1.44	2.20	0.27	3.91
12005	1.97	2.92	0.39	5.28
12006	2.39	3.31	0.47	6.17
12007	2.90	3.48	0.56	6.94

Modifiers (PAR) ▯

Code	Mod 50	Mod 51	Mod 62	Mod 66	Mod 80
12001	0	2	0	0	1
12002	0	2	0	0	1
12004	0	2	0	0	1
12005	0	2	0	0	1
12006	0	2	0	0	1
12007	0	2	1	0	1

Global Period

Code	Days
12001	000
12002	000
12004	000
12005	000
12006	000
12007	000

12020-12021

12020 Treatment of superficial wound dehiscence; simple closure

12021 Treatment of superficial wound dehiscence; with packing

(For extensive or complicated secondary wound closure, use 13160)

AMA Coding Guideline

Repair-Simple Procedures on the Integumentary System

Sum of lengths of repairs for each group of anatomic sites.

Surgical Repair (Closure) Procedures on the Integumentary System

Use the codes in this section to designate wound closure utilizing sutures, staples, or tissue adhesives (eg, 2-cyanoacrylate), either singly or in combination with each other, or in combination with adhesive strips. Chemical cauterization, electrocauterization, or wound closure utilizing adhesive strips as the sole repair material are included in the appropriate E/M code.

Definitions

The repair of wounds may be classified as Simple, Intermediate, or Complex.

Simple repair is used when the wound is superficial (eg, involving primarily epidermis or dermis, or subcutaneous tissues without significant involvement of deeper structures) and requires simple one-layer closure. Hemostasis and local or topical anesthesia, when performed, are not reported separately.

Intermediate repair includes the repair of wounds that, in addition to the above, require layered closure of one or more of the deeper layers of subcutaneous tissue and superficial (non-muscle) fascia, in addition to the skin (epidermal and dermal) closure. It includes limited undermining (defined as a distance less than the maximum width of the defect, measured perpendicular to the closure line, along at least one entire edge of the defect). Single-layer closure of heavily contaminated wounds that have required extensive cleaning or removal of particulate matter also constitutes intermediate repair.

Complex repair includes the repair of wounds that, in addition to the requirements for intermediate repair, require at least one of the following: exposure of bone, cartilage, tendon, or named neurovascular structure; debridement of wound edges (eg, traumatic lacerations or avulsions); extensive undermining (defined as a distance greater than or equal to the maximum width of the defect, measured perpendicular to the closure line along at least one entire edge of the defect); involvement of free margins of helical rim, vermilion border, or nostril rim; placement of retention sutures. Necessary preparation includes creation of a limited defect for repairs or the debridement of complicated lacerations or avulsions. Complex repair does not include excision of benign (11400-11446) or malignant (11600-11646) lesions, excisional preparation of a wound bed (15002-15005) or debridement of an open fracture or open dislocation.

Instructions for listing services at time of wound repair:

1. The repaired wound(s) should be measured and recorded in centimeters, whether curved, angular, or stellate.

2. When multiple wounds are repaired, add together the lengths of those in the same classification (see above) and from all anatomic sites that are grouped together into the same code descriptor. For example, add together the lengths of intermediate repairs to the trunk and extremities. Do not add lengths of repairs from different groupings of anatomic sites (eg, face and extremities). Also, do not add together lengths of different classifications (eg, intermediate and complex repairs).

When more than one classification of wounds is repaired, list the more complicated as the primary procedure and the less complicated as the secondary procedure, using modifier 59.

3. Decontamination and/or debridement: Debridement is considered a separate procedure only when gross contamination requires prolonged cleansing, when appreciable amounts of devitalized or contaminated tissue are removed, or when debridement is carried out separately without immediate primary closure.

4. Involvement of nerves, blood vessels and tendons: Report under appropriate system (Nervous, Cardiovascular, Musculoskeletal) for repair of these structures. The repair of these associated wounds is included in the primary procedure unless it qualifies as a complex repair, in which case modifier 59 applies.

Simple ligation of vessels in an open wound is considered as part of any wound closure.

Simple "exploration" of nerves, blood vessels or tendons exposed in an open wound is also considered part of the essential treatment of the wound and is not a separate procedure unless appreciable dissection is required. If the wound requires enlargement, extension of dissection (to determine penetration), debridement, removal of foreign body(s), ligation or coagulation of minor subcutaneous and/or muscular blood vessel(s) of the subcutaneous tissue, muscle fascia, and/or muscle, not requiring thoracotomy or laparotomy, use codes 20100-20103, as appropriate.

AMA Coding Notes

Surgical Repair (Closure) Procedures on the Integumentary System

(For extensive debridement of soft tissue and/or bone, not associated with open fracture(s) and/or dislocation(s) resulting from penetrating and/or blunt trauma, see 11042-11047.)

(For extensive debridement of subcutaneous tissue, muscle fascia, muscle, and/or bone associated with open fracture(s) and/or dislocation(s), see 11010-11012.)

AMA *CPT® Assistant* ☐

12020: Feb 00: 10, Jan 02: 10, Feb 08: 8

12021: Feb 00: 10, Jan 02: 10, Feb 08: 8

Plain English Description

Wound dehiscence is an opening or splitting of a wound along the suture line. The wound is cleansed. The edges of the wound may be trimmed to initiate bleeding. In 12020, a simple single layer wound closure is performed using sutures, staples, or tissue adhesive. In 12021, the wound is left open and packed with sterile gauze. Packing is typically performed on wounds that are infected. A secondary closure may be performed when the infection has resolved.

Treatment of superficial dehiscence

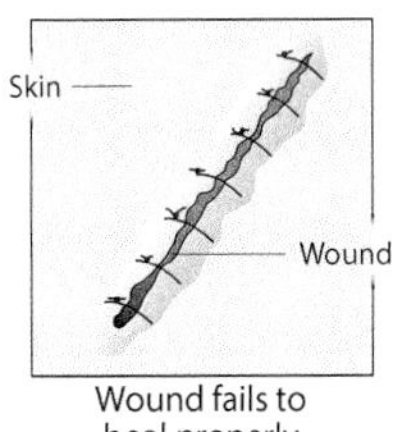

Wound fails to heal properly

Scissors

Skin margins may be trimmed

Needle

Wound is sutured if not infected

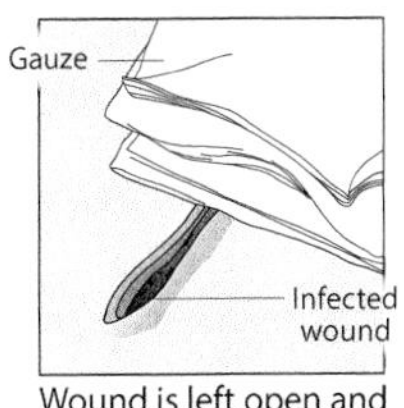

Wound is left open and packed with gauze strips if infected

ICD-10-CM Diagnostic Codes

➐	T81.30	Disruption of wound, unspecified
➐	T81.31	Disruption of external operation (surgical) wound, not elsewhere classified
➐	T81.32	Disruption of internal operation (surgical) wound, not elsewhere classified
➐	T81.33	Disruption of traumatic injury wound repair
➐	T81.41	Infection following a procedure, superficial incisional surgical site

ICD-10-CM Coding Notes

For codes requiring a 7th character extension, refer to your ICD-10-CM book. Review the character descriptions and coding guidelines for proper selection. For some procedures, only certain characters will apply.

CCI Edits

Refer to Appendix A for CCI edits.

Facility RVUs

Code	Work	PE Facility	MP	Total Facility
12020	2.67	2.44	0.41	5.52
12021	1.89	1.95	0.31	4.15

Non-facility RVUs

Code	Work	PE Non-Facility	MP	Total Non-Facility
12020	2.67	5.90	0.41	8.98
12021	1.89	3.08	0.31	5.28

Modifiers (PAR)

Code	Mod 50	Mod 51	Mod 62	Mod 66	Mod 80
12020	0	2	0	0	1
12021	0	2	0	0	1

Global Period

Code	Days
12020	010
12021	010

12041-12047

12041 Repair, intermediate, wounds of neck, hands, feet and/or external genitalia; 2.5 cm or less

12042 Repair, intermediate, wounds of neck, hands, feet and/or external genitalia; 2.6 cm to 7.5 cm

12044 Repair, intermediate, wounds of neck, hands, feet and/or external genitalia; 7.6 cm to 12.5 cm

12045 Repair, intermediate, wounds of neck, hands, feet and/or external genitalia; 12.6 cm to 20.0 cm

12046 Repair, intermediate, wounds of neck, hands, feet and/or external genitalia; 20.1 cm to 30.0 cm

12047 Repair, intermediate, wounds of neck, hands, feet and/or external genitalia; over 30.0 cm

AMA Coding Guideline

Repair-Intermediate Procedures on the Integumentary System

Sum of lengths of repairs for each group of anatomic sites.

Surgical Repair (Closure) Procedures on the Integumentary System

Use the codes in this section to designate wound closure utilizing sutures, staples, or tissue adhesives (eg, 2-cyanoacrylate), either singly or in combination with each other, or in combination with adhesive strips. Chemical cauterization, electrocauterization, or wound closure utilizing adhesive strips as the sole repair material are included in the appropriate E/M code.

Definitions

The repair of wounds may be classified as Simple, Intermediate, or Complex.

Simple repair is used when the wound is superficial (eg, involving primarily epidermis or dermis, or subcutaneous tissues without significant involvement of deeper structures) and requires simple one-layer closure. Hemostasis and local or topical anesthesia, when performed, are not reported separately.

Intermediate repair includes the repair of wounds that, in addition to the above, require layered closure of one or more of the deeper layers of subcutaneous tissue and superficial (non-muscle) fascia, in addition to the skin (epidermal and dermal) closure. It includes limited undermining (defined as a distance less than the maximum width of the defect, measured perpendicular to the closure line, along at least one entire edge of the defect). Single-layer closure of heavily contaminated wounds that have required extensive cleaning or removal of particulate matter also constitutes intermediate repair.

Complex repair includes the repair of wounds that, in addition to the requirements for intermediate repair, require at least one of the following: exposure of bone, cartilage, tendon, or named neurovascular structure; debridement of wound edges (eg, traumatic lacerations or avulsions); extensive undermining (defined as a distance greater than or equal to the maximum width of the defect, measured perpendicular to the closure line along at least one entire edge of the defect); involvement of free margins of helical rim, vermilion border, or nostril rim; placement of retention sutures. Necessary preparation includes creation of a limited defect for repairs or the debridement of complicated lacerations or avulsions. Complex repair does not include excision of benign (11400-11446) or malignant (11600-11646) lesions, excisional preparation of a wound bed (15002-15005) or debridement of an open fracture or open dislocation.

Instructions for listing services at time of wound repair:

1. The repaired wound(s) should be measured and recorded in centimeters, whether curved, angular, or stellate.

2. When multiple wounds are repaired, add together the lengths of those in the same classification (see above) and from all anatomic sites that are grouped together into the same code descriptor. For example, add together the lengths of intermediate repairs to the trunk and extremities. Do not add lengths of repairs from different groupings of anatomic sites (eg, face and extremities). Also, do not add together lengths of different classifications (eg, intermediate and complex repairs).

When more than one classification of wounds is repaired, list the more complicated as the primary procedure and the less complicated as the secondary procedure, using modifier 59.

3. Decontamination and/or debridement: Debridement is considered a separate procedure only when gross contamination requires prolonged cleansing, when appreciable amounts of devitalized or contaminated tissue are removed, or when debridement is carried out separately without immediate primary closure.

4. Involvement of nerves, blood vessels and tendons: Report under appropriate system (Nervous, Cardiovascular, Musculoskeletal) for repair of these structures. The repair of these associated wounds is included in the primary procedure unless it qualifies as a complex repair, in which case modifier 59 applies.

Simple ligation of vessels in an open wound is considered as part of any wound closure.

Simple "exploration" of nerves, blood vessels or tendons exposed in an open wound is also considered part of the essential treatment of the wound and is not a separate procedure unless appreciable dissection is required. If the wound requires enlargement, extension of dissection (to determine penetration), debridement, removal of foreign body(s), ligation or coagulation of minor subcutaneous and/or muscular blood vessel(s) of the subcutaneous tissue, muscle fascia, and/or muscle, not requiring thoracotomy or laparotomy, use codes 20100-20103, as appropriate.

AMA Coding Notes

Surgical Repair (Closure) Procedures on the Integumentary System

(For extensive debridement of soft tissue and/or bone, not associated with open fracture(s) and/or dislocation(s) resulting from penetrating and/or blunt trauma, see 11042-11047.)

(For extensive debridement of subcutaneous tissue, muscle fascia, muscle, and/or bone associated with open fracture(s) and/or dislocation(s), see 11010-11012.)

AMA *CPT® Assistant* ☐

12041: Sep 97: 11, Feb 00: 10, Apr 00: 8, Jan 02: 10, Feb 07: 10, Jan 13: 15, Sep 18: 7

12042: Feb 00: 10, Apr 00: 9, Jan 02: 10, Feb 07: 10, Jan 13: 15, Sep 18: 7

12044: Feb 00: 10, Jan 02: 10, Feb 07: 10, Jan 13: 15, Sep 18: 7

12045: Feb 00: 10, Jan 02: 10, Feb 07: 10, Jan 13: 15, Sep 18: 7

12046: Feb 00: 10, Jan 02: 10, Feb 07: 10, Jan 13: 15, Sep 18: 7

12047: Feb 00: 10, Jan 02: 10, Feb 07: 10, Jan 13: 15, Sep 18: 7

Plain English Description

Intermediate repair of wounds of the neck, hands, feet, and/or external genitalia is performed. The wound is cleansed and a local anesthetic administered. The wound is inspected and determined to involve deeper layers of the subcutaneous tissue and superficial (non-muscle) fascia or to require extensive cleaning and/or removal of particulate matter in a heavily contaminated superficial wound. A layered closure using sutures, staples, and/or tissue adhesive is performed. Tissues are undermined using scissors or scalpel to minimize tension on the wound. Bleeding is controlled by chemical or electrocautery. The deepest layers are then closed with absorbable sutures and the knot is buried. Alternatively, permanent sutures may be used. The superficial layer is closed, taking care to ensure that the wound edges are aligned and everted to prevent depression of the scar. Use 12041 for intermediate repair of a wound 2.5 cm or less; 12042 for a wound 2.6 to 7.5 cm; 12044 for a wound 7.6 to 12.5 cm; 12045 for a wound 12.6 to 20.0 cm; 12046 for a wound 20.1 to 30.0 cm; or 12047 for a wound over 30.0 cm.

Repair, intermediate, wounds of neck, hands, feet and/or external genitalia

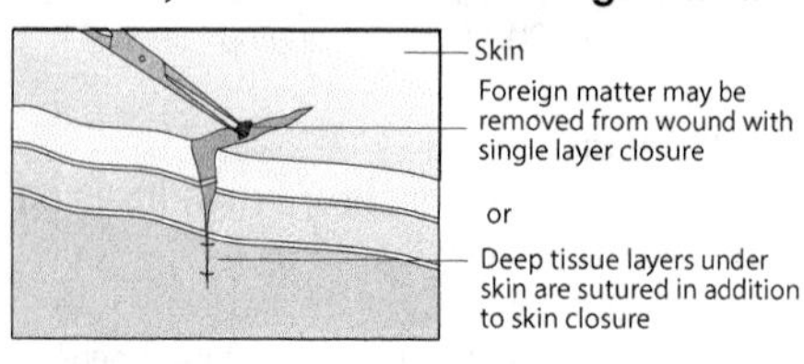

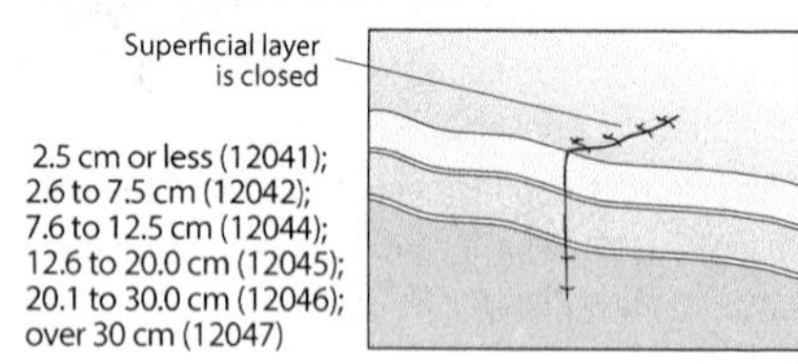

ICD-10-CM Diagnostic Codes

	C60.0	Malignant neoplasm of prepuce ♂
	C60.1	Malignant neoplasm of glans penis ♂
	C60.2	Malignant neoplasm of body of penis ♂
	C60.8	Malignant neoplasm of overlapping sites of penis ♂
	C63.2	Malignant neoplasm of scrotum ♂
	C79.2	Secondary malignant neoplasm of skin
	C79.82	Secondary malignant neoplasm of genital organs
	D07.4	Carcinoma in situ of penis ♂
	D07.61	Carcinoma in situ of scrotum ♂
	D18.01	Hemangioma of skin and subcutaneous tissue
	D29.0	Benign neoplasm of penis ♂
	D29.4	Benign neoplasm of scrotum ♂
	D48.5	Neoplasm of uncertain behavior of skin
❼	S31.21	Laceration without foreign body of penis
❼	S31.22	Laceration with foreign body of penis
❼	S31.23	Puncture wound without foreign body of penis
❼	S31.24	Puncture wound with foreign body of penis
❼	S31.25	Open bite of penis
❼	S31.31	Laceration without foreign body of scrotum and testes
❼	S31.32	Laceration with foreign body of scrotum and testes
❼	S31.33	Puncture wound without foreign body of scrotum and testes
❼	S31.34	Puncture wound with foreign body of scrotum and testes
❼	S31.35	Open bite of scrotum and testes

ICD-10-CM Coding Notes

For codes requiring a 7th character extension, refer to your ICD-10-CM book. Review the character descriptions and coding guidelines for proper selection. For some procedures, only certain characters will apply.

CCI Edits

Refer to Appendix A for CCI edits.

Facility RVUs ▯

Code	Work	PE Facility	MP	Total Facility
12041	2.10	1.86	0.25	4.21
12042	2.79	2.60	0.32	5.71
12044	3.19	2.62	0.43	6.24
12045	3.75	3.58	0.65	7.98
12046	4.30	4.07	1.09	9.46
12047	4.95	4.31	1.25	10.51

Non-facility RVUs ▯

Code	Work	PE Non-Facility	MP	Total Non-Facility
12041	2.10	5.58	0.25	7.93
12042	2.79	6.16	0.32	9.27
12044	3.19	7.77	0.43	11.39
12045	3.75	7.80	0.65	12.20
12046	4.30	9.72	1.09	15.11
12047	4.95	10.32	1.25	16.52

Modifiers (PAR) ▯

Code	Mod 50	Mod 51	Mod 62	Mod 66	Mod 80
12041	0	2	0	0	1
12042	0	2	0	0	1
12044	0	2	0	0	1
12045	0	2	0	0	1
12046	0	2	0	0	0
12047	0	2	1	0	2

Global Period

Code	Days
12041	010
12042	010
12044	010
12045	010
12046	010
12047	010

13131-13133

13131 Repair, complex, forehead, cheeks, chin, mouth, neck, axillae, genitalia, hands and/or feet; 1.1 cm to 2.5 cm

(For 1.0 cm or less, see simple or intermediate repairs)

13132 Repair, complex, forehead, cheeks, chin, mouth, neck, axillae, genitalia, hands and/or feet; 2.6 cm to 7.5 cm

+ **13133 Repair, complex, forehead, cheeks, chin, mouth, neck, axillae, genitalia, hands and/or feet; each additional 5 cm or less (List separately in addition to code for primary procedure)**

(Use 13133 in conjunction with 13132)

(For 1.0 cm or less, see simple or intermediate repairs)

AMA Coding Guideline

Repair-Complex Procedures on the Integumentary System

Reconstructive procedures, complicated wound closure.

Sum of lengths of repairs for each group of anatomic sites.

Surgical Repair (Closure) Procedures on the Integumentary System

Use the codes in this section to designate wound closure utilizing sutures, staples, or tissue adhesives (eg, 2-cyanoacrylate), either singly or in combination with each other, or in combination with adhesive strips. Chemical cauterization, electrocauterization, or wound closure utilizing adhesive strips as the sole repair material are included in the appropriate E/M code.

Definitions

The repair of wounds may be classified as Simple, Intermediate, or Complex.

Simple repair is used when the wound is superficial (eg, involving primarily epidermis or dermis, or subcutaneous tissues without significant involvement of deeper structures) and requires simple one-layer closure. Hemostasis and local or topical anesthesia, when performed, are not reported separately.

Intermediate repair includes the repair of wounds that, in addition to the above, require layered closure of one or more of the deeper layers of subcutaneous tissue and superficial (non-muscle) fascia, in addition to the skin (epidermal and dermal) closure. It includes limited undermining (defined as a distance less than the maximum width of the defect, measured perpendicular to the closure line, along at least one entire edge of the defect). Single-layer closure of heavily contaminated wounds that have required extensive cleaning or removal of particulate matter also constitutes intermediate repair.

Complex repair includes the repair of wounds that, in addition to the requirements for intermediate repair, require at least one of the following: exposure of bone, cartilage, tendon, or named neurovascular structure; debridement of wound edges (eg, traumatic lacerations or avulsions); extensive undermining (defined as a distance greater than or equal to the maximum width of the defect, measured perpendicular to the closure line along at least one entire edge of the defect); involvement of free margins of helical rim, vermilion border, or nostril rim; placement of retention sutures. Necessary preparation includes creation of a limited defect for repairs or the debridement of complicated lacerations or avulsions. Complex repair does not include excision of benign (11400-11446) or malignant (11600-11646) lesions, excisional preparation of a wound bed (15002-15005) or debridement of an open fracture or open dislocation.

Instructions for listing services at time of wound repair:

1. The repaired wound(s) should be measured and recorded in centimeters, whether curved, angular, or stellate.

2. When multiple wounds are repaired, add together the lengths of those in the same classification (see above) and from all anatomic sites that are grouped together into the same code descriptor. For example, add together the lengths of intermediate repairs to the trunk and extremities. Do not add lengths of repairs from different groupings of anatomic sites (eg, face and extremities). Also, do not add together lengths of different classifications (eg, intermediate and complex repairs).

When more than one classification of wounds is repaired, list the more complicated as the primary procedure and the less complicated as the secondary procedure, using modifier 59.

3. Decontamination and/or debridement: Debridement is considered a separate procedure only when gross contamination requires prolonged cleansing, when appreciable amounts of devitalized or contaminated tissue are removed, or when debridement is carried out separately without immediate primary closure.

4. Involvement of nerves, blood vessels and tendons: Report under appropriate system (Nervous, Cardiovascular, Musculoskeletal) for repair of these structures. The repair of these associated wounds is included in the primary procedure unless it qualifies as a complex repair, in which case modifier 59 applies.

Simple ligation of vessels in an open wound is considered as part of any wound closure.

Simple "exploration" of nerves, blood vessels or tendons exposed in an open wound is also considered part of the essential treatment of the wound and is not a separate procedure unless appreciable dissection is required. If the wound requires enlargement, extension of dissection (to determine penetration), debridement, removal of foreign body(s), ligation or coagulation of minor subcutaneous and/or muscular blood vessel(s) of the subcutaneous tissue, muscle fascia, and/or muscle, not requiring thoracotomy or laparotomy, use codes 20100-20103, as appropriate.

AMA Coding Notes

Repair-Complex Procedures on the Integumentary System

(For full thickness repair of lip or eyelid, see respective anatomical subsections)

Surgical Repair (Closure) Procedures on the Integumentary System

(For extensive debridement of soft tissue and/or bone, not associated with open fracture(s) and/or dislocation(s) resulting from penetrating and/or blunt trauma, see 11042-11047.)

(For extensive debridement of subcutaneous tissue, muscle fascia, muscle, and/or bone associated with open fracture(s) and/or dislocation(s), see 11010-11012.)

AMA *CPT® Assistant*

13131: Fall 93: 7, Sep 97: 11, Dec 98: 5, Nov 99: 10, Feb 00: 10, Apr 00: 8, Feb 10: 3, May 11: 4, Jan 12: 8, Dec 12: 6, Jan 13: 15, Apr 17: 9, Sep 18: 7

13132: Fall 93: 7, Dec 98: 5, Nov 99: 10, Dec 99: 10, Feb 00: 10, Apr 00: 9, Aug 00: 9, Feb 10: 3, May 11: 4, Jan 12: 8, Dec 12: 6, Jan 13: 15, Oct 14: 14, Apr 17: 9, Sep 18: 7

13133: Fall 93: 7, Feb 00: 10, Apr 00: 9, Feb 10: 3, May 11: 4, Jan 12: 8, Dec 12: 6, Jan 13: 15, Apr 17: 9, Sep 18: 7

Plain English Description

A complex repair of a wound of the forehead, cheeks, chin, mouth, neck, axillae, genitalia, hands, and/or feet is performed. The wound is cleansed and a local anesthetic administered. The wound is inspected and determined to require more than layered closure. If the complex repair is for scar revision, the scar is excised. If the repair is for a traumatic laceration or avulsion, the wound is cleansed and particulate matter removed. The wound may be debrided using sharp dissection. Tissues may be extensively undermined using scissors or scalpel to minimize tension on the wound. Bleeding is controlled by chemical or electrocautery. Closure of the wound depends on the site and nature of the injury. The deepest layers may be closed with absorbable sutures and the knot buried followed by closure of superficial layers with non-absorbable sutures. If retention sutures are used to hold the edges of the wound together without tension, they are placed through the entire thickness of the wound, a short length of plastic or rubber tubing is threaded over each suture, and each suture is then tied. Stents may also be used to hold tissue in place or maintain the opening of an orifice. Care is taken to carefully align wound edges to prevent scar depression. Use 13131 for complex repair of a wound of the forehead, cheeks, chin, mouth, neck, axillae, genitalia, hands, and/or feet 1.1 to 2.5 cm in length and 13132 for a wound 2.6 to 7.5 cm in length. Use add-on code 13133 for each additional 5 cm or less for wounds over 7.5 cm in length.

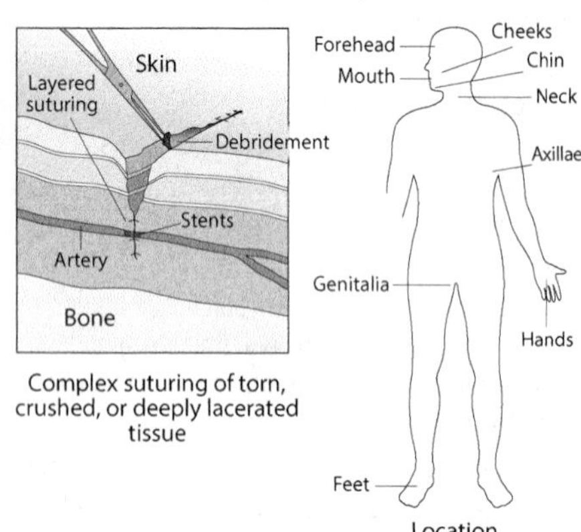

Complex suturing of torn, crushed, or deeply lacerated tissue

ICD-10-CM Diagnostic Codes

	C60.0	Malignant neoplasm of prepuce ♂
	C60.1	Malignant neoplasm of glans penis ♂
	C60.2	Malignant neoplasm of body of penis ♂
	C60.8	Malignant neoplasm of overlapping sites of penis ♂
	C63.8	Malignant neoplasm of overlapping sites of male genital organs ♂
	C79.2	Secondary malignant neoplasm of skin
	C79.82	Secondary malignant neoplasm of genital organs
	D03.59	Melanoma in situ of other part of trunk
	D07.4	Carcinoma in situ of penis ♂
	D07.61	Carcinoma in situ of scrotum ♂
	D07.69	Carcinoma in situ of other male genital organs ♂
	D18.01	Hemangioma of skin and subcutaneous tissue
	D29.0	Benign neoplasm of penis ♂
	D29.4	Benign neoplasm of scrotum ♂
❼	S31.21	Laceration without foreign body of penis
❼	S31.22	Laceration with foreign body of penis
❼	S31.23	Puncture wound without foreign body of penis
❼	S31.24	Puncture wound with foreign body of penis
❼	S31.25	Open bite of penis
❼	S31.31	Laceration without foreign body of scrotum and testes
❼	S31.32	Laceration with foreign body of scrotum and testes
❼	S31.33	Puncture wound without foreign body of scrotum and testes
❼	S31.34	Puncture wound with foreign body of scrotum and testes
❼	S31.35	Open bite of scrotum and testes
❼	S38.232	Partial traumatic amputation of scrotum and testis

ICD-10-CM Coding Notes

For codes requiring a 7th character extension, refer to your ICD-10-CM book. Review the character descriptions and coding guidelines for proper selection. For some procedures, only certain characters will apply.

CCI Edits

Refer to Appendix A for CCI edits.

Facility RVUs ☐

Code	Work	PE Facility	MP	Total Facility
13131	3.73	2.91	0.42	7.06
13132	4.78	3.53	0.52	8.83
13133	2.19	1.21	0.25	3.65

Non-facility RVUs ☐

Code	Work	PE Non-Facility	MP	Total Non-Facility
13131	3.73	7.44	0.42	11.59
13132	4.78	8.77	0.52	14.07
13133	2.19	2.54	0.25	4.98

Modifiers (PAR) ☐

Code	Mod 50	Mod 51	Mod 62	Mod 66	Mod 80
13131	0	2	0	0	1
13132	0	2	0	0	1
13133	0	0	0	0	1

Global Period

Code	Days
13131	010
13132	010
13133	ZZZ

13160

13160 Secondary closure of surgical wound or dehiscence, extensive or complicated

(Do not report 13160 in conjunction with 11960)

(For packing or simple secondary wound closure, see 12020, 12021)

AMA Coding Guideline

Repair-Complex Procedures on the Integumentary System

Reconstructive procedures, complicated wound closure.

Sum of lengths of repairs for each group of anatomic sites.

Surgical Repair (Closure) Procedures on the Integumentary System

Use the codes in this section to designate wound closure utilizing sutures, staples, or tissue adhesives (eg, 2-cyanoacrylate), either singly or in combination with each other, or in combination with adhesive strips. Chemical cauterization, electrocauterization, or wound closure utilizing adhesive strips as the sole repair material are included in the appropriate E/M code.

Definitions

The repair of wounds may be classified as Simple, Intermediate, or Complex.

Simple repair is used when the wound is superficial (eg, involving primarily epidermis or dermis, or subcutaneous tissues without significant involvement of deeper structures) and requires simple one-layer closure. Hemostasis and local or topical anesthesia, when performed, are not reported separately.

Intermediate repair includes the repair of wounds that, in addition to the above, require layered closure of one or more of the deeper layers of subcutaneous tissue and superficial (non-muscle) fascia, in addition to the skin (epidermal and dermal) closure. It includes limited undermining (defined as a distance less than the maximum width of the defect, measured perpendicular to the closure line, along at least one entire edge of the defect). Single-layer closure of heavily contaminated wounds that have required extensive cleaning or removal of particulate matter also constitutes intermediate repair.

Complex repair includes the repair of wounds that, in addition to the requirements for intermediate repair, require at least one of the following: exposure of bone, cartilage, tendon, or named neurovascular structure; debridement of wound edges (eg, traumatic lacerations or avulsions); extensive undermining (defined as a distance greater than or equal to the maximum width of the defect, measured perpendicular to the closure line along at least one entire edge of the defect); involvement of free margins of helical rim, vermilion border, or nostril rim; placement of retention sutures. Necessary preparation includes creation of a limited defect for repairs or the debridement of complicated lacerations or avulsions. Complex repair does not include excision of benign (11400-11446) or malignant (11600-11646) lesions, excisional preparation of a wound bed (15002-15005) or debridement of an open fracture or open dislocation.

Instructions for listing services at time of wound repair:

1. The repaired wound(s) should be measured and recorded in centimeters, whether curved, angular, or stellate.

2. When multiple wounds are repaired, add together the lengths of those in the same classification (see above) and from all anatomic sites that are grouped together into the same code descriptor. For example, add together the lengths of intermediate repairs to the trunk and extremities. Do not add lengths of repairs from different groupings of anatomic sites (eg, face and extremities). Also, do not add together lengths of different classifications (eg, intermediate and complex repairs).

When more than one classification of wounds is repaired, list the more complicated as the primary procedure and the less complicated as the secondary procedure, using modifier 59.

3. Decontamination and/or debridement: Debridement is considered a separate procedure only when gross contamination requires prolonged cleansing, when appreciable amounts of devitalized or contaminated tissue are removed, or when debridement is carried out separately without immediate primary closure.

4. Involvement of nerves, blood vessels and tendons: Report under appropriate system (Nervous, Cardiovascular, Musculoskeletal) for repair of these structures. The repair of these associated wounds is included in the primary procedure unless it qualifies as a complex repair, in which case modifier 59 applies.

Simple ligation of vessels in an open wound is considered as part of any wound closure.

Simple "exploration" of nerves, blood vessels or tendons exposed in an open wound is also considered part of the essential treatment of the wound and is not a separate procedure unless appreciable dissection is required. If the wound requires enlargement, extension of dissection (to determine penetration), debridement, removal of foreign body(s), ligation or coagulation of minor subcutaneous and/or muscular blood vessel(s) of the subcutaneous tissue, muscle fascia, and/or muscle, not requiring thoracotomy or laparotomy, use codes 20100-20103, as appropriate.

AMA Coding Notes

Repair-Complex Procedures on the Integumentary System

(For full thickness repair of lip or eyelid, see respective anatomical subsections)

Surgical Repair (Closure) Procedures on the Integumentary System

(For extensive debridement of soft tissue and/or bone, not associated with open fracture(s) and/or dislocation(s) resulting from penetrating and/or blunt trauma, see 11042-11047.)

(For extensive debridement of subcutaneous tissue, muscle fascia, muscle, and/or bone associated with open fracture(s) and/or dislocation(s), see 11010-11012.)

AMA *CPT® Assistant* ☐

13160: Sep 97: 11, Dec 98: 5, Apr 00: 8, May 11: 4, Dec 12: 6

Plain English Description

Secondary closure of an extensive or complicated surgical wound or wound dehiscence is performed. This procedure covers two scenarios, one in which the surgical wound is not closed at the time of the original surgical procedure, and another in which a surgically closed wound opens along the previous suture line. Secondary surgical wound closure is performed on a date subsequent to the original surgical procedure during a separate surgical session or encounter. The edges of the open surgical wound are trimmed. The deepest layers may be closed with absorbable sutures, and the knot buried followed by closure of superficial layers with non-absorbable sutures. If retention sutures are used to hold the edges of the wound together without tension, they are placed through the entire thickness of the wound, a short length of plastic or rubber tubing is threaded over each suture, and each suture is then tied. Stents may also be used to hold tissue in place or maintain the opening of an orifice. Care is taken to carefully align wound edges to prevent scar depression. Secondary closure of a wound dehiscence is performed on a wound that has opened at the site of the earlier repair. The extent of the wound dehiscence is evaluated. The wound is irrigated with sterile saline or an antibiotic solution. The previously placed sutures are removed and the edges of the wound are trimmed. Any necrotic tissue is debrided. The wound is then repaired as described above.

Secondary closure of complicated surgical wound or dehiscence

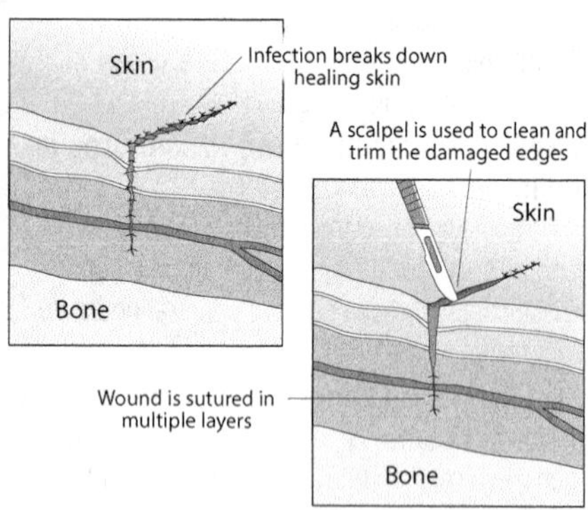
Skin
Infection breaks down healing skin
Bone
A scalpel is used to clean and trim the damaged edges
Skin
Wound is sutured in multiple layers
Bone

ICD-10-CM Diagnostic Codes

➐	T81.30	Disruption of wound, unspecified
➐	T81.31	Disruption of external operation (surgical) wound, not elsewhere classified
➐	T81.32	Disruption of internal operation (surgical) wound, not elsewhere classified
➐	T81.33	Disruption of traumatic injury wound repair
	Z48.1	Encounter for planned postprocedural wound closure

ICD-10-CM Coding Notes

For codes requiring a 7th character extension, refer to your ICD-10-CM book. Review the character descriptions and coding guidelines for proper selection. For some procedures, only certain characters will apply.

CCI Edits

Refer to Appendix A for CCI edits.

Facility RVUs ▯

Code	Work	PE Facility	MP	Total Facility
13160	12.04	9.43	2.09	23.56

Non-facility RVUs ▯

Code	Work	PE Non-Facility	MP	Total Non-Facility
13160	12.04	9.43	2.09	23.56

Modifiers (PAR) ▯

Code	Mod 50	Mod 51	Mod 62	Mod 66	Mod 80
13160	0	2	0	0	1

Global Period

Code	Days
13160	090

17270-17276

17270 Destruction, malignant lesion (eg, laser surgery, electrosurgery, cryosurgery, chemosurgery, surgical curettement), scalp, neck, hands, feet, genitalia; lesion diameter 0.5 cm or less

17271 Destruction, malignant lesion (eg, laser surgery, electrosurgery, cryosurgery, chemosurgery, surgical curettement), scalp, neck, hands, feet, genitalia; lesion diameter 0.6 to 1.0 cm

17272 Destruction, malignant lesion (eg, laser surgery, electrosurgery, cryosurgery, chemosurgery, surgical curettement), scalp, neck, hands, feet, genitalia; lesion diameter 1.1 to 2.0 cm

17273 Destruction, malignant lesion (eg, laser surgery, electrosurgery, cryosurgery, chemosurgery, surgical curettement), scalp, neck, hands, feet, genitalia; lesion diameter 2.1 to 3.0 cm

17274 Destruction, malignant lesion (eg, laser surgery, electrosurgery, cryosurgery, chemosurgery, surgical curettement), scalp, neck, hands, feet, genitalia; lesion diameter 3.1 to 4.0 cm

17276 Destruction, malignant lesion (eg, laser surgery, electrosurgery, cryosurgery, chemosurgery, surgical curettement), scalp, neck, hands, feet, genitalia; lesion diameter over 4.0 cm

AMA Coding Guideline

Destruction Procedures on the Integumentary System

Destruction means the ablation of benign, premalignant or malignant tissues by any method, with or without curettement, including local anesthesia, and not usually requiring closure.

Any method includes electrosurgery, cryosurgery, laser and chemical treatment. Lesions include condylomata, papillomata, molluscum contagiosum, herpetic lesions, warts (ie, common, plantar, flat), milia, or other benign, premalignant (eg, actinic keratoses), or malignant lesions.

AMA Coding Notes

Destruction Procedures on the Integumentary System

(For destruction of lesion(s) in specific anatomic sites, see 40820, 46900-46917, 46924, 54050-54057, 54065, 56501, 56515, 57061, 57065, 67850, 68135)

(For laser treatment for inflammatory skin disease, see 96920-96922)

(For paring or cutting of benign hyperkeratotic lesions (eg, corns or calluses), see 11055-11057)

(For sharp removal or electrosurgical destruction of skin tags and fibrocutaneous tags, see 11200, 11201)

(For cryotherapy of acne, use 17340)

(For initiation or follow-up care of topical chemotherapy (eg, 5-FU or similar agents), see appropriate office visits)

(For shaving of epidermal or dermal lesions, see 11300-11313)

(For excision of cicatricial lesion[s] [eg, full thickness excision, through the dermis], see 11400-11446)

(For incisional removal of burn scar, see 16035, 16036)

(For fractional ablative laser fenestration for functional improvement of traumatic or burn scars, see 0479T, 0480T)

AMA *CPT® Assistant* ☐

17270: Dec 17: 14
17271: Dec 17: 14
17272: Dec 17: 14
17273: Dec 17: 14
17274: Dec 17: 14
17276: Dec 17: 14

Plain English Description

Malignant lesions of the skin include basal cell carcinoma, squamous cell carcinoma, and malignant melanoma. The lesion is examined and the most appropriate form of destruction determined. A local anesthetic is administered as needed. Cryosurgery is performed with liquid nitrogen to freeze the lesion using a series of freeze-thaw cycles. Surgical curettage followed by electrosurgery is another method of destruction. Multiple lesions are more often treated using chemical or pharmacologic agent or laser resurfacing with a carbon dioxide laser. The physician destroys the lesion as well as a surrounding border of normal tissue. Use 17270 for a lesion with diameter of less than 0.5 cm; use 17271 for lesion diameter 0.6-1.0; use 17272 for lesion diameter 1.1-2.0; use 17273 for lesion diameter 2.1-3.0; use 17274 for lesion 3.1-4.0; or use 17276 for lesion diameter over 4.0.

Destruction of a malignant lesion

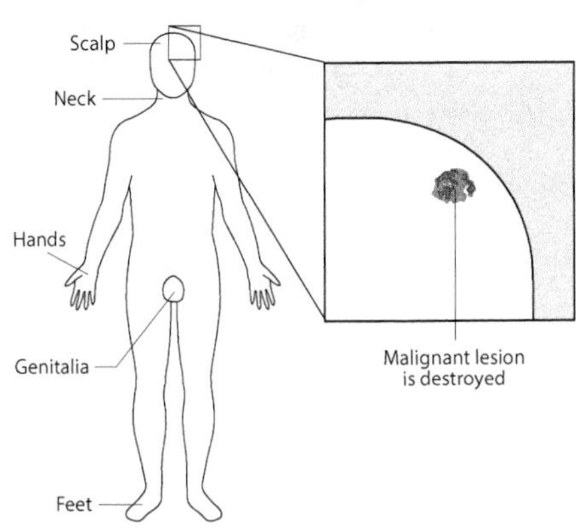

Location of lesion

ICD-10-CM Diagnostic Codes

C51.0	Malignant neoplasm of labium majus ♀
C51.1	Malignant neoplasm of labium minus ♀
C51.2	Malignant neoplasm of clitoris ♀
C51.8	Malignant neoplasm of overlapping sites of vulva ♀
C60.0	Malignant neoplasm of prepuce ♂
C60.1	Malignant neoplasm of glans penis ♂
C60.2	Malignant neoplasm of body of penis ♂
C60.8	Malignant neoplasm of overlapping sites of penis ♂
C63.2	Malignant neoplasm of scrotum ♂
C63.8	Malignant neoplasm of overlapping sites of male genital organs ♂
C79.2	Secondary malignant neoplasm of skin
C79.82	Secondary malignant neoplasm of genital organs

CCI Edits

Refer to Appendix A for CCI edits.

Pub 100

17270: Pub 100-03, 1, 140.5
17271: Pub 100-03, 1, 140.5
17272: Pub 100-03, 1, 140.5
17273: Pub 100-03, 1, 140.5
17274: Pub 100-03, 1, 140.5
17276: Pub 100-03, 1, 140.5

Facility RVUs

Code	Work	PE Facility	MP	Total Facility
17270	1.37	1.25	0.12	2.74
17271	1.54	1.35	0.14	3.03
17272	1.82	1.51	0.19	3.52
17273	2.10	1.67	0.21	3.98
17274	2.64	1.97	0.25	4.86
17276	3.25	2.28	0.33	5.86

Non-facility RVUs

Code	Work	PE Non-Facility	MP	Total Non-Facility
17270	1.37	2.91	0.12	4.40
17271	1.54	3.23	0.14	4.91
17272	1.82	3.59	0.19	5.60
17273	2.10	3.88	0.21	6.19
17274	2.64	4.34	0.25	7.23
17276	3.25	4.83	0.33	8.41

Modifiers (PAR)

Code	Mod 50	Mod 51	Mod 62	Mod 66	Mod 80
17270	0	2	0	0	1
17271	0	2	0	0	1
17272	0	2	0	0	1
17273	0	2	0	0	1
17274	0	2	0	0	1
17276	0	2	0	0	1

Global Period

Code	Days
17270	010
17271	010
17272	010
17273	010
17274	010
17276	010

35800-35860

35800 Exploration for postoperative hemorrhage, thrombosis or infection; neck

35820 Exploration for postoperative hemorrhage, thrombosis or infection; chest

35840 Exploration for postoperative hemorrhage, thrombosis or infection; abdomen

35860 Exploration for postoperative hemorrhage, thrombosis or infection; extremity

AMA Coding Guideline

Surgical Procedures on Arteries and Veins

Primary vascular procedure listings include establishing both inflow and outflow by whatever procedures necessary. Also included is that portion of the operative arteriogram performed by the surgeon, as indicated. Sympathectomy, when done, is included in the listed aortic procedures. For unlisted vascular procedure, use 37799.

Please see the Surgery Guidelines section for the following guidelines:

- *Surgical Procedures on the Cardiovascular System*

AMA *CPT® Assistant*

35840: May 97: 8

35860: Fall 92: 21, Apr 14: 10

Plain English Description

Following a previously performed surgical procedure, the operative wound is re-opened and the surgical site explored for post-operative hemorrhage, thrombosis, or infection. A patient with symptoms indicative of a post-operative hemorrhage, such as low red blood count; thrombosis, such as pain, redness, swelling, and/or shortness of breath; or infection, such as fever, redness, swelling, and/or tenderness over the surgical site is evaluated. If non-surgical measures fail to resolve the symptoms, the patient is returned to the operating room for exploration of the surgical site. The surgical incision is re-opened and thoroughly inspected. Any bleeding is controlled by ligation or cautery. Any blood clots are evacuated. Any evidence of infection is treated by opening abscess pockets and draining pus and fluid. The surgical wound is flushed with normal saline or antibiotic solution. Drains are placed as needed. The surgical wound may be closed or packed with gauze. Use 35800 for post-operative exploration of the neck, 35820 for the chest, 35840 for the abdomen, and 35860 for an extremity.

Exploration for postoperative hemorrhage/thrombosis/infection

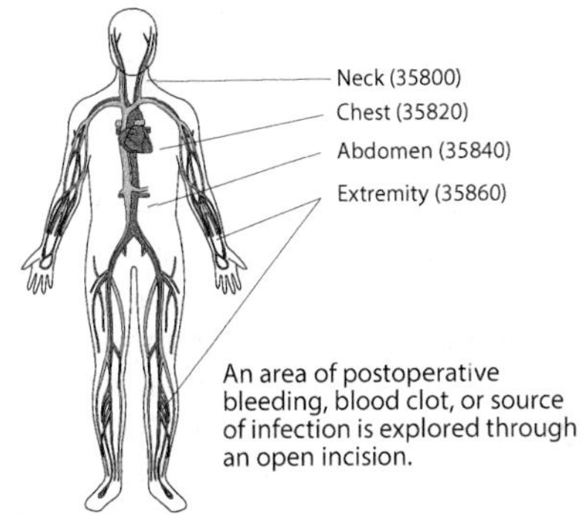

ICD-10-CM Diagnostic Codes

	I77.2	Rupture of artery
	K68.11	Postprocedural retroperitoneal abscess
	N99.510	Cystostomy hemorrhage
	N99.511	Cystostomy infection
	N99.520	Hemorrhage of incontinent external stoma of urinary tract
	N99.521	Infection of incontinent external stoma of urinary tract
	N99.530	Hemorrhage of continent stoma of urinary tract
	N99.531	Infection of continent stoma of urinary tract
	N99.820	Postprocedural hemorrhage of a genitourinary system organ or structure following a genitourinary system procedure
	N99.821	Postprocedural hemorrhage of a genitourinary system organ or structure following other procedure
❼	T81.42	Infection following a procedure, deep incisional surgical site
❼	T81.43	Infection following a procedure, organ and space surgical site
❼	T81.710	Complication of mesenteric artery following a procedure, not elsewhere classified
❼	T81.711	Complication of renal artery following a procedure, not elsewhere classified
❼	T81.718	Complication of other artery following a procedure, not elsewhere classified
❼	T81.719	Complication of unspecified artery following a procedure, not elsewhere classified
❼	T81.72	Complication of vein following a procedure, not elsewhere classified
❼	T88.8	Other specified complications of surgical and medical care, not elsewhere classified

ICD-10-CM Coding Notes

For codes requiring a 7th character extension, refer to your ICD-10-CM book. Review the character descriptions and coding guidelines for proper selection. For some procedures, only certain characters will apply.

CCI Edits

Refer to Appendix A for CCI edits.

Facility RVUs

Code	Work	PE Facility	MP	Total Facility
35800	12.00	7.13	2.38	21.51
35820	36.89	13.51	8.64	59.04
35840	20.75	10.07	4.93	35.75
35860	15.25	5.68	3.74	24.67

Non-facility RVUs

Code	Work	PE Non-Facility	MP	Total Non-Facility
35800	12.00	7.13	2.38	21.51
35820	36.89	13.51	8.64	59.04
35840	20.75	10.07	4.93	35.75
35860	15.25	5.68	3.74	24.67

Modifiers (PAR)

Code	Mod 50	Mod 51	Mod 62	Mod 66	Mod 80
35800	0	2	1	0	2
35820	0	2	1	0	2
35840	0	2	1	0	2
35860	0	2	1	0	2

Global Period

Code	Days
35800	090
35820	090
35840	090
35860	090

36000

36000 Introduction of needle or intracatheter, vein

AMA Coding Guideline

Intravenous Vascular Introduction and Injection Procedures

An intracatheter is a sheathed combination of needle and short catheter.

Vascular Introduction and Injection Procedures

Listed services for injection procedures include necessary local anesthesia, introduction of needles or catheter, injection of contrast media with or without automatic power injection, and/or necessary pre- and postinjection care specifically related to the injection procedure.

Selective vascular catheterization should be coded to include introduction and all lesser order selective catheterization used in the approach (eg, the description for a selective right middle cerebral artery catheterization includes the introduction and placement catheterization of the right common and internal carotid arteries).

Additional second and/or third order arterial catheterization within the same family of arteries or veins supplied by a single first order vessel should be expressed by 36012, 36218, or 36248.

Additional first order or higher catheterization in vascular families supplied by a first order vessel different from a previously selected and coded family should be separately coded using the conventions described above.

Surgical Procedures on Arteries and Veins

Primary vascular procedure listings include establishing both inflow and outflow by whatever procedures necessary. Also included is that portion of the operative arteriogram performed by the surgeon, as indicated. Sympathectomy, when done, is included in the listed aortic procedures. For unlisted vascular procedure, use 37799.

Please see the Surgery Guidelines section for the following guidelines:

- *Surgical Procedures on the Cardiovascular System*

AMA Coding Notes

Vascular Introduction and Injection Procedures

(For radiological supervision and interpretation, see Radiology)

(For injection procedures in conjunction with cardiac catheterization, see 93452-93461, 93563-93568)

(For chemotherapy of malignant disease, see 96401-96549)

AMA *CPT® Assistant* ☐

36000: Summer 95: 2, Apr 98: 1, 3, 7, Jul 98: 1, Apr 03: 26, Oct 03: 2, Jul 06: 4, Feb 07: 10, Jul 07: 1, Dec 08: 7, May 14: 4, Sep 14: 13, Oct 14: 6, Aug 19: 8

Plain English Description

The physician may place a metal needle, such as a butterfly or scalp needle; a plastic catheter mounted on a metal needle, also referred to as a plastic needle; or an intracatheter, which is a catheter inserted through a needle. The planned puncture site is selected and cleansed. The selected device is then introduced into the vein. A butterfly needle can be introduced into smaller veins in the hand. The butterfly shape stabilizes the hub on the skin surface. If a plastic needle is used, the metal tip is introduced into the vein and then removed. The plastic catheter is advanced into the vein. If an intracatheter is used, the metal needle is used to puncture the vein. The catheter is then introduced through the needle into the vein. The needle or intracatheter is secured to the skin with tape.

Introduction of needle or intracatheter, vein

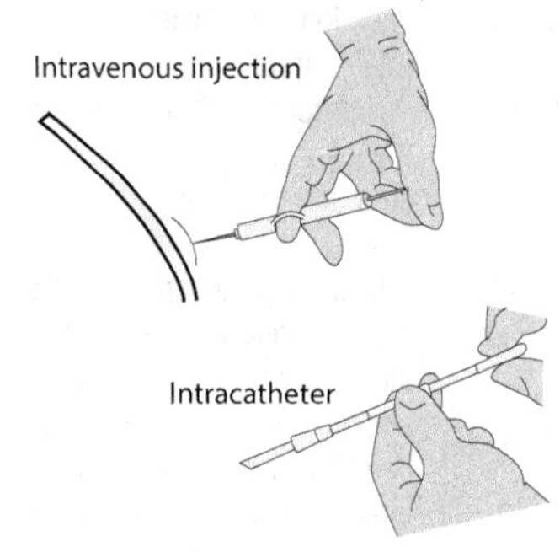

ICD-10-CM Diagnostic Codes

There are too many ICD-10-CM codes to list. Refer to ICD-10-CM code book for associated diagnostic codes.

CCI Edits

Refer to Appendix A for CCI edits.

Pub 100

36000: Pub 100-04, 12, 30.6.12

Facility RVUs ☐

Code	Work	PE Facility	MP	Total Facility
36000	0.18	0.07	0.01	0.26

Non-facility RVUs ☐

Code	Work	PE Non-Facility	MP	Total Non-Facility
36000	0.18	0.70	0.01	0.89

Modifiers (PAR) ☐

Code	Mod 50	Mod 51	Mod 62	Mod 66	Mod 80
36000	9	9	9	9	9

Global Period

Code	Days
36000	XXX

36011-36012

36011 Selective catheter placement, venous system; first order branch (eg, renal vein, jugular vein)

36012 Selective catheter placement, venous system; second order, or more selective, branch (eg, left adrenal vein, petrosal sinus)

AMA Coding Guideline

Intravenous Vascular Introduction and Injection Procedures

An intracatheter is a sheathed combination of needle and short catheter.

Vascular Introduction and Injection Procedures

Listed services for injection procedures include necessary local anesthesia, introduction of needles or catheter, injection of contrast media with or without automatic power injection, and/or necessary pre- and postinjection care specifically related to the injection procedure.

Selective vascular catheterization should be coded to include introduction and all lesser order selective catheterization used in the approach (eg, the description for a selective right middle cerebral artery catheterization includes the introduction and placement catheterization of the right common and internal carotid arteries).

Additional second and/or third order arterial catheterization within the same family of arteries or veins supplied by a single first order vessel should be expressed by 36012, 36218, or 36248.

Additional first order or higher catheterization in vascular families supplied by a first order vessel different from a previously selected and coded family should be separately coded using the conventions described above.

Surgical Procedures on Arteries and Veins

Primary vascular procedure listings include establishing both inflow and outflow by whatever procedures necessary. Also included is that portion of the operative arteriogram performed by the surgeon, as indicated. Sympathectomy, when done, is included in the listed aortic procedures. For unlisted vascular procedure, use 37799.

Please see the Surgery Guidelines section for the following guidelines:

- *Surgical Procedures on the Cardiovascular System*

AMA Coding Notes

Vascular Introduction and Injection Procedures

(For radiological supervision and interpretation, see Radiology)

(For injection procedures in conjunction with cardiac catheterization, see 93452-93461, 93563-93568)

(For chemotherapy of malignant disease, see 96401-96549)

AMA *CPT® Assistant* ▢

36011: Aug 96: 11, Apr 98: 7, Jul 03: 12, Dec 03: 2, Apr 12: 5

36012: Aug 96: 11, Sep 98: 7, Jul 03: 12, Apr 12: 5, Oct 18: 3

Plain English Description

A selective venous catheterization procedure is performed. Common access veins include the brachial and cephalic veins. A small incision is made over the planned puncture site and an introducer sheath placed in the vein. From the brachial or cephalic vein, a guidewire is advanced through the access vein and into the superior vena cava. From there, the catheter is advanced into a venous branch off the superior vena cava, such as the jugular vein, or the catheter may be advanced through the right atrium and into the inferior vena cava and then into a branch off the inferior vena cava, such as the hepatic or renal vein. The catheter may remain in the first-order branch, which is any vein that drains directly into the vena cava, or the catheter may be advanced into a second-order or more selective branch, such as the petrosal sinus or left adrenal vein. Injection of medication and/or radiopaque contrast is performed as needed. Use 36011 for selective catheter placement in a first-order vein branch and 36012 for a second-order or more selective vein branch.

Selective catheter placement, venous system

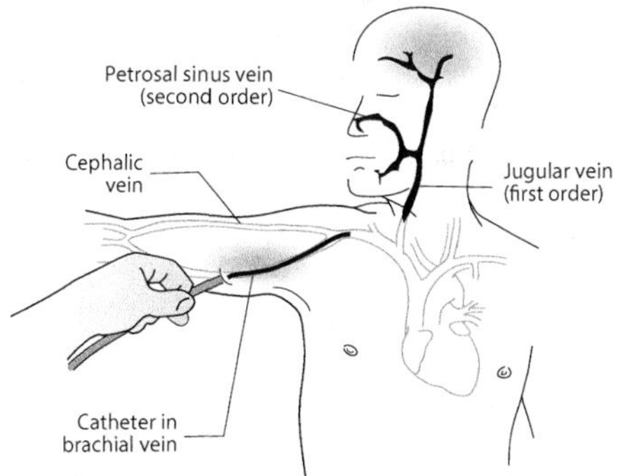

A catheter is placed into first (36011); second (36012) venous order branch.

ICD-10-CM Diagnostic Codes

There are too many ICD-10-CM codes to list. Refer to ICD-10-CM code book for associated diagnostic codes.

CCI Edits

Refer to Appendix A for CCI edits.

Facility RVUs ▢

Code	Work	PE Facility	MP	Total Facility
36011	3.14	0.92	0.52	4.58
36012	3.51	0.98	0.57	5.06

Non-facility RVUs ▢

Code	Work	PE Non-Facility	MP	Total Non-Facility
36011	3.14	21.59	0.52	25.25
36012	3.51	21.75	0.57	25.83

Modifiers (PAR) ▢

Code	Mod 50	Mod 51	Mod 62	Mod 66	Mod 80
36011	1	2	0	0	1
36012	1	2	0	0	1

Global Period

Code	Days
36011	XXX
36012	XXX

36245-36248

36245 Selective catheter placement, arterial system; each first order abdominal, pelvic, or lower extremity artery branch, within a vascular family

36246 Selective catheter placement, arterial system; initial second order abdominal, pelvic, or lower extremity artery branch, within a vascular family

36247 Selective catheter placement, arterial system; initial third order or more selective abdominal, pelvic, or lower extremity artery branch, within a vascular family

+ 36248 Selective catheter placement, arterial system; additional second order, third order, and beyond, abdominal, pelvic, or lower extremity artery branch, within a vascular family (List in addition to code for initial second or third order vessel as appropriate)

(Use 36248 in conjunction with 36246, 36247)

AMA Coding Guideline

Vascular Introduction and Injection Procedures

Listed services for injection procedures include necessary local anesthesia, introduction of needles or catheter, injection of contrast media with or without automatic power injection, and/or necessary pre- and postinjection care specifically related to the injection procedure.

Selective vascular catheterization should be coded to include introduction and all lesser order selective catheterization used in the approach (eg, the description for a selective right middle cerebral artery catheterization includes the introduction and placement catheterization of the right common and internal carotid arteries).

Additional second and/or third order arterial catheterization within the same family of arteries or veins supplied by a single first order vessel should be expressed by 36012, 36218, or 36248.

Additional first order or higher catheterization in vascular families supplied by a first order vessel different from a previously selected and coded family should be separately coded using the conventions described above.

Surgical Procedures on Arteries and Veins

Primary vascular procedure listings include establishing both inflow and outflow by whatever procedures necessary. Also included is that portion of the operative arteriogram performed by the surgeon, as indicated. Sympathectomy, when done, is included in the listed aortic procedures. For unlisted vascular procedure, use 37799.

Please see the Surgery Guidelines section for the following guidelines:

- *Surgical Procedures on the Cardiovascular System*

AMA Coding Notes

Intra-Arterial-Intra-Aortic Vascular Injection Procedures

(For radiological supervision and interpretation, see Radiology)

Vascular Introduction and Injection Procedures

(For radiological supervision and interpretation, see Radiology)

(For injection procedures in conjunction with cardiac catheterization, see 93452-93461, 93563-93568)

(For chemotherapy of malignant disease, see 96401-96549)

AMA *CPT® Assistant* ☐

36245: Fall 93: 15, Aug 96: 3, Jan 01: 14, Jan 07: 7, Dec 07: 10, Jul 11: 5, Oct 11: 9, Apr 12: 4, Nov 13: 14

36246: Fall 93: 15, Aug 96: 3, Jan 01: 14, Jan 07: 7, Dec 07: 10-11, Jul 11: 5, Oct 11: 9, Apr 12: 4, Nov 13: 14

36247: Fall 93: 15, Aug 96: 3, Jan 01: 14, Jan 07: 7, Dec 07: 10, Jul 11: 5, Apr 12: 4, Nov 13: 14, Sep 20: 14

36248: Fall 93: 15, Aug 96: 3, Apr 98: 1, 7, Oct 00: 4, Jan 01: 14, Jan 07: 7, Jul 11: 5, Apr 12: 4, Oct 18: 3

Plain English Description

A selective catheter placement in an abdominal, pelvic, or lower extremity branch of a single vascular family of the arterial system is performed. A catheter is introduced into an extremity artery, with the preferred introduction site being a femoral artery, although an upper extremity artery may also be used. A small skin incision is made over the planned insertion site. An introducer sheath is placed in the artery and a guidewire inserted. If the right femoral artery is used, the guidewire is manipulated through the femoral and iliac arteries and into the aorta. A catheter is advanced over the guidewire into the aorta. The guidewire is advanced as needed and the physician then manipulates the catheter over the guidewire into a first order abdominal, pelvic, or lower extremity branch off the aorta. The physician continues to selectively advance the guidewire and catheter through higher order branches (second, third, and beyond) until the catheter is situated in the highest order branch requiring evaluation. The guidewire is removed. Injection of medication and/or radiopaque contrast media is performed as needed. Use 36245 if a first order branch is the highest order branch catheterized within the vascular family, 36246 if a second order branch is the highest order branch catheterized, 36247 if a third or higher order branch is the highest order branch catheterized. Use 36248 for catheterization of each additional second, third, or higher order abdominal or pelvic, or lower extremity branch within the same vascular family.

Selective catheter placement, arterial system; abdominal/pelvic/lower extremity

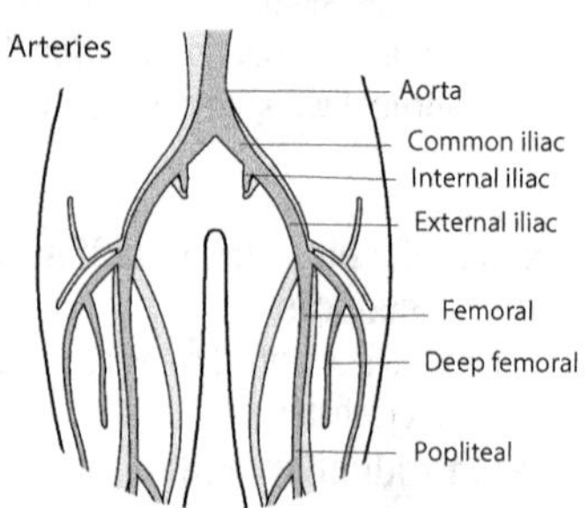

First (36245); initial second (36246); initial third/more selective (32647); additional second/third/beyond (32648) order

ICD-10-CM Diagnostic Codes

There are too many ICD-10-CM codes to list. Refer to ICD-10-CM code book for associated diagnostic codes.

CCI Edits

Refer to Appendix A for CCI edits.

Facility RVUs ☐

Code	Work	PE Facility	MP	Total Facility
36245	4.65	1.42	0.79	6.86
36246	5.02	1.34	1.01	7.37
36247	6.04	1.63	1.02	8.69
36248	1.01	0.28	0.11	1.40

Non-facility RVUs ☐

Code	Work	PE Non-Facility	MP	Total Non-Facility
36245	4.65	33.01	0.79	38.45
36246	5.02	19.75	1.01	25.78
36247	6.04	37.03	1.02	44.09
36248	1.01	2.43	0.11	3.55

Modifiers (PAR) ☐

Code	Mod 50	Mod 51	Mod 62	Mod 66	Mod 80
36245	1	2	0	0	1
36246	1	2	0	0	1
36247	1	2	0	0	1
36248	0	0	0	0	1

Global Period

Code	Days
36245	XXX
36246	000
36247	000
36248	ZZZ

36251-36252

36251 Selective catheter placement (first-order), main renal artery and any accessory renal artery(s) for renal angiography, including arterial puncture and catheter placement(s), fluoroscopy, contrast injection(s), image postprocessing, permanent recording of images, and radiological supervision and interpretation, including pressure gradient measurements when performed, and flush aortogram when performed; unilateral

36252 Selective catheter placement (first-order), main renal artery and any accessory renal artery(s) for renal angiography, including arterial puncture and catheter placement(s), fluoroscopy, contrast injection(s), image postprocessing, permanent recording of images, and radiological supervision and interpretation, including pressure gradient measurements when performed, and flush aortogram when performed; bilateral

AMA Coding Guideline

Vascular Introduction and Injection Procedures

Listed services for injection procedures include necessary local anesthesia, introduction of needles or catheter, injection of contrast media with or without automatic power injection, and/or necessary pre- and postinjection care specifically related to the injection procedure.

Selective vascular catheterization should be coded to include introduction and all lesser order selective catheterization used in the approach (eg, the description for a selective right middle cerebral artery catheterization includes the introduction and placement catheterization of the right common and internal carotid arteries).

Additional second and/or third order arterial catheterization within the same family of arteries or veins supplied by a single first order vessel should be expressed by 36012, 36218, or 36248.

Additional first order or higher catheterization in vascular families supplied by a first order vessel different from a previously selected and coded family should be separately coded using the conventions described above.

Surgical Procedures on Arteries and Veins

Primary vascular procedure listings include establishing both inflow and outflow by whatever procedures necessary. Also included is that portion of the operative arteriogram performed by the surgeon, as indicated. Sympathectomy, when done, is included in the listed aortic procedures. For unlisted vascular procedure, use 37799.

Please see the Surgery Guidelines section for the following guidelines:

- *Surgical Procedures on the Cardiovascular System*

AMA Coding Notes

Intra-Arterial-Intra-Aortic Vascular Injection Procedures

(For radiological supervision and interpretation, see Radiology)

Vascular Introduction and Injection Procedures

(For radiological supervision and interpretation, see Radiology)

(For injection procedures in conjunction with cardiac catheterization, see 93452-93461, 93563-93568)

(For chemotherapy of malignant disease, see 96401-96549)

AMA *CPT® Assistant*

36251: Apr 12: 6, Aug 12: 13, Nov 13: 14
36252: Apr 12: 6

Plain English Description

A selective catheter placement in the main renal artery and any accessory renal arteries is performed for renal angiography. A catheter is introduced into an extremity artery, with the preferred introduction site being a femoral artery in the groin. A small skin incision is made over the planned insertion site. An introducer sheath is placed in the artery and a guidewire is inserted. If the right femoral artery is used, the guidewire is manipulated through the femoral and iliac arteries and into the aorta under fluoroscopic guidance. A catheter is advanced over the guidewire into the aorta. The guidewire is then advanced into the main renal artery and any accessory renal arteries and the physician then manipulates the catheter over the guidewire until the catheter is situated at the desired location. The guidewire is removed. Injection of medication and/or radiopaque contrast media is performed as needed. Pressure gradient measurements may also be obtained to determine if any visualized narrowing in the renal arteries is affecting blood flow to the kidneys. Images are obtained, processed, and permanent recordings are made as needed. The physician reviews the images and recordings and provides a written report of findings. Use 36251 for a selective unilateral renal angiogram. Use 36252 for a selective bilateral study.

Selective catheter placement (first order), renal artery

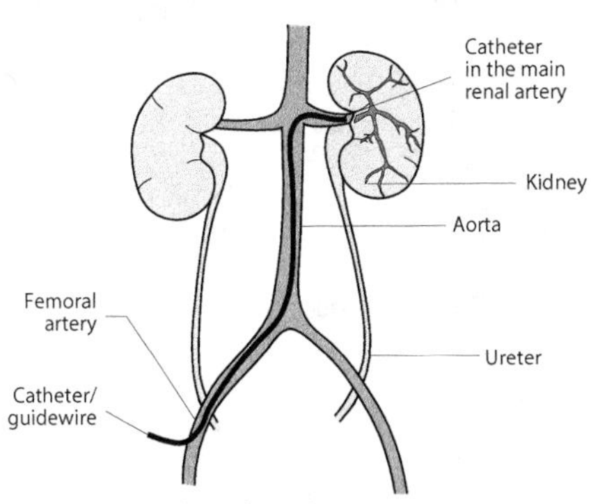

A catheter is brought to the main or an accessory renal artery for angiography. Unilateral (36251); bilateral (36252).

ICD-10-CM Diagnostic Codes

I12.0	Hypertensive chronic kidney disease with stage 5 chronic kidney disease or end stage renal disease
I12.9	Hypertensive chronic kidney disease with stage 1 through stage 4 chronic kidney disease, or unspecified chronic kidney disease
I13.0	Hypertensive heart and chronic kidney disease with heart failure and stage 1 through stage 4 chronic kidney disease, or unspecified chronic kidney disease
I13.10	Hypertensive heart and chronic kidney disease without heart failure, with stage 1 through stage 4 chronic kidney disease, or unspecified chronic kidney disease
I13.11	Hypertensive heart and chronic kidney disease without heart failure, with stage 5 chronic kidney disease, or end stage renal disease
I13.2	Hypertensive heart and chronic kidney disease with heart failure and with stage 5 chronic kidney disease, or end stage renal disease
I15.0	Renovascular hypertension
I15.1	Hypertension secondary to other renal disorders
I70.0	Atherosclerosis of aorta
I70.1	Atherosclerosis of renal artery
I72.2	Aneurysm of renal artery
I75.81	Atheroembolism of kidney
I77.1	Stricture of artery
I77.3	Arterial fibromuscular dysplasia
I77.4	Celiac artery compression syndrome
I77.73	Dissection of renal artery
I82.3	Embolism and thrombosis of renal vein
N05.8	Unspecified nephritic syndrome with other morphologic changes
N08	Glomerular disorders in diseases classified elsewhere
N18.1	Chronic kidney disease, stage 1
N18.2	Chronic kidney disease, stage 2 (mild)
N18.30	Chronic kidney disease, stage 3 unspecified

N18.31	Chronic kidney disease, stage 3a
N18.32	Chronic kidney disease, stage 3b
N18.4	Chronic kidney disease, stage 4 (severe)
N18.5	Chronic kidney disease, stage 5
N18.6	End stage renal disease
N26.9	Renal sclerosis, unspecified
N28.0	Ischemia and infarction of kidney
N28.9	Disorder of kidney and ureter, unspecified
Q27.1	Congenital renal artery stenosis
Q27.2	Other congenital malformations of renal artery

CCI Edits

Refer to Appendix A for CCI edits.

Facility RVUs ▯

Code	Work	PE Facility	MP	Total Facility
36251	5.10	1.49	0.89	7.48
36252	6.74	2.25	1.48	10.47

Non-facility RVUs ▯

Code	Work	PE Non-Facility	MP	Total Non-Facility
36251	5.10	33.88	0.89	39.87
36252	6.74	34.76	1.48	42.98

Modifiers (PAR) ▯

Code	Mod 50	Mod 51	Mod 62	Mod 66	Mod 80
36251	0	2	0	0	1
36252	2	2	0	0	1

Global Period

Code	Days
36251	000
36252	000

36253-36254

36253 Superselective catheter placement (one or more second order or higher renal artery branches) renal artery and any accessory renal artery(s) for renal angiography, including arterial puncture, catheterization, fluoroscopy, contrast injection(s), image postprocessing, permanent recording of images, and radiological supervision and interpretation, including pressure gradient measurements when performed, and flush aortogram when performed; unilateral

(Do not report 36253 in conjunction with 36251 when performed for the same kidney)

36254 Superselective catheter placement (one or more second order or higher renal artery branches) renal artery and any accessory renal artery(s) for renal angiography, including arterial puncture, catheterization, fluoroscopy, contrast injection(s), image postprocessing, permanent recording of images, and radiological supervision and interpretation, including pressure gradient measurements when performed, and flush aortogram when performed; bilateral

(Do not report 36254 in conjunction with 36252)

(Placement of closure device at the vascular access site is not separately reported with 36251-36254)

(Do not report 36251, 36252, 36253, 36254 in conjunction with 0338T, 0339T)

AMA Coding Guideline

Vascular Introduction and Injection Procedures

Listed services for injection procedures include necessary local anesthesia, introduction of needles or catheter, injection of contrast media with or without automatic power injection, and/or necessary pre- and postinjection care specifically related to the injection procedure.

Selective vascular catheterization should be coded to include introduction and all lesser order selective catheterization used in the approach (eg, the description for a selective right middle cerebral artery catheterization includes the introduction and placement catheterization of the right common and internal carotid arteries).

Additional second and/or third order arterial catheterization within the same family of arteries or veins supplied by a single first order vessel should be expressed by 36012, 36218, or 36248. Additional first order or higher catheterization in vascular families supplied by a first order vessel different from a previously selected and coded family should be separately coded using the conventions described above.

Surgical Procedures on Arteries and Veins

Primary vascular procedure listings include establishing both inflow and outflow by whatever procedures necessary. Also included is that portion of the operative arteriogram performed by the surgeon, as indicated. Sympathectomy, when done, is included in the listed aortic procedures. For unlisted vascular procedure, use 37799.

Please see the Surgery Guidelines section for the following guidelines:

- *Surgical Procedures on the Cardiovascular System*

AMA Coding Notes

Intra-Arterial-Intra-Aortic Vascular Injection Procedures

(For radiological supervision and interpretation, see Radiology)

Vascular Introduction and Injection Procedures

(For radiological supervision and interpretation, see Radiology)

(For injection procedures in conjunction with cardiac catheterization, see 93452-93461, 93563-93568)

(For chemotherapy of malignant disease, see 96401-96549)

AMA *CPT® Assistant*

36253: Apr 12: 6, Aug 12: 13, Nov 13: 14
36254: Apr 12: 6, Aug 12: 13

Plain English Description

A super-selective catheter placement in one or more second order or higher renal branches is performed for renal angiography. A catheter is introduced into an extremity artery, with the preferred introduction site being a femoral artery in the groin. A small skin incision is made over the planned insertion site. An introducer sheath is placed in the artery and a guidewire is inserted. If the right femoral artery is used, the guidewire is manipulated through the femoral and iliac arteries and into the aorta under fluoroscopic guidance. A catheter is advanced over the guidewire into the aorta. The guidewire is then advanced into the main renal artery and the physician manipulates the catheter over the guidewire into the main renal artery. The physician continues to selectively advance the guidewire and catheter through higher order branches (second, third, and beyond) until the catheter is situated in the highest order branch requiring evaluation. The guidewire is removed. Injection of medication and/or radiopaque contrast media is performed as needed. Pressure gradient measurements may also be obtained to determine if any visualized narrowing in the renal arteries is affecting blood flow to the kidneys. Images are obtained, processed, and permanent recordings are made as needed. The physician reviews the images and recordings and provides a written report of findings. Use 36253 for a super-selective unilateral renal angiogram. Use 36254 for a super-selective bilateral study.

Superselective catheter placement (second order or higher), renal artery

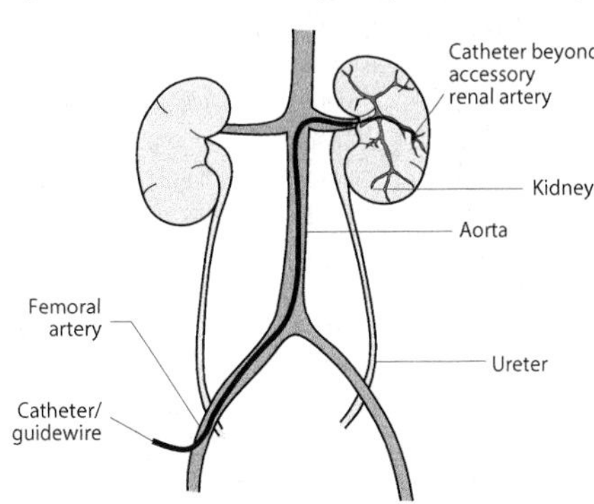

A catheter is brought to second or higher branch renal artery for angiography. Unilateral (36253); bilateral (36254).

ICD-10-CM Diagnostic Codes

I12.0	Hypertensive chronic kidney disease with stage 5 chronic kidney disease or end stage renal disease
I12.9	Hypertensive chronic kidney disease with stage 1 through stage 4 chronic kidney disease, or unspecified chronic kidney disease
I13.0	Hypertensive heart and chronic kidney disease with heart failure and stage 1 through stage 4 chronic kidney disease, or unspecified chronic kidney disease
I13.10	Hypertensive heart and chronic kidney disease without heart failure, with stage 1 through stage 4 chronic kidney disease, or unspecified chronic kidney disease
I13.11	Hypertensive heart and chronic kidney disease without heart failure, with stage 5 chronic kidney disease, or end stage renal disease
I13.2	Hypertensive heart and chronic kidney disease with heart failure and with stage 5 chronic kidney disease, or end stage renal disease
I15.0	Renovascular hypertension
I15.1	Hypertension secondary to other renal disorders
I70.0	Atherosclerosis of aorta
I70.1	Atherosclerosis of renal artery
I72.2	Aneurysm of renal artery
I75.81	Atheroembolism of kidney
I77.1	Stricture of artery
I77.3	Arterial fibromuscular dysplasia
I77.4	Celiac artery compression syndrome

I77.73	Dissection of renal artery
I82.3	Embolism and thrombosis of renal vein
N05.8	Unspecified nephritic syndrome with other morphologic changes
N08	Glomerular disorders in diseases classified elsewhere
N18.1	Chronic kidney disease, stage 1
N18.2	Chronic kidney disease, stage 2 (mild)
N18.30	Chronic kidney disease, stage 3 unspecified
N18.31	Chronic kidney disease, stage 3a
N18.32	Chronic kidney disease, stage 3b
N18.4	Chronic kidney disease, stage 4 (severe)
N18.5	Chronic kidney disease, stage 5
N18.6	End stage renal disease
N28.0	Ischemia and infarction of kidney
N28.9	Disorder of kidney and ureter, unspecified
Q27.1	Congenital renal artery stenosis
Q27.2	Other congenital malformations of renal artery

CCI Edits

Refer to Appendix A for CCI edits.

Facility RVUs 🗆

Code	Work	PE Facility	MP	Total Facility
36253	7.30	2.15	0.85	10.30
36254	7.90	2.50	1.61	12.01

Non-facility RVUs 🗆

Code	Work	PE Non-Facility	MP	Total Non-Facility
36253	7.30	54.16	0.85	62.31
36254	7.90	52.13	1.61	61.64

Modifiers (PAR) 🗆

Code	Mod 50	Mod 51	Mod 62	Mod 66	Mod 80
36253	0	2	0	0	1
36254	2	2	0	0	1

Global Period

Code	Days
36253	000
36254	000

36415-36416

36415 Collection of venous blood by venipuncture

(Do not report modifier 63 in conjunction with 36415)

36416 Collection of capillary blood specimen (eg, finger, heel, ear stick)

AMA Coding Guideline

Venous Procedures

Venipuncture, needle or catheter for diagnostic study or intravenous therapy, percutaneous. These codes are also used to report the therapy as specified. For collection of a specimen from an established catheter, use 36592. For collection of a specimen from a completely implantable venous access device, use 36591.

Vascular Introduction and Injection Procedures

Listed services for injection procedures include necessary local anesthesia, introduction of needles or catheter, injection of contrast media with or without automatic power injection, and/or necessary pre- and postinjection care specifically related to the injection procedure.

Selective vascular catheterization should be coded to include introduction and all lesser order selective catheterization used in the approach (eg, the description for a selective right middle cerebral artery catheterization includes the introduction and placement catheterization of the right common and internal carotid arteries).

Additional second and/or third order arterial catheterization within the same family of arteries or veins supplied by a single first order vessel should be expressed by 36012, 36218, or 36248.

Additional first order or higher catheterization in vascular families supplied by a first order vessel different from a previously selected and coded family should be separately coded using the conventions described above.

Surgical Procedures on Arteries and Veins

Primary vascular procedure listings include establishing both inflow and outflow by whatever procedures necessary. Also included is that portion of the operative arteriogram performed by the surgeon, as indicated. Sympathectomy, when done, is included in the listed aortic procedures. For unlisted vascular procedure, use 37799.

Please see the Surgery Guidelines section for the following guidelines:

- *Surgical Procedures on the Cardiovascular System*

AMA Coding Notes

Vascular Introduction and Injection Procedures

(For radiological supervision and interpretation, see Radiology)

(For injection procedures in conjunction with cardiac catheterization, see 93452-93461, 93563-93568)

(For chemotherapy of malignant disease, see 96401-96549)

AMA *CPT® Assistant* ☐

36415: Jun 96: 10, Mar 98: 10, Oct 99: 11, Aug 00: 2, Feb 07: 10, Jul 07: 1, Dec 08: 7, May 14: 4, Aug 19: 8

Plain English Description

In 36415, an appropriate vein is selected, usually one of the larger antecubital veins such as the median cubital, basilic, or cephalic vein. A tourniquet is placed above the planned puncture site. The site is disinfected with an alcohol pad. A needle is attached to a hub and the vein is punctured. A Vacutainer tube is attached to the hub and the blood specimen is collected. The Vacutainer tube is removed. Depending on the specific blood tests required, multiple Vacutainers may be filled from the same puncture site. In 36416, a blood sample is obtained by capillary puncture usually performed on the fingertip, ear lobe, heel, or toe. Heel and toe sites are typically used only on neonates and infants. The planned puncture site is cleaned with an alcohol pad. A lancet is used to puncture the skin. A drop of blood is allowed to form at the puncture site and is then touched with a capillary tube to collect the specimen.

Collection of blood specimen

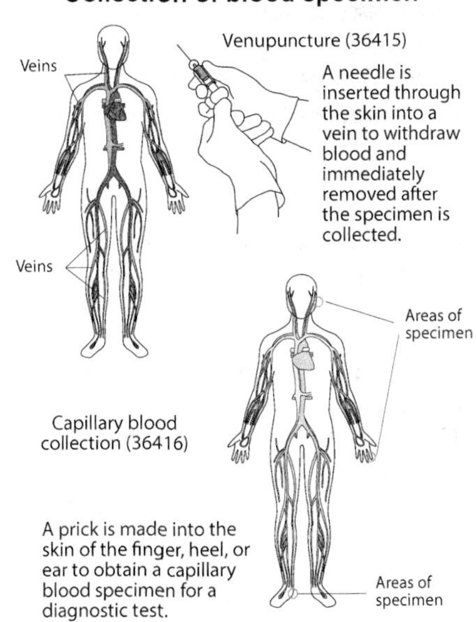

Venupuncture (36415)
Veins
A needle is inserted through the skin into a vein to withdraw blood and immediately removed after the specimen is collected.
Veins
Areas of specimen
Capillary blood collection (36416)
A prick is made into the skin of the finger, heel, or ear to obtain a capillary blood specimen for a diagnostic test.
Areas of specimen

ICD-10-CM Diagnostic Codes

There are too many ICD-10-CM codes to list. Refer to ICD-10-CM code book for associated diagnostic codes.

CCI Edits

Refer to Appendix A for CCI edits.

Pub 100

36415: Pub 100-04, 12, 30.6.12, Pub 100-04, 16, 60.1.4

Facility RVUs ☐

Code	Work	PE Facility	MP	Total Facility
36415	0.00	0.00	0.00	0.00
36416	0.00	0.00	0.00	0.00

Non-facility RVUs ☐

Code	Work	PE Non-Facility	MP	Total Non-Facility
36415	0.00	0.00	0.00	0.00
36416	0.00	0.00	0.00	0.00

Modifiers (PAR) ☐

Code	Mod 50	Mod 51	Mod 62	Mod 66	Mod 80
36415	9	9	9	9	9
36416	9	9	9	9	9

Global Period

Code	Days
36415	XXX
36416	XXX

36593

36593 Declotting by thrombolytic agent of implanted vascular access device or catheter

AMA Coding Guideline

Central Venous Access Procedures

To qualify as a central venous access catheter or device, the tip of the catheter/device must terminate in the subclavian, brachiocephalic (innominate) or iliac veins, the superior or inferior vena cava, or the right atrium. The venous access device may be either centrally inserted (jugular, subclavian, femoral vein or inferior vena cava catheter entry site) or peripherally inserted (eg, basilic, cephalic, or saphenous vein entry site). The device may be accessed for use either via exposed catheter (external to the skin), via a subcutaneous port or via a subcutaneous pump.

The procedures involving these types of devices fall into five categories:

1. Insertion (placement of catheter through a newly established venous access)
2. Repair (fixing device without replacement of either catheter or port/pump, other than pharmacologic or mechanical correction of intracatheter or pericatheter occlusion [see 36595 or 36596])
3. Partial replacement of only the catheter component associated with a port/pump device, but not entire device
4. Complete replacement of entire device via same venous access site (complete exchange)
5. Removal of entire device.

There is no coding distinction between venous access achieved percutaneously versus by cutdown or based on catheter size.

For the repair, partial (catheter only) replacement, complete replacement, or removal of both catheters (placed from separate venous access sites) of a multi-catheter device, with or without subcutaneous ports/pumps, use the appropriate code describing the service with a frequency of two.

If an existing central venous access device is removed and a new one placed via a separate venous access site, appropriate codes for both procedures (removal of old, if code exists, and insertion of new device) should be reported.

When imaging guidance is used for centrally inserted central venous catheters, for gaining access to the venous entry site and/or for manipulating the catheter into final central position, imaging guidance codes (eg, 76937, 77001) may be reported separately. Do not use 76937, 77001 in conjunction with 36568, 36569, 36572, 36573, 36584.

Please see the Surgical Guidelines section for the following table: The Central Venous Access Procedures Table

Vascular Introduction and Injection Procedures

Listed services for injection procedures include necessary local anesthesia, introduction of needles or catheter, injection of contrast media with or without automatic power injection, and/or necessary pre- and postinjection care specifically related to the injection procedure.

Selective vascular catheterization should be coded to include introduction and all lesser order selective catheterization used in the approach (eg, the description for a selective right middle cerebral artery catheterization includes the introduction and placement catheterization of the right common and internal carotid arteries).

Additional second and/or third order arterial catheterization within the same family of arteries or veins supplied by a single first order vessel should be expressed by 36012, 36218, or 36248.

Additional first order or higher catheterization in vascular families supplied by a first order vessel different from a previously selected and coded family should be separately coded using the conventions described above.

Surgical Procedures on Arteries and Veins

Primary vascular procedure listings include establishing both inflow and outflow by whatever procedures necessary. Also included is that portion of the operative arteriogram performed by the surgeon, as indicated. Sympathectomy, when done, is included in the listed aortic procedures. For unlisted vascular procedure, use 37799.

Please see the Surgery Guidelines section for the following guidelines:

- *Surgical Procedures on the Cardiovascular System*

AMA Coding Notes

Central Venous Access Procedures

(For refilling and maintenance of an implantable pump or reservoir for intravenous or intra-arterial drug delivery, use 96522)

Vascular Introduction and Injection Procedures

(For radiological supervision and interpretation, see Radiology)

(For injection procedures in conjunction with cardiac catheterization, see 93452-93461, 93563-93568)

(For chemotherapy of malignant disease, see 96401-96549)

AMA *CPT® Assistant* ▯

36593: Apr 08: 9, Dec 09: 11, Aug 11: 9, Feb 13: 3

Plain English Description

A thrombolytic agent, such as streptokinase, tissue-type plasminogen activator (t-PA), urokinase, or heparin, is instilled into an implanted vascular access device (IVAD) or central venous catheter (CVC) to dissolve a thrombus (blood clot) obstructing the IVAD or catheter. The thrombolytic agent is prepared using the drug manufacturer's protocol. The skin over the IVAD or the catheter hub is cleansed. The thrombolytic agent is instilled into the IVAD or into each lumen of the CVC. The thrombolytic agent is left in the catheter for the required dwell time as indicated by the drug manufacturer. Dwell time may be from 30 to 60 minutes. Patency is checked by attempting to draw blood or infuse fluids. If the IVAD or catheter is still obstructed, a second instillation of the thrombolytic agent may be attempted.

Declotting by thrombolytic agent of implanted vascular access device or catheter

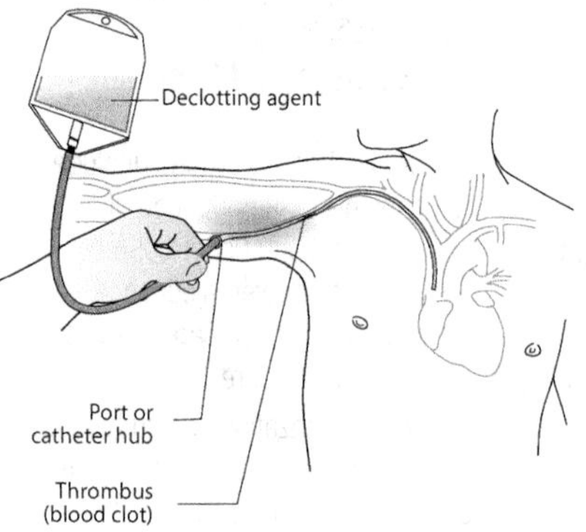

ICD-10-CM Diagnostic Codes

❼	T82.49	Other complication of vascular dialysis catheter
❼	T82.818	Embolism due to vascular prosthetic devices, implants and grafts
❼	T82.868	Thrombosis due to vascular prosthetic devices, implants and grafts
❼	T82.898	Other specified complication of vascular prosthetic devices, implants and grafts
	Z45.2	Encounter for adjustment and management of vascular access device

ICD-10-CM Coding Notes

For codes requiring a 7th character extension, refer to your ICD-10-CM book. Review the character descriptions and coding guidelines for proper selection. For some procedures, only certain characters will apply.

CCI Edits

Refer to Appendix A for CCI edits.

Facility RVUs □

Code	Work	PE Facility	MP	Total Facility
36593	0.00	0.95	0.02	0.97

Non-facility RVUs □

Code	Work	PE Non-Facility	MP	Total Non-Facility
36593	0.00	0.95	0.02	0.97

Modifiers (PAR) □

Code	Mod 50	Mod 51	Mod 62	Mod 66	Mod 80
36593	0	0	0	0	0

Global Period

Code	Days
36593	XXX

CPT® Procedural Coding

36600

36600 Arterial puncture, withdrawal of blood for diagnosis

AMA Coding Guideline

Surgical Procedures on Arteries and Veins

Primary vascular procedure listings include establishing both inflow and outflow by whatever procedures necessary. Also included is that portion of the operative arteriogram performed by the surgeon, as indicated. Sympathectomy, when done, is included in the listed aortic procedures. For unlisted vascular procedure, use 37799.

Please see the Surgery Guidelines section for the following guidelines:

- *Surgical Procedures on the Cardiovascular System*

AMA *CPT® Assistant* ▯

36600: Fall 95: 7, Aug 00: 2, Oct 03: 2, Jul 05: 11, Jul 06: 4, Feb 07: 10, Jul 07: 1, May 14: 4, Aug 19: 8

Plain English Description

The radial artery is the most common site for arterial puncture, with alternative sites being the axillary and femoral arteries. The arterial puncture site is selected. The skin is prepared for sterile entry. The selected artery is punctured and the necessary blood samples obtained for separately reportable laboratory studies. The needle is withdrawn and pressure applied to the puncture site.

Arterial puncture, for blood sampling

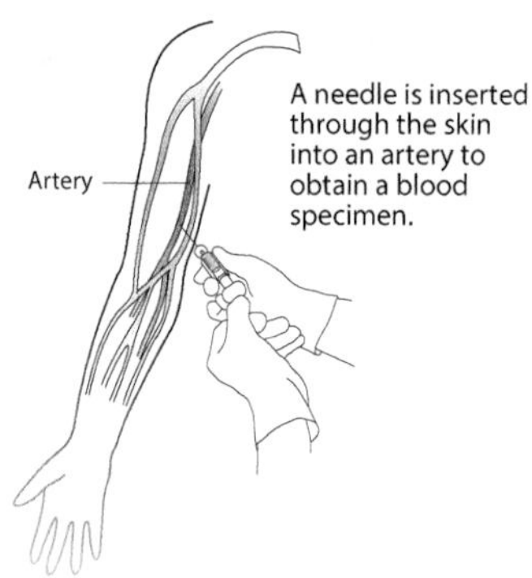
Artery
A needle is inserted through the skin into an artery to obtain a blood specimen.

ICD-10-CM Diagnostic Codes

There are too many ICD-10-CM codes to list. Refer to ICD-10-CM code book for associated diagnostic codes.

CCI Edits

Refer to Appendix A for CCI edits.

Pub 100

36600: Pub 100-04, 12, 30.6.12

Facility RVUs ▯

Code	Work	PE Facility	MP	Total Facility
36600	0.32	0.10	0.04	0.46

Non-facility RVUs ▯

Code	Work	PE Non-Facility	MP	Total Non-Facility
36600	0.32	0.49	0.04	0.85

Modifiers (PAR) ▯

Code	Mod 50	Mod 51	Mod 62	Mod 66	Mod 80
36600	0	2	0	0	1

Global Period

Code	Days
36600	XXX

36800-36815

36800 Insertion of cannula for hemodialysis, other purpose (separate procedure); vein to vein

36810 Insertion of cannula for hemodialysis, other purpose (separate procedure); arteriovenous, external (Scribner type)

36815 Insertion of cannula for hemodialysis, other purpose (separate procedure); arteriovenous, external revision, or closure

AMA Coding Guideline

Surgical Procedures on Arteries and Veins

Primary vascular procedure listings include establishing both inflow and outflow by whatever procedures necessary. Also included is that portion of the operative arteriogram performed by the surgeon, as indicated. Sympathectomy, when done, is included in the listed aortic procedures. For unlisted vascular procedure, use 37799.

Please see the Surgery Guidelines section for the following guidelines:

- *Surgical Procedures on the Cardiovascular System*

AMA *CPT® Assistant* ▯

36800: Fall 93: 3
36810: Fall 93: 3, May 97: 10
36815: Fall 93: 3

Plain English Description

A cannula is inserted for hemodialysis, or other purpose. In 36800, two suitable veins are selected. Veins in the nondominant forearm are preferred. The blood vessels are exposed and incised. One cannula is inserted into the first vein and another into the second vein. The cannulas are secured with sutures. The distal segments of the selected veins are ligated. The two cannulas are connected with synthetic material, which may be partially or completely buried. During dialysis, the cannulas are connected to tubing that is directly connected to the dialysis machine. In 36810, an external Scribner-type arteriovenous cannula is inserted. The Scribner-type cannula is a semi-permanent arteriovenous hemodialysis shunt that is rarely used today. A suitable peripheral artery and vein are selected, usually the radial artery and cephalic vein at the wrist or the tibial artery and saphenous vein at the ankle. The blood vessels are exposed and incised. One cannula is inserted into the selected artery and another into the selected vein. The cannulas are secured with sutures. The distal segments of the selected artery and vein are ligated. The two cannulas are externally connected with a rigid piece of Teflon or other synthetic material placed over a stainless steel arm plate when not in use. During dialysis the Teflon segment is removed and the cannulas are connected to tubing that is directly connected to the dialysis machine. Use 36810 for the initial placement of the shunt. Use 36815 for external revision or closure of the shunt. If the shunt is revised, one or both cannulas are removed and new cannulas inserted. To close the shunt, the skin over the cannulas is opened and the cannulas are exposed. Securing sutures are cut and the cannulas are removed. The vessels are sutured closed and the skin over the cannula sites is closed.

ICD-10-CM Diagnostic Codes

	A41.9	Sepsis, unspecified organism
	E08.22	Diabetes mellitus due to underlying condition with diabetic chronic kidney disease
	E09.22	Drug or chemical induced diabetes mellitus with diabetic chronic kidney disease
	E10.22	Type 1 diabetes mellitus with diabetic chronic kidney disease
	E11.22	Type 2 diabetes mellitus with diabetic chronic kidney disease
	E13.22	Other specified diabetes mellitus with diabetic chronic kidney disease
	I12.0	Hypertensive chronic kidney disease with stage 5 chronic kidney disease or end stage renal disease
	I13.11	Hypertensive heart and chronic kidney disease without heart failure, with stage 5 chronic kidney disease, or end stage renal disease
	I13.2	Hypertensive heart and chronic kidney disease with heart failure and with stage 5 chronic kidney disease, or end stage renal disease
	M35.04	Sjögren syndrome with tubulo-interstitial nephropathy
	M35.81	Multisystem inflammatory syndrome
	N00.2	Acute nephritic syndrome with diffuse membranous glomerulonephritis
	N00.3	Acute nephritic syndrome with diffuse mesangial proliferative glomerulonephritis
	N00.4	Acute nephritic syndrome with diffuse endocapillary proliferative glomerulonephritis
	N00.5	Acute nephritic syndrome with diffuse mesangiocapillary glomerulonephritis
	N00.6	Acute nephritic syndrome with dense deposit disease
	N00.7	Acute nephritic syndrome with diffuse crescentic glomerulonephritis
	N00.8	Acute nephritic syndrome with other morphologic changes
	N01.2	Rapidly progressive nephritic syndrome with diffuse membranous glomerulonephritis
	N01.3	Rapidly progressive nephritic syndrome with diffuse mesangial proliferative glomerulonephritis
	N01.4	Rapidly progressive nephritic syndrome with diffuse endocapillary proliferative glomerulonephritis
	N01.5	Rapidly progressive nephritic syndrome with diffuse mesangiocapillary glomerulonephritis
	N01.6	Rapidly progressive nephritic syndrome with dense deposit disease
	N01.7	Rapidly progressive nephritic syndrome with diffuse crescentic glomerulonephritis
	N01.8	Rapidly progressive nephritic syndrome with other morphologic changes
	N03.2	Chronic nephritic syndrome with diffuse membranous glomerulonephritis
	N03.3	Chronic nephritic syndrome with diffuse mesangial proliferative glomerulonephritis
	N03.4	Chronic nephritic syndrome with diffuse endocapillary proliferative glomerulonephritis
	N03.5	Chronic nephritic syndrome with diffuse mesangiocapillary glomerulonephritis
	N03.6	Chronic nephritic syndrome with dense deposit disease
	N03.7	Chronic nephritic syndrome with diffuse crescentic glomerulonephritis
	N03.8	Chronic nephritic syndrome with other morphologic changes
	N08	Glomerular disorders in diseases classified elsewhere
	N10	Acute pyelonephritis
	N11.0	Nonobstructive reflux-associated chronic pyelonephritis
	N11.1	Chronic obstructive pyelonephritis
	N16	Renal tubulo-interstitial disorders in diseases classified elsewhere
	N17.0	Acute kidney failure with tubular necrosis
	N17.1	Acute kidney failure with acute cortical necrosis
	N17.2	Acute kidney failure with medullary necrosis
	N17.8	Other acute kidney failure
	N17.9	Acute kidney failure, unspecified
	N18.4	Chronic kidney disease, stage 4 (severe)
	N18.5	Chronic kidney disease, stage 5
	N18.6	End stage renal disease
	N28.0	Ischemia and infarction of kidney
	R65.11	Systemic inflammatory response syndrome (SIRS) of non-infectious origin with acute organ dysfunction
	R65.20	Severe sepsis without septic shock
	R65.21	Severe sepsis with septic shock
❼⇄	S37.061	Major laceration of right kidney
❼⇄	S37.062	Major laceration of left kidney
❼	T79.5	Traumatic anuria

ICD-10-CM Coding Notes

For codes requiring a 7th character extension, refer to your ICD-10-CM book. Review the character descriptions and coding guidelines for proper selection. For some procedures, only certain characters will apply.

CCI Edits

Refer to Appendix A for CCI edits.

Facility RVUs ▯

Code	Work	PE Facility	MP	Total Facility
36800	2.43	0.85	0.29	3.57
36810	3.96	1.79	0.43	6.18
36815	2.62	0.69	0.65	3.96

Non-facility RVUs ▯

Code	Work	PE Non-Facility	MP	Total Non-Facility
36800	2.43	0.85	0.29	3.57
36810	3.96	1.79	0.43	6.18
36815	2.62	0.69	0.65	3.96

Modifiers (PAR) ▯

Code	Mod 50	Mod 51	Mod 62	Mod 66	Mod 80
36800	0	2	0	0	1
36810	0	2	0	0	1
36815	0	2	0	0	1

Global Period

Code	Days
36800	000
36810	000
36815	000

36818-36820

36818 Arteriovenous anastomosis, open; by upper arm cephalic vein transposition

(Do not report 36818 in conjunction with 36819, 36820, 36821, 36830 during a unilateral upper extremity procedure. For bilateral upper extremity open arteriovenous anastomoses performed at the same operative session, use modifier 50 or 59 as appropriate)

36819 Arteriovenous anastomosis, open; by upper arm basilic vein transposition

(Do not report 36819 in conjunction with 36818, 36820, 36821, 36830 during a unilateral upper extremity procedure. For bilateral upper extremity open arteriovenous anastomoses performed at the same operative session, use modifier 50 or 59 as appropriate)

36820 Arteriovenous anastomosis, open; by forearm vein transposition

AMA Coding Guideline

Surgical Procedures on Arteries and Veins

Primary vascular procedure listings include establishing both inflow and outflow by whatever procedures necessary. Also included is that portion of the operative arteriogram performed by the surgeon, as indicated. Sympathectomy, when done, is included in the listed aortic procedures. For unlisted vascular procedure, use 37799.

Please see the Surgery Guidelines section for the following guidelines:

- *Surgical Procedures on the Cardiovascular System*

AMA *CPT® Assistant* ▯

36818: Jul 05: 9, Mar 16: 10, Mar 17: 5
36819: Nov 99: 20, Jul 05: 9, Mar 17: 5
36820: Fall 93: 4, Jul 05: 9, Mar 17: 5

Plain English Description

An open arteriovenous anastomosis is performed to provide hemodialysis access by upper arm cephalic vein transposition (36818), upper arm basilic vein transposition (36819), or forearm vein transposition (36820). In 36818, an incision is made medially in the upper arm to expose the brachial artery and a second incision is made laterally to expose the cephalic vein. The cephalic vein is assessed to ensure that it is patent and of adequate size. A subcutaneous tunnel is then created between the two incisions. The cephalic vein is mobilized and branches ligated. The mobilized segment of cephalic vein is transected, taking care to ensure that it is of adequate length for transposition to a more superficial location and tunneling to the brachial artery. The cephalic vein is pulled through the tunnel. An incision is made in the brachial artery and the segment of cephalic vein sutured (anastomosed) to the brachial artery at the arteriotomy site. In 36819, an incision is made in the medial upper arm and the basilic vein and brachial artery exposed. The basilic vein is assessed and if it is found to be patent and of adequate size, the excision is extended, exposing the entire basilic vein up to the point where it joins the axillary vein. The basilic vein is then transected near the elbow, branches are ligated, and the basilic vein is transposed and tunneled subcutaneously to the point where it will be connected to the brachial artery. An incision is made in the brachial artery and the transposed segment of basilic vein is anastomosed to the brachial artery at the arteriotomy site. In 36820, the basilic vein is mobilized from the level of the wrist to the middle of the forearm, transposed and tunneled subcutaneously, and then connected to the radial artery or less commonly to the ulnar artery.

Arteriovenous anastomosis, open cephalic/basilic/forearm vein

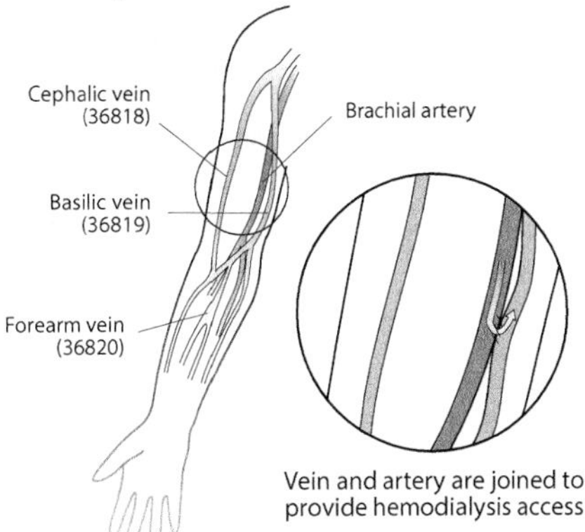

ICD-10-CM Diagnostic Codes

E08.22	Diabetes mellitus due to underlying condition with diabetic chronic kidney disease
E09.22	Drug or chemical induced diabetes mellitus with diabetic chronic kidney disease
E10.22	Type 1 diabetes mellitus with diabetic chronic kidney disease
E11.22	Type 2 diabetes mellitus with diabetic chronic kidney disease
E13.22	Other specified diabetes mellitus with diabetic chronic kidney disease
I12.0	Hypertensive chronic kidney disease with stage 5 chronic kidney disease or end stage renal disease
I13.11	Hypertensive heart and chronic kidney disease without heart failure, with stage 5 chronic kidney disease, or end stage renal disease
I13.2	Hypertensive heart and chronic kidney disease with heart failure and with stage 5 chronic kidney disease, or end stage renal disease
I82.3	Embolism and thrombosis of renal vein
M35.04	Sjögren syndrome with tubulo-interstitial nephropathy
M35.81	Multisystem inflammatory syndrome
N00.2	Acute nephritic syndrome with diffuse membranous glomerulonephritis
N00.3	Acute nephritic syndrome with diffuse mesangial proliferative glomerulonephritis
N00.4	Acute nephritic syndrome with diffuse endocapillary proliferative glomerulonephritis
N00.5	Acute nephritic syndrome with diffuse mesangiocapillary glomerulonephritis
N00.6	Acute nephritic syndrome with dense deposit disease
N00.7	Acute nephritic syndrome with diffuse crescentic glomerulonephritis
N00.8	Acute nephritic syndrome with other morphologic changes
N01.2	Rapidly progressive nephritic syndrome with diffuse membranous glomerulonephritis
N01.3	Rapidly progressive nephritic syndrome with diffuse mesangial proliferative glomerulonephritis
N01.4	Rapidly progressive nephritic syndrome with diffuse endocapillary proliferative glomerulonephritis
N01.5	Rapidly progressive nephritic syndrome with diffuse mesangiocapillary glomerulonephritis
N01.6	Rapidly progressive nephritic syndrome with dense deposit disease
N01.7	Rapidly progressive nephritic syndrome with diffuse crescentic glomerulonephritis
N01.8	Rapidly progressive nephritic syndrome with other morphologic changes
N03.2	Chronic nephritic syndrome with diffuse membranous glomerulonephritis
N03.3	Chronic nephritic syndrome with diffuse mesangial proliferative glomerulonephritis
N03.4	Chronic nephritic syndrome with diffuse endocapillary proliferative glomerulonephritis
N03.5	Chronic nephritic syndrome with diffuse mesangiocapillary glomerulonephritis
N03.6	Chronic nephritic syndrome with dense deposit disease
N03.7	Chronic nephritic syndrome with diffuse crescentic glomerulonephritis
N03.8	Chronic nephritic syndrome with other morphologic changes
N08	Glomerular disorders in diseases classified elsewhere

	N11.0	Nonobstructive reflux-associated chronic pyelonephritis
	N11.1	Chronic obstructive pyelonephritis
	N11.8	Other chronic tubulo-interstitial nephritis
	N16	Renal tubulo-interstitial disorders in diseases classified elsewhere
	N17.0	Acute kidney failure with tubular necrosis
	N17.1	Acute kidney failure with acute cortical necrosis
	N17.2	Acute kidney failure with medullary necrosis
	N17.8	Other acute kidney failure
	N18.4	Chronic kidney disease, stage 4 (severe)
	N18.5	Chronic kidney disease, stage 5
	N18.6	End stage renal disease
	N28.0	Ischemia and infarction of kidney
	R65.11	Systemic inflammatory response syndrome (SIRS) of non-infectious origin with acute organ dysfunction
	R65.20	Severe sepsis without septic shock
	R65.21	Severe sepsis with septic shock
❼⇄	S37.061	Major laceration of right kidney
❼⇄	S37.062	Major laceration of left kidney
❼	T79.5	Traumatic anuria

ICD-10-CM Coding Notes

For codes requiring a 7th character extension, refer to your ICD-10-CM book. Review the character descriptions and coding guidelines for proper selection. For some procedures, only certain characters will apply.

CCI Edits

Refer to Appendix A for CCI edits.

Facility RVUs ▢

Code	Work	PE Facility	MP	Total Facility
36818	12.39	4.83	3.04	20.26
36819	13.29	4.90	3.29	21.48
36820	13.07	4.88	3.18	21.13

Non-facility RVUs ▢

Code	Work	PE Non-Facility	MP	Total Non-Facility
36818	12.39	4.83	3.04	20.26
36819	13.29	4.90	3.29	21.48
36820	13.07	4.88	3.18	21.13

Modifiers (PAR) ▢

Code	Mod 50	Mod 51	Mod 62	Mod 66	Mod 80
36818	0	2	1	0	2
36819	0	2	1	0	2
36820	1	2	1	0	2

Global Period

Code	Days
36818	090
36819	090
36820	090

36821

36821 Arteriovenous anastomosis, open; direct, any site (eg, Cimino type) (separate procedure)

AMA Coding Guideline

Surgical Procedures on Arteries and Veins

Primary vascular procedure listings include establishing both inflow and outflow by whatever procedures necessary. Also included is that portion of the operative arteriogram performed by the surgeon, as indicated. Sympathectomy, when done, is included in the listed aortic procedures. For unlisted vascular procedure, use 37799.

Please see the Surgery Guidelines section for the following guidelines:

- *Surgical Procedures on the Cardiovascular System*

AMA *CPT® Assistant*

36821: Fall 93: 3, Feb 97: 2, Nov 99: 20, Jul 05: 9, Aug 15: 8, Mar 17: 5

Plain English Description

A direct arteriovenous anastomosis is performed using an open technique to provide hemodialysis access. This procedure may also be referred to as a Cimino-type arteriovenous anastomosis or Cimino fistula. The most common site for construction of a Cimino fistula is at the wrist, but other sites in the arm may be used. This procedure is typically performed using a local infiltration anesthetic or a brachial plexus nerve block. The arm pulses are palpated and a blood pressure cuff is applied to the upper arm to restrict blood flow. The veins are marked using indelible ink. A longitudinal incision is made in the skin to expose the radial artery. The cephalic vein is dissected free of subcutaneous fat and any tributaries are ligated. The vein is positioned next to the radial artery, which is then mobilized. The artery and vein are then connected (anastomosed) in one of four configurations including side-to-side, arterial end to vein side, vein end to arterial side, or end-to-end. A fistula is created by incising the vein and/or artery depending on the configuration used and suturing the vein and artery together.

Arteriovenous anastomosis, open; direct, any site

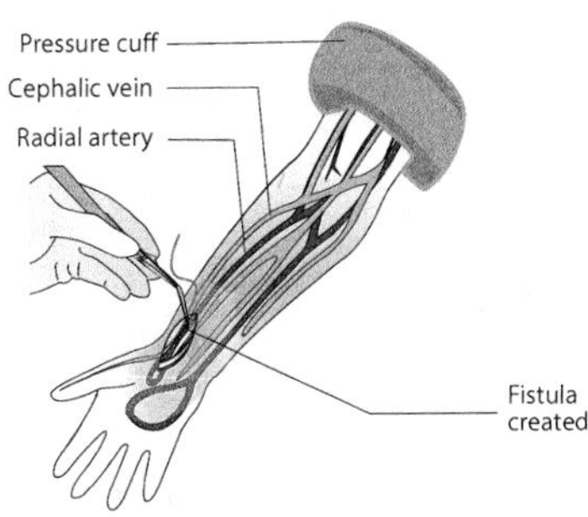

ICD-10-CM Diagnostic Codes

	E08.22	Diabetes mellitus due to underlying condition with diabetic chronic kidney disease
	E09.22	Drug or chemical induced diabetes mellitus with diabetic chronic kidney disease
	E10.22	Type 1 diabetes mellitus with diabetic chronic kidney disease
	E11.22	Type 2 diabetes mellitus with diabetic chronic kidney disease
	E13.22	Other specified diabetes mellitus with diabetic chronic kidney disease
	I12.0	Hypertensive chronic kidney disease with stage 5 chronic kidney disease or end stage renal disease
	I13.11	Hypertensive heart and chronic kidney disease without heart failure, with stage 5 chronic kidney disease, or end stage renal disease
	I13.2	Hypertensive heart and chronic kidney disease with heart failure and with stage 5 chronic kidney disease, or end stage renal disease
	I82.3	Embolism and thrombosis of renal vein
	M35.04	Sjögren syndrome with tubulo-interstitial nephropathy
	M35.81	Multisystem inflammatory syndrome
	N00.2	Acute nephritic syndrome with diffuse membranous glomerulonephritis
	N00.3	Acute nephritic syndrome with diffuse mesangial proliferative glomerulonephritis
	N00.4	Acute nephritic syndrome with diffuse endocapillary proliferative glomerulonephritis
	N00.5	Acute nephritic syndrome with diffuse mesangiocapillary glomerulonephritis
	N00.6	Acute nephritic syndrome with dense deposit disease
	N00.7	Acute nephritic syndrome with diffuse crescentic glomerulonephritis
	N00.8	Acute nephritic syndrome with other morphologic changes
	N01.2	Rapidly progressive nephritic syndrome with diffuse membranous glomerulonephritis
	N01.3	Rapidly progressive nephritic syndrome with diffuse mesangial proliferative glomerulonephritis
	N01.4	Rapidly progressive nephritic syndrome with diffuse endocapillary proliferative glomerulonephritis
	N01.5	Rapidly progressive nephritic syndrome with diffuse mesangiocapillary glomerulonephritis
	N01.6	Rapidly progressive nephritic syndrome with dense deposit disease
	N01.7	Rapidly progressive nephritic syndrome with diffuse crescentic glomerulonephritis
	N01.8	Rapidly progressive nephritic syndrome with other morphologic changes
	N03.2	Chronic nephritic syndrome with diffuse membranous glomerulonephritis
	N03.3	Chronic nephritic syndrome with diffuse mesangial proliferative glomerulonephritis
	N03.4	Chronic nephritic syndrome with diffuse endocapillary proliferative glomerulonephritis
	N03.5	Chronic nephritic syndrome with diffuse mesangiocapillary glomerulonephritis
	N03.6	Chronic nephritic syndrome with dense deposit disease
	N03.7	Chronic nephritic syndrome with diffuse crescentic glomerulonephritis
	N03.8	Chronic nephritic syndrome with other morphologic changes
	N08	Glomerular disorders in diseases classified elsewhere
	N11.0	Nonobstructive reflux-associated chronic pyelonephritis
	N11.1	Chronic obstructive pyelonephritis
	N16	Renal tubulo-interstitial disorders in diseases classified elsewhere
	N17.0	Acute kidney failure with tubular necrosis
	N17.2	Acute kidney failure with medullary necrosis
	N17.8	Other acute kidney failure
	N18.4	Chronic kidney disease, stage 4 (severe)
	N18.5	Chronic kidney disease, stage 5
	N18.6	End stage renal disease
	N28.0	Ischemia and infarction of kidney
	R65.11	Systemic inflammatory response syndrome (SIRS) of non-infectious origin with acute organ dysfunction
	R65.20	Severe sepsis without septic shock
	R65.21	Severe sepsis with septic shock
❼⇄	S37.061	Major laceration of right kidney
❼⇄	S37.062	Major laceration of left kidney
❼	T79.5	Traumatic anuria

ICD-10-CM Coding Notes

For codes requiring a 7th character extension, refer to your ICD-10-CM book. Review the character descriptions and coding guidelines for proper selection. For some procedures, only certain characters will apply.

CCI Edits

Refer to Appendix A for CCI edits.

Facility RVUs

Code	Work	PE Facility	MP	Total Facility
36821	11.90	4.63	2.94	19.47

Non-facility RVUs

Code	Work	PE Non-Facility	MP	Total Non-Facility
36821	11.90	4.63	2.94	19.47

Modifiers (PAR)

Code	Mod 50	Mod 51	Mod 62	Mod 66	Mod 80
36821	0	2	1	0	2

Global Period

Code	Days
36821	090

36825-36830

36825 Creation of arteriovenous fistula by other than direct arteriovenous anastomosis (separate procedure); autogenous graft

(For direct arteriovenous anastomosis, use 36821)

36830 Creation of arteriovenous fistula by other than direct arteriovenous anastomosis (separate procedure); nonautogenous graft (eg, biological collagen, thermoplastic graft)

(For direct arteriovenous anastomosis, use 36821)

AMA Coding Guideline

Surgical Procedures on Arteries and Veins

Primary vascular procedure listings include establishing both inflow and outflow by whatever procedures necessary. Also included is that portion of the operative arteriogram performed by the surgeon, as indicated. Sympathectomy, when done, is included in the listed aortic procedures. For unlisted vascular procedure, use 37799.

Please see the Surgery Guidelines section for the following guidelines:

- *Surgical Procedures on the Cardiovascular System*

AMA *CPT® Assistant*

36825: Fall 93: 3, Feb 97: 2, Jul 05: 9, Mar 17: 5

36830: Fall 93: 3, Feb 97: 2, Jul 05: 9, Jan 15: 13, Mar 17: 5

Plain English Description

The physician creates an arteriovenous (AV) fistula using a technique other than direct arteriovenous anastomosis. An AV fistula is an artificial connection between a vein and an artery, which is created to allow repeated long-term access to the vascular system for hemodialysis. An incision is made in the forearm over the planned AV fistula site. An artery and vein are selected, exposed, and dissected free of surrounding tissue. Vessel loops are placed around the vein and artery to control blood flow. If an autogenous graft is used, a vein segment is harvested, usually from the saphenous vein. An incision is made in the skin of the leg over the section of saphenous vein to be harvested. Soft tissue is dissected off the vein and branches are ligated and divided. The section of saphenous vein to be used is then ligated proximally and distally, divided, and removed from the leg. Alternatively, a nonautogenous graft, such as biological collagen or thermoplastic graft material, may be used. The artery is incised and the graft sutured to the artery. The vein is then incised and the other end of the graft is sutured to the vein. Vessel loops are released and hemostasis checked. Once the artery and vein are joined by the graft, blood flow through to the vein will increase, causing it to become larger and thicker so that it can withstand repeated punctures for vascular access. Use 36825 for AV fistula creation using an autogenous graft and 36830 when a nonautogenous graft is used.

Creation of arteriovenous fistula by other than direct arteriovenous anastomosis

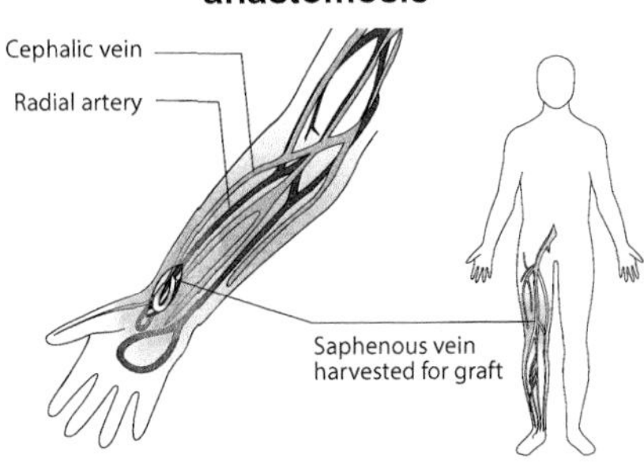

Autogenous graft (36825); nonautogenous graft (36830)

ICD-10-CM Diagnostic Codes

E08.22	Diabetes mellitus due to underlying condition with diabetic chronic kidney disease
E09.22	Drug or chemical induced diabetes mellitus with diabetic chronic kidney disease
E10.22	Type 1 diabetes mellitus with diabetic chronic kidney disease
E11.22	Type 2 diabetes mellitus with diabetic chronic kidney disease
E13.22	Other specified diabetes mellitus with diabetic chronic kidney disease
I12.0	Hypertensive chronic kidney disease with stage 5 chronic kidney disease or end stage renal disease
I13.11	Hypertensive heart and chronic kidney disease without heart failure, with stage 5 chronic kidney disease, or end stage renal disease
I13.2	Hypertensive heart and chronic kidney disease with heart failure and with stage 5 chronic kidney disease, or end stage renal disease
I82.3	Embolism and thrombosis of renal vein
M35.04	Sjögren syndrome with tubulo-interstitial nephropathy
M35.81	Multisystem inflammatory syndrome
N00.2	Acute nephritic syndrome with diffuse membranous glomerulonephritis
N00.3	Acute nephritic syndrome with diffuse mesangial proliferative glomerulonephritis
N00.4	Acute nephritic syndrome with diffuse endocapillary proliferative glomerulonephritis
N00.5	Acute nephritic syndrome with diffuse mesangiocapillary glomerulonephritis
N00.6	Acute nephritic syndrome with dense deposit disease
N00.7	Acute nephritic syndrome with diffuse crescentic glomerulonephritis
N00.8	Acute nephritic syndrome with other morphologic changes
N01.2	Rapidly progressive nephritic syndrome with diffuse membranous glomerulonephritis
N01.3	Rapidly progressive nephritic syndrome with diffuse mesangial proliferative glomerulonephritis
N01.4	Rapidly progressive nephritic syndrome with diffuse endocapillary proliferative glomerulonephritis
N01.5	Rapidly progressive nephritic syndrome with diffuse mesangiocapillary glomerulonephritis
N01.6	Rapidly progressive nephritic syndrome with dense deposit disease
N01.7	Rapidly progressive nephritic syndrome with diffuse crescentic glomerulonephritis
N01.8	Rapidly progressive nephritic syndrome with other morphologic changes
N03.2	Chronic nephritic syndrome with diffuse membranous glomerulonephritis
N03.3	Chronic nephritic syndrome with diffuse mesangial proliferative glomerulonephritis
N03.4	Chronic nephritic syndrome with diffuse endocapillary proliferative glomerulonephritis
N03.5	Chronic nephritic syndrome with diffuse mesangiocapillary glomerulonephritis
N03.6	Chronic nephritic syndrome with dense deposit disease
N03.7	Chronic nephritic syndrome with diffuse crescentic glomerulonephritis
N03.8	Chronic nephritic syndrome with other morphologic changes
N08	Glomerular disorders in diseases classified elsewhere
N11.0	Nonobstructive reflux-associated chronic pyelonephritis
N11.1	Chronic obstructive pyelonephritis
N16	Renal tubulo-interstitial disorders in diseases classified elsewhere
N17.0	Acute kidney failure with tubular necrosis
N17.2	Acute kidney failure with medullary necrosis
N17.8	Other acute kidney failure
N18.4	Chronic kidney disease, stage 4 (severe)
N18.5	Chronic kidney disease, stage 5
N18.6	End stage renal disease
N28.0	Ischemia and infarction of kidney
R65.11	Systemic inflammatory response syndrome (SIRS) of non-infectious origin with acute organ dysfunction
R65.20	Severe sepsis without septic shock
R65.21	Severe sepsis with septic shock

❼⇄	S37.061	Major laceration of right kidney
❼⇄	S37.062	Major laceration of left kidney
❼	T79.5	Traumatic anuria

ICD-10-CM Coding Notes

For codes requiring a 7th character extension, refer to your ICD-10-CM book. Review the character descriptions and coding guidelines for proper selection. For some procedures, only certain characters will apply.

CCI Edits

Refer to Appendix A for CCI edits.

Facility RVUs 🗌

Code	Work	PE Facility	MP	Total Facility
36825	14.17	5.64	3.53	23.34
36830	12.03	4.60	2.97	19.60

Non-facility RVUs 🗌

Code	Work	PE Non-Facility	MP	Total Non-Facility
36825	14.17	5.64	3.53	23.34
36830	12.03	4.60	2.97	19.60

Modifiers (PAR) 🗌

Code	Mod 50	Mod 51	Mod 62	Mod 66	Mod 80
36825	0	2	1	0	2
36830	0	2	1	0	2

Global Period

Code	Days
36825	090
36830	090

36831

36831 Thrombectomy, open, arteriovenous fistula without revision, autogenous or nonautogenous dialysis graft (separate procedure)

AMA Coding Guideline

Surgical Procedures on Arteries and Veins

Primary vascular procedure listings include establishing both inflow and outflow by whatever procedures necessary. Also included is that portion of the operative arteriogram performed by the surgeon, as indicated. Sympathectomy, when done, is included in the listed aortic procedures. For unlisted vascular procedure, use 37799.

Please see the Surgery Guidelines section for the following guidelines:

- *Surgical Procedures on the Cardiovascular System*

AMA *CPT® Assistant* ▢

36831: Nov 98: 14-15, Feb 99: 6, Mar 99: 6, Apr 99: 11, Mar 17: 5

Plain English Description

Following creation of an arteriovenous (AV) fistula, a thrombus may form, causing occlusion. An incision is made over the AV fistula and the artery and vein. The blood vessels and graft are exposed. Vessel loops are placed proximal and distal to the thrombus to control blood flow. The artery, vein, and/or graft are opened and the thrombus (clot) removed by direct exposure. The physician may use arterial back pressure or massage to expel the thrombus. Following removal of the thrombus, a completion angiography may be performed to ensure that the entire clot has been removed and that the AV fistula is patent.

Open thrombectomy, arteriovenous fistula

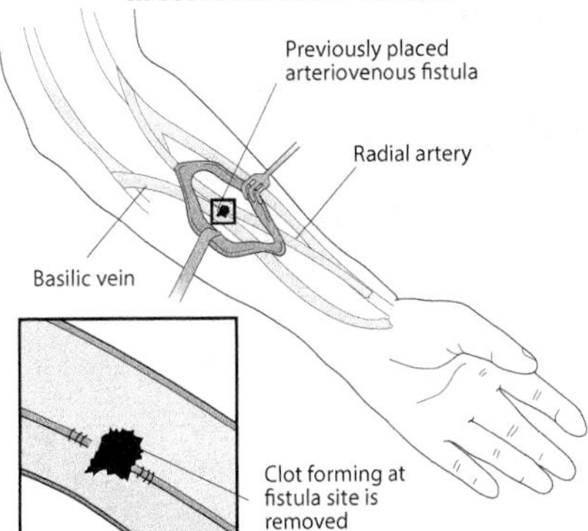

ICD-10-CM Diagnostic Codes

❼	T82.818	Embolism due to vascular prosthetic devices, implants and grafts
❼	T82.828	Fibrosis due to vascular prosthetic devices, implants and grafts
❼	T82.848	Pain due to vascular prosthetic devices, implants and grafts
❼	T82.868	Thrombosis due to vascular prosthetic devices, implants and grafts
❼	T82.898	Other specified complication of vascular prosthetic devices, implants and grafts
	Z45.89	Encounter for adjustment and management of other implanted devices

ICD-10-CM Coding Notes

For codes requiring a 7th character extension, refer to your ICD-10-CM book. Review the character descriptions and coding guidelines for proper selection. For some procedures, only certain characters will apply.

CCI Edits

Refer to Appendix A for CCI edits.

Facility RVUs ▢

Code	Work	PE Facility	MP	Total Facility
36831	11.00	4.37	2.71	18.08

Non-facility RVUs ▢

Code	Work	PE Non-Facility	MP	Total Non-Facility
36831	11.00	4.37	2.71	18.08

Modifiers (PAR) ▢

Code	Mod 50	Mod 51	Mod 62	Mod 66	Mod 80
36831	0	2	1	0	2

Global Period

Code	Days
36831	090

36832-36833

36832 Revision, open, arteriovenous fistula; without thrombectomy, autogenous or nonautogenous dialysis graft (separate procedure)

36833 Revision, open, arteriovenous fistula; with thrombectomy, autogenous or nonautogenous dialysis graft (separate procedure)

(For percutaneous thrombectomy within the dialysis circuit, see 36904, 36905, 36906)

(For central dialysis segment angioplasty in conjunction with 36818-36833, use 36907)

(For central dialysis segment stent placement in conjunction with 36818-36833, use 36908)

(Do not report 36832, 36833 in conjunction with 36901, 36902, 36903, 36904, 36905, 36906 for revision of the dialysis circuit)

AMA Coding Guideline

Surgical Procedures on Arteries and Veins

Primary vascular procedure listings include establishing both inflow and outflow by whatever procedures necessary. Also included is that portion of the operative arteriogram performed by the surgeon, as indicated. Sympathectomy, when done, is included in the listed aortic procedures. For unlisted vascular procedure, use 37799.

Please see the Surgery Guidelines section for the following guidelines:

- *Surgical Procedures on the Cardiovascular System*

AMA *CPT® Assistant* □

36832: Fall 93: 3, Feb 97: 2, Nov 98: 15, Feb 99: 6, Mar 99: 6, Apr 99: 11, Nov 99: 20-21, Mar 17: 5

36833: Nov 98: 15, Feb 99: 6, Apr 99: 11, Mar 17: 5

Plain English Description

An open revision of an arteriovenous (AV) fistula is performed with or without thrombectomy. Stenosis, thrombus formation, and occlusion of an AV fistula created using a graft is a complication requiring operative treatment. An incision is made in skin and soft tissue over the area of stenosis. The graft, artery, and vein are exposed. The blood vessels and graft are dissected free of surrounding tissue. Vessel loops are placed proximal and distal to the stenosed area to control blood flow. If a thrombus is present, it is removed by direct exposure. The artery, vein, and/or graft are opened and the thrombus (clot) removed using arterial back pressure or massage to expel the thrombus. The graft is then revised. Revision may involve incision and placement of a vein patch or excision of the stenosed area with placement of a new segment of autogenous vein or nonautogenous graft material. If the AV fistula is revised using a patch graft, a segment of vein, usually the saphenous, is harvested. An elliptical patch is tailored to fit over the stenosed segment of the graft. The patch graft is inserted within the longitudinal incision and sutured into place. This increases the diameter of the stenosed segment, improving blood flow through the graft. Alternatively, the stenosed segment of the AV fistula may be excised. A tubular segment of new vein is harvested or a nonautogenous graft is prepared and sutured to the remaining proximal and distal segments of graft or blood vessels. Vessel loops are released, hemostasis checked, and a completion angiography performed to ensure that the revised AV fistula is patent.

Revision, open, arteriovenous fistula

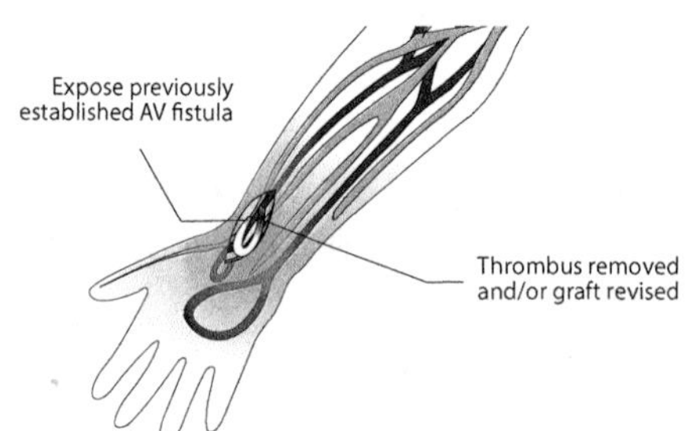
Expose previously established AV fistula
Thrombus removed and/or graft revised

Without thrombectomy, autogenous or nonautogenous dialysis graft (36832); with thrombectomy, autogenous or nonautogenous dialysis graft (36833)

ICD-10-CM Diagnostic Codes

❼	T82.318	Breakdown (mechanical) of other vascular grafts
❼	T82.328	Displacement of other vascular grafts
❼	T82.338	Leakage of other vascular grafts
❼	T82.398	Other mechanical complication of other vascular grafts
❼	T82.510	Breakdown (mechanical) of surgically created arteriovenous fistula
❼	T82.520	Displacement of surgically created arteriovenous fistula
❼	T82.530	Leakage of surgically created arteriovenous fistula
❼	T82.590	Other mechanical complication of surgically created arteriovenous fistula
❼	T82.7	Infection and inflammatory reaction due to other cardiac and vascular devices, implants and grafts
❼	T82.818	Embolism due to vascular prosthetic devices, implants and grafts
❼	T82.828	Fibrosis due to vascular prosthetic devices, implants and grafts
❼	T82.848	Pain due to vascular prosthetic devices, implants and grafts
❼	T82.858	Stenosis of other vascular prosthetic devices, implants and grafts
❼	T82.868	Thrombosis due to vascular prosthetic devices, implants and grafts
❼	T82.898	Other specified complication of vascular prosthetic devices, implants and grafts
	Z45.89	Encounter for adjustment and management of other implanted devices
	Z46.89	Encounter for fitting and adjustment of other specified devices

ICD-10-CM Coding Notes

For codes requiring a 7th character extension, refer to your ICD-10-CM book. Review the character descriptions and coding guidelines for proper selection. For some procedures, only certain characters will apply.

CCI Edits

Refer to Appendix A for CCI edits.

Facility RVUs □

Code	Work	PE Facility	MP	Total Facility
36832	13.50	5.39	3.33	22.22
36833	14.50	5.66	3.60	23.76

Non-facility RVUs □

Code	Work	PE Non-Facility	MP	Total Non-Facility
36832	13.50	5.39	3.33	22.22
36833	14.50	5.66	3.60	23.76

Modifiers (PAR) □

Code	Mod 50	Mod 51	Mod 62	Mod 66	Mod 80
36832	0	2	1	0	2
36833	0	2	1	0	2

Global Period

Code	Days
36832	090
36833	090

36835

36835 Insertion of Thomas shunt (separate procedure)

AMA Coding Guideline

Surgical Procedures on Arteries and Veins

Primary vascular procedure listings include establishing both inflow and outflow by whatever procedures necessary. Also included is that portion of the operative arteriogram performed by the surgeon, as indicated. Sympathectomy, when done, is included in the listed aortic procedures. For unlisted vascular procedure, use 37799.

Please see the Surgery Guidelines section for the following guidelines:

- *Surgical Procedures on the Cardiovascular System*

Plain English Description

A Thomas shunt is inserted to allow repeated long-term access to the vascular system for hemodialysis. The Thomas shunt is a transcutaneously placed external shunt consisting of two silastic cannulas with a Dacron patch at one end. Separate small incisions are made over the femoral artery and vein and the vessels are exposed. The vessels are incised. The Dacron patch at the end of one silastic cannula is sutured to the femoral artery and the other silastic cannula is sutured to the femoral vein using the Dacron patch. Suturing the Dacron patches to the vessels prevents the cannula from occluding the vessels. The two cannulas are tunneled subcutaneously to the anterointernal aspect of the thigh, exiting through two skin incisions. The two external cannula tips are joined with a Teflon connector to form a closed loop. The Teflon connector is removed during the dialysis procedure and the cannulas are connected to the hemodialysis tubing. When hemodialysis is not in use, the Teflon connector is replaced on the silastic cannulas.

Insertion of Thomas shunt

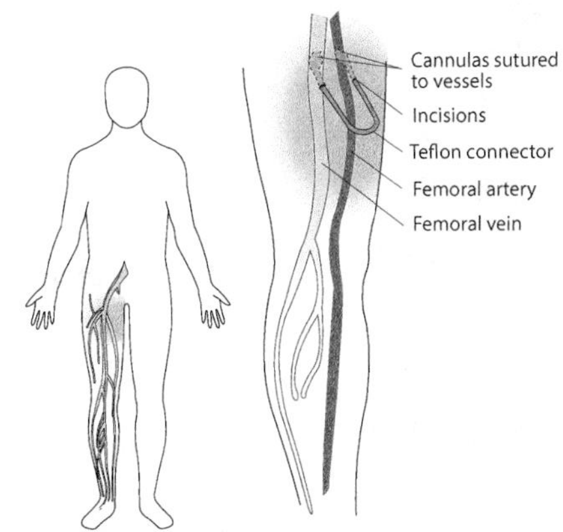

ICD-10-CM Diagnostic Codes

E08.22	Diabetes mellitus due to underlying condition with diabetic chronic kidney disease
E09.22	Drug or chemical induced diabetes mellitus with diabetic chronic kidney disease
E10.22	Type 1 diabetes mellitus with diabetic chronic kidney disease
E11.22	Type 2 diabetes mellitus with diabetic chronic kidney disease
E13.22	Other specified diabetes mellitus with diabetic chronic kidney disease
I12.0	Hypertensive chronic kidney disease with stage 5 chronic kidney disease or end stage renal disease
I13.11	Hypertensive heart and chronic kidney disease without heart failure, with stage 5 chronic kidney disease, or end stage renal disease
I13.2	Hypertensive heart and chronic kidney disease with heart failure and with stage 5 chronic kidney disease, or end stage renal disease
M35.04	Sjögren syndrome with tubulo-interstitial nephropathy
N01.2	Rapidly progressive nephritic syndrome with diffuse membranous glomerulonephritis
N01.3	Rapidly progressive nephritic syndrome with diffuse mesangial proliferative glomerulonephritis
N01.4	Rapidly progressive nephritic syndrome with diffuse endocapillary proliferative glomerulonephritis
N01.5	Rapidly progressive nephritic syndrome with diffuse mesangiocapillary glomerulonephritis
N01.6	Rapidly progressive nephritic syndrome with dense deposit disease
N01.7	Rapidly progressive nephritic syndrome with diffuse crescentic glomerulonephritis
N01.8	Rapidly progressive nephritic syndrome with other morphologic changes
N03.2	Chronic nephritic syndrome with diffuse membranous glomerulonephritis
N03.3	Chronic nephritic syndrome with diffuse mesangial proliferative glomerulonephritis
N03.4	Chronic nephritic syndrome with diffuse endocapillary proliferative glomerulonephritis
N03.5	Chronic nephritic syndrome with diffuse mesangiocapillary glomerulonephritis
N03.6	Chronic nephritic syndrome with dense deposit disease
N03.7	Chronic nephritic syndrome with diffuse crescentic glomerulonephritis
N03.8	Chronic nephritic syndrome with other morphologic changes
N04.2	Nephrotic syndrome with diffuse membranous glomerulonephritis
N04.3	Nephrotic syndrome with diffuse mesangial proliferative glomerulonephritis
N04.4	Nephrotic syndrome with diffuse endocapillary proliferative glomerulonephritis
N04.5	Nephrotic syndrome with diffuse mesangiocapillary glomerulonephritis
N04.6	Nephrotic syndrome with dense deposit disease
N04.7	Nephrotic syndrome with diffuse crescentic glomerulonephritis
N04.8	Nephrotic syndrome with other morphologic changes
N08	Glomerular disorders in diseases classified elsewhere
N11.0	Nonobstructive reflux-associated chronic pyelonephritis
N11.1	Chronic obstructive pyelonephritis
N11.8	Other chronic tubulo-interstitial nephritis
N16	Renal tubulo-interstitial disorders in diseases classified elsewhere
N18.4	Chronic kidney disease, stage 4 (severe)
N18.5	Chronic kidney disease, stage 5
N18.6	End stage renal disease

CCI Edits

Refer to Appendix A for CCI edits.

Facility RVUs

Code	Work	PE Facility	MP	Total Facility
36835	7.51	5.01	1.78	14.30

Non-facility RVUs

Code	Work	PE Non-Facility	MP	Total Non-Facility
36835	7.51	5.01	1.78	14.30

Modifiers (PAR)

Code	Mod 50	Mod 51	Mod 62	Mod 66	Mod 80
36835	0	2	0	0	1

Global Period

Code	Days
36835	090

36838

36838 Distal revascularization and interval ligation (DRIL), upper extremity hemodialysis access (steal syndrome)

(Do not report 36838 in conjunction with 35512, 35522, 35523, 36832, 37607, 37618)

AMA Coding Guideline

Surgical Procedures on Arteries and Veins

Primary vascular procedure listings include establishing both inflow and outflow by whatever procedures necessary. Also included is that portion of the operative arteriogram performed by the surgeon, as indicated. Sympathectomy, when done, is included in the listed aortic procedures. For unlisted vascular procedure, use 37799.

Please see the Surgery Guidelines section for the following guidelines:

- *Surgical Procedures on the Cardiovascular System*

Plain English Description

Steal syndrome is a complication in which the hemodialysis access diverts blood flow from the hand, causing ischemia and hand pain. The physician places a bypass graft in the arm with the proximal anastomosis site above the hemodialysis access site and the distal anastomosis below it. The bypass graft will divert blood around the hemodialysis access site, allowing better perfusion of the hand. An incision is made in the upper arm over the brachial artery, which is exposed and dissected free of surrounding tissue. A second incision is made in the lower arm distal to the hemodialysis access site and the brachial artery exposed. A subcutaneous tunnel is created from the proximal skin incision to the distal skin incision. Vessel loops are placed around the exposed brachial artery. A vein graft is harvested. If a saphenous vein graft is used, an incision is made in the skin of the leg over the section of saphenous vein to be harvested. Soft tissue is dissected off the vein and branches ligated and divided. The section of saphenous vein to be used is then ligated proximally and distally, divided, and removed from the leg. Vascular clamps are placed on the brachial artery in the upper arm. The artery is incised and the vein graft anastomosed. The vein graft is tunneled to the lower arm and anastomosed to the distal aspect of the brachial artery. A segment of brachial artery is isolated above the distal anastomosis of the just-completed bypass graft but below the hemodialysis access. The brachial artery is suture ligated to prevent blood from flowing retrograde into the hemodialysis access. The vascular clamps are removed and hemostasis verified. Blood flow through the graft and hemodialysis access is checked using Doppler and distal pulses are evaluated to ensure patency of the bypass graft.

Distal revascularization and interval ligation (DRIL), upper extremity hemodialysis access (steal syndrome)

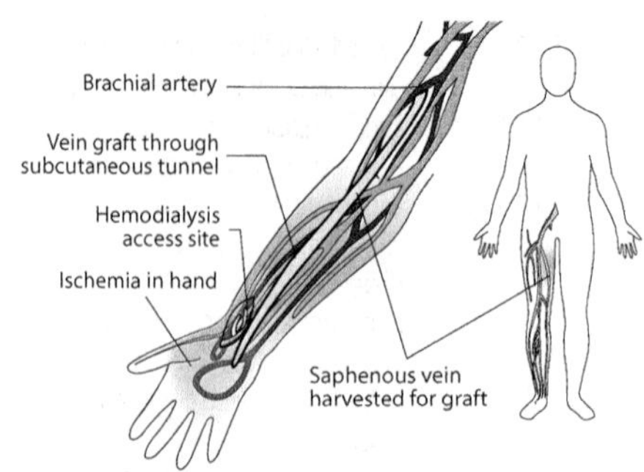

ICD-10-CM Diagnostic Codes

⇄	M79.641	Pain in right hand
⇄	M79.642	Pain in left hand
	N18.5	Chronic kidney disease, stage 5
	N18.6	End stage renal disease
❼	T82.318	Breakdown (mechanical) of other vascular grafts
❼	T82.398	Other mechanical complication of other vascular grafts
❼	T82.41	Breakdown (mechanical) of vascular dialysis catheter
❼	T82.49	Other complication of vascular dialysis catheter
❼	T82.510	Breakdown (mechanical) of surgically created arteriovenous fistula
❼	T82.518	Breakdown (mechanical) of other cardiac and vascular devices and implants
❼	T82.590	Other mechanical complication of surgically created arteriovenous fistula
❼	T82.598	Other mechanical complication of other cardiac and vascular devices and implants
❼	T82.7	Infection and inflammatory reaction due to other cardiac and vascular devices, implants and grafts
❼	T82.818	Embolism due to vascular prosthetic devices, implants and grafts
❼	T82.828	Fibrosis due to vascular prosthetic devices, implants and grafts
❼	T82.848	Pain due to vascular prosthetic devices, implants and grafts
❼	T82.858	Stenosis of other vascular prosthetic devices, implants and grafts
❼	T82.868	Thrombosis due to vascular prosthetic devices, implants and grafts
❼	T82.898	Other specified complication of vascular prosthetic devices, implants and grafts

ICD-10-CM Coding Notes

For codes requiring a 7th character extension, refer to your ICD-10-CM book. Review the character descriptions and coding guidelines for proper selection. For some procedures, only certain characters will apply.

CCI Edits

Refer to Appendix A for CCI edits.

Facility RVUs ▢

Code	Work	PE Facility	MP	Total Facility
36838	21.69	6.45	5.39	33.53

Non-facility RVUs ▢

Code	Work	PE Non-Facility	MP	Total Non-Facility
36838	21.69	6.45	5.39	33.53

Modifiers (PAR) ▢

Code	Mod 50	Mod 51	Mod 62	Mod 66	Mod 80
36838	1	2	1	0	2

Global Period

Code	Days
36838	090

36860-36861

36860 External cannula declotting (separate procedure); without balloon catheter

36861 External cannula declotting (separate procedure); with balloon catheter

(If imaging guidance is performed, use 76000)

AMA Coding Guideline

Surgical Procedures on Arteries and Veins

Primary vascular procedure listings include establishing both inflow and outflow by whatever procedures necessary. Also included is that portion of the operative arteriogram performed by the surgeon, as indicated. Sympathectomy, when done, is included in the listed aortic procedures. For unlisted vascular procedure, use 37799.

Please see the Surgery Guidelines section for the following guidelines:

- *Surgical Procedures on the Cardiovascular System*

AMA *CPT® Assistant* ◻

36860: Fall 93: 3, Feb 97: 2, Nov 98: 15, Feb 99: 6, May 01: 3

36861: Fall 93: 3, Feb 97: 2, May 01: 3

Plain English Description

The physician performs external cannula declotting either without a balloon catheter (36860) or with a balloon catheter (36861). The external cannula is examined and palpated to determine whether the occlusion is due to a thrombus. If the occlusion is due to a small thrombus, the physician first attempts to remove the thrombus by digital manipulation and the injection of a thrombolytic agent (36860). The thrombolytic agent may be administered either in a pulse-spray or a small amount may be injected using a lyse-and-wait technique. In 36861, the physician uses a balloon catheter to declot the cannula. A combination multipurpose catheter and guidewire is passed to the site of the obstruction. The multipurpose catheter is exchanged for a balloon catheter. The balloon catheter is then inflated at the site of the blood clot (thrombus). The balloon catheter is then deflated and blood flow evaluated. The balloon catheter may be inflated-deflated several times and is removed when adequate blood flow is observed.

External cannula declotting

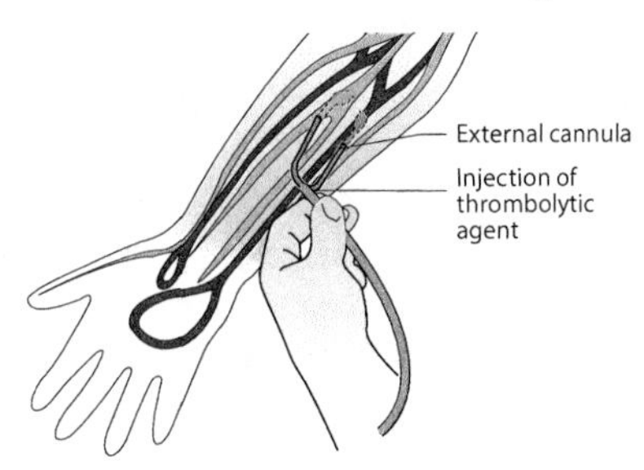

Without balloon catheter (36860); with balloon catheter (36861)

ICD-10-CM Diagnostic Codes

❼	T82.49	Other complication of vascular dialysis catheter
❼	T82.818	Embolism due to vascular prosthetic devices, implants and grafts
❼	T82.828	Fibrosis due to vascular prosthetic devices, implants and grafts
❼	T82.858	Stenosis of other vascular prosthetic devices, implants and grafts
❼	T82.868	Thrombosis due to vascular prosthetic devices, implants and grafts
❼	T82.898	Other specified complication of vascular prosthetic devices, implants and grafts

ICD-10-CM Coding Notes

For codes requiring a 7th character extension, refer to your ICD-10-CM book. Review the character descriptions and coding guidelines for proper selection. For some procedures, only certain characters will apply.

CCI Edits

Refer to Appendix A for CCI edits.

Facility RVUs ◻

Code	Work	PE Facility	MP	Total Facility
36860	2.01	0.75	0.51	3.27
36861	2.52	0.94	0.64	4.10

Non-facility RVUs ◻

Code	Work	PE Non-Facility	MP	Total Non-Facility
36860	2.01	4.50	0.51	7.02
36861	2.52	0.94	0.64	4.10

Modifiers (PAR) ◻

Code	Mod 50	Mod 51	Mod 62	Mod 66	Mod 80
36860	0	2	0	0	1
36861	0	2	0	0	1

Global Period

Code	Days
36860	000
36861	000

36901-36903

36901 Introduction of needle(s) and/or catheter(s), dialysis circuit, with diagnostic angiography of the dialysis circuit, including all direct puncture(s) and catheter placement(s), injection(s) of contrast, all necessary imaging from the arterial anastomosis and adjacent artery through entire venous outflow including the inferior or superior vena cava, fluoroscopic guidance, radiological supervision and interpretation and image documentation and report

(Do not report 36901 in conjunction with 36833, 36902, 36903, 36904, 36905, 36906)

36902 Introduction of needle(s) and/or catheter(s), dialysis circuit, with diagnostic angiography of the dialysis circuit, including all direct puncture(s) and catheter placement(s), injection(s) of contrast, all necessary imaging from the arterial anastomosis and adjacent artery through entire venous outflow including the inferior or superior vena cava, fluoroscopic guidance, radiological supervision and interpretation and image documentation and report; with transluminal balloon angioplasty, peripheral dialysis segment, including all imaging and radiological supervision and interpretation necessary to perform the angioplasty

(Do not report 36902 in conjunction with 36903)

36903 Introduction of needle(s) and/or catheter(s), dialysis circuit, with diagnostic angiography of the dialysis circuit, including all direct puncture(s) and catheter placement(s), injection(s) of contrast, all necessary imaging from the arterial anastomosis and adjacent artery through entire venous outflow including the inferior or superior vena cava, fluoroscopic guidance, radiological supervision and interpretation and image documentation and report; with transcatheter placement of intravascular stent(s), peripheral dialysis segment, including all imaging and radiological supervision and interpretation necessary to perform the stenting, and all angioplasty within the peripheral dialysis segment

(Do not report 36902, 36903 in conjunction with 36833, 36904, 36905, 36906)

(Do not report 36901, 36902, 36903 more than once per operative session)

(For transluminal balloon angioplasty within central vein(s) when performed through dialysis circuit, use 36907)

(For transcatheter placement of intravascular stent(s) within central vein(s) when performed through dialysis circuit, use 36908)

AMA Coding Guideline

Dialysis Circuit Procedures

Definitions

Dialysis circuit: The arteriovenous (AV) dialysis circuit is designed for easy and repetitive access to perform hemodialysis. It begins at the arterial anastomosis and extends to the right atrium. The circuit may be created using either an arterial-venous anastomosis, known as an arteriovenous fistula (AVF), or a prosthetic graft placed between an artery and vein, known as an arteriovenous graft (AVG). The dialysis circuit is comprised of two segments, termed the (1) peripheral dialysis segment and (2) central dialysis segment. Both are defined as follows.

Peripheral dialysis segment: The peripheral dialysis segment is the portion of the dialysis circuit that begins at the arterial anastomosis and extends to the central dialysis segment. In the upper extremity, the peripheral dialysis segment extends through the axillary vein (or entire cephalic vein in the case of cephalic venous outflow). In the lower extremity, the peripheral dialysis segment extends through the common femoral vein. The peripheral dialysis segment includes the historic "peri-anastomotic region" (defined below).

Central dialysis segment: The central dialysis segment includes all draining veins central to the peripheral dialysis segment. In the upper extremity, the central dialysis segment includes the veins central to the axillary and cephalic veins, including the subclavian and innominate veins through the superior vena cava. In the lower extremity, the central dialysis segment includes the veins central to the common femoral vein, including the external iliac and common iliac veins through the inferior vena cava.

Peri-anastomotic region: A historic term referring to the region of a dialysis circuit near the arterial anastomosis encompassing a short segment of the parent artery, the anastomosis, and a short segment of the dialysis circuit immediately adjacent to the anastomosis. The peri-anastomotic region is included within the peripheral segment of the dialysis circuit.

Performed through dialysis circuit: Any diagnostic study or therapeutic intervention within the dialysis circuit that is performed through a direct percutaneous access to the dialysis circuit.

Code 36901 includes direct access and imaging of the entire dialysis circuit. Antegrade and/or retrograde punctures of the dialysis circuit are typically used for imaging, and contrast may be injected directly through a needle or through a catheter placed into the dialysis circuit. All dialysis circuit punctures required to perform the procedure are included in 36901. Occasionally, the catheter needs to be advanced further into the circuit to adequately visualize the arterial anastomosis or the central veins, or selective catheterization of a venous branch may be required. All manipulation(s) of the catheter for diagnostic imaging of the dialysis circuit is included in 36901. Advancement of the catheter to the vena cava to adequately image that segment of the dialysis circuit is included in 36901 and is not separately reported. Code 36901 also includes catheterization of additional venous side branches communicating with the dialysis circuit, known as accessory veins. Advancement of the catheter tip through the arterial anastomosis to adequately visualize the anastomosis is also included in the service described by 36901 and is not separately reported. Evaluation of the peri-anastomotic portion of the inflow is an integral part of the dialysis circuit angiogram and is included in 36901.

For the purposes of reporting dialysis access maintenance services, the arterial inflow to the dialysis circuit is considered a separate vessel. If a more proximal arterial inflow problem separate from the peripheral dialysis segment is suspected, additional catheter placement and imaging required for adequate evaluation of the artery may be separately reported. If a catheter is selectively advanced from the dialysis circuit puncture beyond the peri-anastomotic segment into the inflow artery, an additional catheterization code may be reported. For example, 36215 may be used to report image-guided retrograde catheter placement into the inflow artery and into the aorta, if necessary (36200 is not reported in addition to 36215 in this example). Note that 75710 may also be reported if contrast injection for diagnostic arteriography is performed through this catheter and radiological supervision and interpretation and imaging documentation is performed.

Ultrasound guidance for puncture of the dialysis circuit access is not typically performed and is not included in 36901, 36902, 36903, 36904, 36905, 36906. However, in the case of a new (immature) or failing AVF, ultrasound may be necessary to safely and effectively puncture the dialysis circuit for evaluation, and this may be reported separately with 76937, if all the appropriate elements for reporting 76937 are performed and documented.

For radiological supervision and interpretation of dialysis circuit angiography performed through existing access(es) or catheter-based arterial access, report 36901 with modifier 52.

Dialysis Circuit Interventions (AV Grafts and AV Fistulae): For the purposes of coding interventional procedures in the dialysis circuit (both AVF and AVG), the dialysis circuit is artificially divided into two distinct segments: peripheral dialysis segment and central dialysis segment (see definitions).

Codes 36901, 36902, 36903 and 36904, 36905, 36906 are built on progressive hierarchies that have more intensive services, which include less intensive services. Report only one code (36901, 36902, 36903, 36904, 36905, 36906) for services provided in a dialysis circuit.

Code 36901 describes the diagnostic evaluation of the dialysis circuit, and this service is included in the services described by 36901, 36902, 36903, 36904, 36905, 36906. All catheterizations required to perform diagnostic fistulography are included in 36901. All catheterizations required to perform additional interventional services are included in codes 36902, 36903, 36904, 36905, 36906, 36907, 36908, 36909 and not separately reported. All angiography, fluoroscopic image guidance, roadmapping, and radiological supervision and interpretation required to perform each service are included in each code. Closure of the puncture(s) by any method is included in the service of each individual code.

Code 36902 includes the services in 36901 plus transluminal balloon angioplasty in the peripheral segment of the dialysis circuit. Code 36902 would be reported only once per session to describe all angioplasty services performed in the peripheral segment of the dialysis circuit, regardless of the number of distinct lesions treated within that segment, the number of times the balloon is inflated, or the number of balloon catheters or sizes required to open all lesions, and includes angioplasty of the peri-anastomotic segment when performed. Code 36903 includes the services in 36902 plus transcatheter stent placement in the peripheral segment of the dialysis circuit. Code 36903 is reported only once per session to describe placing stent(s) within the peripheral segment, regardless of the number of stent(s) placed or the number of discrete lesion(s) treated within the peripheral segment. If both angioplasty and stenting are performed in the peripheral segment, including treatment of separate lesions, report 36903 only once.

Code 36904 describes percutaneous transluminal mechanical thrombectomy and/or infusion for thrombolysis in the dialysis circuit (all thrombus treated in both the peripheral and central dialysis circuit segments) and includes diagnostic angiography (36901), fluoroscopic image guidance, catheter placement(s), and all maneuvers required to remove thrombus from the peripheral and/or central segments, including all intraprocedural pharmacological thrombolytic injection(s)/infusion(s). It is never appropriate to report removal of the arterial plug during a declot/thrombectomy procedure as an angioplasty (36905). Removal of the arterial plug is included in a fistula thrombectomy, even if a balloon catheter is used to mechanically dislodge the resistant thrombus. Codes 36905 (angioplasty) and 36906 (stent) describe services in the peripheral circuit when performed in conjunction with thrombolysis/thrombectomy. Code 36905 includes the services in 36904 plus transluminal balloon angioplasty in the peripheral segment of the dialysis circuit. Code 36905 may be reported only once per session to describe all angioplasty performed in the peripheral segment of the dialysis circuit, regardless of the number of distinct lesions treated within that segment, the number of times the balloon is inflated, or the number of balloon catheters required to open all lesions. Code 36906 includes the services in 36905 plus transcatheter stent placement in the peripheral segment of the dialysis circuit. Code 36906 is reported only once per session to describe placing stent(s) within the peripheral segment, regardless of the number of stent(s) placed or the number of discrete lesion(s) treated within the peripheral segment.

Codes 36907 and 36908 describe procedures performed through puncture(s) in the dialysis circuit. Similar procedures performed from a different access (eg, common femoral vein) may be reported using 37248, 37249 or 37238, 37239. Code 36907 is an add-on code used in conjunction with 36901, 36902, 36903, 36904, 36905, 36906 to report angioplasty within the central dialysis segment when performed through puncture of the dialysis circuit, and is reported once per session independent of the number of discrete lesions treated, the number of balloon inflations, and number of balloon catheters or sizes required. These additional services should be clearly documented in the patient record, including the recorded images. Code 36907 may be reported only once per session with 36901, 36902, 36903, 36904, 36905, 36906, as appropriate. Report 36907 once for all angioplasty performed within the central dialysis segment.

Code 36908 is an add-on code used in conjunction with 36901, 36902, 36903, 36904, 36905, 36906 to report stenting lesion(s) in the central dialysis segment when performed through puncture of the dialysis circuit. It is reported once, regardless of the number of discrete lesions treated or the number of stents placed. Code 36908 includes the services in 36907; therefore, 36908 may not be reported with 36907 in the same session. Code 36908 may be reported only once per session with 36901, 36902, 36903, 36904, 36905, 36906, as appropriate.

Code 36909 is an add-on code used to report endovascular embolization or occlusion of the main vessel or side branches arising from (emptying into) the dialysis circuit. Code 36909 may only be reported once per therapeutic session, irrespective of the number of branches embolized or occluded. Embolization or occlusion of the main vessel or these side branches may not be reported with 37241.

If open dialysis circuit creation, revision, and/or thrombectomy (36818-36833) are performed, completion angiography is bundled, as is peripheral segment angioplasty and/or stent placement (36901, 36902, 36903) and, therefore, not separately reported. However, dialysis circuit central segment angioplasty and/or stent placement may be separately reported (36907, 36908).

Surgical Procedures on Arteries and Veins

Primary vascular procedure listings include establishing both inflow and outflow by whatever procedures necessary. Also included is that portion of the operative arteriogram performed by the surgeon, as indicated. Sympathectomy, when done, is included in the listed aortic procedures. For unlisted vascular procedure, use 37799.

Please see the Surgery Guidelines section for the following guidelines:

- *Surgical Procedures on the Cardiovascular System*

AMA *CPT® Assistant* ▢

36901: Mar 17: 3, May 17: 3
36902: Mar 17: 3, May 17: 3
36903: Mar 17: 3, May 17: 3

Plain English Description

A procedure is performed using diagnostic angiography to visualize the hemodialysis circuit, including adjacent artery through the entire venous outflow for stenosis or obstruction causing low blood flow, elevated pre-pump arterial pressure, or high venous return pressure. The dialysis circuit may consist of a central venous catheter (CVC), an arteriovenous (AV) fistula, or a synthetic AV graft. For CVC, a double lumen or 2 separate catheters are inserted into a large vein (vena cava, internal jugular, femoral vein). Blood is withdrawn from one lumen for filtration outside the body and returned via a second lumen. An AV fistula is created by anastomosing an artery to a vein and bypassing the capillaries. A synthetic graft also creates an arteriovenous anastomosis using synthetic material when the vessels are not in close proximity. To facilitate dialysis through an AV fistula or graft, a needle placed "upstream" withdraws blood, circulates it through the dialysis machine, and returns the filtered blood through a needle placed "downstream." The AV fistula and graft may become narrowed over time due to intimal hyperplasia and/or thrombosis. For diagnostic angiography of the entire dialysis circuit (36901), an AV fistula or AV graft is accessed with a small needle, a CVC through the port/catheter lumen. A guidewire is threaded through the needle or port/lumen and the needle exchanged for a vascular sheath. A catheter is placed over the guidewire and contrast dye is injected to visualize the vessels through the entire venous outflow using fluoroscopy. If stenosis is present in the peripheral dialysis segment, balloon angioplasty (36902) may be performed. A balloon-tipped catheter is inserted over the guidewire through the area of stenosis. The balloon is inflated with dilute radiopaque contrast and visualized with fluoroscopy. At the end of the prescribed time, the balloon is deflated and the catheter is removed. A vascular catheter with a working channel is then threaded over the guidewire and angiography is repeated to evaluate for resistant or residual stenosis. If stenosis remains, a fine mesh/wire stent is delivered to the area of stenosis through the working channel of the vascular catheter (36903). The stent expands, placing pressure on the walls of the blood vessel to keep it open. The catheter is removed and a purse string suture may be placed to control bleeding before the vascular sheath is removed. Stent placement in the peripheral dialysis segment includes the angioplasty.

Diagnostic angiography of hemodialysis circuit

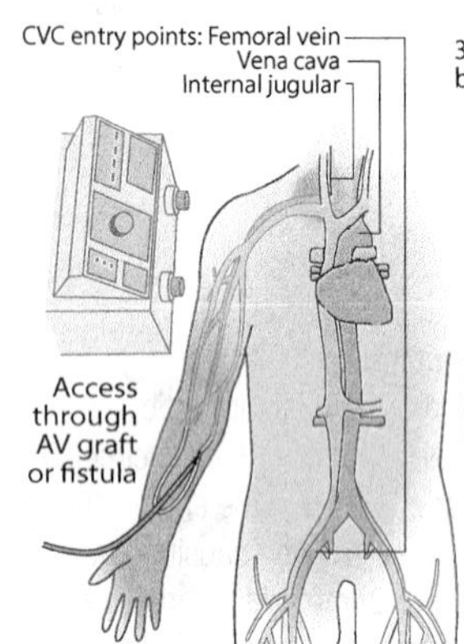

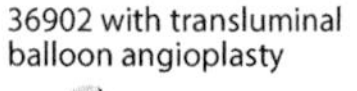

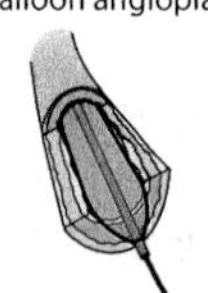

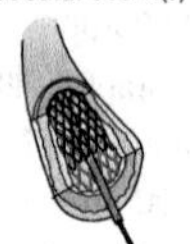

ICD-10-CM Diagnostic Codes

❼	T82.828	Fibrosis due to vascular prosthetic devices, implants and grafts
❼	T82.848	Pain due to vascular prosthetic devices, implants and grafts
❼	T82.858	Stenosis of other vascular prosthetic devices, implants and grafts
	Z45.2	Encounter for adjustment and management of vascular access device

ICD-10-CM Coding Notes

For codes requiring a 7th character extension, refer to your ICD-10-CM book. Review the character descriptions and coding guidelines for proper selection. For some procedures, only certain characters will apply.

CCI Edits

Refer to Appendix A for CCI edits.

Facility RVUs

Code	Work	PE Facility	MP	Total Facility
36901	3.36	1.05	0.50	4.91
36902	4.83	1.47	0.68	6.98
36903	6.39	1.82	0.99	9.20

Non-facility RVUs

Code	Work	PE Non-Facility	MP	Total Non-Facility
36901	3.36	17.91	0.50	21.77
36902	4.83	31.90	0.68	37.41
36903	6.39	127.30	0.99	134.68

Modifiers (PAR)

Code	Mod 50	Mod 51	Mod 62	Mod 66	Mod 80
36901	0	2	0	0	1
36902	0	2	0	0	1
36903	0	2	0	0	1

Global Period

Code	Days
36901	000
36902	000
36903	000

36904-36906

36904 Percutaneous transluminal mechanical thrombectomy and/or infusion for thrombolysis, dialysis circuit, any method, including all imaging and radiological supervision and interpretation, diagnostic angiography, fluoroscopic guidance, catheter placement(s), and intraprocedural pharmacological thrombolytic injection(s)

(For open thrombectomy within the dialysis circuit, see 36831, 36833)

36905 Percutaneous transluminal mechanical thrombectomy and/or infusion for thrombolysis, dialysis circuit, any method, including all imaging and radiological supervision and interpretation, diagnostic angiography, fluoroscopic guidance, catheter placement(s), and intraprocedural pharmacological thrombolytic injection(s); with transluminal balloon angioplasty, peripheral dialysis segment, including all imaging and radiological supervision and interpretation necessary to perform the angioplasty

(Do not report 36905 in conjunction with 36904)

36906 Percutaneous transluminal mechanical thrombectomy and/or infusion for thrombolysis, dialysis circuit, any method, including all imaging and radiological supervision and interpretation, diagnostic angiography, fluoroscopic guidance, catheter placement(s), and intraprocedural pharmacological thrombolytic injection(s); with transcatheter placement of intravascular stent(s), peripheral dialysis segment, including all imaging and radiological supervision and interpretation necessary to perform the stenting, and all angioplasty within the peripheral dialysis circuit

(Do not report 36906 in conjunction with 36901, 36902, 36903, 36904, 36905)

(Do not report 36904, 36905, 36906 more than once per operative session)

(For transluminal balloon angioplasty within central vein(s) when performed through dialysis circuit, use 36907)

(For transcatheter placement of intravascular stent(s) within central vein(s) when performed through dialysis circuit, use 36908)

AMA Coding Guideline

Dialysis Circuit Procedures

Definitions

Dialysis circuit: The arteriovenous (AV) dialysis circuit is designed for easy and repetitive access to perform hemodialysis. It begins at the arterial anastomosis and extends to the right atrium. The circuit may be created using either an arterial-venous anastomosis, known as an arteriovenous fistula (AVF), or a prosthetic graft placed between an artery and vein, known as an arteriovenous graft (AVG). The dialysis circuit is comprised of two segments, termed the (1) peripheral dialysis segment and (2) central dialysis segment. Both are defined as follows.

Peripheral dialysis segment: The peripheral dialysis segment is the portion of the dialysis circuit that begins at the arterial anastomosis and extends to the central dialysis segment. In the upper extremity, the peripheral dialysis segment extends through the axillary vein (or entire cephalic vein in the case of cephalic venous outflow). In the lower extremity, the peripheral dialysis segment extends through the common femoral vein. The peripheral dialysis segment includes the historic "peri-anastomotic region" (defined below).

Central dialysis segment: The central dialysis segment includes all draining veins central to the peripheral dialysis segment. In the upper extremity, the central dialysis segment includes the veins central to the axillary and cephalic veins, including the subclavian and innominate veins through the superior vena cava. In the lower extremity, the central dialysis segment includes the veins central to the common femoral vein, including the external iliac and common iliac veins through the inferior vena cava.

Peri-anastomotic region: A historic term referring to the region of a dialysis circuit near the arterial anastomosis encompassing a short segment of the parent artery, the anastomosis, and a short segment of the dialysis circuit immediately adjacent to the anastomosis. The peri-anastomotic region is included within the peripheral segment of the dialysis circuit.

Performed through dialysis circuit: Any diagnostic study or therapeutic intervention within the dialysis circuit that is performed through a direct percutaneous access to the dialysis circuit.

Code 36901 includes direct access and imaging of the entire dialysis circuit. Antegrade and/or retrograde punctures of the dialysis circuit are typically used for imaging, and contrast may be injected directly through a needle or through a catheter placed into the dialysis circuit. All dialysis circuit punctures required to perform the procedure are included in 36901. Occasionally, the catheter needs to be advanced further into the circuit to adequately visualize the arterial anastomosis or the central veins, or selective catheterization of a venous branch may be required. All manipulation(s) of the catheter for diagnostic imaging of the dialysis circuit is included in 36901. Advancement of the catheter to the vena cava to adequately image that segment of the dialysis circuit is included in 36901 and is not separately reported. Code 36901 also includes catheterization of additional venous side branches communicating with the dialysis circuit, known as accessory veins. Advancement of the catheter tip through the arterial anastomosis to adequately visualize the anastomosis is also included in the service described by 36901 and is not separately reported. Evaluation of the peri-anastomotic portion of the inflow is an integral part of the dialysis circuit angiogram and is included in 36901.

For the purposes of reporting dialysis access maintenance services, the arterial inflow to the dialysis circuit is considered a separate vessel. If a more proximal arterial inflow problem separate from the peripheral dialysis segment is suspected, additional catheter placement and imaging required for adequate evaluation of the artery may be separately reported. If a catheter is selectively advanced from the dialysis circuit puncture beyond the peri-anastomotic segment into the inflow artery, an additional catheterization code may be reported. For example, 36215 may be used to report image-guided retrograde catheter placement into the inflow artery and into the aorta, if necessary (36200 is not reported in addition to 36215 in this example). Note that 75710 may also be reported if contrast injection for diagnostic arteriography is performed through this catheter and radiological supervision and interpretation and imaging documentation is performed.

Ultrasound guidance for puncture of the dialysis circuit access is not typically performed and is not included in 36901, 36902, 36903, 36904, 36905, 36906. However, in the case of a new (immature) or failing AVF, ultrasound may be necessary to safely and effectively puncture the dialysis circuit for evaluation, and this may be reported separately with 76937, if all the appropriate elements for reporting 76937 are performed and documented.

For radiological supervision and interpretation of dialysis circuit angiography performed through existing access(es) or catheter-based arterial access, report 36901 with modifier 52.

Dialysis Circuit Interventions (AV Grafts and AV Fistulae): For the purposes of coding interventional procedures in the dialysis circuit (both AVF and AVG), the dialysis circuit is artificially divided into two distinct segments: peripheral dialysis segment and central dialysis segment (see definitions).

Codes 36901, 36902, 36903 and 36904, 36905, 36906 are built on progressive hierarchies that have more intensive services, which include less intensive services. Report only one code (36901,

36902, 36903, 36904, 36905, 36906) for services provided in a dialysis circuit.

Code 36901 describes the diagnostic evaluation of the dialysis circuit, and this service is included in the services described by 36901, 36902, 36903, 36904, 36905, 36906. All catheterizations required to perform diagnostic fistulography are included in 36901. All catheterizations required to perform additional interventional services are included in codes 36902, 36903, 36904, 36905, 36906, 36907, 36908, 36909 and not separately reported. All angiography, fluoroscopic image guidance, roadmapping, and radiological supervision and interpretation required to perform each service are included in each code. Closure of the puncture(s) by any method is included in the service of each individual code.

Code 36902 includes the services in 36901 plus transluminal balloon angioplasty in the peripheral segment of the dialysis circuit. Code 36902 would be reported only once per session to describe all angioplasty services performed in the peripheral segment of the dialysis circuit, regardless of the number of distinct lesions treated within that segment, the number of times the balloon is inflated, or the number of balloon catheters or sizes required to open all lesions, and includes angioplasty of the peri-anastomotic segment when performed. Code 36903 includes the services in 36902 plus transcatheter stent placement in the peripheral segment of the dialysis circuit. Code 36903 is reported only once per session to describe placing stent(s) within the peripheral segment, regardless of the number of stent(s) placed or the number of discrete lesion(s) treated within the peripheral segment. If both angioplasty and stenting are performed in the peripheral segment, including treatment of separate lesions, report 36903 only once.

Code 36904 describes percutaneous transluminal mechanical thrombectomy and/or infusion for thrombolysis in the dialysis circuit (all thrombus treated in both the peripheral and central dialysis circuit segments) and includes diagnostic angiography (36901), fluoroscopic image guidance, catheter placement(s), and all maneuvers required to remove thrombus from the peripheral and/or central segments, including all intraprocedural pharmacological thrombolytic injection(s)/infusion(s). It is never appropriate to report removal of the arterial plug during a declot/thrombectomy procedure as an angioplasty (36905). Removal of the arterial plug is included in a fistula thrombectomy, even if a balloon catheter is used to mechanically dislodge the resistant thrombus. Codes 36905 (angioplasty) and 36906 (stent) describe services in the peripheral circuit when performed in conjunction with thrombolysis/thrombectomy. Code 36905 includes the services in 36904 plus transluminal balloon angioplasty in the peripheral segment of the dialysis circuit. Code 36905 may be reported only once per session to describe all angioplasty performed in the peripheral segment of the dialysis circuit, regardless of the number of distinct lesions treated within that segment, the number of times the balloon is inflated, or the number of balloon catheters required to open all lesions. Code 36906 includes the services in 36905 plus transcatheter stent placement in the peripheral segment of the dialysis circuit. Code 36906 is reported only once per session to describe placing stent(s) within the peripheral segment, regardless of the number of stent(s) placed or the number of discrete lesion(s) treated within the peripheral segment.

Codes 36907 and 36908 describe procedures performed through puncture(s) in the dialysis circuit. Similar procedures performed from a different access (eg, common femoral vein) may be reported using 37248, 37249 or 37238, 37239. Code 36907 is an add-on code used in conjunction with 36901, 36902, 36903, 36904, 36905, 36906 to report angioplasty within the central dialysis segment when performed through puncture of the dialysis circuit, and is reported once per session independent of the number of discrete lesions treated, the number of balloon inflations, and number of balloon catheters or sizes required. These additional services should be clearly documented in the patient record, including the recorded images. Code 36907 may be reported only once per session with 36901, 36902, 36903, 36904, 36905, 36906, as appropriate. Report 36907 once for all angioplasty performed within the central dialysis segment.

Code 36908 is an add-on code used in conjunction with 36901, 36902, 36903, 36904, 36905, 36906 to report stenting lesion(s) in the central dialysis segment when performed through puncture of the dialysis circuit. It is reported once, regardless of the number of discrete lesions treated or the number of stents placed. Code 36908 includes the services in 36907; therefore, 36908 may not be reported with 36907 in the same session. Code 36908 may be reported only once per session with 36901, 36902, 36903, 36904, 36905, 36906, as appropriate.

Code 36909 is an add-on code used to report endovascular embolization or occlusion of the main vessel or side branches arising from (emptying into) the dialysis circuit. Code 36909 may only be reported once per therapeutic session, irrespective of the number of branches embolized or occluded. Embolization or occlusion of the main vessel or these side branches may not be reported with 37241.

If open dialysis circuit creation, revision, and/or thrombectomy (36818-36833) are performed, completion angiography is bundled, as is peripheral segment angioplasty and/or stent placement (36901, 36902, 36903) and, therefore, not separately reported. However, dialysis circuit central segment angioplasty and/or stent placement may be separately reported (36907, 36908).

Surgical Procedures on Arteries and Veins

Primary vascular procedure listings include establishing both inflow and outflow by whatever procedures necessary. Also included is that portion of the operative arteriogram performed by the surgeon, as indicated. Sympathectomy, when done, is included in the listed aortic procedures. For unlisted vascular procedure, use 37799.

Please see the Surgery Guidelines section for the following guidelines:

- *Surgical Procedures on the Cardiovascular System*

AMA *CPT® Assistant* ☐

36904: Mar 17: 3, May 17: 3
36905: Mar 17: 3, May 17: 3
36906: Mar 17: 3, May 17: 3

Plain English Description

A procedure is performed to dissolve or remove blood clots within the dialysis circuit using percutaneous transluminal mechanical thrombectomy and/or infusion of clot-dissolving pharmaceutical agents. The dialysis circuit may consist of a central venous catheter (CVC), an arteriovenous (AV) fistula, or a synthetic AV graft. The incidence of thrombosis is highest with an AV graft and also common with an AV fistula. Symptoms of dialysis circuit thrombosis include absence of thrill or pulse at the fistula/graft site, vessel swelling or distention, and/or absence of blood flash with needle insertion. Ultrasound or duplex Doppler study may be used to define the length of the thrombus if the vessel is not well distended. To perform thrombectomy (36904) on an AV fistula, needles are placed at either end of the thrombus and guidewires are inserted in a crossed fashion. Crossing sheaths are then placed over the guidewires and the needles are removed. A thrombolytic pharmaceutical agent (heparin, TPA) is injected into the fistula. After a prescribed period of time, if resistant clot remains, a thrombectomy catheter is inserted over the guidewire and the clot is evacuated mechanically. To perform thrombectomy (36904) on an AV graft, the venous segment is accessed first, then the arterial segment, using a needle in downstream venous direction followed by a guidewire threaded through the clot. The needle is exchanged with a vascular sheath and a thrombolytic pharmaceutical agent is injected through the sheath. After a prescribed period of time, if residual clot remains, an embolectomy catheter is inserted over a guidewire and the clot is evacuated mechanically. This procedure is repeated on the arterial side of the graft with the needle directed upstream. Angiography of the dialysis circuit is then performed to visualize residual blood clot and/or vessel stenosis. If stenosis is present in the peripheral dialysis circuit, balloon angioplasty (36905) may be performed. A balloon-tipped catheter is inserted over a guidewire through the stenosed area. The balloon is inflated with dilute radiopaque contrast and visualized with fluoroscopy. The balloon is deflated and the catheter is removed. A vascular catheter with a working channel is then threaded over the guidewire and angiography is repeated to evaluate for resistant or residual stenosis. If stenosis remains, a fine mesh/wire stent is delivered to the area of stenosis through the working channel of the vascular catheter (36906). The stent expands, placing pressure on the walls of the blood vessel to keep it open. The catheter is removed and a purse string suture may be placed to control bleeding before the vascular sheath is removed. Stent placement in the peripheral dialysis segment includes the angioplasty.

Percutaneous transluminal mechanical thrombectomy in dialysis circuit

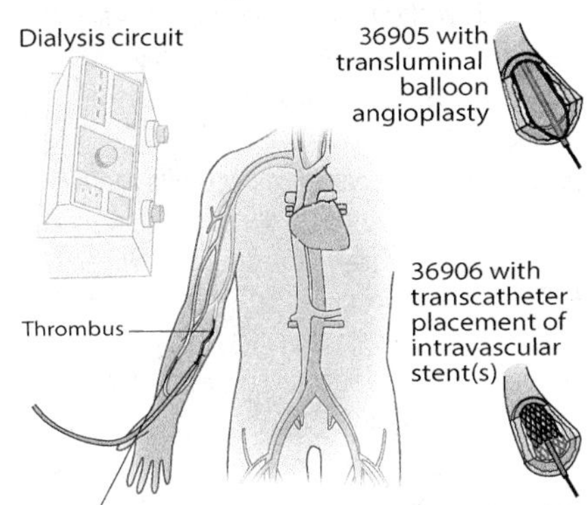

ICD-10-CM Diagnostic Codes

❼	T82.818	Embolism due to vascular prosthetic devices, implants and grafts
❼	T82.828	Fibrosis due to vascular prosthetic devices, implants and grafts
❼	T82.848	Pain due to vascular prosthetic devices, implants and grafts
❼	T82.858	Stenosis of other vascular prosthetic devices, implants and grafts
❼	T82.868	Thrombosis due to vascular prosthetic devices, implants and grafts
❼	T82.898	Other specified complication of vascular prosthetic devices, implants and grafts
	Z45.2	Encounter for adjustment and management of vascular access device

ICD-10-CM Coding Notes

For codes requiring a 7th character extension, refer to your ICD-10-CM book. Review the character descriptions and coding guidelines for proper selection. For some procedures, only certain characters will apply.

CCI Edits

Refer to Appendix A for CCI edits.

Facility RVUs ☐

Code	Work	PE Facility	MP	Total Facility
36904	7.50	2.15	1.04	10.69
36905	9.00	2.72	1.20	12.92
36906	10.42	3.01	1.42	14.85

Non-facility RVUs ☐

Code	Work	PE Non-Facility	MP	Total Non-Facility
36904	7.50	47.32	1.04	55.86
36905	9.00	60.63	1.20	70.83
36906	10.42	158.47	1.42	170.31

Modifiers (PAR) ☐

Code	Mod 50	Mod 51	Mod 62	Mod 66	Mod 80
36904	0	2	1	0	1
36905	0	2	1	0	1
36906	0	2	1	0	1

Global Period

Code	Days
36904	000
36905	000
36906	000

36907-36908

✚ **36907 Transluminal balloon angioplasty, central dialysis segment, performed through dialysis circuit, including all imaging and radiological supervision and interpretation required to perform the angioplasty (List separately in addition to code for primary procedure)**

(Use 36907 in conjunction with 36818-36833, 36901, 36902, 36903, 36904, 36905, 36906)

(Do not report 36907 in conjunction with 36908)

(Report 36907 once for all angioplasty performed within the central dialysis segment)

✚ **36908 Transcatheter placement of intravascular stent(s), central dialysis segment, performed through dialysis circuit, including all imaging and radiological supervision and interpretation required to perform the stenting, and all angioplasty in the central dialysis segment (List separately in addition to code for primary procedure)**

(Use 36908 in conjunction with 36818-36833, 36901, 36902, 36903, 36904, 36905, 36906)

(Do not report 36908 in conjunction with 36907)

(Report 36908 once for all stenting performed within the central dialysis segment)

AMA Coding Guideline
Dialysis Circuit Procedures

Definitions

Dialysis circuit: The arteriovenous (AV) dialysis circuit is designed for easy and repetitive access to perform hemodialysis. It begins at the arterial anastomosis and extends to the right atrium. The circuit may be created using either an arterial-venous anastomosis, known as an arteriovenous fistula (AVF), or a prosthetic graft placed between an artery and vein, known as an arteriovenous graft (AVG). The dialysis circuit is comprised of two segments, termed the (1) peripheral dialysis segment and (2) central dialysis segment. Both are defined as follows.

Peripheral dialysis segment: The peripheral dialysis segment is the portion of the dialysis circuit that begins at the arterial anastomosis and extends to the central dialysis segment. In the upper extremity, the peripheral dialysis segment extends through the axillary vein (or entire cephalic vein in the case of cephalic venous outflow). In the lower extremity, the peripheral dialysis segment extends through the common femoral vein. The peripheral dialysis segment includes the historic "peri-anastomotic region" (defined below).

Central dialysis segment: The central dialysis segment includes all draining veins central to the peripheral dialysis segment. In the upper extremity, the central dialysis segment includes the veins central to the axillary and cephalic veins, including the subclavian and innominate veins through the superior vena cava. In the lower extremity, the central dialysis segment includes the veins central to the common femoral vein, including the external iliac and common iliac veins through the inferior vena cava.

Peri-anastomotic region: A historic term referring to the region of a dialysis circuit near the arterial anastomosis encompassing a short segment of the parent artery, the anastomosis, and a short segment of the dialysis circuit immediately adjacent to the anastomosis. The peri-anastomotic region is included within the peripheral segment of the dialysis circuit.

Performed through dialysis circuit: Any diagnostic study or therapeutic intervention within the dialysis circuit that is performed through a direct percutaneous access to the dialysis circuit.

Code 36901 includes direct access and imaging of the entire dialysis circuit. Antegrade and/or retrograde punctures of the dialysis circuit are typically used for imaging, and contrast may be injected directly through a needle or through a catheter placed into the dialysis circuit. All dialysis circuit punctures required to perform the procedure are included in 36901. Occasionally, the catheter needs to be advanced further into the circuit to adequately visualize the arterial anastomosis or the central veins, or selective catheterization of a venous branch may be required. All manipulation(s) of the catheter for diagnostic imaging of the dialysis circuit is included in 36901. Advancement of the catheter to the vena cava to adequately image that segment of the dialysis circuit is included in 36901 and is not separately reported. Code 36901 also includes catheterization of additional venous side branches communicating with the dialysis circuit, known as accessory veins. Advancement of the catheter tip through the arterial anastomosis to adequately visualize the anastomosis is also included in the service described by 36901 and is not separately reported. Evaluation of the peri-anastomotic portion of the inflow is an integral part of the dialysis circuit angiogram and is included in 36901.

For the purposes of reporting dialysis access maintenance services, the arterial inflow to the dialysis circuit is considered a separate vessel. If a more proximal arterial inflow problem separate from the peripheral dialysis segment is suspected, additional catheter placement and imaging required for adequate evaluation of the artery may be separately reported. If a catheter is selectively advanced from the dialysis circuit puncture beyond the peri-anastomotic segment into the inflow artery, an additional catheterization code may be reported. For example, 36215 may be used to report image-guided retrograde catheter placement into the inflow artery and into the aorta, if necessary (36200 is not reported in addition to 36215 in this example). Note that 75710 may also be reported if contrast injection for diagnostic arteriography is performed through this catheter and radiological supervision and interpretation and imaging documentation is performed.

Ultrasound guidance for puncture of the dialysis circuit access is not typically performed and is not included in 36901, 36902, 36903, 36904, 36905, 36906. However, in the case of a new (immature) or failing AVF, ultrasound may be necessary to safely and effectively puncture the dialysis circuit for evaluation, and this may be reported separately with 76937, if all the appropriate elements for reporting 76937 are performed and documented.

For radiological supervision and interpretation of dialysis circuit angiography performed through existing access(es) or catheter-based arterial access, report 36901 with modifier 52.

Dialysis Circuit Interventions (AV Grafts and AV Fistulae): For the purposes of coding interventional procedures in the dialysis circuit (both AVF and AVG), the dialysis circuit is artificially divided into two distinct segments: peripheral dialysis segment and central dialysis segment (see definitions).

Codes 36901, 36902, 36903 and 36904, 36905, 36906 are built on progressive hierarchies that have more intensive services, which include less intensive services. Report only one code (36901, 36902, 36903, 36904, 36905, 36906) for services provided in a dialysis circuit.

Code 36901 describes the diagnostic evaluation of the dialysis circuit, and this service is included in the services described by 36901, 36902, 36903, 36904, 36905, 36906. All catheterizations required to perform diagnostic fistulography are included in 36901. All catheterizations required to perform additional interventional services are included in codes 36902, 36903, 36904, 36905, 36906, 36907, 36908, 36909 and not separately reported. All angiography, fluoroscopic image guidance, roadmapping, and radiological supervision and interpretation required to perform each service are included in each code. Closure of the puncture(s) by any method is included in the service of each individual code.

Code 36902 includes the services in 36901 plus transluminal balloon angioplasty in the peripheral segment of the dialysis circuit. Code 36902 would be reported only once per session to describe all angioplasty services performed in the peripheral segment of the dialysis circuit, regardless of the number of distinct lesions treated within that segment, the number of times the balloon is inflated, or the number of balloon catheters or sizes required to open all lesions, and includes angioplasty of the peri-anastomotic segment when performed. Code 36903 includes the services in 36902 plus transcatheter stent placement in the peripheral segment of the dialysis circuit. Code 36903 is reported only once per session to describe placing stent(s) within the peripheral segment, regardless of the number of stent(s) placed or the number of discrete lesion(s) treated within the peripheral segment. If both angioplasty and stenting are performed in the peripheral segment, including treatment of separate lesions, report 36903 only once.

Code 36904 describes percutaneous transluminal mechanical thrombectomy and/or infusion for thrombolysis in the dialysis circuit (all thrombus treated in both the peripheral and central dialysis circuit segments) and includes diagnostic angiography (36901), fluoroscopic image guidance, catheter placement(s), and all maneuvers required to remove thrombus from the peripheral and/or central segments, including all intraprocedural pharmacological thrombolytic injection(s)/infusion(s). It is never appropriate to report removal of the arterial plug during a declot/thrombectomy procedure as an angioplasty (36905). Removal of the arterial plug is included in a fistula thrombectomy, even if a balloon catheter is used to mechanically dislodge the resistant thrombus. Codes 36905 (angioplasty) and 36906 (stent) describe services in the peripheral circuit when performed in conjunction with thrombolysis/thrombectomy. Code 36905 includes the services in 36904 plus transluminal balloon angioplasty in the peripheral segment of the dialysis circuit. Code 36905 may be reported only once per session to describe all angioplasty performed in the peripheral segment of the dialysis circuit, regardless of the number of distinct lesions treated within that segment, the number of times the balloon is inflated, or the number of balloon catheters required to open all lesions. Code 36906 includes the services in 36905 plus transcatheter stent placement in the peripheral segment of the dialysis circuit. Code 36906 is reported only once per session to describe placing stent(s) within the peripheral segment, regardless of the number of stent(s) placed or the number of discrete lesion(s) treated within the peripheral segment.

Codes 36907 and 36908 describe procedures performed through puncture(s) in the dialysis circuit. Similar procedures performed from a different access (eg, common femoral vein) may be reported using 37248, 37249 or 37238, 37239. Code 36907 is an add-on code used in conjunction with 36901, 36902, 36903, 36904, 36905, 36906 to report angioplasty within the central dialysis segment when performed through puncture of the dialysis circuit, and is reported once per session independent of the number of discrete lesions treated, the number of balloon inflations, and number of balloon catheters or sizes required. These additional services should be clearly documented in the patient record, including the recorded images. Code 36907 may be reported only once per session with 36901, 36902, 36903, 36904, 36905, 36906, as appropriate. Report 36907 once for all angioplasty performed within the central dialysis segment.

Code 36908 is an add-on code used in conjunction with 36901, 36902, 36903, 36904, 36905, 36906 to report stenting lesion(s) in the central dialysis segment when performed through puncture of the dialysis circuit. It is reported once, regardless of the number of discrete lesions treated or the number of stents placed. Code 36908 includes the services in 36907; therefore, 36908 may not be reported with 36907 in the same session. Code 36908 may be reported only once per session with 36901, 36902, 36903, 36904, 36905, 36906, as appropriate.

Code 36909 is an add-on code used to report endovascular embolization or occlusion of the main vessel or side branches arising from (emptying into) the dialysis circuit. Code 36909 may only be reported once per therapeutic session, irrespective of the number of branches embolized or occluded. Embolization or occlusion of the main vessel or these side branches may not be reported with 37241.

If open dialysis circuit creation, revision, and/or thrombectomy (36818-36833) are performed, completion angiography is bundled, as is peripheral segment angioplasty and/or stent placement (36901, 36902, 36903) and, therefore, not separately reported. However, dialysis circuit central segment angioplasty and/or stent placement may be separately reported (36907, 36908).

Surgical Procedures on Arteries and Veins

Primary vascular procedure listings include establishing both inflow and outflow by whatever procedures necessary. Also included is that portion of the operative arteriogram performed by the surgeon, as indicated. Sympathectomy, when done, is included in the listed aortic procedures. For unlisted vascular procedure, use 37799.

Please see the Surgery Guidelines section for the following guidelines:

- *Surgical Procedures on the Cardiovascular System*

AMA *CPT® Assistant* ☐

36907: Mar 17: 3, May 17: 3
36908: Mar 17: 3, May 17: 3

Plain English Description

A procedure is performed to restore blood flow through a narrowed or obstructed central venous dialysis segment (axillary vein, subclavian vein, innominate vein, vena cava). Symptoms of hemodialysis-related central venous occlusive disease (CVOD) include elevated urea recirculation, elevated venous dialysis pressure, and arm edema. The central venous dialysis segment is accessed via the AV graft/fistula. The AV graft/fistula is punctured with a needle, a guidewire is threaded through the needle, and the needle is exchanged for a vascular sheath. A catheter is placed over the guidewire and angiography is performed to visualize the central venous segments. Transluminal balloon angioplasty (36907) is performed when stenosis of the central vein(s) is identified. A balloon tipped catheter is inserted over the guidewire through the stenosed area. The balloon is inflated with dilute radiopaque contrast and visualized with fluoroscopy. At the end of the prescribed time, the balloon is deflated and the catheter is removed. A vascular catheter with a working channel is then threaded over the guidewire and angiography is repeated to evaluate for resistant or residual stenosis. If stenosis remains, a fine mesh/wire stent is delivered to the area of stenosis in the central venous segment through the working channel of the vascular catheter (36908). The stent expands, placing pressure on the walls of the blood vessel to keep it open. The catheter is removed and a purse string suture may be placed to control bleeding before the vascular sheath is removed. Stent placement in the central dialysis segment includes the angioplasty, all imagining, and radiological supervision and interpretation.

Transluminal balloon angioplasty (36907); transcatheter placement of stent (36908) in central dialysis segment

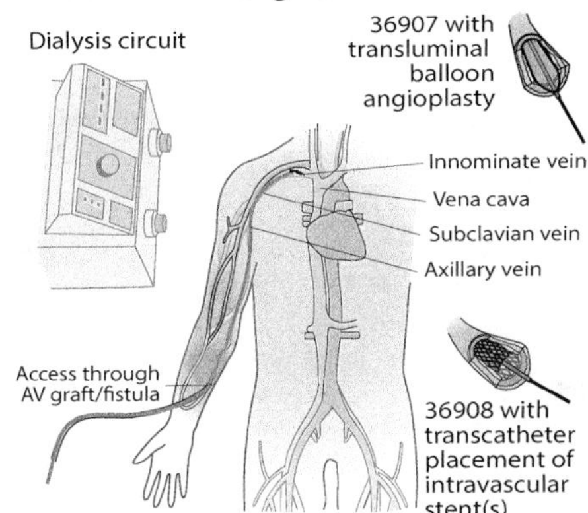

ICD-10-CM Diagnostic Codes

See Primary Procedure code for crosswalks.

CCI Edits

Refer to Appendix A for CCI edits.

Facility RVUs

Code	Work	PE Facility	MP	Total Facility
36907	3.00	0.83	0.42	4.25
36908	4.25	1.11	0.67	6.03

Non-facility RVUs

Code	Work	PE Non-Facility	MP	Total Non-Facility
36907	3.00	14.83	0.42	18.25
36908	4.25	39.30	0.67	44.22

Modifiers (PAR)

Code	Mod 50	Mod 51	Mod 62	Mod 66	Mod 80
36907	0	0	0	0	1
36908	0	0	0	0	1

Global Period

Code	Days
36907	ZZZ
36908	ZZZ

36909

✚ **36909 Dialysis circuit permanent vascular embolization or occlusion (including main circuit or any accessory veins), endovascular, including all imaging and radiological supervision and interpretation necessary to complete the intervention (List separately in addition to code for primary procedure)**

(36909 includes all permanent vascular occlusions within the dialysis circuit and may only be reported once per encounter per day)

(Report 36909 in conjunction with 36901, 36902, 36903, 36904, 36905, 36906)

(For open ligation/occlusion in dialysis access, use 37607)

AMA Coding Guideline

Dialysis Circuit Procedures

Definitions

Dialysis circuit: The arteriovenous (AV) dialysis circuit is designed for easy and repetitive access to perform hemodialysis. It begins at the arterial anastomosis and extends to the right atrium. The circuit may be created using either an arterial-venous anastomosis, known as an arteriovenous fistula (AVF), or a prosthetic graft placed between an artery and vein, known as an arteriovenous graft (AVG). The dialysis circuit is comprised of two segments, termed the (1) peripheral dialysis segment and (2) central dialysis segment. Both are defined as follows.

Peripheral dialysis segment: The peripheral dialysis segment is the portion of the dialysis circuit that begins at the arterial anastomosis and extends to the central dialysis segment. In the upper extremity, the peripheral dialysis segment extends through the axillary vein (or entire cephalic vein in the case of cephalic venous outflow). In the lower extremity, the peripheral dialysis segment extends through the common femoral vein. The peripheral dialysis segment includes the historic "peri-anastomotic region" (defined below).

Central dialysis segment: The central dialysis segment includes all draining veins central to the peripheral dialysis segment. In the upper extremity, the central dialysis segment includes the veins central to the axillary and cephalic veins, including the subclavian and innominate veins through the superior vena cava. In the lower extremity, the central dialysis segment includes the veins central to the common femoral vein, including the external iliac and common iliac veins through the inferior vena cava.

Peri-anastomotic region: A historic term referring to the region of a dialysis circuit near the arterial anastomosis encompassing a short segment of the parent artery, the anastomosis, and a short segment of the dialysis circuit immediately adjacent to the anastomosis. The peri-anastomotic region is included within the peripheral segment of the dialysis circuit.

Performed through dialysis circuit: Any diagnostic study or therapeutic intervention within the dialysis circuit that is performed through a direct percutaneous access to the dialysis circuit.

Code 36901 includes direct access and imaging of the entire dialysis circuit. Antegrade and/or retrograde punctures of the dialysis circuit are typically used for imaging, and contrast may be injected directly through a needle or through a catheter placed into the dialysis circuit. All dialysis circuit punctures required to perform the procedure are included in 36901. Occasionally, the catheter needs to be advanced further into the circuit to adequately visualize the arterial anastomosis or the central veins, or selective catheterization of a venous branch may be required. All manipulation(s) of the catheter for diagnostic imaging of the dialysis circuit is included in 36901. Advancement of the catheter to the vena cava to adequately image that segment of the dialysis circuit is included in 36901 and is not separately reported. Code 36901 also includes catheterization of additional venous side branches communicating with the dialysis circuit, known as accessory veins. Advancement of the catheter tip through the arterial anastomosis to adequately visualize the anastomosis is also included in the service described by 36901 and is not separately reported. Evaluation of the peri-anastomotic portion of the inflow is an integral part of the dialysis circuit angiogram and is included in 36901.

For the purposes of reporting dialysis access maintenance services, the arterial inflow to the dialysis circuit is considered a separate vessel. If a more proximal arterial inflow problem separate from the peripheral dialysis segment is suspected, additional catheter placement and imaging required for adequate evaluation of the artery may be separately reported. If a catheter is selectively advanced from the dialysis circuit puncture beyond the peri-anastomotic segment into the inflow artery, an additional catheterization code may be reported. For example, 36215 may be used to report image-guided retrograde catheter placement into the inflow artery and into the aorta, if necessary (36200 is not reported in addition to 36215 in this example). Note that 75710 may also be reported if contrast injection for diagnostic arteriography is performed through this catheter and radiological supervision and interpretation and imaging documentation is performed.

Ultrasound guidance for puncture of the dialysis circuit access is not typically performed and is not included in 36901, 36902, 36903, 36904, 36905, 36906. However, in the case of a new (immature) or failing AVF, ultrasound may be necessary to safely and effectively puncture the dialysis circuit for evaluation, and this may be reported separately with 76937, if all the appropriate elements for reporting 76937 are performed and documented.

For radiological supervision and interpretation of dialysis circuit angiography performed through existing access(es) or catheter-based arterial access, report 36901 with modifier 52.

Dialysis Circuit Interventions (AV Grafts and AV Fistulae): For the purposes of coding interventional procedures in the dialysis circuit (both AVF and AVG), the dialysis circuit is artificially divided into two distinct segments: peripheral dialysis segment and central dialysis segment (see definitions).

Codes 36901, 36902, 36903 and 36904, 36905, 36906 are built on progressive hierarchies that have more intensive services, which include less intensive services. Report only one code (36901, 36902, 36903, 36904, 36905, 36906) for services provided in a dialysis circuit.

Code 36901 describes the diagnostic evaluation of the dialysis circuit, and this service is included in the services described by 36901, 36902, 36903, 36904, 36905, 36906. All catheterizations required to perform diagnostic fistulography are included in 36901. All catheterizations required to perform additional interventional services are included in codes 36902, 36903, 36904, 36905, 36906, 36907, 36908, 36909 and not separately reported. All angiography, fluoroscopic image guidance, roadmapping, and radiological supervision and interpretation required to perform each service are included in each code. Closure of the puncture(s) by any method is included in the service of each individual code.

Code 36902 includes the services in 36901 plus transluminal balloon angioplasty in the peripheral segment of the dialysis circuit. Code 36902 would be reported only once per session to describe all angioplasty services performed in the peripheral segment of the dialysis circuit, regardless of the number of distinct lesions treated within that segment, the number of times the balloon is inflated, or the number of balloon catheters or sizes required to open all lesions, and includes angioplasty of the peri-anastomotic segment when performed. Code 36903 includes the services in 36902 plus transcatheter stent placement in the peripheral segment of the dialysis circuit. Code 36903 is reported only once per session to describe placing stent(s) within the peripheral segment, regardless of the number of stent(s) placed or the number of discrete lesion(s) treated within the peripheral segment. If both angioplasty and stenting are performed in the peripheral segment, including treatment of separate lesions, report 36903 only once.

Code 36904 describes percutaneous transluminal mechanical thrombectomy and/or infusion for thrombolysis in the dialysis circuit (all thrombus treated in both the peripheral and central dialysis circuit segments) and includes diagnostic angiography (36901), fluoroscopic image guidance, catheter placement(s), and all maneuvers required to remove thrombus from the peripheral and/or central segments, including all intraprocedural pharmacological thrombolytic injection(s)/infusion(s). It is never appropriate to report removal of the arterial plug during a declot/thrombectomy procedure as an angioplasty (36905). Removal of the arterial plug is included in a fistula thrombectomy, even if a balloon catheter is used to mechanically dislodge the resistant thrombus. Codes 36905 (angioplasty) and 36906 (stent) describe services in the peripheral circuit when performed in conjunction with thrombolysis/thrombectomy. Code 36905 includes the services in 36904 plus transluminal balloon angioplasty in the peripheral segment of the dialysis circuit. Code 36905 may be reported only once per session to describe all angioplasty performed in the peripheral segment of the dialysis circuit, regardless of the number of distinct lesions treated within that segment, the number of times the balloon is inflated, or the number of balloon catheters required to open all lesions. Code 36906 includes the services in 36905 plus transcatheter stent placement in the peripheral segment of the dialysis circuit. Code 36906 is reported only once per session to describe placing stent(s) within the peripheral segment, regardless of the number of stent(s) placed or the number of discrete lesion(s) treated within the peripheral segment.

Codes 36907 and 36908 describe procedures performed through puncture(s) in the dialysis circuit. Similar procedures performed from a different access (eg, common femoral vein) may be reported using 37248, 37249 or 37238, 37239. Code 36907 is an add-on code used in conjunction with 36901, 36902, 36903, 36904, 36905, 36906 to report angioplasty within the central dialysis segment when performed through puncture of the dialysis circuit, and is reported once per session independent of the number of discrete lesions treated, the number of balloon inflations, and number of balloon catheters or sizes required. These additional services should be clearly documented in the patient record, including the recorded images. Code 36907 may be reported only once per session with 36901, 36902, 36903, 36904, 36905, 36906, as appropriate. Report 36907 once for all angioplasty performed within the central dialysis segment.

Code 36908 is an add-on code used in conjunction with 36901, 36902, 36903, 36904, 36905, 36906 to report stenting lesion(s) in the central dialysis segment when performed through puncture of the dialysis circuit. It is reported once, regardless of the number of discrete lesions treated or the number of stents placed. Code 36908 includes the services in 36907; therefore, 36908 may not be reported with 36907 in the same session. Code 36908 may be reported only once per session with 36901, 36902, 36903, 36904, 36905, 36906, as appropriate.

Code 36909 is an add-on code used to report endovascular embolization or occlusion of the main vessel or side branches arising from (emptying into) the dialysis circuit. Code 36909 may only be reported once per therapeutic session, irrespective of the number of branches embolized or occluded. Embolization or occlusion of the main vessel or these side branches may not be reported with 37241.

If open dialysis circuit creation, revision, and/or thrombectomy (36818-36833) are performed, completion angiography is bundled, as is peripheral segment angioplasty and/or stent placement (36901, 36902, 36903) and, therefore, not separately reported. However, dialysis circuit central segment angioplasty and/or stent placement may be separately reported (36907, 36908).

Surgical Procedures on Arteries and Veins

Primary vascular procedure listings include establishing both inflow and outflow by whatever procedures necessary. Also included is that portion of the operative arteriogram performed by the surgeon, as indicated. Sympathectomy, when done, is included in the listed aortic procedures. For unlisted vascular procedure, use 37799.

Please see the Surgery Guidelines section for the following guidelines:

- *Surgical Procedures on the Cardiovascular System*

AMA *CPT® Assistant* ▢

36909: Mar 17: 3, May 17: 3

Plain English Description

Permanent vascular embolization or occlusion of the main dialysis circuit or accessory veins may be used to treat dialysis-related steal syndrome, critical hand ischemia, venous aneurysm, central venous occlusion syndrome not amenable to endovascular recanalization, or hyperdynamic heart failure. The dialysis circuit is accessed using a needle and a guidewire is placed through the needle into the vessel. A vascular sheath replaces the needle and a catheter is introduced through the vascular sheath. Contrast dye is injected and the target area of the dialysis circuit/accessory veins is identified using fluoroscopy. An embolization agent (gelfoam, particulate agent, liquid sclerosing agent, liquid glue) or occlusion device (metallic plug/coil) is delivered to the target area through the catheter. Post procedure angiography is obtained to verify that the embolization or occlusion procedure has been successful. The catheter is removed and a purse string suture may be placed to control bleeding before the vascular sheath is removed. Code 36909 includes all imaging and radiological supervision and interpretation necessary to complete the intervention and is reported in addition to the primary procedure.

Permanent vascular embolization or occlusion of the main dialysis circuit or accessory veins

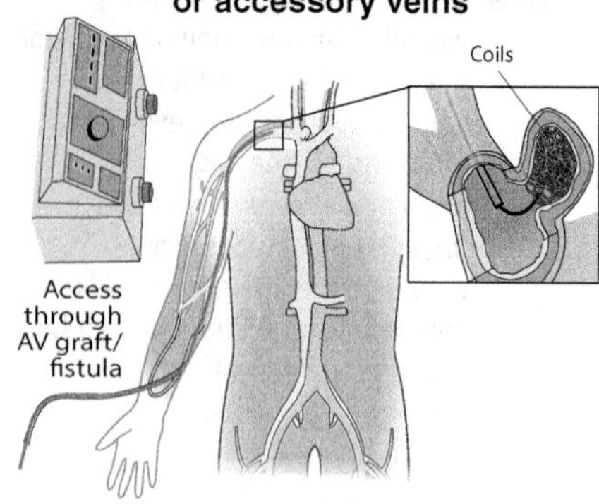

ICD-10-CM Diagnostic Codes

See Primary Procedure code for crosswalks.

CCI Edits

Refer to Appendix A for CCI edits.

Facility RVUs ▢

Code	Work	PE Facility	MP	Total Facility
36909	4.12	1.11	0.64	5.87

Non-facility RVUs ▢

Code	Work	PE Non-Facility	MP	Total Non-Facility
36909	4.12	55.62	0.64	60.38

Modifiers (PAR) ▢

Code	Mod 50	Mod 51	Mod 62	Mod 66	Mod 80
36909	0	0	0	0	1

Global Period

Code	Days
36909	ZZZ

37788

37788 Penile revascularization, artery, with or without vein graft

AMA Coding Guideline

Surgical Procedures on Arteries and Veins

Primary vascular procedure listings include establishing both inflow and outflow by whatever procedures necessary. Also included is that portion of the operative arteriogram performed by the surgeon, as indicated. Sympathectomy, when done, is included in the listed aortic procedures. For unlisted vascular procedure, use 37799.

Please see the Surgery Guidelines section for the following guidelines:

- *Surgical Procedures on the Cardiovascular System*

Plain English Description

Penile revascularization is performed with or without vein graft to increase the cavernosal arterial blood supply to the penis. This procedure is performed on patients with penile arterial insufficiency and resulting erectile dysfunction. Penile arterial insufficiency may be caused by arteriosclerotic disease, trauma to the pelvis or perineum, or other organic disease processes. A number of surgical techniques are used to perform revascularization, which may include direct anastomosis of the inferior epigastric artery to the corpus cavernosum or placement of a saphenous or basilic vein graft between the inferior epigastric or femoral artery and the corpus cavernosum. To perform direct anastomosis of the inferior epigastric artery to the corpus cavernosum, the artery is exposed, dissected free of surrounding tissue up to the level of the umbilicus, and transected. It is then passed through a subcutaneous tunnel to the base of the penis. The tunica albuginea is then exposed and a plug excised. Using microsurgical technique, the artery is anastomosed to the endothelium of the corpus cavernosum. Following anastomosis, the penis is observed for evidence of erection. Surgical incisions are then closed in a layered fashion. If a vein graft is used, the selected vein is harvested. If a saphenous vein graft is used, an incision is made in the skin of the leg over the section of saphenous vein to be harvested. Soft tissue is dissected off the vein and branches ligated and divided. The section of saphenous vein to be used is then ligated proximally and distally, divided, and removed from the leg. The vein graft is then anastomosed in an end-to-side fashion to the inferior epigastric or femoral vein and tunneled to the base of the penis where it is anastomosed to the corpus cavernosum using the same technique described above.

Penile revascularization, artery, with or without vein graft

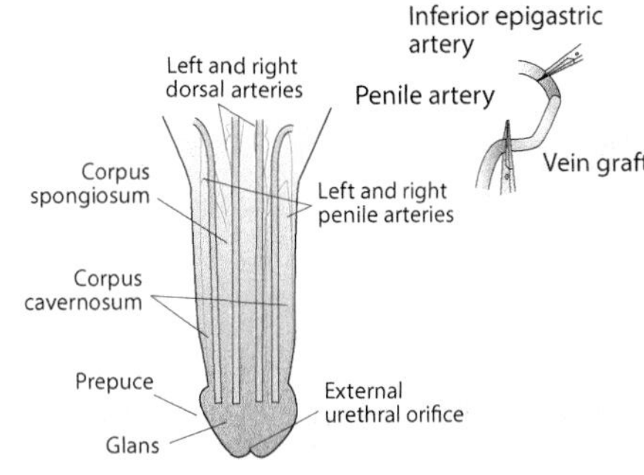

A small incision is made at the base of the penis to access the penile artery and surrounding vessels.

ICD-10-CM Diagnostic Codes

	I70.91	Generalized atherosclerosis
	N50.1	Vascular disorders of male genital organs ♂
	N52.01	Erectile dysfunction due to arterial insufficiency ♂
	N52.03	Combined arterial insufficiency and corporo-venous occlusive erectile dysfunction ♂
	N52.1	Erectile dysfunction due to diseases classified elsewhere ♂
❼	S30.21	Contusion of penis
❼	S31.20	Unspecified open wound of penis

ICD-10-CM Coding Notes

For codes requiring a 7th character extension, refer to your ICD-10-CM book. Review the character descriptions and coding guidelines for proper selection. For some procedures, only certain characters will apply.

CCI Edits

Refer to Appendix A for CCI edits.

Facility RVUs ▢

Code	Work	PE Facility	MP	Total Facility
37788	23.33	10.77	2.78	36.88

Non-facility RVUs ▢

Code	Work	PE Non-Facility	MP	Total Non-Facility
37788	23.33	10.77	2.78	36.88

Modifiers (PAR) ▢

Code	Mod 50	Mod 51	Mod 62	Mod 66	Mod 80
37788	0	2	1	0	2

Global Period

Code	Days
37788	090

37790

37790 Penile venous occlusive procedure

AMA Coding Guideline

Surgical Procedures on Arteries and Veins

Primary vascular procedure listings include establishing both inflow and outflow by whatever procedures necessary. Also included is that portion of the operative arteriogram performed by the surgeon, as indicated. Sympathectomy, when done, is included in the listed aortic procedures. For unlisted vascular procedure, use 37799.

Please see the Surgery Guidelines section for the following guidelines:

- *Surgical Procedures on the Cardiovascular System*

Plain English Description

A penile venous occlusive procedure is performed on a patient with penile venous leakage, penile veno-occlusive insufficiency, or dysfunction. Veno-occlusive dysfunction is a cause of erectile dysfunction that results from a greater outflow of venous blood than inflow. Storage of a sufficient amount of blood in the corpora cavernosa is necessary for penile rigidity, and leakage causes insufficient storage of blood resulting in erectile dysfunction. Veno-occlusive dysfunction may be a result of trauma or due to a congenital disorder. Penile venous ligation is performed on the cavernosal and crural veins. Using microsurgical technique, the penile veins exhibiting leakage are exposed and carefully dissected free of surrounding tissue. The dorsal arteries and nerves are identified and protected. The penile veins exhibiting leakage are individually suture ligated. Following completion of the ligation procedure, the penis is observed for evidence of erection. Surgical wounds are closed in a layered fashion.

Penile venous occlusive procedure

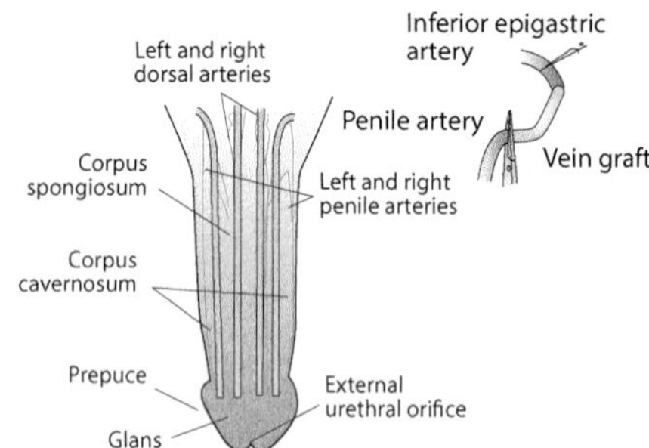

A penile vein is occluded with sutures to either reduce or completely stop blood flow.

ICD-10-CM Diagnostic Codes

N50.1	Vascular disorders of male genital organs ♂
N52.02	Corporo-venous occlusive erectile dysfunction ♂
N52.03	Combined arterial insufficiency and corporo-venous occlusive erectile dysfunction ♂

CCI Edits

Refer to Appendix A for CCI edits.

Facility RVUs ▯

Code	Work	PE Facility	MP	Total Facility
37790	8.43	4.77	1.00	14.20

Non-facility RVUs ▯

Code	Work	PE Non-Facility	MP	Total Non-Facility
37790	8.43	4.77	1.00	14.20

Modifiers (PAR) ▯

Code	Mod 50	Mod 51	Mod 62	Mod 66	Mod 80
37790	0	2	0	0	0

Global Period

Code	Days
37790	090

38500-38505

38500 Biopsy or excision of lymph node(s); open, superficial

(Do not report 38500 with 38700-38780)

38505 Biopsy or excision of lymph node(s); by needle, superficial (eg, cervical, inguinal, axillary)

(If imaging guidance is performed, see 76942, 77002, 77012, 77021)

(For fine needle aspiration biopsy, see 10004, 10005, 10006, 10007, 10008, 10009, 10010, 10011, 10012, 10021)

(For evaluation of fine needle aspirate, see 88172, 88173)

AMA Coding Notes

Excision Procedures on the Lymph Nodes and Lymphatic Channels

(For injection for sentinel node identification, use 38792)

AMA *CPT® Assistant*

38500: Jun 97: 5, Jul 99: 7, Oct 05: 23, Dec 07: 8, Sep 08: 5, Jan 09: 7, Jun 12: 15

38505: Jul 99: 6, Jan 09: 7, Feb 19: 8

Plain English Description

A biopsy or excision of one or more superficial lymph nodes is performed. Superficial cervical, inguinal, and axillary lymph nodes lie close to the surface of the skin and can be accessed with only minimal dissection of overlying tissues. In 38500, an open biopsy or excision is performed. The lymph node to be biopsied is identified by palpation. The skin overlying the node is disinfected and a local anesthetic administered. The skin is incised and the lymph node exposed. If an excisional biopsy is performed, the lymph node is dissected free of surrounding tissue and removed. If an incisional biopsy is performed, a tissue sample is obtained from the lymph node. The lymph node or the tissue sample is then sent for separately reportable laboratory analysis. In 38505, a needle biopsy is obtained. The lymph node is identified by palpation. The skin is cleansed over the planned puncture site and local anesthesia administered. Separately reportable imaging guidance is used as needed. A large-bore needle is then advanced into the lymph node and tissue samples obtained and sent for separately reportable laboratory evaluation.

Biopsy/excision of lymph node(s); superficial

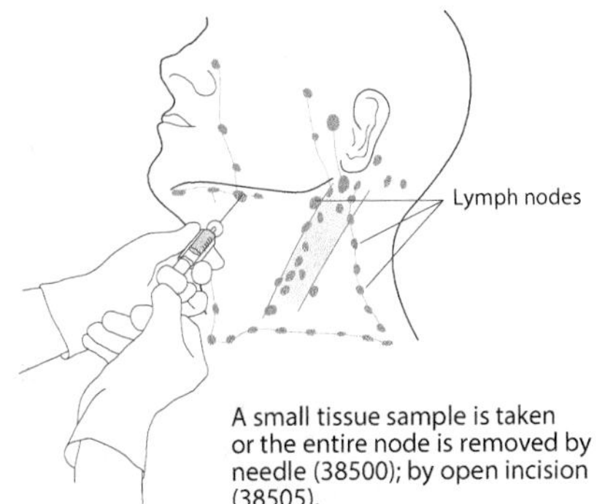

A small tissue sample is taken or the entire node is removed by needle (38500); by open incision (38505).

ICD-10-CM Diagnostic Codes

	C60.0	Malignant neoplasm of prepuce ♂
	C60.1	Malignant neoplasm of glans penis ♂
	C60.2	Malignant neoplasm of body of penis ♂
	C60.8	Malignant neoplasm of overlapping sites of penis ♂
	C61	Malignant neoplasm of prostate ♂
⇄	C62.01	Malignant neoplasm of undescended right testis ♂
⇄	C62.02	Malignant neoplasm of undescended left testis ♂
⇄	C62.11	Malignant neoplasm of descended right testis ♂
⇄	C62.12	Malignant neoplasm of descended left testis ♂
⇄	C63.01	Malignant neoplasm of right epididymis ♂
⇄	C63.02	Malignant neoplasm of left epididymis ♂
⇄	C63.11	Malignant neoplasm of right spermatic cord ♂
⇄	C63.12	Malignant neoplasm of left spermatic cord ♂
	C63.2	Malignant neoplasm of scrotum ♂
	C63.7	Malignant neoplasm of other specified male genital organs ♂
	C67.0	Malignant neoplasm of trigone of bladder
	C67.1	Malignant neoplasm of dome of bladder
	C67.2	Malignant neoplasm of lateral wall of bladder
	C67.3	Malignant neoplasm of anterior wall of bladder
	C67.4	Malignant neoplasm of posterior wall of bladder
	C67.5	Malignant neoplasm of bladder neck
	C67.6	Malignant neoplasm of ureteric orifice
	C67.7	Malignant neoplasm of urachus
	C67.8	Malignant neoplasm of overlapping sites of bladder
	C77.4	Secondary and unspecified malignant neoplasm of inguinal and lower limb lymph nodes

CCI Edits

Refer to Appendix A for CCI edits.

Facility RVUs

Code	Work	PE Facility	MP	Total Facility
38500	3.79	2.93	0.89	7.61
38505	1.59	0.77	0.14	2.50

Non-facility RVUs

Code	Work	PE Non-Facility	MP	Total Non-Facility
38500	3.79	5.45	0.89	10.13
38505	1.59	3.60	0.14	5.33

Modifiers (PAR)

Code	Mod 50	Mod 51	Mod 62	Mod 66	Mod 80
38500	1	2	0	0	1
38505	1	2	0	0	1

Global Period

Code	Days
38500	010
38505	000

38531

38531 Biopsy or excision of lymph node(s); open, inguinofemoral node(s)

(For bilateral procedure, report 38531 with modifier 50)

AMA Coding Notes

Excision Procedures on the Lymph Nodes and Lymphatic Channels

(For injection for sentinel node identification, use 38792)

AMA *CPT® Assistant* ▢

38531: Feb 19: 8

Plain English Description

Open biopsy or excision of inguinofemoral lymph node(s) may be performed to diagnose, treat, or prevent the spread of cancer into the lymph nodes of the groin from cancer cells of the vulva, penis, anus, and even the skin of the torso. Cancerous nodes or nodes with a high chance of becoming cancerous may be removed, or the first node in a chain may be biopsied and tested for the presence of cancerous cells. A chain of approximately 10 superficial lymph nodes located close to the surface in the upper inner thigh drain into 3 to 5 deeper nodes in the connective tissue of the upper thigh. An incision is made in the groin over the involved nodes, which may be only the superficial nodes, or dissection may be carried down through soft tissues to the deep nodes as well, taking care to protect surrounding blood vessels and nerves. One or more node(s) is dissected free of surrounding tissue and removed, or tissue samples of the node(s) are biopsied. A small skin flap may be created to cover the incision and tubes are placed for drainage. The nodes or tissue samples are sent to the laboratory for separately reportable pathological evaluation.

Biopsy or excision of lymph node(s); open, inguinofemoral node(s)

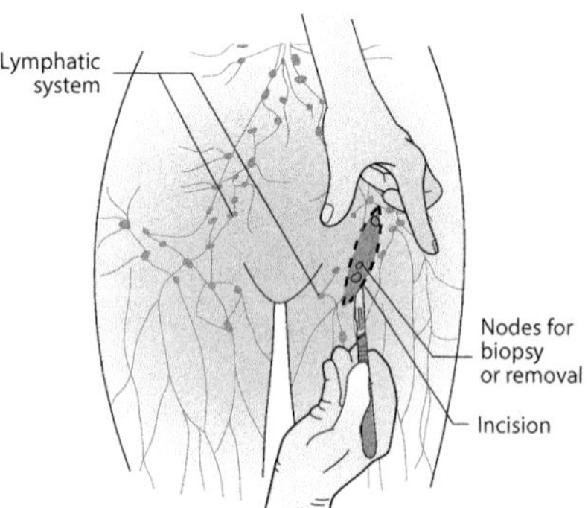

ICD-10-CM Diagnostic Codes

	C43.59	Malignant melanoma of other part of trunk
	C44.529	Squamous cell carcinoma of skin of other part of trunk
	C44.599	Other specified malignant neoplasm of skin of other part of trunk
	C44.82	Squamous cell carcinoma of overlapping sites of skin
	C60.0	Malignant neoplasm of prepuce ♂
	C60.1	Malignant neoplasm of glans penis ♂
	C60.2	Malignant neoplasm of body of penis ♂
	C60.8	Malignant neoplasm of overlapping sites of penis ♂
	C60.9	Malignant neoplasm of penis, unspecified ♂
	C61	Malignant neoplasm of prostate ♂
⇄	C62.01	Malignant neoplasm of undescended right testis ♂
⇄	C62.02	Malignant neoplasm of undescended left testis ♂
⇄	C62.11	Malignant neoplasm of descended right testis ♂
⇄	C62.12	Malignant neoplasm of descended left testis ♂
⇄	C63.01	Malignant neoplasm of right epididymis ♂
⇄	C63.02	Malignant neoplasm of left epididymis ♂
⇄	C63.11	Malignant neoplasm of right spermatic cord ♂
⇄	C63.12	Malignant neoplasm of left spermatic cord ♂
	C63.2	Malignant neoplasm of scrotum ♂
	C63.7	Malignant neoplasm of other specified male genital organs ♂
	C63.8	Malignant neoplasm of overlapping sites of male genital organs ♂
	C77.4	Secondary and unspecified malignant neoplasm of inguinal and lower limb lymph nodes
	D03.59	Melanoma in situ of other part of trunk
	D03.8	Melanoma in situ of other sites
	D07.4	Carcinoma in situ of penis ♂
	D07.5	Carcinoma in situ of prostate ♂
	D07.61	Carcinoma in situ of scrotum ♂
	D07.69	Carcinoma in situ of other male genital organs ♂
	D18.1	Lymphangioma, any site
	D36.0	Benign neoplasm of lymph nodes
	I88.1	Chronic lymphadenitis, except mesenteric
	I88.8	Other nonspecific lymphadenitis
	I88.9	Nonspecific lymphadenitis, unspecified
	R59.0	Localized enlarged lymph nodes
	Z85.46	Personal history of malignant neoplasm of prostate ♂
	Z85.47	Personal history of malignant neoplasm of testis ♂
	Z85.48	Personal history of malignant neoplasm of epididymis ♂
	Z85.49	Personal history of malignant neoplasm of other male genital organs ♂

CCI Edits

Refer to Appendix A for CCI edits.

Facility RVUs ▢

Code	Work	PE Facility	MP	Total Facility
38531	6.74	5.00	1.55	13.29

Non-facility RVUs ▢

Code	Work	PE Non-Facility	MP	Total Non-Facility
38531	6.74	5.00	1.55	13.29

Modifiers (PAR) ▢

Code	Mod 50	Mod 51	Mod 62	Mod 66	Mod 80
38531	1	2	0	0	0

Global Period

Code	Days
38531	090

38562-38564

38562 Limited lymphadenectomy for staging (separate procedure); pelvic and para-aortic

(When combined with prostatectomy, use 55812 or 55842)

(When combined with insertion of radioactive substance into prostate, use 55862)

38564 Limited lymphadenectomy for staging (separate procedure); retroperitoneal (aortic and/or splenic)

AMA *CPT® Assistant* ▯

38562: Mar 01: 10

Plain English Description

The abdomen is incised for a limited staging lymphadenectomy on the pelvic and para-aortic lymph nodes (38562). Before opening the peritoneum, the pelvic lymph nodes are explored and removed. Taking care to preserve the genitofemoral nerve and psoas muscle, fatty tissue is stripped from the mid-portion of both common iliac vessels and along the internal and external iliac vessels to the level of the circumflex iliac vein. Iliac, hypogastric, and obturator nodes are excised bilaterally. The peritoneal cavity is opened and the abdomen and pelvis are explored for evidence of metastatic disease. The para-aortic lymph nodes are exposed. Biopsies are taken and sent for frozen section. Involved para-aortic lymph nodes are excised. For retroperitoneal lymph node staging (38564), the two most common approaches are transabdominal and thoracoabdominal. Typically, the procedure is performed first on the same side as the malignancy. The retroperitoneum is fully exposed. The aortic lymph node dissection begins at the take-off of the renal vessels and then extends laterally to the ureters and inferiorly to the bifurcation of the inferior mesenteric artery. The dissection includes lymph nodes between the aorta and inferior vena cava. Lymph nodes along the splenic artery may also be sampled and positive nodes excised. Frozen section is performed on all lymph node samples to determine the extent of lymph node involvement and the procedure is tailored based on frozen section findings. Depending on the extent of involvement of lymph nodes on the ipsilateral (same) side, lymph nodes on the contralateral (opposite) side may also be sampled and excised.

Limited lymphadenectomy for staging

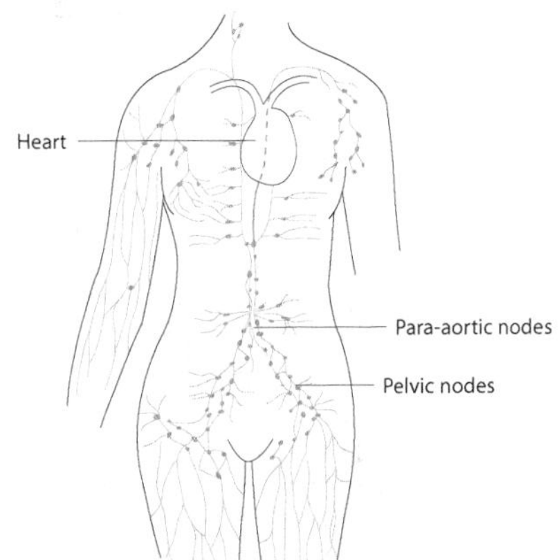

An abdominal incision is made and lymph nodes are removed for staging.

ICD-10-CM Diagnostic Codes

	C60.0	Malignant neoplasm of prepuce ♂
	C60.1	Malignant neoplasm of glans penis ♂
	C60.2	Malignant neoplasm of body of penis ♂
	C60.8	Malignant neoplasm of overlapping sites of penis ♂
	C61	Malignant neoplasm of prostate ♂
⇄	C62.01	Malignant neoplasm of undescended right testis ♂
⇄	C62.02	Malignant neoplasm of undescended left testis ♂
⇄	C62.11	Malignant neoplasm of descended right testis ♂
⇄	C62.12	Malignant neoplasm of descended left testis ♂
⇄	C63.01	Malignant neoplasm of right epididymis ♂
⇄	C63.02	Malignant neoplasm of left epididymis ♂
⇄	C63.11	Malignant neoplasm of right spermatic cord ♂
⇄	C63.12	Malignant neoplasm of left spermatic cord ♂
	C63.2	Malignant neoplasm of scrotum ♂
	C63.7	Malignant neoplasm of other specified male genital organs ♂
	C63.8	Malignant neoplasm of overlapping sites of male genital organs ♂
⇄	C64.1	Malignant neoplasm of right kidney, except renal pelvis
⇄	C64.2	Malignant neoplasm of left kidney, except renal pelvis
⇄	C65.1	Malignant neoplasm of right renal pelvis
⇄	C65.2	Malignant neoplasm of left renal pelvis
⇄	C66.1	Malignant neoplasm of right ureter
⇄	C66.2	Malignant neoplasm of left ureter
	C67.0	Malignant neoplasm of trigone of bladder
	C67.1	Malignant neoplasm of dome of bladder
	C67.2	Malignant neoplasm of lateral wall of bladder
	C67.3	Malignant neoplasm of anterior wall of bladder
	C67.4	Malignant neoplasm of posterior wall of bladder
	C67.5	Malignant neoplasm of bladder neck
	C67.6	Malignant neoplasm of ureteric orifice
	C67.8	Malignant neoplasm of overlapping sites of bladder
	C68.0	Malignant neoplasm of urethra
	C68.1	Malignant neoplasm of paraurethral glands
	C68.8	Malignant neoplasm of overlapping sites of urinary organs
	C78.6	Secondary malignant neoplasm of retroperitoneum and peritoneum
⇄	C79.01	Secondary malignant neoplasm of right kidney and renal pelvis
⇄	C79.02	Secondary malignant neoplasm of left kidney and renal pelvis
	C79.11	Secondary malignant neoplasm of bladder
	C79.19	Secondary malignant neoplasm of other urinary organs
	C7A.093	Malignant carcinoid tumor of the kidney
	C7B.01	Secondary carcinoid tumors of distant lymph nodes
	C7B.04	Secondary carcinoid tumors of peritoneum
	C7B.09	Secondary carcinoid tumors of other sites
	C7B.1	Secondary Merkel cell carcinoma

CCI Edits

Refer to Appendix A for CCI edits.

Facility RVUs ▯

Code	Work	PE Facility	MP	Total Facility
38562	11.06	7.91	1.94	20.91
38564	11.38	7.10	2.50	20.98

Non-facility RVUs ▯

Code	Work	PE Non-Facility	MP	Total Non-Facility
38562	11.06	7.91	1.94	20.91
38564	11.38	7.10	2.50	20.98

Modifiers (PAR) ▯

Code	Mod 50	Mod 51	Mod 62	Mod 66	Mod 80
38562	2	2	1	0	2
38564	0	2	1	0	2

Global Period

Code	Days
38562	090
38564	090

38570

38570 Laparoscopy, surgical; with retroperitoneal lymph node sampling (biopsy), single or multiple

AMA Coding Guideline

Laparoscopic Procedures on the Lymph Nodes and Lymphatic Channels

Surgical laparoscopy always includes diagnostic laparoscopy. To report a diagnostic laparoscopy (peritoneoscopy) (separate procedure), use 49320.

AMA *CPT® Assistant* ▢

38570: Nov 99: 21, Mar 00: 8

Plain English Description

The physician performs laparoscopic retroperitoneal lymph sampling (biopsy). Using a transperitoneal approach, a trocar is placed off the midline just lateral to the umbilicus on the same side as the malignancy and the laparoscope is inserted. Two additional operating trocars are placed above and below the first just lateral to the rectus muscle. Additional trocars are placed as needed. The colon is mobilized to allow full exposure of the retroperitoneum. The lymph node sampling begins along the aorta at the take-off of the renal vessels and then extends laterally to the ureters and inferiorly to the bifurcation of the inferior mesenteric artery. The sampling includes lymph nodes between the aorta and inferior vena cava. Lymph nodes along the splenic artery may also be sampled and positive nodes excised. Frozen section is performed on all lymph node samples to determine the extent of lymph node involvement and the procedure is tailored based on frozen section findings. Depending on the extent of involvement of lymph nodes on the ipsilateral (same) side, lymph nodes on the contralateral (opposite) side may also be sampled. Upon completion of the procedure, surgical instruments are removed along with the laparoscope and incisions are sutured closed.

Laparoscopy, surgical; with retroperitoneal lymph node sampling (biopsy), single or multiple

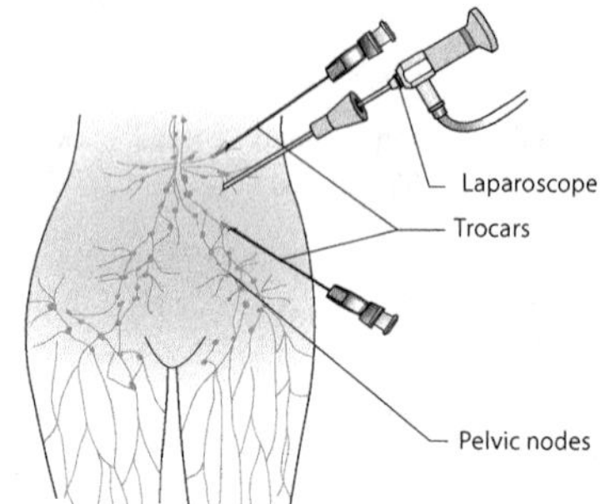

ICD-10-CM Diagnostic Codes

	C48.0	Malignant neoplasm of retroperitoneum
	C48.8	Malignant neoplasm of overlapping sites of retroperitoneum and peritoneum
	C60.0	Malignant neoplasm of prepuce ♂
	C60.1	Malignant neoplasm of glans penis ♂
	C60.2	Malignant neoplasm of body of penis ♂
	C60.8	Malignant neoplasm of overlapping sites of penis ♂
	C61	Malignant neoplasm of prostate ♂
⇄	C62.01	Malignant neoplasm of undescended right testis ♂
⇄	C62.02	Malignant neoplasm of undescended left testis ♂
⇄	C62.11	Malignant neoplasm of descended right testis ♂
⇄	C62.12	Malignant neoplasm of descended left testis ♂
⇄	C63.01	Malignant neoplasm of right epididymis ♂
⇄	C63.02	Malignant neoplasm of left epididymis ♂
⇄	C63.11	Malignant neoplasm of right spermatic cord ♂
⇄	C63.12	Malignant neoplasm of left spermatic cord ♂
	C63.2	Malignant neoplasm of scrotum ♂
	C63.7	Malignant neoplasm of other specified male genital organs ♂
	C63.8	Malignant neoplasm of overlapping sites of male genital organs ♂
⇄	C64.1	Malignant neoplasm of right kidney, except renal pelvis
⇄	C64.2	Malignant neoplasm of left kidney, except renal pelvis
⇄	C65.1	Malignant neoplasm of right renal pelvis
⇄	C65.2	Malignant neoplasm of left renal pelvis
⇄	C66.1	Malignant neoplasm of right ureter
⇄	C66.2	Malignant neoplasm of left ureter
	C67.0	Malignant neoplasm of trigone of bladder
	C67.1	Malignant neoplasm of dome of bladder
	C67.2	Malignant neoplasm of lateral wall of bladder
	C67.3	Malignant neoplasm of anterior wall of bladder
	C67.4	Malignant neoplasm of posterior wall of bladder
	C67.5	Malignant neoplasm of bladder neck
	C67.6	Malignant neoplasm of ureteric orifice
	C67.8	Malignant neoplasm of overlapping sites of bladder
	C68.0	Malignant neoplasm of urethra
	C68.1	Malignant neoplasm of paraurethral glands
	C68.8	Malignant neoplasm of overlapping sites of urinary organs
	C78.6	Secondary malignant neoplasm of retroperitoneum and peritoneum
⇄	C79.01	Secondary malignant neoplasm of right kidney and renal pelvis
⇄	C79.02	Secondary malignant neoplasm of left kidney and renal pelvis
	C79.11	Secondary malignant neoplasm of bladder
	C79.19	Secondary malignant neoplasm of other urinary organs
	C7A.093	Malignant carcinoid tumor of the kidney
	C7B.01	Secondary carcinoid tumors of distant lymph nodes
	C7B.04	Secondary carcinoid tumors of peritoneum
	C7B.09	Secondary carcinoid tumors of other sites
	C7B.1	Secondary Merkel cell carcinoma

CCI Edits

Refer to Appendix A for CCI edits.

Facility RVUs ▢

Code	Work	PE Facility	MP	Total Facility
38570	8.49	5.28	1.47	15.24

Non-facility RVUs ▢

Code	Work	PE Non-Facility	MP	Total Non-Facility
38570	8.49	5.28	1.47	15.24

Modifiers (PAR) ▢

Code	Mod 50	Mod 51	Mod 62	Mod 66	Mod 80
38570	0	3	2	0	2

Global Period

Code	Days
38570	010

38760-38765

38760 Inguinofemoral lymphadenectomy, superficial, including Cloquet's node (separate procedure)

(For bilateral procedure, report 38760 with modifier 50)

38765 Inguinofemoral lymphadenectomy, superficial, in continuity with pelvic lymphadenectomy, including external iliac, hypogastric, and obturator nodes (separate procedure)

(For bilateral procedure, report 38765 with modifier 50)

Inguinofemoral lymphadenectomy, superficial

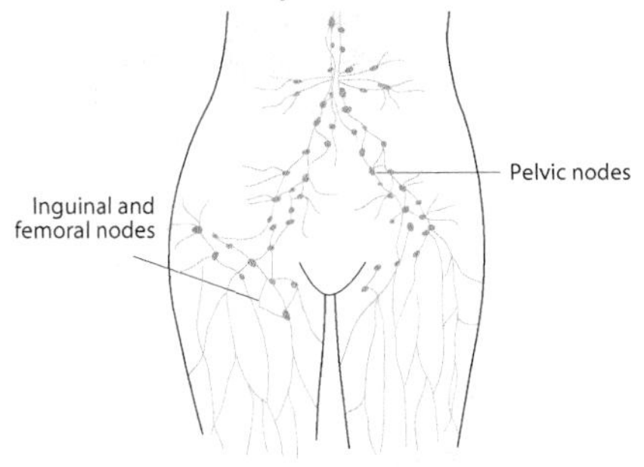

Inguinofemoral lymphadenectomy including Cloquet's node (38760); procedure done in continuity with pelvic nodes (38765)

AMA Coding Notes

Radical Lymphadenectomy (Radical Resection of Lymph Nodes)

(For limited pelvic and retroperitoneal lymphadenectomies, see 38562, 38564)

Plain English Description

A superficial inguinofemoral lymphadenectomy is performed in a separate procedure. In 38760, the procedure is performed with excision of Cloquet's node. Cloquet's node is the deep inguinal lymph node that represents the transitional zone between the inguinal and the iliac regions. An incision is made parallel to the inguinofemoral ligament and carried down to Camper's fascia. Skin flaps are elevated while simultaneously separating the flaps from the underlying fat pad. Deep tissues at the superior aspect of the inguinal region are dissected. Cloquet's node is identified, excised, and frozen section is performed. The fat pad containing nodal tissue is elevated and mobilized down to the inferior margin of the inguinal ligament. Dissection continues into the femoral triangle. The cribriform fascia is opened. Once the nodal tissue over the common femoral vein has been completely freed, the inguinofemoral nodal tissue is removed as a single specimen. In 38765, inguinofemoral lymphadenectomy is performed as described above. If Cloquet's node is positive for malignancy, pelvic lymphadenectomy including excision of external iliac, hypogastric, and obturator nodes is also performed. The abdomen is incised. Without opening the peritoneum, the pelvic lymph nodes on the side of the malignancy are explored. Taking care to preserve the genitofemoral nerve and psoas muscle, fatty tissue is stripped from the mid-portion of the common iliac vessel and along the internal and external iliac vessels to the level of the circumflex iliac vein. Iliac, hypogastric, and obturator nodes are excised and sent for separately reportable pathological evaluation. The groin and abdominal incisions are closed in layers.

ICD-10-CM Diagnostic Codes

	C60.0	Malignant neoplasm of prepuce ♂
	C60.1	Malignant neoplasm of glans penis ♂
	C60.2	Malignant neoplasm of body of penis ♂
	C60.8	Malignant neoplasm of overlapping sites of penis ♂
	C61	Malignant neoplasm of prostate ♂
⇄	C62.01	Malignant neoplasm of undescended right testis ♂
⇄	C62.02	Malignant neoplasm of undescended left testis ♂
⇄	C62.11	Malignant neoplasm of descended right testis ♂
⇄	C62.12	Malignant neoplasm of descended left testis ♂
⇄	C63.01	Malignant neoplasm of right epididymis ♂
⇄	C63.02	Malignant neoplasm of left epididymis ♂
⇄	C63.11	Malignant neoplasm of right spermatic cord ♂
⇄	C63.12	Malignant neoplasm of left spermatic cord ♂
	C63.2	Malignant neoplasm of scrotum ♂
	C63.7	Malignant neoplasm of other specified male genital organs ♂
	C63.8	Malignant neoplasm of overlapping sites of male genital organs ♂
	C67.0	Malignant neoplasm of trigone of bladder
	C67.1	Malignant neoplasm of dome of bladder
	C67.2	Malignant neoplasm of lateral wall of bladder
	C67.3	Malignant neoplasm of anterior wall of bladder
	C67.4	Malignant neoplasm of posterior wall of bladder
	C67.5	Malignant neoplasm of bladder neck
	C67.6	Malignant neoplasm of ureteric orifice
	C67.8	Malignant neoplasm of overlapping sites of bladder
	C68.0	Malignant neoplasm of urethra
	C68.1	Malignant neoplasm of paraurethral glands
	C68.8	Malignant neoplasm of overlapping sites of urinary organs
	C77.4	Secondary and unspecified malignant neoplasm of inguinal and lower limb lymph nodes
	C77.5	Secondary and unspecified malignant neoplasm of intrapelvic lymph nodes
	D36.0	Benign neoplasm of lymph nodes

CCI Edits

Refer to Appendix A for CCI edits.

Facility RVUs ☐

Code	Work	PE Facility	MP	Total Facility
38760	13.62	8.35	2.85	24.82
38765	21.91	12.46	4.45	38.82

Non-facility RVUs ☐

Code	Work	PE Non-Facility	MP	Total Non-Facility
38760	13.62	8.35	2.85	24.82
38765	21.91	12.46	4.45	38.82

Modifiers (PAR) ☐

Code	Mod 50	Mod 51	Mod 62	Mod 66	Mod 80
38760	1	2	1	0	2
38765	1	2	1	0	2

Global Period

Code	Days
38760	090
38765	090

38770

38770 Pelvic lymphadenectomy, including external iliac, hypogastric, and obturator nodes (separate procedure)

(For bilateral procedure, report 38770 with modifier 50)

AMA Coding Notes

Radical Lymphadenectomy (Radical Resection of Lymph Nodes)

(For limited pelvic and retroperitoneal lymphadenectomies, see 38562, 38564)

Plain English Description

The abdomen is incised, and without opening the peritoneum, the pelvic lymph nodes on the side of the malignancy are explored. Taking care to preserve the genitofemoral nerve and psoas muscle, fatty tissue is stripped from the mid-portion of both common iliac vessels and along the internal and external iliac vessels to the level of the circumflex iliac vein. Iliac, hypogastric, and obturator nodes are excised and sent for separately reportable pathological evaluation. The abdominal incision is closed in layers.

Pelvic lymphadenectomy

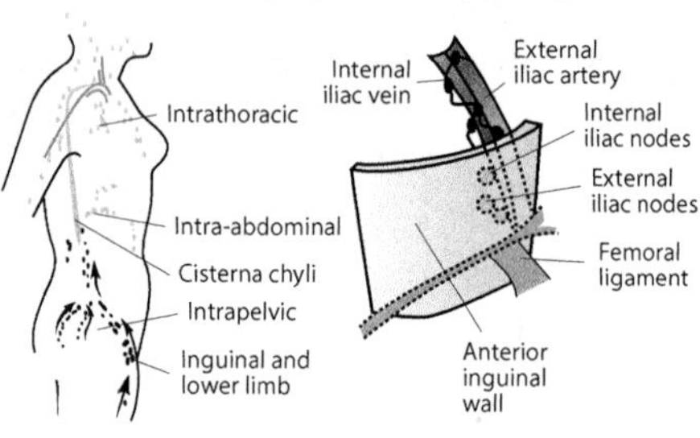

Pelvic nodes are removed, including internal and external iliac nodes.

ICD-10-CM Diagnostic Codes

	C60.0	Malignant neoplasm of prepuce ♂
	C60.1	Malignant neoplasm of glans penis ♂
	C60.2	Malignant neoplasm of body of penis ♂
	C60.8	Malignant neoplasm of overlapping sites of penis ♂
	C61	Malignant neoplasm of prostate ♂
⇄	C62.01	Malignant neoplasm of undescended right testis ♂
⇄	C62.02	Malignant neoplasm of undescended left testis ♂
⇄	C62.11	Malignant neoplasm of descended right testis ♂
⇄	C62.12	Malignant neoplasm of descended left testis ♂
⇄	C63.01	Malignant neoplasm of right epididymis ♂
⇄	C63.02	Malignant neoplasm of left epididymis ♂
⇄	C63.12	Malignant neoplasm of left spermatic cord ♂
	C63.2	Malignant neoplasm of scrotum ♂
	C63.7	Malignant neoplasm of other specified male genital organs ♂
	C63.8	Malignant neoplasm of overlapping sites of male genital organs ♂
⇄	C64.1	Malignant neoplasm of right kidney, except renal pelvis
⇄	C64.2	Malignant neoplasm of left kidney, except renal pelvis
⇄	C65.1	Malignant neoplasm of right renal pelvis
⇄	C65.2	Malignant neoplasm of left renal pelvis
⇄	C66.1	Malignant neoplasm of right ureter
⇄	C66.2	Malignant neoplasm of left ureter
	C67.0	Malignant neoplasm of trigone of bladder
	C67.1	Malignant neoplasm of dome of bladder
	C67.2	Malignant neoplasm of lateral wall of bladder
	C67.3	Malignant neoplasm of anterior wall of bladder
	C67.4	Malignant neoplasm of posterior wall of bladder
	C67.5	Malignant neoplasm of bladder neck
	C67.6	Malignant neoplasm of ureteric orifice
	C67.8	Malignant neoplasm of overlapping sites of bladder
	C68.0	Malignant neoplasm of urethra
	C68.1	Malignant neoplasm of paraurethral glands
	C68.8	Malignant neoplasm of overlapping sites of urinary organs
	C77.5	Secondary and unspecified malignant neoplasm of intrapelvic lymph nodes
	C7A.093	Malignant carcinoid tumor of the kidney
	C7B.01	Secondary carcinoid tumors of distant lymph nodes

CCI Edits

Refer to Appendix A for CCI edits.

Facility RVUs

Code	Work	PE Facility	MP	Total Facility
38770	14.06	7.53	2.07	23.66

Non-facility RVUs

Code	Work	PE Non-Facility	MP	Total Non-Facility
38770	14.06	7.53	2.07	23.66

Modifiers (PAR)

Code	Mod 50	Mod 51	Mod 62	Mod 66	Mod 80
38770	1	2	1	0	2

Global Period

Code	Days
38770	090

38780

38780 Retroperitoneal transabdominal lymphadenectomy, extensive, including pelvic, aortic, and renal nodes (separate procedure)

(For excision and repair of lymphedematous skin and subcutaneous tissue, see 15004-15005, 15570-15650)

AMA Coding Notes

Radical Lymphadenectomy (Radical Resection of Lymph Nodes)

(For limited pelvic and retroperitoneal lymphadenectomies, see 38562, 38564)

Plain English Description

Typically, the procedure is performed first on the same side as the malignancy. Before opening the retroperitoneum, pelvic lymph nodes are explored and removed. Taking care to preserve the genitofemoral nerve and psoas muscle, fatty tissue is stripped from the mid-portion of both common iliac vessels and along the internal and external iliac vessels to the level of the circumflex iliac vein. Iliac, hypogastric, and obturator nodes are excised bilaterally. The retroperitoneum is fully exposed using a transabdominal approach. The retroperitoneum is inspected for evidence of metastatic disease. The aortic lymph node dissection begins at the take-off of the renal vessels and then extends laterally to the ureters and inferiorly to the bifurcation of the inferior mesenteric artery. The dissection includes lymph nodes between the aorta and inferior vena cava. Aortic lymph nodes are excised along with surrounding tissue. Lymph nodes along the renal and splenic arteries may also be excised. Depending on the extent of involvement of lymph nodes on the ipsilateral (same) side, lymph nodes on the contralateral (opposite) side may also be sampled and excised.

Retroperitoneal transabdominal lymphadenectomy

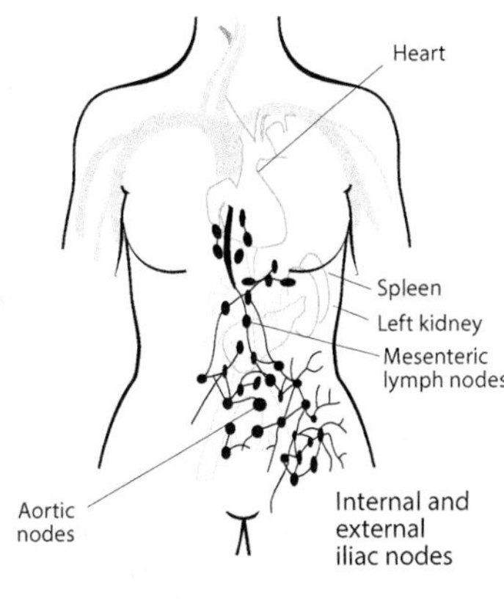

Extensive removal of lymph nodes of the retroperitoneal area is performed.

ICD-10-CM Diagnostic Codes

	C48.0	Malignant neoplasm of retroperitoneum
	C48.1	Malignant neoplasm of specified parts of peritoneum
	C48.8	Malignant neoplasm of overlapping sites of retroperitoneum and peritoneum
	C61	Malignant neoplasm of prostate ♂
⇄	C62.01	Malignant neoplasm of undescended right testis ♂
⇄	C62.02	Malignant neoplasm of undescended left testis ♂
⇄	C62.11	Malignant neoplasm of descended right testis ♂
⇄	C62.12	Malignant neoplasm of descended left testis ♂
⇄	C63.01	Malignant neoplasm of right epididymis ♂
⇄	C63.02	Malignant neoplasm of left epididymis ♂
⇄	C63.11	Malignant neoplasm of right spermatic cord ♂
⇄	C63.12	Malignant neoplasm of left spermatic cord ♂
	C63.7	Malignant neoplasm of other specified male genital organs ♂
	C63.8	Malignant neoplasm of overlapping sites of male genital organs ♂
⇄	C64.1	Malignant neoplasm of right kidney, except renal pelvis
⇄	C64.2	Malignant neoplasm of left kidney, except renal pelvis
⇄	C65.1	Malignant neoplasm of right renal pelvis
⇄	C65.2	Malignant neoplasm of left renal pelvis
⇄	C66.1	Malignant neoplasm of right ureter
⇄	C66.2	Malignant neoplasm of left ureter
	C67.0	Malignant neoplasm of trigone of bladder
	C67.1	Malignant neoplasm of dome of bladder
	C67.2	Malignant neoplasm of lateral wall of bladder
	C67.3	Malignant neoplasm of anterior wall of bladder
	C67.4	Malignant neoplasm of posterior wall of bladder
	C67.5	Malignant neoplasm of bladder neck
	C67.6	Malignant neoplasm of ureteric orifice
	C67.8	Malignant neoplasm of overlapping sites of bladder
	C68.0	Malignant neoplasm of urethra
	C68.1	Malignant neoplasm of paraurethral glands
	C68.8	Malignant neoplasm of overlapping sites of urinary organs
⇄	C74.01	Malignant neoplasm of cortex of right adrenal gland
⇄	C74.02	Malignant neoplasm of cortex of left adrenal gland
⇄	C74.11	Malignant neoplasm of medulla of right adrenal gland
⇄	C74.12	Malignant neoplasm of medulla of left adrenal gland
	C77.2	Secondary and unspecified malignant neoplasm of intra-abdominal lymph nodes
	C77.5	Secondary and unspecified malignant neoplasm of intrapelvic lymph nodes
	C78.6	Secondary malignant neoplasm of retroperitoneum and peritoneum
⇄	C79.01	Secondary malignant neoplasm of right kidney and renal pelvis
⇄	C79.02	Secondary malignant neoplasm of left kidney and renal pelvis
	C79.11	Secondary malignant neoplasm of bladder
	C79.19	Secondary malignant neoplasm of other urinary organs
	C7A.093	Malignant carcinoid tumor of the kidney
	C7B.01	Secondary carcinoid tumors of distant lymph nodes
	C7B.04	Secondary carcinoid tumors of peritoneum
	C7B.09	Secondary carcinoid tumors of other sites
	C7B.1	Secondary Merkel cell carcinoma
	D48.3	Neoplasm of uncertain behavior of retroperitoneum
	D48.4	Neoplasm of uncertain behavior of peritoneum

CCI Edits

Refer to Appendix A for CCI edits.

Facility RVUs ▯

Code	Work	PE Facility	MP	Total Facility
38780	17.70	9.95	3.03	30.68

Non-facility RVUs ▯

Code	Work	PE Non-Facility	MP	Total Non-Facility
38780	17.70	9.95	3.03	30.68

Modifiers (PAR) ▯

Code	Mod 50	Mod 51	Mod 62	Mod 66	Mod 80
38780	0	2	1	0	2

Global Period

Code	Days
38780	090

44660-44661

44660 Closure of enterovesical fistula; without intestinal or bladder resection

44661 Closure of enterovesical fistula; with intestine and/or bladder resection

(For closure of renocolic fistula, see 50525, 50526)

(For closure of gastrocolic fistula, use 43880)

(For closure of rectovesical fistula, see 45800, 45805)

Plain English Description

An enterovesical fistula is an abnormal communication between a segment of intestine and the urinary bladder. The most common cause of enterovesical fistula is diverticular disease of the colon, with other common causes being colon cancer, inflammatory bowel diseases such as Crohn's disease, complications of radiation therapy, or trauma. The abdomen is opened and the fistulous tract located. The fistulous tract is divided and bladder and bowel separated. The tract is examined to determine whether the bowel and bladder can be repaired by primary closure or whether resection is required. In 44660, primary closure is performed. The fistulous tract is excised. The openings in the bowel and bladder are each repaired separately with sutures. In 44661, resection of the bladder and/or intestine is required. The fistulous tract between the bowel and bladder is severed. The bowel is clamped above and below the fistulous tract, transected, and the portion containing the fistulous tract removed. An end-to-end anastomosis is then used to reapproximate the bowel. If the bladder requires resection, the fistulous tract is excised along with a portion of the surrounding bladder. The remaining bladder wall is then reapproximated with sutures. A separately reportable omental flap may be developed and placed between the bowel and bladder to prevent recurrence. Drains are placed in the abdomen and the abdominal incision is closed.

Closure of enterovesical fistula

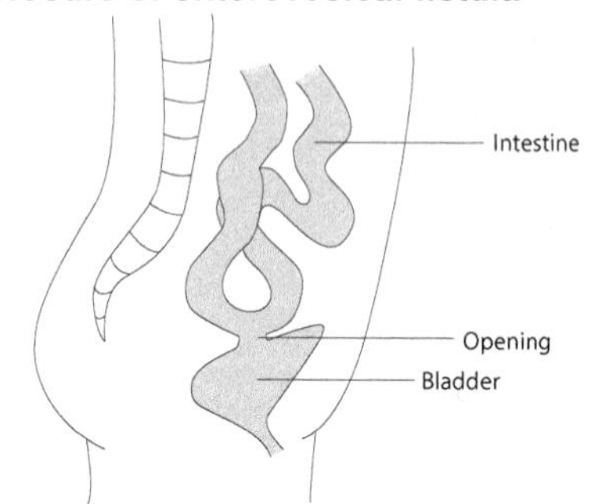

For 44660, an opening between the intestine and bladder is closed. Report 44661 for intestine and/or bladder resection.

ICD-10-CM Diagnostic Codes

K50.013	Crohn's disease of small intestine with fistula
K50.113	Crohn's disease of large intestine with fistula
K50.813	Crohn's disease of both small and large intestine with fistula
K51.013	Ulcerative (chronic) pancolitis with fistula
K51.213	Ulcerative (chronic) proctitis with fistula
K51.313	Ulcerative (chronic) rectosigmoiditis with fistula
K51.413	Inflammatory polyps of colon with fistula
K51.513	Left sided colitis with fistula
K51.813	Other ulcerative colitis with fistula
K56.690	Other partial intestinal obstruction
K56.691	Other complete intestinal obstruction
N32.1	Vesicointestinal fistula
N32.2	Vesical fistula, not elsewhere classified
Q64.79	Other congenital malformations of bladder and urethra
Q64.8	Other specified congenital malformations of urinary system

CCI Edits

Refer to Appendix A for CCI edits.

Facility RVUs

Code	Work	PE Facility	MP	Total Facility
44660	23.91	11.08	4.32	39.31
44661	27.35	12.71	5.68	45.74

Non-facility RVUs

Code	Work	PE Non-Facility	MP	Total Non-Facility
44660	23.91	11.08	4.32	39.31
44661	27.35	12.71	5.68	45.74

Modifiers (PAR)

Code	Mod 50	Mod 51	Mod 62	Mod 66	Mod 80
44660	0	2	1	0	2
44661	0	2	1	0	2

Global Period

Code	Days
44660	090
44661	090

49000-49002

49000 Exploratory laparotomy, exploratory celiotomy with or without biopsy(s) (separate procedure)

(To report wound exploration due to penetrating trauma without laparotomy, use 20102)

49002 Reopening of recent laparotomy

(To report re-exploration of hepatic wound for removal of packing, use 47362)

(To report re-exploration of pelvic wound for removal, including repacking, when performed, use 49014)

AMA *CPT® Assistant*

49000: Fall 92: 23, Mar 01: 10, Nov 08: 7, Sep 12: 11, Jan 20: 6

49002: Fall 92: 23, Nov 08: 7, Jan 20: 6

Plain English Description

The physician performs an exploratory laparotomy or celiotomy with or without biopsies in a separate procedure. The abdomen is incised. Abdominal organs are visually examined for evidence of infection, inflammation, perforations, lesions, or other injuries or diseased conditions. Any abnormalities are noted, including the presence of blood, bile, or other fluids in the abdominal cavity. Fluid or tissue samples may be obtained and sent for separately reportable laboratory analysis. Following examination, abdominal organs are returned to their normal positions and the abdominal incision is closed in layers. In 49002, a laparotomy site is opened and re-explored, as above.

Exploratory laparotomy, exploratory celiotomy with or without biopsy(s)

An access incision is made into the abdominal cavity for exploratory purposes. Biopsy samples may be collected during the surgical session.

ICD-10-CM Diagnostic Codes

	C48.0	Malignant neoplasm of retroperitoneum
⇄	C64.1	Malignant neoplasm of right kidney, except renal pelvis
⇄	C64.2	Malignant neoplasm of left kidney, except renal pelvis
⇄	C65.1	Malignant neoplasm of right renal pelvis
⇄	C65.2	Malignant neoplasm of left renal pelvis
⇄	C66.1	Malignant neoplasm of right ureter
⇄	C66.2	Malignant neoplasm of left ureter
	C67.1	Malignant neoplasm of dome of bladder
	C67.2	Malignant neoplasm of lateral wall of bladder
	C67.3	Malignant neoplasm of anterior wall of bladder
	C67.4	Malignant neoplasm of posterior wall of bladder
	C67.5	Malignant neoplasm of bladder neck
	C67.6	Malignant neoplasm of ureteric orifice
	C67.7	Malignant neoplasm of urachus
	C67.8	Malignant neoplasm of overlapping sites of bladder
	C76.3	Malignant neoplasm of pelvis
	C77.2	Secondary and unspecified malignant neoplasm of intra-abdominal lymph nodes
	C77.8	Secondary and unspecified malignant neoplasm of lymph nodes of multiple regions
	C78.6	Secondary malignant neoplasm of retroperitoneum and peritoneum
⇄	C79.01	Secondary malignant neoplasm of right kidney and renal pelvis
⇄	C79.02	Secondary malignant neoplasm of left kidney and renal pelvis
	C79.11	Secondary malignant neoplasm of bladder
	C79.19	Secondary malignant neoplasm of other urinary organs
	C79.82	Secondary malignant neoplasm of genital organs
	C7B.01	Secondary carcinoid tumors of distant lymph nodes
	C7B.1	Secondary Merkel cell carcinoma
	C80.0	Disseminated malignant neoplasm, unspecified
	K56.51	Intestinal adhesions [bands], with partial obstruction
	K56.52	Intestinal adhesions [bands] with complete obstruction
	K56.690	Other partial intestinal obstruction
	K56.691	Other complete intestinal obstruction
	K65.0	Generalized (acute) peritonitis
	N99.820	Postprocedural hemorrhage of a genitourinary system organ or structure following a genitourinary system procedure
	N99.821	Postprocedural hemorrhage of a genitourinary system organ or structure following other procedure
	R19.07	Generalized intra-abdominal and pelvic swelling, mass and lump
	R19.09	Other intra-abdominal and pelvic swelling, mass and lump
❼	T81.43	Infection following a procedure, organ and space surgical site
❼	T81.44	Sepsis following a procedure
❼	T81.60	Unspecified acute reaction to foreign substance accidentally left during a procedure
❼	T81.61	Aseptic peritonitis due to foreign substance accidentally left during a procedure

ICD-10-CM Coding Notes

For codes requiring a 7th character extension, refer to your ICD-10-CM book. Review the character descriptions and coding guidelines for proper selection. For some procedures, only certain characters will apply.

CCI Edits

Refer to Appendix A for CCI edits.

Facility RVUs

Code	Work	PE Facility	MP	Total Facility
49000	12.54	7.45	2.93	22.92
49002	17.63	9.27	4.16	31.06

Non-facility RVUs

Code	Work	PE Non-Facility	MP	Total Non-Facility
49000	12.54	7.45	2.93	22.92
49002	17.63	9.27	4.16	31.06

Modifiers (PAR)

Code	Mod 50	Mod 51	Mod 62	Mod 66	Mod 80
49000	0	2	1	0	2
49002	0	2	1	0	2

Global Period

Code	Days
49000	090
49002	090

● New ▲ Revised ✚ Add On ⊘Modifier 51 Exempt ★Telemedicine ☐ CPT QuickRef ✗FDA Pending ⇄ Laterality ❼ Seventh Character ♂Male ♀Female

CPT® Procedural Coding

49010

49010 Exploration, retroperitoneal area with or without biopsy(s) (separate procedure)

(To report wound exploration due to penetrating trauma without laparotomy, use 20102)

AMA *CPT® Assistant*

49010: Jan 20: 6

Plain English Description

An exploration of the retroperitoneal area with or without biopsies is performed. The retroperitoneal area lies behind the peritoneum, the sac that lines the abdominopelvic cavity. Organs that lie within the retroperitoneal cavity include the adrenal glands, kidneys, ureters, bladder, aorta, inferior vena cava, and part of the esophagus, rectum, and uterus. The retroperitoneum may be approached anteriorly through a transverse, subcostal, midline rectus or paramedial lateral rectus incision or posteriorly through a flank incision just below the 11th or 12th rib. The retroperitoneal area and organs are visually examined for evidence of infection, inflammation, perforations, lesions, injuries, abnormalities, or other diseased condition. Any abnormalities are noted, including the presence of blood or other fluids in the retroperitoneal space. Fluid or tissue samples may be obtained and sent for separately reportable laboratory analysis. Following examination, the incision is closed in layers.

Exploration, retroperitoneal area with or without biopsy(s) (separate procedure)

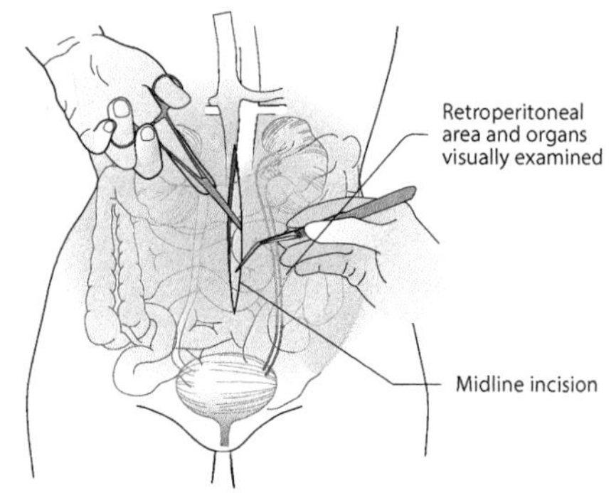

ICD-10-CM Diagnostic Codes

	C48.0	Malignant neoplasm of retroperitoneum
	C48.8	Malignant neoplasm of overlapping sites of retroperitoneum and peritoneum
⇄	C64.1	Malignant neoplasm of right kidney, except renal pelvis
⇄	C64.2	Malignant neoplasm of left kidney, except renal pelvis
⇄	C65.1	Malignant neoplasm of right renal pelvis
⇄	C65.2	Malignant neoplasm of left renal pelvis
⇄	C66.1	Malignant neoplasm of right ureter
⇄	C66.2	Malignant neoplasm of left ureter
	C67.0	Malignant neoplasm of trigone of bladder
	C67.1	Malignant neoplasm of dome of bladder
	C67.2	Malignant neoplasm of lateral wall of bladder
	C67.3	Malignant neoplasm of anterior wall of bladder
	C67.4	Malignant neoplasm of posterior wall of bladder
	C67.5	Malignant neoplasm of bladder neck
	C67.6	Malignant neoplasm of ureteric orifice
	C67.7	Malignant neoplasm of urachus
	C67.8	Malignant neoplasm of overlapping sites of bladder
	C76.2	Malignant neoplasm of abdomen
	C78.6	Secondary malignant neoplasm of retroperitoneum and peritoneum
⇄	C79.01	Secondary malignant neoplasm of right kidney and renal pelvis
⇄	C79.02	Secondary malignant neoplasm of left kidney and renal pelvis
	C79.11	Secondary malignant neoplasm of bladder
	C79.19	Secondary malignant neoplasm of other urinary organs
	C79.82	Secondary malignant neoplasm of genital organs
	D20.0	Benign neoplasm of soft tissue of retroperitoneum
	D48.3	Neoplasm of uncertain behavior of retroperitoneum
	K66.1	Hemoperitoneum
	K68.19	Other retroperitoneal abscess
	K68.9	Other disorders of retroperitoneum
	R10.84	Generalized abdominal pain
	R19.07	Generalized intra-abdominal and pelvic swelling, mass and lump
	R93.5	Abnormal findings on diagnostic imaging of other abdominal regions, including retroperitoneum

CCI Edits

Refer to Appendix A for CCI edits.

Facility RVUs

Code	Work	PE Facility	MP	Total Facility
49010	16.06	7.69	3.71	27.46

Non-facility RVUs

Code	Work	PE Non-Facility	MP	Total Non-Facility
49010	16.06	7.69	3.71	27.46

Modifiers (PAR)

Code	Mod 50	Mod 51	Mod 62	Mod 66	Mod 80
49010	0	2	1	0	2

Global Period

Code	Days
49010	090

49020

49020 Drainage of peritoneal abscess or localized peritonitis, exclusive of appendiceal abscess, open

(For appendiceal abscess, use 44900)

(For percutaneous image-guided drainage of peritoneal abscess or localized peritonitis by catheter, use 49406)

(For transrectal or transvaginal image-guided drainage of peritoneal abscess by catheter, use 49407)

Plain English Description

An abscess is a localized collection of pus. A peritoneal abscess is one contained within the peritoneum and may also be referred to as an intraperitoneal abscess. Localized peritonitis is an inflammation of the peritoneal tissue in a circumscribed region. An incision is made in the abdomen. The entire peritoneal cavity is explored and the abscess is located. Loculations are separated and all debris, which may include pus, blood, and necrotic tissue, is evacuated. The abscess site is vigorously irrigated with sterile saline or antibiotic solution until all debris has been removed. A drain is placed in the abscess cavity and the abdomen is closed around the drain.

Drainage of peritoneal abscess or localized peritonitis

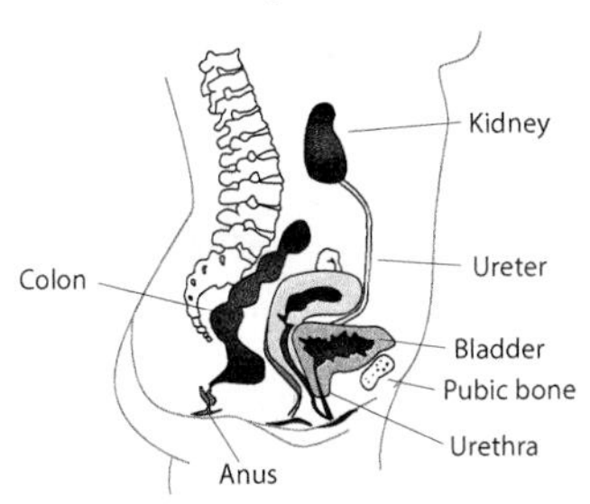

Peritonitis is an infectious irritation of the peritoneum, the lining of internal organs and abdominal walls. A localized irritation may form or an abscess may develop.

ICD-10-CM Diagnostic Codes

A54.85	Gonococcal peritonitis
A74.81	Chlamydial peritonitis
K65.0	Generalized (acute) peritonitis
K65.1	Peritoneal abscess
K65.2	Spontaneous bacterial peritonitis
K65.3	Choleperitonitis
K65.4	Sclerosing mesenteritis
K65.8	Other peritonitis
K65.9	Peritonitis, unspecified
K66.1	Hemoperitoneum
K66.8	Other specified disorders of peritoneum
K67	Disorders of peritoneum in infectious diseases classified elsewhere
K68.11	Postprocedural retroperitoneal abscess
K68.12	Psoas muscle abscess
K68.19	Other retroperitoneal abscess
K68.9	Other disorders of retroperitoneum
❼ T81.43	Infection following a procedure, organ and space surgical site

ICD-10-CM Coding Notes

For codes requiring a 7th character extension, refer to your ICD-10-CM book. Review the character descriptions and coding guidelines for proper selection. For some procedures, only certain characters will apply.

CCI Edits

Refer to Appendix A for CCI edits.

Facility RVUs

Code	Work	PE Facility	MP	Total Facility
49020	26.67	14.60	6.18	47.45

Non-facility RVUs

Code	Work	PE Non-Facility	MP	Total Non-Facility
49020	26.67	14.60	6.18	47.45

Modifiers (PAR)

Code	Mod 50	Mod 51	Mod 62	Mod 66	Mod 80
49020	0	2	0	0	2

Global Period

Code	Days
49020	090

CPT® Procedural Coding

49060

49060 Drainage of retroperitoneal abscess, open

(For percutaneous image-guided drainage of retroperitoneal abscess by catheter, use 49406)

(For transrectal or transvaginal image-guided drainage of retroperitoneal abscess by catheter, use 49407)

AMA *CPT® Assistant*

49060: Nov 97: 18, Nov 99: 24, Jul 01: 11, Aug 01: 10

Plain English Description

A retroperitoneal abscess is a collection of pus that is located in the abdominal cavity behind the peritoneum and may also be referred to as an extraperitoneal abscess. The retroperitoneum is accessed using an open approach through an anterior or posterior subcostal incision, a midline abdominal incision, or a flank incision. The entire retroperitoneal cavity is explored and the abscess located. Loculations are separated and all debris, which may include pus, blood, and necrotic tissue, is evacuated. The abscess site is vigorously irrigated with sterile saline or antibiotic solution until all debris has been removed. A drain is placed in the abscess cavity and the incision is closed around the drain.

Drainage of retroperitoneal abscess

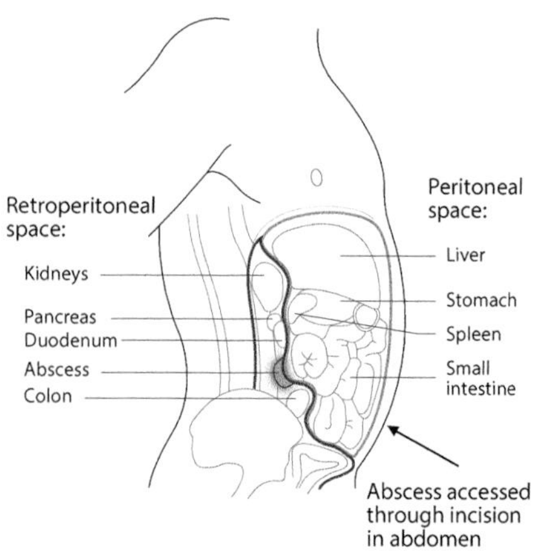

ICD-10-CM Diagnostic Codes

K65.0	Generalized (acute) peritonitis
K65.2	Spontaneous bacterial peritonitis
K65.4	Sclerosing mesenteritis
K65.8	Other peritonitis
K66.8	Other specified disorders of peritoneum
K67	Disorders of peritoneum in infectious diseases classified elsewhere
K68.11	Postprocedural retroperitoneal abscess
K68.12	Psoas muscle abscess
K68.19	Other retroperitoneal abscess
K68.9	Other disorders of retroperitoneum
N15.1	Renal and perinephric abscess
➐ T81.43	Infection following a procedure, organ and space surgical site

ICD-10-CM Coding Notes

For codes requiring a 7th character extension, refer to your ICD-10-CM book. Review the character descriptions and coding guidelines for proper selection. For some procedures, only certain characters will apply.

CCI Edits

Refer to Appendix A for CCI edits.

Facility RVUs

Code	Work	PE Facility	MP	Total Facility
49060	18.53	9.98	4.18	32.69

Non-facility RVUs

Code	Work	PE Non-Facility	MP	Total Non-Facility
49060	18.53	9.98	4.18	32.69

Modifiers (PAR)

Code	Mod 50	Mod 51	Mod 62	Mod 66	Mod 80
49060	0	2	1	0	1

Global Period

Code	Days
49060	090

49082-49083

49082 Abdominal paracentesis (diagnostic or therapeutic); without imaging guidance

49083 Abdominal paracentesis (diagnostic or therapeutic); with imaging guidance

(Do not report 49083 in conjunction with 76942, 77002, 77012, 77021)

(For percutaneous image-guided drainage of retroperitoneal abscess by catheter, use 49406)

AMA *CPT® Assistant* ▯

49082: Dec 12: 9

49083: Dec 12: 9, Mar 14: 14

Plain English Description

An abdominal paracentesis may be performed as a diagnostic procedure to help determine the cause of fluid buildup in the abdominal cavity. It may also be performed therapeutically when fluid buildup causes pain or impairs breathing. The skin over the planned puncture site is cleansed and a local anesthetic is injected. A paracentesis needle attached to a syringe is inserted into the abdominal cavity using imaging guidance as needed. Fluid is aspirated. The fluid is visually examined for evidence of bleeding or other conditions. If the procedure is performed for diagnostic purposes, only a small amount of fluid is withdrawn and the fluid is then sent to the laboratory for separately reportable analysis. If the procedure is performed for therapeutic purposes, fluid continues to be aspirated until as much fluid as possible has been removed from the abdominal cavity. Use 49082 when the procedure is performed without imaging guidance. Use 49083 when imaging guidance is used.

Abdominal paracentesis (diagnostic or therapeutic)

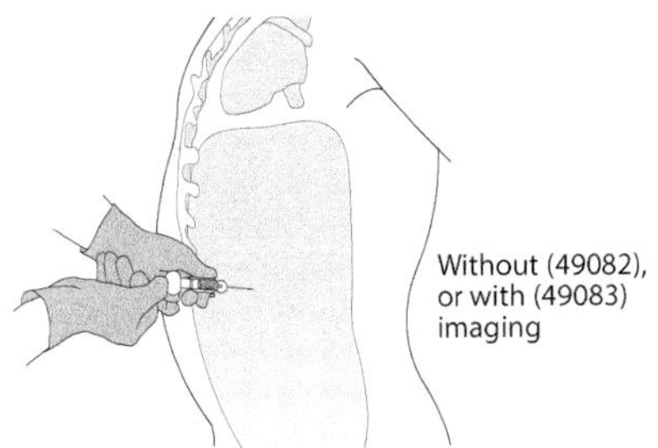

Catheter/needle is inserted into the abdomen/peritoneum. Fluid is withdrawn and analyzed.

ICD-10-CM Diagnostic Codes

	A18.31	Tuberculous peritonitis
	C48.0	Malignant neoplasm of retroperitoneum
	C48.8	Malignant neoplasm of overlapping sites of retroperitoneum and peritoneum
⇄	C64.1	Malignant neoplasm of right kidney, except renal pelvis
⇄	C64.2	Malignant neoplasm of left kidney, except renal pelvis
⇄	C65.1	Malignant neoplasm of right renal pelvis
⇄	C65.2	Malignant neoplasm of left renal pelvis
⇄	C66.1	Malignant neoplasm of right ureter
⇄	C66.2	Malignant neoplasm of left ureter
	C78.6	Secondary malignant neoplasm of retroperitoneum and peritoneum
	E87.70	Fluid overload, unspecified
	E87.79	Other fluid overload
	I89.8	Other specified noninfective disorders of lymphatic vessels and lymph nodes
	K65.0	Generalized (acute) peritonitis
	K65.1	Peritoneal abscess
	K65.2	Spontaneous bacterial peritonitis
	K65.3	Choleperitonitis
	K65.4	Sclerosing mesenteritis
	K65.8	Other peritonitis
	K66.1	Hemoperitoneum
	K67	Disorders of peritoneum in infectious diseases classified elsewhere
	L98.495	Non-pressure chronic ulcer of skin of other sites with muscle involvement without evidence of necrosis
	L98.496	Non-pressure chronic ulcer of skin of other sites with bone involvement without evidence of necrosis
	N18.6	End stage renal disease
	N25.89	Other disorders resulting from impaired renal tubular function
	R18.0	Malignant ascites
	R18.8	Other ascites
❼	S36.81	Injury of peritoneum
❼	S36.892	Contusion of other intra-abdominal organs
❼	S36.893	Laceration of other intra-abdominal organs
❼	S36.898	Other injury of other intra-abdominal organs

ICD-10-CM Coding Notes

For codes requiring a 7th character extension, refer to your ICD-10-CM book. Review the character descriptions and coding guidelines for proper selection. For some procedures, only certain characters will apply.

CCI Edits

Refer to Appendix A for CCI edits.

Facility RVUs ▯

Code	Work	PE Facility	MP	Total Facility
49082	1.24	0.73	0.19	2.16
49083	2.00	0.91	0.19	3.10

Non-facility RVUs ▯

Code	Work	PE Non-Facility	MP	Total Non-Facility
49082	1.24	5.05	0.19	6.48
49083	2.00	6.78	0.19	8.97

Modifiers (PAR) ▯

Code	Mod 50	Mod 51	Mod 62	Mod 66	Mod 80
49082	0	2	0	0	1
49083	0	2	0	0	1

Global Period

Code	Days
49082	000
49083	000

49084

49084 Peritoneal lavage, including imaging guidance, when performed

(Do not report 49084 in conjunction with 76942, 77002, 77012, 77021)

(For percutaneous image-guided drainage of retroperitoneal abscess by catheter, use 49406)

AMA *CPT® Assistant* ▢

49084: Dec 12: 9

Plain English Description

The abdomen is cleansed and a local anesthetic is injected. A small incision is made in the skin and carried down through the abdominal wall. Using imaging guidance as needed, a dialysis-type catheter is inserted into the peritoneal cavity. Fluid is drained from the peritoneal cavity and visually examined for evidence of bleeding or other conditions. The fluid is then sent to a laboratory for separately reportable analysis. A saline solution is instilled into the cavity and withdrawn to flush the cavity of blood clots or debris.

Peritoneal lavage

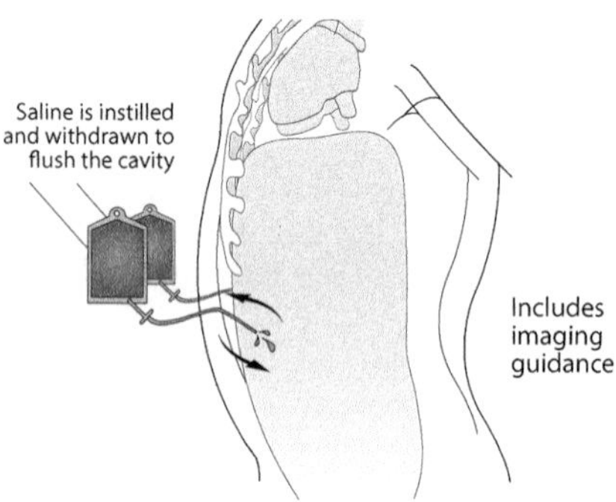
Saline is instilled and withdrawn to flush the cavity
Includes imaging guidance

ICD-10-CM Diagnostic Codes

A18.31	Tuberculous peritonitis
A54.85	Gonococcal peritonitis
C48.1	Malignant neoplasm of specified parts of peritoneum
C48.2	Malignant neoplasm of peritoneum, unspecified
C48.8	Malignant neoplasm of overlapping sites of retroperitoneum and peritoneum
C78.6	Secondary malignant neoplasm of retroperitoneum and peritoneum
I89.8	Other specified noninfective disorders of lymphatic vessels and lymph nodes
K65.0	Generalized (acute) peritonitis
K65.1	Peritoneal abscess
K65.2	Spontaneous bacterial peritonitis
K65.4	Sclerosing mesenteritis
K65.8	Other peritonitis
K66.1	Hemoperitoneum
K67	Disorders of peritoneum in infectious diseases classified elsewhere
❼ S36.81	Injury of peritoneum

ICD-10-CM Coding Notes

For codes requiring a 7th character extension, refer to your ICD-10-CM book. Review the character descriptions and coding guidelines for proper selection. For some procedures, only certain characters will apply.

CCI Edits

Refer to Appendix A for CCI edits.

Facility RVUs ▢

Code	Work	PE Facility	MP	Total Facility
49084	2.00	0.74	0.42	3.16

Non-facility RVUs ▢

Code	Work	PE Non-Facility	MP	Total Non-Facility
49084	2.00	0.74	0.42	3.16

Modifiers (PAR) ▢

Code	Mod 50	Mod 51	Mod 62	Mod 66	Mod 80
49084	0	2	0	0	1

Global Period

Code	Days
49084	000

49180

49180 Biopsy, abdominal or retroperitoneal mass, percutaneous needle

(If imaging guidance is performed, see 76942, 77002, 77012, 77021)

(For fine needle aspiration biopsy, see 10004, 10005, 10006, 10007, 10008, 10009, 10010, 10011, 10012, 10021)

(For evaluation of fine needle aspirate, see 88172, 88173)

AMA Coding Guideline

Excision and Destruction Procedures on the Abdomen, Peritoneum, and Omentum

Code 49185 describes sclerotherapy of a fluid collection (eg, lymphocele, cyst, or seroma) through a percutaneous access. It includes contrast injection(s), sclerosant injection(s), sclerosant dwell time, diagnostic study, imaging guidance (eg, ultrasound, fluoroscopy), and radiological supervision and interpretation, when performed. Code 49185 may be reported once per day for each lesion treated through a separate catheter. Do not report 49185 more than once if treating multiple lesions through the same catheter. Codes for access to and drainage of the collection may be separately reportable according to location (eg, 10030, 10160, 49405, 49406, 49407, 50390).

AMA Coding Notes

Excision and Destruction Procedures on the Abdomen, Peritoneum, and Omentum

(For lysis of intestinal adhesions, use 44005)

AMA *CPT® Assistant* ▢

49180: Fall 93: 11

Plain English Description

This procedure is typically performed using separately reportable imaging guidance to identify the mass and to facilitate accurate placement of the needle within the mass. Using continuous imaging guidance, the core biopsy needle is inserted through the abdomen into the mass. A tissue sample is obtained. The physician may make multiple passes through the same puncture site or may approach the lesion through a different puncture site until an adequate tissue sample is obtained. The tissue sample is then sent to the laboratory for separately reportable histologic evaluation.

Biopsy, abdominal or retroperitoneal mass, percutaneous needle

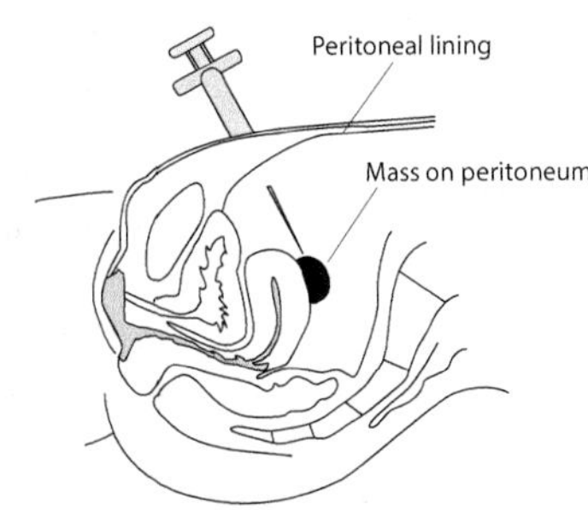

Tissue is taken by a needle from the abdominal cavity, or the area immediately outside of the lining that surrounds the abdominal cavity. The tissue is then used for examination and diagnosis.

ICD-10-CM Diagnostic Codes

	C48.0	Malignant neoplasm of retroperitoneum
	C48.1	Malignant neoplasm of specified parts of peritoneum
	C48.8	Malignant neoplasm of overlapping sites of retroperitoneum and peritoneum
	C49.5	Malignant neoplasm of connective and soft tissue of pelvis
⇄	C64.1	Malignant neoplasm of right kidney, except renal pelvis
⇄	C64.2	Malignant neoplasm of left kidney, except renal pelvis
⇄	C65.1	Malignant neoplasm of right renal pelvis
⇄	C65.2	Malignant neoplasm of left renal pelvis
⇄	C66.1	Malignant neoplasm of right ureter
⇄	C66.2	Malignant neoplasm of left ureter
	C67.0	Malignant neoplasm of trigone of bladder
	C67.1	Malignant neoplasm of dome of bladder
	C67.2	Malignant neoplasm of lateral wall of bladder
	C67.3	Malignant neoplasm of anterior wall of bladder
	C67.4	Malignant neoplasm of posterior wall of bladder
	C67.5	Malignant neoplasm of bladder neck
	C67.6	Malignant neoplasm of ureteric orifice
	C67.7	Malignant neoplasm of urachus
	C67.8	Malignant neoplasm of overlapping sites of bladder
	C68.8	Malignant neoplasm of overlapping sites of urinary organs
	C76.2	Malignant neoplasm of abdomen
	C77.2	Secondary and unspecified malignant neoplasm of intra-abdominal lymph nodes
	C77.5	Secondary and unspecified malignant neoplasm of intrapelvic lymph nodes
	C79.89	Secondary malignant neoplasm of other specified sites
	C7A.1	Malignant poorly differentiated neuroendocrine tumors
	C7B.04	Secondary carcinoid tumors of peritoneum
	D18.03	Hemangioma of intra-abdominal structures
	D20.0	Benign neoplasm of soft tissue of retroperitoneum
	D20.1	Benign neoplasm of soft tissue of peritoneum
	D48.3	Neoplasm of uncertain behavior of retroperitoneum
	D48.4	Neoplasm of uncertain behavior of peritoneum
	L03.314	Cellulitis of groin
	L03.315	Cellulitis of perineum
	L03.324	Acute lymphangitis of groin
	L03.325	Acute lymphangitis of perineum
	R10.30	Lower abdominal pain, unspecified
⇄	R19.01	Right upper quadrant abdominal swelling, mass and lump
⇄	R19.02	Left upper quadrant abdominal swelling, mass and lump
⇄	R19.03	Right lower quadrant abdominal swelling, mass and lump
⇄	R19.04	Left lower quadrant abdominal swelling, mass and lump
	R19.05	Periumbilic swelling, mass or lump
	R19.06	Epigastric swelling, mass or lump
	R19.07	Generalized intra-abdominal and pelvic swelling, mass and lump
	R19.09	Other intra-abdominal and pelvic swelling, mass and lump
	R59.0	Localized enlarged lymph nodes
	R59.1	Generalized enlarged lymph nodes

CCI Edits

Refer to Appendix A for CCI edits.

Facility RVUs ▢

Code	Work	PE Facility	MP	Total Facility
49180	1.73	0.54	0.14	2.41

Non-facility RVUs ▢

Code	Work	PE Non-Facility	MP	Total Non-Facility
49180	1.73	3.35	0.14	5.22

Modifiers (PAR) ▢

Code	Mod 50	Mod 51	Mod 62	Mod 66	Mod 80
49180	0	2	0	0	1

Global Period

Code	Days
49180	000

49185

49185 Sclerotherapy of a fluid collection (eg, lymphocele, cyst, or seroma), percutaneous, including contrast injection(s), sclerosant injection(s), diagnostic study, imaging guidance (eg, ultrasound, fluoroscopy) and radiological supervision and interpretation when performed

(For treatment of multiple lesions in a single day requiring separate access, use modifier 59 for each additional treated lesion)

(For treatment of multiple interconnected lesions treated through a single access, report 49185 once)

(For access/drainage with needle, see 10160, 50390)

(For access/drainage with catheter, see 10030, 49405, 49406, 49407, 50390)

(For exchange of existing catheter, before or after injection of sclerosant, see 49423, 75984)

(For sclerotherapy of a lymphatic/vascular malformation, use 37241)

(For sclerosis of veins or endovenous ablation of incompetent extremity veins, see 36468, 36470, 36471, 36475, 36476, 36478, 36479)

(For pleurodesis, use 32560)

(Do not report 49185 in conjunction with 49424, 76080)

AMA Coding Guideline

Excision and Destruction Procedures on the Abdomen, Peritoneum, and Omentum

Code 49185 describes sclerotherapy of a fluid collection (eg, lymphocele, cyst, or seroma) through a percutaneous access. It includes contrast injection(s), sclerosant injection(s), sclerosant dwell time, diagnostic study, imaging guidance (eg, ultrasound, fluoroscopy), and radiological supervision and interpretation, when performed. Code 49185 may be reported once per day for each lesion treated through a separate catheter. Do not report 49185 more than once if treating multiple lesions through the same catheter. Codes for access to and drainage of the collection may be separately reportable according to location (eg, 10030, 10160, 49405, 49406, 49407, 50390).

AMA Coding Notes

Excision and Destruction Procedures on the Abdomen, Peritoneum, and Omentum

(For lysis of intestinal adhesions, use 44005)

AMA *CPT® Assistant* ▢

49185: Mar 16: 10

Plain English Description

A procedure is performed to remove a collection of fluid, such as from a lymphocele, cyst, or seroma, and instill a chemical sclerosant into the cavity. Sclerotherapy induces inflammatory fibrosis of the cyst or lesion wall to prevent re-accumulation of fluid. A small-bore needle is inserted through the skin into the lesion. A pigtail catheter is inserted over the needle and fluid is aspirated and measured. A sample is sent for laboratory analysis (Gram stain, culture, cytology). Diluted contrast dye is injected through the catheter and observed using fluoroscopy to rule out fistula communication and/or leakage into the peritoneum, blood vessels, biliary system, or renal collecting system. Communication of the cyst or fluid cavity to any of these structures contraindicates injection of a sclerosant. After determining that no leakage is present, approximately 50% of the aspirated volume is replaced with the sclerosant. Ethanol is the most commonly used sclerosant. Other chemicals that may be used include bismuth, povidone-iodine, tetracycline, bleomycin, hypertonic saline, ethanolamine oleate, and acetic acid. The patient's position is rotated to ensure that the entire cyst wall has contact with the sclerosant. After a prescribed period of time, minimally 20 minutes, the sclerosant is removed via aspiration. The catheter is connected to bulb suction and ultrasound or computed tomography is performed to ensure complete evacuation of the sclerosant. The catheter may be removed immediately or be left in place if subsequent treatments are anticipated or planned. Code 49185 includes all imaging guidance and associated supervision and interpretation during sclerotherapy.

ICD-10-CM Diagnostic Codes

B67.0	Echinococcus granulosus infection of liver
B67.5	Echinococcus multilocularis infection of liver
B67.99	Other echinococcosis
D78.33	Postprocedural seroma of the spleen following a procedure on the spleen
D78.34	Postprocedural seroma of the spleen following other procedure
K76.89	Other specified diseases of liver
K86.2	Cyst of pancreas
K91.872	Postprocedural seroma of a digestive system organ or structure following a digestive system procedure
K91.873	Postprocedural seroma of a digestive system organ or structure following other procedure
M79.81	Nontraumatic hematoma of soft tissue
N28.1	Cyst of kidney, acquired
N99.111	Postprocedural bulbous urethral stricture, male ♂
N99.112	Postprocedural membranous urethral stricture, male ♂
N99.842	Postprocedural seroma of a genitourinary system organ or structure following a genitourinary system procedure
N99.843	Postprocedural seroma of a genitourinary system organ or structure following other procedure
Q44.6	Cystic disease of liver
Q45.2	Congenital pancreatic cyst
Q61.01	Congenital single renal cyst
Q61.02	Congenital multiple renal cysts
Q61.11	Cystic dilatation of collecting ducts
Q61.19	Other polycystic kidney, infantile type
Q61.2	Polycystic kidney, adult type
Q61.8	Other cystic kidney diseases
➐ T79.2	Traumatic secondary and recurrent hemorrhage and seroma

ICD-10-CM Coding Notes

For codes requiring a 7th character extension, refer to your ICD-10-CM book. Review the character descriptions and coding guidelines for proper selection. For some procedures, only certain characters will apply.

CCI Edits

Refer to Appendix A for CCI edits.

Facility RVUs ▢

Code	Work	PE Facility	MP	Total Facility
49185	2.35	0.87	0.23	3.45

Non-facility RVUs ▢

Code	Work	PE Non-Facility	MP	Total Non-Facility
49185	2.35	37.00	0.23	39.58

Modifiers (PAR) ▢

Code	Mod 50	Mod 51	Mod 62	Mod 66	Mod 80
49185	0	0	0	0	1

Global Period

Code	Days
49185	000

49320

49320 Laparoscopy, abdomen, peritoneum, and omentum, diagnostic, with or without collection of specimen(s) by brushing or washing (separate procedure)

AMA Coding Guideline

Laparoscopic Procedures on the Abdomen, Peritoneum, and Omentum

Surgical laparoscopy always includes diagnostic laparoscopy. To report a diagnostic laparoscopy (peritoneoscopy), (separate procedure), use 49320.

For laparoscopic fulguration or excision of lesions of the ovary, pelvic viscera, or peritoneal surface use 58662.

AMA *CPT® Assistant* ☐

49320: Nov 99: 24, Mar 00: 9, Apr 06: 19, Mar 07: 4, Nov 07: 1, Dec 08: 7, Jun 10: 7, Dec 15: 18, Apr 17: 7

Plain English Description

A periumbilical port is placed and pneumoperitoneum established by the insufflation of air. The laparoscope is inserted and the entire abdominal cavity, peritoneum, and/or omentum inspected for signs of malignancy, disease, or injury using a video camera. A biopsy brush may be inserted through the laparoscope and cell samples obtained. Alternatively, cells may be obtained by washing, which involves instilling a small amount of sterile saline through the laparoscope and then aspirating the fluid. Brushings or washings are sent to the laboratory for separately reportable cytological evaluation. Following completion of the procedure, the instruments are withdrawn and pressure applied to the abdomen to express any remaining air in the peritoneum. The portal incisions are closed.

Diagnostic laparoscopy

Additional probe

Laparoscope

A laparoscope is inserted into the abdominal cavity through a small incision.

ICD-10-CM Diagnostic Codes

	C48.1	Malignant neoplasm of specified parts of peritoneum
	C48.2	Malignant neoplasm of peritoneum, unspecified
	C48.8	Malignant neoplasm of overlapping sites of retroperitoneum and peritoneum
	C60.8	Malignant neoplasm of overlapping sites of penis ♂
	C61	Malignant neoplasm of prostate ♂
⇄	C62.01	Malignant neoplasm of undescended right testis ♂
⇄	C62.02	Malignant neoplasm of undescended left testis ♂
⇄	C62.11	Malignant neoplasm of descended right testis ♂
⇄	C62.12	Malignant neoplasm of descended left testis ♂
⇄	C63.01	Malignant neoplasm of right epididymis ♂
⇄	C63.02	Malignant neoplasm of left epididymis ♂
⇄	C63.11	Malignant neoplasm of right spermatic cord ♂
⇄	C63.12	Malignant neoplasm of left spermatic cord ♂
	C63.7	Malignant neoplasm of other specified male genital organs ♂
	C63.8	Malignant neoplasm of overlapping sites of male genital organs ♂
⇄	C64.1	Malignant neoplasm of right kidney, except renal pelvis
⇄	C64.2	Malignant neoplasm of left kidney, except renal pelvis
⇄	C65.1	Malignant neoplasm of right renal pelvis
⇄	C65.2	Malignant neoplasm of left renal pelvis
⇄	C66.1	Malignant neoplasm of right ureter
⇄	C66.2	Malignant neoplasm of left ureter
	C67.0	Malignant neoplasm of trigone of bladder
	C67.1	Malignant neoplasm of dome of bladder
	C67.2	Malignant neoplasm of lateral wall of bladder
	C67.3	Malignant neoplasm of anterior wall of bladder
	C67.4	Malignant neoplasm of posterior wall of bladder
	C67.5	Malignant neoplasm of bladder neck
⇄	C74.01	Malignant neoplasm of cortex of right adrenal gland
⇄	C74.02	Malignant neoplasm of cortex of left adrenal gland
⇄	C74.11	Malignant neoplasm of medulla of right adrenal gland
⇄	C74.12	Malignant neoplasm of medulla of left adrenal gland
	C76.2	Malignant neoplasm of abdomen
	C78.6	Secondary malignant neoplasm of retroperitoneum and peritoneum
⇄	C79.01	Secondary malignant neoplasm of right kidney and renal pelvis
⇄	C79.02	Secondary malignant neoplasm of left kidney and renal pelvis
	C79.11	Secondary malignant neoplasm of bladder
	C79.19	Secondary malignant neoplasm of other urinary organs
	C79.82	Secondary malignant neoplasm of genital organs
	D48.3	Neoplasm of uncertain behavior of retroperitoneum
	D48.4	Neoplasm of uncertain behavior of peritoneum

CCI Edits

Refer to Appendix A for CCI edits.

Pub 100

49320: Pub 100-04, 32, 150.2

Facility RVUs ☐

Code	Work	PE Facility	MP	Total Facility
49320	5.14	3.47	1.18	9.79

Non-facility RVUs ☐

Code	Work	PE Non-Facility	MP	Total Non-Facility
49320	5.14	3.47	1.18	9.79

Modifiers (PAR) ☐

Code	Mod 50	Mod 51	Mod 62	Mod 66	Mod 80
49320	0	2	0	0	2

Global Period

Code	Days
49320	010

49321

49321 Laparoscopy, surgical; with biopsy (single or multiple)

AMA Coding Guideline

Laparoscopic Procedures on the Abdomen, Peritoneum, and Omentum

Surgical laparoscopy always includes diagnostic laparoscopy. To report a diagnostic laparoscopy (peritoneoscopy), (separate procedure), use 49320.

For laparoscopic fulguration or excision of lesions of the ovary, pelvic viscera, or peritoneal surface use 58662.

AMA *CPT® Assistant* ▯

49321: Nov 99: 24, Mar 00: 9, Aug 18: 10

Plain English Description

A periumbilical port is placed and pneumoperitoneum established by the insufflation of air. The laparoscope is inserted and the entire abdominal cavity, peritoneum, and/or omentum inspected for signs of malignancy, disease, or injury using a video camera. Biopsy forceps are inserted through the laparoscope and a tissue sample obtained. One or more tissue samples may be obtained from a single or multiple sites. Tissue samples are sent to the laboratory for separately reportable histologic evaluation. Following completion of the procedure, the biopsy sites are inspected for bleeding and any bleeding controlled by laser or electrocautery. The instruments are withdrawn and pressure applied to the abdomen to express any remaining air in the peritoneum. The portal incisions are closed.

Laparoscopy with biopsy

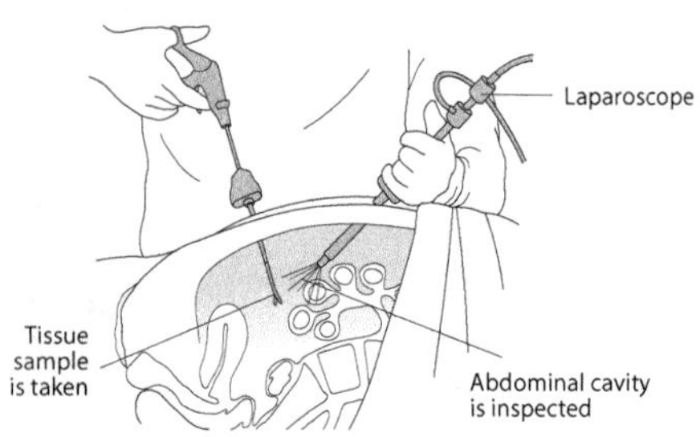

ICD-10-CM Diagnostic Codes

There are too many ICD-10-CM codes to list. Refer to ICD-10-CM code book for associated diagnostic codes.

CCI Edits

Refer to Appendix A for CCI edits.

Facility RVUs ▯

Code	Work	PE Facility	MP	Total Facility
49321	5.44	3.62	1.20	10.26

Non-facility RVUs ▯

Code	Work	PE Non-Facility	MP	Total Non-Facility
49321	5.44	3.62	1.20	10.26

Modifiers (PAR) ▯

Code	Mod 50	Mod 51	Mod 62	Mod 66	Mod 80
49321	0	3	2	0	2

Global Period

Code	Days
49321	010

49324-49325

49324 Laparoscopy, surgical; with insertion of tunneled intraperitoneal catheter

(For subcutaneous extension of intraperitoneal catheter with remote chest exit site, use 49435 in conjunction with 49324)

(For open insertion of tunneled intraperitoneal catheter, use 49421)

49325 Laparoscopy, surgical; with revision of previously placed intraperitoneal cannula or catheter, with removal of intraluminal obstructive material if performed

AMA Coding Guideline

Laparoscopic Procedures on the Abdomen, Peritoneum, and Omentum

Surgical laparoscopy always includes diagnostic laparoscopy. To report a diagnostic laparoscopy (peritoneoscopy), (separate procedure), use 49320.

For laparoscopic fulguration or excision of lesions of the ovary, pelvic viscera, or peritoneal surface use 58662.

Plain English Description

An intraperitoneal catheter is inserted (49324) or revised (49325). A small incision is made in the area of the umbilicus and the laparoscope is inserted. The abdomen is inflated with gas. Two or three additional small incisions are made in the abdomen and trocars are inserted. Surgical instruments are inserted through the trocars. The abdomen is inspected for adhesions and the site of entry for the catheter into the peritoneum is identified. In 49324, the catheter is attached to the tunneler, and the tunneler and catheter are passed into the subcutaneous tissue deep to Scarpa's fascia and through the subcutaneous tissue to the site where the catheter will enter the peritoneum. The tunneler and catheter are passed out through the skin and the tunneler is removed. An introducer needle is placed into the peritoneum adjacent to the catheter under laparoscopic guidance. A guidewire is placed through the introducer into the peritoneum and the introducer is removed. A combined catheter introducer and dilator are advanced over the guidewire into the peritoneum. The guidewire and dilator are removed. The intraperitoneal catheter is then passed into the abdomen through the introducer. Proper positioning of the catheter is verified laparoscopically. The introducer is removed from the abdomen and the gas (pneumoperitoneum) is released. The laparoscope and trocars are removed and portal incisions are closed with sutures. In 49325, a previously placed intraperitoneal catheter is inspected using the laparoscope. The tip of the catheter may be repositioned or obstructive debris that has collected in the catheter may be flushed out of the lumen.

Laparoscopy, with insertion of tunneled intraperitoneal catheter

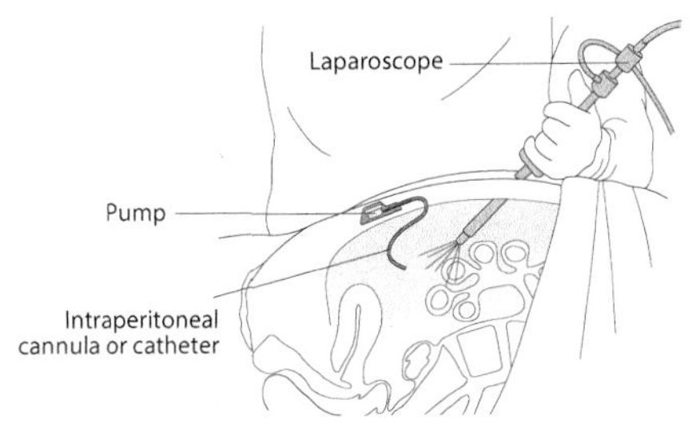

Cannula/catheter is inserted (49324), or revised (49325)

ICD-10-CM Diagnostic Codes

E08.22	Diabetes mellitus due to underlying condition with diabetic chronic kidney disease
E09.22	Drug or chemical induced diabetes mellitus with diabetic chronic kidney disease
E10.22	Type 1 diabetes mellitus with diabetic chronic kidney disease
E11.22	Type 2 diabetes mellitus with diabetic chronic kidney disease
E13.22	Other specified diabetes mellitus with diabetic chronic kidney disease
I12.0	Hypertensive chronic kidney disease with stage 5 chronic kidney disease or end stage renal disease
I13.11	Hypertensive heart and chronic kidney disease without heart failure, with stage 5 chronic kidney disease, or end stage renal disease
I13.2	Hypertensive heart and chronic kidney disease with heart failure and with stage 5 chronic kidney disease, or end stage renal disease
M35.04	Sjögren syndrome with tubulo-interstitial nephropathy
N00.2	Acute nephritic syndrome with diffuse membranous glomerulonephritis
N00.3	Acute nephritic syndrome with diffuse mesangial proliferative glomerulonephritis
N00.4	Acute nephritic syndrome with diffuse endocapillary proliferative glomerulonephritis
N00.5	Acute nephritic syndrome with diffuse mesangiocapillary glomerulonephritis
N00.6	Acute nephritic syndrome with dense deposit disease
N00.7	Acute nephritic syndrome with diffuse crescentic glomerulonephritis
N00.8	Acute nephritic syndrome with other morphologic changes
N01.2	Rapidly progressive nephritic syndrome with diffuse membranous glomerulonephritis
N01.3	Rapidly progressive nephritic syndrome with diffuse mesangial proliferative glomerulonephritis
N01.4	Rapidly progressive nephritic syndrome with diffuse endocapillary proliferative glomerulonephritis
N01.5	Rapidly progressive nephritic syndrome with diffuse mesangiocapillary glomerulonephritis
N01.6	Rapidly progressive nephritic syndrome with dense deposit disease
N01.7	Rapidly progressive nephritic syndrome with diffuse crescentic glomerulonephritis
N01.8	Rapidly progressive nephritic syndrome with other morphologic changes
N03.2	Chronic nephritic syndrome with diffuse membranous glomerulonephritis
N03.3	Chronic nephritic syndrome with diffuse mesangial proliferative glomerulonephritis
N03.4	Chronic nephritic syndrome with diffuse endocapillary proliferative glomerulonephritis
N03.5	Chronic nephritic syndrome with diffuse mesangiocapillary glomerulonephritis
N03.6	Chronic nephritic syndrome with dense deposit disease
N03.7	Chronic nephritic syndrome with diffuse crescentic glomerulonephritis
N03.8	Chronic nephritic syndrome with other morphologic changes
N04.2	Nephrotic syndrome with diffuse membranous glomerulonephritis
N04.3	Nephrotic syndrome with diffuse mesangial proliferative glomerulonephritis
N04.4	Nephrotic syndrome with diffuse endocapillary proliferative glomerulonephritis
N04.5	Nephrotic syndrome with diffuse mesangiocapillary glomerulonephritis
N04.6	Nephrotic syndrome with dense deposit disease
N04.7	Nephrotic syndrome with diffuse crescentic glomerulonephritis
N04.8	Nephrotic syndrome with other morphologic changes
N11.0	Nonobstructive reflux-associated chronic pyelonephritis
N11.1	Chronic obstructive pyelonephritis
N11.8	Other chronic tubulo-interstitial nephritis
N16	Renal tubulo-interstitial disorders in diseases classified elsewhere
N17.0	Acute kidney failure with tubular necrosis
N17.1	Acute kidney failure with acute cortical necrosis
N17.2	Acute kidney failure with medullary necrosis

	N17.8	Other acute kidney failure
	N18.5	Chronic kidney disease, stage 5
	N18.6	End stage renal disease
❼	T85.611	Breakdown (mechanical) of intraperitoneal dialysis catheter
❼	T85.621	Displacement of intraperitoneal dialysis catheter
❼	T85.631	Leakage of intraperitoneal dialysis catheter
❼	T85.691	Other mechanical complication of intraperitoneal dialysis catheter
	Z49.02	Encounter for fitting and adjustment of peritoneal dialysis catheter
	Z49.32	Encounter for adequacy testing for peritoneal dialysis

ICD-10-CM Coding Notes

For codes requiring a 7th character extension, refer to your ICD-10-CM book. Review the character descriptions and coding guidelines for proper selection. For some procedures, only certain characters will apply.

CCI Edits

Refer to Appendix A for CCI edits.

Facility RVUs ▯

Code	Work	PE Facility	MP	Total Facility
49324	6.32	3.70	1.55	11.57
49325	6.82	3.85	1.69	12.36

Non-facility RVUs ▯

Code	Work	PE Non-Facility	MP	Total Non-Facility
49324	6.32	3.70	1.55	11.57
49325	6.82	3.85	1.69	12.36

Modifiers (PAR) ▯

Code	Mod 50	Mod 51	Mod 62	Mod 66	Mod 80
49324	0	3	2	0	2
49325	0	3	2	0	2

Global Period

Code	Days
49324	010
49325	010

49327

+ 49327 Laparoscopy, surgical; with placement of interstitial device(s) for radiation therapy guidance (eg, fiducial markers, dosimeter), intra-abdominal, intrapelvic, and/or retroperitoneum, including imaging guidance, if performed, single or multiple (List separately in addition to code for primary procedure)

(Use 49327 in conjunction with laparoscopic abdominal, pelvic, or retroperitoneal procedure[s] performed concurrently)

(For placement of interstitial device[s] for intra-abdominal, intrapelvic, and/or retroperitoneal radiation therapy guidance concurrent with open procedure, use 49412)

(For percutaneous placement of interstitial device[s] for intra-abdominal, intrapelvic, and/or retroperitoneal radiation therapy guidance, use 49411)

AMA Coding Guideline

Laparoscopic Procedures on the Abdomen, Peritoneum, and Omentum

Surgical laparoscopy always includes diagnostic laparoscopy. To report a diagnostic laparoscopy (peritoneoscopy), (separate procedure), use 49320.

For laparoscopic fulguration or excision of lesions of the ovary, pelvic viscera, or peritoneal surface use 58662.

Plain English Description

Interstitial devices, such as fiducial markers and dosimeters, are placed prior to radiation therapy and are used to locate the tumor or mass and/or measure the radiation dose precisely. Placement of interstitial fiducial markers allows radiation to be directed at the malignant tissue while preventing extensive radiation damage to surrounding tissues and structures. Fiducial markers are gold seeds that are implanted in or around the malignant tumor. Implantable dosimeters measure the amount of radiation at the site of the tumor. During a separately reportable laparoscopic procedure, the planned placement sites in the abdomen, pelvis, or retroperitoneum are identified and measured using imaging guidance. One or more markers are passed through one of the operating ports into the tumor, tumor bed, and/or the tissue surrounding the tumor. The positions of the markers are checked radiographically to ensure that they are properly placed. The same technique is used for placement of an interstitial dosimeter. The laparoscopic procedure is completed; the laparoscope and trocars are removed and portal incisions are closed with sutures.

Surgical laparoscopy with placement of interstitial device(s)

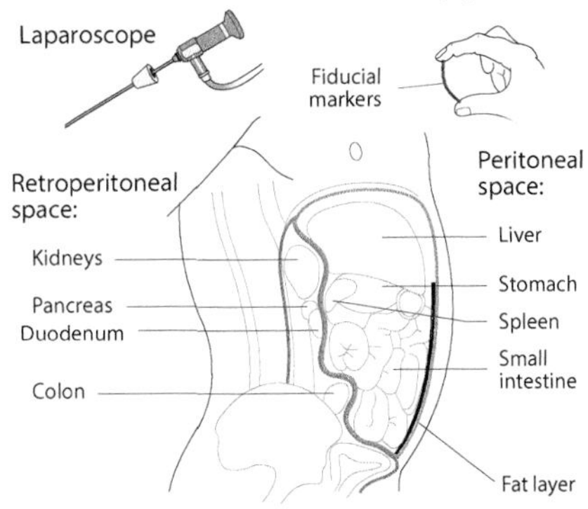

Using a laparoscope, interstitial devices are placed to precisely focus radiation therapy on a tumor.

ICD-10-CM Diagnostic Codes

See Primary Procedure code for crosswalks.

CCI Edits

Refer to Appendix A for CCI edits.

Facility RVUs

Code	Work	PE Facility	MP	Total Facility
49327	2.38	0.89	0.60	3.87

Non-facility RVUs

Code	Work	PE Non-Facility	MP	Total Non-Facility
49327	2.38	0.89	0.60	3.87

Modifiers (PAR)

Code	Mod 50	Mod 51	Mod 62	Mod 66	Mod 80
49327	0	0	1	0	2

Global Period

Code	Days
49327	ZZZ

49400

49400 Injection of air or contrast into peritoneal cavity (separate procedure)

(For radiological supervision and interpretation, use 74190)

AMA *CPT® Assistant*

49400: Dec 10: 13

Plain English Description

Using separately reportable radiographic guidance, a needle is inserted through the abdomen into the peritoneal cavity. The peritoneal cavity is then filled with air to create a pneumoperitoneum or contrast is injected and separately reportable radiographs are obtained.

Injection of air or contrast into peritoneal cavity

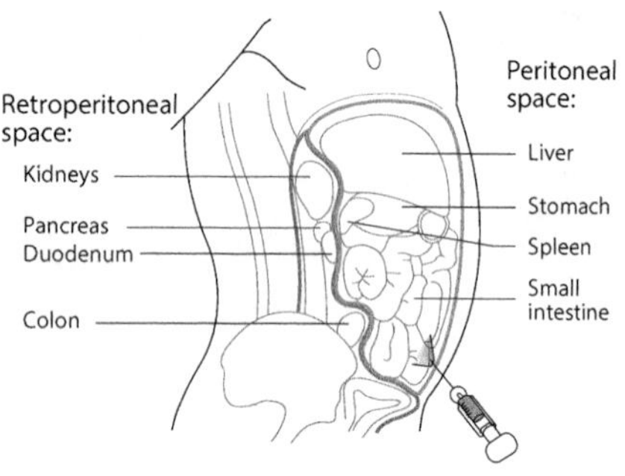

Air or a special dye is injected into the abdominal cavity to show more detail(s) on an X-ray.

ICD-10-CM Diagnostic Codes

There are too many ICD-10-CM codes to list. Refer to ICD-10-CM code book for associated diagnostic codes.

CCI Edits

Refer to Appendix A for CCI edits.

Facility RVUs

Code	Work	PE Facility	MP	Total Facility
49400	1.88	0.57	0.20	2.65

Non-facility RVUs

Code	Work	PE Non-Facility	MP	Total Non-Facility
49400	1.88	2.46	0.20	4.54

Modifiers (PAR)

Code	Mod 50	Mod 51	Mod 62	Mod 66	Mod 80
49400	0	2	0	0	1

Global Period

Code	Days
49400	000

49402

49402 Removal of peritoneal foreign body from peritoneal cavity

(For lysis of intestinal adhesions, use 44005)

(For open or percutaneous peritoneal drainage or lavage, see 49406, 49020, 49040, 49082-49084, as appropriate)

(For percutaneous insertion of a tunneled intraperitoneal catheter without subcutaneous port, use 49418)

Plain English Description

A peritoneal foreign body is removed from the peritoneal cavity. The abdominal wall is incised and the peritoneum is entered to allow the physician to explore the cavity and locate the foreign body, which is removed, and the incision is closed with sutures.

Removal of peritoneal foreign body from peritoneal cavity

Foreign body

ICD-10-CM Diagnostic Codes

- ➐⇄ S31.603 Unspecified open wound of abdominal wall, right lower quadrant with penetration into peritoneal cavity
- ➐⇄ S31.604 Unspecified open wound of abdominal wall, left lower quadrant with penetration into peritoneal cavity
- ➐⇄ S31.605 Unspecified open wound of abdominal wall, periumbilic region with penetration into peritoneal cavity
- ➐⇄ S31.623 Laceration with foreign body of abdominal wall, right lower quadrant with penetration into peritoneal cavity
- ➐⇄ S31.624 Laceration with foreign body of abdominal wall, left lower quadrant with penetration into peritoneal cavity
- ➐⇄ S31.625 Laceration with foreign body of abdominal wall, periumbilic region with penetration into peritoneal cavity
- ➐⇄ S31.643 Puncture wound with foreign body of abdominal wall, right lower quadrant with penetration into peritoneal cavity
- ➐⇄ S31.644 Puncture wound with foreign body of abdominal wall, left lower quadrant with penetration into peritoneal cavity
- ➐⇄ S31.645 Puncture wound with foreign body of abdominal wall, periumbilic region with penetration into peritoneal cavity
- ➐ S36.81 Injury of peritoneum
- ➐ T81.500 Unspecified complication of foreign body accidentally left in body following surgical operation
- ➐ T81.501 Unspecified complication of foreign body accidentally left in body following infusion or transfusion
- ➐ T81.502 Unspecified complication of foreign body accidentally left in body following kidney dialysis
- ➐ T81.504 Unspecified complication of foreign body accidentally left in body following endoscopic examination
- ➐ T81.506 Unspecified complication of foreign body accidentally left in body following aspiration, puncture or other catheterization
- ➐ T81.507 Unspecified complication of foreign body accidentally left in body following removal of catheter or packing
- ➐ T81.508 Unspecified complication of foreign body accidentally left in body following other procedure
- ➐ T81.510 Adhesions due to foreign body accidentally left in body following surgical operation
- ➐ T81.511 Adhesions due to foreign body accidentally left in body following infusion or transfusion
- ➐ T81.512 Adhesions due to foreign body accidentally left in body following kidney dialysis
- ➐ T81.514 Adhesions due to foreign body accidentally left in body following endoscopic examination
- ➐ T81.516 Adhesions due to foreign body accidentally left in body following aspiration, puncture or other catheterization
- ➐ T81.517 Adhesions due to foreign body accidentally left in body following removal of catheter or packing
- ➐ T81.518 Adhesions due to foreign body accidentally left in body following other procedure
- ➐ T81.520 Obstruction due to foreign body accidentally left in body following surgical operation
- ➐ T81.521 Obstruction due to foreign body accidentally left in body following infusion or transfusion
- ➐ T81.522 Obstruction due to foreign body accidentally left in body following kidney dialysis
- ➐ T81.524 Obstruction due to foreign body accidentally left in body following endoscopic examination
- ➐ T81.526 Obstruction due to foreign body accidentally left in body following aspiration, puncture or other catheterization
- ➐ T81.527 Obstruction due to foreign body accidentally left in body following removal of catheter or packing
- ➐ T81.528 Obstruction due to foreign body accidentally left in body following other procedure
- ➐ T81.530 Perforation due to foreign body accidentally left in body following surgical operation
- ➐ T81.531 Perforation due to foreign body accidentally left in body following infusion or transfusion
- ➐ T81.532 Perforation due to foreign body accidentally left in body following kidney dialysis
- ➐ T81.534 Perforation due to foreign body accidentally left in body following endoscopic examination
- ➐ T81.536 Perforation due to foreign body accidentally left in body following aspiration, puncture or other catheterization
- ➐ T81.537 Perforation due to foreign body accidentally left in body following removal of catheter or packing
- ➐ T81.538 Perforation due to foreign body accidentally left in body following other procedure
- ➐ T81.590 Other complications of foreign body accidentally left in body following surgical operation
- ➐ T81.591 Other complications of foreign body accidentally left in body following infusion or transfusion
- ➐ T81.592 Other complications of foreign body accidentally left in body following kidney dialysis
- ➐ T81.594 Other complications of foreign body accidentally left in body following endoscopic examination
- ➐ T81.596 Other complications of foreign body accidentally left in body following aspiration, puncture or other catheterization
- ➐ T81.597 Other complications of foreign body accidentally left in body following removal of catheter or packing
- ➐ T81.598 Other complications of foreign body accidentally left in body following other procedure
- ➐ T85.611 Breakdown (mechanical) of intraperitoneal dialysis catheter
- ➐ T85.621 Displacement of intraperitoneal dialysis catheter
- ➐ T85.631 Leakage of intraperitoneal dialysis catheter
- ➐ T85.691 Other mechanical complication of intraperitoneal dialysis catheter

ICD-10-CM Coding Notes

For codes requiring a 7th character extension, refer to your ICD-10-CM book. Review the character descriptions and coding guidelines for proper selection. For some procedures, only certain characters will apply.

CCI Edits

Refer to Appendix A for CCI edits.

Facility RVUs

Code	Work	PE Facility	MP	Total Facility
49402	14.09	8.01	3.34	25.44

Non-facility RVUs

Code	Work	PE Non-Facility	MP	Total Non-Facility
49402	14.09	8.01	3.34	25.44

Modifiers (PAR)

Code	Mod 50	Mod 51	Mod 62	Mod 66	Mod 80
49402	0	2	1	0	1

Global Period

Code	Days
49402	090

49405-49407

49405 Image-guided fluid collection drainage by catheter (eg, abscess, hematoma, seroma, lymphocele, cyst); visceral (eg, kidney, liver, spleen, lung/mediastinum), percutaneous

(Do not report 49405 in conjunction with 75989, 76942, 77002, 77003, 77012, 77021)

(For percutaneous cholecystostomy, use 47490)

(For pneumonostomy, use 32200)

(For thoracentesis, see 32554, 32555)

(For percutaneous pleural drainage, see 32556, 32557)

(For open visceral drainage, see 32200 [lung abscess or cyst], 47010 [liver abscess or cyst], 48510 [pseudocyst of pancreas], 50020 [perirenal or renal abscess])

49406 Image-guided fluid collection drainage by catheter (eg, abscess, hematoma, seroma, lymphocele, cyst); peritoneal or retroperitoneal, percutaneous

(Do not report 49406 in conjunction with 75989, 76942, 77002, 77003, 77012, 77021)

(For abdominal paracentesis [diagnostic or therapeutic], see 49082, 49083)

(For transrectal or transvaginal image-guided peritoneal or retroperitoneal fluid collection drainage by catheter, use 49407)

(For open transrectal drainage of pelvic abscess, use 45000)

(For open peritoneal or retroperitoneal drainage, see 44900 [appendiceal abscess], 49020 [peritoneal abscess or localized peritonitis], 49040 [subdiaphragmatic or subphrenic abscess], 49060 [retroperitoneal abscess], 49062 [extraperitoneal lymphocele], 49084 [peritoneal lavage], 50020 [perirenal or renal abscess], 58805 [ovarian cyst], 58822 [ovarian abscess])

(For percutaneous paracentesis, see 49082, 49083)

(For percutaneous insertion of a tunneled intraperitoneal catheter without subcutaneous port, use 49418)

49407 Image-guided fluid collection drainage by catheter (eg, abscess, hematoma, seroma, lymphocele, cyst); peritoneal or retroperitoneal, transvaginal or transrectal

(Do not report 49407 in conjunction with 75989, 76942, 77002, 77003, 77012, 77021)

(Report 49405, 49406, 49407 separately for each individual collection drained with a separate catheter)

(For open transrectal or transvaginal drainage, see 45000 [pelvic abscess], 58800 [ovarian cyst], 58820 [ovarian abscess])

(For percutaneous image-guided fluid collection drainage by catheter [eg, abscess, hematoma, seroma, lymphocele, cyst] for soft tissue [eg, extremity, abdominal wall, neck], use 10030)

AMA *CPT® Assistant* □

49405: May 14: 9, Feb 20: 13
49406: May 14: 9, Feb 20: 13
49407: May 14: 9

Plain English Description

The physician performs image-guided drainage of a fluid collection, such as an abscess, hematoma, seroma, lymphocele, or cyst of the digestive, respiratory, urogenital, or endocrine system or in the spleen, heart, or great vessels. Using fluoroscopic, ultrasonic, or computed tomographic guidance, the fluid collection is identified. A catheter with a sheath is introduced into the mediastinal, pleural, peritoneal, or retroperitoneal cavity. The catheter and sheath are passed through the organ that contains the fluid collection and into the fluid-filled cavity. The fluid collection is then drained. The fluid-filled cavity may be flushed with sterile saline or antibiotic solution to clear all pus, blood, and other fluid from the site. The catheter may be removed or left in place to provide continuous drainage. For code 49405, access is gained using a needle, and localization is confirmed by imaging. Then a wire is advanced into the cavity, and a dilator is used to perform a fascial dilatation to accommodate the drainage catheter. A catheter is advanced over the wire into the fluid collection, the wire is removed, and the catheter is locked. Use code 49406 for a percutaneous approach to a fluid collection contained in the peritoneal and retroperitoneal cavity and located in the digestive system, urogenital system, or endocrine system including the kidney, liver, or spleen. Use 49407 for a transvaginal or transrectal approach to a fluid collection contained in the peritoneal or retroperitoneal cavity. A transvaginal or transrectal approach is most commonly performed for drainage of fluid collections of urogenital organs such as the ovary or a pericolic fluid collection. A transvaginal approach uses an ultrasound probe with a drainage catheter mounted in the transducer groove that is placed in the vagina. The catheter tip is positioned over the fluid collection site. The stylet is inserted through the catheter tip and advanced through the vaginal wall into the fluid collection. A trocar is then advanced into the center of the fluid collection and it is drained. The catheter may be removed once the fluid is completely drained or it may be left in place to provide continuous drainage. If it is left in place, the stylet is removed and the catheter is attached to a drainage bag or to wall suction. A transrectal approach is performed in the same manner except that the catheter is introduced through the rectum using radiological guidance.

Image-guided fluid collection drainage by catheter

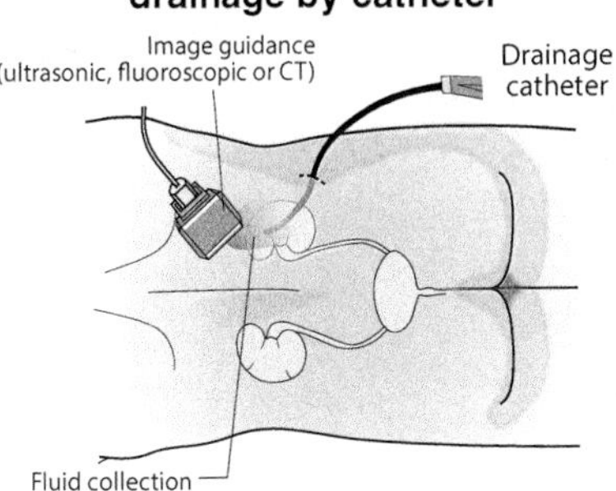

Visceral-percutaneous (49405); peritoneal or retroperitoneal-percutaneous (49406); peritoneal or retroperitoneal-transvaginal or transrectal (49407)

ICD-10-CM Diagnostic Codes

K65.1	Peritoneal abscess
K68.11	Postprocedural retroperitoneal abscess
K68.19	Other retroperitoneal abscess
N15.1	Renal and perinephric abscess
N28.1	Cyst of kidney, acquired
N34.0	Urethral abscess
N41.2	Abscess of prostate ♂
N99.840	Postprocedural hematoma of a genitourinary system organ or structure following a genitourinary system procedure
N99.841	Postprocedural hematoma of a genitourinary system organ or structure following other procedure
N99.842	Postprocedural seroma of a genitourinary system organ or structure following a genitourinary system procedure
N99.843	Postprocedural seroma of a genitourinary system organ or structure following other procedure
Q61.01	Congenital single renal cyst
Q61.02	Congenital multiple renal cysts
Q61.1	Polycystic kidney, infantile type
Q61.2	Polycystic kidney, adult type
Q61.3	Polycystic kidney, unspecified
Q61.8	Other cystic kidney diseases
Q61.9	Cystic kidney disease, unspecified

CCI Edits

Refer to Appendix A for CCI edits.

Facility RVUs

Code	Work	PE Facility	MP	Total Facility
49405	4.00	1.31	0.35	5.66
49406	4.00	1.30	0.35	5.65
49407	4.25	1.33	0.41	5.99

Non-facility RVUs

Code	Work	PE Non-Facility	MP	Total Non-Facility
49405	4.00	23.06	0.35	27.41
49406	4.00	23.05	0.35	27.40
49407	4.25	18.40	0.41	23.06

Modifiers (PAR)

Code	Mod 50	Mod 51	Mod 62	Mod 66	Mod 80
49405	0	2	0	0	1
49406	0	2	0	0	1
49407	0	2	0	0	1

Global Period

Code	Days
49405	000
49406	000
49407	000

49411-49412

49411 Placement of interstitial device(s) for radiation therapy guidance (eg, fiducial markers, dosimeter), percutaneous, intra-abdominal, intra-pelvic (except prostate), and/or retroperitoneum, single or multiple

(Report supply of device separately)

(For imaging guidance, see 76942, 77002, 77012, 77021)

(For percutaneous placement of interstitial device[s] for intra-thoracic radiation therapy guidance, use 32553)

✚ **49412 Placement of interstitial device(s) for radiation therapy guidance (eg, fiducial markers, dosimeter), open, intra-abdominal, intrapelvic, and/or retroperitoneum, including image guidance, if performed, single or multiple (List separately in addition to code for primary procedure)**

(Use 49412 in conjunction with open abdominal, pelvic, or retroperitoneal procedure[s] performed concurrently)

(For placement of interstitial device[s] for intra-abdominal, intrapelvic, and/or retroperitoneal radiation therapy guidance concurrent with laparoscopic procedure, use 49327)

(For percutaneous placement of interstitial device[s] for intra-abdominal, intrapelvic, and/or retroperitoneal radiation therapy guidance, use 49411)

AMA *CPT® Assistant* ▢

49411: Feb 10: 7, Jun 16: 3

Plain English Description

Interstitial devices, such as fiducial markers and dosimeters, are placed prior to radiation therapy and are used to locate the tumor or mass and/or measure the radiation dose precisely. Placement of interstitial fiducial markers allows radiation to be directed at the malignant tissue while preventing extensive radiation damage to surrounding tissues and structures. Fiducial markers are gold seeds that are implanted in or around the malignant tumor. Implantable dosimeters measure the amount of radiation at the site of the tumor. In 49411, the planned placement sites in the abdomen, pelvis, or retroperitoneum are identified and measured using separately reportable imaging guidance. A local anesthetic is administered to numb tissue along the planned insertion sites. Using radiologic guidance, one or more markers are passed through an introducer needle into the tumor and/or the tissue surrounding the tumor. The positions of the markers are checked radiographically to ensure that they are properly placed. The same technique is used for placement of an interstitial dosimeter. In 49412, the interstitial devices are placed during a separately reportable open procedure. The sites for placement of fiducial markers and/or a dosimeter are selected. The markers and/or dosimeter are advanced into any remaining tumor tissue, the tumor bed, and/or surrounding tissues. Imaging guidance is used as needed to ensure proper placement of the devices. The open procedure is completed and the operative wound is closed.

Placement of interstitial device(s)

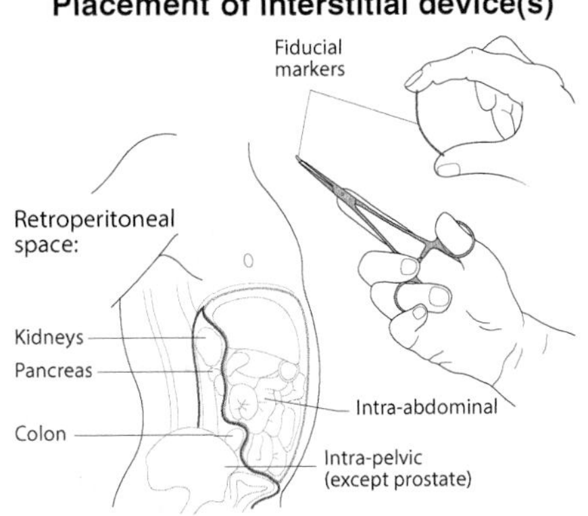

Interstitial devices are placed to precisely focus radiation therapy on a tumor; percutaneous (49411); open with image guidance (49412).

ICD-10-CM Diagnostic Codes

	C48.0	Malignant neoplasm of retroperitoneum
	C48.8	Malignant neoplasm of overlapping sites of retroperitoneum and peritoneum
⇄	C62.01	Malignant neoplasm of undescended right testis ♂
⇄	C62.02	Malignant neoplasm of undescended left testis ♂
⇄	C64.1	Malignant neoplasm of right kidney, except renal pelvis
⇄	C64.2	Malignant neoplasm of left kidney, except renal pelvis
⇄	C65.1	Malignant neoplasm of right renal pelvis
⇄	C65.2	Malignant neoplasm of left renal pelvis
⇄	C66.1	Malignant neoplasm of right ureter
⇄	C66.2	Malignant neoplasm of left ureter
	C68.0	Malignant neoplasm of urethra
	C68.1	Malignant neoplasm of paraurethral glands
	C68.8	Malignant neoplasm of overlapping sites of urinary organs
⇄	C74.01	Malignant neoplasm of cortex of right adrenal gland
⇄	C74.02	Malignant neoplasm of cortex of left adrenal gland
⇄	C74.12	Malignant neoplasm of medulla of left adrenal gland
	C78.6	Secondary malignant neoplasm of retroperitoneum and peritoneum
⇄	C79.01	Secondary malignant neoplasm of right kidney and renal pelvis
⇄	C79.02	Secondary malignant neoplasm of left kidney and renal pelvis
	C79.19	Secondary malignant neoplasm of other urinary organs
⇄	C79.71	Secondary malignant neoplasm of right adrenal gland
⇄	C79.72	Secondary malignant neoplasm of left adrenal gland
	C79.82	Secondary malignant neoplasm of genital organs
	C7A.093	Malignant carcinoid tumor of the kidney
	C7B.09	Secondary carcinoid tumors of other sites
	C7B.1	Secondary Merkel cell carcinoma

CCI Edits

Refer to Appendix A for CCI edits.

Facility RVUs ▢

Code	Work	PE Facility	MP	Total Facility
49411	3.57	1.45	0.31	5.33
49412	1.50	0.56	0.39	2.45

Non-facility RVUs ▢

Code	Work	PE Non-Facility	MP	Total Non-Facility
49411	3.57	10.70	0.31	14.58
49412	1.50	0.56	0.39	2.45

Modifiers (PAR) ▢

Code	Mod 50	Mod 51	Mod 62	Mod 66	Mod 80
49411	0	2	0	0	0
49412	0	0	1	0	0

Global Period

Code	Days
49411	000
49412	ZZZ

49418

49418 Insertion of tunneled intraperitoneal catheter (eg, dialysis, intraperitoneal chemotherapy instillation, management of ascites), complete procedure, including imaging guidance, catheter placement, contrast injection when performed, and radiological supervision and interpretation, percutaneous

Plain English Description

A tunneled intraperitoneal catheter is inserted using percutaneous technique. Using imaging guidance, the sites for the catheter insertion into the skin and the puncture site for insertion into the peritoneum are selected and marked on the skin. The catheter is attached to the tunneler, and the tunneler and catheter are passed into the subcutaneous tissue deep to Scarpa's fascia at the skin insertion site. The tunneler and catheter are then passed through the subcutaneous tissue to the site where the catheter will enter the peritoneum, and the tunneler and catheter are passed out through the skin. The tunneler is removed. An introducer needle is placed into the peritoneum adjacent to the catheter using imaging guidance. A guidewire is placed through the introducer into the peritoneum and the introducer is removed. A combined catheter introducer and dilator are advanced over the guidewire and into the peritoneum. The guidewire and dilator are removed. The catheter is passed into the abdomen through the introducer. A small amount of contrast may be injected through the catheter and observed radiographically to ensure proper positioning of the catheter. The introducer is removed from the abdomen.

Insertion of tunneled intraperitoneal catheter, complete procedure

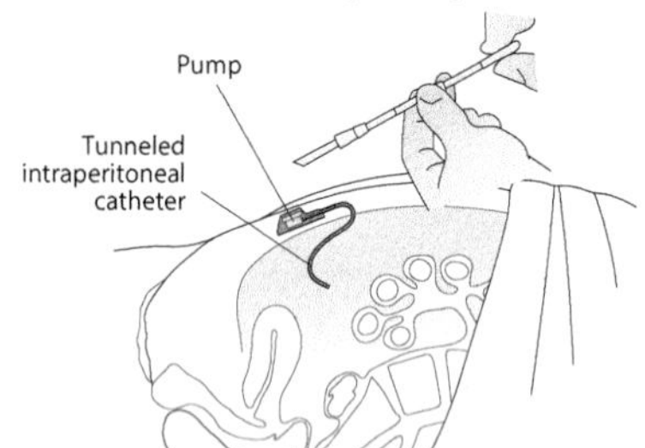

A complete catheter procedure (e.g., dialysis, chemotherapy, management of ascites).

ICD-10-CM Diagnostic Codes

E08.22	Diabetes mellitus due to underlying condition with diabetic chronic kidney disease
E09.22	Drug or chemical induced diabetes mellitus with diabetic chronic kidney disease
E10.22	Type 1 diabetes mellitus with diabetic chronic kidney disease
E11.22	Type 2 diabetes mellitus with diabetic chronic kidney disease
E13.22	Other specified diabetes mellitus with diabetic chronic kidney disease
I12.0	Hypertensive chronic kidney disease with stage 5 chronic kidney disease or end stage renal disease
I13.11	Hypertensive heart and chronic kidney disease without heart failure, with stage 5 chronic kidney disease, or end stage renal disease
I13.2	Hypertensive heart and chronic kidney disease with heart failure and with stage 5 chronic kidney disease, or end stage renal disease
M35.04	Sjögren syndrome with tubulo-interstitial nephropathy
N00.2	Acute nephritic syndrome with diffuse membranous glomerulonephritis
N00.3	Acute nephritic syndrome with diffuse mesangial proliferative glomerulonephritis
N00.4	Acute nephritic syndrome with diffuse endocapillary proliferative glomerulonephritis
N00.5	Acute nephritic syndrome with diffuse mesangiocapillary glomerulonephritis
N00.6	Acute nephritic syndrome with dense deposit disease
N00.7	Acute nephritic syndrome with diffuse crescentic glomerulonephritis
N00.8	Acute nephritic syndrome with other morphologic changes
N01.2	Rapidly progressive nephritic syndrome with diffuse membranous glomerulonephritis
N01.3	Rapidly progressive nephritic syndrome with diffuse mesangial proliferative glomerulonephritis
N01.4	Rapidly progressive nephritic syndrome with diffuse endocapillary proliferative glomerulonephritis
N01.5	Rapidly progressive nephritic syndrome with diffuse mesangiocapillary glomerulonephritis
N01.6	Rapidly progressive nephritic syndrome with dense deposit disease
N01.7	Rapidly progressive nephritic syndrome with diffuse crescentic glomerulonephritis
N01.8	Rapidly progressive nephritic syndrome with other morphologic changes
N03.2	Chronic nephritic syndrome with diffuse membranous glomerulonephritis
N03.3	Chronic nephritic syndrome with diffuse mesangial proliferative glomerulonephritis
N03.4	Chronic nephritic syndrome with diffuse endocapillary proliferative glomerulonephritis
N03.5	Chronic nephritic syndrome with diffuse mesangiocapillary glomerulonephritis
N03.6	Chronic nephritic syndrome with dense deposit disease
N03.7	Chronic nephritic syndrome with diffuse crescentic glomerulonephritis
N03.8	Chronic nephritic syndrome with other morphologic changes
N04.2	Nephrotic syndrome with diffuse membranous glomerulonephritis
N04.3	Nephrotic syndrome with diffuse mesangial proliferative glomerulonephritis
N04.4	Nephrotic syndrome with diffuse endocapillary proliferative glomerulonephritis
N04.5	Nephrotic syndrome with diffuse mesangiocapillary glomerulonephritis
N04.6	Nephrotic syndrome with dense deposit disease
N04.7	Nephrotic syndrome with diffuse crescentic glomerulonephritis
N04.8	Nephrotic syndrome with other morphologic changes
N11.0	Nonobstructive reflux-associated chronic pyelonephritis
N11.1	Chronic obstructive pyelonephritis
N11.8	Other chronic tubulo-interstitial nephritis
N16	Renal tubulo-interstitial disorders in diseases classified elsewhere
N17.0	Acute kidney failure with tubular necrosis
N17.2	Acute kidney failure with medullary necrosis
N17.8	Other acute kidney failure
N18.5	Chronic kidney disease, stage 5
N18.6	End stage renal disease
N28.0	Ischemia and infarction of kidney

CCI Edits

Refer to Appendix A for CCI edits.

Facility RVUs

Code	Work	PE Facility	MP	Total Facility
49418	3.96	1.49	0.40	5.85

Non-facility RVUs

Code	Work	PE Non-Facility	MP	Total Non-Facility
49418	3.96	26.16	0.40	30.52

Modifiers (PAR)

Code	Mod 50	Mod 51	Mod 62	Mod 66	Mod 80
49418	0	2	0	0	0

Global Period

Code	Days
49418	000

49419

49419 Insertion of tunneled intraperitoneal catheter, with subcutaneous port (ie, totally implantable)

(For removal, use 49422)

Plain English Description

A tunneled intraperitoneal catheter with a subcutaneous port is completely indwelling without any external access ports. This may be used for infusion of intra-abdominal chemotherapeutic agents as well as intraperitoneal dialysis. An incision is made in the upper abdomen and carried down through the peritoneum. Any adhesions are lysed and the bowel is dissected as needed to provide a cavity in the peritoneum that is not obstructed by other structures. The skin and subcutaneous tissue over the rectus fascia are incised and a subcutaneous pocket is created. The port is then sutured to the fascia and filled with heparinized saline. A catheter or cannula is tunneled through the subcutaneous tissue and to the site where the catheter will enter the peritoneal cavity. The peritoneum is punctured and the catheter is advanced into the peritoneum. The port and catheter are checked to ensure that medication or other fluid flows freely into the cavity. The upper abdominal incision is closed and the skin pocket is closed over the reservoir.

Insertion of intraperitoneal catheter with subcutaneous port

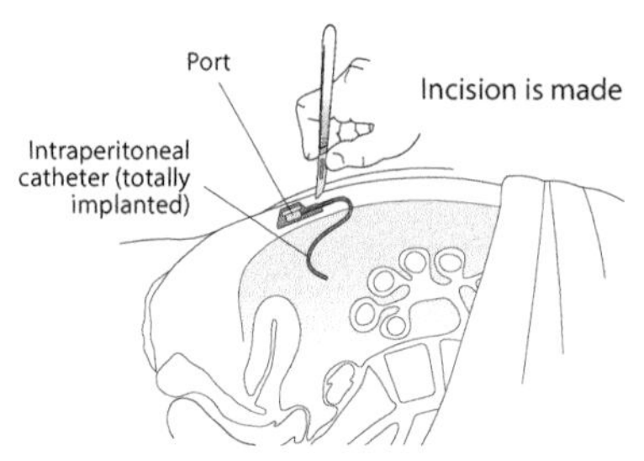

A tube for continually delivering drugs into a patient's abdominal cavity is implanted just under the skin.

ICD-10-CM Diagnostic Codes

E08.22	Diabetes mellitus due to underlying condition with diabetic chronic kidney disease
E09.22	Drug or chemical induced diabetes mellitus with diabetic chronic kidney disease
E10.22	Type 1 diabetes mellitus with diabetic chronic kidney disease
E11.22	Type 2 diabetes mellitus with diabetic chronic kidney disease
E13.22	Other specified diabetes mellitus with diabetic chronic kidney disease
I12.0	Hypertensive chronic kidney disease with stage 5 chronic kidney disease or end stage renal disease
I13.11	Hypertensive heart and chronic kidney disease without heart failure, with stage 5 chronic kidney disease, or end stage renal disease
I13.2	Hypertensive heart and chronic kidney disease with heart failure and with stage 5 chronic kidney disease, or end stage renal disease
M35.04	Sjögren syndrome with tubulo-interstitial nephropathy
N00.2	Acute nephritic syndrome with diffuse membranous glomerulonephritis
N00.3	Acute nephritic syndrome with diffuse mesangial proliferative glomerulonephritis
N00.4	Acute nephritic syndrome with diffuse endocapillary proliferative glomerulonephritis
N00.5	Acute nephritic syndrome with diffuse mesangiocapillary glomerulonephritis
N00.6	Acute nephritic syndrome with dense deposit disease
N00.7	Acute nephritic syndrome with diffuse crescentic glomerulonephritis
N00.8	Acute nephritic syndrome with other morphologic changes
N01.2	Rapidly progressive nephritic syndrome with diffuse membranous glomerulonephritis
N01.3	Rapidly progressive nephritic syndrome with diffuse mesangial proliferative glomerulonephritis
N01.4	Rapidly progressive nephritic syndrome with diffuse endocapillary proliferative glomerulonephritis
N01.5	Rapidly progressive nephritic syndrome with diffuse mesangiocapillary glomerulonephritis
N01.6	Rapidly progressive nephritic syndrome with dense deposit disease
N01.7	Rapidly progressive nephritic syndrome with diffuse crescentic glomerulonephritis
N01.8	Rapidly progressive nephritic syndrome with other morphologic changes
N03.2	Chronic nephritic syndrome with diffuse membranous glomerulonephritis
N03.3	Chronic nephritic syndrome with diffuse mesangial proliferative glomerulonephritis
N03.4	Chronic nephritic syndrome with diffuse endocapillary proliferative glomerulonephritis
N03.5	Chronic nephritic syndrome with diffuse mesangiocapillary glomerulonephritis
N03.6	Chronic nephritic syndrome with dense deposit disease
N03.7	Chronic nephritic syndrome with diffuse crescentic glomerulonephritis
N03.8	Chronic nephritic syndrome with other morphologic changes
N04.2	Nephrotic syndrome with diffuse membranous glomerulonephritis
N04.3	Nephrotic syndrome with diffuse mesangial proliferative glomerulonephritis
N04.4	Nephrotic syndrome with diffuse endocapillary proliferative glomerulonephritis
N04.5	Nephrotic syndrome with diffuse mesangiocapillary glomerulonephritis
N04.6	Nephrotic syndrome with dense deposit disease
N04.7	Nephrotic syndrome with diffuse crescentic glomerulonephritis
N04.8	Nephrotic syndrome with other morphologic changes
N11.0	Nonobstructive reflux-associated chronic pyelonephritis
N11.1	Chronic obstructive pyelonephritis
N11.8	Other chronic tubulo-interstitial nephritis
N16	Renal tubulo-interstitial disorders in diseases classified elsewhere
N17.0	Acute kidney failure with tubular necrosis
N17.2	Acute kidney failure with medullary necrosis
N17.8	Other acute kidney failure
N18.5	Chronic kidney disease, stage 5
N18.6	End stage renal disease
N28.0	Ischemia and infarction of kidney

CCI Edits

Refer to Appendix A for CCI edits.

Facility RVUs ▢

Code	Work	PE Facility	MP	Total Facility
49419	7.08	4.14	1.41	12.63

Non-facility RVUs ▢

Code	Work	PE Non-Facility	MP	Total Non-Facility
49419	7.08	4.14	1.41	12.63

Modifiers (PAR) ▢

Code	Mod 50	Mod 51	Mod 62	Mod 66	Mod 80
49419	0	2	0	0	1

Global Period

Code	Days
49419	090

49421-49422

49421 Insertion of tunneled intraperitoneal catheter for dialysis, open

(For laparoscopic insertion of tunneled intraperitoneal catheter, use 49324)

(For subcutaneous extension of intraperitoneal catheter with remote chest exit site, use 49435 in conjunction with 49421)

49422 Removal of tunneled intraperitoneal catheter

(For removal of a non-tunneled catheter, use appropriate E/M code)

AMA *CPT® Assistant*

49421: Fall 93: 2, Jul 06: 19

Plain English Description

A tunneled intraperitoneal catheter is inserted (49421) or removed (49422). Open insertion of a cannula or catheter is performed by making an incision in the upper abdomen carried down through the peritoneum. Any adhesions are lysed and the bowel is dissected as needed to provide a cavity in the peritoneum that is not obstructed by other structures. The catheter or cannula is inserted and clamped or connected to an external port. The upper abdominal incision is closed. In 49422, a tunneled intraperitoneal catheter is removed. The area around the insertion site is cleansed and a local anesthetic is injected. Using blunt dissection as needed, the catheter is freed from the tunnel and removed. Bleeding is controlled with pressure; the insertion site is closed as needed; and a pressure dressing is applied.

Insertion/removal of intraperitoneal cannula/catheter for drainage/dialysis

Intraperitoneal cannula or catheter

Incision

A tube is placed in the abdominal cavity to drain fluid through to the tube to the outside of the body. This tube can also be used for dialysis treatment. Report (49422) for removal of catheter.

ICD-10-CM Diagnostic Codes

	E08.22	Diabetes mellitus due to underlying condition with diabetic chronic kidney disease
	E09.22	Drug or chemical induced diabetes mellitus with diabetic chronic kidney disease
	E10.22	Type 1 diabetes mellitus with diabetic chronic kidney disease
	E11.22	Type 2 diabetes mellitus with diabetic chronic kidney disease
	E13.22	Other specified diabetes mellitus with diabetic chronic kidney disease
	I12.0	Hypertensive chronic kidney disease with stage 5 chronic kidney disease or end stage renal disease
	I13.11	Hypertensive heart and chronic kidney disease without heart failure, with stage 5 chronic kidney disease, or end stage renal disease
	I13.2	Hypertensive heart and chronic kidney disease with heart failure and with stage 5 chronic kidney disease, or end stage renal disease
	K56.50	Intestinal adhesions [bands], unspecified as to partial versus complete obstruction
	K56.51	Intestinal adhesions [bands], with partial obstruction
	K56.52	Intestinal adhesions [bands] with complete obstruction
	M35.04	Sjögren syndrome with tubulo-interstitial nephropathy
	N00.2	Acute nephritic syndrome with diffuse membranous glomerulonephritis
	N00.3	Acute nephritic syndrome with diffuse mesangial proliferative glomerulonephritis
	N00.4	Acute nephritic syndrome with diffuse endocapillary proliferative glomerulonephritis
	N00.5	Acute nephritic syndrome with diffuse mesangiocapillary glomerulonephritis
	N00.6	Acute nephritic syndrome with dense deposit disease
	N00.7	Acute nephritic syndrome with diffuse crescentic glomerulonephritis
	N00.8	Acute nephritic syndrome with other morphologic changes
	N01.2	Rapidly progressive nephritic syndrome with diffuse membranous glomerulonephritis
	N01.3	Rapidly progressive nephritic syndrome with diffuse mesangial proliferative glomerulonephritis
	N01.4	Rapidly progressive nephritic syndrome with diffuse endocapillary proliferative glomerulonephritis
	N01.5	Rapidly progressive nephritic syndrome with diffuse mesangiocapillary glomerulonephritis
	N01.6	Rapidly progressive nephritic syndrome with dense deposit disease
	N01.7	Rapidly progressive nephritic syndrome with diffuse crescentic glomerulonephritis
	N01.8	Rapidly progressive nephritic syndrome with other morphologic changes
	N03.2	Chronic nephritic syndrome with diffuse membranous glomerulonephritis
	N03.3	Chronic nephritic syndrome with diffuse mesangial proliferative glomerulonephritis
	N03.4	Chronic nephritic syndrome with diffuse endocapillary proliferative glomerulonephritis
	N03.5	Chronic nephritic syndrome with diffuse mesangiocapillary glomerulonephritis
	N03.6	Chronic nephritic syndrome with dense deposit disease
	N03.7	Chronic nephritic syndrome with diffuse crescentic glomerulonephritis
	N03.8	Chronic nephritic syndrome with other morphologic changes
	N04.2	Nephrotic syndrome with diffuse membranous glomerulonephritis
	N04.3	Nephrotic syndrome with diffuse mesangial proliferative glomerulonephritis
	N04.4	Nephrotic syndrome with diffuse endocapillary proliferative glomerulonephritis
	N04.5	Nephrotic syndrome with diffuse mesangiocapillary glomerulonephritis
	N04.6	Nephrotic syndrome with dense deposit disease
	N04.7	Nephrotic syndrome with diffuse crescentic glomerulonephritis
	N04.8	Nephrotic syndrome with other morphologic changes
	N11.0	Nonobstructive reflux-associated chronic pyelonephritis
	N11.1	Chronic obstructive pyelonephritis
	N11.8	Other chronic tubulo-interstitial nephritis
	N16	Renal tubulo-interstitial disorders in diseases classified elsewhere
	N17.0	Acute kidney failure with tubular necrosis
	N17.2	Acute kidney failure with medullary necrosis
	N17.8	Other acute kidney failure
	N18.5	Chronic kidney disease, stage 5
	N18.6	End stage renal disease
	N28.0	Ischemia and infarction of kidney
❼	T85.611	Breakdown (mechanical) of intraperitoneal dialysis catheter
❼	T85.621	Displacement of intraperitoneal dialysis catheter
❼	T85.631	Leakage of intraperitoneal dialysis catheter
❼	T85.691	Other mechanical complication of intraperitoneal dialysis catheter
❼	T85.71	Infection and inflammatory reaction due to peritoneal dialysis catheter
❼	T85.818	Embolism due to other internal prosthetic devices, implants and grafts
❼	T85.828	Fibrosis due to other internal prosthetic devices, implants and grafts

➐	T85.838	Hemorrhage due to other internal prosthetic devices, implants and grafts
➐	T85.848	Pain due to other internal prosthetic devices, implants and grafts
➐	T85.858	Stenosis due to other internal prosthetic devices, implants and grafts
➐	T85.868	Thrombosis due to other internal prosthetic devices, implants and grafts
➐	T85.898	Other specified complication of other internal prosthetic devices, implants and grafts
	Z49.02	Encounter for fitting and adjustment of peritoneal dialysis catheter

ICD-10-CM Coding Notes

For codes requiring a 7th character extension, refer to your ICD-10-CM book. Review the character descriptions and coding guidelines for proper selection. For some procedures, only certain characters will apply.

CCI Edits

Refer to Appendix A for CCI edits.

Facility RVUs ▯

Code	Work	PE Facility	MP	Total Facility
49421	4.21	1.52	0.99	6.72
49422	4.00	1.63	0.94	6.57

Non-facility RVUs ▯

Code	Work	PE Non-Facility	MP	Total Non-Facility
49421	4.21	1.52	0.99	6.72
49422	4.00	1.63	0.94	6.57

Modifiers (PAR) ▯

Code	Mod 50	Mod 51	Mod 62	Mod 66	Mod 80
49421	0	2	0	0	1
49422	0	2	0	0	1

Global Period

Code	Days
49421	000
49422	000

49423-49424

49423 Exchange of previously placed abscess or cyst drainage catheter under radiological guidance (separate procedure)

(For radiological supervision and interpretation, use 75984)

49424 Contrast injection for assessment of abscess or cyst via previously placed drainage catheter or tube (separate procedure)

(For radiological supervision and interpretation, use 76080)

AMA *CPT® Assistant* ☐

49423: Nov 97: 19, Mar 98: 8
49424: Nov 97: 19, Mar 98: 8, Nov 03: 14

Plain English Description

A contrast injection is performed through a previously placed drainage catheter to assess an abscess or cyst (49424). The draining abscess or cyst is evaluated to determine the size and location of the abscess pocket or cyst. Contrast media is injected through the existing catheter and distribution of the contrast material is observed radiographically. Separately reportable radiographic supervision and interpretation are performed during the injection procedure. In 49423, a previously placed abscess or cyst drainage catheter is exchanged. Using continuous radiological guidance throughout the procedure, a guidewire is placed into the existing catheter, which is removed over the guidewire. A replacement catheter is then placed over the guidewire and advanced through the existing tract into the abscess pocket or cyst. The guidewire is removed.

ICD-10-CM Diagnostic Codes

	K65.1	Peritoneal abscess
	K68.11	Postprocedural retroperitoneal abscess
	K68.19	Other retroperitoneal abscess
	N15.1	Renal and perinephric abscess
	N28.1	Cyst of kidney, acquired
	N28.84	Pyelitis cystica
	N28.85	Pyeloureteritis cystica
	N28.86	Ureteritis cystica
	N30.80	Other cystitis without hematuria
	N30.81	Other cystitis with hematuria
	N34.0	Urethral abscess
	N41.2	Abscess of prostate ♂
	Q61.01	Congenital single renal cyst
	Q61.02	Congenital multiple renal cysts
	Q61.2	Polycystic kidney, adult type
	Q61.8	Other cystic kidney diseases
	Q61.9	Cystic kidney disease, unspecified
❼	T85.628	Displacement of other specified internal prosthetic devices, implants and grafts
❼	T85.698	Other mechanical complication of other specified internal prosthetic devices, implants and grafts
❼	T85.838	Hemorrhage due to other internal prosthetic devices, implants and grafts
❼	T85.848	Pain due to other internal prosthetic devices, implants and grafts
❼	T85.898	Other specified complication of other internal prosthetic devices, implants and grafts

ICD-10-CM Coding Notes

For codes requiring a 7th character extension, refer to your ICD-10-CM book. Review the character descriptions and coding guidelines for proper selection. For some procedures, only certain characters will apply.

CCI Edits

Refer to Appendix A for CCI edits.

Facility RVUs ☐

Code	Work	PE Facility	MP	Total Facility
49423	1.46	0.45	0.12	2.03
49424	0.76	0.26	0.08	1.10

Non-facility RVUs ☐

Code	Work	PE Non-Facility	MP	Total Non-Facility
49423	1.46	16.88	0.12	18.46
49424	0.76	4.82	0.08	5.66

Modifiers (PAR) ☐

Code	Mod 50	Mod 51	Mod 62	Mod 66	Mod 80
49423	0	2	0	0	0
49424	0	2	0	0	0

Global Period

Code	Days
49423	000
49424	000

49435

✚ **49435 Insertion of subcutaneous extension to intraperitoneal cannula or catheter with remote chest exit site (List separately in addition to code for primary procedure)**

(Use 49435 in conjunction with 49324, 49421)

Plain English Description

As an add-on procedure, the physician inserts an additional extension to an abdominal cannula/catheter subcutaneously, beginning in the peritoneum. The external site is threaded through, exiting through a remote site in the chest.

Insertion of subcutaneous extension to intraperitoneal cannula or catheter with remote chest exit site

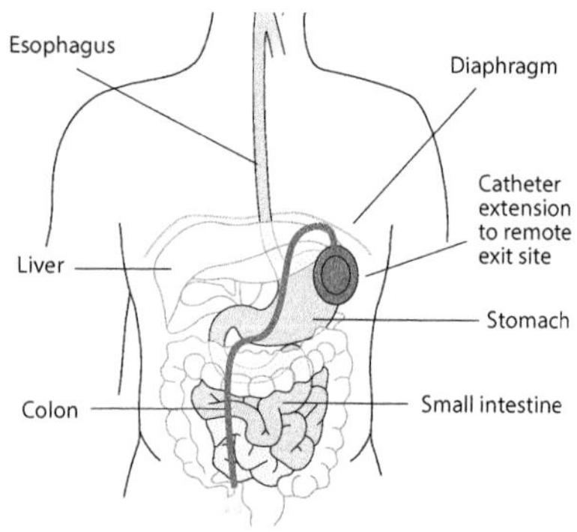

ICD-10-CM Diagnostic Codes

See Primary Procedure code for crosswalks.

CCI Edits

Refer to Appendix A for CCI edits.

Facility RVUs

Code	Work	PE Facility	MP	Total Facility
49435	2.25	0.72	0.56	3.53

Non-facility RVUs

Code	Work	PE Non-Facility	MP	Total Non-Facility
49435	2.25	0.72	0.56	3.53

Modifiers (PAR)

Code	Mod 50	Mod 51	Mod 62	Mod 66	Mod 80
49435	0	0	1	0	2

Global Period

Code	Days
49435	ZZZ

49436

49436 Delayed creation of exit site from embedded subcutaneous segment of intraperitoneal cannula or catheter

Plain English Description

After another procedure, the physician creates an embedded portion of an abdominal cannula/catheter subcutaneously, beginning in the peritoneum. The external site is threaded through, exiting through a remote site in the chest.

Delayed creation of exit site from embedded subcutaneous segment of intraperitoneal cannula/catheter

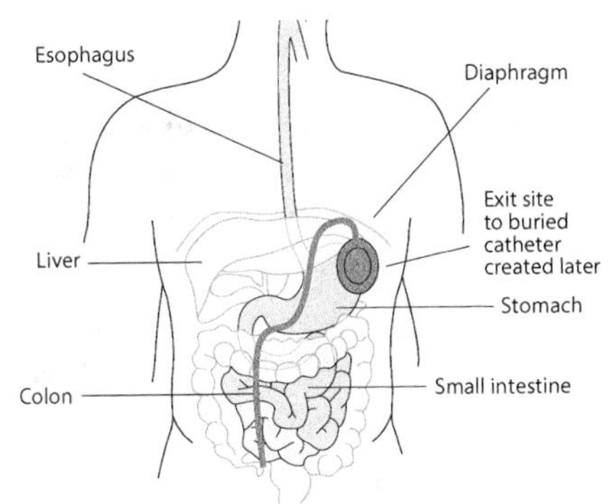

ICD-10-CM Diagnostic Codes

	L03.311	Cellulitis of abdominal wall
	L03.321	Acute lymphangitis of abdominal wall
	R18.8	Other ascites
	R60.0	Localized edema
	R60.1	Generalized edema
❼⇄	S31.602	Unspecified open wound of abdominal wall, epigastric region with penetration into peritoneal cavity
❼⇄	S31.603	Unspecified open wound of abdominal wall, right lower quadrant with penetration into peritoneal cavity
❼⇄	S31.604	Unspecified open wound of abdominal wall, left lower quadrant with penetration into peritoneal cavity
❼⇄	S31.605	Unspecified open wound of abdominal wall, periumbilic region with penetration into peritoneal cavity
❼⇄	S31.609	Unspecified open wound of abdominal wall, unspecified quadrant with penetration into peritoneal cavity
❼	T85.611	Breakdown (mechanical) of intraperitoneal dialysis catheter
❼	T85.621	Displacement of intraperitoneal dialysis catheter
❼	T85.631	Leakage of intraperitoneal dialysis catheter
❼	T85.691	Other mechanical complication of intraperitoneal dialysis catheter
❼	T85.71	Infection and inflammatory reaction due to peritoneal dialysis catheter
❼	T85.818	Embolism due to other internal prosthetic devices, implants and grafts
❼	T85.828	Fibrosis due to other internal prosthetic devices, implants and grafts
❼	T85.838	Hemorrhage due to other internal prosthetic devices, implants and grafts
❼	T85.848	Pain due to other internal prosthetic devices, implants and grafts
❼	T85.858	Stenosis due to other internal prosthetic devices, implants and grafts
❼	T85.868	Thrombosis due to other internal prosthetic devices, implants and grafts
❼	T85.898	Other specified complication of other internal prosthetic devices, implants and grafts

ICD-10-CM Coding Notes

For codes requiring a 7th character extension, refer to your ICD-10-CM book. Review the character descriptions and coding guidelines for proper selection. For some procedures, only certain characters will apply.

CCI Edits

Refer to Appendix A for CCI edits.

Facility RVUs ☐

Code	Work	PE Facility	MP	Total Facility
49436	2.72	2.23	0.67	5.62

Non-facility RVUs ☐

Code	Work	PE Non-Facility	MP	Total Non-Facility
49436	2.72	2.23	0.67	5.62

Modifiers (PAR) ☐

Code	Mod 50	Mod 51	Mod 62	Mod 66	Mod 80
49436	0	2	1	0	2

Global Period

Code	Days
49436	010

50010

50010 Renal exploration, not necessitating other specific procedures

(For laparoscopic ablation of renal mass lesion(s), use 50542)

AMA Coding Notes

Incision Procedures on the Kidney

(For retroperitoneal exploration, abscess, tumor, or cyst, see 49010, 49060, 49203-49205)

Surgical Procedures on the Urinary System

(For provision of chemotherapeutic agents, report both the specific service in addition to code(s) for the specific substance(s) or drug(s) provided)

Plain English Description

Renal exploration may be performed following blunt or penetrating renal trauma, particularly when there is evidence of persistent hemorrhage, the presence of devitalized renal tissue, or persistent urinary leakage. The approach depends on whether there are other intra-abdominal injuries that require exploration. The renal artery is exposed and a loop is placed around the artery to prevent hemorrhage. Gerota's fascia is incised and perirenal fat is dissected. The kidney is exposed and visually examined to determine the extent of injury. The surgical wound is irrigated and perioperative drains are placed as needed. No additional surgical interventions are required in this procedure. Once the kidney and surrounding tissue have been thoroughly explored, Gerota's fascia is closed, vessel loops are removed, and the incision is closed in layers. Perirenal drains may be left in place.

Renal exploration

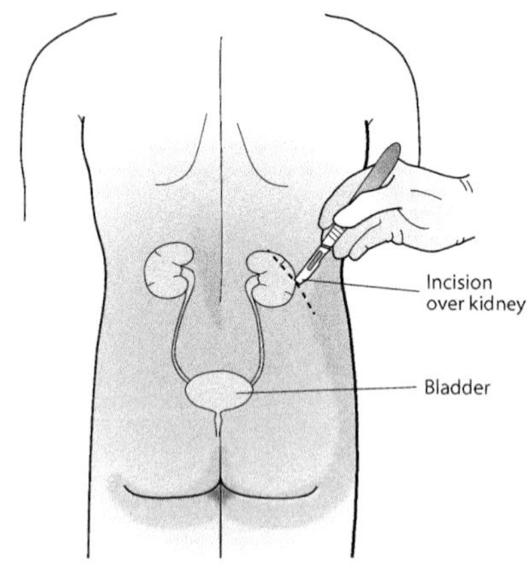

ICD-10-CM Diagnostic Codes

⇄ C64.1 Malignant neoplasm of right kidney, except renal pelvis
⇄ C64.2 Malignant neoplasm of left kidney, except renal pelvis
⇄ C65.1 Malignant neoplasm of right renal pelvis
⇄ C65.2 Malignant neoplasm of left renal pelvis
⇄ C79.01 Secondary malignant neoplasm of right kidney and renal pelvis
⇄ C79.02 Secondary malignant neoplasm of left kidney and renal pelvis
C7A.093 Malignant carcinoid tumor of the kidney
C80.2 Malignant neoplasm associated with transplanted organ
D09.19 Carcinoma in situ of other urinary organs
⇄ D30.01 Benign neoplasm of right kidney
⇄ D30.02 Benign neoplasm of left kidney
⇄ D30.11 Benign neoplasm of right renal pelvis
⇄ D30.12 Benign neoplasm of left renal pelvis
D3A.093 Benign carcinoid tumor of the kidney
⇄ D41.01 Neoplasm of uncertain behavior of right kidney
⇄ D41.02 Neoplasm of uncertain behavior of left kidney
⇄ D41.11 Neoplasm of uncertain behavior of right renal pelvis
⇄ D41.12 Neoplasm of uncertain behavior of left renal pelvis
⇄ D49.511 Neoplasm of unspecified behavior of right kidney
⇄ D49.512 Neoplasm of unspecified behavior of left kidney
N13.0 Hydronephrosis with ureteropelvic junction obstruction
N13.1 Hydronephrosis with ureteral stricture, not elsewhere classified
N13.2 Hydronephrosis with renal and ureteral calculous obstruction
N13.39 Other hydronephrosis
N28.0 Ischemia and infarction of kidney
N28.1 Cyst of kidney, acquired
N28.81 Hypertrophy of kidney
N28.83 Nephroptosis
N28.89 Other specified disorders of kidney and ureter
N29 Other disorders of kidney and ureter in diseases classified elsewhere
Q61.01 Congenital single renal cyst
Q61.02 Congenital multiple renal cysts
Q61.19 Other polycystic kidney, infantile type
Q61.2 Polycystic kidney, adult type
Q61.4 Renal dysplasia
Q61.5 Medullary cystic kidney
Q61.8 Other cystic kidney diseases
Q62.0 Congenital hydronephrosis
Q62.39 Other obstructive defects of renal pelvis and ureter
R31.0 Gross hematuria
R31.9 Hematuria, unspecified
➐⇄ S37.021 Major contusion of right kidney
➐⇄ S37.022 Major contusion of left kidney
➐⇄ S37.031 Laceration of right kidney, unspecified degree
➐⇄ S37.032 Laceration of left kidney, unspecified degree
➐⇄ S37.051 Moderate laceration of right kidney
➐⇄ S37.052 Moderate laceration of left kidney
➐⇄ S37.061 Major laceration of right kidney
➐⇄ S37.062 Major laceration of left kidney
➐⇄ S37.091 Other injury of right kidney
➐⇄ S37.092 Other injury of left kidney
➐ T79.5 Traumatic anuria

ICD-10-CM Coding Notes

For codes requiring a 7th character extension, refer to your ICD-10-CM book. Review the character descriptions and coding guidelines for proper selection. For some procedures, only certain characters will apply.

CCI Edits

Refer to Appendix A for CCI edits.

Facility RVUs ▯

Code	Work	PE Facility	MP	Total Facility
50010	12.28	6.88	1.47	20.63

Non-facility RVUs ▯

Code	Work	PE Non-Facility	MP	Total Non-Facility
50010	12.28	6.88	1.47	20.63

Modifiers (PAR) ▯

Code	Mod 50	Mod 51	Mod 62	Mod 66	Mod 80
50010	1	2	1	0	2

Global Period

Code	Days
50010	090

50020

50020 Drainage of perirenal or renal abscess, open

(For percutaneous image-guided fluid collection drainage by catheter of perirenal/renal abscess, use 49405)

AMA Coding Notes

Incision Procedures on the Kidney

(For retroperitoneal exploration, abscess, tumor, or cyst, see 49010, 49060, 49203-49205)

Surgical Procedures on the Urinary System

(For provision of chemotherapeutic agents, report both the specific service in addition to code(s) for the specific substance(s) or drug(s) provided)

AMA *CPT® Assistant* ▯

50020: Nov 97: 19, Oct 01: 8, May 14: 9

Plain English Description

Perirenal abscess, renal abscess, or infected urinoma resulting from blunt or penetrating trauma or other cause is treated with open drainage. The skin is incised and underlying soft tissues are dissected. Gerota's fascia is incised and perirenal fat is dissected. The abscess is located and incised. Loculations are separated and all debris, which may include pus, blood, and necrotic tissue, is evacuated. The abscess site is vigorously irrigated with sterile saline or antibiotic solution until all debris has been cleared from the abscess pocket. A drain is placed in the abscess cavity and incisions are closed in layers around the drain.

Drainage of perirenal abscess

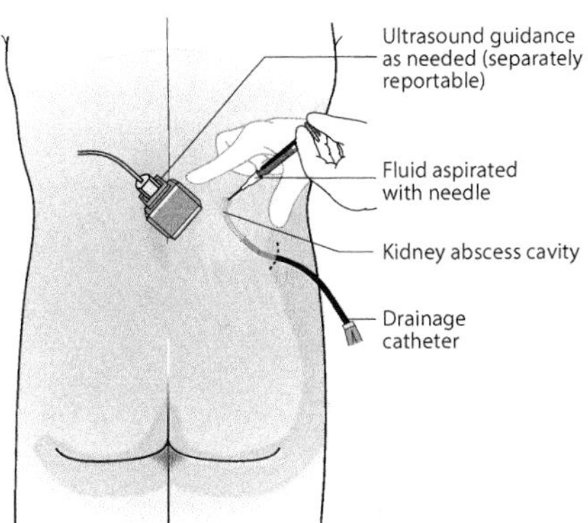

ICD-10-CM Diagnostic Codes

N15.1	Renal and perinephric abscess

CCI Edits

Refer to Appendix A for CCI edits.

Facility RVUs ▯

Code	Work	PE Facility	MP	Total Facility
50020	18.08	9.43	2.17	29.68

Non-facility RVUs ▯

Code	Work	PE Non-Facility	MP	Total Non-Facility
50020	18.08	9.43	2.17	29.68

Modifiers (PAR) ▯

Code	Mod 50	Mod 51	Mod 62	Mod 66	Mod 80
50020	0	2	1	0	1

Global Period

Code	Days
50020	090

50040

50040 Nephrostomy, nephrotomy with drainage

AMA Coding Notes

Incision Procedures on the Kidney

(For retroperitoneal exploration, abscess, tumor, or cyst, see 49010, 49060, 49203-49205)

Surgical Procedures on the Urinary System

(For provision of chemotherapeutic agents, report both the specific service in addition to code(s) for the specific substance(s) or drug(s) provided)

AMA *CPT® Assistant* ▢

50040: Spring 93: 35, Oct 01: 8

Plain English Description

Open nephrostomy or nephrotomy may be performed to drain urine from the kidney when the ureter is blocked due to a kidney stone or tumor, when the ureter or bladder has been injured causing urine to leak into the retroperitoneal or peritoneal cavity, or as a diagnostic procedure to assess kidney anatomy and function. A skin incision is made over the kidney and soft tissues are dissected. Gerota's fascia is incised and perirenal fat is dissected. Blood vessels are identified and controlled by placing a loop around each vessel. The kidney is exposed and visually examined. A small incision (pyelotomy) is made in the kidney to open the renal pelvis. A small drainage catheter or tube is placed through the renal pelvis to the calyces and cortex to drain urine from the kidney. The catheter or tube is passed through the skin incision or separate stab incision in the flank and secured with sutures. The incisions and overlying tissues are closed around the drainage device.

Nephrostomy/nephrotomy

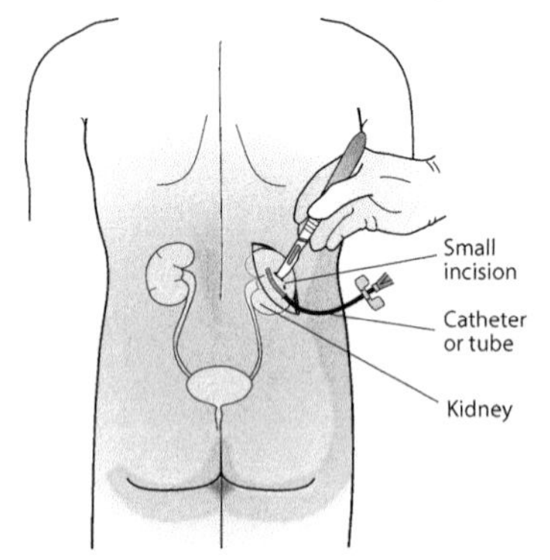

Nephrostomy, nephrotomy with drainage (50040); nephrotomy, with exploration (50045)

ICD-10-CM Diagnostic Codes

	N10	Acute pyelonephritis
	N11.1	Chronic obstructive pyelonephritis
	N13.0	Hydronephrosis with ureteropelvic junction obstruction
	N13.1	Hydronephrosis with ureteral stricture, not elsewhere classified
	N13.2	Hydronephrosis with renal and ureteral calculous obstruction
	N13.39	Other hydronephrosis
	N13.6	Pyonephrosis
	N13.71	Vesicoureteral-reflux without reflux nephropathy
	N13.721	Vesicoureteral-reflux with reflux nephropathy without hydroureter, unilateral
	N13.722	Vesicoureteral-reflux with reflux nephropathy without hydroureter, bilateral
	N13.731	Vesicoureteral-reflux with reflux nephropathy with hydroureter, unilateral
	N13.732	Vesicoureteral-reflux with reflux nephropathy with hydroureter, bilateral
	N13.8	Other obstructive and reflux uropathy
	N15.1	Renal and perinephric abscess
	N20.0	Calculus of kidney
	N20.2	Calculus of kidney with calculus of ureter
	N28.1	Cyst of kidney, acquired
	N28.89	Other specified disorders of kidney and ureter
	Q61.01	Congenital single renal cyst
	Q61.02	Congenital multiple renal cysts
	Q61.11	Cystic dilatation of collecting ducts
	Q61.19	Other polycystic kidney, infantile type
	Q61.2	Polycystic kidney, adult type
	Q61.5	Medullary cystic kidney
	Q61.8	Other cystic kidney diseases
	Q62.0	Congenital hydronephrosis
	Q62.11	Congenital occlusion of ureteropelvic junction
	Q62.12	Congenital occlusion of ureterovesical orifice
	Q62.39	Other obstructive defects of renal pelvis and ureter
	Q63.1	Lobulated, fused and horseshoe kidney
	Q63.8	Other specified congenital malformations of kidney
➐⇄	S37.021	Major contusion of right kidney
➐⇄	S37.022	Major contusion of left kidney
➐	T79.5	Traumatic anuria

ICD-10-CM Coding Notes

For codes requiring a 7th character extension, refer to your ICD-10-CM book. Review the character descriptions and coding guidelines for proper selection. For some procedures, only certain characters will apply.

CCI Edits

Refer to Appendix A for CCI edits.

Facility RVUs ▢

Code	Work	PE Facility	MP	Total Facility
50040	16.68	8.37	1.99	27.04

Non-facility RVUs ▢

Code	Work	PE Non-Facility	MP	Total Non-Facility
50040	16.68	8.37	1.99	27.04

Modifiers (PAR) ▢

Code	Mod 50	Mod 51	Mod 62	Mod 66	Mod 80
50040	1	2	1	0	1

Global Period

Code	Days
50040	090

50045

50045 Nephrotomy, with exploration

(For renal endoscopy performed in conjunction with this procedure, see 50570-50580)

AMA Coding Notes

Incision Procedures on the Kidney

(For retroperitoneal exploration, abscess, tumor, or cyst, see 49010, 49060, 49203-49205)

Surgical Procedures on the Urinary System

(For provision of chemotherapeutic agents, report both the specific service in addition to code(s) for the specific substance(s) or drug(s) provided)

AMA *CPT® Assistant* ▯

50045: Oct 01: 8

Plain English Description

Open nephrotomy is performed for exploring the kidney internally. A skin incision is made over the kidney and soft tissues are dissected. Part of the lower rib(s) may need to be removed. Gerota's fascia is incised and perirenal fat is dissected. Blood vessels are identified and controlled by placing a loop around each vessel. The kidney is exposed and visually examined by making a small incision in the kidney and retracting the edges of the incision. After exploration of the kidney is complete, a drainage catheter or tube is placed, as needed, out through the skin and secured. Gerota's fascia is closed, vessel loops are removed, and the incision is closed in layers.

ICD-10-CM Diagnostic Codes

⇄	C64.1	Malignant neoplasm of right kidney, except renal pelvis
⇄	C64.2	Malignant neoplasm of left kidney, except renal pelvis
⇄	C65.1	Malignant neoplasm of right renal pelvis
⇄	C65.2	Malignant neoplasm of left renal pelvis
⇄	C79.01	Secondary malignant neoplasm of right kidney and renal pelvis
⇄	C79.02	Secondary malignant neoplasm of left kidney and renal pelvis
	C7A.093	Malignant carcinoid tumor of the kidney
	C80.2	Malignant neoplasm associated with transplanted organ
	D09.19	Carcinoma in situ of other urinary organs
⇄	D30.01	Benign neoplasm of right kidney
⇄	D30.02	Benign neoplasm of left kidney
⇄	D30.11	Benign neoplasm of right renal pelvis
⇄	D30.12	Benign neoplasm of left renal pelvis
	D3A.093	Benign carcinoid tumor of the kidney
⇄	D41.01	Neoplasm of uncertain behavior of right kidney
⇄	D41.02	Neoplasm of uncertain behavior of left kidney
⇄	D41.11	Neoplasm of uncertain behavior of right renal pelvis
⇄	D41.12	Neoplasm of uncertain behavior of left renal pelvis
	N13.0	Hydronephrosis with ureteropelvic junction obstruction
	N13.1	Hydronephrosis with ureteral stricture, not elsewhere classified
	N13.2	Hydronephrosis with renal and ureteral calculous obstruction
	N13.39	Other hydronephrosis
	N20.0	Calculus of kidney
	N28.0	Ischemia and infarction of kidney
	N28.1	Cyst of kidney, acquired
	N28.81	Hypertrophy of kidney
	N28.83	Nephroptosis
	N28.89	Other specified disorders of kidney and ureter
	N29	Other disorders of kidney and ureter in diseases classified elsewhere
	Q61.01	Congenital single renal cyst
	Q61.02	Congenital multiple renal cysts
	Q61.19	Other polycystic kidney, infantile type
	Q61.2	Polycystic kidney, adult type
	Q61.4	Renal dysplasia
	Q61.5	Medullary cystic kidney
	Q61.8	Other cystic kidney diseases
	Q62.0	Congenital hydronephrosis
	Q62.39	Other obstructive defects of renal pelvis and ureter
	R31.0	Gross hematuria
❼⇄	S37.021	Major contusion of right kidney
❼⇄	S37.022	Major contusion of left kidney
❼⇄	S37.051	Moderate laceration of right kidney
❼⇄	S37.052	Moderate laceration of left kidney
❼⇄	S37.061	Major laceration of right kidney
❼⇄	S37.062	Major laceration of left kidney
❼⇄	S37.091	Other injury of right kidney
❼⇄	S37.092	Other injury of left kidney
❼	T79.5	Traumatic anuria

ICD-10-CM Coding Notes

For codes requiring a 7th character extension, refer to your ICD-10-CM book. Review the character descriptions and coding guidelines for proper selection. For some procedures, only certain characters will apply.

CCI Edits

Refer to Appendix A for CCI edits.

Facility RVUs ▯

Code	Work	PE Facility	MP	Total Facility
50045	16.82	8.42	2.01	27.25

Non-facility RVUs ▯

Code	Work	PE Non-Facility	MP	Total Non-Facility
50045	16.82	8.42	2.01	27.25

Modifiers (PAR) ▯

Code	Mod 50	Mod 51	Mod 62	Mod 66	Mod 80
50045	1	2	1	0	2

Global Period

Code	Days
50045	090

50060-50065

50060 Nephrolithotomy; removal of calculus

50065 Nephrolithotomy; secondary surgical operation for calculus

AMA Coding Notes

Incision Procedures on the Kidney

(For retroperitoneal exploration, abscess, tumor, or cyst, see 49010, 49060, 49203-49205)

Surgical Procedures on the Urinary System

(For provision of chemotherapeutic agents, report both the specific service in addition to code(s) for the specific substance(s) or drug(s) provided)

AMA *CPT® Assistant* ▯

50060: Oct 01: 8

50065: Oct 01: 8

Plain English Description

Open nephrolithotomy is performed to remove a renal calculus. A skin incision is made over the kidney and soft tissues are dissected. Gerota's fascia is incised and perirenal fat is dissected. Blood vessels are identified and controlled by placing a loop around each vessel. The kidney is exposed and visually examined. An incision is made in the kidney over the site of the renal calculus. The calculus is located and removed and sent to the laboratory for separately reportable analysis. Drains are placed as needed, Gerota's fascia is closed, vessel loops are removed, and the incision is closed in layers. Use 50060 for the primary surgical procedure to remove the renal calculus. Use 50065 if this is a secondary surgical operation to remove the calculus.

Nephrolithotomy

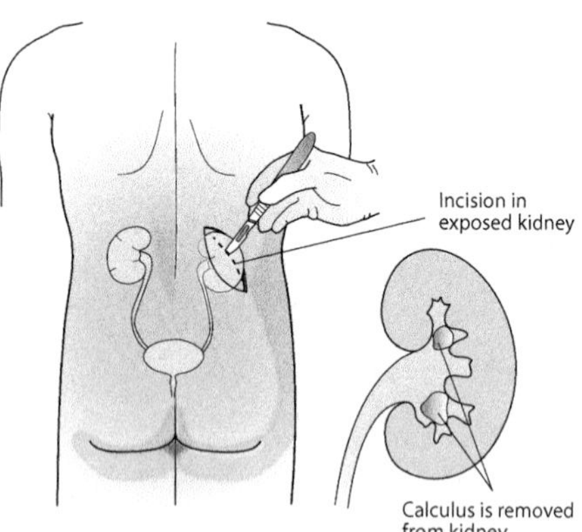

Removal of calculus (50060); secondary surgical operation for calculus (50065)

ICD-10-CM Diagnostic Codes

N20.0	Calculus of kidney
N20.2	Calculus of kidney with calculus of ureter
N22	Calculus of urinary tract in diseases classified elsewhere

CCI Edits

Refer to Appendix A for CCI edits.

Pub 100

50060: Pub 100-03, 1, 230.1

50065: Pub 100-03, 1, 230.1

Facility RVUs ▯

Code	Work	PE Facility	MP	Total Facility
50060	20.95	9.81	2.49	33.25
50065	22.32	10.27	2.66	35.25

Non-facility RVUs ▯

Code	Work	PE Non-Facility	MP	Total Non-Facility
50060	20.95	9.81	2.49	33.25
50065	22.32	10.27	2.66	35.25

Modifiers (PAR) ▯

Code	Mod 50	Mod 51	Mod 62	Mod 66	Mod 80
50060	1	2	1	0	2
50065	1	2	0	0	2

Global Period

Code	Days
50060	090
50065	090

50070-50075

50070 Nephrolithotomy; complicated by congenital kidney abnormality

50075 Nephrolithotomy; removal of large staghorn calculus filling renal pelvis and calyces (including anatrophic pyelolithotomy)

AMA Coding Notes

Incision Procedures on the Kidney

(For retroperitoneal exploration, abscess, tumor, or cyst, see 49010, 49060, 49203-49205)

Surgical Procedures on the Urinary System

(For provision of chemotherapeutic agents, report both the specific service in addition to code(s) for the specific substance(s) or drug(s) provided)

AMA *CPT® Assistant*

50070: Oct 01: 8

50075: Oct 01: 8

Plain English Description

Open nephrolithotomy is performed to remove a renal calculus in a procedure complicated by congenital kidney abnormality or by removal of a large staghorn calculus. A skin incision is made over the kidney and soft tissues are dissected. Gerota's fascia is incised and perirenal fat is dissected. Blood vessels are identified and controlled by placing a loop around each vessel. The kidney is exposed and visually examined. An incision is made in the kidney over the site of the renal calculus. Use 50070 for open removal of a renal calculus when the patient has a congenital kidney abnormality such as parenchymal disease, congenital obstruction of the ureteropelvic junction with or without hydronephrosis, or polycystic kidneys. The calculus is located and removed and sent to the laboratory for separately reportable analysis. Drains are placed as needed, Gerota's fascia is closed, vessel loops are removed, and the incision is closed in layers. Use 50075 if the patient has a large staghorn calculus, which may also be referred to as a struvite calculus. To be classified as a staghorn calculus, the stone must involve the renal pelvis and extend into at least two calyces. In order to completely expose and excise the stone, the kidney is bivalved along the lateral aspect, which is also referred to as anatrophic nephrolithotomy, or the renal pelvis is opened, which is also referred to as anatrophic pyelolithotomy. The staghorn calculus is then carefully dissected free of the renal parenchyma and removed. The renal pelvis and calyces are carefully inspected to ensure that all stone fragments are removed.

Nephrolithotomy

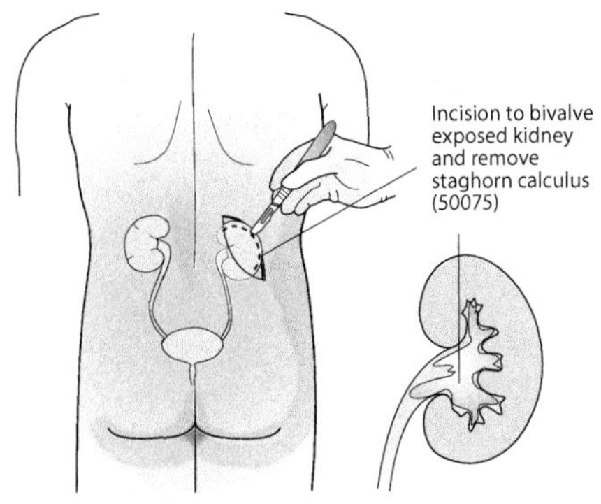

Complicated by congenital kidney abnormality (50070); removal of large staghorn calculus (50075)

ICD-10-CM Diagnostic Codes

N20.0	Calculus of kidney
N20.2	Calculus of kidney with calculus of ureter
N22	Calculus of urinary tract in diseases classified elsewhere
Q63.0	Accessory kidney
Q63.1	Lobulated, fused and horseshoe kidney
Q63.2	Ectopic kidney
Q63.3	Hyperplastic and giant kidney
Q63.8	Other specified congenital malformations of kidney

CCI Edits

Refer to Appendix A for CCI edits.

Pub 100

50070: Pub 100-03, 1, 230.1

50075: Pub 100-03, 1, 230.1

Facility RVUs

Code	Work	PE Facility	MP	Total Facility
50070	21.85	10.11	2.62	34.58
50075	27.09	12.17	3.23	42.49

Non-facility RVUs

Code	Work	PE Non-Facility	MP	Total Non-Facility
50070	21.85	10.11	2.62	34.58
50075	27.09	12.17	3.23	42.49

Modifiers (PAR)

Code	Mod 50	Mod 51	Mod 62	Mod 66	Mod 80
50070	1	2	1	0	2
50075	1	2	1	0	2

Global Period

Code	Days
50070	090
50075	090

50080-50081

50080 Percutaneous nephrostolithotomy or pyelostolithotomy, with or without dilation, endoscopy, lithotripsy, stenting, or basket extraction; up to 2 cm

50081 Percutaneous nephrostolithotomy or pyelostolithotomy, with or without dilation, endoscopy, lithotripsy, stenting, or basket extraction; over 2 cm

(For establishment of nephrostomy without nephrostolithotomy, see 50040, 50432, 50433, 52334)

(For fluoroscopic guidance, use 76000)

(Do not report 50080, 50081 in conjunction with 50436, 50437, when performed by the same physician or other qualified health care professional)

AMA Coding Notes

Incision Procedures on the Kidney

(For retroperitoneal exploration, abscess, tumor, or cyst, see 49010, 49060, 49203-49205)

Surgical Procedures on the Urinary System

(For provision of chemotherapeutic agents, report both the specific service in addition to code(s) for the specific substance(s) or drug(s) provided)

AMA *CPT® Assistant*

50080: Oct 01: 8, Dec 08: 7, Jun 09: 10
50081: Oct 01: 8, Dec 08: 7, Jun 09: 10

Plain English Description

A renal calculus is removed by percutaneous technique. The skin over the planned puncture site is cleansed and a local anesthetic is injected. The skin is punctured and a needle is advanced into the kidney to the site of the calculus using separately reportable fluoroscopic guidance. A guidewire is then advanced through the needle and the needle is removed. A rigid and/or flexible nephroscope is introduced over the guidewire and the guidewire is removed. The calculus is visualized. If the calculus is large, a series of dilators may be passed through the nephroscope to widen the tract and provide better access to the calculus. A permanent indwelling stent may be placed to maintain the opening. Lithotripsy is performed as needed using ultrasound, an electrohydraulic device, pneumatic lithotrites, and/or laser to fragment the stone. A basket extraction device may be used to remove the calculus. Once the calculus and any fragments have been completely removed, a nephrostomy tube is placed to ensure good post-procedural drainage of the kidney. A large branched staghorn calculus may require multiple percutaneous nephrolithotomy or pyelolithotomy tracts for complete removal of the calculus. Use 50080 for a calculus up to 2 cm. Use 50081 if the calculus is over 2 cm.

Percutaneous nephrostolithotomy or pyelostolithotomy

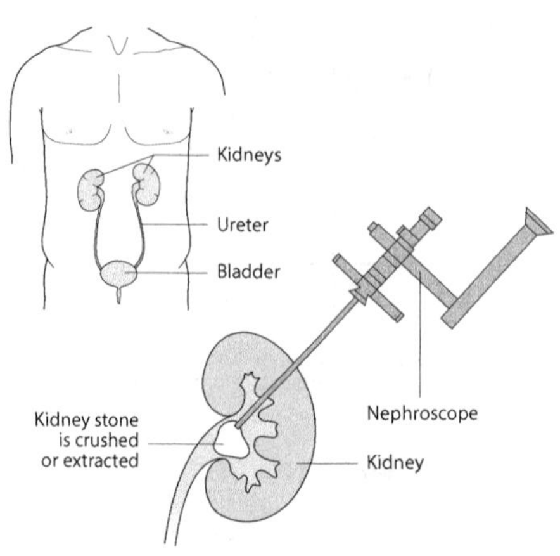

ICD-10-CM Diagnostic Codes

N20.0	Calculus of kidney
N20.2	Calculus of kidney with calculus of ureter
N22	Calculus of urinary tract in diseases classified elsewhere

CCI Edits

Refer to Appendix A for CCI edits.

Pub 100

50080: Pub 100-03, 1, 230.1
50081: Pub 100-03, 1, 230.1

Facility RVUs

Code	Work	PE Facility	MP	Total Facility
50080	15.74	7.76	1.86	25.36
50081	23.50	10.98	2.82	37.30

Non-facility RVUs

Code	Work	PE Non-Facility	MP	Total Non-Facility
50080	15.74	7.76	1.86	25.36
50081	23.50	10.98	2.82	37.30

Modifiers (PAR)

Code	Mod 50	Mod 51	Mod 62	Mod 66	Mod 80
50080	1	2	0	0	1
50081	1	2	1	0	2

Global Period

Code	Days
50080	090
50081	090

50100

50100 Transection or repositioning of aberrant renal vessels (separate procedure)

AMA Coding Notes

Incision Procedures on the Kidney

(For retroperitoneal exploration, abscess, tumor, or cyst, see 49010, 49060, 49203-49205)

Surgical Procedures on the Urinary System

(For provision of chemotherapeutic agents, report both the specific service in addition to code(s) for the specific substance(s) or drug(s) provided)

AMA *CPT® Assistant* ▢

50100: Oct 01: 8

Plain English Description

Aberrant renal blood vessels are one cause of ureteropelvic junction (UPJ) obstruction. This occurs when the renal arteries and/or veins at the inferior pole of the kidney cross anterior to the ureter, causing obstruction and hydronephrosis. An anterior approach is used to expose the aberrant blood vessels, ureter, and kidney. The aberrant blood vessels are dissected free of surrounding tissue. If the kidney has adequate blood supply from other renal vessels, the aberrant vessels are ligated and transected. If the aberrant blood vessels must be preserved, vessel loops are placed superior and inferior to the planned transection site. The vessels are transected between the vessel loops and repositioned so that they no longer obstruct the UPJ. The vessels are anastomosed. The vessel loops are removed and the operative wound is closed in layers.

Transection or repositioning of aberrant renal vessels

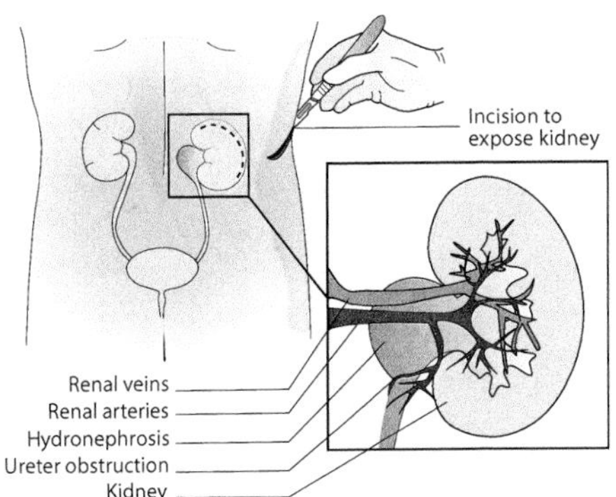

ICD-10-CM Diagnostic Codes

N11.1	Chronic obstructive pyelonephritis
N13.0	Hydronephrosis with ureteropelvic junction obstruction
N13.1	Hydronephrosis with ureteral stricture, not elsewhere classified
N13.5	Crossing vessel and stricture of ureter without hydronephrosis
N28.0	Ischemia and infarction of kidney
Q27.1	Congenital renal artery stenosis
Q27.2	Other congenital malformations of renal artery
Q27.34	Arteriovenous malformation of renal vessel
Q62.0	Congenital hydronephrosis
Q62.11	Congenital occlusion of ureteropelvic junction
Q62.39	Other obstructive defects of renal pelvis and ureter
Q63.0	Accessory kidney
Q63.1	Lobulated, fused and horseshoe kidney
Q63.2	Ectopic kidney
Q63.8	Other specified congenital malformations of kidney

CCI Edits

Refer to Appendix A for CCI edits.

Facility RVUs ▢

Code	Work	PE Facility	MP	Total Facility
50100	17.45	10.48	4.42	32.35

Non-facility RVUs ▢

Code	Work	PE Non-Facility	MP	Total Non-Facility
50100	17.45	10.48	4.42	32.35

Modifiers (PAR) ▢

Code	Mod 50	Mod 51	Mod 62	Mod 66	Mod 80
50100	1	2	1	0	2

Global Period

Code	Days
50100	090

50120-50135

50120 Pyelotomy; with exploration

(For renal endoscopy performed in conjunction with this procedure, see 50570-50580)

50125 Pyelotomy; with drainage, pyelostomy

50130 Pyelotomy; with removal of calculus (pyelolithotomy, pelviolithotomy, including coagulum pyelolithotomy)

50135 Pyelotomy; complicated (eg, secondary operation, congenital kidney abnormality)

(For supply of anticarcinogenic agents, use 99070 in addition to code for primary procedure)

AMA Coding Notes

Incision Procedures on the Kidney

(For retroperitoneal exploration, abscess, tumor, or cyst, see 49010, 49060, 49203-49205)

Surgical Procedures on the Urinary System

(For provision of chemotherapeutic agents, report both the specific service in addition to code(s) for the specific substance(s) or drug(s) provided)

AMA *CPT® Assistant*

50120: Oct 01: 8
50125: Oct 01: 8
50130: Oct 01: 8
50135: Oct 01: 8

Plain English Description

A pyelotomy is an incision into the renal pelvis, the large cavity in the center of the kidney where urine is collected. The renal pelvis collects urine from the calyces. Urine drains from the renal pelvis into the ureter. A skin incision is made over the kidney. Gerota's fascia is incised and perirenal fat is dissected. Blood vessels are identified and controlled by placing a loop around each vessel. The kidney and ureter are exposed and visually examined. The ureter is traced upwards to the ureteropelvic junction (UPJ) and the renal pelvis is located. The posterior aspect of the renal pelvis is exposed and incised. In 50120, the renal pelvis is carefully explored for signs of disease or injury. In 50125, the renal pelvis is incised and a pyelostomy tube is placed into the pelvis to drain urine. A purse-string suture is placed around the pyelostomy tube to secure it to the renal pelvis. The surgical wound is closed in layers around the tube and a pyelostomy bag is attached to the tube to collect urine. In 50130, a calculus is removed from the renal pelvis. A single stone is removed using stone forceps. A coagulum pyelolithotomy may be used to remove multiple small stones. This involves creating a coagulum (clot) that envelops the small stones. For coagulum pyelolithotomy, a noncrushing clamp is placed around the ureter at the UPJ. Prior to incising the renal pelvis, thrombin and calcium chloride solution are injected into the renal pelvis to precipitate clot formation. Once the clot has formed, the renal pelvis is incised and the clot containing the small stones is removed. In 50135, a complicated pyelotomy is performed on a patient who has had previous surgery on the kidney or a patient who has a congenital kidney abnormality, such as parenchymal disease, congenital obstruction of the ureteropelvic junction with or without hydronephrosis, or polycystic kidneys. The physician may explore the renal pelvis, place a pyelostomy tube, or remove a calculus. Upon completion of the procedure, drains are placed as needed and the surgical wound is closed in layers.

Pyelotomy

With exploration (50120); with drainage, pyelostomy (50125); with removal of calculus (50130); complicated (50135)

ICD-10-CM Diagnostic Codes

⇄	C65.1	Malignant neoplasm of right renal pelvis
⇄	C65.2	Malignant neoplasm of left renal pelvis
⇄	C79.01	Secondary malignant neoplasm of right kidney and renal pelvis
⇄	C79.02	Secondary malignant neoplasm of left kidney and renal pelvis
	D09.19	Carcinoma in situ of other urinary organs
⇄	D30.11	Benign neoplasm of right renal pelvis
⇄	D30.12	Benign neoplasm of left renal pelvis
⇄	D41.11	Neoplasm of uncertain behavior of right renal pelvis
⇄	D41.12	Neoplasm of uncertain behavior of left renal pelvis
	M35.04	Sjögren syndrome with tubulo-interstitial nephropathy
	N10	Acute pyelonephritis
	N11.0	Nonobstructive reflux-associated chronic pyelonephritis
	N11.1	Chronic obstructive pyelonephritis
	N11.8	Other chronic tubulo-interstitial nephritis
	N12	Tubulo-interstitial nephritis, not specified as acute or chronic
	N15.1	Renal and perinephric abscess
	N16	Renal tubulo-interstitial disorders in diseases classified elsewhere
	N20.0	Calculus of kidney
	N20.2	Calculus of kidney with calculus of ureter
	N22	Calculus of urinary tract in diseases classified elsewhere
	N28.84	Pyelitis cystica
	N28.85	Pyeloureteritis cystica
	N28.89	Other specified disorders of kidney and ureter
	Q62.39	Other obstructive defects of renal pelvis and ureter
	Q63.0	Accessory kidney
	Q63.1	Lobulated, fused and horseshoe kidney
	Q63.2	Ectopic kidney
	Q63.8	Other specified congenital malformations of kidney

CCI Edits

Refer to Appendix A for CCI edits.

Pub 100

50130: Pub 100-03, 1, 230.1
50135: Pub 100-03, 1, 230.1

Facility RVUs

Code	Work	PE Facility	MP	Total Facility
50120	17.21	8.48	2.04	27.73
50125	17.82	8.76	2.14	28.72
50130	18.82	9.10	2.23	30.15
50135	20.59	9.69	2.46	32.74

Non-facility RVUs

Code	Work	PE Non-Facility	MP	Total Non-Facility
50120	17.21	8.48	2.04	27.73
50125	17.82	8.76	2.14	28.72
50130	18.82	9.10	2.23	30.15
50135	20.59	9.69	2.46	32.74

Modifiers (PAR)

Code	Mod 50	Mod 51	Mod 62	Mod 66	Mod 80
50120	1	2	1	0	2
50125	1	2	1	0	2
50130	1	2	1	0	2
50135	1	2	1	0	2

Global Period

Code	Days
50120	090
50125	090
50130	090
50135	090

CPT® Procedural Coding

50200-50205

50200 Renal biopsy; percutaneous, by trocar or needle

(For radiological supervision and interpretation, see 76942, 77002, 77012, 77021)

(For fine needle aspiration biopsy, see 10005, 10006, 10007, 10008, 10009, 10010, 10011, 10012)

(For evaluation of fine needle aspirate, see 88172, 88173)

50205 Renal biopsy; by surgical exposure of kidney

AMA Coding Notes

Excision Procedures on the Kidney

(For excision of retroperitoneal tumor or cyst, see 49203-49205)

(For laparoscopic ablation of renal mass lesion(s), use 50542)

Surgical Procedures on the Urinary System

(For provision of chemotherapeutic agents, report both the specific service in addition to code(s) for the specific substance(s) or drug(s) provided)

AMA *CPT® Assistant*

50200: Fall 93: 13, Oct 01: 8, Feb 10: 7
50205: Oct 01: 8

Plain English Description

In 50200, a percutaneous trocar or needle biopsy is performed using separately reportable radiological guidance. The patient is sedated and a local anesthetic administered. The patient is placed prone on top of pillows or folded sheets to compress the abdomen and upper ribs, allowing better access to the kidney. The kidneys are visualized using ultrasound, fluoroscopy, CT, or MRI, with the most common modality being ultrasound. The trocar or needle is then placed through the skin over the kidney and advanced under direct vision to the renal capsule. A tissue sample is obtained. In 50205, an open biopsy is performed by surgical exposure of the kidney. A small incision is made in the back over the kidney and the renal capsule exposed. A tissue sample is obtained and sent for separately reportable pathological evaluation.

Renal biopsy

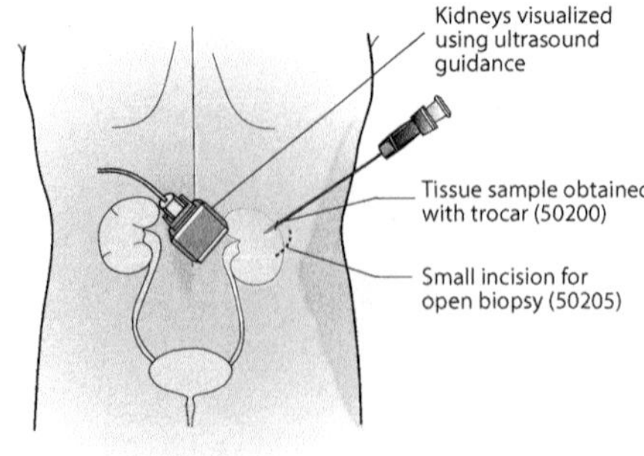

Percutaneous by trocar or needle (50200); by surgical exposure of kidney (50205)

ICD-10-CM Diagnostic Codes

	Code	Description
	A02.25	Salmonella pyelonephritis
	B58.83	Toxoplasma tubulo-interstitial nephropathy
⇄	C64.1	Malignant neoplasm of right kidney, except renal pelvis
⇄	C64.2	Malignant neoplasm of left kidney, except renal pelvis
⇄	C65.1	Malignant neoplasm of right renal pelvis
⇄	C65.2	Malignant neoplasm of left renal pelvis
⇄	C79.01	Secondary malignant neoplasm of right kidney and renal pelvis
⇄	C79.02	Secondary malignant neoplasm of left kidney and renal pelvis
	C7A.093	Malignant carcinoid tumor of the kidney
	C80.2	Malignant neoplasm associated with transplanted organ
	D09.19	Carcinoma in situ of other urinary organs
⇄	D30.01	Benign neoplasm of right kidney
⇄	D30.02	Benign neoplasm of left kidney
⇄	D30.11	Benign neoplasm of right renal pelvis
⇄	D30.12	Benign neoplasm of left renal pelvis
	D3A.093	Benign carcinoid tumor of the kidney
⇄	D41.01	Neoplasm of uncertain behavior of right kidney
⇄	D41.02	Neoplasm of uncertain behavior of left kidney
⇄	D41.11	Neoplasm of uncertain behavior of right renal pelvis
⇄	D41.12	Neoplasm of uncertain behavior of left renal pelvis
	D86.84	Sarcoid pyelonephritis
	E08.21	Diabetes mellitus due to underlying condition with diabetic nephropathy
	E08.22	Diabetes mellitus due to underlying condition with diabetic chronic kidney disease
	E08.29	Diabetes mellitus due to underlying condition with other diabetic kidney complication
	E09.21	Drug or chemical induced diabetes mellitus with diabetic nephropathy
	E09.22	Drug or chemical induced diabetes mellitus with diabetic chronic kidney disease
	E09.29	Drug or chemical induced diabetes mellitus with other diabetic kidney complication
	E10.21	Type 1 diabetes mellitus with diabetic nephropathy
	E10.22	Type 1 diabetes mellitus with diabetic chronic kidney disease
	E10.29	Type 1 diabetes mellitus with other diabetic kidney complication
	E11.21	Type 2 diabetes mellitus with diabetic nephropathy
	E11.22	Type 2 diabetes mellitus with diabetic chronic kidney disease
	E11.29	Type 2 diabetes mellitus with other diabetic kidney complication
	E13.21	Other specified diabetes mellitus with diabetic nephropathy
	E13.22	Other specified diabetes mellitus with diabetic chronic kidney disease
	E13.29	Other specified diabetes mellitus with other diabetic kidney complication
	E85.0	Non-neuropathic heredofamilial amyloidosis
	E85.3	Secondary systemic amyloidosis
	E85.4	Organ-limited amyloidosis
	E85.81	Light chain (AL) amyloidosis
	E85.82	Wild-type transthyretin-related (ATTR) amyloidosis
	I75.81	Atheroembolism of kidney
	M32.14	Glomerular disease in systemic lupus erythematosus
	M32.15	Tubulo-interstitial nephropathy in systemic lupus erythematosus
	M35.04	Sjögren syndrome with tubulo-interstitial nephropathy
	N00.0	Acute nephritic syndrome with minor glomerular abnormality
	N00.1	Acute nephritic syndrome with focal and segmental glomerular lesions
	N00.2	Acute nephritic syndrome with diffuse membranous glomerulonephritis
	N00.3	Acute nephritic syndrome with diffuse mesangial proliferative glomerulonephritis
	N00.4	Acute nephritic syndrome with diffuse endocapillary proliferative glomerulonephritis
	N00.5	Acute nephritic syndrome with diffuse mesangiocapillary glomerulonephritis
	N00.6	Acute nephritic syndrome with dense deposit disease
	N00.7	Acute nephritic syndrome with diffuse crescentic glomerulonephritis
	N00.8	Acute nephritic syndrome with other morphologic changes
	N00.9	Acute nephritic syndrome with unspecified morphologic changes
	N00.A	Acute nephritic syndrome with C3 glomerulonephritis

N02.0 Recurrent and persistent hematuria with minor glomerular abnormality
N02.1 Recurrent and persistent hematuria with focal and segmental glomerular lesions
N02.2 Recurrent and persistent hematuria with diffuse membranous glomerulonephritis
N02.3 Recurrent and persistent hematuria with diffuse mesangial proliferative glomerulonephritis
N02.4 Recurrent and persistent hematuria with diffuse endocapillary proliferative glomerulonephritis
N02.5 Recurrent and persistent hematuria with diffuse mesangiocapillary glomerulonephritis
N02.6 Recurrent and persistent hematuria with dense deposit disease
N02.7 Recurrent and persistent hematuria with diffuse crescentic glomerulonephritis
N02.8 Recurrent and persistent hematuria with other morphologic changes
N02.9 Recurrent and persistent hematuria with unspecified morphologic changes
N02.A Recurrent and persistent hematuria with C3 glomerulonephritis
N03.0 Chronic nephritic syndrome with minor glomerular abnormality
N03.1 Chronic nephritic syndrome with focal and segmental glomerular lesions
N03.2 Chronic nephritic syndrome with diffuse membranous glomerulonephritis
N03.3 Chronic nephritic syndrome with diffuse mesangial proliferative glomerulonephritis
N03.4 Chronic nephritic syndrome with diffuse endocapillary proliferative glomerulonephritis
N03.5 Chronic nephritic syndrome with diffuse mesangiocapillary glomerulonephritis
N03.6 Chronic nephritic syndrome with dense deposit disease
N03.7 Chronic nephritic syndrome with diffuse crescentic glomerulonephritis
N03.8 Chronic nephritic syndrome with other morphologic changes
N03.9 Chronic nephritic syndrome with unspecified morphologic changes
N03.A Chronic nephritic syndrome with C3 glomerulonephritis
N04.0 Nephrotic syndrome with minor glomerular abnormality
N04.1 Nephrotic syndrome with focal and segmental glomerular lesions
N04.2 Nephrotic syndrome with diffuse membranous glomerulonephritis
N04.3 Nephrotic syndrome with diffuse mesangial proliferative glomerulonephritis
N04.4 Nephrotic syndrome with diffuse endocapillary proliferative glomerulonephritis
N04.5 Nephrotic syndrome with diffuse mesangiocapillary glomerulonephritis
N04.6 Nephrotic syndrome with dense deposit disease
N04.7 Nephrotic syndrome with diffuse crescentic glomerulonephritis
N04.8 Nephrotic syndrome with other morphologic changes
N04.9 Nephrotic syndrome with unspecified morphologic changes
N04.A Nephrotic syndrome with C3 glomerulonephritis
N06.0 Isolated proteinuria with minor glomerular abnormality
N06.1 Isolated proteinuria with focal and segmental glomerular lesions
N06.2 Isolated proteinuria with diffuse membranous glomerulonephritis
N06.3 Isolated proteinuria with diffuse mesangial proliferative glomerulonephritis
N06.5 Isolated proteinuria with diffuse mesangiocapillary glomerulonephritis
N06.6 Isolated proteinuria with dense deposit disease
N06.7 Isolated proteinuria with diffuse crescentic glomerulonephritis
N06.8 Isolated proteinuria with other morphologic lesion
N06.9 Isolated proteinuria with unspecified morphologic lesion
N06.A Isolated proteinuria with C3 glomerulonephritis
N08 Glomerular disorders in diseases classified elsewhere
N13.721 Vesicoureteral-reflux with reflux nephropathy without hydroureter, unilateral
N13.722 Vesicoureteral-reflux with reflux nephropathy without hydroureter, bilateral
N13.731 Vesicoureteral-reflux with reflux nephropathy with hydroureter, unilateral
N13.732 Vesicoureteral-reflux with reflux nephropathy with hydroureter, bilateral
N16 Renal tubulo-interstitial disorders in diseases classified elsewhere
N17.0 Acute kidney failure with tubular necrosis
N17.1 Acute kidney failure with acute cortical necrosis
N17.2 Acute kidney failure with medullary necrosis
N17.8 Other acute kidney failure
N17.9 Acute kidney failure, unspecified
N18.1 Chronic kidney disease, stage 1
N18.2 Chronic kidney disease, stage 2 (mild)
N18.30 Chronic kidney disease, stage 3 unspecified
N18.31 Chronic kidney disease, stage 3a
N18.32 Chronic kidney disease, stage 3b
N18.4 Chronic kidney disease, stage 4 (severe)
N18.5 Chronic kidney disease, stage 5
N18.6 End stage renal disease
N28.9 Disorder of kidney and ureter, unspecified
N29 Other disorders of kidney and ureter in diseases classified elsewhere
Q60.3 Renal hypoplasia, unilateral
Q60.4 Renal hypoplasia, bilateral
Q60.6 Potter's syndrome
R31.0 Gross hematuria
R77.0 Abnormality of albumin
R77.8 Other specified abnormalities of plasma proteins
R80.1 Persistent proteinuria, unspecified
R80.8 Other proteinuria
R80.9 Proteinuria, unspecified
R82.6 Abnormal urine levels of substances chiefly nonmedicinal as to source
R82.991 Hypocitraturia
R82.992 Hyperoxaluria
R82.993 Hyperuricosuria
R82.994 Hypercalciuria
R82.998 Other abnormal findings in urine
T86.10 Unspecified complication of kidney transplant
T86.11 Kidney transplant rejection
T86.12 Kidney transplant failure
T86.13 Kidney transplant infection
T86.19 Other complication of kidney transplant

CCI Edits

Refer to Appendix A for CCI edits.

Facility RVUs ☐

Code	Work	PE Facility	MP	Total Facility
50200	2.38	1.10	0.22	3.70
50205	12.29	7.29	2.85	22.43

Non-facility RVUs ☐

Code	Work	PE Non-Facility	MP	Total Non-Facility
50200	2.38	13.33	0.22	15.93
50205	12.29	7.29	2.85	22.43

Modifiers (PAR) ☐

Code	Mod 50	Mod 51	Mod 62	Mod 66	Mod 80
50200	1	2	0	0	1
50205	1	2	1	0	2

Global Period

Code	Days
50200	000
50205	090

50220-50225

50220 Nephrectomy, including partial ureterectomy, any open approach including rib resection

50225 Nephrectomy, including partial ureterectomy, any open approach including rib resection; complicated because of previous surgery on same kidney

AMA Coding Notes

Excision Procedures on the Kidney

(For excision of retroperitoneal tumor or cyst, see 49203-49205)

(For laparoscopic ablation of renal mass lesion(s), use 50542)

Surgical Procedures on the Urinary System

(For provision of chemotherapeutic agents, report both the specific service in addition to code(s) for the specific substance(s) or drug(s) provided)

AMA *CPT® Assistant*

50220: Oct 01: 8, Nov 02: 3, Aug 08: 7

50225: Oct 01: 8, Nov 02: 3

Plain English Description

An open nephrectomy is performed including partial ureterectomy and rib resection when needed. A wide flank incision is made immediately below the lower border of the ribs or near the 11th or 12th rib. The 11th and/or 12th ribs are removed as needed to allow surgical access to the kidney. Alternatively, an anterior subcostal approach may be utilized. The kidney and ureter are exposed. The renal artery and vein are isolated, ligated, and divided. The kidney is dissected free from surrounding tissue. A section of ureter is removed by first dissecting the involved section of ureter free of surrounding tissue. The ureter is then divided and the diseased section removed along with the kidney. Bleeding is controlled, drains are placed as needed, and the incisions are closed. Report 50225 when the procedure is complicated by previous surgery on the same kidney.

Nephrectomy

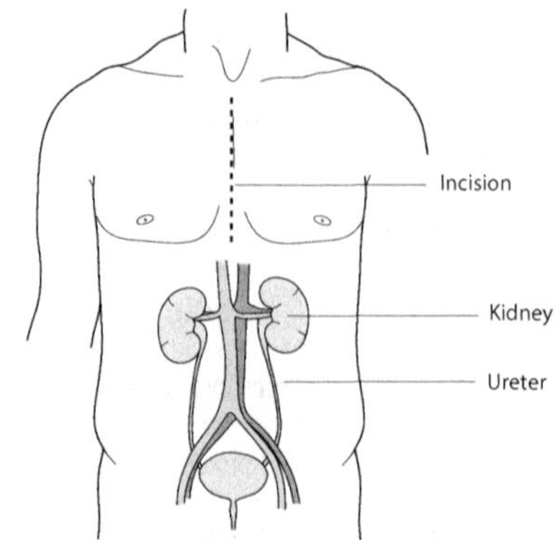

For 50220, an incision is made in the chest or back to remove a kidney, along with the section of ureter that was connected to the kidney. Report 50225 if the surgery was done previously.

ICD-10-CM Diagnostic Codes

	Code	Description
⇄	C64.1	Malignant neoplasm of right kidney, except renal pelvis
⇄	C64.2	Malignant neoplasm of left kidney, except renal pelvis
⇄	C65.1	Malignant neoplasm of right renal pelvis
⇄	C65.2	Malignant neoplasm of left renal pelvis
⇄	C66.1	Malignant neoplasm of right ureter
⇄	C66.2	Malignant neoplasm of left ureter
	C68.8	Malignant neoplasm of overlapping sites of urinary organs
⇄	C79.01	Secondary malignant neoplasm of right kidney and renal pelvis
⇄	C79.02	Secondary malignant neoplasm of left kidney and renal pelvis
	C79.19	Secondary malignant neoplasm of other urinary organs
	C7A.093	Malignant carcinoid tumor of the kidney
	D09.19	Carcinoma in situ of other urinary organs
⇄	D30.21	Benign neoplasm of right ureter
⇄	D30.22	Benign neoplasm of left ureter
	D3A.093	Benign carcinoid tumor of the kidney
⇄	D41.01	Neoplasm of uncertain behavior of right kidney
⇄	D41.02	Neoplasm of uncertain behavior of left kidney
⇄	D41.11	Neoplasm of uncertain behavior of right renal pelvis
⇄	D41.12	Neoplasm of uncertain behavior of left renal pelvis
⇄	D41.21	Neoplasm of uncertain behavior of right ureter
⇄	D41.22	Neoplasm of uncertain behavior of left ureter
	I12.0	Hypertensive chronic kidney disease with stage 5 chronic kidney disease or end stage renal disease
	I75.81	Atheroembolism of kidney
	N00.1	Acute nephritic syndrome with focal and segmental glomerular lesions
	N00.2	Acute nephritic syndrome with diffuse membranous glomerulonephritis
	N00.3	Acute nephritic syndrome with diffuse mesangial proliferative glomerulonephritis
	N00.4	Acute nephritic syndrome with diffuse endocapillary proliferative glomerulonephritis
	N00.5	Acute nephritic syndrome with diffuse mesangiocapillary glomerulonephritis
	N00.6	Acute nephritic syndrome with dense deposit disease
	N00.7	Acute nephritic syndrome with diffuse crescentic glomerulonephritis
	N00.8	Acute nephritic syndrome with other morphologic changes
	N03.1	Chronic nephritic syndrome with focal and segmental glomerular lesions
	N03.2	Chronic nephritic syndrome with diffuse membranous glomerulonephritis
	N03.3	Chronic nephritic syndrome with diffuse mesangial proliferative glomerulonephritis
	N03.4	Chronic nephritic syndrome with diffuse endocapillary proliferative glomerulonephritis
	N03.5	Chronic nephritic syndrome with diffuse mesangiocapillary glomerulonephritis
	N03.6	Chronic nephritic syndrome with dense deposit disease
	N03.8	Chronic nephritic syndrome with other morphologic changes
	N04.1	Nephrotic syndrome with focal and segmental glomerular lesions
	N04.2	Nephrotic syndrome with diffuse membranous glomerulonephritis
	N04.3	Nephrotic syndrome with diffuse mesangial proliferative glomerulonephritis
	N04.4	Nephrotic syndrome with diffuse endocapillary proliferative glomerulonephritis
	N04.5	Nephrotic syndrome with diffuse mesangiocapillary glomerulonephritis
	N04.6	Nephrotic syndrome with dense deposit disease
	N04.7	Nephrotic syndrome with diffuse crescentic glomerulonephritis
	N04.8	Nephrotic syndrome with other morphologic changes
	N08	Glomerular disorders in diseases classified elsewhere
	N11.0	Nonobstructive reflux-associated chronic pyelonephritis
	N11.1	Chronic obstructive pyelonephritis
	N13.0	Hydronephrosis with ureteropelvic junction obstruction
	N13.1	Hydronephrosis with ureteral stricture, not elsewhere classified
	N13.2	Hydronephrosis with renal and ureteral calculous obstruction
	N13.4	Hydroureter

N13.5	Crossing vessel and stricture of ureter without hydronephrosis
N13.6	Pyonephrosis
N13.721	Vesicoureteral-reflux with reflux nephropathy without hydroureter, unilateral
N13.722	Vesicoureteral-reflux with reflux nephropathy without hydroureter, bilateral
N13.731	Vesicoureteral-reflux with reflux nephropathy with hydroureter, unilateral
N13.732	Vesicoureteral-reflux with reflux nephropathy with hydroureter, bilateral
N17.0	Acute kidney failure with tubular necrosis
N17.1	Acute kidney failure with acute cortical necrosis
N17.2	Acute kidney failure with medullary necrosis
N18.4	Chronic kidney disease, stage 4 (severe)
N18.5	Chronic kidney disease, stage 5
N18.6	End stage renal disease
N20.0	Calculus of kidney
N20.2	Calculus of kidney with calculus of ureter
N26.1	Atrophy of kidney (terminal)
N26.2	Page kidney
N26.9	Renal sclerosis, unspecified
N28.0	Ischemia and infarction of kidney
N28.1	Cyst of kidney, acquired
N28.81	Hypertrophy of kidney
N28.82	Megaloureter
Q60.3	Renal hypoplasia, unilateral
Q60.4	Renal hypoplasia, bilateral
Q60.6	Potter's syndrome
Q61.01	Congenital single renal cyst
Q61.02	Congenital multiple renal cysts
Q61.11	Cystic dilatation of collecting ducts
Q61.2	Polycystic kidney, adult type
Q61.4	Renal dysplasia
Q61.5	Medullary cystic kidney
Q62.0	Congenital hydronephrosis
Q62.11	Congenital occlusion of ureteropelvic junction
Q62.2	Congenital megaureter
Q62.31	Congenital ureterocele, orthotopic
Q62.39	Other obstructive defects of renal pelvis and ureter
❼⇄ S37.061	Major laceration of right kidney
❼⇄ S37.062	Major laceration of left kidney
❼⇄ S37.091	Other injury of right kidney
❼⇄ S37.092	Other injury of left kidney

ICD-10-CM Coding Notes

For codes requiring a 7th character extension, refer to your ICD-10-CM book. Review the character descriptions and coding guidelines for proper selection. For some procedures, only certain characters will apply.

CCI Edits

Refer to Appendix A for CCI edits.

Facility RVUs ▯

Code	Work	PE Facility	MP	Total Facility
50220	18.68	9.40	2.85	30.93
50225	21.88	10.25	3.06	35.19

Non-facility RVUs ▯

Code	Work	PE Non-Facility	MP	Total Non-Facility
50220	18.68	9.40	2.85	30.93
50225	21.88	10.25	3.06	35.19

Modifiers (PAR) ▯

Code	Mod 50	Mod 51	Mod 62	Mod 66	Mod 80
50220	1	2	1	0	2
50225	1	2	1	0	2

Global Period

Code	Days
50220	090
50225	090

50230

50230 Nephrectomy, including partial ureterectomy, any open approach including rib resection; radical, with regional lymphadenectomy and/or vena caval thrombectomy

(When vena caval resection with reconstruction is necessary, use 37799)

AMA Coding Notes

Excision Procedures on the Kidney

(For excision of retroperitoneal tumor or cyst, see 49203-49205)

(For laparoscopic ablation of renal mass lesion(s), use 50542)

Surgical Procedures on the Urinary System

(For provision of chemotherapeutic agents, report both the specific service in addition to code(s) for the specific substance(s) or drug(s) provided)

AMA *CPT® Assistant* ▢

50230: Oct 01: 8, Nov 02: 3

Plain English Description

An open radical nephrectomy is performed including partial ureterectomy, regional lymph node excision, vena caval thrombectomy, and rib resection, when needed. A wide flank incision is made immediately below the lower border of the ribs or near the 11th or 12th rib. The 11th and/or 12th ribs are removed as needed to allow surgical access to the kidney. Alternatively, an anterior subcostal approach may be utilized. The kidney and ureter are exposed. The aortocaval space is entered and regional lymph nodes are excised. The renal artery is isolated, ligated, and divided and the renal vein is palpated to identify any evidence of tumor thrombus. If tumor thrombus is present, the thrombus is milked back toward the kidney and the renal vein is ligated near the vena cava. If this is not possible, the renal vein is divided, the vena cava is incised, and the thrombus is resected. The Gerota's fascia is dissected free from surrounding structures and the lymphatic vessels are ligated. The gonadal vein is mobilized, clamped, and ligated. The ureter is dissected free of surrounding tissue and divided. The kidney is then mobilized and retracted to expose the adrenal gland. The adrenal gland is dissected free of surrounding tissue and removed along with the kidney. Bleeding is controlled, drains are placed as needed, and the incision is closed with sutures.

Nephrectomy with regional lymphadenectomy and/or vena caval thrombectomy

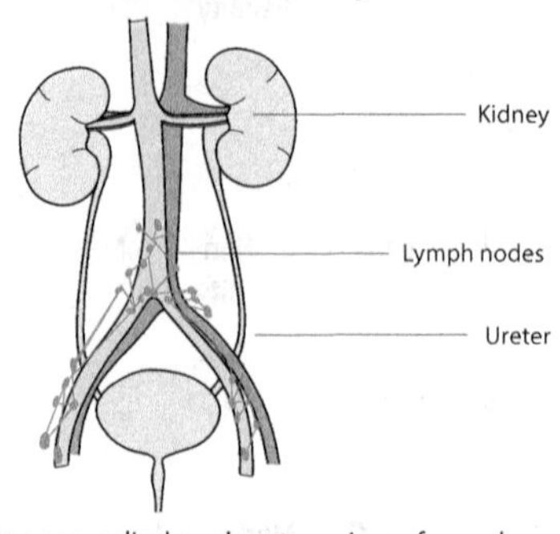

An open radical nephrectomy is performed including partial reterectomy, regional lymph node excision, vena caval thrombectomy, and rib resection, when needed.

ICD-10-CM Diagnostic Codes

	Code	Description
⇄	C64.1	Malignant neoplasm of right kidney, except renal pelvis
⇄	C64.2	Malignant neoplasm of left kidney, except renal pelvis
⇄	C65.1	Malignant neoplasm of right renal pelvis
⇄	C65.2	Malignant neoplasm of left renal pelvis
⇄	C66.1	Malignant neoplasm of right ureter
⇄	C66.2	Malignant neoplasm of left ureter
	C68.8	Malignant neoplasm of overlapping sites of urinary organs
	C77.2	Secondary and unspecified malignant neoplasm of intra-abdominal lymph nodes
	C77.5	Secondary and unspecified malignant neoplasm of intrapelvic lymph nodes
	C77.8	Secondary and unspecified malignant neoplasm of lymph nodes of multiple regions
⇄	C79.01	Secondary malignant neoplasm of right kidney and renal pelvis
⇄	C79.02	Secondary malignant neoplasm of left kidney and renal pelvis
	C79.19	Secondary malignant neoplasm of other urinary organs
	C7A.093	Malignant carcinoid tumor of the kidney
	C80.2	Malignant neoplasm associated with transplanted organ
	D3A.093	Benign carcinoid tumor of the kidney
	I12.0	Hypertensive chronic kidney disease with stage 5 chronic kidney disease or end stage renal disease
	I75.81	Atheroembolism of kidney
	I82.220	Acute embolism and thrombosis of inferior vena cava
	I82.221	Chronic embolism and thrombosis of inferior vena cava
	N00.1	Acute nephritic syndrome with focal and segmental glomerular lesions
	N00.2	Acute nephritic syndrome with diffuse membranous glomerulonephritis
	N00.3	Acute nephritic syndrome with diffuse mesangial proliferative glomerulonephritis
	N00.4	Acute nephritic syndrome with diffuse endocapillary proliferative glomerulonephritis
	N00.5	Acute nephritic syndrome with diffuse mesangiocapillary glomerulonephritis
	N00.6	Acute nephritic syndrome with dense deposit disease
	N00.7	Acute nephritic syndrome with diffuse crescentic glomerulonephritis
	N00.8	Acute nephritic syndrome with other morphologic changes
	N03.1	Chronic nephritic syndrome with focal and segmental glomerular lesions
	N03.2	Chronic nephritic syndrome with diffuse membranous glomerulonephritis
	N03.3	Chronic nephritic syndrome with diffuse mesangial proliferative glomerulonephritis
	N03.4	Chronic nephritic syndrome with diffuse endocapillary proliferative glomerulonephritis
	N03.5	Chronic nephritic syndrome with diffuse mesangiocapillary glomerulonephritis
	N03.6	Chronic nephritic syndrome with dense deposit disease
	N03.7	Chronic nephritic syndrome with diffuse crescentic glomerulonephritis
	N03.8	Chronic nephritic syndrome with other morphologic changes
	N04.1	Nephrotic syndrome with focal and segmental glomerular lesions
	N04.2	Nephrotic syndrome with diffuse membranous glomerulonephritis
	N04.3	Nephrotic syndrome with diffuse mesangial proliferative glomerulonephritis
	N04.4	Nephrotic syndrome with diffuse endocapillary proliferative glomerulonephritis
	N04.5	Nephrotic syndrome with diffuse mesangiocapillary glomerulonephritis
	N04.6	Nephrotic syndrome with dense deposit disease
	N04.7	Nephrotic syndrome with diffuse crescentic glomerulonephritis
	N04.8	Nephrotic syndrome with other morphologic changes
	N08	Glomerular disorders in diseases classified elsewhere
	N11.0	Nonobstructive reflux-associated chronic pyelonephritis
	N11.1	Chronic obstructive pyelonephritis
	N13.0	Hydronephrosis with ureteropelvic junction obstruction
	N13.1	Hydronephrosis with ureteral stricture, not elsewhere classified
	N13.2	Hydronephrosis with renal and ureteral calculous obstruction
	N13.4	Hydroureter

N13.5	Crossing vessel and stricture of ureter without hydronephrosis
N13.6	Pyonephrosis
N13.721	Vesicoureteral-reflux with reflux nephropathy without hydroureter, unilateral
N13.722	Vesicoureteral-reflux with reflux nephropathy without hydroureter, bilateral
N13.731	Vesicoureteral-reflux with reflux nephropathy with hydroureter, unilateral
N13.732	Vesicoureteral-reflux with reflux nephropathy with hydroureter, bilateral
N17.0	Acute kidney failure with tubular necrosis
N17.1	Acute kidney failure with acute cortical necrosis
N17.2	Acute kidney failure with medullary necrosis
N18.4	Chronic kidney disease, stage 4 (severe)
N18.5	Chronic kidney disease, stage 5
N18.6	End stage renal disease
N20.0	Calculus of kidney
N20.2	Calculus of kidney with calculus of ureter
N26.1	Atrophy of kidney (terminal)
N26.2	Page kidney
N28.0	Ischemia and infarction of kidney
N28.1	Cyst of kidney, acquired
N28.81	Hypertrophy of kidney
N28.82	Megaloureter
Q60.3	Renal hypoplasia, unilateral
Q60.4	Renal hypoplasia, bilateral
Q60.6	Potter's syndrome
Q61.01	Congenital single renal cyst
Q61.02	Congenital multiple renal cysts
Q61.11	Cystic dilatation of collecting ducts
Q61.2	Polycystic kidney, adult type
Q61.4	Renal dysplasia
Q61.5	Medullary cystic kidney
Q62.0	Congenital hydronephrosis
Q62.11	Congenital occlusion of ureteropelvic junction
Q62.2	Congenital megaureter
Q62.31	Congenital ureterocele, orthotopic
Q62.39	Other obstructive defects of renal pelvis and ureter
➐⇄ S37.061	Major laceration of right kidney
➐⇄ S37.062	Major laceration of left kidney
➐⇄ S37.091	Other injury of right kidney
➐⇄ S37.092	Other injury of left kidney

ICD-10-CM Coding Notes

For codes requiring a 7th character extension, refer to your ICD-10-CM book. Review the character descriptions and coding guidelines for proper selection. For some procedures, only certain characters will apply.

CCI Edits

Refer to Appendix A for CCI edits.

Facility RVUs ▯

Code	Work	PE Facility	MP	Total Facility
50230	23.81	10.47	3.12	37.40

Non-facility RVUs ▯

Code	Work	PE Non-Facility	MP	Total Non-Facility
50230	23.81	10.47	3.12	37.40

Modifiers (PAR) ▯

Code	Mod 50	Mod 51	Mod 62	Mod 66	Mod 80
50230	1	2	2	0	2

Global Period

Code	Days
50230	090

50234-50236

50234 Nephrectomy with total ureterectomy and bladder cuff; through same incision

50236 Nephrectomy with total ureterectomy and bladder cuff; through separate incision

AMA Coding Notes

Excision Procedures on the Kidney

(For excision of retroperitoneal tumor or cyst, see 49203-49205)

(For laparoscopic ablation of renal mass lesion(s), use 50542)

Surgical Procedures on the Urinary System

(For provision of chemotherapeutic agents, report both the specific service in addition to code(s) for the specific substance(s) or drug(s) provided)

AMA *CPT® Assistant* ▢

50234: Oct 01: 8, Nov 02: 3

50236: Oct 01: 8, Nov 02: 3

Plain English Description

An open nephrectomy with total ureterectomy and excision of the bladder cuff is performed. A Foley catheter is placed and the bladder is drained. A wide flank incision is made immediately below the lower border of the ribs or near the 11th or 12th rib. Alternatively, an anterior subcostal approach may be utilized. The kidney and ureter are exposed. The renal artery and vein are isolated, ligated and divided. The kidney is dissected free from surrounding tissue and removed. The entire ureter along with a section of bladder at the ureterovesical junction (UVJ) are removed by first dissecting the ureter free from surrounding tissue. The bladder is then incised just below the UVJ and the bladder cuff removed. The bladder incision is closed. Bleeding is controlled, drains placed as needed, and the incisions closed. Report 50234 when the procedure is performed through a single incision; report 50236 when the kidney is removed through a subcostal or flank incision and a separate incision is used to remove the ureter and bladder cuff.

Nephrectomy with total ureterectomy and bladder cuff

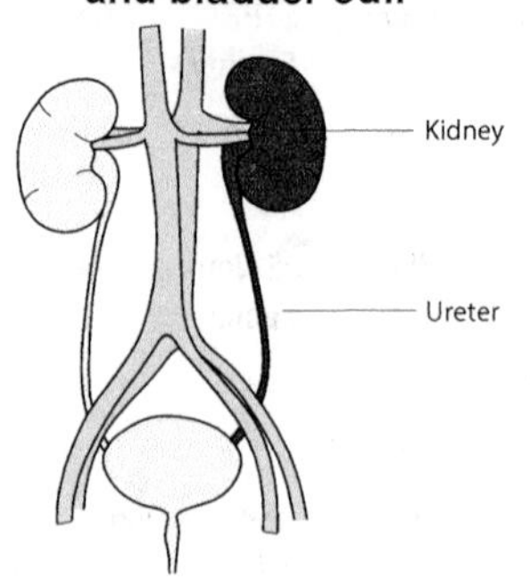

For 50234, the kidney, along with the entire length of the ureter from the kidney to the bladder, is removed through same incision. Report 50236 if two separate incisions are used.

ICD-10-CM Diagnostic Codes

	Code	Description
⇄	C64.1	Malignant neoplasm of right kidney, except renal pelvis
⇄	C64.2	Malignant neoplasm of left kidney, except renal pelvis
⇄	C65.1	Malignant neoplasm of right renal pelvis
⇄	C65.2	Malignant neoplasm of left renal pelvis
⇄	C66.1	Malignant neoplasm of right ureter
⇄	C66.2	Malignant neoplasm of left ureter
	C68.8	Malignant neoplasm of overlapping sites of urinary organs
⇄	C79.01	Secondary malignant neoplasm of right kidney and renal pelvis
⇄	C79.02	Secondary malignant neoplasm of left kidney and renal pelvis
	C79.19	Secondary malignant neoplasm of other urinary organs
	C7A.093	Malignant carcinoid tumor of the kidney
	D09.19	Carcinoma in situ of other urinary organs
⇄	D30.01	Benign neoplasm of right kidney
⇄	D30.02	Benign neoplasm of left kidney
⇄	D30.11	Benign neoplasm of right renal pelvis
⇄	D30.12	Benign neoplasm of left renal pelvis
⇄	D30.21	Benign neoplasm of right ureter
⇄	D30.22	Benign neoplasm of left ureter
	D3A.093	Benign carcinoid tumor of the kidney
⇄	D41.01	Neoplasm of uncertain behavior of right kidney
⇄	D41.02	Neoplasm of uncertain behavior of left kidney
⇄	D41.11	Neoplasm of uncertain behavior of right renal pelvis
⇄	D41.12	Neoplasm of uncertain behavior of left renal pelvis
⇄	D41.21	Neoplasm of uncertain behavior of right ureter
⇄	D41.22	Neoplasm of uncertain behavior of left ureter
	I12.0	Hypertensive chronic kidney disease with stage 5 chronic kidney disease or end stage renal disease
	I75.81	Atheroembolism of kidney
	N00.1	Acute nephritic syndrome with focal and segmental glomerular lesions
	N00.2	Acute nephritic syndrome with diffuse membranous glomerulonephritis
	N00.3	Acute nephritic syndrome with diffuse mesangial proliferative glomerulonephritis
	N00.4	Acute nephritic syndrome with diffuse endocapillary proliferative glomerulonephritis
	N00.5	Acute nephritic syndrome with diffuse mesangiocapillary glomerulonephritis
	N00.6	Acute nephritic syndrome with dense deposit disease
	N00.7	Acute nephritic syndrome with diffuse crescentic glomerulonephritis
	N00.8	Acute nephritic syndrome with other morphologic changes
	N03.1	Chronic nephritic syndrome with focal and segmental glomerular lesions
	N03.2	Chronic nephritic syndrome with diffuse membranous glomerulonephritis
	N03.3	Chronic nephritic syndrome with diffuse mesangial proliferative glomerulonephritis
	N03.4	Chronic nephritic syndrome with diffuse endocapillary proliferative glomerulonephritis
	N03.5	Chronic nephritic syndrome with diffuse mesangiocapillary glomerulonephritis
	N03.6	Chronic nephritic syndrome with dense deposit disease
	N03.7	Chronic nephritic syndrome with diffuse crescentic glomerulonephritis
	N03.8	Chronic nephritic syndrome with other morphologic changes
	N04.1	Nephrotic syndrome with focal and segmental glomerular lesions
	N04.2	Nephrotic syndrome with diffuse membranous glomerulonephritis
	N04.3	Nephrotic syndrome with diffuse mesangial proliferative glomerulonephritis
	N04.4	Nephrotic syndrome with diffuse endocapillary proliferative glomerulonephritis
	N04.5	Nephrotic syndrome with diffuse mesangiocapillary glomerulonephritis
	N04.6	Nephrotic syndrome with dense deposit disease
	N04.7	Nephrotic syndrome with diffuse crescentic glomerulonephritis
	N04.8	Nephrotic syndrome with other morphologic changes
	N08	Glomerular disorders in diseases classified elsewhere
	N11.0	Nonobstructive reflux-associated chronic pyelonephritis
	N11.1	Chronic obstructive pyelonephritis

N13.0 Hydronephrosis with ureteropelvic junction obstruction
N13.1 Hydronephrosis with ureteral stricture, not elsewhere classified
N13.2 Hydronephrosis with renal and ureteral calculous obstruction
N13.4 Hydroureter
N13.5 Crossing vessel and stricture of ureter without hydronephrosis
N13.6 Pyonephrosis
N13.721 Vesicoureteral-reflux with reflux nephropathy without hydroureter, unilateral
N13.722 Vesicoureteral-reflux with reflux nephropathy without hydroureter, bilateral
N13.731 Vesicoureteral-reflux with reflux nephropathy with hydroureter, unilateral
N13.732 Vesicoureteral-reflux with reflux nephropathy with hydroureter, bilateral
N17.0 Acute kidney failure with tubular necrosis
N17.1 Acute kidney failure with acute cortical necrosis
N17.2 Acute kidney failure with medullary necrosis
N18.4 Chronic kidney disease, stage 4 (severe)
N18.5 Chronic kidney disease, stage 5
N18.6 End stage renal disease
N20.2 Calculus of kidney with calculus of ureter
N26.1 Atrophy of kidney (terminal)
N26.2 Page kidney
N28.0 Ischemia and infarction of kidney
N28.1 Cyst of kidney, acquired
N28.81 Hypertrophy of kidney
N28.82 Megaloureter
Q60.3 Renal hypoplasia, unilateral
Q60.4 Renal hypoplasia, bilateral
Q60.6 Potter's syndrome
Q61.01 Congenital single renal cyst
Q61.02 Congenital multiple renal cysts
Q61.11 Cystic dilatation of collecting ducts
Q61.2 Polycystic kidney, adult type
Q61.4 Renal dysplasia
Q61.5 Medullary cystic kidney
Q62.0 Congenital hydronephrosis
Q62.11 Congenital occlusion of ureteropelvic junction
Q62.2 Congenital megaureter
Q62.31 Congenital ureterocele, orthotopic
Q62.39 Other obstructive defects of renal pelvis and ureter

CCI Edits

Refer to Appendix A for CCI edits.

Facility RVUs

Code	Work	PE Facility	MP	Total Facility
50234	24.05	10.96	3.12	38.13
50236	26.94	12.57	3.27	42.78

Non-facility RVUs

Code	Work	PE Non-Facility	MP	Total Non-Facility
50234	24.05	10.96	3.12	38.13
50236	26.94	12.57	3.27	42.78

Modifiers (PAR)

Code	Mod 50	Mod 51	Mod 62	Mod 66	Mod 80
50234	1	2	1	0	2
50236	1	2	1	0	2

Global Period

Code	Days
50234	090
50236	090

50240

50240 Nephrectomy, partial

(For laparoscopic partial nephrectomy, use 50543)

AMA Coding Notes

Excision Procedures on the Kidney

(For excision of retroperitoneal tumor or cyst, see 49203-49205)

(For laparoscopic ablation of renal mass lesion(s), use 50542)

Surgical Procedures on the Urinary System

(For provision of chemotherapeutic agents, report both the specific service in addition to code(s) for the specific substance(s) or drug(s) provided)

AMA *CPT® Assistant* ▯

50240: Oct 01: 8, Nov 02: 3, Jan 03: 20, Apr 05: 10, 12, Aug 08: 7

Plain English Description

An open partial nephrectomy is performed. A wide flank incision is made immediately below the lower border of the ribs. Alternatively, an anterior subcostal approach may be utilized. The kidney and ureter are exposed, taking care to preserve the kidney vasculature. The renal artery is isolated and a vascular loop placed. Perirenal fat is dissected free of the kidney. The kidney lesion is located. Small lesions are enucleated and excised using blunt and sharp dissection. Large lesions require diuresis, temporary occlusion of the renal artery supplying the tumor site, and renal hypothermia. The renal mass is then resected by blunt and sharp dissection. Bleeding is controlled by suture-ligation of bleeding arteries and veins. The parenchymal defect in the kidney is closed.

Nephrectomy

An open partial nephrectomy is performed. A wide flank incision is made immediately below the lower border of the ribs.

ICD-10-CM Diagnostic Codes

	Code	Description
⇄	C64.1	Malignant neoplasm of right kidney, except renal pelvis
⇄	C64.2	Malignant neoplasm of left kidney, except renal pelvis
⇄	C65.1	Malignant neoplasm of right renal pelvis
⇄	C65.2	Malignant neoplasm of left renal pelvis
⇄	C79.01	Secondary malignant neoplasm of right kidney and renal pelvis
⇄	C79.02	Secondary malignant neoplasm of left kidney and renal pelvis
	C7A.093	Malignant carcinoid tumor of the kidney
	D09.19	Carcinoma in situ of other urinary organs
⇄	D30.01	Benign neoplasm of right kidney
⇄	D30.02	Benign neoplasm of left kidney
⇄	D30.11	Benign neoplasm of right renal pelvis
⇄	D30.12	Benign neoplasm of left renal pelvis
	D3A.093	Benign carcinoid tumor of the kidney
⇄	D41.01	Neoplasm of uncertain behavior of right kidney
⇄	D41.02	Neoplasm of uncertain behavior of left kidney
⇄	D41.11	Neoplasm of uncertain behavior of right renal pelvis
⇄	D41.12	Neoplasm of uncertain behavior of left renal pelvis
	I12.0	Hypertensive chronic kidney disease with stage 5 chronic kidney disease or end stage renal disease
	I13.11	Hypertensive heart and chronic kidney disease without heart failure, with stage 5 chronic kidney disease, or end stage renal disease
	N00.1	Acute nephritic syndrome with focal and segmental glomerular lesions
	N00.2	Acute nephritic syndrome with diffuse membranous glomerulonephritis
	N00.3	Acute nephritic syndrome with diffuse mesangial proliferative glomerulonephritis
	N00.4	Acute nephritic syndrome with diffuse endocapillary proliferative glomerulonephritis
	N00.5	Acute nephritic syndrome with diffuse mesangiocapillary glomerulonephritis
	N00.6	Acute nephritic syndrome with dense deposit disease
	N00.7	Acute nephritic syndrome with diffuse crescentic glomerulonephritis
	N00.8	Acute nephritic syndrome with other morphologic changes
	N03.1	Chronic nephritic syndrome with focal and segmental glomerular lesions
	N03.2	Chronic nephritic syndrome with diffuse membranous glomerulonephritis
	N03.3	Chronic nephritic syndrome with diffuse mesangial proliferative glomerulonephritis
	N03.4	Chronic nephritic syndrome with diffuse endocapillary proliferative glomerulonephritis
	N03.5	Chronic nephritic syndrome with diffuse mesangiocapillary glomerulonephritis
	N03.6	Chronic nephritic syndrome with dense deposit disease
	N03.7	Chronic nephritic syndrome with diffuse crescentic glomerulonephritis
	N03.8	Chronic nephritic syndrome with other morphologic changes
	N04.1	Nephrotic syndrome with focal and segmental glomerular lesions
	N04.2	Nephrotic syndrome with diffuse membranous glomerulonephritis
	N04.3	Nephrotic syndrome with diffuse mesangial proliferative glomerulonephritis
	N04.4	Nephrotic syndrome with diffuse endocapillary proliferative glomerulonephritis
	N04.5	Nephrotic syndrome with diffuse mesangiocapillary glomerulonephritis
	N04.6	Nephrotic syndrome with dense deposit disease
	N04.7	Nephrotic syndrome with diffuse crescentic glomerulonephritis
	N04.8	Nephrotic syndrome with other morphologic changes
	N11.0	Nonobstructive reflux-associated chronic pyelonephritis
	N11.1	Chronic obstructive pyelonephritis
	N11.8	Other chronic tubulo-interstitial nephritis
	N13.0	Hydronephrosis with ureteropelvic junction obstruction
	N13.1	Hydronephrosis with ureteral stricture, not elsewhere classified
	N13.2	Hydronephrosis with renal and ureteral calculous obstruction
	N13.4	Hydroureter
	N13.6	Pyonephrosis
	N13.721	Vesicoureteral-reflux with reflux nephropathy without hydroureter, unilateral
	N13.722	Vesicoureteral-reflux with reflux nephropathy without hydroureter, bilateral
	N13.731	Vesicoureteral-reflux with reflux nephropathy with hydroureter, unilateral
	N13.732	Vesicoureteral-reflux with reflux nephropathy with hydroureter, bilateral
	N13.8	Other obstructive and reflux uropathy
	N17.0	Acute kidney failure with tubular necrosis
	N17.1	Acute kidney failure with acute cortical necrosis
	N17.2	Acute kidney failure with medullary necrosis
	N18.4	Chronic kidney disease, stage 4 (severe)
	N18.5	Chronic kidney disease, stage 5
	N18.6	End stage renal disease
	N20.0	Calculus of kidney
	N20.2	Calculus of kidney with calculus of ureter
	N26.1	Atrophy of kidney (terminal)
	N26.2	Page kidney
	N28.0	Ischemia and infarction of kidney

	N28.1	Cyst of kidney, acquired
	N28.81	Hypertrophy of kidney
	Q60.3	Renal hypoplasia, unilateral
	Q60.4	Renal hypoplasia, bilateral
	Q60.6	Potter's syndrome
	Q61.01	Congenital single renal cyst
	Q61.02	Congenital multiple renal cysts
	Q61.11	Cystic dilatation of collecting ducts
	Q61.19	Other polycystic kidney, infantile type
	Q61.2	Polycystic kidney, adult type
	Q61.4	Renal dysplasia
	Q61.5	Medullary cystic kidney
	Q62.0	Congenital hydronephrosis
	Q62.11	Congenital occlusion of ureteropelvic junction
❼⇄	S37.061	Major laceration of right kidney
❼⇄	S37.062	Major laceration of left kidney
❼⇄	S37.091	Other injury of right kidney
❼⇄	S37.092	Other injury of left kidney

ICD-10-CM Coding Notes

For codes requiring a 7th character extension, refer to your ICD-10-CM book. Review the character descriptions and coding guidelines for proper selection. For some procedures, only certain characters will apply.

CCI Edits

Refer to Appendix A for CCI edits.

Facility RVUs ▯

Code	Work	PE Facility	MP	Total Facility
50240	24.21	11.56	2.98	38.75

Non-facility RVUs ▯

Code	Work	PE Non-Facility	MP	Total Non-Facility
50240	24.21	11.56	2.98	38.75

Modifiers (PAR) ▯

Code	Mod 50	Mod 51	Mod 62	Mod 66	Mod 80
50240	1	2	1	0	2

Global Period

Code	Days
50240	090

50250

50250 Ablation, open, 1 or more renal mass lesion(s), cryosurgical, including intraoperative ultrasound guidance and monitoring, if performed

(For laparoscopic ablation of renal mass lesions, use 50542)

(For percutaneous ablation of renal tumors, see 50592, 50593)

AMA Coding Notes

Excision Procedures on the Kidney

(For excision of retroperitoneal tumor or cyst, see 49203-49205)

(For laparoscopic ablation of renal mass lesion(s), use 50542)

Surgical Procedures on the Urinary System

(For provision of chemotherapeutic agents, report both the specific service in addition to code(s) for the specific substance(s) or drug(s) provided)

AMA *CPT® Assistant* ▯

50250: May 06: 17

Plain English Description

The physician performs an open procedure to destroy (ablate) one or more lesions in the kidney using cryosurgery with intraoperative ultrasound guidance as needed. A wide flank incision is made over the affected kidney. The kidney is exposed and the lesion is identified. One or more cryosurgical probes are then inserted into the lesion and the first freeze-thaw cycle is initiated. The ice ball created during the freeze cycle is monitored using ultrasound to ensure adequate extension of the ice ball beyond the lesion margins. A second freeze-thaw cycle is performed in the same manner. Additional lesions are treated in the same manner. The probes are removed, bleeding is controlled, drains are placed, and the incision is closed around the drains.

Ablation, renal mass lesion, cryosurgical

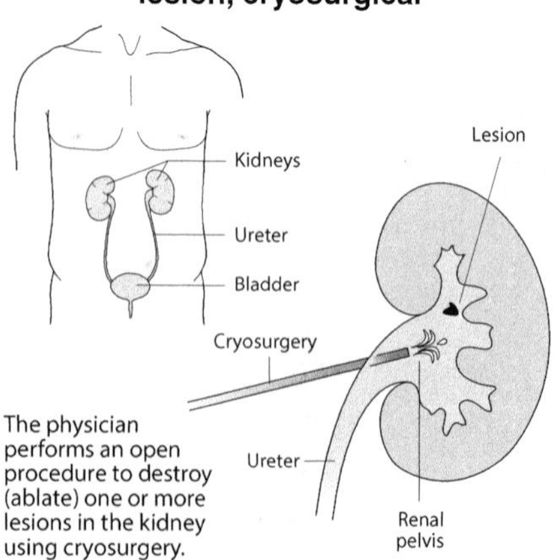
Kidneys
Ureter
Bladder
Lesion
Cryosurgery
Ureter
Renal pelvis
The physician performs an open procedure to destroy (ablate) one or more lesions in the kidney using cryosurgery.

ICD-10-CM Diagnostic Codes

	Code	Description
⇄	C64.1	Malignant neoplasm of right kidney, except renal pelvis
⇄	C64.2	Malignant neoplasm of left kidney, except renal pelvis
⇄	C65.1	Malignant neoplasm of right renal pelvis
⇄	C65.2	Malignant neoplasm of left renal pelvis
⇄	C79.01	Secondary malignant neoplasm of right kidney and renal pelvis
⇄	C79.02	Secondary malignant neoplasm of left kidney and renal pelvis
	C7A.093	Malignant carcinoid tumor of the kidney
	C80.2	Malignant neoplasm associated with transplanted organ
	D09.19	Carcinoma in situ of other urinary organs
⇄	D30.01	Benign neoplasm of right kidney
⇄	D30.02	Benign neoplasm of left kidney
⇄	D30.11	Benign neoplasm of right renal pelvis
⇄	D30.12	Benign neoplasm of left renal pelvis
	D3A.093	Benign carcinoid tumor of the kidney
⇄	D41.01	Neoplasm of uncertain behavior of right kidney
⇄	D41.02	Neoplasm of uncertain behavior of left kidney
⇄	D41.11	Neoplasm of uncertain behavior of right renal pelvis
⇄	D41.12	Neoplasm of uncertain behavior of left renal pelvis
	N28.1	Cyst of kidney, acquired
	N28.89	Other specified disorders of kidney and ureter
	Q61.01	Congenital single renal cyst
	Q61.02	Congenital multiple renal cysts
	Q61.11	Cystic dilatation of collecting ducts
	Q61.19	Other polycystic kidney, infantile type
	Q61.2	Polycystic kidney, adult type
	Q61.4	Renal dysplasia
	Q61.5	Medullary cystic kidney
	Q61.8	Other cystic kidney diseases

CCI Edits

Refer to Appendix A for CCI edits.

Facility RVUs ▯

Code	Work	PE Facility	MP	Total Facility
50250	22.22	10.65	2.66	35.53

Non-facility RVUs ▯

Code	Work	PE Non-Facility	MP	Total Non-Facility
50250	22.22	10.65	2.66	35.53

Modifiers (PAR) ▯

Code	Mod 50	Mod 51	Mod 62	Mod 66	Mod 80
50250	0	2	1	0	2

Global Period

Code	Days
50250	090

50280

50280 Excision or unroofing of cyst(s) of kidney

(For laparoscopic ablation of renal cysts, use 50541)

AMA Coding Notes

Excision Procedures on the Kidney

(For excision of retroperitoneal tumor or cyst, see 49203-49205)

(For laparoscopic ablation of renal mass lesion(s), use 50542)

Surgical Procedures on the Urinary System

(For provision of chemotherapeutic agents, report both the specific service in addition to code(s) for the specific substance(s) or drug(s) provided)

AMA *CPT® Assistant* ▯

50280: Nov 99: 25, Oct 01: 8

Plain English Description

One or more cysts of the kidney are treated by open surgical excision or unroofing of the cyst(s). A wide flank incision is made over the affected kidney and the kidney is exposed. The cyst is then opened and the fluid is drained. The redundant cyst wall is excised in its entirety using blunt and sharp dissection. The base of the cyst is fulgurated to prevent recurrence and the defect is filled with perirenal fat. Alternatively, an unroofing procedure may be performed, which involves creating a window in the cyst wall or partially resecting the cyst wall and then marsupializing the cyst, creating an open pocket of the remaining cyst wall. Drains may be placed in the window to facilitate drainage and the remaining cyst wall is closed around the drains. Bleeding is controlled and incisions are closed.

Excision or unroofing of cyst(s) of kidney

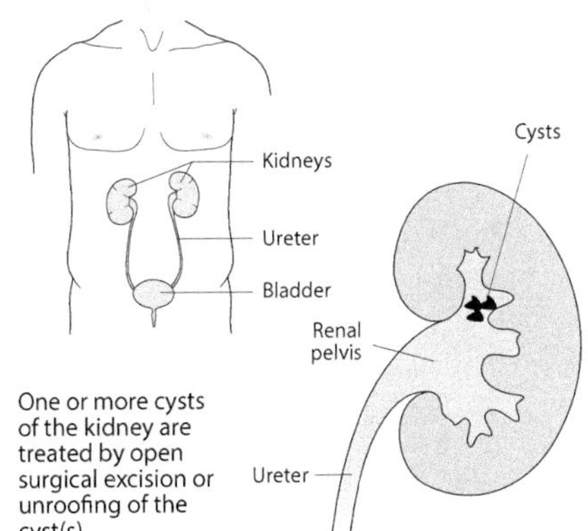
Kidneys
Ureter
Bladder
Cysts
Renal pelvis
Ureter
One or more cysts of the kidney are treated by open surgical excision or unroofing of the cyst(s).

ICD-10-CM Diagnostic Codes

N28.1	Cyst of kidney, acquired
Q61.00	Congenital renal cyst, unspecified
Q61.01	Congenital single renal cyst
Q61.02	Congenital multiple renal cysts
Q61.11	Cystic dilatation of collecting ducts
Q61.19	Other polycystic kidney, infantile type
Q61.2	Polycystic kidney, adult type
Q61.3	Polycystic kidney, unspecified
Q61.8	Other cystic kidney diseases

CCI Edits

Refer to Appendix A for CCI edits.

Facility RVUs ▯

Code	Work	PE Facility	MP	Total Facility
50280	17.09	8.67	2.37	28.13

Non-facility RVUs ▯

Code	Work	PE Non-Facility	MP	Total Non-Facility
50280	17.09	8.67	2.37	28.13

Modifiers (PAR) ▯

Code	Mod 50	Mod 51	Mod 62	Mod 66	Mod 80
50280	1	2	1	0	2

Global Period

Code	Days
50280	090

50290

50290 Excision of perinephric cyst

AMA Coding Notes

Excision Procedures on the Kidney

(For excision of retroperitoneal tumor or cyst, see 49203-49205)

(For laparoscopic ablation of renal mass lesion(s), use 50542)

Surgical Procedures on the Urinary System

(For provision of chemotherapeutic agents, report both the specific service in addition to code(s) for the specific substance(s) or drug(s) provided)

AMA *CPT® Assistant* ▢

50290: Oct 01: 8

Plain English Description

The physician performs an excision of a perinephric cyst. Perinephric cysts, also referred to as perirenal cysts, occur on the exterior surface of the kidney in the space surrounding it. A wide flank incision is made over the affected kidney. Gerota's fascia is dissected off the surface of the cyst and excised along with perinephric fat overlying the cyst. The cyst is exposed and may be decompressed by aspirating the fluid or it may be left intact and dissected free from the surface of the kidney to facilitate identification of the margins. If the cyst has been decompressed, the redundant cyst wall is then excised in its entirety using blunt and sharp dissection. Depending on the location of the cyst, the base may be fulgurated to prevent recurrence. If the base of the cyst is in close proximity to the renal pelvis or hilum, fulguration may not be performed due to the risk of damage to surrounding vasculature. The defect is filled with perirenal fat. Bleeding is controlled and incisions are closed.

Excision of perinephric cyst

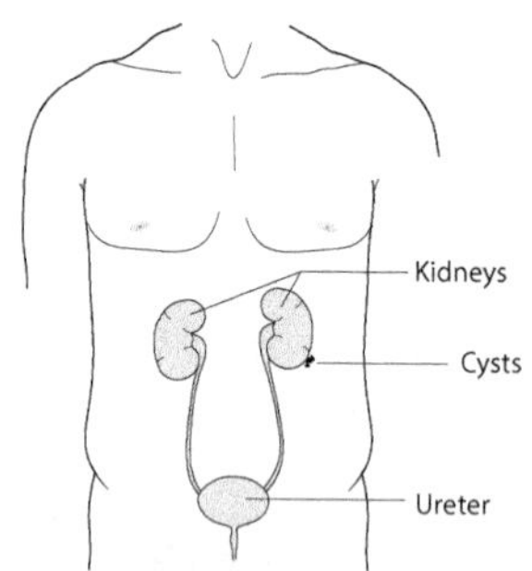

The physician performs an excision of a perinephric cyst. Perinephric cysts, also referred to as perirenal cysts, occur on the exterior surface of the kidney in the space surrounding it.

ICD-10-CM Diagnostic Codes

N28.1	Cyst of kidney, acquired
Q61.00	Congenital renal cyst, unspecified
Q61.01	Congenital single renal cyst
Q61.02	Congenital multiple renal cysts
Q61.11	Cystic dilatation of collecting ducts
Q61.19	Other polycystic kidney, infantile type
Q61.2	Polycystic kidney, adult type
Q61.3	Polycystic kidney, unspecified
Q61.8	Other cystic kidney diseases

CCI Edits

Refer to Appendix A for CCI edits.

Facility RVUs ▢

Code	Work	PE Facility	MP	Total Facility
50290	16.15	8.19	1.94	26.28

Non-facility RVUs ▢

Code	Work	PE Non-Facility	MP	Total Non-Facility
50290	16.15	8.19	1.94	26.28

Modifiers (PAR) ▢

Code	Mod 50	Mod 51	Mod 62	Mod 66	Mod 80
50290	0	2	1	0	2

Global Period

Code	Days
50290	090

50300

50300 Donor nephrectomy (including cold preservation); from cadaver donor, unilateral or bilateral

AMA Coding Guideline

Renal Transplantation Procedures

Renal autotransplantation includes reimplantation of the autograft as the primary procedure, along with secondary extra-corporeal procedure(s) (eg, partial nephrectomy, nephrolithotomy) reported with modifier 51 (see 50380 and applicable secondary procedure(s)).

Renal allotransplantation involves three distinct components of physician work:

1. Cadaver donor nephrectomy, unilateral or bilateral, which includes harvesting the graft(s) and cold preservation of the graft(s) (perfusing with cold preservation solution and cold maintenance) (use 50300). Living donor nephrectomy, which includes harvesting the graft, cold preservation of the graft (perfusing with cold preservation solution and cold maintenance), and care of the donor (see 50320, 50547).

2. Backbench work:

Standard preparation of a cadaver donor renal allograft prior to transplantation including dissection and removal of perinephric fat, diaphragmatic and retroperitoneal attachments; excision of adrenal gland; and preparation of ureter(s), renal vein(s), and renal artery(s), ligating branches, as necessary (use 50323).

Standard preparation of a living donor renal allograft (open or laparoscopic) prior to transplantation including dissection and removal of perinephric fat and preparation of ureter(s), renal vein(s), and renal artery(s), ligating branches, as necessary (use 50325).

Additional reconstruction of a cadaver or living donor renal allograft prior to transplantation may include venous, arterial, and/or ureteral anastomosis(es) necessary for implantation (see 50327-50329).

3. Recipient renal allotransplantation, which includes transplantation of the allograft (with or without recipient nephrectomy) and care of the recipient (see 50360, 50365).

AMA Coding Notes

Renal Transplantation Procedures

(For dialysis, see 90935-90999)

(For laparoscopic donor nephrectomy, use 50547)

(For laparoscopic drainage of lymphocele to peritoneal cavity, use 49323)

Surgical Procedures on the Urinary System

(For provision of chemotherapeutic agents, report both the specific service in addition to code(s) for the specific substance(s) or drug(s) provided)

AMA *CPT® Assistant* ▯

50300: Nov 99: 25, Apr 05: 10, 12

Plain English Description

One or both kidneys are harvested from a deceased (cadaver) donor that has been maintained medically until the surgical transplant team arrives. The inferior vena cava, aorta, and both renal pedicles are dissected free of surrounding structures. The gonadal, lumbar, and adrenal veins are clipped and divided. The renal artery is identified and dissected free of surrounding tissue. Lateral, posterior, and inferior kidney attachments are left intact to prevent torsion of the kidney and damage to its vascular pedicle. The ureter is dissected free of surrounding tissue to the level of the iliac vessels and divided. The kidney is dissected free from the remaining lateral and inferior attachments. The lower pole of the kidney is elevated and dissected free of posterior attachments. The vascular pedicle containing the renal artery and vein is divided. If cardiocirculatory arrest is initiated, retrograde cannulation of the aorta above the renal arteries is performed and the kidneys are cooled in situ by perfusing them with cold preservation solution. The kidneys and ureters are then removed and packed in ice and delivered to the recipient transplant team(s).

Donor nephrectomy from cadaver donor

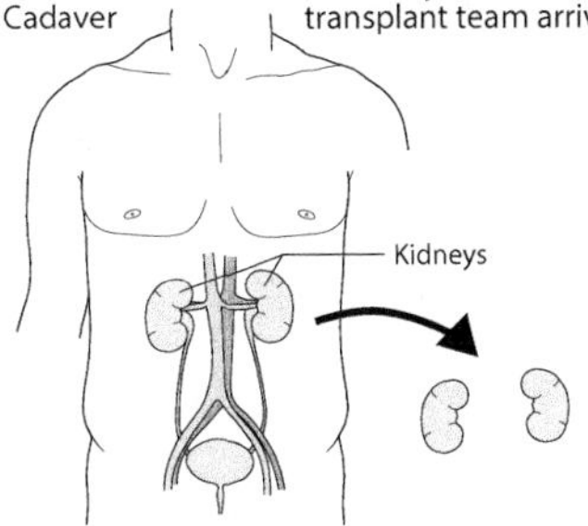

One or both kidneys are harvested from a deceased donor that has been maintained medically until the surgical transplant team arrives.
Cadaver
Kidneys

ICD-10-CM Diagnostic Codes

Z52.4 Kidney donor

CCI Edits

Refer to Appendix A for CCI edits.

Pub 100

50300: Pub 100-04, 3, 90.1-90.6

Facility RVUs ▯

Code	Work	PE Facility	MP	Total Facility
50300	0.00	0.00	0.00	0.00

Non-facility RVUs ▯

Code	Work	PE Non-Facility	MP	Total Non-Facility
50300	0.00	0.00	0.00	0.00

Modifiers (PAR) ▯

Code	Mod 50	Mod 51	Mod 62	Mod 66	Mod 80
50300	9	9	9	9	9

Global Period

Code	Days
50300	XXX

50320

50320 Donor nephrectomy (including cold preservation); open, from living donor

AMA Coding Guideline

Renal Transplantation Procedures

Renal autotransplantation includes reimplantation of the autograft as the primary procedure, along with secondary extra-corporeal procedure(s) (eg, partial nephrectomy, nephrolithotomy) reported with modifier 51 (see 50380 and applicable secondary procedure(s)).

Renal allotransplantation involves three distinct components of physician work:

1. Cadaver donor nephrectomy, unilateral or bilateral, which includes harvesting the graft(s) and cold preservation of the graft(s) (perfusing with cold preservation solution and cold maintenance) (use 50300). Living donor nephrectomy, which includes harvesting the graft, cold preservation of the graft (perfusing with cold preservation solution and cold maintenance), and care of the donor (see 50320, 50547).

2. Backbench work:

Standard preparation of a cadaver donor renal allograft prior to transplantation including dissection and removal of perinephric fat, diaphragmatic and retroperitoneal attachments; excision of adrenal gland; and preparation of ureter(s), renal vein(s), and renal artery(s), ligating branches, as necessary (use 50323).

Standard preparation of a living donor renal allograft (open or laparoscopic) prior to transplantation including dissection and removal of perinephric fat and preparation of ureter(s), renal vein(s), and renal artery(s), ligating branches, as necessary (use 50325).

Additional reconstruction of a cadaver or living donor renal allograft prior to transplantation may include venous, arterial, and/or ureteral anastomosis(es) necessary for implantation (see 50327-50329).

3. Recipient renal allotransplantation, which includes transplantation of the allograft (with or without recipient nephrectomy) and care of the recipient (see 50360, 50365).

AMA Coding Notes

Renal Transplantation Procedures

(For dialysis, see 90935-90999)

(For laparoscopic donor nephrectomy, use 50547)

(For laparoscopic drainage of lymphocele to peritoneal cavity, use 49323)

Surgical Procedures on the Urinary System

(For provision of chemotherapeutic agents, report both the specific service in addition to code(s) for the specific substance(s) or drug(s) provided)

AMA *CPT® Assistant*

50320: Nov 99: 25, May 00: 4

Plain English Description

A living donor nephrectomy inclusive of cold preservation of the donor kidney is performed via an open approach. The lateral line of Toldt is identified and incised. The peritoneum over the kidney is mobilized and the anterior surface of the kidney is visualized. The colon is mobilized and rolled medially. The colorenal ligaments are divided and Gerota's fascia is exposed. The ureter and surrounding vascular structures are identified and retracted to expose the lower pole of the kidney and the renal hilum. The lower pole is partially mobilized. The kidney is retracted laterally and superiorly to allow access to the renal hilum. The renal hilum is dissected free of the surrounding structures. The renal vein is exposed. The gonadal, lumbar, and adrenal veins are clipped and divided. The renal artery is identified and dissected free of surrounding tissue. Lateral, posterior, and inferior kidney attachments are left intact to prevent torsion of the kidney and damage to its vascular pedicle. The ureter is dissected free of surrounding tissue to the level of the iliac vessels and divided. The kidney is dissected free from the remaining lateral and inferior attachments. The lower pole of the kidney is elevated and dissected free of posterior attachments. The vascular pedicle containing the renal artery and vein is divided. The kidney and ureter are then removed. The kidney may be perfused with cold preservation solution and/or placed on ice and delivered to the recipient surgical team.

Donor nephrectomy; open

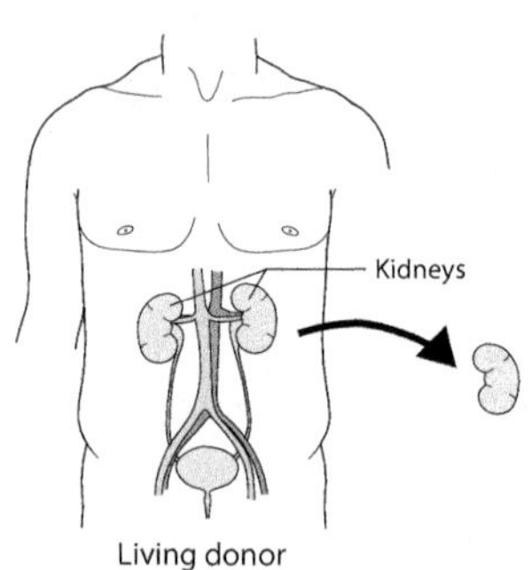

A living donor nephrectomy inclusive of cold preservation of the donor kidney is performed via an open approach.

ICD-10-CM Diagnostic Codes

Z52.4 Kidney donor

CCI Edits

Refer to Appendix A for CCI edits.

Pub 100

50320: Pub 100-04, 3, 90.1-90.6

Facility RVUs

Code	Work	PE Facility	MP	Total Facility
50320	22.43	17.16	5.65	45.24

Non-facility RVUs

Code	Work	PE Non-Facility	MP	Total Non-Facility
50320	22.43	17.16	5.65	45.24

Modifiers (PAR)

Code	Mod 50	Mod 51	Mod 62	Mod 66	Mod 80
50320	1	2	1	0	2

Global Period

Code	Days
50320	090

● New ▲ Revised ✚ Add On ⊘Modifier 51 Exempt ★Telemedicine ▢ CPT QuickRef ⁄⁄FDA Pending ⇄ Laterality ❼ Seventh Character ♂Male ♀Female

50323-50325

50323 Backbench standard preparation of cadaver donor renal allograft prior to transplantation, including dissection and removal of perinephric fat, diaphragmatic and retroperitoneal attachments, excision of adrenal gland, and preparation of ureter(s), renal vein(s), and renal artery(s), ligating branches, as necessary

(Do not report 50323 in conjunction with 60540, 60545)

50325 Backbench standard preparation of living donor renal allograft (open or laparoscopic) prior to transplantation, including dissection and removal of perinephric fat and preparation of ureter(s), renal vein(s), and renal artery(s), ligating branches, as necessary

AMA Coding Guideline

Renal Transplantation Procedures

Renal autotransplantation includes reimplantation of the autograft as the primary procedure, along with secondary extra-corporeal procedure(s) (eg, partial nephrectomy, nephrolithotomy) reported with modifier 51 (see 50380 and applicable secondary procedure(s)).

Renal allotransplantation involves three distinct components of physician work:

1. Cadaver donor nephrectomy, unilateral or bilateral, which includes harvesting the graft(s) and cold preservation of the graft(s) (perfusing with cold preservation solution and cold maintenance) (use 50300). Living donor nephrectomy, which includes harvesting the graft, cold preservation of the graft (perfusing with cold preservation solution and cold maintenance), and care of the donor (see 50320, 50547).

2. Backbench work:

Standard preparation of a cadaver donor renal allograft prior to transplantation including dissection and removal of perinephric fat, diaphragmatic and retroperitoneal attachments; excision of adrenal gland; and preparation of ureter(s), renal vein(s), and renal artery(s), ligating branches, as necessary (use 50323).

Standard preparation of a living donor renal allograft (open or laparoscopic) prior to transplantation including dissection and removal of perinephric fat and preparation of ureter(s), renal vein(s), and renal artery(s), ligating branches, as necessary (use 50325).

Additional reconstruction of a cadaver or living donor renal allograft prior to transplantation may include venous, arterial, and/or ureteral anastomosis(es) necessary for implantation (see 50327-50329).

3. Recipient renal allotransplantation, which includes transplantation of the allograft (with or without recipient nephrectomy) and care of the recipient (see 50360, 50365).

AMA Coding Notes

Renal Transplantation Procedures

(For dialysis, see 90935-90999)

(For laparoscopic donor nephrectomy, use 50547)

(For laparoscopic drainage of lymphocele to peritoneal cavity, use 49323)

Surgical Procedures on the Urinary System

(For provision of chemotherapeutic agents, report both the specific service in addition to code(s) for the specific substance(s) or drug(s) provided)

AMA *CPT® Assistant* □

50323: Apr 05: 10-11

Plain English Description

Standard backbench (back table) preparation of a kidney harvested from a cadaver or living donor is performed prior to transplant. The kidney is unpackaged and transferred to a back table basin and placed in iced Ringers lactate solution. Cultures are taken of the preservation fluid and sent to the laboratory. Fat and surrounding tissue are dissected off the external surface of the kidney. The adrenal gland is excised. The kidney is inspected and all open ends of small blood vessels are suture ligated to prevent post-transplant bleeding. Lymphatic vessels are also suture ligated to prevent post-transplant lymphocele formation. Large blood vessels are then addressed. The gonadal, adrenal, and any lumbar vein branches are divided and ligated. The renal vein is trimmed. If any reconstruction of the renal vein is required, it is reported separately. The renal arteries are evaluated. Some donors have only a single renal artery and others have multiple renal arteries. The renal arteries are trimmed and branches ligated as needed. If any reconstruction is required on the renal arteries, it is reported separately. The ureter is then prepared, leaving as much surrounding tissue as possible undisturbed to prevent damage to the vascular structures. The renal vessels are then flushed with Ringers lactate to identify any vascular defects or leaks that may require additional preparation or repair. Report 50323 for back bench preparation on a cadaver donor kidney and 50325 for back bench preparation on a living donor kidney.

Backbench standard preparation of cadaver donor renal allograft prior to transplantation

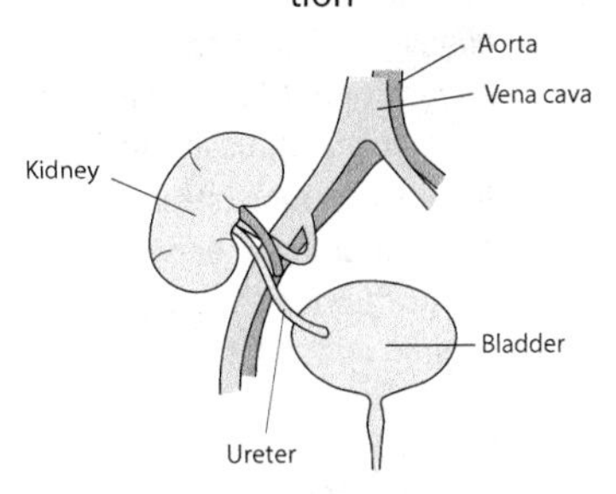

For 50323, a donor kidney is prepared for transplant from a cadaver donor. Report 50325, for removal of excess tissue and fat from the kidney(s) to be transplanted.

ICD-10-CM Diagnostic Codes

Z52.4	Kidney donor

CCI Edits

Refer to Appendix A for CCI edits.

Pub 100

50323: Pub 100-04, 3, 90.1-90.6
50325: Pub 100-04, 3, 90.1-90.6

Facility RVUs □

Code	Work	PE Facility	MP	Total Facility
50323	0.00	0.00	0.00	0.00
50325	0.00	0.00	0.00	0.00

Non-facility RVUs □

Code	Work	PE Non-Facility	MP	Total Non-Facility
50323	0.00	0.00	0.00	0.00
50325	0.00	0.00	0.00	0.00

Modifiers (PAR) □

Code	Mod 50	Mod 51	Mod 62	Mod 66	Mod 80
50323	0	2	1	0	2
50325	0	2	1	0	2

Global Period

Code	Days
50323	XXX
50325	XXX

50327-50328

50327 Backbench reconstruction of cadaver or living donor renal allograft prior to transplantation; venous anastomosis, each

50328 Backbench reconstruction of cadaver or living donor renal allograft prior to transplantation; arterial anastomosis, each

AMA Coding Guideline

Renal Transplantation Procedures

Renal autotransplantation includes reimplantation of the autograft as the primary procedure, along with secondary extra-corporeal procedure(s) (eg, partial nephrectomy, nephrolithotomy) reported with modifier 51 (see 50380 and applicable secondary procedure(s)).

Renal allotransplantation involves three distinct components of physician work:

1. Cadaver donor nephrectomy, unilateral or bilateral, which includes harvesting the graft(s) and cold preservation of the graft(s) (perfusing with cold preservation solution and cold maintenance) (use 50300). Living donor nephrectomy, which includes harvesting the graft, cold preservation of the graft (perfusing with cold preservation solution and cold maintenance), and care of the donor (see 50320, 50547).

2. Backbench work:

Standard preparation of a cadaver donor renal allograft prior to transplantation including dissection and removal of perinephric fat, diaphragmatic and retroperitoneal attachments; excision of adrenal gland; and preparation of ureter(s), renal vein(s), and renal artery(s), ligating branches, as necessary (use 50323).

Standard preparation of a living donor renal allograft (open or laparoscopic) prior to transplantation including dissection and removal of perinephric fat and preparation of ureter(s), renal vein(s), and renal artery(s), ligating branches, as necessary (use 50325).

Additional reconstruction of a cadaver or living donor renal allograft prior to transplantation may include venous, arterial, and/or ureteral anastomosis(es) necessary for implantation (see 50327-50329).

3. Recipient renal allotransplantation, which includes transplantation of the allograft (with or without recipient nephrectomy) and care of the recipient (see 50360, 50365).

AMA Coding Notes

Renal Transplantation Procedures

(For dialysis, see 90935-90999)

(For laparoscopic donor nephrectomy, use 50547)

(For laparoscopic drainage of lymphocele to peritoneal cavity, use 49323)

Surgical Procedures on the Urinary System

(For provision of chemotherapeutic agents, report both the specific service in addition to code(s) for the specific substance(s) or drug(s) provided)

Plain English Description

Backbench venous or arterial reconstruction is performed on a cadaver or living donor kidney. In 50327, the renal vein is reconstructed using a section of the vena cava or a vein graft. The renal vein is trimmed. The section of vena cava or vein graft is then fashioned to the correct length and width and anastomosed to the renal vein. If multiple renal vein branches are present, these may be anastomosed to form a single vein or each may be prepared separately. Report 50327 for each venous anastomosis performed. In 50328, one or more renal arteries are reconstructed using the gonadal vein obtained from the harvested kidney. The donor gonadal vein is used to create a patch or graft when a single renal artery requires repair or lengthening. When multiple renal artery branches are present, the renal arteries may be anastomosed to each other in a side-to-side fashion to create a single renal artery or each artery may be prepared separately with a venous graft. Report 50328 for each arterial anastomosis performed.

Backbench reconstruction of cadaver or living donor renal allograft prior to transplantation

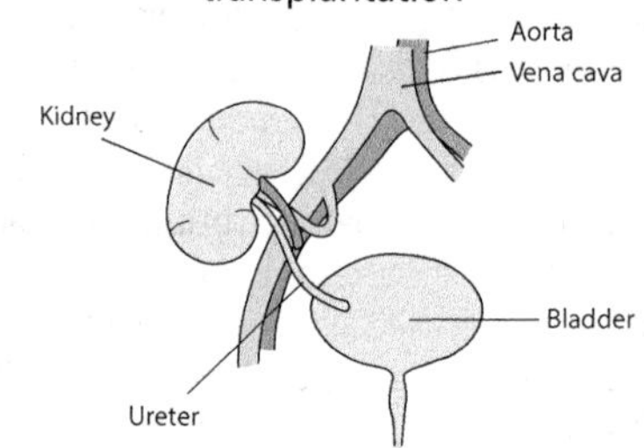

For 50327, a donor kidney is prepared for transplant from a cadaver or living donor. Report 50238 for removal of excess tissue and fat from the kidney(s) to be transplanted.

ICD-10-CM Diagnostic Codes

Z52.4 Kidney donor

CCI Edits

Refer to Appendix A for CCI edits.

Pub 100

50327: Pub 100-04, 3, 90.1-90.6

50328: Pub 100-04, 3, 90.1-90.6

Facility RVUs

Code	Work	PE Facility	MP	Total Facility
50327	4.00	1.46	0.95	6.41
50328	3.50	1.29	0.83	5.62

Non-facility RVUs

Code	Work	PE Non-Facility	MP	Total Non-Facility
50327	4.00	1.46	0.95	6.41
50328	3.50	1.29	0.83	5.62

Modifiers (PAR)

Code	Mod 50	Mod 51	Mod 62	Mod 66	Mod 80
50327	0	2	1	0	2
50328	0	2	1	0	2

Global Period

Code	Days
50327	XXX
50328	XXX

50329

50329 Backbench reconstruction of cadaver or living donor renal allograft prior to transplantation; ureteral anastomosis, each

AMA Coding Guideline

Renal Transplantation Procedures

Renal autotransplantation includes reimplantation of the autograft as the primary procedure, along with secondary extra-corporeal procedure(s) (eg, partial nephrectomy, nephrolithotomy) reported with modifier 51 (see 50380 and applicable secondary procedure(s)).

Renal allotransplantation involves three distinct components of physician work:

1. Cadaver donor nephrectomy, unilateral or bilateral, which includes harvesting the graft(s) and cold preservation of the graft(s) (perfusing with cold preservation solution and cold maintenance) (use 50300). Living donor nephrectomy, which includes harvesting the graft, cold preservation of the graft (perfusing with cold preservation solution and cold maintenance), and care of the donor (see 50320, 50547).

2. Backbench work:

Standard preparation of a cadaver donor renal allograft prior to transplantation including dissection and removal of perinephric fat, diaphragmatic and retroperitoneal attachments; excision of adrenal gland; and preparation of ureter(s), renal vein(s), and renal artery(s), ligating branches, as necessary (use 50323).

Standard preparation of a living donor renal allograft (open or laparoscopic) prior to transplantation including dissection and removal of perinephric fat and preparation of ureter(s), renal vein(s), and renal artery(s), ligating branches, as necessary (use 50325).

Additional reconstruction of a cadaver or living donor renal allograft prior to transplantation may include venous, arterial, and/or ureteral anastomosis(es) necessary for implantation (see 50327-50329).

3. Recipient renal allotransplantation, which includes transplantation of the allograft (with or without recipient nephrectomy) and care of the recipient (see 50360, 50365).

AMA Coding Notes

Renal Transplantation Procedures

(For dialysis, see 90935-90999)

(For laparoscopic donor nephrectomy, use 50547)

(For laparoscopic drainage of lymphocele to peritoneal cavity, use 49323)

Surgical Procedures on the Urinary System

(For provision of chemotherapeutic agents, report both the specific service in addition to code(s) for the specific substance(s) or drug(s) provided)

Plain English Description

Backbench reconstruction of the ureter is performed on a cadaver or living donor renal allograft prior to transplant. This may be required when the donor kidney has an anomaly, such as the presence of double ureters. The ureter is carefully dissected free of surrounding tissue, taking care not to compromise the vascular supply. A patch or graft is then prepared, usually with a section of ureter from the transplant recipient, and anastomosed to the ureter. When double ureters are present, they may be anastomosed to each other or each ureter may require separate preparation with graft anastomosis. Report 50329 for each ureteral anastomosis performed.

Backbench reconstruction of cadaver or living donor renal allograft prior to transplantation

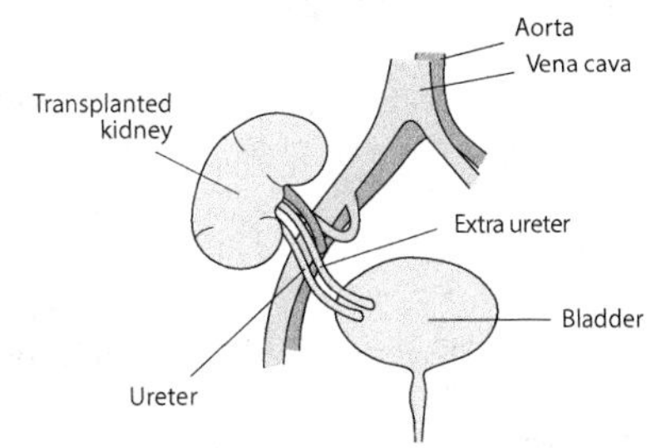

Backbench reconstruction of the ureter is performed on a cadaver or living donor renal allograft prior to transplant. This may be required when the donor kidney has an anomaly, such as the presence of double ureters. The ureter is carefully dissected free of surrounding tissue, taking care not to compromise the vascular supply.

ICD-10-CM Diagnostic Codes

Z52.4	Kidney donor

CCI Edits

Refer to Appendix A for CCI edits.

Pub 100

50329: Pub 100-04, 3, 90.1-90.6

Facility RVUs ☐

Code	Work	PE Facility	MP	Total Facility
50329	3.34	1.23	0.75	5.32

Non-facility RVUs ☐

Code	Work	PE Non-Facility	MP	Total Non-Facility
50329	3.34	1.23	0.75	5.32

Modifiers (PAR) ☐

Code	Mod 50	Mod 51	Mod 62	Mod 66	Mod 80
50329	0	2	1	0	2

Global Period

Code	Days
50329	XXX

50340

50340 Recipient nephrectomy (separate procedure)

(For bilateral procedure, report 50340 with modifier 50)

AMA Coding Guideline

Renal Transplantation Procedures

Renal autotransplantation includes reimplantation of the autograft as the primary procedure, along with secondary extra-corporeal procedure(s) (eg, partial nephrectomy, nephrolithotomy) reported with modifier 51 (see 50380 and applicable secondary procedure(s)).

Renal allotransplantation involves three distinct components of physician work:

1. Cadaver donor nephrectomy, unilateral or bilateral, which includes harvesting the graft(s) and cold preservation of the graft(s) (perfusing with cold preservation solution and cold maintenance) (use 50300). Living donor nephrectomy, which includes harvesting the graft, cold preservation of the graft (perfusing with cold preservation solution and cold maintenance), and care of the donor (see 50320, 50547).

2. Backbench work:

Standard preparation of a cadaver donor renal allograft prior to transplantation including dissection and removal of perinephric fat, diaphragmatic and retroperitoneal attachments; excision of adrenal gland; and preparation of ureter(s), renal vein(s), and renal artery(s), ligating branches, as necessary (use 50323).

Standard preparation of a living donor renal allograft (open or laparoscopic) prior to transplantation including dissection and removal of perinephric fat and preparation of ureter(s), renal vein(s), and renal artery(s), ligating branches, as necessary (use 50325).

Additional reconstruction of a cadaver or living donor renal allograft prior to transplantation may include venous, arterial, and/or ureteral anastomosis(es) necessary for implantation (see 50327-50329).

3. Recipient renal allotransplantation, which includes transplantation of the allograft (with or without recipient nephrectomy) and care of the recipient (see 50360, 50365).

AMA Coding Notes

Renal Transplantation Procedures

(For dialysis, see 90935-90999)

(For laparoscopic donor nephrectomy, use 50547)

(For laparoscopic drainage of lymphocele to peritoneal cavity, use 49323)

Surgical Procedures on the Urinary System

(For provision of chemotherapeutic agents, report both the specific service in addition to code(s) for the specific substance(s) or drug(s) provided)

Plain English Description

A kidney is removed from the donor recipient prior to transplantation in a separate procedure. A wide flank incision is made immediately below the lower border of the ribs or near the 11th or 12th rib. Alternatively, an anterior subcostal approach may be utilized. The peritoneum over the kidney is mobilized and the anterior surface of the kidney is visualized. The colon is mobilized and rolled medially. The colorenal ligaments are divided and Gerota's fascia is exposed. The ureter and surrounding vascular structures are identified and retracted to expose the lower pole of the kidney and the renal hilum. The lower pole is partially mobilized. The kidney is retracted laterally and superiorly to allow access to the renal hilum. The renal hilum is dissected free of the surrounding structures. The renal vein is exposed. The gonadal, lumbar, and adrenal veins are clipped and divided. The renal artery is identified and dissected free of surrounding tissue. Lateral, posterior, and inferior kidney attachments are left intact to prevent torsion of the kidney and damage to its vascular pedicle. The ureter is dissected free of surrounding tissue to the level of the iliac vessels and divided. The kidney is dissected free from the remaining lateral and inferior attachments. The lower pole of the kidney is elevated and dissected free of posterior attachments. The vascular pedicle containing the renal artery and vein is divided. The kidney is removed and the intact segment of ureter is closed. Bleeding is controlled, drains placed as needed, and the incisions closed.

Recipient nephrectomy

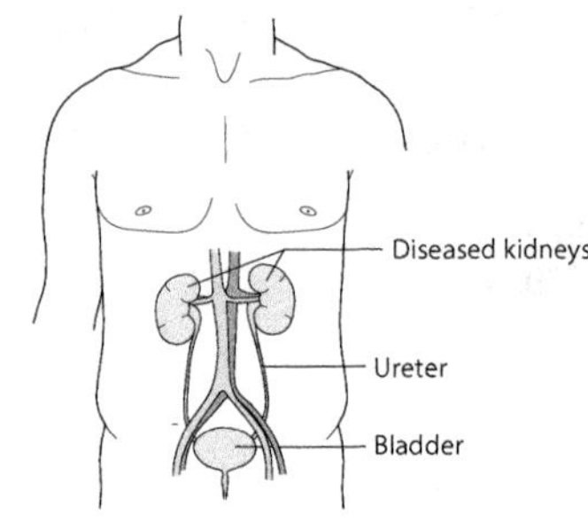

A kidney is removed from the donor recipient prior to transplantation in a separate procedure.

ICD-10-CM Diagnostic Codes

⇄	C64.1	Malignant neoplasm of right kidney, except renal pelvis
⇄	C64.2	Malignant neoplasm of left kidney, except renal pelvis
⇄	C65.1	Malignant neoplasm of right renal pelvis
⇄	C65.2	Malignant neoplasm of left renal pelvis
⇄	C79.01	Secondary malignant neoplasm of right kidney and renal pelvis
⇄	C79.02	Secondary malignant neoplasm of left kidney and renal pelvis
	C7A.093	Malignant carcinoid tumor of the kidney
	E08.22	Diabetes mellitus due to underlying condition with diabetic chronic kidney disease
	E08.29	Diabetes mellitus due to underlying condition with other diabetic kidney complication
	E09.22	Drug or chemical induced diabetes mellitus with diabetic chronic kidney disease
	E09.29	Drug or chemical induced diabetes mellitus with other diabetic kidney complication
	E10.22	Type 1 diabetes mellitus with diabetic chronic kidney disease
	E10.29	Type 1 diabetes mellitus with other diabetic kidney complication
	E11.22	Type 2 diabetes mellitus with diabetic chronic kidney disease
	E11.29	Type 2 diabetes mellitus with other diabetic kidney complication
	E13.22	Other specified diabetes mellitus with diabetic chronic kidney disease
	E13.29	Other specified diabetes mellitus with other diabetic kidney complication
	E85.4	Organ-limited amyloidosis
	E85.81	Light chain (AL) amyloidosis
	I12.0	Hypertensive chronic kidney disease with stage 5 chronic kidney disease or end stage renal disease
	I75.81	Atheroembolism of kidney
	M31.31	Wegener's granulomatosis with renal involvement
	M32.14	Glomerular disease in systemic lupus erythematosus
	M32.15	Tubulo-interstitial nephropathy in systemic lupus erythematosus
	N00.1	Acute nephritic syndrome with focal and segmental glomerular lesions
	N00.2	Acute nephritic syndrome with diffuse membranous glomerulonephritis
	N00.3	Acute nephritic syndrome with diffuse mesangial proliferative glomerulonephritis
	N00.4	Acute nephritic syndrome with diffuse endocapillary proliferative glomerulonephritis
	N00.5	Acute nephritic syndrome with diffuse mesangiocapillary glomerulonephritis
	N00.6	Acute nephritic syndrome with dense deposit disease
	N00.7	Acute nephritic syndrome with diffuse crescentic glomerulonephritis
	N00.8	Acute nephritic syndrome with other morphologic changes
	N03.1	Chronic nephritic syndrome with focal and segmental glomerular lesions
	N03.2	Chronic nephritic syndrome with diffuse membranous glomerulonephritis

N03.3 Chronic nephritic syndrome with diffuse mesangial proliferative glomerulonephritis
N03.4 Chronic nephritic syndrome with diffuse endocapillary proliferative glomerulonephritis
N03.5 Chronic nephritic syndrome with diffuse mesangiocapillary glomerulonephritis
N03.6 Chronic nephritic syndrome with dense deposit disease
N03.7 Chronic nephritic syndrome with diffuse crescentic glomerulonephritis
N03.8 Chronic nephritic syndrome with other morphologic changes
N04.1 Nephrotic syndrome with focal and segmental glomerular lesions
N04.2 Nephrotic syndrome with diffuse membranous glomerulonephritis
N04.3 Nephrotic syndrome with diffuse mesangial proliferative glomerulonephritis
N04.4 Nephrotic syndrome with diffuse endocapillary proliferative glomerulonephritis
N04.5 Nephrotic syndrome with diffuse mesangiocapillary glomerulonephritis
N04.6 Nephrotic syndrome with dense deposit disease
N04.7 Nephrotic syndrome with diffuse crescentic glomerulonephritis
N04.8 Nephrotic syndrome with other morphologic changes
N08 Glomerular disorders in diseases classified elsewhere
N11.0 Nonobstructive reflux-associated chronic pyelonephritis
N11.1 Chronic obstructive pyelonephritis
N11.8 Other chronic tubulo-interstitial nephritis
N13.0 Hydronephrosis with ureteropelvic junction obstruction
N13.1 Hydronephrosis with ureteral stricture, not elsewhere classified
N13.2 Hydronephrosis with renal and ureteral calculous obstruction
N13.39 Other hydronephrosis
N13.6 Pyonephrosis
N13.721 Vesicoureteral-reflux with reflux nephropathy without hydroureter, unilateral
N13.722 Vesicoureteral-reflux with reflux nephropathy without hydroureter, bilateral
N13.731 Vesicoureteral-reflux with reflux nephropathy with hydroureter, unilateral
N13.732 Vesicoureteral-reflux with reflux nephropathy with hydroureter, bilateral
N13.8 Other obstructive and reflux uropathy
N16 Renal tubulo-interstitial disorders in diseases classified elsewhere
N17.0 Acute kidney failure with tubular necrosis
N17.1 Acute kidney failure with acute cortical necrosis
N17.2 Acute kidney failure with medullary necrosis
N18.4 Chronic kidney disease, stage 4 (severe)
N18.5 Chronic kidney disease, stage 5
N18.6 End stage renal disease
N20.0 Calculus of kidney
N20.2 Calculus of kidney with calculus of ureter
N26.1 Atrophy of kidney (terminal)
N26.2 Page kidney
N28.0 Ischemia and infarction of kidney
N28.1 Cyst of kidney, acquired
N28.81 Hypertrophy of kidney
N28.89 Other specified disorders of kidney and ureter
N29 Other disorders of kidney and ureter in diseases classified elsewhere
Q60.3 Renal hypoplasia, unilateral
Q60.4 Renal hypoplasia, bilateral
Q60.6 Potter's syndrome
Q61.02 Congenital multiple renal cysts
Q61.11 Cystic dilatation of collecting ducts
Q61.19 Other polycystic kidney, infantile type
Q61.2 Polycystic kidney, adult type
Q61.4 Renal dysplasia
Q61.5 Medullary cystic kidney
Q61.8 Other cystic kidney diseases
Q62.0 Congenital hydronephrosis
Q62.11 Congenital occlusion of ureteropelvic junction
Q62.39 Other obstructive defects of renal pelvis and ureter
Q63.8 Other specified congenital malformations of kidney
❼⇄ S37.061 Major laceration of right kidney
❼⇄ S37.062 Major laceration of left kidney
❼ T79.5 Traumatic anuria

ICD-10-CM Coding Notes

For codes requiring a 7th character extension, refer to your ICD-10-CM book. Review the character descriptions and coding guidelines for proper selection. For some procedures, only certain characters will apply.

CCI Edits

Refer to Appendix A for CCI edits.

Pub 100

50340: Pub 100-04, 3, 90.1-90.6

Facility RVUs ▯

Code	Work	PE Facility	MP	Total Facility
50340	14.04	10.99	3.55	28.58

Non-facility RVUs ▯

Code	Work	PE Non-Facility	MP	Total Non-Facility
50340	14.04	10.99	3.55	28.58

Modifiers (PAR) ▯

Code	Mod 50	Mod 51	Mod 62	Mod 66	Mod 80
50340	1	2	1	0	2

Global Period

Code	Days
50340	090

50360-50365

50360 Renal allotransplantation, implantation of graft; without recipient nephrectomy

50365 Renal allotransplantation, implantation of graft; with recipient nephrectomy

(For bilateral procedure, report 50365 with modifier 50)

AMA Coding Guideline
Renal Transplantation Procedures

Renal autotransplantation includes reimplantation of the autograft as the primary procedure, along with secondary extra-corporeal procedure(s) (eg, partial nephrectomy, nephrolithotomy) reported with modifier 51 (see 50380 and applicable secondary procedure(s)).

Renal allotransplantation involves three distinct components of physician work:

1. Cadaver donor nephrectomy, unilateral or bilateral, which includes harvesting the graft(s) and cold preservation of the graft(s) (perfusing with cold preservation solution and cold maintenance) (use 50300). Living donor nephrectomy, which includes harvesting the graft, cold preservation of the graft (perfusing with cold preservation solution and cold maintenance), and care of the donor (see 50320, 50547).

2. Backbench work:

Standard preparation of a cadaver donor renal allograft prior to transplantation including dissection and removal of perinephric fat, diaphragmatic and retroperitoneal attachments; excision of adrenal gland; and preparation of ureter(s), renal vein(s), and renal artery(s), ligating branches, as necessary (use 50323).

Standard preparation of a living donor renal allograft (open or laparoscopic) prior to transplantation including dissection and removal of perinephric fat and preparation of ureter(s), renal vein(s), and renal artery(s), ligating branches, as necessary (use 50325).

Additional reconstruction of a cadaver or living donor renal allograft prior to transplantation may include venous, arterial, and/or ureteral anastomosis(es) necessary for implantation (see 50327-50329).

3. Recipient renal allotransplantation, which includes transplantation of the allograft (with or without recipient nephrectomy) and care of the recipient (see 50360, 50365).

AMA Coding Notes
Renal Transplantation Procedures

(For dialysis, see 90935-90999)

(For laparoscopic donor nephrectomy, use 50547)

(For laparoscopic drainage of lymphocele to peritoneal cavity, use 49323)

Surgical Procedures on the Urinary System

(For provision of chemotherapeutic agents, report both the specific service in addition to code(s) for the specific substance(s) or drug(s) provided)

AMA *CPT® Assistant* ▯

50365: Apr 05: 10-11

Plain English Description

The physician transplants the prepared kidney obtained from a cadaver or living donor in the transplant recipient. An incision is made in the lower abdomen. The transversalis fascia is incised and the retroperitoneal space entered. The peritoneum is retracted medially to allow exposure of the iliac blood vessels. Lymphatic vessels surrounding the iliac blood vessels are ligated and divided. The iliac blood vessels are dissected free of surrounding tissue from the region immediately above the iliac lymph nodes to the bifurcation of the external and internal iliac artery. Vascular clamps are applied. The external iliac vein is incised and the prepared renal vein in the renal allograft is anastomosed to the external iliac vein. If more than one renal vein is present in the allograft, these are anastomosed separately to the external iliac vein. The prepared renal artery is then anastomosed to the internal or external iliac artery. If more than one renal artery is present, separate incisions are made and each artery is anastomosed to a separate site in the internal or external iliac artery. Vascular clamps are released, the anastomosis sites inspected, and any bleeding controlled. The ureter in the donor kidney is now prepared for anastomosis. The dome of the bladder is exposed and incised. The ureter is trimmed to the correct length and the end spatulated to match the opening in the bladder. The mucosa of the bladder and ureter are anastomosed followed by closure of the detrusor muscle layer over the ureter. A temporary stent may be placed to ensure patency at the anastomosis site. The kidney is then placed in the parapsoas fossa, taking care to avoid any kinking of the blood vessels or ureter. Incisions are closed. Report 50360 when the kidney transplant is performed as described above leaving the recipient kidney intact. Report 50365 when the recipient kidney is removed at the time of the transplant procedure. A wide flank incision is made immediately below the lower border of the ribs or near the 11th or 12th rib. Alternatively, an anterior subcostal approach may be utilized. The kidney and ureter are exposed. The renal artery and vein are isolated, ligated, and divided. The kidney is dissected free from surrounding tissue. The ureter is divided and the intact segment of ureter closed. Bleeding is controlled, drains placed as needed, and the incisions closed. The physician then proceeds with the transplant procedure as described above.

Renal allotransplantation, with/without recipient nephrectomy

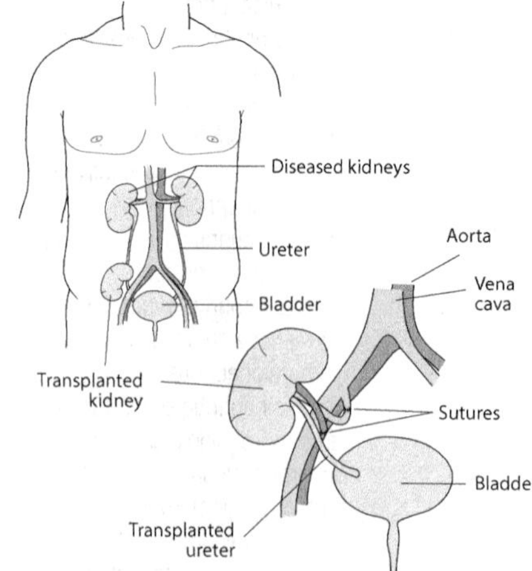

Without (50360), or with (50365) recipient nephrectomy

ICD-10-CM Diagnostic Codes

E08.22	Diabetes mellitus due to underlying condition with diabetic chronic kidney disease
E08.29	Diabetes mellitus due to underlying condition with other diabetic kidney complication
E09.22	Drug or chemical induced diabetes mellitus with diabetic chronic kidney disease
E09.29	Drug or chemical induced diabetes mellitus with other diabetic kidney complication
E10.22	Type 1 diabetes mellitus with diabetic chronic kidney disease
E10.29	Type 1 diabetes mellitus with other diabetic kidney complication
E11.22	Type 2 diabetes mellitus with diabetic chronic kidney disease
E11.29	Type 2 diabetes mellitus with other diabetic kidney complication
E13.22	Other specified diabetes mellitus with diabetic chronic kidney disease
E13.29	Other specified diabetes mellitus with other diabetic kidney complication
E85.4	Organ-limited amyloidosis
E85.81	Light chain (AL) amyloidosis
I12.0	Hypertensive chronic kidney disease with stage 5 chronic kidney disease or end stage renal disease
I13.11	Hypertensive heart and chronic kidney disease without heart failure, with stage 5 chronic kidney disease, or end stage renal disease
I75.81	Atheroembolism of kidney
M31.31	Wegener's granulomatosis with renal involvement
M32.14	Glomerular disease in systemic lupus erythematosus
M32.15	Tubulo-interstitial nephropathy in systemic lupus erythematosus
N00.1	Acute nephritic syndrome with focal and segmental glomerular lesions

N00.2 Acute nephritic syndrome with diffuse membranous glomerulonephritis
N00.3 Acute nephritic syndrome with diffuse mesangial proliferative glomerulonephritis
N00.4 Acute nephritic syndrome with diffuse endocapillary proliferative glomerulonephritis
N00.5 Acute nephritic syndrome with diffuse mesangiocapillary glomerulonephritis
N00.6 Acute nephritic syndrome with dense deposit disease
N00.7 Acute nephritic syndrome with diffuse crescentic glomerulonephritis
N00.8 Acute nephritic syndrome with other morphologic changes
N03.1 Chronic nephritic syndrome with focal and segmental glomerular lesions
N03.2 Chronic nephritic syndrome with diffuse membranous glomerulonephritis
N03.3 Chronic nephritic syndrome with diffuse mesangial proliferative glomerulonephritis
N03.4 Chronic nephritic syndrome with diffuse endocapillary proliferative glomerulonephritis
N03.5 Chronic nephritic syndrome with diffuse mesangiocapillary glomerulonephritis
N03.6 Chronic nephritic syndrome with dense deposit disease
N03.7 Chronic nephritic syndrome with diffuse crescentic glomerulonephritis
N03.8 Chronic nephritic syndrome with other morphologic changes
N04.1 Nephrotic syndrome with focal and segmental glomerular lesions
N04.2 Nephrotic syndrome with diffuse membranous glomerulonephritis
N04.3 Nephrotic syndrome with diffuse mesangial proliferative glomerulonephritis
N04.5 Nephrotic syndrome with diffuse mesangiocapillary glomerulonephritis
N04.6 Nephrotic syndrome with dense deposit disease
N04.7 Nephrotic syndrome with diffuse crescentic glomerulonephritis
N04.8 Nephrotic syndrome with other morphologic changes
N08 Glomerular disorders in diseases classified elsewhere
N11.0 Nonobstructive reflux-associated chronic pyelonephritis
N11.1 Chronic obstructive pyelonephritis
N11.8 Other chronic tubulo-interstitial nephritis
N13.0 Hydronephrosis with ureteropelvic junction obstruction
N13.1 Hydronephrosis with ureteral stricture, not elsewhere classified
N13.2 Hydronephrosis with renal and ureteral calculous obstruction
N13.39 Other hydronephrosis
N13.6 Pyonephrosis
N13.721 Vesicoureteral-reflux with reflux nephropathy without hydroureter, unilateral
N13.722 Vesicoureteral-reflux with reflux nephropathy without hydroureter, bilateral
N13.731 Vesicoureteral-reflux with reflux nephropathy with hydroureter, unilateral
N13.732 Vesicoureteral-reflux with reflux nephropathy with hydroureter, bilateral
N13.8 Other obstructive and reflux uropathy
N16 Renal tubulo-interstitial disorders in diseases classified elsewhere
N17.0 Acute kidney failure with tubular necrosis
N17.1 Acute kidney failure with acute cortical necrosis
N17.2 Acute kidney failure with medullary necrosis
N18.4 Chronic kidney disease, stage 4 (severe)
N18.5 Chronic kidney disease, stage 5
N18.6 End stage renal disease
N20.0 Calculus of kidney
N20.2 Calculus of kidney with calculus of ureter
N26.1 Atrophy of kidney (terminal)
N26.2 Page kidney
N27.1 Small kidney, bilateral
N28.0 Ischemia and infarction of kidney
N28.1 Cyst of kidney, acquired
N28.81 Hypertrophy of kidney
N29 Other disorders of kidney and ureter in diseases classified elsewhere
Q60.3 Renal hypoplasia, unilateral
Q60.4 Renal hypoplasia, bilateral
Q60.6 Potter's syndrome
Q61.01 Congenital single renal cyst
Q61.02 Congenital multiple renal cysts
Q61.11 Cystic dilatation of collecting ducts
Q61.19 Other polycystic kidney, infantile type
Q61.2 Polycystic kidney, adult type
Q61.4 Renal dysplasia
Q61.5 Medullary cystic kidney
Q61.8 Other cystic kidney diseases
Q62.0 Congenital hydronephrosis
Q62.11 Congenital occlusion of ureteropelvic junction
Q62.39 Other obstructive defects of renal pelvis and ureter
Q63.8 Other specified congenital malformations of kidney

CCI Edits

Refer to Appendix A for CCI edits.

Pub 100

50360: Pub 100-04, 3, 90.1-90.6
50365: Pub 100-04, 3, 90.1-90.6

Facility RVUs ▫

Code	Work	PE Facility	MP	Total Facility
50360	39.88	22.73	9.60	72.21
50365	46.13	29.03	10.97	86.13

Non-facility RVUs ▫

Code	Work	PE Non-Facility	MP	Total Non-Facility
50360	39.88	22.73	9.60	72.21
50365	46.13	29.03	10.97	86.13

Modifiers (PAR) ▫

Code	Mod 50	Mod 51	Mod 62	Mod 66	Mod 80
50360	0	2	2	2	2
50365	1	2	2	2	2

Global Period

Code	Days
50360	090
50365	090

50370

50370 Removal of transplanted renal allograft

AMA Coding Guideline

Renal Transplantation Procedures

Renal autotransplantation includes reimplantation of the autograft as the primary procedure, along with secondary extra-corporeal procedure(s) (eg, partial nephrectomy, nephrolithotomy) reported with modifier 51 (see 50380 and applicable secondary procedure(s)).

Renal allotransplantation involves three distinct components of physician work:

1. Cadaver donor nephrectomy, unilateral or bilateral, which includes harvesting the graft(s) and cold preservation of the graft(s) (perfusing with cold preservation solution and cold maintenance) (use 50300). Living donor nephrectomy, which includes harvesting the graft, cold preservation of the graft (perfusing with cold preservation solution and cold maintenance), and care of the donor (see 50320, 50547).

2. Backbench work:

Standard preparation of a cadaver donor renal allograft prior to transplantation including dissection and removal of perinephric fat, diaphragmatic and retroperitoneal attachments; excision of adrenal gland; and preparation of ureter(s), renal vein(s), and renal artery(s), ligating branches, as necessary (use 50323).

Standard preparation of a living donor renal allograft (open or laparoscopic) prior to transplantation including dissection and removal of perinephric fat and preparation of ureter(s), renal vein(s), and renal artery(s), ligating branches, as necessary (use 50325).

Additional reconstruction of a cadaver or living donor renal allograft prior to transplantation may include venous, arterial, and/or ureteral anastomosis(es) necessary for implantation (see 50327-50329).

3. Recipient renal allotransplantation, which includes transplantation of the allograft (with or without recipient nephrectomy) and care of the recipient (see 50360, 50365).

AMA Coding Notes

Renal Transplantation Procedures

(For dialysis, see 90935-90999)

(For laparoscopic donor nephrectomy, use 50547)

(For laparoscopic drainage of lymphocele to peritoneal cavity, use 49323)

Surgical Procedures on the Urinary System

(For provision of chemotherapeutic agents, report both the specific service in addition to code(s) for the specific substance(s) or drug(s) provided)

Plain English Description

The physician removes a previously transplanted donor kidney. An incision is made in the lower abdomen. The transversalis fascia is incised and the retroperitoneal space is entered. The peritoneum is retracted medially and the transplanted kidney is exposed, then dissected free of surrounding tissue. The anastomosis sites of the transplanted ureter and renal vessels are exposed. The ureter is dissected free of surrounding tissue, ligated, and divided. The renal vessels are dissected free of surrounding tissues, ligated, and divided. The transplanted kidney is removed, bleeding is controlled, and incisions are closed.

Removal of transplanted renal allograft

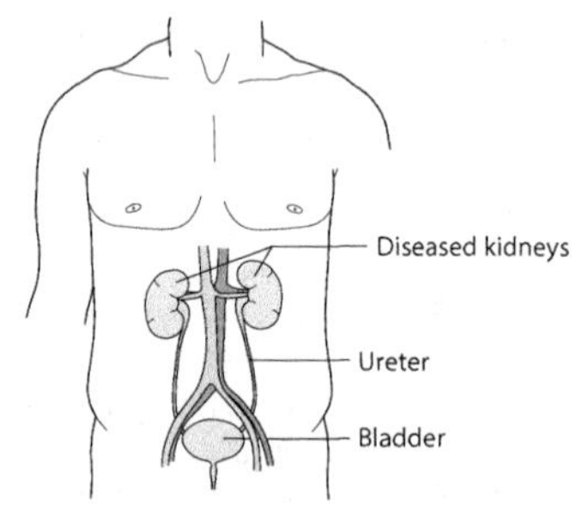

The physician removes a previously transplanted donor kidney.

ICD-10-CM Diagnostic Codes

C80.2	Malignant neoplasm associated with transplanted organ
D89.810	Acute graft-versus-host disease
D89.811	Chronic graft-versus-host disease
D89.812	Acute on chronic graft-versus-host disease
N18.6	End stage renal disease
T86.10	Unspecified complication of kidney transplant
T86.11	Kidney transplant rejection
T86.12	Kidney transplant failure
T86.13	Kidney transplant infection
T86.19	Other complication of kidney transplant
Z94.0	Kidney transplant status

CCI Edits

Refer to Appendix A for CCI edits.

Pub 100

50370: Pub 100-04, 3, 90.1-90.6

Facility RVUs ☐

Code	Work	PE Facility	MP	Total Facility
50370	18.88	12.81	4.46	36.15

Non-facility RVUs ☐

Code	Work	PE Non-Facility	MP	Total Non-Facility
50370	18.88	12.81	4.46	36.15

Modifiers (PAR) ☐

Code	Mod 50	Mod 51	Mod 62	Mod 66	Mod 80
50370	0	2	1	0	2

Global Period

Code	Days
50370	090

50380

50380 Renal autotransplantation, reimplantation of kidney

(For renal autotransplantation extra-corporeal [bench] surgery, use autotransplantation as the primary procedure and report secondary procedure[s] [eg, partial nephrectomy, nephrolithotomy] with modifier 51)

AMA Coding Guideline
Renal Transplantation Procedures

Renal autotransplantation includes reimplantation of the autograft as the primary procedure, along with secondary extra-corporeal procedure(s) (eg, partial nephrectomy, nephrolithotomy) reported with modifier 51 (see 50380 and applicable secondary procedure(s)).

Renal allotransplantation involves three distinct components of physician work:

1. Cadaver donor nephrectomy, unilateral or bilateral, which includes harvesting the graft(s) and cold preservation of the graft(s) (perfusing with cold preservation solution and cold maintenance) (use 50300). Living donor nephrectomy, which includes harvesting the graft, cold preservation of the graft (perfusing with cold preservation solution and cold maintenance), and care of the donor (see 50320, 50547).

2. Backbench work:

Standard preparation of a cadaver donor renal allograft prior to transplantation including dissection and removal of perinephric fat, diaphragmatic and retroperitoneal attachments; excision of adrenal gland; and preparation of ureter(s), renal vein(s), and renal artery(s), ligating branches, as necessary (use 50323).

Standard preparation of a living donor renal allograft (open or laparoscopic) prior to transplantation including dissection and removal of perinephric fat and preparation of ureter(s), renal vein(s), and renal artery(s), ligating branches, as necessary (use 50325).

Additional reconstruction of a cadaver or living donor renal allograft prior to transplantation may include venous, arterial, and/or ureteral anastomosis(es) necessary for implantation (see 50327-50329).

3. Recipient renal allotransplantation, which includes transplantation of the allograft (with or without recipient nephrectomy) and care of the recipient (see 50360, 50365).

AMA Coding Notes
Renal Transplantation Procedures

(For dialysis, see 90935-90999)

(For laparoscopic donor nephrectomy, use 50547)

(For laparoscopic drainage of lymphocele to peritoneal cavity, use 49323)

Surgical Procedures on the Urinary System

(For provision of chemotherapeutic agents, report both the specific service in addition to code(s) for the specific substance(s) or drug(s) provided)

AMA *CPT® Assistant* ☐

50380: Apr 05: 10, 12, Sep 19: 11

Plain English Description

The physician removes the patient's kidney from the normal anatomic location and reimplants it in the parapsoas fossa or other site. The lateral line of Toldt is identified and incised. The peritoneum over the kidney is mobilized and the anterior surface of the kidney is visualized. The colon is mobilized and rolled medially. The colorenal ligaments are divided and Gerota's fascia is exposed. The ureter and surrounding vascular structures are identified and retracted to expose the lower pole of the kidney and the renal hilum. The lower pole is partially mobilized. The kidney is retracted laterally and superiorly to allow access to the renal hilum, which is dissected free of the surrounding structures. The renal vein is exposed. The gonadal, lumbar, and adrenal veins are clipped and divided. The renal artery is identified and dissected free of surrounding tissue. Lateral, posterior, and inferior kidney attachments are left intact to prevent torsion of the kidney and damage to its vascular pedicle. The ureter is dissected free of surrounding tissue to the level of the iliac vessels and divided. The kidney is dissected free from the remaining lateral and inferior attachments. The lower pole of the kidney is elevated and dissected free of posterior attachments. The vascular pedicle containing the renal artery and vein is divided. The kidney and ureter are removed. The kidney is prepared for reimplantation into the parapsoas fossa or other site. For implantation into the parapsoas fossa, an incision is made in the lower abdomen. The transversalis fascia is incised and the retroperitoneal space is entered. The peritoneum is retracted medially to allow exposure of the iliac vessels. Surrounding lymphatic vessels are ligated and divided. The iliac vessels are dissected free of surrounding tissue from the region immediately above the iliac lymph nodes to the bifurcation of the external and internal iliac artery. Vascular clamps are applied. The external iliac vein is incised and the prepared renal vein in the renal autograft is anastomosed to the external iliac vein. If more than one renal vein is present, they are anastomosed separately to the external iliac vein. The prepared renal artery is then anastomosed to the internal or external iliac artery. If more than one renal artery is present, separate incisions are made and each artery is anastomosed to a separate site in the internal or external iliac artery. Vascular clamps are released and the anastomosis sites are inspected. The ureter is prepared for anastomosis. The dome of the bladder is exposed and incised. The ureter is trimmed to the correct length and the end is spatulated to match the opening in the bladder. The mucosa of the bladder and ureter are anastomosed, followed by closure of the detrusor muscle layer over the ureter. A temporary stent may be placed to ensure patency at the anastomosis site. The kidney is then placed in the parapsoas fossa, taking care to avoid any kinking of the blood vessels or ureter. Drains are placed as needed and incisions are closed.

Renal autotransplantation, reimplantation of kidney

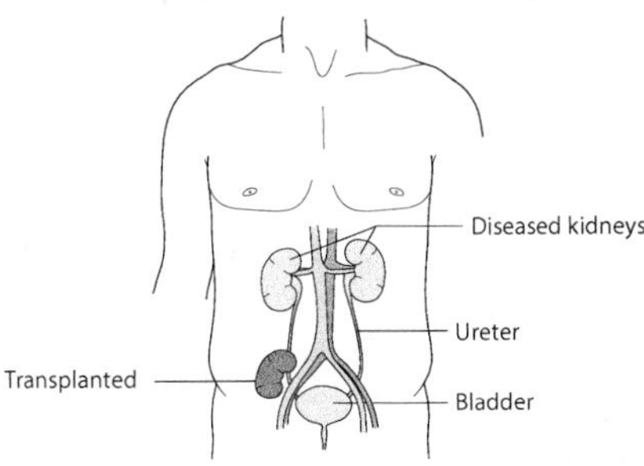

The physician removes the patient's kidney from the normal anatomic location and reimplants it in the parapsoas fossa or other site.

ICD-10-CM Diagnostic Codes

⇄	C64.1	Malignant neoplasm of right kidney, except renal pelvis
⇄	C64.2	Malignant neoplasm of left kidney, except renal pelvis
⇄	C65.1	Malignant neoplasm of right renal pelvis
⇄	C65.2	Malignant neoplasm of left renal pelvis
⇄	C66.1	Malignant neoplasm of right ureter
⇄	C66.2	Malignant neoplasm of left ureter
⇄	C79.01	Secondary malignant neoplasm of right kidney and renal pelvis
⇄	C79.02	Secondary malignant neoplasm of left kidney and renal pelvis
	C7A.093	Malignant carcinoid tumor of the kidney
	D09.19	Carcinoma in situ of other urinary organs
⇄	D30.01	Benign neoplasm of right kidney
⇄	D30.02	Benign neoplasm of left kidney
⇄	D30.11	Benign neoplasm of right renal pelvis
⇄	D30.12	Benign neoplasm of left renal pelvis
⇄	D30.21	Benign neoplasm of right ureter
⇄	D30.22	Benign neoplasm of left ureter
	D3A.093	Benign carcinoid tumor of the kidney
⇄	D41.01	Neoplasm of uncertain behavior of right kidney
⇄	D41.02	Neoplasm of uncertain behavior of left kidney
⇄	D41.11	Neoplasm of uncertain behavior of right renal pelvis
⇄	D41.12	Neoplasm of uncertain behavior of left renal pelvis
⇄	D41.21	Neoplasm of uncertain behavior of right ureter
⇄	D41.22	Neoplasm of uncertain behavior of left ureter
	I15.0	Renovascular hypertension

	Code	Description
	I70.1	Atherosclerosis of renal artery
	I72.2	Aneurysm of renal artery
	I75.81	Atheroembolism of kidney
	I77.3	Arterial fibromuscular dysplasia
	I77.73	Dissection of renal artery
	I82.3	Embolism and thrombosis of renal vein
	N13.5	Crossing vessel and stricture of ureter without hydronephrosis
	N20.0	Calculus of kidney
	N28.0	Ischemia and infarction of kidney
	Q27.1	Congenital renal artery stenosis
	Q27.2	Other congenital malformations of renal artery
	Q27.34	Arteriovenous malformation of renal vessel
	Q62.11	Congenital occlusion of ureteropelvic junction
	Q62.31	Congenital ureterocele, orthotopic
	Q62.39	Other obstructive defects of renal pelvis and ureter
❼⇄	S35.401	Unspecified injury of right renal artery
❼⇄	S35.402	Unspecified injury of left renal artery
❼⇄	S35.404	Unspecified injury of right renal vein
❼⇄	S35.405	Unspecified injury of left renal vein
❼⇄	S35.411	Laceration of right renal artery
❼⇄	S35.412	Laceration of left renal artery
❼⇄	S35.414	Laceration of right renal vein
❼⇄	S35.415	Laceration of left renal vein
❼⇄	S35.491	Other specified injury of right renal artery
❼⇄	S35.492	Other specified injury of left renal artery
❼⇄	S35.494	Other specified injury of right renal vein
❼⇄	S35.495	Other specified injury of left renal vein
❼	T81.711	Complication of renal artery following a procedure, not elsewhere classified

ICD-10-CM Coding Notes

For codes requiring a 7th character extension, refer to your ICD-10-CM book. Review the character descriptions and coding guidelines for proper selection. For some procedures, only certain characters will apply.

CCI Edits

Refer to Appendix A for CCI edits.

Pub 100

50380: Pub 100-04, 3, 90.1-90.6

Facility RVUs ▯

Code	Work	PE Facility	MP	Total Facility
50380	30.11	22.96	7.61	60.68

Non-facility RVUs ▯

Code	Work	PE Non-Facility	MP	Total Non-Facility
50380	30.11	22.96	7.61	60.68

Modifiers (PAR) ▯

Code	Mod 50	Mod 51	Mod 62	Mod 66	Mod 80
50380	0	2	1	0	2

Global Period

Code	Days
50380	090

50382-50384

50382 Removal (via snare/capture) and replacement of internally dwelling ureteral stent via percutaneous approach, including radiological supervision and interpretation

(For bilateral procedure, use modifier 50)

(For removal and replacement of an internally dwelling ureteral stent via a transurethral approach, use 50385)

50384 Removal (via snare/capture) of internally dwelling ureteral stent via percutaneous approach, including radiological supervision and interpretation

(For bilateral procedure, use modifier 50)

(Do not report 50382, 50384 in conjunction with 50436, 50437)

(For removal of an internally dwelling ureteral stent via a transurethral approach, use 50386)

AMA Coding Notes

Surgical Procedures on the Urinary System

(For provision of chemotherapeutic agents, report both the specific service in addition to code(s) for the specific substance(s) or drug(s) provided)

AMA *CPT® Assistant*

50382: Sep 06: 1, 16, Oct 08: 8, Dec 09: 4, Jan 16: 3

50384: Sep 06: 2, 16, Oct 08: 8, Jan 16: 3

Plain English Description

The physician removes and replaces an indwelling ureteral stent via a percutaneous approach using radiographic guidance. A small skin incision is made over the selected entry site in the kidney. A needle is inserted into the renal calyx and positioned using radiographic guidance. Contrast media is injected and fluoroscopy performed. The kidney and ureter are visualized. A guidewire is introduced into the renal pelvis, the needle is removed, and the tract is dilated. A sheath is placed over the guidewire and into the renal pelvis. A snare device is then passed through the renal pelvis and into the ureter to capture the indwelling stent. The stent is retracted until the proximal end is exposed. A guidewire is placed through the partially externalized stent and positioned in the ureter. The stent is then removed. leaving the guidewire in place. The replacement stent is advanced over the guidewire and the distal end of the stent positioned in the bladder. Correct positioning of the replacement stent is verified radiographically. All surgical instruments are removed. A final set of radiographs are obtained to document correct positioning of the stent. Use 50382 to report removal and replacement of an indwelling ureteral stent. Use 50384 to report removal only.

Removal of internally dwelling ureteral stent via percutaneous approach

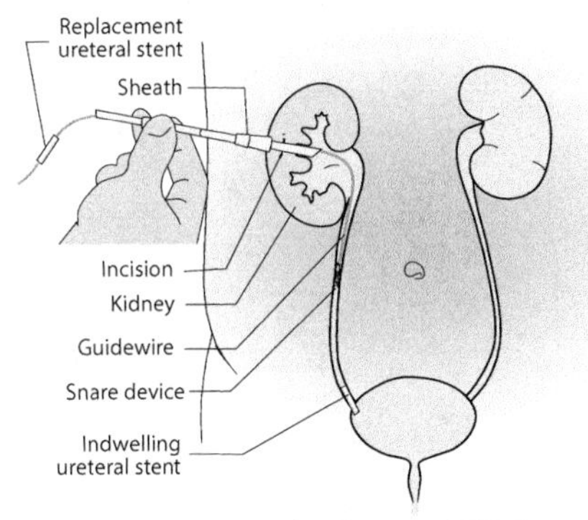

For removal and replacement (50382); for removal only (50384)

ICD-10-CM Diagnostic Codes

	Code	Description
➐	T83.112	Breakdown (mechanical) of indwelling ureteral stent
➐	T83.122	Displacement of indwelling ureteral stent
➐	T83.192	Other mechanical complication of indwelling ureteral stent
➐	T83.592	Infection and inflammatory reaction due to indwelling ureteral stent
➐	T83.81	Embolism due to genitourinary prosthetic devices, implants and grafts
➐	T83.82	Fibrosis due to genitourinary prosthetic devices, implants and grafts
➐	T83.83	Hemorrhage due to genitourinary prosthetic devices, implants and grafts
➐	T83.84	Pain due to genitourinary prosthetic devices, implants and grafts
➐	T83.85	Stenosis due to genitourinary prosthetic devices, implants and grafts
➐	T83.86	Thrombosis due to genitourinary prosthetic devices, implants and grafts
➐	T83.89	Other specified complication of genitourinary prosthetic devices, implants and grafts

ICD-10-CM Coding Notes

For codes requiring a 7th character extension, refer to your ICD-10-CM book. Review the character descriptions and coding guidelines for proper selection. For some procedures, only certain characters will apply.

CCI Edits

Refer to Appendix A for CCI edits.

Facility RVUs

Code	Work	PE Facility	MP	Total Facility
50382	5.25	1.57	0.50	7.32
50384	4.75	1.37	0.44	6.56

Non-facility RVUs

Code	Work	PE Non-Facility	MP	Total Non-Facility
50382	5.25	25.41	0.50	31.16
50384	4.75	21.44	0.44	26.63

Modifiers (PAR)

Code	Mod 50	Mod 51	Mod 62	Mod 66	Mod 80
50382	1	2	0	0	1
50384	1	2	0	0	1

Global Period

Code	Days
50382	000
50384	000

50385-50386

50385 Removal (via snare/capture) and replacement of internally dwelling ureteral stent via transurethral approach, without use of cystoscopy, including radiological supervision and interpretation

50386 Removal (via snare/capture) of internally dwelling ureteral stent via transurethral approach, without use of cystoscopy, including radiological supervision and interpretation

AMA Coding Notes

Surgical Procedures on the Urinary System

(For provision of chemotherapeutic agents, report both the specific service in addition to code(s) for the specific substance(s) or drug(s) provided)

AMA *CPT® Assistant* ▢

50385: Oct 08: 8, Dec 09: 4, Jan 16: 3

50386: Oct 08: 8, Jan 16: 3

Plain English Description

An internally dwelling ureteral stent is removed via snare or other capture device and replaced using a transurethral catheter approach under fluoroscopic guidance without the use of cystoscopy. This procedure includes radiological supervision and interpretation. A ureteral stent is a soft, hollow tube about the size of a strand of spaghetti that holds the ureter open to allow urine to drain from the kidney to the bladder in cases of obstruction or blockage. Most stents are left in place only until the obstruction has been relieved, which typically takes from a few weeks to a few months. A catheter is advanced into the bladder and contrast is injected for visualization. A guidewire is advanced into the bladder, the first catheter is replaced with a larger catheter, and the snare or other capture device is introduced and advanced to the distal pigtail portion of the ureteral stent in the bladder. The stent is grasped and pulled into the bladder and urethra until it is exposed. A guidewire is then introduced through the stent and advanced into the renal pelvis using fluoroscopic guidance. The stent is then removed and a catheter is advanced over the guidewire. Additional contrast is injected, the catheter is removed, and a new stent is passed over the guidewire and positioned with the proximal pigtail in the renal pelvis and the distal pigtail in the bladder. The guidewire is then removed. Stent position is confirmed by fluoroscopy and X-ray images are obtained to document correct placement. Use 50386 if the ureteral stent is removed without being replaced.

Removal of internally dwelling ureteral stent

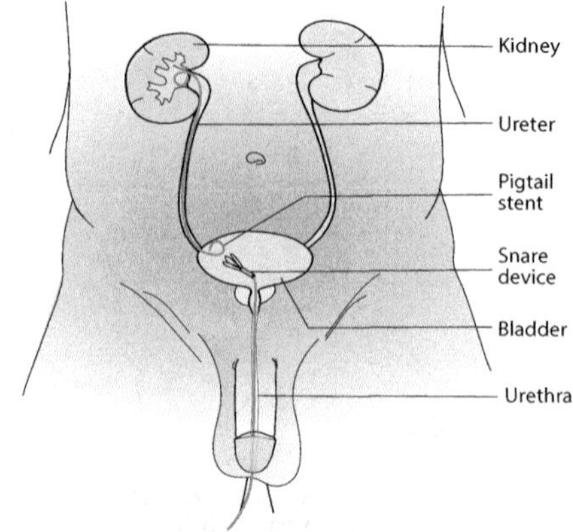

With stent replacement (50385); without replacement (50386)

ICD-10-CM Diagnostic Codes

	Code	Description
❼	T83.112	Breakdown (mechanical) of indwelling ureteral stent
❼	T83.122	Displacement of indwelling ureteral stent
❼	T83.192	Other mechanical complication of indwelling ureteral stent
❼	T83.592	Infection and inflammatory reaction due to indwelling ureteral stent
❼	T83.81	Embolism due to genitourinary prosthetic devices, implants and grafts
❼	T83.82	Fibrosis due to genitourinary prosthetic devices, implants and grafts
❼	T83.83	Hemorrhage due to genitourinary prosthetic devices, implants and grafts
❼	T83.84	Pain due to genitourinary prosthetic devices, implants and grafts
❼	T83.85	Stenosis due to genitourinary prosthetic devices, implants and grafts
❼	T83.86	Thrombosis due to genitourinary prosthetic devices, implants and grafts
❼	T83.89	Other specified complication of genitourinary prosthetic devices, implants and grafts

ICD-10-CM Coding Notes

For codes requiring a 7th character extension, refer to your ICD-10-CM book. Review the character descriptions and coding guidelines for proper selection. For some procedures, only certain characters will apply.

CCI Edits

Refer to Appendix A for CCI edits.

Facility RVUs ▢

Code	Work	PE Facility	MP	Total Facility
50385	4.19	1.65	0.44	6.28
50386	3.05	1.30	0.34	4.69

Non-facility RVUs ▢

Code	Work	PE Non-Facility	MP	Total Non-Facility
50385	4.19	26.65	0.44	31.28
50386	3.05	19.70	0.34	23.09

Modifiers (PAR) ▢

Code	Mod 50	Mod 51	Mod 62	Mod 66	Mod 80
50385	1	2	0	0	0
50386	1	2	0	0	0

Global Period

Code	Days
50385	000
50386	000

50387

50387 Removal and replacement of externally accessible nephroureteral catheter (eg, external/internal stent) requiring fluoroscopic guidance, including radiological supervision and interpretation

(For bilateral procedure, use modifier 50)

(For removal and replacement of externally accessible ureteral stent via ureterostomy or ileal conduit, use 50688)

(For removal without replacement of an externally accessible ureteral stent not requiring fluoroscopic guidance, see Evaluation and Management services codes)

AMA Coding Notes

Surgical Procedures on the Urinary System

(For provision of chemotherapeutic agents, report both the specific service in addition to code(s) for the specific substance(s) or drug(s) provided)

AMA *CPT® Assistant* ▢

50387: Sep 06: 2, 4, 16, Dec 09: 4, Mar 12: 3, Jan 16: 3, Mar 16: 10

Plain English Description

An externally accessible nephroureteral catheter is a thin flexible tube that extends from the kidney through the ureter and into the bladder with a hub exiting the skin over the kidney. For removal and replacement of the nephroureteral catheter, contrast is injected as needed through the existing external/internal stent to enhance fluoroscopic visualization of the kidney, ureter, bladder, and the existing stent. Using continuous fluoroscopic guidance, the proximal suture fixing the stent to the kidney is cut. A guidewire is inserted through the stent and advanced into the bladder. The existing stent is removed over the guidewire. A new stent is advanced over the guidewire into the bladder. Once the stent is properly positioned in the bladder, the guidewire is partially removed and the stent is visualized to ensure that the stent has coiled in the bladder. The coil, which is referred to as a pigtail, is necessary to prevent accidental dislodgement of the stent from the bladder. The remaining length of stent is assessed to ensure that it is long enough to coil properly in the renal pelvis. The guidewire is removed. A suture is placed to secure the proximal aspect of the stent in the kidney. Contrast is injected as needed to ensure that the stent is patent and functioning properly. The stent hub is secured to the skin with sutures and capped or a drainage device is attached to allow external drainage of urine. Final radiographic images are obtained to ensure that the stent is properly positioned. Code 50387 includes the radiologic supervision and interpretation required for stent removal and replacement.

Removal and replacement transnephric ureteral stent

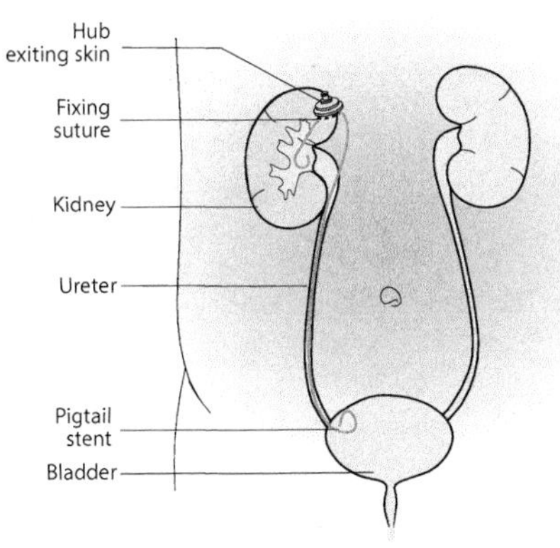

ICD-10-CM Diagnostic Codes

	Code	Description
➐	T83.113	Breakdown (mechanical) of other urinary stents
➐	T83.123	Displacement of other urinary stents
➐	T83.193	Other mechanical complication of other urinary stent
➐	T83.593	Infection and inflammatory reaction due to other urinary stents
➐	T83.81	Embolism due to genitourinary prosthetic devices, implants and grafts
➐	T83.82	Fibrosis due to genitourinary prosthetic devices, implants and grafts
➐	T83.83	Hemorrhage due to genitourinary prosthetic devices, implants and grafts
➐	T83.84	Pain due to genitourinary prosthetic devices, implants and grafts
➐	T83.85	Stenosis due to genitourinary prosthetic devices, implants and grafts
➐	T83.86	Thrombosis due to genitourinary prosthetic devices, implants and grafts
➐	T83.89	Other specified complication of genitourinary prosthetic devices, implants and grafts

ICD-10-CM Coding Notes

For codes requiring a 7th character extension, refer to your ICD-10-CM book. Review the character descriptions and coding guidelines for proper selection. For some procedures, only certain characters will apply.

CCI Edits

Refer to Appendix A for CCI edits.

Facility RVUs ▢

Code	Work	PE Facility	MP	Total Facility
50387	1.75	0.50	0.17	2.42

Non-facility RVUs ▢

Code	Work	PE Non-Facility	MP	Total Non-Facility
50387	1.75	15.44	0.17	17.36

Modifiers (PAR) ▢

Code	Mod 50	Mod 51	Mod 62	Mod 66	Mod 80
50387	1	2	0	0	0

Global Period

Code	Days
50387	000

50389

50389 Removal of nephrostomy tube, requiring fluoroscopic guidance (eg, with concurrent indwelling ureteral stent)

(Removal of nephrostomy tube not requiring fluoroscopic guidance is considered inherent to E/M services. Report the appropriate level of E/M service provided)

AMA Coding Notes

Surgical Procedures on the Urinary System

(For provision of chemotherapeutic agents, report both the specific service in addition to code(s) for the specific substance(s) or drug(s) provided)

AMA *CPT® Assistant*

50389: Sep 06: 1-2, 4, Jan 16: 3

Plain English Description

A nephrostomy tube, also referred to as a stent or catheter, is a tube that passes through the skin into the renal pelvis or a calyx of the kidney. It may be used alone or with a concurrent indwelling ureteral stent. For removal of the tube, contrast is injected as needed into the nephrostomy tube to enhance fluoroscopic visualization of the kidney, ureter, bladder, and any existing stent. Using continuous fluoroscopic guidance, the suture fixing the tube to the kidney is cut. A guidewire is inserted through the tube into the renal pelvis, taking care to avoid accidentally hooking any existing indwelling ureteral stent or the stent retention suture. The nephrostomy tube is removed over the guidewire and the guidewire is then removed. Final radiographic images are obtained to ensure that any existing stent remains properly positioned.

Removal of nephrostomy tube, requiring fluoroscopic guidance

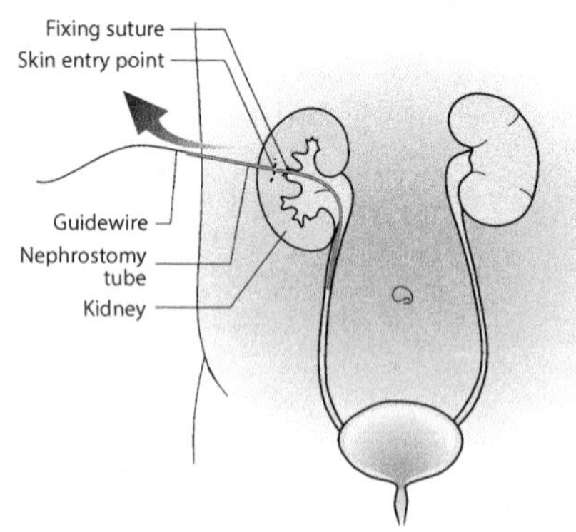

ICD-10-CM Diagnostic Codes

❼	T83.012	Breakdown (mechanical) of nephrostomy catheter
❼	T83.022	Displacement of nephrostomy catheter
❼	T83.032	Leakage of nephrostomy catheter
❼	T83.092	Other mechanical complication of nephrostomy catheter
❼	T83.512	Infection and inflammatory reaction due to nephrostomy catheter
❼	T83.81	Embolism due to genitourinary prosthetic devices, implants and grafts
❼	T83.82	Fibrosis due to genitourinary prosthetic devices, implants and grafts
❼	T83.83	Hemorrhage due to genitourinary prosthetic devices, implants and grafts
❼	T83.84	Pain due to genitourinary prosthetic devices, implants and grafts
❼	T83.85	Stenosis due to genitourinary prosthetic devices, implants and grafts
❼	T83.86	Thrombosis due to genitourinary prosthetic devices, implants and grafts
❼	T83.89	Other specified complication of genitourinary prosthetic devices, implants and grafts

ICD-10-CM Coding Notes

For codes requiring a 7th character extension, refer to your ICD-10-CM book. Review the character descriptions and coding guidelines for proper selection. For some procedures, only certain characters will apply.

CCI Edits

Refer to Appendix A for CCI edits.

Facility RVUs

Code	Work	PE Facility	MP	Total Facility
50389	1.10	0.34	0.10	1.54

Non-facility RVUs

Code	Work	PE Non-Facility	MP	Total Non-Facility
50389	1.10	11.78	0.10	12.98

Modifiers (PAR)

Code	Mod 50	Mod 51	Mod 62	Mod 66	Mod 80
50389	1	2	0	0	1

Global Period

Code	Days
50389	000

50390

50390 Aspiration and/or injection of renal cyst or pelvis by needle, percutaneous

(For radiological supervision and interpretation, see 74425, 74470, 76942, 77002, 77012, 77021)

(For antegrade nephrostogram and/ or antegrade pyelogram, see 50430, 50431)

AMA Coding Guideline

Other Renal Introduction (Injection/ Change/Removal) Procedures

Percutaneous genitourinary procedures are performed with imaging guidance (eg, fluoroscopy and/or ultrasound). Diagnostic nephrostogram and/or ureterogram are typically performed with percutaneous genitourinary procedures and are included in 50432, 50433, 50434, 50435, 50436, 50437, 50693, 50694, 50695.

Code 50436 describes enlargement of an existing percutaneous tract to the renal collecting system to accommodate large instruments used in an endourologic procedure. Code 50436 includes predilation urinary tract imaging, postprocedure nephrostomy tube placement, when performed, and includes all radiological supervision and interpretation and imaging guidance (eg, ultrasound, fluoroscopy). Code 50436 may not be reported with 50432, 50433, 52334 for basic dilation of a percutaneous tract during initial placement of a catheter or device.

Code 50437 includes all elements of 50436, but also includes new access into the renal collecting system performed in the same session when a pre-existing tract is not present.

Codes 50430 and 50431 are diagnostic procedure codes that include injection(s) of contrast material, all associated radiological supervision and interpretation, and procedural imaging guidance (eg, ultrasound and/or fluoroscopy). Code 50430 also includes accessing the collecting system and/ or associated ureter with a needle and/or catheter. Codes 50430 or 50431 may not be reported together with 50432, 50433, 50434, 50435, 50693, 50694, 50695.

Codes 50432, 50433, 50434, 50435 represent therapeutic procedures describing catheter placement or exchange, and include the elements of access, drainage catheter manipulations, and imaging guidance (eg, ultrasonography and/ or fluoroscopy), as well as diagnostic imaging supervision and interpretation, when performed.

Code 50433 describes percutaneous nephrostomy with the additional accessing of the ureter/bladder to ultimately place a nephroureteral catheter (a single transnephric catheter with nephrostomy and ureteral components that allows drainage internally, externally, or both).

For codes 50430, 50431, 50432, 50433, 50434, 50435,50606, 50693, 50694, 50695, 50705, and 50706, the renal pelvis and its associated ureter are considered a single entity for reporting purposes. Codes 50430, 50431, 50432, 50433, 50434, 50435, 50606, 50693, 50694, 50695, 50705, and 50706 may be reported once for each renal collecting system/ureter accessed (eg, two separate codes would be reported for bilateral nephrostomy tube placement or for unilateral duplicated collecting system/ureter requiring two separate procedures).

AMA Coding Notes

Surgical Procedures on the Urinary System

(For provision of chemotherapeutic agents, report both the specific service in addition to code(s) for the specific substance(s) or drug(s) provided)

AMA *CPT® Assistant* ▯

50390: Fall 93: 14, Dec 97: 7, Oct 01: 8, Oct 05: 18, Oct 08: 8

Plain English Description

Aspiration and/or injection is performed to treat a renal cyst or to remove fluid from the renal pelvis. Kidney cysts are fluid filled sacs that form in the kidneys. Simple cysts are typically benign and asymptomatic. When a kidney cyst causes flank pain, frequent urination, or blood in the urine, aspiration is performed followed by injection of a sclerotic solution. The skin in the flank region over the kidney is cleansed. A local anesthetic is infiltrated as a needle is passed under separately reportable radiologic supervision to the site of the planned aspiration and/or injection. If the procedure is a simple aspiration of urine from the renal pelvis, a needle is advanced into the renal pelvis and urine is removed. If the procedure is for treatment of a real cyst, the needle is advanced into the renal cyst. Cystic fluid is aspirated and sent for separately reportable laboratory evaluation. Contrast is then injected into the cystic lesion to determine if there is any communication (opening) between the cyst and the collecting system. If there is no communication, a sclerosing solution, usually 95% ethanol, is injected into the cyst. The sclerosing solution is left in the cyst for several minutes and then removed.

Aspiration and/or injection of renal cyst or pelvis by needle, percutaneous

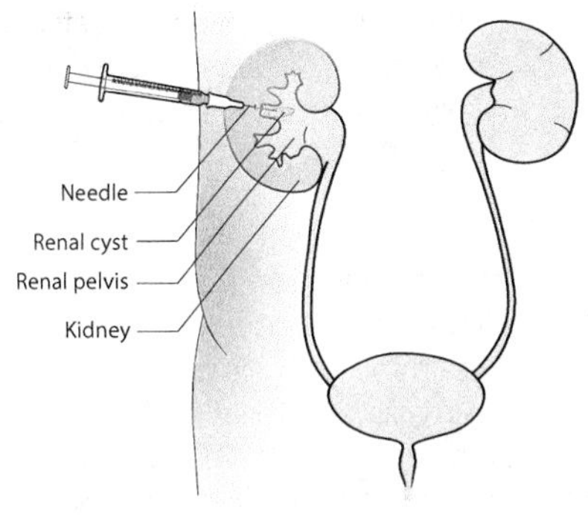

ICD-10-CM Diagnostic Codes

N13.0	Hydronephrosis with ureteropelvic junction obstruction
N13.1	Hydronephrosis with ureteral stricture, not elsewhere classified
N13.2	Hydronephrosis with renal and ureteral calculous obstruction
N13.39	Other hydronephrosis
N13.6	Pyonephrosis
N15.1	Renal and perinephric abscess
N28.1	Cyst of kidney, acquired
Q61.01	Congenital single renal cyst
Q61.02	Congenital multiple renal cysts
Q61.11	Cystic dilatation of collecting ducts
Q61.19	Other polycystic kidney, infantile type
Q61.2	Polycystic kidney, adult type
Q61.8	Other cystic kidney diseases
Q62.0	Congenital hydronephrosis

CCI Edits

Refer to Appendix A for CCI edits.

Pub 100

50390: Pub 100-03, 1, 220.5

Facility RVUs ▯

Code	Work	PE Facility	MP	Total Facility
50390	1.96	0.62	0.19	2.77

Non-facility RVUs ▯

Code	Work	PE Non-Facility	MP	Total Non-Facility
50390	1.96	0.62	0.19	2.77

Modifiers (PAR) ▯

Code	Mod 50	Mod 51	Mod 62	Mod 66	Mod 80
50390	1	2	0	0	1

Global Period

Code	Days
50390	000

50391

50391 Instillation(s) of therapeutic agent into renal pelvis and/or ureter through established nephrostomy, pyelostomy or ureterostomy tube (eg, anticarcinogenic or antifungal agent)

AMA Coding Guideline

Other Renal Introduction (Injection/ Change/Removal) Procedures

Percutaneous genitourinary procedures are performed with imaging guidance (eg, fluoroscopy and/or ultrasound). Diagnostic nephrostogram and/or ureterogram are typically performed with percutaneous genitourinary procedures and are included in 50432, 50433, 50434, 50435, 50436, 50437, 50693, 50694, 50695.

Code 50436 describes enlargement of an existing percutaneous tract to the renal collecting system to accommodate large instruments used in an endourologic procedure. Code 50436 includes predilation urinary tract imaging, postprocedure nephrostomy tube placement, when performed, and includes all radiological supervision and interpretation and imaging guidance (eg, ultrasound, fluoroscopy). Code 50436 may not be reported with 50432, 50433, 52334 for basic dilation of a percutaneous tract during initial placement of a catheter or device.

Code 50437 includes all elements of 50436, but also includes new access into the renal collecting system performed in the same session when a pre-existing tract is not present.

Codes 50430 and 50431 are diagnostic procedure codes that include injection(s) of contrast material, all associated radiological supervision and interpretation, and procedural imaging guidance (eg, ultrasound and/or fluoroscopy). Code 50430 also includes accessing the collecting system and/ or associated ureter with a needle and/or catheter. Codes 50430 or 50431 may not be reported together with 50432, 50433, 50434, 50435, 50693, 50694, 50695.

Codes 50432, 50433, 50434, 50435 represent therapeutic procedures describing catheter placement or exchange, and include the elements of access, drainage catheter manipulations, and imaging guidance (eg, ultrasonography and/ or fluoroscopy), as well as diagnostic imaging supervision and interpretation, when performed.

Code 50433 describes percutaneous nephrostomy with the additional accessing of the ureter/bladder to ultimately place a nephroureteral catheter (a single transnephric catheter with nephrostomy and ureteral components that allows drainage internally, externally, or both).

For codes 50430, 50431, 50432, 50433, 50434, 50435,50606, 50693, 50694, 50695, 50705, and 50706, the renal pelvis and its associated ureter are considered a single entity for reporting purposes. Codes 50430, 50431, 50432, 50433, 50434, 50435, 50606, 50693, 50694, 50695, 50705, and 50706 may be reported once for each renal collecting system/ureter accessed (eg, two separate codes would be reported for bilateral nephrostomy tube placement or for unilateral duplicated collecting system/ureter requiring two separate procedures).

AMA Coding Notes

Surgical Procedures on the Urinary System

(For provision of chemotherapeutic agents, report both the specific service in addition to code(s) for the specific substance(s) or drug(s) provided)

AMA *CPT® Assistant* □

50391: Oct 05: 18

Plain English Description

A therapeutic agent, such as an anticarcinogenic or antifungal agent, is instilled into the renal pelvis and/or ureter through an established nephrostomy, pyelostomy, or ureterostomy tube. This procedure is usually performed to treat malignancy of the epithelial lining of the urinary tract. It may also be used to treat fungal infection of the renal pelvis caused by Candida albicans. Using separately reportable fluoroscopic guidance, the position of the previously placed nephrostomy, pyelostomy, or ureterostomy tube is checked. The anticarcinogenic, antifungal, or other agent is prepared and placed in a syringe, which is connected to the ostomy tube, and instilled into the kidney or ureter. The agent is left in the kidney or ureter for the appropriate amount of time and then drained and disposed of properly. The ostomy tube is then reconnected to the drainage system.

Instillation(s) of therapeutic agent into renal pelvis and/or ureter

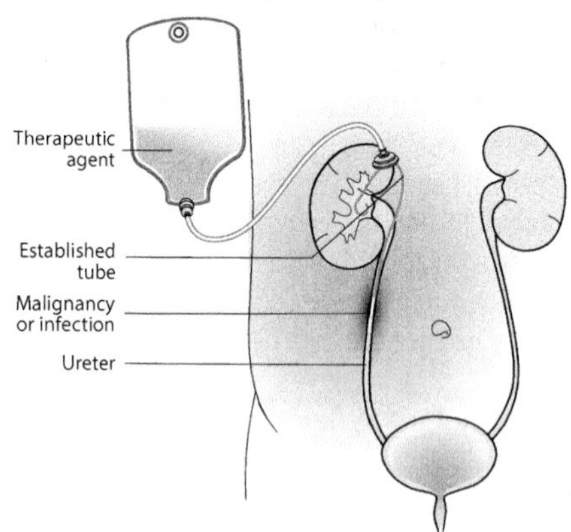

ICD-10-CM Diagnostic Codes

	Code	Description
	B37.49	Other urogenital candidiasis
	B38.89	Other forms of coccidioidomycosis
	B40.89	Other forms of blastomycosis
	B44.89	Other forms of aspergillosis
	B45.8	Other forms of cryptococcosis
	B48.8	Other specified mycoses
⇄	C64.1	Malignant neoplasm of right kidney, except renal pelvis
⇄	C64.2	Malignant neoplasm of left kidney, except renal pelvis
⇄	C65.1	Malignant neoplasm of right renal pelvis
⇄	C65.2	Malignant neoplasm of left renal pelvis
⇄	C66.1	Malignant neoplasm of right ureter
⇄	C66.2	Malignant neoplasm of left ureter
	C67.6	Malignant neoplasm of ureteric orifice
⇄	C79.01	Secondary malignant neoplasm of right kidney and renal pelvis
⇄	C79.02	Secondary malignant neoplasm of left kidney and renal pelvis
	C79.11	Secondary malignant neoplasm of bladder
	C79.19	Secondary malignant neoplasm of other urinary organs
	C7A.093	Malignant carcinoid tumor of the kidney
	D09.0	Carcinoma in situ of bladder
	D09.19	Carcinoma in situ of other urinary organs
⇄	D41.01	Neoplasm of uncertain behavior of right kidney
⇄	D41.02	Neoplasm of uncertain behavior of left kidney
⇄	D41.11	Neoplasm of uncertain behavior of right renal pelvis
⇄	D41.12	Neoplasm of uncertain behavior of left renal pelvis
⇄	D41.21	Neoplasm of uncertain behavior of right ureter
⇄	D41.22	Neoplasm of uncertain behavior of left ureter
	D41.4	Neoplasm of uncertain behavior of bladder
	M35.04	Sjögren syndrome with tubulo-interstitial nephropathy
	N08	Glomerular disorders in diseases classified elsewhere
	N16	Renal tubulo-interstitial disorders in diseases classified elsewhere

CCI Edits

Refer to Appendix A for CCI edits.

Pub 100

50391: Pub 100-02, 15, 50.4.5-50.4.5.1

Facility RVUs

Code	Work	PE Facility	MP	Total Facility
50391	1.96	0.66	0.23	2.85

Non-facility RVUs

Code	Work	PE Non-Facility	MP	Total Non-Facility
50391	1.96	1.50	0.23	3.69

Modifiers (PAR)

Code	Mod 50	Mod 51	Mod 62	Mod 66	Mod 80
50391	1	2	0	0	1

Global Period

Code	Days
50391	000

CPT® Procedural Coding

50396

50396 Manometric studies through nephrostomy or pyelostomy tube, or indwelling ureteral catheter

(For radiological supervision and interpretation, use 74425)

AMA Coding Guideline

Other Renal Introduction (Injection/Change/Removal) Procedures

Percutaneous genitourinary procedures are performed with imaging guidance (eg, fluoroscopy and/or ultrasound). Diagnostic nephrostogram and/or ureterogram are typically performed with percutaneous genitourinary procedures and are included in 50432, 50433, 50434, 50435, 50436, 50437, 50693, 50694, 50695.

Code 50436 describes enlargement of an existing percutaneous tract to the renal collecting system to accommodate large instruments used in an endourologic procedure. Code 50436 includes predilation urinary tract imaging, postprocedure nephrostomy tube placement, when performed, and includes all radiological supervision and interpretation and imaging guidance (eg, ultrasound, fluoroscopy). Code 50436 may not be reported with 50432, 50433, 52334 for basic dilation of a percutaneous tract during initial placement of a catheter or device.

Code 50437 includes all elements of 50436, but also includes new access into the renal collecting system performed in the same session when a pre-existing tract is not present.

Codes 50430 and 50431 are diagnostic procedure codes that include injection(s) of contrast material, all associated radiological supervision and interpretation, and procedural imaging guidance (eg, ultrasound and/or fluoroscopy). Code 50430 also includes accessing the collecting system and/or associated ureter with a needle and/or catheter. Codes 50430 or 50431 may not be reported together with 50432, 50433, 50434, 50435, 50693, 50694, 50695.

Codes 50432, 50433, 50434, 50435 represent therapeutic procedures describing catheter placement or exchange, and include the elements of access, drainage catheter manipulations, and imaging guidance (eg, ultrasonography and/or fluoroscopy), as well as diagnostic imaging supervision and interpretation, when performed.

Code 50433 describes percutaneous nephrostomy with the additional accessing of the ureter/bladder to ultimately place a nephroureteral catheter (a single transnephric catheter with nephrostomy and ureteral components that allows drainage internally, externally, or both).

For codes 50430, 50431, 50432, 50433, 50434, 50435,50606, 50693, 50694, 50695, 50705, and 50706, the renal pelvis and its associated ureter are considered a single entity for reporting purposes. Codes 50430, 50431, 50432, 50433, 50434, 50435, 50606, 50693, 50694, 50695, 50705, and 50706 may be reported once for each renal collecting system/ureter accessed (eg, two separate codes would be reported for bilateral nephrostomy tube placement or for unilateral duplicated collecting system/ureter requiring two separate procedures).

AMA Coding Notes

Surgical Procedures on the Urinary System

(For provision of chemotherapeutic agents, report both the specific service in addition to code(s) for the specific substance(s) or drug(s) provided)

AMA *CPT® Assistant*

50396: Fall 93: 16, Dec 97: 7, Oct 01: 8

Plain English Description

Manometric studies of the renal pelvis and/or ureter are also referred to as a Whitaker test. The procedure may be performed to evaluate persistent upper urinary tract dilatation, particularly in patients who have undergone previous operative intervention to relieve obstruction of the upper urinary tract. The procedure may also be performed to evaluate patency of an indwelling ureteral catheter. A bladder catheter is inserted through the urethra. The skin around an existing nephrostomy or pyelostomy tube insertion site and the external tube components are cleansed with antibacterial solution. The drainage bag is disconnected from the nephrostomy tube. The nephrostomy tube and bladder catheter are connected to a pressure transducer and baseline pressures are obtained. Saline or a contrast dilution is slowly perfused into the kidney and serial pressures in the kidney and bladder are obtained. Upon completion of the manometric studies, the manometer is disconnected from the nephrostomy tube and bladder catheter; the external drainage bag is connected to the tube; and the bladder catheter is removed. The physician reviews the manometry recording and provides a written interpretation of the studies.

Manometric studies through nephrostomy or pyelostomy tube

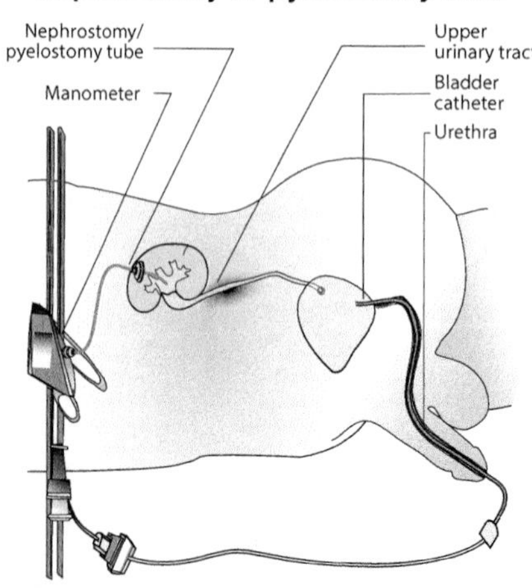

ICD-10-CM Diagnostic Codes

Code	Description
N11.1	Chronic obstructive pyelonephritis
N13.0	Hydronephrosis with ureteropelvic junction obstruction
N13.1	Hydronephrosis with ureteral stricture, not elsewhere classified
N13.2	Hydronephrosis with renal and ureteral calculous obstruction
N13.39	Other hydronephrosis
N13.4	Hydroureter
N13.5	Crossing vessel and stricture of ureter without hydronephrosis
N13.6	Pyonephrosis
N13.731	Vesicoureteral-reflux with reflux nephropathy with hydroureter, unilateral
N13.732	Vesicoureteral-reflux with reflux nephropathy with hydroureter, bilateral
N13.8	Other obstructive and reflux uropathy
N13.9	Obstructive and reflux uropathy, unspecified
N39.41	Urge incontinence
N39.45	Continuous leakage
N39.46	Mixed incontinence
Q62.0	Congenital hydronephrosis
Q62.11	Congenital occlusion of ureteropelvic junction
Q62.12	Congenital occlusion of ureterovesical orifice
Q62.2	Congenital megaureter
Q62.31	Congenital ureterocele, orthotopic
Q62.39	Other obstructive defects of renal pelvis and ureter
R33.8	Other retention of urine
R34	Anuria and oliguria

CCI Edits

Refer to Appendix A for CCI edits.

Facility RVUs

Code	Work	PE Facility	MP	Total Facility
50396	2.09	1.11	0.18	3.38

Non-facility RVUs

Code	Work	PE Non-Facility	MP	Total Non-Facility
50396	2.09	1.11	0.18	3.38

Modifiers (PAR)

Code	Mod 50	Mod 51	Mod 62	Mod 66	Mod 80
50396	1	2	0	0	0

Global Period

Code	Days
50396	000

50400-50405

50400 Pyeloplasty (Foley Y-pyeloplasty), plastic operation on renal pelvis, with or without plastic operation on ureter, nephropexy, nephrostomy, pyelostomy, or ureteral splinting; simple

50405 Pyeloplasty (Foley Y-pyeloplasty), plastic operation on renal pelvis, with or without plastic operation on ureter, nephropexy, nephrostomy, pyelostomy, or ureteral splinting; complicated (congenital kidney abnormality, secondary pyeloplasty, solitary kidney, calycoplasty)

(For laparoscopic approach, use 50544)

AMA Coding Notes

Surgical Procedures on the Urinary System

(For provision of chemotherapeutic agents, report both the specific service in addition to code(s) for the specific substance(s) or drug(s) provided)

AMA *CPT® Assistant*

50400: Nov 99: 25, May 00: 4, Oct 01: 8

50405: Nov 99: 25, May 00: 4, Oct 01: 8

Plain English Description

Pyeloplasty is a plastic operation on the kidney typically performed to treat congenital high insertion of the ureter into the renal pelvis with obstruction. Foley Y-pyeloplasty, one of the more common surgical techniques, is described here. A skin incision is made over the kidney. Gerota's fascia is incised and perirenal fat is dissected. Blood vessels are identified and controlled by placing a loop around each vessel. The kidney and ureter are exposed and visually examined. Because of the upper urinary tract obstruction, the renal pelvis is typically extremely dilated. A Y-shaped incision is made in the dilated renal pelvis beginning with an anterior incision at the ureteropelvic junction that is extended laterally and downward toward the hilum of the kidney, creating the first arm of the Y incision. A posterior incision is then made in the renal pelvis in the same fashion, creating the second arm of the Y. Next, the ureter is incised longitudinally in the lateral aspect, which is the side facing the renal pelvis. The renal pelvis flap is trimmed as needed. Prior to repositioning and anastomosis of the ureter, a nephrostomy or pyelostomy tube may be placed and/or a ureteral splint (stent) may be introduced to maintain the diameter of the ureter. The ureter is then positioned along the incision lines in the renal pelvis and anastomosed. Drains are placed as needed and the operative wound is closed around the drains. Use 50400 for a simple pyeloplasty. Use 50405 when the procedure is complicated by other congenital kidney abnormalities, or previous surgery on the kidney or ureter such as a previous pyeloplasty or repair of the renal calyces (calycoplasty).

Pyeloplasty (Foley Y-pyeloplasty) plastic operation on renal pelvis

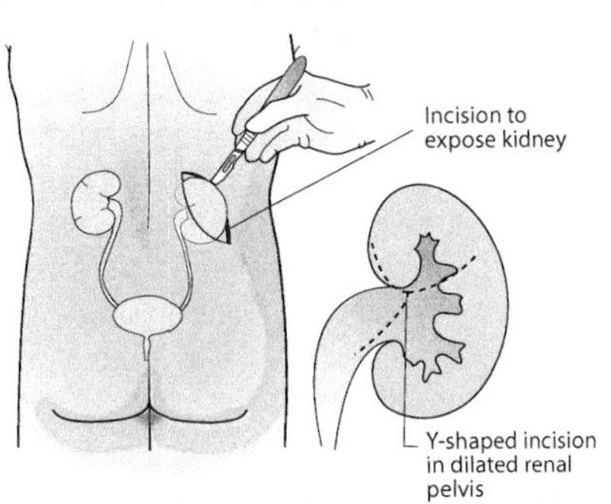

Simple (50400); complicated (50405)

ICD-10-CM Diagnostic Codes

N11.1	Chronic obstructive pyelonephritis
N13.0	Hydronephrosis with ureteropelvic junction obstruction
N13.1	Hydronephrosis with ureteral stricture, not elsewhere classified
N13.2	Hydronephrosis with renal and ureteral calculous obstruction
N13.39	Other hydronephrosis
N13.4	Hydroureter
N13.5	Crossing vessel and stricture of ureter without hydronephrosis
N13.71	Vesicoureteral-reflux without reflux nephropathy
N13.721	Vesicoureteral-reflux with reflux nephropathy without hydroureter, unilateral
N13.722	Vesicoureteral-reflux with reflux nephropathy without hydroureter, bilateral
N13.731	Vesicoureteral-reflux with reflux nephropathy with hydroureter, unilateral
N13.732	Vesicoureteral-reflux with reflux nephropathy with hydroureter, bilateral
N13.8	Other obstructive and reflux uropathy
N20.0	Calculus of kidney
N20.1	Calculus of ureter
N20.2	Calculus of kidney with calculus of ureter
N28.83	Nephroptosis
Q62.0	Congenital hydronephrosis
Q62.11	Congenital occlusion of ureteropelvic junction
Q62.12	Congenital occlusion of ureterovesical orifice
Q62.2	Congenital megaureter
Q62.31	Congenital ureterocele, orthotopic
Q62.39	Other obstructive defects of renal pelvis and ureter
Q62.5	Duplication of ureter
Q62.61	Deviation of ureter
Q62.62	Displacement of ureter
Q62.63	Anomalous implantation of ureter
Q62.69	Other malposition of ureter
Q62.7	Congenital vesico-uretero-renal reflux
Q62.8	Other congenital malformations of ureter
Q63.1	Lobulated, fused and horseshoe kidney
Q63.2	Ectopic kidney
Q63.3	Hyperplastic and giant kidney
Q63.8	Other specified congenital malformations of kidney

CCI Edits

Refer to Appendix A for CCI edits.

Facility RVUs

Code	Work	PE Facility	MP	Total Facility
50400	21.27	9.92	2.54	33.73
50405	25.86	11.76	3.06	40.68

Non-facility RVUs

Code	Work	PE Non-Facility	MP	Total Non-Facility
50400	21.27	9.92	2.54	33.73
50405	25.86	11.76	3.06	40.68

Modifiers (PAR)

Code	Mod 50	Mod 51	Mod 62	Mod 66	Mod 80
50400	1	2	1	0	2
50405	1	2	1	0	2

Global Period

Code	Days
50400	090
50405	090

CPT® Procedural Coding

50430-50431

50430 Injection procedure for antegrade nephrostogram and/or ureterogram, complete diagnostic procedure including imaging guidance (eg, ultrasound and fluoroscopy) and all associated radiological supervision and interpretation; new access

50431 Injection procedure for antegrade nephrostogram and/or ureterogram, complete diagnostic procedure including imaging guidance (eg, ultrasound and fluoroscopy) and all associated radiological supervision and interpretation; existing access

(Do not report 50430, 50431 in conjunction with 50432, 50433, 50434, 50435, 50693, 50694, 50695, 74425 for the same renal collecting system and/or associated ureter)

AMA Coding Guideline

Other Renal Introduction (Injection/Change/Removal) Procedures

Percutaneous genitourinary procedures are performed with imaging guidance (eg, fluoroscopy and/or ultrasound). Diagnostic nephrostogram and/or ureterogram are typically performed with percutaneous genitourinary procedures and are included in 50432, 50433, 50434, 50435, 50436, 50437, 50693, 50694, 50695.

Code 50436 describes enlargement of an existing percutaneous tract to the renal collecting system to accommodate large instruments used in an endourologic procedure. Code 50436 includes predilation urinary tract imaging, postprocedure nephrostomy tube placement, when performed, and includes all radiological supervision and interpretation and imaging guidance (eg, ultrasound, fluoroscopy). Code 50436 may not be reported with 50432, 50433, 52334 for basic dilation of a percutaneous tract during initial placement of a catheter or device.

Code 50437 includes all elements of 50436, but also includes new access into the renal collecting system performed in the same session when a pre-existing tract is not present.

Codes 50430 and 50431 are diagnostic procedure codes that include injection(s) of contrast material, all associated radiological supervision and interpretation, and procedural imaging guidance (eg, ultrasound and/or fluoroscopy). Code 50430 also includes accessing the collecting system and/or associated ureter with a needle and/or catheter. Codes 50430 or 50431 may not be reported together with 50432, 50433, 50434, 50435, 50693, 50694, 50695.

Codes 50432, 50433, 50434, 50435 represent therapeutic procedures describing catheter placement or exchange, and include the elements of access, drainage catheter manipulations, and imaging guidance (eg, ultrasonography and/or fluoroscopy), as well as diagnostic imaging supervision and interpretation, when performed.

Code 50433 describes percutaneous nephrostomy with the additional accessing of the ureter/bladder to ultimately place a nephroureteral catheter (a single transnephric catheter with nephrostomy and ureteral components that allows drainage internally, externally, or both).

For codes 50430, 50431, 50432, 50433, 50434, 50435,50606, 50693, 50694, 50695, 50705, and 50706, the renal pelvis and its associated ureter are considered a single entity for reporting purposes. Codes 50430, 50431, 50432, 50433, 50434, 50435, 50606, 50693, 50694, 50695, 50705, and 50706 may be reported once for each renal collecting system/ureter accessed (eg, two separate codes would be reported for bilateral nephrostomy tube placement or for unilateral duplicated collecting system/ureter requiring two separate procedures).

AMA Coding Notes

Surgical Procedures on the Urinary System

(For provision of chemotherapeutic agents, report both the specific service in addition to code(s) for the specific substance(s) or drug(s) provided)

AMA *CPT® Assistant* ▢

50430: Oct 15: 5, Jan 16: 3
50431: Oct 15: 5, Jan 16: 3

Plain English Description

Antegrade nephrostogram and/or ureterogram is performed to visualize the kidney and/or ureter and detect urinary tract obstruction caused by strictures, stones, blood clots, or tumors, or to assess kidney and ureter function prior to or following surgical treatment. When a nephrostomy or pyelostomy tube is already in place, this procedure may be performed to check for tube patency, blockage, or leakage. To establish a new access, the patient is positioned prone, a local anesthetic is injected, and a needle is inserted and advanced to the ureter/renal pelvis under ultrasound and/or fluoroscopic guidance. Contrast dye is injected and a series of X-rays are taken to visualize movement through the tube and urinary tract. A thin wire may be threaded through the needle to facilitate placement of a catheter or nephrostomy tube. The needle and wire are then removed. If placement of a catheter/tube is not indicated, the needle is simply removed after completion of the procedure. To perform the nephrostogram/ureterogram through an existing access, the tube and surrounding skin are first washed with an antibacterial solution and contrast is injected through the catheter/tube. A series of X-rays are taken to monitor and record the movement of contrast through the tube and the urinary tract. At the conclusion of the study, the catheter/tube may be plugged or connected to drainage. These codes include the injection, imaging guidance, and associated radiologic supervision and interpretation for new access in 50430 or an existing access in 50431.

ICD-10-CM Diagnostic Codes

	Code	Description
⇄	C64.1	Malignant neoplasm of right kidney, except renal pelvis
⇄	C64.2	Malignant neoplasm of left kidney, except renal pelvis
⇄	C65.1	Malignant neoplasm of right renal pelvis
⇄	C65.2	Malignant neoplasm of left renal pelvis
⇄	C66.1	Malignant neoplasm of right ureter
⇄	C66.2	Malignant neoplasm of left ureter
⇄	C79.01	Secondary malignant neoplasm of right kidney and renal pelvis
⇄	C79.02	Secondary malignant neoplasm of left kidney and renal pelvis
	C79.19	Secondary malignant neoplasm of other urinary organs
	C7A.093	Malignant carcinoid tumor of the kidney
	D09.19	Carcinoma in situ of other urinary organs
⇄	D30.01	Benign neoplasm of right kidney
⇄	D30.02	Benign neoplasm of left kidney
⇄	D30.11	Benign neoplasm of right renal pelvis
⇄	D30.12	Benign neoplasm of left renal pelvis
⇄	D30.21	Benign neoplasm of right ureter
⇄	D30.22	Benign neoplasm of left ureter
	D3A.093	Benign carcinoid tumor of the kidney
	D41	Neoplasm of uncertain behavior of urinary organs
⇄	D41.01	Neoplasm of uncertain behavior of right kidney
⇄	D41.02	Neoplasm of uncertain behavior of left kidney
⇄	D41.11	Neoplasm of uncertain behavior of right renal pelvis
⇄	D41.12	Neoplasm of uncertain behavior of left renal pelvis
⇄	D41.21	Neoplasm of uncertain behavior of right ureter
⇄	D41.22	Neoplasm of uncertain behavior of left ureter
	E08.21	Diabetes mellitus due to underlying condition with diabetic nephropathy
	E09.21	Drug or chemical induced diabetes mellitus with diabetic nephropathy
	E10.21	Type 1 diabetes mellitus with diabetic nephropathy
	E11.21	Type 2 diabetes mellitus with diabetic nephropathy
	E13.21	Other specified diabetes mellitus with diabetic nephropathy
	E85.0	Non-neuropathic heredofamilial amyloidosis
	E85.81	Light chain (AL) amyloidosis

● New ▲ Revised ✚ Add On ⊘Modifier 51 Exempt ★Telemedicine ▢ CPT QuickRef ⁄⁄FDA Pending ⇄ Laterality ❼ Seventh Character ♂Male ♀Female

E85.82 Wild-type transthyretin-related (ATTR) amyloidosis
M31.0 Hypersensitivity angiitis
M31.31 Wegener's granulomatosis with renal involvement
M32 Systemic lupus erythematosus (SLE)
M32.14 Glomerular disease in systemic lupus erythematosus
M32.15 Tubulo-interstitial nephropathy in systemic lupus erythematosus
M35.04 Sjögren syndrome with tubulo-interstitial nephropathy
N08 Glomerular disorders in diseases classified elsewhere
N11.0 Nonobstructive reflux-associated chronic pyelonephritis
N11.1 Chronic obstructive pyelonephritis
N11.8 Other chronic tubulo-interstitial nephritis
N13.0 Hydronephrosis with ureteropelvic junction obstruction
N13.1 Hydronephrosis with ureteral stricture, not elsewhere classified
N13.2 Hydronephrosis with renal and ureteral calculous obstruction
N13.39 Other hydronephrosis
N13.4 Hydroureter
N13.5 Crossing vessel and stricture of ureter without hydronephrosis
N13.71 Vesicoureteral-reflux without reflux nephropathy
N13.721 Vesicoureteral-reflux with reflux nephropathy without hydroureter, unilateral
N13.722 Vesicoureteral-reflux with reflux nephropathy without hydroureter, bilateral
N13.731 Vesicoureteral-reflux with reflux nephropathy with hydroureter, unilateral
N13.732 Vesicoureteral-reflux with reflux nephropathy with hydroureter, bilateral
N13.8 Other obstructive and reflux uropathy
N13.9 Obstructive and reflux uropathy, unspecified
N16 Renal tubulo-interstitial disorders in diseases classified elsewhere
N19 Unspecified kidney failure
N20.0 Calculus of kidney
N20.1 Calculus of ureter
N20.2 Calculus of kidney with calculus of ureter
N22 Calculus of urinary tract in diseases classified elsewhere
N23 Unspecified renal colic
N25.89 Other disorders resulting from impaired renal tubular function
N27.0 Small kidney, unilateral
N27.1 Small kidney, bilateral
N27.9 Small kidney, unspecified
N28.0 Ischemia and infarction of kidney
N28.1 Cyst of kidney, acquired
N28.81 Hypertrophy of kidney
N28.82 Megaloureter
N28.84 Pyelitis cystica
N28.85 Pyeloureteritis cystica
N28.86 Ureteritis cystica
N28.89 Other specified disorders of kidney and ureter
N29 Other disorders of kidney and ureter in diseases classified elsewhere
N99.0 Postprocedural (acute) (chronic) kidney failure
N99.71 Accidental puncture and laceration of a genitourinary system organ or structure during a genitourinary system procedure
N99.72 Accidental puncture and laceration of a genitourinary system organ or structure during other procedure
N99.820 Postprocedural hemorrhage of a genitourinary system organ or structure following a genitourinary system procedure
N99.821 Postprocedural hemorrhage of a genitourinary system organ or structure following other procedure
N99.840 Postprocedural hematoma of a genitourinary system organ or structure following a genitourinary system procedure
N99.841 Postprocedural hematoma of a genitourinary system organ or structure following other procedure
N99.842 Postprocedural seroma of a genitourinary system organ or structure following a genitourinary system procedure
N99.843 Postprocedural seroma of a genitourinary system organ or structure following other procedure
N99.89 Other postprocedural complications and disorders of genitourinary system
Q60.3 Renal hypoplasia, unilateral
Q60.4 Renal hypoplasia, bilateral
Q60.6 Potter's syndrome
Q61.01 Congenital single renal cyst
Q61.02 Congenital multiple renal cysts
Q61.11 Cystic dilatation of collecting ducts
Q61.19 Other polycystic kidney, infantile type
Q61.2 Polycystic kidney, adult type
Q61.3 Polycystic kidney, unspecified
Q61.4 Renal dysplasia
Q61.5 Medullary cystic kidney
Q61.8 Other cystic kidney diseases
Q61.9 Cystic kidney disease, unspecified
Q62.0 Congenital hydronephrosis
Q62.11 Congenital occlusion of ureteropelvic junction
Q62.12 Congenital occlusion of ureterovesical orifice
Q62.2 Congenital megaureter
Q62.31 Congenital ureterocele, orthotopic
Q62.32 Cecoureterocele
Q62.39 Other obstructive defects of renal pelvis and ureter
Q62.4 Agenesis of ureter
Q62.5 Duplication of ureter
Q62.61 Deviation of ureter
Q62.62 Displacement of ureter
Q62.63 Anomalous implantation of ureter
Q62.69 Other malposition of ureter
Q62.8 Other congenital malformations of ureter
Q63.8 Other specified congenital malformations of kidney

CCI Edits

Refer to Appendix A for CCI edits.

Pub 100

50430: Pub 100-03, 1, 220.5
50431: Pub 100-03, 1, 220.5

Facility RVUs ▢

Code	Work	PE Facility	MP	Total Facility
50430	2.90	1.27	0.28	4.45
50431	1.10	0.69	0.10	1.89

Non-facility RVUs ▢

Code	Work	PE Non-Facility	MP	Total Non-Facility
50430	2.90	16.23	0.28	19.41
50431	1.10	8.78	0.10	9.98

Modifiers (PAR) ▢

Code	Mod 50	Mod 51	Mod 62	Mod 66	Mod 80
50430	1	2	0	0	0
50431	1	2	0	0	1

Global Period

Code	Days
50430	000
50431	000

50432-50433

50432 Placement of nephrostomy catheter, percutaneous, including diagnostic nephrostogram and/or ureterogram when performed, imaging guidance (eg, ultrasound and/or fluoroscopy) and all associated radiological supervision and interpretation

(Do not report 50432 in conjunction with 50430, 50431, 50433, 50436, 50437, 50694, 50695, 74425, for the same renal collecting system and/or associated ureter)

(Do not report 50432 in conjunction with 50436, 50437, for dilation of the nephrostomy tube tract)

50433 Placement of nephroureteral catheter, percutaneous, including diagnostic nephrostogram and/or ureterogram when performed, imaging guidance (eg, ultrasound and/or fluoroscopy) and all associated radiological supervision and interpretation, new access

(Do not report 50433 in conjunction with 50430, 50431, 50432, 50693, 50694, 50695, 74425 for the same renal collecting system and/or associated ureter)

(Do not report 50433 in conjunction with 50436, 50437, for dilation of the nephroureteral catheter tract)

(For nephroureteral catheter removal and replacement, use 50387)

AMA Coding Guideline

Other Renal Introduction (Injection/Change/Removal) Procedures

Percutaneous genitourinary procedures are performed with imaging guidance (eg, fluoroscopy and/or ultrasound). Diagnostic nephrostogram and/or ureterogram are typically performed with percutaneous genitourinary procedures and are included in 50432, 50433, 50434, 50435, 50436, 50437, 50693, 50694, 50695.

Code 50436 describes enlargement of an existing percutaneous tract to the renal collecting system to accommodate large instruments used in an endourologic procedure. Code 50436 includes predilation urinary tract imaging, postprocedure nephrostomy tube placement, when performed, and includes all radiological supervision and interpretation and imaging guidance (eg, ultrasound, fluoroscopy). Code 50436 may not be reported with 50432, 50433, 52334 for basic dilation of a percutaneous tract during initial placement of a catheter or device.

Code 50437 includes all elements of 50436, but also includes new access into the renal collecting system performed in the same session when a pre-existing tract is not present.

Codes 50430 and 50431 are diagnostic procedure codes that include injection(s) of contrast material, all associated radiological supervision and interpretation, and procedural imaging guidance (eg, ultrasound and/or fluoroscopy). Code 50430 also includes accessing the collecting system and/or associated ureter with a needle and/or catheter. Codes 50430 or 50431 may not be reported together with 50432, 50433, 50434, 50435, 50693, 50694, 50695.

Codes 50432, 50433, 50434, 50435 represent therapeutic procedures describing catheter placement or exchange, and include the elements of access, drainage catheter manipulations, and imaging guidance (eg, ultrasonography and/or fluoroscopy), as well as diagnostic imaging supervision and interpretation, when performed. Code 50433 describes percutaneous nephrostomy with the additional accessing of the ureter/bladder to ultimately place a nephroureteral catheter (a single transnephric catheter with nephrostomy and ureteral components that allows drainage internally, externally, or both).

For codes 50430, 50431, 50432, 50433, 50434, 50435,50606, 50693, 50694, 50695, 50705, and 50706, the renal pelvis and its associated ureter are considered a single entity for reporting purposes. Codes 50430, 50431, 50432, 50433, 50434, 50435, 50606, 50693, 50694, 50695, 50705, and 50706 may be reported once for each renal collecting system/ureter accessed (eg, two separate codes would be reported for bilateral nephrostomy tube placement or for unilateral duplicated collecting system/ureter requiring two separate procedures).

AMA Coding Notes

Surgical Procedures on the Urinary System

(For provision of chemotherapeutic agents, report both the specific service in addition to code(s) for the specific substance(s) or drug(s) provided)

AMA *CPT® Assistant* ◻

50432: Oct 15: 5, Jan 16: 3, Mar 18: 11
50433: Oct 15: 5, Jan 16: 3, Mar 18: 11

Plain English Description

Percutaneous placement of a nephrostomy catheter (50432) or nephroureteral catheter (50433) is performed to treat urinary obstruction caused by stones, tumors, or strictures; diagnose urinary conditions; provide access for therapeutic interventions; or divert urine in the presence of traumatic injury, leaks, fistulas, or hemorrhagic cystitis. A single or double needle technique may be employed. Under ultrasound and/or fluoroscopic guidance, a single trocar or Chiba needle is inserted below the 12th rib to minimize the risk of puncturing the pleura. The needle is advanced into the posterior mid or lower pole calyx and urine is aspirated to verify location and decompress the system. Contrast dye is injected and a series of X-rays are taken to visualize movement of dye through the urinary tract. Once satisfactory placement of the needle has been established, a thin wire is threaded through the needle into the proximal ureter (nephroureteral) or upper pole of the calyx (nephrostomy). A self-restraining nephrostomy or nephroureteral catheter is inserted over the wire and the wire is then removed. For double needle technique, the first needle is inserted directly into the renal pelvis and contrast dye is injected to obtain a series of X-rays. A small amount of air or CO2 may be injected after the contrast to enhance visualization of the posterior calyces. A clamp applied to the skin is used to mark the entry site of the second needle placed under the 12th rib in the posterior axillary line. The insertion of the second needle and placement of the catheter are identical to the single needle technique. The first needle is removed at the end of the procedure. These codes include the percutaneous placement of the catheter, any diagnostic nephrostogram and/or ureterogram, the imaging guidance, and all associated radiologic supervision and interpretation.

ICD-10-CM Diagnostic Codes

⇄	C64.1	Malignant neoplasm of right kidney, except renal pelvis
⇄	C64.2	Malignant neoplasm of left kidney, except renal pelvis
⇄	C65.1	Malignant neoplasm of right renal pelvis
⇄	C65.2	Malignant neoplasm of left renal pelvis
⇄	C66.1	Malignant neoplasm of right ureter
⇄	C66.2	Malignant neoplasm of left ureter
⇄	C79.01	Secondary malignant neoplasm of right kidney and renal pelvis
⇄	C79.02	Secondary malignant neoplasm of left kidney and renal pelvis
	C79.19	Secondary malignant neoplasm of other urinary organs
	C7A.093	Malignant carcinoid tumor of the kidney
	D09.19	Carcinoma in situ of other urinary organs
⇄	D30.01	Benign neoplasm of right kidney
⇄	D30.02	Benign neoplasm of left kidney
⇄	D30.11	Benign neoplasm of right renal pelvis
⇄	D30.12	Benign neoplasm of left renal pelvis
⇄	D30.21	Benign neoplasm of right ureter
⇄	D30.22	Benign neoplasm of left ureter
	D3A.093	Benign carcinoid tumor of the kidney
⇄	D41.01	Neoplasm of uncertain behavior of right kidney
⇄	D41.02	Neoplasm of uncertain behavior of left kidney
⇄	D41.11	Neoplasm of uncertain behavior of right renal pelvis
⇄	D41.12	Neoplasm of uncertain behavior of left renal pelvis

⇄ D41.21 Neoplasm of uncertain behavior of right ureter
⇄ D41.22 Neoplasm of uncertain behavior of left ureter
M35.04 Sjögren syndrome with tubulo-interstitial nephropathy
N08 Glomerular disorders in diseases classified elsewhere
N10 Acute pyelonephritis
N11.0 Nonobstructive reflux-associated chronic pyelonephritis
N11.1 Chronic obstructive pyelonephritis
N11.8 Other chronic tubulo-interstitial nephritis
N12 Tubulo-interstitial nephritis, not specified as acute or chronic
N13.0 Hydronephrosis with ureteropelvic junction obstruction
N13.1 Hydronephrosis with ureteral stricture, not elsewhere classified
N13.2 Hydronephrosis with renal and ureteral calculous obstruction
N13.3 Other and unspecified hydronephrosis
N13.4 Hydroureter
N13.5 Crossing vessel and stricture of ureter without hydronephrosis
N13.6 Pyonephrosis
N13.721 Vesicoureteral-reflux with reflux nephropathy without hydroureter, unilateral
N13.722 Vesicoureteral-reflux with reflux nephropathy without hydroureter, bilateral
N13.731 Vesicoureteral-reflux with reflux nephropathy with hydroureter, unilateral
N13.732 Vesicoureteral-reflux with reflux nephropathy with hydroureter, bilateral
N13.8 Other obstructive and reflux uropathy
N15.1 Renal and perinephric abscess
N15.8 Other specified renal tubulo-interstitial diseases
N16 Renal tubulo-interstitial disorders in diseases classified elsewhere
N20 Calculus of kidney and ureter
N20.0 Calculus of kidney
N20.1 Calculus of ureter
N20.2 Calculus of kidney with calculus of ureter
N22 Calculus of urinary tract in diseases classified elsewhere
N25.89 Other disorders resulting from impaired renal tubular function
N28.82 Megaloureter
N28.84 Pyelitis cystica
N28.85 Pyeloureteritis cystica
N28.86 Ureteritis cystica
N28.89 Other specified disorders of kidney and ureter
N99.89 Other postprocedural complications and disorders of genitourinary system
Q61.01 Congenital single renal cyst
Q61.02 Congenital multiple renal cysts
Q61.11 Cystic dilatation of collecting ducts
Q61.19 Other polycystic kidney, infantile type
Q61.2 Polycystic kidney, adult type
Q61.5 Medullary cystic kidney
Q61.8 Other cystic kidney diseases
Q62.0 Congenital hydronephrosis
Q62.11 Congenital occlusion of ureteropelvic junction
Q62.12 Congenital occlusion of ureterovesical orifice
Q62.2 Congenital megaureter
Q62.39 Other obstructive defects of renal pelvis and ureter
Q62.5 Duplication of ureter
Q62.61 Deviation of ureter
Q62.62 Displacement of ureter
Q62.63 Anomalous implantation of ureter
Q62.69 Other malposition of ureter
Q62.8 Other congenital malformations of ureter

CCI Edits

Refer to Appendix A for CCI edits.

Facility RVUs ▯

Code	Work	PE Facility	MP	Total Facility
50432	4.00	1.56	0.35	5.91
50433	5.05	1.83	0.45	7.33

Non-facility RVUs ▯

Code	Work	PE Non-Facility	MP	Total Non-Facility
50432	4.00	23.66	0.35	28.01
50433	5.05	29.40	0.45	34.90

Modifiers (PAR) ▯

Code	Mod 50	Mod 51	Mod 62	Mod 66	Mod 80
50432	1	2	0	0	1
50433	1	2	0	0	1

Global Period

Code	Days
50432	000
50433	000

50434-50435

50434 Convert nephrostomy catheter to nephroureteral catheter, percutaneous, including diagnostic nephrostogram and/or ureterogram when performed, imaging guidance (eg, ultrasound and/or fluoroscopy) and all associated radiological supervision and interpretation, via pre-existing nephrostomy tract

(Do not report 50434 in conjunction with 50430, 50431, 50435, 50684, 50693, 74425 for the same renal collecting system and/or associated ureter)

50435 Exchange nephrostomy catheter, percutaneous, including diagnostic nephrostogram and/or ureterogram when performed, imaging guidance (eg, ultrasound and/or fluoroscopy) and all associated radiological supervision and interpretation

(Do not report 50435 in conjunction with 50430, 50431, 50434, 50693, 74425 for the same renal collecting system and/or associated ureter)

(For removal of nephrostomy catheter requiring fluoroscopic guidance, use 50389)

AMA Coding Guideline

Other Renal Introduction (Injection/ Change/Removal) Procedures

Percutaneous genitourinary procedures are performed with imaging guidance (eg, fluoroscopy and/or ultrasound). Diagnostic nephrostogram and/or ureterogram are typically performed with percutaneous genitourinary procedures and are included in 50432, 50433, 50434, 50435, 50436, 50437, 50693, 50694, 50695.

Code 50436 describes enlargement of an existing percutaneous tract to the renal collecting system to accommodate large instruments used in an endourologic procedure. Code 50436 includes predilation urinary tract imaging, postprocedure nephrostomy tube placement, when performed, and includes all radiological supervision and interpretation and imaging guidance (eg, ultrasound, fluoroscopy). Code 50436 may not be reported with 50432, 50433, 52334 for basic dilation of a percutaneous tract during initial placement of a catheter or device.

Code 50437 includes all elements of 50436, but also includes new access into the renal collecting system performed in the same session when a pre-existing tract is not present.

Codes 50430 and 50431 are diagnostic procedure codes that include injection(s) of contrast material, all associated radiological supervision and interpretation, and procedural imaging guidance (eg, ultrasound and/or fluoroscopy). Code 50430 also includes accessing the collecting system and/ or associated ureter with a needle and/or catheter. Codes 50430 or 50431 may not be reported together with 50432, 50433, 50434, 50435, 50693, 50694, 50695.

Codes 50432, 50433, 50434, 50435 represent therapeutic procedures describing catheter placement or exchange, and include the elements of access, drainage catheter manipulations, and imaging guidance (eg, ultrasonography and/ or fluoroscopy), as well as diagnostic imaging supervision and interpretation, when performed.

Code 50433 describes percutaneous nephrostomy with the additional accessing of the ureter/bladder to ultimately place a nephroureteral catheter (a single transnephric catheter with nephrostomy and ureteral components that allows drainage internally, externally, or both).

For codes 50430, 50431, 50432, 50433, 50434, 50435,50606, 50693, 50694, 50695, 50705, and 50706, the renal pelvis and its associated ureter are considered a single entity for reporting purposes. Codes 50430, 50431, 50432, 50433, 50434, 50435, 50606, 50693, 50694, 50695, 50705, and 50706 may be reported once for each renal collecting system/ureter accessed (eg, two separate codes would be reported for bilateral nephrostomy tube placement or for unilateral duplicated collecting system/ureter requiring two separate procedures).

AMA Coding Notes

Surgical Procedures on the Urinary System

(For provision of chemotherapeutic agents, report both the specific service in addition to code(s) for the specific substance(s) or drug(s) provided)

AMA *CPT® Assistant* ▯

50434: Oct 15: 5, Jan 16: 3
50435: Oct 15: 5, Jan 16: 3, Mar 18: 11

Plain English Description

A procedure is performed to convert an existing percutaneous nephrostomy catheter to a nephroureteral catheter (50434) or to exchange an existing nephrostomy catheter with a new catheter (50435). A nephrostomy or nephroureteral catheter may be used to restore or maintain the flow of urine through the kidney/ ureter when strictures, leaks, or fistulas are present. With the patient positioned prone, contrast dye may be injected through the existing catheter and a series of X-rays taken to monitor contrast movement through the tube and urinary tract. For conversion to a nephroureteral catheter, a guidewire is inserted through the exiting nephrostomy catheter into the kidney and advanced into the proximal ureter. The catheter is then removed and a new catheter is inserted over the guidewire and advanced to the new position. Once placement has been confirmed with fluoroscopy, the guidewire is removed. For nephrostomy catheter exchange, a guidewire is advanced through the catheter into the renal pelvis. The old catheter is removed over the guidewire and replaced with a new catheter. Once the position has been confirmed with fluoroscopy, the guidewire is removed. These codes include any diagnostic nephrostogram and/or ureterogram, imaging guidance, and associated radiologic supervision and interpretation.

ICD-10-CM Diagnostic Codes

	Code	Description
⇄	C64.1	Malignant neoplasm of right kidney, except renal pelvis
⇄	C64.2	Malignant neoplasm of left kidney, except renal pelvis
⇄	C65.1	Malignant neoplasm of right renal pelvis
⇄	C65.2	Malignant neoplasm of left renal pelvis
⇄	C66.1	Malignant neoplasm of right ureter
⇄	C66.2	Malignant neoplasm of left ureter
⇄	C79.01	Secondary malignant neoplasm of right kidney and renal pelvis
⇄	C79.02	Secondary malignant neoplasm of left kidney and renal pelvis
	C79.19	Secondary malignant neoplasm of other urinary organs
	C7A.093	Malignant carcinoid tumor of the kidney
	D09.19	Carcinoma in situ of other urinary organs
⇄	D30.01	Benign neoplasm of right kidney
⇄	D30.02	Benign neoplasm of left kidney
⇄	D30.11	Benign neoplasm of right renal pelvis
⇄	D30.12	Benign neoplasm of left renal pelvis
⇄	D30.21	Benign neoplasm of right ureter
⇄	D30.22	Benign neoplasm of left ureter
	D3A.093	Benign carcinoid tumor of the kidney
⇄	D41.01	Neoplasm of uncertain behavior of right kidney
⇄	D41.02	Neoplasm of uncertain behavior of left kidney
⇄	D41.11	Neoplasm of uncertain behavior of right renal pelvis
⇄	D41.12	Neoplasm of uncertain behavior of left renal pelvis
⇄	D41.21	Neoplasm of uncertain behavior of right ureter
⇄	D41.22	Neoplasm of uncertain behavior of left ureter
	N11.0	Nonobstructive reflux-associated chronic pyelonephritis
	N11.1	Chronic obstructive pyelonephritis
	N11.8	Other chronic tubulo-interstitial nephritis
	N13.0	Hydronephrosis with ureteropelvic junction obstruction
	N13.1	Hydronephrosis with ureteral stricture, not elsewhere classified
	N13.2	Hydronephrosis with renal and ureteral calculous obstruction
	N13.39	Other hydronephrosis

N13.4 Hydroureter
N13.5 Crossing vessel and stricture of ureter without hydronephrosis
N13.71 Vesicoureteral-reflux without reflux nephropathy
N13.721 Vesicoureteral-reflux with reflux nephropathy without hydroureter, unilateral
N13.722 Vesicoureteral-reflux with reflux nephropathy without hydroureter, bilateral
N13.731 Vesicoureteral-reflux with reflux nephropathy with hydroureter, unilateral
N13.732 Vesicoureteral-reflux with reflux nephropathy with hydroureter, bilateral
N13.8 Other obstructive and reflux uropathy
N20.0 Calculus of kidney
N20.1 Calculus of ureter
N20.2 Calculus of kidney with calculus of ureter
N28.82 Megaloureter
N28.84 Pyelitis cystica
N28.85 Pyeloureteritis cystica
N28.86 Ureteritis cystica
N28.89 Other specified disorders of kidney and ureter
Q61.01 Congenital single renal cyst
Q61.02 Congenital multiple renal cysts
Q61.11 Cystic dilatation of collecting ducts
Q61.19 Other polycystic kidney, infantile type
Q61.2 Polycystic kidney, adult type
Q61.3 Polycystic kidney, unspecified
Q61.4 Renal dysplasia
Q61.5 Medullary cystic kidney
Q61.8 Other cystic kidney diseases
Q62.0 Congenital hydronephrosis
Q62.11 Congenital occlusion of ureteropelvic junction
Q62.12 Congenital occlusion of ureterovesical orifice
Q62.2 Congenital megaureter
Q62.31 Congenital ureterocele, orthotopic
Q62.39 Other obstructive defects of renal pelvis and ureter
Q62.5 Duplication of ureter
Q62.61 Deviation of ureter
Q62.62 Displacement of ureter
Q62.63 Anomalous implantation of ureter
Q62.69 Other malposition of ureter
Q62.7 Congenital vesico-uretero-renal reflux
Q62.8 Other congenital malformations of ureter
❼ T83.012 Breakdown (mechanical) of nephrostomy catheter
❼ T83.022 Displacement of nephrostomy catheter
❼ T83.032 Leakage of nephrostomy catheter
❼ T83.092 Other mechanical complication of nephrostomy catheter
❼ T83.512 Infection and inflammatory reaction due to nephrostomy catheter
❼ T83.81 Embolism due to genitourinary prosthetic devices, implants and grafts
❼ T83.82 Fibrosis due to genitourinary prosthetic devices, implants and grafts
❼ T83.83 Hemorrhage due to genitourinary prosthetic devices, implants and grafts
❼ T83.84 Pain due to genitourinary prosthetic devices, implants and grafts
❼ T83.85 Stenosis due to genitourinary prosthetic devices, implants and grafts
❼ T83.86 Thrombosis due to genitourinary prosthetic devices, implants and grafts
❼ T83.89 Other specified complication of genitourinary prosthetic devices, implants and grafts

ICD-10-CM Coding Notes

For codes requiring a 7th character extension, refer to your ICD-10-CM book. Review the character descriptions and coding guidelines for proper selection. For some procedures, only certain characters will apply.

CCI Edits

Refer to Appendix A for CCI edits.

Facility RVUs ☐

Code	Work	PE Facility	MP	Total Facility
50434	3.75	1.42	0.34	5.51
50435	1.82	0.89	0.18	2.89

Non-facility RVUs ☐

Code	Work	PE Non-Facility	MP	Total Non-Facility
50434	3.75	23.98	0.34	28.07
50435	1.82	16.69	0.18	18.69

Modifiers (PAR) ☐

Code	Mod 50	Mod 51	Mod 62	Mod 66	Mod 80
50434	1	2	0	0	1
50435	1	2	0	0	1

Global Period

Code	Days
50434	000
50435	000

50436-50437

50436 Dilation of existing tract, percutaneous, for an endourologic procedure including imaging guidance (eg, ultrasound and/or fluoroscopy) and all associated radiological supervision and interpretation, with postprocedure tube placement, when performed

50437 Dilation of existing tract, percutaneous, for an endourologic procedure including imaging guidance (eg, ultrasound and/or fluoroscopy) and all associated radiological supervision and interpretation, with postprocedure tube placement, when performed; including new access into the renal collecting system

(For nephrostolithotomy, see 50080, 50081)

(For retrograde percutaneous nephrostomy, use 52334)

(For endoscopic surgery, see 50551-50561)

(Do not report 50436, 50437 in conjunction with 50080, 50081, 50382, 50384, 50430, 50431, 50432, 50433, 52334, 74485)

AMA Coding Guideline

Other Renal Introduction (Injection/Change/Removal) Procedures

Percutaneous genitourinary procedures are performed with imaging guidance (eg, fluoroscopy and/or ultrasound). Diagnostic nephrostogram and/or ureterogram are typically performed with percutaneous genitourinary procedures and are included in 50432, 50433, 50434, 50435, 50436, 50437, 50693, 50694, 50695.

Code 50436 describes enlargement of an existing percutaneous tract to the renal collecting system to accommodate large instruments used in an endourologic procedure. Code 50436 includes predilation urinary tract imaging, postprocedure nephrostomy tube placement, when performed, and includes all radiological supervision and interpretation and imaging guidance (eg, ultrasound, fluoroscopy). Code 50436 may not be reported with 50432, 50433, 52334 for basic dilation of a percutaneous tract during initial placement of a catheter or device.

Code 50437 includes all elements of 50436, but also includes new access into the renal collecting system performed in the same session when a pre-existing tract is not present.

Codes 50430 and 50431 are diagnostic procedure codes that include injection(s) of contrast material, all associated radiological supervision and interpretation, and procedural imaging guidance (eg, ultrasound and/or fluoroscopy). Code 50430 also includes accessing the collecting system and/or associated ureter with a needle and/or catheter. Codes 50430 or 50431 may not be reported together with 50432, 50433, 50434, 50435, 50693, 50694, 50695.

Codes 50432, 50433, 50434, 50435 represent therapeutic procedures describing catheter placement or exchange, and include the elements of access, drainage catheter manipulations, and imaging guidance (eg, ultrasonography and/or fluoroscopy), as well as diagnostic imaging supervision and interpretation, when performed.

Code 50433 describes percutaneous nephrostomy with the additional accessing of the ureter/bladder to ultimately place a nephroureteral catheter (a single transnephric catheter with nephrostomy and ureteral components that allows drainage internally, externally, or both).

For codes 50430, 50431, 50432, 50433, 50434, 50435,50606, 50693, 50694, 50695, 50705, and 50706, the renal pelvis and its associated ureter are considered a single entity for reporting purposes. Codes 50430, 50431, 50432, 50433, 50434, 50435, 50606, 50693, 50694, 50695, 50705, and 50706 may be reported once for each renal collecting system/ureter accessed (eg, two separate codes would be reported for bilateral nephrostomy tube placement or for unilateral duplicated collecting system/ureter requiring two separate procedures).

AMA Coding Notes

Surgical Procedures on the Urinary System

(For provision of chemotherapeutic agents, report both the specific service in addition to code(s) for the specific substance(s) or drug(s) provided)

Plain English Description

A percutaneous renal tract may exist to provide urine drainage or diversion from the kidney due to conditions such as obstruction, leaks, or stones. To dilate an existing percutaneous tract (50436), a guide catheter is inserted into the tract under ultrasound and/or fluoroscopic guidance and advanced to the selected renal calyx and intrarenal collecting system. Serial dilators are then introduced through the catheter until the desired diameter has been reached and the catheter is withdrawn. A nephrostomy tube may be placed through the tract to maintain patency, if indicated. New access into the renal collecting system may be necessary following percutaneous dilation of the existing tract (50437). A percutaneous access needle is placed through the skin of the back or flank and advanced to the posterior renal calyces. A catheter or nephrostomy tube is then passed through the needle, into the renal calyx and intrarenal collecting system under ultrasound and/or fluoroscopic guidance, and the needle is withdrawn. Codes 50436 and 50437 include all associated radiologic supervision and interpretation.

ICD-10-CM Diagnostic Codes

There are too many ICD-10-CM codes to list. Refer to ICD-10-CM code book for associated diagnostic codes.

CCI Edits

Refer to Appendix A for CCI edits.

Facility RVUs

Code	Work	PE Facility	MP	Total Facility
50436	2.78	1.31	0.27	4.36
50437	4.85	1.92	0.43	7.20

Non-facility RVUs

Code	Work	PE Non-Facility	MP	Total Non-Facility
50436	2.78	1.31	0.27	4.36
50437	4.85	1.92	0.43	7.20

Modifiers (PAR)

Code	Mod 50	Mod 51	Mod 62	Mod 66	Mod 80
50436	1	2	0	0	1
50437	1	2	0	0	1

Global Period

Code	Days
50436	000
50437	000

50500

50500 Nephrorrhaphy, suture of kidney wound or injury

AMA Coding Notes

Surgical Procedures on the Urinary System

(For provision of chemotherapeutic agents, report both the specific service in addition to code(s) for the specific substance(s) or drug(s) provided)

Plain English Description

The physician performs an open procedure to suture repair a wound or injury to the kidney. A flank incision is made, the injured kidney is exposed, and the area of the lesion is identified. The wound or injury is repaired with sutures. The operative site is irrigated and inspected for any additional injuries, which are also repaired. Any bleeding is controlled. Drains may be placed in the operative site and the surgical wound is closed around the drains.

Nephrorrhaphy, suture of kidney wound or injury

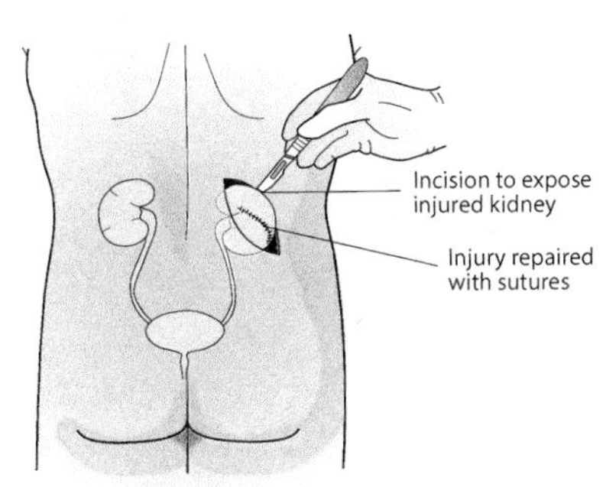

ICD-10-CM Diagnostic Codes

	Code	Description
	N99.71	Accidental puncture and laceration of a genitourinary system organ or structure during a genitourinary system procedure
	N99.72	Accidental puncture and laceration of a genitourinary system organ or structure during other procedure
⑦⇄	S37.031	Laceration of right kidney, unspecified degree
⑦⇄	S37.032	Laceration of left kidney, unspecified degree
⑦⇄	S37.041	Minor laceration of right kidney
⑦⇄	S37.042	Minor laceration of left kidney
⑦⇄	S37.051	Moderate laceration of right kidney
⑦⇄	S37.052	Moderate laceration of left kidney
⑦⇄	S37.061	Major laceration of right kidney
⑦⇄	S37.062	Major laceration of left kidney
⑦⇄	S37.091	Other injury of right kidney
⑦⇄	S37.092	Other injury of left kidney

ICD-10-CM Coding Notes

For codes requiring a 7th character extension, refer to your ICD-10-CM book. Review the character descriptions and coding guidelines for proper selection. For some procedures, only certain characters will apply.

CCI Edits

Refer to Appendix A for CCI edits.

Facility RVUs ☐

Code	Work	PE Facility	MP	Total Facility
50500	21.22	11.17	4.68	37.07

Non-facility RVUs ☐

Code	Work	PE Non-Facility	MP	Total Non-Facility
50500	21.22	11.17	4.68	37.07

Modifiers (PAR) ☐

Code	Mod 50	Mod 51	Mod 62	Mod 66	Mod 80
50500	0	2	1	0	2

Global Period

Code	Days
50500	090

50520

50520 Closure of nephrocutaneous or pyelocutaneous fistula

AMA Coding Notes

Surgical Procedures on the Urinary System

(For provision of chemotherapeutic agents, report both the specific service in addition to code(s) for the specific substance(s) or drug(s) provided)

Plain English Description

A fistulous (sinus) tract from the kidney or ureteropelvic junction (UPJ) leading out to the skin is surgically closed. Fistulous tracts are most often caused by kidney stones or tuberculosis, but may also be caused by injury during percutaneous procedures or lithotripsy. The termination site of the fistulous tract in the abdomen is identified by injecting the fistula with a radiopaque substance. Suture ligation is then used to close the open sinus tract, along with fulguration or injection of fibrin glue.

Closure of nephrocutaneous or pyelocutaneous fistula

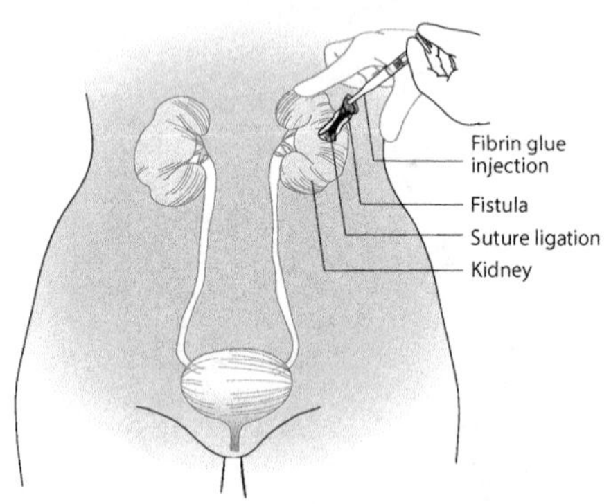

ICD-10-CM Diagnostic Codes

There are too many ICD-10-CM codes to list. Refer to ICD-10-CM code book for associated diagnostic codes.

CCI Edits

Refer to Appendix A for CCI edits.

Facility RVUs ▯

Code	Work	PE Facility	MP	Total Facility
50520	18.88	11.01	4.77	34.66

Non-facility RVUs ▯

Code	Work	PE Non-Facility	MP	Total Non-Facility
50520	18.88	11.01	4.77	34.66

Modifiers (PAR) ▯

Code	Mod 50	Mod 51	Mod 62	Mod 66	Mod 80
50520	0	2	1	0	2

Global Period

Code	Days
50520	090

50525-50526

50525 Closure of nephrovisceral fistula (eg, renocolic), including visceral repair; abdominal approach

50526 Closure of nephrovisceral fistula (eg, renocolic), including visceral repair; thoracic approach

AMA Coding Notes

Surgical Procedures on the Urinary System

(For provision of chemotherapeutic agents, report both the specific service in addition to code(s) for the specific substance(s) or drug(s) provided)

Plain English Description

A fistulous (sinus) tract from the kidney to another internal organ is closed and the involved organ is repaired as needed. Fistulous tracts are most often caused by renal stones or tuberculosis, but may also be caused by injury during percutaneous procedures or lithotripsy. An abdominal or thoracic surgical approach may be employed depending on the location of the fistulous tract. The kidney and ureter are exposed. A catheter is inserted into the ureter and a radiopaque substance injected to identify the fistulous tract. The fistula is followed down to where it enters the involved organ, such as the colon, and is suture ligated and divided. The involved organ is repaired. The origin of the fistula in the kidney is closed. Use 50525 for an abdominal approach and 50526 for a thoracic approach.

Closure of nephrovisceral fistula including visceral repair

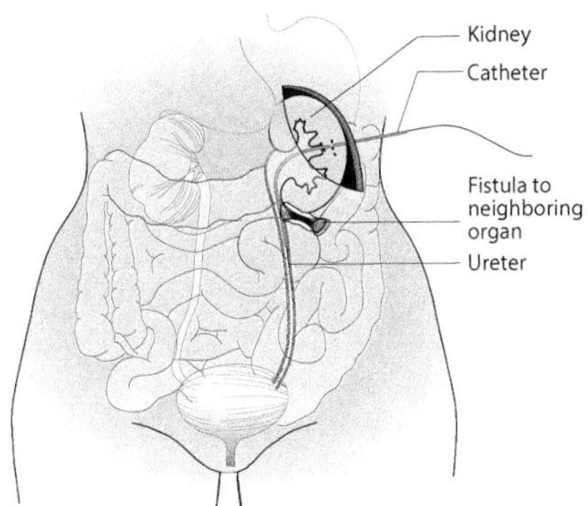

Abdominal approach (50525), or thoracic approach (50526)

ICD-10-CM Diagnostic Codes

N28.89 Other specified disorders of kidney and ureter

CCI Edits

Refer to Appendix A for CCI edits.

Facility RVUs

Code	Work	PE Facility	MP	Total Facility
50525	24.39	13.39	6.17	43.95
50526	26.31	14.10	6.64	47.05

Non-facility RVUs

Code	Work	PE Non-Facility	MP	Total Non-Facility
50525	24.39	13.39	6.17	43.95
50526	26.31	14.10	6.64	47.05

Modifiers (PAR)

Code	Mod 50	Mod 51	Mod 62	Mod 66	Mod 80
50525	0	2	1	0	2
50526	0	2	0	0	2

Global Period

Code	Days
50525	090
50526	090

50540

50540 Symphysiotomy for horseshoe kidney with or without pyeloplasty and/or other plastic procedure, unilateral or bilateral (1 operation)

AMA Coding Notes

Surgical Procedures on the Urinary System

(For provision of chemotherapeutic agents, report both the specific service in addition to code(s) for the specific substance(s) or drug(s) provided)

Plain English Description

The physician performs an open procedure to divide the isthmus (symphysiotomy) connecting the lower poles of a horseshoe kidney. A unilateral or bilateral pyeloplasty or other plastic repair of the kidney may also be performed. A horseshoe kidney is a type of renal fusion anomaly consisting of two distinct functioning kidneys connected at the lower poles by an isthmus of functioning renal or fibrous tissue at the midline. A midline abdominal incision is typically employed to allow access to both sides of the horseshoe kidney and its anomalous vasculature. The isthmus is dissected free of surrounding tissue and divided, taking care to preserve the vasculature to both sides of the horseshoe kidney. If the ureter is obstructed at the ureteropelvic junction (UPJ), a pyeloplasty or other plastic procedure is performed to treat the blockage or narrowing. The ureter and surrounding vascular structures are identified and retracted to expose the lower poles of the horseshoe kidney and the UPJ. The UPJ defect is repaired. One or both ureters may be repaired. A stent is then placed in the ureter bridging the repair to facilitate healing and allow drainage of urine. Drains are placed in the surgical wound. The site is irrigated and inspected, bleeding is controlled, surgical instruments are removed, and incisions are closed.

Symphysiotomy for horseshoe kidney with or without pyeloplasty

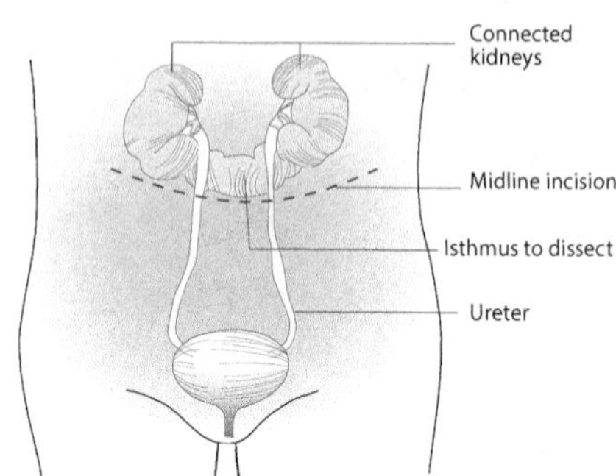

ICD-10-CM Diagnostic Codes

Q63.1 Lobulated, fused and horseshoe kidney

CCI Edits

Refer to Appendix A for CCI edits.

Facility RVUs ▯

Code	Work	PE Facility	MP	Total Facility
50540	21.10	9.86	2.50	33.46

Non-facility RVUs ▯

Code	Work	PE Non-Facility	MP	Total Non-Facility
50540	21.10	9.86	2.50	33.46

Modifiers (PAR) ▯

Code	Mod 50	Mod 51	Mod 62	Mod 66	Mod 80
50540	2	2	1	0	2

Global Period

Code	Days
50540	090

50541-50542

50541 Laparoscopy, surgical; ablation of renal cysts

50542 Laparoscopy, surgical; ablation of renal mass lesion(s), including intraoperative ultrasound guidance and monitoring, when performed

(For open procedure, use 50250)

(For percutaneous ablation of renal tumors, see 50592, 50593)

AMA Coding Guideline

Laparoscopic Procedures on the Kidney

Surgical laparoscopy always includes diagnostic laparoscopy. To report a diagnostic laparoscopy (peritoneoscopy) (separate procedure), use 49320.

AMA Coding Notes

Surgical Procedures on the Urinary System

(For provision of chemotherapeutic agents, report both the specific service in addition to code(s) for the specific substance(s) or drug(s) provided)

AMA *CPT® Assistant* ☐

50541: Nov 99: 25, May 00: 4, Oct 01: 8, Nov 02: 3, Jan 03: 20

50542: Nov 02: 3, Jan 03: 21, Aug 04: 12

Plain English Description

The physician performs a laparoscopic procedure to destroy (ablate) cysts or mass lesions in the kidney. The lesion(s) may be destroyed using any of a number of techniques including cryoablation, radiofrequency ablation (RFA), high-intensity focused ultrasound (HIFU), laser thermal ablation, or other method. Pneumoperitoneum is achieved and trocars are placed. The laparoscope is inserted through the umbilical port. The peritoneum over the kidney is mobilized and the anterior surface of the kidney is visualized. The kidney lesion is identified. One or more cryosurgical probes or other ablation instruments are inserted into the lesion. If cryoablation is the technique used, the first freeze-thaw cycle is initiated. The ice ball created during the freeze cycle is monitored using ultrasound to ensure adequate extension of the ice ball beyond the margins of the lesion. A second freeze-thaw cycle is performed in the same manner. Additional lesions are treated in the same manner. RFA is a thermal technique that heats the lesion and surrounding tissue. If RFA is performed, the appropriate electrode needle or array is selected based on the size and shape of the cyst or lesion. The RFA device is activated and the lesion is ablated. Laser thermal ablation uses a laser to produce heat and destroy the lesion. HIFU uses focused sound waves to produce heat and cavitation. Following ablation of all lesions, the surgical instruments are removed, bleeding is controlled, drains are placed, and portal incisions are closed around the drains. Report 50541 for ablation of renal cysts and 50542 for ablation of other renal mass lesions.

Surgical laparoscopy; ablation of renal cysts/mass lesion(s)

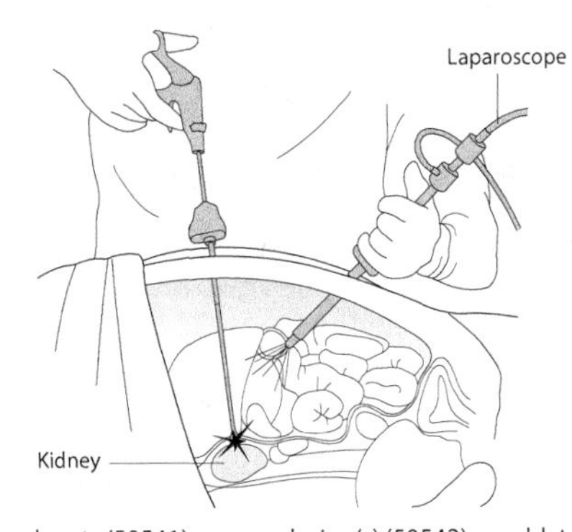

Renal cysts (50541), or mass lesion(s) (50542) are ablated.

ICD-10-CM Diagnostic Codes

	Code	Description
⇄	C64.1	Malignant neoplasm of right kidney, except renal pelvis
⇄	C64.2	Malignant neoplasm of left kidney, except renal pelvis
⇄	C65.1	Malignant neoplasm of right renal pelvis
⇄	C65.2	Malignant neoplasm of left renal pelvis
⇄	C79.01	Secondary malignant neoplasm of right kidney and renal pelvis
⇄	C79.02	Secondary malignant neoplasm of left kidney and renal pelvis
	C7A.093	Malignant carcinoid tumor of the kidney
	D09.19	Carcinoma in situ of other urinary organs
⇄	D30.01	Benign neoplasm of right kidney
⇄	D30.02	Benign neoplasm of left kidney
⇄	D30.11	Benign neoplasm of right renal pelvis
⇄	D30.12	Benign neoplasm of left renal pelvis
	D3A.093	Benign carcinoid tumor of the kidney
⇄	D41.01	Neoplasm of uncertain behavior of right kidney
⇄	D41.02	Neoplasm of uncertain behavior of left kidney
⇄	D41.11	Neoplasm of uncertain behavior of right renal pelvis
⇄	D41.12	Neoplasm of uncertain behavior of left renal pelvis
	N28.1	Cyst of kidney, acquired
	N28.89	Other specified disorders of kidney and ureter
	Q61.01	Congenital single renal cyst
	Q61.02	Congenital multiple renal cysts
	Q61.11	Cystic dilatation of collecting ducts
	Q61.19	Other polycystic kidney, infantile type
	Q61.3	Polycystic kidney, unspecified
	Q61.5	Medullary cystic kidney
	Q61.8	Other cystic kidney diseases

CCI Edits

Refer to Appendix A for CCI edits.

Facility RVUs ☐

Code	Work	PE Facility	MP	Total Facility
50541	16.86	7.87	2.05	26.78
50542	21.36	10.11	2.61	34.08

Non-facility RVUs ☐

Code	Work	PE Non-Facility	MP	Total Non-Facility
50541	16.86	7.87	2.05	26.78
50542	21.36	10.11	2.61	34.08

Modifiers (PAR) ☐

Code	Mod 50	Mod 51	Mod 62	Mod 66	Mod 80
50541	1	2	1	0	2
50542	1	2	1	0	2

Global Period

Code	Days
50541	090
50542	090

50543

50543 Laparoscopy, surgical; partial nephrectomy
(For open procedure, use 50240)

AMA Coding Guideline

Laparoscopic Procedures on the Kidney

Surgical laparoscopy always includes diagnostic laparoscopy. To report a diagnostic laparoscopy (peritoneoscopy) (separate procedure), use 49320.

AMA Coding Notes

Surgical Procedures on the Urinary System

(For provision of chemotherapeutic agents, report both the specific service in addition to code(s) for the specific substance(s) or drug(s) provided)

AMA *CPT® Assistant* ▢

50543: Nov 02: 3, Jan 03: 21

Plain English Description

The physician performs a partial nephrectomy via a laparoscopic approach. Small portal incisions are made and pneumoperitoneum is achieved by insufflating the abdomen with air. Trocars are placed and the laparoscope is inserted through an umbilical port. The lateral line of Toldt is identified and incised. The peritoneum over the kidney is mobilized and the anterior surface of the kidney is visualized. The colon is mobilized and rolled medially. The ureter and surrounding vascular structures are identified and retracted to expose the lower pole of the kidney and the renal hilum. The kidney mass is identified and dissected free from surrounding healthy kidney tissue. The defect left after removal is repaired using sutures and sealant glue. The laparoscope is removed from the umbilical port and inserted into the lateral port. A bag is inserted through the umbilical port and the excised kidney mass is placed in the bag. The umbilical incision is extended and the bag containing the kidney mass is removed. The surgical site is inspected, bleeding is controlled, surgical instruments are removed, and incisions are closed.

Laparoscopy, surgical; partial nephrectomy

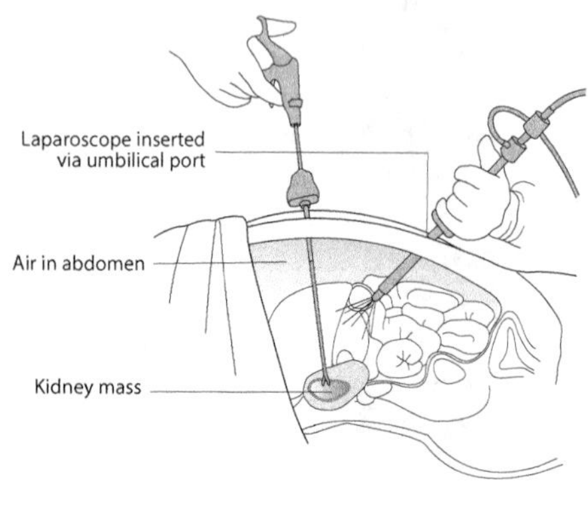

ICD-10-CM Diagnostic Codes

	Code	Description
⇄	C64.1	Malignant neoplasm of right kidney, except renal pelvis
⇄	C64.2	Malignant neoplasm of left kidney, except renal pelvis
⇄	C65.1	Malignant neoplasm of right renal pelvis
⇄	C65.2	Malignant neoplasm of left renal pelvis
⇄	C79.01	Secondary malignant neoplasm of right kidney and renal pelvis
⇄	C79.02	Secondary malignant neoplasm of left kidney and renal pelvis
	C7A.093	Malignant carcinoid tumor of the kidney
	D09.19	Carcinoma in situ of other urinary organs
⇄	D30.01	Benign neoplasm of right kidney
⇄	D30.02	Benign neoplasm of left kidney
⇄	D30.11	Benign neoplasm of right renal pelvis
⇄	D30.12	Benign neoplasm of left renal pelvis
	D3A.093	Benign carcinoid tumor of the kidney
⇄	D41.01	Neoplasm of uncertain behavior of right kidney
⇄	D41.02	Neoplasm of uncertain behavior of left kidney
⇄	D41.11	Neoplasm of uncertain behavior of right renal pelvis
⇄	D41.12	Neoplasm of uncertain behavior of left renal pelvis
	I12.0	Hypertensive chronic kidney disease with stage 5 chronic kidney disease or end stage renal disease
	I13.11	Hypertensive heart and chronic kidney disease without heart failure, with stage 5 chronic kidney disease, or end stage renal disease
	N00.2	Acute nephritic syndrome with diffuse membranous glomerulonephritis
	N00.3	Acute nephritic syndrome with diffuse mesangial proliferative glomerulonephritis
	N00.4	Acute nephritic syndrome with diffuse endocapillary proliferative glomerulonephritis
	N00.5	Acute nephritic syndrome with diffuse mesangiocapillary glomerulonephritis
	N00.6	Acute nephritic syndrome with dense deposit disease
	N00.7	Acute nephritic syndrome with diffuse crescentic glomerulonephritis
	N00.8	Acute nephritic syndrome with other morphologic changes
	N03.1	Chronic nephritic syndrome with focal and segmental glomerular lesions
	N03.2	Chronic nephritic syndrome with diffuse membranous glomerulonephritis
	N03.3	Chronic nephritic syndrome with diffuse mesangial proliferative glomerulonephritis
	N03.4	Chronic nephritic syndrome with diffuse endocapillary proliferative glomerulonephritis
	N03.5	Chronic nephritic syndrome with diffuse mesangiocapillary glomerulonephritis
	N03.6	Chronic nephritic syndrome with dense deposit disease
	N03.7	Chronic nephritic syndrome with diffuse crescentic glomerulonephritis
	N03.8	Chronic nephritic syndrome with other morphologic changes
	N04.1	Nephrotic syndrome with focal and segmental glomerular lesions
	N04.2	Nephrotic syndrome with diffuse membranous glomerulonephritis
	N04.3	Nephrotic syndrome with diffuse mesangial proliferative glomerulonephritis
	N04.4	Nephrotic syndrome with diffuse endocapillary proliferative glomerulonephritis
	N04.5	Nephrotic syndrome with diffuse mesangiocapillary glomerulonephritis
	N04.6	Nephrotic syndrome with dense deposit disease
	N04.7	Nephrotic syndrome with diffuse crescentic glomerulonephritis
	N04.8	Nephrotic syndrome with other morphologic changes
	N11.0	Nonobstructive reflux-associated chronic pyelonephritis
	N11.1	Chronic obstructive pyelonephritis
	N13.0	Hydronephrosis with ureteropelvic junction obstruction
	N13.1	Hydronephrosis with ureteral stricture, not elsewhere classified
	N13.2	Hydronephrosis with renal and ureteral calculous obstruction
	N13.39	Other hydronephrosis
	N13.4	Hydroureter
	N13.5	Crossing vessel and stricture of ureter without hydronephrosis
	N13.6	Pyonephrosis
	N13.71	Vesicoureteral-reflux without reflux nephropathy
	N13.721	Vesicoureteral-reflux with reflux nephropathy without hydroureter, unilateral
	N13.722	Vesicoureteral-reflux with reflux nephropathy without hydroureter, bilateral
	N13.731	Vesicoureteral-reflux with reflux nephropathy with hydroureter, unilateral
	N13.732	Vesicoureteral-reflux with reflux nephropathy with hydroureter, bilateral
	N13.8	Other obstructive and reflux uropathy
	N17.0	Acute kidney failure with tubular necrosis
	N17.1	Acute kidney failure with acute cortical necrosis
	N17.2	Acute kidney failure with medullary necrosis
	N17.8	Other acute kidney failure

N18.4	Chronic kidney disease, stage 4 (severe)
N18.5	Chronic kidney disease, stage 5
N18.6	End stage renal disease
N20	Calculus of kidney and ureter
N20.0	Calculus of kidney
N20.1	Calculus of ureter
N20.2	Calculus of kidney with calculus of ureter
N28.0	Ischemia and infarction of kidney
N28.1	Cyst of kidney, acquired
N28.81	Hypertrophy of kidney
N28.89	Other specified disorders of kidney and ureter
Q60.3	Renal hypoplasia, unilateral
Q60.4	Renal hypoplasia, bilateral
Q60.6	Potter's syndrome
Q61.01	Congenital single renal cyst
Q61.02	Congenital multiple renal cysts
Q61.11	Cystic dilatation of collecting ducts
Q61.19	Other polycystic kidney, infantile type
Q61.2	Polycystic kidney, adult type
Q61.4	Renal dysplasia
Q61.5	Medullary cystic kidney
Q62.0	Congenital hydronephrosis
Q62.11	Congenital occlusion of ureteropelvic junction
❼⇄ S37.061	Major laceration of right kidney
❼⇄ S37.062	Major laceration of left kidney
❼⇄ S37.091	Other injury of right kidney
❼⇄ S37.092	Other injury of left kidney

ICD-10-CM Coding Notes

For codes requiring a 7th character extension, refer to your ICD-10-CM book. Review the character descriptions and coding guidelines for proper selection. For some procedures, only certain characters will apply.

CCI Edits

Refer to Appendix A for CCI edits.

Facility RVUs ▢

Code	Work	PE Facility	MP	Total Facility
50543	27.41	12.77	3.31	43.49

Non-facility RVUs ▢

Code	Work	PE Non-Facility	MP	Total Non-Facility
50543	27.41	12.77	3.31	43.49

Modifiers (PAR) ▢

Code	Mod 50	Mod 51	Mod 62	Mod 66	Mod 80
50543	1	2	1	0	2

Global Period

Code	Days
50543	090

50544

50544 Laparoscopy, surgical; pyeloplasty

AMA Coding Guideline

Laparoscopic Procedures on the Kidney

Surgical laparoscopy always includes diagnostic laparoscopy. To report a diagnostic laparoscopy (peritoneoscopy) (separate procedure), use 49320.

AMA Coding Notes

Surgical Procedures on the Urinary System

(For provision of chemotherapeutic agents, report both the specific service in addition to code(s) for the specific substance(s) or drug(s) provided)

AMA *CPT® Assistant* ▢

50544: Nov 99: 25, May 00: 4, Oct 01: 8

Plain English Description

The physician performs a pyeloplasty via a laparoscopic approach. Pyeloplasty is a reconstructive operation performed to treat blockage or narrowing of the ureter at the ureteropelvic junction (UPJ). Small portal incisions are made and pneumoperitoneum is achieved by insufflating the abdomen with air. Trocars are placed and the laparoscope is inserted through an umbilical port. The lateral line of Toldt is identified and incised. The peritoneum over the kidney is mobilized and the anterior surface of the kidney is visualized. The colon is mobilized and rolled medially. The ureter and surrounding vascular structures are identified. The ureter is dissected free of surrounding tissue, taking care to ensure adequate fat is maintained around the ureter. The ureteropelvic junction (UPJ) is exposed and the lower pole of the kidney is mobilized. The UPJ is isolated and any aberrant blood vessels impinging on the UPJ are identified and dissected free. The obstructed segment of the UPJ is then dissected free and excised. The renal pelvis is trimmed as needed and the ureteral stump is examined and spatulated. A stent is placed through the ureter into the bladder. The posterior wall of the UPJ is anastomosed, followed by closure of the renal pelvis. The proximal end of the ureteral stent is then placed in the renal pelvis and the anterior UPJ incision is closed. A drain may be placed. The surgical site is inspected, bleeding is controlled, surgical instruments are removed, and incisions are closed.

Laparoscopy, surgical; pyeloplasty

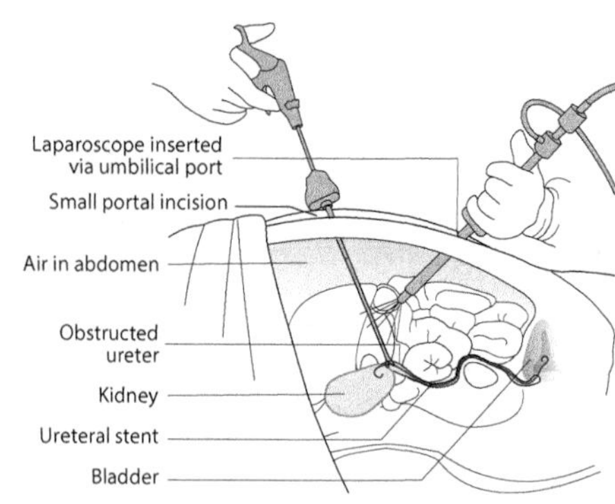

ICD-10-CM Diagnostic Codes

N11.1	Chronic obstructive pyelonephritis
N13.0	Hydronephrosis with ureteropelvic junction obstruction
N13.1	Hydronephrosis with ureteral stricture, not elsewhere classified
N13.2	Hydronephrosis with renal and ureteral calculous obstruction
N13.39	Other hydronephrosis
N13.4	Hydroureter
N13.5	Crossing vessel and stricture of ureter without hydronephrosis
N13.71	Vesicoureteral-reflux without reflux nephropathy
N13.721	Vesicoureteral-reflux with reflux nephropathy without hydroureter, unilateral
N13.722	Vesicoureteral-reflux with reflux nephropathy without hydroureter, bilateral
N13.731	Vesicoureteral-reflux with reflux nephropathy with hydroureter, unilateral
N13.732	Vesicoureteral-reflux with reflux nephropathy with hydroureter, bilateral
N20.0	Calculus of kidney
N20.1	Calculus of ureter
N20.2	Calculus of kidney with calculus of ureter
Q62.11	Congenital occlusion of ureteropelvic junction
Q62.12	Congenital occlusion of ureterovesical orifice
Q62.2	Congenital megaureter
Q62.31	Congenital ureterocele, orthotopic
Q62.32	Cecoureterocele
Q62.39	Other obstructive defects of renal pelvis and ureter

CCI Edits

Refer to Appendix A for CCI edits.

Facility RVUs ▢

Code	Work	PE Facility	MP	Total Facility
50544	23.37	10.05	2.82	36.24

Non-facility RVUs ▢

Code	Work	PE Non-Facility	MP	Total Non-Facility
50544	23.37	10.05	2.82	36.24

Modifiers (PAR) ▢

Code	Mod 50	Mod 51	Mod 62	Mod 66	Mod 80
50544	1	2	1	0	2

Global Period

Code	Days
50544	090

50545

50545 Laparoscopy, surgical; radical nephrectomy (includes removal of Gerota's fascia and surrounding fatty tissue, removal of regional lymph nodes, and adrenalectomy)

(For open procedure, use 50230)

AMA Coding Guideline

Laparoscopic Procedures on the Kidney

Surgical laparoscopy always includes diagnostic laparoscopy. To report a diagnostic laparoscopy (peritoneoscopy) (separate procedure), use 49320.

AMA Coding Notes

Surgical Procedures on the Urinary System

(For provision of chemotherapeutic agents, report both the specific service in addition to code(s) for the specific substance(s) or drug(s) provided)

AMA *CPT® Assistant* ▯

50545: Oct 01: 8

Plain English Description

The physician performs a radical nephrectomy including removal of Gerota's fascia, surrounding fatty tissue, regional lymph nodes, and adrenal glands via a laparoscopic approach. Small portal incisions are made and pneumoperitoneum is achieved by insufflating the abdomen with air. Trocars are placed and the laparoscope is inserted through an umbilical port. The lateral line of Toldt is identified and incised. The peritoneum over the kidney is mobilized and the anterior surface of the kidney visualized. The colon is mobilized and rolled medially. The colorenal ligaments are divided and Gerota's fascia is exposed. Regional lymph nodes are excised, the Gerota's fascia is dissected free from surrounding structures, and the lymphatic vessels are ligated. The ureter and surrounding vascular structures are identified and retracted to expose the lower pole of the kidney and the renal hilum. The lower pole is dissected free of surrounding structures. The kidney is retracted laterally and superiorly to allow access to the renal hilum, which is dissected free of surrounding structures. The renal artery and vein are identified, divided, and ligated. Dissection continues medially along the inferior vena cava to the adrenal vein, which is divided and ligated. The adrenal gland is dissected free of surrounding tissue and the adrenal arteries are divided. The kidney is dissected free from any remaining lateral and superior attachments and the ureter is divided. The laparoscope is removed from the umbilical port and inserted into the lateral port. A bag is inserted through the umbilical port and the kidney, Gerota's fascia, surrounding fatty tissue, regional lymph nodes, and the adrenal gland are placed in the bag for removal. The umbilical incision is extended and the bag containing the kidney and surrounding structures is removed. The surgical site is inspected, bleeding is controlled, surgical instruments are removed, and incisions are closed.

Laparoscopy, surgical; radical nephrectomy

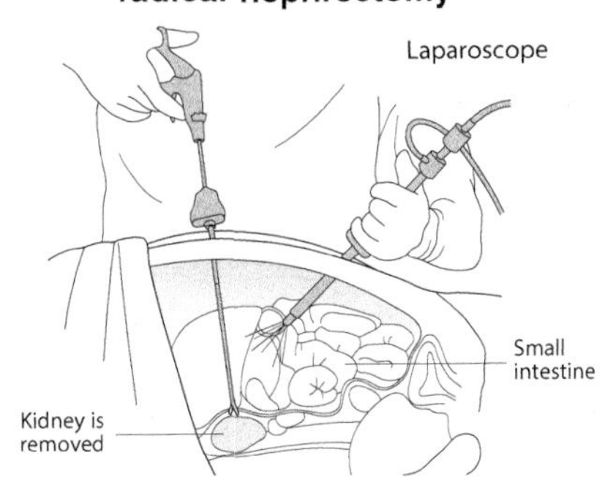

ICD-10-CM Diagnostic Codes

	Code	Description
⇄	C64.1	Malignant neoplasm of right kidney, except renal pelvis
⇄	C64.2	Malignant neoplasm of left kidney, except renal pelvis
⇄	C65.1	Malignant neoplasm of right renal pelvis
⇄	C65.2	Malignant neoplasm of left renal pelvis
⇄	C74.01	Malignant neoplasm of cortex of right adrenal gland
⇄	C74.02	Malignant neoplasm of cortex of left adrenal gland
⇄	C74.11	Malignant neoplasm of medulla of right adrenal gland
⇄	C74.12	Malignant neoplasm of medulla of left adrenal gland
	C77.2	Secondary and unspecified malignant neoplasm of intra-abdominal lymph nodes
	C77.5	Secondary and unspecified malignant neoplasm of intrapelvic lymph nodes
	C77.8	Secondary and unspecified malignant neoplasm of lymph nodes of multiple regions
⇄	C79.01	Secondary malignant neoplasm of right kidney and renal pelvis
⇄	C79.02	Secondary malignant neoplasm of left kidney and renal pelvis
⇄	C79.71	Secondary malignant neoplasm of right adrenal gland
⇄	C79.72	Secondary malignant neoplasm of left adrenal gland
	C7A.093	Malignant carcinoid tumor of the kidney
	D09.19	Carcinoma in situ of other urinary organs
	D3A.093	Benign carcinoid tumor of the kidney
⇄	D41.01	Neoplasm of uncertain behavior of right kidney
⇄	D41.02	Neoplasm of uncertain behavior of left kidney
⇄	D41.11	Neoplasm of uncertain behavior of right renal pelvis
⇄	D41.12	Neoplasm of uncertain behavior of left renal pelvis
⇄	D44.11	Neoplasm of uncertain behavior of right adrenal gland
⇄	D44.12	Neoplasm of uncertain behavior of left adrenal gland
	I12.0	Hypertensive chronic kidney disease with stage 5 chronic kidney disease or end stage renal disease
	I13.11	Hypertensive heart and chronic kidney disease without heart failure, with stage 5 chronic kidney disease, or end stage renal disease
	I75.81	Atheroembolism of kidney
	N00.1	Acute nephritic syndrome with focal and segmental glomerular lesions
	N00.2	Acute nephritic syndrome with diffuse membranous glomerulonephritis
	N00.3	Acute nephritic syndrome with diffuse mesangial proliferative glomerulonephritis
	N00.4	Acute nephritic syndrome with diffuse endocapillary proliferative glomerulonephritis
	N00.5	Acute nephritic syndrome with diffuse mesangiocapillary glomerulonephritis
	N00.6	Acute nephritic syndrome with dense deposit disease
	N00.7	Acute nephritic syndrome with diffuse crescentic glomerulonephritis
	N00.8	Acute nephritic syndrome with other morphologic changes
	N03.1	Chronic nephritic syndrome with focal and segmental glomerular lesions
	N03.2	Chronic nephritic syndrome with diffuse membranous glomerulonephritis
	N03.3	Chronic nephritic syndrome with diffuse mesangial proliferative glomerulonephritis
	N03.4	Chronic nephritic syndrome with diffuse endocapillary proliferative glomerulonephritis
	N03.5	Chronic nephritic syndrome with diffuse mesangiocapillary glomerulonephritis
	N03.6	Chronic nephritic syndrome with dense deposit disease
	N03.7	Chronic nephritic syndrome with diffuse crescentic glomerulonephritis
	N03.8	Chronic nephritic syndrome with other morphologic changes
	N04.1	Nephrotic syndrome with focal and segmental glomerular lesions
	N04.2	Nephrotic syndrome with diffuse membranous glomerulonephritis
	N04.3	Nephrotic syndrome with diffuse mesangial proliferative glomerulonephritis
	N04.4	Nephrotic syndrome with diffuse endocapillary proliferative glomerulonephritis
	N04.5	Nephrotic syndrome with diffuse mesangiocapillary glomerulonephritis

	N04.6	Nephrotic syndrome with dense deposit disease
	N04.7	Nephrotic syndrome with diffuse crescentic glomerulonephritis
	N04.8	Nephrotic syndrome with other morphologic changes
	N11.0	Nonobstructive reflux-associated chronic pyelonephritis
	N11.1	Chronic obstructive pyelonephritis
	N13.0	Hydronephrosis with ureteropelvic junction obstruction
	N13.1	Hydronephrosis with ureteral stricture, not elsewhere classified
	N13.2	Hydronephrosis with renal and ureteral calculous obstruction
	N13.6	Pyonephrosis
	N13.721	Vesicoureteral-reflux with reflux nephropathy without hydroureter, unilateral
	N13.722	Vesicoureteral-reflux with reflux nephropathy without hydroureter, bilateral
	N13.731	Vesicoureteral-reflux with reflux nephropathy with hydroureter, unilateral
	N13.732	Vesicoureteral-reflux with reflux nephropathy with hydroureter, bilateral
	N17.0	Acute kidney failure with tubular necrosis
	N17.1	Acute kidney failure with acute cortical necrosis
	N17.2	Acute kidney failure with medullary necrosis
	N18.4	Chronic kidney disease, stage 4 (severe)
	N18.5	Chronic kidney disease, stage 5
	N18.6	End stage renal disease
	N26.1	Atrophy of kidney (terminal)
	N26.2	Page kidney
	N28.0	Ischemia and infarction of kidney
	N28.1	Cyst of kidney, acquired
	N28.81	Hypertrophy of kidney
	Q60.3	Renal hypoplasia, unilateral
	Q60.4	Renal hypoplasia, bilateral
	Q60.6	Potter's syndrome
	Q61.02	Congenital multiple renal cysts
	Q61.11	Cystic dilatation of collecting ducts
	Q61.2	Polycystic kidney, adult type
	Q61.4	Renal dysplasia
	Q61.5	Medullary cystic kidney
	Q62.0	Congenital hydronephrosis
	Q62.11	Congenital occlusion of ureteropelvic junction
	Q62.39	Other obstructive defects of renal pelvis and ureter
❼⇄	S37.061	Major laceration of right kidney
❼⇄	S37.062	Major laceration of left kidney

ICD-10-CM Coding Notes

For codes requiring a 7th character extension, refer to your ICD-10-CM book. Review the character descriptions and coding guidelines for proper selection. For some procedures, only certain characters will apply.

CCI Edits

Refer to Appendix A for CCI edits.

Facility RVUs ▯

Code	Work	PE Facility	MP	Total Facility
50545	25.06	10.85	3.03	38.94

Non-facility RVUs ▯

Code	Work	PE Non-Facility	MP	Total Non-Facility
50545	25.06	10.85	3.03	38.94

Modifiers (PAR) ▯

Code	Mod 50	Mod 51	Mod 62	Mod 66	Mod 80
50545	1	2	1	0	2

Global Period

Code	Days
50545	090

50546

50546 Laparoscopy, surgical; nephrectomy, including partial ureterectomy

AMA Coding Guideline

Laparoscopic Procedures on the Kidney

Surgical laparoscopy always includes diagnostic laparoscopy. To report a diagnostic laparoscopy (peritoneoscopy) (separate procedure), use 49320.

AMA Coding Notes

Surgical Procedures on the Urinary System

(For provision of chemotherapeutic agents, report both the specific service in addition to code(s) for the specific substance(s) or drug(s) provided)

AMA *CPT® Assistant* ▯

50546: Nov 99: 25, May 00: 4, Oct 01: 8

Plain English Description

The physician performs a nephrectomy with partial ureterectomy via a laparoscopic approach. Small portal incisions are made and pneumoperitoneum is achieved by insufflating the abdomen with air. Trocars are placed and the laparoscope is inserted through an umbilical port. The lateral line of Toldt is identified and incised. The peritoneum over the kidney is mobilized and the anterior surface of the kidney is visualized. The colon is mobilized and rolled medially. The ureter and surrounding vascular structures are identified and retracted to expose the lower pole of the kidney and the renal hilum. The lower pole is then dissected free of surrounding structures. The kidney is retracted laterally and superiorly to allow access to the renal hilum, which is dissected free of surrounding structures. The renal artery and vein are identified and divided. The diseased section of ureter is also dissected and divided. The kidney is mobilized from any remaining lateral and superior attachments. The laparoscope is removed from the umbilical port and inserted into the lateral port. A bag is inserted through the umbilical port. The kidney, along with the section of diseased ureter, is placed in the bag. The umbilical incision is extended and the bag containing the kidney and ureter is removed. The surgical site is inspected, bleeding is controlled, surgical instruments are removed, and incisions are closed.

Laparoscopy, surgical; nephrectomy, including partial ureterectomy

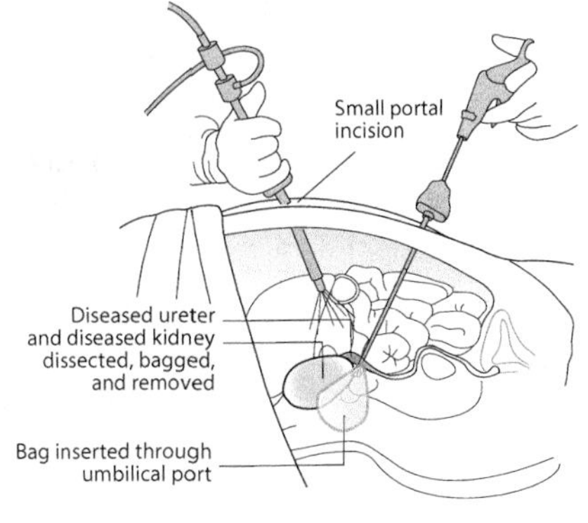

ICD-10-CM Diagnostic Codes

	Code	Description
⇄	C64.1	Malignant neoplasm of right kidney, except renal pelvis
⇄	C64.2	Malignant neoplasm of left kidney, except renal pelvis
⇄	C65.1	Malignant neoplasm of right renal pelvis
⇄	C65.2	Malignant neoplasm of left renal pelvis
⇄	C66.1	Malignant neoplasm of right ureter
⇄	C66.2	Malignant neoplasm of left ureter
	C68.8	Malignant neoplasm of overlapping sites of urinary organs
⇄	C79.01	Secondary malignant neoplasm of right kidney and renal pelvis
⇄	C79.02	Secondary malignant neoplasm of left kidney and renal pelvis
	C79.19	Secondary malignant neoplasm of other urinary organs
	C7A.093	Malignant carcinoid tumor of the kidney
	D09.19	Carcinoma in situ of other urinary organs
	D3A.093	Benign carcinoid tumor of the kidney
⇄	D41.01	Neoplasm of uncertain behavior of right kidney
⇄	D41.02	Neoplasm of uncertain behavior of left kidney
⇄	D41.11	Neoplasm of uncertain behavior of right renal pelvis
⇄	D41.12	Neoplasm of uncertain behavior of left renal pelvis
⇄	D41.21	Neoplasm of uncertain behavior of right ureter
⇄	D41.22	Neoplasm of uncertain behavior of left ureter
	I12.0	Hypertensive chronic kidney disease with stage 5 chronic kidney disease or end stage renal disease
	I13.11	Hypertensive heart and chronic kidney disease without heart failure, with stage 5 chronic kidney disease, or end stage renal disease
	I75.81	Atheroembolism of kidney
	N00.1	Acute nephritic syndrome with focal and segmental glomerular lesions
	N00.2	Acute nephritic syndrome with diffuse membranous glomerulonephritis
	N00.3	Acute nephritic syndrome with diffuse mesangial proliferative glomerulonephritis
	N00.4	Acute nephritic syndrome with diffuse endocapillary proliferative glomerulonephritis
	N00.5	Acute nephritic syndrome with diffuse mesangiocapillary glomerulonephritis
	N00.6	Acute nephritic syndrome with dense deposit disease
	N00.7	Acute nephritic syndrome with diffuse crescentic glomerulonephritis
	N00.8	Acute nephritic syndrome with other morphologic changes
	N03.1	Chronic nephritic syndrome with focal and segmental glomerular lesions
	N03.2	Chronic nephritic syndrome with diffuse membranous glomerulonephritis
	N03.3	Chronic nephritic syndrome with diffuse mesangial proliferative glomerulonephritis
	N03.4	Chronic nephritic syndrome with diffuse endocapillary proliferative glomerulonephritis
	N03.5	Chronic nephritic syndrome with diffuse mesangiocapillary glomerulonephritis
	N03.6	Chronic nephritic syndrome with dense deposit disease
	N03.7	Chronic nephritic syndrome with diffuse crescentic glomerulonephritis
	N03.8	Chronic nephritic syndrome with other morphologic changes
	N04.1	Nephrotic syndrome with focal and segmental glomerular lesions
	N04.2	Nephrotic syndrome with diffuse membranous glomerulonephritis
	N04.3	Nephrotic syndrome with diffuse mesangial proliferative glomerulonephritis
	N04.4	Nephrotic syndrome with diffuse endocapillary proliferative glomerulonephritis
	N04.5	Nephrotic syndrome with diffuse mesangiocapillary glomerulonephritis
	N04.6	Nephrotic syndrome with dense deposit disease
	N04.7	Nephrotic syndrome with diffuse crescentic glomerulonephritis
	N04.8	Nephrotic syndrome with other morphologic changes
	N08	Glomerular disorders in diseases classified elsewhere
	N11.0	Nonobstructive reflux-associated chronic pyelonephritis
	N11.1	Chronic obstructive pyelonephritis
	N13.0	Hydronephrosis with ureteropelvic junction obstruction
	N13.1	Hydronephrosis with ureteral stricture, not elsewhere classified

N13.2	Hydronephrosis with renal and ureteral calculous obstruction
N13.4	Hydroureter
N13.5	Crossing vessel and stricture of ureter without hydronephrosis
N13.6	Pyonephrosis
N13.721	Vesicoureteral-reflux with reflux nephropathy without hydroureter, unilateral
N13.722	Vesicoureteral-reflux with reflux nephropathy without hydroureter, bilateral
N13.731	Vesicoureteral-reflux with reflux nephropathy with hydroureter, unilateral
N13.732	Vesicoureteral-reflux with reflux nephropathy with hydroureter, bilateral
N17.0	Acute kidney failure with tubular necrosis
N17.1	Acute kidney failure with acute cortical necrosis
N17.2	Acute kidney failure with medullary necrosis
N18.4	Chronic kidney disease, stage 4 (severe)
N18.5	Chronic kidney disease, stage 5
N18.6	End stage renal disease
N20.2	Calculus of kidney with calculus of ureter
N26.9	Renal sclerosis, unspecified
N28.0	Ischemia and infarction of kidney
N28.1	Cyst of kidney, acquired
N28.81	Hypertrophy of kidney
N28.82	Megaloureter
Q60.3	Renal hypoplasia, unilateral
Q60.4	Renal hypoplasia, bilateral
Q60.6	Potter's syndrome
Q61.01	Congenital single renal cyst
Q61.02	Congenital multiple renal cysts
Q61.11	Cystic dilatation of collecting ducts
Q61.2	Polycystic kidney, adult type
Q61.4	Renal dysplasia
Q61.5	Medullary cystic kidney
Q62.0	Congenital hydronephrosis
Q62.11	Congenital occlusion of ureteropelvic junction
Q62.2	Congenital megaureter
Q62.31	Congenital ureterocele, orthotopic
Q62.32	Cecoureterocele
Q62.39	Other obstructive defects of renal pelvis and ureter
❼⇄ S37.061	Major laceration of right kidney
❼⇄ S37.062	Major laceration of left kidney
❼⇄ S37.091	Other injury of right kidney
❼⇄ S37.092	Other injury of left kidney

ICD-10-CM Coding Notes

For codes requiring a 7th character extension, refer to your ICD-10-CM book. Review the character descriptions and coding guidelines for proper selection. For some procedures, only certain characters will apply.

CCI Edits

Refer to Appendix A for CCI edits.

Facility RVUs ▯

Code	Work	PE Facility	MP	Total Facility
50546	21.87	10.46	2.85	35.18

Non-facility RVUs ▯

Code	Work	PE Non-Facility	MP	Total Non-Facility
50546	21.87	10.46	2.85	35.18

Modifiers (PAR) ▯

Code	Mod 50	Mod 51	Mod 62	Mod 66	Mod 80
50546	1	2	1	0	2

Global Period

Code	Days
50546	090

50547

50547 Laparoscopy, surgical; donor nephrectomy (including cold preservation), from living donor

(For open procedure, use 50320)

(For backbench renal allograft standard preparation prior to transplantation, use 50325)

(For backbench renal allograft reconstruction prior to transplantation, see 50327-50329)

AMA Coding Guideline

Laparoscopic Procedures on the Kidney

Surgical laparoscopy always includes diagnostic laparoscopy. To report a diagnostic laparoscopy (peritoneoscopy) (separate procedure), use 49320.

AMA Coding Notes

Surgical Procedures on the Urinary System

(For provision of chemotherapeutic agents, report both the specific service in addition to code(s) for the specific substance(s) or drug(s) provided)

AMA *CPT® Assistant* ▢

50547: Nov 99: 25, May 00: 4, Oct 01: 8

Plain English Description

A living donor nephrectomy inclusive of cold preservation of the donor kidney is performed via a laparoscopic approach. Small portal incisions are made and pneumoperitoneum is achieved by insufflating the abdomen with air. Trocars are placed and the laparoscope is inserted through an umbilical port. The lateral line of Toldt is identified and incised. The peritoneum over the kidney is mobilized and the anterior surface of the kidney is visualized. The colon is mobilized and rolled medially. The colorenal ligaments are divided and Gerota's fascia is exposed. The ureter and surrounding vascular structures are identified and retracted to expose the lower pole of the kidney and the renal hilum. The lower pole is partially mobilized. The kidney is retracted laterally and superiorly to allow access to the renal hilum, which is dissected free of surrounding structures. The renal vein is exposed. The gonadal, lumbar, and adrenal veins are clipped and divided. The renal artery is identified and dissected free of surrounding tissue. Lateral, posterior, and inferior kidney attachments are left intact to prevent torsion of the kidney and damage to its vascular pedicle. The ureter is dissected free of surrounding tissue to the level of the iliac vessels and divided. The kidney is dissected free from the remaining lateral and inferior attachments. The lower pole of the kidney is elevated and dissected free of the remaining posterior attachments. The periumbilical incision is extended, taking care to keep the peritoneum intact and preserve the pneumoperitoneum. The vascular pedicle containing the renal artery and vein is divided. The laparoscope is removed from the umbilical port and inserted into the lateral port. A bag is inserted through the umbilical port and the kidney is placed in the bag. The peritoneum is opened and the kidney is delivered. The kidney may be perfused with cold preservation solution and/or placed on ice and is then delivered to the recipient surgical team.

Laparoscopy, surgical; donor nephrectomy, from living donor

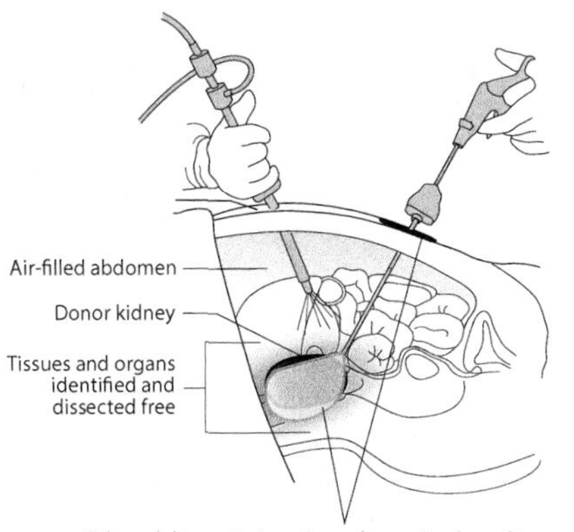

Kidney delivered in bag through opening in peritoneum

ICD-10-CM Diagnostic Codes

Z52.4	Kidney donor

CCI Edits

Refer to Appendix A for CCI edits.

Facility RVUs ▢

Code	Work	PE Facility	MP	Total Facility
50547	26.34	15.71	5.94	47.99

Non-facility RVUs ▢

Code	Work	PE Non-Facility	MP	Total Non-Facility
50547	26.34	15.71	5.94	47.99

Modifiers (PAR) ▢

Code	Mod 50	Mod 51	Mod 62	Mod 66	Mod 80
50547	1	2	1	0	2

Global Period

Code	Days
50547	090

50548

50548 Laparoscopy, surgical; nephrectomy with total ureterectomy

(For open procedure, see 50234, 50236)

AMA Coding Guideline

Laparoscopic Procedures on the Kidney

Surgical laparoscopy always includes diagnostic laparoscopy. To report a diagnostic laparoscopy (peritoneoscopy) (separate procedure), use 49320.

AMA Coding Notes

Surgical Procedures on the Urinary System

(For provision of chemotherapeutic agents, report both the specific service in addition to code(s) for the specific substance(s) or drug(s) provided)

AMA *CPT® Assistant* ▯

50548: Nov 99: 25, May 00: 4, Oct 01: 8

Plain English Description

The physician performs a nephrectomy with total ureterectomy via a laparoscopic approach. Small portal incisions are made and pneumoperitoneum is achieved by insufflating the abdomen with air. Trocars are placed and the laparoscope is inserted through an umbilical port. The lateral line of Toldt is identified and incised. The peritoneum over the kidney is mobilized and the anterior surface of the kidney is visualized. The colon is mobilized and rolled medially. The ureter and surrounding vascular structures are identified and retracted to expose the lower pole of the kidney and the renal hilum. The lower pole is dissected free of surrounding structures. The kidney is retracted laterally and superiorly to allow access to the renal hilum, which is dissected free of surrounding structures. The renal artery and vein are identified and divided. The entire ureter is dissected free of surrounding tissue and divided just above the ureterovesical junction (UVJ). The kidney is dissected free from any remaining lateral and superior attachments. The laparoscope is removed from the umbilical port and inserted into the lateral port. A bag is inserted through the umbilical port and the kidney and ureter are placed in the bag. The umbilical incision is extended and the bag containing the kidney and ureter is removed. The surgical site is inspected, bleeding is controlled, surgical instruments are removed, and incisions are closed.

Laparoscopy, surgical; nephrectomy, with total ureterectomy

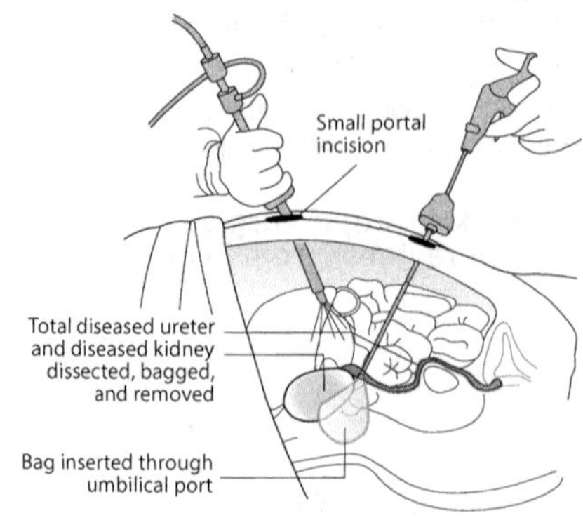

ICD-10-CM Diagnostic Codes

⇄ C64.1 Malignant neoplasm of right kidney, except renal pelvis
⇄ C64.2 Malignant neoplasm of left kidney, except renal pelvis
⇄ C65.1 Malignant neoplasm of right renal pelvis
⇄ C65.2 Malignant neoplasm of left renal pelvis
⇄ C66.1 Malignant neoplasm of right ureter
⇄ C66.2 Malignant neoplasm of left ureter
C68.8 Malignant neoplasm of overlapping sites of urinary organs
⇄ C79.01 Secondary malignant neoplasm of right kidney and renal pelvis
⇄ C79.02 Secondary malignant neoplasm of left kidney and renal pelvis
C79.19 Secondary malignant neoplasm of other urinary organs
C7A.093 Malignant carcinoid tumor of the kidney
D09.19 Carcinoma in situ of other urinary organs
⇄ D30.01 Benign neoplasm of right kidney
⇄ D30.02 Benign neoplasm of left kidney
⇄ D30.11 Benign neoplasm of right renal pelvis
⇄ D30.12 Benign neoplasm of left renal pelvis
⇄ D30.21 Benign neoplasm of right ureter
⇄ D30.22 Benign neoplasm of left ureter
D3A.093 Benign carcinoid tumor of the kidney
⇄ D41.01 Neoplasm of uncertain behavior of right kidney
⇄ D41.02 Neoplasm of uncertain behavior of left kidney
⇄ D41.11 Neoplasm of uncertain behavior of right renal pelvis
⇄ D41.12 Neoplasm of uncertain behavior of left renal pelvis
⇄ D41.21 Neoplasm of uncertain behavior of right ureter
⇄ D41.22 Neoplasm of uncertain behavior of left ureter
I12.0 Hypertensive chronic kidney disease with stage 5 chronic kidney disease or end stage renal disease
I13.11 Hypertensive heart and chronic kidney disease without heart failure, with stage 5 chronic kidney disease, or end stage renal disease
I75.81 Atheroembolism of kidney
N00.1 Acute nephritic syndrome with focal and segmental glomerular lesions
N00.2 Acute nephritic syndrome with diffuse membranous glomerulonephritis
N00.3 Acute nephritic syndrome with diffuse mesangial proliferative glomerulonephritis
N00.4 Acute nephritic syndrome with diffuse endocapillary proliferative glomerulonephritis
N00.5 Acute nephritic syndrome with diffuse mesangiocapillary glomerulonephritis
N00.6 Acute nephritic syndrome with dense deposit disease
N00.7 Acute nephritic syndrome with diffuse crescentic glomerulonephritis
N00.8 Acute nephritic syndrome with other morphologic changes
N03.1 Chronic nephritic syndrome with focal and segmental glomerular lesions
N03.2 Chronic nephritic syndrome with diffuse membranous glomerulonephritis
N03.3 Chronic nephritic syndrome with diffuse mesangial proliferative glomerulonephritis
N03.4 Chronic nephritic syndrome with diffuse endocapillary proliferative glomerulonephritis
N03.5 Chronic nephritic syndrome with diffuse mesangiocapillary glomerulonephritis
N03.6 Chronic nephritic syndrome with dense deposit disease
N03.7 Chronic nephritic syndrome with diffuse crescentic glomerulonephritis
N03.8 Chronic nephritic syndrome with other morphologic changes
N04.1 Nephrotic syndrome with focal and segmental glomerular lesions
N04.2 Nephrotic syndrome with diffuse membranous glomerulonephritis
N04.3 Nephrotic syndrome with diffuse mesangial proliferative glomerulonephritis
N04.4 Nephrotic syndrome with diffuse endocapillary proliferative glomerulonephritis
N04.5 Nephrotic syndrome with diffuse mesangiocapillary glomerulonephritis
N04.6 Nephrotic syndrome with dense deposit disease
N04.7 Nephrotic syndrome with diffuse crescentic glomerulonephritis
N04.8 Nephrotic syndrome with other morphologic changes

N08	Glomerular disorders in diseases classified elsewhere
N11.0	Nonobstructive reflux-associated chronic pyelonephritis
N11.1	Chronic obstructive pyelonephritis
N13.0	Hydronephrosis with ureteropelvic junction obstruction
N13.1	Hydronephrosis with ureteral stricture, not elsewhere classified
N13.2	Hydronephrosis with renal and ureteral calculous obstruction
N13.4	Hydroureter
N13.5	Crossing vessel and stricture of ureter without hydronephrosis
N13.6	Pyonephrosis
N13.721	Vesicoureteral-reflux with reflux nephropathy without hydroureter, unilateral
N13.722	Vesicoureteral-reflux with reflux nephropathy without hydroureter, bilateral
N13.731	Vesicoureteral-reflux with reflux nephropathy with hydroureter, unilateral
N13.732	Vesicoureteral-reflux with reflux nephropathy with hydroureter, bilateral
N17.0	Acute kidney failure with tubular necrosis
N17.1	Acute kidney failure with acute cortical necrosis
N17.2	Acute kidney failure with medullary necrosis
N18.4	Chronic kidney disease, stage 4 (severe)
N18.5	Chronic kidney disease, stage 5
N18.6	End stage renal disease
N20.2	Calculus of kidney with calculus of ureter
N26.1	Atrophy of kidney (terminal)
N26.2	Page kidney
N28.0	Ischemia and infarction of kidney
N28.1	Cyst of kidney, acquired
N28.81	Hypertrophy of kidney
N28.82	Megaloureter
Q60.3	Renal hypoplasia, unilateral
Q60.4	Renal hypoplasia, bilateral
Q60.6	Potter's syndrome
Q61.01	Congenital single renal cyst
Q61.02	Congenital multiple renal cysts
Q61.11	Cystic dilatation of collecting ducts
Q61.2	Polycystic kidney, adult type
Q61.4	Renal dysplasia
Q61.5	Medullary cystic kidney
Q62.0	Congenital hydronephrosis
Q62.11	Congenital occlusion of ureteropelvic junction
Q62.2	Congenital megaureter
Q62.31	Congenital ureterocele, orthotopic
Q62.39	Other obstructive defects of renal pelvis and ureter
❼⇄ S37.061	Major laceration of right kidney
❼⇄ S37.062	Major laceration of left kidney
❼⇄ S37.091	Other injury of right kidney
❼⇄ S37.092	Other injury of left kidney

ICD-10-CM Coding Notes

For codes requiring a 7th character extension, refer to your ICD-10-CM book. Review the character descriptions and coding guidelines for proper selection. For some procedures, only certain characters will apply.

CCI Edits

Refer to Appendix A for CCI edits.

Facility RVUs ☐

Code	Work	PE Facility	MP	Total Facility
50548	25.36	10.74	3.06	39.16

Non-facility RVUs ☐

Code	Work	PE Non-Facility	MP	Total Non-Facility
50548	25.36	10.74	3.06	39.16

Modifiers (PAR) ☐

Code	Mod 50	Mod 51	Mod 62	Mod 66	Mod 80
50548	1	2	1	0	2

Global Period

Code	Days
50548	090

CPT® Procedural Coding

50551-50553

50551 Renal endoscopy through established nephrostomy or pyelostomy, with or without irrigation, instillation, or ureteropyelography, exclusive of radiologic service

50553 Renal endoscopy through established nephrostomy or pyelostomy, with or without irrigation, instillation, or ureteropyelography, exclusive of radiologic service; with ureteral catheterization, with or without dilation of ureter

(For image-guided dilation of ureter without endoscopic guidance, use 50706)

AMA Coding Notes

Endoscopy Procedures on the Kidney

(For supplies and materials, use 99070)

Surgical Procedures on the Urinary System

(For provision of chemotherapeutic agents, report both the specific service in addition to code(s) for the specific substance(s) or drug(s) provided)

AMA *CPT® Assistant*

50551: Oct 01: 8, Jan 03: 21
50553: Oct 01: 8

Plain English Description

To perform endoscopy through an existing nephrostomy, the external drainage bag is removed from the nephrostomy or pyelostomy tube. A guidewire is advanced through the tube and the nephrostomy tube is removed over the guidewire. A series of dilators are then advanced over the guidewire and the tract is dilated to allow insertion of the endoscope. The renal endoscope is inserted into the kidney through the established nephrostomy or pyelostomy tract. The kidney is carefully examined. In 50551, sterile saline or other solution may be used to irrigate the kidney; a diagnostic or therapeutic solution may be instilled into the kidney; or contrast may be instilled for separately reportable radiopyelography. In 50553, ureteral catheterization is performed in addition to the procedures described above. A ureteral catheter is advanced through the endoscope and into the ureter, which is carefully examined for obstruction or stenosis. If stenosis is present, a balloon-tipped catheter is introduced to the site of the stenosis and inflated. The balloon may be deflated and inflated several times until the stenotic region is adequately dilated. All instruments are then removed, the nephrostomy tube is replaced, and the external drainage bag is reattached to the nephrostomy tube.

Renal endoscopy through established nephrostomy or pyelostomy

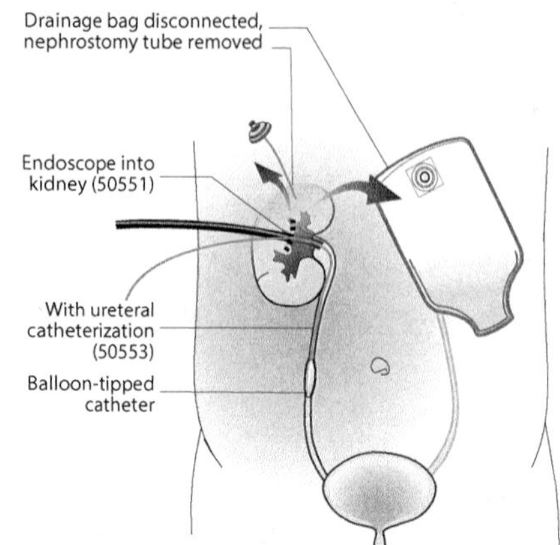

ICD-10-CM Diagnostic Codes

	Code	Description
⇄	C64.1	Malignant neoplasm of right kidney, except renal pelvis
⇄	C64.2	Malignant neoplasm of left kidney, except renal pelvis
⇄	C65.1	Malignant neoplasm of right renal pelvis
⇄	C65.2	Malignant neoplasm of left renal pelvis
⇄	C66.1	Malignant neoplasm of right ureter
⇄	C66.2	Malignant neoplasm of left ureter
	C67.6	Malignant neoplasm of ureteric orifice
⇄	C79.01	Secondary malignant neoplasm of right kidney and renal pelvis
⇄	C79.02	Secondary malignant neoplasm of left kidney and renal pelvis
	C79.19	Secondary malignant neoplasm of other urinary organs
	C7A.093	Malignant carcinoid tumor of the kidney
	D09.19	Carcinoma in situ of other urinary organs
⇄	D30.01	Benign neoplasm of right kidney
⇄	D30.02	Benign neoplasm of left kidney
⇄	D30.11	Benign neoplasm of right renal pelvis
⇄	D30.12	Benign neoplasm of left renal pelvis
⇄	D30.21	Benign neoplasm of right ureter
⇄	D30.22	Benign neoplasm of left ureter
	D3A.093	Benign carcinoid tumor of the kidney
	N02.0	Recurrent and persistent hematuria with minor glomerular abnormality
	N02.8	Recurrent and persistent hematuria with other morphologic changes
	N02.9	Recurrent and persistent hematuria with unspecified morphologic changes
	N11.1	Chronic obstructive pyelonephritis
	N13.0	Hydronephrosis with ureteropelvic junction obstruction
	N13.1	Hydronephrosis with ureteral stricture, not elsewhere classified
	N13.2	Hydronephrosis with renal and ureteral calculous obstruction
	N13.39	Other hydronephrosis
	N13.4	Hydroureter
	N13.5	Crossing vessel and stricture of ureter without hydronephrosis
	N13.8	Other obstructive and reflux uropathy
	N15.1	Renal and perinephric abscess
	N20.0	Calculus of kidney
	N20.1	Calculus of ureter
	N20.2	Calculus of kidney with calculus of ureter
	N28.0	Ischemia and infarction of kidney
	N28.1	Cyst of kidney, acquired
	N28.84	Pyelitis cystica
	N28.85	Pyeloureteritis cystica
	N28.86	Ureteritis cystica
	N28.89	Other specified disorders of kidney and ureter
	Q61.01	Congenital single renal cyst
	Q61.02	Congenital multiple renal cysts
	Q61.11	Cystic dilatation of collecting ducts
	Q61.2	Polycystic kidney, adult type
	Q61.3	Polycystic kidney, unspecified
	Q61.4	Renal dysplasia
	Q61.5	Medullary cystic kidney
	Q61.8	Other cystic kidney diseases
	Q61.9	Cystic kidney disease, unspecified
	Q62.0	Congenital hydronephrosis
	Q62.10	Congenital occlusion of ureter, unspecified
	Q62.11	Congenital occlusion of ureteropelvic junction
	Q62.12	Congenital occlusion of ureterovesical orifice
	Q62.31	Congenital ureterocele, orthotopic
	Q62.39	Other obstructive defects of renal pelvis and ureter
	R31.0	Gross hematuria
	R31.9	Hematuria, unspecified

CCI Edits

Refer to Appendix A for CCI edits.

Facility RVUs

Code	Work	PE Facility	MP	Total Facility
50551	5.59	2.28	0.66	8.53
50553	5.98	2.41	0.72	9.11

Non-facility RVUs

Code	Work	PE Non-Facility	MP	Total Non-Facility
50551	5.59	4.35	0.66	10.60
50553	5.98	4.66	0.72	11.36

Modifiers (PAR)

Code	Mod 50	Mod 51	Mod 62	Mod 66	Mod 80
50551	1	2	0	0	0
50553	1	2	0	0	1

Global Period

Code	Days
50551	000
50553	000

50555-50557

50555 Renal endoscopy through established nephrostomy or pyelostomy, with or without irrigation, instillation, or ureteropyelography, exclusive of radiologic service; with biopsy

(For image-guided biopsy of ureter and/or renal pelvis without endoscopic guidance, use 50606)

50557 Renal endoscopy through established nephrostomy or pyelostomy, with or without irrigation, instillation, or ureteropyelography, exclusive of radiologic service; with fulguration and/or incision, with or without biopsy

AMA Coding Notes

Endoscopy Procedures on the Kidney

(For supplies and materials, use 99070)

Surgical Procedures on the Urinary System

(For provision of chemotherapeutic agents, report both the specific service in addition to code(s) for the specific substance(s) or drug(s) provided)

AMA *CPT® Assistant* ▯

50555: Oct 01: 8
50557: Oct 01: 8

Plain English Description

To obtain a biopsy or fulgurate lesions of the kidney endoscopically through an existing nephrostomy, the external drainage bag is first removed from the nephrostomy or pyelostomy tube. A guidewire is advanced through the tube and the nephrostomy tube is removed over the guidewire. A series of dilators are then advanced over the guidewire and the tract is dilated to allow insertion of the endoscope. A renal endoscope is inserted into the kidney through the established nephrostomy or pyelostomy tract. The kidney is carefully examined. Sterile saline or other solution may be used to irrigate the kidney; a diagnostic or therapeutic solution may be instilled into the kidney; or contrast may be instilled for separately reportable radiopyelography. In 50555, following the endoscopic examination of the kidney, biopsy forceps are introduced through the endoscope and one or more tissue samples are obtained. In 50557, following endoscopic examination, an electrocautery tool is introduced through the endoscope and lesions or tissue in the kidney are destroyed and/or the renal pelvis or calyces may be incised. Tissue samples may also be obtained. All instruments are then removed; the nephrostomy tube is replaced; and the external drainage bag is reattached to the nephrostomy tube.

Renal endoscopy through established nephrostomy or pyelostomy

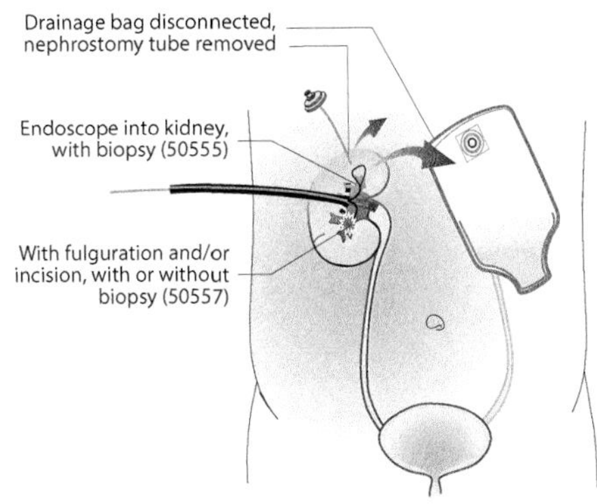

ICD-10-CM Diagnostic Codes

	Code	Description
⇄	C64.1	Malignant neoplasm of right kidney, except renal pelvis
⇄	C64.2	Malignant neoplasm of left kidney, except renal pelvis
⇄	C65.1	Malignant neoplasm of right renal pelvis
⇄	C65.2	Malignant neoplasm of left renal pelvis
⇄	C66.1	Malignant neoplasm of right ureter
⇄	C66.2	Malignant neoplasm of left ureter
	C67.6	Malignant neoplasm of ureteric orifice
	C68.8	Malignant neoplasm of overlapping sites of urinary organs
⇄	C79.01	Secondary malignant neoplasm of right kidney and renal pelvis
⇄	C79.02	Secondary malignant neoplasm of left kidney and renal pelvis
	C79.19	Secondary malignant neoplasm of other urinary organs
	C7A.093	Malignant carcinoid tumor of the kidney
	C80.2	Malignant neoplasm associated with transplanted organ
	D09.19	Carcinoma in situ of other urinary organs
⇄	D30.01	Benign neoplasm of right kidney
⇄	D30.02	Benign neoplasm of left kidney
⇄	D30.11	Benign neoplasm of right renal pelvis
⇄	D30.12	Benign neoplasm of left renal pelvis
⇄	D30.21	Benign neoplasm of right ureter
⇄	D30.22	Benign neoplasm of left ureter
	D3A.093	Benign carcinoid tumor of the kidney
⇄	D41.01	Neoplasm of uncertain behavior of right kidney
⇄	D41.02	Neoplasm of uncertain behavior of left kidney
⇄	D41.11	Neoplasm of uncertain behavior of right renal pelvis
⇄	D41.12	Neoplasm of uncertain behavior of left renal pelvis
⇄	D41.21	Neoplasm of uncertain behavior of right ureter
⇄	D41.22	Neoplasm of uncertain behavior of left ureter
	N13.0	Hydronephrosis with ureteropelvic junction obstruction
	N13.1	Hydronephrosis with ureteral stricture, not elsewhere classified
	N13.2	Hydronephrosis with renal and ureteral calculous obstruction
	N13.3	Other and unspecified hydronephrosis
	N13.4	Hydroureter
	N13.721	Vesicoureteral-reflux with reflux nephropathy without hydroureter, unilateral
	N13.722	Vesicoureteral-reflux with reflux nephropathy without hydroureter, bilateral
	N13.731	Vesicoureteral-reflux with reflux nephropathy with hydroureter, unilateral
	N13.732	Vesicoureteral-reflux with reflux nephropathy with hydroureter, bilateral
	N13.8	Other obstructive and reflux uropathy
	N17.0	Acute kidney failure with tubular necrosis
	N17.1	Acute kidney failure with acute cortical necrosis
	N17.2	Acute kidney failure with medullary necrosis
	N20.0	Calculus of kidney
	N20.1	Calculus of ureter
	N20.2	Calculus of kidney with calculus of ureter
	N28.0	Ischemia and infarction of kidney
	N28.1	Cyst of kidney, acquired
	N28.81	Hypertrophy of kidney
	N28.84	Pyelitis cystica
	N28.85	Pyeloureteritis cystica
	N28.86	Ureteritis cystica
	Q61.01	Congenital single renal cyst
	Q61.02	Congenital multiple renal cysts
	Q61.11	Cystic dilatation of collecting ducts
	Q61.2	Polycystic kidney, adult type
	Q61.3	Polycystic kidney, unspecified
	Q61.4	Renal dysplasia
	Q61.5	Medullary cystic kidney
	Q62.0	Congenital hydronephrosis
	Q62.11	Congenital occlusion of ureteropelvic junction
	Q62.12	Congenital occlusion of ureterovesical orifice
	Q62.2	Congenital megaureter
	Q62.31	Congenital ureterocele, orthotopic
	Q62.39	Other obstructive defects of renal pelvis and ureter
	Z94.0	Kidney transplant status

CCI Edits

Refer to Appendix A for CCI edits.

Facility RVUs

Code	Work	PE Facility	MP	Total Facility
50555	6.52	2.59	0.77	9.88
50557	6.61	2.62	0.78	10.01

Non-facility RVUs

Code	Work	PE Non-Facility	MP	Total Non-Facility
50555	6.52	4.80	0.77	12.09
50557	6.61	4.91	0.78	12.30

Modifiers (PAR)

Code	Mod 50	Mod 51	Mod 62	Mod 66	Mod 80
50555	1	3	0	0	0
50557	1	3	0	0	0

Global Period

Code	Days
50555	000
50557	000

50561

50561 Renal endoscopy through established nephrostomy or pyelostomy, with or without irrigation, instillation, or ureteropyelography, exclusive of radiologic service; with removal of foreign body or calculus

AMA Coding Notes

Endoscopy Procedures on the Kidney

(For supplies and materials, use 99070)

Surgical Procedures on the Urinary System

(For provision of chemotherapeutic agents, report both the specific service in addition to code(s) for the specific substance(s) or drug(s) provided)

AMA *CPT® Assistant* ▯

50561: Oct 01: 8, Jan 03: 21

Plain English Description

To remove a foreign body or stone endoscopically through an existing nephrostomy, the external drainage bag is first removed from the nephrostomy or pyelostomy tube. A guidewire is advanced through the tube and the nephrostomy tube is removed over the guidewire. A series of dilators are then advanced over the guidewire and the tract is dilated to allow insertion of the endoscope. A renal endoscope (nephroscope) is inserted into the kidney through the established nephrostomy or pyelostomy tract. The kidney is carefully examined and the foreign body or calculus is located. Sterile saline or other solution may be used to irrigate the kidney; a diagnostic or therapeutic solution may be instilled into the kidney; or contrast may be instilled for separately reportable radiopyelography. An endograsper is introduced through the nephroscope and the foreign body or calculus is grasped and removed through the endoscope. The renal pelvis and calyces are again inspected to ensure that all foreign body or calculus fragments have been removed. All instruments are removed; the nephrostomy tube is replaced; and the external drainage bag is reattached to the nephrostomy tube.

Renal endoscopy through established nephrostomy or pyelostomy

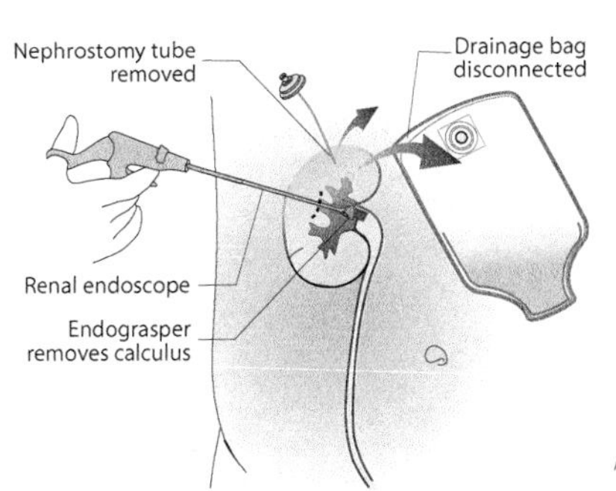

ICD-10-CM Diagnostic Codes

	Code	Description
	N13.2	Hydronephrosis with renal and ureteral calculous obstruction
	N13.6	Pyonephrosis
	N13.8	Other obstructive and reflux uropathy
	N20.0	Calculus of kidney
	N20.1	Calculus of ureter
	N20.2	Calculus of kidney with calculus of ureter
	N20.9	Urinary calculus, unspecified
	N22	Calculus of urinary tract in diseases classified elsewhere
❼	T19.8	Foreign body in other parts of genitourinary tract
❼	T81.500	Unspecified complication of foreign body accidentally left in body following surgical operation
❼	T81.504	Unspecified complication of foreign body accidentally left in body following endoscopic examination
❼	T81.510	Adhesions due to foreign body accidentally left in body following surgical operation
❼	T81.514	Adhesions due to foreign body accidentally left in body following endoscopic examination
❼	T81.520	Obstruction due to foreign body accidentally left in body following surgical operation
❼	T81.524	Obstruction due to foreign body accidentally left in body following endoscopic examination
❼	T81.530	Perforation due to foreign body accidentally left in body following surgical operation
❼	T81.534	Perforation due to foreign body accidentally left in body following endoscopic examination
❼	T81.590	Other complications of foreign body accidentally left in body following surgical operation
❼	T81.594	Other complications of foreign body accidentally left in body following endoscopic examination
❼	T83.012	Breakdown (mechanical) of nephrostomy catheter
❼	T83.022	Displacement of nephrostomy catheter
❼	T83.032	Leakage of nephrostomy catheter
❼	T83.092	Other mechanical complication of nephrostomy catheter
❼	T83.512	Infection and inflammatory reaction due to nephrostomy catheter
❼	T83.84	Pain due to genitourinary prosthetic devices, implants and grafts

ICD-10-CM Coding Notes

For codes requiring a 7th character extension, refer to your ICD-10-CM book. Review the character descriptions and coding guidelines for proper selection. For some procedures, only certain characters will apply.

CCI Edits

Refer to Appendix A for CCI edits.

Facility RVUs ▯

Code	Work	PE Facility	MP	Total Facility
50561	7.58	2.95	0.90	11.43

Non-facility RVUs ▯

Code	Work	PE Non-Facility	MP	Total Non-Facility
50561	7.58	5.46	0.90	13.94

Modifiers (PAR) ▯

Code	Mod 50	Mod 51	Mod 62	Mod 66	Mod 80
50561	1	3	0	0	0

Global Period

Code	Days
50561	000

50562

50562 Renal endoscopy through established nephrostomy or pyelostomy, with or without irrigation, instillation, or ureteropyelography, exclusive of radiologic service; with resection of tumor

(When procedures 50570-50580 provide a significant identifiable service, they may be added to 50045 and 50120)

AMA Coding Notes

Endoscopy Procedures on the Kidney

(For supplies and materials, use 99070)

Surgical Procedures on the Urinary System

(For provision of chemotherapeutic agents, report both the specific service in addition to code(s) for the specific substance(s) or drug(s) provided)

AMA *CPT® Assistant*

50562: Jan 03: 21

Plain English Description

The external drainage bag is removed from the existing nephrostomy or pyelostomy tube. A guidewire is advanced through the nephrostomy tube and the tube is removed. A series of dilators are then advanced over the guidewire and the tract is dilated to allow insertion of the endoscope. A renal endoscope is inserted into the kidney through the established nephrostomy or pyelostomy tract. The kidney is carefully examined and the tumor is located. Sterile saline or other solution may be used to irrigate the kidney; a diagnostic or therapeutic solution may be instilled into the kidney; or contrast may be instilled for separately reportable radiopyelography. The nephroscope is exchanged for a resectoscope and the renal tumor is resected and removed using irrigation and an endoscopic evacuation device. The kidney is then re-examined to ensure that all of the tumor has been removed. Bleeding is controlled by fulguration. The resectoscope is removed. The nephrostomy tube is replaced and the external drainage bag is reattached to the nephrostomy tube.

Renal endoscopy through established nephrostomy or pyelostomy

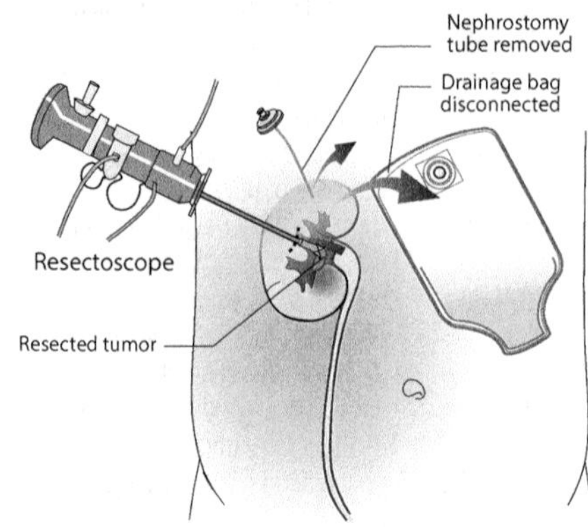

ICD-10-CM Diagnostic Codes

	Code	Description
⇄	C64.1	Malignant neoplasm of right kidney, except renal pelvis
⇄	C64.2	Malignant neoplasm of left kidney, except renal pelvis
⇄	C65.1	Malignant neoplasm of right renal pelvis
⇄	C65.2	Malignant neoplasm of left renal pelvis
⇄	C79.01	Secondary malignant neoplasm of right kidney and renal pelvis
⇄	C79.02	Secondary malignant neoplasm of left kidney and renal pelvis
	C7A.093	Malignant carcinoid tumor of the kidney
	C80.2	Malignant neoplasm associated with transplanted organ
	D09.19	Carcinoma in situ of other urinary organs
⇄	D30.01	Benign neoplasm of right kidney
⇄	D30.02	Benign neoplasm of left kidney
⇄	D30.11	Benign neoplasm of right renal pelvis
⇄	D30.12	Benign neoplasm of left renal pelvis
	D3A.093	Benign carcinoid tumor of the kidney
⇄	D41.01	Neoplasm of uncertain behavior of right kidney
⇄	D41.02	Neoplasm of uncertain behavior of left kidney
⇄	D41.11	Neoplasm of uncertain behavior of right renal pelvis
⇄	D41.12	Neoplasm of uncertain behavior of left renal pelvis
	Z94.0	Kidney transplant status

CCI Edits

Refer to Appendix A for CCI edits.

Facility RVUs

Code	Work	PE Facility	MP	Total Facility
50562	10.90	4.59	1.29	16.78

Non-facility RVUs

Code	Work	PE Non-Facility	MP	Total Non-Facility
50562	10.90	4.59	1.29	16.78

Modifiers (PAR)

Code	Mod 50	Mod 51	Mod 62	Mod 66	Mod 80
50562	0	2	1	0	2

Global Period

Code	Days
50562	090

50570-50572

50570 Renal endoscopy through nephrotomy or pyelotomy, with or without irrigation, instillation, or ureteropyelography, exclusive of radiologic service

(For nephrotomy, use 50045)

(For pyelotomy, use 50120)

50572 Renal endoscopy through nephrotomy or pyelotomy, with or without irrigation, instillation, or ureteropyelography, exclusive of radiologic service; with ureteral catheterization, with or without dilation of ureter

(For image-guided dilation of ureter without endoscopic guidance, use 50706)

AMA Coding Notes

Endoscopy Procedures on the Kidney

(For supplies and materials, use 99070)

Surgical Procedures on the Urinary System

(For provision of chemotherapeutic agents, report both the specific service in addition to code(s) for the specific substance(s) or drug(s) provided)

AMA *CPT® Assistant*

50570: Oct 01: 8

50572: Oct 01: 8

Plain English Description

A small incision is made in the kidney. A renal endoscope is inserted into the kidney through the incision and the kidney is carefully examined. In 50570, sterile saline or other solution may be used to irrigate the kidney; a diagnostic or therapeutic solution may be instilled into the kidney; or contrast may be instilled for separately reportable radiopyelography. In 50572, a ureteral catheterization is also performed in addition to the endoscopic examination with or without irrigation, instillation, or ureteropyelography. Following renal endoscopy, a ureteral catheter is advanced through the endoscope and into the ureter. The ureter is carefully examined for obstruction or stenosis. If stenosis is present, a balloon-tipped catheter is introduced to the site of the stenosis and inflated. This balloon may be deflated and inflated several times until the stenotic region is adequately dilated. All instruments are then removed. A nephrostomy tube is placed as needed and the incision is closed.

Renal endoscopy through nephrotomy or pyelotomy

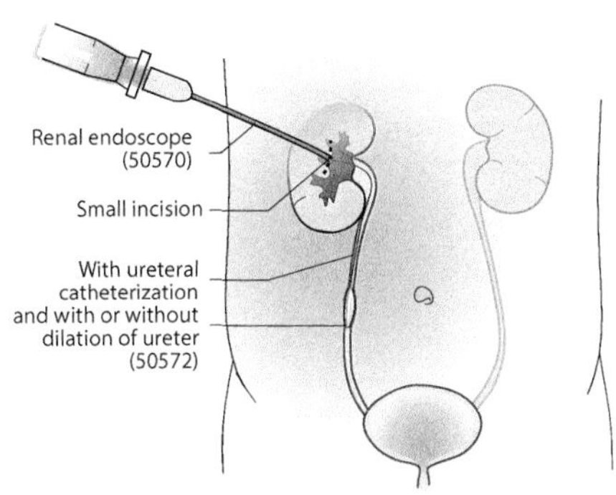

ICD-10-CM Diagnostic Codes

	Code	Description
⇄	C64.1	Malignant neoplasm of right kidney, except renal pelvis
⇄	C64.2	Malignant neoplasm of left kidney, except renal pelvis
⇄	C65.1	Malignant neoplasm of right renal pelvis
⇄	C65.2	Malignant neoplasm of left renal pelvis
⇄	C66.1	Malignant neoplasm of right ureter
⇄	C66.2	Malignant neoplasm of left ureter
	C67.6	Malignant neoplasm of ureteric orifice
⇄	C79.01	Secondary malignant neoplasm of right kidney and renal pelvis
⇄	C79.02	Secondary malignant neoplasm of left kidney and renal pelvis
	C79.19	Secondary malignant neoplasm of other urinary organs
	C7A.093	Malignant carcinoid tumor of the kidney
	D09.19	Carcinoma in situ of other urinary organs
⇄	D30.01	Benign neoplasm of right kidney
⇄	D30.02	Benign neoplasm of left kidney
⇄	D30.11	Benign neoplasm of right renal pelvis
⇄	D30.12	Benign neoplasm of left renal pelvis
⇄	D30.21	Benign neoplasm of right ureter
⇄	D30.22	Benign neoplasm of left ureter
	D3A.093	Benign carcinoid tumor of the kidney
⇄	D41.01	Neoplasm of uncertain behavior of right kidney
⇄	D41.02	Neoplasm of uncertain behavior of left kidney
⇄	D41.11	Neoplasm of uncertain behavior of right renal pelvis
⇄	D41.12	Neoplasm of uncertain behavior of left renal pelvis
⇄	D41.21	Neoplasm of uncertain behavior of right ureter
⇄	D41.22	Neoplasm of uncertain behavior of left ureter
	N02.9	Recurrent and persistent hematuria with unspecified morphologic changes
	N13.0	Hydronephrosis with ureteropelvic junction obstruction
	N13.1	Hydronephrosis with ureteral stricture, not elsewhere classified
	N13.2	Hydronephrosis with renal and ureteral calculous obstruction
	N13.39	Other hydronephrosis
	N13.4	Hydroureter
	N13.5	Crossing vessel and stricture of ureter without hydronephrosis
	N13.6	Pyonephrosis
	N13.8	Other obstructive and reflux uropathy
	N15.1	Renal and perinephric abscess
	N20.0	Calculus of kidney
	N20.1	Calculus of ureter
	N20.2	Calculus of kidney with calculus of ureter
	N22	Calculus of urinary tract in diseases classified elsewhere
	N23	Unspecified renal colic
	N28.0	Ischemia and infarction of kidney
	N28.1	Cyst of kidney, acquired
	N28.81	Hypertrophy of kidney
	N28.84	Pyelitis cystica
	N28.85	Pyeloureteritis cystica
	N28.86	Ureteritis cystica
	N28.9	Disorder of kidney and ureter, unspecified
	Q61.01	Congenital single renal cyst
	Q61.02	Congenital multiple renal cysts
	Q61.11	Cystic dilatation of collecting ducts
	Q61.2	Polycystic kidney, adult type
	Q61.3	Polycystic kidney, unspecified
	Q61.4	Renal dysplasia
	Q61.5	Medullary cystic kidney
	Q61.9	Cystic kidney disease, unspecified
	Q62.0	Congenital hydronephrosis
	Q62.10	Congenital occlusion of ureter, unspecified
	Q62.11	Congenital occlusion of ureteropelvic junction
	Q62.12	Congenital occlusion of ureterovesical orifice
	Q62.31	Congenital ureterocele, orthotopic
	Q62.39	Other obstructive defects of renal pelvis and ureter
	R34	Anuria and oliguria

CCI Edits

Refer to Appendix A for CCI edits.

Facility RVUs

Code	Work	PE Facility	MP	Total Facility
50570	9.53	3.57	1.12	14.22
50572	10.33	3.84	1.22	15.39

Non-facility RVUs

Code	Work	PE Non-Facility	MP	Total Non-Facility
50570	9.53	3.57	1.12	14.22
50572	10.33	3.84	1.22	15.39

Modifiers (PAR)

Code	Mod 50	Mod 51	Mod 62	Mod 66	Mod 80
50570	1	2	0	0	0
50572	1	3	0	0	0

Global Period

Code	Days
50570	000
50572	000

50574

50574 Renal endoscopy through nephrotomy or pyelotomy, with or without irrigation, instillation, or ureteropyelography, exclusive of radiologic service; with biopsy

(For image-guided biopsy of ureter and/or renal pelvis without endoscopic guidance, use 50606)

AMA Coding Notes

Endoscopy Procedures on the Kidney

(For supplies and materials, use 99070)

Surgical Procedures on the Urinary System

(For provision of chemotherapeutic agents, report both the specific service in addition to code(s) for the specific substance(s) or drug(s) provided)

AMA *CPT® Assistant* ▢

50574: Oct 01: 8

Plain English Description

A small incision is made in the kidney. A renal endoscope is inserted into the kidney through the incision and the kidney is carefully examined. Sterile saline or other solution may be used to irrigate the kidney; a diagnostic or therapeutic solution may be instilled into the kidney; or contrast may be instilled for separately reportable radiopyelography. Biopsy forceps are introduced through the endoscope and one or more tissue samples are obtained from the kidney. All instruments are then removed. A nephrostomy tube is placed as needed and the incision is closed.

Renal endoscopy through nephrotomy or pyelotomy
(exclusive of radiologic service; with biopsy)

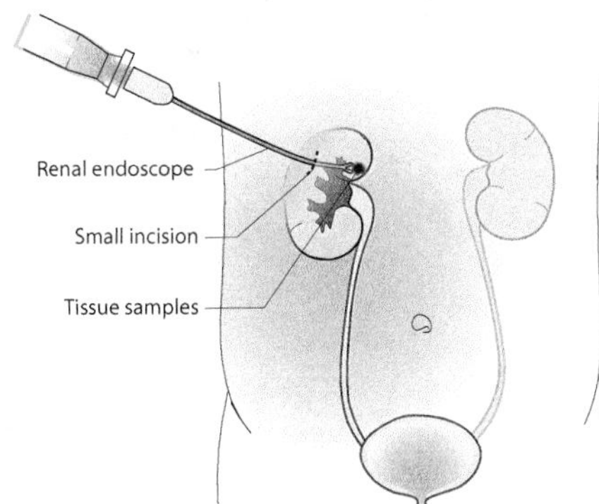

ICD-10-CM Diagnostic Codes

⇄	C64.1	Malignant neoplasm of right kidney, except renal pelvis
⇄	C64.2	Malignant neoplasm of left kidney, except renal pelvis
⇄	C65.1	Malignant neoplasm of right renal pelvis
⇄	C65.2	Malignant neoplasm of left renal pelvis
⇄	C79.01	Secondary malignant neoplasm of right kidney and renal pelvis
⇄	C79.02	Secondary malignant neoplasm of left kidney and renal pelvis
	C7A.093	Malignant carcinoid tumor of the kidney
	C80.2	Malignant neoplasm associated with transplanted organ
	D09.19	Carcinoma in situ of other urinary organs
⇄	D30.01	Benign neoplasm of right kidney
⇄	D30.02	Benign neoplasm of left kidney
⇄	D30.11	Benign neoplasm of right renal pelvis
⇄	D30.12	Benign neoplasm of left renal pelvis
	D3A.093	Benign carcinoid tumor of the kidney
⇄	D41.01	Neoplasm of uncertain behavior of right kidney
⇄	D41.02	Neoplasm of uncertain behavior of left kidney
⇄	D41.11	Neoplasm of uncertain behavior of right renal pelvis
⇄	D41.12	Neoplasm of uncertain behavior of left renal pelvis
	M32.14	Glomerular disease in systemic lupus erythematosus
	M32.15	Tubulo-interstitial nephropathy in systemic lupus erythematosus
	M35.04	Sjögren syndrome with tubulo-interstitial nephropathy
	N00.2	Acute nephritic syndrome with diffuse membranous glomerulonephritis
	N00.3	Acute nephritic syndrome with diffuse mesangial proliferative glomerulonephritis
	N00.4	Acute nephritic syndrome with diffuse endocapillary proliferative glomerulonephritis
	N00.5	Acute nephritic syndrome with diffuse mesangiocapillary glomerulonephritis
	N00.6	Acute nephritic syndrome with dense deposit disease
	N00.7	Acute nephritic syndrome with diffuse crescentic glomerulonephritis
	N00.8	Acute nephritic syndrome with other morphologic changes
	N00.9	Acute nephritic syndrome with unspecified morphologic changes
	N04.1	Nephrotic syndrome with focal and segmental glomerular lesions
	N04.2	Nephrotic syndrome with diffuse membranous glomerulonephritis
	N04.3	Nephrotic syndrome with diffuse mesangial proliferative glomerulonephritis
	N04.4	Nephrotic syndrome with diffuse endocapillary proliferative glomerulonephritis
	N04.5	Nephrotic syndrome with diffuse mesangiocapillary glomerulonephritis
	N04.6	Nephrotic syndrome with dense deposit disease
	N04.7	Nephrotic syndrome with diffuse crescentic glomerulonephritis
	N04.8	Nephrotic syndrome with other morphologic changes
	N04.9	Nephrotic syndrome with unspecified morphologic changes
	N08	Glomerular disorders in diseases classified elsewhere
	N10	Acute pyelonephritis
	N11.0	Nonobstructive reflux-associated chronic pyelonephritis
	N11.8	Other chronic tubulo-interstitial nephritis
	N13.39	Other hydronephrosis
	N13.6	Pyonephrosis
	N16	Renal tubulo-interstitial disorders in diseases classified elsewhere
	N17.0	Acute kidney failure with tubular necrosis
	N17.1	Acute kidney failure with acute cortical necrosis
	N17.2	Acute kidney failure with medullary necrosis
	N17.8	Other acute kidney failure
	N17.9	Acute kidney failure, unspecified
	N18.1	Chronic kidney disease, stage 1
	N18.2	Chronic kidney disease, stage 2 (mild)
	N18.30	Chronic kidney disease, stage 3 unspecified
	N18.31	Chronic kidney disease, stage 3a
	N18.32	Chronic kidney disease, stage 3b
	N18.4	Chronic kidney disease, stage 4 (severe)
	N18.5	Chronic kidney disease, stage 5
	N18.6	End stage renal disease
	N26.9	Renal sclerosis, unspecified
	N28.1	Cyst of kidney, acquired
	N28.81	Hypertrophy of kidney
	N28.84	Pyelitis cystica
	N28.85	Pyeloureteritis cystica
	N28.86	Ureteritis cystica
	N28.89	Other specified disorders of kidney and ureter
	N28.9	Disorder of kidney and ureter, unspecified
	Q61.01	Congenital single renal cyst
	Q61.02	Congenital multiple renal cysts
	Q61.2	Polycystic kidney, adult type
	Q61.4	Renal dysplasia
	Q61.5	Medullary cystic kidney
	Q61.8	Other cystic kidney diseases
	Q61.9	Cystic kidney disease, unspecified
	Z76.82	Awaiting organ transplant status
	Z94.0	Kidney transplant status

CCI Edits

Refer to Appendix A for CCI edits.

Facility RVUs

Code	Work	PE Facility	MP	Total Facility
50574	11.00	4.06	1.30	16.36

Non-facility RVUs

Code	Work	PE Non-Facility	MP	Total Non-Facility
50574	11.00	4.06	1.30	16.36

Modifiers (PAR)

Code	Mod 50	Mod 51	Mod 62	Mod 66	Mod 80
50574	1	3	0	0	0

Global Period

Code	Days
50574	000

50575

50575 Renal endoscopy through nephrotomy or pyelotomy, with or without irrigation, instillation, or ureteropyelography, exclusive of radiologic service; with endopyelotomy (includes cystoscopy, ureteroscopy, dilation of ureter and ureteral pelvic junction, incision of ureteral pelvic junction and insertion of endopyelotomy stent)

AMA Coding Notes

Endoscopy Procedures on the Kidney

(For supplies and materials, use 99070)

Surgical Procedures on the Urinary System

(For provision of chemotherapeutic agents, report both the specific service in addition to code(s) for the specific substance(s) or drug(s) provided)

AMA *CPT® Assistant*

50575: Oct 01: 8, Aug 02: 11

Plain English Description

A small incision is made in the kidney. A renal endoscope is inserted into the kidney through the incision and the kidney is carefully examined. Sterile saline or other solution may be used to irrigate the kidney; a diagnostic or therapeutic solution may be instilled into the kidney; or contrast may be instilled for separately reportable radiopyelography to assess a narrowed ureteropelvic junction. A cystoscope is introduced through the urethra and the bladder is examined. A guidewire is passed through the ureter and obstructed region of the renal pelvis in a retrograde fashion. A ureteroscope is advanced into the ureter over the guidewire and the ureter is examined. A second guidewire may be passed from the renal pelvis into the ureter in an antegrade fashion. Using endoscopic surgical tools such as an electrode device or laser, an endopyelotomy incision is made in the inner (tunica mucosa) and middle layers (tunica muscularis) of the ureteral pelvic junction. The outer fibrous layer (tunica adventitia) is left intact. A balloon dilator may then be used to increase the diameter of the tunica adventitia at the site of the stricture. An endopyelotomy stent is placed to maintain patency while the incision heals. Guidewires and surgical instruments are removed. A nephrostomy tube is placed as needed and the kidney incision is closed.

Renal endoscopy through nephrotomy or pyelotomy

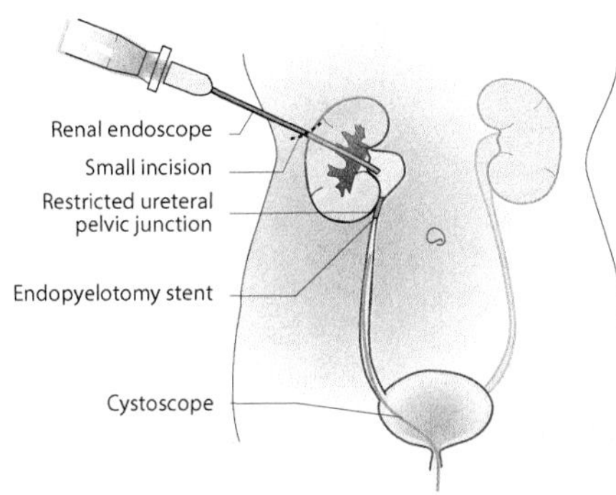

ICD-10-CM Diagnostic Codes

	Code	Description
⇄	C65.1	Malignant neoplasm of right renal pelvis
⇄	C65.2	Malignant neoplasm of left renal pelvis
⇄	C66.1	Malignant neoplasm of right ureter
⇄	C66.2	Malignant neoplasm of left ureter
⇄	C79.01	Secondary malignant neoplasm of right kidney and renal pelvis
⇄	C79.02	Secondary malignant neoplasm of left kidney and renal pelvis
	C7A.093	Malignant carcinoid tumor of the kidney
	D09.19	Carcinoma in situ of other urinary organs
⇄	D30.11	Benign neoplasm of right renal pelvis
⇄	D30.12	Benign neoplasm of left renal pelvis
⇄	D30.21	Benign neoplasm of right ureter
⇄	D30.22	Benign neoplasm of left ureter
	D3A.093	Benign carcinoid tumor of the kidney
⇄	D41.11	Neoplasm of uncertain behavior of right renal pelvis
⇄	D41.12	Neoplasm of uncertain behavior of left renal pelvis
⇄	D41.21	Neoplasm of uncertain behavior of right ureter
⇄	D41.22	Neoplasm of uncertain behavior of left ureter
	N11.1	Chronic obstructive pyelonephritis
	N13.0	Hydronephrosis with ureteropelvic junction obstruction
	N13.1	Hydronephrosis with ureteral stricture, not elsewhere classified
	N13.2	Hydronephrosis with renal and ureteral calculous obstruction
	N13.39	Other hydronephrosis
	N13.4	Hydroureter
	N13.8	Other obstructive and reflux uropathy
	N20.0	Calculus of kidney
	N20.1	Calculus of ureter
	N20.2	Calculus of kidney with calculus of ureter
	N28.9	Disorder of kidney and ureter, unspecified
	Q62.0	Congenital hydronephrosis
	Q62.11	Congenital occlusion of ureteropelvic junction
	Q62.31	Congenital ureterocele, orthotopic
	Q62.32	Cecoureterocele
	Q62.39	Other obstructive defects of renal pelvis and ureter

CCI Edits

Refer to Appendix A for CCI edits.

Facility RVUs

Code	Work	PE Facility	MP	Total Facility
50575	13.96	5.06	1.66	20.68

Non-facility RVUs

Code	Work	PE Non-Facility	MP	Total Non-Facility
50575	13.96	5.06	1.66	20.68

Modifiers (PAR)

Code	Mod 50	Mod 51	Mod 62	Mod 66	Mod 80
50575	1	3	0	0	1

Global Period

Code	Days
50575	000

50576

50576 Renal endoscopy through nephrotomy or pyelotomy, with or without irrigation, instillation, or ureteropyelography, exclusive of radiologic service; with fulguration and/or incision, with or without biopsy

AMA Coding Notes

Endoscopy Procedures on the Kidney

(For supplies and materials, use 99070)

Surgical Procedures on the Urinary System

(For provision of chemotherapeutic agents, report both the specific service in addition to code(s) for the specific substance(s) or drug(s) provided)

AMA *CPT® Assistant*

50576: Oct 01: 8

Plain English Description

A small incision is made in the kidney. A renal endoscope is inserted into the kidney through the incision and the kidney is carefully examined. Sterile saline or other solution may be used to irrigate the kidney; a diagnostic or therapeutic solution may be instilled into the kidney; or contrast may be instilled for separately reportable radiopyelography. Following endoscopic examination, an electrocautery tool is introduced through the endoscope and lesions or tissue in the kidney are destroyed and/or the renal pelvis or calyces may be incised. Biopsy forceps may also be introduced and one or more tissue samples obtained. All instruments are then removed. A nephrostomy tube is placed as needed and the incision is closed.

Renal endoscopy through nephrotomy or pyelotomy, with fulguration, with or without biopsy

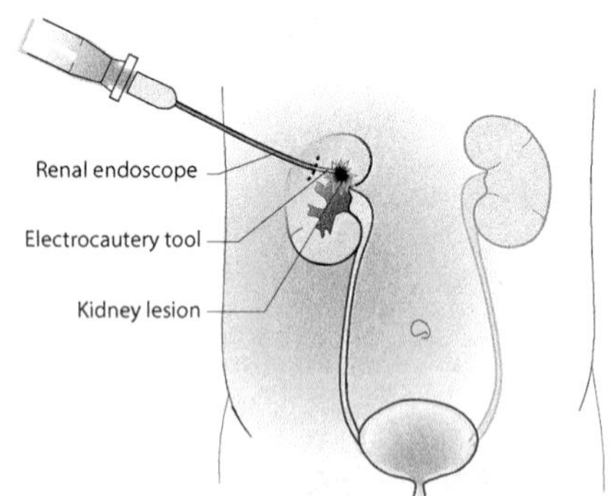

ICD-10-CM Diagnostic Codes

⇄ C64.1 Malignant neoplasm of right kidney, except renal pelvis
⇄ C64.2 Malignant neoplasm of left kidney, except renal pelvis
⇄ C65.1 Malignant neoplasm of right renal pelvis
⇄ C65.2 Malignant neoplasm of left renal pelvis
C68.8 Malignant neoplasm of overlapping sites of urinary organs
⇄ C79.01 Secondary malignant neoplasm of right kidney and renal pelvis
⇄ C79.02 Secondary malignant neoplasm of left kidney and renal pelvis
C79.19 Secondary malignant neoplasm of other urinary organs
C7A.093 Malignant carcinoid tumor of the kidney
C80.2 Malignant neoplasm associated with transplanted organ
D09.19 Carcinoma in situ of other urinary organs
⇄ D30.01 Benign neoplasm of right kidney
⇄ D30.02 Benign neoplasm of left kidney
⇄ D30.11 Benign neoplasm of right renal pelvis
⇄ D30.12 Benign neoplasm of left renal pelvis
D3A.093 Benign carcinoid tumor of the kidney
⇄ D41.01 Neoplasm of uncertain behavior of right kidney
⇄ D41.02 Neoplasm of uncertain behavior of left kidney
⇄ D41.11 Neoplasm of uncertain behavior of right renal pelvis
⇄ D41.12 Neoplasm of uncertain behavior of left renal pelvis
N15.1 Renal and perinephric abscess
N28.0 Ischemia and infarction of kidney
N28.1 Cyst of kidney, acquired
N28.84 Pyelitis cystica
N28.85 Pyeloureteritis cystica
N28.86 Ureteritis cystica
N28.89 Other specified disorders of kidney and ureter
N29 Other disorders of kidney and ureter in diseases classified elsewhere
Q61.01 Congenital single renal cyst
Q61.02 Congenital multiple renal cysts
Q61.11 Cystic dilatation of collecting ducts
Q61.2 Polycystic kidney, adult type
Q61.5 Medullary cystic kidney

CCI Edits

Refer to Appendix A for CCI edits.

Facility RVUs

Code	Work	PE Facility	MP	Total Facility
50576	10.97	4.05	1.30	16.32

Non-facility RVUs

Code	Work	PE Non-Facility	MP	Total Non-Facility
50576	10.97	4.05	1.30	16.32

Modifiers (PAR)

Code	Mod 50	Mod 51	Mod 62	Mod 66	Mod 80
50576	1	3	0	0	0

Global Period

Code	Days
50576	000

50580

50580 Renal endoscopy through nephrotomy or pyelotomy, with or without irrigation, instillation, or ureteropyelography, exclusive of radiologic service; with removal of foreign body or calculus

AMA Coding Notes

Endoscopy Procedures on the Kidney

(For supplies and materials, use 99070)

Surgical Procedures on the Urinary System

(For provision of chemotherapeutic agents, report both the specific service in addition to code(s) for the specific substance(s) or drug(s) provided)

AMA *CPT® Assistant* ☐

50580: Oct 01: 8

Plain English Description

A small incision is made in the kidney. A renal endoscope is inserted into the kidney through the incision and the kidney is carefully examined. The foreign body or calculus is located. Sterile saline or other solution may be used to irrigate the kidney; a diagnostic or therapeutic solution may be instilled into the kidney; or contrast may be instilled for separately reportable radiopyelography. An endograsper is introduced through the nephroscope and the foreign body or calculus is grasped and removed through the endoscope. The renal pelvis and calyces are again inspected to ensure that all foreign body or calculus fragments have been removed. All instruments are then removed. A nephrostomy tube is placed as needed and the incision is closed.

Renal endoscopy through nephrotomy or pyelotomy
(with removal of foreign body or calculus)

ICD-10-CM Diagnostic Codes

	Code	Description
	N20.0	Calculus of kidney
	N20.1	Calculus of ureter
	N20.2	Calculus of kidney with calculus of ureter
	N20.9	Urinary calculus, unspecified
	N22	Calculus of urinary tract in diseases classified elsewhere
➐	T19.8	Foreign body in other parts of genitourinary tract
➐	T81.500	Unspecified complication of foreign body accidentally left in body following surgical operation
➐	T81.504	Unspecified complication of foreign body accidentally left in body following endoscopic examination
➐	T81.506	Unspecified complication of foreign body accidentally left in body following aspiration, puncture or other catheterization
➐	T81.507	Unspecified complication of foreign body accidentally left in body following removal of catheter or packing
➐	T81.508	Unspecified complication of foreign body accidentally left in body following other procedure
➐	T81.520	Obstruction due to foreign body accidentally left in body following surgical operation
➐	T81.524	Obstruction due to foreign body accidentally left in body following endoscopic examination
➐	T81.526	Obstruction due to foreign body accidentally left in body following aspiration, puncture or other catheterization
➐	T81.527	Obstruction due to foreign body accidentally left in body following removal of catheter or packing
➐	T81.528	Obstruction due to foreign body accidentally left in body following other procedure
➐	T81.530	Perforation due to foreign body accidentally left in body following surgical operation
➐	T81.534	Perforation due to foreign body accidentally left in body following endoscopic examination
➐	T81.536	Perforation due to foreign body accidentally left in body following aspiration, puncture or other catheterization
➐	T81.537	Perforation due to foreign body accidentally left in body following removal of catheter or packing
➐	T81.538	Perforation due to foreign body accidentally left in body following other procedure
➐	T81.590	Other complications of foreign body accidentally left in body following surgical operation
➐	T81.594	Other complications of foreign body accidentally left in body following endoscopic examination
➐	T81.596	Other complications of foreign body accidentally left in body following aspiration, puncture or other catheterization
➐	T81.597	Other complications of foreign body accidentally left in body following removal of catheter or packing
➐	T81.598	Other complications of foreign body accidentally left in body following other procedure

ICD-10-CM Coding Notes

For codes requiring a 7th character extension, refer to your ICD-10-CM book. Review the character descriptions and coding guidelines for proper selection. For some procedures, only certain characters will apply.

CCI Edits

Refer to Appendix A for CCI edits.

Pub 100

50580: Pub 100-03, 1, 230.1

Facility RVUs ☐

Code	Work	PE Facility	MP	Total Facility
50580	11.84	4.34	1.40	17.58

Non-facility RVUs ☐

Code	Work	PE Non-Facility	MP	Total Non-Facility
50580	11.84	4.34	1.40	17.58

Modifiers (PAR) ☐

Code	Mod 50	Mod 51	Mod 62	Mod 66	Mod 80
50580	1	3	0	0	0

Global Period

Code	Days
50580	000

50590

50590 Lithotripsy, extracorporeal shock wave

AMA Coding Notes

Surgical Procedures on the Urinary System

(For provision of chemotherapeutic agents, report both the specific service in addition to code(s) for the specific substance(s) or drug(s) provided)

AMA *CPT® Assistant* ▢

50590: Jul 01: 11, Aug 01: 10, Oct 01: 8, Jul 03: 16, Aug 03: 14

Plain English Description

Extracorporeal shock wave lithotripsy (ESWL) is the preferred method of treatment for renal and ureteral stones (calculi). Lithotripsy machines have four basic components: a shock-wave generator, a focusing system, a coupling mechanism, and an imaging unit that localizes the stone and monitors fragmentation. Most lithotripsy machines are powered with an electromagnetic shock-wave generator. The focusing system is used to concentrate the shock waves on the target, which is the stone. The coupling mechanism consists of water contained in a silicone membrane. These small water-filled drums, or cushions on the shock tube, provide air-free contact between the patient's skin and the tube. The imaging unit is required for localizing the stone and monitoring the fragmentation. Depending on the location of the stone, the patient is placed either on the back or abdomen on the treatment table. Using fluoroscopic or ultrasound imaging, the stone is positioned in the focus of the shock wave. Coupling gel is applied on the skin at the site where the shock tube is to be placed. The shock tube is pressed against the skin and shock waves are then delivered through the tube at rates of up to 120 per minute. Stone fragmentation is monitored radiographically as the ESWL treatment is delivered. Once the stone fragments are small enough to allow them to pass through the kidney and ureter, ESWL is terminated.

Lithotripsy, extracorporeal shock wave

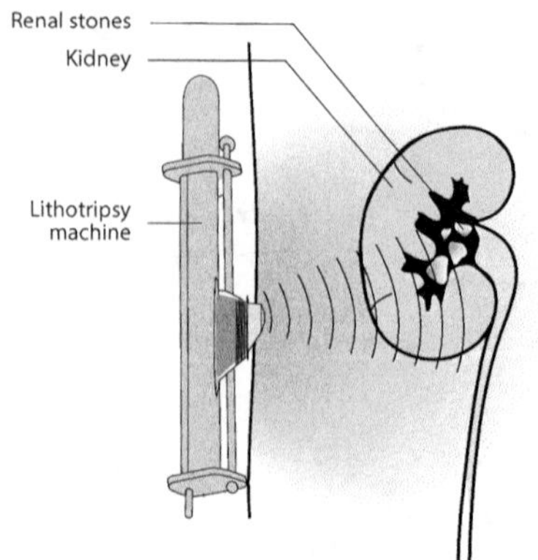

ICD-10-CM Diagnostic Codes

N20.0	Calculus of kidney
N20.1	Calculus of ureter
N20.2	Calculus of kidney with calculus of ureter
N22	Calculus of urinary tract in diseases classified elsewhere

CCI Edits

Refer to Appendix A for CCI edits.

Pub 100

50590: Pub 100-03, 1, 230.1

Facility RVUs ▢

Code	Work	PE Facility	MP	Total Facility
50590	9.77	5.78	1.17	16.72

Non-facility RVUs ▢

Code	Work	PE Non-Facility	MP	Total Non-Facility
50590	9.77	11.05	1.17	21.99

Modifiers (PAR) ▢

Code	Mod 50	Mod 51	Mod 62	Mod 66	Mod 80
50590	1	2	0	0	1

Global Period

Code	Days
50590	090

50592

50592 Ablation, 1 or more renal tumor(s), percutaneous, unilateral, radiofrequency

(50592 is a unilateral procedure. For bilateral procedure, report 50592 with modifier 50)

(For imaging guidance and monitoring, see 76940, 77013, 77022)

AMA Coding Notes

Surgical Procedures on the Urinary System

(For provision of chemotherapeutic agents, report both the specific service in addition to code(s) for the specific substance(s) or drug(s) provided)

Plain English Description

One or more renal tumors of the right or left kidney are destroyed (ablated) by radiofrequency using percutaneous technique. Radiofrequency uses electrical currents in the range of radiofrequency waves. The electrical currents produce heat around the needle to destroy tumor tissue. The heat also cauterizes blood vessels, which reduces the risk of bleeding. Grounding pads are placed on the back and thighs. Using separately reportable ultrasound, CT, or MRI guidance, the tumor is located. The optimal track and placement of the electrode needle are determined. The electrode needle is inserted through the skin and into the tumor using continuous imaging guidance, taking care to avoid other organs and major blood vessels. The location of the needle tip is confirmed and the electrode needle is connected to the radiofrequency generator, which is activated. Imaging guidance is used to monitor and assess tumor destruction. For multiple or very large tumors, more than one needle may be used. Alternatively, the needle may be partially withdrawn and repositioned following each radiofrequency application. When treatment is complete, the needle is withdrawn and pressure is applied to prevent bleeding along the needle track.

Ablation, one or more renal tumor(s), percutaneous, unilateral

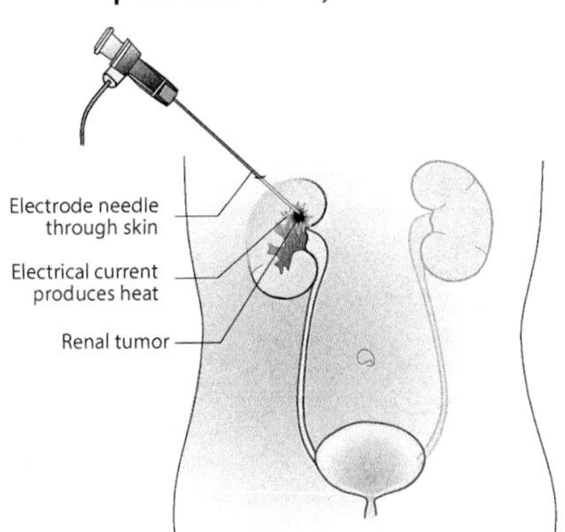

ICD-10-CM Diagnostic Codes

	Code	Description
⇄	C64.1	Malignant neoplasm of right kidney, except renal pelvis
⇄	C64.2	Malignant neoplasm of left kidney, except renal pelvis
⇄	C65.1	Malignant neoplasm of right renal pelvis
⇄	C65.2	Malignant neoplasm of left renal pelvis
	C68.8	Malignant neoplasm of overlapping sites of urinary organs
⇄	C79.01	Secondary malignant neoplasm of right kidney and renal pelvis
⇄	C79.02	Secondary malignant neoplasm of left kidney and renal pelvis
	C7A.093	Malignant carcinoid tumor of the kidney
	C80.2	Malignant neoplasm associated with transplanted organ
	D09.19	Carcinoma in situ of other urinary organs
⇄	D30.01	Benign neoplasm of right kidney
⇄	D30.02	Benign neoplasm of left kidney
⇄	D30.11	Benign neoplasm of right renal pelvis
⇄	D30.12	Benign neoplasm of left renal pelvis
	D3A.093	Benign carcinoid tumor of the kidney
⇄	D41.01	Neoplasm of uncertain behavior of right kidney
⇄	D41.02	Neoplasm of uncertain behavior of left kidney
⇄	D41.11	Neoplasm of uncertain behavior of right renal pelvis
⇄	D41.12	Neoplasm of uncertain behavior of left renal pelvis

CCI Edits

Refer to Appendix A for CCI edits.

Facility RVUs ▯

Code	Work	PE Facility	MP	Total Facility
50592	6.55	2.80	0.60	9.95

Non-facility RVUs ▯

Code	Work	PE Non-Facility	MP	Total Non-Facility
50592	6.55	81.32	0.60	88.47

Modifiers (PAR) ▯

Code	Mod 50	Mod 51	Mod 62	Mod 66	Mod 80
50592	1	2	0	0	1

Global Period

Code	Days
50592	010

50593

50593 Ablation, renal tumor(s), unilateral, percutaneous, cryotherapy

(50593 is a unilateral procedure. For bilateral procedure, report 50593 with modifier 50)

(For imaging guidance and monitoring, see codes 76940, 77013, 77022)

AMA Coding Notes

Surgical Procedures on the Urinary System

(For provision of chemotherapeutic agents, report both the specific service in addition to code(s) for the specific substance(s) or drug(s) provided)

AMA *CPT® Assistant* ▢

50593: May 17: 3

Plain English Description

One or more renal tumors are destroyed (ablated) by cryotherapy using percutaneous technique. Cryotherapy uses extreme cold to freeze and destroy tissue. The tumor(s) is identified using separately reportable ultrasound, CT, or MRI guidance. Most tumors require placement of multiple probes to ensure complete tumor destruction and allow sufficient margins. The entry sites for cryotherapy probe placement are determined and small incisions are made to facilitate placement. The probes are inserted into the center of the tumor(s) using imaging guidance and taking care to avoid other organs and major blood vessels. The location of the probe tips is confirmed and the cryoablation unit is activated. The probes are filled with argon gas, resulting in rapid freezing at temperatures as low as -100 degrees centigrade. This is followed by a thawing cycle that is initiated by replacing the argon with helium. Imaging guidance is used to monitor the creation of the cryoablation sphere (ice ball) and assess tumor destruction (necrosis). Complete destruction typically requires two freeze/thaw cycles. When treatment is complete, the probes are withdrawn, the skin incisions are cleansed, and a dressing is applied.

Ablation, renal tumor(s), unilateral, percutaneous, cryotherapy

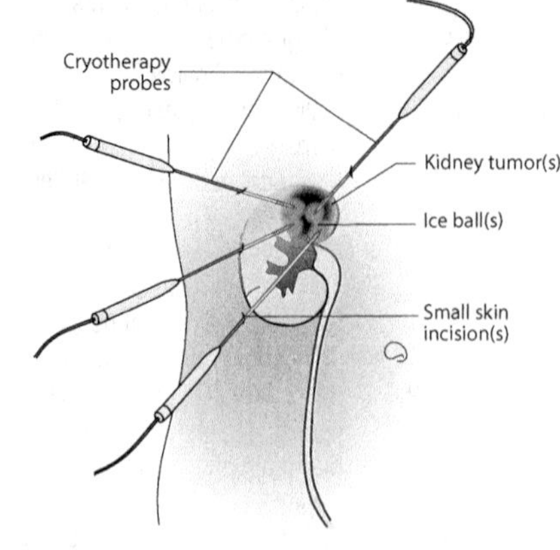

ICD-10-CM Diagnostic Codes

	Code	Description
⇄	C64.1	Malignant neoplasm of right kidney, except renal pelvis
⇄	C64.2	Malignant neoplasm of left kidney, except renal pelvis
⇄	C65.1	Malignant neoplasm of right renal pelvis
⇄	C65.2	Malignant neoplasm of left renal pelvis
	C68.8	Malignant neoplasm of overlapping sites of urinary organs
⇄	C79.01	Secondary malignant neoplasm of right kidney and renal pelvis
⇄	C79.02	Secondary malignant neoplasm of left kidney and renal pelvis
	C7A.093	Malignant carcinoid tumor of the kidney
	C80.2	Malignant neoplasm associated with transplanted organ
	D09.19	Carcinoma in situ of other urinary organs
⇄	D30.01	Benign neoplasm of right kidney
⇄	D30.02	Benign neoplasm of left kidney
⇄	D30.11	Benign neoplasm of right renal pelvis
⇄	D30.12	Benign neoplasm of left renal pelvis
	D3A.093	Benign carcinoid tumor of the kidney
⇄	D41.01	Neoplasm of uncertain behavior of right kidney
⇄	D41.02	Neoplasm of uncertain behavior of left kidney
⇄	D41.11	Neoplasm of uncertain behavior of right renal pelvis
⇄	D41.12	Neoplasm of uncertain behavior of left renal pelvis

CCI Edits

Refer to Appendix A for CCI edits.

Facility RVUs ▢

Code	Work	PE Facility	MP	Total Facility
50593	8.88	3.56	0.79	13.23

Non-facility RVUs ▢

Code	Work	PE Non-Facility	MP	Total Non-Facility
50593	8.88	108.61	0.79	118.28

Modifiers (PAR) ▢

Code	Mod 50	Mod 51	Mod 62	Mod 66	Mod 80
50593	1	2	0	0	2

Global Period

Code	Days
50593	010

50600

50600 Ureterotomy with exploration or drainage (separate procedure)

(For ureteral endoscopy performed in conjunction with this procedure, see 50970-50980)

AMA Coding Guideline

Incision/Biopsy Procedures on the Ureter

Code 50606 is an add-on code describing endoluminal biopsy (eg, brush) using non-endoscopic imaging guidance, which may be reported once per ureter per day. This code includes the work of the biopsy and the imaging guidance and radiological supervision and interpretation required to accomplish the biopsy. The biopsy may be performed through de novo transrenal access, an existing renal/ureteral access, transurethral access, an ileal conduit, or ureterostomy. The service of gaining access may be reported separately. Diagnostic pyelography/ureterography is not included in the work of 50606 and may be reported separately. Other interventions or catheter placements performed at the same setting as the biopsy may be reported separately.

For codes 50430, 50431, 50432, 50433, 50434, 50435, 50606, 50693, 50694, 50695, 50705, and 50706, the renal pelvis and its associated ureter are considered a single entity for reporting purposes. Codes 50430, 50431, 50432, 50433, 50434, 50435, 50606, 50693, 50694, 50695, 50705, and 50706 may be reported once for each renal collecting system/ureter accessed (eg, two separate codes would be reported for bilateral nephrostomy tube placement or for unilateral duplicated collecting system/ureter requiring two separate procedures).

AMA Coding Notes

Surgical Procedures on the Urinary System

(For provision of chemotherapeutic agents, report both the specific service in addition to code(s) for the specific substance(s) or drug(s) provided)

Plain English Description

Ureterotomy with exploration or drainage is performed. An incision is made in the abdomen over the upper, middle, or lower ureter depending on the nature of the exploration or drainage procedure. Muscles of the abdominal wall are divided and the peritoneum is pushed aside. The ureter is identified and dissected free of the serosa and periureteral fat and then incised. Exploration is performed to identify any disease or abnormalities. A soft Penrose drainage or suction tube is placed and the ureter is drained and flushed with irrigation solution. The drainage tube is left in place and incisions are closed around the drain.

Ureterotomy with exploration or drainage (separate procedure)

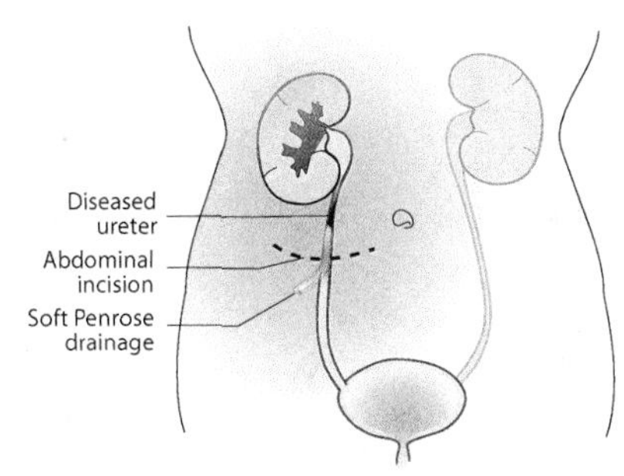

ICD-10-CM Diagnostic Codes

	Code	Description
⇄	C66.1	Malignant neoplasm of right ureter
⇄	C66.2	Malignant neoplasm of left ureter
	C79.19	Secondary malignant neoplasm of other urinary organs
	D09.19	Carcinoma in situ of other urinary organs
⇄	D30.21	Benign neoplasm of right ureter
⇄	D30.22	Benign neoplasm of left ureter
⇄	D41.21	Neoplasm of uncertain behavior of right ureter
⇄	D41.22	Neoplasm of uncertain behavior of left ureter
	N11.1	Chronic obstructive pyelonephritis
	N13.0	Hydronephrosis with ureteropelvic junction obstruction
	N13.1	Hydronephrosis with ureteral stricture, not elsewhere classified
	N13.2	Hydronephrosis with renal and ureteral calculous obstruction
	N13.4	Hydroureter
	N13.5	Crossing vessel and stricture of ureter without hydronephrosis
	N13.8	Other obstructive and reflux uropathy
	N28.86	Ureteritis cystica
	N28.89	Other specified disorders of kidney and ureter
	N29	Other disorders of kidney and ureter in diseases classified elsewhere
	N99.71	Accidental puncture and laceration of a genitourinary system organ or structure during a genitourinary system procedure
	N99.72	Accidental puncture and laceration of a genitourinary system organ or structure during other procedure
	Q62.10	Congenital occlusion of ureter, unspecified
	Q62.11	Congenital occlusion of ureteropelvic junction
	Q62.12	Congenital occlusion of ureterovesical orifice
	Q62.31	Congenital ureterocele, orthotopic
	Q62.39	Other obstructive defects of renal pelvis and ureter
	Q62.5	Duplication of ureter
	Q62.60	Malposition of ureter, unspecified
	Q62.61	Deviation of ureter
	Q62.62	Displacement of ureter
	Q62.63	Anomalous implantation of ureter
	Q62.69	Other malposition of ureter
❼	S37.12	Contusion of ureter
❼	S37.13	Laceration of ureter
❼	S37.19	Other injury of ureter

ICD-10-CM Coding Notes

For codes requiring a 7th character extension, refer to your ICD-10-CM book. Review the character descriptions and coding guidelines for proper selection. For some procedures, only certain characters will apply.

CCI Edits

Refer to Appendix A for CCI edits.

Facility RVUs ▢

Code	Work	PE Facility	MP	Total Facility
50600	17.17	8.17	2.04	27.38

Non-facility RVUs ▢

Code	Work	PE Non-Facility	MP	Total Non-Facility
50600	17.17	8.17	2.04	27.38

Modifiers (PAR) ▢

Code	Mod 50	Mod 51	Mod 62	Mod 66	Mod 80
50600	1	2	1	0	2

Global Period

Code	Days
50600	090

50605

50605 Ureterotomy for insertion of indwelling stent, all types

AMA Coding Guideline

Incision/Biopsy Procedures on the Ureter

Code 50606 is an add-on code describing endoluminal biopsy (eg, brush) using non-endoscopic imaging guidance, which may be reported once per ureter per day. This code includes the work of the biopsy and the imaging guidance and radiological supervision and interpretation required to accomplish the biopsy. The biopsy may be performed through de novo transrenal access, an existing renal/ureteral access, transurethral access, an ileal conduit, or ureterostomy. The service of gaining access may be reported separately. Diagnostic pyelography/ureterography is not included in the work of 50606 and may be reported separately. Other interventions or catheter placements performed at the same setting as the biopsy may be reported separately.

For codes 50430, 50431, 50432, 50433, 50434, 50435, 50606, 50693, 50694, 50695, 50705, and 50706, the renal pelvis and its associated ureter are considered a single entity for reporting purposes. Codes 50430, 50431, 50432, 50433, 50434, 50435, 50606, 50693, 50694, 50695, 50705, and 50706 may be reported once for each renal collecting system/ureter accessed (eg, two separate codes would be reported for bilateral nephrostomy tube placement or for unilateral duplicated collecting system/ureter requiring two separate procedures).

AMA Coding Notes

Surgical Procedures on the Urinary System

(For provision of chemotherapeutic agents, report both the specific service in addition to code(s) for the specific substance(s) or drug(s) provided)

AMA *CPT® Assistant*

50605: Oct 01: 8, Dec 09: 4, Apr 12: 18

Plain English Description

Ureterotomy with stent placement is performed. An incision is made in the abdomen over the upper, middle, or lower ureter depending on the location of the stricture or other abnormality. Muscles of the abdominal wall are divided and the peritoneum is pushed aside. The ureter is identified and dissected free of the serosa and periureteral fat. The ureter is then incised and explored. A soft Penrose drainage or suction tube is placed above the site of the stricture or other abnormality and the ureter is drained and flushed with irrigation solution. A double J stent is placed in the ureter at the stricture site. The ureterotomy site may be left open with a drainage tube in place. Abdominal and skin incisions are closed around the drain.

Ureterotomy for insertion of indwelling stent, all types

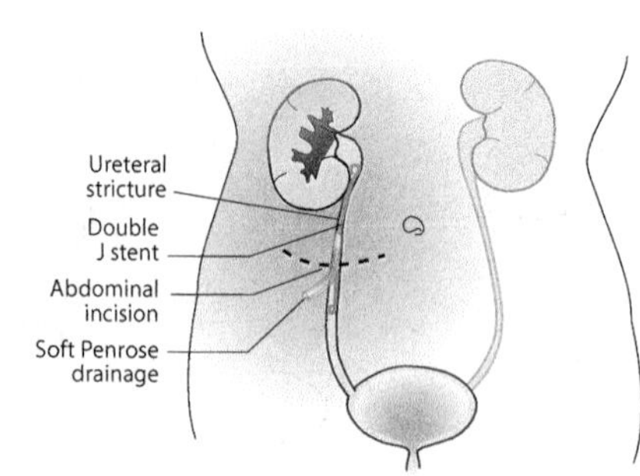

ICD-10-CM Diagnostic Codes

	Code	Description
⇄	C66.1	Malignant neoplasm of right ureter
⇄	C66.2	Malignant neoplasm of left ureter
	C79.19	Secondary malignant neoplasm of other urinary organs
	D09.19	Carcinoma in situ of other urinary organs
⇄	D30.21	Benign neoplasm of right ureter
⇄	D30.22	Benign neoplasm of left ureter
⇄	D41.21	Neoplasm of uncertain behavior of right ureter
⇄	D41.22	Neoplasm of uncertain behavior of left ureter
	N11.1	Chronic obstructive pyelonephritis
	N13.0	Hydronephrosis with ureteropelvic junction obstruction
	N13.1	Hydronephrosis with ureteral stricture, not elsewhere classified
	N13.2	Hydronephrosis with renal and ureteral calculous obstruction
	N13.4	Hydroureter
	N13.5	Crossing vessel and stricture of ureter without hydronephrosis
	N13.8	Other obstructive and reflux uropathy
	N28.86	Ureteritis cystica
	N28.89	Other specified disorders of kidney and ureter
	N29	Other disorders of kidney and ureter in diseases classified elsewhere

CCI Edits

Refer to Appendix A for CCI edits.

Facility RVUs

Code	Work	PE Facility	MP	Total Facility
50605	16.79	9.26	3.75	29.80

Non-facility RVUs

Code	Work	PE Non-Facility	MP	Total Non-Facility
50605	16.79	9.26	3.75	29.80

Modifiers (PAR)

Code	Mod 50	Mod 51	Mod 62	Mod 66	Mod 80
50605	1	2	1	0	2

Global Period

Code	Days
50605	090

50606

✚ **50606 Endoluminal biopsy of ureter and/or renal pelvis, non-endoscopic, including imaging guidance (eg, ultrasound and/or fluoroscopy) and all associated radiological supervision and interpretation (List separately in addition to code for primary procedure)**

(Use 50606 in conjunction with 50382, 50384, 50385, 50386, 50387, 50389, 50430, 50431, 50432, 50433, 50434, 50435, 50684, 50688, 50690, 50693, 50694, 50695, 51610)

(Do not report 50606 in conjunction with 50555, 50574, 50955, 50974, 52007, 74425 for the same renal collecting system and/or associated ureter)

AMA Coding Guideline

Incision/Biopsy Procedures on the Ureter

Code 50606 is an add-on code describing endoluminal biopsy (eg, brush) using non-endoscopic imaging guidance, which may be reported once per ureter per day. This code includes the work of the biopsy and the imaging guidance and radiological supervision and interpretation required to accomplish the biopsy. The biopsy may be performed through de novo transrenal access, an existing renal/ureteral access, transurethral access, an ileal conduit, or ureterostomy. The service of gaining access may be reported separately. Diagnostic pyelography/ureterography is not included in the work of 50606 and may be reported separately. Other interventions or catheter placements performed at the same setting as the biopsy may be reported separately.

For codes 50430, 50431, 50432, 50433, 50434, 50435, 50606, 50693, 50694, 50695, 50705, and 50706, the renal pelvis and its associated ureter are considered a single entity for reporting purposes. Codes 50430, 50431, 50432, 50433, 50434, 50435, 50606, 50693, 50694, 50695, 50705, and 50706 may be reported once for each renal collecting system/ureter accessed (eg, two separate codes would be reported for bilateral nephrostomy tube placement or for unilateral duplicated collecting system/ureter requiring two separate procedures).

AMA Coding Notes

Surgical Procedures on the Urinary System

(For provision of chemotherapeutic agents, report both the specific service in addition to code(s) for the specific substance(s) or drug(s) provided)

AMA *CPT® Assistant* ▯

50606: Jan 16: 3

Plain English Description

Endoluminal biopsy taken of the ureter and/or renal pelvis is performed in conjunction with other genitourinary procedures. Through a previously positioned catheter, such as for nephrostogram or ureterogram, a guidewire is placed and the ureteropelvic junction is explored. The ureter is accessed and the suspect area to be biopsied is located. The catheter and guidewire are manipulated past the lesion or area of stricture and the catheter is removed, leaving the guidewire in position. A sheath is advanced over the guidewire to a point just past the target area. A special brush biopsy catheter is then advanced through the sheath over the guidewire; the sheath is retracted to a point just proximal to the target lesion area; and the cytology brush then takes several brushings of the target lesion or mass. The brush biopsy catheter is removed, and the brush with the samplings is placed in a container to be sent to the laboratory. The sheath and guidewire are then removed. This is an add-on code reported in conjunction with the primary procedure. All radiological guidance, imaging, and interpretation necessary for the endoluminal biopsy are included.

ICD-10-CM Diagnostic Codes

See Primary Procedure code for crosswalks.

CCI Edits

Refer to Appendix A for CCI edits.

Pub 100

50606: Pub 100-03, 1, 220.5

Facility RVUs ▯

Code	Work	PE Facility	MP	Total Facility
50606	3.16	0.52	0.32	4.00

Non-facility RVUs ▯

Code	Work	PE Non-Facility	MP	Total Non-Facility
50606	3.16	11.31	0.32	14.79

Modifiers (PAR) ▯

Code	Mod 50	Mod 51	Mod 62	Mod 66	Mod 80
50606	1	0	0	0	1

Global Period

Code	Days
50606	ZZZ

CPT® Procedural Coding

50610-50630

50610 Ureterolithotomy; upper one-third of ureter

50620 Ureterolithotomy; middle one-third of ureter

50630 Ureterolithotomy; lower one-third of ureter

(For laparoscopic approach, use 50945)

(For transvesical ureterolithotomy, use 51060)

(For cystotomy with stone basket extraction of ureteral calculus, use 51065)

(For endoscopic extraction or manipulation of ureteral calculus, see 50080, 50081, 50561, 50961, 50980, 52320-52330, 52352, 52353, 52356)

AMA Coding Guideline

Incision/Biopsy Procedures on the Ureter

Code 50606 is an add-on code describing endoluminal biopsy (eg, brush) using non-endoscopic imaging guidance, which may be reported once per ureter per day. This code includes the work of the biopsy and the imaging guidance and radiological supervision and interpretation required to accomplish the biopsy. The biopsy may be performed through de novo transrenal access, an existing renal/ureteral access, transurethral access, an ileal conduit, or ureterostomy. The service of gaining access may be reported separately. Diagnostic pyelography/ureterography is not included in the work of 50606 and may be reported separately. Other interventions or catheter placements performed at the same setting as the biopsy may be reported separately.

For codes 50430, 50431, 50432, 50433, 50434, 50435, 50606, 50693, 50694, 50695, 50705, and 50706, the renal pelvis and its associated ureter are considered a single entity for reporting purposes. Codes 50430, 50431, 50432, 50433, 50434, 50435, 50606, 50693, 50694, 50695, 50705, and 50706 may be reported once for each renal collecting system/ureter accessed (eg, two separate codes would be reported for bilateral nephrostomy tube placement or for unilateral duplicated collecting system/ureter requiring two separate procedures).

AMA Coding Notes

Surgical Procedures on the Urinary System

(For provision of chemotherapeutic agents, report both the specific service in addition to code(s) for the specific substance(s) or drug(s) provided)

AMA *CPT® Assistant*

50610: Nov 99: 26, Oct 01: 8

50620: Nov 99: 26, Oct 01: 8

50630: Nov 99: 26, Oct 01: 8, May 14: 3

Plain English Description

An ureterolithotomy is performed to remove a calculus or stone from the ureter. An incision is made in the abdomen over the upper, middle, or lower ureter depending on the location of the stone. Muscles of the abdominal wall are divided and the peritoneum is pushed aside. The ureter is identified and dissected free of the serosa and periureteral fat. The site of the stone is identified visually by noting a bulge in the ureter or manually by palpating the ureter. The stone is immobilized by placement of vascular loops above and below the stone. The ureter is incised over the stone and the stone is removed. A catheter is placed in the ureter, the ureter is irrigated, and any stone fragments are removed. A soft Penrose drainage tube or suction tube is placed and the ureter drained. The incision in the ureter is closed, taking care not to constrict the ureter. A drainage tube is placed and the abdomen is closed around the drain. Report 50610 for removal of a stone from the upper one-third of the ureter, 50620 for removal from the middle one-third of the ureter, and 50630 for removal from the lower one-third of the ureter.

Ureterolithotomy

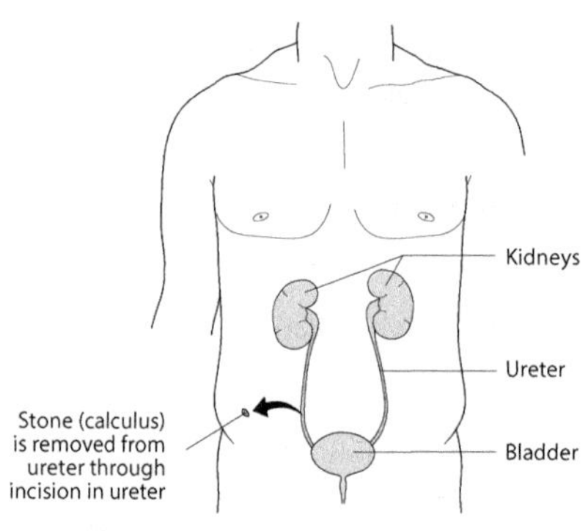

ICD-10-CM Diagnostic Codes

N20.1	Calculus of ureter
N20.2	Calculus of kidney with calculus of ureter
N22	Calculus of urinary tract in diseases classified elsewhere

CCI Edits

Refer to Appendix A for CCI edits.

Facility RVUs

Code	Work	PE Facility	MP	Total Facility
50610	17.25	8.27	2.05	27.57
50620	16.43	7.99	1.95	26.37
50630	16.21	7.92	1.94	26.07

Non-facility RVUs

Code	Work	PE Non-Facility	MP	Total Non-Facility
50610	17.25	8.27	2.05	27.57
50620	16.43	7.99	1.95	26.37
50630	16.21	7.92	1.94	26.07

Modifiers (PAR)

Code	Mod 50	Mod 51	Mod 62	Mod 66	Mod 80
50610	1	2	1	0	2
50620	1	2	1	0	2
50630	1	2	1	0	2

Global Period

Code	Days
50610	090
50620	090
50630	090

50650

50650 Ureterectomy, with bladder cuff (separate procedure)

AMA Coding Notes

Excision Procedures on the Ureter

(For ureterocele, see 51535, 52300)

Surgical Procedures on the Urinary System

(For provision of chemotherapeutic agents, report both the specific service in addition to code(s) for the specific substance(s) or drug(s) provided)

Plain English Description

The distal ureter is excised along with a section of bladder at the site of the ureteral orifice. A Foley catheter is placed and the bladder is drained. An incision is made in the abdomen over the affected ureter and bladder, which are exposed and inspected. The distal ureter and bladder cuff are then excised by first transecting the ureter above the site of the abnormality or lesion and then incising the bladder just below the ureterovesical junction (UVJ) and removing the bladder cuff. The opening in the bladder is repaired and a drainage tube is placed. The incisions are closed around the drain.

Ureterectomy, with bladder cuff (separate procedure)

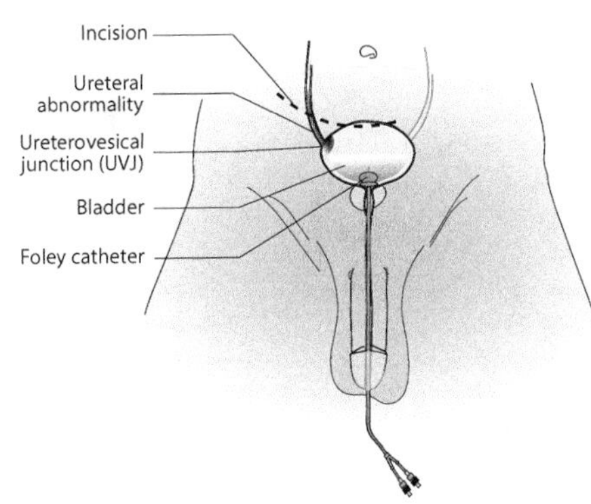

ICD-10-CM Diagnostic Codes

	Code	Description
⇄	C66.1	Malignant neoplasm of right ureter
⇄	C66.2	Malignant neoplasm of left ureter
	C67.0	Malignant neoplasm of trigone of bladder
	C67.1	Malignant neoplasm of dome of bladder
	C67.2	Malignant neoplasm of lateral wall of bladder
	C67.3	Malignant neoplasm of anterior wall of bladder
	C67.4	Malignant neoplasm of posterior wall of bladder
	C67.5	Malignant neoplasm of bladder neck
	C67.6	Malignant neoplasm of ureteric orifice
	C67.7	Malignant neoplasm of urachus
	C79.11	Secondary malignant neoplasm of bladder
	C79.19	Secondary malignant neoplasm of other urinary organs
	D09.19	Carcinoma in situ of other urinary organs
⇄	D30.21	Benign neoplasm of right ureter
⇄	D30.22	Benign neoplasm of left ureter
⇄	D41.21	Neoplasm of uncertain behavior of right ureter
⇄	D41.22	Neoplasm of uncertain behavior of left ureter
	N13.8	Other obstructive and reflux uropathy
	N28.82	Megaloureter
	N28.89	Other specified disorders of kidney and ureter
❼	S37.12	Contusion of ureter
❼	S37.13	Laceration of ureter
❼	S37.19	Other injury of ureter

ICD-10-CM Coding Notes

For codes requiring a 7th character extension, refer to your ICD-10-CM book. Review the character descriptions and coding guidelines for proper selection. For some procedures, only certain characters will apply.

CCI Edits

Refer to Appendix A for CCI edits.

Facility RVUs ☐

Code	Work	PE Facility	MP	Total Facility
50650	18.82	9.19	2.36	30.37

Non-facility RVUs ☐

Code	Work	PE Non-Facility	MP	Total Non-Facility
50650	18.82	9.19	2.36	30.37

Modifiers (PAR) ☐

Code	Mod 50	Mod 51	Mod 62	Mod 66	Mod 80
50650	1	2	1	0	2

Global Period

Code	Days
50650	090

50660

50660 Ureterectomy, total, ectopic ureter, combination abdominal, vaginal and/or perineal approach

AMA Coding Notes

Excision Procedures on the Ureter

(For ureterocele, see 51535, 52300)

Surgical Procedures on the Urinary System

(For provision of chemotherapeutic agents, report both the specific service in addition to code(s) for the specific substance(s) or drug(s) provided)

Plain English Description

An ectopic ureter is excised by a combined abdominal, vaginal, and/or perineal approach. An ectopic ureter is one that terminates in an abnormal location. An ectopic ureter may terminate in the epididymis, vas deferens, ejaculatory duct, seminal vesicle, urethra, or utriculus in males or in the Gartner's duct, upper vagina, cervix, uterus, or urethra in females. Less commonly, it may terminate in the rectum in both sexes. A Foley catheter is placed and the bladder is drained. An incision is made in the abdomen over the ureter. The ureter is exposed and inspected. A second incision may be made in the vagina or perineum at the site where the ureter terminates. The ureter is excised.

Total ureterectomy

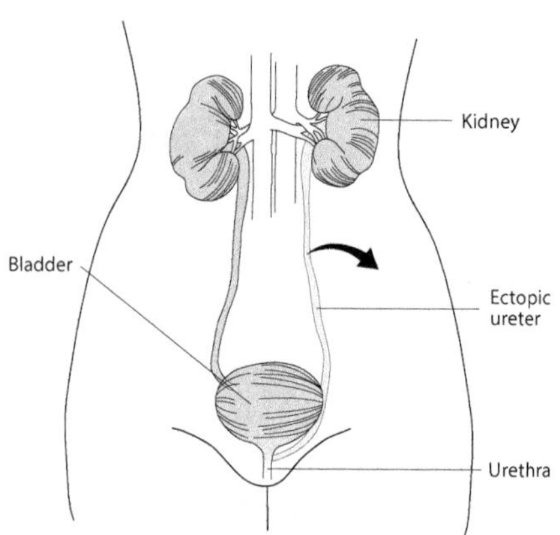

An ectopic ureter is removed.

ICD-10-CM Diagnostic Codes

N11.1	Chronic obstructive pyelonephritis
N13.1	Hydronephrosis with ureteral stricture, not elsewhere classified
N13.5	Crossing vessel and stricture of ureter without hydronephrosis
Q62.0	Congenital hydronephrosis
Q62.11	Congenital occlusion of ureteropelvic junction
Q62.12	Congenital occlusion of ureterovesical orifice
Q62.2	Congenital megaureter
Q62.39	Other obstructive defects of renal pelvis and ureter
Q62.4	Agenesis of ureter
Q62.5	Duplication of ureter
Q62.61	Deviation of ureter
Q62.62	Displacement of ureter
Q62.63	Anomalous implantation of ureter
Q62.69	Other malposition of ureter
Q62.7	Congenital vesico-uretero-renal reflux
Q62.8	Other congenital malformations of ureter

CCI Edits

Refer to Appendix A for CCI edits.

Facility RVUs ▢

Code	Work	PE Facility	MP	Total Facility
50660	21.02	9.83	2.50	33.35

Non-facility RVUs ▢

Code	Work	PE Non-Facility	MP	Total Non-Facility
50660	21.02	9.83	2.50	33.35

Modifiers (PAR) ▢

Code	Mod 50	Mod 51	Mod 62	Mod 66	Mod 80
50660	0	2	1	0	2

Global Period

Code	Days
50660	090

50684

50684 Injection procedure for ureterography or ureteropyelography through ureterostomy or indwelling ureteral catheter

(Do not report 50684 in conjunction with 50433, 50434, 50693, 50694, 50695)

(For radiological supervision and interpretation, use 74425)

AMA Coding Guideline

Other Introduction (Injection/Change/Removal) Procedures on the Ureter

Codes 50693, 50694, 50695 are therapeutic procedure codes describing percutaneous placement of ureteral stents. These codes include access, drainage, catheter manipulations, diagnostic nephrostogram and/or ureterogram, when performed, imaging guidance (eg, ultrasonography and/or fluoroscopy), and all associated radiological supervision and interpretation. When a separate ureteral stent and a nephrostomy catheter are placed into a ureter and its associated renal pelvis during the same session through a new percutaneous renal access, use 50695 to report the procedure.

AMA Coding Notes

Surgical Procedures on the Urinary System

(For provision of chemotherapeutic agents, report both the specific service in addition to code(s) for the specific substance(s) or drug(s) provided)

AMA *CPT® Assistant* ☐

50684: Jan 16: 3

Plain English Description

An injection procedure is performed through a previously created ureterostomy or a previously placed indwelling ureteral catheter to visualize the ureter and/or renal pelvis. A catheter is placed through the stoma in the skin into the ureter or through the indwelling ureteral catheter. Radiographic contrast media is injected through the catheter into the ureter and renal pelvis. Following the injection procedure, separately reportable radiographs of the ureter and renal pelvis are obtained.

Injection procedure for ureterography through ureterostomy or indwelling ureteral catheter

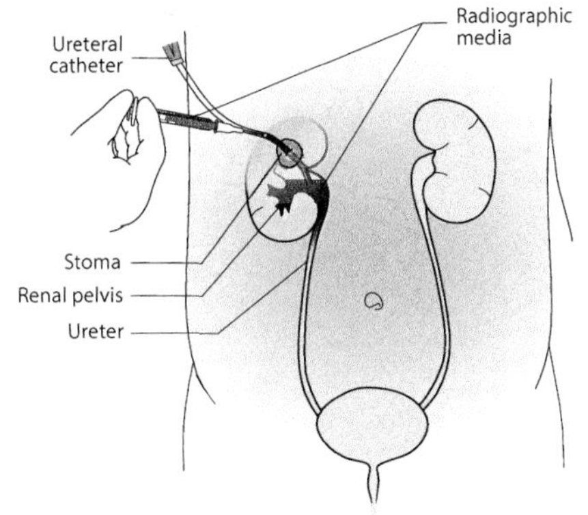

ICD-10-CM Diagnostic Codes

	Code	Description
⇄	C64.1	Malignant neoplasm of right kidney, except renal pelvis
⇄	C64.2	Malignant neoplasm of left kidney, except renal pelvis
⇄	C65.1	Malignant neoplasm of right renal pelvis
⇄	C65.2	Malignant neoplasm of left renal pelvis
⇄	C66.1	Malignant neoplasm of right ureter
⇄	C66.2	Malignant neoplasm of left ureter
	C68.8	Malignant neoplasm of overlapping sites of urinary organs
⇄	C79.01	Secondary malignant neoplasm of right kidney and renal pelvis
⇄	C79.02	Secondary malignant neoplasm of left kidney and renal pelvis
	C79.11	Secondary malignant neoplasm of bladder
	C79.19	Secondary malignant neoplasm of other urinary organs
	C7A.093	Malignant carcinoid tumor of the kidney
	C80.2	Malignant neoplasm associated with transplanted organ
	D09.19	Carcinoma in situ of other urinary organs
⇄	D30.01	Benign neoplasm of right kidney
⇄	D30.02	Benign neoplasm of left kidney
⇄	D30.11	Benign neoplasm of right renal pelvis
⇄	D30.12	Benign neoplasm of left renal pelvis
⇄	D30.21	Benign neoplasm of right ureter
⇄	D30.22	Benign neoplasm of left ureter
	D3A.093	Benign carcinoid tumor of the kidney
⇄	D41.01	Neoplasm of uncertain behavior of right kidney
⇄	D41.02	Neoplasm of uncertain behavior of left kidney
⇄	D41.11	Neoplasm of uncertain behavior of right renal pelvis
⇄	D41.12	Neoplasm of uncertain behavior of left renal pelvis
⇄	D41.21	Neoplasm of uncertain behavior of right ureter
⇄	D41.22	Neoplasm of uncertain behavior of left ureter
	D47.Z1	Post-transplant lymphoproliferative disorder (PTLD)
⇄	D49.511	Neoplasm of unspecified behavior of right kidney
⇄	D49.512	Neoplasm of unspecified behavior of left kidney
	G63	Polyneuropathy in diseases classified elsewhere
	N11.0	Nonobstructive reflux-associated chronic pyelonephritis
	N11.1	Chronic obstructive pyelonephritis
	N11.8	Other chronic tubulo-interstitial nephritis
	N13.1	Hydronephrosis with ureteral stricture, not elsewhere classified
	N13.2	Hydronephrosis with renal and ureteral calculous obstruction
	N13.39	Other hydronephrosis
	N13.4	Hydroureter
	N13.5	Crossing vessel and stricture of ureter without hydronephrosis
	N13.71	Vesicoureteral-reflux without reflux nephropathy
	N13.721	Vesicoureteral-reflux with reflux nephropathy without hydroureter, unilateral
	N13.722	Vesicoureteral-reflux with reflux nephropathy without hydroureter, bilateral
	N13.731	Vesicoureteral-reflux with reflux nephropathy with hydroureter, unilateral
	N13.732	Vesicoureteral-reflux with reflux nephropathy with hydroureter, bilateral
	N13.8	Other obstructive and reflux uropathy
	N20.0	Calculus of kidney
	N20.2	Calculus of kidney with calculus of ureter
	N22	Calculus of urinary tract in diseases classified elsewhere
	N23	Unspecified renal colic
	N25.81	Secondary hyperparathyroidism of renal origin
	N25.89	Other disorders resulting from impaired renal tubular function
	N26.1	Atrophy of kidney (terminal)
	N28.1	Cyst of kidney, acquired
	N28.82	Megaloureter
	N28.84	Pyelitis cystica
	N28.85	Pyeloureteritis cystica
	N28.86	Ureteritis cystica
	N28.89	Other specified disorders of kidney and ureter
	N29	Other disorders of kidney and ureter in diseases classified elsewhere
	N39.3	Stress incontinence (female) (male)
	N39.41	Urge incontinence
	N39.42	Incontinence without sensory awareness
	N39.43	Post-void dribbling
	N39.44	Nocturnal enuresis
	N39.45	Continuous leakage
	N39.46	Mixed incontinence
	N39.490	Overflow incontinence
	N39.498	Other specified urinary incontinence

N41.1	Chronic prostatitis ♂
N99.0	Postprocedural (acute) (chronic) kidney failure
N99.81	Other intraoperative complications of genitourinary system
N99.89	Other postprocedural complications and disorders of genitourinary system
Q60.3	Renal hypoplasia, unilateral
Q60.4	Renal hypoplasia, bilateral
Q60.6	Potter's syndrome
Q61.01	Congenital single renal cyst
Q61.02	Congenital multiple renal cysts
Q61.11	Cystic dilatation of collecting ducts
Q61.19	Other polycystic kidney, infantile type
Q61.2	Polycystic kidney, adult type
Q61.4	Renal dysplasia
Q61.5	Medullary cystic kidney
Q61.8	Other cystic kidney diseases
Q62.0	Congenital hydronephrosis
Q62.11	Congenital occlusion of ureteropelvic junction
Q62.12	Congenital occlusion of ureterovesical orifice
Q62.2	Congenital megaureter
Q62.31	Congenital ureterocele, orthotopic
Q62.32	Cecoureterocele
Q62.39	Other obstructive defects of renal pelvis and ureter
Q64.8	Other specified congenital malformations of urinary system
Q84.8	Other specified congenital malformations of integument

CCI Edits

Refer to Appendix A for CCI edits.

Facility RVUs

Code	Work	PE Facility	MP	Total Facility
50684	0.76	0.61	0.09	1.46

Non-facility RVUs

Code	Work	PE Non-Facility	MP	Total Non-Facility
50684	0.76	2.99	0.09	3.84

Modifiers (PAR)

Code	Mod 50	Mod 51	Mod 62	Mod 66	Mod 80
50684	1	2	0	0	1

Global Period

Code	Days
50684	000

50686

50686 Manometric studies through ureterostomy or indwelling ureteral catheter

AMA Coding Guideline

Other Introduction (Injection/Change/Removal) Procedures on the Ureter

Codes 50693, 50694, 50695 are therapeutic procedure codes describing percutaneous placement of ureteral stents. These codes include access, drainage, catheter manipulations, diagnostic nephrostogram and/or ureterogram, when performed, imaging guidance (eg, ultrasonography and/or fluoroscopy), and all associated radiological supervision and interpretation. When a separate ureteral stent and a nephrostomy catheter are placed into a ureter and its associated renal pelvis during the same session through a new percutaneous renal access, use 50695 to report the procedure.

AMA Coding Notes

Surgical Procedures on the Urinary System

(For provision of chemotherapeutic agents, report both the specific service in addition to code(s) for the specific substance(s) or drug(s) provided)

Plain English Description

Manometric studies are performed through a previously created ureterostomy or previously placed indwelling ureteral catheter to evaluate ureteral function and diagnose ureteral reflux. Ureteral reflux occurs when the direction of the flow of urine is reversed and travels back into the kidneys. This may occur when the muscular attachments of the ureter to the bladder that create the valve-like mechanism that closes the ureteric opening when urine is stored and voided fails to function. The reasons may be anatomical or functional. Manometry measures the strength of an organ's muscles. A catheter with a specialized manometer sensor is placed within the ureter, either through the stoma opening or the indwelling ureteral catheter. The pressure sensor in the catheter transmits muscle impulses to a computer and pressure recordings are obtained and analyzed.

Manometric studies through ureterostomy or indwelling ureteral catheter

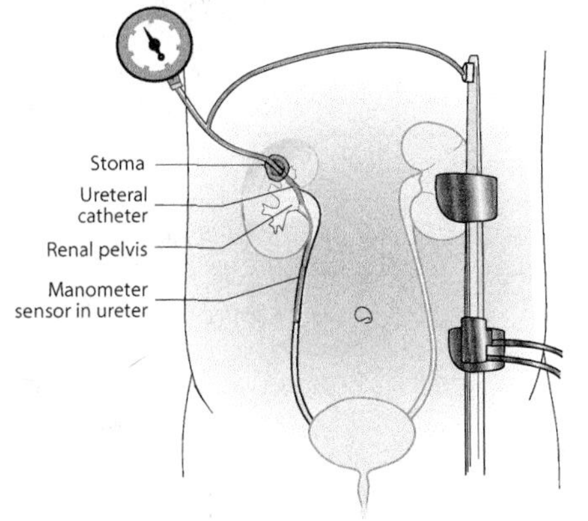

ICD-10-CM Diagnostic Codes

N11.1	Chronic obstructive pyelonephritis
N13.1	Hydronephrosis with ureteral stricture, not elsewhere classified
N13.2	Hydronephrosis with renal and ureteral calculous obstruction
N13.39	Other hydronephrosis
N13.5	Crossing vessel and stricture of ureter without hydronephrosis
N13.70	Vesicoureteral-reflux, unspecified
N13.71	Vesicoureteral-reflux without reflux nephropathy
N13.721	Vesicoureteral-reflux with reflux nephropathy without hydroureter, unilateral
N13.722	Vesicoureteral-reflux with reflux nephropathy without hydroureter, bilateral
N13.729	Vesicoureteral-reflux with reflux nephropathy without hydroureter, unspecified
Q62.0	Congenital hydronephrosis
Q62.11	Congenital occlusion of ureteropelvic junction
Q62.12	Congenital occlusion of ureterovesical orifice
Q62.2	Congenital megaureter
Q62.31	Congenital ureterocele, orthotopic
Q62.32	Cecoureterocele
Q62.39	Other obstructive defects of renal pelvis and ureter

CCI Edits

Refer to Appendix A for CCI edits.

Facility RVUs ▢

Code	Work	PE Facility	MP	Total Facility
50686	1.51	0.87	0.19	2.57

Non-facility RVUs ▢

Code	Work	PE Non-Facility	MP	Total Non-Facility
50686	1.51	2.54	0.19	4.24

Modifiers (PAR) ▢

Code	Mod 50	Mod 51	Mod 62	Mod 66	Mod 80
50686	0	2	0	0	0

Global Period

Code	Days
50686	000

50688

50688 Change of ureterostomy tube or externally accessible ureteral stent via ileal conduit

(If imaging guidance is performed, use 75984)

AMA Coding Guideline

Other Introduction (Injection/Change/Removal) Procedures on the Ureter

Codes 50693, 50694, 50695 are therapeutic procedure codes describing percutaneous placement of ureteral stents. These codes include access, drainage, catheter manipulations, diagnostic nephrostogram and/or ureterogram, when performed, imaging guidance (eg, ultrasonography and/or fluoroscopy), and all associated radiological supervision and interpretation. When a separate ureteral stent and a nephrostomy catheter are placed into a ureter and its associated renal pelvis during the same session through a new percutaneous renal access, use 50695 to report the procedure.

AMA Coding Notes

Surgical Procedures on the Urinary System

(For provision of chemotherapeutic agents, report both the specific service in addition to code(s) for the specific substance(s) or drug(s) provided)

AMA *CPT® Assistant* ▢

50688: Jan 16: 3

Plain English Description

The physician changes a ureterostomy tube or an externally accessible ureteral stent via a previously created ileal conduit. Under separately reportable radiographic guidance, a guidewire and sheath are introduced through the previously created ileal conduit. The ureterostomy tube or externally accessible stent is grasped and removed through the sheath. The replacement tube or stent is then loaded and advanced over the guidewire into the ureter. Correct positioning is verified radiographically before the guidewire is removed.

Change of ureterostomy tube or externally accessible ureteral stent via ileal conduit

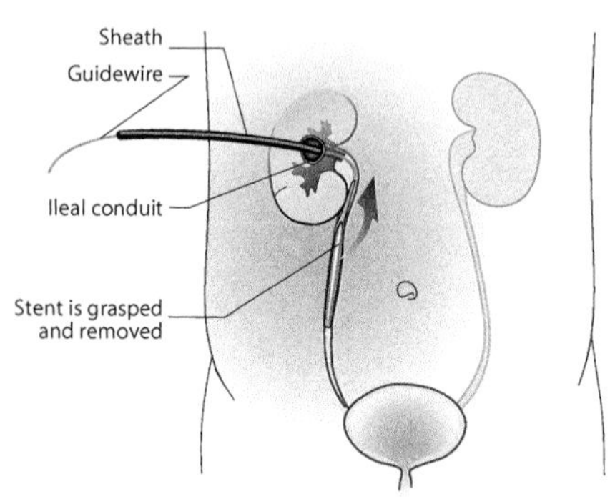

ICD-10-CM Diagnostic Codes

	Code	Description
	N99.89	Other postprocedural complications and disorders of genitourinary system
❼	T83.112	Breakdown (mechanical) of indwelling ureteral stent
❼	T83.118	Breakdown (mechanical) of other urinary devices and implants
❼	T83.122	Displacement of indwelling ureteral stent
❼	T83.128	Displacement of other urinary devices and implants
❼	T83.192	Other mechanical complication of indwelling ureteral stent
❼	T83.198	Other mechanical complication of other urinary devices and implants
❼	T83.593	Infection and inflammatory reaction due to other urinary stents
❼	T83.81	Embolism due to genitourinary prosthetic devices, implants and grafts
❼	T83.82	Fibrosis due to genitourinary prosthetic devices, implants and grafts
❼	T83.83	Hemorrhage due to genitourinary prosthetic devices, implants and grafts
❼	T83.84	Pain due to genitourinary prosthetic devices, implants and grafts
❼	T83.85	Stenosis due to genitourinary prosthetic devices, implants and grafts
❼	T83.86	Thrombosis due to genitourinary prosthetic devices, implants and grafts
❼	T83.89	Other specified complication of genitourinary prosthetic devices, implants and grafts
	Z43.6	Encounter for attention to other artificial openings of urinary tract

ICD-10-CM Coding Notes

For codes requiring a 7th character extension, refer to your ICD-10-CM book. Review the character descriptions and coding guidelines for proper selection. For some procedures, only certain characters will apply.

CCI Edits

Refer to Appendix A for CCI edits.

Facility RVUs ▢

Code	Work	PE Facility	MP	Total Facility
50688	1.20	0.93	0.11	2.24

Non-facility RVUs ▢

Code	Work	PE Non-Facility	MP	Total Non-Facility
50688	1.20	0.93	0.11	2.24

Modifiers (PAR) ▢

Code	Mod 50	Mod 51	Mod 62	Mod 66	Mod 80
50688	0	2	0	0	1

Global Period

Code	Days
50688	010

50690

50690 Injection procedure for visualization of ileal conduit and/or ureteropyelography, exclusive of radiologic service

(For radiological supervision and interpretation, see 74420 for retrograde or 74425 for antegrade injection)

AMA Coding Guideline

Other Introduction (Injection/Change/Removal) Procedures on the Ureter

Codes 50693, 50694, 50695 are therapeutic procedure codes describing percutaneous placement of ureteral stents. These codes include access, drainage, catheter manipulations, diagnostic nephrostogram and/or ureterogram, when performed, imaging guidance (eg, ultrasonography and/or fluoroscopy), and all associated radiological supervision and interpretation. When a separate ureteral stent and a nephrostomy catheter are placed into a ureter and its associated renal pelvis during the same session through a new percutaneous renal access, use 50695 to report the procedure.

AMA Coding Notes

Surgical Procedures on the Urinary System

(For provision of chemotherapeutic agents, report both the specific service in addition to code(s) for the specific substance(s) or drug(s) provided)

AMA *CPT® Assistant* ▯

50690: Jan 16: 3

Plain English Description

An injection procedure is performed to visualize a previously created ileal conduit and/or for ureteropyelography. A catheter is placed in the ileal conduit. Radiographic contrast media is injected through the catheter into the ileal conduit, ureter, and renal pelvis. Following the injection, separately reportable radiographs of the ileal conduit, ureter, and renal pelvis are obtained.

Injection procedure for visualization of ileal conduit and/or ureteropyelography, exclusive of radiologic service

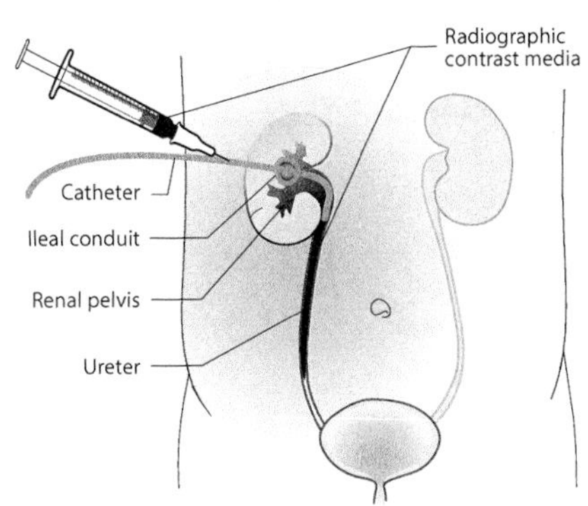

ICD-10-CM Diagnostic Codes

	Code	Description
⇄	C64.1	Malignant neoplasm of right kidney, except renal pelvis
⇄	C64.2	Malignant neoplasm of left kidney, except renal pelvis
⇄	C65.1	Malignant neoplasm of right renal pelvis
⇄	C65.2	Malignant neoplasm of left renal pelvis
⇄	C66.1	Malignant neoplasm of right ureter
⇄	C66.2	Malignant neoplasm of left ureter
	C68.8	Malignant neoplasm of overlapping sites of urinary organs
⇄	C79.01	Secondary malignant neoplasm of right kidney and renal pelvis
⇄	C79.02	Secondary malignant neoplasm of left kidney and renal pelvis
	C79.11	Secondary malignant neoplasm of bladder
	C79.19	Secondary malignant neoplasm of other urinary organs
	C7A.093	Malignant carcinoid tumor of the kidney
	C80.2	Malignant neoplasm associated with transplanted organ
⇄	D30.01	Benign neoplasm of right kidney
⇄	D30.02	Benign neoplasm of left kidney
⇄	D30.11	Benign neoplasm of right renal pelvis
⇄	D30.12	Benign neoplasm of left renal pelvis
⇄	D30.21	Benign neoplasm of right ureter
⇄	D30.22	Benign neoplasm of left ureter
	D3A.093	Benign carcinoid tumor of the kidney
⇄	D41.01	Neoplasm of uncertain behavior of right kidney
⇄	D41.02	Neoplasm of uncertain behavior of left kidney
⇄	D41.11	Neoplasm of uncertain behavior of right renal pelvis
⇄	D41.12	Neoplasm of uncertain behavior of left renal pelvis
⇄	D41.21	Neoplasm of uncertain behavior of right ureter
⇄	D41.22	Neoplasm of uncertain behavior of left ureter
	D47.Z1	Post-transplant lymphoproliferative disorder (PTLD)
	N11.1	Chronic obstructive pyelonephritis
	N13.39	Other hydronephrosis
	N13.5	Crossing vessel and stricture of ureter without hydronephrosis
	N13.8	Other obstructive and reflux uropathy
	N13.9	Obstructive and reflux uropathy, unspecified
	N20.0	Calculus of kidney
	N20.1	Calculus of ureter
	N20.2	Calculus of kidney with calculus of ureter
	N21.0	Calculus in bladder
	N22	Calculus of urinary tract in diseases classified elsewhere
	N29	Other disorders of kidney and ureter in diseases classified elsewhere
	N30.10	Interstitial cystitis (chronic) without hematuria
	N30.11	Interstitial cystitis (chronic) with hematuria
	N30.20	Other chronic cystitis without hematuria
	N30.21	Other chronic cystitis with hematuria
	N31.0	Uninhibited neuropathic bladder, not elsewhere classified
	N31.1	Reflex neuropathic bladder, not elsewhere classified
	N31.2	Flaccid neuropathic bladder, not elsewhere classified
	N31.8	Other neuromuscular dysfunction of bladder
	N31.9	Neuromuscular dysfunction of bladder, unspecified
	N32.0	Bladder-neck obstruction
	N32.3	Diverticulum of bladder
	N32.81	Overactive bladder
	N99.0	Postprocedural (acute) (chronic) kidney failure
	N99.520	Hemorrhage of incontinent external stoma of urinary tract
	N99.521	Infection of incontinent external stoma of urinary tract
	N99.522	Malfunction of incontinent external stoma of urinary tract
	N99.528	Other complication of incontinent external stoma of urinary tract
	N99.530	Hemorrhage of continent stoma of urinary tract
	N99.531	Infection of continent stoma of urinary tract
	N99.532	Malfunction of continent stoma of urinary tract
	N99.538	Other complication of continent stoma of urinary tract
	N99.81	Other intraoperative complications of genitourinary system
	N99.89	Other postprocedural complications and disorders of genitourinary system
	Q64.11	Supravesical fissure of urinary bladder
	Q64.5	Congenital absence of bladder and urethra
	Q64.6	Congenital diverticulum of bladder
	Q64.70	Unspecified congenital malformation of bladder and urethra
	Q64.71	Congenital prolapse of urethra
	Q64.72	Congenital prolapse of urinary meatus
	Q64.73	Congenital urethrorectal fistula
	Q64.79	Other congenital malformations of bladder and urethra
	Q64.8	Other specified congenital malformations of urinary system
❼	T83.010	Breakdown (mechanical) of cystostomy catheter
❼	T83.020	Displacement of cystostomy catheter
❼	T83.030	Leakage of cystostomy catheter
❼	T83.090	Other mechanical complication of cystostomy catheter
❼	T83.110	Breakdown (mechanical) of urinary electronic stimulator device
❼	T83.111	Breakdown (mechanical) of implanted urinary sphincter

❼	T83.112	Breakdown (mechanical) of indwelling ureteral stent
❼	T83.118	Breakdown (mechanical) of other urinary devices and implants
❼	T83.592	Infection and inflammatory reaction due to indwelling ureteral stent
❼	T83.85	Stenosis due to genitourinary prosthetic devices, implants and grafts
	Z85.51	Personal history of malignant neoplasm of bladder
	Z93.6	Other artificial openings of urinary tract status

ICD-10-CM Coding Notes

For codes requiring a 7th character extension, refer to your ICD-10-CM book. Review the character descriptions and coding guidelines for proper selection. For some procedures, only certain characters will apply.

CCI Edits

Refer to Appendix A for CCI edits.

Facility RVUs ▢

Code	Work	PE Facility	MP	Total Facility
50690	1.16	0.75	0.11	2.02

Non-facility RVUs ▢

Code	Work	PE Non-Facility	MP	Total Non-Facility
50690	1.16	2.30	0.11	3.57

Modifiers (PAR) ▢

Code	Mod 50	Mod 51	Mod 62	Mod 66	Mod 80
50690	0	2	0	0	1

Global Period

Code	Days
50690	000

50693

50693 Placement of ureteral stent, percutaneous, including diagnostic nephrostogram and/or ureterogram when performed, imaging guidance (eg, ultrasound and/or fluoroscopy), and all associated radiological supervision and interpretation; pre-existing nephrostomy tract

AMA Coding Guideline

Other Introduction (Injection/Change/Removal) Procedures on the Ureter

Codes 50693, 50694, 50695 are therapeutic procedure codes describing percutaneous placement of ureteral stents. These codes include access, drainage, catheter manipulations, diagnostic nephrostogram and/or ureterogram, when performed, imaging guidance (eg, ultrasonography and/or fluoroscopy), and all associated radiological supervision and interpretation. When a separate ureteral stent and a nephrostomy catheter are placed into a ureter and its associated renal pelvis during the same session through a new percutaneous renal access, use 50695 to report the procedure.

AMA Coding Notes

Surgical Procedures on the Urinary System

(For provision of chemotherapeutic agents, report both the specific service in addition to code(s) for the specific substance(s) or drug(s) provided)

AMA *CPT® Assistant* ▢

50693: Oct 15: 5, Jan 16: 3

Plain English Description

A procedure is performed to place a ureteral stent through a pre-existing nephrostomy tract. A ureteral stent may be required to facilitate the flow of urine from the kidney to the bladder through the ureter in the presence of strictures, leaks, or fistulas. With the patient positioned prone, contrast dye is injected through the pre-existing nephrostomy catheter and the urinary system is visualized using ultrasound and/or fluoroscopy. A guidewire is inserted through the catheter into the renal collecting system, coiled through the renal pelvis, and advanced down the ureter and into the bladder. The old nephrostomy catheter is removed and the stent is inserted over the guidewire and advanced into position. The proximal end remains outside the body with the distal pigtail threaded through the kidney, down the ureter, and into the bladder. This includes any diagnostic nephrostogram and/or ureterogram prepared, imaging guidance, and all associated radiologic supervision and interpretation.

ICD-10-CM Diagnostic Codes

	Code	Description
⇄	C64.1	Malignant neoplasm of right kidney, except renal pelvis
⇄	C64.2	Malignant neoplasm of left kidney, except renal pelvis
⇄	C65.1	Malignant neoplasm of right renal pelvis
⇄	C65.2	Malignant neoplasm of left renal pelvis
⇄	C66.1	Malignant neoplasm of right ureter
⇄	C66.2	Malignant neoplasm of left ureter
⇄	C79.01	Secondary malignant neoplasm of right kidney and renal pelvis
⇄	C79.02	Secondary malignant neoplasm of left kidney and renal pelvis
	C79.19	Secondary malignant neoplasm of other urinary organs
	C7A.093	Malignant carcinoid tumor of the kidney
	D09.19	Carcinoma in situ of other urinary organs
⇄	D30.11	Benign neoplasm of right renal pelvis
⇄	D30.21	Benign neoplasm of right ureter
⇄	D30.22	Benign neoplasm of left ureter
⇄	D41.01	Neoplasm of uncertain behavior of right kidney
⇄	D41.02	Neoplasm of uncertain behavior of left kidney
⇄	D41.11	Neoplasm of uncertain behavior of right renal pelvis
⇄	D41.12	Neoplasm of uncertain behavior of left renal pelvis
⇄	D41.21	Neoplasm of uncertain behavior of right ureter
⇄	D41.22	Neoplasm of uncertain behavior of left ureter
	N10	Acute pyelonephritis
	N11.0	Nonobstructive reflux-associated chronic pyelonephritis
	N11.1	Chronic obstructive pyelonephritis
	N11.8	Other chronic tubulo-interstitial nephritis
	N12	Tubulo-interstitial nephritis, not specified as acute or chronic
	N13.1	Hydronephrosis with ureteral stricture, not elsewhere classified
	N13.2	Hydronephrosis with renal and ureteral calculous obstruction
	N13.39	Other hydronephrosis
	N13.4	Hydroureter
	N13.5	Crossing vessel and stricture of ureter without hydronephrosis
	N13.721	Vesicoureteral-reflux with reflux nephropathy without hydroureter, unilateral
	N13.722	Vesicoureteral-reflux with reflux nephropathy without hydroureter, bilateral
	N13.731	Vesicoureteral-reflux with reflux nephropathy with hydroureter, unilateral
	N13.732	Vesicoureteral-reflux with reflux nephropathy with hydroureter, bilateral
	N13.8	Other obstructive and reflux uropathy
	N20.0	Calculus of kidney
	N20.1	Calculus of ureter
	N20.2	Calculus of kidney with calculus of ureter
	N25.81	Secondary hyperparathyroidism of renal origin
	N25.89	Other disorders resulting from impaired renal tubular function
	N28.82	Megaloureter
	N28.84	Pyelitis cystica
	N28.85	Pyeloureteritis cystica
	N28.86	Ureteritis cystica
	N28.89	Other specified disorders of kidney and ureter
	N39.3	Stress incontinence (female) (male)
	N39.41	Urge incontinence
	N39.42	Incontinence without sensory awareness
	N39.43	Post-void dribbling
	N39.44	Nocturnal enuresis
	N39.45	Continuous leakage
	N39.46	Mixed incontinence
	N39.490	Overflow incontinence
	N39.498	Other specified urinary incontinence
	N39.8	Other specified disorders of urinary system
	N82.1	Other female urinary-genital tract fistulae ♀
	Q62.0	Congenital hydronephrosis
	Q62.11	Congenital occlusion of ureteropelvic junction
	Q62.12	Congenital occlusion of ureterovesical orifice
	Q62.2	Congenital megaureter
	Q62.31	Congenital ureterocele, orthotopic
	Q62.32	Cecoureterocele
	Q62.39	Other obstructive defects of renal pelvis and ureter
	Q62.5	Duplication of ureter
	Q62.61	Deviation of ureter
	Q62.62	Displacement of ureter
	Q62.63	Anomalous implantation of ureter
	Q62.69	Other malposition of ureter
	Q62.8	Other congenital malformations of ureter

CCI Edits

Refer to Appendix A for CCI edits.

Facility RVUs

Code	Work	PE Facility	MP	Total Facility
50693	3.96	1.56	0.35	5.87

Non-facility RVUs

Code	Work	PE Non-Facility	MP	Total Non-Facility
50693	3.96	26.44	0.35	30.75

Modifiers (PAR)

Code	Mod 50	Mod 51	Mod 62	Mod 66	Mod 80
50693	1	2	0	0	1

Global Period

Code	Days
50693	000

50694-50695

50694 Placement of ureteral stent, percutaneous, including diagnostic nephrostogram and/or ureterogram when performed, imaging guidance (eg, ultrasound and/or fluoroscopy), and all associated radiological supervision and interpretation; new access, without separate nephrostomy catheter

50695 Placement of ureteral stent, percutaneous, including diagnostic nephrostogram and/or ureterogram when performed, imaging guidance (eg, ultrasound and/or fluoroscopy), and all associated radiological supervision and interpretation; new access, with separate nephrostomy catheter

(Do not report 50693, 50694, 50695 in conjunction with 50430, 50431, 50432, 50433, 50434, 50435, 50684, 74425 for the same renal collecting system and/or associated ureter)

AMA Coding Guideline

Other Introduction (Injection/Change/Removal) Procedures on the Ureter

Codes 50693, 50694, 50695 are therapeutic procedure codes describing percutaneous placement of ureteral stents. These codes include access, drainage, catheter manipulations, diagnostic nephrostogram and/or ureterogram, when performed, imaging guidance (eg, ultrasonography and/or fluoroscopy), and all associated radiological supervision and interpretation. When a separate ureteral stent and a nephrostomy catheter are placed into a ureter and its associated renal pelvis during the same session through a new percutaneous renal access, use 50695 to report the procedure.

AMA Coding Notes

Surgical Procedures on the Urinary System

(For provision of chemotherapeutic agents, report both the specific service in addition to code(s) for the specific substance(s) or drug(s) provided)

AMA *CPT® Assistant* ☐

50694: Oct 15: 5, Jan 16: 3
50695: Oct 15: 5, Jan 16: 3

Plain English Description

Percutaneous placement of a ureteral stent with or without placement of a separate nephrostomy catheter may be performed to treat urinary obstruction caused by stones, tumors, or strictures; diagnose urinary conditions; provide access for therapeutic interventions; or divert urine in the presence of traumatic injury, leaks, fistulas, or hemorrhagic cystitis. A single or double needle technique may be employed. Under ultrasound and/or fluoroscopic guidance, a single trocar or Chiba needle is inserted below the 12th rib to minimize the risk of puncturing the pleura. The needle is advanced into the renal pelvis, and urine is aspirated to verify location and decompress the system. Contrast dye is then injected and a series of X-rays are taken to visualize movement of dye through the urinary tract. Once satisfactory needle placement has been established, a thin wire is threaded through the needle into the renal pelvis and advanced down the ureter into the bladder. The stent is inserted over the guidewire and advanced into position. The proximal end is coiled within the renal pelvis with the distal pigtail in the bladder. If a separate nephrostomy catheter is not inserted (50694), the proximal end of the stent may remain outside the body or lie entirely inside the renal system. When a separate nephrostomy catheter is inserted (50695), the catheter is threaded over the guidewire into the upper pole of the calyx with the end outside the body. For double needle technique, the first needle is inserted directly into the renal pelvis and contrast dye is injected to obtain a series of X-rays. A small amount of air or CO2 may be injected to enhance visualization of the posterior calyces. A clamp applied to the skin is used to mark the entry site of the second needle placed under the 12th rib in the posterior axillary line. Insertion of the second needle and placement of the stent/catheter are identical to the single needle technique. These codes include any diagnostic nephrostogram and/or ureterogram, imaging guidance, and all associated radiologic supervision and interpretation.

ICD-10-CM Diagnostic Codes

⇄	C64.1	Malignant neoplasm of right kidney, except renal pelvis
⇄	C64.2	Malignant neoplasm of left kidney, except renal pelvis
⇄	C65.1	Malignant neoplasm of right renal pelvis
⇄	C65.2	Malignant neoplasm of left renal pelvis
⇄	C66.1	Malignant neoplasm of right ureter
⇄	C66.2	Malignant neoplasm of left ureter
⇄	C79.01	Secondary malignant neoplasm of right kidney and renal pelvis
⇄	C79.02	Secondary malignant neoplasm of left kidney and renal pelvis
	C79.19	Secondary malignant neoplasm of other urinary organs
	C7A.093	Malignant carcinoid tumor of the kidney
	D09.19	Carcinoma in situ of other urinary organs
⇄	D30.11	Benign neoplasm of right renal pelvis
⇄	D30.12	Benign neoplasm of left renal pelvis
⇄	D30.21	Benign neoplasm of right ureter
⇄	D30.22	Benign neoplasm of left ureter
⇄	D41.01	Neoplasm of uncertain behavior of right kidney
⇄	D41.02	Neoplasm of uncertain behavior of left kidney
⇄	D41.11	Neoplasm of uncertain behavior of right renal pelvis
⇄	D41.12	Neoplasm of uncertain behavior of left renal pelvis
⇄	D41.21	Neoplasm of uncertain behavior of right ureter
⇄	D41.22	Neoplasm of uncertain behavior of left ureter
	N10	Acute pyelonephritis
	N11	Chronic tubulo-interstitial nephritis
	N11.0	Nonobstructive reflux-associated chronic pyelonephritis
	N11.1	Chronic obstructive pyelonephritis
	N11.8	Other chronic tubulo-interstitial nephritis
	N12	Tubulo-interstitial nephritis, not specified as acute or chronic
	N13.2	Hydronephrosis with renal and ureteral calculous obstruction
	N13.39	Other hydronephrosis
	N13.4	Hydroureter
	N13.5	Crossing vessel and stricture of ureter without hydronephrosis
	N13.721	Vesicoureteral-reflux with reflux nephropathy without hydroureter, unilateral
	N13.722	Vesicoureteral-reflux with reflux nephropathy without hydroureter, bilateral
	N13.731	Vesicoureteral-reflux with reflux nephropathy with hydroureter, unilateral
	N13.732	Vesicoureteral-reflux with reflux nephropathy with hydroureter, bilateral
	N13.8	Other obstructive and reflux uropathy
	N20.0	Calculus of kidney
	N20.1	Calculus of ureter
	N20.2	Calculus of kidney with calculus of ureter
	N28.81	Hypertrophy of kidney
	N28.82	Megaloureter
	N28.84	Pyelitis cystica
	N28.85	Pyeloureteritis cystica
	N28.86	Ureteritis cystica
	N28.89	Other specified disorders of kidney and ureter
	N39.3	Stress incontinence (female) (male)
	N39.41	Urge incontinence
	N39.42	Incontinence without sensory awareness
	N39.43	Post-void dribbling
	N39.44	Nocturnal enuresis
	N39.45	Continuous leakage
	N39.46	Mixed incontinence
	N39.490	Overflow incontinence
	N39.498	Other specified urinary incontinence
	N39.8	Other specified disorders of urinary system
	N82.1	Other female urinary-genital tract fistulae ♀
	Q62.0	Congenital hydronephrosis

Q62.11	Congenital occlusion of ureteropelvic junction
Q62.12	Congenital occlusion of ureterovesical orifice
Q62.2	Congenital megaureter
Q62.31	Congenital ureterocele, orthotopic
Q62.32	Cecoureterocele
Q62.39	Other obstructive defects of renal pelvis and ureter
Q62.5	Duplication of ureter
Q62.61	Deviation of ureter
Q62.62	Displacement of ureter
Q62.63	Anomalous implantation of ureter
Q62.69	Other malposition of ureter
Q62.8	Other congenital malformations of ureter

CCI Edits

Refer to Appendix A for CCI edits.

Facility RVUs ▯

Code	Work	PE Facility	MP	Total Facility
50694	5.25	1.97	0.45	7.67
50695	6.80	2.48	0.60	9.88

Non-facility RVUs ▯

Code	Work	PE Non-Facility	MP	Total Non-Facility
50694	5.25	28.70	0.45	34.40
50695	6.80	33.93	0.60	41.33

Modifiers (PAR) ▯

Code	Mod 50	Mod 51	Mod 62	Mod 66	Mod 80
50694	1	2	0	0	1
50695	1	2	0	0	1

Global Period

Code	Days
50694	000
50695	000

50700

50700 Ureteroplasty, plastic operation on ureter (eg, stricture)

AMA Coding Guideline

Repair Procedures on the Ureter

Codes 50705, 50706 are add-on codes describing embolization and balloon dilation of the ureter using non-endoscopic imaging guidance, and each may be reported once per ureter per day. These codes include embolization or dilation plus imaging guidance and radiological supervision and interpretation required to accomplish the embolization or dilation. These procedures may be performed through de novo transrenal access, an existing renal/ureteral access, transurethral access, an ileal conduit, or ureterostomy. The service of gaining access may be reported separately. Diagnostic pyelography/ureterography is not included in 50705 and 50706 and may be reported separately. Other interventions or catheter placements performed at the same setting as the embolization/dilation may be reported separately.

AMA Coding Notes

Surgical Procedures on the Urinary System

(For provision of chemotherapeutic agents, report both the specific service in addition to code(s) for the specific substance(s) or drug(s) provided)

Plain English Description

The ureter is exposed and the narrowed, injured, or diseased portion is isolated. Plastic repair of the ureter depends on the exact nature of the ureteral abnormality. One type of repair involves the use of a Z-plasty. Horizontal and oblique incisions are made over the narrowed or injured portion of the ureter. The flaps are then rotated and re-anastomosed. This type of repair increases the lumen diameter at the site of the narrowing or injury.

Ureteroplasty, plastic operation on ureter

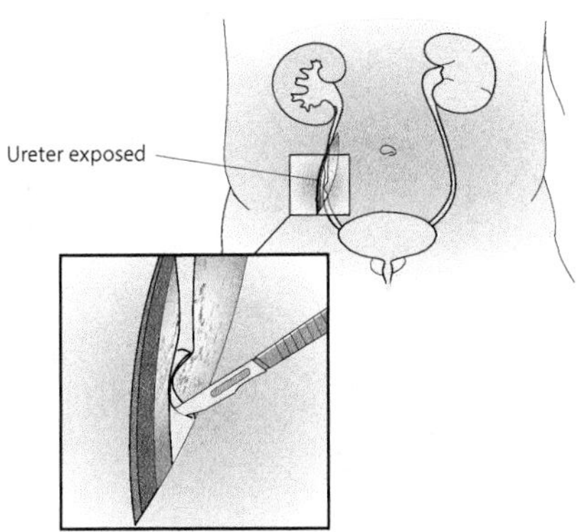

ICD-10-CM Diagnostic Codes

	N11.1	Chronic obstructive pyelonephritis
	N13.30	Unspecified hydronephrosis
	N13.4	Hydroureter
	N13.5	Crossing vessel and stricture of ureter without hydronephrosis
	N13.8	Other obstructive and reflux uropathy
	N20.1	Calculus of ureter
	N28.82	Megaloureter
	N28.89	Other specified disorders of kidney and ureter
	Q62.11	Congenital occlusion of ureteropelvic junction
	Q62.12	Congenital occlusion of ureterovesical orifice
	Q62.2	Congenital megaureter
	Q62.31	Congenital ureterocele, orthotopic
	Q62.32	Cecoureterocele
	Q62.39	Other obstructive defects of renal pelvis and ureter
❼	S37.10	Unspecified injury of ureter
❼	S37.13	Laceration of ureter
❼	S37.19	Other injury of ureter

ICD-10-CM Coding Notes

For codes requiring a 7th character extension, refer to your ICD-10-CM book. Review the character descriptions and coding guidelines for proper selection. For some procedures, only certain characters will apply.

CCI Edits

Refer to Appendix A for CCI edits.

Facility RVUs ▯

Code	Work	PE Facility	MP	Total Facility
50700	16.69	8.38	1.99	27.06

Non-facility RVUs ▯

Code	Work	PE Non-Facility	MP	Total Non-Facility
50700	16.69	8.38	1.99	27.06

Modifiers (PAR) ▯

Code	Mod 50	Mod 51	Mod 62	Mod 66	Mod 80
50700	1	2	1	0	2

Global Period

Code	Days
50700	090

50705

+ 50705 Ureteral embolization or occlusion, including imaging guidance (eg, ultrasound and/or fluoroscopy) and all associated radiological supervision and interpretation (List separately in addition to code for primary procedure)

(Use 50705 in conjunction with 50382, 50384, 50385, 50386, 50387, 50389, 50430, 50431, 50432, 50433, 50434, 50435, 50684, 50688, 50690, 50693, 50694, 50695, 51610)

AMA Coding Guideline

Repair Procedures on the Ureter

Codes 50705, 50706 are add-on codes describing embolization and balloon dilation of the ureter using non-endoscopic imaging guidance, and each may be reported once per ureter per day. These codes include embolization or dilation plus imaging guidance and radiological supervision and interpretation required to accomplish the embolization or dilation. These procedures may be performed through de novo transrenal access, an existing renal/ureteral access, transurethral access, an ileal conduit, or ureterostomy. The service of gaining access may be reported separately. Diagnostic pyelography/ureterography is not included in 50705 and 50706 and may be reported separately. Other interventions or catheter placements performed at the same setting as the embolization/dilation may be reported separately.

AMA Coding Notes

Surgical Procedures on the Urinary System

(For provision of chemotherapeutic agents, report both the specific service in addition to code(s) for the specific substance(s) or drug(s) provided)

AMA *CPT® Assistant* ▯

50705: Jan 16: 3

Plain English Description

Ureteral embolization or occlusion may be used to interrupt the flow of urine from the kidney(s) to the bladder when chronic or refractory lower urinary tract fistulas are present. The development of fistulas can be due to trauma, malignancy, or radiation. If percutaneous access is first required, a trocar or Chiba needle is inserted below the 12th rib under ultrasound and/or fluoroscopic guidance to minimize the risk of puncturing the pleura. The needle is advanced into the renal pelvis and urine is aspirated to verify location and decompress the system. After satisfactory placement of the needle, a thin wire is threaded through the needle into the distal ureter.
A guidewire may also be placed through an existing percutaneous tube or catheter into the ureter.
A delivery catheter or access sheath is inserted over the wire; and the wire is removed. The delivery catheter or access sheath may also be introduced through a cystoscope/ureteroscope. Stainless steel coils and gelatin sponge pledgets are inserted through the catheter/sheath to occlude the ureter. Additional images are obtained to confirm ureteral occlusion. This includes imaging guidance and associated radiologic supervision and interpretation for ureteral embolization or occlusion prepared in conjunction with a separate primary procedure.

ICD-10-CM Diagnostic Codes

See Primary Procedure code for crosswalks.

CCI Edits

Refer to Appendix A for CCI edits.

Facility RVUs ▯

Code	Work	PE Facility	MP	Total Facility
50705	4.03	0.66	0.40	5.09

Non-facility RVUs ▯

Code	Work	PE Non-Facility	MP	Total Non-Facility
50705	4.03	52.88	0.40	57.31

Modifiers (PAR) ▯

Code	Mod 50	Mod 51	Mod 62	Mod 66	Mod 80
50705	1	0	0	0	1

Global Period

Code	Days
50705	ZZZ

50706

✚ **50706 Balloon dilation, ureteral stricture, including imaging guidance (eg, ultrasound and/or fluoroscopy) and all associated radiological supervision and interpretation (List separately in addition to code for primary procedure)**

(Use 50706 in conjunction with 50382, 50384, 50385, 50386, 50387, 50389, 50430, 50431, 50432, 50433, 50434, 50435, 50684, 50688, 50690, 50693, 50694, 50695, 51610)

(Do not report 50706 in conjunction with 50553, 50572, 50953, 50972, 52341, 52344, 52345, 74485)

(For percutaneous nephrostomy, nephroureteral catheter, and/or ureteral catheter placement use 50385, 50387, 50432, 50433, 50434, 50435, 50693, 50694, 50695)

AMA Coding Guideline

Repair Procedures on the Ureter

Codes 50705, 50706 are add-on codes describing embolization and balloon dilation of the ureter using non-endoscopic imaging guidance, and each may be reported once per ureter per day. These codes include embolization or dilation plus imaging guidance and radiological supervision and interpretation required to accomplish the embolization or dilation. These procedures may be performed through de novo transrenal access, an existing renal/ureteral access, transurethral access, an ileal conduit, or ureterostomy. The service of gaining access may be reported separately. Diagnostic pyelography/ureterography is not included in 50705 and 50706 and may be reported separately. Other interventions or catheter placements performed at the same setting as the embolization/dilation may be reported separately.

AMA Coding Notes

Surgical Procedures on the Urinary System

(For provision of chemotherapeutic agents, report both the specific service in addition to code(s) for the specific substance(s) or drug(s) provided)

AMA *CPT® Assistant* ☐

50706: Jan 16: 3

Plain English Description

Balloon dilation of a ureteral stricture may be performed through a percutaneously placed catheter or through the bladder and ureteroscope. Radiologic guidance is required for either approach to ensure that the balloon is centered directly over the stricture. Strictures are narrowed segments of the ureteral lumen that obstruct urine flow. Common causes include tumors and fibrosis. If percutaneous access is first required, a trocar or Chiba needle is inserted below the 12th rib under ultrasound and/or fluoroscopic guidance to minimize the risk of puncturing the pleura. The needle is advanced into the renal pelvis and urine is aspirated to verify location and decompress the system. After satisfactory placement of the needle has been established, a thin wire is threaded through the needle to the location of the ureteral stricture. A guidewire may also be placed through an existing percutaneous tube or catheter to the stricture. The balloon catheter is placed over the guidewire and the guidewire is removed. Once the balloon is positioned directly over the stricture, the balloon is serially dilated until the narrowed area is open. A stent may be inserted following dilation to maintain patency of the ureter. Additional imaging may confirm that the ureter is patent. The balloon catheter may also be introduced through a cystoscope/ureteroscope and placed directly over the stricture, confirmed by fluoroscopy. The balloon is serially dilated until the narrowed ureteral lumen is open. A stent may be inserted following the balloon dilation to maintain patency of the ureter. Urethrogram images confirm that the ureter is patent. The balloon catheter is removed. Code 50706 includes imaging guidance and associated radiologic supervision and interpretation for balloon dilation of a ureteral stricture prepared in conjunction with a separate primary procedure.

ICD-10-CM Diagnostic Codes

See Primary Procedure code for crosswalks.

CCI Edits

Refer to Appendix A for CCI edits.

Facility RVUs ☐

Code	Work	PE Facility	MP	Total Facility
50706	3.80	1.09	0.34	5.23

Non-facility RVUs ☐

Code	Work	PE Non-Facility	MP	Total Non-Facility
50706	3.80	21.82	0.34	25.96

Modifiers (PAR) ☐

Code	Mod 50	Mod 51	Mod 62	Mod 66	Mod 80
50706	1	0	0	0	1

Global Period

Code	Days
50706	ZZZ

CPT® Procedural Coding

50715

50715 Ureterolysis, with or without repositioning of ureter for retroperitoneal fibrosis

(For bilateral procedure, report 50715 with modifier 50)

AMA Coding Guideline

Repair Procedures on the Ureter

Codes 50705, 50706 are add-on codes describing embolization and balloon dilation of the ureter using non-endoscopic imaging guidance, and each may be reported once per ureter per day. These codes include embolization or dilation plus imaging guidance and radiological supervision and interpretation required to accomplish the embolization or dilation. These procedures may be performed through de novo transrenal access, an existing renal/ureteral access, transurethral access, an ileal conduit, or ureterostomy. The service of gaining access may be reported separately. Diagnostic pyelography/ureterography is not included in 50705 and 50706 and may be reported separately. Other interventions or catheter placements performed at the same setting as the embolization/dilation may be reported separately.

AMA Coding Notes

Surgical Procedures on the Urinary System

(For provision of chemotherapeutic agents, report both the specific service in addition to code(s) for the specific substance(s) or drug(s) provided)

Plain English Description

An open ureterolysis is performed on an obstructed ureter that is entrapped by fibrous tissue in the retroperitoneum. This condition is referred to as retroperitoneal fibrosis (RPF). RPF is a rare condition characterized by chronic inflammation of the retroperitoneal structures, including the ureters. The ureter is approached using a flank incision. The colon is mobilized medially to the level of the vena cava and iliac vessels and the retroperitoneum and ureter are exposed. The extent of fibrosis is evaluated and the ureter is then dissected free of the fibrotic mass, which is biopsied for analysis. The ureter may be divided and the normal distal segment repositioned and reattached to the kidney, or the ureter may be left intact and wrapped in omentum.

Ureterolysis, with/without repositioning of ureter

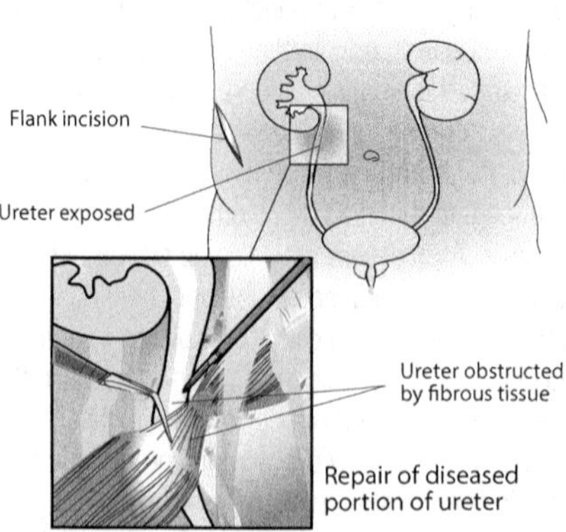

ICD-10-CM Diagnostic Codes

N11.1	Chronic obstructive pyelonephritis
N13.5	Crossing vessel and stricture of ureter without hydronephrosis
N13.8	Other obstructive and reflux uropathy
N28.82	Megaloureter
N28.89	Other specified disorders of kidney and ureter

CCI Edits

Refer to Appendix A for CCI edits.

Facility RVUs

Code	Work	PE Facility	MP	Total Facility
50715	20.64	11.34	3.48	35.46

Non-facility RVUs

Code	Work	PE Non-Facility	MP	Total Non-Facility
50715	20.64	11.34	3.48	35.46

Modifiers (PAR)

Code	Mod 50	Mod 51	Mod 62	Mod 66	Mod 80
50715	1	2	1	0	2

Global Period

Code	Days
50715	090

50722-50725

50722 Ureterolysis for ovarian vein syndrome

50725 Ureterolysis for retrocaval ureter, with reanastomosis of upper urinary tract or vena cava

AMA Coding Guideline

Repair Procedures on the Ureter

Codes 50705, 50706 are add-on codes describing embolization and balloon dilation of the ureter using non-endoscopic imaging guidance, and each may be reported once per ureter per day. These codes include embolization or dilation plus imaging guidance and radiological supervision and interpretation required to accomplish the embolization or dilation. These procedures may be performed through de novo transrenal access, an existing renal/ureteral access, transurethral access, an ileal conduit, or ureterostomy. The service of gaining access may be reported separately. Diagnostic pyelography/ureterography is not included in 50705 and 50706 and may be reported separately. Other interventions or catheter placements performed at the same setting as the embolization/dilation may be reported separately.

AMA Coding Notes

Surgical Procedures on the Urinary System

(For provision of chemotherapeutic agents, report both the specific service in addition to code(s) for the specific substance(s) or drug(s) provided)

Plain English Description

An open ureterolysis is performed on an obstructed ureter that has become entrapped due to ovarian vein syndrome or retrocaval ureter. In 50722, the ureteral obstruction is due to ovarian vein syndrome. Ovarian vein syndrome occurs when an enlarged or tortuous ovarian vein compresses the ureter. An incision is made in the abdomen and the enlarged ovarian vein exposed. Adhesions between the ureter, ovarian vein, or other structures are severed. The ovarian vein may be divided and the enlarged section excised to release the entrapped ureter. In 50725, the ureteral obstruction is due to a retrocaval ureter. Retrocaval ureter, also referred to as circumcaval ureter, is a rare congenital anomaly resulting from persistence of the posterior cardinal veins. This causes malposition of the ureter behind the inferior vena cava where it can become compressed and obstructed between the inferior vena cava and aorta. The retrocaval ureter is exposed by a subcostal incision. The ureter is dissected free of surrounding tissues and mobilized. The compressed segment of ureter is excised. The distal and proximal ends of ureter are spatulated and continuity of the ureter restored by anastomosis. A temporary double J stent is placed to maintain patency and facilitate healing of the ureter. External drainage tubes may be placed in the operative wound. Bleeding is controlled and incisions closed. Alternatively, the vena cava may be divided, the ureter repositioned, and the vena cava reanastomosed.

Ureterolysis

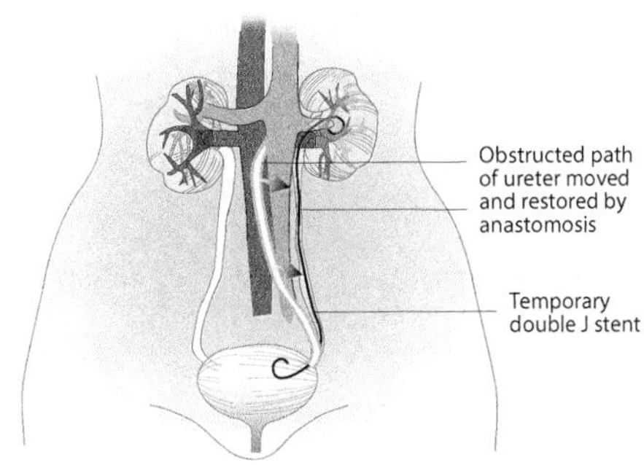

For ovarian vein syndrome (50722); for retrocaval ureter, with reanastomosis of upper urinary tract or vena cava (50725)

ICD-10-CM Diagnostic Codes

N13.8	Other obstructive and reflux uropathy
Q62.4	Agenesis of ureter
Q62.5	Duplication of ureter
Q62.61	Deviation of ureter
Q62.62	Displacement of ureter
Q62.63	Anomalous implantation of ureter
Q62.69	Other malposition of ureter
Q62.7	Congenital vesico-uretero-renal reflux
Q62.8	Other congenital malformations of ureter

CCI Edits

Refer to Appendix A for CCI edits.

Facility RVUs

Code	Work	PE Facility	MP	Total Facility
50722	17.95	9.32	2.94	30.21
50725	20.20	9.55	2.39	32.14

Non-facility RVUs

Code	Work	PE Non-Facility	MP	Total Non-Facility
50722	17.95	9.32	2.94	30.21
50725	20.20	9.55	2.39	32.14

Modifiers (PAR)

Code	Mod 50	Mod 51	Mod 62	Mod 66	Mod 80
50722	0	2	1	0	2
50725	0	2	1	0	2

Global Period

Code	Days
50722	090
50725	090

50727-50728

50727 Revision of urinary-cutaneous anastomosis (any type urostomy)

50728 Revision of urinary-cutaneous anastomosis (any type urostomy); with repair of fascial defect and hernia

AMA Coding Guideline

Repair Procedures on the Ureter

Codes 50705, 50706 are add-on codes describing embolization and balloon dilation of the ureter using non-endoscopic imaging guidance, and each may be reported once per ureter per day. These codes include embolization or dilation plus imaging guidance and radiological supervision and interpretation required to accomplish the embolization or dilation. These procedures may be performed through de novo transrenal access, an existing renal/ureteral access, transurethral access, an ileal conduit, or ureterostomy. The service of gaining access may be reported separately. Diagnostic pyelography/ureterography is not included in 50705 and 50706 and may be reported separately. Other interventions or catheter placements performed at the same setting as the embolization/dilation may be reported separately.

AMA Coding Notes

Surgical Procedures on the Urinary System

(For provision of chemotherapeutic agents, report both the specific service in addition to code(s) for the specific substance(s) or drug(s) provided)

Plain English Description

A previously created urostomy is revised. The exact nature of the procedure depends on the type of urostomy, which may be a cutaneous ureterostomy, cystostomy, or nephrostomy. Revision may be necessary if the stoma becomes constricted or obstructed; if the urinary tract tissue prolapses through the stoma or if it retracts, causing the stoma to sink below the level of the skin, or even detaches from the skin; if necrosis occurs; or if the patient develops a parastomal hernia. In 50727, a skin incision is made around the entire circumference of the urostomy. Local release of scar tissue (adhesions) around the stoma may be performed. Alternatively, dissection may continue down through fascia and peritoneum and the distal portion of the urinary tissue may be resected, then everted, and sutured back to the skin and subcutaneous tissue. If the stoma needs to be relocated, the abdomen is opened at the new stoma site. Adhesions are lysed and the exteriorized urinary tissue is mobilized. Any necrotic tissue is excised. The terminal end of the urinary tissue is brought through the abdominal wall, folded back on itself (everted), and sutured to the skin and subcutaneous tissue. In 50728, a urostomy fascial defect and hernia are repaired. An incision is made over the hernia and the hernia is reduced. Overlying fascia is then repaired with sutures or a mesh implant.

Revision of urinary-cutaneous anastomosis

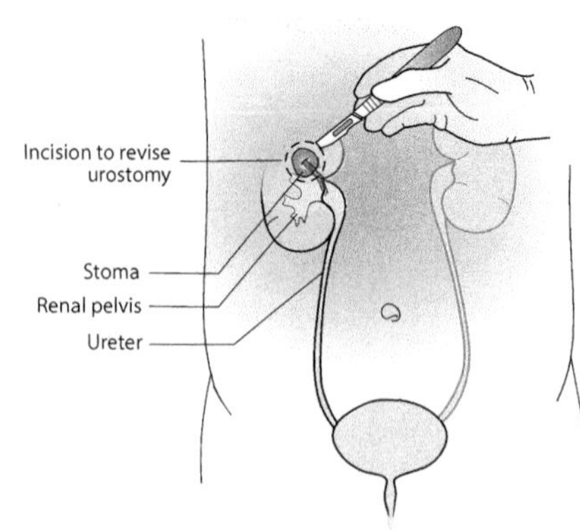

Any type urostomy (50727); with repair of fascial defect and hernia (50728)

ICD-10-CM Diagnostic Codes

K94.09	Other complications of colostomy
K94.11	Enterostomy hemorrhage
K94.12	Enterostomy infection
K94.13	Enterostomy malfunction
K94.19	Other complications of enterostomy
L02.211	Cutaneous abscess of abdominal wall
L02.214	Cutaneous abscess of groin
L03.311	Cellulitis of abdominal wall
L03.314	Cellulitis of groin
L03.319	Cellulitis of trunk, unspecified
L03.321	Acute lymphangitis of abdominal wall
L03.324	Acute lymphangitis of groin
L03.329	Acute lymphangitis of trunk, unspecified
N73.6	Female pelvic peritoneal adhesions (postinfective) ♀
N99.0	Postprocedural (acute) (chronic) kidney failure
N99.510	Cystostomy hemorrhage
N99.511	Cystostomy infection
N99.512	Cystostomy malfunction
N99.518	Other cystostomy complication
N99.520	Hemorrhage of incontinent external stoma of urinary tract
N99.521	Infection of incontinent external stoma of urinary tract
N99.522	Malfunction of incontinent external stoma of urinary tract
N99.528	Other complication of incontinent external stoma of urinary tract
N99.531	Infection of continent stoma of urinary tract
N99.532	Malfunction of continent stoma of urinary tract
N99.538	Other complication of continent stoma of urinary tract
Z43.6	Encounter for attention to other artificial openings of urinary tract

CCI Edits

Refer to Appendix A for CCI edits.

Facility RVUs ▢

Code	Work	PE Facility	MP	Total Facility
50727	8.28	5.66	1.10	15.04
50728	12.18	7.39	1.99	21.56

Non-facility RVUs ▢

Code	Work	PE Non-Facility	MP	Total Non-Facility
50727	8.28	5.66	1.10	15.04
50728	12.18	7.39	1.99	21.56

Modifiers (PAR) ▢

Code	Mod 50	Mod 51	Mod 62	Mod 66	Mod 80
50727	0	2	2	0	2
50728	0	2	2	0	2

Global Period

Code	Days
50727	090
50728	090

50740-50750

50740 Ureteropyelostomy, anastomosis of ureter and renal pelvis
50750 Ureterocalycostomy, anastomosis of ureter to renal calyx

AMA Coding Guideline

Repair Procedures on the Ureter

Codes 50705, 50706 are add-on codes describing embolization and balloon dilation of the ureter using non-endoscopic imaging guidance, and each may be reported once per ureter per day. These codes include embolization or dilation plus imaging guidance and radiological supervision and interpretation required to accomplish the embolization or dilation. These procedures may be performed through de novo transrenal access, an existing renal/ureteral access, transurethral access, an ileal conduit, or ureterostomy. The service of gaining access may be reported separately. Diagnostic pyelography/ureterography is not included in 50705 and 50706 and may be reported separately. Other interventions or catheter placements performed at the same setting as the embolization/dilation may be reported separately.

AMA Coding Notes

Surgical Procedures on the Urinary System

(For provision of chemotherapeutic agents, report both the specific service in addition to code(s) for the specific substance(s) or drug(s) provided)

AMA *CPT® Assistant* ▯

50740: Oct 01: 8
50750: Oct 01: 8

Plain English Description

Ureteropyelostomy is a procedure that joins the upper aspect of the ureter to the lower aspect of the renal pelvis while ureterocalycostomy joins the ureter to the calyces at a point above the lower aspect of the renal pelvis. These procedures are performed to treat ureteropelvic junction (UPJ) obstruction or a long proximal ureteral stricture. Ureterocalycostomy is performed when the renal pelvis is severely fibrosed or scarred. The ureter is exposed and mobilized, taking care to preserve periureteral tissue. The ureter is divided just distal to the narrowed region. The proximal ureteral stump is ligated. The kidney is exposed and mobilized. In 50740, the lower aspect of the renal pelvis is excised at a point above the narrowed or obstructed portion. The proximal aspect of the remaining segment of healthy ureter is spatulated. A stent is placed and the ureteropelvic anastomosis is performed over the stent. The repair is reinforced with perinephric fat or omentum. In 50750, the procedure is performed as described above except that the lower pole calyx is exposed and the parenchyma over the lower pole is resected. Any remaining fibrotic or diseased tissue is excised. The proximal ureter is spatulated. A stent is placed and the ureterocalyceal anastomosis is performed over the stent.

ICD-10-CM Diagnostic Codes

⇄	C64.1	Malignant neoplasm of right kidney, except renal pelvis
⇄	C64.2	Malignant neoplasm of left kidney, except renal pelvis
⇄	C65.1	Malignant neoplasm of right renal pelvis
⇄	C65.2	Malignant neoplasm of left renal pelvis
⇄	C66.1	Malignant neoplasm of right ureter
⇄	C66.2	Malignant neoplasm of left ureter
	C68.8	Malignant neoplasm of overlapping sites of urinary organs
⇄	C79.01	Secondary malignant neoplasm of right kidney and renal pelvis
⇄	C79.02	Secondary malignant neoplasm of left kidney and renal pelvis
	C79.19	Secondary malignant neoplasm of other urinary organs
	C7A.093	Malignant carcinoid tumor of the kidney
	C80.2	Malignant neoplasm associated with transplanted organ
⇄	D30.01	Benign neoplasm of right kidney
⇄	D30.02	Benign neoplasm of left kidney
⇄	D30.11	Benign neoplasm of right renal pelvis
⇄	D30.12	Benign neoplasm of left renal pelvis
	D3A.093	Benign carcinoid tumor of the kidney
⇄	D41.01	Neoplasm of uncertain behavior of right kidney
⇄	D41.02	Neoplasm of uncertain behavior of left kidney
⇄	D41.11	Neoplasm of uncertain behavior of right renal pelvis
⇄	D41.12	Neoplasm of uncertain behavior of left renal pelvis
⇄	D41.21	Neoplasm of uncertain behavior of right ureter
⇄	D41.22	Neoplasm of uncertain behavior of left ureter
	N11.1	Chronic obstructive pyelonephritis
	N13.1	Hydronephrosis with ureteral stricture, not elsewhere classified
	N13.2	Hydronephrosis with renal and ureteral calculous obstruction
	N13.39	Other hydronephrosis
	N13.5	Crossing vessel and stricture of ureter without hydronephrosis
	N13.8	Other obstructive and reflux uropathy
	N20.0	Calculus of kidney
	N20.1	Calculus of ureter
	N20.2	Calculus of kidney with calculus of ureter
	N28.89	Other specified disorders of kidney and ureter
	N99.89	Other postprocedural complications and disorders of genitourinary system
	Q61.00	Congenital renal cyst, unspecified
	Q61.02	Congenital multiple renal cysts
	Q61.8	Other cystic kidney diseases
	Q62.0	Congenital hydronephrosis
	Q62.11	Congenital occlusion of ureteropelvic junction
	Q62.31	Congenital ureterocele, orthotopic
	Q62.32	Cecoureterocele
	Q62.39	Other obstructive defects of renal pelvis and ureter
❼	S37.10	Unspecified injury of ureter

ICD-10-CM Coding Notes

For codes requiring a 7th character extension, refer to your ICD-10-CM book. Review the character descriptions and coding guidelines for proper selection. For some procedures, only certain characters will apply.

CCI Edits

Refer to Appendix A for CCI edits.

Facility RVUs ▯

Code	Work	PE Facility	MP	Total Facility
50740	20.07	11.46	5.06	36.59
50750	21.22	9.90	2.51	33.63

Non-facility RVUs ▯

Code	Work	PE Non-Facility	MP	Total Non-Facility
50740	20.07	11.46	5.06	36.59
50750	21.22	9.90	2.51	33.63

Modifiers (PAR) ▯

Code	Mod 50	Mod 51	Mod 62	Mod 66	Mod 80
50740	1	2	1	0	2
50750	1	2	0	0	2

Global Period

Code	Days
50740	090
50750	090

50760-50770

50760 Ureteroureterostomy

50770 Transureteroureterostomy, anastomosis of ureter to contralateral ureter

(Codes 50780-50785 include minor procedures to prevent vesicoureteral reflux)

AMA Coding Guideline

Repair Procedures on the Ureter

Codes 50705, 50706 are add-on codes describing embolization and balloon dilation of the ureter using non-endoscopic imaging guidance, and each may be reported once per ureter per day. These codes include embolization or dilation plus imaging guidance and radiological supervision and interpretation required to accomplish the embolization or dilation. These procedures may be performed through de novo transrenal access, an existing renal/ureteral access, transurethral access, an ileal conduit, or ureterostomy. The service of gaining access may be reported separately. Diagnostic pyelography/ureterography is not included in 50705 and 50706 and may be reported separately. Other interventions or catheter placements performed at the same setting as the embolization/dilation may be reported separately.

AMA Coding Notes

Surgical Procedures on the Urinary System

(For provision of chemotherapeutic agents, report both the specific service in addition to code(s) for the specific substance(s) or drug(s) provided)

AMA *CPT® Assistant*

50760: Oct 01: 8

Plain English Description

Ureteroureterostomy is a procedure that joins two segments of the same ureter while transureteroureterostomy joins one ureter to the contralateral ureter. These procedures are performed to treat ureteral stenosis, obstruction, or injury. In 50760, the ureter is exposed and the narrowed or injured portion is identified. The ureter is dissected free of surrounding tissues and mobilized between soft rubber loops. Care is taken to preserve periureteral tissues and blood supply. The narrowed or damaged portion is excised. A ureteral catheter is inserted extending from the renal pelvis to the bladder. The two segments of ureter are anastomosed over the ureteral catheter. A drain is placed in the abdomen adjacent to the anastomosis. The surgical wound is closed in layers. In 50770, both ureters are exposed and mobility and length are evaluated. The diseased ureter is mobilized above the area of the diseased portion up to the ureteropelvic junction (UPJ), taking care to preserve periureteral tissue and blood supply. A retroperitoneal tunnel is created. The diseased ureter is transected above the diseased segment. The proximal healthy segment of the ureter is brought across the midline through the tunnel to the opposite ureter. The recipient ureter is mobilized. The transposed ureter is spatulated. An incision is made in the recipient ureter and the transposed ureter is sutured to the recipient ureter. Ureteral stenting is performed as needed. A drain is placed in the abdomen and the surgical wound is closed.

Ureteroureterostomy/ transureteroureterostomy

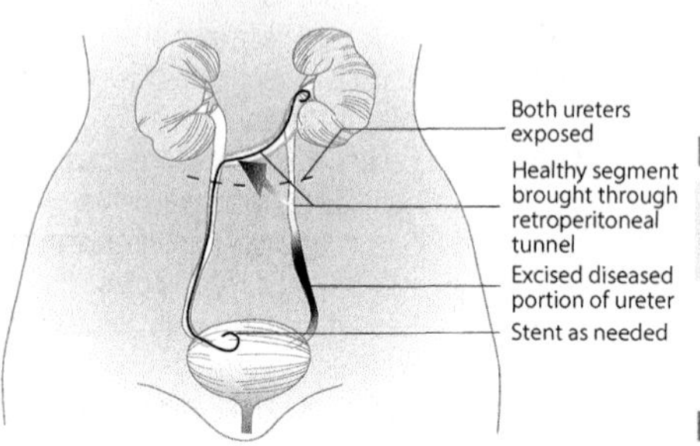

For ureteroureterostomy (50760); for transureteroureterostomy, anastomosis of ureter to contralateral ureter (50770)

ICD-10-CM Diagnostic Codes

⇄	C66.1	Malignant neoplasm of right ureter
⇄	C66.2	Malignant neoplasm of left ureter
	N11.1	Chronic obstructive pyelonephritis
	N13.5	Crossing vessel and stricture of ureter without hydronephrosis
	N13.71	Vesicoureteral-reflux without reflux nephropathy
	N13.721	Vesicoureteral-reflux with reflux nephropathy without hydroureter, unilateral
	N13.722	Vesicoureteral-reflux with reflux nephropathy without hydroureter, bilateral
	N13.731	Vesicoureteral-reflux with reflux nephropathy with hydroureter, unilateral
	N13.732	Vesicoureteral-reflux with reflux nephropathy with hydroureter, bilateral
	N13.8	Other obstructive and reflux uropathy
	Q62.0	Congenital hydronephrosis
	Q62.11	Congenital occlusion of ureteropelvic junction
	Q62.12	Congenital occlusion of ureterovesical orifice
	Q62.2	Congenital megaureter
	Q62.31	Congenital ureterocele, orthotopic
	Q62.32	Cecoureterocele
	Q62.39	Other obstructive defects of renal pelvis and ureter
	Q62.61	Deviation of ureter
	Q62.62	Displacement of ureter
	Q62.63	Anomalous implantation of ureter
	Q62.69	Other malposition of ureter
	Q62.7	Congenital vesico-uretero-renal reflux
	Q62.8	Other congenital malformations of ureter
❼	S37.12	Contusion of ureter
❼	S37.13	Laceration of ureter
❼	S37.19	Other injury of ureter

ICD-10-CM Coding Notes

For codes requiring a 7th character extension, refer to your ICD-10-CM book. Review the character descriptions and coding guidelines for proper selection. For some procedures, only certain characters will apply.

CCI Edits

Refer to Appendix A for CCI edits.

Facility RVUs

Code	Work	PE Facility	MP	Total Facility
50760	20.07	10.04	3.29	33.40
50770	21.22	9.90	2.51	33.63

Non-facility RVUs

Code	Work	PE Non-Facility	MP	Total Non-Facility
50760	20.07	10.04	3.29	33.40
50770	21.22	9.90	2.51	33.63

Modifiers (PAR)

Code	Mod 50	Mod 51	Mod 62	Mod 66	Mod 80
50760	1	2	1	0	2
50770	0	2	1	0	2

Global Period

Code	Days
50760	090
50770	090

50780-50785

50780 Ureteroneocystostomy; anastomosis of single ureter to bladder
(For bilateral procedure, report 50780 with modifier 50)
(When combined with cystourethroplasty or vesical neck revision, use 51820)

50782 Ureteroneocystostomy; anastomosis of duplicated ureter to bladder

50783 Ureteroneocystostomy; with extensive ureteral tailoring

50785 Ureteroneocystostomy; with vesico-psoas hitch or bladder flap
(For bilateral procedure, report 50785 with modifier 50)

AMA Coding Guideline
Repair Procedures on the Ureter

Codes 50705, 50706 are add-on codes describing embolization and balloon dilation of the ureter using non-endoscopic imaging guidance, and each may be reported once per ureter per day. These codes include embolization or dilation plus imaging guidance and radiological supervision and interpretation required to accomplish the embolization or dilation. These procedures may be performed through de novo transrenal access, an existing renal/ureteral access, transurethral access, an ileal conduit, or ureterostomy. The service of gaining access may be reported separately. Diagnostic pyelography/ureterography is not included in 50705 and 50706 and may be reported separately. Other interventions or catheter placements performed at the same setting as the embolization/dilation may be reported separately.

AMA Coding Notes
Surgical Procedures on the Urinary System

(For provision of chemotherapeutic agents, report both the specific service in addition to code(s) for the specific substance(s) or drug(s) provided)

AMA *CPT® Assistant* ▯

50780: Oct 01: 8, Feb 18: 11
50782: Oct 01: 8
50783: Oct 01: 8
50785: Oct 01: 8

Plain English Description

An open ureteroneocystostomy is performed. The distal ureter is divided at or near the ureterovesical junction (UVJ). An incision is then made in the dome of the bladder wall to the level of the mucosa. A smaller incision is made in the bladder mucosa. The detached segment of ureter is trimmed and the end spatulated. The full thickness of the ureter is anastomosed to the bladder mucosa. The bladder wall is then closed over a 2-3 cm segment of ureter to create a tunnel for the ureter to help prevent reflux. The opening at the UVJ is closed. A temporary ureteral stent may be placed to ensure patency and facilitate healing. Report 50780 when the procedure is performed on a single ureter. Report 50782 when the procedure is performed on a duplicated (double) ureter. Duplicated ureters are the result of a duplicated collecting system in a single kidney with two ureters that may be fused into a single ureter or may each empty separately into the bladder. Report 50783 when extensive ureteral tailoring or reconstruction is required prior to implantation into the bladder. Report 50785 when the procedure is performed with a vesico-psoas hitch or bladder flap. The procedure is performed as described above; however, prior to implantation of the ureter, the bladder is mobilized and sutured (fixed) to the psoas muscle. The bladder is then incised at the point of fixation to the psoas muscle and the ureter implanted in the immobile bladder portion along the line of fixation using a long submucosal tunnel. Alternatively, a bladder flap, also referred to as a Boari flap, may be used when the distal ureteral segment is too short to reach the bladder.

Ureteroneocystostomy

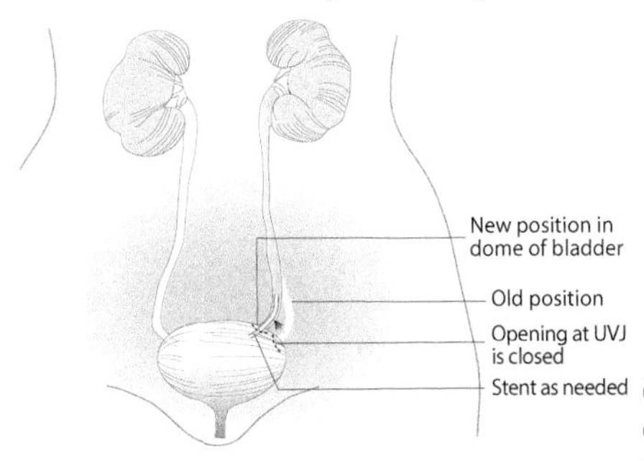

Anastomosis of single ureter (50780); anastomosis of duplicated ureter (50782); with extensive ureteral tailoring (50783); with vesico-psoas hitch or bladder flap (50785)

ICD-10-CM Diagnostic Codes

⇄	C66.1	Malignant neoplasm of right ureter
⇄	C66.2	Malignant neoplasm of left ureter
	C79.19	Secondary malignant neoplasm of other urinary organs
⇄	D30.21	Benign neoplasm of right ureter
⇄	D30.22	Benign neoplasm of left ureter
⇄	D41.11	Neoplasm of uncertain behavior of right renal pelvis
⇄	D41.12	Neoplasm of uncertain behavior of left renal pelvis
⇄	D41.21	Neoplasm of uncertain behavior of right ureter
⇄	D41.22	Neoplasm of uncertain behavior of left ureter
	D41.8	Neoplasm of uncertain behavior of other specified urinary organs
	D47.Z1	Post-transplant lymphoproliferative disorder (PTLD)
	N11.1	Chronic obstructive pyelonephritis
	N13.5	Crossing vessel and stricture of ureter without hydronephrosis
	N13.721	Vesicoureteral-reflux with reflux nephropathy without hydroureter, unilateral
	N13.722	Vesicoureteral-reflux with reflux nephropathy without hydroureter, bilateral
	N13.731	Vesicoureteral-reflux with reflux nephropathy with hydroureter, unilateral
	N13.732	Vesicoureteral-reflux with reflux nephropathy with hydroureter, bilateral
	N13.8	Other obstructive and reflux uropathy
	N28.82	Megaloureter
	N28.89	Other specified disorders of kidney and ureter
	Q62	Congenital obstructive defects of renal pelvis and congenital malformations of ureter
	Q62.0	Congenital hydronephrosis
	Q62.11	Congenital occlusion of ureteropelvic junction
	Q62.12	Congenital occlusion of ureterovesical orifice
	Q62.2	Congenital megaureter
	Q62.31	Congenital ureterocele, orthotopic
	Q62.32	Cecoureterocele
	Q62.39	Other obstructive defects of renal pelvis and ureter
	Q62.5	Duplication of ureter
	Q62.61	Deviation of ureter
	Q62.62	Displacement of ureter
	Q62.63	Anomalous implantation of ureter
	Q62.69	Other malposition of ureter
	Q62.7	Congenital vesico-uretero-renal reflux
	Q62.8	Other congenital malformations of ureter
	Q64.8	Other specified congenital malformations of urinary system
❼	S37.12	Contusion of ureter
❼	S37.13	Laceration of ureter
❼	S37.19	Other injury of ureter
	T86.11	Kidney transplant rejection
	T86.12	Kidney transplant failure
	T86.13	Kidney transplant infection
	T86.19	Other complication of kidney transplant

ICD-10-CM Coding Notes

For codes requiring a 7th character extension, refer to your ICD-10-CM book. Review the character descriptions and coding guidelines for proper selection. For some procedures, only certain characters will apply.

CCI Edits

Refer to Appendix A for CCI edits.

Facility RVUs

Code	Work	PE Facility	MP	Total Facility
50780	19.95	9.75	2.82	32.52
50782	19.66	9.38	2.33	31.37
50783	20.70	9.72	2.47	32.89
50785	22.23	10.40	2.82	35.45

Non-facility RVUs

Code	Work	PE Non-Facility	MP	Total Non-Facility
50780	19.95	9.75	2.82	32.52
50782	19.66	9.38	2.33	31.37
50783	20.70	9.72	2.47	32.89
50785	22.23	10.40	2.82	35.45

Modifiers (PAR)

Code	Mod 50	Mod 51	Mod 62	Mod 66	Mod 80
50780	1	2	1	0	2
50782	1	2	2	0	2
50783	1	2	2	0	2
50785	1	2	1	0	2

Global Period

Code	Days
50780	090
50782	090
50783	090
50785	090

50800

50800 Ureteroenterostomy, direct anastomosis of ureter to intestine

(For bilateral procedure, report 50800 with modifier 50)

AMA Coding Guideline

Repair Procedures on the Ureter

Codes 50705, 50706 are add-on codes describing embolization and balloon dilation of the ureter using non-endoscopic imaging guidance, and each may be reported once per ureter per day. These codes include embolization or dilation plus imaging guidance and radiological supervision and interpretation required to accomplish the embolization or dilation. These procedures may be performed through de novo transrenal access, an existing renal/ureteral access, transurethral access, an ileal conduit, or ureterostomy. The service of gaining access may be reported separately. Diagnostic pyelography/ureterography is not included in 50705 and 50706 and may be reported separately. Other interventions or catheter placements performed at the same setting as the embolization/dilation may be reported separately.

AMA Coding Notes

Surgical Procedures on the Urinary System

(For provision of chemotherapeutic agents, report both the specific service in addition to code(s) for the specific substance(s) or drug(s) provided)

AMA *CPT® Assistant*

50800: Oct 01: 8

Plain English Description

A diseased or injured segment of the middle or distal ureter is excised and the healthy proximal ureteral segment is anastomosed to the intestine. The abdomen is incised in the midline and the peritoneum is opened. The small bowel is isolated and packed out of the surgical field. The ureter is exposed and mobilized, taking care to preserve perirenal tissue and blood supply. The diseased segment of ureter is excised and the distal ureteral stump is ligated at the ureterovesical junction. A segment of intestine, usually ileum, is selected and mobilized as needed. The ureter is spatulated, stented, and anastomosed to the intestine in an end-to-side fashion. A nephrostomy tube is placed as needed. The surgical wound is closed in layers.

Ureteroenterostomy, direct anastomosis of ureter to intestine

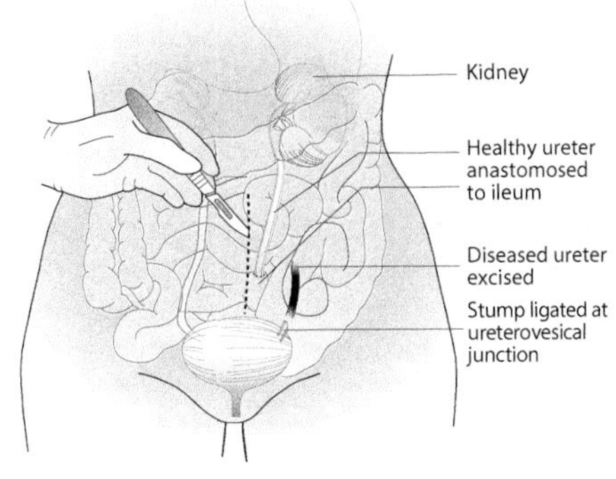

ICD-10-CM Diagnostic Codes

C67.0	Malignant neoplasm of trigone of bladder
C67.1	Malignant neoplasm of dome of bladder
C67.2	Malignant neoplasm of lateral wall of bladder
C67.3	Malignant neoplasm of anterior wall of bladder
C67.4	Malignant neoplasm of posterior wall of bladder
C67.5	Malignant neoplasm of bladder neck
C67.6	Malignant neoplasm of ureteric orifice
C67.8	Malignant neoplasm of overlapping sites of bladder
C79.11	Secondary malignant neoplasm of bladder
C79.19	Secondary malignant neoplasm of other urinary organs
D09.0	Carcinoma in situ of bladder
D41.4	Neoplasm of uncertain behavior of bladder
N11.1	Chronic obstructive pyelonephritis
N13.5	Crossing vessel and stricture of ureter without hydronephrosis
N13.8	Other obstructive and reflux uropathy
N20.1	Calculus of ureter
N20.2	Calculus of kidney with calculus of ureter
N21.0	Calculus in bladder
N99.520	Hemorrhage of incontinent external stoma of urinary tract
N99.521	Infection of incontinent external stoma of urinary tract
N99.522	Malfunction of incontinent external stoma of urinary tract
N99.528	Other complication of incontinent external stoma of urinary tract
N99.530	Hemorrhage of continent stoma of urinary tract
N99.531	Infection of continent stoma of urinary tract
N99.532	Malfunction of continent stoma of urinary tract
N99.538	Other complication of continent stoma of urinary tract
N99.81	Other intraoperative complications of genitourinary system
N99.89	Other postprocedural complications and disorders of genitourinary system
Q64.8	Other specified congenital malformations of urinary system
Q64.9	Congenital malformation of urinary system, unspecified
R80.2	Orthostatic proteinuria, unspecified
❼ S37.22	Contusion of bladder
❼ S37.23	Laceration of bladder
❼ S37.29	Other injury of bladder

ICD-10-CM Coding Notes

For codes requiring a 7th character extension, refer to your ICD-10-CM book. Review the character descriptions and coding guidelines for proper selection. For some procedures, only certain characters will apply.

CCI Edits

Refer to Appendix A for CCI edits.

Facility RVUs

Code	Work	PE Facility	MP	Total Facility
50800	16.41	8.60	2.01	27.02

Non-facility RVUs

Code	Work	PE Non-Facility	MP	Total Non-Facility
50800	16.41	8.60	2.01	27.02

Modifiers (PAR)

Code	Mod 50	Mod 51	Mod 62	Mod 66	Mod 80
50800	1	2	1	0	2

Global Period

Code	Days
50800	090

50810

50810 Ureterosigmoidostomy, with creation of sigmoid bladder and establishment of abdominal or perineal colostomy, including intestine anastomosis

AMA Coding Guideline

Repair Procedures on the Ureter

Codes 50705, 50706 are add-on codes describing embolization and balloon dilation of the ureter using non-endoscopic imaging guidance, and each may be reported once per ureter per day. These codes include embolization or dilation plus imaging guidance and radiological supervision and interpretation required to accomplish the embolization or dilation. These procedures may be performed through de novo transrenal access, an existing renal/ureteral access, transurethral access, an ileal conduit, or ureterostomy. The service of gaining access may be reported separately. Diagnostic pyelography/ureterography is not included in 50705 and 50706 and may be reported separately. Other interventions or catheter placements performed at the same setting as the embolization/dilation may be reported separately.

AMA Coding Notes

Surgical Procedures on the Urinary System

(For provision of chemotherapeutic agents, report both the specific service in addition to code(s) for the specific substance(s) or drug(s) provided)

AMA *CPT® Assistant* ☐

50810: Oct 01: 8

Plain English Description

Ureterosigmoidostomy is one type of urinary diversion that may be performed on patients with bladder cancer, neurogenic bladder, radiation injury to the bladder, intractable incontinence, as well as other conditions. The abdomen is incised in the midline and the peritoneum is opened. The small bowel is isolated and packed out of the surgical field. The ureters are exposed, mobilized, and divided distally near the ureterovesical junction. The ureteral stumps are ligated. A segment of sigmoid colon is selected and mobilized. The segment from which the sigmoid bladder is to be constructed is isolated. The sigmoid colon is divided and an appropriately sized segment is isolated. The remaining distal and proximal portions of the sigmoid colon are then anastomosed and bowel continuity is restored. The sigmoid bladder is fashioned. A tunnel is created from the sigmoid bladder to the ureters. The ureters are pulled through the tunnel to the sigmoid bladder and into the lumen of the sigmoid. The ends of the ureters are spatulated along the anterior aspect. Stents are placed in both ureters. The ureters are anastomosed to the sigmoid colon approximately 3 cm apart. A separate abdominal or perineal incision is made for creation of the stoma through which urine will be expelled. The sigmoid bladder is exteriorized through the stoma, folded back on itself (everted), and sutured to the skin or subcutaneous tissue, creating either an abdominal or perineal colostomy. An ostomy bag is secured over the sigmoidostomy site or a catheter is placed in the stoma. Drains are placed as needed and surgical incisions are closed in layers.

Ureterosigmoidostomy

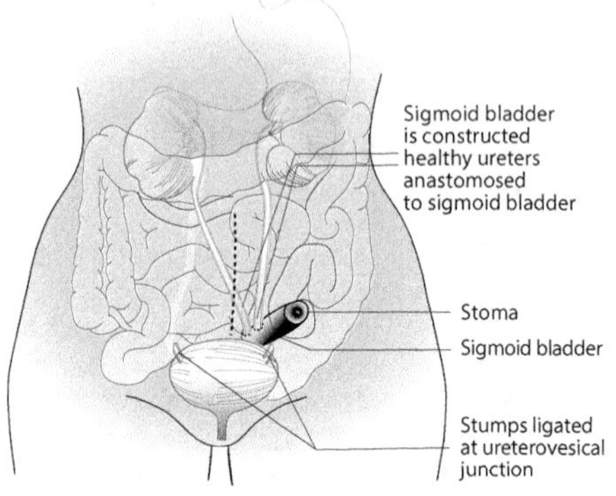

ICD-10-CM Diagnostic Codes

	C67.0	Malignant neoplasm of trigone of bladder
	C67.1	Malignant neoplasm of dome of bladder
	C67.2	Malignant neoplasm of lateral wall of bladder
	C67.3	Malignant neoplasm of anterior wall of bladder
	C67.4	Malignant neoplasm of posterior wall of bladder
	C67.5	Malignant neoplasm of bladder neck
	C67.6	Malignant neoplasm of ureteric orifice
	C67.7	Malignant neoplasm of urachus
	C67.8	Malignant neoplasm of overlapping sites of bladder
	C79.11	Secondary malignant neoplasm of bladder
	D09.0	Carcinoma in situ of bladder
	D41.4	Neoplasm of uncertain behavior of bladder
	G83.4	Cauda equina syndrome
	N11.1	Chronic obstructive pyelonephritis
	N13.8	Other obstructive and reflux uropathy
	N21.0	Calculus in bladder
	N30.40	Irradiation cystitis without hematuria
	N30.80	Other cystitis without hematuria
	N30.81	Other cystitis with hematuria
	N31.0	Uninhibited neuropathic bladder, not elsewhere classified
	N31.1	Reflex neuropathic bladder, not elsewhere classified
	N31.9	Neuromuscular dysfunction of bladder, unspecified
	N32.0	Bladder-neck obstruction
	N32.1	Vesicointestinal fistula
	N32.3	Diverticulum of bladder
	N32.89	Other specified disorders of bladder
	N33	Bladder disorders in diseases classified elsewhere
	N99.520	Hemorrhage of incontinent external stoma of urinary tract
	N99.521	Infection of incontinent external stoma of urinary tract
	N99.522	Malfunction of incontinent external stoma of urinary tract
	N99.528	Other complication of incontinent external stoma of urinary tract
	N99.530	Hemorrhage of continent stoma of urinary tract
	N99.531	Infection of continent stoma of urinary tract
	N99.532	Malfunction of continent stoma of urinary tract
	N99.538	Other complication of continent stoma of urinary tract
	N99.81	Other intraoperative complications of genitourinary system
	N99.89	Other postprocedural complications and disorders of genitourinary system
	Q64.11	Supravesical fissure of urinary bladder
	Q64.12	Cloacal exstrophy of urinary bladder
	Q64.19	Other exstrophy of urinary bladder
	Q64.5	Congenital absence of bladder and urethra
	Q64.6	Congenital diverticulum of bladder
	Q64.79	Other congenital malformations of bladder and urethra
❼	S37.22	Contusion of bladder
❼	S37.23	Laceration of bladder
❼	S37.29	Other injury of bladder

ICD-10-CM Coding Notes

For codes requiring a 7th character extension, refer to your ICD-10-CM book. Review the character descriptions and coding guidelines for proper selection. For some procedures, only certain characters will apply.

CCI Edits

Refer to Appendix A for CCI edits.

Facility RVUs

Code	Work	PE Facility	MP	Total Facility
50810	22.61	13.68	5.72	42.01

Non-facility RVUs

Code	Work	PE Non-Facility	MP	Total Non-Facility
50810	22.61	13.68	5.72	42.01

Modifiers (PAR)

Code	Mod 50	Mod 51	Mod 62	Mod 66	Mod 80
50810	0	2	1	0	2

Global Period

Code	Days
50810	090

50815-50820

50815 Ureterocolon conduit, including intestine anastomosis

(For bilateral procedure, report 50815 with modifier 50)

50820 Ureteroileal conduit (ileal bladder), including intestine anastomosis (Bricker operation)

(For bilateral procedure, report 50820 with modifier 50)

(For combination of 50800-50820 with cystectomy, see 51580-51595)

AMA Coding Guideline

Repair Procedures on the Ureter

Codes 50705, 50706 are add-on codes describing embolization and balloon dilation of the ureter using non-endoscopic imaging guidance, and each may be reported once per ureter per day. These codes include embolization or dilation plus imaging guidance and radiological supervision and interpretation required to accomplish the embolization or dilation. These procedures may be performed through de novo transrenal access, an existing renal/ureteral access, transurethral access, an ileal conduit, or ureterostomy. The service of gaining access may be reported separately. Diagnostic pyelography/ureterography is not included in 50705 and 50706 and may be reported separately. Other interventions or catheter placements performed at the same setting as the embolization/dilation may be reported separately.

AMA Coding Notes

Surgical Procedures on the Urinary System

(For provision of chemotherapeutic agents, report both the specific service in addition to code(s) for the specific substance(s) or drug(s) provided)

AMA *CPT® Assistant* ▢

50815: Oct 01: 8

50820: Oct 01: 8

Plain English Description

Ureterocolon and ureteroileal conduits are types of urinary diversions that may be performed on patients with bladder cancer, neurogenic bladder, radiation injury to the bladder, and intractable incontinence, as well as other conditions. The abdomen is incised in the midline and the peritoneum is opened. The small bowel is isolated and packed out of the surgical field. The ureters are exposed and mobilized. The ureters are divided distally near the ureterovesical junction and the ureteral stumps are ligated. The portion of colon or ileum to be used for the conduit is identified and isolated. The remaining segments of bowel distal and proximal to the isolated segment are anastomosed and bowel continuity is restored. A stoma site is selected and the skin is incised. Dissection is carried down to the anterior rectus fascia, which is incised. The rectus muscle is divided using blunt dissection. The distal end of the conduit is pulled through the abdominal wall, everted, and sutured to skin or subcutaneous tissues to create the stoma. The proximal end of the conduit is closed with sutures. A tunnel is created from the conduit to the ureters. The ureters are pulled through the tunnel to the conduit. The ends of the ureters are spatulated. Stents are placed in both ureters. Small incisions are made in the conduit and the ureters are anastomosed to the conduit approximately 3 cm apart. Drains are placed as needed and surgical incisions are closed in layers. An ostomy bag is placed over the ostomy site to collect urine. Use 50815 when the conduit is created using a portion of the colon; use 50820 when a portion of the ileum is used.

Ureterocolon conduit, ureteroileal conduit

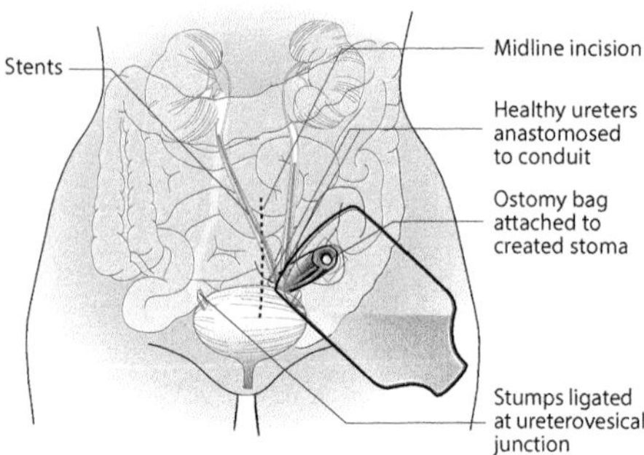

Including intestine anastomosis (50815); ileal bladder, including intestine anastomosis (50820)

ICD-10-CM Diagnostic Codes

C67.0	Malignant neoplasm of trigone of bladder
C67.1	Malignant neoplasm of dome of bladder
C67.2	Malignant neoplasm of lateral wall of bladder
C67.3	Malignant neoplasm of anterior wall of bladder
C67.4	Malignant neoplasm of posterior wall of bladder
C67.5	Malignant neoplasm of bladder neck
C67.6	Malignant neoplasm of ureteric orifice
C67.7	Malignant neoplasm of urachus
C67.8	Malignant neoplasm of overlapping sites of bladder
C79.11	Secondary malignant neoplasm of bladder
D09.0	Carcinoma in situ of bladder
G83.4	Cauda equina syndrome
N11.1	Chronic obstructive pyelonephritis
N13.8	Other obstructive and reflux uropathy
N21.0	Calculus in bladder
N30.40	Irradiation cystitis without hematuria
N30.41	Irradiation cystitis with hematuria
N30.80	Other cystitis without hematuria
N30.81	Other cystitis with hematuria
N31.0	Uninhibited neuropathic bladder, not elsewhere classified
N31.1	Reflex neuropathic bladder, not elsewhere classified
N31.9	Neuromuscular dysfunction of bladder, unspecified
N32.0	Bladder-neck obstruction
N32.3	Diverticulum of bladder
N32.89	Other specified disorders of bladder
N33	Bladder disorders in diseases classified elsewhere
Q64.11	Supravesical fissure of urinary bladder
Q64.12	Cloacal exstrophy of urinary bladder
Q64.19	Other exstrophy of urinary bladder
Q64.75	Double urinary meatus
Q64.79	Other congenital malformations of bladder and urethra
❼ S37.22	Contusion of bladder
❼ S37.23	Laceration of bladder
❼ S37.29	Other injury of bladder

ICD-10-CM Coding Notes

For codes requiring a 7th character extension, refer to your ICD-10-CM book. Review the character descriptions and coding guidelines for proper selection. For some procedures, only certain characters will apply.

CCI Edits

Refer to Appendix A for CCI edits.

Facility RVUs ▢

Code	Work	PE Facility	MP	Total Facility
50815	22.26	10.84	2.66	35.76
50820	24.07	11.25	3.00	38.32

Non-facility RVUs ▢

Code	Work	PE Non-Facility	MP	Total Non-Facility
50815	22.26	10.84	2.66	35.76
50820	24.07	11.25	3.00	38.32

Modifiers (PAR) ▢

Code	Mod 50	Mod 51	Mod 62	Mod 66	Mod 80
50815	1	2	1	0	2
50820	1	2	1	0	2

Global Period

Code	Days
50815	090
50820	090

50825

50825 Continent diversion, including intestine anastomosis using any segment of small and/or large intestine (Kock pouch or Camey enterocystoplasty)

AMA Coding Guideline

Repair Procedures on the Ureter

Codes 50705, 50706 are add-on codes describing embolization and balloon dilation of the ureter using non-endoscopic imaging guidance, and each may be reported once per ureter per day. These codes include embolization or dilation plus imaging guidance and radiological supervision and interpretation required to accomplish the embolization or dilation. These procedures may be performed through de novo transrenal access, an existing renal/ureteral access, transurethral access, an ileal conduit, or ureterostomy. The service of gaining access may be reported separately. Diagnostic pyelography/ureterography is not included in 50705 and 50706 and may be reported separately. Other interventions or catheter placements performed at the same setting as the embolization/dilation may be reported separately.

AMA Coding Notes

Surgical Procedures on the Urinary System

(For provision of chemotherapeutic agents, report both the specific service in addition to code(s) for the specific substance(s) or drug(s) provided)

AMA *CPT® Assistant* ▢

50825: Oct 01: 8

Plain English Description

A continent urinary diversion procedure is performed. Continent urinary diversion differs from other urinary diversion procedures in that the patient may void normally through the urethra. Alternatively, a stoma may be created with a valve mechanism using intussuscepted colon that prevents leakage of urine. With this type of stoma, the patient removes urine by periodically catheterizing the pouch. The abdomen in incised in the midline. The small bowel is isolated and packed out of the surgical field. The ureters are exposed, mobilized, and divided distally near the ureterovesical junction. The ureteral stumps are ligated. A segment of small or large intestine is selected and mobilized. The segment, usually 30-35 cm of intestine from which the pouch is to be constructed, is isolated. The intestine is divided, leaving the isolated segment attached to the mesenteric pedicle, keeping the blood supply intact. The remaining distal and proximal portions of the intestine are then anastomosed and bowel continuity is restored. The intestinal pouch is fashioned by arranging the isolated segment in a U or W configuration. The segment is incised longitudinally along the mesenteric border to detubularize it. The intestine is fashioned into a pouch. A tunnel is created from the pouch to the ureters. The ureters are pulled through the tunnel to the pouch. The ends of the ureters are spatulated along the anterior aspect. The ureters are anastomosed to the pouch approximately 3 cm apart. The distal aspect of the pouch may be incised and anastomosed to the bladder neck in females or the proximal urethra in males. Alternatively, a stoma may be created through a separate incision. When a stoma is created, the pouch is configured and detubularized as described above except for the portion of intestine that will be used to form the valve. The remaining tubular segment is scarified using electrocautery and adjacent mesentery is excised. The scarified segment is telescoped (intussuscepted) into the pouch and secured with sutures, creating the valve. The valve component is then sutured to the previously prepared stoma site in the abdominal wall. A catheter is placed through the valve into the stoma. Drains are placed as needed and surgical incisions are closed in layers.

Ureterocolon conduit, ureteroileal conduit

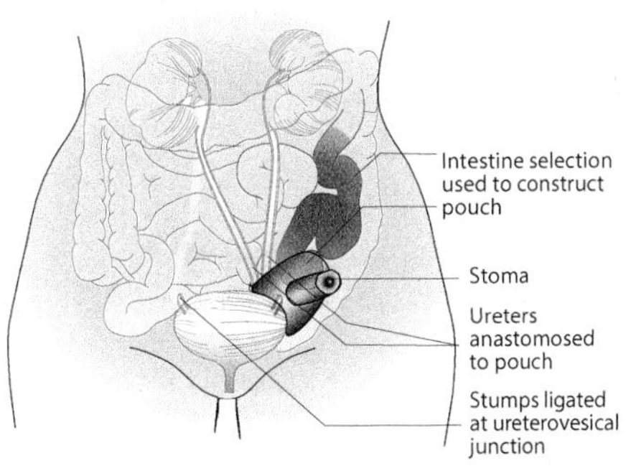

ICD-10-CM Diagnostic Codes

C67.0	Malignant neoplasm of trigone of bladder
C67.1	Malignant neoplasm of dome of bladder
C67.2	Malignant neoplasm of lateral wall of bladder
C67.3	Malignant neoplasm of anterior wall of bladder
C67.4	Malignant neoplasm of posterior wall of bladder
C67.5	Malignant neoplasm of bladder neck
C67.6	Malignant neoplasm of ureteric orifice
C67.7	Malignant neoplasm of urachus
C68.0	Malignant neoplasm of urethra
C79.11	Secondary malignant neoplasm of bladder
D09.0	Carcinoma in situ of bladder
D41.4	Neoplasm of uncertain behavior of bladder
N21.0	Calculus in bladder
N30.40	Irradiation cystitis without hematuria
N30.41	Irradiation cystitis with hematuria
N30.80	Other cystitis without hematuria
N30.81	Other cystitis with hematuria
N31.0	Uninhibited neuropathic bladder, not elsewhere classified
N31.1	Reflex neuropathic bladder, not elsewhere classified
N32.0	Bladder-neck obstruction
N32.3	Diverticulum of bladder
N32.89	Other specified disorders of bladder
N33	Bladder disorders in diseases classified elsewhere
Q64.11	Supravesical fissure of urinary bladder
Q64.12	Cloacal exstrophy of urinary bladder
Q64.19	Other exstrophy of urinary bladder
Q64.31	Congenital bladder neck obstruction
Q64.39	Other atresia and stenosis of urethra and bladder neck
Q64.75	Double urinary meatus
Q64.79	Other congenital malformations of bladder and urethra
❼ S37.22	Contusion of bladder
❼ S37.23	Laceration of bladder
❼ S37.29	Other injury of bladder

ICD-10-CM Coding Notes

For codes requiring a 7th character extension, refer to your ICD-10-CM book. Review the character descriptions and coding guidelines for proper selection. For some procedures, only certain characters will apply.

CCI Edits

Refer to Appendix A for CCI edits.

Facility RVUs ▢

Code	Work	PE Facility	MP	Total Facility
50825	30.68	13.68	3.66	48.02

Non-facility RVUs ▢

Code	Work	PE Non-Facility	MP	Total Non-Facility
50825	30.68	13.68	3.66	48.02

Modifiers (PAR) ▢

Code	Mod 50	Mod 51	Mod 62	Mod 66	Mod 80
50825	0	2	1	0	2

Global Period

Code	Days
50825	090

50830

50830 Urinary undiversion (eg, taking down of ureteroileal conduit, ureterosigmoidostomy or ureteroenterostomy with ureteroureterostomy or ureteroneocystostomy)

AMA Coding Guideline

Repair Procedures on the Ureter

Codes 50705, 50706 are add-on codes describing embolization and balloon dilation of the ureter using non-endoscopic imaging guidance, and each may be reported once per ureter per day. These codes include embolization or dilation plus imaging guidance and radiological supervision and interpretation required to accomplish the embolization or dilation. These procedures may be performed through de novo transrenal access, an existing renal/ureteral access, transurethral access, an ileal conduit, or ureterostomy. The service of gaining access may be reported separately. Diagnostic pyelography/ureterography is not included in 50705 and 50706 and may be reported separately. Other interventions or catheter placements performed at the same setting as the embolization/dilation may be reported separately.

AMA Coding Notes

Surgical Procedures on the Urinary System

(For provision of chemotherapeutic agents, report both the specific service in addition to code(s) for the specific substance(s) or drug(s) provided)

AMA *CPT® Assistant* ▢

50830: Oct 01: 8

Plain English Description

A urinary undiversion or take-down procedure is performed to restore the continuity of the urinary tract. This procedure is performed primarily on patients with previous injury to the ureter or bladder that required temporary diversion, and children with urologic conditions that require temporary diversion until the condition can be surgically corrected or until it resolves. The exact procedure performed depends on the type of urinary diversion and the patient's anatomy. The abdomen is incised in the midline and the peritoneum is opened. The small bowel is isolated and packed out of the surgical field. Adhesions are lysed and the previously reconfigured anatomy is evaluated, including the remaining proximal ureteral segments, ureteral anastomosis sites, any distal ureteral segments, urinary bladder, and the ileal conduit, if present. The proximal ureters are exposed and dissected free of surrounding tissue, taking care to preserve surrounding periureteral tissue and blood supply. If ureterosigmoidostomy or ureteroenterostomy has been performed, the ureters are disconnected from the bowel, stents are removed, and the anastomosis sites in the bowel are repaired. The proximal ureteral segments are then reconnected to the distal ureteral segments, if present, or to the bladder. Reconnecting the ureters may require mobilization of the renal pelvis in order to achieve reimplantation of the ureters in the bladder. Stents are placed in the ureters as needed. If an ileal conduit has been used, the cutaneous connection is severed. The ileal conduit is mobilized, taking care to preserve blood supply. The bladder is incised and a submucosal tunnel is created in the internal bladder wall. The distal aspect of the ileal conduit is passed through the tunnel and anchored to the bladder muscle. The conduit exits the bladder mucosa near the bladder trigone. Stents are placed in the ureters as needed. The cutaneous stoma is closed. Drains are placed and the abdominal incision is closed in layers.

Urinary undiversion

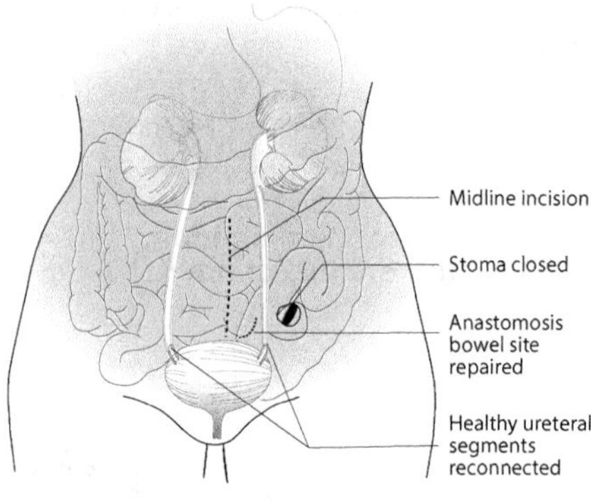

ICD-10-CM Diagnostic Codes

N31.0	Uninhibited neuropathic bladder, not elsewhere classified
N31.1	Reflex neuropathic bladder, not elsewhere classified
N31.2	Flaccid neuropathic bladder, not elsewhere classified
N31.8	Other neuromuscular dysfunction of bladder
Q62.12	Congenital occlusion of ureterovesical orifice
Q62.2	Congenital megaureter
Z43.6	Encounter for attention to other artificial openings of urinary tract
Z85.51	Personal history of malignant neoplasm of bladder

CCI Edits

Refer to Appendix A for CCI edits.

Facility RVUs ▢

Code	Work	PE Facility	MP	Total Facility
50830	33.77	14.72	4.01	52.50

Non-facility RVUs ▢

Code	Work	PE Non-Facility	MP	Total Non-Facility
50830	33.77	14.72	4.01	52.50

Modifiers (PAR) ▢

Code	Mod 50	Mod 51	Mod 62	Mod 66	Mod 80
50830	0	2	1	0	2

Global Period

Code	Days
50830	090

50840

50840 Replacement of all or part of ureter by intestine segment, including intestine anastomosis

(For bilateral procedure, report 50840 with modifier 50)

AMA Coding Guideline

Repair Procedures on the Ureter

Codes 50705, 50706 are add-on codes describing embolization and balloon dilation of the ureter using non-endoscopic imaging guidance, and each may be reported once per ureter per day. These codes include embolization or dilation plus imaging guidance and radiological supervision and interpretation required to accomplish the embolization or dilation. These procedures may be performed through de novo transrenal access, an existing renal/ureteral access, transurethral access, an ileal conduit, or ureterostomy. The service of gaining access may be reported separately. Diagnostic pyelography/ureterography is not included in 50705 and 50706 and may be reported separately. Other interventions or catheter placements performed at the same setting as the embolization/dilation may be reported separately.

AMA Coding Notes

Surgical Procedures on the Urinary System

(For provision of chemotherapeutic agents, report both the specific service in addition to code(s) for the specific substance(s) or drug(s) provided)

AMA *CPT® Assistant*

50840: Oct 01: 8

Plain English Description

A diseased or injured segment of the ureter is excised and any remaining healthy proximal ureteral segment is anastomosed to the intestine as a ureteral replacement. The abdomen is incised in the midline and the peritoneum is opened. The small bowel is isolated and packed out of the surgical field. The ureter is exposed and mobilized. The diseased segment of ureter is excised and the distal ureteral stump is ligated at the ureterovesical junction. A segment of intestine, usually ileum, is selected and mobilized. The length of intestine required for ureteral replacement is determined. The intestine is divided and a segment of the required length is isolated. The intestinal segments proximal and distal to the isolated segment are then anastomosed and bowel continuity is restored. The isolated segment of intestine is prepared for anastomosis to the ureter and bladder. The proximal end of the isolated segment of intestine is closed with sutures. The ureter is spatulated, stented, and anastomosed to the proximal end of the isolated segment of intestine in an end-to-side fashion. The distal end of isolated intestine is anastomosed to the bladder. An incision is made in the bladder wall usually 1-2 cm posterolateral to the native ureteral orifice. A full-thickness segment of bladder wall matching the diameter of the distal segment of intestine is excised. The distal segment of intestine is anastomosed to the bladder. A nephrostomy tube is placed as needed. The surgical wound is closed in layers.

Replacement of all or part of ureter

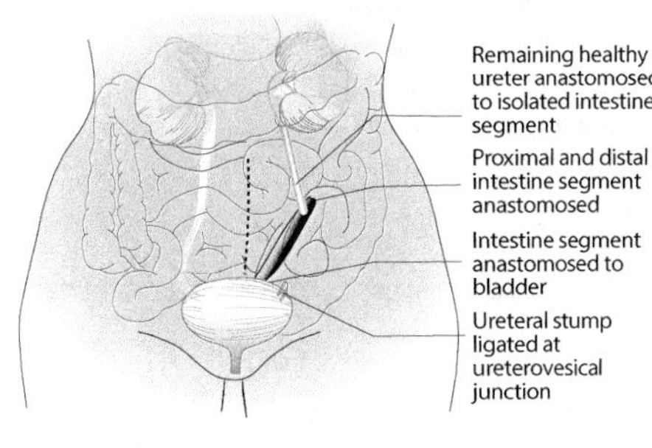

ICD-10-CM Diagnostic Codes

⇄	C66.1	Malignant neoplasm of right ureter
⇄	C66.2	Malignant neoplasm of left ureter
⇄	D41.21	Neoplasm of uncertain behavior of right ureter
⇄	D41.22	Neoplasm of uncertain behavior of left ureter
	G83.4	Cauda equina syndrome
	N11.1	Chronic obstructive pyelonephritis
	N13.5	Crossing vessel and stricture of ureter without hydronephrosis
	N13.8	Other obstructive and reflux uropathy
	N20.1	Calculus of ureter
	N20.2	Calculus of kidney with calculus of ureter
	N99.520	Hemorrhage of incontinent external stoma of urinary tract
	N99.521	Infection of incontinent external stoma of urinary tract
	N99.522	Malfunction of incontinent external stoma of urinary tract
	N99.528	Other complication of incontinent external stoma of urinary tract
	N99.530	Hemorrhage of continent stoma of urinary tract
	N99.531	Infection of continent stoma of urinary tract
	N99.532	Malfunction of continent stoma of urinary tract
	N99.538	Other complication of continent stoma of urinary tract
	N99.81	Other intraoperative complications of genitourinary system
	N99.89	Other postprocedural complications and disorders of genitourinary system
	Q62.11	Congenital occlusion of ureteropelvic junction
	Q62.12	Congenital occlusion of ureterovesical orifice
	Q62.2	Congenital megaureter
❼	S37.12	Contusion of ureter
❼	S37.13	Laceration of ureter
❼	S37.19	Other injury of ureter

ICD-10-CM Coding Notes

For codes requiring a 7th character extension, refer to your ICD-10-CM book. Review the character descriptions and coding guidelines for proper selection. For some procedures, only certain characters will apply.

CCI Edits

Refer to Appendix A for CCI edits.

Facility RVUs

Code	Work	PE Facility	MP	Total Facility
50840	22.39	10.88	2.67	35.94

Non-facility RVUs

Code	Work	PE Non-Facility	MP	Total Non-Facility
50840	22.39	10.88	2.67	35.94

Modifiers (PAR)

Code	Mod 50	Mod 51	Mod 62	Mod 66	Mod 80
50840	1	2	1	0	2

Global Period

Code	Days
50840	090

CPT® Procedural Coding

50845

50845 Cutaneous appendico-vesicostomy

AMA Coding Guideline

Repair Procedures on the Ureter

Codes 50705, 50706 are add-on codes describing embolization and balloon dilation of the ureter using non-endoscopic imaging guidance, and each may be reported once per ureter per day. These codes include embolization or dilation plus imaging guidance and radiological supervision and interpretation required to accomplish the embolization or dilation. These procedures may be performed through de novo transrenal access, an existing renal/ureteral access, transurethral access, an ileal conduit, or ureterostomy. The service of gaining access may be reported separately. Diagnostic pyelography/ureterography is not included in 50705 and 50706 and may be reported separately. Other interventions or catheter placements performed at the same setting as the embolization/dilation may be reported separately.

AMA Coding Notes

Surgical Procedures on the Urinary System

(For provision of chemotherapeutic agents, report both the specific service in addition to code(s) for the specific substance(s) or drug(s) provided)

Plain English Description

Appendico-vesicostomy is performed primarily in children and young adults to treat conditions such as neuropathic bladder due to myelomeningocele, exstrophy-epispadias, cloacal anomalies, prune belly syndrome, and posterior urethral valves. The procedure involves creation of an appendiceal channel, referred to as a Mitrofanoff channel, within the bladder. The appendiceal channel extends from the bladder to the skin. This type of channel is easy to catheterize and durable enough to last a lifetime. The right colon is mobilized beyond the hepatic flexure. The appendix and bladder are mobilized. The appendix is detached from the cecum and the cecum is closed. The terminal aspect of the appendix is incised and dilated as needed to increase the size of the lumen. The bladder is incised. A submucosal bladder tunnel is created. The terminal aspect of the appendix is passed into the bladder, through the submucosal tunnel, spatulated, and sutured to the bladder, making sure that the sutures pass through the detrusor muscle and mucosa at the distal aspect of the bladder tunnel. The appendix is also secured at the proximal aspect where it enters the bladder. The appendiceal channel is catheterized to ensure that a catheter can pass easily into the bladder. A stoma site is selected, usually at the umbilicus or in the right lower quadrant. The skin is incised and underlying soft tissues are dissected to the level of the fascia. The fascia is incised and widened until the opening is large enough to allow passage of the index finger. The appendix is brought through the opening to the skin until the bladder is positioned against the posterior fascial wall. The appendix and bladder are sutured to the fascia. The cecal end of the appendix is spatulated and any redundant appendix is trimmed. The spatulated appendix is then sutured to the skin or subcutaneous tissues at the stoma site. A temporary indwelling catheter is placed until the surgical wounds have healed sufficiently to allow intermittent catheterization through the stoma. Abdominal drains are placed as needed and the abdominal incision is closed in layers.

Cutaneous appendico-vesicostomy

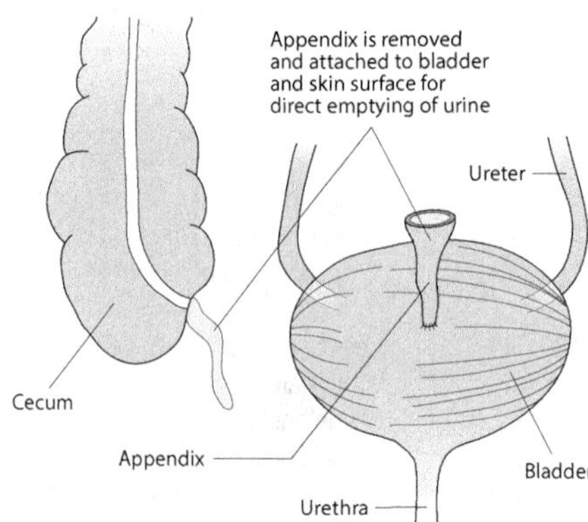

ICD-10-CM Diagnostic Codes

C67.5	Malignant neoplasm of bladder neck
C68.0	Malignant neoplasm of urethra
C68.8	Malignant neoplasm of overlapping sites of urinary organs
D30.3	Benign neoplasm of bladder
D30.4	Benign neoplasm of urethra
D41.3	Neoplasm of uncertain behavior of urethra
G83.4	Cauda equina syndrome
N21.1	Calculus in urethra
N31.0	Uninhibited neuropathic bladder, not elsewhere classified
N31.1	Reflex neuropathic bladder, not elsewhere classified
N31.2	Flaccid neuropathic bladder, not elsewhere classified
N31.8	Other neuromuscular dysfunction of bladder
N31.9	Neuromuscular dysfunction of bladder, unspecified
N32.0	Bladder-neck obstruction
N32.81	Overactive bladder
N34.0	Urethral abscess
N34.1	Nonspecific urethritis
N34.2	Other urethritis
N35.011	Post-traumatic bulbous urethral stricture ♂
N35.012	Post-traumatic membranous urethral stricture ♂
N35.013	Post-traumatic anterior urethral stricture ♂
N35.016	Post-traumatic urethral stricture, male, overlapping sites ♂
N35.021	Urethral stricture due to childbirth ♀
N35.028	Other post-traumatic urethral stricture, female ♀
N35.112	Postinfective bulbous urethral stricture, not elsewhere classified, male ♂
N35.113	Postinfective membranous urethral stricture, not elsewhere classified, male ♂
N35.114	Postinfective anterior urethral stricture, not elsewhere classified, male ♂
N35.116	Postinfective urethral stricture, not elsewhere classified, male, overlapping sites ♂
N35.12	Postinfective urethral stricture, not elsewhere classified, female ♀
N35.812	Other urethral bulbous stricture, male ♂
N35.813	Other membranous urethral stricture, male ♂
N35.814	Other anterior urethral stricture, male ♂
N35.816	Other urethral stricture, male, overlapping sites ♂
N35.82	Other urethral stricture, female ♀
N36.0	Urethral fistula
N36.1	Urethral diverticulum
N36.8	Other specified disorders of urethra
N37	Urethral disorders in diseases classified elsewhere
N99.111	Postprocedural bulbous urethral stricture, male ♂
N99.112	Postprocedural membranous urethral stricture, male ♂
N99.113	Postprocedural anterior bulbous urethral stricture, male ♂
N99.115	Postprocedural fossa navicularis urethral stricture ♂
N99.116	Postprocedural urethral stricture, male, overlapping sites ♂
N99.12	Postprocedural urethral stricture, female ♀
Q05.7	Lumbar spina bifida without hydrocephalus
Q05.8	Sacral spina bifida without hydrocephalus
Q07.00	Arnold-Chiari syndrome without spina bifida or hydrocephalus
Q07.01	Arnold-Chiari syndrome with spina bifida
Q64.0	Epispadias
Q64.2	Congenital posterior urethral valves
Q64.31	Congenital bladder neck obstruction
Q64.32	Congenital stricture of urethra
Q64.33	Congenital stricture of urinary meatus
Q64.71	Congenital prolapse of urethra
Q64.72	Congenital prolapse of urinary meatus
Q79.4	Prune belly syndrome
Q79.51	Congenital hernia of bladder

CCI Edits

Refer to Appendix A for CCI edits.

Facility RVUs

Code	Work	PE Facility	MP	Total Facility
50845	22.46	11.50	2.68	36.64

Non-facility RVUs

Code	Work	PE Non-Facility	MP	Total Non-Facility
50845	22.46	11.50	2.68	36.64

Modifiers (PAR)

Code	Mod 50	Mod 51	Mod 62	Mod 66	Mod 80
50845	0	2	1	0	2

Global Period

Code	Days
50845	090

50860

50860 Ureterostomy, transplantation of ureter to skin

(For bilateral procedure, report 50860 with modifier 50)

AMA Coding Guideline

Repair Procedures on the Ureter

Codes 50705, 50706 are add-on codes describing embolization and balloon dilation of the ureter using non-endoscopic imaging guidance, and each may be reported once per ureter per day. These codes include embolization or dilation plus imaging guidance and radiological supervision and interpretation required to accomplish the embolization or dilation. These procedures may be performed through de novo transrenal access, an existing renal/ureteral access, transurethral access, an ileal conduit, or ureterostomy. The service of gaining access may be reported separately. Diagnostic pyelography/ureterography is not included in 50705 and 50706 and may be reported separately. Other interventions or catheter placements performed at the same setting as the embolization/dilation may be reported separately.

AMA Coding Notes

Surgical Procedures on the Urinary System

(For provision of chemotherapeutic agents, report both the specific service in addition to code(s) for the specific substance(s) or drug(s) provided)

Plain English Description

A cutaneous ureterostomy is performed. A lateral incision is made in the abdomen, overlying muscle is divided, and the peritoneum is retracted to expose the ureter, which is divided as close to the ureterovesical junction (UVJ) as possible. The distal stump of the ureter is ligated. The proximal ureter is then dissected free of surrounding tissue and brought up into the surgical wound. A catheter is passed through the ureter into the renal pelvis to drain the kidney. The catheter may be left in place and sutured to the abdominal wall. Alternatively, an artificial opening, or stoma, may be created on the surface of the abdomen with the ureter sutured to the stoma to divert the passage of urine from the bladder out through the abdomen. A drain is inserted into the abdominal wound and the wound is closed around the drain.

Ureterostomy, transplantation of ureter to skin

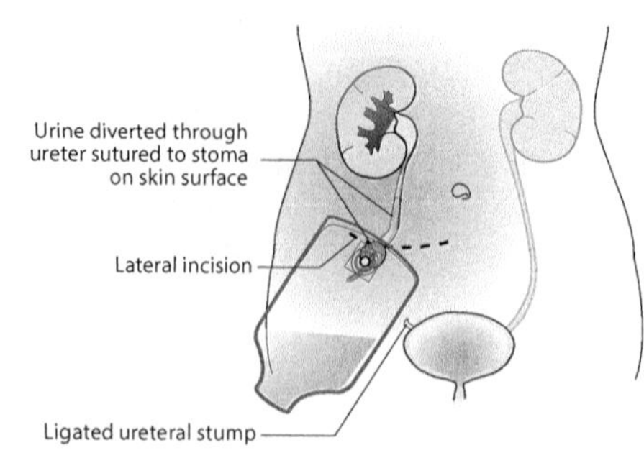

ICD-10-CM Diagnostic Codes

C67.0	Malignant neoplasm of trigone of bladder
C67.1	Malignant neoplasm of dome of bladder
C67.2	Malignant neoplasm of lateral wall of bladder
C67.3	Malignant neoplasm of anterior wall of bladder
C67.4	Malignant neoplasm of posterior wall of bladder
C67.5	Malignant neoplasm of bladder neck
C67.6	Malignant neoplasm of ureteric orifice
C67.7	Malignant neoplasm of urachus
C67.8	Malignant neoplasm of overlapping sites of bladder
C68.0	Malignant neoplasm of urethra
C79.11	Secondary malignant neoplasm of bladder
D09.0	Carcinoma in situ of bladder
D41.4	Neoplasm of uncertain behavior of bladder
G83.4	Cauda equina syndrome
N11.1	Chronic obstructive pyelonephritis
N13.8	Other obstructive and reflux uropathy
N20.1	Calculus of ureter
N21.0	Calculus in bladder
N30.40	Irradiation cystitis without hematuria
N30.41	Irradiation cystitis with hematuria
N30.80	Other cystitis without hematuria
N30.81	Other cystitis with hematuria
N31.0	Uninhibited neuropathic bladder, not elsewhere classified
N31.1	Reflex neuropathic bladder, not elsewhere classified
N31.2	Flaccid neuropathic bladder, not elsewhere classified
N31.8	Other neuromuscular dysfunction of bladder
N32.0	Bladder-neck obstruction
N32.3	Diverticulum of bladder
N32.89	Other specified disorders of bladder
N33	Bladder disorders in diseases classified elsewhere
Q62.0	Congenital hydronephrosis
Q62.11	Congenital occlusion of ureteropelvic junction
Q62.12	Congenital occlusion of ureterovesical orifice
Q62.2	Congenital megaureter
Q62.39	Other obstructive defects of renal pelvis and ureter
Q64.11	Supravesical fissure of urinary bladder
Q64.12	Cloacal exstrophy of urinary bladder
Q64.2	Congenital posterior urethral valves
Q64.31	Congenital bladder neck obstruction
Q64.32	Congenital stricture of urethra
Q64.33	Congenital stricture of urinary meatus
Q64.39	Other atresia and stenosis of urethra and bladder neck
Q64.5	Congenital absence of bladder and urethra
Q64.6	Congenital diverticulum of bladder
Q64.79	Other congenital malformations of bladder and urethra
➐ S37.22	Contusion of bladder
➐ S37.23	Laceration of bladder
➐ S37.29	Other injury of bladder
➐ S37.32	Contusion of urethra
➐ S37.33	Laceration of urethra
➐ S37.39	Other injury of urethra

ICD-10-CM Coding Notes

For codes requiring a 7th character extension, refer to your ICD-10-CM book. Review the character descriptions and coding guidelines for proper selection. For some procedures, only certain characters will apply.

CCI Edits

Refer to Appendix A for CCI edits.

Facility RVUs ▢

Code	Work	PE Facility	MP	Total Facility
50860	17.08	8.51	2.03	27.62

Non-facility RVUs ▢

Code	Work	PE Non-Facility	MP	Total Non-Facility
50860	17.08	8.51	2.03	27.62

Modifiers (PAR) ▢

Code	Mod 50	Mod 51	Mod 62	Mod 66	Mod 80
50860	1	2	1	0	2

Global Period

Code	Days
50860	090

● New ▲ Revised ✚ Add On ⊘Modifier 51 Exempt ★Telemedicine ▢ CPT QuickRef ⁄FDA Pending ⇄ Laterality ➐ Seventh Character ♂Male ♀Female

50900

50900 Ureterorrhaphy, suture of ureter (separate procedure)

AMA Coding Guideline

Repair Procedures on the Ureter

Codes 50705, 50706 are add-on codes describing embolization and balloon dilation of the ureter using non-endoscopic imaging guidance, and each may be reported once per ureter per day. These codes include embolization or dilation plus imaging guidance and radiological supervision and interpretation required to accomplish the embolization or dilation. These procedures may be performed through de novo transrenal access, an existing renal/ureteral access, transurethral access, an ileal conduit, or ureterostomy. The service of gaining access may be reported separately. Diagnostic pyelography/ureterography is not included in 50705 and 50706 and may be reported separately. Other interventions or catheter placements performed at the same setting as the embolization/dilation may be reported separately.

AMA Coding Notes

Surgical Procedures on the Urinary System

(For provision of chemotherapeutic agents, report both the specific service in addition to code(s) for the specific substance(s) or drug(s) provided)

Plain English Description

Suture repair of a ureter is performed in a separate procedure. The damaged ureter is exposed. The injury is located, inspected, and determined to be minor and suitable for suture repair alone. The edges of the ureteral laceration are approximated and fine sutures are placed. Drains are placed as needed and the surgical wound is closed in layers.

Ureterorrhaphy, suture of ureter (separate procedure)

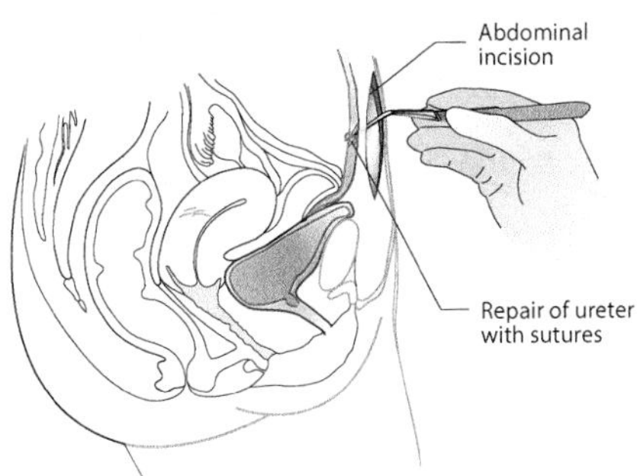

ICD-10-CM Diagnostic Codes

❼	S37.12	Contusion of ureter
❼	S37.13	Laceration of ureter
❼	S37.19	Other injury of ureter

ICD-10-CM Coding Notes

For codes requiring a 7th character extension, refer to your ICD-10-CM book. Review the character descriptions and coding guidelines for proper selection. For some procedures, only certain characters will apply.

CCI Edits

Refer to Appendix A for CCI edits.

Facility RVUs ☐

Code	Work	PE Facility	MP	Total Facility
50900	15.04	7.82	1.80	24.66

Non-facility RVUs ☐

Code	Work	PE Non-Facility	MP	Total Non-Facility
50900	15.04	7.82	1.80	24.66

Modifiers (PAR) ☐

Code	Mod 50	Mod 51	Mod 62	Mod 66	Mod 80
50900	1	2	1	0	2

Global Period

Code	Days
50900	090

50920-50930

50920 Closure of ureterocutaneous fistula

50930 Closure of ureterovisceral fistula (including visceral repair)

AMA Coding Guideline

Repair Procedures on the Ureter

Codes 50705, 50706 are add-on codes describing embolization and balloon dilation of the ureter using non-endoscopic imaging guidance, and each may be reported once per ureter per day. These codes include embolization or dilation plus imaging guidance and radiological supervision and interpretation required to accomplish the embolization or dilation. These procedures may be performed through de novo transrenal access, an existing renal/ureteral access, transurethral access, an ileal conduit, or ureterostomy. The service of gaining access may be reported separately. Diagnostic pyelography/ureterography is not included in 50705 and 50706 and may be reported separately. Other interventions or catheter placements performed at the same setting as the embolization/dilation may be reported separately.

AMA Coding Notes

Surgical Procedures on the Urinary System

(For provision of chemotherapeutic agents, report both the specific service in addition to code(s) for the specific substance(s) or drug(s) provided)

Plain English Description

A urethrocutaneous fistula is an abnormal communication between a ureter and the skin while a ureterovisceral fistula is an abnormal communication between a ureter and a hollow multilayered walled organ. The ureter is exposed and the abnormal communication is located. The fistula tract is followed from the ureter to the skin or the visceral organ and excised. The fistulous opening in the ureter is debrided as needed and closed with sutures. In 50920, the skin and subcutaneous tissues in the skin are also debrided and closed with sutures. In 50930, the opening in the visceral organ is debrided and closed with sutures or repaired by another technique. The operative wound is closed in layers.

Closure of ureterocutaneous/ ureterovisceral fistula

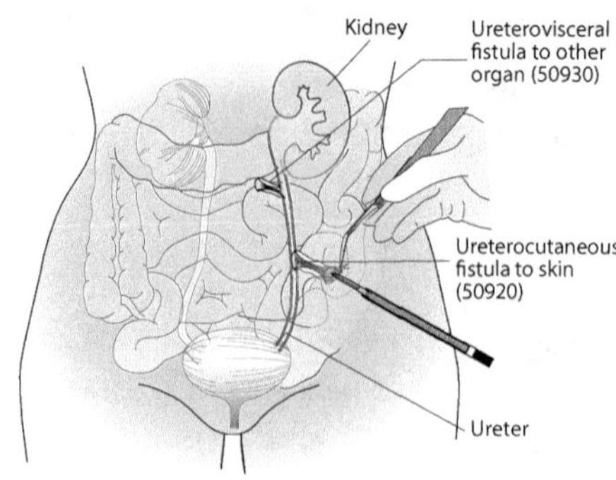

ICD-10-CM Diagnostic Codes

N28.89 Other specified disorders of kidney and ureter

CCI Edits

Refer to Appendix A for CCI edits.

Facility RVUs ▢

Code	Work	PE Facility	MP	Total Facility
50920	15.81	8.08	1.87	25.76
50930	20.19	9.55	2.39	32.13

Non-facility RVUs ▢

Code	Work	PE Non-Facility	MP	Total Non-Facility
50920	15.81	8.08	1.87	25.76
50930	20.19	9.55	2.39	32.13

Modifiers (PAR) ▢

Code	Mod 50	Mod 51	Mod 62	Mod 66	Mod 80
50920	0	2	1	0	2
50930	0	2	1	0	2

Global Period

Code	Days
50920	090
50930	090

50940

50940 Deligation of ureter

(For ureteroplasty, ureterolysis, see 50700-50860)

AMA Coding Guideline

Repair Procedures on the Ureter

Codes 50705, 50706 are add-on codes describing embolization and balloon dilation of the ureter using non-endoscopic imaging guidance, and each may be reported once per ureter per day. These codes include embolization or dilation plus imaging guidance and radiological supervision and interpretation required to accomplish the embolization or dilation. These procedures may be performed through de novo transrenal access, an existing renal/ureteral access, transurethral access, an ileal conduit, or ureterostomy. The service of gaining access may be reported separately. Diagnostic pyelography/ureterography is not included in 50705 and 50706 and may be reported separately. Other interventions or catheter placements performed at the same setting as the embolization/dilation may be reported separately.

AMA Coding Notes

Surgical Procedures on the Urinary System

(For provision of chemotherapeutic agents, report both the specific service in addition to code(s) for the specific substance(s) or drug(s) provided)

Plain English Description

The physician performs deligation of the ureter. Deligation is performed to remove a ligature from a ureter that has been unintentionally tied off during an abdominal or retroperitoneal procedure. This can happen when blood vessels around the ureter are ligated and the ureter is inadvertently caught in the ligature. Inadvertent ligation of the ureter causes complete or partial obstruction. The ureter is exposed by a retroperitoneal or transperitoneal approach. The health of the ureter is evaluated to determine whether blood supply to the ureter is intact. If the ureter is healthy, the ligature is removed to relieve the obstruction.

Deligation of ureter

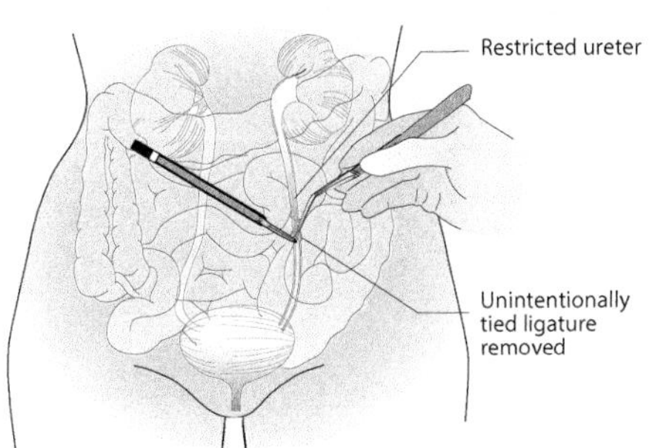

ICD-10-CM Diagnostic Codes

Y65.2	Failure in suture or ligature during surgical operation
Z48.02	Encounter for removal of sutures
Z48.89	Encounter for other specified surgical aftercare

CCI Edits

Refer to Appendix A for CCI edits.

Facility RVUs

Code	Work	PE Facility	MP	Total Facility
50940	15.93	8.12	1.90	25.95

Non-facility RVUs

Code	Work	PE Non-Facility	MP	Total Non-Facility
50940	15.93	8.12	1.90	25.95

Modifiers (PAR)

Code	Mod 50	Mod 51	Mod 62	Mod 66	Mod 80
50940	1	2	1	0	2

Global Period

Code	Days
50940	090

50945

50945 Laparoscopy, surgical; ureterolithotomy

AMA Coding Guideline

Laparoscopic Procedures on the Ureter

Surgical laparoscopy always includes diagnostic laparoscopy. To report a diagnostic laparoscopy (peritoneoscopy) (separate procedure), use 49320.

AMA Coding Notes

Surgical Procedures on the Urinary System

(For provision of chemotherapeutic agents, report both the specific service in addition to code(s) for the specific substance(s) or drug(s) provided)

AMA *CPT® Assistant* ▯

50945: Nov 99: 26, May 00: 4, Oct 01: 8, Sep 06: 13

Plain English Description

Ureterolithotomy is performed to remove a ureteral stone (calculus) from the ureter. The laparoscopic procedure can be performed using a retroperitoneal or transperitoneal approach. Using a retroperitoneal approach, the laparoscope is introduced either through an incision below the tip of the 12th rib if the ureteral stone is in the upper ureter or through an incision medial to the anterosuperior iliac spine if the stone is in the lower ureter. Muscles are split and the peritoneum separated from the abdominal wall with blunt dissection. Additional portal incisions are made for the introduction of surgical instruments. The ureter is identified and the stone, which is seen as a bulge in the ureter, located. Forceps are used to grasp the ureter at the site of the stone to prevent it from moving. The ureter is dissected and incised. The stone is extracted from the ureter using forceps and carefully removed through one of the portal incisions. A double J stent may be placed if needed through the ureteral incision. The ureter is repaired, the laparoscopic and surgical instruments removed, and the abdomen closed.

Laparoscopy, surgical; ureterolithotomy

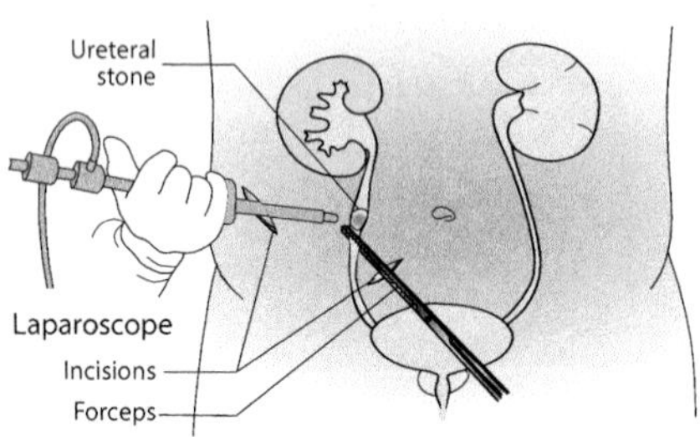

ICD-10-CM Diagnostic Codes

N20.1	Calculus of ureter
N20.2	Calculus of kidney with calculus of ureter

CCI Edits

Refer to Appendix A for CCI edits.

Facility RVUs ▯

Code	Work	PE Facility	MP	Total Facility
50945	17.97	8.22	2.17	28.36

Non-facility RVUs ▯

Code	Work	PE Non-Facility	MP	Total Non-Facility
50945	17.97	8.22	2.17	28.36

Modifiers (PAR) ▯

Code	Mod 50	Mod 51	Mod 62	Mod 66	Mod 80
50945	1	2	1	0	2

Global Period

Code	Days
50945	090

50947-50948

50947 Laparoscopy, surgical; ureteroneocystostomy with cystoscopy and ureteral stent placement

50948 Laparoscopy, surgical; ureteroneocystostomy without cystoscopy and ureteral stent placement

(For open ureteroneocystostomy, see 50780-50785)

AMA Coding Guideline

Laparoscopic Procedures on the Ureter

Surgical laparoscopy always includes diagnostic laparoscopy. To report a diagnostic laparoscopy (peritoneoscopy) (separate procedure), use 49320.

AMA Coding Notes

Surgical Procedures on the Urinary System

(For provision of chemotherapeutic agents, report both the specific service in addition to code(s) for the specific substance(s) or drug(s) provided)

AMA *CPT® Assistant* ▢

50947: Oct 01: 8

50948: Oct 01: 8

Plain English Description

Ureteroneocystostomy is performed by laparoscopic approach. In 50948, a small incision is made inferior to the umbilicus. A trocar is placed into the peritoneal cavity; the laparoscope is introduced through the trocar; and the abdomen is insufflated. Several additional portal incisions are made for the introduction of surgical instruments. Dissection is then performed under laparoscopic control to mobilize the ureter, beginning proximal to the broad ligament and carried down to the ureterovesical junction. An incision is made in the muscular wall of the bladder (detrusor muscle) to create a trough at the planned ureteral transplant site along the lateral aspect of the bladder. An incision is made in the bladder and the ureter is inserted into the detrusor trough. The ureter is anastomosed to the detrusor edges and the trough is closed around the ureter. In 50947, ureteroneocystostomy is performed as described above followed by cystoscopy and ureteral stent placement. A cystoscope is inserted through the urethra and into the urinary bladder. The opening in the ureter is identified. A guidewire is advanced into the ureter and a stent is then advanced over the guidewire and positioned in the ureter under laparoscopic visualization. Following completion of the procedure, a urethral catheter is placed; the cystoscope and laparoscope are removed; and the abdominal incisions are closed.

Laparoscopy, surgical; ureteroneocystostomy

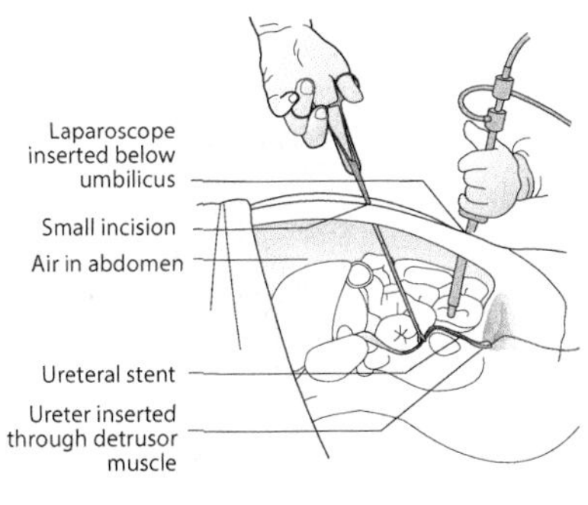

With cystoscopy and ureteral stent placement (50947); without cystoscopy and ureteral stent placement (50948)

ICD-10-CM Diagnostic Codes

⇄	C66.1	Malignant neoplasm of right ureter
⇄	C66.2	Malignant neoplasm of left ureter
	C79.19	Secondary malignant neoplasm of other urinary organs
⇄	D30.21	Benign neoplasm of right ureter
⇄	D30.22	Benign neoplasm of left ureter
⇄	D41.11	Neoplasm of uncertain behavior of right renal pelvis
⇄	D41.12	Neoplasm of uncertain behavior of left renal pelvis
⇄	D41.21	Neoplasm of uncertain behavior of right ureter
⇄	D41.22	Neoplasm of uncertain behavior of left ureter
	D41.8	Neoplasm of uncertain behavior of other specified urinary organs
	D47.Z1	Post-transplant lymphoproliferative disorder (PTLD)
	N11.1	Chronic obstructive pyelonephritis
	N13.5	Crossing vessel and stricture of ureter without hydronephrosis
	N13.71	Vesicoureteral-reflux without reflux nephropathy
	N13.721	Vesicoureteral-reflux with reflux nephropathy without hydroureter, unilateral
	N13.722	Vesicoureteral-reflux with reflux nephropathy without hydroureter, bilateral
	N13.732	Vesicoureteral-reflux with reflux nephropathy with hydroureter, bilateral
	N13.8	Other obstructive and reflux uropathy
	Q62.0	Congenital hydronephrosis
	Q62.11	Congenital occlusion of ureteropelvic junction
	Q62.12	Congenital occlusion of ureterovesical orifice
	Q62.2	Congenital megaureter
	Q62.31	Congenital ureterocele, orthotopic
	Q62.32	Cecoureterocele
	Q62.39	Other obstructive defects of renal pelvis and ureter
	Q62.61	Deviation of ureter
	Q62.62	Displacement of ureter
	Q62.63	Anomalous implantation of ureter
	Q62.69	Other malposition of ureter
	Q62.7	Congenital vesico-uretero-renal reflux
	Q62.8	Other congenital malformations of ureter
	Q64.8	Other specified congenital malformations of urinary system
❼	S37.12	Contusion of ureter
❼	S37.13	Laceration of ureter
❼	S37.19	Other injury of ureter
	T86.11	Kidney transplant rejection
	T86.12	Kidney transplant failure
	T86.13	Kidney transplant infection
	T86.19	Other complication of kidney transplant

ICD-10-CM Coding Notes

For codes requiring a 7th character extension, refer to your ICD-10-CM book. Review the character descriptions and coding guidelines for proper selection. For some procedures, only certain characters will apply.

CCI Edits

Refer to Appendix A for CCI edits.

Facility RVUs ▢

Code	Work	PE Facility	MP	Total Facility
50947	25.78	11.50	3.13	40.41
50948	23.82	10.44	2.94	37.20

Non-facility RVUs ▢

Code	Work	PE Non-Facility	MP	Total Non-Facility
50947	25.78	11.50	3.13	40.41
50948	23.82	10.44	2.94	37.20

Modifiers (PAR) ▢

Code	Mod 50	Mod 51	Mod 62	Mod 66	Mod 80
50947	1	2	1	0	2
50948	1	2	1	0	2

Global Period

Code	Days
50947	090
50948	090

CPT® Procedural Coding

50951-50953

50951 Ureteral endoscopy through established ureterostomy, with or without irrigation, instillation, or ureteropyelography, exclusive of radiologic service

50953 Ureteral endoscopy through established ureterostomy, with or without irrigation, instillation, or ureteropyelography, exclusive of radiologic service; with ureteral catheterization, with or without dilation of ureter

(For image-guided dilation of ureter without endoscopic guidance, use 50706)

AMA Coding Notes

Surgical Procedures on the Urinary System

(For provision of chemotherapeutic agents, report both the specific service in addition to code(s) for the specific substance(s) or drug(s) provided)

AMA *CPT® Assistant* ▯

50951: Oct 01: 8

50953: Oct 01: 8

Plain English Description

Ureteral endoscopy is performed through an existing ureteral stoma or ureteral catheter exiting the skin. The ureteroscope is introduced through the ureterostomy. In 50951, the ureter is inspected and any obstruction, stenosis, stricture, or other abnormal condition is noted. The ureter may be irrigated with normal saline or diagnostic or therapeutic solution may be instilled. Contrast material may be injected and separately reportable ureteropyelography performed. In 50953, following visual examination, a ureteral catheter is advanced through the ureteroscope. If stenosis is present, a balloon-tipped catheter is introduced to the site of the stenosis and inflated. This balloon may be deflated and inflated several times until the stenotic region is adequately dilated. The ureter may be irrigated with normal saline or diagnostic or therapeutic solution may be instilled. Contrast material may be injected and separately reportable ureteropyelography performed. All instruments are then removed.

Ureteral endoscopy through established ureterostomy

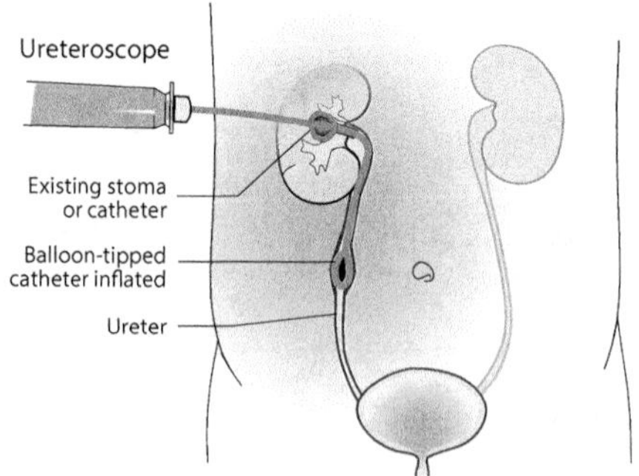

Without ureteral catheterization (50951); with ureteral catheterization, with or without dilation of ureter (50953)

ICD-10-CM Diagnostic Codes

⇄	C64.1	Malignant neoplasm of right kidney, except renal pelvis
⇄	C64.2	Malignant neoplasm of left kidney, except renal pelvis
⇄	C65.1	Malignant neoplasm of right renal pelvis
⇄	C65.2	Malignant neoplasm of left renal pelvis
⇄	C66.1	Malignant neoplasm of right ureter
⇄	C66.2	Malignant neoplasm of left ureter
	C67.6	Malignant neoplasm of ureteric orifice
⇄	C79.01	Secondary malignant neoplasm of right kidney and renal pelvis
⇄	C79.02	Secondary malignant neoplasm of left kidney and renal pelvis
	C79.11	Secondary malignant neoplasm of bladder
	C79.19	Secondary malignant neoplasm of other urinary organs
	C7A.093	Malignant carcinoid tumor of the kidney
	C80.2	Malignant neoplasm associated with transplanted organ
	D09.0	Carcinoma in situ of bladder
	D09.19	Carcinoma in situ of other urinary organs
⇄	D30.01	Benign neoplasm of right kidney
⇄	D30.11	Benign neoplasm of right renal pelvis
⇄	D30.12	Benign neoplasm of left renal pelvis
⇄	D30.21	Benign neoplasm of right ureter
⇄	D30.22	Benign neoplasm of left ureter
	D3A.093	Benign carcinoid tumor of the kidney
⇄	D41.01	Neoplasm of uncertain behavior of right kidney
⇄	D41.02	Neoplasm of uncertain behavior of left kidney
⇄	D41.11	Neoplasm of uncertain behavior of right renal pelvis
⇄	D41.12	Neoplasm of uncertain behavior of left renal pelvis
⇄	D41.21	Neoplasm of uncertain behavior of right ureter
⇄	D41.22	Neoplasm of uncertain behavior of left ureter
	D41.4	Neoplasm of uncertain behavior of bladder
	N11.1	Chronic obstructive pyelonephritis
	N13.1	Hydronephrosis with ureteral stricture, not elsewhere classified
	N13.2	Hydronephrosis with renal and ureteral calculous obstruction
	N13.39	Other hydronephrosis
	N13.4	Hydroureter
	N13.5	Crossing vessel and stricture of ureter without hydronephrosis
	N13.8	Other obstructive and reflux uropathy
	N15.1	Renal and perinephric abscess
	N20.0	Calculus of kidney
	N20.1	Calculus of ureter
	N20.2	Calculus of kidney with calculus of ureter
	N22	Calculus of urinary tract in diseases classified elsewhere
	N25.81	Secondary hyperparathyroidism of renal origin
	N28.0	Ischemia and infarction of kidney
	N28.1	Cyst of kidney, acquired
	N28.81	Hypertrophy of kidney
	N28.82	Megaloureter
	N28.83	Nephroptosis
	N28.89	Other specified disorders of kidney and ureter
	N29	Other disorders of kidney and ureter in diseases classified elsewhere
	Q61.01	Congenital single renal cyst
	Q61.02	Congenital multiple renal cysts
	Q61.19	Other polycystic kidney, infantile type
	Q61.2	Polycystic kidney, adult type
	Q61.4	Renal dysplasia
	Q61.5	Medullary cystic kidney
	Q61.8	Other cystic kidney diseases
	Q62.0	Congenital hydronephrosis
	Q62.11	Congenital occlusion of ureteropelvic junction
	Q62.12	Congenital occlusion of ureterovesical orifice
	Q62.2	Congenital megaureter
	Q62.31	Congenital ureterocele, orthotopic
	Q62.32	Cecoureterocele
	Q62.39	Other obstructive defects of renal pelvis and ureter

CCI Edits

Refer to Appendix A for CCI edits.

Pub 100

50953: Pub 100-03, 1, 230.1, Pub 100-04, 20, 130.1

Facility RVUs

Code	Work	PE Facility	MP	Total Facility
50951	5.83	2.37	0.68	8.88
50953	6.23	2.49	0.73	9.45

Non-facility RVUs

Code	Work	PE Non-Facility	MP	Total Non-Facility
50951	5.83	4.60	0.68	11.11
50953	6.23	4.79	0.73	11.75

Modifiers (PAR)

Code	Mod 50	Mod 51	Mod 62	Mod 66	Mod 80
50951	1	2	0	0	0
50953	1	3	0	0	0

Global Period

Code	Days
50951	000
50953	000

50955-50961

50955 Ureteral endoscopy through established ureterostomy, with or without irrigation, instillation, or ureteropyelography, exclusive of radiologic service; with biopsy

(For image-guided biopsy of ureter and/or renal pelvis without endoscopic guidance, use 50606)

50957 Ureteral endoscopy through established ureterostomy, with or without irrigation, instillation, or ureteropyelography, exclusive of radiologic service; with fulguration and/or incision, with or without biopsy

50961 Ureteral endoscopy through established ureterostomy, with or without irrigation, instillation, or ureteropyelography, exclusive of radiologic service; with removal of foreign body or calculus

AMA Coding Notes

Surgical Procedures on the Urinary System

(For provision of chemotherapeutic agents, report both the specific service in addition to code(s) for the specific substance(s) or drug(s) provided)

AMA *CPT® Assistant*

50955: Oct 01: 8
50957: Oct 01: 8
50961: Oct 01: 8, Mar 07: 10, Apr 07: 12

Plain English Description

Ureteral endoscopy is performed through an existing ureteral stoma or ureteral catheter exiting the skin. The ureteroscope is introduced through the ureterostomy. The ureter is inspected for abnormal tissue, foreign body, or calculus. The ureter may be irrigated with normal saline or diagnostic or therapeutic solution may be instilled. Contrast material may be injected and separately reportable ureteropyelography performed. In 50955, a biopsy is performed. Biopsy forceps are inserted through the ureteroscope and one or more tissue samples are obtained. In 50957, fulguration and/or incision of abnormal tissue is performed. A biopsy may be performed prior to the fulguration procedure as described above. To destroy abnormal tissue, an electrocautery device is advanced through the ureteroscope to the site of the lesion. The device is activated and the abnormal tissue is destroyed. Alternatively, a laser or cryoprobe may be used to destroy the abnormal tissue. The physician may introduce a blade and incise the abnormal tissue instead of, or in addition to, the fulguration procedure. In 50961, the ureter is inspected and a foreign body, such as a stent or calculus, is located. A grasping device or basket is advanced through the working channel of the ureteroscope and the foreign body or calculus is captured and removed. The ureter is re-inspected to ensure that there has not been any injury to the ureter during the procedure.

Ureteral endoscopy through established ureterostomy

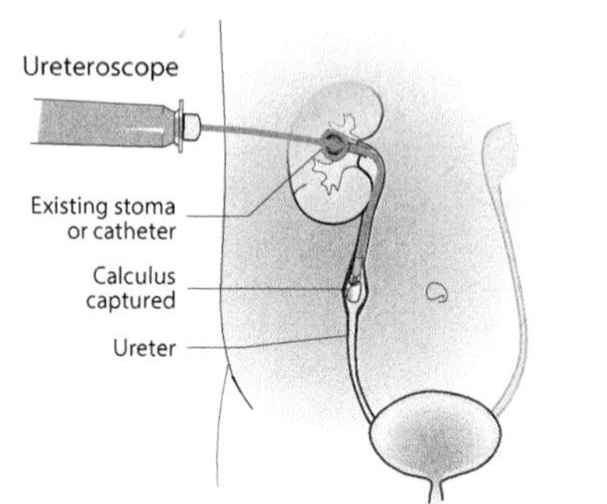

With biopsy (50955); with fulguration and/or incision, with or without biopsy (50957); with removal of foreign body or calculus (50961)

ICD-10-CM Diagnostic Codes

⇄	C64.1	Malignant neoplasm of right kidney, except renal pelvis
⇄	C64.2	Malignant neoplasm of left kidney, except renal pelvis
⇄	C65.1	Malignant neoplasm of right renal pelvis
⇄	C65.2	Malignant neoplasm of left renal pelvis
⇄	C66.1	Malignant neoplasm of right ureter
⇄	C66.2	Malignant neoplasm of left ureter
	C67.6	Malignant neoplasm of ureteric orifice
⇄	C79.01	Secondary malignant neoplasm of right kidney and renal pelvis
⇄	C79.02	Secondary malignant neoplasm of left kidney and renal pelvis
	C79.11	Secondary malignant neoplasm of bladder
	C79.19	Secondary malignant neoplasm of other urinary organs
	C7A.093	Malignant carcinoid tumor of the kidney
	C80.2	Malignant neoplasm associated with transplanted organ
	D09.0	Carcinoma in situ of bladder
	D09.19	Carcinoma in situ of other urinary organs
⇄	D30.01	Benign neoplasm of right kidney
⇄	D30.02	Benign neoplasm of left kidney
⇄	D30.11	Benign neoplasm of right renal pelvis
⇄	D30.12	Benign neoplasm of left renal pelvis
⇄	D30.21	Benign neoplasm of right ureter
⇄	D30.22	Benign neoplasm of left ureter
	D3A.093	Benign carcinoid tumor of the kidney
⇄	D41.01	Neoplasm of uncertain behavior of right kidney
⇄	D41.02	Neoplasm of uncertain behavior of left kidney
⇄	D41.11	Neoplasm of uncertain behavior of right renal pelvis
⇄	D41.12	Neoplasm of uncertain behavior of left renal pelvis
⇄	D41.21	Neoplasm of uncertain behavior of right ureter
⇄	D41.22	Neoplasm of uncertain behavior of left ureter
	D41.4	Neoplasm of uncertain behavior of bladder
	N11.1	Chronic obstructive pyelonephritis
	N13.1	Hydronephrosis with ureteral stricture, not elsewhere classified
	N13.2	Hydronephrosis with renal and ureteral calculous obstruction
	N13.39	Other hydronephrosis
	N13.4	Hydroureter
	N13.5	Crossing vessel and stricture of ureter without hydronephrosis
	N13.8	Other obstructive and reflux uropathy
	N15.1	Renal and perinephric abscess
	N20.2	Calculus of kidney with calculus of ureter
	N22	Calculus of urinary tract in diseases classified elsewhere
	N25.81	Secondary hyperparathyroidism of renal origin
	N28.0	Ischemia and infarction of kidney
	N28.1	Cyst of kidney, acquired
	N28.81	Hypertrophy of kidney
	N28.82	Megaloureter
	N28.83	Nephroptosis
	N28.89	Other specified disorders of kidney and ureter
	N29	Other disorders of kidney and ureter in diseases classified elsewhere
	Q61.01	Congenital single renal cyst
	Q61.02	Congenital multiple renal cysts
	Q61.19	Other polycystic kidney, infantile type
	Q61.2	Polycystic kidney, adult type
	Q61.4	Renal dysplasia
	Q61.5	Medullary cystic kidney
	Q61.8	Other cystic kidney diseases
	Q62.0	Congenital hydronephrosis
	Q62.11	Congenital occlusion of ureteropelvic junction
	Q62.12	Congenital occlusion of ureterovesical orifice
	Q62.2	Congenital megaureter
	Q62.31	Congenital ureterocele, orthotopic
	Q62.32	Cecoureterocele
	Q62.39	Other obstructive defects of renal pelvis and ureter
❼	T19.8	Foreign body in other parts of genitourinary tract
❼	T81.510	Adhesions due to foreign body accidentally left in body following surgical operation
❼	T81.512	Adhesions due to foreign body accidentally left in body following kidney dialysis
❼	T81.514	Adhesions due to foreign body accidentally left in body following endoscopic examination
❼	T81.516	Adhesions due to foreign body accidentally left in body following aspiration, puncture or other catheterization

➐	T81.517	Adhesions due to foreign body accidentally left in body following removal of catheter or packing
➐	T81.518	Adhesions due to foreign body accidentally left in body following other procedure
➐	T81.520	Obstruction due to foreign body accidentally left in body following surgical operation
➐	T81.522	Obstruction due to foreign body accidentally left in body following kidney dialysis
➐	T81.524	Obstruction due to foreign body accidentally left in body following endoscopic examination
➐	T81.526	Obstruction due to foreign body accidentally left in body following aspiration, puncture or other catheterization
➐	T81.527	Obstruction due to foreign body accidentally left in body following removal of catheter or packing
➐	T81.528	Obstruction due to foreign body accidentally left in body following other procedure
➐	T81.530	Perforation due to foreign body accidentally left in body following surgical operation
➐	T81.534	Perforation due to foreign body accidentally left in body following endoscopic examination
➐	T81.536	Perforation due to foreign body accidentally left in body following aspiration, puncture or other catheterization
➐	T81.537	Perforation due to foreign body accidentally left in body following removal of catheter or packing
➐	T81.538	Perforation due to foreign body accidentally left in body following other procedure
➐	T81.590	Other complications of foreign body accidentally left in body following surgical operation
➐	T81.592	Other complications of foreign body accidentally left in body following kidney dialysis
➐	T81.594	Other complications of foreign body accidentally left in body following endoscopic examination
➐	T81.598	Other complications of foreign body accidentally left in body following other procedure

ICD-10-CM Coding Notes

For codes requiring a 7th character extension, refer to your ICD-10-CM book. Review the character descriptions and coding guidelines for proper selection. For some procedures, only certain characters will apply.

CCI Edits

Refer to Appendix A for CCI edits.

Pub 100

50955: Pub 100-03, 1, 230.1, Pub 100-04, 20, 130.1

50957: Pub 100-03, 1, 230.1, Pub 100-04, 20, 130.1

50961: Pub 100-03, 1, 230.1, Pub 100-04, 20, 130.1

Facility RVUs ☐

Code	Work	PE Facility	MP	Total Facility
50955	6.74	2.66	0.79	10.19
50957	6.78	2.68	0.79	10.25
50961	6.04	2.43	0.73	9.20

Non-facility RVUs ☐

Code	Work	PE Non-Facility	MP	Total Non-Facility
50955	6.74	4.99	0.79	12.52
50957	6.78	5.06	0.79	12.63
50961	6.04	4.66	0.73	11.43

Modifiers (PAR) ☐

Code	Mod 50	Mod 51	Mod 62	Mod 66	Mod 80
50955	1	3	0	0	0
50957	1	3	0	0	0
50961	1	3	0	0	0

Global Period

Code	Days
50955	000
50957	000
50961	000

50970-50972

50970 Ureteral endoscopy through ureterotomy, with or without irrigation, instillation, or ureteropyelography, exclusive of radiologic service

(For ureterotomy, use 50600)

50972 Ureteral endoscopy through ureterotomy, with or without irrigation, instillation, or ureteropyelography, exclusive of radiologic service; with ureteral catheterization, with or without dilation of ureter

(For image-guided dilation of ureter without endoscopic guidance, use 50706)

AMA Coding Notes

Surgical Procedures on the Urinary System

(For provision of chemotherapeutic agents, report both the specific service in addition to code(s) for the specific substance(s) or drug(s) provided)

AMA *CPT® Assistant*

50970: Oct 01: 8

50972: Oct 01: 8

Plain English Description

Ureteral endoscopy is performed through an incision in the ureter. An incision is made to expose the ureter. A small incision is made in the ureter and the ureteroscope is introduced. In 50970, the ureter is inspected and any obstruction, stenosis, stricture, or other abnormal condition is noted. The ureter may be irrigated with normal saline or diagnostic or therapeutic solution may be instilled. Contrast material may be injected and separately reportable ureteropyelography performed. In 50972, following visual examination, a ureteral catheter is advanced through the ureteroscope. If stenosis is present, a balloon-tipped catheter is introduced to the site of the stenosis and inflated. This balloon may be deflated and inflated several times until the stenotic region is adequately dilated. The ureter may be irrigated with normal saline or diagnostic or therapeutic solution may be instilled. Contrast material may be injected and separately reportable ureteropyelography performed. All instruments are removed and the ureterotomy is closed with sutures.

Ureteral endoscopy through ureterotomy

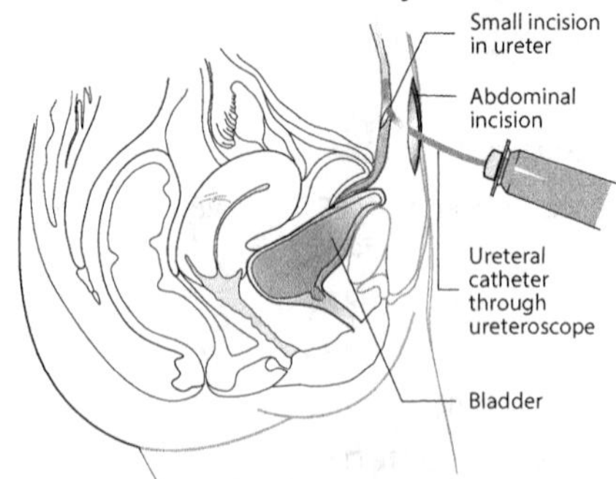

Without ureteral catheterization (50970); with ureteral catheterization, with or without dilation of ureter (50972)

ICD-10-CM Diagnostic Codes

⇄	C64.1	Malignant neoplasm of right kidney, except renal pelvis
⇄	C64.2	Malignant neoplasm of left kidney, except renal pelvis
⇄	C65.1	Malignant neoplasm of right renal pelvis
⇄	C65.2	Malignant neoplasm of left renal pelvis
⇄	C66.1	Malignant neoplasm of right ureter
⇄	C66.2	Malignant neoplasm of left ureter
	C67.6	Malignant neoplasm of ureteric orifice
⇄	C79.01	Secondary malignant neoplasm of right kidney and renal pelvis
⇄	C79.02	Secondary malignant neoplasm of left kidney and renal pelvis
	C79.11	Secondary malignant neoplasm of bladder
	C79.19	Secondary malignant neoplasm of other urinary organs
	C7A.093	Malignant carcinoid tumor of the kidney
	C80.2	Malignant neoplasm associated with transplanted organ
	D09.0	Carcinoma in situ of bladder
	D09.19	Carcinoma in situ of other urinary organs
⇄	D30.01	Benign neoplasm of right kidney
⇄	D30.02	Benign neoplasm of left kidney
⇄	D30.11	Benign neoplasm of right renal pelvis
⇄	D30.12	Benign neoplasm of left renal pelvis
⇄	D30.21	Benign neoplasm of right ureter
⇄	D30.22	Benign neoplasm of left ureter
	D3A.093	Benign carcinoid tumor of the kidney
⇄	D41.01	Neoplasm of uncertain behavior of right kidney
⇄	D41.02	Neoplasm of uncertain behavior of left kidney
⇄	D41.11	Neoplasm of uncertain behavior of right renal pelvis
⇄	D41.12	Neoplasm of uncertain behavior of left renal pelvis
⇄	D41.21	Neoplasm of uncertain behavior of right ureter
⇄	D41.22	Neoplasm of uncertain behavior of left ureter
	D41.4	Neoplasm of uncertain behavior of bladder
	N11.1	Chronic obstructive pyelonephritis
	N13.1	Hydronephrosis with ureteral stricture, not elsewhere classified
	N13.2	Hydronephrosis with renal and ureteral calculous obstruction
	N13.39	Other hydronephrosis
	N13.4	Hydroureter
	N13.5	Crossing vessel and stricture of ureter without hydronephrosis
	N13.8	Other obstructive and reflux uropathy
	N15.1	Renal and perinephric abscess
	N20.1	Calculus of ureter
	N20.2	Calculus of kidney with calculus of ureter
	N22	Calculus of urinary tract in diseases classified elsewhere
	N25.81	Secondary hyperparathyroidism of renal origin
	N28.0	Ischemia and infarction of kidney
	N28.1	Cyst of kidney, acquired
	N28.81	Hypertrophy of kidney
	N28.82	Megaloureter
	N28.83	Nephroptosis
	N28.89	Other specified disorders of kidney and ureter
	N29	Other disorders of kidney and ureter in diseases classified elsewhere
	Q61.01	Congenital single renal cyst
	Q61.02	Congenital multiple renal cysts
	Q61.19	Other polycystic kidney, infantile type
	Q61.2	Polycystic kidney, adult type
	Q61.4	Renal dysplasia
	Q61.5	Medullary cystic kidney
	Q61.8	Other cystic kidney diseases
	Q62.0	Congenital hydronephrosis
	Q62.11	Congenital occlusion of ureteropelvic junction
	Q62.12	Congenital occlusion of ureterovesical orifice
	Q62.2	Congenital megaureter
	Q62.31	Congenital ureterocele, orthotopic
	Q62.32	Cecoureterocele
	Q62.39	Other obstructive defects of renal pelvis and ureter

CCI Edits

Refer to Appendix A for CCI edits.

Facility RVUs

Code	Work	PE Facility	MP	Total Facility
50970	7.13	2.76	0.86	10.75
50972	6.88	2.68	0.83	10.39

Non-facility RVUs

Code	Work	PE Non-Facility	MP	Total Non-Facility
50970	7.13	2.76	0.86	10.75
50972	6.88	2.68	0.83	10.39

Modifiers (PAR)

Code	Mod 50	Mod 51	Mod 62	Mod 66	Mod 80
50970	1	2	0	0	0
50972	1	2	0	0	0

Global Period

Code	Days
50970	000
50972	000

50974-50980

50974 Ureteral endoscopy through ureterotomy, with or without irrigation, instillation, or ureteropyelography, exclusive of radiologic service; with biopsy

(For image-guided biopsy of ureter and/or renal pelvis without endoscopic guidance, use 50606)

50976 Ureteral endoscopy through ureterotomy, with or without irrigation, instillation, or ureteropyelography, exclusive of radiologic service; with fulguration and/or incision, with or without biopsy

50980 Ureteral endoscopy through ureterotomy, with or without irrigation, instillation, or ureteropyelography, exclusive of radiologic service; with removal of foreign body or calculus

AMA Coding Notes

Surgical Procedures on the Urinary System

(For provision of chemotherapeutic agents, report both the specific service in addition to code(s) for the specific substance(s) or drug(s) provided)

AMA *CPT® Assistant* ▯

50974: Oct 01: 8
50976: Oct 01: 8
50980: Oct 01: 8

Plain English Description

Ureteral endoscopy is performed through an incision in the ureter. An incision is made to expose the ureter. A small incision is made in the ureter and the ureteroscope is introduced. The ureter is inspected for abnormal tissue, foreign body, or calculus. The ureter may be irrigated with normal saline, or diagnostic or therapeutic solution may be instilled. Contrast material may be injected and separately reportable ureteropyelography performed. In 50974, a biopsy is performed. Biopsy forceps are inserted through the ureteroscope and one or more tissue samples are obtained. In 50976, fulguration and/or incision of abnormal tissue is performed. A biopsy may be performed prior to the fulguration procedure as described above. To destroy abnormal tissue, an electrocautery device is advanced through the ureteroscope to the site of the lesion. The device is activated and the abnormal tissue is destroyed. Alternatively, a laser or cryoprobe may be used to destroy the abnormal tissue. The physician may introduce a blade and incise the abnormal tissue instead of, or in addition to, the fulguration procedure. In 50980, the ureter is inspected and a foreign body, such as a stent or calculus, is located. A grasping device or basket is advanced through the working channel of the ureteroscope and the foreign body or calculus is captured and removed. The ureter is re-inspected to ensure that there has not been any injury to the ureter during the procedure.

Ureteral endoscopy through ureterotomy

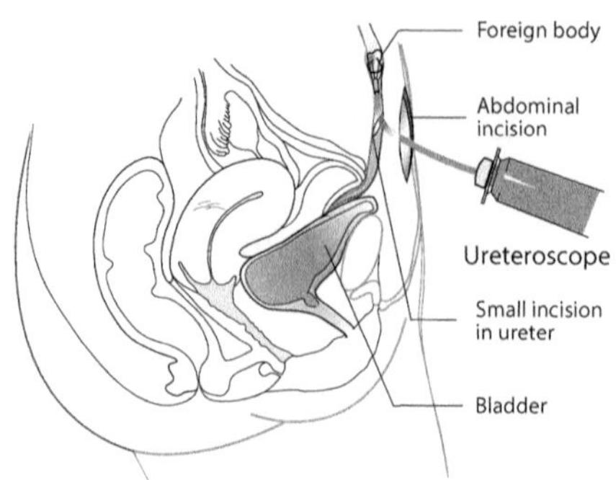

With biopsy (50974); with fulguration and/or incision, with or without biopsy (50976); with removal of foreign body or calculus (50980)

ICD-10-CM Diagnostic Codes

⇄	C64.1	Malignant neoplasm of right kidney, except renal pelvis
⇄	C64.2	Malignant neoplasm of left kidney, except renal pelvis
⇄	C65.1	Malignant neoplasm of right renal pelvis
⇄	C65.2	Malignant neoplasm of left renal pelvis
⇄	C66.1	Malignant neoplasm of right ureter
⇄	C66.2	Malignant neoplasm of left ureter
	C67.6	Malignant neoplasm of ureteric orifice
⇄	C79.01	Secondary malignant neoplasm of right kidney and renal pelvis
⇄	C79.02	Secondary malignant neoplasm of left kidney and renal pelvis
	C79.11	Secondary malignant neoplasm of bladder
	C79.19	Secondary malignant neoplasm of other urinary organs
	C7A.093	Malignant carcinoid tumor of the kidney
	C80.2	Malignant neoplasm associated with transplanted organ
	D09.0	Carcinoma in situ of bladder
	D09.19	Carcinoma in situ of other urinary organs
⇄	D30.01	Benign neoplasm of right kidney
⇄	D30.02	Benign neoplasm of left kidney
⇄	D30.11	Benign neoplasm of right renal pelvis
⇄	D30.12	Benign neoplasm of left renal pelvis
⇄	D30.21	Benign neoplasm of right ureter
⇄	D30.22	Benign neoplasm of left ureter
	D3A.093	Benign carcinoid tumor of the kidney
⇄	D41.01	Neoplasm of uncertain behavior of right kidney
⇄	D41.02	Neoplasm of uncertain behavior of left kidney
⇄	D41.11	Neoplasm of uncertain behavior of right renal pelvis
⇄	D41.12	Neoplasm of uncertain behavior of left renal pelvis
⇄	D41.21	Neoplasm of uncertain behavior of right ureter
⇄	D41.22	Neoplasm of uncertain behavior of left ureter
	D41.4	Neoplasm of uncertain behavior of bladder
	N11.1	Chronic obstructive pyelonephritis
	N13.1	Hydronephrosis with ureteral stricture, not elsewhere classified
	N13.2	Hydronephrosis with renal and ureteral calculous obstruction
	N13.39	Other hydronephrosis
	N13.4	Hydroureter
	N13.5	Crossing vessel and stricture of ureter without hydronephrosis
	N13.8	Other obstructive and reflux uropathy
	N15.1	Renal and perinephric abscess
	N20.0	Calculus of kidney
	N20.1	Calculus of ureter
	N20.2	Calculus of kidney with calculus of ureter
	N22	Calculus of urinary tract in diseases classified elsewhere
	N25.81	Secondary hyperparathyroidism of renal origin
	N28.0	Ischemia and infarction of kidney
	N28.1	Cyst of kidney, acquired
	N28.81	Hypertrophy of kidney
	N28.83	Nephroptosis
	N28.89	Other specified disorders of kidney and ureter
	N29	Other disorders of kidney and ureter in diseases classified elsewhere
	Q61.01	Congenital single renal cyst
	Q61.02	Congenital multiple renal cysts
	Q61.19	Other polycystic kidney, infantile type
	Q61.2	Polycystic kidney, adult type
	Q61.4	Renal dysplasia
	Q61.5	Medullary cystic kidney
	Q61.8	Other cystic kidney diseases
	Q62.0	Congenital hydronephrosis
	Q62.11	Congenital occlusion of ureteropelvic junction
	Q62.12	Congenital occlusion of ureterovesical orifice
	Q62.2	Congenital megaureter
	Q62.31	Congenital ureterocele, orthotopic
	Q62.32	Cecoureterocele
	Q62.39	Other obstructive defects of renal pelvis and ureter

CCI Edits

Refer to Appendix A for CCI edits.

Facility RVUs

Code	Work	PE Facility	MP	Total Facility
50974	9.16	3.45	1.09	13.70
50976	9.03	3.40	1.07	13.50
50980	6.84	2.66	0.83	10.33

Non-facility RVUs

Code	Work	PE Non-Facility	MP	Total Non-Facility
50974	9.16	3.45	1.09	13.70
50976	9.03	3.40	1.07	13.50
50980	6.84	2.66	0.83	10.33

Modifiers (PAR)

Code	Mod 50	Mod 51	Mod 62	Mod 66	Mod 80
50974	1	3	0	0	0
50976	1	3	0	0	0
50980	1	2	0	0	0

Global Period

Code	Days
50974	000
50976	000
50980	000

51020-51030

51020 Cystotomy or cystostomy; with fulguration and/or insertion of radioactive material

51030 Cystotomy or cystostomy; with cryosurgical destruction of intravesical lesion

AMA Coding Notes

Surgical Procedures on the Urinary System

(For provision of chemotherapeutic agents, report both the specific service in addition to code(s) for the specific substance(s) or drug(s) provided)

Plain English Description

The urinary bladder is exposed and incised. Alternatively, a small incision is made over the bladder and the bladder wall is punctured to provide surgical access to the internal lumen. In 51020, abnormal tissue is destroyed by fulguration or radioactive material is inserted into a lesion. To destroy abnormal tissue, an electrocautery device is advanced through the incision to the site where the abnormal tissue is located. The device is activated and the lesion is destroyed. Alternatively, a laser may be used to destroy the abnormal tissue. If a radioactive material is used to treat a lesion, the delivery device is inserted into the bladder and positioned at the site of the lesion or abnormal tissue. The radioactive pellet is then embedded in the mucosa or bladder wall at the site of the lesion or abnormal tissue. In 51030, a cryoprobe is introduced through the incision and abnormal tissue is frozen. Several freeze-thaw cycles may be required to completely destroy all abnormal tissue.

Cystotomy or cystostomy

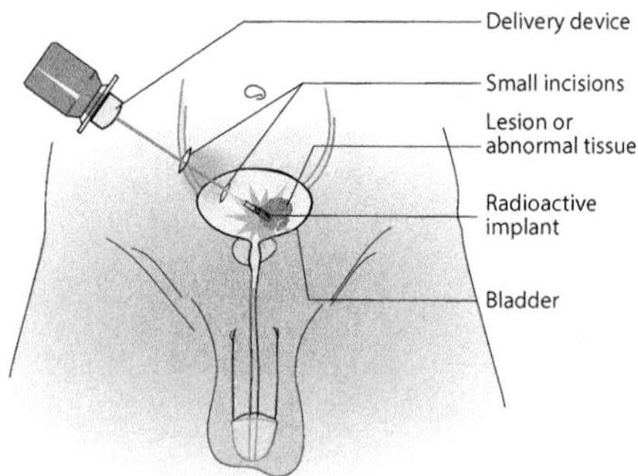

With fulguration and/or insertion of radioactive material (51020); with cryosurgical destruction of intravesical lesion (51030)

ICD-10-CM Diagnostic Codes

C67.0	Malignant neoplasm of trigone of bladder
C67.1	Malignant neoplasm of dome of bladder
C67.2	Malignant neoplasm of lateral wall of bladder
C67.3	Malignant neoplasm of anterior wall of bladder
C67.4	Malignant neoplasm of posterior wall of bladder
C67.5	Malignant neoplasm of bladder neck
C67.6	Malignant neoplasm of ureteric orifice
C67.7	Malignant neoplasm of urachus
C67.8	Malignant neoplasm of overlapping sites of bladder
C79.11	Secondary malignant neoplasm of bladder
D09.0	Carcinoma in situ of bladder
D30.3	Benign neoplasm of bladder
D41.4	Neoplasm of uncertain behavior of bladder
N30.10	Interstitial cystitis (chronic) without hematuria
N30.11	Interstitial cystitis (chronic) with hematuria
N32.89	Other specified disorders of bladder

CCI Edits

Refer to Appendix A for CCI edits.

Facility RVUs ▢

Code	Work	PE Facility	MP	Total Facility
51020	7.69	5.18	0.93	13.80
51030	7.81	5.15	0.94	13.90

Non-facility RVUs ▢

Code	Work	PE Non-Facility	MP	Total Non-Facility
51020	7.69	5.18	0.93	13.80
51030	7.81	5.15	0.94	13.90

Modifiers (PAR) ▢

Code	Mod 50	Mod 51	Mod 62	Mod 66	Mod 80
51020	0	2	1	0	2
51030	0	2	0	0	0

Global Period

Code	Days
51020	090
51030	090

51040

51040 Cystostomy, cystotomy with drainage

AMA Coding Notes

Surgical Procedures on the Urinary System

(For provision of chemotherapeutic agents, report both the specific service in addition to code(s) for the specific substance(s) or drug(s) provided)

Plain English Description

A cystostomy or cystotomy with drainage is performed. The skin over the lower abdomen is cleansed. An incision is made in the abdominal wall and into the bladder. A drainage tube (catheter) is inserted and secured to the abdomen to facilitate drainage, and a sterile dressing is applied.

Cystostomy, cystotomy with drainage

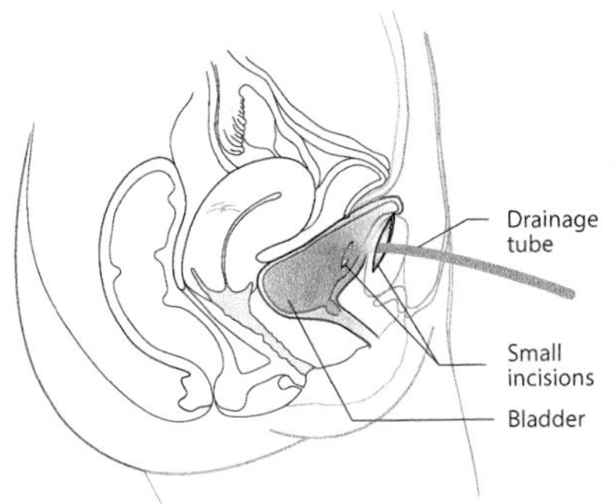

ICD-10-CM Diagnostic Codes

A56.01	Chlamydial cystitis and urethritis
C61	Malignant neoplasm of prostate ♂
C67.0	Malignant neoplasm of trigone of bladder
C67.2	Malignant neoplasm of lateral wall of bladder
C67.3	Malignant neoplasm of anterior wall of bladder
C67.4	Malignant neoplasm of posterior wall of bladder
C67.5	Malignant neoplasm of bladder neck
C67.6	Malignant neoplasm of ureteric orifice
D07.5	Carcinoma in situ of prostate ♂
D40.0	Neoplasm of uncertain behavior of prostate ♂
G83.4	Cauda equina syndrome
N11.0	Nonobstructive reflux-associated chronic pyelonephritis
N11.8	Other chronic tubulo-interstitial nephritis
N13.71	Vesicoureteral-reflux without reflux nephropathy
N16	Renal tubulo-interstitial disorders in diseases classified elsewhere
N21.1	Calculus in urethra
N28.84	Pyelitis cystica
N28.85	Pyeloureteritis cystica
N28.86	Ureteritis cystica
N30.00	Acute cystitis without hematuria
N30.01	Acute cystitis with hematuria
N30.10	Interstitial cystitis (chronic) without hematuria
N30.11	Interstitial cystitis (chronic) with hematuria
N30.30	Trigonitis without hematuria
N30.31	Trigonitis with hematuria
N30.80	Other cystitis without hematuria
N30.81	Other cystitis with hematuria
N31.8	Other neuromuscular dysfunction of bladder
N31.9	Neuromuscular dysfunction of bladder, unspecified
N32.0	Bladder-neck obstruction
N32.1	Vesicointestinal fistula
N32.3	Diverticulum of bladder
N32.81	Overactive bladder
N36.0	Urethral fistula
N39.0	Urinary tract infection, site not specified
N39.3	Stress incontinence (female) (male)
N40.0	Benign prostatic hyperplasia without lower urinary tract symptoms ♂
N40.1	Benign prostatic hyperplasia with lower urinary tract symptoms ♂
N40.3	Nodular prostate with lower urinary tract symptoms ♂
N81.11	Cystocele, midline ♀
N81.12	Cystocele, lateral ♀
N82.0	Vesicovaginal fistula ♀
P39.3	Neonatal urinary tract infection
Q64.2	Congenital posterior urethral valves
Q64.31	Congenital bladder neck obstruction
Q64.32	Congenital stricture of urethra
Q64.33	Congenital stricture of urinary meatus
Q64.39	Other atresia and stenosis of urethra and bladder neck
R31	Hematuria
R31.0	Gross hematuria
R31.1	Benign essential microscopic hematuria
R33.8	Other retention of urine
R33.9	Retention of urine, unspecified
R39.14	Feeling of incomplete bladder emptying
➐ S37.22	Contusion of bladder
➐ S37.23	Laceration of bladder
➐ S37.32	Contusion of urethra
➐ S37.33	Laceration of urethra

ICD-10-CM Coding Notes

For codes requiring a 7th character extension, refer to your ICD-10-CM book. Review the character descriptions and coding guidelines for proper selection. For some procedures, only certain characters will apply.

CCI Edits

Refer to Appendix A for CCI edits.

Facility RVUs ▢

Code	Work	PE Facility	MP	Total Facility
51040	4.49	3.51	0.55	8.55

Non-facility RVUs ▢

Code	Work	PE Non-Facility	MP	Total Non-Facility
51040	4.49	3.51	0.55	8.55

Modifiers (PAR) ▢

Code	Mod 50	Mod 51	Mod 62	Mod 66	Mod 80
51040	0	2	1	0	2

Global Period

Code	Days
51040	090

51045

51045 Cystotomy, with insertion of ureteral catheter or stent (separate procedure)

AMA Coding Notes

Surgical Procedures on the Urinary System

(For provision of chemotherapeutic agents, report both the specific service in addition to code(s) for the specific substance(s) or drug(s) provided)

Plain English Description

The urinary bladder is exposed and a small incision is made in the bladder wall. A guidewire is introduced through the incision and advanced through the ureter to the renal pelvis. A catheter is advanced over the guidewire to the renal pelvis. The guidewire is removed. The ureter may be irrigated with normal saline, or diagnostic or therapeutic solution may be instilled. Alternatively, a ureteral stent may be placed over the guidewire. The stent is advanced over the guidewire and the proximal end is positioned in the renal pelvis. The guidewire is slowly withdrawn, taking care not to dislodge the stent. The distal end of the stent is positioned in the urinary bladder.

Cystotomy, with insertion of ureteral catheter or stent

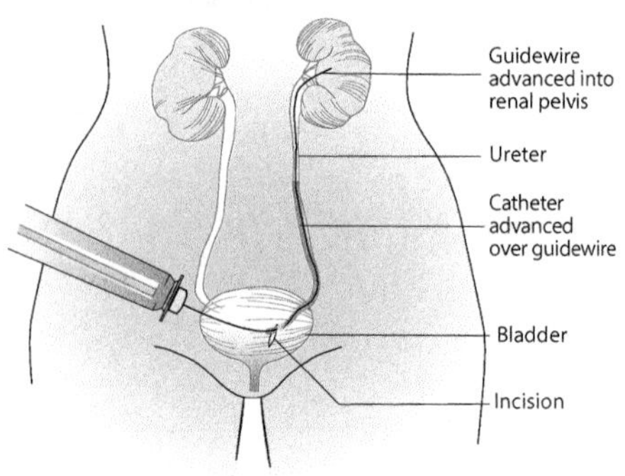

ICD-10-CM Diagnostic Codes

⇄	C66.1	Malignant neoplasm of right ureter
⇄	C66.2	Malignant neoplasm of left ureter
⇄	D30.21	Benign neoplasm of right ureter
⇄	D30.22	Benign neoplasm of left ureter
⇄	D41.21	Neoplasm of uncertain behavior of right ureter
⇄	D41.22	Neoplasm of uncertain behavior of left ureter
	N11.1	Chronic obstructive pyelonephritis
	N13.4	Hydroureter
	N13.5	Crossing vessel and stricture of ureter without hydronephrosis
	N13.8	Other obstructive and reflux uropathy
	N20.1	Calculus of ureter
	N28.89	Other specified disorders of kidney and ureter
	Q62.0	Congenital hydronephrosis
	Q62.11	Congenital occlusion of ureteropelvic junction
	Q62.12	Congenital occlusion of ureterovesical orifice
	Q62.2	Congenital megaureter
	Q62.31	Congenital ureterocele, orthotopic
	Q62.32	Cecoureterocele
	Q62.39	Other obstructive defects of renal pelvis and ureter
❼	S37.12	Contusion of ureter
❼	S37.13	Laceration of ureter
❼	S37.19	Other injury of ureter

ICD-10-CM Coding Notes

For codes requiring a 7th character extension, refer to your ICD-10-CM book. Review the character descriptions and coding guidelines for proper selection. For some procedures, only certain characters will apply.

CCI Edits

Refer to Appendix A for CCI edits.

Facility RVUs ▯

Code	Work	PE Facility	MP	Total Facility
51045	7.81	5.75	1.39	14.95

Non-facility RVUs ▯

Code	Work	PE Non-Facility	MP	Total Non-Facility
51045	7.81	5.75	1.39	14.95

Modifiers (PAR) ▯

Code	Mod 50	Mod 51	Mod 62	Mod 66	Mod 80
51045	0	2	0	0	2

Global Period

Code	Days
51045	090

51050

51050 Cystolithotomy, cystotomy with removal of calculus, without vesical neck resection

AMA Coding Notes

Surgical Procedures on the Urinary System

(For provision of chemotherapeutic agents, report both the specific service in addition to code(s) for the specific substance(s) or drug(s) provided)

Plain English Description

A skin incision is made in the lower abdomen over the urinary bladder. Tissues are dissected down to the anterior rectus muscle sheath. The rectus abdominus and pyramidalis muscles are separated and retracted. The peritoneum is reflected. The urinary bladder is exposed and an incision is made in the bladder wall to perform a cystotomy and remove a calculus from the bladder. Two stay sutures are placed in the bladder wall lateral to the planned incision site. The stay sutures are pulled to tent the bladder. A stab incision is made between the stay sutures in the tented portion of the bladder. The incision is enlarged until it is wide enough to accommodate extraction of the calculus. Grasping forceps are introduced and the calculus is captured and removed. The bladder incision is closed followed by layered closure of the abdominal incision.

Cystolithotomy, cystotomy with removal of calculus, without vesical neck resection

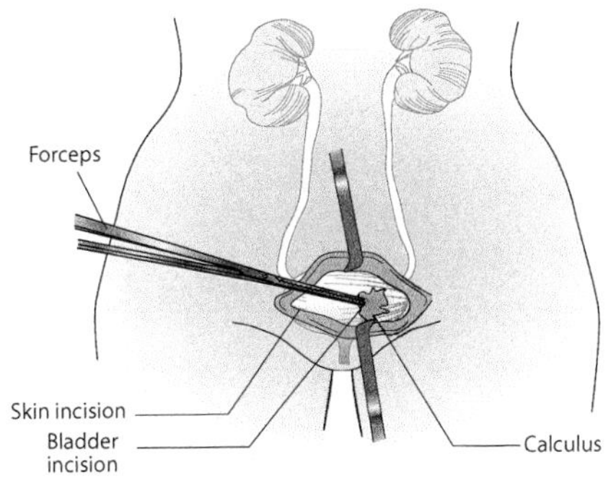

ICD-10-CM Diagnostic Codes

N21.0	Calculus in bladder
N21.1	Calculus in urethra
N21.8	Other lower urinary tract calculus

CCI Edits

Refer to Appendix A for CCI edits.

Facility RVUs

Code	Work	PE Facility	MP	Total Facility
51050	7.97	4.90	0.95	13.82

Non-facility RVUs

Code	Work	PE Non-Facility	MP	Total Non-Facility
51050	7.97	4.90	0.95	13.82

Modifiers (PAR)

Code	Mod 50	Mod 51	Mod 62	Mod 66	Mod 80
51050	0	2	1	0	2

Global Period

Code	Days
51050	090

51060

51060 Transvesical ureterolithotomy

AMA Coding Notes

Surgical Procedures on the Urinary System

(For provision of chemotherapeutic agents, report both the specific service in addition to code(s) for the specific substance(s) or drug(s) provided)

Plain English Description

A skin incision is made in the lower abdomen over the urinary bladder. Tissues are dissected down to the anterior rectus muscle sheath. The rectus abdominus and pyramidalis muscles are separated and retracted. The peritoneum is reflected. The urinary bladder is exposed and an incision is made in the bladder wall. Two stay sutures are placed in the bladder wall lateral to the planned incision site. The stay sutures are pulled to tent the bladder. A stab incision is made between the stay sutures in the tented portion of the bladder. The incision is enlarged until the ureteral orifice is visible. A second incision is made through the bladder wall near the ureter. The calculus in the distal aspect of the ureter is located. The ureter is incised and the calculus extracted through the bladder. The ureteral incision is closed, followed by the proximal bladder incision. The anterior wall of the bladder is closed, followed by layered closure of the abdominal incision.

Transvesical ureterolithotomy

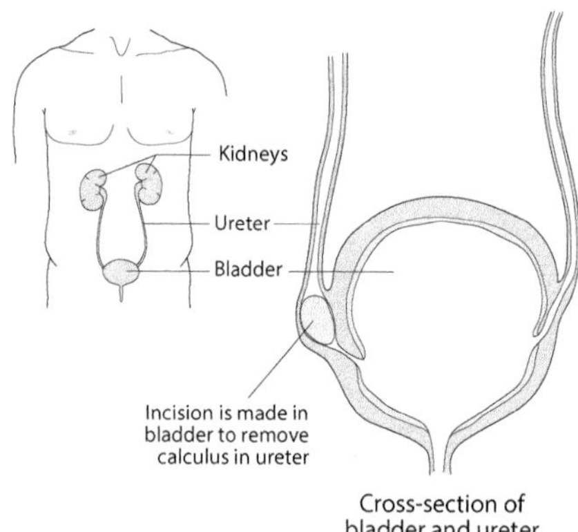

ICD-10-CM Diagnostic Codes

N20.1	Calculus of ureter
N20.2	Calculus of kidney with calculus of ureter

CCI Edits

Refer to Appendix A for CCI edits.

Facility RVUs

Code	Work	PE Facility	MP	Total Facility
51060	9.95	5.95	1.18	17.08

Non-facility RVUs

Code	Work	PE Non-Facility	MP	Total Non-Facility
51060	9.95	5.95	1.18	17.08

Modifiers (PAR)

Code	Mod 50	Mod 51	Mod 62	Mod 66	Mod 80
51060	0	2	1	0	2

Global Period

Code	Days
51060	090

51065

51065 Cystotomy, with calculus basket extraction and/or ultrasonic or electrohydraulic fragmentation of ureteral calculus

AMA Coding Notes

Surgical Procedures on the Urinary System

(For provision of chemotherapeutic agents, report both the specific service in addition to code(s) for the specific substance(s) or drug(s) provided)

Plain English Description

A skin incision is made in the lower abdomen over the urinary bladder. Tissues are dissected down to the anterior rectus muscle sheath. The rectus abdominus and pyramidalis muscles are separated and retracted. The peritoneum is reflected. The urinary bladder is then exposed and an incision is made in the bladder wall to perform a cystotomy for basket extraction and/or fragmentation of a ureteral calculus. Two stay sutures are placed in the bladder wall lateral to the planned incision site. The stay sutures are pulled to tent the bladder. A stab incision is made between the stay sutures in the tented portion of the bladder. The incision is enlarged until the ureteral orifice is visible. The basket extraction device is advanced through the bladder and into the ureter. The calculus is captured and removed. Lithotripsy may be performed using ultrasound or an electrohydraulic device to fragment the ureteral calculus prior to, or instead of, basket extraction. Once all stone fragments have been removed, the bladder incision is closed, followed by the abdominal incision, which is closed in layers.

Cystotomy, with calculus basket extraction and/or ultrasonic or electrohydraulic fragmentation of ureteral calculus

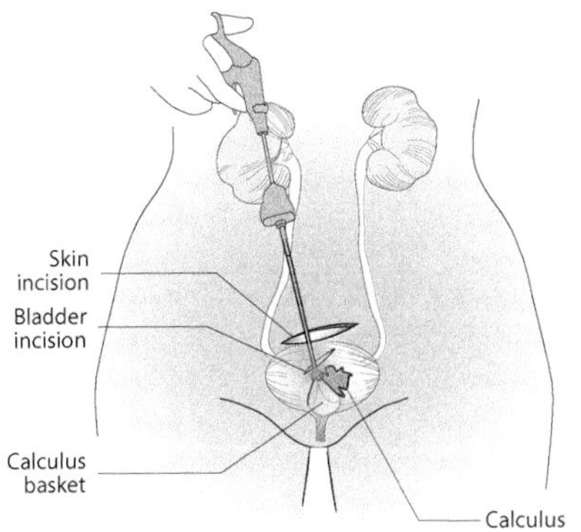

ICD-10-CM Diagnostic Codes

N20.1	Calculus of ureter
N20.2	Calculus of kidney with calculus of ureter

CCI Edits

Refer to Appendix A for CCI edits.

Facility RVUs

Code	Work	PE Facility	MP	Total Facility
51065	9.95	5.88	1.18	17.01

Non-facility RVUs

Code	Work	PE Non-Facility	MP	Total Non-Facility
51065	9.95	5.88	1.18	17.01

Modifiers (PAR)

Code	Mod 50	Mod 51	Mod 62	Mod 66	Mod 80
51065	0	2	0	0	0

Global Period

Code	Days
51065	090

51080

51080 Drainage of perivesical or prevesical space abscess

(For percutaneous image-guided fluid collection drainage by catheter of perivesicular or prevesicular space abscess, use 49406)

AMA Coding Notes

Surgical Procedures on the Urinary System

(For provision of chemotherapeutic agents, report both the specific service in addition to code(s) for the specific substance(s) or drug(s) provided)

Plain English Description

The physician drains fluid from an abscess located in the tissue around the bladder. A skin incision is made in the lower abdomen over the urinary bladder. Tissues are dissected down to the anterior rectus muscle sheath. The rectus abdominus and pyramidalis muscles are separated and retracted. The peritoneum is reflected. An abscess in the perivesical or prevesical space is located. The abscess cavity is opened and drained. Blunt dissection is used to break up loculations. The cavity is flushed with sterile saline or antibiotic solution, and a drain is placed. The incision is closed over the drain.

Drainage of perivesical or prevesical space abscess

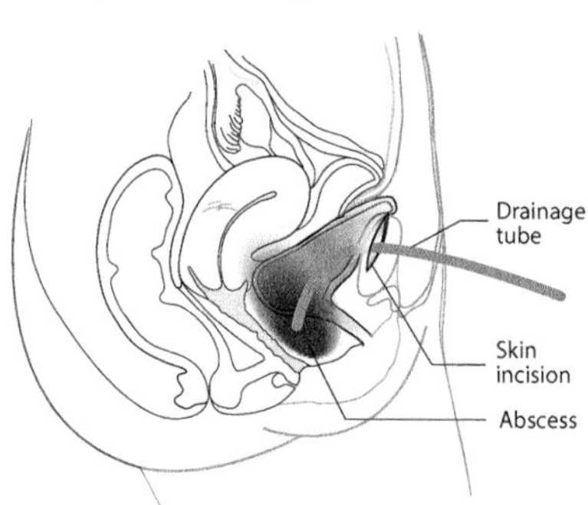

ICD-10-CM Diagnostic Codes

K65	Peritonitis
K65.1	Peritoneal abscess
K68.11	Postprocedural retroperitoneal abscess
K68.19	Other retroperitoneal abscess
N30.80	Other cystitis without hematuria
N30.81	Other cystitis with hematuria
R31.0	Gross hematuria
R31.1	Benign essential microscopic hematuria

CCI Edits

Refer to Appendix A for CCI edits.

Facility RVUs ▯

Code	Work	PE Facility	MP	Total Facility
51080	6.71	4.48	0.79	11.98

Non-facility RVUs ▯

Code	Work	PE Non-Facility	MP	Total Non-Facility
51080	6.71	4.48	0.79	11.98

Modifiers (PAR) ▯

Code	Mod 50	Mod 51	Mod 62	Mod 66	Mod 80
51080	0	2	1	0	2

Global Period

Code	Days
51080	090

51100-51102

51100 Aspiration of bladder; by needle
51101 Aspiration of bladder; by trocar or intracatheter
51102 Aspiration of bladder; with insertion of suprapubic catheter
(For imaging guidance, see 76942, 77002, 77012)

AMA Coding Notes
Surgical Procedures on the Urinary System
(For provision of chemotherapeutic agents, report both the specific service in addition to code(s) for the specific substance(s) or drug(s) provided)

AMA *CPT® Assistant*
51100: Jun 08: 11
51101: Jun 08: 11
51102: Jun 08: 11

Plain English Description
A needle aspiration of the bladder is performed in 51100. A needle is inserted through the skin in the suprapubic region and advanced into the bladder. A small amount of urine is aspirated. This procedure is usually performed for urinalysis and culture for suspected urinary tract infection and requires a minimum of 2 mL of urine. Use 51101 for bladder aspiration using a trocar or intracatheter. A small incision is made in the skin over the suprapubic region. A trocar or intracatheter is inserted into the bladder and urine is aspirated. Use 51102 for bladder aspiration with insertion of a suprapubic catheter. A needle aspiration is performed as described above prior to insertion of the suprapubic catheter. The syringe is then removed and a guidewire is placed through the needle. The needle is removed and a small incision is made adjacent to the guidewire. A peel-away sheath introducer is placed over the guidewire and the guidewire is removed. A Foley catheter is advanced through the sheath introducer into the bladder and the balloon is deployed. The sheath introducer is removed and the catheter pulled back until resistance is met. The catheter tubing is secured on the abdominal wall and a drainage bag is attached.

Aspiration of bladder

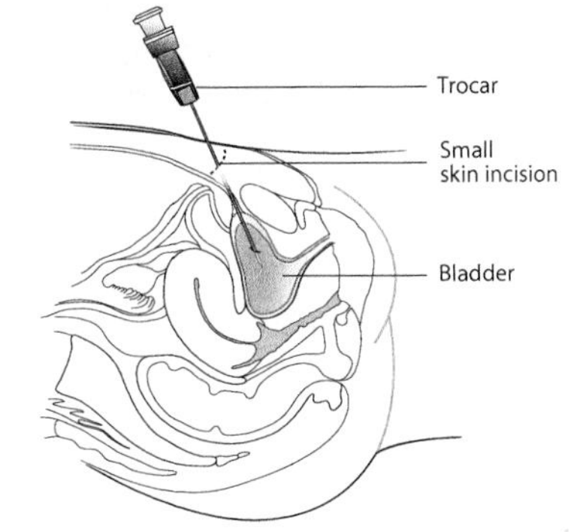

By needle (51100); by trocar or intracatheter (51101); with insertion of suprapubic catheter (51102)

ICD-10-CM Diagnostic Codes

A56.01	Chlamydial cystitis and urethritis
N28.84	Pyelitis cystica
N28.85	Pyeloureteritis cystica
N28.86	Ureteritis cystica
N30.00	Acute cystitis without hematuria
N30.01	Acute cystitis with hematuria
N30.10	Interstitial cystitis (chronic) without hematuria
N30.11	Interstitial cystitis (chronic) with hematuria
N30.30	Trigonitis without hematuria
N30.31	Trigonitis with hematuria
N32.0	Bladder-neck obstruction
N39.0	Urinary tract infection, site not specified
P39.3	Neonatal urinary tract infection

CCI Edits
Refer to Appendix A for CCI edits.

Facility RVUs

Code	Work	PE Facility	MP	Total Facility
51100	0.78	0.26	0.09	1.13
51101	1.02	0.35	0.11	1.48
51102	2.70	1.22	0.29	4.21

Non-facility RVUs

Code	Work	PE Non-Facility	MP	Total Non-Facility
51100	0.78	1.32	0.09	2.19
51101	1.02	3.57	0.11	4.70
51102	2.70	4.24	0.29	7.23

Modifiers (PAR)

Code	Mod 50	Mod 51	Mod 62	Mod 66	Mod 80
51100	0	2	0	0	1
51101	0	2	0	0	1
51102	0	2	0	0	1

Global Period

Code	Days
51100	000
51101	000
51102	000

51500

51500 Excision of urachal cyst or sinus, with or without umbilical hernia repair

AMA Coding Notes

Surgical Procedures on the Urinary System

(For provision of chemotherapeutic agents, report both the specific service in addition to code(s) for the specific substance(s) or drug(s) provided)

Plain English Description

The urachus is a duct present in the fetus that is usually obliterated between the 2nd and 4th month of gestation, becoming the median umbilical ligament. However, in some individuals this duct persists as a sinus that communicates with the umbilicus and bladder, or as a cyst. A persistent urachal sinus or cyst is usually asymptomatic and is not surgically excised unless infection occurs. A catheter is placed through the urethra and into the bladder. The skin is incised over the midline of the abdomen beginning just below the umbilicus and extending over the bladder. Underlying tissues are dissected; the anterior rectus abdominus muscle is divided; and the sinus or cyst is exposed. Usually a portion of the median umbilical ligament has begun to form and this is detached from the umbilicus. The sinus or cyst is mobilized using sharp dissection down towards the bladder. The bladder is filled with sterile saline. The peritoneum is incised and mobilization of the sinus or cyst continues down to the bladder dome. All connections between the sinus or cyst and the bladder dome are severed. This may require resection of the bladder cuff, which is then repaired with sutures. The sinus or cyst is completely excised. If an umbilical hernia is present, it is repaired. The hernia sac is exposed. The neck of the sac is incised and lifted away from the abdominal wall. The hernia contents are extracted and inspected. Any adhesions are severed. The bowel is returned to the abdomen. The hernia sac is excised. The defect in the abdominal wall is closed with sutures and/or a mesh implant is applied. Skin and subcutaneous tissues are closed is layers.

Excision of urachal cyst or sinus, with or without umbilical hernia repair

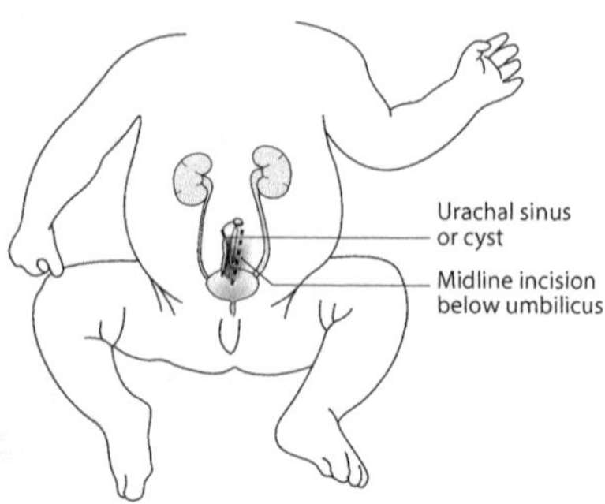

ICD-10-CM Diagnostic Codes

K42.0	Umbilical hernia with obstruction, without gangrene
K42.1	Umbilical hernia with gangrene
K42.9	Umbilical hernia without obstruction or gangrene
Q64.4	Malformation of urachus

CCI Edits

Refer to Appendix A for CCI edits.

Facility RVUs

Code	Work	PE Facility	MP	Total Facility
51500	11.05	6.31	1.32	18.68

Non-facility RVUs

Code	Work	PE Non-Facility	MP	Total Non-Facility
51500	11.05	6.31	1.32	18.68

Modifiers (PAR)

Code	Mod 50	Mod 51	Mod 62	Mod 66	Mod 80
51500	0	2	1	0	2

Global Period

Code	Days
51500	090

51520-51530

51520 Cystotomy; for simple excision of vesical neck (separate procedure)

51525 Cystotomy; for excision of bladder diverticulum, single or multiple (separate procedure)

51530 Cystotomy; for excision of bladder tumor

(For transurethral resection, see 52234-52240, 52305)

AMA Coding Notes

Surgical Procedures on the Urinary System

(For provision of chemotherapeutic agents, report both the specific service in addition to code(s) for the specific substance(s) or drug(s) provided)

Plain English Description

A midline extraperitoneal abdominal approach is used to expose the bladder. The rectus and transversalis fascia are divided and the incision is carried down through the space of Retzius. The anterior bladder wall and vesical neck are identified. The bladder dome is incised and the bladder wall is inspected including the trigone, ureteral orifices, and bladder neck. In 51520, the bladder (vesical) neck is excised. The bladder neck is mobilized and resected. Visceral bladder fascia is used to reconstruct the neck. In 51525, one or more bladder diverticula are excised. A bladder diverticulum is a protrusion of mucosal tissue through the detrusor muscles of the bladder and into the abdominal cavity. Intravesical excision involves pulling the diverticulum into the bladder. Tension is then applied to the everted diverticulum and it is excised or divided at its base using electrocautery. If the diverticulum cannot be pulled into the bladder due to adhesions, the mucosa around the diverticular orifice is divided. Adhesions are lysed and the diverticulum is then pulled into the bladder and removed. The defect in the bladder wall is repaired. In 51530, a bladder tumor is excised. The tumor is excised along with a margin of healthy tissue using sharp dissection. The defect in the bladder is repaired with sutures. The bladder incision is closed. The abdominal incision is closed in layers.

Cystotomy

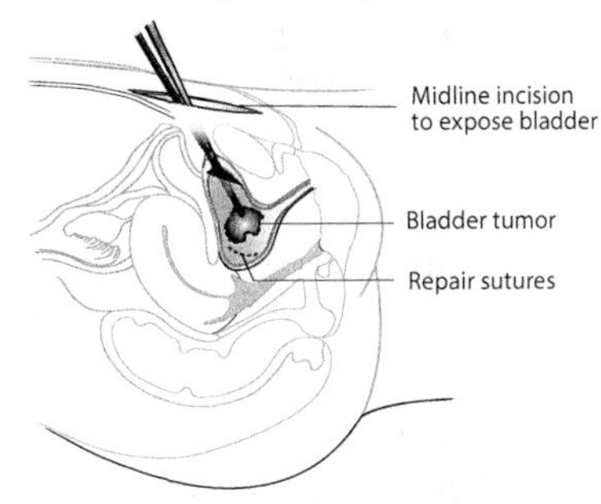

For simple excision of vesical neck (51520); for excision of bladder diverticulum, single or multiple (separate procedure) (51525); for excision of bladder tumor (51530)

ICD-10-CM Diagnostic Codes

C67.0	Malignant neoplasm of trigone of bladder
C67.1	Malignant neoplasm of dome of bladder
C67.2	Malignant neoplasm of lateral wall of bladder
C67.3	Malignant neoplasm of anterior wall of bladder
C67.4	Malignant neoplasm of posterior wall of bladder
C67.5	Malignant neoplasm of bladder neck
C67.6	Malignant neoplasm of ureteric orifice
C67.7	Malignant neoplasm of urachus
C79.11	Secondary malignant neoplasm of bladder
C79.19	Secondary malignant neoplasm of other urinary organs
D09.0	Carcinoma in situ of bladder
D30.3	Benign neoplasm of bladder
D41	Neoplasm of uncertain behavior of urinary organs
D49.4	Neoplasm of unspecified behavior of bladder
N32.0	Bladder-neck obstruction
N32.3	Diverticulum of bladder
N32.89	Other specified disorders of bladder
Q64.31	Congenital bladder neck obstruction
Q64.39	Other atresia and stenosis of urethra and bladder neck

CCI Edits

Refer to Appendix A for CCI edits.

Facility RVUs

Code	Work	PE Facility	MP	Total Facility
51520	10.21	6.04	1.21	17.46
51525	15.42	7.84	1.87	25.13
51530	13.71	7.20	1.64	22.55

Non-facility RVUs

Code	Work	PE Non-Facility	MP	Total Non-Facility
51520	10.21	6.04	1.21	17.46
51525	15.42	7.84	1.87	25.13
51530	13.71	7.20	1.64	22.55

Modifiers (PAR)

Code	Mod 50	Mod 51	Mod 62	Mod 66	Mod 80
51520	0	2	1	0	2
51525	0	2	1	0	2
51530	0	2	1	0	2

Global Period

Code	Days
51520	090
51525	090
51530	090

51535

51535 Cystotomy for excision, incision, or repair of ureterocele

(For bilateral procedure, report 51535 with modifier 50)

(For transurethral excision, use 52300)

AMA Coding Notes

Surgical Procedures on the Urinary System

(For provision of chemotherapeutic agents, report both the specific service in addition to code(s) for the specific substance(s) or drug(s) provided)

Plain English Description

A ureterocele is a congenital cystic dilation of the submucosa of the ureter occurring in the distal aspect near the ureterovesical junction and protruding into the bladder. A midline extraperitoneal abdominal approach is used to expose the bladder. The rectus and transversalis fascia are divided and the incision is carried down through the space of Retzius. The anterior bladder wall and vesical neck are identified. The bladder dome is incised and the bladder wall is inspected including the trigone, ureteral orifices, and bladder neck. The ureterocele is identified. One of three surgical interventions is then used to treat the ureterocele: excision, incision, or repair. Excision involves making a circumferential incision around the ureterocele using electrocautery and removing the dilated submucosal tissue. Incision is used to deflate the ureterocele. The full-thickness incision begins at the roof of the ureterocele. The incision is extended to the base of the defect. Repair involves excision of the ureterocele using electrocautery and then repairing any defects in the ureteral or bladder wall associated with the ureterocele.

Cystotomy for excision, incision, or repair of ureterocele

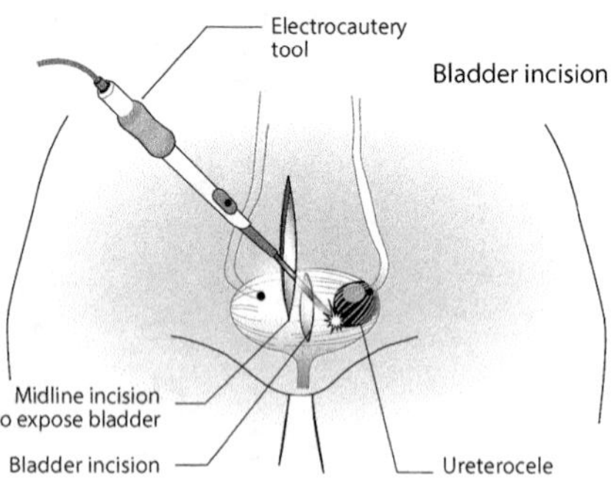

ICD-10-CM Diagnostic Codes

Q62.31	Congenital ureterocele, orthotopic
Q62.32	Cecoureterocele

CCI Edits

Refer to Appendix A for CCI edits.

Facility RVUs

Code	Work	PE Facility	MP	Total Facility
51535	13.90	7.26	1.65	22.81

Non-facility RVUs

Code	Work	PE Non-Facility	MP	Total Non-Facility
51535	13.90	7.26	1.65	22.81

Modifiers (PAR)

Code	Mod 50	Mod 51	Mod 62	Mod 66	Mod 80
51535	1	2	1	0	2

Global Period

Code	Days
51535	090

51550-51565

51550 Cystectomy, partial; simple
51555 Cystectomy, partial; complicated (eg, postradiation, previous surgery, difficult location)
51565 Cystectomy, partial, with reimplantation of ureter(s) into bladder (ureteroneocystostomy)

AMA Coding Notes

Surgical Procedures on the Urinary System

(For provision of chemotherapeutic agents, report both the specific service in addition to code(s) for the specific substance(s) or drug(s) provided)

Plain English Description

Partial cystectomy is typically performed for localized malignant neoplasm of the bladder. The bladder is exposed using a low midline or transverse suprapubic incision. Lesions in the posterior bladder are typically approached intraperitoneally while lesions in the dome or anterior bladder are approached extraperitoneally. Separately reportable pelvic lymph node dissection is performed as needed. The bladder is then mobilized. Stay sutures are strategically placed at a site distant from the lesion. The bladder is incised between the stay sutures and enlarged to allow good visualization of the lesion. The portion of the bladder containing the lesion is then excised along with overlying perivesical fat and peritoneum, taking care to remove a margin of healthy tissue as well. The submucosa and muscle of the bladder wall are closed in layers. For 51550, a simple partial cystectomy is performed, which includes initial bladder procedures and/or those where the lesion is easily accessible. For 51555, a complicated procedure is performed, which includes those where a previous bladder surgery has been performed, the patient has received radiation treatment affecting the lower abdomen or bladder, or lesions are difficult to access. For 51565, ureteral re-implantation is also performed. Ureteral re-implantation is required when the ureteral orifice must be sacrificed in order to ensure complete removal of the lesion. The site for the re-implantation is selected and incised. A submucosal tunnel is created from the incision site to the desired exit site of the ureter. The ureter is passed through the tunnel and secured with sutures.

Cystectomy, partial

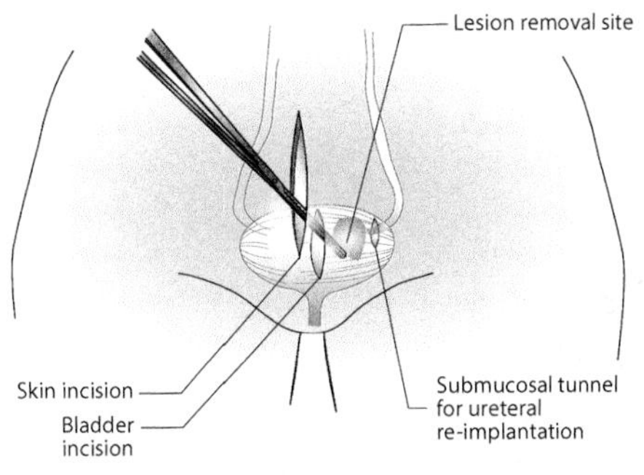

Simple (51550); complicated (51555); with reimplantation of ureter(s) into bladder (51565)

ICD-10-CM Diagnostic Codes

C67.0	Malignant neoplasm of trigone of bladder
C67.1	Malignant neoplasm of dome of bladder
C67.2	Malignant neoplasm of lateral wall of bladder
C67.3	Malignant neoplasm of anterior wall of bladder
C67.4	Malignant neoplasm of posterior wall of bladder
C67.5	Malignant neoplasm of bladder neck
C67.6	Malignant neoplasm of ureteric orifice
C67.8	Malignant neoplasm of overlapping sites of bladder
C79.11	Secondary malignant neoplasm of bladder
D09.0	Carcinoma in situ of bladder

CCI Edits

Refer to Appendix A for CCI edits.

Facility RVUs

Code	Work	PE Facility	MP	Total Facility
51550	17.23	8.65	2.33	28.21
51555	23.18	10.73	2.98	36.89
51565	23.68	11.12	2.83	37.63

Non-facility RVUs

Code	Work	PE Non-Facility	MP	Total Non-Facility
51550	17.23	8.65	2.33	28.21
51555	23.18	10.73	2.98	36.89
51565	23.68	11.12	2.83	37.63

Modifiers (PAR)

Code	Mod 50	Mod 51	Mod 62	Mod 66	Mod 80
51550	0	2	1	0	2
51555	0	2	1	0	2
51565	0	2	1	0	2

Global Period

Code	Days
51550	090
51555	090
51565	090

51570-51575

51570 Cystectomy, complete; (separate procedure)

51575 Cystectomy, complete; with bilateral pelvic lymphadenectomy, including external iliac, hypogastric, and obturator nodes

AMA Coding Notes

Surgical Procedures on the Urinary System

(For provision of chemotherapeutic agents, report both the specific service in addition to code(s) for the specific substance(s) or drug(s) provided)

AMA *CPT® Assistant*

51570: Spring 93: 35

51575: Spring 93: 35

Plain English Description

Complete cystectomy is performed for conditions such as malignant neoplasm, severe radiation or chemical cystitis, refractory interstitial cystitis, hemorrhagic cystitis, neurogenic bladder disease, severe incontinence, trauma, fistula, upper urinary tract obstruction, or refractory urethral stricture. When urinary diversion has been performed during a previous surgical encounter, an extraperitoneal approach is typically used. The bladder is exposed using a low midline or transverse suprapubic incision. Overlying fascia is divided and the space of Retzius is entered. Pelvic lymph node dissection is performed as needed. Fatty tissue is stripped from the mid-portion of the common iliac vessels bilaterally and from the internal and external iliac vessels to the level of the circumflex iliac vein. Iliac, hypogastric, and obturator nodes are excised bilaterally. Following pelvic lymphadenectomy, blunt and sharp dissection is used to separate the parietal peritoneum from the dome and posterior wall of the bladder. The superior bladder (vesical) pedicles are clamped and divided. Any remaining portions of the distal ureters are freed from surrounding structures. Dissection of the posterior bladder, bladder neck, and base of the bladder continues until the entire bladder is completely freed from all surrounding structures. The lateral vascular pedicles are ligated and divided. The urethra is divided and the bladder is removed. If complete cystectomy is performed without pelvic lymphadenectomy, use code 51570; if pelvic lymphadenectomy is performed, use code 51575.

Cystectomy, complete

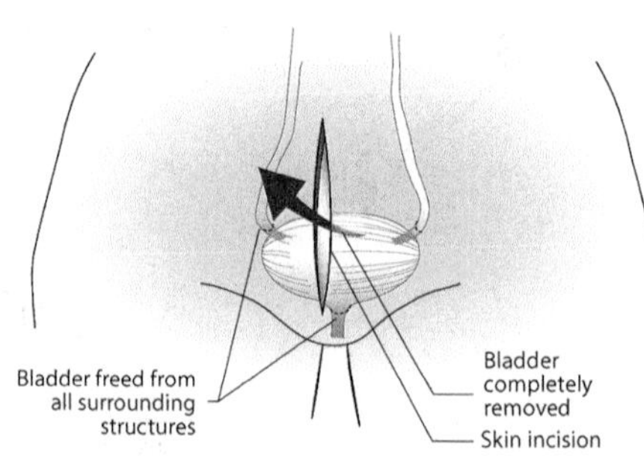

For separate procedure (51570); with bilateral pelvic lymphadenectomy, including external iliac, hypogastric, and obturator nodes (51575)

ICD-10-CM Diagnostic Codes

C67.0	Malignant neoplasm of trigone of bladder
C67.1	Malignant neoplasm of dome of bladder
C67.2	Malignant neoplasm of lateral wall of bladder
C67.3	Malignant neoplasm of anterior wall of bladder
C67.4	Malignant neoplasm of posterior wall of bladder
C67.5	Malignant neoplasm of bladder neck
C67.6	Malignant neoplasm of ureteric orifice
C67.8	Malignant neoplasm of overlapping sites of bladder
C77.5	Secondary and unspecified malignant neoplasm of intrapelvic lymph nodes
C79.11	Secondary malignant neoplasm of bladder
D09.0	Carcinoma in situ of bladder
N30.10	Interstitial cystitis (chronic) without hematuria
N30.11	Interstitial cystitis (chronic) with hematuria

CCI Edits

Refer to Appendix A for CCI edits.

Facility RVUs

Code	Work	PE Facility	MP	Total Facility
51570	27.46	12.11	3.34	42.91
51575	34.18	14.73	4.20	53.11

Non-facility RVUs

Code	Work	PE Non-Facility	MP	Total Non-Facility
51570	27.46	12.11	3.34	42.91
51575	34.18	14.73	4.20	53.11

Modifiers (PAR)

Code	Mod 50	Mod 51	Mod 62	Mod 66	Mod 80
51570	0	2	1	0	2
51575	2	2	1	0	2

Global Period

Code	Days
51570	090
51575	090

51580-51585

51580 Cystectomy, complete, with ureterosigmoidostomy or ureterocutaneous transplantations

51585 Cystectomy, complete, with ureterosigmoidostomy or ureterocutaneous transplantations; with bilateral pelvic lymphadenectomy, including external iliac, hypogastric, and obturator nodes

AMA Coding Notes

Surgical Procedures on the Urinary System

(For provision of chemotherapeutic agents, report both the specific service in addition to code(s) for the specific substance(s) or drug(s) provided)

Plain English Description

The entire bladder is removed, and the ureters are connected to the large intestine or the skin surface to drain urine. When urinary diversion is performed in conjunction with complete cystectomy, an intraperitoneal approach is used. The abdomen is incised in the midline. Prior to opening the peritoneum, pelvic lymph nodes are dissected as needed. Fatty tissue is stripped from the mid-portion of the common iliac vessels bilaterally and from the internal and external iliac vessels to the level of the circumflex iliac vein. Iliac, hypogastric, and obturator nodes are excised bilaterally. The peritoneum opened. The small bowel is isolated and packed out of the surgical field. The ureters are exposed and mobilized, taking care to preserve perirenal tissue and blood supply. The ureters are divided as close to the ureterovesical junction as possible. A segment of the sigmoid colon is selected and mobilized. A tunnel is created from the sigmoid colon to the ureters. The ureters are pulled through the tunnel and into the lumen of the sigmoid colon. The ends of the ureters are spatulated along the anterior aspect. Stents are placed in both ureters. The ureters are anastomosed to the sigmoid colon. The stents are then pulled through the colon exiting through the anus. Alternatively, the ureters may be transplanted to the skin. Following mobilization of the ureters, a catheter is passed through each ureter and into the renal pelvis. The catheters may be left in place and attached to the skin or a stoma may be created the ureters sutured to the stoma. Following completion of the urinary diversion procedure, blunt and sharp dissection is used to mobilize the bladder. The superior bladder (vesical) pedicles are clamped and divided. Any remaining portions of the distal ureters are freed from surrounding structures. Dissection continues until the entire bladder is completely freed from all surrounding structures. The lateral vascular pedicles are ligated and divided. The urethra is divided and the bladder is removed. Drains are placed as needed and surgical incisions are closed in layers. If the procedure is performed without pelvic lymphadenectomy, use code 51580; if pelvic lymphadenectomy is performed, use code 51585.

Cystectomy, complete

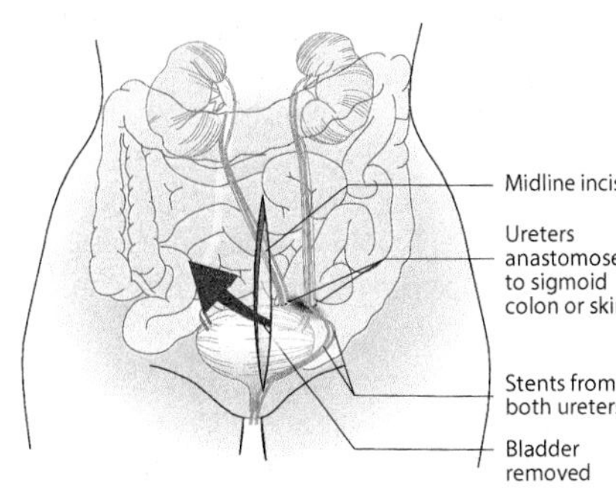

With ureterosigmoidostomy or ureterocutaneous transplantations (51580); with bilateral pelvic lymphadenectomy, including external iliac, hypogastric, and obturator nodes (51585)

ICD-10-CM Diagnostic Codes

C67.0	Malignant neoplasm of trigone of bladder
C67.1	Malignant neoplasm of dome of bladder
C67.2	Malignant neoplasm of lateral wall of bladder
C67.3	Malignant neoplasm of anterior wall of bladder
C67.4	Malignant neoplasm of posterior wall of bladder
C67.5	Malignant neoplasm of bladder neck
C67.7	Malignant neoplasm of urachus
C67.8	Malignant neoplasm of overlapping sites of bladder
C77.5	Secondary and unspecified malignant neoplasm of intrapelvic lymph nodes
C79.11	Secondary malignant neoplasm of bladder
D09.0	Carcinoma in situ of bladder

CCI Edits

Refer to Appendix A for CCI edits.

Facility RVUs

Code	Work	PE Facility	MP	Total Facility
51580	35.37	15.69	4.22	55.28
51585	39.64	17.13	4.74	61.51

Non-facility RVUs

Code	Work	PE Non-Facility	MP	Total Non-Facility
51580	35.37	15.69	4.22	55.28
51585	39.64	17.13	4.74	61.51

Modifiers (PAR)

Code	Mod 50	Mod 51	Mod 62	Mod 66	Mod 80
51580	0	2	1	0	2
51585	2	2	1	0	2

Global Period

Code	Days
51580	090
51585	090

51590-51595

51590 Cystectomy, complete, with ureteroileal conduit or sigmoid bladder, including intestine anastomosis

51595 Cystectomy, complete, with ureteroileal conduit or sigmoid bladder, including intestine anastomosis; with bilateral pelvic lymphadenectomy, including external iliac, hypogastric, and obturator nodes

AMA Coding Notes

Surgical Procedures on the Urinary System

(For provision of chemotherapeutic agents, report both the specific service in addition to code(s) for the specific substance(s) or drug(s) provided)

Plain English Description

When urinary diversion is performed in conjunction with complete cystectomy, an intraperitoneal approach is used. The abdomen is incised in the midline. Prior to opening the peritoneum, pelvic lymph nodes are dissected as needed. Fatty tissue is stripped from the mid-portion of the common iliac vessels bilaterally and from the internal and external iliac vessels to the level of the circumflex iliac vein. Iliac, hypogastric, and obturator nodes are excised bilaterally. The peritoneum is opened. The small bowel is isolated and packed out of the surgical field. The ureters are exposed and mobilized, taking care to preserve perirenal tissue and blood supply. The ureters are divided as close to the ureterovesical junction as possible. Either a segment of ileum or sigmoid colon is isolated depending on whether a ureteroileal conduit or sigmoid bladder is constructed. The remaining bowel segments distal and proximal to the isolated segment are anastomosed and bowel continuity is resorted. A separate abdominal or perineal incision is made for creation of the stoma through which urine will be expelled. Dissection is carried down to the anterior rectus fascia, which is incised. The rectus muscle is divided using blunt dissection. If an ileal conduit is constructed, the distal end of the conduit is pulled through the abdominal wall, everted, and sutured to skin or subcutaneous tissues to create the stoma. The proximal end of the conduit is closed with sutures. A tunnel is created from the conduit to the ureters. The ureters are pulled through the tunnel to the conduit. The ends of the ureters are spatulated. Stents are placed in both ureters. Small incisions are made in the conduit and the ureters are anastomosed to the conduit approximately 3 cm apart.

If a sigmoid bladder is constructed, the sigmoid bladder is fashioned. A tunnel is created from the sigmoid bladder to the ureters. The ureters are pulled through the tunnel to the sigmoid bladder and into the lumen of the sigmoid. The ends of the ureters are spatulated along the anterior aspect. Stents are placed in both ureters. The ureters are anastomosed to the sigmoid bladder approximately 3 cm apart. The sigmoid bladder is exteriorized through the stomal incision, folded back on itself (everted), and sutured to the skin or subcutaneous tissue, creating either an abdominal or perineal colostomy. An ostomy bag is secured over the ostomy site. Following completion of the urinary diversion procedure, blunt and sharp dissection is used to mobilize the bladder. The superior bladder (vesical) pedicles are clamped and divided. Any remaining portions of the distal ureters are freed from surrounding structures. Dissection continues until the entire bladder is completely freed from all surrounding structures. The lateral vascular pedicles are ligated and divided. The urethra is divided and the bladder is removed. Drains are placed as needed and surgical incisions are closed in layers. If the procedure is performed without pelvic lymphadenectomy, use code 51590; if pelvic lymphadenectomy is performed, use code 51595.

Cystectomy, complete

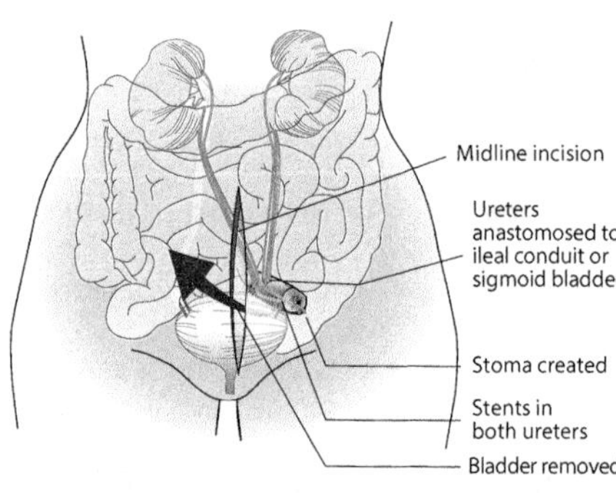

With ureteroileal conduit or sigmoid bladder, including intestine anastomosis (51590); with pelvic lymphadenectomy (51595)

ICD-10-CM Diagnostic Codes

C67.0	Malignant neoplasm of trigone of bladder
C67.1	Malignant neoplasm of dome of bladder
C67.2	Malignant neoplasm of lateral wall of bladder
C67.3	Malignant neoplasm of anterior wall of bladder
C67.4	Malignant neoplasm of posterior wall of bladder
C67.5	Malignant neoplasm of bladder neck
C67.6	Malignant neoplasm of ureteric orifice
C67.8	Malignant neoplasm of overlapping sites of bladder
C77.5	Secondary and unspecified malignant neoplasm of intrapelvic lymph nodes
C79.11	Secondary malignant neoplasm of bladder
D09.0	Carcinoma in situ of bladder

CCI Edits

Refer to Appendix A for CCI edits.

Facility RVUs ☐

Code	Work	PE Facility	MP	Total Facility
51590	36.33	15.50	4.50	56.33
51595	41.32	17.38	5.00	63.70

Non-facility RVUs ☐

Code	Work	PE Non-Facility	MP	Total Non-Facility
51590	36.33	15.50	4.50	56.33
51595	41.32	17.38	5.00	63.70

Modifiers (PAR) ☐

Code	Mod 50	Mod 51	Mod 62	Mod 66	Mod 80
51590	0	2	1	0	2
51595	2	2	1	0	2

Global Period

Code	Days
51590	090
51595	090

51596

51596 Cystectomy, complete, with continent diversion, any open technique, using any segment of small and/or large intestine to construct neobladder

AMA Coding Notes

Surgical Procedures on the Urinary System

(For provision of chemotherapeutic agents, report both the specific service in addition to code(s) for the specific substance(s) or drug(s) provided)

Plain English Description

Bladder resection is performed in conjunction with continent urinary diversion. Continent urinary diversion differs from other urinary diversion procedures in that the patient may void normally through the urethra. Alternatively, a stoma may be created with a valve mechanism using intussuscepted colon that prevents leakage of urine. With this type of stoma, the patient removes urine by periodically catheterizing the pouch. The abdomen is incised in the midline. The small bowel is isolated and packed out of the surgical field. The ureters are exposed, mobilized, and divided distally near the ureterovesical junction and the ureteral stumps are ligated. Blunt and sharp dissection is used to mobilize the bladder. The superior bladder (vesical) pedicles are clamped and divided. Any remaining portions of the distal ureters are freed from surrounding structures. Dissection continues until the entire bladder is completely freed from all surrounding structures. The lateral vascular pedicles are ligated and divided. The urethra is divided and the bladder is removed. A segment of small or large intestine is selected and mobilized. The segment, usually 30-35 cm of intestine, from which the pouch is to be constructed, is isolated. The intestine is divided, leaving the isolated segment attached to the mesenteric pedicle and keeping blood supply intact. The remaining distal and proximal portions of the intestine are then anastomosed and bowel continuity is restored. The intestinal pouch is fashioned by arranging the isolated segment in a U or W configuration. The segment is incised longitudinally along the mesenteric border to detubularize it. The intestine is fashioned into a pouch. A tunnel is created from the pouch to the ureters. The ureters are pulled through the tunnel to the pouch. The ends of the ureters are spatulated along the anterior aspect and anastomosed to the pouch approximately 3 cm apart. The distal aspect of the pouch may be incised and anastomosed to the bladder neck in females or the proximal urethra in males. Alternatively, a stoma may be created through a separate incision. When a stoma is created, the pouch is configured and detubularized as described above except for the portion of intestine that will be used to form the valve. The remaining tubular segment is scarified using electrocautery and adjacent mesentery is excised. The scarified segment is telescoped (intussuscepted) into the pouch and secured with sutures, creating the valve. The valve component is then sutured to the previously prepared stoma site in the abdominal wall. A catheter is placed through the valve into the stoma. Drains are placed as needed and surgical incisions are closed in layers.

Cystectomy, complete, with continent diversion, any open technique, neobladder construction

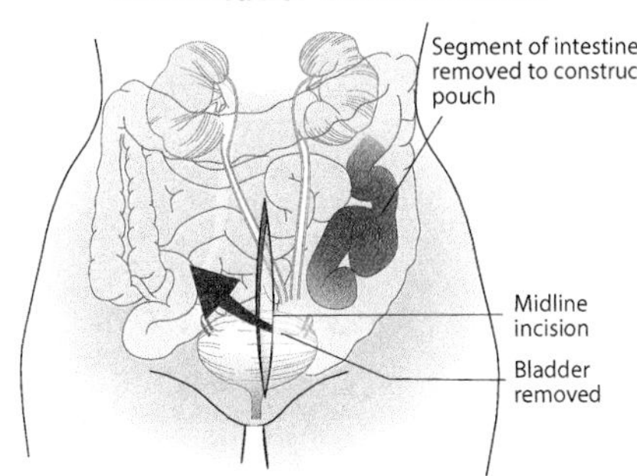

ICD-10-CM Diagnostic Codes

C67.0	Malignant neoplasm of trigone of bladder
C67.1	Malignant neoplasm of dome of bladder
C67.2	Malignant neoplasm of lateral wall of bladder
C67.3	Malignant neoplasm of anterior wall of bladder
C67.4	Malignant neoplasm of posterior wall of bladder
C67.5	Malignant neoplasm of bladder neck
C67.6	Malignant neoplasm of ureteric orifice
C67.8	Malignant neoplasm of overlapping sites of bladder
D09.0	Carcinoma in situ of bladder
D30.3	Benign neoplasm of bladder
N13.0	Hydronephrosis with ureteropelvic junction obstruction
N30.10	Interstitial cystitis (chronic) without hematuria
N30.11	Interstitial cystitis (chronic) with hematuria

CCI Edits

Refer to Appendix A for CCI edits.

Facility RVUs ☐

Code	Work	PE Facility	MP	Total Facility
51596	44.26	18.97	5.39	68.62

Non-facility RVUs ☐

Code	Work	PE Non-Facility	MP	Total Non-Facility
51596	44.26	18.97	5.39	68.62

Modifiers (PAR) ☐

Code	Mod 50	Mod 51	Mod 62	Mod 66	Mod 80
51596	0	2	1	0	2

Global Period

Code	Days
51596	090

51597

51597 Pelvic exenteration, complete, for vesical, prostatic or urethral malignancy, with removal of bladder and ureteral transplantations, with or without hysterectomy and/or abdominoperineal resection of rectum and colon and colostomy, or any combination thereof

(For pelvic exenteration for gynecologic malignancy, use 58240)

AMA Coding Notes

Surgical Procedures on the Urinary System

(For provision of chemotherapeutic agents, report both the specific service in addition to code(s) for the specific substance(s) or drug(s) provided)

Plain English Description

Pelvic exenteration is performed to treat a primary bladder, prostatic, and/or urethral malignancy that has spread to other pelvic tissues or organs. The extent of the procedure depends on which organs have metastatic disease. The procedure includes removal of the bladder with urinary diversion and resection of the rectum and colon with colostomy as needed. Reproductive organs may also be removed if they have not been removed during a previous surgery. Females will have the uterus, ovaries, fallopian tubes, and cervix removed. Males will have the prostate removed. The abdomen is opened and explored. The liver, peritoneum, bowel, and aortic and pelvic lymph nodes are inspected. Biopsies are taken as needed. The pararectal, paravesical, and Retzius spaces are opened. If a total hysterectomy is needed, the round ligaments are cut and tied. The broad ligaments are opened. The infundibulopelvic ligaments are clamped, cut, and tied along with the ovarian vessels. If a prostatectomy is needed, the prostate is dissected free of surrounding tissues and removed. The retroperitoneal space is opened and the ureters are exposed. The hypogastric artery is identified and divided. The cardinal ligaments are divided. The ureters are dissected free of surrounding tissue, ligated, and divided. The rectal space between the rectosigmoid colon and the sacrum/coccyx is developed. The sigmoid arcade and superior vessels are ligated. The rectosigmoid colon is divided. The rectum is elevated and freed from surrounding tissues. The bladder is freed from the pubic symphysis. The urethra, rectum, and vagina are divided below the level of the malignancy. All involved pelvic organs are removed, including some or all of the following: ovaries, tubes, uterus, cervix, bladder, distal ureters, rectum, and colon. Following removal of involved organs, the rectum and colon are anastomosed or a colostomy is performed. The proximal ureters are then transplanted to provide urinary diversion. If noncontinent diversion is employed, a ureteroileal conduit may be created by implanting the ureters in a segment of ileum that is then brought out in a cutaneous stoma. Alternatively, a continent pouch using the right colon may be developed. The exenterated pelvis is reconstructed using omental, myocutaneous, and/or muscle flaps.

Complete pelvic exenteration

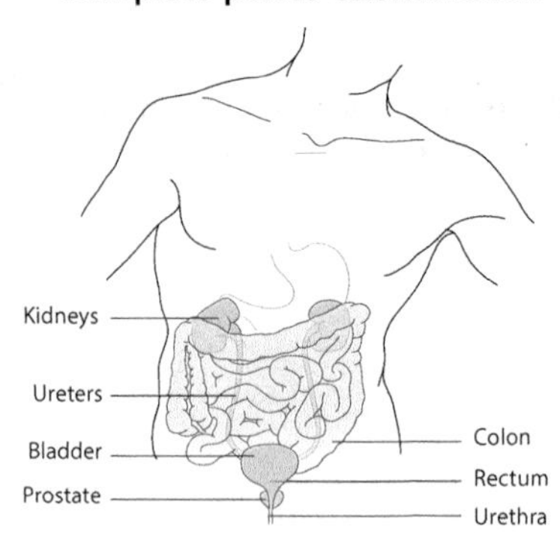

Lower urinary system is removed, including lower ureters, urethra, prostate, and lymph nodes. All or part of the uterus, rectum, or colon may also be removed.

ICD-10-CM Diagnostic Codes

C61	Malignant neoplasm of prostate ♂
C67.0	Malignant neoplasm of trigone of bladder
C67.1	Malignant neoplasm of dome of bladder
C67.2	Malignant neoplasm of lateral wall of bladder
C67.3	Malignant neoplasm of anterior wall of bladder
C67.4	Malignant neoplasm of posterior wall of bladder
C67.5	Malignant neoplasm of bladder neck
C67.6	Malignant neoplasm of ureteric orifice
C67.8	Malignant neoplasm of overlapping sites of bladder
C68.0	Malignant neoplasm of urethra
C68.1	Malignant neoplasm of paraurethral glands
C77.2	Secondary and unspecified malignant neoplasm of intra-abdominal lymph nodes
C77.4	Secondary and unspecified malignant neoplasm of inguinal and lower limb lymph nodes
C77.5	Secondary and unspecified malignant neoplasm of intrapelvic lymph nodes
C78.6	Secondary malignant neoplasm of retroperitoneum and peritoneum
C79.10	Secondary malignant neoplasm of unspecified urinary organs
C79.11	Secondary malignant neoplasm of bladder
C79.19	Secondary malignant neoplasm of other urinary organs
C79.82	Secondary malignant neoplasm of genital organs

CCI Edits

Refer to Appendix A for CCI edits.

Facility RVUs ☐

Code	Work	PE Facility	MP	Total Facility
51597	42.86	18.74	5.43	67.03

Non-facility RVUs ☐

Code	Work	PE Non-Facility	MP	Total Non-Facility
51597	42.86	18.74	5.43	67.03

Modifiers (PAR) ☐

Code	Mod 50	Mod 51	Mod 62	Mod 66	Mod 80
51597	0	2	1	0	2

Global Period

Code	Days
51597	090

51600

51600 Injection procedure for cystography or voiding urethrocystography

(For radiological supervision and interpretation, see 74430, 74455)

AMA Coding Notes

Surgical Procedures on the Urinary System

(For provision of chemotherapeutic agents, report both the specific service in addition to code(s) for the specific substance(s) or drug(s) provided)

AMA *CPT® Assistant*

51600: Oct 19: 11

Plain English Description

Contrast media is instilled into the bladder using a technique other than retrograde injection of contrast. For example, if the patient has a suprapubic catheter, contrast is injected through the existing catheter. For cystography, separately reportable radiographs are taken of the bladder as it is filled with contrast. Any filling abnormalities are noted. For voiding cystourethrography, separately reportable radiographs are taken as the bladder is filled and additional radiographs are obtained of the bladder and urethra as the bladder is emptied.

Injection procedure for cystography or voiding urethrocystography

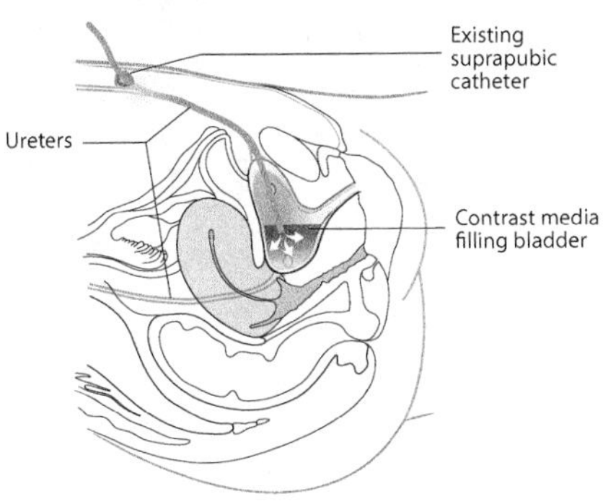

ICD-10-CM Diagnostic Codes

N13.0	Hydronephrosis with ureteropelvic junction obstruction
N13.1	Hydronephrosis with ureteral stricture, not elsewhere classified
N39.3	Stress incontinence (female) (male)
N39.41	Urge incontinence
N39.42	Incontinence without sensory awareness
N39.43	Post-void dribbling
N39.44	Nocturnal enuresis
N39.45	Continuous leakage
N39.46	Mixed incontinence
N39.490	Overflow incontinence
N39.491	Coital incontinence
N39.492	Postural (urinary) incontinence
N39.498	Other specified urinary incontinence
Q64.31	Congenital bladder neck obstruction
Q64.39	Other atresia and stenosis of urethra and bladder neck
Q64.79	Other congenital malformations of bladder and urethra
Q64.8	Other specified congenital malformations of urinary system
R31.0	Gross hematuria
R31.1	Benign essential microscopic hematuria
R31.21	Asymptomatic microscopic hematuria
R31.29	Other microscopic hematuria
R33.0	Drug induced retention of urine
R33.8	Other retention of urine

CCI Edits

Refer to Appendix A for CCI edits.

Pub 100

51600: Pub 100-03, 1, 220.5

Facility RVUs

Code	Work	PE Facility	MP	Total Facility
51600	0.88	0.31	0.09	1.28

Non-facility RVUs

Code	Work	PE Non-Facility	MP	Total Non-Facility
51600	0.88	5.56	0.09	6.53

Modifiers (PAR)

Code	Mod 50	Mod 51	Mod 62	Mod 66	Mod 80
51600	0	2	0	0	1

Global Period

Code	Days
51600	000

51605

51605 Injection procedure and placement of chain for contrast and/or chain urethrocystography

(For radiological supervision and interpretation, use 74430)

AMA Coding Notes

Surgical Procedures on the Urinary System

(For provision of chemotherapeutic agents, report both the specific service in addition to code(s) for the specific substance(s) or drug(s) provided)

Plain English Description

A tube containing a beaded chain and catheter are introduced through the urethra. Contrast is injected. Separately reportable radiographs are obtained. Chain cystourethrography is an outdated diagnostic procedure that was used to evaluate stress incontinence in women. The chain allowed assessment of urethral hypermobility and the degree of bladder descent. This procedure has largely been replaced by video urodynamic studies.

Injection procedure and placement of chain for contrast and/or chain urethrocystography

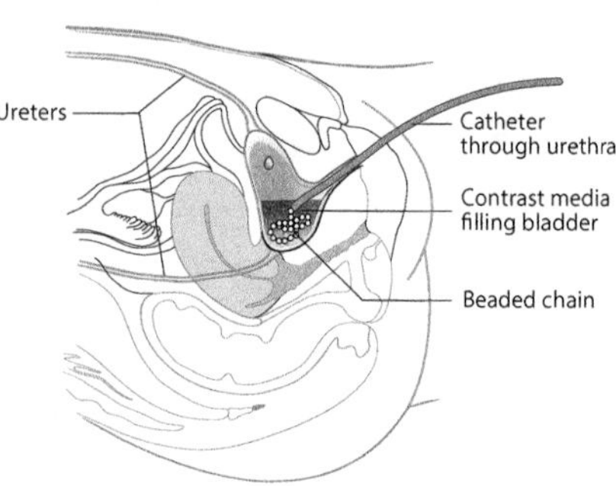

ICD-10-CM Diagnostic Codes

N30.00	Acute cystitis without hematuria
N30.01	Acute cystitis with hematuria
N30.20	Other chronic cystitis without hematuria
N30.21	Other chronic cystitis with hematuria
N30.30	Trigonitis without hematuria
N30.31	Trigonitis with hematuria
N30.40	Irradiation cystitis without hematuria
N30.41	Irradiation cystitis with hematuria
N30.80	Other cystitis without hematuria
N30.81	Other cystitis with hematuria
N32.2	Vesical fistula, not elsewhere classified
N32.81	Overactive bladder
N35.021	Urethral stricture due to childbirth ♀
N36.8	Other specified disorders of urethra
N37	Urethral disorders in diseases classified elsewhere
N39.3	Stress incontinence (female) (male)
N39.41	Urge incontinence
N39.42	Incontinence without sensory awareness
N39.43	Post-void dribbling
N39.44	Nocturnal enuresis
N39.45	Continuous leakage
N39.46	Mixed incontinence
N39.490	Overflow incontinence
N39.498	Other specified urinary incontinence
N39.8	Other specified disorders of urinary system
Q64.31	Congenital bladder neck obstruction
Q64.39	Other atresia and stenosis of urethra and bladder neck
Q64.71	Congenital prolapse of urethra
Q64.72	Congenital prolapse of urinary meatus
Q64.79	Other congenital malformations of bladder and urethra
Q64.8	Other specified congenital malformations of urinary system

CCI Edits

Refer to Appendix A for CCI edits.

Facility RVUs ☐

Code	Work	PE Facility	MP	Total Facility
51605	0.64	0.40	0.09	1.13

Non-facility RVUs ☐

Code	Work	PE Non-Facility	MP	Total Non-Facility
51605	0.64	0.40	0.09	1.13

Modifiers (PAR) ☐

Code	Mod 50	Mod 51	Mod 62	Mod 66	Mod 80
51605	0	2	0	0	1

Global Period

Code	Days
51605	000

51610

51610 Injection procedure for retrograde urethrocystography

(For radiological supervision and interpretation, use 74450)

AMA Coding Notes

Surgical Procedures on the Urinary System

(For provision of chemotherapeutic agents, report both the specific service in addition to code(s) for the specific substance(s) or drug(s) provided)

AMA *CPT® Assistant* ◻

51610: Jan 16: 3, Oct 19: 11, Jan 21: 11

Plain English Description

Retrograde cystourethrography is performed to evaluate the size, shape, and capacity of the bladder and urethra. The physician also evaluates whether there is any vesicoureteral reflux, which is reverse flow of urine back into the ureters and kidneys. The urethral orifice is cleansed with antiseptic. A sterile catheter is inserted through the urethra into the bladder. Contrast media is then instilled into the bladder. Separately reportable radiographs are taken of the bladder as it is filled with contrast. Any filling abnormalities are noted. The patient may be asked to strain, or pressure may be applied to the abdomen to see if there is any reflux into the ureters and kidneys. The head of the X-ray table may be lowered and additional radiographs taken. The catheter is then removed and additional radiographs are obtained of the bladder and urethra as the bladder is emptied.

Injection procedure for retrograde urethrocystography

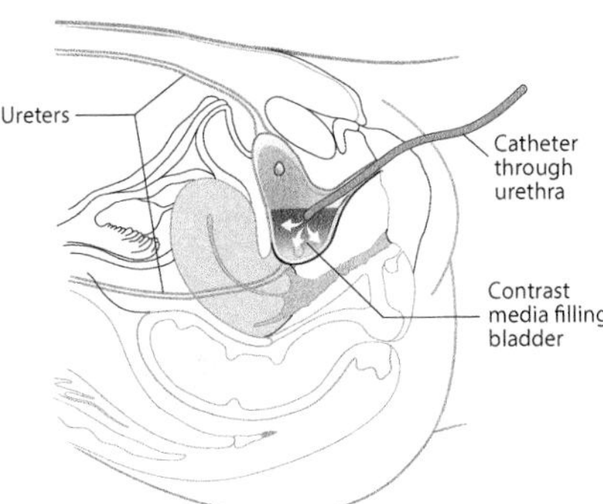

ICD-10-CM Diagnostic Codes

C67.0	Malignant neoplasm of trigone of bladder
C67.1	Malignant neoplasm of dome of bladder
C67.2	Malignant neoplasm of lateral wall of bladder
C67.3	Malignant neoplasm of anterior wall of bladder
C67.4	Malignant neoplasm of posterior wall of bladder
C67.5	Malignant neoplasm of bladder neck
C67.8	Malignant neoplasm of overlapping sites of bladder
D30.3	Benign neoplasm of bladder
D30.4	Benign neoplasm of urethra
D30.8	Benign neoplasm of other specified urinary organs
D49.4	Neoplasm of unspecified behavior of bladder
N13.0	Hydronephrosis with ureteropelvic junction obstruction
N13.1	Hydronephrosis with ureteral stricture, not elsewhere classified
N13.2	Hydronephrosis with renal and ureteral calculous obstruction
N13.39	Other hydronephrosis
N13.71	Vesicoureteral-reflux without reflux nephropathy
N13.721	Vesicoureteral-reflux with reflux nephropathy without hydroureter, unilateral
N13.722	Vesicoureteral-reflux with reflux nephropathy without hydroureter, bilateral
N13.731	Vesicoureteral-reflux with reflux nephropathy with hydroureter, unilateral
N13.732	Vesicoureteral-reflux with reflux nephropathy with hydroureter, bilateral
N13.8	Other obstructive and reflux uropathy
N31.1	Reflex neuropathic bladder, not elsewhere classified
N31.2	Flaccid neuropathic bladder, not elsewhere classified
N32.3	Diverticulum of bladder
N32.81	Overactive bladder
N34.2	Other urethritis
N35.010	Post-traumatic urethral stricture, male, meatal ♂
N35.011	Post-traumatic bulbous urethral stricture ♂
N35.012	Post-traumatic membranous urethral stricture ♂
N35.013	Post-traumatic anterior urethral stricture ♂
N35.016	Post-traumatic urethral stricture, male, overlapping sites ♂
N35.021	Urethral stricture due to childbirth ♀
N35.028	Other post-traumatic urethral stricture, female ♀
N35.111	Postinfective urethral stricture, not elsewhere classified, male, meatal ♂
N35.112	Postinfective bulbous urethral stricture, not elsewhere classified, male ♂
N35.113	Postinfective membranous urethral stricture, not elsewhere classified, male ♂
N35.114	Postinfective anterior urethral stricture, not elsewhere classified, male ♂
N35.116	Postinfective urethral stricture, not elsewhere classified, male, overlapping sites ♂
N35.12	Postinfective urethral stricture, not elsewhere classified, female ♀
N35.811	Other urethral stricture, male, meatal ♂
N35.812	Other urethral bulbous stricture, male ♂
N35.813	Other membranous urethral stricture, male ♂
N35.814	Other anterior urethral stricture, male ♂
N35.816	Other urethral stricture, male, overlapping sites ♂
N36.0	Urethral fistula
N36.8	Other specified disorders of urethra
N37	Urethral disorders in diseases classified elsewhere
N39.0	Urinary tract infection, site not specified
N39.3	Stress incontinence (female) (male)
N39.43	Post-void dribbling
N39.44	Nocturnal enuresis
N39.45	Continuous leakage
N39.46	Mixed incontinence
N39.490	Overflow incontinence
N39.491	Coital incontinence
N39.492	Postural (urinary) incontinence
N39.498	Other specified urinary incontinence
N39.8	Other specified disorders of urinary system
N40.1	Benign prostatic hyperplasia with lower urinary tract symptoms ♂
N40.3	Nodular prostate with lower urinary tract symptoms ♂
N42.89	Other specified disorders of prostate ♂
N81.0	Urethrocele ♀
N81.11	Cystocele, midline ♀
N81.12	Cystocele, lateral ♀
N99.110	Postprocedural urethral stricture, male, meatal ♂
N99.111	Postprocedural bulbous urethral stricture, male ♂
N99.112	Postprocedural membranous urethral stricture, male ♂
N99.113	Postprocedural anterior bulbous urethral stricture, male ♂
N99.115	Postprocedural fossa navicularis urethral stricture ♂
N99.116	Postprocedural urethral stricture, male, overlapping sites ♂
N99.89	Other postprocedural complications and disorders of genitourinary system
Q64.2	Congenital posterior urethral valves
Q64.31	Congenital bladder neck obstruction
Q64.39	Other atresia and stenosis of urethra and bladder neck
Q64.71	Congenital prolapse of urethra
Q64.72	Congenital prolapse of urinary meatus
Q64.74	Double urethra
Q64.75	Double urinary meatus
Q64.79	Other congenital malformations of bladder and urethra
Q64.8	Other specified congenital malformations of urinary system

CCI Edits

Refer to Appendix A for CCI edits.

Facility RVUs ▯

Code	Work	PE Facility	MP	Total Facility
51610	1.05	0.70	0.11	1.86

Non-facility RVUs ▯

Code	Work	PE Non-Facility	MP	Total Non-Facility
51610	1.05	2.73	0.11	3.89

Modifiers (PAR) ▯

Code	Mod 50	Mod 51	Mod 62	Mod 66	Mod 80
51610	0	2	0	0	1

Global Period

Code	Days
51610	000

51700

51700 Bladder irrigation, simple, lavage and/or instillation

(Codes 51701-51702 are reported only when performed independently. Do not report 51701-51702 when catheter insertion is an inclusive component of another procedure.)

AMA Coding Notes

Surgical Procedures on the Urinary System

(For provision of chemotherapeutic agents, report both the specific service in addition to code(s) for the specific substance(s) or drug(s) provided)

AMA *CPT® Assistant*

51700: Jan 21: 11

Plain English Description

A lavage procedure, which involves instillation and removal of fluid or only an instillation procedure, may be performed. A catheter is inserted into the bladder. If a lavage is being performed for bladder irrigation, normal saline is instilled and then removed from the bladder. Lavage is performed to help prevent or treat blood clots in the bladder. Instillation may be performed with normal saline or a medication such as an antibiotic. Antibiotic instillation may be performed over a period of time as a continuous drip into the bladder. Once the lavage and/or instillation procedure is completed, the catheter may be removed from the bladder or left in place to drain urine.

Bladder irrigation, simple, lavage and/or instillation

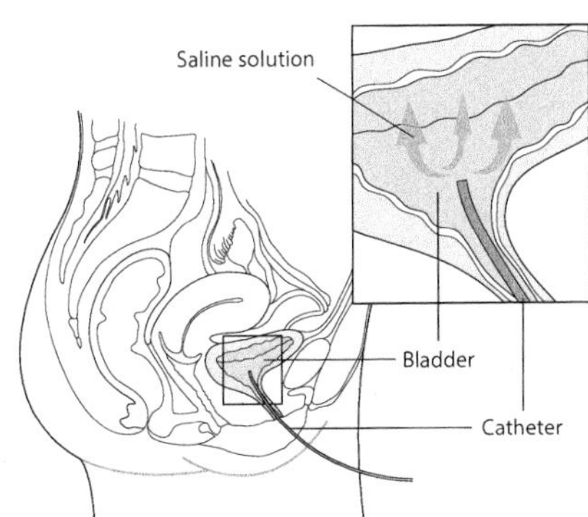

The bladder is washed with saline solution and/or medication.

ICD-10-CM Diagnostic Codes

A56.01	Chlamydial cystitis and urethritis
C67.0	Malignant neoplasm of trigone of bladder
C67.1	Malignant neoplasm of dome of bladder
C67.2	Malignant neoplasm of lateral wall of bladder
C67.3	Malignant neoplasm of anterior wall of bladder
C67.4	Malignant neoplasm of posterior wall of bladder
C67.5	Malignant neoplasm of bladder neck
C67.8	Malignant neoplasm of overlapping sites of bladder
D09.0	Carcinoma in situ of bladder
G83.4	Cauda equina syndrome
N11.1	Chronic obstructive pyelonephritis
N13.1	Hydronephrosis with ureteral stricture, not elsewhere classified
N13.5	Crossing vessel and stricture of ureter without hydronephrosis
N30.00	Acute cystitis without hematuria
N30.01	Acute cystitis with hematuria
N30.10	Interstitial cystitis (chronic) without hematuria
N30.11	Interstitial cystitis (chronic) with hematuria
N30.20	Other chronic cystitis without hematuria
N30.21	Other chronic cystitis with hematuria
N30.30	Trigonitis without hematuria
N30.31	Trigonitis with hematuria
N30.40	Irradiation cystitis without hematuria
N30.41	Irradiation cystitis with hematuria
N30.80	Other cystitis without hematuria
N30.81	Other cystitis with hematuria
N31.2	Flaccid neuropathic bladder, not elsewhere classified
N32.0	Bladder-neck obstruction
N32.89	Other specified disorders of bladder
N33	Bladder disorders in diseases classified elsewhere
N34.1	Nonspecific urethritis
N34.2	Other urethritis
N35.010	Post-traumatic urethral stricture, male, meatal ♂
N35.011	Post-traumatic bulbous urethral stricture ♂
N35.012	Post-traumatic membranous urethral stricture ♂
N35.013	Post-traumatic anterior urethral stricture ♂
N35.016	Post-traumatic urethral stricture, male, overlapping sites ♂
N35.021	Urethral stricture due to childbirth ♀
N35.028	Other post-traumatic urethral stricture, female ♀
N35.111	Postinfective urethral stricture, not elsewhere classified, male, meatal ♂
N35.112	Postinfective bulbous urethral stricture, not elsewhere classified, male ♂
N35.113	Postinfective membranous urethral stricture, not elsewhere classified, male ♂
N35.114	Postinfective anterior urethral stricture, not elsewhere classified, male ♂
N35.116	Postinfective urethral stricture, not elsewhere classified, male, overlapping sites ♂
N35.12	Postinfective urethral stricture, not elsewhere classified, female ♀
N35.811	Other urethral stricture, male, meatal ♂
N35.812	Other urethral bulbous stricture, male ♂
N35.813	Other membranous urethral stricture, male ♂
N35.814	Other anterior urethral stricture, male ♂
N35.816	Other urethral stricture, male, overlapping sites ♂
N37	Urethral disorders in diseases classified elsewhere
N39.0	Urinary tract infection, site not specified
N40.1	Benign prostatic hyperplasia with lower urinary tract symptoms ♂
N40.3	Nodular prostate with lower urinary tract symptoms ♂
N41.1	Chronic prostatitis ♂
N42.83	Cyst of prostate ♂
N81.0	Urethrocele ♀
N99.110	Postprocedural urethral stricture, male, meatal ♂
N99.111	Postprocedural bulbous urethral stricture, male ♂
N99.112	Postprocedural membranous urethral stricture, male ♂
N99.113	Postprocedural anterior bulbous urethral stricture, male ♂
N99.116	Postprocedural urethral stricture, male, overlapping sites ♂
N99.12	Postprocedural urethral stricture, female ♀
R31.0	Gross hematuria
R31.1	Benign essential microscopic hematuria
R31.21	Asymptomatic microscopic hematuria
R31.29	Other microscopic hematuria
R33.0	Drug induced retention of urine
R82.71	Bacteriuria
Z43.5	Encounter for attention to cystostomy

CCI Edits

Refer to Appendix A for CCI edits.

Facility RVUs

Code	Work	PE Facility	MP	Total Facility
51700	0.60	0.21	0.09	0.90

Non-facility RVUs

Code	Work	PE Non-Facility	MP	Total Non-Facility
51700	0.60	1.60	0.09	2.29

Modifiers (PAR)

Code	Mod 50	Mod 51	Mod 62	Mod 66	Mod 80
51700	0	2	0	0	1

Global Period

Code	Days
51700	000

51701

51701 Insertion of non-indwelling bladder catheter (eg, straight catheterization for residual urine)

AMA Coding Notes

Surgical Procedures on the Urinary System

(For provision of chemotherapeutic agents, report both the specific service in addition to code(s) for the specific substance(s) or drug(s) provided)

AMA *CPT® Assistant*

51701: Jul 06: 4, Jan 07: 31, Jul 07: 1, Jan 21: 11

Plain English Description

A non-indwelling catheter is inserted into the bladder. This may be referred to as straight catheterization. Straight catheterization is performed to empty the bladder of urine or to test for residual urine following urination, which indicates incomplete emptying of the bladder. If the patient is being checked for residual urine, the patient first empties the bladder into a container and the amount is measured. A catheter kit is prepared. The urethra is cleansed with antiseptic solution. A sterile catheter is then inserted through the urethra into the bladder. Urine is drained from the bladder and the amount of residual urine is measured.

Insertion of non-indwelling catheter

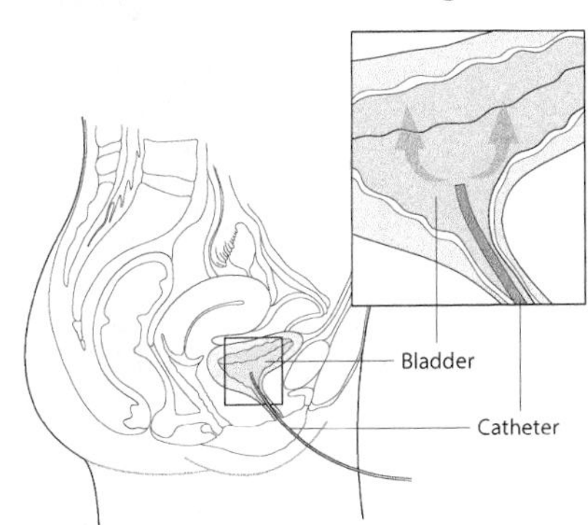

Straight catheterization is done to empty the bladder of residual urine.

ICD-10-CM Diagnostic Codes

	A56.01	Chlamydial cystitis and urethritis
	C61	Malignant neoplasm of prostate ♂
⇄	C64.1	Malignant neoplasm of right kidney, except renal pelvis
⇄	C64.2	Malignant neoplasm of left kidney, except renal pelvis
⇄	C65.1	Malignant neoplasm of right renal pelvis
⇄	C65.2	Malignant neoplasm of left renal pelvis
⇄	C66.1	Malignant neoplasm of right ureter
⇄	C66.2	Malignant neoplasm of left ureter
	C67.0	Malignant neoplasm of trigone of bladder
	C67.1	Malignant neoplasm of dome of bladder
	C67.2	Malignant neoplasm of lateral wall of bladder
	C67.3	Malignant neoplasm of anterior wall of bladder
	C67.4	Malignant neoplasm of posterior wall of bladder
	C67.5	Malignant neoplasm of bladder neck
	C67.6	Malignant neoplasm of ureteric orifice
	C67.7	Malignant neoplasm of urachus
	C68.0	Malignant neoplasm of urethra
	C68.1	Malignant neoplasm of paraurethral glands
	C7A.093	Malignant carcinoid tumor of the kidney
	D09.0	Carcinoma in situ of bladder
	G83.4	Cauda equina syndrome
	N11.1	Chronic obstructive pyelonephritis
	N13.5	Crossing vessel and stricture of ureter without hydronephrosis
	N21.0	Calculus in bladder
	N21.1	Calculus in urethra
	N30.01	Acute cystitis with hematuria
	N30.10	Interstitial cystitis (chronic) without hematuria
	N30.11	Interstitial cystitis (chronic) with hematuria
	N30.20	Other chronic cystitis without hematuria
	N30.21	Other chronic cystitis with hematuria
	N30.30	Trigonitis without hematuria
	N30.31	Trigonitis with hematuria
	N31.2	Flaccid neuropathic bladder, not elsewhere classified
	N32.81	Overactive bladder
	N34.1	Nonspecific urethritis
	N35.010	Post-traumatic urethral stricture, male, meatal ♂
	N35.011	Post-traumatic bulbous urethral stricture ♂
	N35.012	Post-traumatic membranous urethral stricture ♂
	N35.021	Urethral stricture due to childbirth ♀
	N35.111	Postinfective urethral stricture, not elsewhere classified, male, meatal ♂
	N35.112	Postinfective bulbous urethral stricture, not elsewhere classified, male ♂
	N35.113	Postinfective membranous urethral stricture, not elsewhere classified, male ♂
	N35.114	Postinfective anterior urethral stricture, not elsewhere classified, male ♂
	N35.12	Postinfective urethral stricture, not elsewhere classified, female ♀
	N36.0	Urethral fistula
	N36.1	Urethral diverticulum
	N36.2	Urethral caruncle
	N36.5	Urethral false passage
	N37	Urethral disorders in diseases classified elsewhere
	N39.3	Stress incontinence (female) (male)
	N39.45	Continuous leakage
	N39.490	Overflow incontinence
	N40.1	Benign prostatic hyperplasia with lower urinary tract symptoms ♂
	N40.3	Nodular prostate with lower urinary tract symptoms ♂
	N41.1	Chronic prostatitis ♂
	N42.83	Cyst of prostate ♂
	N81.0	Urethrocele ♀
	N81.11	Cystocele, midline ♀
	N81.12	Cystocele, lateral ♀
	N81.81	Perineocele ♀
	N81.82	Incompetence or weakening of pubocervical tissue ♀
	N81.83	Incompetence or weakening of rectovaginal tissue ♀
	N81.84	Pelvic muscle wasting ♀
	N99.0	Postprocedural (acute) (chronic) kidney failure
	N99.110	Postprocedural urethral stricture, male, meatal ♂
	N99.111	Postprocedural bulbous urethral stricture, male ♂
	N99.112	Postprocedural membranous urethral stricture, male ♂
	N99.113	Postprocedural anterior bulbous urethral stricture, male ♂
	N99.12	Postprocedural urethral stricture, female ♀
	N99.520	Hemorrhage of incontinent external stoma of urinary tract
	N99.521	Infection of incontinent external stoma of urinary tract
	N99.522	Malfunction of incontinent external stoma of urinary tract
	N99.530	Hemorrhage of continent stoma of urinary tract
	N99.531	Infection of continent stoma of urinary tract
	N99.532	Malfunction of continent stoma of urinary tract
	R30.0	Dysuria
	R30.1	Vesical tenesmus
	R31.0	Gross hematuria
	R31.1	Benign essential microscopic hematuria
	R33.0	Drug induced retention of urine
	R35.0	Frequency of micturition
	R39.14	Feeling of incomplete bladder emptying
	R39.2	Extrarenal uremia
	R39.81	Functional urinary incontinence
❼	S34.3	Injury of cauda equina
❼	S37.22	Contusion of bladder
❼	S37.23	Laceration of bladder
❼	S37.32	Contusion of urethra
❼	S37.33	Laceration of urethra

ICD-10-CM Coding Notes

For codes requiring a 7th character extension, refer to your ICD-10-CM book. Review the character descriptions and coding guidelines for proper selection. For some procedures, only certain characters will apply.

CCI Edits

Refer to Appendix A for CCI edits.

Facility RVUs

Code	Work	PE Facility	MP	Total Facility
51701	0.50	0.18	0.08	0.76

Non-facility RVUs

Code	Work	PE Non-Facility	MP	Total Non-Facility
51701	0.50	0.75	0.08	1.33

Modifiers (PAR)

Code	Mod 50	Mod 51	Mod 62	Mod 66	Mod 80
51701	0	2	0	0	1

Global Period

Code	Days
51701	000

51702-51703

51702 Insertion of temporary indwelling bladder catheter; simple (eg, Foley)

(Do not report 51702 in conjunction with 0071T, 0072T)

51703 Insertion of temporary indwelling bladder catheter; complicated (eg, altered anatomy, fractured catheter/balloon)

AMA Coding Notes

Surgical Procedures on the Urinary System

(For provision of chemotherapeutic agents, report both the specific service in addition to code(s) for the specific substance(s) or drug(s) provided)

AMA *CPT® Assistant*

51702: Oct 03: 10, Jul 06: 4, Jan 07: 31, Jul 07: 1, May 14: 3, Jan 21: 11

51703: Jan 07: 31, Jan 21: 11

Plain English Description

A temporary indwelling catheter is inserted into the bladder. This may be referred to as Foley catheterization. A catheter kit is prepared. The urethra is cleansed with antiseptic solution. A sterile Foley catheter is inserted through the urethra into the bladder. The balloon is then inflated with about 10 cc of water to keep it in place. The catheter is attached to a sterile drainage bag and urine is continuously drained from the bladder. Use 51702 for a simple catheterization procedure and 51703 for a procedure complicated by altered anatomy or a fractured catheter or balloon.

Insertion of temporary indwelling bladder catheter

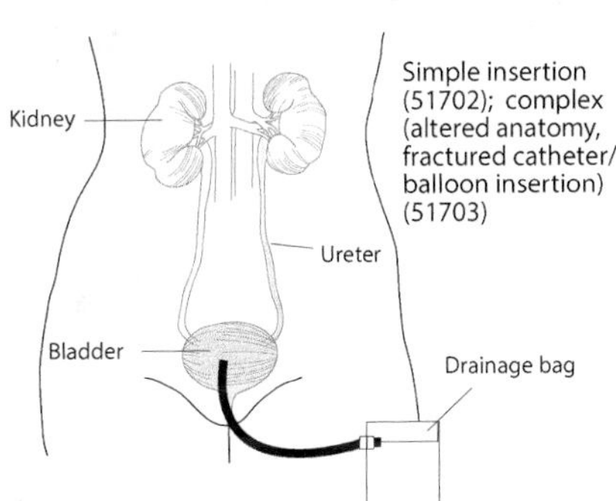

A tube is inserted through the urethra into the bladder to drain urine. The tube is connected to a drainage bag and remains in place for a short while.

ICD-10-CM Diagnostic Codes

	A56.01	Chlamydial cystitis and urethritis
	C61	Malignant neoplasm of prostate ♂
⇄	C64.1	Malignant neoplasm of right kidney, except renal pelvis
⇄	C64.2	Malignant neoplasm of left kidney, except renal pelvis
⇄	C65.1	Malignant neoplasm of right renal pelvis
⇄	C65.2	Malignant neoplasm of left renal pelvis
⇄	C66.1	Malignant neoplasm of right ureter
⇄	C66.2	Malignant neoplasm of left ureter
	C67.0	Malignant neoplasm of trigone of bladder
	C67.1	Malignant neoplasm of dome of bladder
	C67.2	Malignant neoplasm of lateral wall of bladder
	C67.3	Malignant neoplasm of anterior wall of bladder
	C67.4	Malignant neoplasm of posterior wall of bladder
	C67.5	Malignant neoplasm of bladder neck
	C67.6	Malignant neoplasm of ureteric orifice
	C67.7	Malignant neoplasm of urachus
	C68.0	Malignant neoplasm of urethra
	C68.1	Malignant neoplasm of paraurethral glands
	C7A.093	Malignant carcinoid tumor of the kidney
	D09.0	Carcinoma in situ of bladder
	G83.4	Cauda equina syndrome
	N13.1	Hydronephrosis with ureteral stricture, not elsewhere classified
	N13.5	Crossing vessel and stricture of ureter without hydronephrosis
	N21.0	Calculus in bladder
	N21.1	Calculus in urethra
	N30.00	Acute cystitis without hematuria
	N30.01	Acute cystitis with hematuria
	N30.10	Interstitial cystitis (chronic) without hematuria
	N30.11	Interstitial cystitis (chronic) with hematuria
	N30.20	Other chronic cystitis without hematuria
	N30.21	Other chronic cystitis with hematuria
	N30.30	Trigonitis without hematuria
	N30.31	Trigonitis with hematuria
	N31.2	Flaccid neuropathic bladder, not elsewhere classified
	N32.81	Overactive bladder
	N34.1	Nonspecific urethritis
	N35.010	Post-traumatic urethral stricture, male, meatal ♂
	N35.011	Post-traumatic bulbous urethral stricture ♂
	N35.012	Post-traumatic membranous urethral stricture ♂
	N35.021	Urethral stricture due to childbirth ♀
	N35.111	Postinfective urethral stricture, not elsewhere classified, male, meatal ♂
	N35.112	Postinfective bulbous urethral stricture, not elsewhere classified, male ♂
	N35.113	Postinfective membranous urethral stricture, not elsewhere classified, male ♂
	N35.114	Postinfective anterior urethral stricture, not elsewhere classified, male ♂
	N35.12	Postinfective urethral stricture, not elsewhere classified, female ♀
	N36.0	Urethral fistula
	N36.1	Urethral diverticulum
	N36.2	Urethral caruncle
	N36.5	Urethral false passage
	N37	Urethral disorders in diseases classified elsewhere
	N39.3	Stress incontinence (female) (male)
	N39.45	Continuous leakage
	N39.490	Overflow incontinence
	N39.491	Coital incontinence
	N39.492	Postural (urinary) incontinence
	N40.1	Benign prostatic hyperplasia with lower urinary tract symptoms ♂
	N40.3	Nodular prostate with lower urinary tract symptoms ♂
	N41	Inflammatory diseases of prostate
	N41.1	Chronic prostatitis ♂
	N42.83	Cyst of prostate ♂
	N81.0	Urethrocele ♀
	N81.11	Cystocele, midline ♀
	N81.12	Cystocele, lateral ♀
	N99.0	Postprocedural (acute) (chronic) kidney failure
	N99.110	Postprocedural urethral stricture, male, meatal ♂
	N99.111	Postprocedural bulbous urethral stricture, male ♂
	N99.112	Postprocedural membranous urethral stricture, male ♂
	N99.113	Postprocedural anterior bulbous urethral stricture, male ♂
	N99.12	Postprocedural urethral stricture, female ♀
	N99.520	Hemorrhage of incontinent external stoma of urinary tract
	N99.521	Infection of incontinent external stoma of urinary tract
	N99.522	Malfunction of incontinent external stoma of urinary tract
	N99.530	Hemorrhage of continent stoma of urinary tract
	N99.531	Infection of continent stoma of urinary tract
	N99.532	Malfunction of continent stoma of urinary tract
	R31.0	Gross hematuria
	R31.1	Benign essential microscopic hematuria
	R33.0	Drug induced retention of urine
	R35.0	Frequency of micturition
	R39.14	Feeling of incomplete bladder emptying
	R39.2	Extrarenal uremia
	R39.81	Functional urinary incontinence
❼	S34.3	Injury of cauda equina
❼	S37.22	Contusion of bladder
❼	S37.23	Laceration of bladder
❼	S37.32	Contusion of urethra
❼	S37.33	Laceration of urethra

ICD-10-CM Coding Notes

For codes requiring a 7th character extension, refer to your ICD-10-CM book. Review the character descriptions and coding guidelines for proper selection. For some procedures, only certain characters will apply.

CCI Edits

Refer to Appendix A for CCI edits.

Facility RVUs ▯

Code	Work	PE Facility	MP	Total Facility
51702	0.50	0.18	0.07	0.75
51703	1.47	0.58	0.19	2.24

Non-facility RVUs ▯

Code	Work	PE Non-Facility	MP	Total Non-Facility
51702	0.50	1.28	0.07	1.85
51703	1.47	2.84	0.19	4.50

Modifiers (PAR) ▯

Code	Mod 50	Mod 51	Mod 62	Mod 66	Mod 80
51702	0	2	0	0	1
51703	0	2	0	0	1

Global Period

Code	Days
51702	000
51703	000

51705-51710

51705 Change of cystostomy tube; simple

51710 Change of cystostomy tube; complicated

(If imaging guidance is performed, use 75984)

AMA Coding Notes

Surgical Procedures on the Urinary System

(For provision of chemotherapeutic agents, report both the specific service in addition to code(s) for the specific substance(s) or drug(s) provided)

AMA *CPT® Assistant*

51705: Dec 07: 13, Jan 21: 11

51710: Dec 07: 13

Plain English Description

The physician changes a previously placed cystostomy tube. The cystostomy tube is changed periodically to prevent encrustation of the tube. Separately reportable imaging guidance may be used. A guidewire is inserted through the existing cystostomy tube. The purse-string suture securing the existing catheter is removed. The existing tube is removed. A new cystostomy tube is passed over the guidewire and into the bladder. The new tube is secured with a purse-string suture. Use 51705 if the tube change is simple and 51710 if it is complicated, such as a procedure performed on a patient with altered anatomy or when the tube has adhered to the cystostomy tunnel.

Change of cystostomy tube

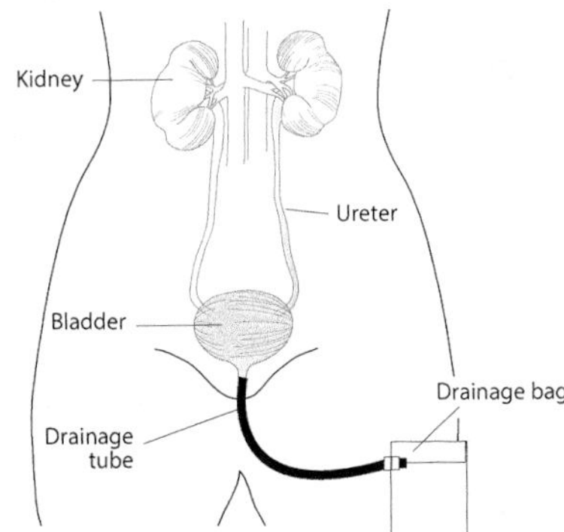

The physician replaces a drainage tube in the bladder. Use 51710 for a complicated exchange.

ICD-10-CM Diagnostic Codes

➐	T83.010	Breakdown (mechanical) of cystostomy catheter
➐	T83.020	Displacement of cystostomy catheter
➐	T83.030	Leakage of cystostomy catheter
➐	T83.090	Other mechanical complication of cystostomy catheter
➐	T83.510	Infection and inflammatory reaction due to cystostomy catheter
➐	T83.81	Embolism due to genitourinary prosthetic devices, implants and grafts
➐	T83.82	Fibrosis due to genitourinary prosthetic devices, implants and grafts
➐	T83.83	Hemorrhage due to genitourinary prosthetic devices, implants and grafts
➐	T83.84	Pain due to genitourinary prosthetic devices, implants and grafts
➐	T83.85	Stenosis due to genitourinary prosthetic devices, implants and grafts
➐	T83.86	Thrombosis due to genitourinary prosthetic devices, implants and grafts
➐	T83.89	Other specified complication of genitourinary prosthetic devices, implants and grafts
	Z43.5	Encounter for attention to cystostomy

ICD-10-CM Coding Notes

For codes requiring a 7th character extension, refer to your ICD-10-CM book. Review the character descriptions and coding guidelines for proper selection. For some procedures, only certain characters will apply.

CCI Edits

Refer to Appendix A for CCI edits.

Facility RVUs

Code	Work	PE Facility	MP	Total Facility
51705	0.90	0.49	0.11	1.50
51710	1.35	0.80	0.17	2.32

Non-facility RVUs

Code	Work	PE Non-Facility	MP	Total Non-Facility
51705	0.90	1.87	0.11	2.88
51710	1.35	2.54	0.17	4.06

Modifiers (PAR)

Code	Mod 50	Mod 51	Mod 62	Mod 66	Mod 80
51705	0	2	0	0	1
51710	0	2	0	0	1

Global Period

Code	Days
51705	000
51710	000

51715

51715 Endoscopic injection of implant material into the submucosal tissues of the urethra and/or bladder neck

AMA Coding Notes

Surgical Procedures on the Urinary System

(For provision of chemotherapeutic agents, report both the specific service in addition to code(s) for the specific substance(s) or drug(s) provided)

Plain English Description

This procedure is performed to treat mild incontinence due to thinning of tissues at the bladder outlet. A cystourethroscope is placed at the bladder outlet so that the outlet can be visualized while the injection procedure is performed. The physician then injects implant material, usually collagen or a newer material composed of water-based gel containing carbon-coated beads. The implant material is injected into the submucosal tissues surrounding the urethra and/or bladder neck. Once the bladder outlet tissues have been plumped up and any floppiness of the bladder outlet valve relieved, the cystourethroscope is removed. The injection procedure may need to be repeated two to three times over the course of several weeks to achieve the desired level of valve closure and prevent incontinence.

Endoscopic injection of implant material, submucosal tissues of urethra/bladder neck

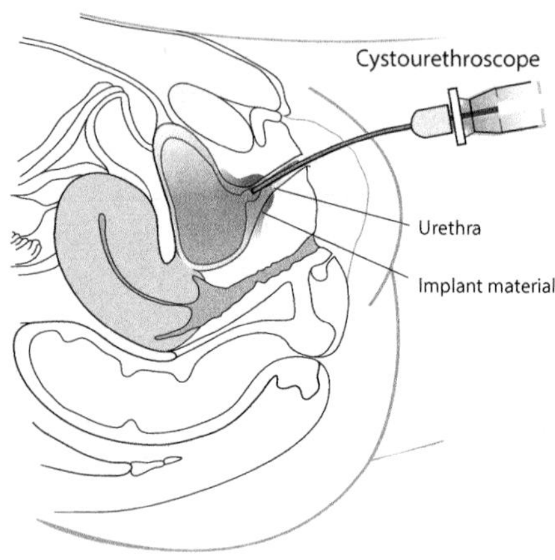

ICD-10-CM Diagnostic Codes

N31.9	Neuromuscular dysfunction of bladder, unspecified
N36.41	Hypermobility of urethra
N36.42	Intrinsic sphincter deficiency (ISD)
N36.43	Combined hypermobility of urethra and intrinsic sphincter deficiency
N36.44	Muscular disorders of urethra
N39.41	Urge incontinence
N39.42	Incontinence without sensory awareness
N39.43	Post-void dribbling
N39.44	Nocturnal enuresis
N39.45	Continuous leakage
N39.46	Mixed incontinence
N39.490	Overflow incontinence
N39.498	Other specified urinary incontinence
R35.0	Frequency of micturition

CCI Edits

Refer to Appendix A for CCI edits.

Pub 100

51715: Pub 100-03, 1, 230.10

Facility RVUs ▢

Code	Work	PE Facility	MP	Total Facility
51715	3.73	1.59	0.50	5.82

Non-facility RVUs ▢

Code	Work	PE Non-Facility	MP	Total Non-Facility
51715	3.73	6.99	0.50	11.22

Modifiers (PAR) ▢

Code	Mod 50	Mod 51	Mod 62	Mod 66	Mod 80
51715	0	2	0	0	0

Global Period

Code	Days
51715	000

51720

51720 Bladder instillation of anticarcinogenic agent (including retention time)

AMA Coding Notes

Surgical Procedures on the Urinary System

(For provision of chemotherapeutic agents, report both the specific service in addition to code(s) for the specific substance(s) or drug(s) provided)

AMA *CPT® Assistant*

51720: Nov 02: 11

Plain English Description

An anticarcinogenic agent is prepared per the manufacturer's instructions. The urethral orifice is cleansed and a catheter is inserted through the urethra into the bladder. The bladder is drained of urine. The anticarcinogenic agent is instilled into the bladder through the catheter and the catheter is removed. The patient is then repositioned, periodically rotating from the right side, back, left side, and stomach to ensure that the anticarcinogenic agent comes in contact with all bladder surfaces over the course of the treatment period, which may be as long as 2 hours. Upon completion of the treatment, the patient empties the bladder into the toilet.

Bladder instillation of anticarcinogenic agent

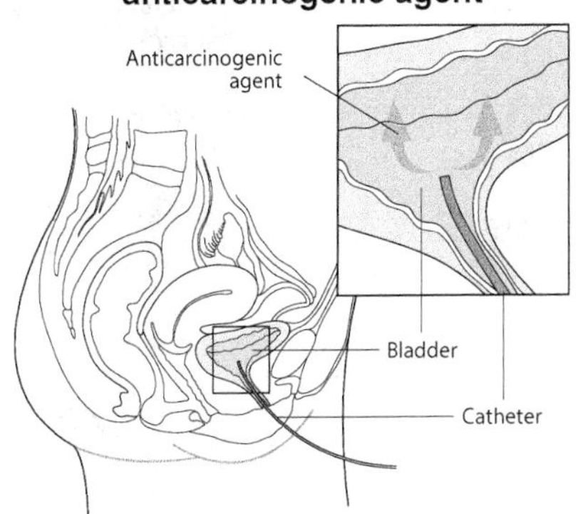

ICD-10-CM Diagnostic Codes

C67.0	Malignant neoplasm of trigone of bladder
C67.1	Malignant neoplasm of dome of bladder
C67.2	Malignant neoplasm of lateral wall of bladder
C67.3	Malignant neoplasm of anterior wall of bladder
C67.4	Malignant neoplasm of posterior wall of bladder
C67.5	Malignant neoplasm of bladder neck
C67.6	Malignant neoplasm of ureteric orifice
C67.7	Malignant neoplasm of urachus
C67.8	Malignant neoplasm of overlapping sites of bladder
C79.11	Secondary malignant neoplasm of bladder
D09.0	Carcinoma in situ of bladder
Z51.11	Encounter for antineoplastic chemotherapy

CCI Edits

Refer to Appendix A for CCI edits.

Pub 100

51720: Pub 100-02, 15, 50.4.5-50.4.5.1

Facility RVUs

Code	Work	PE Facility	MP	Total Facility
51720	0.87	0.30	0.10	1.27

Non-facility RVUs

Code	Work	PE Non-Facility	MP	Total Non-Facility
51720	0.87	1.62	0.10	2.59

Modifiers (PAR)

Code	Mod 50	Mod 51	Mod 62	Mod 66	Mod 80
51720	0	2	0	0	1

Global Period

Code	Days
51720	000

51725

51725 Simple cystometrogram (CMG) (eg, spinal manometer)

AMA Coding Guideline

Urodynamic Procedures on the Bladder

The following section (51725-51798) lists procedures that may be used separately or in many and varied combinations.

When multiple procedures are performed in the same investigative session, modifier 51 should be employed.

All procedures in this section imply that these services are performed by, or are under the direct supervision of, a physician or other qualified health care professional and that all instruments, equipment, fluids, gases, probes, catheters, technician's fees, medications, gloves, trays, tubing, and other sterile supplies be provided by that individual. When the individual only interprets the results and/or operates the equipment, a professional component, modifier 26, should be used to identify these services.

AMA Coding Notes

Surgical Procedures on the Urinary System

(For provision of chemotherapeutic agents, report both the specific service in addition to code(s) for the specific substance(s) or drug(s) provided)

AMA *CPT® Assistant*

51725: Sep 02: 6, Feb 10: 7

Plain English Description

A cystometrogram (CMG) is performed to measure bladder capacity and bladder storage pressures. CMG is used to evaluate conditions such as urinary incontinence, difficulty with urination, and neurogenic bladder. Prior to the CMG, the patient empties the bladder and the amount is measured. The urethra is cleansed with antiseptic solution. A sterile catheter with a sensor is then inserted through the urethra into the bladder. The bladder is then filled with sterile saline and the physician queries the patient about the sensations experienced during the filling process including fullness, pain, urgency, and leakage. Simple CMG (51725) measures bladder capacity and storage pressures using a spinal manometer or by simply observing the column of fluid entering the bladder. The patient may be asked to cough or strain to increase abdominal pressure, which allows the physician to evaluate any stress incontinence. Complex CMG (51726) uses calibrated electronic equipment and measures intra-abdominal, total bladder and true detrusor pressures simultaneously. The detrusor is the muscular wall of the bladder. Complex CMG can differentiate between involuntary detrusor contraction and reversed bladder compliance due to increased intra-abdominal pressure. Emptying pressures are not measured during simple or complex CMG. Only bladder capacity and storage pressures are measured.

Simple cystometrogram (CMG) (eg, spinal manometer)

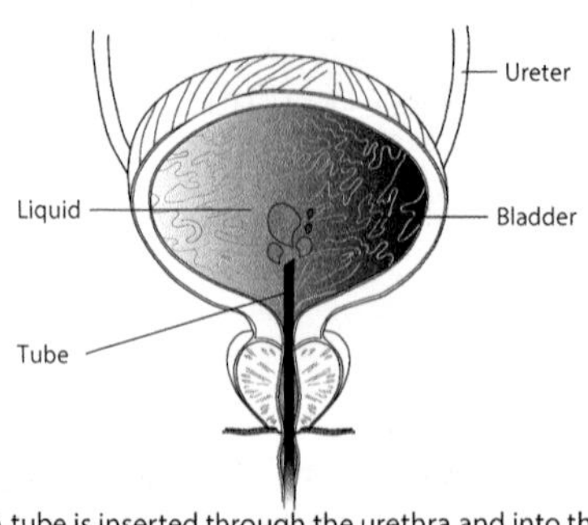

A tube is inserted through the urethra and into the bladder. The bladder is then filled with liquid so that the physician can measure the volume, rate of discharge, and other factors relating to the elimination of urine.

ICD-10-CM Diagnostic Codes

G83.4	Cauda equina syndrome
N13.721	Vesicoureteral-reflux with reflux nephropathy without hydroureter, unilateral
N13.722	Vesicoureteral-reflux with reflux nephropathy without hydroureter, bilateral
N13.731	Vesicoureteral-reflux with reflux nephropathy with hydroureter, unilateral
N13.732	Vesicoureteral-reflux with reflux nephropathy with hydroureter, bilateral
N31.0	Uninhibited neuropathic bladder, not elsewhere classified
N31.1	Reflex neuropathic bladder, not elsewhere classified
N31.2	Flaccid neuropathic bladder, not elsewhere classified
N32.0	Bladder-neck obstruction
N32.1	Vesicointestinal fistula
N32.2	Vesical fistula, not elsewhere classified
N32.3	Diverticulum of bladder
N32.81	Overactive bladder
N35.010	Post-traumatic urethral stricture, male, meatal ♂
N35.011	Post-traumatic bulbous urethral stricture ♂
N35.012	Post-traumatic membranous urethral stricture ♂
N35.013	Post-traumatic anterior urethral stricture ♂
N35.021	Urethral stricture due to childbirth ♀
N35.111	Postinfective urethral stricture, not elsewhere classified, male, meatal ♂
N35.112	Postinfective bulbous urethral stricture, not elsewhere classified, male ♂
N35.113	Postinfective membranous urethral stricture, not elsewhere classified, male ♂
N35.114	Postinfective anterior urethral stricture, not elsewhere classified, male ♂
N35.12	Postinfective urethral stricture, not elsewhere classified, female ♀
N36.44	Muscular disorders of urethra
N39.3	Stress incontinence (female) (male)
N39.41	Urge incontinence
N39.42	Incontinence without sensory awareness
N39.43	Post-void dribbling
N39.44	Nocturnal enuresis
N39.45	Continuous leakage
N39.46	Mixed incontinence
N39.490	Overflow incontinence
N40.1	Benign prostatic hyperplasia with lower urinary tract symptoms ♂
N40.3	Nodular prostate with lower urinary tract symptoms ♂
N41.1	Chronic prostatitis ♂
N42.83	Cyst of prostate ♂
N81.0	Urethrocele ♀
N81.11	Cystocele, midline ♀
N81.12	Cystocele, lateral ♀
N81.84	Pelvic muscle wasting ♀
N99.110	Postprocedural urethral stricture, male, meatal ♂
N99.111	Postprocedural bulbous urethral stricture, male ♂
N99.112	Postprocedural membranous urethral stricture, male ♂
N99.113	Postprocedural anterior bulbous urethral stricture, male ♂
N99.12	Postprocedural urethral stricture, female ♀
Q64.2	Congenital posterior urethral valves
Q64.31	Congenital bladder neck obstruction
Q64.32	Congenital stricture of urethra
Q64.33	Congenital stricture of urinary meatus
R30.0	Dysuria
R30.1	Vesical tenesmus
R31.0	Gross hematuria
R31.1	Benign essential microscopic hematuria
R33.0	Drug induced retention of urine
R35.0	Frequency of micturition
R35.1	Nocturia
R39.1	Other difficulties with micturition
R39.11	Hesitancy of micturition
R39.12	Poor urinary stream
R39.13	Splitting of urinary stream
R39.14	Feeling of incomplete bladder emptying
R39.15	Urgency of urination
R39.16	Straining to void
R39.81	Functional urinary incontinence
R39.82	Chronic bladder pain

CCI Edits

Refer to Appendix A for CCI edits.

Facility RVUs

Code	Work	PE Facility	MP	Total Facility
51725	1.51	5.22	0.16	6.89

Non-facility RVUs

Code	Work	PE Non-Facility	MP	Total Non-Facility
51725	1.51	5.22	0.16	6.89

Modifiers (PAR)

Code	Mod 50	Mod 51	Mod 62	Mod 66	Mod 80
51725	0	2	0	0	0

Global Period

Code	Days
51725	000

51726-51729

51726 Complex cystometrogram (ie, calibrated electronic equipment)
51727 Complex cystometrogram (ie, calibrated electronic equipment); with urethral pressure profile studies (ie, urethral closure pressure profile), any technique
51728 Complex cystometrogram (ie, calibrated electronic equipment); with voiding pressure studies (ie, bladder voiding pressure), any technique
51729 Complex cystometrogram (ie, calibrated electronic equipment); with voiding pressure studies (ie, bladder voiding pressure) and urethral pressure profile studies (ie, urethral closure pressure profile), any technique

AMA Coding Guideline

Urodynamic Procedures on the Bladder

The following section (51725-51798) lists procedures that may be used separately or in many and varied combinations.

When multiple procedures are performed in the same investigative session, modifier 51 should be employed.

All procedures in this section imply that these services are performed by, or are under the direct supervision of, a physician or other qualified health care professional and that all instruments, equipment, fluids, gases, probes, catheters, technician's fees, medications, gloves, trays, tubing, and other sterile supplies be provided by that individual. When the individual only interprets the results and/or operates the equipment, a professional component, modifier 26, should be used to identify these services.

AMA Coding Notes

Surgical Procedures on the Urinary System

(For provision of chemotherapeutic agents, report both the specific service in addition to code(s) for the specific substance(s) or drug(s) provided)

AMA *CPT® Assistant* ▯

51726: Sep 02: 6, Feb 10: 7
51727: Feb 10: 7
51728: Feb 10: 7
51729: Feb 10: 7

Plain English Description

A cystometrogram (CMG) is performed to measure bladder capacity and bladder storage pressures. CMG is used to evaluate conditions such as urinary incontinence, difficulty with urination, and neurogenic bladder. Prior to the CMG, the patient empties the bladder and the amount is measured. The urethra is cleansed with antiseptic solution. A sterile catheter with a sensor is then inserted through the urethra into the bladder. The bladder is then filled with sterile saline and the physician queries the patient about the sensations experienced during the filling process including fullness, pain, urgency, and leakage. In 51726, a complex CMG is performed using calibrated electronic equipment that measures intra-abdominal, total bladder, and true detrusor pressures simultaneously. The detrusor is the muscular wall of the bladder. Complex CMG can differentiate between involuntary detrusor contraction and reversed bladder compliance due to increased intra-abdominal pressure. In 51727, a complex CMG is performed as described above with urethral pressure profile studies that provide information on the ability of the urethra to prevent leakage of urine. A fluid-filled catheter with multiple radial lumen openings is advanced into the bladder. The catheter is continuously perfused with saline solution as the catheter is pulled through the urethra at a slow continuous rate. The catheter contains a sensor that is connected to a recording device. As the catheter is removed, urethral pressures are recorded and a tracing of the pressures provided. In 51728, a complex CMG is performed with voiding pressure studies (VP) using any technique. A catheter is inserted into the bladder and the bladder filled with fluid. A device is used to measure the amount of pressure the bladder can generate and the flow of urine. After filling the bladder with fluid, the patient is asked to void. Sensors record pressures prior to voiding, sphincter opening pressure and opening time, maximum voiding pressure, pressure at maximum flow, and flow during and after bladder contractions. Multiple bladder fills may be necessary to accurately evaluate bladder voiding pressure. In 51729, a complex CMG is performed with urethral pressure profile and voiding pressure studies as described above. Following completion of the complex CMG and additional studies, the physician interprets the studies and provides a written report.

Complex cystometrogram (CMG) (eg, calibrated electronic equipment)

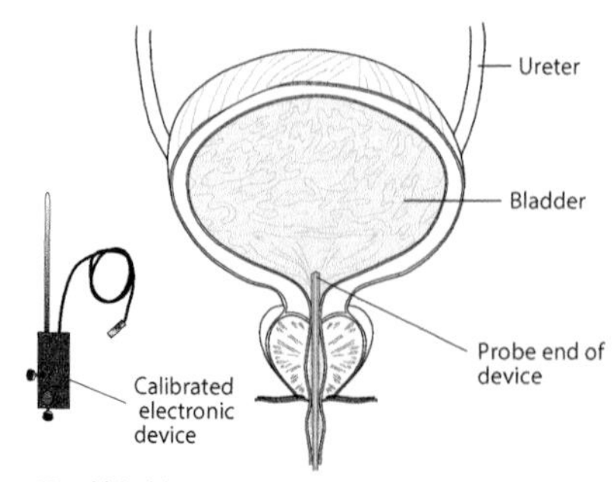

Total bladder/true detrusor pressure are measured (51726); with urethral pressure (51727); with voiding pressure (51728); with both urethral and voiding pressure studies (51729)

ICD-10-CM Diagnostic Codes

G83.4	Cauda equina syndrome
N13.721	Vesicoureteral-reflux with reflux nephropathy without hydroureter, unilateral
N13.722	Vesicoureteral-reflux with reflux nephropathy without hydroureter, bilateral
N13.731	Vesicoureteral-reflux with reflux nephropathy with hydroureter, unilateral
N13.732	Vesicoureteral-reflux with reflux nephropathy with hydroureter, bilateral
N31.0	Uninhibited neuropathic bladder, not elsewhere classified
N31.1	Reflex neuropathic bladder, not elsewhere classified
N31.2	Flaccid neuropathic bladder, not elsewhere classified
N32.0	Bladder-neck obstruction
N32.1	Vesicointestinal fistula
N32.2	Vesical fistula, not elsewhere classified
N32.3	Diverticulum of bladder
N32.81	Overactive bladder
N35.010	Post-traumatic urethral stricture, male, meatal ♂
N35.011	Post-traumatic bulbous urethral stricture ♂
N35.012	Post-traumatic membranous urethral stricture ♂
N35.013	Post-traumatic anterior urethral stricture ♂
N35.021	Urethral stricture due to childbirth ♀
N35.111	Postinfective urethral stricture, not elsewhere classified, male, meatal ♂
N35.112	Postinfective bulbous urethral stricture, not elsewhere classified, male ♂
N35.113	Postinfective membranous urethral stricture, not elsewhere classified, male ♂
N35.114	Postinfective anterior urethral stricture, not elsewhere classified, male ♂
N35.12	Postinfective urethral stricture, not elsewhere classified, female ♀
N36.44	Muscular disorders of urethra
N39.3	Stress incontinence (female) (male)
N39.41	Urge incontinence
N39.42	Incontinence without sensory awareness
N39.43	Post-void dribbling
N39.44	Nocturnal enuresis
N39.45	Continuous leakage
N39.46	Mixed incontinence
N39.490	Overflow incontinence
N40.1	Benign prostatic hyperplasia with lower urinary tract symptoms ♂
N40.2	Nodular prostate without lower urinary tract symptoms ♂
N40.3	Nodular prostate with lower urinary tract symptoms ♂
N41.1	Chronic prostatitis ♂
N42.83	Cyst of prostate ♂
N81.0	Urethrocele ♀
N81.11	Cystocele, midline ♀
N81.12	Cystocele, lateral ♀

N81.84	Pelvic muscle wasting ♀
N99.110	Postprocedural urethral stricture, male, meatal ♂
N99.111	Postprocedural bulbous urethral stricture, male ♂
N99.112	Postprocedural membranous urethral stricture, male ♂
N99.113	Postprocedural anterior bulbous urethral stricture, male ♂
N99.12	Postprocedural urethral stricture, female ♀
Q64.2	Congenital posterior urethral valves
Q64.3	Other atresia and stenosis of urethra and bladder neck
Q64.31	Congenital bladder neck obstruction
Q64.32	Congenital stricture of urethra
Q64.33	Congenital stricture of urinary meatus
Q64.71	Congenital prolapse of urethra
Q64.72	Congenital prolapse of urinary meatus
R30.0	Dysuria
R30.1	Vesical tenesmus
R31.0	Gross hematuria
R31.1	Benign essential microscopic hematuria
R33.0	Drug induced retention of urine
R35.0	Frequency of micturition
R35.1	Nocturia
R39.11	Hesitancy of micturition
R39.12	Poor urinary stream
R39.13	Splitting of urinary stream
R39.14	Feeling of incomplete bladder emptying
R39.15	Urgency of urination
R39.16	Straining to void
R39.81	Functional urinary incontinence
R39.82	Chronic bladder pain

CCI Edits

Refer to Appendix A for CCI edits.

Facility RVUs ▯

Code	Work	PE Facility	MP	Total Facility
51726	1.71	7.24	0.16	9.11
51727	2.11	8.66	0.23	11.00
51728	2.11	8.76	0.21	11.08
51729	2.51	8.93	0.27	11.71

Non-facility RVUs ▯

Code	Work	PE Non-Facility	MP	Total Non-Facility
51726	1.71	7.24	0.16	9.11
51727	2.11	8.66	0.23	11.00
51728	2.11	8.76	0.21	11.08
51729	2.51	8.93	0.27	11.71

Modifiers (PAR) ▯

Code	Mod 50	Mod 51	Mod 62	Mod 66	Mod 80
51726	0	2	0	0	1
51727	0	2	0	0	0
51728	0	2	0	0	0
51729	0	2	0	0	0

Global Period

Code	Days
51726	000
51727	000
51728	000
51729	000

51736-51741

51736 Simple uroflowmetry (UFR) (eg, stop-watch flow rate, mechanical uroflowmeter)
51741 Complex uroflowmetry (eg, calibrated electronic equipment)

AMA Coding Guideline

Urodynamic Procedures on the Bladder

The following section (51725-51798) lists procedures that may be used separately or in many and varied combinations.

When multiple procedures are performed in the same investigative session, modifier 51 should be employed.

All procedures in this section imply that these services are performed by, or are under the direct supervision of, a physician or other qualified health care professional and that all instruments, equipment, fluids, gases, probes, catheters, technician's fees, medications, gloves, trays, tubing, and other sterile supplies be provided by that individual. When the individual only interprets the results and/or operates the equipment, a professional component, modifier 26, should be used to identify these services.

AMA Coding Notes

Surgical Procedures on the Urinary System

(For provision of chemotherapeutic agents, report both the specific service in addition to code(s) for the specific substance(s) or drug(s) provided)

AMA *CPT® Assistant* ☐

51736: Sep 02: 6, Feb 10: 7
51741: Sep 02: 6, Feb 10: 7, Sep 14: 14

Plain English Description

Simple (51736) or complex (51741) uroflowmetry (UFR) is performed to measure urine flow rate. This test evaluates detrusor muscle contraction and bladder neck and urethral function. The detrusor muscle is the muscular wall of the bladder that contracts during urination. Contraction of the detrusor works in conjunction with gravity and increased intra-abdominal pressure to facilitate emptying of the bladder. Decreased flow rate may be caused by poor detrusor function due to neurological lesions, obstruction due to benign prostatic hypertrophy, or bladder prolapse (cystocele). Increased flow rate may be due to urethral sphincter dysfunction. In 51736, the flow of urine is visually observed to gauge the flow and a stopwatch may be used to determine how long it takes to empty the bladder. In 51741, calibrated electronic equipment is used to measure the flow of urine.

Uroflowmetry (UFR)

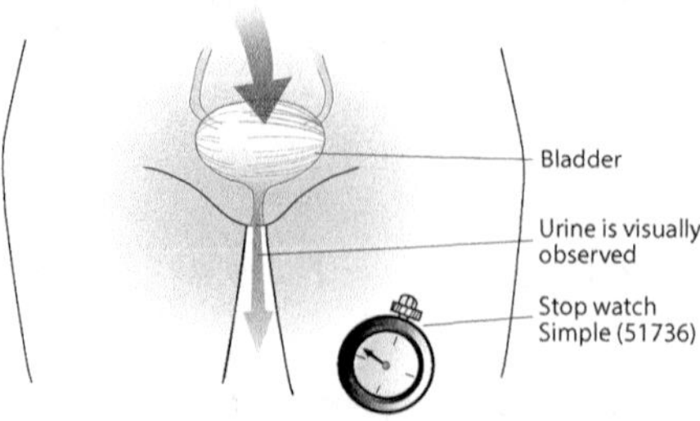

Complex (calibrated electronic equipment) (51741)

ICD-10-CM Diagnostic Codes

A56.01	Chlamydial cystitis and urethritis
C61	Malignant neoplasm of prostate ♂
G83.4	Cauda equina syndrome
N30.10	Interstitial cystitis (chronic) without hematuria
N30.20	Other chronic cystitis without hematuria
N30.21	Other chronic cystitis with hematuria
N31.0	Uninhibited neuropathic bladder, not elsewhere classified
N31.1	Reflex neuropathic bladder, not elsewhere classified
N31.2	Flaccid neuropathic bladder, not elsewhere classified
N32.0	Bladder-neck obstruction
N32.1	Vesicointestinal fistula
N32.2	Vesical fistula, not elsewhere classified
N32.3	Diverticulum of bladder
N32.81	Overactive bladder
N33	Bladder disorders in diseases classified elsewhere
N35.010	Post-traumatic urethral stricture, male, meatal ♂
N35.011	Post-traumatic bulbous urethral stricture ♂
N35.012	Post-traumatic membranous urethral stricture ♂
N35.013	Post-traumatic anterior urethral stricture ♂
N35.021	Urethral stricture due to childbirth ♀
N35.111	Postinfective urethral stricture, not elsewhere classified, male, meatal ♂
N35.112	Postinfective bulbous urethral stricture, not elsewhere classified, male ♂
N35.113	Postinfective membranous urethral stricture, not elsewhere classified, male ♂
N35.114	Postinfective anterior urethral stricture, not elsewhere classified, male ♂
N35.12	Postinfective urethral stricture, not elsewhere classified, female ♀
N36.0	Urethral fistula
N36.1	Urethral diverticulum
N36.41	Hypermobility of urethra
N36.42	Intrinsic sphincter deficiency (ISD)
N36.43	Combined hypermobility of urethra and intrinsic sphincter deficiency
N36.44	Muscular disorders of urethra
N39.3	Stress incontinence (female) (male)
N39.41	Urge incontinence
N39.42	Incontinence without sensory awareness
N39.43	Post-void dribbling
N39.44	Nocturnal enuresis
N39.45	Continuous leakage
N39.46	Mixed incontinence
N39.490	Overflow incontinence
N40.1	Benign prostatic hyperplasia with lower urinary tract symptoms ♂
N40.3	Nodular prostate with lower urinary tract symptoms ♂
N41.1	Chronic prostatitis ♂
N81.84	Pelvic muscle wasting ♀
N99.110	Postprocedural urethral stricture, male, meatal ♂
N99.111	Postprocedural bulbous urethral stricture, male ♂
N99.112	Postprocedural membranous urethral stricture, male ♂
N99.113	Postprocedural anterior bulbous urethral stricture, male ♂
N99.12	Postprocedural urethral stricture, female ♀
R30.0	Dysuria
R30.1	Vesical tenesmus
R31.0	Gross hematuria
R31.1	Benign essential microscopic hematuria
R35.0	Frequency of micturition
R35.1	Nocturia
R39.11	Hesitancy of micturition
R39.12	Poor urinary stream
R39.13	Splitting of urinary stream
R39.14	Feeling of incomplete bladder emptying
R39.15	Urgency of urination
R39.16	Straining to void
R39.2	Extrarenal uremia
R39.81	Functional urinary incontinence

CCI Edits

Refer to Appendix A for CCI edits.

Pub 100

51736: Pub 100-03, 1, 230.2
51741: Pub 100-03, 1, 230.2

Facility RVUs

Code	Work	PE Facility	MP	Total Facility
51736	0.17	0.20	0.02	0.39
51741	0.17	0.21	0.03	0.41

Non-facility RVUs

Code	Work	PE Non-Facility	MP	Total Non-Facility
51736	0.17	0.20	0.02	0.39
51741	0.17	0.21	0.03	0.41

Modifiers (PAR)

Code	Mod 50	Mod 51	Mod 62	Mod 66	Mod 80
51736	0	2	0	0	0
51741	0	2	0	0	1

Global Period

Code	Days
51736	XXX
51741	XXX

51784-51785

51784 Electromyography studies (EMG) of anal or urethral sphincter, other than needle, any technique

(Do not report 51784 in conjunction with 51792)

51785 Needle electromyography studies (EMG) of anal or urethral sphincter, any technique

AMA Coding Guideline

Urodynamic Procedures on the Bladder

The following section (51725-51798) lists procedures that may be used separately or in many and varied combinations.

When multiple procedures are performed in the same investigative session, modifier 51 should be employed.

All procedures in this section imply that these services are performed by, or are under the direct supervision of, a physician or other qualified health care professional and that all instruments, equipment, fluids, gases, probes, catheters, technician's fees, medications, gloves, trays, tubing, and other sterile supplies be provided by that individual. When the individual only interprets the results and/or operates the equipment, a professional component, modifier 26, should be used to identify these services.

AMA Coding Notes

Surgical Procedures on the Urinary System

(For provision of chemotherapeutic agents, report both the specific service in addition to code(s) for the specific substance(s) or drug(s) provided)

AMA *CPT® Assistant* ▯

51784: Sep 02: 6, Feb 10: 7, Feb 14: 11, Sep 14: 14

51785: Apr 02: 6, Sep 02: 6, Jul 04: 13, Feb 10: 7

Plain English Description

Electromyography (EMG) measures the electrical activity in the anal or urethral sphincter muscles. Muscles and nerves generate electrical impulses that facilitate sphincter contraction and relaxation. If electrical impulses are impaired, the sphincter will not open and close properly. In 51784, an EMG electrode patch is placed around the urethral sphincter or anal sphincter and muscle impulses recorded. EMG of the anal or urethral sphincter using an electrode patch is performed at the time of separately reportable complex cystometrogram (CMG) or voiding pressure (VP) studies. Electrical activity is recorded during filling and emptying of the bladder. In 51785, needles are placed in the urethral or anal sphincter to obtain information on pelvic floor muscle activity. This test is performed during separately reportable complex CMG in patients with neurological disease to record electrical impulses during filling and emptying of the bladder.

Electromyography studies (EMG) of anal or urethral sphincter

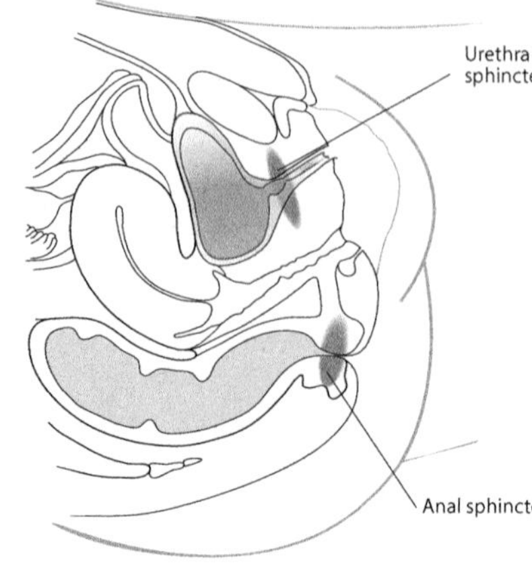

Other than needle, any technique (51784); needle, any technique (51785)

ICD-10-CM Diagnostic Codes

G54.1	Lumbosacral plexus disorders
G63	Polyneuropathy in diseases classified elsewhere
G83.4	Cauda equina syndrome
G95.89	Other specified diseases of spinal cord
M62.58	Muscle wasting and atrophy, not elsewhere classified, other site
N31.0	Uninhibited neuropathic bladder, not elsewhere classified
N31.1	Reflex neuropathic bladder, not elsewhere classified
N31.2	Flaccid neuropathic bladder, not elsewhere classified
N31.8	Other neuromuscular dysfunction of bladder
N31.9	Neuromuscular dysfunction of bladder, unspecified
N32.81	Overactive bladder
N36.41	Hypermobility of urethra
N36.42	Intrinsic sphincter deficiency (ISD)
N36.43	Combined hypermobility of urethra and intrinsic sphincter deficiency
N36.44	Muscular disorders of urethra
N39.3	Stress incontinence (female) (male)
N39.41	Urge incontinence
N39.42	Incontinence without sensory awareness
N39.44	Nocturnal enuresis
N39.45	Continuous leakage
N39.46	Mixed incontinence
N39.490	Overflow incontinence
N39.491	Coital incontinence
N39.492	Postural (urinary) incontinence
N39.498	Other specified urinary incontinence
N81.82	Incompetence or weakening of pubocervical tissue ♀
N81.83	Incompetence or weakening of rectovaginal tissue ♀
N81.84	Pelvic muscle wasting ♀
N99.89	Other postprocedural complications and disorders of genitourinary system
R15.0	Incomplete defecation
R15.1	Fecal smearing
R15.2	Fecal urgency
R15.9	Full incontinence of feces
R30.0	Dysuria
R30.1	Vesical tenesmus
R33.8	Other retention of urine
R33.9	Retention of urine, unspecified
R35.0	Frequency of micturition
R35.1	Nocturia
R39.11	Hesitancy of micturition
R39.14	Feeling of incomplete bladder emptying
R39.15	Urgency of urination
R39.81	Functional urinary incontinence

CCI Edits

Refer to Appendix A for CCI edits.

Facility RVUs ▯

Code	Work	PE Facility	MP	Total Facility
51784	0.75	1.06	0.09	1.90
51785	1.53	11.43	0.49	13.45

Non-facility RVUs ▯

Code	Work	PE Non-Facility	MP	Total Non-Facility
51784	0.75	1.06	0.09	1.90
51785	1.53	11.43	0.49	13.45

Modifiers (PAR) ▯

Code	Mod 50	Mod 51	Mod 62	Mod 66	Mod 80
51784	0	2	0	0	1
51785	0	2	0	0	0

Global Period

Code	Days
51784	XXX
51785	XXX

● New ▲ Revised ✚ Add On ⊘Modifier 51 Exempt ★Telemedicine ▯ CPT QuickRef ⁄ FDA Pending ⇄ Laterality ❼ Seventh Character ♂Male ♀Female

51792

51792 Stimulus evoked response (eg, measurement of bulbocavernosus reflex latency time)

(Do not report 51792 in conjunction with 51784)

AMA Coding Guideline

Urodynamic Procedures on the Bladder

The following section (51725-51798) lists procedures that may be used separately or in many and varied combinations.

When multiple procedures are performed in the same investigative session, modifier 51 should be employed.

All procedures in this section imply that these services are performed by, or are under the direct supervision of, a physician or other qualified health care professional and that all instruments, equipment, fluids, gases, probes, catheters, technician's fees, medications, gloves, trays, tubing, and other sterile supplies be provided by that individual. When the individual only interprets the results and/or operates the equipment, a professional component, modifier 26, should be used to identify these services.

AMA Coding Notes

Surgical Procedures on the Urinary System

(For provision of chemotherapeutic agents, report both the specific service in addition to code(s) for the specific substance(s) or drug(s) provided)

AMA *CPT® Assistant* ☐

51792: Apr 02: 6, Sep 02: 6, Feb 10: 7, Feb 14: 11

Plain English Description

Stimulus evoked response is performed to measure bulbocavernosus reflex latency time. In men, the bulbocavernosus muscle constricts the bulbous urethra during urination, allowing the last drops of urine to be expelled. In women, the bulbocavernosus muscle helps support the pelvic floor. Stimulus evoked response is used to help evaluate cauda equina syndrome. The glans penis or clitoris is stimulated, which in turn stimulates the sacral reflex arch (S2-S4). As the sacral reflex arch is stimulated, motor activity of the urethral sphincter in men or the pelvic floor in women is evaluated.

Stimulus evoked response

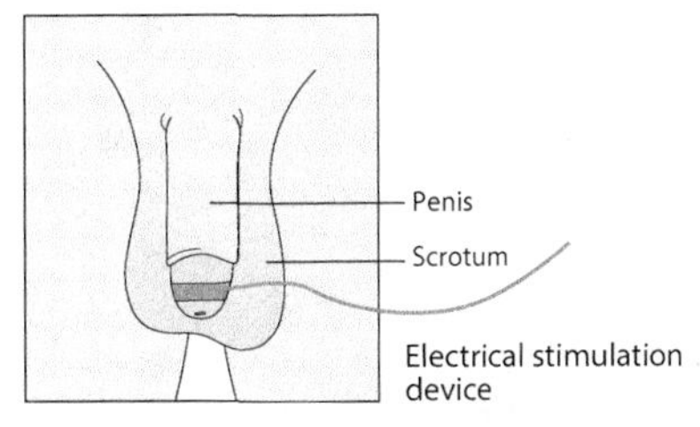

The head of the penis is electrically stimulated so that the physician can measure the response times of the pelvic nerves.

ICD-10-CM Diagnostic Codes

C61	Malignant neoplasm of prostate ♂
D07.5	Carcinoma in situ of prostate ♂
D29.1	Benign neoplasm of prostate ♂
G83.4	Cauda equina syndrome
N31.0	Uninhibited neuropathic bladder, not elsewhere classified
N31.1	Reflex neuropathic bladder, not elsewhere classified
N31.2	Flaccid neuropathic bladder, not elsewhere classified
N31.8	Other neuromuscular dysfunction of bladder
N31.9	Neuromuscular dysfunction of bladder, unspecified
N36.42	Intrinsic sphincter deficiency (ISD)
N36.43	Combined hypermobility of urethra and intrinsic sphincter deficiency
N39.3	Stress incontinence (female) (male)
N39.41	Urge incontinence
N39.43	Post-void dribbling
N39.44	Nocturnal enuresis
N39.45	Continuous leakage
N39.46	Mixed incontinence
N39.498	Other specified urinary incontinence
N52.01	Erectile dysfunction due to arterial insufficiency ♂
N52.02	Corporo-venous occlusive erectile dysfunction ♂
N52.03	Combined arterial insufficiency and corporo-venous occlusive erectile dysfunction ♂
N52.1	Erectile dysfunction due to diseases classified elsewhere ♂
N52.2	Drug-induced erectile dysfunction ♂
N52.31	Erectile dysfunction following radical prostatectomy ♂
N52.32	Erectile dysfunction following radical cystectomy ♂
N52.33	Erectile dysfunction following urethral surgery ♂
N52.34	Erectile dysfunction following simple prostatectomy ♂
N52.39	Other and unspecified postprocedural erectile dysfunction ♂
N52.8	Other male erectile dysfunction ♂
R32	Unspecified urinary incontinence
R33.0	Drug induced retention of urine
R33.8	Other retention of urine
R35.0	Frequency of micturition
R35.1	Nocturia
R35.89	Other polyuria
R39.14	Feeling of incomplete bladder emptying
R39.15	Urgency of urination

CCI Edits

Refer to Appendix A for CCI edits.

Facility RVUs ☐

Code	Work	PE Facility	MP	Total Facility
51792	1.10	6.98	0.13	8.21

Non-facility RVUs ☐

Code	Work	PE Non-Facility	MP	Total Non-Facility
51792	1.10	6.98	0.13	8.21

Modifiers (PAR) ☐

Code	Mod 50	Mod 51	Mod 62	Mod 66	Mod 80
51792	0	2	0	0	0

Global Period

Code	Days
51792	000

51797

+ **51797 Voiding pressure studies, intra-abdominal (ie, rectal, gastric, intraperitoneal) (List separately in addition to code for primary procedure)**

(Use 51797 in conjunction with 51728, 51729)

AMA Coding Guideline

Urodynamic Procedures on the Bladder

The following section (51725-51798) lists procedures that may be used separately or in many and varied combinations.

When multiple procedures are performed in the same investigative session, modifier 51 should be employed.

All procedures in this section imply that these services are performed by, or are under the direct supervision of, a physician or other qualified health care professional and that all instruments, equipment, fluids, gases, probes, catheters, technician's fees, medications, gloves, trays, tubing, and other sterile supplies be provided by that individual. When the individual only interprets the results and/or operates the equipment, a professional component, modifier 26, should be used to identify these services.

AMA Coding Notes

Surgical Procedures on the Urinary System

(For provision of chemotherapeutic agents, report both the specific service in addition to code(s) for the specific substance(s) or drug(s) provided)

AMA *CPT® Assistant*

51797: Dec 01: 7, Sep 02: 6, Oct 09: 7, Feb 10: 7

Plain English Description

Abdominal voiding pressure measures how much the patient must strain to void. A catheter is inserted into the rectum and a device used to measure intra-abdominal pressure. The bladder is filled with fluid. Intra-abdominal pressure is recorded as the patient voids. Multiple bladder fills may be necessary to accurately evaluate intra-abdominal pressure. The physician then interprets the intra-abdominal voiding pressure and compares it to the total bladder (intravesical) voiding pressure to obtain the true intravesical pressure during voiding. Intra-abdominal voiding pressure (AP) (rectal, gastric, intraperitoneal) is evaluated at the time of a separately reportable bladder voiding pressure study.

Voiding pressure studies, intra-abdominal

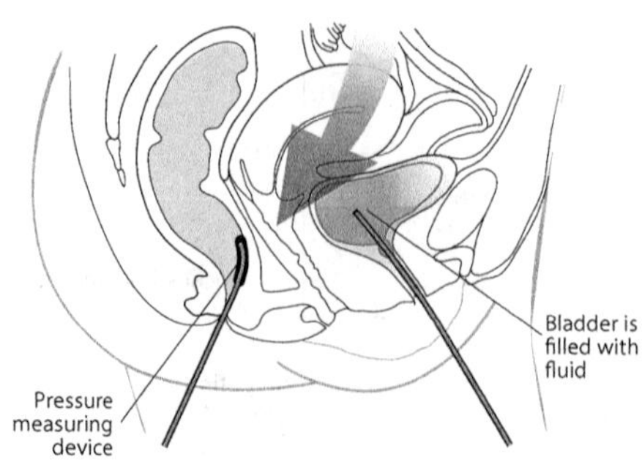

ICD-10-CM Diagnostic Codes

See Primary Procedure code for crosswalks.

CCI Edits

Refer to Appendix A for CCI edits.

Facility RVUs

Code	Work	PE Facility	MP	Total Facility
51797	0.80	5.04	0.08	5.92

Non-facility RVUs

Code	Work	PE Non-Facility	MP	Total Non-Facility
51797	0.80	5.04	0.08	5.92

Modifiers (PAR)

Code	Mod 50	Mod 51	Mod 62	Mod 66	Mod 80
51797	0	0	0	0	0

Global Period

Code	Days
51797	ZZZ

51798

51798 Measurement of post-voiding residual urine and/or bladder capacity by ultrasound, non-imaging

AMA Coding Guideline

Urodynamic Procedures on the Bladder

The following section (51725-51798) lists procedures that may be used separately or in many and varied combinations.

When multiple procedures are performed in the same investigative session, modifier 51 should be employed.

All procedures in this section imply that these services are performed by, or are under the direct supervision of, a physician or other qualified health care professional and that all instruments, equipment, fluids, gases, probes, catheters, technician's fees, medications, gloves, trays, tubing, and other sterile supplies be provided by that individual. When the individual only interprets the results and/or operates the equipment, a professional component, modifier 26, should be used to identify these services.

AMA Coding Notes

Surgical Procedures on the Urinary System

(For provision of chemotherapeutic agents, report both the specific service in addition to code(s) for the specific substance(s) or drug(s) provided)

AMA *CPT® Assistant*

51798: Dec 05: 3, Feb 10: 7, Jun 18: 11

Plain English Description

Post-voiding residual urine and/or bladder capacity is measured using nonimaging ultrasound. An ultrasound probe, which may be part of a hand-held unit or a larger conventional ultrasound unit, is placed on the patient's abdomen over the bladder. Sound waves are transmitted from the transducer to the bladder and reflected back from the bladder to the transducer. Data from multiple cross-sectional scans are then transmitted to a computer within the ultrasound unit and the computer calculates bladder capacity including bladder volume measurements. When post-voiding residual is measured, the patient is asked to urinate and the amount of urine remaining in the bladder after urination is then measured using the ultrasound device and computer calculations.

Measurement of residual urine and/or bladder capacity

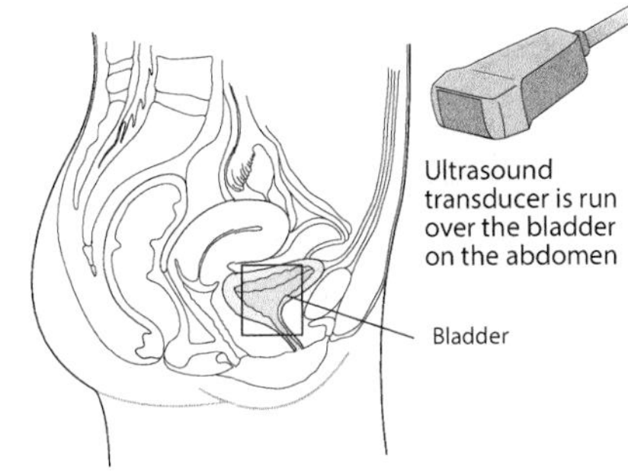

After a patient has expelled urine, an ultrasound device is used to scan the bladder and measure how much urine is left in the bladder and/or the bladder's total volume capacity.

ICD-10-CM Diagnostic Codes

N31.0	Uninhibited neuropathic bladder, not elsewhere classified
N31.1	Reflex neuropathic bladder, not elsewhere classified
N31.2	Flaccid neuropathic bladder, not elsewhere classified
N39.3	Stress incontinence (female) (male)
N39.41	Urge incontinence
N39.43	Post-void dribbling
N39.44	Nocturnal enuresis
N39.45	Continuous leakage
N39.46	Mixed incontinence
N39.490	Overflow incontinence
N39.498	Other specified urinary incontinence
N40.0	Benign prostatic hyperplasia without lower urinary tract symptoms ♂
N40.1	Benign prostatic hyperplasia with lower urinary tract symptoms ♂
R30.1	Vesical tenesmus
R33.0	Drug induced retention of urine
R33.8	Other retention of urine
R34	Anuria and oliguria
R35.0	Frequency of micturition
R35.1	Nocturia
R35.81	Nocturnal polyuria
R35.89	Other polyuria
R36.0	Urethral discharge without blood
R39.0	Extravasation of urine
R39.11	Hesitancy of micturition
R39.12	Poor urinary stream
R39.13	Splitting of urinary stream
R39.14	Feeling of incomplete bladder emptying
R39.15	Urgency of urination
R39.16	Straining to void
R39.191	Need to immediately re-void
R39.192	Position dependent micturition
R39.198	Other difficulties with micturition
R39.2	Extrarenal uremia
R39.81	Functional urinary incontinence
R39.89	Other symptoms and signs involving the genitourinary system

CCI Edits

Refer to Appendix A for CCI edits.

Pub 100

51798: Pub 100-03, 1, 220.5

Facility RVUs

Code	Work	PE Facility	MP	Total Facility
51798	0.00	0.30	0.01	0.31

Non-facility RVUs

Code	Work	PE Non-Facility	MP	Total Non-Facility
51798	0.00	0.30	0.01	0.31

Modifiers (PAR)

Code	Mod 50	Mod 51	Mod 62	Mod 66	Mod 80
51798	0	0	0	0	0

Global Period

Code	Days
51798	XXX

51800-51820

51800 Cystoplasty or cystourethroplasty, plastic operation on bladder and/or vesical neck (anterior Y-plasty, vesical fundus resection), any procedure, with or without wedge resection of posterior vesical neck

51820 Cystourethroplasty with unilateral or bilateral ureteroneocystostomy

AMA Coding Notes

Surgical Procedures on the Urinary System

(For provision of chemotherapeutic agents, report both the specific service in addition to code(s) for the specific substance(s) or drug(s) provided)

Plain English Description

Plastic reconstruction of the bladder, which may also include reconstruction of the vesical neck and urethra, is performed. Plastic reconstruction may be performed for congenital anomalies, scarring or acquired deformities due to previous surgery, or traumatic injuries. There are a number of different reconstruction techniques that may be employed depending on the condition being treated. The bladder is exposed using a low midline or transverse suprapubic incision. A defect in the posterior bladder is typically approached intraperitoneally while defects in the dome, anterior bladder, vesical neck, and/or urethra are approached extraperitoneally. In 51800, the bladder is incised and the bladder defect is inspected. Portions of the bladder, bladder neck, or urethra may be excised. The bladder wall is reconfigured as needed. For example, to reconfigure an enlarged bladder trigone, the wall of the bladder neck may be plicated or a Y-plasty may be performed. In 51820, the bladder defect is located near one or both ureteral orifices, and a ureteroneocystostomy is performed in conjunction with the cystourethroplasty. One or both ureters are ligated and transected at the ureterovesical junction. The bladder defect is then repaired and the ureters are transplanted to a new site in the bladder. An incision is made in the muscular wall of the bladder and a trough is created. The ureter(s) is placed in the trough in the detrusor muscle. An incision is made in the bladder mucosa at the distal aspect of the trough. The ureter(s) is secured to the interior aspect of the bladder with sutures. The trough is closed over the proximal aspect of the ureter(s).

Cystoplasty or cystourethroplasty

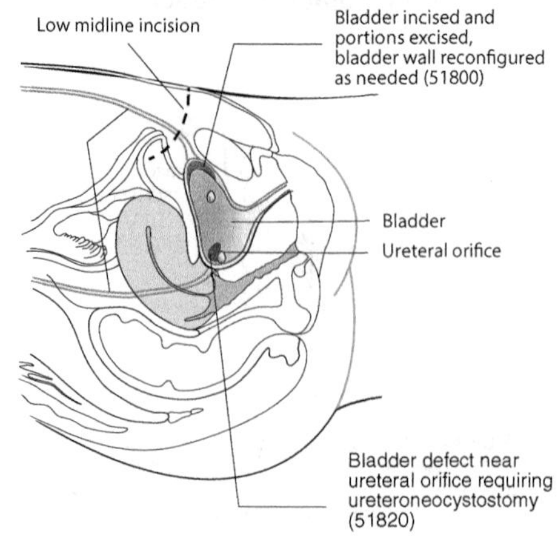

ICD-10-CM Diagnostic Codes

	N32.0	Bladder-neck obstruction
	N32.89	Other specified disorders of bladder
	N35.012	Post-traumatic membranous urethral stricture ♂
	N35.021	Urethral stricture due to childbirth ♀
	N35.028	Other post-traumatic urethral stricture, female ♀
	N35.113	Postinfective membranous urethral stricture, not elsewhere classified, male ♂
	N35.12	Postinfective urethral stricture, not elsewhere classified, female ♀
	N35.813	Other membranous urethral stricture, male ♂
	N39.3	Stress incontinence (female) (male)
	N39.41	Urge incontinence
	N39.42	Incontinence without sensory awareness
	N39.46	Mixed incontinence
	N99.112	Postprocedural membranous urethral stricture, male ♂
	N99.12	Postprocedural urethral stricture, female ♀
	Q64.11	Supravesical fissure of urinary bladder
	Q64.12	Cloacal exstrophy of urinary bladder
	Q64.19	Other exstrophy of urinary bladder
	Q64.31	Congenital bladder neck obstruction
	Q64.39	Other atresia and stenosis of urethra and bladder neck
	Q64.6	Congenital diverticulum of bladder
	Q64.71	Congenital prolapse of urethra
	Q64.73	Congenital urethrorectal fistula
	Q64.79	Other congenital malformations of bladder and urethra
❼	S37.23	Laceration of bladder
❼	S37.29	Other injury of bladder
❼	S37.33	Laceration of urethra
❼	S37.39	Other injury of urethra

ICD-10-CM Coding Notes

For codes requiring a 7th character extension, refer to your ICD-10-CM book. Review the character descriptions and coding guidelines for proper selection. For some procedures, only certain characters will apply.

CCI Edits

Refer to Appendix A for CCI edits.

Facility RVUs □

Code	Work	PE Facility	MP	Total Facility
51800	18.89	9.19	2.23	30.31
51820	19.59	9.78	2.33	31.70

Non-facility RVUs □

Code	Work	PE Non-Facility	MP	Total Non-Facility
51800	18.89	9.19	2.23	30.31
51820	19.59	9.78	2.33	31.70

Modifiers (PAR) □

Code	Mod 50	Mod 51	Mod 62	Mod 66	Mod 80
51800	0	2	1	0	2
51820	2	2	1	0	2

Global Period

Code	Days
51800	090
51820	090

51840-51841

51840 Anterior vesicourethropexy, or urethropexy (eg, Marshall-Marchetti-Krantz, Burch); simple

51841 Anterior vesicourethropexy, or urethropexy (eg, Marshall-Marchetti-Krantz, Burch); complicated (eg, secondary repair)

(For urethropexy (Pereyra type), use 57289)

AMA Coding Notes

Surgical Procedures on the Urinary System

(For provision of chemotherapeutic agents, report both the specific service in addition to code(s) for the specific substance(s) or drug(s) provided)

AMA *CPT® Assistant*

51840: Jan 97: 1, Nov 97: 19, Apr 98: 15, Jun 02: 7, May 06: 17, Jun 10: 6, Aug 12: 13

51841: Jan 97: 1, Jun 02: 7, Jun 10: 6, Aug 12: 13

Plain English Description

The physician performs an anterior vesicourethropexy or urethropexy, also referred to as a Marshall-Marchetti-Krantz or Burch procedure, or an abdominal bladder suspension. This procedure is performed to treat incontinence in women caused by stretching of the pelvic ligaments with vaginal wall prolapse. An incision is made in the abdomen, and the bladder neck and urethra are exposed. The prolapsed vaginal wall and urethra are then suspended. Two sutures are placed through the paravaginal fascia, one on each side of the urethrovesical junction, and oriented perpendicular to the vaginal axis. The sutures are then passed through the Cooper's ligament, pelvic fascia, or pubic bone and tied to provide suspension and support to the bladder and urethra. If additional suspension is required, a second set of sutures may be placed along the base of the bladder. Use 51840 for simple bladder suspension in patients who have not been operated on previously (primary bladder suspension or repair). Use code 51841 for a complex procedure in patients with a failed suspension procedure requiring secondary repair.

Anterior vesicourethropexy, or urethropexy

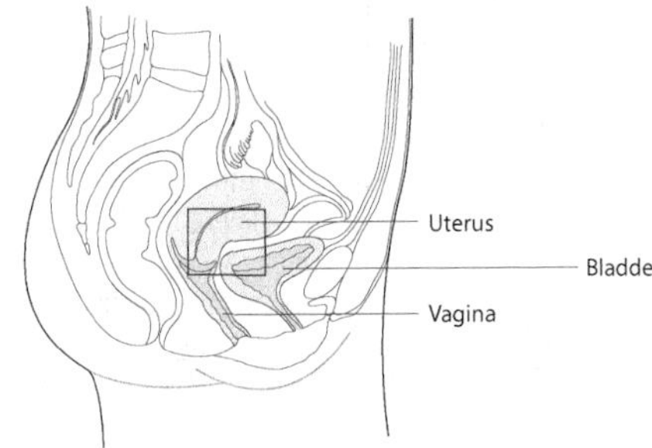

The bladder is sutured to the pubic bone or the wall of the vagina.

ICD-10-CM Diagnostic Codes

N39.3	Stress incontinence (female) (male)
N39.41	Urge incontinence
N39.42	Incontinence without sensory awareness
N39.43	Post-void dribbling
N39.44	Nocturnal enuresis
N39.45	Continuous leakage
N39.46	Mixed incontinence
N39.490	Overflow incontinence
N39.498	Other specified urinary incontinence
N81.0	Urethrocele ♀
N81.11	Cystocele, midline ♀
N81.12	Cystocele, lateral ♀
N81.2	Incomplete uterovaginal prolapse ♀
N81.3	Complete uterovaginal prolapse ♀
N81.5	Vaginal enterocele ♀
N81.6	Rectocele ♀
N81.81	Perineocele ♀
N81.82	Incompetence or weakening of pubocervical tissue ♀
N81.84	Pelvic muscle wasting ♀
N81.85	Cervical stump prolapse ♀
N81.89	Other female genital prolapse ♀
N99.3	Prolapse of vaginal vault after hysterectomy ♀

CCI Edits

Refer to Appendix A for CCI edits.

Facility RVUs

Code	Work	PE Facility	MP	Total Facility
51840	11.36	7.73	1.48	20.57
51841	13.68	8.43	1.63	23.74

Non-facility RVUs

Code	Work	PE Non-Facility	MP	Total Non-Facility
51840	11.36	7.73	1.48	20.57
51841	13.68	8.43	1.63	23.74

Modifiers (PAR)

Code	Mod 50	Mod 51	Mod 62	Mod 66	Mod 80
51840	0	2	1	0	2
51841	0	2	1	0	2

Global Period

Code	Days
51840	090
51841	090

51860-51865

51860 Cystorrhaphy, suture of bladder wound, injury or rupture; simple

51865 Cystorrhaphy, suture of bladder wound, injury or rupture; complicated

AMA Coding Notes

Surgical Procedures on the Urinary System

(For provision of chemotherapeutic agents, report both the specific service in addition to code(s) for the specific substance(s) or drug(s) provided)

Plain English Description

A cystorrhaphy is performed for suture repair of a bladder wound, injury, or rupture. Types of bladder injuries include contusion with tear of the bladder mucosa, intraperitoneal laceration or rupture, interstitial injury, extraperitoneal laceration or rupture, or a combination of these types of injuries. A Foley catheter is inserted and the bladder drained. A vertical midline incision is made in the abdomen. The pelvic viscera, ureters, bowel, and blood vessels are inspected. The exterior of the bladder is inspected. The dome of the bladder is opened and the interior of the bladder inspected. Any foreign bodies are removed. The ureteral orifices are inspected to ensure that they are intact. The bladder injury is localized and any nonviable tissue debrided. The bladder injury is closed in layers in a watertight fashion. Omental fat may be interposed on the closure to cushion the bladder from associated pelvic fractures. Following closure, water or saline is instilled through the Foley catheter to ensure that no leakage occurs at the repair site. A suprapubic catheter may be placed through a separate incision along with a drain in the perivesical space. The abdomen is then closed in layers. Use code 51860 for a simple suture repair and code 51865 for a complicated repair. Complicated repairs include bladder injuries with foreign body, debris, extensive nonviable tissue, and pelvic fracture or other injury that complicates the cystorrhaphy.

Cystorrhaphy

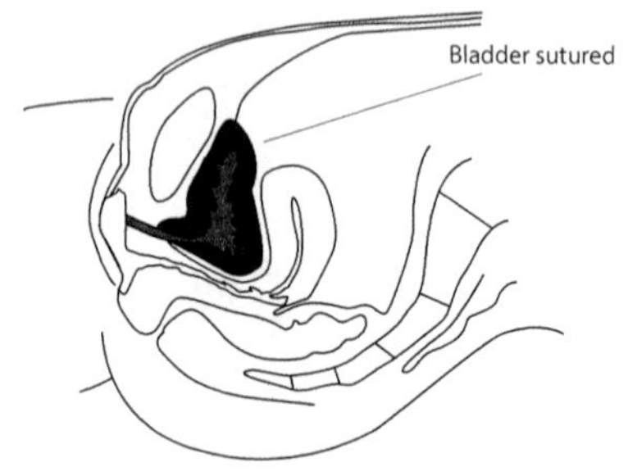

For 51860, a simple wound to the bladder is repaired. For 51865, a complicated wound to the bladder is repaired.

ICD-10-CM Diagnostic Codes

	N32.89	Other specified disorders of bladder
	N99.71	Accidental puncture and laceration of a genitourinary system organ or structure during a genitourinary system procedure
	N99.72	Accidental puncture and laceration of a genitourinary system organ or structure during other procedure
	O03.34	Damage to pelvic organs following incomplete spontaneous abortion ♀
	O03.84	Damage to pelvic organs following complete or unspecified spontaneous abortion ♀
	O04.84	Damage to pelvic organs following (induced) termination of pregnancy ♀
	O07.34	Damage to pelvic organs following failed attempted termination of pregnancy ♀
➐	S37.23	Laceration of bladder
➐	S37.29	Other injury of bladder

ICD-10-CM Coding Notes

For codes requiring a 7th character extension, refer to your ICD-10-CM book. Review the character descriptions and coding guidelines for proper selection. For some procedures, only certain characters will apply.

CCI Edits

Refer to Appendix A for CCI edits.

Facility RVUs ▢

Code	Work	PE Facility	MP	Total Facility
51860	12.60	7.44	1.93	21.97
51865	15.80	8.38	2.17	26.35

Non-facility RVUs ▢

Code	Work	PE Non-Facility	MP	Total Non-Facility
51860	12.60	7.44	1.93	21.97
51865	15.80	8.38	2.17	26.35

Modifiers (PAR) ▢

Code	Mod 50	Mod 51	Mod 62	Mod 66	Mod 80
51860	0	2	1	0	2
51865	0	2	1	0	2

Global Period

Code	Days
51860	090
51865	090

51880

51880 Closure of cystostomy (separate procedure)

AMA Coding Notes

Surgical Procedures on the Urinary System

(For provision of chemotherapeutic agents, report both the specific service in addition to code(s) for the specific substance(s) or drug(s) provided)

Plain English Description

The physician closes a cystostomy, a surgically created opening through the abdomen into the bladder through which a catheter is inserted for drainage. The drainage catheter is removed and the surgically created opening in the bladder is closed in a layered fashion. The opening in the abdominal wall and skin are also closed.

Closure of cystostomy

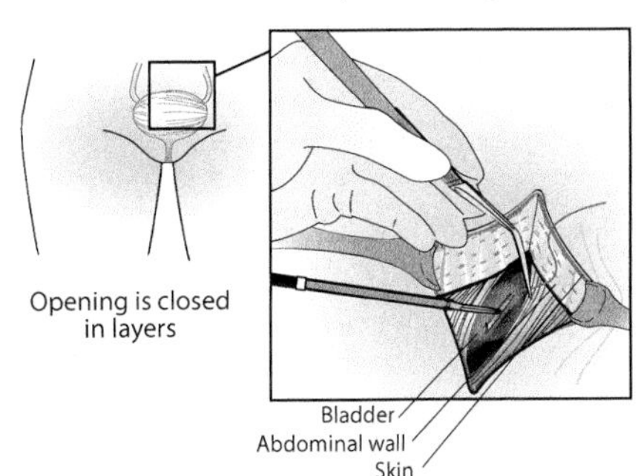

ICD-10-CM Diagnostic Codes

	N99.510	Cystostomy hemorrhage
	N99.511	Cystostomy infection
	N99.512	Cystostomy malfunction
	N99.518	Other cystostomy complication
❼	T83.010	Breakdown (mechanical) of cystostomy catheter
❼	T83.020	Displacement of cystostomy catheter
❼	T83.030	Leakage of cystostomy catheter
❼	T83.090	Other mechanical complication of cystostomy catheter
❼	T83.84	Pain due to genitourinary prosthetic devices, implants and grafts
❼	T83.85	Stenosis due to genitourinary prosthetic devices, implants and grafts
❼	T83.86	Thrombosis due to genitourinary prosthetic devices, implants and grafts

ICD-10-CM Coding Notes

For codes requiring a 7th character extension, refer to your ICD-10-CM book. Review the character descriptions and coding guidelines for proper selection. For some procedures, only certain characters will apply.

CCI Edits

Refer to Appendix A for CCI edits.

Facility RVUs ▯

Code	Work	PE Facility	MP	Total Facility
51880	7.87	4.76	1.04	13.67

Non-facility RVUs ▯

Code	Work	PE Non-Facility	MP	Total Non-Facility
51880	7.87	4.76	1.04	13.67

Modifiers (PAR) ▯

Code	Mod 50	Mod 51	Mod 62	Mod 66	Mod 80
51880	0	2	1	0	2

Global Period

Code	Days
51880	090

51900

51900 Closure of vesicovaginal fistula, abdominal approach

(For vaginal approach, see 57320-57330)

AMA Coding Notes

Surgical Procedures on the Urinary System

(For provision of chemotherapeutic agents, report both the specific service in addition to code(s) for the specific substance(s) or drug(s) provided)

Plain English Description

A vesicovaginal fistula is an abnormal passage between the bladder and vagina through which urine is passing into the vaginal vault. The abdomen is incised and the bladder is exposed. An incision is made in the bladder, the ureters are catheterized, and the fistula tract is located. Stay sutures are placed around the fistula tract, which is then excised along with any scar tissue or necrotic tissue. The bladder wall is dissected free of the endopelvic fascia and vaginal wall. The vaginal wall defect is closed. The bladder wall defect is closed. The ureteral catheters are removed and the cystotomy is closed.

Closure of vesicovaginal fistula, abdominal approach

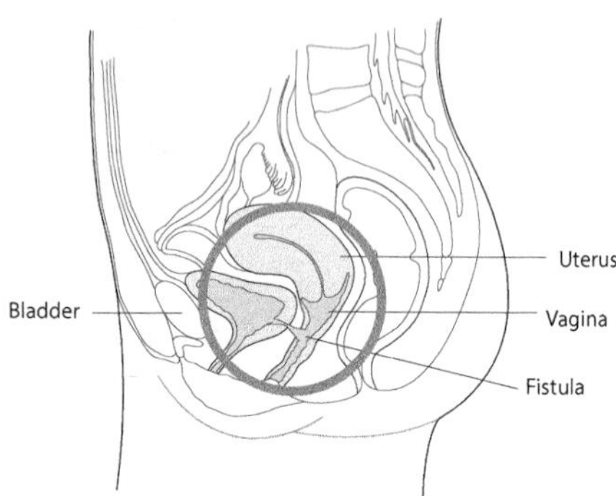

A vesicovaginal fistula is closed using an abdominal approach.

ICD-10-CM Diagnostic Codes

N82.0	Vesicovaginal fistula ♀
N82.1	Other female urinary-genital tract fistulae ♀

CCI Edits

Refer to Appendix A for CCI edits.

Facility RVUs

Code	Work	PE Facility	MP	Total Facility
51900	14.63	7.74	1.73	24.10

Non-facility RVUs

Code	Work	PE Non-Facility	MP	Total Non-Facility
51900	14.63	7.74	1.73	24.10

Modifiers (PAR)

Code	Mod 50	Mod 51	Mod 62	Mod 66	Mod 80
51900	0	2	1	0	2

Global Period

Code	Days
51900	090

51920-51925

51920 Closure of vesicouterine fistula

51925 Closure of vesicouterine fistula; with hysterectomy

(For closure of vesicoenteric fistula, see 44660, 44661)

(For closure of rectovesical fistula, see 45800-45805)

AMA Coding Notes

Surgical Procedures on the Urinary System

(For provision of chemotherapeutic agents, report both the specific service in addition to code(s) for the specific substance(s) or drug(s) provided)

Plain English Description

The physician closes a vesicouterine fistula. An incision is made in the lower abdomen and the abdomen and pelvis are inspected. The vesicouterine space is dissected using sharp and blunt dissection. The fistulous tract is located and excised. The fistulous opening in the bladder is closed. The fistulous opening in the uterus is closed and omentum interposed between the bladder and uterus. The bladder is filled in a retrograde fashion and watertight repair of the bladder wall verified. The abdominal wall and skin are closed in a layered fashion. In 51925, the vesicouterine fistula is closed and a hysterectomy is performed. The fistula is excised and the bladder wall defect is closed as described above. The abdominal hysterectomy is then performed. The infundibulopelvic and round ligaments are identified, suture ligated, and divided. The bladder is reflected away from the cervix. Uterine and cervical vessels are cross clamped, divided, and ligated. The vagina is incised and the cervix separated from the vagina. The vaginal cuff is closed. The uterus and cervix are removed, bleeding is controlled, and the abdominal incision is closed in a layered fashion.

Closure of vesicouterine fistula

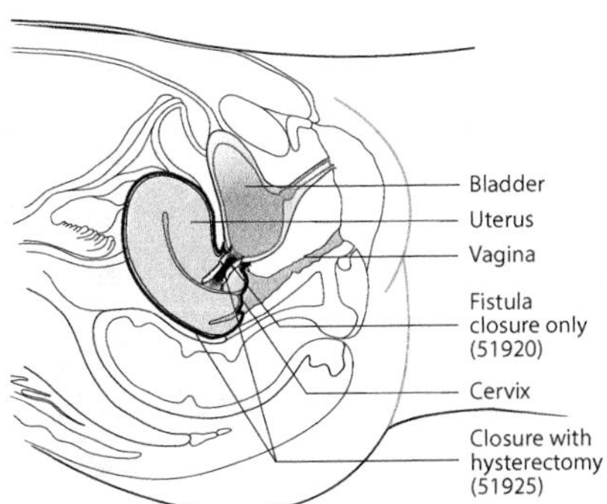

ICD-10-CM Diagnostic Codes

N82.1 Other female urinary-genital tract fistulae ♀

CCI Edits

Refer to Appendix A for CCI edits.

Pub 100

51925: Pub 100-03, 1, 230.3

Facility RVUs ▯

Code	Work	PE Facility	MP	Total Facility
51920	13.41	7.33	1.60	22.34
51925	17.53	11.75	2.88	32.16

Non-facility RVUs ▯

Code	Work	PE Non-Facility	MP	Total Non-Facility
51920	13.41	7.33	1.60	22.34
51925	17.53	11.75	2.88	32.16

Modifiers (PAR) ▯

Code	Mod 50	Mod 51	Mod 62	Mod 66	Mod 80
51920	0	2	1	0	2
51925	0	2	1	0	2

Global Period

Code	Days
51920	090
51925	090

51940

51940 Closure, exstrophy of bladder
(See also 54390)

AMA Coding Notes
Surgical Procedures on the Urinary System

(For provision of chemotherapeutic agents, report both the specific service in addition to code(s) for the specific substance(s) or drug(s) provided)

Plain English Description

Bladder exstrophy is a congenital defect in which the bladder is flat instead of round and exposed outside the body. The defect also affects the abdominal wall, pelvic bones, bladder neck, perineum, urethra, and external genitalia. The abdominal wall is open. The symphysis pubis is widely separated at the midline with bony deficits at the anterior pubic rami as well as anterior rotation of the posterior and anterior aspects of the pelvis. There is also a shortening of the distance between the umbilicus and the anus due to shortening and broadening of the perineum. The musculature at the bladder neck does not form properly, affecting bladder control. There is shortening and broadening of the perineum. In girls, the urethra and vagina are shorter than normal and the labia are widely separated with a bifid clitoris. In boys, the penis appears shorter than normal because the base of the penis remains attached to the pubic bones internally. The failure of the pubic bones to fuse causes the base of the penis to spread apart internally. The procedure begins by bringing the pelvic bones together. Minor pelvic bone separation may be treated by medial rotation of the greater trochanters, which will bring the pubic bones together at the midline. If the pelvic bones are widely separated, osteotomy may be required. Bilateral transverse anterior innominate bone and anterior vertical iliac bone osteotomies are performed with pin placement to close the separation at the symphysis pubis. Next, the bladder, posterior urethra, and abdominal wall are closed. An incision is made around the umbilicus and bladder and carried down to the urethral plate. The umbilical vessels are doubly ligated and transected. The bladder dome is separated from the peritoneum. The retropubic space is developed and the bladder is separated from the rectus sheath and muscle. In males, the prostrate is freed from the rectus muscle. The upper border of the urogenital diaphragm fibers between the bladder neck, posterior urethra, and pubic bone are sharply incised and separated down to the pelvic floor. In males, the prostate and anterior corpus are freed from the pubis by deep incision. Ureteral stents are placed; the bladder neck and urethra are reconstructed as needed; and the bladder wall is closed. The pubic bones are approximated using nylon sutures placed between the fibrous cartilages of the pubic rami. A drain is placed near the umbilicus and the abdominal wall is closed in layers.

Closure, exstrophy of bladder

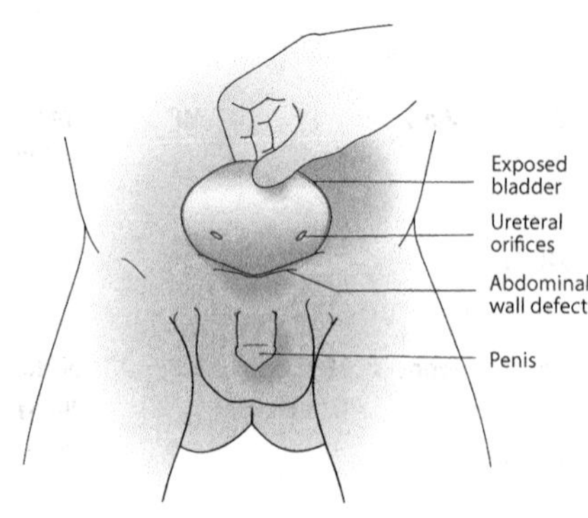

ICD-10-CM Diagnostic Codes

Q64.12	Cloacal exstrophy of urinary bladder
Q64.19	Other exstrophy of urinary bladder

CCI Edits

Refer to Appendix A for CCI edits.

Facility RVUs ☐

Code	Work	PE Facility	MP	Total Facility
51940	30.66	13.54	3.66	47.86

Non-facility RVUs ☐

Code	Work	PE Non-Facility	MP	Total Non-Facility
51940	30.66	13.54	3.66	47.86

Modifiers (PAR) ☐

Code	Mod 50	Mod 51	Mod 62	Mod 66	Mod 80
51940	0	2	1	0	2

Global Period

Code	Days
51940	090

51960

51960 Enterocystoplasty, including intestinal anastomosis

AMA Coding Notes

Surgical Procedures on the Urinary System

(For provision of chemotherapeutic agents, report both the specific service in addition to code(s) for the specific substance(s) or drug(s) provided)

Plain English Description

Enterocystoplasty, also referred to as bladder augmentation, uses a segment of intestine to enlarge the bladder and reduce intravesical pressure in patients with bladder neuropathy and high-pressure detrusor contractions. Cystoscopic examination of the bladder is performed. Internal ureteral stents or external ureteral catheters are placed. The cystoscope is removed and a Foley catheter is placed. The abdomen is incised in the midline and the peritoneum is opened. The small bowel is isolated and packed out of the surgical field. The ureters are identified and protected. The portion of colon or ileum to be used for the augmentation is isolated and harvested. The remaining segments of bowel distal and proximal to the isolated segment are anastomosed and bowel continuity is restored. The harvested segment of bowel is detubularized and reconfigured into a U-, S-, or W-shaped graft. The bladder is bivalved. A large-caliber suprapubic catheter is placed in addition to the Foley catheter. The intestinal graft is sutured to the bladder. Drains are placed as needed and the abdomen is closed around the drains.

Enterocystoplasty, including intestinal anastomosis

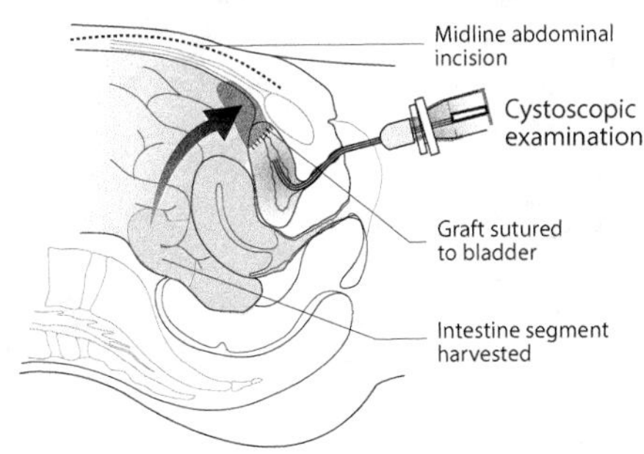

ICD-10-CM Diagnostic Codes

G83.4	Cauda equina syndrome
N30.10	Interstitial cystitis (chronic) without hematuria
N30.11	Interstitial cystitis (chronic) with hematuria
N30.40	Irradiation cystitis without hematuria
N30.41	Irradiation cystitis with hematuria
N31.0	Uninhibited neuropathic bladder, not elsewhere classified
N31.1	Reflex neuropathic bladder, not elsewhere classified
N31.8	Other neuromuscular dysfunction of bladder
N31.9	Neuromuscular dysfunction of bladder, unspecified
N32.89	Other specified disorders of bladder
N99.89	Other postprocedural complications and disorders of genitourinary system
Q64.0	Epispadias
Q64.12	Cloacal exstrophy of urinary bladder
Q64.19	Other exstrophy of urinary bladder
Q64.2	Congenital posterior urethral valves

CCI Edits

Refer to Appendix A for CCI edits.

Facility RVUs

Code	Work	PE Facility	MP	Total Facility
51960	25.40	11.99	3.02	40.41

Non-facility RVUs

Code	Work	PE Non-Facility	MP	Total Non-Facility
51960	25.40	11.99	3.02	40.41

Modifiers (PAR)

Code	Mod 50	Mod 51	Mod 62	Mod 66	Mod 80
51960	0	2	1	0	2

Global Period

Code	Days
51960	090

CPT® Procedural Coding

51980

51980 Cutaneous vesicostomy

AMA Coding Notes

Surgical Procedures on the Urinary System

(For provision of chemotherapeutic agents, report both the specific service in addition to code(s) for the specific substance(s) or drug(s) provided)

Plain English Description

Cutaneous vesicostomy, also referred to as cutaneous cystostomy, involves incising the bladder and creating a stoma on the skin to allow drainage of urine. The abdomen is incised and the rectus fascia is exposed. A triangular segment of fascia is excised. The rectus muscle is divided and the space of Retzius is entered. The dome of the bladder is exposed. The bladder is incised. The bladder wall is sutured to the rectus fascia. The bladder epithelium is sutured to the skin. An ostomy bag is placed over the stoma.

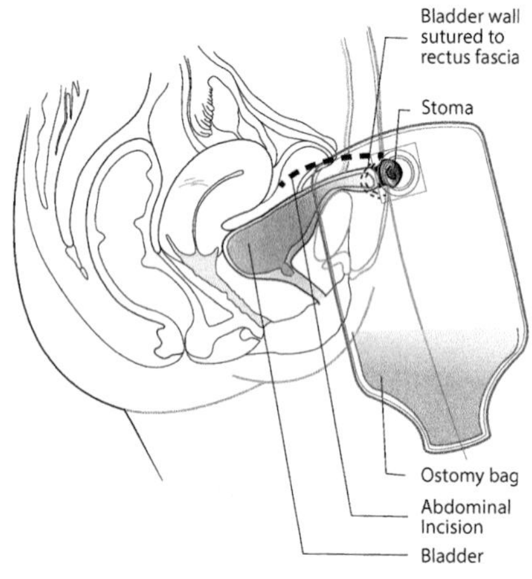

ICD-10-CM Diagnostic Codes

⇄	C65.9	Malignant neoplasm of unspecified renal pelvis
	C67.6	Malignant neoplasm of ureteric orifice
	C67.9	Malignant neoplasm of bladder, unspecified
	D07.5	Carcinoma in situ of prostate ♂
	G83.4	Cauda equina syndrome
	N13.71	Vesicoureteral-reflux without reflux nephropathy
	N13.721	Vesicoureteral-reflux with reflux nephropathy without hydroureter, unilateral
	N13.722	Vesicoureteral-reflux with reflux nephropathy without hydroureter, bilateral
	N13.731	Vesicoureteral-reflux with reflux nephropathy with hydroureter, unilateral
	N13.732	Vesicoureteral-reflux with reflux nephropathy with hydroureter, bilateral
	N13.8	Other obstructive and reflux uropathy
	N31.0	Uninhibited neuropathic bladder, not elsewhere classified
	N31.1	Reflex neuropathic bladder, not elsewhere classified
	N31.8	Other neuromuscular dysfunction of bladder
	N31.9	Neuromuscular dysfunction of bladder, unspecified
	N99.89	Other postprocedural complications and disorders of genitourinary system
	Q64.11	Supravesical fissure of urinary bladder
	Q64.12	Cloacal exstrophy of urinary bladder
	Q64.19	Other exstrophy of urinary bladder
	R33.9	Retention of urine, unspecified

CCI Edits

Refer to Appendix A for CCI edits.

Facility RVUs ▯

Code	Work	PE Facility	MP	Total Facility
51980	12.57	6.83	1.49	20.89

Non-facility RVUs ▯

Code	Work	PE Non-Facility	MP	Total Non-Facility
51980	12.57	6.83	1.49	20.89

Modifiers (PAR) ▯

Code	Mod 50	Mod 51	Mod 62	Mod 66	Mod 80
51980	0	2	1	0	2

Global Period

Code	Days
51980	090

51990

51990 Laparoscopy, surgical; urethral suspension for stress incontinence

AMA Coding Guideline

Laparoscopic Procedures on the Bladder

Surgical laparoscopy always includes diagnostic laparoscopy. To report a diagnostic laparoscopy (peritoneoscopy) (separate procedure), use 49320.

AMA Coding Notes

Surgical Procedures on the Urinary System

(For provision of chemotherapeutic agents, report both the specific service in addition to code(s) for the specific substance(s) or drug(s) provided)

AMA *CPT® Assistant* ▢

51990: Nov 99: 26, May 00: 4, Jun 10: 6, Mar 12: 10, Aug 12: 13

Plain English Description

A urethral suspension procedure for stress incontinence is performed via a laparoscopic approach. A small incision is made just below the umbilicus and the laparoscope is introduced. Two or three additional small incisions are made in the abdomen to allow introduction of surgical instruments. The intraperitoneal cavity is inspected. The space of Retzius is dissected and the paravaginal fascia is identified and elevated. Two endoscopic sutures are then placed through the paravaginal fascia, one on each side of the urethrovesical junction, and oriented perpendicular to the vaginal axis. The sutures are passed through Cooper's ligament and tied. This elevates the urethrovesical angle and provides a platform on which the bladder neck rests. The suspension is then checked visually, manually, or by cystoscopy to ensure that it is adequate. If additional suspension is required, a second set of sutures may be placed along the base of the bladder. The laparoscope and surgical instruments are removed and the abdominal incisions are closed.

Laparoscopy, surgical; urethral suspension for stress incontinence

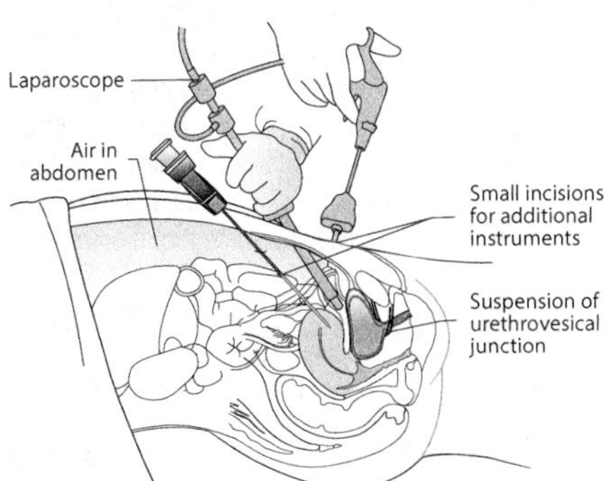

ICD-10-CM Diagnostic Codes

N36.41	Hypermobility of urethra
N36.42	Intrinsic sphincter deficiency (ISD)
N36.43	Combined hypermobility of urethra and intrinsic sphincter deficiency
N39.3	Stress incontinence (female) (male)
N39.46	Mixed incontinence
N81.0	Urethrocele ♀
N81.11	Cystocele, midline ♀
N81.12	Cystocele, lateral ♀

CCI Edits

Refer to Appendix A for CCI edits.

Facility RVUs ▢

Code	Work	PE Facility	MP	Total Facility
51990	13.36	6.83	1.64	21.83

Non-facility RVUs ▢

Code	Work	PE Non-Facility	MP	Total Non-Facility
51990	13.36	6.83	1.64	21.83

Modifiers (PAR) ▢

Code	Mod 50	Mod 51	Mod 62	Mod 66	Mod 80
51990	0	2	1	0	2

Global Period

Code	Days
51990	090

CPT® Procedural Coding

52000

52000 Cystourethroscopy (separate procedure)

(Do not report 52000 in conjunction with 52001, 52320, 52325, 52327, 52330, 52332, 52334, 52341, 52342, 52343, 52356)

(Do not report 52000 in conjunction with 57240, 57260, 57265)

AMA Coding Guideline

Endoscopy-Cystoscopy, Urethroscopy, Cystourethroscopy Procedures on the Bladder

Endoscopic descriptions are listed so that the main procedure can be identified without having to list all the minor related functions performed at the same time. For example: meatotomy, urethral calibration and/or dilation, urethroscopy, and cystoscopy prior to a transurethral resection of prostate; ureteral catheterization following extraction of ureteral calculus; internal urethrotomy and bladder neck fulguration when performing a cystourethroscopy for the female urethral syndrome. When the secondary procedure requires significant additional time and effort, it may be identified by the addition of modifier 22.

For example: urethrotomy performed for a documented pre-existing stricture or bladder neck contracture.

Because cutaneous urinary diversions utilizing ileum or colon serve as functional replacements of a native bladder, endoscopy of such bowel segments, as well as performance of secondary procedures can be captured by using the cystourethroscopy codes. For example, endoscopy of an ileal loop with removal of ureteral calculus would be coded as cystourethroscopy (including ureteral catheterization); with removal of ureteral calculus (52320).

AMA Coding Notes

Surgical Procedures on the Urinary System

(For provision of chemotherapeutic agents, report both the specific service in addition to code(s) for the specific substance(s) or drug(s) provided)

AMA *CPT® Assistant*

52000: Oct 00: 7, May 01: 5, Sep 04: 11, Oct 05: 23, Nov 07: 9, Mar 13: 14, May 14: 3, Oct 17: 9, Nov 18: 10

Plain English Description

A cystourethroscopy is performed to visualize the inside of the bladder and urethra in a separate procedure. The urethra is cleansed with antiseptic solution. A rigid or flexible cystoscope consisting of a thin, telescope-like tube with a light and camera is introduced through the urethra into the bladder. The camera allows images of the urethra and bladder to be viewed on a computer or television monitor. The bladder may be filled with sterile saline or water to improve visualization of the bladder wall. Once the procedure is complete, the saline or water is drained from the bladder and the cystoscope is removed.

Cystourethroscopy

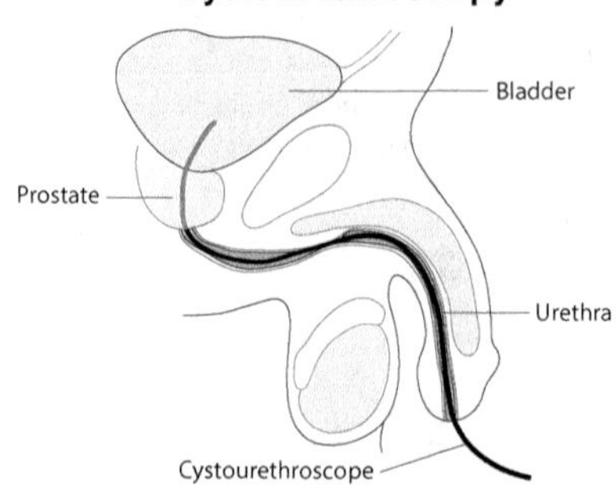

A cystourethroscope is inserted into the urethra and up into the bladder for diagnostic visualization.

ICD-10-CM Diagnostic Codes

C67.0	Malignant neoplasm of trigone of bladder
C67.1	Malignant neoplasm of dome of bladder
C67.2	Malignant neoplasm of lateral wall of bladder
C67.3	Malignant neoplasm of anterior wall of bladder
C67.4	Malignant neoplasm of posterior wall of bladder
C67.5	Malignant neoplasm of bladder neck
C67.6	Malignant neoplasm of ureteric orifice
C67.8	Malignant neoplasm of overlapping sites of bladder
C68.0	Malignant neoplasm of urethra
C79.11	Secondary malignant neoplasm of bladder
C79.19	Secondary malignant neoplasm of other urinary organs
D09.0	Carcinoma in situ of bladder
D09.19	Carcinoma in situ of other urinary organs
D30.3	Benign neoplasm of bladder
D30.4	Benign neoplasm of urethra
D41.3	Neoplasm of uncertain behavior of urethra
D41.4	Neoplasm of uncertain behavior of bladder
D49.4	Neoplasm of unspecified behavior of bladder
N11.0	Nonobstructive reflux-associated chronic pyelonephritis
N13.2	Hydronephrosis with renal and ureteral calculous obstruction
N21.0	Calculus in bladder
N30.10	Interstitial cystitis (chronic) without hematuria
N30.11	Interstitial cystitis (chronic) with hematuria
N30.30	Trigonitis without hematuria
N30.31	Trigonitis with hematuria
N30.40	Irradiation cystitis without hematuria
N30.41	Irradiation cystitis with hematuria
N31.9	Neuromuscular dysfunction of bladder, unspecified
N32.0	Bladder-neck obstruction
N32.1	Vesicointestinal fistula
N32.2	Vesical fistula, not elsewhere classified
N32.3	Diverticulum of bladder
N32.81	Overactive bladder
N32.89	Other specified disorders of bladder
N34.0	Urethral abscess
N34.1	Nonspecific urethritis
N34.2	Other urethritis
N34.3	Urethral syndrome, unspecified
N35.010	Post-traumatic urethral stricture, male, meatal ♂
N35.011	Post-traumatic bulbous urethral stricture ♂
N35.012	Post-traumatic membranous urethral stricture ♂
N35.013	Post-traumatic anterior urethral stricture ♂
N35.016	Post-traumatic urethral stricture, male, overlapping sites ♂
N35.021	Urethral stricture due to childbirth ♀
N35.111	Postinfective urethral stricture, not elsewhere classified, male, meatal ♂
N35.112	Postinfective bulbous urethral stricture, not elsewhere classified, male ♂
N35.113	Postinfective membranous urethral stricture, not elsewhere classified, male ♂
N35.114	Postinfective anterior urethral stricture, not elsewhere classified, male ♂
N35.116	Postinfective urethral stricture, not elsewhere classified, male, overlapping sites ♂
N35.811	Other urethral stricture, male, meatal ♂
N35.812	Other urethral bulbous stricture, male ♂
N35.813	Other membranous urethral stricture, male ♂
N35.814	Other anterior urethral stricture, male ♂
N35.816	Other urethral stricture, male, overlapping sites ♂
N35.82	Other urethral stricture, female ♀
N35.92	Unspecified urethral stricture, female ♀
N36.0	Urethral fistula
N36.1	Urethral diverticulum
N36.2	Urethral caruncle
N36.41	Hypermobility of urethra
N36.42	Intrinsic sphincter deficiency (ISD)
N36.43	Combined hypermobility of urethra and intrinsic sphincter deficiency
N36.44	Muscular disorders of urethra
N36.5	Urethral false passage
N37	Urethral disorders in diseases classified elsewhere
N39.0	Urinary tract infection, site not specified
N39.3	Stress incontinence (female) (male)
N39.41	Urge incontinence
N39.42	Incontinence without sensory awareness

N39.43 Post-void dribbling
N39.44 Nocturnal enuresis
N39.45 Continuous leakage
N39.46 Mixed incontinence
N39.490 Overflow incontinence
N39.491 Coital incontinence
N39.492 Postural (urinary) incontinence
N39.498 Other specified urinary incontinence
N40.0 Benign prostatic hyperplasia without lower urinary tract symptoms ♂
N40.1 Benign prostatic hyperplasia with lower urinary tract symptoms ♂
N40.2 Nodular prostate without lower urinary tract symptoms ♂
N40.3 Nodular prostate with lower urinary tract symptoms ♂
N41.0 Acute prostatitis ♂
N41.1 Chronic prostatitis ♂
N41.3 Prostatocystitis ♂
N41.4 Granulomatous prostatitis ♂
N42.0 Calculus of prostate ♂
N42.1 Congestion and hemorrhage of prostate ♂
N42.30 Unspecified dysplasia of prostate ♂
N42.31 Prostatic intraepithelial neoplasia ♂
N42.32 Atypical small acinar proliferation of prostate ♂
N42.39 Other dysplasia of prostate ♂
N42.81 Prostatodynia syndrome ♂
N42.82 Prostatosis syndrome ♂
N42.83 Cyst of prostate ♂
N82.0 Vesicovaginal fistula ♀
N99.110 Postprocedural urethral stricture, male, meatal ♂
N99.111 Postprocedural bulbous urethral stricture, male ♂
N99.112 Postprocedural membranous urethral stricture, male ♂
N99.113 Postprocedural anterior bulbous urethral stricture, male ♂
N99.115 Postprocedural fossa navicularis urethral stricture ♂
N99.116 Postprocedural urethral stricture, male, overlapping sites ♂
N99.12 Postprocedural urethral stricture, female ♀
Q64.11 Supravesical fissure of urinary bladder
Q64.12 Cloacal exstrophy of urinary bladder
Q64.2 Congenital posterior urethral valves
Q64.31 Congenital bladder neck obstruction
Q64.32 Congenital stricture of urethra
Q64.33 Congenital stricture of urinary meatus
Q64.5 Congenital absence of bladder and urethra
Q64.6 Congenital diverticulum of bladder
Q64.71 Congenital prolapse of urethra
Q64.72 Congenital prolapse of urinary meatus
Q64.73 Congenital urethrorectal fistula
Q64.74 Double urethra
Q64.75 Double urinary meatus
R31.0 Gross hematuria
R31.9 Hematuria, unspecified
R33.8 Other retention of urine
R35.0 Frequency of micturition
R35.1 Nocturia
R36.0 Urethral discharge without blood
R36.1 Hematospermia ♂
R36.9 Urethral discharge, unspecified
R39.12 Poor urinary stream
R39.14 Feeling of incomplete bladder emptying
R39.15 Urgency of urination
R39.16 Straining to void
Z85.51 Personal history of malignant neoplasm of bladder

CCI Edits

Refer to Appendix A for CCI edits.

Facility RVUs ☐

Code	Work	PE Facility	MP	Total Facility
52000	1.53	0.63	0.19	2.35

Non-facility RVUs ☐

Code	Work	PE Non-Facility	MP	Total Non-Facility
52000	1.53	5.59	0.19	7.31

Modifiers (PAR) ☐

Code	Mod 50	Mod 51	Mod 62	Mod 66	Mod 80
52000	0	2	0	0	1

Global Period

Code	Days
52000	000

52001

52001 Cystourethroscopy with irrigation and evacuation of multiple obstructing clots

(Do not report 52001 in conjunction with 52000)

AMA Coding Guideline

Endoscopy-Cystoscopy, Urethroscopy, Cystourethroscopy Procedures on the Bladder

Endoscopic descriptions are listed so that the main procedure can be identified without having to list all the minor related functions performed at the same time. For example: meatotomy, urethral calibration and/or dilation, urethroscopy, and cystoscopy prior to a transurethral resection of prostate; ureteral catheterization following extraction of ureteral calculus; internal urethrotomy and bladder neck fulguration when performing a cystourethroscopy for the female urethral syndrome. When the secondary procedure requires significant additional time and effort, it may be identified by the addition of modifier 22.

For example: urethrotomy performed for a documented pre-existing stricture or bladder neck contracture.

Because cutaneous urinary diversions utilizing ileum or colon serve as functional replacements of a native bladder, endoscopy of such bowel segments, as well as performance of secondary procedures can be captured by using the cystourethroscopy codes. For example, endoscopy of an ileal loop with removal of ureteral calculus would be coded as cystourethroscopy (including ureteral catheterization); with removal of ureteral calculus (52320).

AMA Coding Notes

Surgical Procedures on the Urinary System

(For provision of chemotherapeutic agents, report both the specific service in addition to code(s) for the specific substance(s) or drug(s) provided)

Plain English Description

Cystourethroscopy is performed to visualize the inside of the bladder and urethra and remove obstructing blood clots. The urethra is cleansed with antiseptic solution. A rigid or flexible cystoscope is introduced through the urethra into the bladder. The bladder is inspected and obstructing blood clots are noted. The cystoscope is removed and a resectoscope is introduced into the bladder. The clots are broken up and evacuated. The bladder is flushed with sterile saline and inspected for any residual blood clots or bleeding. The resectoscope is removed. A catheter is inserted as needed for continuous bladder irrigation and/or drainage.

Cystourethroscopy with irrigation and evacuation of clots

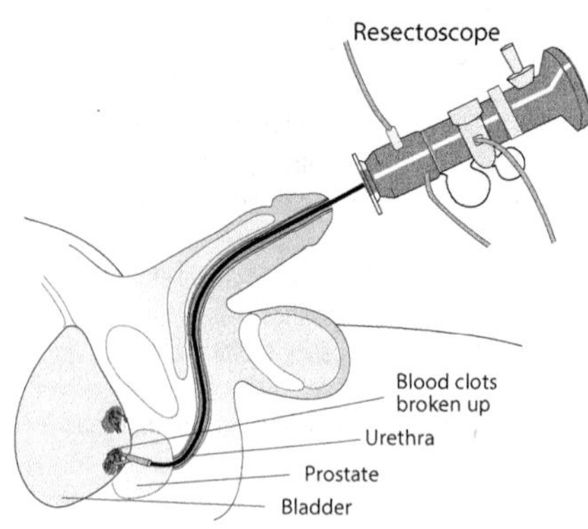

ICD-10-CM Diagnostic Codes

C67.9	Malignant neoplasm of bladder, unspecified
N21.0	Calculus in bladder
N30.40	Irradiation cystitis without hematuria
N30.41	Irradiation cystitis with hematuria
N32.0	Bladder-neck obstruction
N32.89	Other specified disorders of bladder
N36.8	Other specified disorders of urethra
N40.0	Benign prostatic hyperplasia without lower urinary tract symptoms ♂
R31.0	Gross hematuria
R31.9	Hematuria, unspecified
R33.9	Retention of urine, unspecified
R39.14	Feeling of incomplete bladder emptying

CCI Edits

Refer to Appendix A for CCI edits.

Facility RVUs ☐

Code	Work	PE Facility	MP	Total Facility
52001	5.44	2.23	0.65	8.32

Non-facility RVUs ☐

Code	Work	PE Non-Facility	MP	Total Non-Facility
52001	5.44	7.08	0.65	13.17

Modifiers (PAR) ☐

Code	Mod 50	Mod 51	Mod 62	Mod 66	Mod 80
52001	0	3	0	0	1

Global Period

Code	Days
52001	000

52005-52007

52005 Cystourethroscopy, with ureteral catheterization, with or without irrigation, instillation, or ureteropyelography, exclusive of radiologic service

52007 Cystourethroscopy, with ureteral catheterization, with or without irrigation, instillation, or ureteropyelography, exclusive of radiologic service; with brush biopsy of ureter and/or renal pelvis

(For image-guided biopsy of ureter and/or renal pelvis without endoscopic guidance, use 50606)

AMA Coding Guideline

Endoscopy-Cystoscopy, Urethroscopy, Cystourethroscopy Procedures on the Bladder

Endoscopic descriptions are listed so that the main procedure can be identified without having to list all the minor related functions performed at the same time. For example: meatotomy, urethral calibration and/or dilation, urethroscopy, and cystoscopy prior to a transurethral resection of prostate; ureteral catheterization following extraction of ureteral calculus; internal urethrotomy and bladder neck fulguration when performing a cystourethroscopy for the female urethral syndrome. When the secondary procedure requires significant additional time and effort, it may be identified by the addition of modifier 22.

For example: urethrotomy performed for a documented pre-existing stricture or bladder neck contracture.

Because cutaneous urinary diversions utilizing ileum or colon serve as functional replacements of a native bladder, endoscopy of such bowel segments, as well as performance of secondary procedures can be captured by using the cystourethroscopy codes. For example, endoscopy of an ileal loop with removal of ureteral calculus would be coded as cystourethroscopy (including ureteral catheterization); with removal of ureteral calculus (52320).

AMA Coding Notes

Surgical Procedures on the Urinary System

(For provision of chemotherapeutic agents, report both the specific service in addition to code(s) for the specific substance(s) or drug(s) provided)

AMA *CPT® Assistant* ☐

52005: Sep 00: 11, Jan 01: 13, May 01: 5, Oct 01: 8, Dec 10: 15, Mar 19: 11

52007: May 01: 5, Oct 01: 8

Plain English Description

Cystourethroscopy is performed to visualize the inside of the bladder and urethra with catheterization of the ureters. The urethra is cleansed with antiseptic solution. A rigid or flexible cystoscope is introduced through the urethra into the bladder. The bladder may be filled with sterile saline to allow better visualization of the bladder wall. In 52005, following inspection of the bladder, the ureters are catheterized. A guidewire is introduced through the cystoscope and advanced into the first ureter and through the ureter to the renal pelvis. A catheter is advanced over the guidewire to the renal pelvis. The ureter may be irrigated with normal saline, or diagnostic or therapeutic solution may be instilled. Contrast material may be injected and separately reportable ureteropyelography performed. The procedure may be repeated on the opposite ureter. Upon completion of the procedure, the catheter and guidewire are removed. In 52007, the ureters are catheterized as described above and tissue samples are obtained using a nylon or steel brush.

Cystourethroscopy, with ureteral catheterization

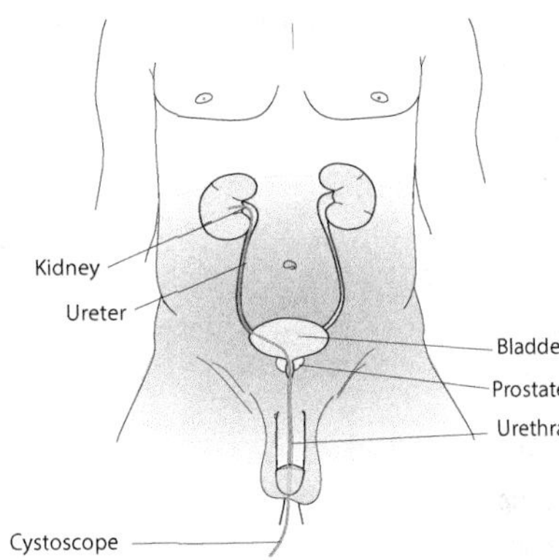

Exclusive of radiologic service (52005); with brush biopsy of ureter and/or renal pelvis (52007)

ICD-10-CM Diagnostic Codes

	C61	Malignant neoplasm of prostate ♂
⇄	C65.1	Malignant neoplasm of right renal pelvis
⇄	C65.2	Malignant neoplasm of left renal pelvis
⇄	C66.1	Malignant neoplasm of right ureter
⇄	C66.2	Malignant neoplasm of left ureter
	C67.0	Malignant neoplasm of trigone of bladder
	C67.1	Malignant neoplasm of dome of bladder
	C67.2	Malignant neoplasm of lateral wall of bladder
	C67.3	Malignant neoplasm of anterior wall of bladder
	C67.4	Malignant neoplasm of posterior wall of bladder
	C67.5	Malignant neoplasm of bladder neck
	C67.6	Malignant neoplasm of ureteric orifice
	C67.8	Malignant neoplasm of overlapping sites of bladder
	C68.0	Malignant neoplasm of urethra
⇄	C79.01	Secondary malignant neoplasm of right kidney and renal pelvis
⇄	C79.02	Secondary malignant neoplasm of left kidney and renal pelvis
	C79.11	Secondary malignant neoplasm of bladder
	D09.0	Carcinoma in situ of bladder
	D29.1	Benign neoplasm of prostate ♂
⇄	D30.01	Benign neoplasm of right kidney
⇄	D30.02	Benign neoplasm of left kidney
⇄	D30.11	Benign neoplasm of right renal pelvis
⇄	D30.12	Benign neoplasm of left renal pelvis
	D30.3	Benign neoplasm of bladder
	D30.4	Benign neoplasm of urethra
	D40.0	Neoplasm of uncertain behavior of prostate ♂
	D41.4	Neoplasm of uncertain behavior of bladder
	N11.1	Chronic obstructive pyelonephritis
	N13.1	Hydronephrosis with ureteral stricture, not elsewhere classified
	N13.2	Hydronephrosis with renal and ureteral calculous obstruction
	N13.4	Hydroureter
	N13.5	Crossing vessel and stricture of ureter without hydronephrosis
	N13.71	Vesicoureteral-reflux without reflux nephropathy
	N13.721	Vesicoureteral-reflux with reflux nephropathy without hydroureter, unilateral
	N13.722	Vesicoureteral-reflux with reflux nephropathy without hydroureter, bilateral
	N13.731	Vesicoureteral-reflux with reflux nephropathy with hydroureter, unilateral
	N13.732	Vesicoureteral-reflux with reflux nephropathy with hydroureter, bilateral
	N13.8	Other obstructive and reflux uropathy
	N20.0	Calculus of kidney
	N20.1	Calculus of ureter
	N20.2	Calculus of kidney with calculus of ureter
	N21.0	Calculus in bladder
	N28.0	Ischemia and infarction of kidney
	N28.1	Cyst of kidney, acquired
	N28.81	Hypertrophy of kidney
	N28.82	Megaloureter
	N28.83	Nephroptosis
	N30.10	Interstitial cystitis (chronic) without hematuria
	N30.11	Interstitial cystitis (chronic) with hematuria
	N30.20	Other chronic cystitis without hematuria
	N30.21	Other chronic cystitis with hematuria
	N30.30	Trigonitis without hematuria
	N30.31	Trigonitis with hematuria
	N30.40	Irradiation cystitis without hematuria

N30.41 Irradiation cystitis with hematuria
N30.80 Other cystitis without hematuria
N30.81 Other cystitis with hematuria
N32.0 Bladder-neck obstruction
N32.1 Vesicointestinal fistula
N32.3 Diverticulum of bladder
N32.81 Overactive bladder
N39.0 Urinary tract infection, site not specified
N39.3 Stress incontinence (female) (male)
N39.41 Urge incontinence
N39.42 Incontinence without sensory awareness
N39.43 Post-void dribbling
N39.44 Nocturnal enuresis
N39.45 Continuous leakage
N39.46 Mixed incontinence
N39.490 Overflow incontinence
N39.491 Coital incontinence
N39.492 Postural (urinary) incontinence
N40.0 Benign prostatic hyperplasia without lower urinary tract symptoms ♂
N40.1 Benign prostatic hyperplasia with lower urinary tract symptoms ♂
N40.2 Nodular prostate without lower urinary tract symptoms ♂
N40.3 Nodular prostate with lower urinary tract symptoms ♂
N41.0 Acute prostatitis ♂
N41.1 Chronic prostatitis ♂
N41.4 Granulomatous prostatitis ♂
N42.83 Cyst of prostate ♂
Q60.0 Renal agenesis, unilateral
Q60.1 Renal agenesis, bilateral
Q60.3 Renal hypoplasia, unilateral
Q60.4 Renal hypoplasia, bilateral
Q61.11 Cystic dilatation of collecting ducts
Q61.2 Polycystic kidney, adult type
Q61.4 Renal dysplasia
Q61.5 Medullary cystic kidney
Q62.0 Congenital hydronephrosis
Q62.11 Congenital occlusion of ureteropelvic junction
Q62.12 Congenital occlusion of ureterovesical orifice
Q62.2 Congenital megaureter
Q62.31 Congenital ureterocele, orthotopic
Q62.32 Cecoureterocele
Q62.61 Deviation of ureter
Q62.62 Displacement of ureter
Q62.63 Anomalous implantation of ureter
Q62.7 Congenital vesico-uretero-renal reflux
Q63.0 Accessory kidney
Q63.1 Lobulated, fused and horseshoe kidney
Q63.2 Ectopic kidney
Q63.3 Hyperplastic and giant kidney
Q64.11 Supravesical fissure of urinary bladder
Q64.12 Cloacal exstrophy of urinary bladder
Q64.2 Congenital posterior urethral valves
Q64.31 Congenital bladder neck obstruction
Q64.32 Congenital stricture of urethra
Q64.33 Congenital stricture of urinary meatus
Q64.5 Congenital absence of bladder and urethra
Q64.6 Congenital diverticulum of bladder
Q64.71 Congenital prolapse of urethra
Q64.72 Congenital prolapse of urinary meatus
Q64.73 Congenital urethrorectal fistula
Q64.74 Double urethra
Q64.75 Double urinary meatus
R33.9 Retention of urine, unspecified

CCI Edits

Refer to Appendix A for CCI edits.

Pub 100

52005: Pub 100-04, 12, 30.2

Facility RVUs ▯

Code	Work	PE Facility	MP	Total Facility
52005	2.37	1.20	0.28	3.85
52007	3.02	1.41	0.37	4.80

Non-facility RVUs ▯

Code	Work	PE Non-Facility	MP	Total Non-Facility
52005	2.37	6.56	0.28	9.21
52007	3.02	10.37	0.37	13.76

Modifiers (PAR) ▯

Code	Mod 50	Mod 51	Mod 62	Mod 66	Mod 80
52005	0	3	0	0	1
52007	1	3	0	0	1

Global Period

Code	Days
52005	000
52007	000

52010

52010 Cystourethroscopy, with ejaculatory duct catheterization, with or without irrigation, instillation, or duct radiography, exclusive of radiologic service

(For radiological supervision and interpretation, use 74440)

AMA Coding Guideline

Endoscopy-Cystoscopy, Urethroscopy, Cystourethroscopy Procedures on the Bladder

Endoscopic descriptions are listed so that the main procedure can be identified without having to list all the minor related functions performed at the same time. For example: meatotomy, urethral calibration and/or dilation, urethroscopy, and cystoscopy prior to a transurethral resection of prostate; ureteral catheterization following extraction of ureteral calculus; internal urethrotomy and bladder neck fulguration when performing a cystourethroscopy for the female urethral syndrome. When the secondary procedure requires significant additional time and effort, it may be identified by the addition of modifier 22.

For example: urethrotomy performed for a documented pre-existing stricture or bladder neck contracture.

Because cutaneous urinary diversions utilizing ileum or colon serve as functional replacements of a native bladder, endoscopy of such bowel segments, as well as performance of secondary procedures can be captured by using the cystourethroscopy codes. For example, endoscopy of an ileal loop with removal of ureteral calculus would be coded as cystourethroscopy (including ureteral catheterization); with removal of ureteral calculus (52320).

AMA Coding Notes

Surgical Procedures on the Urinary System

(For provision of chemotherapeutic agents, report both the specific service in addition to code(s) for the specific substance(s) or drug(s) provided)

AMA *CPT® Assistant* ▢

52010: May 01: 5

Plain English Description

Cystourethroscopy is performed to visualize the inside of the bladder and urethra with catheterization of the ejaculatory ducts. The urethra is cleansed with antiseptic solution. A rigid or flexible cystoscope is introduced through the urethra into the bladder. The bladder may be filled with sterile saline to allow better visualization of the bladder wall. The bladder is inspected and the ureteral orifices are identified and examined. The cystoscope is pulled back into the proximal urethra, which is inspected, and the ejaculatory ducts are located. Guidewires are advanced through the urethra and into the ejaculatory ducts. A catheter is threaded through each ejaculatory duct and the guidewires are removed. The ducts may be flushed with sterile saline or contrast injected for separately reportable ejaculatory duct radiography. Upon completion of the procedure, the catheters are removed. The bladder, urethra, and ejaculatory duct orifices are re-inspected with the cystoscope, which is then removed.

Cystourethroscopy, with ejaculatory duct catheterization

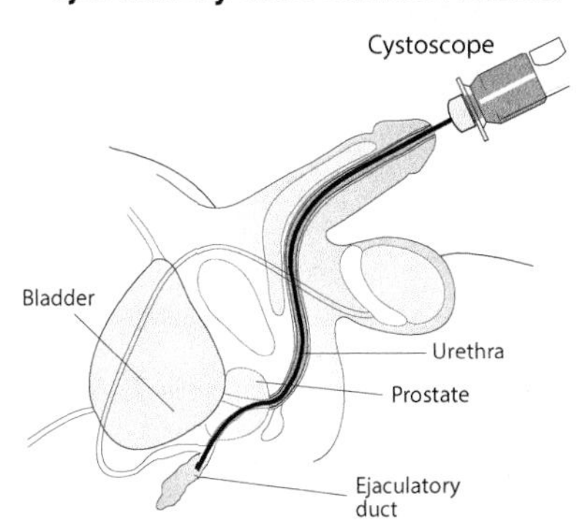

ICD-10-CM Diagnostic Codes

N13.0	Hydronephrosis with ureteropelvic junction obstruction
N30.80	Other cystitis without hematuria
N30.81	Other cystitis with hematuria
N31.0	Uninhibited neuropathic bladder, not elsewhere classified
N31.2	Flaccid neuropathic bladder, not elsewhere classified
N39.498	Other specified urinary incontinence
N40.0	Benign prostatic hyperplasia without lower urinary tract symptoms ♂
N40.1	Benign prostatic hyperplasia with lower urinary tract symptoms ♂
N40.2	Nodular prostate without lower urinary tract symptoms ♂
N40.3	Nodular prostate with lower urinary tract symptoms ♂
N42.83	Cyst of prostate ♂
N46.029	Azoospermia due to other extratesticular causes ♂
N46.8	Other male infertility ♂
N50.89	Other specified disorders of the male genital organs ♂
N52.01	Erectile dysfunction due to arterial insufficiency ♂
N52.02	Corporo-venous occlusive erectile dysfunction ♂
N52.03	Combined arterial insufficiency and corporo-venous occlusive erectile dysfunction ♂
N52.1	Erectile dysfunction due to diseases classified elsewhere ♂
N52.31	Erectile dysfunction following radical prostatectomy ♂
N52.32	Erectile dysfunction following radical cystectomy ♂
N52.33	Erectile dysfunction following urethral surgery ♂
N52.34	Erectile dysfunction following simple prostatectomy ♂
N52.35	Erectile dysfunction following radiation therapy ♂
N52.36	Erectile dysfunction following interstitial seed therapy ♂
N52.37	Erectile dysfunction following prostate ablative therapy ♂
N52.39	Other and unspecified postprocedural erectile dysfunction ♂
N52.8	Other male erectile dysfunction ♂
Q55.4	Other congenital malformations of vas deferens, epididymis, seminal vesicles and prostate ♂
Q64.8	Other specified congenital malformations of urinary system
R31.0	Gross hematuria
R31.9	Hematuria, unspecified
R36.1	Hematospermia ♂

CCI Edits

Refer to Appendix A for CCI edits.

Facility RVUs ▢

Code	Work	PE Facility	MP	Total Facility
52010	3.02	1.41	0.35	4.78

Non-facility RVUs ▢

Code	Work	PE Non-Facility	MP	Total Non-Facility
52010	3.02	8.21	0.35	11.58

Modifiers (PAR) ▢

Code	Mod 50	Mod 51	Mod 62	Mod 66	Mod 80
52010	0	3	0	0	1

Global Period

Code	Days
52010	000

52204

52204 Cystourethroscopy, with biopsy(s)

AMA Coding Notes

Surgical Procedures on the Urinary System

(For provision of chemotherapeutic agents, report both the specific service in addition to code(s) for the specific substance(s) or drug(s) provided)

AMA *CPT® Assistant*

52204: May 01: 5, Sep 01: 1, Sep 03: 16, Aug 09: 6, May 16: 12

Plain English Description

Cystourethroscopy is performed to visualize the inside of the bladder and urethra and tissue samples are obtained. The urethra is cleansed with antiseptic solution. A rigid or flexible cystoscope is introduced through the urethra into the bladder. The bladder may be filled with sterile saline to allow better visualization of the bladder wall. The bladder is inspected and the ureteral orifices are identified and examined. Biopsy forceps are introduced through the cystoscope and tissue samples are obtained. The bladder and urethra are re-inspected following biopsy and any bleeding is controlled. The cystoscope is removed.

Cystourethroscopy, with biopsy(s)

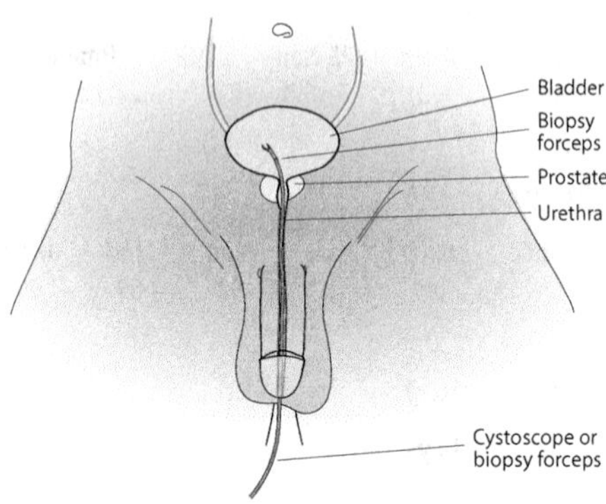

ICD-10-CM Diagnostic Codes

C67.0	Malignant neoplasm of trigone of bladder
C67.1	Malignant neoplasm of dome of bladder
C67.2	Malignant neoplasm of lateral wall of bladder
C67.3	Malignant neoplasm of anterior wall of bladder
C67.4	Malignant neoplasm of posterior wall of bladder
C67.5	Malignant neoplasm of bladder neck
C67.6	Malignant neoplasm of ureteric orifice
C67.8	Malignant neoplasm of overlapping sites of bladder
C68.0	Malignant neoplasm of urethra
C79.11	Secondary malignant neoplasm of bladder
C79.19	Secondary malignant neoplasm of other urinary organs
D09.0	Carcinoma in situ of bladder
D09.19	Carcinoma in situ of other urinary organs
D30.3	Benign neoplasm of bladder
D30.4	Benign neoplasm of urethra
D41.3	Neoplasm of uncertain behavior of urethra
D41.4	Neoplasm of uncertain behavior of bladder
N21.0	Calculus in bladder
N22	Calculus of urinary tract in diseases classified elsewhere
N30.00	Acute cystitis without hematuria
N30.01	Acute cystitis with hematuria
N30.10	Interstitial cystitis (chronic) without hematuria
N30.11	Interstitial cystitis (chronic) with hematuria
N30.20	Other chronic cystitis without hematuria
N30.21	Other chronic cystitis with hematuria
N30.30	Trigonitis without hematuria
N30.31	Trigonitis with hematuria
N30.40	Irradiation cystitis without hematuria
N30.41	Irradiation cystitis with hematuria
N30.80	Other cystitis without hematuria
N30.81	Other cystitis with hematuria
N31.2	Flaccid neuropathic bladder, not elsewhere classified
N31.9	Neuromuscular dysfunction of bladder, unspecified
N32.0	Bladder-neck obstruction
N32.3	Diverticulum of bladder
N32.81	Overactive bladder
N32.89	Other specified disorders of bladder
N33	Bladder disorders in diseases classified elsewhere
N34.0	Urethral abscess
N34.1	Nonspecific urethritis
N34.2	Other urethritis
N36.2	Urethral caruncle
N36.8	Other specified disorders of urethra
N39.0	Urinary tract infection, site not specified
N39.45	Continuous leakage
N39.46	Mixed incontinence
N39.498	Other specified urinary incontinence
N82.0	Vesicovaginal fistula ♀
N82.1	Other female urinary-genital tract fistulae ♀
Q62.31	Congenital ureterocele, orthotopic
Q64.10	Exstrophy of urinary bladder, unspecified
Q64.19	Other exstrophy of urinary bladder
Q64.2	Congenital posterior urethral valves
Q64.31	Congenital bladder neck obstruction
Q64.32	Congenital stricture of urethra
Q64.33	Congenital stricture of urinary meatus
Q64.5	Congenital absence of bladder and urethra
Q64.6	Congenital diverticulum of bladder
Q64.71	Congenital prolapse of urethra
Q64.73	Congenital urethrorectal fistula
Q64.74	Double urethra
Q64.75	Double urinary meatus
Q64.79	Other congenital malformations of bladder and urethra
Q64.9	Congenital malformation of urinary system, unspecified
R31.0	Gross hematuria
R31.9	Hematuria, unspecified
R33.8	Other retention of urine
R35.0	Frequency of micturition
R39.0	Extravasation of urine
R39.12	Poor urinary stream
R39.14	Feeling of incomplete bladder emptying
R39.15	Urgency of urination
R39.16	Straining to void
R89.7	Abnormal histological findings in specimens from other organs, systems and tissues
Z12.6	Encounter for screening for malignant neoplasm of bladder
Z80.51	Family history of malignant neoplasm of kidney
Z80.52	Family history of malignant neoplasm of bladder

CCI Edits

Refer to Appendix A for CCI edits.

Facility RVUs

Code	Work	PE Facility	MP	Total Facility
52204	2.59	1.20	0.31	4.10

Non-facility RVUs

Code	Work	PE Non-Facility	MP	Total Non-Facility
52204	2.59	8.63	0.31	11.53

Modifiers (PAR)

Code	Mod 50	Mod 51	Mod 62	Mod 66	Mod 80
52204	0	3	0	0	1

Global Period

Code	Days
52204	000

52214

52214 Cystourethroscopy, with fulguration (including cryosurgery or laser surgery) of trigone, bladder neck, prostatic fossa, urethra, or periurethral glands

(For transurethral fulguration of prostate tissue performed within the postoperative period of 52601 or 52630 performed by the same physician, append modifier 78)

(For transurethral fulguration of prostate tissue performed within the postoperative period of a related procedure performed by the same physician, append modifier 78)

(For transurethral fulguration of prostate for postoperative bleeding performed by the same physician, append modifier 78)

AMA Coding Notes

Surgical Procedures on the Urinary System

(For provision of chemotherapeutic agents, report both the specific service in addition to code(s) for the specific substance(s) or drug(s) provided)

AMA *CPT® Assistant* 🗆

52214: May 01: 5, Sep 01: 1, Aug 09: 6, May 16: 12

Plain English Description

Cystourethroscopy is performed to visualize the inside of the bladder and urethra. Abnormal tissue in the distal aspect of the bladder (bladder trigone), bladder neck, prostatic fossa, urethra, or periurethral glands is destroyed using a high-frequency electrical current. The urethral orifice is cleansed with antiseptic solution. A rigid or flexible cystoscope is introduced through the urethra into the bladder. The bladder may be filled with sterile saline to allow better visualization of the bladder wall. The bladder is inspected and the ureteral orifices are identified and examined. The cystoscope is withdrawn and the prostatic fossa, urethra, and periurethral glands are examined and any abnormal tissue is noted. An electrocautery device is then advanced through the urethroscope to the site where the abnormal tissue is located. The device is activated and the lesion is destroyed. Alternatively, a laser or cryoprobe may be used to destroy the abnormal tissue. Upon completion of the procedure, the bladder trigone and neck, prostatic fossa, urethra, and periurethral glands are re-inspected to ensure that all abnormal tissue has been destroyed. The cystoscope is then removed.

Cystourethroscopy, with fulguration

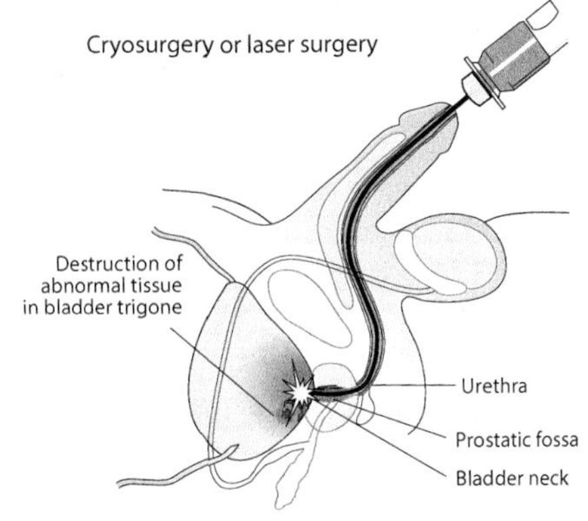

ICD-10-CM Diagnostic Codes

C67.0	Malignant neoplasm of trigone of bladder
C67.1	Malignant neoplasm of dome of bladder
C67.5	Malignant neoplasm of bladder neck
C68.0	Malignant neoplasm of urethra
C79.11	Secondary malignant neoplasm of bladder
D09.0	Carcinoma in situ of bladder
D30.3	Benign neoplasm of bladder
D30.4	Benign neoplasm of urethra
D41.3	Neoplasm of uncertain behavior of urethra
D41.4	Neoplasm of uncertain behavior of bladder
D49.4	Neoplasm of unspecified behavior of bladder
N30.10	Interstitial cystitis (chronic) without hematuria
N30.11	Interstitial cystitis (chronic) with hematuria
N30.20	Other chronic cystitis without hematuria
N30.21	Other chronic cystitis with hematuria
N30.30	Trigonitis without hematuria
N30.31	Trigonitis with hematuria
N32.0	Bladder-neck obstruction
N32.89	Other specified disorders of bladder
N33	Bladder disorders in diseases classified elsewhere
N36.1	Urethral diverticulum
N36.2	Urethral caruncle
N36.8	Other specified disorders of urethra
R31.0	Gross hematuria
R31.9	Hematuria, unspecified

CCI Edits

Refer to Appendix A for CCI edits.

Pub 100

52214: Pub 100-03, 1, 140.5

Facility RVUs 🗆

Code	Work	PE Facility	MP	Total Facility
52214	3.50	1.19	0.41	5.10

Non-facility RVUs 🗆

Code	Work	PE Non-Facility	MP	Total Non-Facility
52214	3.50	19.10	0.41	23.01

Modifiers (PAR) 🗆

Code	Mod 50	Mod 51	Mod 62	Mod 66	Mod 80
52214	0	3	0	0	1

Global Period

Code	Days
52214	000

52224-52240

52224 Cystourethroscopy, with fulguration (including cryosurgery or laser surgery) or treatment of MINOR (less than 0.5 cm) lesion(s) with or without biopsy

52234 Cystourethroscopy, with fulguration (including cryosurgery or laser surgery) and/or resection of; SMALL bladder tumor(s) (0.5 up to 2.0 cm)

52235 Cystourethroscopy, with fulguration (including cryosurgery or laser surgery) and/or resection of; MEDIUM bladder tumor(s) (2.0 to 5.0 cm)

52240 Cystourethroscopy, with fulguration (including cryosurgery or laser surgery) and/or resection of; LARGE bladder tumor(s)

AMA Coding Notes

Surgical Procedures on the Urinary System

(For provision of chemotherapeutic agents, report both the specific service in addition to code(s) for the specific substance(s) or drug(s) provided)

AMA *CPT® Assistant* ▢

52224: May 01: 5, Sep 01: 1, Dec 07: 7, Jun 09: 10, Aug 09: 6, May 16: 12

52234: May 01: 5, Sep 01: 1, Oct 02: 12, Jan 03: 21, Jun 09: 10, Aug 09: 6, May 16: 12

52235: May 01: 5, Sep 01: 1, Oct 02: 12, Jan 03: 21, Jun 09: 10, Aug 09: 6, May 16: 12

52240: May 01: 5, Sep 01: 1, Jun 09: 10, Aug 09: 6, May 16: 12

Plain English Description

Cystourethroscopy is performed to visualize the inside of the bladder and urethra and bladder tumors are destroyed using a high-frequency electrical current. The urethral orifice is cleansed with antiseptic solution. A rigid or flexible cystoscope is introduced through the urethra into the bladder. The bladder may be filled with sterile saline to allow better visualization of the bladder wall. The bladder is inspected and the ureteral orifices are identified and examined. Bladder tumors are located. An electrocautery device is then advanced through the urethroscope to the site where the tumors are located. The device is activated and the tumors are destroyed. Alternatively, a laser or cryoprobe may be used to destroy the tumors. Upon completion of the procedure, the bladder is re-inspected to ensure that all tumors have been destroyed. The cystoscope is then removed. In 52224, a minor lesion less than 0.5 cm is destroyed. In 52234, 52235, or 52240, larger bladder tumors are destroyed as described above, or resected.
If resection is performed, the tumors are located as described above. The cystoscope is removed, a resectoscope is advanced to the site of the tumor, and the tumor is resected. The tumor is removed using irrigation and a cystoscopic evacuation device. This is repeated until all tumors have been removed. Bleeding is controlled as needed using electrocoagulation or laser coagulation. Use 52234 for one or more small bladder tumors measuring 0.5 up to 2.0 cm in greatest diameter, use 52235 for medium bladder tumors measuring 2 to 5 cm, or 52240 for large bladder tumors measuring greater than 5 cm.

Cystourethroscopy, with fulguration

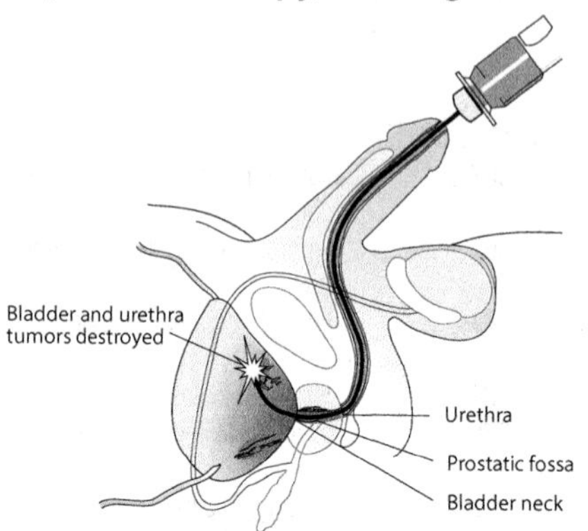

Minor lesion(s) (less than 0.5 cm) (52224); small tumor(s) (0.5 up to 2.0 cm) (52234); medium tumor(s) (2.0 to 5.0 cm) (52235); large tumor(s) (52240)

ICD-10-CM Diagnostic Codes

C67.0	Malignant neoplasm of trigone of bladder
C67.1	Malignant neoplasm of dome of bladder
C67.2	Malignant neoplasm of lateral wall of bladder
C67.3	Malignant neoplasm of anterior wall of bladder
C67.4	Malignant neoplasm of posterior wall of bladder
C67.5	Malignant neoplasm of bladder neck
C67.6	Malignant neoplasm of ureteric orifice
C67.8	Malignant neoplasm of overlapping sites of bladder
C79.11	Secondary malignant neoplasm of bladder
D09.0	Carcinoma in situ of bladder
D30.3	Benign neoplasm of bladder
D41.4	Neoplasm of uncertain behavior of bladder
D49.4	Neoplasm of unspecified behavior of bladder

CCI Edits

Refer to Appendix A for CCI edits.

Pub 100

52224: Pub 100-03, 1, 140.5

52234: Pub 100-03, 1, 140.5, Pub 100-04, 12, 30.2

52235: Pub 100-03, 1, 140.5, Pub 100-04, 12, 30.2

52240: Pub 100-03, 1, 140.5, Pub 100-04, 12, 30.2

Facility RVUs ▢

Code	Work	PE Facility	MP	Total Facility
52224	4.05	1.36	0.50	5.91
52234	4.62	1.95	0.56	7.13
52235	5.44	2.26	0.65	8.35
52240	7.50	2.96	0.90	11.36

Non-facility RVUs ▢

Code	Work	PE Non-Facility	MP	Total Non-Facility
52224	4.05	19.48	0.50	24.03
52234	4.62	1.95	0.56	7.13
52235	5.44	2.26	0.65	8.35
52240	7.50	2.96	0.90	11.36

Modifiers (PAR) ▢

Code	Mod 50	Mod 51	Mod 62	Mod 66	Mod 80
52224	0	3	0	0	1
52234	0	3	0	0	1
52235	0	3	0	0	1
52240	0	3	0	0	1

Global Period

Code	Days
52224	000
52234	000
52235	000
52240	000

52250

52250 Cystourethroscopy with insertion of radioactive substance, with or without biopsy or fulguration

AMA Coding Notes

Surgical Procedures on the Urinary System

(For provision of chemotherapeutic agents, report both the specific service in addition to code(s) for the specific substance(s) or drug(s) provided)

AMA *CPT® Assistant* ☐

52250: May 01: 5, Sep 01: 1

Plain English Description

Cystourethroscopy is performed to visualize the inside of the bladder and urethra and bladder tumors are destroyed using a radioactive substance inserted at the tumor site. The urethral orifice is cleansed with antiseptic solution. A rigid or flexible cystoscope is introduced through the urethra into the bladder. The bladder may be filled with sterile saline to allow better visualization of the bladder wall. The bladder is inspected and the ureteral orifices are identified and examined. The bladder tumors are located. A tissue sample may be obtained using biopsy forceps. Tissue may also be destroyed by electrocautery, laser, or other technique. If electrocautery is used, an electrocautery device is advanced through the urethroscope to the site where the tumor is located. The device is activated and the tumor is destroyed. The radioactive substance is then loaded into a delivery device and implanted into the bladder at the site of the malignancy. All surgical tools are removed along with the cystoscope. The radioactive implant may be left in the bladder for several days. When the internal radiation treatment is completed, the implant is removed using the cystoscope.

Cystourethroscopy with insertion of radioactive substance

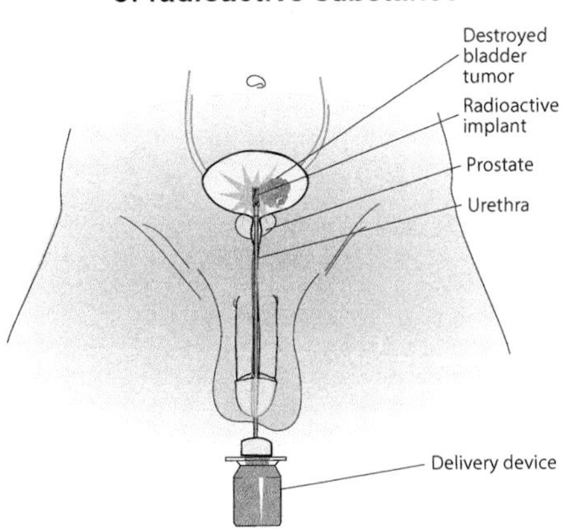

ICD-10-CM Diagnostic Codes

C67.0	Malignant neoplasm of trigone of bladder
C67.1	Malignant neoplasm of dome of bladder
C67.2	Malignant neoplasm of lateral wall of bladder
C67.3	Malignant neoplasm of anterior wall of bladder
C67.4	Malignant neoplasm of posterior wall of bladder
C67.5	Malignant neoplasm of bladder neck
C67.6	Malignant neoplasm of ureteric orifice
C67.7	Malignant neoplasm of urachus
C67.8	Malignant neoplasm of overlapping sites of bladder
C79.11	Secondary malignant neoplasm of bladder
D09.0	Carcinoma in situ of bladder
D09.19	Carcinoma in situ of other urinary organs
D41.4	Neoplasm of uncertain behavior of bladder
D49.4	Neoplasm of unspecified behavior of bladder

CCI Edits

Refer to Appendix A for CCI edits.

Facility RVUs ☐

Code	Work	PE Facility	MP	Total Facility
52250	4.49	1.90	0.55	6.94

Non-facility RVUs ☐

Code	Work	PE Non-Facility	MP	Total Non-Facility
52250	4.49	1.90	0.55	6.94

Modifiers (PAR) ☐

Code	Mod 50	Mod 51	Mod 62	Mod 66	Mod 80
52250	0	3	0	0	1

Global Period

Code	Days
52250	000

52260-52265

52260 Cystourethroscopy, with dilation of bladder for interstitial cystitis; general or conduction (spinal) anesthesia

52265 Cystourethroscopy, with dilation of bladder for interstitial cystitis; local anesthesia

AMA Coding Notes

Surgical Procedures on the Urinary System

(For provision of chemotherapeutic agents, report both the specific service in addition to code(s) for the specific substance(s) or drug(s) provided)

AMA *CPT® Assistant* ☐

52260: May 01: 5, Sep 01: 1, Oct 05: 23
52265: May 01: 5, Sep 01: 1

Plain English Description

Interstitial cystitis (IC), also referred to as painful bladder syndrome, is characterized by recurring bladder and pelvic pain that may be accompanied by frequent urination. Cystourethroscopy is performed to visualize the inside of the bladder and urethra. The urethral orifice is cleansed with antiseptic solution. A rigid or flexible cystoscope is introduced through the urethra into the bladder. The bladder is inspected and the ureteral orifices are identified and examined. Areas of inflammation, scarring, and fibrosis are noted. Any ulcerations in the bladder wall are also noted. Bladder distention is then performed to dilate the urinary bladder. This is accomplished by inserting a catheter and filling the bladder with normal saline or gas. If normal saline is used, it may be mixed with a local anesthetic agent. The saline or gas is left in the bladder for 10-15 minutes and then removed. The catheter is removed. The bladder and urethra may be re-examined using the cystoscope, which is then removed. Use 52260 when the procedure is performed using general or conduction (spinal anesthesia); use 52265 when local anesthesia is used.

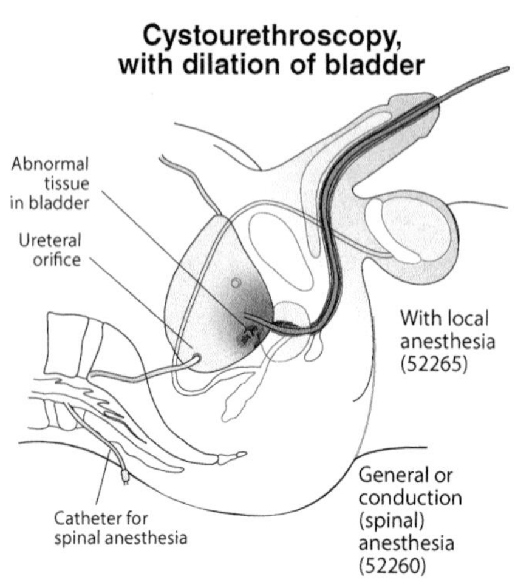

ICD-10-CM Diagnostic Codes

N30.10	Interstitial cystitis (chronic) without hematuria
N30.11	Interstitial cystitis (chronic) with hematuria
N30.20	Other chronic cystitis without hematuria
N30.21	Other chronic cystitis with hematuria
N30.30	Trigonitis without hematuria
N30.31	Trigonitis with hematuria
N30.90	Cystitis, unspecified without hematuria
N30.91	Cystitis, unspecified with hematuria
R31.0	Gross hematuria
R31.9	Hematuria, unspecified

CCI Edits

Refer to Appendix A for CCI edits.

Facility RVUs ☐

Code	Work	PE Facility	MP	Total Facility
52260	3.91	1.71	0.50	6.12
52265	2.94	1.39	0.39	4.72

Non-facility RVUs ☐

Code	Work	PE Non-Facility	MP	Total Non-Facility
52260	3.91	1.71	0.50	6.12
52265	2.94	8.06	0.39	11.39

Modifiers (PAR) ☐

Code	Mod 50	Mod 51	Mod 62	Mod 66	Mod 80
52260	0	3	0	0	1
52265	0	3	0	0	1

Global Period

Code	Days
52260	000
52265	000

52270-52276

52270 Cystourethroscopy, with internal urethrotomy; female
52275 Cystourethroscopy, with internal urethrotomy; male
52276 Cystourethroscopy with direct vision internal urethrotomy

AMA Coding Notes

Surgical Procedures on the Urinary System

(For provision of chemotherapeutic agents, report both the specific service in addition to code(s) for the specific substance(s) or drug(s) provided)

AMA *CPT® Assistant*

52270: May 01: 5, Sep 01: 1
52275: May 01: 5, Sep 01: 1
52276: May 01: 5, Sep 01: 1, May 09: 8, Feb 10: 7

Plain English Description

Internal urethrotomy is performed to treat internal urethral stricture. Cystourethroscopy is performed to visualize the inside of the bladder and urethra and identify the area of urethral stricture. The urethral orifice is cleansed with antiseptic solution. A rigid or flexible cystoscope is introduced through the urethra into the bladder. The bladder is inspected and the ureteral orifices are identified and examined. The cystoscope is slowly removed and the area of stricture is identified. A cold knife incision is made at 12 o'clock or multiple radial incisions are made at the site of the stricture. If multiple areas of stricture are noted, the procedure is repeated until all narrowed portions of the urethra have been incised. The urethra is then re-examined using the cystoscope. The cystoscope is removed and a Foley catheter is placed through the urethra and into the bladder to help maintain the diameter of the treated areas. Use 52270 for incision of a female urethral stricture; use 52275 for a male; and use 52276 for direct vision urethrotomy. Direct vision urethrotomy is performed by inserting a special telescope that allows the physician to see the stricture and make incisions while visualizing the stricture.

Cystourethroscopy

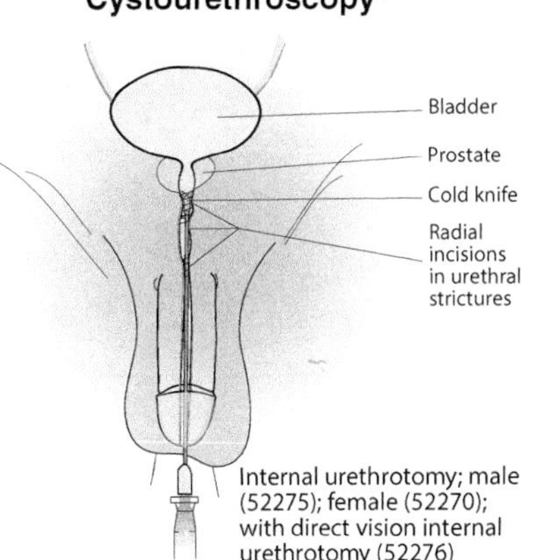

ICD-10-CM Diagnostic Codes

N30.30	Trigonitis without hematuria
N34.2	Other urethritis
N34.3	Urethral syndrome, unspecified
N35.021	Urethral stricture due to childbirth ♀
N35.028	Other post-traumatic urethral stricture, female ♀
N35.12	Postinfective urethral stricture, not elsewhere classified, female ♀
N35.82	Other urethral stricture, female ♀
N35.92	Unspecified urethral stricture, female ♀
N37	Urethral disorders in diseases classified elsewhere
N99.115	Postprocedural fossa navicularis urethral stricture ♂
N99.12	Postprocedural urethral stricture, female ♀
Q64.32	Congenital stricture of urethra
Q64.33	Congenital stricture of urinary meatus
Q64.39	Other atresia and stenosis of urethra and bladder neck
R39.14	Feeling of incomplete bladder emptying

CCI Edits

Refer to Appendix A for CCI edits.

Facility RVUs

Code	Work	PE Facility	MP	Total Facility
52270	3.36	1.50	0.40	5.26
52275	4.69	1.95	0.56	7.20
52276	4.99	2.07	0.60	7.66

Non-facility RVUs

Code	Work	PE Non-Facility	MP	Total Non-Facility
52270	3.36	9.04	0.40	12.80
52275	4.69	11.17	0.56	16.42
52276	4.99	2.07	0.60	7.66

Modifiers (PAR)

Code	Mod 50	Mod 51	Mod 62	Mod 66	Mod 80
52270	0	3	0	0	1
52275	0	3	0	0	1
52276	0	3	0	0	1

Global Period

Code	Days
52270	000
52275	000
52276	000

52277

52277 Cystourethroscopy, with resection of external sphincter (sphincterotomy)

AMA Coding Notes

Surgical Procedures on the Urinary System

(For provision of chemotherapeutic agents, report both the specific service in addition to code(s) for the specific substance(s) or drug(s) provided)

AMA *CPT® Assistant* ▢

52277: May 01: 5, Sep 01: 1

Plain English Description

The external urethral sphincter is a ring-like muscle in the urethra that controls emptying of the bladder. Cystourethroscopy is performed to visualize the inside of the bladder and urethra and identify the area of the external sphincter. The urethral orifice is cleansed with antiseptic solution. A rigid or flexible cystoscope is introduced through the urethra into the bladder. The bladder is inspected and the ureteral orifices are identified and examined. The cystoscope is slowly removed and the area of the urethral sphincter is identified. Multiple radial incisions are made in the external urethral sphincter to help relax it and allow urine to pass more easily. The urethra is then re-examined using the cystoscope and any bleeding is controlled. The cystoscope is removed and a Foley catheter is placed through the urethra and into the bladder to help maintain the diameter of the urethral sphincter.

Cystourethroscopy, with sphincterotomy

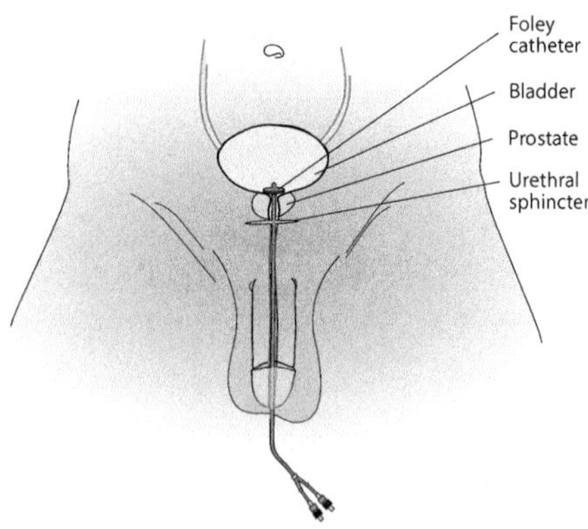

ICD-10-CM Diagnostic Codes

G83.4	Cauda equina syndrome
N31.0	Uninhibited neuropathic bladder, not elsewhere classified
N31.1	Reflex neuropathic bladder, not elsewhere classified
N31.8	Other neuromuscular dysfunction of bladder
N32.0	Bladder-neck obstruction
N36.44	Muscular disorders of urethra
N40.0	Benign prostatic hyperplasia without lower urinary tract symptoms ♂
N40.1	Benign prostatic hyperplasia with lower urinary tract symptoms ♂
R33.8	Other retention of urine

CCI Edits

Refer to Appendix A for CCI edits.

Facility RVUs ▢

Code	Work	PE Facility	MP	Total Facility
52277	6.16	2.47	0.73	9.36

Non-facility RVUs ▢

Code	Work	PE Non-Facility	MP	Total Non-Facility
52277	6.16	2.47	0.73	9.36

Modifiers (PAR) ▢

Code	Mod 50	Mod 51	Mod 62	Mod 66	Mod 80
52277	0	3	0	0	0

Global Period

Code	Days
52277	000

52281

52281 Cystourethroscopy, with calibration and/or dilation of urethral stricture or stenosis, with or without meatotomy, with or without injection procedure for cystography, male or female

(To report cystourethroscopy with urethral therapeutic drug delivery, use 0499T)

AMA Coding Notes

Surgical Procedures on the Urinary System

(For provision of chemotherapeutic agents, report both the specific service in addition to code(s) for the specific substance(s) or drug(s) provided)

AMA *CPT® Assistant* ▯

52281: Nov 97: 20, May 01: 5, Sep 01: 1, Jun 07: 10, Oct 17: 9

Plain English Description

Urethral calibration involves measuring the diameter of the narrowed portion of the urethra. Calibration and/or dilation of a urethral stricture or stenosis is typically performed only when the narrowed portion is at the distal aspect of the urethra or the urethral opening, called the urethral meatus. A series of cone-shaped instruments of increasing diameter called bougies are advanced into the tip of the urethra and then withdrawn. The physician begins with the smallest size, usually an 8 French bougie. If this size can be easily inserted and withdrawn, progressively larger-diameter bougies are inserted until resistance is felt. The largest bougie that can be inserted determines the diameter of the distal urethra. Once the diameter of the narrowed distal segment has been determined, the physician then examines the urethra using a cystourethroscope. Following visualization through the urethroscope, the physician determines the best treatment method. The stricture may be dilated using progressively larger sounds, a filiform and progressively larger followers, or a balloon catheter that is inflated and deflated at the site of the stricture. The urethral meatus may be incised in a radial fashion to open the narrowed portion. Contrast material may also be injected through the urethra and into the bladder and separately reportable cystography performed.

Cystourethroscopy, with calibration and/or dilation

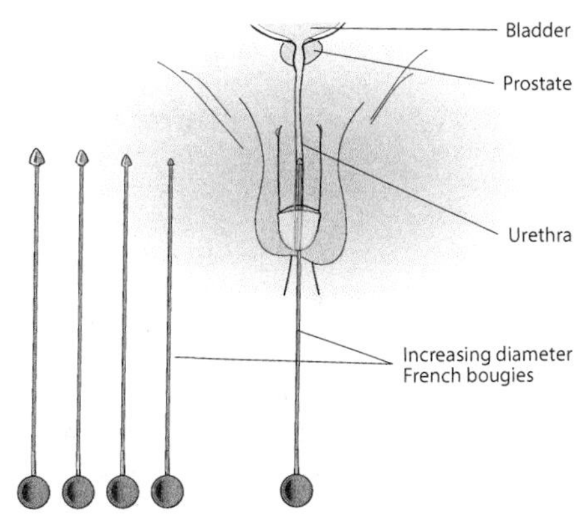

ICD-10-CM Diagnostic Codes

N32.0	Bladder-neck obstruction
N35.010	Post-traumatic urethral stricture, male, meatal ♂
N35.011	Post-traumatic bulbous urethral stricture ♂
N35.012	Post-traumatic membranous urethral stricture ♂
N35.013	Post-traumatic anterior urethral stricture ♂
N35.016	Post-traumatic urethral stricture, male, overlapping sites ♂
N35.021	Urethral stricture due to childbirth ♀
N35.028	Other post-traumatic urethral stricture, female ♀
N35.111	Postinfective urethral stricture, not elsewhere classified, male, meatal ♂
N35.112	Postinfective bulbous urethral stricture, not elsewhere classified, male ♂
N35.113	Postinfective membranous urethral stricture, not elsewhere classified, male ♂
N35.114	Postinfective anterior urethral stricture, not elsewhere classified, male ♂
N35.116	Postinfective urethral stricture, not elsewhere classified, male, overlapping sites ♂
N35.12	Postinfective urethral stricture, not elsewhere classified, female ♀
N35.811	Other urethral stricture, male, meatal ♂
N35.812	Other urethral bulbous stricture, male ♂
N35.813	Other membranous urethral stricture, male ♂
N35.814	Other anterior urethral stricture, male ♂
N35.816	Other urethral stricture, male, overlapping sites ♂
N35.82	Other urethral stricture, female ♀
N37	Urethral disorders in diseases classified elsewhere
N40.0	Benign prostatic hyperplasia without lower urinary tract symptoms ♂
N40.1	Benign prostatic hyperplasia with lower urinary tract symptoms ♂
N40.2	Nodular prostate without lower urinary tract symptoms ♂
N40.3	Nodular prostate with lower urinary tract symptoms ♂
N99.110	Postprocedural urethral stricture, male, meatal ♂
N99.111	Postprocedural bulbous urethral stricture, male ♂
N99.112	Postprocedural membranous urethral stricture, male ♂
N99.113	Postprocedural anterior bulbous urethral stricture, male ♂
N99.115	Postprocedural fossa navicularis urethral stricture ♂
N99.116	Postprocedural urethral stricture, male, overlapping sites ♂
N99.12	Postprocedural urethral stricture, female ♀
Q62.12	Congenital occlusion of ureterovesical orifice
Q64.32	Congenital stricture of urethra
Q64.33	Congenital stricture of urinary meatus
Q64.39	Other atresia and stenosis of urethra and bladder neck

CCI Edits

Refer to Appendix A for CCI edits.

Facility RVUs ▯

Code	Work	PE Facility	MP	Total Facility
52281	2.75	1.33	0.33	4.41

Non-facility RVUs ▯

Code	Work	PE Non-Facility	MP	Total Non-Facility
52281	2.75	6.81	0.33	9.89

Modifiers (PAR) ▯

Code	Mod 50	Mod 51	Mod 62	Mod 66	Mod 80
52281	0	3	0	0	1

Global Period

Code	Days
52281	000

52282

52282 Cystourethroscopy, with insertion of permanent urethral stent

(For placement of temporary prostatic urethral stent, use 53855)

AMA Coding Notes

Surgical Procedures on the Urinary System

(For provision of chemotherapeutic agents, report both the specific service in addition to code(s) for the specific substance(s) or drug(s) provided)

AMA *CPT® Assistant*

52282: Nov 97: 20, May 01: 5, Sep 01: 1, Feb 10: 7, Jun 15: 5

Plain English Description

A permanent urethral stent is used to treat a persistent stricture or narrowing of the urethra. The urethral orifice is cleansed with antiseptic solution. A rigid or flexible cystoscope consisting of a thin, telescope-like tube with a light and camera is introduced through the urethra into the bladder. The camera allows images of the urethra and bladder to be viewed on a computer or television monitor. The bladder may be filled with sterile saline or water to improve visualization of the bladder wall. The saline or water is drained from the bladder and the narrowed portion of the urethra evaluated. An appropriately sized permanent urethral stent is selected and introduced into the urethra through the working channel of the cystoscope. The stent is positioned in the narrowed segment and deployed. The cystoscope is then removed.

Cystourethroscopy, with insertion of urethral stent

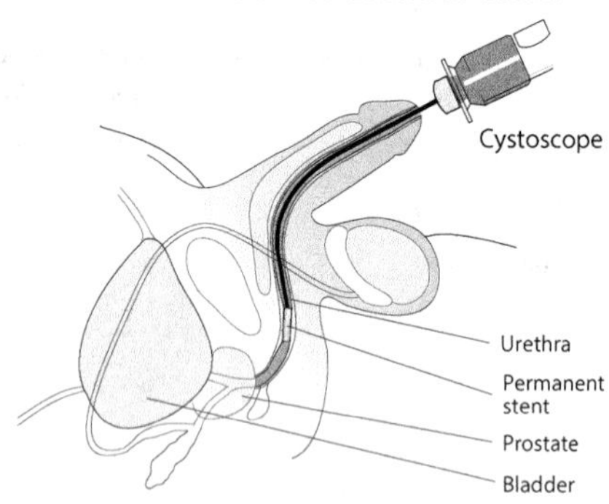

ICD-10-CM Diagnostic Codes

N32.0	Bladder-neck obstruction
N35.011	Post-traumatic bulbous urethral stricture ♂
N35.012	Post-traumatic membranous urethral stricture ♂
N35.013	Post-traumatic anterior urethral stricture ♂
N35.016	Post-traumatic urethral stricture, male, overlapping sites ♂
N35.021	Urethral stricture due to childbirth ♀
N35.028	Other post-traumatic urethral stricture, female ♀
N35.112	Postinfective bulbous urethral stricture, not elsewhere classified, male ♂
N35.113	Postinfective membranous urethral stricture, not elsewhere classified, male ♂
N35.114	Postinfective anterior urethral stricture, not elsewhere classified, male ♂
N35.116	Postinfective urethral stricture, not elsewhere classified, male, overlapping sites ♂
N35.12	Postinfective urethral stricture, not elsewhere classified, female ♀
N35.812	Other urethral bulbous stricture, male ♂
N35.813	Other membranous urethral stricture, male ♂
N35.814	Other anterior urethral stricture, male ♂
N35.816	Other urethral stricture, male, overlapping sites ♂
N37	Urethral disorders in diseases classified elsewhere
N99.111	Postprocedural bulbous urethral stricture, male ♂
N99.112	Postprocedural membranous urethral stricture, male ♂
N99.113	Postprocedural anterior bulbous urethral stricture, male ♂
N99.115	Postprocedural fossa navicularis urethral stricture ♂
N99.116	Postprocedural urethral stricture, male, overlapping sites ♂
N99.12	Postprocedural urethral stricture, female ♀
Q64.32	Congenital stricture of urethra
Q64.33	Congenital stricture of urinary meatus
Q64.39	Other atresia and stenosis of urethra and bladder neck

CCI Edits

Refer to Appendix A for CCI edits.

Facility RVUs

Code	Work	PE Facility	MP	Total Facility
52282	6.39	2.58	0.76	9.73

Non-facility RVUs

Code	Work	PE Non-Facility	MP	Total Non-Facility
52282	6.39	2.58	0.76	9.73

Modifiers (PAR)

Code	Mod 50	Mod 51	Mod 62	Mod 66	Mod 80
52282	0	3	0	0	1

Global Period

Code	Days
52282	000

52283

52283 Cystourethroscopy, with steroid injection into stricture

AMA Coding Notes

Surgical Procedures on the Urinary System

(For provision of chemotherapeutic agents, report both the specific service in addition to code(s) for the specific substance(s) or drug(s) provided)

AMA *CPT® Assistant* ▢

52283: May 01: 5, Sep 01: 1, Mar 15: 9

Plain English Description

Steroid injection is performed to treat urethral stricture. Steroid injection is typically reserved for strictures of the distal urethra or meatus, strictures that occur following radical prostatectomy, or for patients who have had multiple urethroplasties. Cystourethroscopy is performed to visualize the urethra and identify the area of stricture. The urethral orifice is cleansed with antiseptic solution. A rigid or flexible cystoscope is introduced through the urethra and advanced to the area of the stricture. The narrowed portion of the urethra is injected with a steroid medication, and the cystoscope is removed.

Cystourethroscopy, with steroid injection into stricture

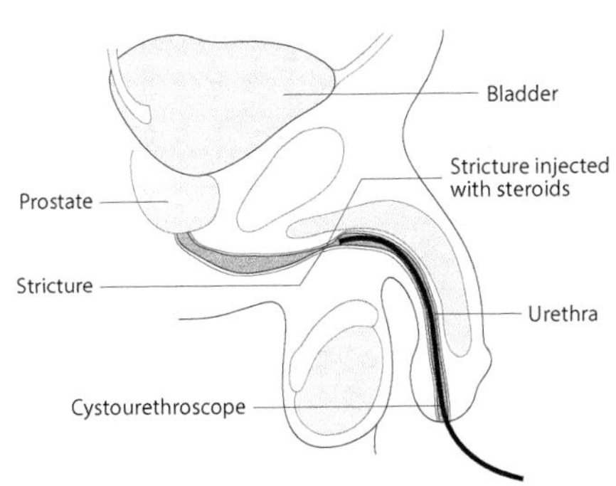

ICD-10-CM Diagnostic Codes

N32.0 Bladder-neck obstruction
N35.011 Post-traumatic bulbous urethral stricture ♂
N35.012 Post-traumatic membranous urethral stricture ♂
N35.013 Post-traumatic anterior urethral stricture ♂
N35.016 Post-traumatic urethral stricture, male, overlapping sites ♂
N35.021 Urethral stricture due to childbirth ♀
N35.028 Other post-traumatic urethral stricture, female ♀
N35.112 Postinfective bulbous urethral stricture, not elsewhere classified, male ♂
N35.113 Postinfective membranous urethral stricture, not elsewhere classified, male ♂
N35.114 Postinfective anterior urethral stricture, not elsewhere classified, male ♂
N35.116 Postinfective urethral stricture, not elsewhere classified, male, overlapping sites ♂
N35.12 Postinfective urethral stricture, not elsewhere classified, female ♀
N35.812 Other urethral bulbous stricture, male ♂
N35.813 Other membranous urethral stricture, male ♂
N35.814 Other anterior urethral stricture, male ♂
N35.816 Other urethral stricture, male, overlapping sites ♂
N37 Urethral disorders in diseases classified elsewhere
N99.111 Postprocedural bulbous urethral stricture, male ♂
N99.112 Postprocedural membranous urethral stricture, male ♂
N99.113 Postprocedural anterior bulbous urethral stricture, male ♂
N99.115 Postprocedural fossa navicularis urethral stricture ♂
N99.116 Postprocedural urethral stricture, male, overlapping sites ♂
N99.12 Postprocedural urethral stricture, female ♀
Q64.32 Congenital stricture of urethra
Q64.33 Congenital stricture of urinary meatus
Q64.39 Other atresia and stenosis of urethra and bladder neck

CCI Edits

Refer to Appendix A for CCI edits.

Facility RVUs ▢

Code	Work	PE Facility	MP	Total Facility
52283	3.73	1.66	0.43	5.82

Non-facility RVUs ▢

Code	Work	PE Non-Facility	MP	Total Non-Facility
52283	3.73	6.50	0.43	10.66

Modifiers (PAR) ▢

Code	Mod 50	Mod 51	Mod 62	Mod 66	Mod 80
52283	0	3	0	0	1

Global Period

Code	Days
52283	000

52285

52285 Cystourethroscopy for treatment of the female urethral syndrome with any or all of the following: urethral meatotomy, urethral dilation, internal urethrotomy, lysis of urethrovaginal septal fibrosis, lateral incisions of the bladder neck, and fulguration of polyp(s) of urethra, bladder neck, and/or trigone

AMA Coding Notes

Surgical Procedures on the Urinary System

(For provision of chemotherapeutic agents, report both the specific service in addition to code(s) for the specific substance(s) or drug(s) provided)

AMA *CPT® Assistant* ▯

52285: May 01: 5, Sep 01: 1

Plain English Description

Female urethral syndrome is characterized by urinary frequency and pain on urination without the presence of a urinary tract infection or other urinary tract abnormality. The urethral orifice is cleansed with antiseptic solution. A rigid or flexible cystoscope is introduced through the urethra into the bladder. The bladder may be filled with sterile saline to allow better visualization of the bladder wall. The bladder is inspected and the ureteral orifices are identified and examined. The cystoscope is slowly withdrawn and the urethra is inspected. The physician may perform one or more therapeutic procedures depending on the cystoscopic findings, including urethral meatotomy or dilation, internal urethrotomy, lysis of urethrovaginal septum fibrosis, lateral incisions of the bladder neck, and/or fulguration of polyps. If the meatus is stenosed, a meatotomy may be performed by incising the urethral meatus. A urethral stricture may be dilated using progressively larger sounds, a filiform and progressively larger followers, or a balloon catheter. Polyps of the urethra, bladder neck, and/or trigone may be treated using an electrocautery device that is advanced through the urethroscope to the site where the polyps are located. The device is activated and the polyps are destroyed. Alternatively, a laser or cryoprobe may be used to destroy the polyps. Fibrotic adhesions at the urethrovaginal septum are severed as needed. Transurethral relaxing incisions are made at the bladder neck as needed. Upon completion of the procedure, the bladder trigone, neck, and urethra are re-inspected with the cystoscope and any bleeding is controlled. The cystoscope is then removed.

Cystourethroscopy, with treatment of female urethral syndrome

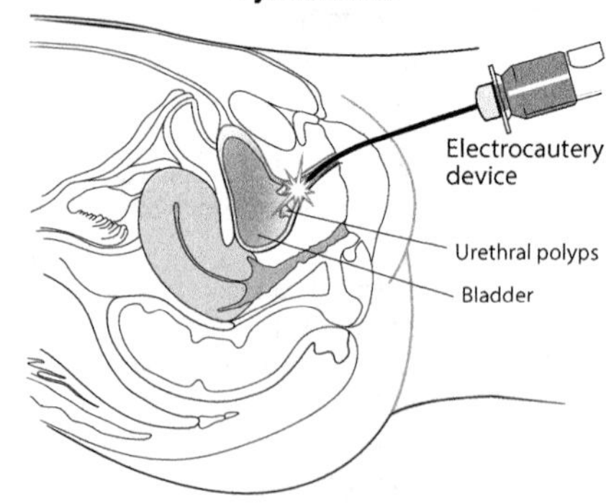

ICD-10-CM Diagnostic Codes

N13.8	Other obstructive and reflux uropathy
N30.10	Interstitial cystitis (chronic) without hematuria
N30.11	Interstitial cystitis (chronic) with hematuria
N30.20	Other chronic cystitis without hematuria
N30.21	Other chronic cystitis with hematuria
N30.90	Cystitis, unspecified without hematuria
N30.91	Cystitis, unspecified with hematuria
N32.0	Bladder-neck obstruction
N34.0	Urethral abscess
N34.1	Nonspecific urethritis
N34.2	Other urethritis
N34.3	Urethral syndrome, unspecified
N36.2	Urethral caruncle
N36.8	Other specified disorders of urethra
N37	Urethral disorders in diseases classified elsewhere
R33.9	Retention of urine, unspecified
R35.0	Frequency of micturition
R39.14	Feeling of incomplete bladder emptying

CCI Edits

Refer to Appendix A for CCI edits.

Facility RVUs ▯

Code	Work	PE Facility	MP	Total Facility
52285	3.60	1.63	0.43	5.66

Non-facility RVUs ▯

Code	Work	PE Non-Facility	MP	Total Non-Facility
52285	3.60	6.52	0.43	10.55

Modifiers (PAR) ▯

Code	Mod 50	Mod 51	Mod 62	Mod 66	Mod 80
52285	0	3	0	0	1

Global Period

Code	Days
52285	000

52287

52287 Cystourethroscopy, with injection(s) for chemodenervation of the bladder

(The supply of the chemodenervation agent is reported separately)

AMA Coding Notes

Surgical Procedures on the Urinary System

(For provision of chemotherapeutic agents, report both the specific service in addition to code(s) for the specific substance(s) or drug(s) provided)

Plain English Description

Chemodenervation involves the injection of a toxin (type A botulinum) directly into a muscle to produce temporary muscle paralysis by blocking the release of acetylcholine. Multiple injections are often required to achieve denervation. Chemical denervation begins within 2 to 3 days of the injection and lasts approximately 3 to 6 months. After anesthetizing the urethra and bladder, the physician places the cystoscope and begins injecting Botox across the back of the trigone and in a radial fashion from the trigone up the posterior wall and toward the dome of the bladder. Treatment of urinary incontinence due to detrusor overactivity involves Botox injected cystoscopically into the detrusor muscle at 30 different locations. Intravesical or sphincteric injections of Botox A are used to treat overactive bladder and functional outlet obstruction.

Cystourethroscopy, with injection(s) for chemodenervation of the bladder

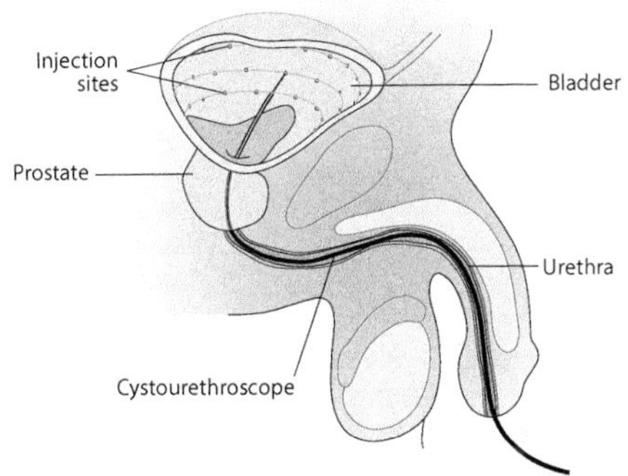

ICD-10-CM Diagnostic Codes

G83.4	Cauda equina syndrome
N31.8	Other neuromuscular dysfunction of bladder
N31.9	Neuromuscular dysfunction of bladder, unspecified
N32.0	Bladder-neck obstruction
N32.81	Overactive bladder

CCI Edits

Refer to Appendix A for CCI edits.

Facility RVUs

Code	Work	PE Facility	MP	Total Facility
52287	3.20	1.32	0.40	4.92

Non-facility RVUs

Code	Work	PE Non-Facility	MP	Total Non-Facility
52287	3.20	8.19	0.40	11.79

Modifiers (PAR)

Code	Mod 50	Mod 51	Mod 62	Mod 66	Mod 80
52287	0	3	0	0	1

Global Period

Code	Days
52287	000

52290

52290 Cystourethroscopy; with ureteral meatotomy, unilateral or bilateral

AMA Coding Notes

Surgical Procedures on the Urinary System

(For provision of chemotherapeutic agents, report both the specific service in addition to code(s) for the specific substance(s) or drug(s) provided)

AMA *CPT® Assistant* □

52290: May 01: 5, Sep 01: 1

Plain English Description

Cystourethroscopy is performed to visualize the inside of the bladder, ureteral orifices, and urethra and incise restricted ureteral opening(s). The urethral orifice is cleansed with antiseptic solution. A rigid or flexible cystoscope is introduced through the urethra into the bladder. The bladder is inspected and the ureteral orifices are identified and examined. A retractable blade is introduced through the cystoscope and advanced to the ureteral orifice. The blade is exposed and the intravesical ureteral orifice is incised. The procedure is repeated on the opposite side as needed. The incisions are inspected with the cystoscope and bleeding is controlled. The cystoscope is removed.

Cystourethroscopy, with ureteral meatotomy

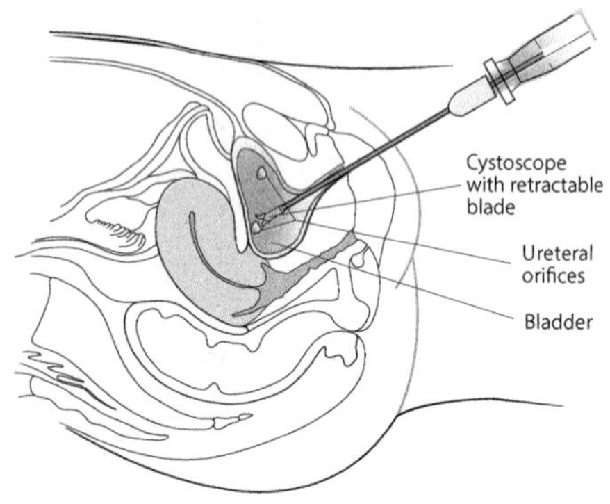

ICD-10-CM Diagnostic Codes

⇄	C66.1	Malignant neoplasm of right ureter
⇄	C66.2	Malignant neoplasm of left ureter
⇄	D30.21	Benign neoplasm of right ureter
⇄	D30.22	Benign neoplasm of left ureter
	N11.1	Chronic obstructive pyelonephritis
	N13.0	Hydronephrosis with ureteropelvic junction obstruction
	N13.1	Hydronephrosis with ureteral stricture, not elsewhere classified
	N13.2	Hydronephrosis with renal and ureteral calculous obstruction
	N13.5	Crossing vessel and stricture of ureter without hydronephrosis
	N13.8	Other obstructive and reflux uropathy
	N20.0	Calculus of kidney
	N20.1	Calculus of ureter
	N21.0	Calculus in bladder
	N28.82	Megaloureter
	N28.89	Other specified disorders of kidney and ureter
	Q62.10	Congenital occlusion of ureter, unspecified
	Q62.11	Congenital occlusion of ureteropelvic junction
	Q62.12	Congenital occlusion of ureterovesical orifice
	Q62.31	Congenital ureterocele, orthotopic
	Q62.32	Cecoureterocele
	Q62.39	Other obstructive defects of renal pelvis and ureter
	Q62.4	Agenesis of ureter
	Q62.5	Duplication of ureter
	Q62.61	Deviation of ureter
	Q62.62	Displacement of ureter
	Q62.63	Anomalous implantation of ureter
	Q62.8	Other congenital malformations of ureter

CCI Edits

Refer to Appendix A for CCI edits.

Pub 100

52290: Pub 100-04, 12, 40.7

Facility RVUs □

Code	Work	PE Facility	MP	Total Facility
52290	4.58	1.93	0.56	7.07

Non-facility RVUs □

Code	Work	PE Non-Facility	MP	Total Non-Facility
52290	4.58	1.93	0.56	7.07

Modifiers (PAR) □

Code	Mod 50	Mod 51	Mod 62	Mod 66	Mod 80
52290	2	3	0	0	1

Global Period

Code	Days
52290	000

52300-52301

52300 Cystourethroscopy; with resection or fulguration of orthotopic ureterocele(s), unilateral or bilateral

52301 Cystourethroscopy; with resection or fulguration of ectopic ureterocele(s), unilateral or bilateral

AMA Coding Notes

Surgical Procedures on the Urinary System

(For provision of chemotherapeutic agents, report both the specific service in addition to code(s) for the specific substance(s) or drug(s) provided)

AMA *CPT® Assistant* ▯

52300: May 01: 5, Sep 01: 1

52301: May 01: 5, Sep 01: 1

Plain English Description

This procedure may also be referred to as endoscopic or transurethral resection or fulguration of ureterocele. An ureterocele is a saccular outpouching of the distal ureter that protrudes into the urinary bladder. An orthotopic ureterocele has its orifice located in the normal anatomic position in the bladder. An ectopic ureterocele has its orifice located in an abnormal position, often in the bladder neck or urethra. Cystourethroscopy is performed to visualize the inside of the bladder and ureteral orifices. The urethral orifice is cleansed with antiseptic solution. A rigid or flexible cystoscope is introduced through the urethra into the bladder. The bladder may be filled with sterile saline to allow better visualization of the bladder wall. The bladder is inspected and the ureterocele is identified and examined. If the ureterocele is fulgurated, an electrocautery device is then advanced through the urethroscope to the ureterocele. The device is activated and the out-pouching is destroyed. Alternatively, a laser or cryoprobe may be used to destroy the ureterocele. If resection is performed, the cystoscope is removed and a resectoscope is advanced to the site of the ureterocele, which is resected. Tissue is removed using irrigation and a cystoscopic evacuation device. Bleeding is controlled as needed using electrocoagulation or laser coagulation. The procedure is repeated on the contralateral ureter as needed. Upon completion of the procedure, the bladder and ureteral orifices are re-inspected to ensure that the abnormal portion of the ureter has been completely resected or destroyed. Use 52300 for unilateral or bilateral orthotopic ureteroceles; use 52301 for unilateral or bilateral ectopic ureteroceles.

Cystourethroscopy, with resection or fulguration of ureterocele

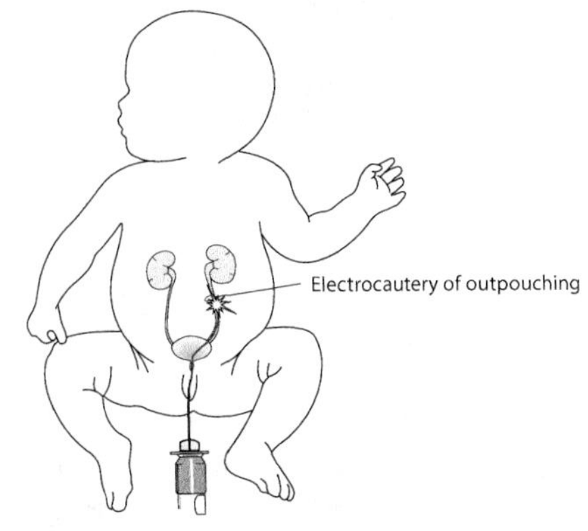

Orthotopic ureterocele (52300); ectopic ureterocele (52301)

ICD-10-CM Diagnostic Codes

N28.82	Megaloureter
N28.89	Other specified disorders of kidney and ureter
N32.3	Diverticulum of bladder
Q62.31	Congenital ureterocele, orthotopic
Q62.32	Cecoureterocele
Q62.5	Duplication of ureter

CCI Edits

Refer to Appendix A for CCI edits.

Facility RVUs ▯

Code	Work	PE Facility	MP	Total Facility
52300	5.30	2.18	0.62	8.10
52301	5.50	2.24	0.65	8.39

Non-facility RVUs ▯

Code	Work	PE Non-Facility	MP	Total Non-Facility
52300	5.30	2.18	0.62	8.10
52301	5.50	2.24	0.65	8.39

Modifiers (PAR) ▯

Code	Mod 50	Mod 51	Mod 62	Mod 66	Mod 80
52300	2	3	0	0	0
52301	2	3	0	0	0

Global Period

Code	Days
52300	000
52301	000

52305

52305 Cystourethroscopy; with incision or resection of orifice of bladder diverticulum, single or multiple

AMA Coding Notes

Surgical Procedures on the Urinary System

(For provision of chemotherapeutic agents, report both the specific service in addition to code(s) for the specific substance(s) or drug(s) provided)

AMA *CPT® Assistant* ▢

52305: May 01: 5, Sep 01: 1

Plain English Description

A bladder diverticulum is a pouch in the bladder wall that may be congenital or acquired. Diverticula may cause ureteral obstruction or vesicoureteral reflux, recurrent urinary tract infections, or stone formation in the bladder. Cystourethroscopy is performed to visualize the inside of the bladder, ureteral orifices, or urethra. The urethral orifice is cleansed with antiseptic solution. A rigid or flexible cystoscope is introduced through the urethra into the bladder. The bladder may be filled with sterile saline to allow better visualization of the bladder wall. The bladder is inspected and the diverticulum is identified and examined. If the diverticulum is incised, a retractable blade is introduced through the cystoscope, the blade is exposed, and the diverticulum is incised. If resection is performed, the cystoscope is removed and a resectoscope is advanced to the site of the diverticulum, which is resected. Tissue is removed using irrigation and a cystoscopic evacuation device. Bleeding is controlled as needed using electrocoagulation or laser coagulation. If multiple diverticula are present, the procedure is repeated until all diverticula have been treated.

Cystourethroscopy;
incision or resection of bladder diverticulum

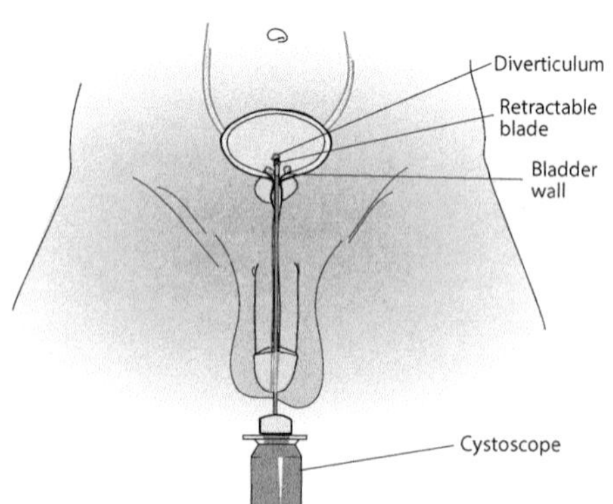

ICD-10-CM Diagnostic Codes

N28.82	Megaloureter
N28.89	Other specified disorders of kidney and ureter
N32.3	Diverticulum of bladder
Q62.31	Congenital ureterocele, orthotopic
Q62.32	Cecoureterocele
Q62.5	Duplication of ureter

CCI Edits

Refer to Appendix A for CCI edits.

Facility RVUs ▢

Code	Work	PE Facility	MP	Total Facility
52305	5.30	2.13	0.62	8.05

Non-facility RVUs ▢

Code	Work	PE Non-Facility	MP	Total Non-Facility
52305	5.30	2.13	0.62	8.05

Modifiers (PAR) ▢

Code	Mod 50	Mod 51	Mod 62	Mod 66	Mod 80
52305	0	3	0	0	1

Global Period

Code	Days
52305	000

52310-52315

52310 Cystourethroscopy, with removal of foreign body, calculus, or ureteral stent from urethra or bladder (separate procedure); simple

52315 Cystourethroscopy, with removal of foreign body, calculus, or ureteral stent from urethra or bladder (separate procedure); complicated

AMA Coding Notes

Surgical Procedures on the Urinary System

(For provision of chemotherapeutic agents, report both the specific service in addition to code(s) for the specific substance(s) or drug(s) provided)

AMA *CPT® Assistant* ▯

52310: May 01: 5, Sep 01: 1

52315: May 01: 5, Sep 01: 1

Plain English Description

Cystourethroscopy is performed to visualize the inside of the bladder, ureteral orifices, and urethra. The urethral orifice is cleansed with antiseptic solution. A rigid or flexible cystoscope is introduced through the urethra into the bladder. The bladder is inspected and foreign body or calculus or ureteral stent is located. A grasping device is advanced through the working channel of the cystoscope and the foreign body, calculus, or ureteral stent is captured and removed from the bladder. The bladder and ureteral orifices are re-inspected to ensure that there has not been any injury to the bladder or ureters. The cystoscope is removed. Use 52310 for a simple removal; use 52315 for a complicated removal.

Cystourethroscopy, with removal of foreign body

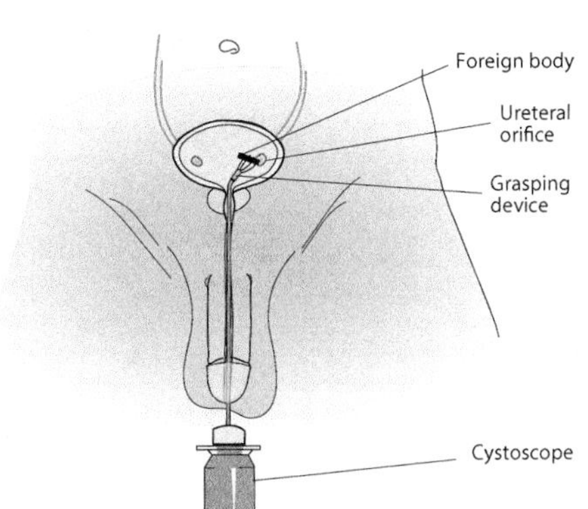

Simple removal (52310); complicated removal (52315)

ICD-10-CM Diagnostic Codes

	N13.5	Crossing vessel and stricture of ureter without hydronephrosis
	N13.8	Other obstructive and reflux uropathy
	N21.0	Calculus in bladder
	N21.1	Calculus in urethra
	N32.0	Bladder-neck obstruction
➐	T19.0	Foreign body in urethra
➐	T19.1	Foreign body in bladder
➐	T83.112	Breakdown (mechanical) of indwelling ureteral stent
➐	T83.122	Displacement of indwelling ureteral stent
➐	T83.192	Other mechanical complication of indwelling ureteral stent
➐	T83.81	Embolism due to genitourinary prosthetic devices, implants and grafts
➐	T83.82	Fibrosis due to genitourinary prosthetic devices, implants and grafts
➐	T83.83	Hemorrhage due to genitourinary prosthetic devices, implants and grafts
➐	T83.84	Pain due to genitourinary prosthetic devices, implants and grafts
➐	T83.85	Stenosis due to genitourinary prosthetic devices, implants and grafts
➐	T83.86	Thrombosis due to genitourinary prosthetic devices, implants and grafts
➐	T83.89	Other specified complication of genitourinary prosthetic devices, implants and grafts

ICD-10-CM Coding Notes

For codes requiring a 7th character extension, refer to your ICD-10-CM book. Review the character descriptions and coding guidelines for proper selection. For some procedures, only certain characters will apply.

CCI Edits

Refer to Appendix A for CCI edits.

Facility RVUs ▯

Code	Work	PE Facility	MP	Total Facility
52310	2.81	1.24	0.34	4.39
52315	5.20	2.13	0.62	7.95

Non-facility RVUs ▯

Code	Work	PE Non-Facility	MP	Total Non-Facility
52310	2.81	6.45	0.34	9.60
52315	5.20	8.28	0.62	14.10

Modifiers (PAR) ▯

Code	Mod 50	Mod 51	Mod 62	Mod 66	Mod 80
52310	0	3	0	0	1
52315	0	3	0	0	1

Global Period

Code	Days
52310	000
52315	000

52317-52318

52317 Litholapaxy: crushing or fragmentation of calculus by any means in bladder and removal of fragments; simple or small (less than 2.5 cm)

52318 Litholapaxy: crushing or fragmentation of calculus by any means in bladder and removal of fragments; complicated or large (over 2.5 cm)

AMA Coding Notes

Surgical Procedures on the Urinary System

(For provision of chemotherapeutic agents, report both the specific service in addition to code(s) for the specific substance(s) or drug(s) provided)

AMA *CPT® Assistant* ▢

52317: May 01: 5, Sep 01: 1, Feb 12: 11
52318: May 01: 5, Sep 01: 1, Feb 12: 11

Plain English Description

A scope is inserted into the bladder and the stone is visualized. To remove the stone by litholapaxy, a crushing instrument or mechanical disintegration probe or laser is inserted through the urethra into the bladder. The stone is then fragmented into smaller and smaller pieces until the remaining fragments are small enough to pass through an evacuation catheter, which is then inserted through the urethra and into the bladder. The bladder is irrigated with sterile saline or other solution and the stone fragments are flushed out of the bladder through the catheter. The bladder is re-inspected with the scope to ensure that all stones have been pulverized and that all fragments have been flushed from the bladder. Use 52317 for simple litholapaxy or small stones less than 2.5 cm; use 52318 for complicated litholapaxy or large stones over 2.5 cm.

Litholapaxy
Crushing or fragmentation of calculus by any means in bladder and removal of fragments

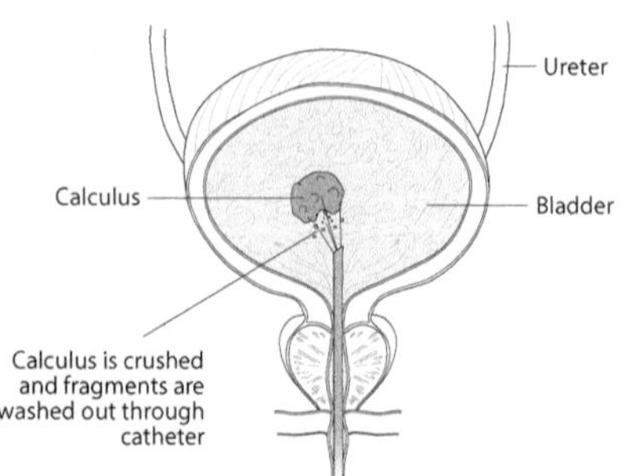
Ureter
Calculus
Bladder
Calculus is crushed and fragments are washed out through catheter

ICD-10-CM Diagnostic Codes

N20.1	Calculus of ureter
N21.0	Calculus in bladder

CCI Edits

Refer to Appendix A for CCI edits.

Facility RVUs ▢

Code	Work	PE Facility	MP	Total Facility
52317	6.71	2.55	0.79	10.05
52318	9.18	3.44	1.09	13.71

Non-facility RVUs ▢

Code	Work	PE Non-Facility	MP	Total Non-Facility
52317	6.71	19.51	0.79	27.01
52318	9.18	3.44	1.09	13.71

Modifiers (PAR) ▢

Code	Mod 50	Mod 51	Mod 62	Mod 66	Mod 80
52317	0	3	0	0	1
52318	0	3	0	0	1

Global Period

Code	Days
52317	000
52318	000

52320-52325

52320 Cystourethroscopy (including ureteral catheterization); with removal of ureteral calculus

52325 Cystourethroscopy (including ureteral catheterization); with fragmentation of ureteral calculus (eg, ultrasonic or electro-hydraulic technique)

AMA Coding Guideline

Ureter and Pelvis Transurethral Surgical Procedures

Therapeutic cystourethroscopy always includes diagnostic cystourethroscopy. To report a diagnostic cystourethroscopy, use 52000. Therapeutic cystourethroscopy with ureteroscopy and/or pyeloscopy always includes diagnostic cystourethroscopy with ureteroscopy and/or pyeloscopy. To report a diagnostic cystourethroscopy with ureteroscopy and/or pyeloscopy, use 52351.

Do not report 52000 in conjunction with 52320-52343, 52356.

Do not report 52351 in conjunction with 52344-52346, 52352-52356.

The insertion and removal of a temporary ureteral catheter (52005) during diagnostic or therapeutic cystourethroscopy with ureteroscopy and/or pyeloscopy is included in 52320-52356 and should not be reported separately.

To report insertion of a self-retaining, indwelling stent performed during diagnostic or therapeutic cystourethroscopy with ureteroscopy and/or pyeloscopy, report 52332, in addition to primary procedure(s) performed (52320-52330, 52334-52352, 52354, 52355), and append modifier 51. Code 52332 is used to report a unilateral procedure unless otherwise specified.

For bilateral insertion of self-retaining, indwelling ureteral stents, use code 52332, and append modifier 50.

To report cystourethroscopic removal of a self-retaining, indwelling ureteral stent, see 52310, 52315, and append modifier 58, if appropriate.

AMA Coding Notes

Surgical Procedures on the Urinary System

(For provision of chemotherapeutic agents, report both the specific service in addition to code(s) for the specific substance(s) or drug(s) provided)

AMA *CPT® Assistant*

52320: Mar 96: 1, May 96: 11, Jan 01: 13, May 01: 5, Sep 01: 1, Oct 01: 8, May 14: 3

52325: Mar 96: 1, May 96: 11, May 01: 5, Sep 01: 1, Oct 01: 8, Dec 07: 13

Plain English Description

The urethra is cleansed with antiseptic solution. A rigid or flexible cystoscope is introduced through the urethra into the bladder for cystourethroscopy to remove a stone from the ureter. The bladder may be filled with sterile saline to allow better visualization of the bladder wall. Following inspection of the bladder, the ureters are catheterized. A guidewire is introduced through the cystoscope and advanced through the ureter into the renal pelvis. In 52320, a grasping or retrieval device is advanced through the cystoscope over the guidewire to the calculus in the ureter, and the calculus is captured and removed. In 52325, the calculus is first fragmented using an ultrasonic or electrohydraulic technique. The ultrasonic or electrohydraulic probe is advanced through the cystoscope to the ureteral stone. The probe is activated and shock waves are generated, causing fragmentation of the calculus. Following retrieval or fragmentation of the calculus, a catheter may be advanced over the guidewire to the renal pelvis and the ureter may be irrigated to remove calculus fragments. Diagnostic or therapeutic solution may also be instilled into the ureter through the catheter. Upon completion of the procedure, the catheter, guidewire, and cystoscope are removed.

Cystourethroscopy, with removal of ureteral calculus

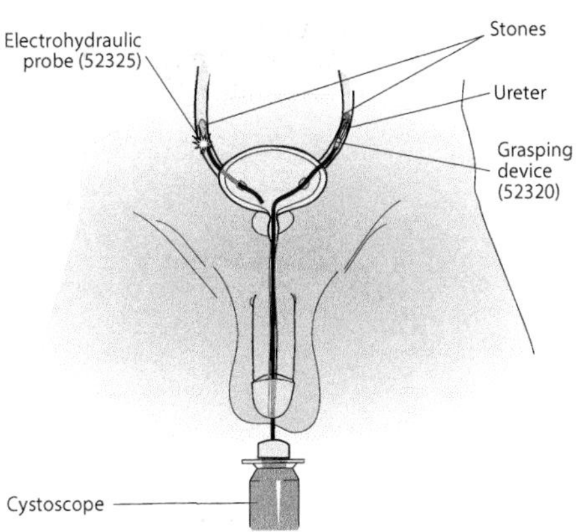

ICD-10-CM Diagnostic Codes

N20.1	Calculus of ureter
N20.2	Calculus of kidney with calculus of ureter

CCI Edits

Refer to Appendix A for CCI edits.

Facility RVUs

Code	Work	PE Facility	MP	Total Facility
52320	4.69	1.89	0.56	7.14
52325	6.15	2.39	0.73	9.27

Non-facility RVUs

Code	Work	PE Non-Facility	MP	Total Non-Facility
52320	4.69	1.89	0.56	7.14
52325	6.15	2.39	0.73	9.27

Modifiers (PAR)

Code	Mod 50	Mod 51	Mod 62	Mod 66	Mod 80
52320	1	3	0	0	1
52325	1	3	0	0	1

Global Period

Code	Days
52320	000
52325	000

52327

52327 Cystourethroscopy (including ureteral catheterization); with subureteric injection of implant material

AMA Coding Guideline

Ureter and Pelvis Transurethral Surgical Procedures

Therapeutic cystourethroscopy always includes diagnostic cystourethroscopy. To report a diagnostic cystourethroscopy, use 52000. Therapeutic cystourethroscopy with ureteroscopy and/or pyeloscopy always includes diagnostic cystourethroscopy with ureteroscopy and/or pyeloscopy. To report a diagnostic cystourethroscopy with ureteroscopy and/or pyeloscopy, use 52351.

Do not report 52000 in conjunction with 52320-52343, 52356.

Do not report 52351 in conjunction with 52344-52346, 52352-52356.

The insertion and removal of a temporary ureteral catheter (52005) during diagnostic or therapeutic cystourethroscopy with ureteroscopy and/or pyeloscopy is included in 52320-52356 and should not be reported separately.

To report insertion of a self-retaining, indwelling stent performed during diagnostic or therapeutic cystourethroscopy with ureteroscopy and/or pyeloscopy, report 52332, in addition to primary procedure(s) performed (52320-52330, 52334-52352, 52354, 52355), and append modifier 51. Code 52332 is used to report a unilateral procedure unless otherwise specified.

For bilateral insertion of self-retaining, indwelling ureteral stents, use code 52332, and append modifier 50.

To report cystourethroscopic removal of a self-retaining, indwelling ureteral stent, see 52310, 52315, and append modifier 58, if appropriate.

AMA Coding Notes

Surgical Procedures on the Urinary System

(For provision of chemotherapeutic agents, report both the specific service in addition to code(s) for the specific substance(s) or drug(s) provided)

AMA *CPT® Assistant* ▢

52327: Mar 96: 1, May 96: 11, May 01: 5, Sep 01: 1, Oct 01: 8

Plain English Description

The physician performs cystourethroscopy with subureteric injection of implant material including any required ureteral catheterization. This procedure may also be referred to as a subureteral transurethral injection (STING) procedure.
A modification of the STING procedure is the hydrodistention-implantation technique, also referred to as a HIT procedure. A catheter is used to drain urine from the bladder. A cystourethroscope is inserted into the urethra and advanced into the bladder. The bladder is then partially filled with fluid in a retrograde fashion to allow better visualization of the ureteral orifice. The scope is advanced to the ureteral orifice. The ureter may be distended using a pressurized stream of irrigation fluid directed into the ureter. If ureteral catheterization is required, a couple of techniques may be employed.
If guidewires are used, two are required. A safety guidewire is passed into the ureter first. A semirigid or flexible ureteroscope is then passed alongside the safety guidewire over a working guidewire and the ureter is catheterized by passing a temporary ureteral catheter over the working guidewire and positioning it in the ureter. Alternatively, a wireless or "no touch" technique may be used to position the catheter in the ureter. The ureteroscope is removed and a needle is passed through the cystourethroscope into the submucosa below the ureteral orifice. Implant material is then injected to elevate and narrow the ureteral orifice and support the ureter. The scope is withdrawn to the level of the bladder neck and the implant site is visualized to ensure that the implant material has been properly placed. The bladder is then emptied and the scope is withdrawn.

Cystourethroscopy, with subureteric injection of implant material

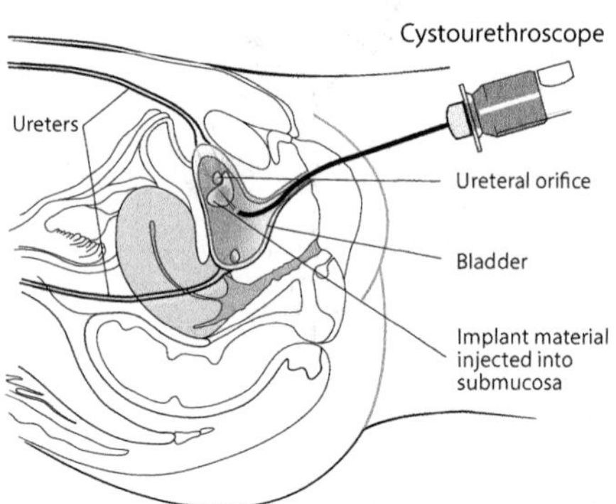

ICD-10-CM Diagnostic Codes

N20.1	Calculus of ureter
N20.2	Calculus of kidney with calculus of ureter

CCI Edits

Refer to Appendix A for CCI edits.

Facility RVUs ▢

Code	Work	PE Facility	MP	Total Facility
52327	5.18	1.79	0.67	7.64

Non-facility RVUs ▢

Code	Work	PE Non-Facility	MP	Total Non-Facility
52327	5.18	1.79	0.67	7.64

Modifiers (PAR) ▢

Code	Mod 50	Mod 51	Mod 62	Mod 66	Mod 80
52327	1	3	0	0	1

Global Period

Code	Days
52327	000

52330

52330 Cystourethroscopy (including ureteral catheterization); with manipulation, without removal of ureteral calculus

(Do not report 52320, 52325, 52327, 52330 in conjunction with 52000)

AMA Coding Guideline

Ureter and Pelvis Transurethral Surgical Procedures

Therapeutic cystourethroscopy always includes diagnostic cystourethroscopy. To report a diagnostic cystourethroscopy, use 52000. Therapeutic cystourethroscopy with ureteroscopy and/or pyeloscopy always includes diagnostic cystourethroscopy with ureteroscopy and/or pyeloscopy. To report a diagnostic cystourethroscopy with ureteroscopy and/or pyeloscopy, use 52351.

Do not report 52000 in conjunction with 52320-52343, 52356.

Do not report 52351 in conjunction with 52344-52346, 52352-52356.

The insertion and removal of a temporary ureteral catheter (52005) during diagnostic or therapeutic cystourethroscopy with ureteroscopy and/or pyeloscopy is included in 52320-52356 and should not be reported separately.

To report insertion of a self-retaining, indwelling stent performed during diagnostic or therapeutic cystourethroscopy with ureteroscopy and/or pyeloscopy, report 52332, in addition to primary procedure(s) performed (52320-52330, 52334-52352, 52354, 52355), and append modifier 51. Code 52332 is used to report a unilateral procedure unless otherwise specified.

For bilateral insertion of self-retaining, indwelling ureteral stents, use code 52332, and append modifier 50.

To report cystourethroscopic removal of a self-retaining, indwelling ureteral stent, see 52310, 52315, and append modifier 58, if appropriate.

AMA Coding Notes

Surgical Procedures on the Urinary System

(For provision of chemotherapeutic agents, report both the specific service in addition to code(s) for the specific substance(s) or drug(s) provided)

AMA *CPT® Assistant* ☐

52330: Mar 96: 1, May 96: 11, Sep 00: 11, May 01: 5, Sep 01: 1, Oct 01: 8, May 14: 3

Plain English Description

The urethra is cleansed with antiseptic solution. A rigid or flexible cystoscope is introduced through the urethra into the bladder. The bladder may be filled with sterile saline to allow better visualization of the bladder wall. Following inspection of the bladder, the ureter is catheterized. A guidewire is introduced through the cystoscope and advanced into the ureter and through the ureter to the renal pelvis. A grasping device is advanced through the cystoscope and the calculus is grasped and manipulated into a different location without removal. The ureter may be irrigated with normal saline. Upon completion of the procedure, the catheter, guidewire, and cystoscope are removed.

Cystourethroscopy, without removal of calculus

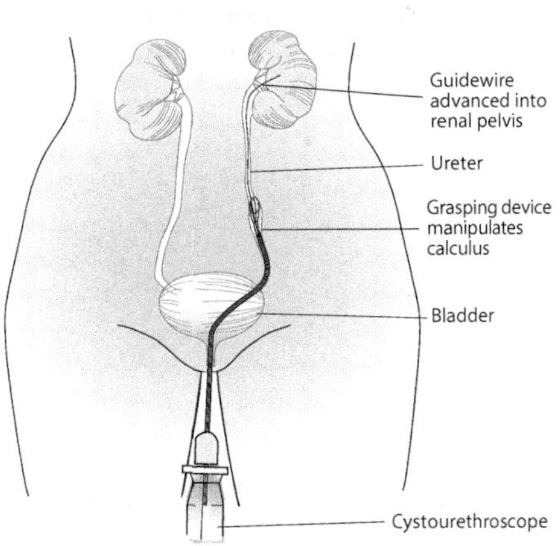

ICD-10-CM Diagnostic Codes

N20.1	Calculus of ureter
N20.2	Calculus of kidney with calculus of ureter

CCI Edits

Refer to Appendix A for CCI edits.

Facility RVUs ☐

Code	Work	PE Facility	MP	Total Facility
52330	5.03	2.00	0.60	7.63

Non-facility RVUs ☐

Code	Work	PE Non-Facility	MP	Total Non-Facility
52330	5.03	12.71	0.60	18.34

Modifiers (PAR) ☐

Code	Mod 50	Mod 51	Mod 62	Mod 66	Mod 80
52330	1	3	0	0	1

Global Period

Code	Days
52330	000

52332

52332 Cystourethroscopy, with insertion of indwelling ureteral stent (eg, Gibbons or double-J type)

(Do not report 52332 in conjunction with 52000, 52353, 52356 when performed together on the same side)

AMA Coding Guideline

Ureter and Pelvis Transurethral Surgical Procedures

Therapeutic cystourethroscopy always includes diagnostic cystourethroscopy. To report a diagnostic cystourethroscopy, use 52000. Therapeutic cystourethroscopy with ureteroscopy and/or pyeloscopy always includes diagnostic cystourethroscopy with ureteroscopy and/or pyeloscopy. To report a diagnostic cystourethroscopy with ureteroscopy and/or pyeloscopy, use 52351.

Do not report 52000 in conjunction with 52320-52343, 52356.

Do not report 52351 in conjunction with 52344-52346, 52352-52356.

The insertion and removal of a temporary ureteral catheter (52005) during diagnostic or therapeutic cystourethroscopy with ureteroscopy and/or pyeloscopy is included in 52320-52356 and should not be reported separately.

To report insertion of a self-retaining, indwelling stent performed during diagnostic or therapeutic cystourethroscopy with ureteroscopy and/or pyeloscopy, report 52332, in addition to primary procedure(s) performed (52320-52330, 52334-52352, 52354, 52355), and append modifier 51. Code 52332 is used to report a unilateral procedure unless otherwise specified.

For bilateral insertion of self-retaining, indwelling ureteral stents, use code 52332, and append modifier 50.

To report cystourethroscopic removal of a self-retaining, indwelling ureteral stent, see 52310, 52315, and append modifier 58, if appropriate.

AMA Coding Notes

Surgical Procedures on the Urinary System

(For provision of chemotherapeutic agents, report both the specific service in addition to code(s) for the specific substance(s) or drug(s) provided)

AMA *CPT® Assistant* ▢

52332: Mar 96: 1, May 96: 11, Nov 96: 8, Jan 01: 13, May 01: 5, Sep 01: 1, Oct 01: 8, Oct 05: 18, Dec 09: 4, 12, May 14: 3

Plain English Description

The urethra is cleansed with antiseptic solution. A rigid or flexible cystoscope is introduced through the urethra into the bladder. The bladder may be filled with sterile saline to allow better visualization of the bladder wall. Following inspection of the bladder, the ureter is catheterized. A guidewire is introduced through the cystoscope and advanced into the ureter and through the ureter to the renal pelvis. A stent is then advanced through the cystoscope, over the guidewire, and positioned within the ureter. The guidewire is removed, leaving the stent in place. The bladder is re-inspected and the position of the distal tail of the stent is inspected to ensure that it is properly positioned in the bladder. Upon completion of the procedure, the cystoscope is removed.

Cystourethroscopy, with insertion of ureteral stent

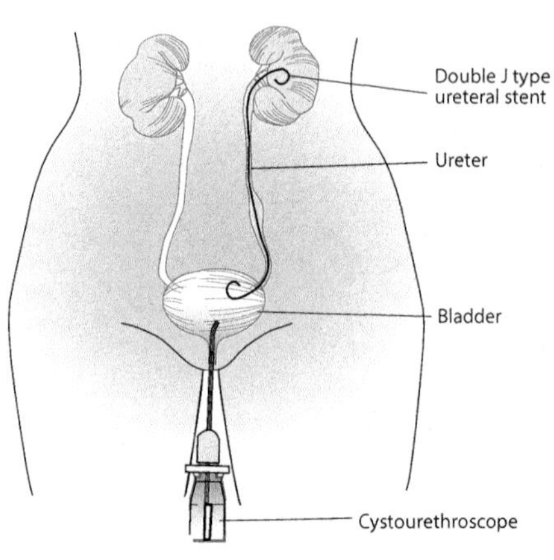

ICD-10-CM Diagnostic Codes

⇄	C66.1	Malignant neoplasm of right ureter
⇄	C66.2	Malignant neoplasm of left ureter
⇄	D30.21	Benign neoplasm of right ureter
⇄	D30.22	Benign neoplasm of left ureter
⇄	D41.21	Neoplasm of uncertain behavior of right ureter
⇄	D41.22	Neoplasm of uncertain behavior of left ureter
	N11.1	Chronic obstructive pyelonephritis
	N13.1	Hydronephrosis with ureteral stricture, not elsewhere classified
	N13.2	Hydronephrosis with renal and ureteral calculous obstruction
	N13.39	Other hydronephrosis
	N13.5	Crossing vessel and stricture of ureter without hydronephrosis
	N13.8	Other obstructive and reflux uropathy
	N20.0	Calculus of kidney
	N20.1	Calculus of ureter
	N20.2	Calculus of kidney with calculus of ureter
	N28.82	Megaloureter
	N28.89	Other specified disorders of kidney and ureter
	Q62.10	Congenital occlusion of ureter, unspecified
	Q62.11	Congenital occlusion of ureteropelvic junction
	Q62.12	Congenital occlusion of ureterovesical orifice
	Q62.2	Congenital megaureter
	Q62.39	Other obstructive defects of renal pelvis and ureter
	Q62.7	Congenital vesico-uretero-renal reflux
	Q62.8	Other congenital malformations of ureter

CCI Edits

Refer to Appendix A for CCI edits.

Facility RVUs ▢

Code	Work	PE Facility	MP	Total Facility
52332	2.82	1.35	0.34	4.51

Non-facility RVUs ▢

Code	Work	PE Non-Facility	MP	Total Non-Facility
52332	2.82	9.07	0.34	12.23

Modifiers (PAR) ▢

Code	Mod 50	Mod 51	Mod 62	Mod 66	Mod 80
52332	1	3	0	0	1

Global Period

Code	Days
52332	000

52334

52334 Cystourethroscopy with insertion of ureteral guide wire through kidney to establish a percutaneous nephrostomy, retrograde

(For percutaneous nephrostolithotomy, see 50080, 50081; for establishment of percutaneous nephrostomy, see 50432, 50433)

(For cystourethroscopy, with ureteroscopy and/or pyeloscopy, see 52351-52356)

(For cystourethroscopy with incision, fulguration, or resection of congenital posterior urethral valves or obstructive hypertrophic mucosal folds, use 52400)

(Do not report 52334 in conjunction with 50437, 52000, 52351)

AMA Coding Guideline

Ureter and Pelvis Transurethral Surgical Procedures

Therapeutic cystourethroscopy always includes diagnostic cystourethroscopy. To report a diagnostic cystourethroscopy, use 52000. Therapeutic cystourethroscopy with ureteroscopy and/or pyeloscopy always includes diagnostic cystourethroscopy with ureteroscopy and/or pyeloscopy. To report a diagnostic cystourethroscopy with ureteroscopy and/or pyeloscopy, use 52351.

Do not report 52000 in conjunction with 52320-52343, 52356.

Do not report 52351 in conjunction with 52344-52346, 52352-52356.

The insertion and removal of a temporary ureteral catheter (52005) during diagnostic or therapeutic cystourethroscopy with ureteroscopy and/or pyeloscopy is included in 52320-52356 and should not be reported separately.

To report insertion of a self-retaining, indwelling stent performed during diagnostic or therapeutic cystourethroscopy with ureteroscopy and/or pyeloscopy, report 52332, in addition to primary procedure(s) performed (52320-52330, 52334-52352, 52354, 52355), and append modifier 51. Code 52332 is used to report a unilateral procedure unless otherwise specified.

For bilateral insertion of self-retaining, indwelling ureteral stents, use code 52332, and append modifier 50.

To report cystourethroscopic removal of a self-retaining, indwelling ureteral stent, see 52310, 52315, and append modifier 58, if appropriate.

AMA Coding Notes

Surgical Procedures on the Urinary System

(For provision of chemotherapeutic agents, report both the specific service in addition to code(s) for the specific substance(s) or drug(s) provided)

AMA *CPT® Assistant* ▯

52334: Mar 96: 11, May 96: 11, May 01: 5, Sep 01: 1, Oct 01: 8, May 14: 3

Plain English Description

A nephrostomy is created endoscopically by means of a controlled, retrograde fine wire puncture from within the renal pelvis or calyx to provide percutaneous access to the kidney. The urethra is cleansed with antiseptic solution. A rigid or flexible cystoscope is introduced through the urethra into the bladder. The bladder may be filled with sterile saline to allow better visualization of the bladder wall. Following inspection of the bladder, the ureter is catheterized. A guidewire is introduced through the cystoscope and advanced into the ureter and through the ureter to the renal pelvis or desired calyx. A nephrostomy catheter is then advanced over the guidewire into the renal pelvis and then into the desired calyx. The guidewire is removed, leaving the nephrostomy catheter in place. A sheathed needle is then advanced through the catheter. The needle is exposed and advanced through the calyx until it exits the skin. The nephrostomy tract is dilated over the needle. Once the desired diameter has been achieved, a nephrostomy tube is placed and secured with sutures. The needle, cystoscope, and other surgical devices are removed.

Cystourethroscopy, with percutaneous nephrostomy

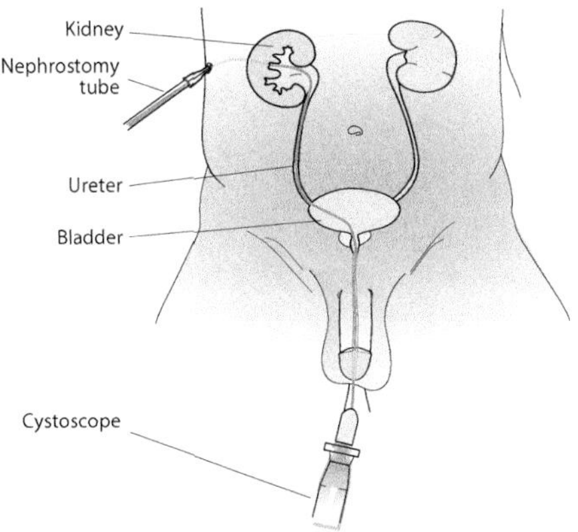

ICD-10-CM Diagnostic Codes

⇄	C64.1	Malignant neoplasm of right kidney, except renal pelvis
⇄	C64.2	Malignant neoplasm of left kidney, except renal pelvis
⇄	C65.1	Malignant neoplasm of right renal pelvis
⇄	C65.2	Malignant neoplasm of left renal pelvis
	C67.0	Malignant neoplasm of trigone of bladder
	C67.1	Malignant neoplasm of dome of bladder
	C67.2	Malignant neoplasm of lateral wall of bladder
	C67.3	Malignant neoplasm of anterior wall of bladder
	C67.4	Malignant neoplasm of posterior wall of bladder
	C67.5	Malignant neoplasm of bladder neck
	C67.6	Malignant neoplasm of ureteric orifice
	C67.8	Malignant neoplasm of overlapping sites of bladder
	C7A.093	Malignant carcinoid tumor of the kidney
	D41.4	Neoplasm of uncertain behavior of bladder
	N00.8	Acute nephritic syndrome with other morphologic changes
	N00.9	Acute nephritic syndrome with unspecified morphologic changes
	N02.8	Recurrent and persistent hematuria with other morphologic changes
	N02.9	Recurrent and persistent hematuria with unspecified morphologic changes
	N03.0	Chronic nephritic syndrome with minor glomerular abnormality
	N03.8	Chronic nephritic syndrome with other morphologic changes
	N03.9	Chronic nephritic syndrome with unspecified morphologic changes
	N04.7	Nephrotic syndrome with diffuse crescentic glomerulonephritis
	N04.8	Nephrotic syndrome with other morphologic changes
	N11.1	Chronic obstructive pyelonephritis
	N13.1	Hydronephrosis with ureteral stricture, not elsewhere classified
	N13.2	Hydronephrosis with renal and ureteral calculous obstruction
	N13.39	Other hydronephrosis
	N13.5	Crossing vessel and stricture of ureter without hydronephrosis
	N13.6	Pyonephrosis
	N13.8	Other obstructive and reflux uropathy
	N15.1	Renal and perinephric abscess
	N15.8	Other specified renal tubulo-interstitial diseases
	N20.0	Calculus of kidney
	N20.1	Calculus of ureter
	N20.2	Calculus of kidney with calculus of ureter
	N28.82	Megaloureter
	N28.84	Pyelitis cystica
	N28.85	Pyeloureteritis cystica
	N28.86	Ureteritis cystica
	N28.89	Other specified disorders of kidney and ureter
	N32.89	Other specified disorders of bladder
	N33	Bladder disorders in diseases classified elsewhere
	N39.42	Incontinence without sensory awareness
	N39.46	Mixed incontinence
	Q62.0	Congenital hydronephrosis
	Q62.11	Congenital occlusion of ureteropelvic junction
	Q62.12	Congenital occlusion of ureterovesical orifice
	Q62.2	Congenital megaureter

Q62.39	Other obstructive defects of renal pelvis and ureter
Q63.1	Lobulated, fused and horseshoe kidney
Q63.2	Ectopic kidney
Q63.3	Hyperplastic and giant kidney
Q63.8	Other specified congenital malformations of kidney
Z85.53	Personal history of malignant neoplasm of renal pelvis

CCI Edits

Refer to Appendix A for CCI edits.

Facility RVUs

Code	Work	PE Facility	MP	Total Facility
52334	3.37	1.52	0.40	5.29

Non-facility RVUs

Code	Work	PE Non-Facility	MP	Total Non-Facility
52334	3.37	1.52	0.40	5.29

Modifiers (PAR)

Code	Mod 50	Mod 51	Mod 62	Mod 66	Mod 80
52334	0	3	0	0	1

Global Period

Code	Days
52334	000

52341-52343

52341 Cystourethroscopy; with treatment of ureteral stricture (eg, balloon dilation, laser, electrocautery, and incision)

52342 Cystourethroscopy; with treatment of ureteropelvic junction stricture (eg, balloon dilation, laser, electrocautery, and incision)

52343 Cystourethroscopy; with treatment of intra-renal stricture (eg, balloon dilation, laser, electrocautery, and incision)

(Do not report 52341, 52342, 52343 in conjunction with 52000, 52351)

(For image-guided dilation of ureter, ureteropelvic junction stricture without endoscopic guidance, use 50706)

(For radiological supervision and interpretation, use 74485)

AMA Coding Guideline

Ureter and Pelvis Transurethral Surgical Procedures

Therapeutic cystourethroscopy always includes diagnostic cystourethroscopy. To report a diagnostic cystourethroscopy, use 52000. Therapeutic cystourethroscopy with ureteroscopy and/or pyeloscopy always includes diagnostic cystourethroscopy with ureteroscopy and/or pyeloscopy. To report a diagnostic cystourethroscopy with ureteroscopy and/or pyeloscopy, use 52351.

Do not report 52000 in conjunction with 52320-52343, 52356.

Do not report 52351 in conjunction with 52344-52346, 52352-52356.

The insertion and removal of a temporary ureteral catheter (52005) during diagnostic or therapeutic cystourethroscopy with ureteroscopy and/or pyeloscopy is included in 52320-52356 and should not be reported separately.

To report insertion of a self-retaining, indwelling stent performed during diagnostic or therapeutic cystourethroscopy with ureteroscopy and/or pyeloscopy, report 52332, in addition to primary procedure(s) performed (52320-52330, 52334-52352, 52354, 52355), and append modifier 51. Code 52332 is used to report a unilateral procedure unless otherwise specified.

For bilateral insertion of self-retaining, indwelling ureteral stents, use code 52332, and append modifier 50.

To report cystourethroscopic removal of a self-retaining, indwelling ureteral stent, see 52310, 52315, and append modifier 58, if appropriate.

AMA Coding Notes

Surgical Procedures on the Urinary System

(For provision of chemotherapeutic agents, report both the specific service in addition to code(s) for the specific substance(s) or drug(s) provided)

AMA *CPT® Assistant*

52341: Nov 96: 9, Apr 01: 4, May 01: 5, Sep 01: 1, Oct 01: 8

52342: Apr 01: 4, May 01: 5, Sep 01: 1, Oct 01: 8, Aug 02: 11

52343: Apr 01: 4, May 01: 5, Sep 01: 1, Oct 01: 8, May 14: 3

Plain English Description

The physician performs cystourethroscopy to treat a ureteral, ureteropelvic junction (UPJ), or intra-renal stricture using balloon dilation, laser, electrocautery, and/or incision. A cystourethroscope is inserted into the urethra and advanced through the bladder and into the ureter. A guidewire is passed under ureteroscopic control through the area of the stricture. A semi-rigid or flexible ureteroscope is then passed alongside the guidewire to the area of the stricture. A balloon dilator may be advanced and inflated to dilate the stricture. This may be followed by incision of the stricture using an endoincision technique with a laser fiber, electrocautery, or other endoscopic surgical tool. Incisions are made through the full thickness of the ureter or UPJ until periureteric or perirenal fat is encountered. Dilation and/or incisions are made along the length of the stricture until the ureteroscope can be passed through the area of the stricture. A temporary indwelling stent is then placed across the surgical site and surgical instruments are removed. Report 52341 for treatment of a ureteral stricture, 52342 for treatment of a UPJ stricture, and 52343 for treatment of an intra-renal stricture.

Cystourethroscopy, with treatment of stricture

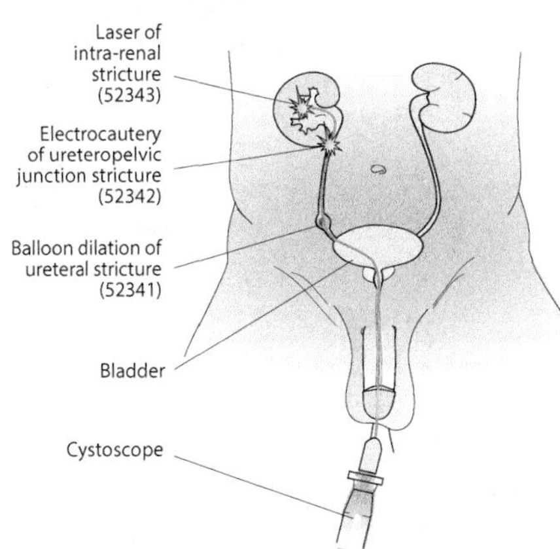

ICD-10-CM Diagnostic Codes

	A18.11	Tuberculosis of kidney and ureter
⇄	C66.1	Malignant neoplasm of right ureter
⇄	C66.2	Malignant neoplasm of left ureter
⇄	D30.21	Benign neoplasm of right ureter
⇄	D30.22	Benign neoplasm of left ureter
	N11.1	Chronic obstructive pyelonephritis
	N13.0	Hydronephrosis with ureteropelvic junction obstruction
	N13.1	Hydronephrosis with ureteral stricture, not elsewhere classified
	N13.2	Hydronephrosis with renal and ureteral calculous obstruction
	N13.5	Crossing vessel and stricture of ureter without hydronephrosis
	N13.8	Other obstructive and reflux uropathy
	N20.1	Calculus of ureter
	N20.2	Calculus of kidney with calculus of ureter
	N28.82	Megaloureter
	N28.89	Other specified disorders of kidney and ureter
	N99.111	Postprocedural bulbous urethral stricture, male ♂
	N99.112	Postprocedural membranous urethral stricture, male ♂
	N99.113	Postprocedural anterior bulbous urethral stricture, male ♂

CCI Edits

Refer to Appendix A for CCI edits.

Pub 100

52341: Pub 100-03, 1, 140.5

52342: Pub 100-03, 1, 140.5

52343: Pub 100-03, 1, 140.5

Facility RVUs

Code	Work	PE Facility	MP	Total Facility
52341	5.35	2.23	0.64	8.22
52342	5.85	2.40	0.70	8.95
52343	6.55	2.64	0.77	9.96

Non-facility RVUs

Code	Work	PE Non-Facility	MP	Total Non-Facility
52341	5.35	2.23	0.64	8.22
52342	5.85	2.40	0.70	8.95
52343	6.55	2.64	0.77	9.96

Modifiers (PAR)

Code	Mod 50	Mod 51	Mod 62	Mod 66	Mod 80
52341	1	3	0	0	1
52342	1	3	0	0	1
52343	1	3	0	0	1

Global Period

Code	Days
52341	000
52342	000
52343	000

52344-52346

52344 Cystourethroscopy with ureteroscopy; with treatment of ureteral stricture (eg, balloon dilation, laser, electrocautery, and incision)

52345 Cystourethroscopy with ureteroscopy; with treatment of ureteropelvic junction stricture (eg, balloon dilation, laser, electrocautery, and incision)

52346 Cystourethroscopy with ureteroscopy; with treatment of intra-renal stricture (eg, balloon dilation, laser, electrocautery, and incision)

(For transurethral resection or incision of ejaculatory ducts, use 52402)

(Do not report 52344, 52345, 52346 in conjunction with 52351)

(For image-guided dilation of ureter, ureteropelvic junction stricture without endoscopic guidance, use 50706)

(For radiological supervision and interpretation, use 74485)

AMA Coding Guideline

Ureter and Pelvis Transurethral Surgical Procedures

Therapeutic cystourethroscopy always includes diagnostic cystourethroscopy. To report a diagnostic cystourethroscopy, use 52000. Therapeutic cystourethroscopy with ureteroscopy and/or pyeloscopy always includes diagnostic cystourethroscopy with ureteroscopy and/or pyeloscopy. To report a diagnostic cystourethroscopy with ureteroscopy and/or pyeloscopy, use 52351.

Do not report 52000 in conjunction with 52320-52343, 52356.

Do not report 52351 in conjunction with 52344-52346, 52352-52356.

The insertion and removal of a temporary ureteral catheter (52005) during diagnostic or therapeutic cystourethroscopy with ureteroscopy and/or pyeloscopy is included in 52320-52356 and should not be reported separately.

To report insertion of a self-retaining, indwelling stent performed during diagnostic or therapeutic cystourethroscopy with ureteroscopy and/or pyeloscopy, report 52332, in addition to primary procedure(s) performed (52320-52330, 52334-52352, 52354, 52355), and append modifier 51. Code 52332 is used to report a unilateral procedure unless otherwise specified.

For bilateral insertion of self-retaining, indwelling ureteral stents, use code 52332, and append modifier 50.

To report cystourethroscopic removal of a self-retaining, indwelling ureteral stent, see 52310, 52315, and append modifier 58, if appropriate.

AMA Coding Notes

Surgical Procedures on the Urinary System

(For provision of chemotherapeutic agents, report both the specific service in addition to code(s) for the specific substance(s) or drug(s) provided)

AMA *CPT® Assistant*

52344: Apr 01: 4, May 01: 5, Sep 01: 1, Oct 01: 8
52345: Apr 01: 4, May 01: 5, Sep 01: 1, Oct 01: 8
52346: Apr 01: 4, May 01: 5, Sep 01: 1, Oct 01: 8, May 14: 3

Plain English Description

Cystourethroscopy with ureteroscopy is performed to treat a ureteral stricture (52344), ureteropelvic junction stricture (52345), or intra-renal stricture (52346) using balloon dilation, laser, electrocautery, and/or incision. Cystoscopy with ureteroscopy uses an ureteroscope that is passed through the urethra into the bladder and then into the ureter. The ureteroscope is used to directly visualize the ureter, pass guidewires, and direct the use of laser, balloons, or incisional or electrocautery devices. In 52344, the ureteroscope is passed from the bladder into the ureter to the site of the stricture. The stricture is visualized. A guidewire is then passed through the stricture. If a balloon catheter is used, it is advanced over the guidewire, inflated at the site of the narrowing, deflated, and removed. If a laser is used, the laser fiber is passed to the site of the stricture and fired to incise the narrowed area. Electrocautery and/or incision may also be performed via the ureteroscope to open the narrowed area. In 52345, the ureteroscope is advanced into the upper ureter. The ureteropelvic junction is visualized. A guidewire is passed through the stricture at the ureteropelvic junction and the stricture is treated as described above. In 52346, the ureteroscope is passed further up into the renal pelvis; a guidewire is passed through the stricture; and the narrowing is treated as described above.

Cystourethroscopy with ureteroscopy, with treatment of stricture

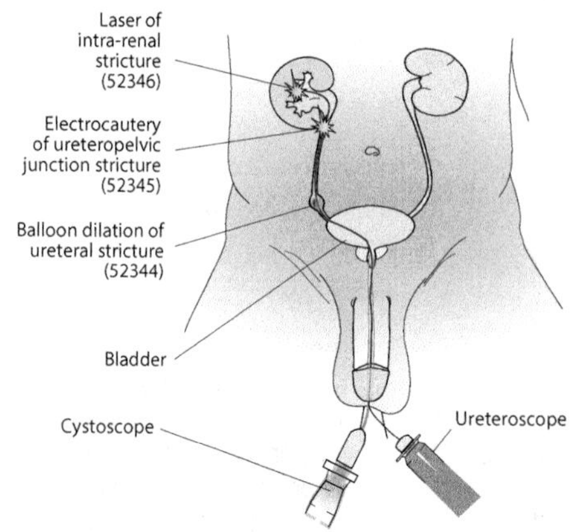

ICD-10-CM Diagnostic Codes

	A18.11	Tuberculosis of kidney and ureter
⇄	C66.1	Malignant neoplasm of right ureter
⇄	C66.2	Malignant neoplasm of left ureter
⇄	D30.21	Benign neoplasm of right ureter
⇄	D30.22	Benign neoplasm of left ureter
	N11.1	Chronic obstructive pyelonephritis
	N13.0	Hydronephrosis with ureteropelvic junction obstruction
	N13.1	Hydronephrosis with ureteral stricture, not elsewhere classified
	N13.2	Hydronephrosis with renal and ureteral calculous obstruction
	N13.5	Crossing vessel and stricture of ureter without hydronephrosis
	N13.6	Pyonephrosis
	N13.8	Other obstructive and reflux uropathy
	N20.1	Calculus of ureter
	N20.2	Calculus of kidney with calculus of ureter
	N28.82	Megaloureter
	N28.89	Other specified disorders of kidney and ureter
	N99.111	Postprocedural bulbous urethral stricture, male ♂
	N99.112	Postprocedural membranous urethral stricture, male ♂
	N99.113	Postprocedural anterior bulbous urethral stricture, male ♂
	Q62.11	Congenital occlusion of ureteropelvic junction
	Q62.12	Congenital occlusion of ureterovesical orifice

CCI Edits

Refer to Appendix A for CCI edits.

Pub 100

52344: Pub 100-03, 1, 140.5
52345: Pub 100-03, 1, 140.5
52346: Pub 100-03, 1, 140.5

Facility RVUs

Code	Work	PE Facility	MP	Total Facility
52344	7.05	2.81	0.85	10.71
52345	7.55	2.97	0.90	11.42
52346	8.58	3.34	1.00	12.92

Non-facility RVUs

Code	Work	PE Non-Facility	MP	Total Non-Facility
52344	7.05	2.81	0.85	10.71
52345	7.55	2.97	0.90	11.42
52346	8.58	3.34	1.00	12.92

Modifiers (PAR)

Code	Mod 50	Mod 51	Mod 62	Mod 66	Mod 80
52344	1	3	0	0	1
52345	1	3	0	0	0
52346	1	3	0	0	0

Global Period

Code	Days
52344	000
52345	000
52346	000

52351

52351 Cystourethroscopy, with ureteroscopy and/or pyeloscopy; diagnostic

(Do not report 52351 in conjunction with 52341, 52342, 52343, 52344, 52345, 52346, 52352-52356)

AMA Coding Guideline

Ureter and Pelvis Transurethral Surgical Procedures

Therapeutic cystourethroscopy always includes diagnostic cystourethroscopy. To report a diagnostic cystourethroscopy, use 52000. Therapeutic cystourethroscopy with ureteroscopy and/or pyeloscopy always includes diagnostic cystourethroscopy with ureteroscopy and/or pyeloscopy. To report a diagnostic cystourethroscopy with ureteroscopy and/or pyeloscopy, use 52351.

Do not report 52000 in conjunction with 52320-52343, 52356.

Do not report 52351 in conjunction with 52344-52346, 52352-52356.

The insertion and removal of a temporary ureteral catheter (52005) during diagnostic or therapeutic cystourethroscopy with ureteroscopy and/or pyeloscopy is included in 52320-52356 and should not be reported separately.

To report insertion of a self-retaining, indwelling stent performed during diagnostic or therapeutic cystourethroscopy with ureteroscopy and/or pyeloscopy, report 52332, in addition to primary procedure(s) performed (52320-52330, 52334-52352, 52354, 52355), and append modifier 51. Code 52332 is used to report a unilateral procedure unless otherwise specified.

For bilateral insertion of self-retaining, indwelling ureteral stents, use code 52332, and append modifier 50.

To report cystourethroscopic removal of a self-retaining, indwelling ureteral stent, see 52310, 52315, and append modifier 58, if appropriate.

AMA Coding Notes

Surgical Procedures on the Urinary System

(For provision of chemotherapeutic agents, report both the specific service in addition to code(s) for the specific substance(s) or drug(s) provided)

AMA *CPT® Assistant*

52351: Apr 01: 4, May 01: 5, Sep 01: 1, Oct 01: 8, May 14: 3

Plain English Description

The urethra is cleansed with antiseptic solution. A rigid or flexible cystoscope is introduced through the urethra into the bladder. The bladder may be filled with sterile saline to allow better visualization of the bladder wall. Following inspection of the bladder, a guidewire is introduced through the cystoscope and advanced into the first ureter and through the ureter to the renal pelvis. The cystoscope is removed. A ureteroscope is then advanced over the guidewire and into the renal pelvis. The guidewire is removed. The renal pelvis is inspected and any abnormalities are noted. The ureteroscope is slowly withdrawn and the entire length of the ureter is inspected. The diagnostic ureteroscopy and/or pyeloscopy is repeated on the opposite ureter as needed. Upon completion of the procedure, the ureteroscope is removed.

Cystourethroscopy with ureteroscopy and/or pyeloscopy; diagnostic

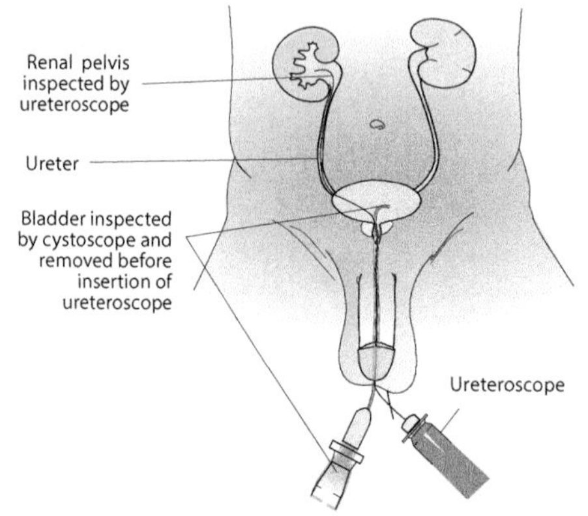

ICD-10-CM Diagnostic Codes

⇄	C65.1	Malignant neoplasm of right renal pelvis
⇄	C65.2	Malignant neoplasm of left renal pelvis
⇄	C66.1	Malignant neoplasm of right ureter
⇄	C66.2	Malignant neoplasm of left ureter
	C67.0	Malignant neoplasm of trigone of bladder
	C67.1	Malignant neoplasm of dome of bladder
	C67.2	Malignant neoplasm of lateral wall of bladder
	C67.3	Malignant neoplasm of anterior wall of bladder
	C67.4	Malignant neoplasm of posterior wall of bladder
	C67.5	Malignant neoplasm of bladder neck
	C67.6	Malignant neoplasm of ureteric orifice
	C67.7	Malignant neoplasm of urachus
	C67.8	Malignant neoplasm of overlapping sites of bladder
⇄	C79.01	Secondary malignant neoplasm of right kidney and renal pelvis
⇄	C79.02	Secondary malignant neoplasm of left kidney and renal pelvis
	C79.11	Secondary malignant neoplasm of bladder
	C79.19	Secondary malignant neoplasm of other urinary organs
	D09.0	Carcinoma in situ of bladder
	D09.19	Carcinoma in situ of other urinary organs
⇄	D30.11	Benign neoplasm of right renal pelvis
⇄	D30.12	Benign neoplasm of left renal pelvis
⇄	D30.21	Benign neoplasm of right ureter
⇄	D30.22	Benign neoplasm of left ureter
	D30.3	Benign neoplasm of bladder
⇄	D41.11	Neoplasm of uncertain behavior of right renal pelvis
⇄	D41.12	Neoplasm of uncertain behavior of left renal pelvis
⇄	D41.21	Neoplasm of uncertain behavior of right ureter
⇄	D41.22	Neoplasm of uncertain behavior of left ureter
	D49.1	Neoplasm of unspecified behavior of respiratory system
	D49.4	Neoplasm of unspecified behavior of bladder
	N11.0	Nonobstructive reflux-associated chronic pyelonephritis
	N11.1	Chronic obstructive pyelonephritis
	N11.8	Other chronic tubulo-interstitial nephritis
	N13.0	Hydronephrosis with ureteropelvic junction obstruction
	N13.1	Hydronephrosis with ureteral stricture, not elsewhere classified
	N13.2	Hydronephrosis with renal and ureteral calculous obstruction
	N13.39	Other hydronephrosis
	N13.4	Hydroureter
	N13.5	Crossing vessel and stricture of ureter without hydronephrosis
	N13.8	Other obstructive and reflux uropathy
	N20.0	Calculus of kidney
	N20.1	Calculus of ureter
	N20.2	Calculus of kidney with calculus of ureter
	N21.0	Calculus in bladder
	N22	Calculus of urinary tract in diseases classified elsewhere
	N28.82	Megaloureter
	N28.89	Other specified disorders of kidney and ureter
	N30.10	Interstitial cystitis (chronic) without hematuria
	N30.11	Interstitial cystitis (chronic) with hematuria
	N30.20	Other chronic cystitis without hematuria
	N30.21	Other chronic cystitis with hematuria
	N30.30	Trigonitis without hematuria
	N30.31	Trigonitis with hematuria
	N30.40	Irradiation cystitis without hematuria
	N30.41	Irradiation cystitis with hematuria
	N30.80	Other cystitis without hematuria
	N30.81	Other cystitis with hematuria
	N31.0	Uninhibited neuropathic bladder, not elsewhere classified
	N31.1	Reflex neuropathic bladder, not elsewhere classified
	N31.2	Flaccid neuropathic bladder, not elsewhere classified

N31.8	Other neuromuscular dysfunction of bladder
N32.0	Bladder-neck obstruction
N32.1	Vesicointestinal fistula
N32.2	Vesical fistula, not elsewhere classified
N32.3	Diverticulum of bladder
N32.81	Overactive bladder
N32.89	Other specified disorders of bladder
N33	Bladder disorders in diseases classified elsewhere
N39.0	Urinary tract infection, site not specified
N39.3	Stress incontinence (female) (male)
N39.41	Urge incontinence
N39.42	Incontinence without sensory awareness
N39.43	Post-void dribbling
N39.44	Nocturnal enuresis
N39.45	Continuous leakage
N39.46	Mixed incontinence
N39.490	Overflow incontinence
N39.491	Coital incontinence
N39.492	Postural (urinary) incontinence
N39.498	Other specified urinary incontinence
N39.8	Other specified disorders of urinary system
N82.0	Vesicovaginal fistula ♀
N82.1	Other female urinary-genital tract fistulae ♀
N99.111	Postprocedural bulbous urethral stricture, male ♂
N99.112	Postprocedural membranous urethral stricture, male ♂
N99.113	Postprocedural anterior bulbous urethral stricture, male ♂
Q62.0	Congenital hydronephrosis
Q62.11	Congenital occlusion of ureteropelvic junction
Q62.12	Congenital occlusion of ureterovesical orifice
Q62.2	Congenital megaureter
Q62.31	Congenital ureterocele, orthotopic
Q62.32	Cecoureterocele
Q62.39	Other obstructive defects of renal pelvis and ureter
Q64.11	Supravesical fissure of urinary bladder
Q64.12	Cloacal exstrophy of urinary bladder
Q64.19	Other exstrophy of urinary bladder
Q64.31	Congenital bladder neck obstruction
Q64.33	Congenital stricture of urinary meatus
Q64.39	Other atresia and stenosis of urethra and bladder neck
Q64.5	Congenital absence of bladder and urethra
Q64.6	Congenital diverticulum of bladder
Q64.72	Congenital prolapse of urinary meatus
Q64.73	Congenital urethrorectal fistula
Q64.79	Other congenital malformations of bladder and urethra

CCI Edits

Refer to Appendix A for CCI edits.

Facility RVUs ☐

Code	Work	PE Facility	MP	Total Facility
52351	5.75	2.33	0.68	8.76

Non-facility RVUs ☐

Code	Work	PE Non-Facility	MP	Total Non-Facility
52351	5.75	2.33	0.68	8.76

Modifiers (PAR) ☐

Code	Mod 50	Mod 51	Mod 62	Mod 66	Mod 80
52351	0	2	0	0	1

Global Period

Code	Days
52351	000

52352-52353

52352 Cystourethroscopy, with ureteroscopy and/or pyeloscopy; with removal or manipulation of calculus (ureteral catheterization is included)

52353 Cystourethroscopy, with ureteroscopy and/or pyeloscopy; with lithotripsy (ureteral catheterization is included)

(Do not report 52353 in conjunction with 52332, 52356 when performed together on the same side)

AMA Coding Guideline

Ureter and Pelvis Transurethral Surgical Procedures

Therapeutic cystourethroscopy always includes diagnostic cystourethroscopy. To report a diagnostic cystourethroscopy, use 52000. Therapeutic cystourethroscopy with ureteroscopy and/or pyeloscopy always includes diagnostic cystourethroscopy with ureteroscopy and/or pyeloscopy. To report a diagnostic cystourethroscopy with ureteroscopy and/or pyeloscopy, use 52351.

Do not report 52000 in conjunction with 52320-52343, 52356.

Do not report 52351 in conjunction with 52344-52346, 52352-52356.

The insertion and removal of a temporary ureteral catheter (52005) during diagnostic or therapeutic cystourethroscopy with ureteroscopy and/or pyeloscopy is included in 52320-52356 and should not be reported separately.

To report insertion of a self-retaining, indwelling stent performed during diagnostic or therapeutic cystourethroscopy with ureteroscopy and/or pyeloscopy, report 52332, in addition to primary procedure(s) performed (52320-52330, 52334-52352, 52354, 52355), and append modifier 51. Code 52332 is used to report a unilateral procedure unless otherwise specified.

For bilateral insertion of self-retaining, indwelling ureteral stents, use code 52332, and append modifier 50.

To report cystourethroscopic removal of a self-retaining, indwelling ureteral stent, see 52310, 52315, and append modifier 58, if appropriate.

AMA Coding Notes

Surgical Procedures on the Urinary System

(For provision of chemotherapeutic agents, report both the specific service in addition to code(s) for the specific substance(s) or drug(s) provided)

AMA *CPT® Assistant* ▢

52352: Apr 01: 4, May 01: 5, Sep 01: 1, Oct 01: 8, Jun 07: 10, Feb 10: 13, May 14: 3, Dec 19: 12

52353: Apr 01: 4, May 01: 5, Sep 01: 1, Oct 01: 8, Dec 07: 13, Apr 09: 8, May 14: 3, Dec 19: 12

Plain English Description

The urethra is cleansed with antiseptic solution. A rigid or flexible cystoscope is introduced through the urethra into the bladder. The bladder may be filled with sterile saline to allow better visualization of the bladder wall. Following inspection of the bladder, the ureters are catheterized. A guidewire is introduced through the cystoscope and advanced into the ureter and through the ureter to the site of the calculus within the ureter or renal pelvis. The cystoscope is removed. A ureteroscope is then advanced over the guidewire to the site of the calculus.
In 52352, the calculus is manipulated or removed. A grasping or retrieval device is advanced through the cystoscope over the guidewire to the calculus, which is captured and extracted. Alternatively, the calculus may be grasped and manipulated into a different location without removal. In 52353, the calculus is fragmented with lithotripsy, using an ultrasonic or electrohydraulic technique. The ultrasonic or electrohydraulic probe is advanced through the ureteroscope to the ureter. The probe is activated and shock waves are generated, causing fragmentation of the calculus. Following retrieval, manipulation, or fragmentation of the calculus, a catheter may be advanced over the guidewire to the renal pelvis and the ureter may be irrigated to remove the calculus fragments. Diagnostic or therapeutic solution may also be instilled into the ureter through the catheter. The ureteroscope may be advanced into the renal pelvis and the renal pelvis and ureter examined again as the ureteroscope is slowly withdrawn.

Cystourethroscopy with ureteroscopy and/or pyeloscopy

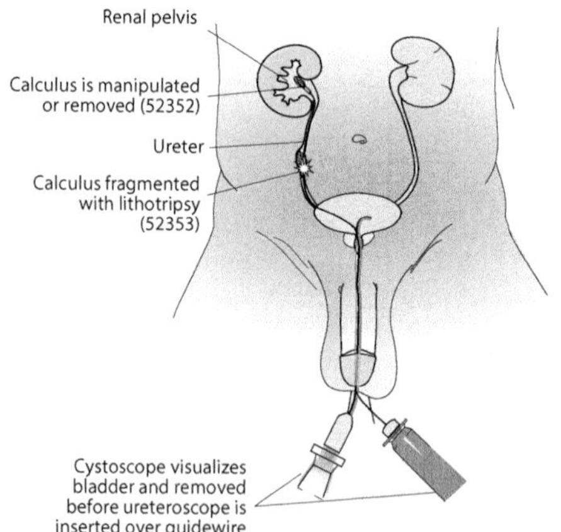

ICD-10-CM Diagnostic Codes

N13.0	Hydronephrosis with ureteropelvic junction obstruction
N13.2	Hydronephrosis with renal and ureteral calculous obstruction
N20.0	Calculus of kidney
N20.1	Calculus of ureter
N20.2	Calculus of kidney with calculus of ureter
N21.0	Calculus in bladder
N21.1	Calculus in urethra
N21.8	Other lower urinary tract calculus

CCI Edits

Refer to Appendix A for CCI edits.

Pub 100

52352: Pub 100-03, 1, 230.1
52353: Pub 100-03, 1, 230.1

Facility RVUs ▢

Code	Work	PE Facility	MP	Total Facility
52352	6.75	2.71	0.79	10.25
52353	7.50	2.96	0.90	11.36

Non-facility RVUs ▢

Code	Work	PE Non-Facility	MP	Total Non-Facility
52352	6.75	2.71	0.79	10.25
52353	7.50	2.96	0.90	11.36

Modifiers (PAR) ▢

Code	Mod 50	Mod 51	Mod 62	Mod 66	Mod 80
52352	1	3	0	0	1
52353	1	3	0	0	1

Global Period

Code	Days
52352	000
52353	000

52354-52355

52354 Cystourethroscopy, with ureteroscopy and/or pyeloscopy; with biopsy and/or fulguration of ureteral or renal pelvic lesion

(For image-guided biopsy of ureter and/or renal pelvis without endoscopic guidance, use 50606)

52355 Cystourethroscopy, with ureteroscopy and/or pyeloscopy; with resection of ureteral or renal pelvic tumor

AMA Coding Guideline

Ureter and Pelvis Transurethral Surgical Procedures

Therapeutic cystourethroscopy always includes diagnostic cystourethroscopy. To report a diagnostic cystourethroscopy, use 52000. Therapeutic cystourethroscopy with ureteroscopy and/or pyeloscopy always includes diagnostic cystourethroscopy with ureteroscopy and/or pyeloscopy. To report a diagnostic cystourethroscopy with ureteroscopy and/or pyeloscopy, use 52351.

Do not report 52000 in conjunction with 52320-52343, 52356.

Do not report 52351 in conjunction with 52344-52346, 52352-52356.

The insertion and removal of a temporary ureteral catheter (52005) during diagnostic or therapeutic cystourethroscopy with ureteroscopy and/or pyeloscopy is included in 52320-52356 and should not be reported separately.

To report insertion of a self-retaining, indwelling stent performed during diagnostic or therapeutic cystourethroscopy with ureteroscopy and/or pyeloscopy, report 52332, in addition to primary procedure(s) performed (52320-52330, 52334-52352, 52354, 52355), and append modifier 51. Code 52332 is used to report a unilateral procedure unless otherwise specified.

For bilateral insertion of self-retaining, indwelling ureteral stents, use code 52332, and append modifier 50.

To report cystourethroscopic removal of a self-retaining, indwelling ureteral stent, see 52310, 52315, and append modifier 58, if appropriate.

AMA Coding Notes

Surgical Procedures on the Urinary System

(For provision of chemotherapeutic agents, report both the specific service in addition to code(s) for the specific substance(s) or drug(s) provided)

AMA *CPT® Assistant* □

52354: Apr 01: 4, May 01: 5, Sep 01: 1, Oct 01: 8, May 14: 3

52355: Apr 01: 4, May 01: 5, Sep 01: 1, Oct 01: 8, Jan 03: 21, May 14: 3

Plain English Description

The urethra is cleansed with antiseptic solution. A rigid or flexible cystoscope is introduced through the urethra into the bladder. The bladder may be filled with sterile saline to allow better visualization of the bladder wall. Following inspection of the bladder, the ureters are catheterized. A guidewire is introduced through the cystoscope and advanced into the ureter or renal pelvis to the site of the lesion or abnormal tissue. The cystoscope is removed. A ureteroscope is then advanced over the guidewire to the site of the tumor or lesion. In 52354, biopsy forceps are introduced through the ureteroscope and tissue samples are obtained. The renal pelvis and/or ureter are re-inspected following biopsy and any bleeding is controlled. Alternatively, an electrocautery device, laser, or cryoprobe is advanced through the ureteroscope to the site of the lesion. The device is activated and the abnormal tissue is destroyed by fulguration. In 52355, the renal pelvis and/or ureteral tumor is located and a resectoscope is advanced to the site of the tumor, which is then resected. The tumor is removed using irrigation and an endoscopic evacuation device. Bleeding is controlled as needed using electrocoagulation or laser coagulation. Following biopsy, fulguration, or tumor resection, a catheter may be advanced over the guidewire to the renal pelvis and the ureter and renal pelvis may be irrigated. Diagnostic or therapeutic solution may also be instilled through the catheter. The ureteroscope may be advanced into the renal pelvis and the renal pelvis and ureter examined as the ureteroscope is slowly withdrawn.

Cystourethroscopy, with ureteroscopy and/or pyeloscopy

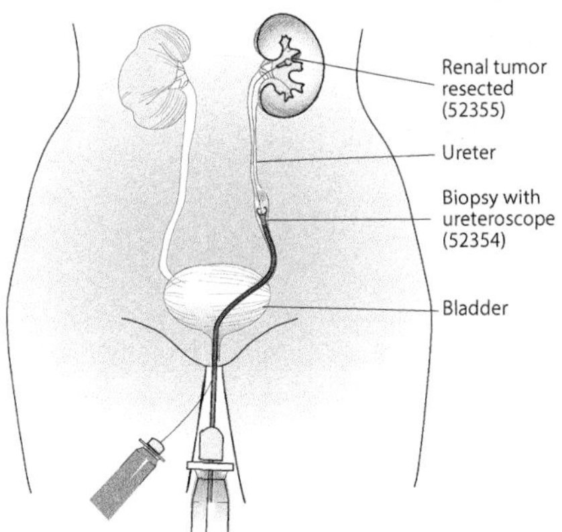

The cystoscope visualizes the bladder and is removed before a ureteroscope is inserted over a guidewire.

ICD-10-CM Diagnostic Codes

There are too many ICD-10-CM codes to list. Refer to ICD-10-CM code book for associated diagnostic codes.

CCI Edits

Refer to Appendix A for CCI edits.

Facility RVUs □

Code	Work	PE Facility	MP	Total Facility
52354	8.00	3.13	0.95	12.08
52355	9.00	3.46	1.06	13.52

Non-facility RVUs □

Code	Work	PE Non-Facility	MP	Total Non-Facility
52354	8.00	3.13	0.95	12.08
52355	9.00	3.46	1.06	13.52

Modifiers (PAR) □

Code	Mod 50	Mod 51	Mod 62	Mod 66	Mod 80
52354	1	3	0	0	1
52355	1	3	0	0	1

Global Period

Code	Days
52354	000
52355	000

52356

52356 Cystourethroscopy, with ureteroscopy and/or pyeloscopy; with lithotripsy including insertion of indwelling ureteral stent (eg, Gibbons or double-J type)

(Do not report 52356 in conjunction with 52332, 52353 when performed together on the same side)

AMA Coding Guideline

Ureter and Pelvis Transurethral Surgical Procedures

Therapeutic cystourethroscopy always includes diagnostic cystourethroscopy. To report a diagnostic cystourethroscopy, use 52000. Therapeutic cystourethroscopy with ureteroscopy and/or pyeloscopy always includes diagnostic cystourethroscopy with ureteroscopy and/or pyeloscopy. To report a diagnostic cystourethroscopy with ureteroscopy and/or pyeloscopy, use 52351.

Do not report 52000 in conjunction with 52320-52343, 52356.

Do not report 52351 in conjunction with 52344-52346, 52352-52356.

The insertion and removal of a temporary ureteral catheter (52005) during diagnostic or therapeutic cystourethroscopy with ureteroscopy and/or pyeloscopy is included in 52320-52356 and should not be reported separately.

To report insertion of a self-retaining, indwelling stent performed during diagnostic or therapeutic cystourethroscopy with ureteroscopy and/or pyeloscopy, report 52332, in addition to primary procedure(s) performed (52320-52330, 52334-52352, 52354, 52355), and append modifier 51. Code 52332 is used to report a unilateral procedure unless otherwise specified.

For bilateral insertion of self-retaining, indwelling ureteral stents, use code 52332, and append modifier 50.

To report cystourethroscopic removal of a self-retaining, indwelling ureteral stent, see 52310, 52315, and append modifier 58, if appropriate.

AMA Coding Notes

Surgical Procedures on the Urinary System

(For provision of chemotherapeutic agents, report both the specific service in addition to code(s) for the specific substance(s) or drug(s) provided)

AMA *CPT® Assistant* ▢

52356: May 14: 3, Dec 19: 12

Plain English Description

The urethra is cleansed with antiseptic solution. A rigid or flexible cystoscope is introduced through the urethra and into the bladder. The bladder may be filled with sterile saline to allow better visualization of the bladder wall. Following inspection of the bladder, the ureters are catheterized. A guidewire is introduced through the cystoscope and advanced into and through the ureter to the site of the calculus in the ureter or renal pelvis. A ureteroscope is then advanced over the guidewire to the site of the calculus, which is fragmented using lithotripsy by either ultrasonic or electrohydraulic technique. The ultrasonic or electrohydraulic probe is advanced through the ureteroscope to the calculus. The probe is activated and shock waves are generated to fragment the calculus. The probe is withdrawn and a catheter is advanced over the guidewire. The ureter and/or renal pelvis are irrigated to help flush out the calculus fragments. The catheter is removed and the ureteroscope is again advanced through the ureter to the renal pelvis. The renal pelvis and ureter are examined prior to stent placement as the ureteroscope is slowly withdrawn. A stent is advanced over the guidewire and positioned in the ureter. The guidewire is removed, leaving the stent in place. The bladder is inspected again using the cystoscope and the position of the distal tail of the stent in the bladder is noted. Upon completion of the procedure, the cystoscope is removed.

ICD-10-CM Diagnostic Codes

N13.2	Hydronephrosis with renal and ureteral calculous obstruction
N20.0	Calculus of kidney
N20.1	Calculus of ureter
N20.2	Calculus of kidney with calculus of ureter
N21.0	Calculus in bladder
N21.1	Calculus in urethra
N21.8	Other lower urinary tract calculus

CCI Edits

Refer to Appendix A for CCI edits.

Pub 100

52356: Pub 100-03, 1, 230.1

Facility RVUs ▢

Code	Work	PE Facility	MP	Total Facility
52356	8.00	3.09	0.95	12.04

Non-facility RVUs ▢

Code	Work	PE Non-Facility	MP	Total Non-Facility
52356	8.00	3.09	0.95	12.04

Modifiers (PAR) ▢

Code	Mod 50	Mod 51	Mod 62	Mod 66	Mod 80
52356	1	3	0	0	1

Global Period

Code	Days
52356	000

52400

52400 Cystourethroscopy with incision, fulguration, or resection of congenital posterior urethral valves, or congenital obstructive hypertrophic mucosal folds

AMA Coding Notes

Surgical Procedures on the Urinary System

(For provision of chemotherapeutic agents, report both the specific service in addition to code(s) for the specific substance(s) or drug(s) provided)

AMA *CPT® Assistant*

52400: Apr 01: 4

Plain English Description

Cystourethroscopy is performed with incision, fulguration, or resection of posterior urethral valves or obstructive hypertrophic mucosal folds. Both posterior urethral valves and obstructive hypertrophic mucosal folds are congenital anomalies of the urethra characterized by an obstructing membrane in the posterior segment of the male urethra causing bladder outlet obstruction. A cystourethroscope is inserted into the urethra and advanced into the bladder. The valves or mucosal folds are then incised, ablated (fulgurated), or resected through the cystourethroscope using cold knife, electrocautery, or laser energy.

Cystourethroscopy with incision, fulguration, or resection

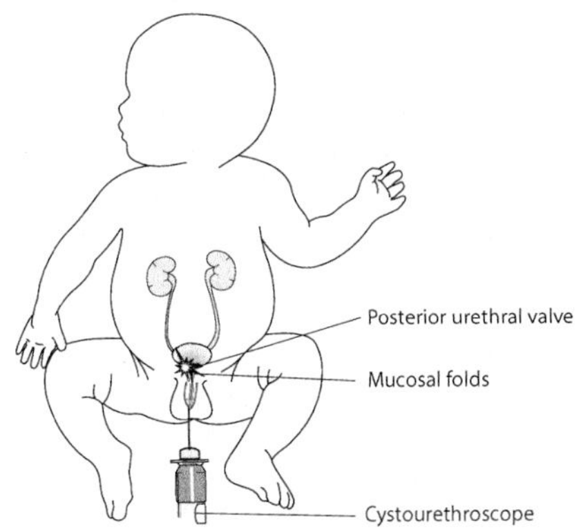

ICD-10-CM Diagnostic Codes

N32.89	Other specified disorders of bladder
N33	Bladder disorders in diseases classified elsewhere
Q64.11	Supravesical fissure of urinary bladder
Q64.2	Congenital posterior urethral valves
Q64.31	Congenital bladder neck obstruction
Q64.32	Congenital stricture of urethra
Q64.39	Other atresia and stenosis of urethra and bladder neck
Q64.6	Congenital diverticulum of bladder
Q64.71	Congenital prolapse of urethra
Q64.79	Other congenital malformations of bladder and urethra

CCI Edits

Refer to Appendix A for CCI edits.

Facility RVUs

Code	Work	PE Facility	MP	Total Facility
52400	8.69	4.20	1.04	13.93

Non-facility RVUs

Code	Work	PE Non-Facility	MP	Total Non-Facility
52400	8.69	4.20	1.04	13.93

Modifiers (PAR)

Code	Mod 50	Mod 51	Mod 62	Mod 66	Mod 80
52400	0	3	0	0	1

Global Period

Code	Days
52400	090

52402

52402 Cystourethroscopy with transurethral resection or incision of ejaculatory ducts

AMA Coding Notes

Surgical Procedures on the Urinary System

(For provision of chemotherapeutic agents, report both the specific service in addition to code(s) for the specific substance(s) or drug(s) provided)

Plain English Description

The physician performs a cystourethroscopy with transurethral resection or incision of ejaculatory ducts to treat an obstruction caused by scar tissue, prostatic cysts, or stones. This procedure may also be referred to as a TURED (transurethral resection of ejaculatory ducts), TUIED (transurethral incision of ejaculatory ducts), or a resection of the verumontanum. The verumontanum is a small protuberance in the distal end of the prostatic urethra where the ejaculatory ducts enter the urethra. A cystourethroscope is inserted into the urethra and the urethra and bladder are examined endoscopically with careful attention to the region of the prostatic urethra and the ejaculatory duct orifices at the verumontanum. A resectoscope is then inserted and a hook electrode is used to incise one or both ejaculatory ducts. Alternatively, a loop electrode may be used to perform a resection of the verumontanum. This may require several passes of the cutting loop. Adequate incision or resection of the ejaculatory ducts is verified endoscopically by visualization of fluid refluxing from the opened ducts. Bleeding is controlled by cauterization of blood vessels, taking care to avoid damage to the duct openings. The surgical instruments are then removed along with the cystourethroscope and a Foley catheter is placed in the bladder for 24-48 hours.

Cystourethroscopy with transurethral resection or incision of ejaculatory ducts

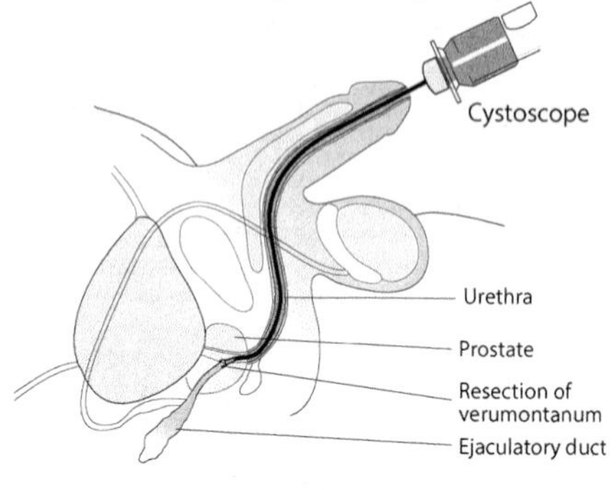

ICD-10-CM Diagnostic Codes

⇄ C63.11 Malignant neoplasm of right spermatic cord ♂
⇄ C63.12 Malignant neoplasm of left spermatic cord ♂
C63.7 Malignant neoplasm of other specified male genital organs ♂
C79.82 Secondary malignant neoplasm of genital organs
D07.69 Carcinoma in situ of other male genital organs ♂
D17.6 Benign lipomatous neoplasm of spermatic cord ♂
D29.8 Benign neoplasm of other specified male genital organs ♂
D30.4 Benign neoplasm of urethra
D40.8 Neoplasm of uncertain behavior of other specified male genital organs ♂
N35.111 Postinfective urethral stricture, not elsewhere classified, male, meatal ♂
N40.0 Benign prostatic hyperplasia without lower urinary tract symptoms ♂
N40.1 Benign prostatic hyperplasia with lower urinary tract symptoms ♂
N43.41 Spermatocele of epididymis, single ♂
N43.42 Spermatocele of epididymis, multiple ♂
N44.01 Extravaginal torsion of spermatic cord ♂
N44.02 Intravaginal torsion of spermatic cord ♂
N50.3 Cyst of epididymis ♂
N50.89 Other specified disorders of the male genital organs ♂
N51 Disorders of male genital organs in diseases classified elsewhere ♂
N53.12 Painful ejaculation ♂
N53.14 Retrograde ejaculation ♂
P83.81 Umbilical granuloma
Q53.111 Unilateral intraabdominal testis ♂
Q53.112 Unilateral inguinal testis ♂
Q53.13 Unilateral high scrotal testis ♂
Q53.211 Bilateral intraabdominal testes ♂
Q53.212 Bilateral inguinal testes ♂
Q53.23 Bilateral high scrotal testes ♂
Q55.4 Other congenital malformations of vas deferens, epididymis, seminal vesicles and prostate ♂
R33.9 Retention of urine, unspecified
R36.1 Hematospermia ♂
R39.83 Unilateral non-palpable testicle ♂
R39.84 Bilateral non-palpable testicles ♂

CCI Edits

Refer to Appendix A for CCI edits.

Pub 100

52402: Pub 100-03, 1, 230.3

Facility RVUs ▢

Code	Work	PE Facility	MP	Total Facility
52402	5.27	1.82	0.62	7.71

Non-facility RVUs ▢

Code	Work	PE Non-Facility	MP	Total Non-Facility
52402	5.27	1.82	0.62	7.71

Modifiers (PAR) ▢

Code	Mod 50	Mod 51	Mod 62	Mod 66	Mod 80
52402	0	3	0	0	1

Global Period

Code	Days
52402	000

52441-52442

52441 Cystourethroscopy, with insertion of permanent adjustable transprostatic implant; single implant

+ 52442 Cystourethroscopy, with insertion of permanent adjustable transprostatic implant; each additional permanent adjustable transprostatic implant (List separately in addition to code for primary procedure)

(Use 52442 in conjunction with 52441)

(To report removal of implant[s], use 52310)

(For insertion of a permanent urethral stent, use 52282. For insertion of a temporary prostatic urethral stent, use 53855)

AMA Coding Notes

Surgical Procedures on the Urinary System

(For provision of chemotherapeutic agents, report both the specific service in addition to code(s) for the specific substance(s) or drug(s) provided)

AMA *CPT® Assistant*

52441: Jun 15: 5

52442: Jun 15: 5

Plain English Description

A permanent adjustable transprostatic implant is inserted via cystourethroscopy to retract obstructing lateral lobes of an enlarged prostate and expand the urethral lumen. This minimally invasive procedure can provide rapid relief of lower urinary symptoms associated with benign prostatic hypertrophy. A rigid cystoscope is inserted into the urethra and, under visualization, the implant delivery device is advanced into the sheath and angled anterolaterally to compress the obstructive lobe. A needle loaded with a monofilament and metallic tab is deployed through the prostate lobe and the needle is retracted, leaving the tab engaged and the monofilament tensioned. The implant is delivered by attaching the urethral end-piece to the monofilament, which is then cut. The urethral end-piece invaginates into the urethral wall, causing focal injury and epithelialization. Code 52441 is reported for a single implant and code 52442 is reported for each additional implant.

ICD-10-CM Diagnostic Codes

C61	Malignant neoplasm of prostate ♂
C63.8	Malignant neoplasm of overlapping sites of male genital organs ♂
C79.82	Secondary malignant neoplasm of genital organs
D07.5	Carcinoma in situ of prostate ♂
D29.1	Benign neoplasm of prostate ♂
D29.8	Benign neoplasm of other specified male genital organs ♂
D40.0	Neoplasm of uncertain behavior of prostate ♂
D40.8	Neoplasm of uncertain behavior of other specified male genital organs ♂
N32.0	Bladder-neck obstruction
N40.0	Benign prostatic hyperplasia without lower urinary tract symptoms ♂
N40.1	Benign prostatic hyperplasia with lower urinary tract symptoms ♂
N40.2	Nodular prostate without lower urinary tract symptoms ♂
N40.3	Nodular prostate with lower urinary tract symptoms ♂
N41.2	Abscess of prostate ♂
N41.3	Prostatocystitis ♂
N41.4	Granulomatous prostatitis ♂
N41.8	Other inflammatory diseases of prostate ♂
N42.83	Cyst of prostate ♂
N42.89	Other specified disorders of prostate ♂
R33.8	Other retention of urine
R39.14	Feeling of incomplete bladder emptying

CCI Edits

Refer to Appendix A for CCI edits.

Facility RVUs

Code	Work	PE Facility	MP	Total Facility
52441	4.00	1.61	0.47	6.08
52442	1.01	0.34	0.11	1.46

Non-facility RVUs

Code	Work	PE Non-Facility	MP	Total Non-Facility
52441	4.00	34.78	0.47	39.25
52442	1.01	25.86	0.11	26.98

Modifiers (PAR)

Code	Mod 50	Mod 51	Mod 62	Mod 66	Mod 80
52441	0	3	0	0	1
52442	0	0	0	0	1

Global Period

Code	Days
52441	000
52442	ZZZ

52450

52450 Transurethral incision of prostate

AMA Coding Notes

Surgical Procedures on the Urinary System

(For provision of chemotherapeutic agents, report both the specific service in addition to code(s) for the specific substance(s) or drug(s) provided)

AMA *CPT® Assistant*

52450: Apr 01: 4, Jul 05: 15, Jun 15: 5

Plain English Description

The physician performs a transurethral incision of the prostate (TUIP). An incision is made through the urethra using electrocautery or a laser beam at the site where the prostate meets the bladder. The incision is carried down through the muscle tissue and into the prostate where one or two small incisions or grooves are made in the prostate. No tissue is removed. This is performed to release the tension on the urethra, allowing urine to flow out of the bladder more easily.

Cystourethroscopy with fulguration

ICD-10-CM Diagnostic Codes

N40.0	Benign prostatic hyperplasia without lower urinary tract symptoms ♂
N40.1	Benign prostatic hyperplasia with lower urinary tract symptoms ♂
N40.2	Nodular prostate without lower urinary tract symptoms ♂
N40.3	Nodular prostate with lower urinary tract symptoms ♂
N42.30	Unspecified dysplasia of prostate ♂
N42.31	Prostatic intraepithelial neoplasia ♂
N42.32	Atypical small acinar proliferation of prostate ♂
N42.39	Other dysplasia of prostate ♂
N42.89	Other specified disorders of prostate ♂
R33.8	Other retention of urine
R39.14	Feeling of incomplete bladder emptying

CCI Edits

Refer to Appendix A for CCI edits.

Facility RVUs

Code	Work	PE Facility	MP	Total Facility
52450	7.78	5.17	0.94	13.89

Non-facility RVUs

Code	Work	PE Non-Facility	MP	Total Non-Facility
52450	7.78	5.17	0.94	13.89

Modifiers (PAR)

Code	Mod 50	Mod 51	Mod 62	Mod 66	Mod 80
52450	0	2	0	0	1

Global Period

Code	Days
52450	090

52500

52500 Transurethral resection of bladder neck (separate procedure)

AMA Coding Notes

Surgical Procedures on the Urinary System

(For provision of chemotherapeutic agents, report both the specific service in addition to code(s) for the specific substance(s) or drug(s) provided)

AMA *CPT® Assistant*

52500: Apr 01: 4, Jan 04: 27, Jul 05: 15, May 09: 8

Plain English Description

The physician performs transurethral resection of the bladder neck. A cystourethroscope is inserted into the urethra and the urethra and bladder are examined endoscopically with careful attention to the region of the prostatic urethra and bladder neck. Meatotomy or urethrotomy are performed as needed prior to insertion of the resectoscope. An irrigating resectoscope is then introduced and the prostate is resected at 4 and 8 o'clock to the level of the prostate capsule. The prostate is incised using a diathermy loop and the incision is carried down to the level of the extracapsular fat. The incision is then extended from the verumontanum to the level immediately below the bladder trigone. Bleeding is controlled, surgical instruments and the cystourethroscope are removed, and the resected prostate chips are submitted for pathological examination.

Transurethral resection of bladder neck (separate procedure)

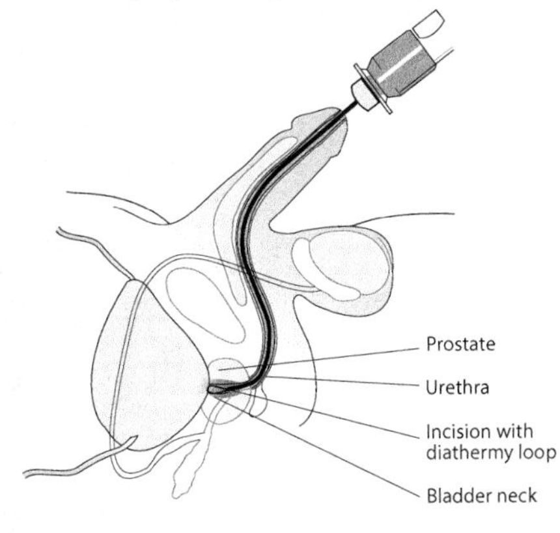

ICD-10-CM Diagnostic Codes

C67.5	Malignant neoplasm of bladder neck
C79.11	Secondary malignant neoplasm of bladder
D09.0	Carcinoma in situ of bladder
D30.3	Benign neoplasm of bladder
D30.8	Benign neoplasm of other specified urinary organs
D41.4	Neoplasm of uncertain behavior of bladder
D49.4	Neoplasm of unspecified behavior of bladder
N21.0	Calculus in bladder
N31.0	Uninhibited neuropathic bladder, not elsewhere classified
N31.1	Reflex neuropathic bladder, not elsewhere classified
N31.9	Neuromuscular dysfunction of bladder, unspecified
N32.0	Bladder-neck obstruction
N32.89	Other specified disorders of bladder
N33	Bladder disorders in diseases classified elsewhere
N36.2	Urethral caruncle
N36.8	Other specified disorders of urethra
N40.0	Benign prostatic hyperplasia without lower urinary tract symptoms ♂
N40.1	Benign prostatic hyperplasia with lower urinary tract symptoms ♂
N40.2	Nodular prostate without lower urinary tract symptoms ♂
N40.3	Nodular prostate with lower urinary tract symptoms ♂
R30.9	Painful micturition, unspecified
R33.9	Retention of urine, unspecified
R39.12	Poor urinary stream
R39.14	Feeling of incomplete bladder emptying
R39.16	Straining to void
R39.192	Position dependent micturition
R39.198	Other difficulties with micturition
Z85.51	Personal history of malignant neoplasm of bladder

CCI Edits

Refer to Appendix A for CCI edits.

Facility RVUs

Code	Work	PE Facility	MP	Total Facility
52500	8.14	5.29	0.96	14.39

Non-facility RVUs

Code	Work	PE Non-Facility	MP	Total Non-Facility
52500	8.14	5.29	0.96	14.39

Modifiers (PAR)

Code	Mod 50	Mod 51	Mod 62	Mod 66	Mod 80
52500	0	2	0	0	1

Global Period

Code	Days
52500	090

52601

52601 Transurethral electrosurgical resection of prostate, including control of postoperative bleeding, complete (vasectomy, meatotomy, cystourethroscopy, urethral calibration and/or dilation, and internal urethrotomy are included)

(For transurethral waterjet ablation of prostate, use 0421T)

(For other approaches, see 55801-55845)

AMA Coding Notes

Surgical Procedures on the Urinary System

(For provision of chemotherapeutic agents, report both the specific service in addition to code(s) for the specific substance(s) or drug(s) provided)

AMA *CPT® Assistant*

52601: Nov 97: 20, Apr 01: 4, Jun 03: 6, Oct 11: 10, Jun 15: 5

Plain English Description

The physician performs a complete transurethral electrosurgical resection of the prostate (TURP). The following procedures may also be performed and are included: vasectomy, meatotomy, cystourethroscopy, urethral calibration, urethral dilation, internal urethrotomy, and control of postoperative bleeding. A cystourethroscope is inserted into the urethra and the urethra and bladder are examined endoscopically, with careful attention to the region of the prostatic urethra and prostate. The physician may need to incise the urethral meatus (meatotomy), dilate and/or calibrate the urethra, or incise the internal urethra (internal urethrotomy) for better surgical access prior to insertion of the resectoscope. An irrigating resectoscope is introduced and the prostate is completely resected using an electrical loop that simultaneously cuts or vaporizes the obstructive tissue and cauterizes the blood vessels. The prostate is irrigated and the chips of prostate tissue are flushed from the prostate and into the bladder. A vasectomy may also be performed by resecting the vas deferens along with the prostate. Following completion of the procedure, the irrigation fluid, prostatic tissue, and surgical debris are flushed from the bladder. Bleeding is controlled, surgical instruments and cystourethroscope are removed, and the resected prostate chips are submitted for pathological examination. Postoperative bleeding is monitored and any excessive bleeding may require a return to the operating room for cystourethroscopy and cauterization of blood vessels.

Transurethral electrosurgical resection of prostate (TURP)

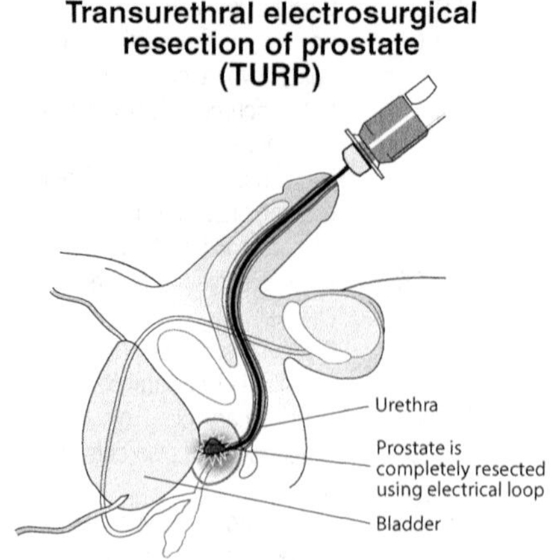

Urethra
Prostate is completely resected using electrical loop
Bladder

ICD-10-CM Diagnostic Codes

C61	Malignant neoplasm of prostate ♂
D07.5	Carcinoma in situ of prostate ♂
D29.1	Benign neoplasm of prostate ♂
D40.0	Neoplasm of uncertain behavior of prostate ♂
N40.0	Benign prostatic hyperplasia without lower urinary tract symptoms ♂
N40.1	Benign prostatic hyperplasia with lower urinary tract symptoms ♂
N40.2	Nodular prostate without lower urinary tract symptoms ♂
N40.3	Nodular prostate with lower urinary tract symptoms ♂
N42.0	Calculus of prostate ♂
N42.30	Unspecified dysplasia of prostate ♂
N42.31	Prostatic intraepithelial neoplasia ♂
N42.32	Atypical small acinar proliferation of prostate ♂
N42.39	Other dysplasia of prostate ♂
N42.89	Other specified disorders of prostate ♂
R33.9	Retention of urine, unspecified

CCI Edits

Refer to Appendix A for CCI edits.

Pub 100

52601: Pub 100-03, 1, 230.3

Facility RVUs

Code	Work	PE Facility	MP	Total Facility
52601	13.16	6.58	1.55	21.29

Non-facility RVUs

Code	Work	PE Non-Facility	MP	Total Non-Facility
52601	13.16	6.58	1.55	21.29

Modifiers (PAR)

Code	Mod 50	Mod 51	Mod 62	Mod 66	Mod 80
52601	0	2	0	0	1

Global Period

Code	Days
52601	090

52630

52630 Transurethral resection; residual or regrowth of obstructive prostate tissue including control of postoperative bleeding, complete (vasectomy, meatotomy, cystourethroscopy, urethral calibration and/or dilation, and internal urethrotomy are included)

(For resection of residual prostate tissue performed within the postoperative period of a related procedure performed by the same physician, append modifier 78)

(For transurethral waterjet ablation of prostate, use 0421T)

Transurethral resection; residual or regrowth of obstructive prostate tissue

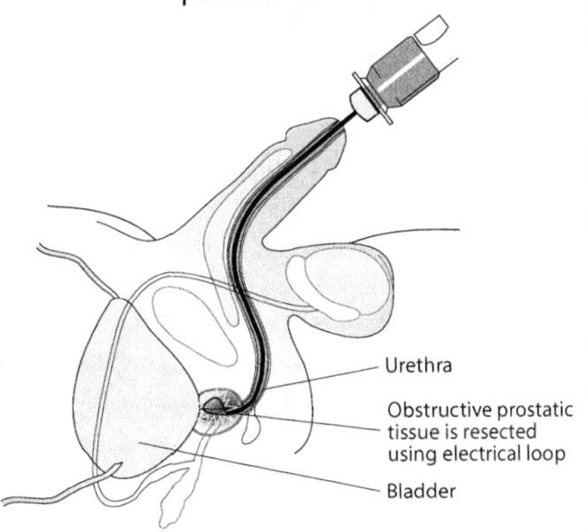
Urethra
Obstructive prostatic tissue is resected using electrical loop
Bladder

AMA Coding Notes

Surgical Procedures on the Urinary System

(For provision of chemotherapeutic agents, report both the specific service in addition to code(s) for the specific substance(s) or drug(s) provided)

AMA *CPT® Assistant* ▢

52630: Apr 01: 4

Plain English Description

The physician performs a transurethral resection of residual obstructive tissue or regrowth following a previous resection of the prostate. A cystourethroscope is inserted into the urethra, and the urethra and bladder are examined endoscopically with careful attention to the region of the prostatic urethra and prostate. The physician may need to incise the urethral meatus (meatotomy), dilate and/or calibrate the urethra, and incise the internal urethra (internal urethrotomy) for better surgical access prior to insertion of the resectoscope. An irrigating resectoscope is introduced, and the obstructive regrowth of prostatic tissue is resected using an electrical loop that simultaneously cuts or vaporizes the obstructive tissue and cauterizes the blood vessels. The prostate is irrigated and the chips of prostatic tissue are flushed from the prostate into the bladder. Following completion of the procedure, the irrigation fluid, prostatic tissue, and surgical debris are flushed from the bladder. Bleeding is controlled, surgical instruments and the cystourethroscope are removed, and the resected prostate chips are submitted for pathological examination.

ICD-10-CM Diagnostic Codes

C61	Malignant neoplasm of prostate ♂
D07.5	Carcinoma in situ of prostate ♂
D29.1	Benign neoplasm of prostate ♂
D40.0	Neoplasm of uncertain behavior of prostate ♂
N40.1	Benign prostatic hyperplasia with lower urinary tract symptoms ♂
N40.3	Nodular prostate with lower urinary tract symptoms ♂
N41.4	Granulomatous prostatitis ♂
N42.30	Unspecified dysplasia of prostate ♂
N42.31	Prostatic intraepithelial neoplasia ♂
N42.32	Atypical small acinar proliferation of prostate ♂
N42.39	Other dysplasia of prostate ♂
N42.83	Cyst of prostate ♂
N99.112	Postprocedural membranous urethral stricture, male ♂

CCI Edits

Refer to Appendix A for CCI edits.

Pub 100

52630: Pub 100-03, 1, 230.3

Facility RVUs ▢

Code	Work	PE Facility	MP	Total Facility
52630	6.55	4.54	0.77	11.86

Non-facility RVUs ▢

Code	Work	PE Non-Facility	MP	Total Non-Facility
52630	6.55	4.54	0.77	11.86

Modifiers (PAR) ▢

Code	Mod 50	Mod 51	Mod 62	Mod 66	Mod 80
52630	0	2	0	0	1

Global Period

Code	Days
52630	090

52640

52640 Transurethral resection; of postoperative bladder neck contracture

AMA Coding Notes

Surgical Procedures on the Urinary System

(For provision of chemotherapeutic agents, report both the specific service in addition to code(s) for the specific substance(s) or drug(s) provided)

AMA *CPT® Assistant* ▢

52640: Apr 01: 4

Plain English Description

The physician performs transurethral resection of a postoperative contracture of the bladder neck. A cystourethroscope is inserted into the urethra and both the urethra and bladder are examined endoscopically with careful attention to the bladder neck regions. Meatotomy or urethrotomy are performed as needed prior to insertion of the resectoscope. An irrigating resectoscope is then introduced into the bladder neck region and scar tissue is incised and resected. Bleeding is controlled and the surgical instruments and cystourethroscope are removed.

Transurethral resection of postoperative bladder neck contracture

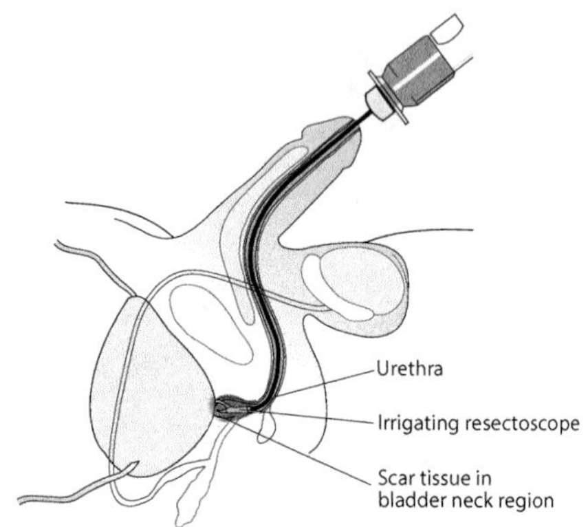

ICD-10-CM Diagnostic Codes

N32.0 Bladder-neck obstruction

CCI Edits

Refer to Appendix A for CCI edits.

Facility RVUs ▢

Code	Work	PE Facility	MP	Total Facility
52640	4.79	4.05	0.57	9.41

Non-facility RVUs ▢

Code	Work	PE Non-Facility	MP	Total Non-Facility
52640	4.79	4.05	0.57	9.41

Modifiers (PAR) ▢

Code	Mod 50	Mod 51	Mod 62	Mod 66	Mod 80
52640	0	2	0	0	1

Global Period

Code	Days
52640	090

52647

52647 Laser coagulation of prostate, including control of postoperative bleeding, complete (vasectomy, meatotomy, cystourethroscopy, urethral calibration and/or dilation, and internal urethrotomy are included if performed)

AMA Coding Notes

Surgical Procedures on the Urinary System

(For provision of chemotherapeutic agents, report both the specific service in addition to code(s) for the specific substance(s) or drug(s) provided)

AMA *CPT® Assistant* ▢

52647: Nov 97: 20, Mar 98: 11, Apr 01: 4, Nov 06: 21

Plain English Description

A complete laser coagulation of the prostate is performed including control of postoperative bleeding. This procedure is also referred to as transurethral ultrasound-guided laser prostatectomy (TULIP) using a free fiber or free-fiber visually guided laser ablation of the prostate (VLAP). TULIP and VLAP result in gradual sloughing of necrotic prostate tissue. The following procedures may also be performed and are included: vasectomy, meatotomy, cystourethroscopy, urethral calibration, urethral dilation, internal urethrotomy, and control of postoperative bleeding. A cystourethroscope is inserted into the urethra and both the urethra and bladder are examined endoscopically with careful attention to the prostatic region. The physician may need to incise the urethral meatus (meatotomy), dilate and/or calibrate the urethra, and/or incise the internal urethra (internal urethrotomy) for better surgical access. The laser probe is advanced through the endoscope to the base of the middle lobe of the prostate. The laser is activated, the temperature is increased to 85 degrees centigrade, and the middle lobe is coagulated. The probe is held in position for up to 3 minutes using direct visualization or fluoroscopic video guidance. An irrigation tube is used to continuously flush blood and debris from the surgical site into the bladder. The bladder is drained and irrigated as needed to maintain good visibility. The probe is then retracted and placed in each lateral lobe and the laser coagulation procedure is repeated. When all lobes of the prostate have been treated, bleeding is controlled, the surgical tools and cystourethroscope are removed, and a Foley catheter is inserted.

Laser coagulation of prostate (including control of bleeding)

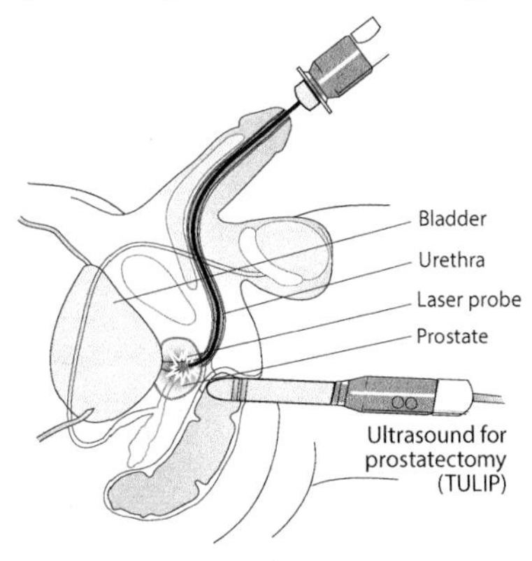

ICD-10-CM Diagnostic Codes

C61	Malignant neoplasm of prostate ♂
D07.5	Carcinoma in situ of prostate ♂
D29.1	Benign neoplasm of prostate ♂
N40.0	Benign prostatic hyperplasia without lower urinary tract symptoms ♂
N40.1	Benign prostatic hyperplasia with lower urinary tract symptoms ♂
N40.2	Nodular prostate without lower urinary tract symptoms ♂
N40.3	Nodular prostate with lower urinary tract symptoms ♂
N41.1	Chronic prostatitis ♂
N41.2	Abscess of prostate ♂
N42.30	Unspecified dysplasia of prostate ♂
N42.31	Prostatic intraepithelial neoplasia ♂
N42.32	Atypical small acinar proliferation of prostate ♂
N42.39	Other dysplasia of prostate ♂
N42.83	Cyst of prostate ♂

CCI Edits

Refer to Appendix A for CCI edits.

Pub 100

52647: Pub 100-03, 1, 140.5, Pub 100-03, 1, 230.3

Facility RVUs ▢

Code	Work	PE Facility	MP	Total Facility
52647	11.30	6.36	1.33	18.99

Non-facility RVUs ▢

Code	Work	PE Non-Facility	MP	Total Non-Facility
52647	11.30	34.95	1.33	47.58

Modifiers (PAR) ▢

Code	Mod 50	Mod 51	Mod 62	Mod 66	Mod 80
52647	0	2	0	0	1

Global Period

Code	Days
52647	090

52648

52648 Laser vaporization of prostate, including control of postoperative bleeding, complete (vasectomy, meatotomy, cystourethroscopy, urethral calibration and/or dilation, internal urethrotomy and transurethral resection of prostate are included if performed)

AMA Coding Notes

Surgical Procedures on the Urinary System

(For provision of chemotherapeutic agents, report both the specific service in addition to code(s) for the specific substance(s) or drug(s) provided)

AMA *CPT® Assistant* ▯

52648: Mar 98: 11, Apr 01: 5, Jul 05: 15, Nov 06: 21, Jun 15: 5

Plain English Description

A complete laser vaporization of the prostate is performed including control of postoperative bleeding. This procedure may also be referred to as interstitial laser coagulation of the prostate (ILCP) or contact laser ablation of the prostate (CLAP). ILCP and CLAP result in immediate laser destruction and vaporization of prostate tissue. The following procedures may also be performed and are included: vasectomy, meatotomy, cystourethroscopy, urethral calibration, urethral dilation, internal urethrotomy, and control of postoperative bleeding. A cystourethroscope is inserted into the urethra and both the urethra and bladder are examined endoscopically, with careful attention to anatomy of the urethral sphincter and prostate. The position of the ureters and bladder neck is also noted. The physician may need to incise the urethral meatus (meatotomy), dilate and/or calibrate the urethra, and/or incise the internal urethra (internal urethrotomy) for better surgical access. The laser fiber is introduced and positioned, taking care to avoid direct contact with the prostate tissue. The laser is fired perpendicularly using slow side-to-side sweeping movements. Effective vaporization of prostate tissue results in formation of bubbles. When all lobes of the prostate have been treated, the bladder is emptied and the surgical cavity is inspected to verify that sufficient tissue has been removed. The bladder neck should be visible from the verumontanum. The integrity of the ureters is also verified. Any bleeding is controlled. The surgical tools and cystourethroscope are removed. Generally, little postoperative bleeding occurs following laser vaporization and a Foley catheter is not typically required.

Laser vaporization of prostate (ILCP or CLAP)

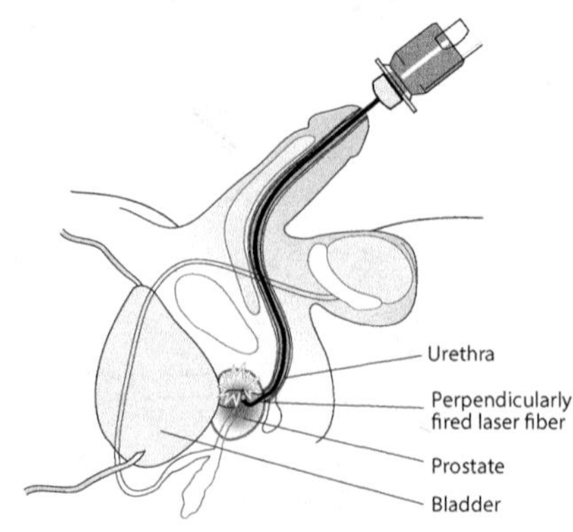

ICD-10-CM Diagnostic Codes

C61	Malignant neoplasm of prostate ♂
D07.5	Carcinoma in situ of prostate ♂
D29.1	Benign neoplasm of prostate ♂
N40.0	Benign prostatic hyperplasia without lower urinary tract symptoms ♂
N40.1	Benign prostatic hyperplasia with lower urinary tract symptoms ♂
N40.2	Nodular prostate without lower urinary tract symptoms ♂
N40.3	Nodular prostate with lower urinary tract symptoms ♂
N41.1	Chronic prostatitis ♂
N41.2	Abscess of prostate ♂
N42.30	Unspecified dysplasia of prostate ♂
N42.31	Prostatic intraepithelial neoplasia ♂
N42.32	Atypical small acinar proliferation of prostate ♂
N42.39	Other dysplasia of prostate ♂
N42.83	Cyst of prostate ♂

CCI Edits

Refer to Appendix A for CCI edits.

Pub 100

52648: Pub 100-03, 1, 140.5, Pub 100-03, 1, 230.3

Facility RVUs ▯

Code	Work	PE Facility	MP	Total Facility
52648	12.15	6.66	1.43	20.24

Non-facility RVUs ▯

Code	Work	PE Non-Facility	MP	Total Non-Facility
52648	12.15	35.48	1.43	49.06

Modifiers (PAR) ▯

Code	Mod 50	Mod 51	Mod 62	Mod 66	Mod 80
52648	0	2	0	0	1

Global Period

Code	Days
52648	090

52649

52649 Laser enucleation of the prostate with morcellation, including control of postoperative bleeding, complete (vasectomy, meatotomy, cystourethroscopy, urethral calibration and/or dilation, internal urethrotomy and transurethral resection of prostate are included if performed)

(Do not report 52649 in conjunction with 52000, 52276, 52281, 52601, 52647, 52648, 53020, 55250)

AMA Coding Notes

Surgical Procedures on the Urinary System

(For provision of chemotherapeutic agents, report both the specific service in addition to code(s) for the specific substance(s) or drug(s) provided)

AMA *CPT® Assistant*

52649: Jun 15: 5

Plain English Description

A complete laser enucleation of the prostate is performed with morcellation including control of postoperative bleeding. Morcellation of the prostate involves dividing it into smaller pieces so that it can be more easily removed. Also included in this procedure are a vasectomy, meatotomy, cystourethroscopy (cystoscopy), urethral calibration and/or dilation, internal urethrotomy, and transurethral resection of the prostate, if performed. Prior to the laser enucleation procedure, a cystoscopy is performed to examine the bladder for the presence of any tumors or masses. The urethra is then calibrated and dilated using a series of sounds. If the meatus is narrowed, it is incised (meatotomy). A continuous flow resectoscope sheath is placed, followed by a laser fiber stabilizing catheter, video system, and lastly the laser fiber. Normal saline irrigant is then run through the resection tubing into the resectoscope. The resectoscope is then used to visualize the anatomy and determine the extent of each lobe's enlargement. Each lobe of the prostate is then sequentially enucleated and resected, usually beginning with the median lobe. This process begins by first cutting a groove with the laser along the sulcus just lateral to the verumontanum (seminal colliculus). The groove is then deepened, undermined, and widened to separate it from the lateral lobe. A second groove may be created by repeating this process. All attachments in the median lobe are divided and the median lobe is enucleated. Dissection of the right lateral lobe is then performed, freeing it from the capsular floor by moving the laser in a side-to-side, transverse fashion. When the floor of the right lobe is dissected free of all attachments, an anterior groove is created along the anterior commissure to separate the right lateral lobe from the roof of the capsule. The remaining lateral attachments at the apex of the right lateral lobe are identified and cut with the laser. Enucleation of the right lobe is completed by dividing any remaining attachments at the bladder neck. Attention is then directed to the left lateral lobe and the left lateral lobe is enucleated in the same fashion as the right. Once all three lobes of the prostate have been enucleated and pushed into the bladder, bleeding is controlled by laser coagulation. The inner sheath of the resectoscope, the laser fiber, and the stabilizing catheter are removed. A morcellator is introduced. Inflow tubing with normal saline is used to distend the bladder. Prostate tissue from one of the lobes that has been pushed into the bladder is isolated and the morcellator blades activated. The prostate tissue is cut into smaller pieces by the morcellator and these smaller pieces of prostate tissue are removed by suction. This is repeated until the bladder is cleared of all prostate tissue.

Laser enucleation of prostate with morcellation

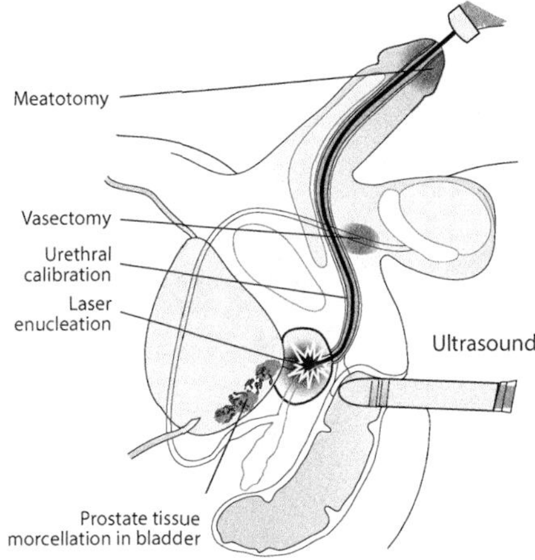

ICD-10-CM Diagnostic Codes

C61	Malignant neoplasm of prostate ♂
D07.5	Carcinoma in situ of prostate ♂
D29.1	Benign neoplasm of prostate ♂
N40.0	Benign prostatic hyperplasia without lower urinary tract symptoms ♂
N40.1	Benign prostatic hyperplasia with lower urinary tract symptoms ♂
N40.2	Nodular prostate without lower urinary tract symptoms ♂
N40.3	Nodular prostate with lower urinary tract symptoms ♂
N41.1	Chronic prostatitis ♂
N41.2	Abscess of prostate ♂
N42.30	Unspecified dysplasia of prostate ♂
N42.31	Prostatic intraepithelial neoplasia ♂
N42.32	Atypical small acinar proliferation of prostate ♂
N42.39	Other dysplasia of prostate ♂
N42.83	Cyst of prostate ♂

CCI Edits

Refer to Appendix A for CCI edits.

Pub 100

52649: Pub 100-03, 1, 140.5, Pub 100-03, 1, 230.3

Facility RVUs

Code	Work	PE Facility	MP	Total Facility
52649	14.56	7.87	1.72	24.15

Non-facility RVUs

Code	Work	PE Non-Facility	MP	Total Non-Facility
52649	14.56	7.87	1.72	24.15

Modifiers (PAR)

Code	Mod 50	Mod 51	Mod 62	Mod 66	Mod 80
52649	0	2	0	0	0

Global Period

Code	Days
52649	090

52700

52700 Transurethral drainage of prostatic abscess

(For litholapaxy, use 52317, 52318)

AMA Coding Notes

Surgical Procedures on the Urinary System

(For provision of chemotherapeutic agents, report both the specific service in addition to code(s) for the specific substance(s) or drug(s) provided)

AMA *CPT® Assistant*

52700: Apr 01: 4

Plain English Description

The physician performs transurethral drainage of a prostatic abscess. The abscess is located using digital rectal exam (DRE) and/or separately reportable transrectal ultrasound (TRUS) guidance. A cystourethroscope is inserted into the urethra and both the urethra and bladder are examined. A needle is used to puncture the abscess and a small amount of fluid is aspirated and sent to the laboratory for culture. An incision is then made in the abscess wall and the abscess is drained.

Transurethral drainage of prostatic abscess

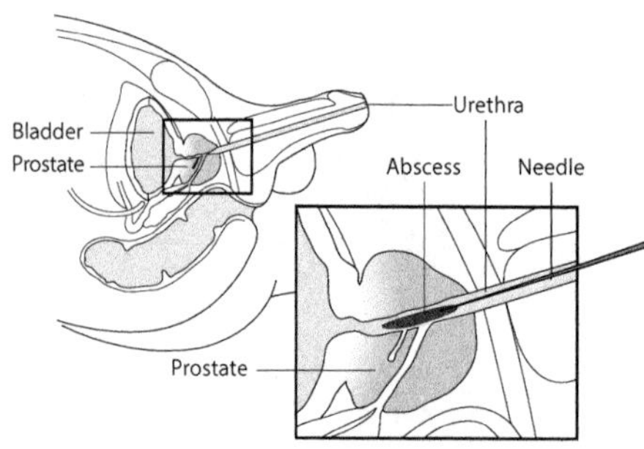

A prostatic abscess is drained by going up through the urethra.

ICD-10-CM Diagnostic Codes

A54.22	Gonococcal prostatitis ♂
N41.2	Abscess of prostate ♂
N41.3	Prostatocystitis ♂
N41.4	Granulomatous prostatitis ♂
N41.8	Other inflammatory diseases of prostate ♂

CCI Edits

Refer to Appendix A for CCI edits.

Facility RVUs

Code	Work	PE Facility	MP	Total Facility
52700	7.49	4.56	0.90	12.95

Non-facility RVUs

Code	Work	PE Non-Facility	MP	Total Non-Facility
52700	7.49	4.56	0.90	12.95

Modifiers (PAR)

Code	Mod 50	Mod 51	Mod 62	Mod 66	Mod 80
52700	0	2	0	0	0

Global Period

Code	Days
52700	090

53000-53010

53000 Urethrotomy or urethrostomy, external (separate procedure); pendulous urethra

53010 Urethrotomy or urethrostomy, external (separate procedure); perineal urethra, external

AMA Coding Notes

Surgical Procedures on the Urethra

(For endoscopy, see cystoscopy, urethroscopy, cystourethroscopy, 52000-52700)

(For injection procedure for urethrocystography, see 51600-51610)

Surgical Procedures on the Urinary System

(For provision of chemotherapeutic agents, report both the specific service in addition to code(s) for the specific substance(s) or drug(s) provided)

Plain English Description

Urethrotomy or urethrostomy is performed to allow access to the penile or perineal urethra, bladder neck, and/or bladder. In males, the urethra is divided into anterior and posterior segments. The anterior urethra includes the meatus, fossa navicularis, penile or pendulous urethra, and bulbar urethra. The posterior urethra includes the membranous and prostatic urethra, which may also be referred to as the perineal urethra. In 53000, the spongiosum is incised and the pendulous urethra is exposed and incised. A catheter is placed into the bladder through the incision in the pendulous urethra to provide drainage of urine. In 53010, the perineum is incised and the perineal urethra is exposed. A catheter is placed into the bladder through the incision in the perineal urethra to provide drainage of urine.

Urethrotomy or urethrostomy, external

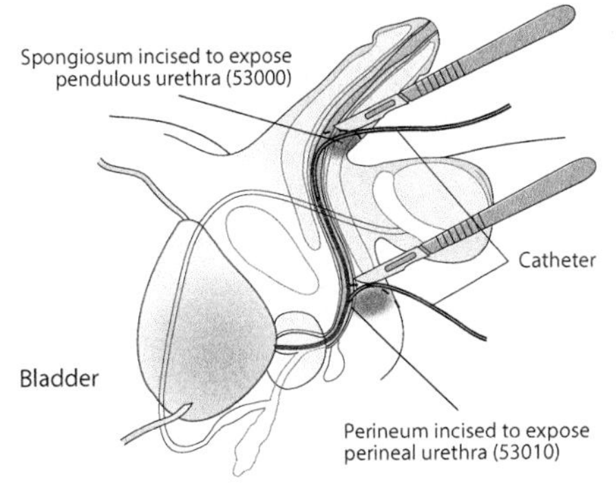

ICD-10-CM Diagnostic Codes

C68.0	Malignant neoplasm of urethra
N35.010	Post-traumatic urethral stricture, male, meatal ♂
N35.011	Post-traumatic bulbous urethral stricture ♂
N35.012	Post-traumatic membranous urethral stricture ♂
N35.013	Post-traumatic anterior urethral stricture ♂
N35.016	Post-traumatic urethral stricture, male, overlapping sites ♂
N35.111	Postinfective urethral stricture, not elsewhere classified, male, meatal ♂
N35.112	Postinfective bulbous urethral stricture, not elsewhere classified, male ♂
N35.113	Postinfective membranous urethral stricture, not elsewhere classified, male ♂
N35.114	Postinfective anterior urethral stricture, not elsewhere classified, male ♂
N35.116	Postinfective urethral stricture, not elsewhere classified, male, overlapping sites ♂
N35.811	Other urethral stricture, male, meatal ♂
N35.812	Other urethral bulbous stricture, male ♂
N35.813	Other membranous urethral stricture, male ♂
N35.814	Other anterior urethral stricture, male ♂
N35.816	Other urethral stricture, male, overlapping sites ♂
N36.8	Other specified disorders of urethra
N37	Urethral disorders in diseases classified elsewhere
N99.110	Postprocedural urethral stricture, male, meatal ♂
N99.111	Postprocedural bulbous urethral stricture, male ♂
N99.112	Postprocedural membranous urethral stricture, male ♂
N99.113	Postprocedural anterior bulbous urethral stricture, male ♂
N99.115	Postprocedural fossa navicularis urethral stricture ♂
N99.116	Postprocedural urethral stricture, male, overlapping sites ♂
Q54.1	Hypospadias, penile ♂
Q54.2	Hypospadias, penoscrotal ♂
Q64.32	Congenital stricture of urethra
Q64.39	Other atresia and stenosis of urethra and bladder neck
S31.21XS	Laceration without foreign body of penis, sequela ♂
S31.22XS	Laceration with foreign body of penis, sequela ♂
Z90.79	Acquired absence of other genital organ(s)

CCI Edits

Refer to Appendix A for CCI edits.

Facility RVUs

Code	Work	PE Facility	MP	Total Facility
53000	2.33	1.74	0.27	4.34
53010	4.45	3.71	0.54	8.70

Non-facility RVUs

Code	Work	PE Non-Facility	MP	Total Non-Facility
53000	2.33	1.74	0.27	4.34
53010	4.45	3.71	0.54	8.70

Modifiers (PAR)

Code	Mod 50	Mod 51	Mod 62	Mod 66	Mod 80
53000	0	2	0	0	1
53010	0	2	0	0	1

Global Period

Code	Days
53000	010
53010	090

53020-53025

53020 Meatotomy, cutting of meatus (separate procedure); except infant

53025 Meatotomy, cutting of meatus (separate procedure); infant

(Do not report modifier 63 in conjunction with 53025)

AMA Coding Notes

Surgical Procedures on the Urethra

(For endoscopy, see cystoscopy, urethroscopy, cystourethroscopy, 52000-52700)

(For injection procedure for urethrocystography, see 51600-51610)

Surgical Procedures on the Urinary System

(For provision of chemotherapeutic agents, report both the specific service in addition to code(s) for the specific substance(s) or drug(s) provided)

Plain English Description

The external urethral meatus is the most distal aspect of the urethra, also referred to as the external urethral orifice. Meatotomy is performed to enlarge the orifice. The urethral meatus is cleansed. A local anesthetic is administered. The meatus is incised. Use 53020 when meatotomy is performed on a child older than an infant, an adolescent, or adult. Use 53025 when meatotomy is performed on an infant.

Meatotomy

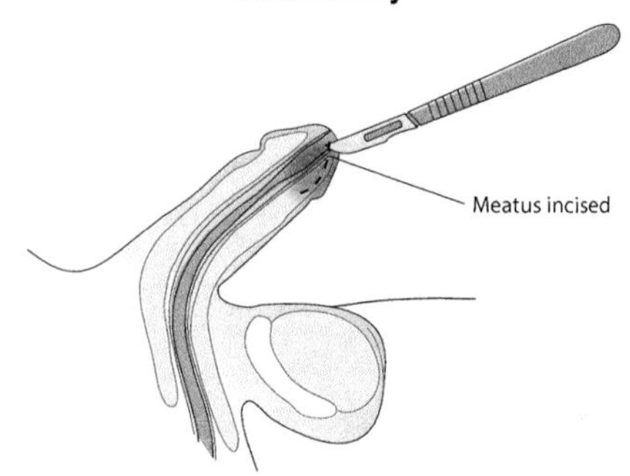

Except infant (53020); infant (53025)

ICD-10-CM Diagnostic Codes

N35.010	Post-traumatic urethral stricture, male, meatal ♂
N35.111	Postinfective urethral stricture, not elsewhere classified, male, meatal ♂
N35.811	Other urethral stricture, male, meatal ♂
N47.6	Balanoposthitis ♂
N48.1	Balanitis ♂
N99.110	Postprocedural urethral stricture, male, meatal ♂
R33.9	Retention of urine, unspecified

CCI Edits

Refer to Appendix A for CCI edits.

Facility RVUs

Code	Work	PE Facility	MP	Total Facility
53020	1.77	0.83	0.21	2.81
53025	1.13	0.72	0.12	1.97

Non-facility RVUs

Code	Work	PE Non-Facility	MP	Total Non-Facility
53020	1.77	0.83	0.21	2.81
53025	1.13	0.72	0.12	1.97

Modifiers (PAR)

Code	Mod 50	Mod 51	Mod 62	Mod 66	Mod 80
53020	0	2	0	0	1
53025	0	2	0	0	0

Global Period

Code	Days
53020	000
53025	000

53040

53040 Drainage of deep periurethral abscess

(For subcutaneous abscess, see 10060, 10061)

AMA Coding Notes

Surgical Procedures on the Urethra

(For endoscopy, see cystoscopy, urethroscopy, cystourethroscopy, 52000-52700)

(For injection procedure for urethrocystography, see 51600-51610)

Surgical Procedures on the Urinary System

(For provision of chemotherapeutic agents, report both the specific service in addition to code(s) for the specific substance(s) or drug(s) provided)

Plain English Description

A deep periurethral abscess is an infection that frequently occurs as a complication of gonococcal infection, urethral stricture, or urethral catheterization. The perineum is incised over the abscess site. The abscess pocket is opened and pus is drained. Loculations are broken up using finger dissection. The abscess pocket is flushed with sterile saline or antibiotic solution. The abscess pocket may be packed with gauze or a drain may be placed.

Drainage of deep periurethral abscess

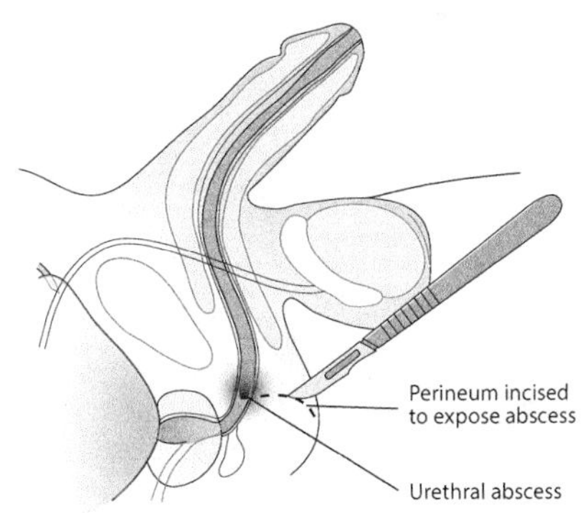

ICD-10-CM Diagnostic Codes

A54.01	Gonococcal cystitis and urethritis, unspecified
A54.1	Gonococcal infection of lower genitourinary tract with periurethral and accessory gland abscess
N34.0	Urethral abscess
N34.1	Nonspecific urethritis
N34.2	Other urethritis
N36.8	Other specified disorders of urethra

CCI Edits

Refer to Appendix A for CCI edits.

Facility RVUs 🗆

Code	Work	PE Facility	MP	Total Facility
53040	6.55	4.17	0.77	11.49

Non-facility RVUs 🗆

Code	Work	PE Non-Facility	MP	Total Non-Facility
53040	6.55	4.17	0.77	11.49

Modifiers (PAR) 🗆

Code	Mod 50	Mod 51	Mod 62	Mod 66	Mod 80
53040	0	2	0	0	0

Global Period

Code	Days
53040	090

53060

53060 Drainage of Skene's gland abscess or cyst

AMA Coding Notes

Surgical Procedures on the Urethra

(For endoscopy, see cystoscopy, urethroscopy, cystourethroscopy, 52000-52700)

(For injection procedure for urethrocystography, see 51600-51610)

Surgical Procedures on the Urinary System

(For provision of chemotherapeutic agents, report both the specific service in addition to code(s) for the specific substance(s) or drug(s) provided)

Plain English Description

Skene's glands are small mucus glands located adjacent to the distal urethra, also known as periurethral glands, which deliver secretions into the female urethra near the urethral meatus. Cysts form when the Skene's ducts become obstructed. The cysts can become infected and turn into abscesses. The cyst or abscess is located by palpation. The cyst or abscess is then incised and drained.

Drainage of Skene's gland abscess or cyst

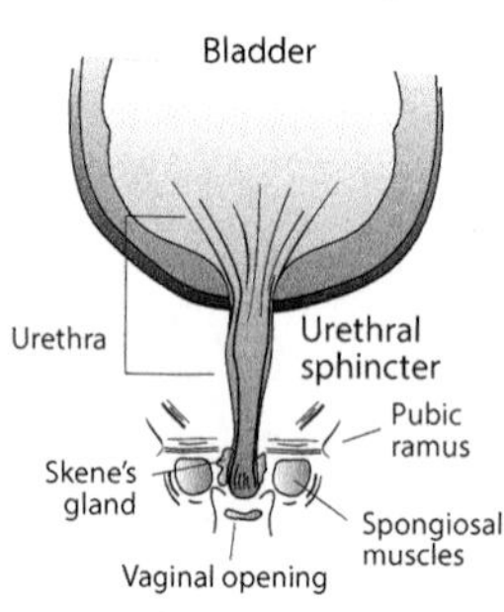

Fluid is drained from an abscess or cyst located just inside of and on the back side of the urethra in the female.

ICD-10-CM Diagnostic Codes

N34.0	Urethral abscess
N36.8	Other specified disorders of urethra

CCI Edits

Refer to Appendix A for CCI edits.

Facility RVUs

Code	Work	PE Facility	MP	Total Facility
53060	2.68	1.78	0.42	4.88

Non-facility RVUs

Code	Work	PE Non-Facility	MP	Total Non-Facility
53060	2.68	2.49	0.42	5.59

Modifiers (PAR)

Code	Mod 50	Mod 51	Mod 62	Mod 66	Mod 80
53060	0	2	0	0	1

Global Period

Code	Days
53060	010

53080-53085

53080 Drainage of perineal urinary extravasation; uncomplicated (separate procedure)

53085 Drainage of perineal urinary extravasation; complicated

AMA Coding Notes

Surgical Procedures on the Urethra

(For endoscopy, see cystoscopy, urethroscopy, cystourethroscopy, 52000-52700)

(For injection procedure for urethrocystography, see 51600-51610)

Surgical Procedures on the Urinary System

(For provision of chemotherapeutic agents, report both the specific service in addition to code(s) for the specific substance(s) or drug(s) provided)

Plain English Description

Perineal urinary extravasation occurs when there is a disruption in the continuity of the perineal urethra and urine leaks out into the perineal tissue, which causes it to become red, tender, and edematous. The disruption may be caused by rupture of the urethra due to a stricture in the distal end or traumatic injury. The urethra cannot be repaired until the urine has been drained from the perineal tissue. In 53080, uncomplicated drainage is performed using multiple incisions in the superficial perineal tissue to allow drainage of the urine. In 53085, complicated drainage is performed, which may be required when there is a traumatic injury to the urethra or when dissection of deeper tissues is required to allow drainage of urine.

Drainage of perineal urinary extravasation

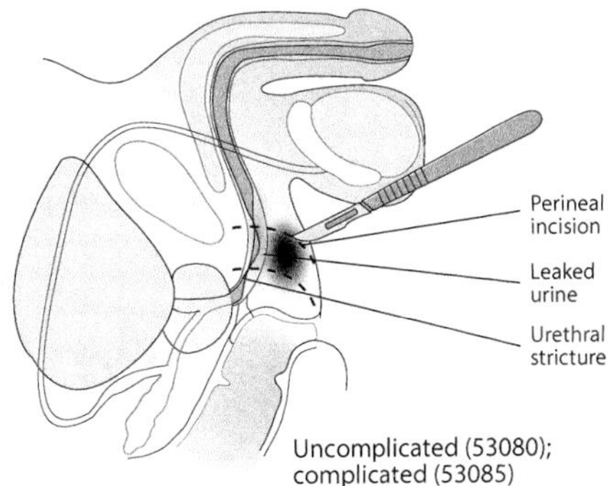

ICD-10-CM Diagnostic Codes

R39.0 Extravasation of urine

CCI Edits

Refer to Appendix A for CCI edits.

Facility RVUs

Code	Work	PE Facility	MP	Total Facility
53080	6.92	4.58	0.84	12.34
53085	11.18	6.51	1.33	19.02

Non-facility RVUs

Code	Work	PE Non-Facility	MP	Total Non-Facility
53080	6.92	4.58	0.84	12.34
53085	11.18	6.51	1.33	19.02

Modifiers (PAR)

Code	Mod 50	Mod 51	Mod 62	Mod 66	Mod 80
53080	0	2	0	0	1
53085	0	2	1	0	2

Global Period

Code	Days
53080	090
53085	090

53200

53200 Biopsy of urethra

AMA Coding Notes

Surgical Procedures on the Urethra

(For endoscopy, see cystoscopy, urethroscopy, cystourethroscopy, 52000-52700)

(For injection procedure for urethrocystography, see 51600-51610)

Surgical Procedures on the Urinary System

(For provision of chemotherapeutic agents, report both the specific service in addition to code(s) for the specific substance(s) or drug(s) provided)

Plain English Description

The lesion on the external aspect of the urethra is visually inspected. The surgical site is cleansed and a local anesthetic administered as needed. One or more tissue samples are obtained. The tissue samples are then prepared and examined by a pathologist in a separately reportable procedure to determine if cancer or other abnormal cells are present.

Biopsy of urethra

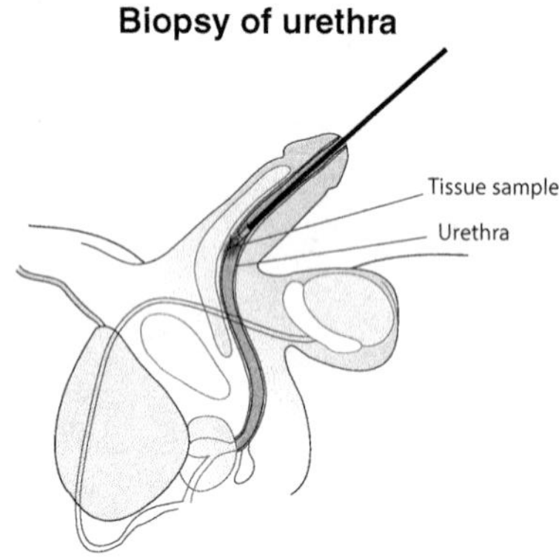

ICD-10-CM Diagnostic Codes

C67.5	Malignant neoplasm of bladder neck
C68.0	Malignant neoplasm of urethra
C68.1	Malignant neoplasm of paraurethral glands
C79.11	Secondary malignant neoplasm of bladder
C79.19	Secondary malignant neoplasm of other urinary organs
D09.0	Carcinoma in situ of bladder
D09.19	Carcinoma in situ of other urinary organs
D30.3	Benign neoplasm of bladder
D30.4	Benign neoplasm of urethra
D41.3	Neoplasm of uncertain behavior of urethra
D41.4	Neoplasm of uncertain behavior of bladder
D49.4	Neoplasm of unspecified behavior of bladder
N34.0	Urethral abscess
N34.1	Nonspecific urethritis
N34.2	Other urethritis
N34.3	Urethral syndrome, unspecified
N36.2	Urethral caruncle
N36.8	Other specified disorders of urethra
N37	Urethral disorders in diseases classified elsewhere
N40.0	Benign prostatic hyperplasia without lower urinary tract symptoms ♂
N40.1	Benign prostatic hyperplasia with lower urinary tract symptoms ♂
R36.0	Urethral discharge without blood
R36.9	Urethral discharge, unspecified
❼ T19.0	Foreign body in urethra

ICD-10-CM Coding Notes

For codes requiring a 7th character extension, refer to your ICD-10-CM book. Review the character descriptions and coding guidelines for proper selection. For some procedures, only certain characters will apply.

CCI Edits

Refer to Appendix A for CCI edits.

Facility RVUs ▯

Code	Work	PE Facility	MP	Total Facility
53200	2.59	1.21	0.33	4.13

Non-facility RVUs ▯

Code	Work	PE Non-Facility	MP	Total Non-Facility
53200	2.59	1.72	0.33	4.64

Modifiers (PAR) ▯

Code	Mod 50	Mod 51	Mod 62	Mod 66	Mod 80
53200	0	2	0	0	1

Global Period

Code	Days
53200	000

53210

53210 Urethrectomy, total, including cystostomy; female

AMA Coding Notes

Surgical Procedures on the Urethra

(For endoscopy, see cystoscopy, urethroscopy, cystourethroscopy, 52000-52700)

(For injection procedure for urethrocystography, see 51600-51610)

Surgical Procedures on the Urinary System

(For provision of chemotherapeutic agents, report both the specific service in addition to code(s) for the specific substance(s) or drug(s) provided)

Plain English Description

The urethra in women is located in the pelvic floor (perineum), in front of and above the vagina. A total urethrectomy is the complete removal of the urethra from the bladder to the perineum. A urethral catheter is inserted. An incision is made around the external urethra and the urethra is dissected free of surrounding tissue. The pubourethral ligament is exposed and transected. The posterior aspect of the urethra is dissected free of the vaginal septum. The right and left urethropelvic ligaments are exposed, isolated, and transected. Once the urethra is completely free of all surrounding tissue from the external meatus to the bladder neck, an incision is made just above the pubis. The completely isolated urethra is pulled into the pelvis and the bladder neck is dissected from surrounding tissue. The urethra is excised at the level of the bladder neck and removed along with the urethral catheter. The bladder neck is closed with sutures. An opening called a cystostomy, also referred to as an epicystostomy or vesicostomy, is surgically created in the lower abdomen to facilitate urine drainage from the bladder. This is accomplished by making an incision in the lower abdomen to the level of the rectus fascia. A triangular section of the rectus fascia is completely excised. The rectus muscle is incised and the dome of the bladder is exposed. The bladder is opened and the bladder wall secured to the opening in the rectus fascia with sutures. The bladder epithelium is then secured to the skin. A catheter or tube is inserted and secured to the abdominal wall with sutures.

Urethrectomy, total, including cystostomy

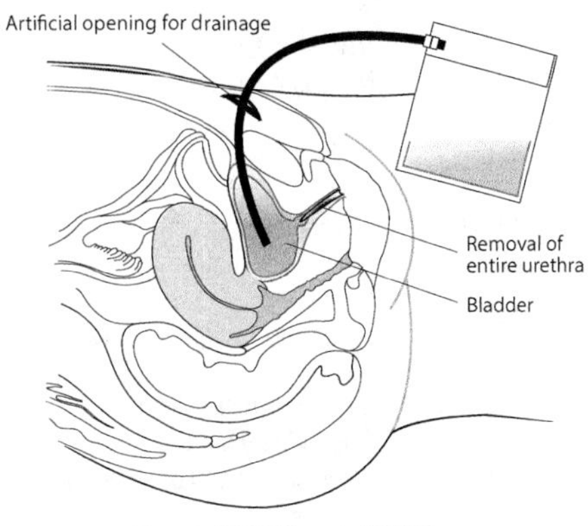

Female (53210); male (53215)

ICD-10-CM Diagnostic Codes

C67.5	Malignant neoplasm of bladder neck
C68.0	Malignant neoplasm of urethra
C68.1	Malignant neoplasm of paraurethral glands
C79.11	Secondary malignant neoplasm of bladder
C79.19	Secondary malignant neoplasm of other urinary organs
D09.0	Carcinoma in situ of bladder
D09.19	Carcinoma in situ of other urinary organs
D41.3	Neoplasm of uncertain behavior of urethra
D41.4	Neoplasm of uncertain behavior of bladder
D49.4	Neoplasm of unspecified behavior of bladder
N34.0	Urethral abscess
N34.3	Urethral syndrome, unspecified
N35.011	Post-traumatic bulbous urethral stricture ♂
N35.012	Post-traumatic membranous urethral stricture ♂
N35.013	Post-traumatic anterior urethral stricture ♂
N35.021	Urethral stricture due to childbirth ♀
N35.028	Other post-traumatic urethral stricture, female ♀
N35.12	Postinfective urethral stricture, not elsewhere classified, female ♀
N36.8	Other specified disorders of urethra
Q64.2	Congenital posterior urethral valves
Q64.31	Congenital bladder neck obstruction
Q64.32	Congenital stricture of urethra
Q64.33	Congenital stricture of urinary meatus
Q64.39	Other atresia and stenosis of urethra and bladder neck

CCI Edits

Refer to Appendix A for CCI edits.

Facility RVUs ☐

Code	Work	PE Facility	MP	Total Facility
53210	13.72	7.33	1.68	22.73

Non-facility RVUs ☐

Code	Work	PE Non-Facility	MP	Total Non-Facility
53210	13.72	7.33	1.68	22.73

Modifiers (PAR) ☐

Code	Mod 50	Mod 51	Mod 62	Mod 66	Mod 80
53210	0	2	1	0	2

Global Period

Code	Days
53210	090

53215

53215 Urethrectomy, total, including cystostomy; male

AMA Coding Notes

Surgical Procedures on the Urethra

(For endoscopy, see cystoscopy, urethroscopy, cystourethroscopy, 52000-52700)

(For injection procedure for urethrocystography, see 51600-51610)

Surgical Procedures on the Urinary System

(For provision of chemotherapeutic agents, report both the specific service in addition to code(s) for the specific substance(s) or drug(s) provided)

Plain English Description

The urethra in men is located centrally down the shaft of the penis. A total urethrectomy is performed by making an incision in the perineum and removing the urethra from the prostate area to the tip of the penis. A Foley catheter or urethral sound is inserted into the urethra. An incision is made in the lower abdomen and the bladder neck exposed. The bulbocavernosus muscle is exposed and incised in the midline. The bulbar urethra is dissected free of surrounding tissue. Buck's fascia is incised and a window created between Buck's fascia and the corpora cavernosa to allow mobilization of the cavernous urethra. The cavernous urethra is dissected from surrounding tissue as tension is applied to the urethra drawing the urethra into the pelvic incision. Dissection continues distally. Tension is applied and the glans penis is inverted. The urethra is mobilized to the level of the coronal sulcus in the glans penis. The glans penis is returned to its normal orientation and a traction suture placed in the glans. An incision is made over the frenulum and the mobilized portion of the urethra captured using umbilical tape or a vessel loop. An incision is made around the external urethral meatus and carried up to the incision over the frenulum. The urethra is dissected free of the glans penis. Once the distal aspect of the urethra has been completely mobilized, the urethra is brought into the pelvis and excised at the level of the bladder neck. The urethra and catheter are removed and the bladder neck is closed. Incisions in the penis are closed in layers. A drain or catheter may be left in place to facilitate drainage from the area. An opening called a cystostomy, also referred to as an epicystostomy or vesicostomy, is surgically created in the lower abdomen to facilitate urine drainage from the bladder. This is accomplished by making an incision in the lower abdomen to the level of the rectus fascia. A triangular section of the rectus fascia is completely excised. The rectus muscle is incised and the dome of the bladder is exposed. The bladder is opened and the bladder wall secured to the opening in the rectus fascia with sutures. The bladder epithelium is then secured to the skin. A catheter or tube is inserted and secured to the abdominal wall with sutures.

ICD-10-CM Diagnostic Codes

C61	Malignant neoplasm of prostate ♂
C67.5	Malignant neoplasm of bladder neck
C68.0	Malignant neoplasm of urethra
C68.1	Malignant neoplasm of paraurethral glands
C79.11	Secondary malignant neoplasm of bladder
C79.19	Secondary malignant neoplasm of other urinary organs
D09.19	Carcinoma in situ of other urinary organs
D30.4	Benign neoplasm of urethra
D41.3	Neoplasm of uncertain behavior of urethra
N34.0	Urethral abscess
N35.016	Post-traumatic urethral stricture, male, overlapping sites ♂
N35.116	Postinfective urethral stricture, not elsewhere classified, male, overlapping sites ♂
N36.42	Intrinsic sphincter deficiency (ISD)
N36.8	Other specified disorders of urethra
N36.9	Urethral disorder, unspecified
N99.116	Postprocedural urethral stricture, male, overlapping sites ♂

CCI Edits

Refer to Appendix A for CCI edits.

Facility RVUs ▯

Code	Work	PE Facility	MP	Total Facility
53215	16.85	8.24	2.03	27.12

Non-facility RVUs ▯

Code	Work	PE Non-Facility	MP	Total Non-Facility
53215	16.85	8.24	2.03	27.12

Modifiers (PAR) ▯

Code	Mod 50	Mod 51	Mod 62	Mod 66	Mod 80
53215	0	2	1	0	2

Global Period

Code	Days
53215	090

53220

53220 Excision or fulguration of carcinoma of urethra

AMA Coding Notes

Surgical Procedures on the Urethra

(For endoscopy, see cystoscopy, urethroscopy, cystourethroscopy, 52000-52700)

(For injection procedure for urethrocystography, see 51600-51610)

Surgical Procedures on the Urinary System

(For provision of chemotherapeutic agents, report both the specific service in addition to code(s) for the specific substance(s) or drug(s) provided)

Plain English Description

Treatment of external urethral cancers in both men and women may be performed by excision or fulguration, also referred to as electrocautery, electroresection, or laser destruction. The lesion on the external urethra may have been previously diagnosed or biopsied and diagnosed during the same surgical session. If excision is performed, the lesion along with a margin of healthy tissue is sharply excised. The specimen is evaluated in a separately reportable procedure by a pathologist to ensure that the margins are free of malignant tissue. If any malignant tissue is identified, the margins are widened until they are completely free of malignancy. Fulguration may be performed using an electrocautery device or laser. The electrocautery device or laser is activated and the abnormal tissue is destroyed.

Excision or fulguration of carcinoma of urethra

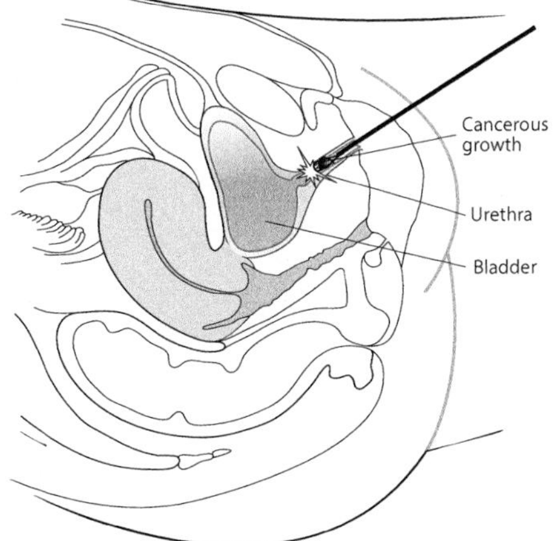

ICD-10-CM Diagnostic Codes

C68.0	Malignant neoplasm of urethra
C79.19	Secondary malignant neoplasm of other urinary organs
D09.19	Carcinoma in situ of other urinary organs

CCI Edits

Refer to Appendix A for CCI edits.

Facility RVUs

Code	Work	PE Facility	MP	Total Facility
53220	7.63	4.70	0.90	13.23

Non-facility RVUs

Code	Work	PE Non-Facility	MP	Total Non-Facility
53220	7.63	4.70	0.90	13.23

Modifiers (PAR)

Code	Mod 50	Mod 51	Mod 62	Mod 66	Mod 80
53220	0	2	0	0	0

Global Period

Code	Days
53220	090

CPT® Procedural Coding

53230

53230 Excision of urethral diverticulum (separate procedure); female

AMA Coding Notes

Surgical Procedures on the Urethra

(For endoscopy, see cystoscopy, urethroscopy, cystourethroscopy, 52000-52700)

(For injection procedure for urethrocystography, see 51600-51610)

Surgical Procedures on the Urinary System

(For provision of chemotherapeutic agents, report both the specific service in addition to code(s) for the specific substance(s) or drug(s) provided)

Plain English Description

Partial ablation and total excision are the most effective treatment when urethral diverticulum is in the middle or proximal area of the female urethra. A percutaneous suprapubic catheter is inserted as needed. The vagina is prepared and draped, a Foley catheter placed transurethrally. A vaginal incision is made via midline vertical, transverse, or U-shape with the apex distal to the diverticulum. In partial ablation, the periurethral fascia is exposed and dissected into proximal and distal flaps exposing the diverticular sac. The body of the diverticular sac is then entered and the sac excised from the periurethral fascia. A metal probe is placed through the ostia to identify the opening and the bulk of the sac excised leaving attenuated tissue around the ostia. The probe is removed and the attenuated tissue is sewn closed in multiple layers. Total excision or urethral diverticulectomy removes the diverticular sac and the surrounding mucosal lining. The vaginal flap is dissected using scissors preserving the periurethral fascia. The periurethral fascia is opened in proximal and distal flaps exposing the diverticular sac. The sac is not entered. The diverticulum is dissected circumferentially to the ostia. Attenuated tissue at the ostia is excised and the entire sac removed. The muscular and mucosal layers of the urethral defect are closed vertically over the catheter. In both procedures, the periurethral fascia is closed transversely and the anterior vaginal wall is also sutured. The urethral catheter is left in place. The suprapubic catheter, if used, may be removed or left in place.

Excision of urethral diverticulum; female

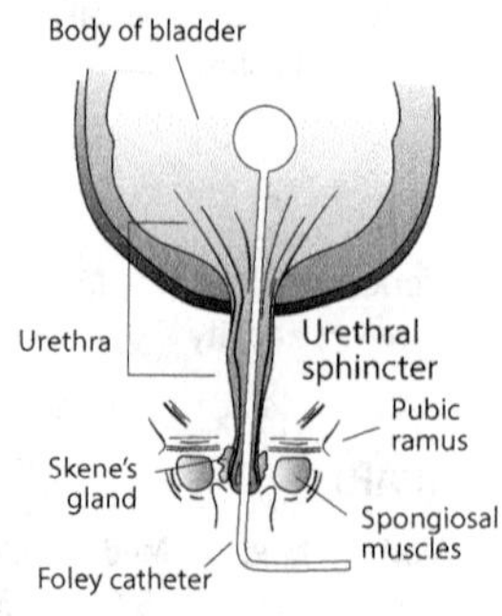

An abnormal sac or pouch is removed from the urethra.

ICD-10-CM Diagnostic Codes

N36.1	Urethral diverticulum

CCI Edits

Refer to Appendix A for CCI edits.

Facility RVUs

Code	Work	PE Facility	MP	Total Facility
53230	10.44	6.13	1.34	17.91

Non-facility RVUs

Code	Work	PE Non-Facility	MP	Total Non-Facility
53230	10.44	6.13	1.34	17.91

Modifiers (PAR)

Code	Mod 50	Mod 51	Mod 62	Mod 66	Mod 80
53230	0	2	1	0	2

Global Period

Code	Days
53230	090

53235

53235 Excision of urethral diverticulum (separate procedure); male

AMA Coding Notes

Surgical Procedures on the Urethra

(For endoscopy, see cystoscopy, urethroscopy, cystourethroscopy, 52000-52700)

(For injection procedure for urethrocystography, see 51600-51610)

Surgical Procedures on the Urinary System

(For provision of chemotherapeutic agents, report both the specific service in addition to code(s) for the specific substance(s) or drug(s) provided)

Plain English Description

Male urethral diverticula are quite rare but can be found in the proximal part of the penile urethra and distal part of the bulbous urethra. With the patient prepped and the penis and scrotum draped, a catheter is placed transurethrally. An incision is made in the skin exposing the corpus spongiosum. The diverticular sac is dissected free of the corpus spongiosum including the attenuated tissue at the ostia. The muscular and mucosal layers of the urethral defect are closed vertically over the catheter. Drains may be placed and the corpus spongiosum closed with sutures followed by closure of the skin. The urethral catheter is left in place.

Excision of urethral diverticulum

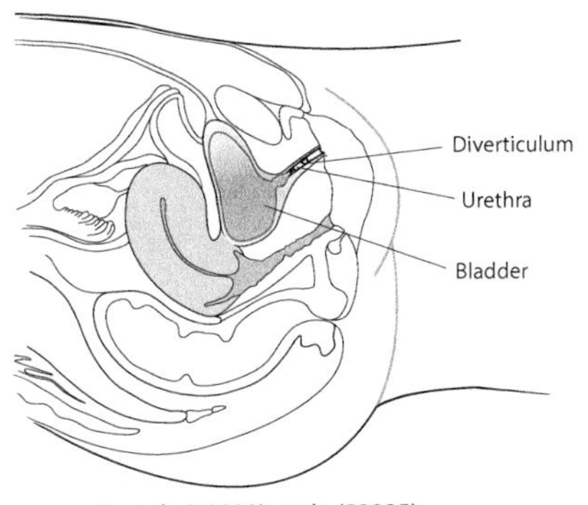

Female (53230); male (53235)

ICD-10-CM Diagnostic Codes

N36.1 Urethral diverticulum

CCI Edits

Refer to Appendix A for CCI edits.

Facility RVUs

Code	Work	PE Facility	MP	Total Facility
53235	10.99	6.28	1.30	18.57

Non-facility RVUs

Code	Work	PE Non-Facility	MP	Total Non-Facility
53235	10.99	6.28	1.30	18.57

Modifiers (PAR)

Code	Mod 50	Mod 51	Mod 62	Mod 66	Mod 80
53235	0	2	1	0	2

Global Period

Code	Days
53235	090

53240

53240 Marsupialization of urethral diverticulum, male or female

AMA Coding Notes

Surgical Procedures on the Urethra

(For endoscopy, see cystoscopy, urethroscopy, cystourethroscopy, 52000-52700)

(For injection procedure for urethrocystography, see 51600-51610)

Surgical Procedures on the Urinary System

(For provision of chemotherapeutic agents, report both the specific service in addition to code(s) for the specific substance(s) or drug(s) provided)

Plain English Description

Marsupialization or Spence procedure is performed on women when the diverticulum is located in the distal urethra, away from the bladder neck. A transurethral catheter is placed and the bladder emptied. The catheter is then withdrawn. Using straight Mayo scissors, one blade in the urethra and the second along the anterior wall of the vagina, an incision is made midline beneath the posterior wall of the urethra and the diverticular sac entered. The incision is enlarged as needed. The diverticulum is inspected for suspicious-appearing tissue. If a biopsy is performed to rule out malignancy, tissue samples are prepared and examined by a pathologist in a separately reportable procedure. The urethral and diverticular epithelial lining is then sutured to the incised vaginal epithelial lining exteriorizing the urinary tract epithelium and creating a large posterior meatotomy. A similar meatotomy is performed in men with distal diverticulum close to the penile tip. The diverticulum and meatus are opened together with scalpel or scissors to form a single, large meatal opening. Spontaneous voiding can be expected following either procedure and a urinary catheter is not usually necessary.

Marsupialization of urethral diverticulum, male or female

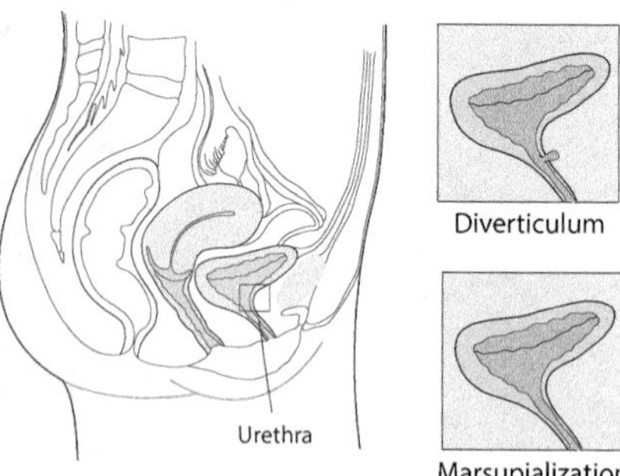

An abnormal sac or pouch located on the urethra is emptied of fluid. The edges are then raised to the skin surface, allowing it to drain and close. This code can be used on a male or a female.

ICD-10-CM Diagnostic Codes

N36.1 Urethral diverticulum

CCI Edits

Refer to Appendix A for CCI edits.

Facility RVUs

Code	Work	PE Facility	MP	Total Facility
53240	7.08	4.53	0.86	12.47

Non-facility RVUs

Code	Work	PE Non-Facility	MP	Total Non-Facility
53240	7.08	4.53	0.86	12.47

Modifiers (PAR)

Code	Mod 50	Mod 51	Mod 62	Mod 66	Mod 80
53240	0	2	0	0	1

Global Period

Code	Days
53240	090

53250

53250 Excision of bulbourethral gland (Cowper's gland)

AMA Coding Notes

Surgical Procedures on the Urethra

(For endoscopy, see cystoscopy, urethroscopy, cystourethroscopy, 52000-52700)

(For injection procedure for urethrocystography, see 51600-51610)

Surgical Procedures on the Urinary System

(For provision of chemotherapeutic agents, report both the specific service in addition to code(s) for the specific substance(s) or drug(s) provided)

Plain English Description

The bulbourethral or Cowper's gland is located at the base of the penis, posterior and lateral to the membranous portion of the urethra. A horizontal curved incision is made in the skin of the perineum above the anal opening and carried down through the superficial Camper's fascia and then the deep Colles' fascia. The rectus urethralis muscular band is then transected allowing entry into the urogenital diaphragm. The perirectal fascia, which makes up the posterior layer of Denonvilliers' fascia, is identified and opened and the bulbourethral gland is located and dissected free. The ductal opening of the gland into the urethra is identified and ligated. The gland and surrounding tissue are removed and inspected. Tissue samples may be prepared and examined by a pathologist in a separately reportable procedure. The incision is closed in layers with absorbable sutures, skin edges are approximated with interrupted sutures. A Penrose drain may be left in place.

Excision of bulbourethral gland (Cowper's gland)

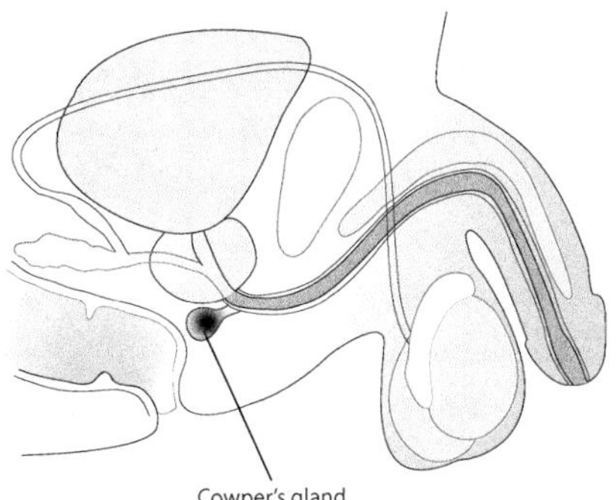

ICD-10-CM Diagnostic Codes

C68.0	Malignant neoplasm of urethra
C79.19	Secondary malignant neoplasm of other urinary organs
D09.19	Carcinoma in situ of other urinary organs
D30.4	Benign neoplasm of urethra
D41.3	Neoplasm of uncertain behavior of urethra
N34.0	Urethral abscess
N34.2	Other urethritis
N36.8	Other specified disorders of urethra

CCI Edits

Refer to Appendix A for CCI edits.

Facility RVUs

Code	Work	PE Facility	MP	Total Facility
53250	6.52	4.32	0.77	11.61

Non-facility RVUs

Code	Work	PE Non-Facility	MP	Total Non-Facility
53250	6.52	4.32	0.77	11.61

Modifiers (PAR)

Code	Mod 50	Mod 51	Mod 62	Mod 66	Mod 80
53250	0	2	0	0	1

Global Period

Code	Days
53250	090

53260

53260 Excision or fulguration; urethral polyp(s), distal urethra
(For endoscopic approach, see 52214, 52224)

AMA Coding Notes

Surgical Procedures on the Urethra

(For endoscopy, see cystoscopy, urethroscopy, cystourethroscopy, 52000-52700)

(For injection procedure for urethrocystography, see 51600-51610)

Surgical Procedures on the Urinary System

(For provision of chemotherapeutic agents, report both the specific service in addition to code(s) for the specific substance(s) or drug(s) provided)

Plain English Description

Open excision to remove polyps in the distal urethra is most often performed when the polyp is large or has reoccurred. With the female patient in dorsal lithotomy position, the vulva, vagina, and perineum are prepared and draped. The male patient is positioned supine and the penis prepared and draped. The urinary meatus and urethra may be dilated using a catheter or balloon to aid with visualization of the polyp. The polyp is grasped using a clamp or forceps and pulled out to elongate the stalk and expose the base of the polyp where it attaches to the urethra. The polyp is completely excised from the urethra by fulguration at the base using an electrocautery device or laser. The polyp is removed and inspected. Tissue samples are prepared and examined by a pathologist in a separately reportable procedure. The patient may have a Foley catheter placed following the procedure.

Excision or fulguration; urethral polyp(s) distal urethra

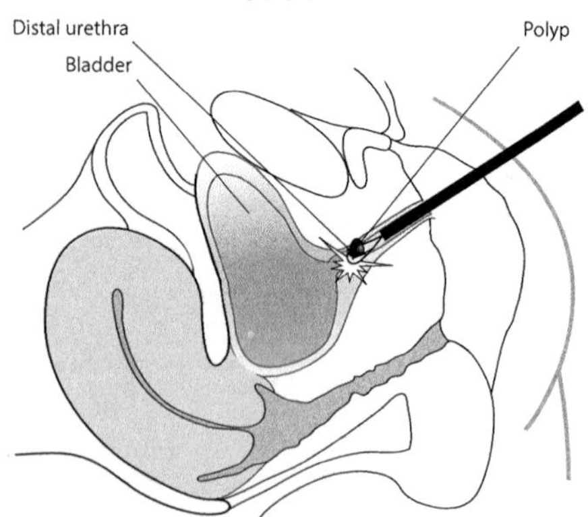

ICD-10-CM Diagnostic Codes

N36.2 Urethral caruncle

CCI Edits

Refer to Appendix A for CCI edits.

Facility RVUs

Code	Work	PE Facility	MP	Total Facility
53260	3.03	1.89	0.40	5.32

Non-facility RVUs

Code	Work	PE Non-Facility	MP	Total Non-Facility
53260	3.03	2.68	0.40	6.11

Modifiers (PAR)

Code	Mod 50	Mod 51	Mod 62	Mod 66	Mod 80
53260	0	2	0	0	1

Global Period

Code	Days
53260	010

53265

53265 Excision or fulguration; urethral caruncle

AMA Coding Notes

Surgical Procedures on the Urethra

(For endoscopy, see cystoscopy, urethroscopy, cystourethroscopy, 52000-52700)

(For injection procedure for urethrocystography, see 51600-51610)

Surgical Procedures on the Urinary System

(For provision of chemotherapeutic agents, report both the specific service in addition to code(s) for the specific substance(s) or drug(s) provided)

Plain English Description

Removal of external urethral caruncle in both men and women may be performed by excision or fulguration, also referred to as electrocautery, electroresection, or laser destruction. With the female in dorsal lithotomy position, the vulva and perineum are prepared and draped. The male is positioned supine and the penis is prepared and draped. Using an Allis clamp, the caruncle is grasped and retracted with slight pressure forward. A scalpel is then used to excise part of the vestibular epithelium and the urethra is transected proximally to the caruncle. The urethral mucosa and vestibular epithelium are now exposed. The two layers are closed using interrupted absorbable sutures, sewing the urethral mucosa to the vestibular epithelium. Fulguration may be performed using an electrocautery device or laser. The electrocautery device or laser is activated and the abnormal tissue is destroyed. A Foley catheter may be placed transurethrally following the procedures.

Excision or fulguration; urethral caruncle

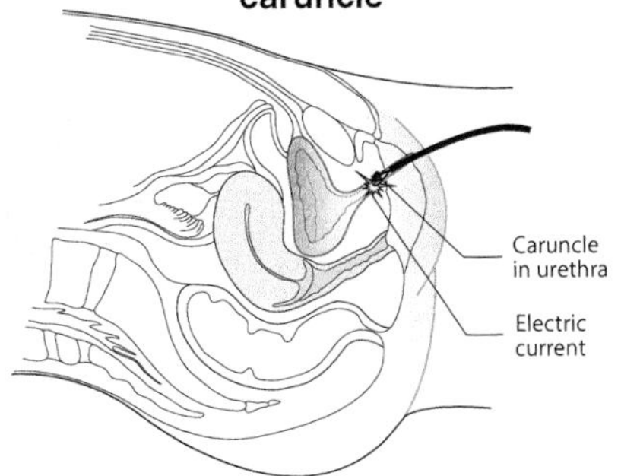

ICD-10-CM Diagnostic Codes

N36.2	Urethral caruncle

CCI Edits

Refer to Appendix A for CCI edits.

Facility RVUs

Code	Work	PE Facility	MP	Total Facility
53265	3.17	1.94	0.42	5.53

Non-facility RVUs

Code	Work	PE Non-Facility	MP	Total Non-Facility
53265	3.17	3.18	0.42	6.77

Modifiers (PAR)

Code	Mod 50	Mod 51	Mod 62	Mod 66	Mod 80
53265	0	2	0	0	1

Global Period

Code	Days
53265	010

53270

53270 Excision or fulguration; Skene's glands

AMA Coding Notes

Surgical Procedures on the Urethra

(For endoscopy, see cystoscopy, urethroscopy, cystourethroscopy, 52000-52700)

(For injection procedure for urethrocystography, see 51600-51610)

Surgical Procedures on the Urinary System

(For provision of chemotherapeutic agents, report both the specific service in addition to code(s) for the specific substance(s) or drug(s) provided)

Plain English Description

Skene's glands, also referred to as lesser vestibular glands, periurethral glands, or paraurethral glands, are located along the sides of the female urethra. Glands that are enlarged due to cysts or infection may be excised by marsupialization or electrocoagulation technique. The glands are located by visualization and/or palpation and an incision made using straight Mayo scissors, one blade in the urethra and the second in the sac of the periurethral gland. The incision is enlarged as needed. The gland is dissected free of surrounding tissue. Tissue samples are prepared and examined by a pathologist as needed in a separately reportable procedure. The incision is closed in layers. The urethral lining and the epithelial lining of the gland are repaired with sutures. Exteriorization of the urinary tract epithelium may result in an enlarged urethral meatus. Fulguration may be performed using an electrocautery device or laser. The electrocautery device or laser is activated and the abnormal tissue is destroyed.

Excision or fulguration; Skene's glands

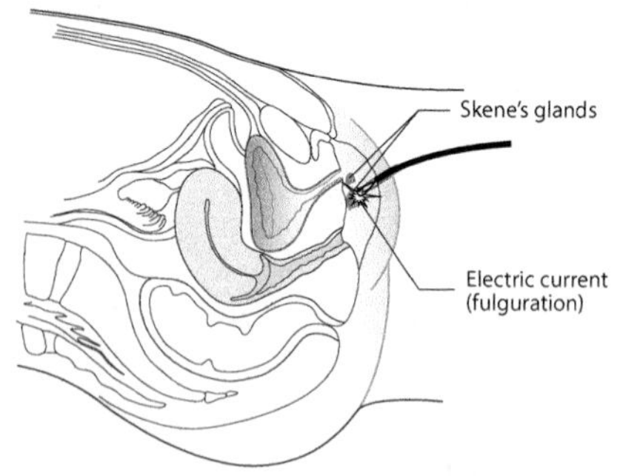

ICD-10-CM Diagnostic Codes

N34.0	Urethral abscess
N34.2	Other urethritis
N36.8	Other specified disorders of urethra
N39.8	Other specified disorders of urinary system

CCI Edits

Refer to Appendix A for CCI edits.

Facility RVUs

Code	Work	PE Facility	MP	Total Facility
53270	3.14	1.90	0.37	5.41

Non-facility RVUs

Code	Work	PE Non-Facility	MP	Total Non-Facility
53270	3.14	2.72	0.37	6.23

Modifiers (PAR)

Code	Mod 50	Mod 51	Mod 62	Mod 66	Mod 80
53270	0	2	0	0	1

Global Period

Code	Days
53270	010

53275

53275 Excision or fulguration; urethral prolapse

AMA Coding Notes

Surgical Procedures on the Urethra

(For endoscopy, see cystoscopy, urethroscopy, cystourethroscopy, 52000-52700)

(For injection procedure for urethrocystography, see 51600-51610)

Surgical Procedures on the Urinary System

(For provision of chemotherapeutic agents, report both the specific service in addition to code(s) for the specific substance(s) or drug(s) provided)

Plain English Description

Several surgical procedures are acceptable to correct a urethral prolapse or urethrocele. Using the Lowe technique, a meatotomy is performed to release constriction of the meatal ring and the prolapsed mucosa is manually reduced. The mucosa and urethra are then tied to the periurethral vestibule using multiple mattress sutures. With the Kelly-Burnham technique, a Foley catheter is placed transurethrally and the prolapsed mucosa is excised circumferentially around it. The edges of the urethral mucosa and introital mucosa are approximated and the incision is closed with interrupted sutures. This technique may be modified by placing holding sutures in the prolapsed mucosa to form quadrants around the urethra. The mucosa is then excised in sections. Prolapsed urethral mucosa may also be removed by fulguration, also referred to as electrocautery, electroresection, or laser destruction. Using an electrocautery device or laser, the device or laser is activated and the abnormal tissue destroyed.

Excision or fulguration; urethral prolapse

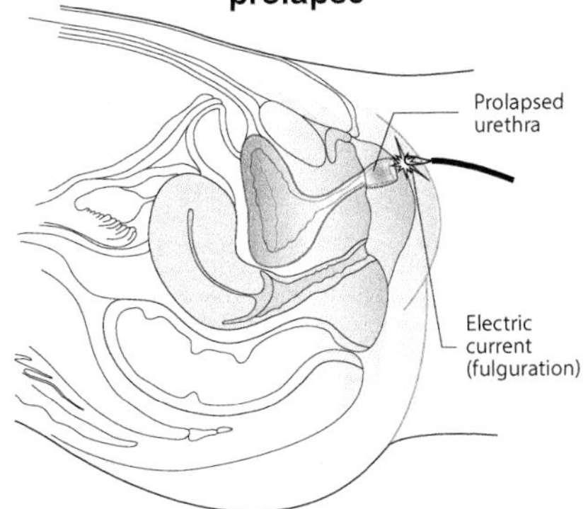

ICD-10-CM Diagnostic Codes

N36.8	Other specified disorders of urethra
Q64.71	Congenital prolapse of urethra

CCI Edits

Refer to Appendix A for CCI edits.

Facility RVUs

Code	Work	PE Facility	MP	Total Facility
53275	4.57	2.56	0.60	7.73

Non-facility RVUs

Code	Work	PE Non-Facility	MP	Total Non-Facility
53275	4.57	2.56	0.60	7.73

Modifiers (PAR)

Code	Mod 50	Mod 51	Mod 62	Mod 66	Mod 80
53275	0	2	0	0	1

Global Period

Code	Days
53275	010

53400-53405

53400 Urethroplasty; first stage, for fistula, diverticulum, or stricture (eg, Johannsen type)

53405 Urethroplasty; second stage (formation of urethra), including urinary diversion

AMA Coding Notes

Repair Procedures on the Urethra

(For hypospadias, see 54300-54352)

Surgical Procedures on the Urethra

(For endoscopy, see cystoscopy, urethroscopy, cystourethroscopy, 52000-52700)

(For injection procedure for urethrocystography, see 51600-51610)

Surgical Procedures on the Urinary System

(For provision of chemotherapeutic agents, report both the specific service in addition to code(s) for the specific substance(s) or drug(s) provided)

Plain English Description

Urethroplasty is performed in two stages. In 53400, the first stage is performed. A skin graft is harvested. In an uncircumcised male, the foreskin can be used. The coronal ridge is marked with ink circumferentially. The prepuce is retracted and adhesions between the glans and prepuce epithelium are lysed. A clamp may be placed with one blade inside the preputial sac and the second on the outer skin creating a crush area at the dorsal midline of the prepuce. The clamp is removed after a few minutes and the crush line is incised using scissors. The prepuce tissue is dissected free of the penis circumferentially along the coronal ridge. Hemostasis is maintained with electrocautery and absorbable sutures are placed to join the skin and preputial epithelium. Alternatively, skin from the inside thigh, groin above the hairline, buttocks, or buccal mucosa is harvested. After the graft has been harvested and prepared, the skin on the penile shaft is incised with a scalpel to expose the urethra. The urethra in incised along the length of the stricture, diverticulum, or fistula until healthy tissue has been exposed proximally and distally. The ostia are calibrated at each end. The prepared graft tissue is laid around the marsupialized urethra and sewn medially to the urethral margin and laterally to the edge of the penile skin with interrupted absorbable sutures. A catheter is placed transurethrally. A percutaneous suprapubic catheter may also be placed into the bladder to divert urine during the postoperative period. In 53405, the second stage is performed once the graft has healed and the epithelium has vascularized. The vascularized epithelial tissue is excised using longitudinal incisions on each side. The proximal and distal ostia are calibrated. If narrowing has occurred, revision of the graft may be performed. The vascularized epithelial tissue is formed into a tubular neourethral structure over a transurethral catheter or stent. The tubular graft is secured using midline anastomosis with a running suture, interspersed with interlocking sutures and the wound is closed in layers. The catheter or stent is left in place.

Urethroplasty; first stage, for fistula, diverticulum, or stricture

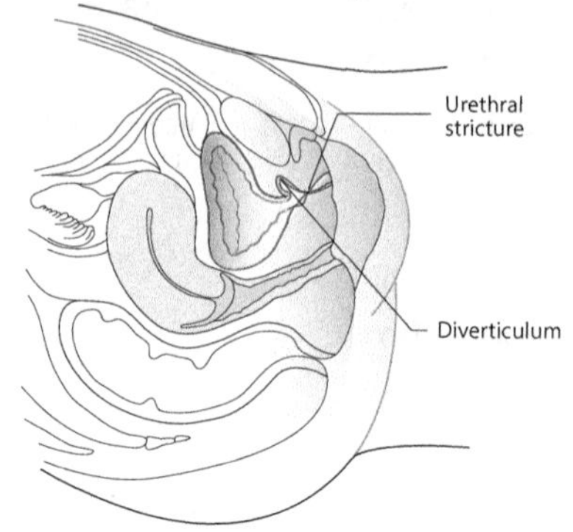

Urethroplasty; first stage for fistula, diverticulum, or stricture (53400); urethroplasty; second stage (formation of urethra), including urinary diversion (53405)

ICD-10-CM Diagnostic Codes

N35.010	Post-traumatic urethral stricture, male, meatal ♂
N35.011	Post-traumatic bulbous urethral stricture ♂
N35.012	Post-traumatic membranous urethral stricture ♂
N35.013	Post-traumatic anterior urethral stricture ♂
N35.016	Post-traumatic urethral stricture, male, overlapping sites ♂
N35.111	Postinfective urethral stricture, not elsewhere classified, male, meatal ♂
N35.112	Postinfective bulbous urethral stricture, not elsewhere classified, male ♂
N35.113	Postinfective membranous urethral stricture, not elsewhere classified, male ♂
N35.114	Postinfective anterior urethral stricture, not elsewhere classified, male ♂
N35.116	Postinfective urethral stricture, not elsewhere classified, male, overlapping sites ♂
N35.811	Other urethral stricture, male, meatal ♂
N35.812	Other urethral bulbous stricture, male ♂
N35.813	Other membranous urethral stricture, male ♂
N35.814	Other anterior urethral stricture, male ♂
N35.816	Other urethral stricture, male, overlapping sites ♂
N36.0	Urethral fistula
N36.1	Urethral diverticulum
N36.8	Other specified disorders of urethra
N37	Urethral disorders in diseases classified elsewhere
N99.110	Postprocedural urethral stricture, male, meatal ♂
N99.111	Postprocedural bulbous urethral stricture, male ♂
N99.112	Postprocedural membranous urethral stricture, male ♂
N99.113	Postprocedural anterior bulbous urethral stricture, male ♂
N99.115	Postprocedural fossa navicularis urethral stricture ♂
N99.116	Postprocedural urethral stricture, male, overlapping sites ♂
N99.89	Other postprocedural complications and disorders of genitourinary system
Q64.32	Congenital stricture of urethra
Q64.39	Other atresia and stenosis of urethra and bladder neck

CCI Edits

Refer to Appendix A for CCI edits.

Facility RVUs □

Code	Work	PE Facility	MP	Total Facility
53400	14.13	7.57	1.70	23.40
53405	15.66	8.01	1.85	25.52

Non-facility RVUs □

Code	Work	PE Non-Facility	MP	Total Non-Facility
53400	14.13	7.57	1.70	23.40
53405	15.66	8.01	1.85	25.52

Modifiers (PAR) □

Code	Mod 50	Mod 51	Mod 62	Mod 66	Mod 80
53400	0	2	1	0	2
53405	0	2	1	0	2

Global Period

Code	Days
53400	090
53405	090

53410

53410 Urethroplasty, 1-stage reconstruction of male anterior urethra

AMA Coding Notes

Repair Procedures on the Urethra

(For hypospadias, see 54300-54352)

Surgical Procedures on the Urethra

(For endoscopy, see cystoscopy, urethroscopy, cystourethroscopy, 52000-52700)

(For injection procedure for urethrocystography, see 51600-51610)

Surgical Procedures on the Urinary System

(For provision of chemotherapeutic agents, report both the specific service in addition to code(s) for the specific substance(s) or drug(s) provided)

Plain English Description

A single stage urethroplasty on the male anterior urethra is most often indicated following trauma or injury. The anterior urethra extends distally from the membranous urethra in three segments. The bulbar segment extends through the proximal corpus spongiosum, ischial cavernosum, and bulbospongiosum until it reaches the penile plane. The penile segment runs the length of the pendulous penis into the third segment, the fossa navicularis in the glans penis. A catheter or urethral sound is used to locate the level of the stricture. A Foley catheter is placed transurethrally into the bladder. A midline incision is made along the ventral penile plane and dissection extended through Buck's fascia until the urethra is identified and adequately exposed. An incision is made along the urethral stricture over the catheter and extended at least 1 cm distally and proximally into healthy urethral tissue is encountered. Using an onlay flap technique, one skin margin is excised to a width not exceeding 25 mm and carried down into the subcutaneous connective tissue. The flap is tapered at each end with the length corresponding to the size of the urethral deficit. At this point the skin edges are checked for approximation to ensure that minimal tension will occur during wound closure. The medial border of the flap is sutured to the incised urethra creating an anchor and then beginning at the distal margin, the flap and the urethral epithelium are sutured together with a running stitch to form a lateral suture line. The free edge of the flap is then rolled and secured to the contralateral margin creating a urethral lumen and a running stitch is made along that margin. Drains may be placed. The subcutaneous connective tissue is closed over the urethral suture lines without injuring the pedicle of the flap. The skin is approximated with minimal tension and closed with a running stitch. The transurethral catheter remains in place.

Urethroplasty, 1-stage reconstruction of male anterior urethra

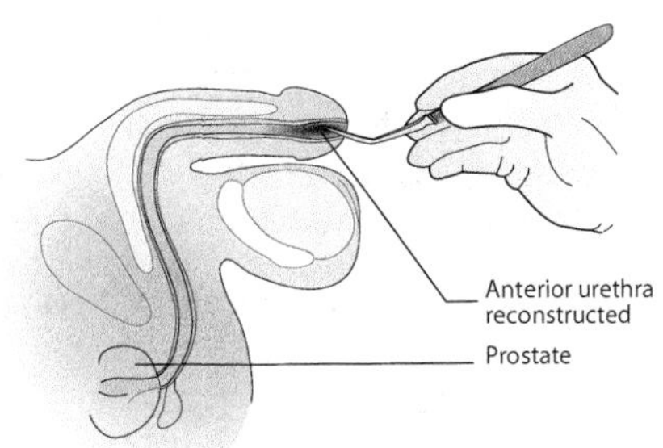

ICD-10-CM Diagnostic Codes

N34.0	Urethral abscess
N34.2	Other urethritis
N35.010	Post-traumatic urethral stricture, male, meatal ♂
N35.011	Post-traumatic bulbous urethral stricture ♂
N35.013	Post-traumatic anterior urethral stricture ♂
N35.016	Post-traumatic urethral stricture, male, overlapping sites ♂
N35.111	Postinfective urethral stricture, not elsewhere classified, male, meatal ♂
N35.112	Postinfective bulbous urethral stricture, not elsewhere classified, male ♂
N35.114	Postinfective anterior urethral stricture, not elsewhere classified, male ♂
N35.116	Postinfective urethral stricture, not elsewhere classified, male, overlapping sites ♂
N35.811	Other urethral stricture, male, meatal ♂
N35.812	Other urethral bulbous stricture, male ♂
N35.814	Other anterior urethral stricture, male ♂
N35.816	Other urethral stricture, male, overlapping sites ♂
N36.0	Urethral fistula
N36.1	Urethral diverticulum
N36.8	Other specified disorders of urethra
N37	Urethral disorders in diseases classified elsewhere
N99.110	Postprocedural urethral stricture, male, meatal ♂
N99.111	Postprocedural bulbous urethral stricture, male ♂
N99.113	Postprocedural anterior bulbous urethral stricture, male ♂
N99.115	Postprocedural fossa navicularis urethral stricture ♂
N99.116	Postprocedural urethral stricture, male, overlapping sites ♂
N99.89	Other postprocedural complications and disorders of genitourinary system
Q64.32	Congenital stricture of urethra
Q64.39	Other atresia and stenosis of urethra and bladder neck

CCI Edits

Refer to Appendix A for CCI edits.

Facility RVUs ▢

Code	Work	PE Facility	MP	Total Facility
53410	17.68	8.84	2.14	28.66

Non-facility RVUs ▢

Code	Work	PE Non-Facility	MP	Total Non-Facility
53410	17.68	8.84	2.14	28.66

Modifiers (PAR) ▢

Code	Mod 50	Mod 51	Mod 62	Mod 66	Mod 80
53410	0	2	1	0	2

Global Period

Code	Days
53410	090

53415

53415 Urethroplasty, transpubic or perineal, 1-stage, for reconstruction or repair of prostatic or membranous urethra

AMA Coding Notes

Repair Procedures on the Urethra

(For hypospadias, see 54300-54352)

Surgical Procedures on the Urethra

(For endoscopy, see cystoscopy, urethroscopy, cystourethroscopy, 52000-52700)

(For injection procedure for urethrocystography, see 51600-51610)

Surgical Procedures on the Urinary System

(For provision of chemotherapeutic agents, report both the specific service in addition to code(s) for the specific substance(s) or drug(s) provided)

Plain English Description

A single-stage repair or reconstruction of the posterior urethra can be accomplished through a transpubic and perineal approach. It is most often indicated following injury or trauma such as pelvic fracture. The posterior urethra is comprised of the prostatic and membranous segments and extends from the bladder neck through the prostate gland, between the prostatic apex and perineal membrane until it connects to the anterior urethra at the bulbar segment. A midline incision is made in the perineum, bifurcating at the posterior end. Dissection continues through the bulbospongiosum muscle, exposing the corpus spongiosum until the urethra is located and mobilized. Proceeding in the direction of the bulbar urethra, the proximal point of obliteration is identified using a catheter and the distal point as far as the suspensory ligament to the penis is assessed. A sound is passed via a previously created suprapubic cystotomy tract through the bladder neck and into the prostatic urethra. Beginning at the level of the crus and working distally, the right and left corporal bodies are separated in the midline for a distance of 4-5 cm allowing the urethra to move upwards and shortening the distance between the urethral ends. If urethral tension remains after separating the corporal bodies, dissection continues by displacing or ligating the penile vessels laterally. Then using bone rongeurs or an osteotome, a wedge of bone is removed from the pubis at the inferior aspect creating a groove for the urethra to settle into and adding 1-2 cm of urethral length. If anastomosis is still not possible due to urethral tension, the urethra is rerouted around the corporal body through a larger resection of the pubic bone by circumferentially mobilizing one of the corporal bodies proximal to the suspensory penile ligament. The distal urethral stump is spatulated and brought down from a 12-o'clock position and the proximal urethral stump is also spatulated and lifted from the 6-o'clock position, healthy tissue is identified along with the seminal ducts in the verumontanum of the prostatic urethra. Anastomosis of the two ends of the urethra is accomplished by placing 8-10 sutures through the urethral mucosa. A fenestrated French catheter is placed transurethrally. The incision is closed in layers and the suprapubic catheter is replaced.

Urethroplasty, transpubic or perineal 1-stage

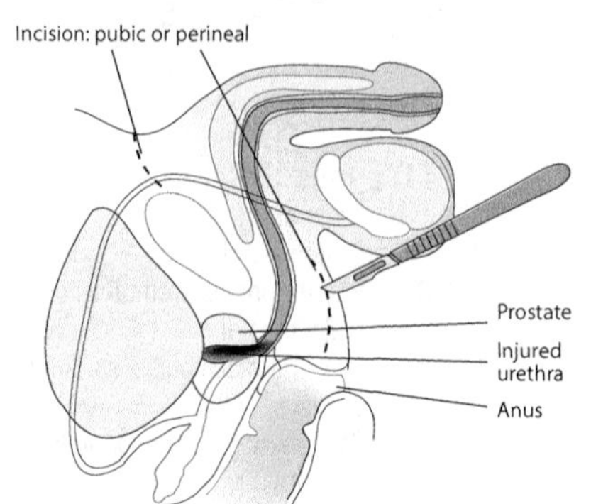

ICD-10-CM Diagnostic Codes

N35.012	Post-traumatic membranous urethral stricture ♂
N35.113	Postinfective membranous urethral stricture, not elsewhere classified, male ♂
N35.813	Other membranous urethral stricture, male ♂
N36.0	Urethral fistula
N36.8	Other specified disorders of urethra
N37	Urethral disorders in diseases classified elsewhere
N40.1	Benign prostatic hyperplasia with lower urinary tract symptoms ♂
N40.3	Nodular prostate with lower urinary tract symptoms ♂
N99.112	Postprocedural membranous urethral stricture, male ♂
N99.113	Postprocedural anterior bulbous urethral stricture, male ♂
Q64.32	Congenital stricture of urethra
Q64.39	Other atresia and stenosis of urethra and bladder neck

CCI Edits

Refer to Appendix A for CCI edits.

Facility RVUs ☐

Code	Work	PE Facility	MP	Total Facility
53415	20.70	9.83	2.48	33.01

Non-facility RVUs ☐

Code	Work	PE Non-Facility	MP	Total Non-Facility
53415	20.70	9.83	2.48	33.01

Modifiers (PAR) ☐

Code	Mod 50	Mod 51	Mod 62	Mod 66	Mod 80
53415	0	2	1	0	2

Global Period

Code	Days
53415	090

53420-53425

53420 Urethroplasty, 2-stage reconstruction or repair of prostatic or membranous urethra; first stage

53425 Urethroplasty, 2-stage reconstruction or repair of prostatic or membranous urethra; second stage

AMA Coding Notes

Repair Procedures on the Urethra

(For hypospadias, see 54300-54352)

Surgical Procedures on the Urethra

(For endoscopy, see cystoscopy, urethroscopy, cystourethroscopy, 52000-52700)

(For injection procedure for urethrocystography, see 51600-51610)

Surgical Procedures on the Urinary System

(For provision of chemotherapeutic agents, report both the specific service in addition to code(s) for the specific substance(s) or drug(s) provided)

Plain English Description

A 2-stage repair of the prostatic or membranous urethra is typically indicated following injury or trauma such as pelvic fracture, prostate surgery, or radiation therapy. In 53420, the first stage is performed using a perineal approach. The prostatic and membranous urethral segments extend from the bladder neck through the prostate gland, between the prostatic apex and perineal membrane, and terminate at the bulbar segment. A previously placed suprapubic catheter is not usually left in place. A midline perineal incision is made. Dissection continues through the bulbospongiosum muscle, exposing the corpus spongiosum until the urethra is located. In the instance of a stricture, the urethra is opened and resected to expose healthy urethral tissue at the distal and proximal ends. If complete transection of the urethra has occurred, the distal and proximal ends are identified and brought to the midline. A previously prepared buccal mucosal graft is used to line the urethral deficit or encase the urethral stumps. The graft is sutured to the perineal skin edges and around the urethral stumps. Urine remains diverted by the suprapubic catheter. In 53425, the second stage of a 2-stage repair is carried out after the graft has vascularized and adequate epithelial tissue is visualized at the perineum. A previously placed suprapubic catheter is left in place. The graft is incised circumferentially from the perineal edge and mobilized laterally. A Foley catheter is placed transurethrally into the bladder and the graft is rolled into a tubular structure around the catheter to form a neourethra. The graft is fixed with sutures at the proximal and distal edges of the stricture opening or the urethral stumps. Drains may be placed and the corpus spongiosum is closed over the newly formed urethra followed by closure of the bulbospongiosum muscle and, finally, closure of the skin. The suprapubic catheter is left in place along with the transurethral catheter.

Urethroplasty, 2-stage repair prostatic or membranous urethra

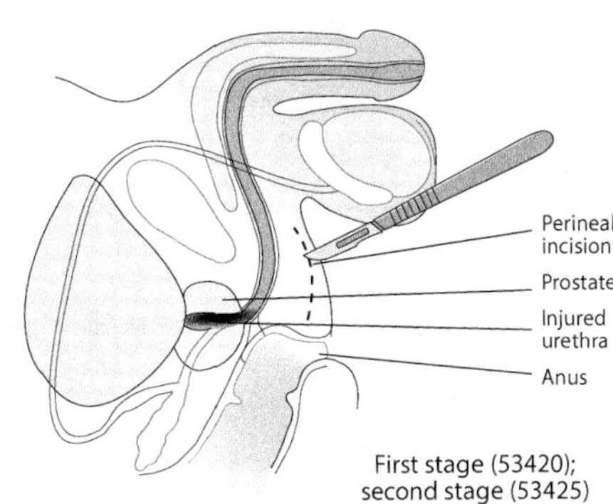

First stage (53420); second stage (53425)

ICD-10-CM Diagnostic Codes

N35.012	Post-traumatic membranous urethral stricture ♂
N35.016	Post-traumatic urethral stricture, male, overlapping sites ♂
N35.113	Postinfective membranous urethral stricture, not elsewhere classified, male ♂
N35.116	Postinfective urethral stricture, not elsewhere classified, male, overlapping sites ♂
N35.816	Other urethral stricture, male, overlapping sites ♂
N36.0	Urethral fistula
N36.8	Other specified disorders of urethra
N37	Urethral disorders in diseases classified elsewhere
N99.112	Postprocedural membranous urethral stricture, male ♂
N99.116	Postprocedural urethral stricture, male, overlapping sites ♂
Q64.32	Congenital stricture of urethra
Q64.39	Other atresia and stenosis of urethra and bladder neck

CCI Edits

Refer to Appendix A for CCI edits.

Facility RVUs ☐

Code	Work	PE Facility	MP	Total Facility
53420	15.17	7.62	1.81	24.60
53425	17.07	8.27	2.03	27.37

Non-facility RVUs ☐

Code	Work	PE Non-Facility	MP	Total Non-Facility
53420	15.17	7.62	1.81	24.60
53425	17.07	8.27	2.03	27.37

Modifiers (PAR) ☐

Code	Mod 50	Mod 51	Mod 62	Mod 66	Mod 80
53420	0	2	1	0	1
53425	0	2	1	0	2

Global Period

Code	Days
53420	090
53425	090

53430

53430 Urethroplasty, reconstruction of female urethra

AMA Coding Notes

Repair Procedures on the Urethra

(For hypospadias, see 54300-54352)

Surgical Procedures on the Urethra

(For endoscopy, see cystoscopy, urethroscopy, cystourethroscopy, 52000-52700)

(For injection procedure for urethrocystography, see 51600-51610)

Surgical Procedures on the Urinary System

(For provision of chemotherapeutic agents, report both the specific service in addition to code(s) for the specific substance(s) or drug(s) provided)

Plain English Description

There are a number of accepted techniques for reconstruction of the female urethra. A Foley catheter is inserted transurethrally. A suprapubic catheter may also be inserted. Using an inverted U-shaped incision on the anterior wall of the vagina, the urethral defect is identified. An incision is made over one of the labia forming a flap that includes the labial fat pad. The urethra is repaired using a Martius flap, which includes the labial flap and the fat pad. The flap is sutured under the urethral repair to provide support. If there is limited periurethral or vaginal tissue, a technique that allows for rotation of the flap may be used. Using a U-shaped anterior vaginal incision, the flap is mobilized from the vaginal wall, rotated distally, and sutured as a dorsal onlay flap creating a tubular neourethra over the Foley catheter. The vaginal wall harvest site is closed with sutures. In both procedures, drains may be placed and the vaginal mucosa is then closed in layers with absorbable sutures. A less frequently used technique involves a dorsal approach and a buccal mucosal graft. The dorsal area of the urethral meatus is exposed using a U-shaped incision. The vulvar mucosa is dissected from the urethral channel to develop a plane between the urethra and the cavernous tissue of the clitoris. The anterior portion of the urethral sphincter is identified and carefully moved upward. The bladder neck is located and identified with a stitch and an incision made lengthwise in the urethra. The prepared buccal mucosal graft is sutured to the right and left sides of the urethral opening. The reinforced dorsal urethra is sutured to the clitoral body forming the new urethral roof. The graft tissue is tailored to make a normal meatal opening. The vulvar incision is closed with absorbable sutures. The Foley catheter remains in place.

Reconstruction of female urethra

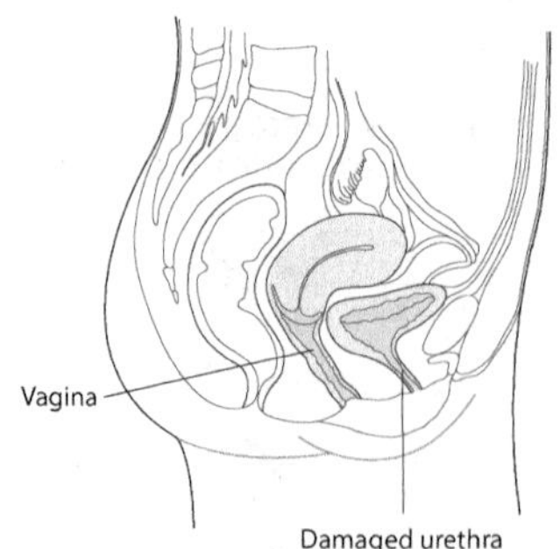

The physician reconstructs the urethra of a female patient.

ICD-10-CM Diagnostic Codes

	N35.021	Urethral stricture due to childbirth ♀
	N35.028	Other post-traumatic urethral stricture, female ♀
	N35.12	Postinfective urethral stricture, not elsewhere classified, female ♀
	N35.82	Other urethral stricture, female ♀
	N35.92	Unspecified urethral stricture, female ♀
	N99.12	Postprocedural urethral stricture, female ♀
➐	S37.30	Unspecified injury of urethra
➐	S37.33	Laceration of urethra
➐	S37.39	Other injury of urethra

ICD-10-CM Coding Notes

For codes requiring a 7th character extension, refer to your ICD-10-CM book. Review the character descriptions and coding guidelines for proper selection. For some procedures, only certain characters will apply.

CCI Edits

Refer to Appendix A for CCI edits.

Facility RVUs ▯

Code	Work	PE Facility	MP	Total Facility
53430	17.43	8.73	2.37	28.53

Non-facility RVUs ▯

Code	Work	PE Non-Facility	MP	Total Non-Facility
53430	17.43	8.73	2.37	28.53

Modifiers (PAR) ▯

Code	Mod 50	Mod 51	Mod 62	Mod 66	Mod 80
53430	0	2	1	0	2

Global Period

Code	Days
53430	090

53431

53431 Urethroplasty with tubularization of posterior urethra and/or lower bladder for incontinence (eg, Tenago, Leadbetter procedure)

AMA Coding Notes

Repair Procedures on the Urethra

(For hypospadias, see 54300-54352)

Surgical Procedures on the Urethra

(For endoscopy, see cystoscopy, urethroscopy, cystourethroscopy, 52000-52700)

(For injection procedure for urethrocystography, see 51600-51610)

Surgical Procedures on the Urinary System

(For provision of chemotherapeutic agents, report both the specific service in addition to code(s) for the specific substance(s) or drug(s) provided)

Plain English Description

The physician lengthens the urethra or the lower part of the bladder with muscle tissue from the bladder. This procedure is performed to relieve a condition in which the patient cannot control the release of urine.

Urethroplasty with tubularization of posterior urethra and/or lower bladder for incontinence

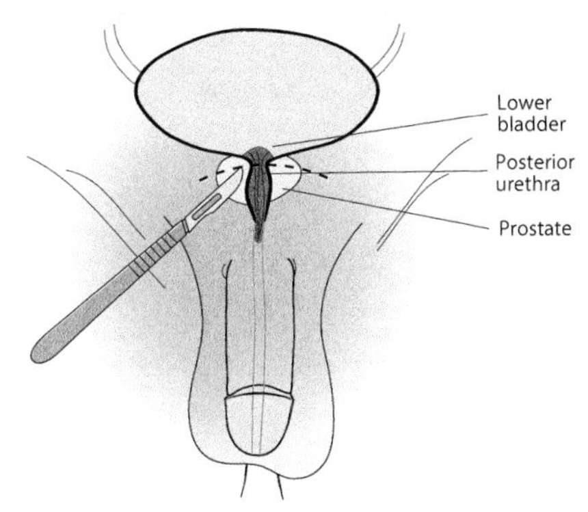

ICD-10-CM Diagnostic Codes

N31.0	Uninhibited neuropathic bladder, not elsewhere classified
N31.1	Reflex neuropathic bladder, not elsewhere classified
N31.2	Flaccid neuropathic bladder, not elsewhere classified
N31.8	Other neuromuscular dysfunction of bladder
N31.9	Neuromuscular dysfunction of bladder, unspecified
N36.41	Hypermobility of urethra
N36.42	Intrinsic sphincter deficiency (ISD)
N36.43	Combined hypermobility of urethra and intrinsic sphincter deficiency
N36.44	Muscular disorders of urethra
N39.3	Stress incontinence (female) (male)
N39.41	Urge incontinence
N39.42	Incontinence without sensory awareness
N39.43	Post-void dribbling
N39.44	Nocturnal enuresis
N39.45	Continuous leakage
N39.490	Overflow incontinence
N39.498	Other specified urinary incontinence

CCI Edits

Refer to Appendix A for CCI edits.

Facility RVUs ▯

Code	Work	PE Facility	MP	Total Facility
53431	21.18	9.95	2.51	33.64

Non-facility RVUs ▯

Code	Work	PE Non-Facility	MP	Total Non-Facility
53431	21.18	9.95	2.51	33.64

Modifiers (PAR) ▯

Code	Mod 50	Mod 51	Mod 62	Mod 66	Mod 80
53431	0	2	1	0	2

Global Period

Code	Days
53431	090

53440

53440 Sling operation for correction of male urinary incontinence (eg, fascia or synthetic)

AMA Coding Notes

Repair Procedures on the Urethra

(For hypospadias, see 54300-54352)

Surgical Procedures on the Urethra

(For endoscopy, see cystoscopy, urethroscopy, cystourethroscopy, 52000-52700)

(For injection procedure for urethrocystography, see 51600-51610)

Surgical Procedures on the Urinary System

(For provision of chemotherapeutic agents, report both the specific service in addition to code(s) for the specific substance(s) or drug(s) provided)

Plain English Description

The sling procedure to correct male urinary incontinence is accomplished by using an allograft, xenograft, or synthetic mesh graft. A Foley catheter is inserted transurethrally. A transverse suprapubic incision is made and the rectus fascia exposed. The rectus fascia is incised allowing access to the retropubic space. A U-shaped perineal incision is made in the skin and carried down through the bulbospongiosum muscle to the corpus spongiosum. Dissection continues until the urethra is identified. The urethra is dissected and the retropubic space entered on both sides of the urethra. A ligature passer is inserted into the retropubic space through the suprapubic incision, the endopelvic fascia is perforated, and the ligature passer then exits through the perineal incision on one side of the urethra. A sling graft is placed under the urethra and one end attached to the ligature passer. The graft is then pulled through the endopelvic fascia into the retropubic space. The graft is detached from the ligature passer and the ligature passer is again passed through the suprapubic incision and endopelvic fascia exiting on the opposite side of the urethra. The other end of the sling graft is attached to the ligature passer and pulled into the retropubic space. The sling is now seated under the urethra. Tension of the sling is adjusted to provide adequate support without obstructing the urethra. The perineal wound is closed. The sling sutures are tunneled through the rectus fascia. The rectus fascia is closed and the sling sutures are tied down over the closed fascia. The suprapubic fascia is closed. Alternatively, the graft may be secured to the pubic rami. Using a bone drill, three screws with sutures are driven into each side of the pubic rami proximally at the level of the bulbar urethra and distally below the pubic symphysis. The graft material is secured to the bone on one side with sutures and on the other with temporary pass through sutures. The tension on the sling is adjusted. The sutures are securely tied. The incision is closed in layers.

Sling operation for correction of male urinary incontinence

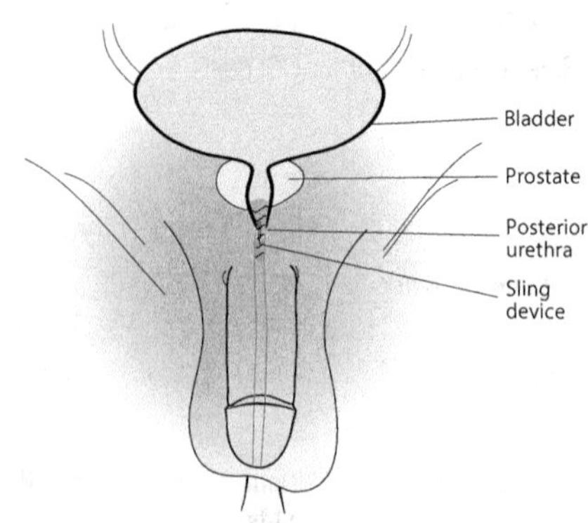

ICD-10-CM Diagnostic Codes

N36.41	Hypermobility of urethra
N36.42	Intrinsic sphincter deficiency (ISD)
N36.43	Combined hypermobility of urethra and intrinsic sphincter deficiency
N36.44	Muscular disorders of urethra
N39.3	Stress incontinence (female) (male)
N39.490	Overflow incontinence
N39.491	Coital incontinence
N39.492	Postural (urinary) incontinence
N39.498	Other specified urinary incontinence

CCI Edits

Refer to Appendix A for CCI edits.

Facility RVUs

Code	Work	PE Facility	MP	Total Facility
53440	13.36	7.08	1.59	22.03

Non-facility RVUs

Code	Work	PE Non-Facility	MP	Total Non-Facility
53440	13.36	7.08	1.59	22.03

Modifiers (PAR)

Code	Mod 50	Mod 51	Mod 62	Mod 66	Mod 80
53440	0	2	1	0	2

Global Period

Code	Days
53440	090

53442

53442 Removal or revision of sling for male urinary incontinence (eg, fascia or synthetic)

AMA Coding Notes

Repair Procedures on the Urethra

(For hypospadias, see 54300-54352)

Surgical Procedures on the Urethra

(For endoscopy, see cystoscopy, urethroscopy, cystourethroscopy, 52000-52700)

(For injection procedure for urethrocystography, see 51600-51610)

Surgical Procedures on the Urinary System

(For provision of chemotherapeutic agents, report both the specific service in addition to code(s) for the specific substance(s) or drug(s) provided)

Plain English Description

Removal or revision of the urethral sling in males is rarely necessary, but may be performed for failure of the sling, pain, or infection. A transurethral catheter is inserted into the bladder. The perineum is incised under the scrotum. Dissection is carried down to the bulbospongiosus muscles and continues until the urethra and sling are exposed. If the sling is revised, it is freed from surrounding tissue and tension readjusted as needed. If the sling is removed, the sling is freed from the surrounding tissue, taking care not to cause further injury to the urethra or surrounding blood vessels. The sling is mobilized up to the endopelvic fascia on both sides of the pelvis. The abdomen is incised just above the pubic bone and the abdominal ends of the sling identified. The rectus fascia is incised and the sling mobilized within the retropubic space down to the endopelvic fascia. Alternatively, if the sling has been secured to the pubic rami, the bone screws are removed. When the sling is completely mobilized, it is removed through the perineal incision. Eroded urethral tissue is debrided and the urethra closed. The abdominal and perineal wounds are irrigated with antibiotic solution. Drains are placed as needed. The abdominal and perineal incisions are individually closed around the drains.

Removal or revision of sling for male urinary incontinence

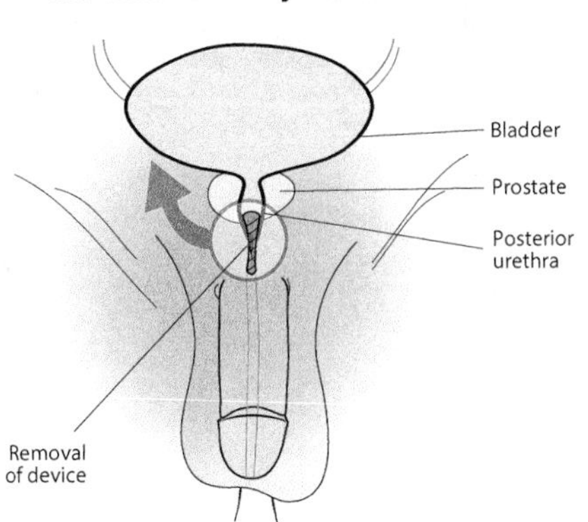

ICD-10-CM Diagnostic Codes

- ➐ T83.111 Breakdown (mechanical) of implanted urinary sphincter
- ➐ T83.121 Displacement of implanted urinary sphincter
- ➐ T83.191 Other mechanical complication of implanted urinary sphincter
- ➐ T83.69 Infection and inflammatory reaction due to other prosthetic device, implant and graft in genital tract
- ➐ T83.719 Erosion of other prosthetic materials to surrounding organ or tissue
- ➐ T83.81 Embolism due to genitourinary prosthetic devices, implants and grafts
- ➐ T83.82 Fibrosis due to genitourinary prosthetic devices, implants and grafts
- ➐ T83.83 Hemorrhage due to genitourinary prosthetic devices, implants and grafts
- ➐ T83.84 Pain due to genitourinary prosthetic devices, implants and grafts
- ➐ T83.85 Stenosis due to genitourinary prosthetic devices, implants and grafts
- ➐ T83.86 Thrombosis due to genitourinary prosthetic devices, implants and grafts
- ➐ T83.89 Other specified complication of genitourinary prosthetic devices, implants and grafts

ICD-10-CM Coding Notes

For codes requiring a 7th character extension, refer to your ICD-10-CM book. Review the character descriptions and coding guidelines for proper selection. For some procedures, only certain characters will apply.

CCI Edits

Refer to Appendix A for CCI edits.

Facility RVUs ☐

Code	Work	PE Facility	MP	Total Facility
53442	13.49	7.89	1.61	22.99

Non-facility RVUs ☐

Code	Work	PE Non-Facility	MP	Total Non-Facility
53442	13.49	7.89	1.61	22.99

Modifiers (PAR) ☐

Code	Mod 50	Mod 51	Mod 62	Mod 66	Mod 80
53442	0	2	0	0	2

Global Period

Code	Days
53442	090

53444

53444 Insertion of tandem cuff (dual cuff)

AMA Coding Notes

Repair Procedures on the Urethra

(For hypospadias, see 54300-54352)

Surgical Procedures on the Urethra

(For endoscopy, see cystoscopy, urethroscopy, cystourethroscopy, 52000-52700)

(For injection procedure for urethrocystography, see 51600-51610)

Surgical Procedures on the Urinary System

(For provision of chemotherapeutic agents, report both the specific service in addition to code(s) for the specific substance(s) or drug(s) provided)

Plain English Description

Insertion of a tandem or dual cuff following insertion of an artificial urinary sphincter (AUS) system is performed when there is failure with the originally placed cuff. An incision is made at the level of the bulbous urethra where the cuff is located. The cuff is exposed and mobilized. The cuff and tubing are freed from the urethra. The tubing is clamped and the existing cuff removed. The urethral diameter is sized. Two appropriately sized cuffs are then placed around the urethra and connected to the existing tubing. The AUS system is activated. The bladder is filled and the cuffs evaluated for leakage. Once it has been determined that the AUS system is functioning properly without leakage, the surgical wound is closed.

Insertion of tandem cuff (dual cuff)

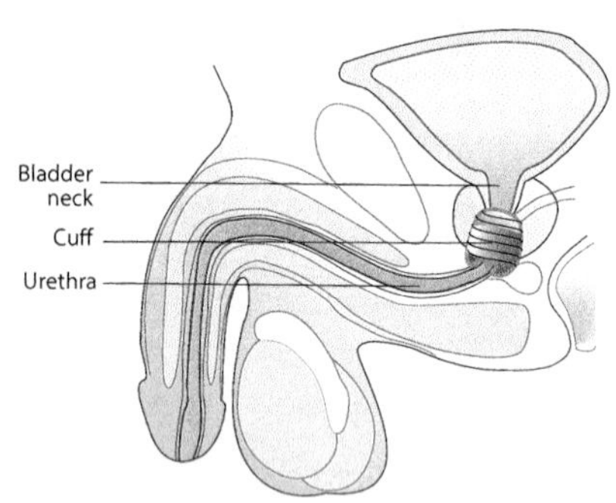

ICD-10-CM Diagnostic Codes

N39.3	Stress incontinence (female) (male)
N39.41	Urge incontinence
N39.42	Incontinence without sensory awareness
N39.43	Post-void dribbling
N39.46	Mixed incontinence
N39.490	Overflow incontinence
N39.491	Coital incontinence
N39.492	Postural (urinary) incontinence
N39.498	Other specified urinary incontinence

CCI Edits

Refer to Appendix A for CCI edits.

Facility RVUs ☐

Code	Work	PE Facility	MP	Total Facility
53444	14.19	7.34	1.68	23.21

Non-facility RVUs ☐

Code	Work	PE Non-Facility	MP	Total Non-Facility
53444	14.19	7.34	1.68	23.21

Modifiers (PAR) ☐

Code	Mod 50	Mod 51	Mod 62	Mod 66	Mod 80
53444	0	2	1	0	2

Global Period

Code	Days
53444	090

53445

53445 Insertion of inflatable urethral/bladder neck sphincter, including placement of pump, reservoir, and cuff

AMA Coding Notes

Repair Procedures on the Urethra

(For hypospadias, see 54300-54352)

Surgical Procedures on the Urethra

(For endoscopy, see cystoscopy, urethroscopy, cystourethroscopy, 52000-52700)

(For injection procedure for urethrocystography, see 51600-51610)

Surgical Procedures on the Urinary System

(For provision of chemotherapeutic agents, report both the specific service in addition to code(s) for the specific substance(s) or drug(s) provided)

Plain English Description

An artificial urinary sphincter (AUS) is used to control the flow of urine from the bladder through the urethra and can be implanted in both men and women. A catheter is placed transurethrally. In male patients, a midline incision is made in the perineum just below the scrotum, carried down through the Colles' fascia and the bulbocavernosus muscle. The urethra is freed circumferentially from surrounding tissue. The catheter is removed so that an accurate circumference of the urethra can be measured. The urethra is measured and an appropriately sized urethral sphincter cuff is chosen. The cuff is prepared and filled with an iso-osmotic solution and passed tab first around the urethra, snapped in place and the tab rotated dorsally. The cuff tubing is then routed through a subcutaneous tunnel to the abdomen. The perineal incision is closed in layers and the surgeon begins the next phase of the surgery through the abdomen. A midline or transverse suprapubic incision is made in the skin and carried down to divide the rectus fascia. The linea alba is opened and the prevesical space is accessed creating a pocket large enough to accommodate the balloon. The balloon is prepared and filled with the iso-osmotic solution and the tubing clamped. The balloon is positioned in the prevesical space and the tubing routed through the rectus fascia to the abdominal incision. The pump is prepared with the iso-osmotic solution. From the abdominal incision, dissection is carried down to the chosen hemiscrotum creating a dependent subdartos pouch. The pump is placed in the pouch with the locking button facing out. The pump tubing should remain above the rectus muscle and fascia in the abdominal incision. After the components are in place, the connecting tubing is trimmed and ends sealed with sutureless connectors. The device is cycled 2 or 3 times to check for fluid leaks and functionality and the cuff is then locked in open position. The abdominal incision is closed in layers and a catheter is again inserted transurethrally. Implantation of an AUS in women is accomplished through a transverse midline incision in the lower abdomen with or without a U-shaped anterior wall incision in the vagina. The abdomen is incised and the rectus muscle separated to enter the retropubic space. The bladder is separated from the pubic symphysis. Bilateral tunnels are created through the endopelvic fascia extending below the urethra and exiting in the anterior wall of the vagina. If the procedure is performed with an anterior vaginal wall incision, the retro pubic space is entered laterally from the undersurface of the pubic bone. The bladder neck and urethra are mobilized. The cuff, tubing, and balloon are placed as described above and the pump is placed in the labia majora. The device is tested as described above and the incisions are closed.

Insertion of inflatable urethral/bladder neck sphincter

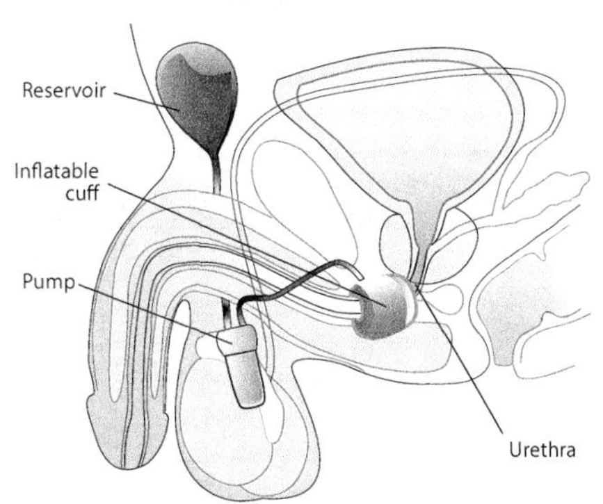

ICD-10-CM Diagnostic Codes

N36.42	Intrinsic sphincter deficiency (ISD)
N36.44	Muscular disorders of urethra
N39.3	Stress incontinence (female) (male)
N39.42	Incontinence without sensory awareness
N39.43	Post-void dribbling
N39.44	Nocturnal enuresis
N39.45	Continuous leakage
N39.46	Mixed incontinence
N39.490	Overflow incontinence
N39.491	Coital incontinence
N39.492	Postural (urinary) incontinence
N39.498	Other specified urinary incontinence

CCI Edits

Refer to Appendix A for CCI edits.

Pub 100

53445: Pub 100-03, 1, 230.10

Facility RVUs ☐

Code	Work	PE Facility	MP	Total Facility
53445	13.00	7.60	1.54	22.14

Non-facility RVUs ☐

Code	Work	PE Non-Facility	MP	Total Non-Facility
53445	13.00	7.60	1.54	22.14

Modifiers (PAR) ☐

Code	Mod 50	Mod 51	Mod 62	Mod 66	Mod 80
53445	0	2	1	0	2

Global Period

Code	Days
53445	090

53446-53448

53446 Removal of inflatable urethral/bladder neck sphincter, including pump, reservoir, and cuff

53447 Removal and replacement of inflatable urethral/bladder neck sphincter including pump, reservoir, and cuff at the same operative session

53448 Removal and replacement of inflatable urethral/bladder neck sphincter including pump, reservoir, and cuff through an infected field at the same operative session including irrigation and debridement of infected tissue

(Do not report 11042, 11043 in addition to 53448)

AMA Coding Notes

Repair Procedures on the Urethra

(For hypospadias, see 54300-54352)

Surgical Procedures on the Urethra

(For endoscopy, see cystoscopy, urethroscopy, cystourethroscopy, 52000-52700)

(For injection procedure for urethrocystography, see 51600-51610)

Surgical Procedures on the Urinary System

(For provision of chemotherapeutic agents, report both the specific service in addition to code(s) for the specific substance(s) or drug(s) provided)

Plain English Description

The artificial urinary sphincter, or AUS, is removed through the same incision site(s) used to implant the device. In 53446, the AUS is removed without replacement. A catheter is placed transurethrally. In male patients, a midline incision is made in the perineum just below the scrotum, carried down through the Colles' fascia and the bulbocavernosus muscle. The tubing is clamped and the cuff is freed from the urethra and surrounding tissue. The tubing is tracked through the subcutaneous tunnel to the abdomen and dissected free from surrounding tissue. A midline or transverse suprapubic incision is made in the skin and carried down to divide the rectus fascia. The linea alba is opened and the balloon and tubing dissected free from the tissue in the prevesical space. The tubing is then tracked to the subdartos pouch in the hemiscrotum and the pump and tubing are dissected free from the surrounding tissue. In women, removal is accomplished through an incision in the lower abdomen with or without a separate anterior wall incision in the vagina. The abdomen is incised and the rectus muscle separated to enter the retropubic space. The balloon is located and dissected free from surrounding tissue, tubing is tracked and dissected to the endopelvic fascia and the anterior wall of the vagina. In a transvaginal approach, tubing is tracked and dissected upwards to the retropubic space. The cuff is located and dissected free from the urethra followed by tracking of tubing and dissection to the pump in the labia majora. In both men and women, the tubing is then clamped to avoid fluid leakage into the surgical wound and the device is removed through the incisions. Drains may be placed and the abdominal and perineal/vaginal incisions are closed in layers. In 53447, the removal is performed as described above and replaced with a new AUS system. A flexible cuff is placed around the bladder neck or urethra. A reservoir of liquid is placed next to the cuff and attached to the cuff with tubing. A pump is placed in the scrotum in males or the labia majora in females. The AUS system is tested for functionality and the incisions are closed. Use 53448 if the removal and replacement are performed on a patient with an infection due to the device. The procedure is performed as described above except that the wound is copiously irrigated with an antibiotic solution and extra care must be taken to ensure that all infected and necrotic tissue has been debrided.

Removal of inflatable urethral/bladder neck sphincter including pump, reservoir, and cuff

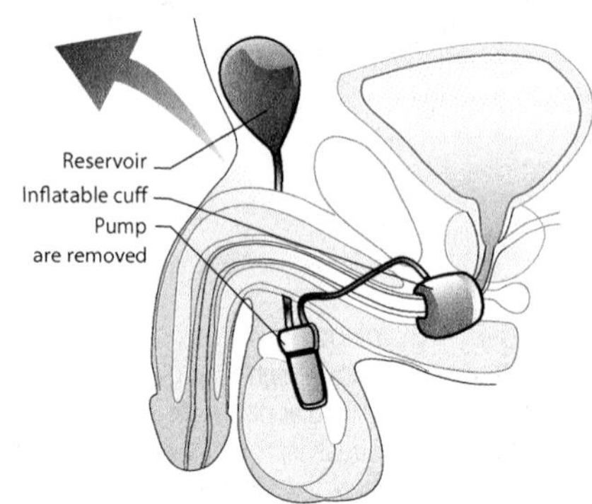

ICD-10-CM Diagnostic Codes

	N99.81	Other intraoperative complications of genitourinary system
	N99.840	Postprocedural hematoma of a genitourinary system organ or structure following a genitourinary system procedure
	N99.842	Postprocedural seroma of a genitourinary system organ or structure following a genitourinary system procedure
	N99.89	Other postprocedural complications and disorders of genitourinary system
❼	T83.111	Breakdown (mechanical) of implanted urinary sphincter
❼	T83.121	Displacement of implanted urinary sphincter
❼	T83.191	Other mechanical complication of implanted urinary sphincter
❼	T83.591	Infection and inflammatory reaction due to implanted urinary sphincter
❼	T83.69	Infection and inflammatory reaction due to other prosthetic device, implant and graft in genital tract
❼	T83.81	Embolism due to genitourinary prosthetic devices, implants and grafts
❼	T83.82	Fibrosis due to genitourinary prosthetic devices, implants and grafts
❼	T83.83	Hemorrhage due to genitourinary prosthetic devices, implants and grafts
❼	T83.84	Pain due to genitourinary prosthetic devices, implants and grafts
❼	T83.85	Stenosis due to genitourinary prosthetic devices, implants and grafts
❼	T83.86	Thrombosis due to genitourinary prosthetic devices, implants and grafts
❼	T83.89	Other specified complication of genitourinary prosthetic devices, implants and grafts

ICD-10-CM Coding Notes

For codes requiring a 7th character extension, refer to your ICD-10-CM book. Review the character descriptions and coding guidelines for proper selection. For some procedures, only certain characters will apply.

CCI Edits

Refer to Appendix A for CCI edits.

Pub 100

53446: Pub 100-03, 1, 230.10

53448: Pub 100-03, 1, 230.10

Facility RVUs

Code	Work	PE Facility	MP	Total Facility
53446	11.02	6.50	1.32	18.84
53447	14.28	7.63	1.70	23.61
53448	23.44	11.03	2.80	37.27

Non-facility RVUs

Code	Work	PE Non-Facility	MP	Total Non-Facility
53446	11.02	6.50	1.32	18.84
53447	14.28	7.63	1.70	23.61
53448	23.44	11.03	2.80	37.27

Modifiers (PAR)

Code	Mod 50	Mod 51	Mod 62	Mod 66	Mod 80
53446	0	2	1	0	2
53447	0	2	1	0	2
53448	0	2	1	0	2

Global Period

Code	Days
53446	090
53447	090
53448	090

53449

53449 Repair of inflatable urethral/ bladder neck sphincter, including pump, reservoir, and cuff

AMA Coding Notes

Repair Procedures on the Urethra

(For hypospadias, see 54300-54352)

Surgical Procedures on the Urethra

(For endoscopy, see cystoscopy, urethroscopy, cystourethroscopy, 52000-52700)

(For injection procedure for urethrocystography, see 51600-51610)

Surgical Procedures on the Urinary System

(For provision of chemotherapeutic agents, report both the specific service in addition to code(s) for the specific substance(s) or drug(s) provided)

Plain English Description

Mechanical failure of the artificial urinary sphincter (AUS) is most often due to depressurization such as loss of fluid or disconnection but may also result from obstruction caused by tubing kinks or inadequate position of the pump. Physical examination or radiologic or urodynamic studies are employed first to try and diagnose the problem. If surgical intervention is necessary, small incisions are made in the lower abdomen to access the balloon and tubing that connects the balloon to the cuff and pump. The tubing is disconnected and using a syringe, iso-osmotic fluid is injected into the balloon to visually inspect for leaks. Next, a syringe is used to inject 1-2 mL of solution into the cuff to check for leaks. After a minute has elapsed, the same amount of fluid should be drawn back out if no leak is present. Pump function is assessed by attaching syringes to the tubing coming from the cuff and balloon and with external manipulation of the pump, fluid is observed shifting between the two syringes. This manipulation may remove air bubbles or debris, which could be the cause of pump malfunction. If any component of the device is found to be defective, it is replaced. Tubing that is kinked is shortened or rerouted in a straighter pathway. Tubing is reconnected and the device is cycled a few times before the small surgical incisions are closed in layers.

Repair of inflatable urethral/bladder neck sphincter

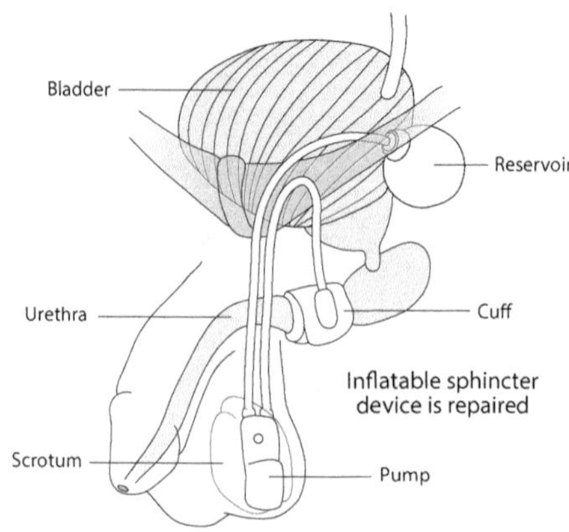

ICD-10-CM Diagnostic Codes

T83.111A	Breakdown (mechanical) of implanted urinary sphincter, initial encounter
T83.121A	Displacement of implanted urinary sphincter, initial encounter
T83.191A	Other mechanical complication of implanted urinary sphincter, initial encounter
T83.89XA	Other specified complication of genitourinary prosthetic devices, implants and grafts, initial encounter

CCI Edits

Refer to Appendix A for CCI edits.

Pub 100

53449: Pub 100-03, 1, 230.10

Facility RVUs

Code	Work	PE Facility	MP	Total Facility
53449	10.56	6.14	1.27	17.97

Non-facility RVUs

Code	Work	PE Non-Facility	MP	Total Non-Facility
53449	10.56	6.14	1.27	17.97

Modifiers (PAR)

Code	Mod 50	Mod 51	Mod 62	Mod 66	Mod 80
53449	0	2	1	0	2

Global Period

Code	Days
53449	090

53450

53450 Urethromeatoplasty, with mucosal advancement

(For meatotomy, see 53020, 53025)

AMA Coding Notes

Repair Procedures on the Urethra

(For hypospadias, see 54300-54352)

Surgical Procedures on the Urethra

(For endoscopy, see cystoscopy, urethroscopy, cystourethroscopy, 52000-52700)

(For injection procedure for urethrocystography, see 51600-51610)

Surgical Procedures on the Urinary System

(For provision of chemotherapeutic agents, report both the specific service in addition to code(s) for the specific substance(s) or drug(s) provided)

AMA *CPT® Assistant* ☐

53450: Sep 12: 16

Plain English Description

Urethromeatoplasty is a procedure to enlarge or reconstruct the opening of the urethra at the distal tip of the penis to improve urination. The urethra is the hollow tube extending from the bladder to the meatus through which urine drains and sperm is ejaculated. The most common cause of urethral narrowing is scarring of the mucosal tissue due to irritation, inflammation, infection, or injury. Meatal stenosis may also be congenital. Symptoms of urethral narrowing can include painful urination, frequent urination, inability to empty the bladder, and upward or sideways urine flow. In 53450, the urethral meatus is opened and a mucosal flap is formed and sutured to the glans. In 53460, a ventral incision in the penis is made and skin is freed from the shaft. Fibrous tissue causing narrowing within the distal urethra is removed and the opening is repaired.

ICD-10-CM Diagnostic Codes

N34.2	Other urethritis
N34.3	Urethral syndrome, unspecified
N35.010	Post-traumatic urethral stricture, male, meatal ♂
N35.028	Other post-traumatic urethral stricture, female ♀
N35.111	Postinfective urethral stricture, not elsewhere classified, male, meatal ♂
N35.12	Postinfective urethral stricture, not elsewhere classified, female ♀
N35.82	Other urethral stricture, female ♀
N36.1	Urethral diverticulum
N36.2	Urethral caruncle
N36.8	Other specified disorders of urethra
N37	Urethral disorders in diseases classified elsewhere
N47.6	Balanoposthitis ♂
N48.0	Leukoplakia of penis ♂
N48.1	Balanitis ♂
N49.8	Inflammatory disorders of other specified male genital organs ♂
N81.0	Urethrocele ♀
N99.110	Postprocedural urethral stricture, male, meatal ♂
N99.115	Postprocedural fossa navicularis urethral stricture ♂
Q64.33	Congenital stricture of urinary meatus
R33.8	Other retention of urine
R35.0	Frequency of micturition
R39.12	Poor urinary stream
R39.14	Feeling of incomplete bladder emptying

CCI Edits

Refer to Appendix A for CCI edits.

Facility RVUs ☐

Code	Work	PE Facility	MP	Total Facility
53450	6.77	4.44	0.79	12.00

Non-facility RVUs ☐

Code	Work	PE Non-Facility	MP	Total Non-Facility
53450	6.77	4.44	0.79	12.00

Modifiers (PAR) ☐

Code	Mod 50	Mod 51	Mod 62	Mod 66	Mod 80
53450	0	2	0	0	1

Global Period

Code	Days
53450	090

53451-53454

● **53451 Periurethral transperineal adjustable balloon continence device; bilateral insertion, including cystourethroscopy and imaging guidance**

(Do not report 53451 in conjunction with 52000, 53452, 53453, 53454, 76000)

● **53452 Periurethral transperineal adjustable balloon continence device; unilateral insertion, including cystourethroscopy and imaging guidance**

(Do not report 53452 in conjunction with 52000, 53451, 53453, 53454, 76000)

● **53453 Periurethral transperineal adjustable balloon continence device; removal, each balloon**

(Do not report 53453 in conjunction with 53451, 53452, 53454)

● **53454 Periurethral transperineal adjustable balloon continence device; percutaneous adjustment of balloon(s) fluid volume**

(Do not report 53454 in conjunction with 53451, 53452, 53453)

(Report 53454 only once per patient encounter)

AMA Coding Notes

Repair Procedures on the Urethra

(For hypospadias, see 54300-54352)

Surgical Procedures on the Urethra

(For endoscopy, see cystoscopy, urethroscopy, cystourethroscopy, 52000-52700)

(For injection procedure for urethrocystography, see 51600-51610)

Surgical Procedures on the Urinary System

(For provision of chemotherapeutic agents, report both the specific service in addition to code(s) for the specific substance(s) or drug(s) provided)

Plain English Description

A transperineal periurethral balloon incontinence device may be used to treat men with urinary incontinence following prostate surgery and/or radiation therapy to restore normal pelvic pressure and urinary continence. A cystoscope is passed though the urethra into the bladder. A sharp tipped trocar and sheath are assembled and a small incision is made in the perineum. Under fluoroscopic guidance, the trocar and sheath are inserted through the incision and advanced through the pelvic floor. The sharp tip trocar is replaced with a blunt tip trocar and advancement continues to the level of the bladder. The trocar is removed and the deflated balloon device is advanced through the sheath to the desired location. The sheath is partially retracted and the balloon is inflated with a small amount of fluid to anchor it in place. The sheath is removed and the perineum is closed (53452). For bilateral placement, the procedure is repeated on the opposite side (53451). After a few weeks of recovery, the device may be accessed using a needle inserted through the perineum and additional fluid added to adjust the balloon volume for adequate pressure (53454). Fluid may be added multiple times until the optimal balloon inflation volume has been reached. To remove the device (53453), a small incision is made in the perineum and the balloon is deflated. The device is dissected free from surrounding tissue and removed.

ICD-10-CM Diagnostic Codes

C61	Malignant neoplasm of prostate ♂
N39.3	Stress incontinence (female) (male)
N39.46	Mixed incontinence
N39.498	Other specified urinary incontinence
N99.89	Other postprocedural complications and disorders of genitourinary system
Y84.2	Radiological procedure and radiotherapy as the cause of abnormal reaction of the patient, or of later complication, without mention of misadventure at the time of the procedure
Z85.46	Personal history of malignant neoplasm of prostate ♂
Z86.002	Personal history of in-situ neoplasm of other and unspecified genital organs
Z87.430	Personal history of prostatic dysplasia ♂
Z98.890	Other specified postprocedural states

CCI Edits

Refer to Appendix A for CCI edits.

Facility RVUs ▯

Code	Work	PE Facility	MP	Total Facility
53451	0.00	0.00	0.00	0.00
53452	0.00	0.00	0.00	0.00
53453	0.00	0.00	0.00	0.00
53454	0.00	0.00	0.00	0.00

Non-facility RVUs ▯

Code	Work	PE Non-Facility	MP	Total Non-Facility
53451	0.00	0.00	0.00	0.00
53452	0.00	0.00	0.00	0.00
53453	0.00	0.00	0.00	0.00
53454	0.00	0.00	0.00	0.00

Modifiers (PAR) ▯

Code	Mod 50	Mod 51	Mod 62	Mod 66	Mod 80
53451					
53452					
53453					
53454					

Global Period

Code	Days
53451	010
53452	010
53453	000
53454	000

53460

53460 Urethromeatoplasty, with partial excision of distal urethral segment (Richardson type procedure)

AMA Coding Notes

Repair Procedures on the Urethra

(For hypospadias, see 54300-54352)

Surgical Procedures on the Urethra

(For endoscopy, see cystoscopy, urethroscopy, cystourethroscopy, 52000-52700)

(For injection procedure for urethrocystography, see 51600-51610)

Surgical Procedures on the Urinary System

(For provision of chemotherapeutic agents, report both the specific service in addition to code(s) for the specific substance(s) or drug(s) provided)

Plain English Description

Urethromeatoplasty is a procedure to enlarge or reconstruct the opening of the urethra at the distal tip of the penis to improve urination. The urethra is the hollow tube extending from the bladder to the meatus through which urine drains and sperm is ejaculated. The most common cause of urethral narrowing is scarring of the mucosal tissue due to irritation, inflammation, infection, or injury. Meatal stenosis may also be congenital. Symptoms of urethral narrowing can include painful urination, frequent urination, inability to empty the bladder, and upward or sideways urine flow. In 53450, the urethral meatus is opened and a mucosal flap is formed and sutured to the glans. In 53460, a ventral incision in the penis is made and skin is freed from the shaft. Fibrous tissue causing narrowing within the distal urethra is removed and the opening is repaired.

CCI Edits

Refer to Appendix A for CCI edits.

Facility RVUs ☐

Code	Work	PE Facility	MP	Total Facility
53460	7.75	4.74	0.94	13.43

Non-facility RVUs ☐

Code	Work	PE Non-Facility	MP	Total Non-Facility
53460	7.75	4.74	0.94	13.43

Modifiers (PAR) ☐

Code	Mod 50	Mod 51	Mod 62	Mod 66	Mod 80
53460	0	2	0	0	0

Global Period

Code	Days
53460	090

CPT® Procedural Coding

53500

53500 Urethrolysis, transvaginal, secondary, open, including cystourethroscopy (eg, postsurgical obstruction, scarring)

(For urethrolysis by retropubic approach, use 53899)

(Do not report 53500 in conjunction with 52000)

AMA Coding Notes

Repair Procedures on the Urethra

(For hypospadias, see 54300-54352)

Surgical Procedures on the Urethra

(For endoscopy, see cystoscopy, urethroscopy, cystourethroscopy, 52000-52700)

(For injection procedure for urethrocystography, see 51600-51610)

Surgical Procedures on the Urinary System

(For provision of chemotherapeutic agents, report both the specific service in addition to code(s) for the specific substance(s) or drug(s) provided)

AMA *CPT® Assistant* ▢

53500: Sep 04: 11

Plain English Description

To identify postoperative obstruction, or scarring and determine if urethrolysis is necessary, cystourethroscopy is performed first. The cystourethroscope is inserted through the urethral meatus and advanced toward the bladder as the surgeon searches for areas of tissue erosion, scarring, stenosis, obstruction or fistula formation. The scope is removed and the procedure continues by making a midline or U-shaped incision in the anterior wall of the vagina. Dissection continues along the surface of the periurethral fascia to the pubic bone. Retracting the endopelvic fascia, periurethral fascia, and vaginal wall laterally exposes the retropubic space, which is entered between the attachment of the endopelvic fascia to the obturator fascia. The urethra is then dissected free of the proximal bladder at the underside of the pubic bone. Any adhesions are lysed. Previously placed sutures may be cut to allow mobility of the bladder and urethra. Once the urethra is completely freed of adhesions and scar tissue, the wound is closed in layers. A catheter may be placed transurethrally following the procedure.

Urethrolysis, transvaginal

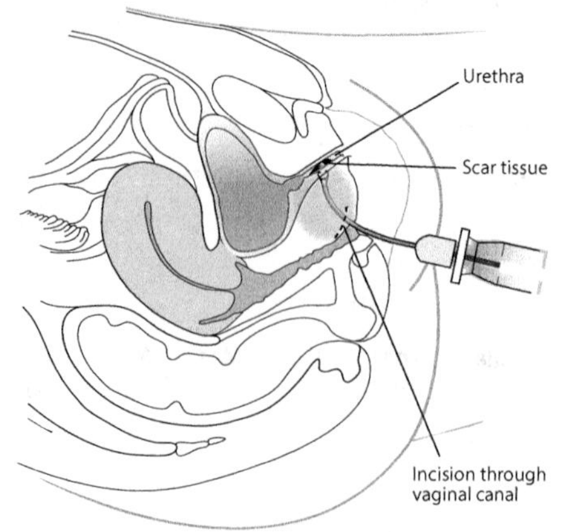

ICD-10-CM Diagnostic Codes

N32	Other disorders of bladder
N35.021	Urethral stricture due to childbirth ♀
N35.028	Other post-traumatic urethral stricture, female ♀
N35.12	Postinfective urethral stricture, not elsewhere classified, female ♀
N35.82	Other urethral stricture, female ♀
N35.92	Unspecified urethral stricture, female ♀
N36.8	Other specified disorders of urethra
N37	Urethral disorders in diseases classified elsewhere
N39.8	Other specified disorders of urinary system
N81.9	Female genital prolapse, unspecified ♀
N99.12	Postprocedural urethral stricture, female ♀

CCI Edits

Refer to Appendix A for CCI edits.

Facility RVUs ▢

Code	Work	PE Facility	MP	Total Facility
53500	13.00	7.18	1.82	22.00

Non-facility RVUs ▢

Code	Work	PE Non-Facility	MP	Total Non-Facility
53500	13.00	7.18	1.82	22.00

Modifiers (PAR) ▢

Code	Mod 50	Mod 51	Mod 62	Mod 66	Mod 80
53500	0	2	1	0	2

Global Period

Code	Days
53500	090

53502

53502 Urethrorrhaphy, suture of urethral wound or injury, female

AMA Coding Notes

Repair Procedures on the Urethra

(For hypospadias, see 54300-54352)

Surgical Procedures on the Urethra

(For endoscopy, see cystoscopy, urethroscopy, cystourethroscopy, 52000-52700)

(For injection procedure for urethrocystography, see 51600-51610)

Surgical Procedures on the Urinary System

(For provision of chemotherapeutic agents, report both the specific service in addition to code(s) for the specific substance(s) or drug(s) provided)

Plain English Description

Surgical repair of a urethral wound or injury in a female is performed. With the patient in dorsal lithotomy position, the vagina, vulva, and perineum are prepared and draped. A midline or U-shaped incision is made in the anterior vaginal wall. The periurethral fascia is dissected and the urethra identified. The mucosal and muscular layers of the urethral defect are closed over a previously placed transurethral catheter. The periurethral fascia is closed with absorbable sutures followed by the vaginal wall. The urethral catheter is left in place.

Urethrorrhaphy, female

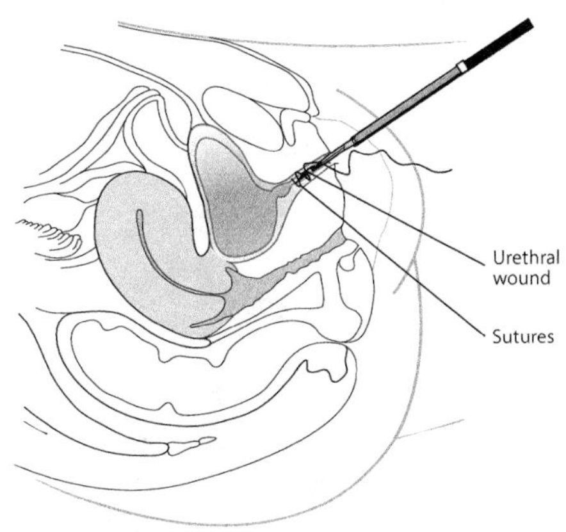

ICD-10-CM Diagnostic Codes

	N99.71	Accidental puncture and laceration of a genitourinary system organ or structure during a genitourinary system procedure
	N99.72	Accidental puncture and laceration of a genitourinary system organ or structure during other procedure
	O71.5	Other obstetric injury to pelvic organs ♀
❼	S37.32	Contusion of urethra
❼	S37.33	Laceration of urethra
❼	S37.39	Other injury of urethra

ICD-10-CM Coding Notes

For codes requiring a 7th character extension, refer to your ICD-10-CM book. Review the character descriptions and coding guidelines for proper selection. For some procedures, only certain characters will apply.

CCI Edits

Refer to Appendix A for CCI edits.

Facility RVUs ▯

Code	Work	PE Facility	MP	Total Facility
53502	8.26	5.00	0.99	14.25

Non-facility RVUs ▯

Code	Work	PE Non-Facility	MP	Total Non-Facility
53502	8.26	5.00	0.99	14.25

Modifiers (PAR) ▯

Code	Mod 50	Mod 51	Mod 62	Mod 66	Mod 80
53502	0	2	0	0	1

Global Period

Code	Days
53502	090

53505-53510

53505 Urethrorrhaphy, suture of urethral wound or injury; penile
53510 Urethrorrhaphy, suture of urethral wound or injury; perineal

AMA Coding Notes

Repair Procedures on the Urethra

(For hypospadias, see 54300-54352)

Surgical Procedures on the Urethra

(For endoscopy, see cystoscopy, urethroscopy, cystourethroscopy, 52000-52700)

(For injection procedure for urethrocystography, see 51600-51610)

Surgical Procedures on the Urinary System

(For provision of chemotherapeutic agents, report both the specific service in addition to code(s) for the specific substance(s) or drug(s) provided)

Plain English Description

Surgical repair of an injury to the male urethra is performed. In 53505, surgical repair of the penile urethra is accomplished with the patient supine or in low lithotomy position. The penis, scrotum, and perineal area are prepared and draped. For a penetrating injury, the wound is cleaned, corpus spongiosum or corpus cavernosum debrided, and the area is examined for associated injuries. The urethral wound is repaired with sutures over a catheter previously placed transurethrally into the bladder. Drains may be placed if the wound is large or contaminated. The corpus spongiosum or corpus cavernosum is closed with absorbable sutures followed by closure of the skin. In 53510, surgical repair of an injury to the bulbar urethra is approached through a midline perineal incision. The bulbocavernosus muscle is divided and corpus spongiosum entered at the site of the injury. The wound is cleaned and corpus spongiosum debrided if necessary. The urethra is exposed and examined. The technique for repair is similar to a urethroplasty for strictures. For a urethral defect of <25 mm, the repair is accomplished by anastomosis. To repair a longer defect, the urethra is dissected distally from the corpus spongiosum to maximize the length. The distal end is spatulated dorsally, the proximal end ventrally. Anastomosis of the urethral ends is accomplished with a single layer suture through the urethral mucosa and spongiosal adventitia on the dorsal surface and two layers of sutures on the ventral surface. Drains may be placed if the wound is large or contaminated. The corpus spongiosum is closed followed by the bulbocavernosus muscle and the skin. A catheter may be placed transurethrally into the bladder at the end of the procedure.

Urethrorrhaphy, suture of urethral wound or injury; penile

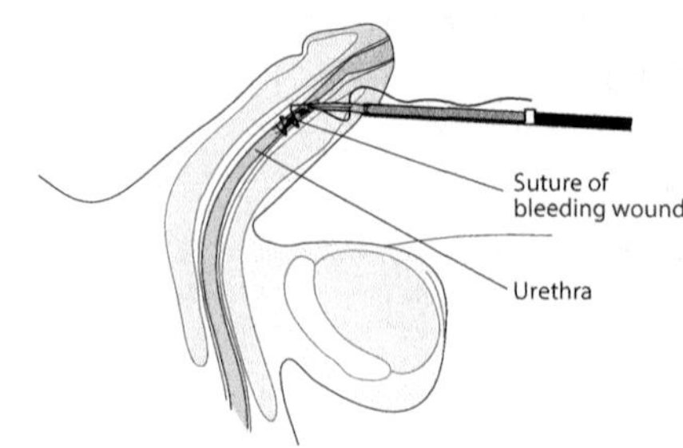

ICD-10-CM Diagnostic Codes

	N99.71	Accidental puncture and laceration of a genitourinary system organ or structure during a genitourinary system procedure
	N99.72	Accidental puncture and laceration of a genitourinary system organ or structure during other procedure
➐	S31.22	Laceration with foreign body of penis
➐	S37.32	Contusion of urethra
➐	S37.33	Laceration of urethra
➐	S37.39	Other injury of urethra

ICD-10-CM Coding Notes

For codes requiring a 7th character extension, refer to your ICD-10-CM book. Review the character descriptions and coding guidelines for proper selection. For some procedures, only certain characters will apply.

CCI Edits

Refer to Appendix A for CCI edits.

Facility RVUs ▢

Code	Work	PE Facility	MP	Total Facility
53505	8.26	4.99	0.99	14.24
53510	10.96	6.27	1.30	18.53

Non-facility RVUs ▢

Code	Work	PE Non-Facility	MP	Total Non-Facility
53505	8.26	4.99	0.99	14.24
53510	10.96	6.27	1.30	18.53

Modifiers (PAR) ▢

Code	Mod 50	Mod 51	Mod 62	Mod 66	Mod 80
53505	0	2	0	0	2
53510	0	2	1	0	2

Global Period

Code	Days
53505	090
53510	090

53515

53515 Urethrorrhaphy, suture of urethral wound or injury; prostatomembranous

AMA Coding Notes

Repair Procedures on the Urethra

(For hypospadias, see 54300-54352)

Surgical Procedures on the Urethra

(For endoscopy, see cystoscopy, urethroscopy, cystourethroscopy, 52000-52700)

(For injection procedure for urethrocystography, see 51600-51610)

Surgical Procedures on the Urinary System

(For provision of chemotherapeutic agents, report both the specific service in addition to code(s) for the specific substance(s) or drug(s) provided)

Plain English Description

Surgical repair of an injury to the prostatomembranous urethra may be attempted immediately if the patient requires exploratory surgery to identify rectal or vascular injuries but is most often delayed as long as 6-12 weeks to allow for absorption of a hematoma. In either case, a suprapubic catheter is necessary and can be placed percutaneously or with open cystotomy. The surgical technique for immediate repair will vary depending on other injuries sustained by the patient. For delayed repair, a midline perineal incision is made and the bulbospongiosus muscle divided. Dissection continues through the corpus spongiosum until the urethra is located. Proceeding in the direction of the bulbar urethra, the proximal point of obliteration is identified using a catheter and the distal point as far as the suspensory ligament to the penis is assessed. A sound is then passed via the suprapubic cystotomy tract through the bladder neck and into the prostatic urethra. Beginning at the level of the crus and working distally, the right and left corporal bodies are separated in the midline for a distance of 4-5 cm allowing the urethra to move upwards and shortening the distance between the urethral ends. If urethral tension remains after separating the corporal bodies, dissection continues by displacing or ligating the penile vessels laterally. Then using bone rongeurs or an osteotome, a wedge of bone is removed from the pubis at the inferior aspect creating a groove for the urethra to settle into and adding 1-2 cm of urethral length. If anastomosis is still not possible due to urethral tension, the urethra is rerouted around the corporal body through a larger resection of the pubic bone by circumferentially mobilizing one of the corporal bodies proximal to the suspensory penile ligament and dissecting away from the surface to avoid injury to neurovascular tissue. The distal urethral stump is spatulated and brought down from a 12-o'clock position and the proximal urethral stump is also spatulated and lifted from the 6-o'clock position, healthy tissue is identified along with the seminal ducts in the verumontanum of the prostatic urethra. Anastomosis of the two ends of the urethra is accomplished by placing sutures through the urethral mucosa and tying them after all have been placed. A fenestrated catheter is placed transurethrally. The corpus spongiosum is closed followed by the bulbospongiosus muscle. The perineal skin is sutured and the suprapubic catheter is replaced.

Urethrorrhaphy, suture of urethral wound or injury; prostatomembranous

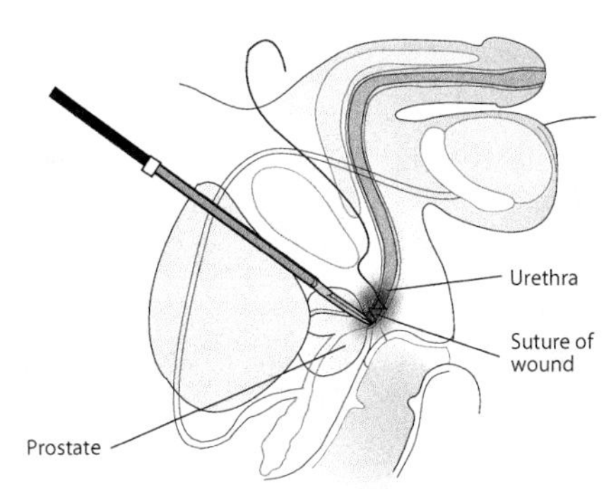

ICD-10-CM Diagnostic Codes

	N99.71	Accidental puncture and laceration of a genitourinary system organ or structure during a genitourinary system procedure
	N99.72	Accidental puncture and laceration of a genitourinary system organ or structure during other procedure
❼	S37.32	Contusion of urethra
❼	S37.33	Laceration of urethra
❼	S37.39	Other injury of urethra

ICD-10-CM Coding Notes

For codes requiring a 7th character extension, refer to your ICD-10-CM book. Review the character descriptions and coding guidelines for proper selection. For some procedures, only certain characters will apply.

CCI Edits

Refer to Appendix A for CCI edits.

Facility RVUs □

Code	Work	PE Facility	MP	Total Facility
53515	14.22	7.36	1.69	23.27

Non-facility RVUs □

Code	Work	PE Non-Facility	MP	Total Non-Facility
53515	14.22	7.36	1.69	23.27

Modifiers (PAR) □

Code	Mod 50	Mod 51	Mod 62	Mod 66	Mod 80
53515	0	2	1	0	2

Global Period

Code	Days
53515	090

53520

53520 Closure of urethrostomy or urethrocutaneous fistula, male (separate procedure)

(For closure of urethrovaginal fistula, use 57310)

(For closure of urethrorectal fistula, see 45820, 45825)

AMA Coding Notes

Repair Procedures on the Urethra

(For hypospadias, see 54300-54352)

Surgical Procedures on the Urethra

(For endoscopy, see cystoscopy, urethroscopy, cystourethroscopy, 52000-52700)

(For injection procedure for urethrocystography, see 51600-51610)

Surgical Procedures on the Urinary System

(For provision of chemotherapeutic agents, report both the specific service in addition to code(s) for the specific substance(s) or drug(s) provided)

Plain English Description

To close an urethrostomy or urethrocutaneous fistula as a separate procedure in males, a catheter is placed transurethrally. A midline incision is made along the urethral opening in the penile skin and the epithelialized fistula/urethrostomy is excised, inverting the urethral mucosa and closing the defect over the catheter. Next, the skin layer of the penile incision is extended proximally toward the scrotum until the subcutaneous dartos muscle is visualized. The scrotal skin is undermined and a flap marked in the dartos muscle. The flap is excised along the marks, elevated, and flipped over the fistula/urethrostomy. Needle point cautery is used to control bleeding. The edges of the flap are sutured over the urethral repair. The dartos muscle is approximated in the scrotum and sutured. A drain may be placed. The scrotal skin is closed. The penile skin is closed without tension over the dartos flap and the Foley catheter is left in place.

Closure of urethrostomy or urethrocutaneous fistula, male

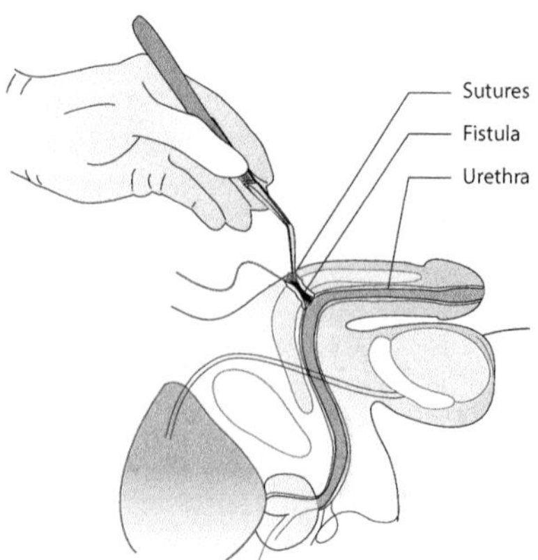

ICD-10-CM Diagnostic Codes

	N36.0	Urethral fistula
❼	T81.83	Persistent postprocedural fistula

ICD-10-CM Coding Notes

For codes requiring a 7th character extension, refer to your ICD-10-CM book. Review the character descriptions and coding guidelines for proper selection. For some procedures, only certain characters will apply.

CCI Edits

Refer to Appendix A for CCI edits.

Facility RVUs ▯

Code	Work	PE Facility	MP	Total Facility
53520	9.48	5.77	1.11	16.36

Non-facility RVUs ▯

Code	Work	PE Non-Facility	MP	Total Non-Facility
53520	9.48	5.77	1.11	16.36

Modifiers (PAR) ▯

Code	Mod 50	Mod 51	Mod 62	Mod 66	Mod 80
53520	0	2	0	0	1

Global Period

Code	Days
53520	090

53600-53601

53600 Dilation of urethral stricture by passage of sound or urethral dilator, male; initial

53601 Dilation of urethral stricture by passage of sound or urethral dilator, male; subsequent

AMA Coding Notes

Manipulation Procedures on the Urethra

(For radiological supervision and interpretation, use 74485)

Surgical Procedures on the Urethra

(For endoscopy, see cystoscopy, urethroscopy, cystourethroscopy, 52000-52700)

(For injection procedure for urethrocystography, see 51600-51610)

Surgical Procedures on the Urinary System

(For provision of chemotherapeutic agents, report both the specific service in addition to code(s) for the specific substance(s) or drug(s) provided)

Plain English Description

A urethral stricture in a male is dilated by passage of a sound or urethral dilator. A urethral stricture is a narrowing of the urethra typically due to infection or trauma. A series of increasingly larger sounds are inserted. Sounds are rods with rounded ends. Alternatively, a special balloon catheter may be used to dilate the stricture. Some balloon dilators have an integral urinary drainage catheter that can be left in the bladder. If sounds are used to dilate the stricture, a urinary catheter may be inserted following dilation to maintain the opening. Use 53600 for the initial dilation using a sound or urethral dilator and 53601 for subsequent procedures.

Dilation of urethral stricture by passage of sound or urethral dilator

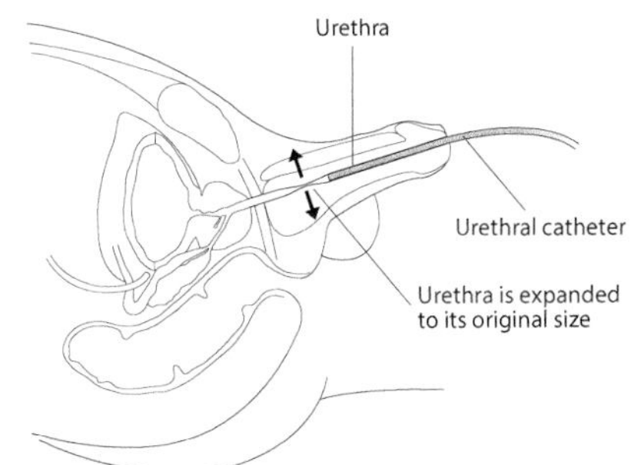

ICD-10-CM Diagnostic Codes

N35.010	Post-traumatic urethral stricture, male, meatal ♂
N35.011	Post-traumatic bulbous urethral stricture ♂
N35.012	Post-traumatic membranous urethral stricture ♂
N35.013	Post-traumatic anterior urethral stricture ♂
N35.016	Post-traumatic urethral stricture, male, overlapping sites ♂
N35.111	Postinfective urethral stricture, not elsewhere classified, male, meatal ♂
N35.112	Postinfective bulbous urethral stricture, not elsewhere classified, male ♂
N35.113	Postinfective membranous urethral stricture, not elsewhere classified, male ♂
N35.114	Postinfective anterior urethral stricture, not elsewhere classified, male ♂
N35.116	Postinfective urethral stricture, not elsewhere classified, male, overlapping sites ♂
N35.812	Other urethral bulbous stricture, male ♂
N35.813	Other membranous urethral stricture, male ♂
N35.814	Other anterior urethral stricture, male ♂
N35.816	Other urethral stricture, male, overlapping sites ♂
N37	Urethral disorders in diseases classified elsewhere
N40.1	Benign prostatic hyperplasia with lower urinary tract symptoms ♂
N40.3	Nodular prostate with lower urinary tract symptoms ♂
N99.110	Postprocedural urethral stricture, male, meatal ♂
N99.111	Postprocedural bulbous urethral stricture, male ♂
N99.112	Postprocedural membranous urethral stricture, male ♂
N99.113	Postprocedural anterior bulbous urethral stricture, male ♂
N99.115	Postprocedural fossa navicularis urethral stricture ♂
N99.116	Postprocedural urethral stricture, male, overlapping sites ♂
Q64.32	Congenital stricture of urethra
Q64.33	Congenital stricture of urinary meatus
Q64.39	Other atresia and stenosis of urethra and bladder neck
R39.12	Poor urinary stream

CCI Edits

Refer to Appendix A for CCI edits.

Facility RVUs ▯

Code	Work	PE Facility	MP	Total Facility
53600	1.21	0.49	0.14	1.84
53601	0.98	0.45	0.11	1.54

Non-facility RVUs ▯

Code	Work	PE Non-Facility	MP	Total Non-Facility
53600	1.21	1.26	0.14	2.61
53601	0.98	1.41	0.11	2.50

Modifiers (PAR) ▯

Code	Mod 50	Mod 51	Mod 62	Mod 66	Mod 80
53600	0	2	0	0	1
53601	0	2	0	0	1

Global Period

Code	Days
53600	000
53601	000

CPT® Procedural Coding

53605

53605 Dilation of urethral stricture or vesical neck by passage of sound or urethral dilator, male, general or conduction (spinal) anesthesia

(For dilation of urethral stricture, male, performed under local anesthesia, see 53600, 53601, 53620, 53621)

AMA Coding Notes

Manipulation Procedures on the Urethra

(For radiological supervision and interpretation, use 74485)

Surgical Procedures on the Urethra

(For endoscopy, see cystoscopy, urethroscopy, cystourethroscopy, 52000-52700)

(For injection procedure for urethrocystography, see 51600-51610)

Surgical Procedures on the Urinary System

(For provision of chemotherapeutic agents, report both the specific service in addition to code(s) for the specific substance(s) or drug(s) provided)

Plain English Description

After satisfactory induction of general or regional anesthesia, the male patient is placed in dorsal lithotomy position and the penis and scrotum are prepared and draped. Serial dilation of the urethral stricture or vesical neck is accomplished using urethral sounds or S-curve urethral dilators of increasing size and thickness until the narrowed area of the urethra or vesical neck has widened. A catheter is placed transurethrally following the procedure.

Dilation of urethral stricture or vesical neck by passage of sound or urethral dilator

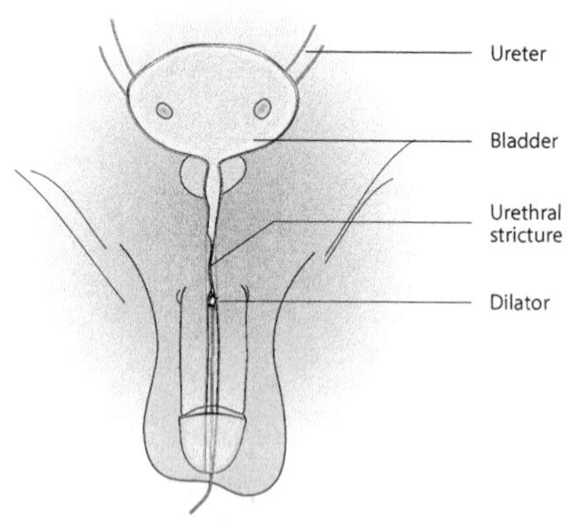

ICD-10-CM Diagnostic Codes

N35.010	Post-traumatic urethral stricture, male, meatal ♂
N35.011	Post-traumatic bulbous urethral stricture ♂
N35.012	Post-traumatic membranous urethral stricture ♂
N35.013	Post-traumatic anterior urethral stricture ♂
N35.016	Post-traumatic urethral stricture, male, overlapping sites ♂
N35.112	Postinfective bulbous urethral stricture, not elsewhere classified, male ♂
N35.113	Postinfective membranous urethral stricture, not elsewhere classified, male ♂
N35.114	Postinfective anterior urethral stricture, not elsewhere classified, male ♂
N35.116	Postinfective urethral stricture, not elsewhere classified, male, overlapping sites ♂
N35.811	Other urethral stricture, male, meatal ♂
N35.812	Other urethral bulbous stricture, male ♂
N35.813	Other membranous urethral stricture, male ♂
N35.814	Other anterior urethral stricture, male ♂
N35.816	Other urethral stricture, male, overlapping sites ♂
N37	Urethral disorders in diseases classified elsewhere
N40.1	Benign prostatic hyperplasia with lower urinary tract symptoms ♂
N40.3	Nodular prostate with lower urinary tract symptoms ♂
N99.110	Postprocedural urethral stricture, male, meatal ♂
N99.111	Postprocedural bulbous urethral stricture, male ♂
N99.112	Postprocedural membranous urethral stricture, male ♂
N99.113	Postprocedural anterior bulbous urethral stricture, male ♂
N99.115	Postprocedural fossa navicularis urethral stricture ♂
N99.116	Postprocedural urethral stricture, male, overlapping sites ♂
Q64.32	Congenital stricture of urethra
Q64.33	Congenital stricture of urinary meatus
Q64.39	Other atresia and stenosis of urethra and bladder neck
R39.12	Poor urinary stream

CCI Edits

Refer to Appendix A for CCI edits.

Facility RVUs 🗆

Code	Work	PE Facility	MP	Total Facility
53605	1.28	0.43	0.14	1.85

Non-facility RVUs 🗆

Code	Work	PE Non-Facility	MP	Total Non-Facility
53605	1.28	0.43	0.14	1.85

Modifiers (PAR) 🗆

Code	Mod 50	Mod 51	Mod 62	Mod 66	Mod 80
53605	0	2	0	0	1

Global Period

Code	Days
53605	000

53620-53621

53620 Dilation of urethral stricture by passage of filiform and follower, male; initial

53621 Dilation of urethral stricture by passage of filiform and follower, male; subsequent

AMA Coding Notes

Manipulation Procedures on the Urethra

(For radiological supervision and interpretation, use 74485)

Surgical Procedures on the Urethra

(For endoscopy, see cystoscopy, urethroscopy, cystourethroscopy, 52000-52700)

(For injection procedure for urethrocystography, see 51600-51610)

Surgical Procedures on the Urinary System

(For provision of chemotherapeutic agents, report both the specific service in addition to code(s) for the specific substance(s) or drug(s) provided)

Plain English Description

A urethral stricture in a male is dilated by passage of a filiform and follower. A urethral stricture is a narrowing of the urethra typically due to infection or trauma. There are two types of filiform dilators available. One type uses a filiform wire guide with a series of followers, which are threadlike instruments. The wire guide is inserted into the urethra. Followers of increasing diameter are then inserted over the wire guide to expand the narrowed portion of the urethra. A second type is an integral filiform urethral dilator that eliminates the need for followers. Use 53620 for the initial dilation using a filiform and follower and 53621 for subsequent procedures.

Dilation of urethral stricture by passage of filiform and follower, male

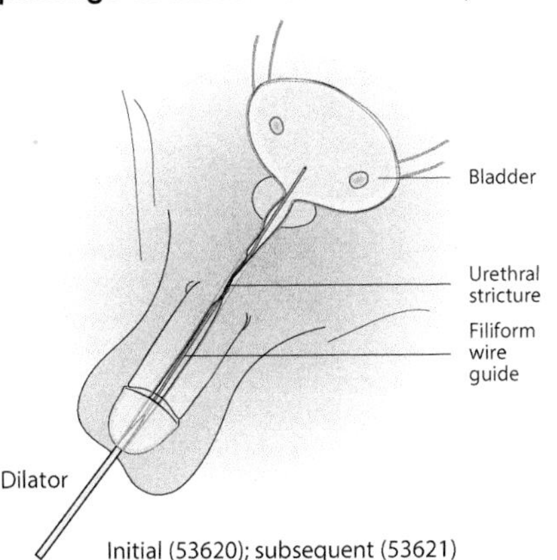

ICD-10-CM Diagnostic Codes

N35.010	Post-traumatic urethral stricture, male, meatal ♂
N35.011	Post-traumatic bulbous urethral stricture ♂
N35.012	Post-traumatic membranous urethral stricture ♂
N35.013	Post-traumatic anterior urethral stricture ♂
N35.016	Post-traumatic urethral stricture, male, overlapping sites ♂
N35.111	Postinfective urethral stricture, not elsewhere classified, male, meatal ♂
N35.112	Postinfective bulbous urethral stricture, not elsewhere classified, male ♂
N35.113	Postinfective membranous urethral stricture, not elsewhere classified, male ♂
N35.114	Postinfective anterior urethral stricture, not elsewhere classified, male ♂
N35.116	Postinfective urethral stricture, not elsewhere classified, male, overlapping sites ♂
N37	Urethral disorders in diseases classified elsewhere
N40.1	Benign prostatic hyperplasia with lower urinary tract symptoms ♂
N40.3	Nodular prostate with lower urinary tract symptoms ♂
N99.110	Postprocedural urethral stricture, male, meatal ♂
N99.111	Postprocedural bulbous urethral stricture, male ♂
N99.112	Postprocedural membranous urethral stricture, male ♂
N99.113	Postprocedural anterior bulbous urethral stricture, male ♂
N99.115	Postprocedural fossa navicularis urethral stricture ♂
N99.116	Postprocedural urethral stricture, male, overlapping sites ♂
Q64.32	Congenital stricture of urethra
Q64.33	Congenital stricture of urinary meatus
Q64.39	Other atresia and stenosis of urethra and bladder neck
R39.1	Other difficulties with micturition
R39.12	Poor urinary stream

CCI Edits

Refer to Appendix A for CCI edits.

Facility RVUs ☐

Code	Work	PE Facility	MP	Total Facility
53620	1.62	0.72	0.20	2.54
53621	1.35	0.58	0.17	2.10

Non-facility RVUs ☐

Code	Work	PE Non-Facility	MP	Total Non-Facility
53620	1.62	3.34	0.20	5.16
53621	1.35	3.40	0.17	4.92

Modifiers (PAR) ☐

Code	Mod 50	Mod 51	Mod 62	Mod 66	Mod 80
53620	0	2	0	0	1
53621	0	2	0	0	1

Global Period

Code	Days
53620	000
53621	000

53660-53665

53660 Dilation of female urethra including suppository and/or instillation; initial

53661 Dilation of female urethra including suppository and/or instillation; subsequent

53665 Dilation of female urethra, general or conduction (spinal) anesthesia

(For urethral catheterization, see 51701-51703)

(For dilation of urethra performed under local anesthesia, female, see 53660, 53661)

AMA Coding Notes

Manipulation Procedures on the Urethra

(For radiological supervision and interpretation, use 74485)

Surgical Procedures on the Urethra

(For endoscopy, see cystoscopy, urethroscopy, cystourethroscopy, 52000-52700)

(For injection procedure for urethrocystography, see 51600-51610)

Surgical Procedures on the Urinary System

(For provision of chemotherapeutic agents, report both the specific service in addition to code(s) for the specific substance(s) or drug(s) provided)

Plain English Description

Dilation of the female urethra is performed. This procedure is performed to treat a narrowing or stricture of the urethra caused by injury, scarring, congenital anomaly, or other conditions. The urethral opening is cleansed. A local anesthetic is applied in the form of a suppository, jelly, or liquid to numb the urethra. Alternatively, general or conduction (spinal) anesthesia may be used. A series of tubes or dilators are then passed through the urethral opening to the urethrovesical junction to increase the diameter of the narrowed segment of urethra. A urethroscope may be used to guide the dilators. Following the dilation procedure, a catheter may be inserted and left in place to drain the bladder. Use 53660 for initial dilation or 53661 for subsequent dilation performed under local anesthesia. Use 53665 for dilation (initial or subsequent) performed under general or conduction (spinal) anesthesia.

Dilation of female urethra, general or conduction (spinal) anesthesia

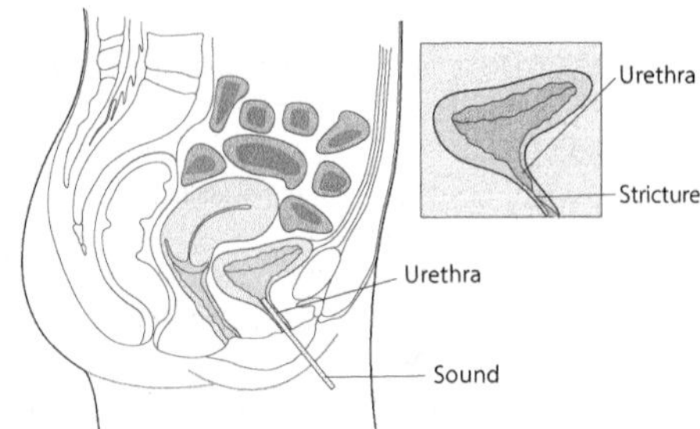

A device is inserted into the urethra of a female patient to widen a section of the urethra that has become constricted.

ICD-10-CM Diagnostic Codes

N13.9	Obstructive and reflux uropathy, unspecified
N34.1	Nonspecific urethritis
N34.2	Other urethritis
N34.3	Urethral syndrome, unspecified
N35.021	Urethral stricture due to childbirth ♀
N35.028	Other post-traumatic urethral stricture, female ♀
N35.12	Postinfective urethral stricture, not elsewhere classified, female ♀
N35.82	Other urethral stricture, female ♀
N35.92	Unspecified urethral stricture, female ♀
N36.42	Intrinsic sphincter deficiency (ISD)
N37	Urethral disorders in diseases classified elsewhere
N39.8	Other specified disorders of urinary system
N99.12	Postprocedural urethral stricture, female ♀
Q64.31	Congenital bladder neck obstruction
Q64.32	Congenital stricture of urethra
Q64.39	Other atresia and stenosis of urethra and bladder neck
R33.9	Retention of urine, unspecified
R35.0	Frequency of micturition
R39.12	Poor urinary stream
R39.14	Feeling of incomplete bladder emptying

CCI Edits

Refer to Appendix A for CCI edits.

Facility RVUs 🗆

Code	Work	PE Facility	MP	Total Facility
53660	0.71	0.41	0.09	1.21
53661	0.72	0.36	0.09	1.17
53665	0.76	0.26	0.10	1.12

Non-facility RVUs 🗆

Code	Work	PE Non-Facility	MP	Total Non-Facility
53660	0.71	1.43	0.09	2.23
53661	0.72	1.38	0.09	2.19
53665	0.76	0.26	0.10	1.12

Modifiers (PAR) 🗆

Code	Mod 50	Mod 51	Mod 62	Mod 66	Mod 80
53660	0	2	0	0	1
53661	0	2	0	0	1
53665	0	2	0	0	1

Global Period

Code	Days
53660	000
53661	000
53665	000

53850

53850 Transurethral destruction of prostate tissue; by microwave thermotherapy

AMA Coding Notes

Other Procedures on the Urethra

(For 2 or 3 glass urinalysis, use 81020)

Surgical Procedures on the Urethra

(For endoscopy, see cystoscopy, urethroscopy, cystourethroscopy, 52000-52700)

(For injection procedure for urethrocystography, see 51600-51610)

Surgical Procedures on the Urinary System

(For provision of chemotherapeutic agents, report both the specific service in addition to code(s) for the specific substance(s) or drug(s) provided)

AMA *CPT® Assistant* ☐

53850: Nov 97: 20, Apr 01: 6, Feb 10: 7, Jun 15: 5, Nov 18: 10

Plain English Description

Transurethral microwave thermotherapy (TUMT) is used to treat benign prostatic hypertrophy (BPH). With the patient awake and positioned supine, the penis is prepared with an antiseptic solution and 10-20 mL of 1-2% lidocaine gel is instilled into the urethra for local anesthesia. A special catheter is inserted through the urethra to the bladder and anchored in place with a balloon tip. The catheter contains a microwave antenna which is positioned within the prostatic urethra. Position of the catheter may be verified using separately reportable transrectal ultrasound. A probe is then placed in the rectum to monitor temperature during the procedure. The machine is activated and treatment begins. Microwave currents raise the temperature to above 45 degrees centigrade in the prostate gland, destroying excess tissue. At the same time, water flows through the catheter and cools the urethra to prevent damage to surrounding tissue. The patient is monitored throughout the 30-60 minute procedure for pain or discomfort. At the end of the procedure, the treatment catheter is removed and replaced by a Foley catheter inserted transurethrally.

Transurethral destruction of prostate tissue; by microwave thermotherapy

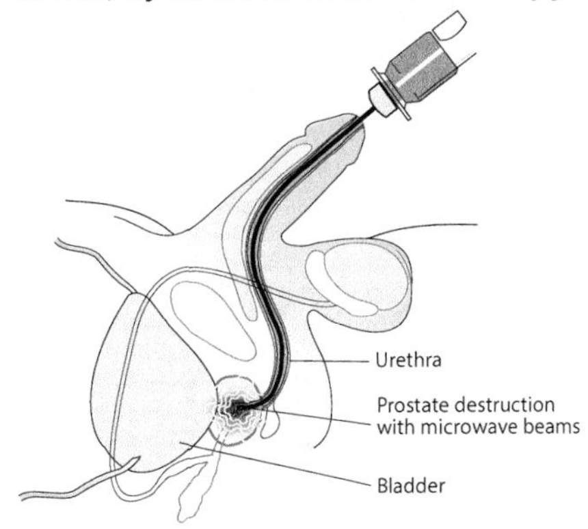

ICD-10-CM Diagnostic Codes

C61	Malignant neoplasm of prostate ♂
C79.82	Secondary malignant neoplasm of genital organs
D07.5	Carcinoma in situ of prostate ♂
D29.1	Benign neoplasm of prostate ♂
D40.0	Neoplasm of uncertain behavior of prostate ♂
N40.0	Benign prostatic hyperplasia without lower urinary tract symptoms ♂
N40.1	Benign prostatic hyperplasia with lower urinary tract symptoms ♂
N40.2	Nodular prostate without lower urinary tract symptoms ♂
N40.3	Nodular prostate with lower urinary tract symptoms ♂
N41.4	Granulomatous prostatitis ♂
N41.8	Other inflammatory diseases of prostate ♂
N42.30	Unspecified dysplasia of prostate ♂
N42.31	Prostatic intraepithelial neoplasia ♂
N42.32	Atypical small acinar proliferation of prostate ♂
N42.39	Other dysplasia of prostate ♂
N42.83	Cyst of prostate ♂
N42.89	Other specified disorders of prostate ♂
R33.8	Other retention of urine
R33.9	Retention of urine, unspecified
R39.12	Poor urinary stream
R39.14	Feeling of incomplete bladder emptying

CCI Edits

Refer to Appendix A for CCI edits.

Facility RVUs ☐

Code	Work	PE Facility	MP	Total Facility
53850	5.42	4.31	0.65	10.38

Non-facility RVUs ☐

Code	Work	PE Non-Facility	MP	Total Non-Facility
53850	5.42	37.52	0.65	43.59

Modifiers (PAR) ☐

Code	Mod 50	Mod 51	Mod 62	Mod 66	Mod 80
53850	0	2	0	0	1

Global Period

Code	Days
53850	090

53852

53852 Transurethral destruction of prostate tissue; by radiofrequency thermotherapy

AMA Coding Notes

Other Procedures on the Urethra

(For 2 or 3 glass urinalysis, use 81020)

Surgical Procedures on the Urethra

(For endoscopy, see cystoscopy, urethroscopy, cystourethroscopy, 52000-52700)

(For injection procedure for urethrocystography, see 51600-51610)

Surgical Procedures on the Urinary System

(For provision of chemotherapeutic agents, report both the specific service in addition to code(s) for the specific substance(s) or drug(s) provided)

AMA *CPT® Assistant* ▯

53852: Nov 97: 20, Apr 01: 6, Jun 15: 5, Nov 18: 10

Plain English Description

Transurethral radiofrequency thermotherapy, also known as transurethral needle ablation (TUNA), is used to treat benign prostatic hypertrophy (BPH). With the patient awake and in a dorsal lithotomy position, the penis is prepared with an antiseptic solution and 10-20 mL of 1-2% lidocaine gel is instilled into the urethra for local anesthesia. A rectal probe may be placed to monitor temperature during the procedure. A special catheter is inserted to the level of the prostatic urethra and an interstitial radiofrequency needle is deployed through the urethral wall into the prostatic tissue. Bipolar electrodes in the needle are activated by a machine. The low-wave radiofrequency energy produces heat to between 60 and 100 degrees centigrade destroying excess prostatic tissue within minutes. At the same time, water flows through the catheter and cools the urethra to prevent damage to surrounding tissue. The needle is withdrawn and repositioned a few centimeters away and the machine is activated again until all lobes of the prostate have been treated. At the end of the procedure, the treatment catheter is removed and may be replaced by a Foley catheter inserted transurethrally.

Transurethral destruction of prostate tissue; by radiofrequency thermotherapy

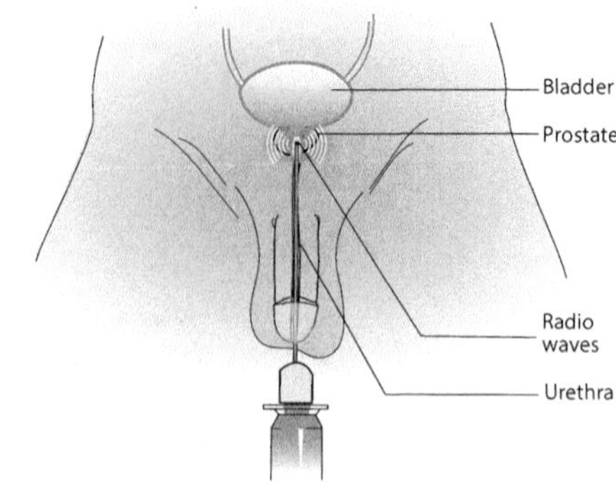

ICD-10-CM Diagnostic Codes

C61	Malignant neoplasm of prostate ♂
C79.82	Secondary malignant neoplasm of genital organs
D07.5	Carcinoma in situ of prostate ♂
D29.1	Benign neoplasm of prostate ♂
D40.0	Neoplasm of uncertain behavior of prostate ♂
N40.0	Benign prostatic hyperplasia without lower urinary tract symptoms ♂
N40.1	Benign prostatic hyperplasia with lower urinary tract symptoms ♂
N40.2	Nodular prostate without lower urinary tract symptoms ♂
N40.3	Nodular prostate with lower urinary tract symptoms ♂
N41.4	Granulomatous prostatitis ♂
N41.8	Other inflammatory diseases of prostate ♂
N42.30	Unspecified dysplasia of prostate ♂
N42.31	Prostatic intraepithelial neoplasia ♂
N42.32	Atypical small acinar proliferation of prostate ♂
N42.39	Other dysplasia of prostate ♂
N42.83	Cyst of prostate ♂
N42.89	Other specified disorders of prostate ♂
R33.8	Other retention of urine
R33.9	Retention of urine, unspecified
R39.12	Poor urinary stream
R39.14	Feeling of incomplete bladder emptying

CCI Edits

Refer to Appendix A for CCI edits.

Facility RVUs ▯

Code	Work	PE Facility	MP	Total Facility
53852	5.93	4.48	0.72	11.13

Non-facility RVUs ▯

Code	Work	PE Non-Facility	MP	Total Non-Facility
53852	5.93	35.87	0.72	42.52

Modifiers (PAR) ▯

Code	Mod 50	Mod 51	Mod 62	Mod 66	Mod 80
53852	0	2	0	0	1

Global Period

Code	Days
53852	090

53854

53854 Transurethral destruction of prostate tissue; by radiofrequency generated water vapor thermotherapy

(For transurethral ablation of malignant prostate tissue by high-energy water vapor thermotherapy, including intraoperative imaging and needle guidance, use 0582T)

AMA Coding Notes

Other Procedures on the Urethra

(For 2 or 3 glass urinalysis, use 81020)

Surgical Procedures on the Urethra

(For endoscopy, see cystoscopy, urethroscopy, cystourethroscopy, 52000-52700)

(For injection procedure for urethrocystography, see 51600-51610)

Surgical Procedures on the Urinary System

(For provision of chemotherapeutic agents, report both the specific service in addition to code(s) for the specific substance(s) or drug(s) provided)

AMA *CPT® Assistant* ▢

53854: Nov 18: 10

Plain English Description

Transurethral water vapor thermotherapy uses the thermal energy in steam to treat benign prostatic hyperplasia (BPH) and its accompanying lower urinary tract symptoms. Tissue is ablated in a minimally invasive way using radiofrequency to generate wet thermal energy and employ convective vs. conductive heat transfer. Most patients are given an oral pain medication/anxiolytic or conscious sedation. A prostate block may also be used. With the patient in the lithotomy position, the hand-held delivery device containing a lens allowing for direct cystoscopic visualization is inserted into the urethra. The needle is positioned within the hypertrophied prostatic tissue of the lateral or median lobes. A generator applies radiofrequency current to the inductive coil within the device and converts a few drops of water into steam. The water vapor is injected into the prostate tissue through the retractable needle with small emitter holes spaced circumferentially around the tip. The vapor immediately turns back to water, releasing the energy stored in the vapor into the cell membranes, causing instant cell death. The needle is retracted and repositioned after each treatment until the prostatic tissue is ablated. Over time, this ablated tissue is reabsorbed by the body, reducing the volume of tissue and allowing the urethra to open.

Transurethral destruction of prostate tissue; by radiofrequency generated water vapor thermotherapy

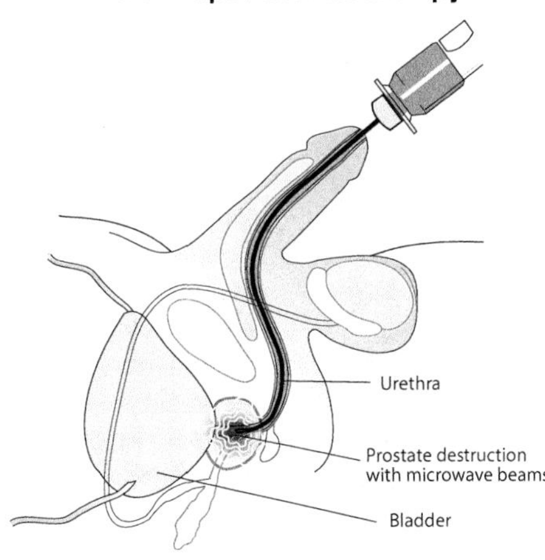

ICD-10-CM Diagnostic Codes

C61	Malignant neoplasm of prostate ♂
C79.82	Secondary malignant neoplasm of genital organs
D07.5	Carcinoma in situ of prostate ♂
D29.1	Benign neoplasm of prostate ♂
D40.0	Neoplasm of uncertain behavior of prostate ♂
N40.0	Benign prostatic hyperplasia without lower urinary tract symptoms ♂
N40.1	Benign prostatic hyperplasia with lower urinary tract symptoms ♂
N40.2	Nodular prostate without lower urinary tract symptoms ♂
N40.3	Nodular prostate with lower urinary tract symptoms ♂
N41.4	Granulomatous prostatitis ♂
N41.8	Other inflammatory diseases of prostate ♂
N42.30	Unspecified dysplasia of prostate ♂
N42.31	Prostatic intraepithelial neoplasia ♂
N42.32	Atypical small acinar proliferation of prostate ♂
N42.39	Other dysplasia of prostate ♂
N42.83	Cyst of prostate ♂
N42.89	Other specified disorders of prostate ♂
R33.8	Other retention of urine
R33.9	Retention of urine, unspecified
R39.12	Poor urinary stream
R39.14	Feeling of incomplete bladder emptying

CCI Edits

Refer to Appendix A for CCI edits.

Facility RVUs ▢

Code	Work	PE Facility	MP	Total Facility
53854	5.93	4.49	0.72	11.14

Non-facility RVUs ▢

Code	Work	PE Non-Facility	MP	Total Non-Facility
53854	5.93	44.92	0.72	51.57

Modifiers (PAR) ▢

Code	Mod 50	Mod 51	Mod 62	Mod 66	Mod 80
53854	0	2	0	0	1

Global Period

Code	Days
53854	090

53855

53855 Insertion of a temporary prostatic urethral stent, including urethral measurement

(For insertion of permanent urethral stent, use 52282)

AMA Coding Notes

Other Procedures on the Urethra

(For 2 or 3 glass urinalysis, use 81020)

Surgical Procedures on the Urethra

(For endoscopy, see cystoscopy, urethroscopy, cystourethroscopy, 52000-52700)

(For injection procedure for urethrocystography, see 51600-51610)

Surgical Procedures on the Urinary System

(For provision of chemotherapeutic agents, report both the specific service in addition to code(s) for the specific substance(s) or drug(s) provided)

AMA *CPT® Assistant* ▯

53855: Feb 10: 7, Nov 18: 10

Plain English Description

A temporary urethral stent is used to treat obstruction of the prostatic urethra due to benign prostatic hyperplasia (BPH) or following surgical treatment for BPH, prostatic cancer, or radiation therapy. Temporary stenting of the prostatic urethra is used as an alternative to placement of a Foley catheter and allows the patient to urinate normally. One type of stent consists of a proximal balloon to prevent migration or displacement of the stent, a urine port is situated above the balloon, a stent that spans the prostatic urethra, an anchor in the distal meatus, and a retrieval string for removal of the temporary stent. The urethral orifice is cleansed with antiseptic solution. An introducer is inserted into the urethra and the stent device advanced until the tip is in the bladder and the stent positioned in the prostatic urethra above the urethral sphincter. The balloon is inflated with sterile water to secure the soft tip in the bladder. The introducer is removed. The stent holds the prostatic urethra open so that urine can be passed normally.

Insertion of a temporary prostatic urethral stent

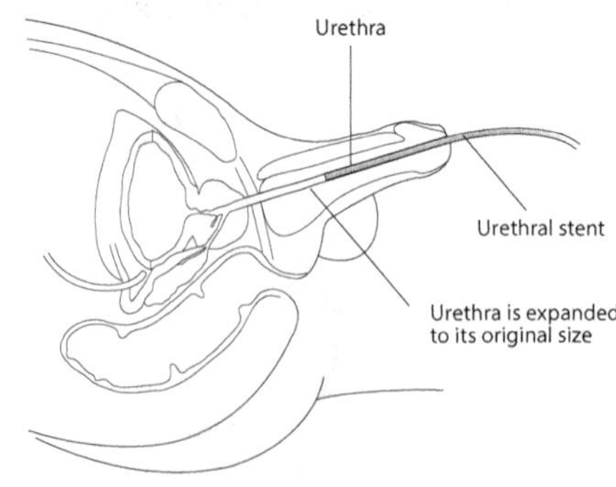

A temporary urethral stent is used to treat obstruction of the prostatic urethra due to benign prostatic hyperplasia (BPH) or following surgical treatment for BPH, prostatic cancer, or radiation therapy.

ICD-10-CM Diagnostic Codes

C61	Malignant neoplasm of prostate ♂
C68.0	Malignant neoplasm of urethra
C79.11	Secondary malignant neoplasm of bladder
C79.19	Secondary malignant neoplasm of other urinary organs
D07.5	Carcinoma in situ of prostate ♂
D29.1	Benign neoplasm of prostate ♂
D40.0	Neoplasm of uncertain behavior of prostate ♂
N32.0	Bladder-neck obstruction
N35.012	Post-traumatic membranous urethral stricture ♂
N35.113	Postinfective membranous urethral stricture, not elsewhere classified, male ♂
N35.813	Other membranous urethral stricture, male ♂
N36.8	Other specified disorders of urethra
N37	Urethral disorders in diseases classified elsewhere
N40.0	Benign prostatic hyperplasia without lower urinary tract symptoms ♂
N40.1	Benign prostatic hyperplasia with lower urinary tract symptoms ♂
N40.2	Nodular prostate without lower urinary tract symptoms ♂
N40.3	Nodular prostate with lower urinary tract symptoms ♂
N99.112	Postprocedural membranous urethral stricture, male ♂
N99.115	Postprocedural fossa navicularis urethral stricture ♂
Q64.31	Congenital bladder neck obstruction
Q64.32	Congenital stricture of urethra
Q64.33	Congenital stricture of urinary meatus
Q64.39	Other atresia and stenosis of urethra and bladder neck

CCI Edits

Refer to Appendix A for CCI edits.

Facility RVUs ▯

Code	Work	PE Facility	MP	Total Facility
53855	1.64	0.56	0.20	2.40

Non-facility RVUs ▯

Code	Work	PE Non-Facility	MP	Total Non-Facility
53855	1.64	18.47	0.20	20.31

Modifiers (PAR) ▯

Code	Mod 50	Mod 51	Mod 62	Mod 66	Mod 80
53855	0	2	0	0	0

Global Period

Code	Days
53855	000

53860

53860 Transurethral radiofrequency micro-remodeling of the female bladder neck and proximal urethra for stress urinary incontinence

AMA Coding Notes

Other Procedures on the Urethra

(For 2 or 3 glass urinalysis, use 81020)

Surgical Procedures on the Urethra

(For endoscopy, see cystoscopy, urethroscopy, cystourethroscopy, 52000-52700)

(For injection procedure for urethrocystography, see 51600-51610)

Surgical Procedures on the Urinary System

(For provision of chemotherapeutic agents, report both the specific service in addition to code(s) for the specific substance(s) or drug(s) provided)

Plain English Description

The physician performs transurethral radiofrequency micro-remodeling of the female bladder neck and proximal urethra for urinary stress incontinence due to hypermobility. Low-temperature radiofrequency energy is used to remodel the submucosal tissue of the bladder neck and urethra and change the luminal function without causing narrowing or thickening of the lumen. A local anesthetic is administered. The transurethral probe is inserted into the urethra, and controlled radiofrequency energy is applied to heat the submucosal tissue at target sites in the lower urinary tract. This results in collagen denaturation at the multiple small treatment sites. When the tissue heals, the treated sites have increased resistance to intra-abdominal pressure, which reduces or eliminates involuntary leakage of urine.

Transurethral radiofrequency micro-remodeling of the female bladder neck and proximal urethra

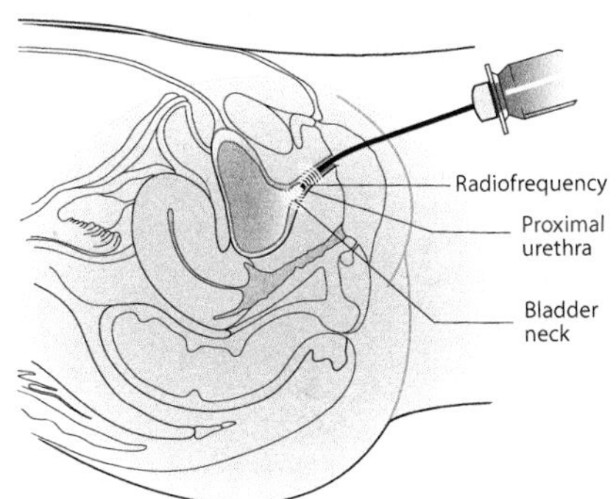

ICD-10-CM Diagnostic Codes

N36.41	Hypermobility of urethra
N36.43	Combined hypermobility of urethra and intrinsic sphincter deficiency
N39.3	Stress incontinence (female) (male)
N39.46	Mixed incontinence

CCI Edits

Refer to Appendix A for CCI edits.

Facility RVUs

Code	Work	PE Facility	MP	Total Facility
53860	3.97	2.05	0.45	6.47

Non-facility RVUs

Code	Work	PE Non-Facility	MP	Total Non-Facility
53860	3.97	69.78	0.45	74.20

Modifiers (PAR)

Code	Mod 50	Mod 51	Mod 62	Mod 66	Mod 80
53860	0	2	0	0	0

Global Period

Code	Days
53860	090

54000-54001

54000 Slitting of prepuce, dorsal or lateral (separate procedure); newborn

(Do not report modifier 63 in conjunction with 54000)

54001 Slitting of prepuce, dorsal or lateral (separate procedure); except newborn

AMA Coding Notes

Incision Procedures on the Penis

(For abdominal perineal gangrene debridement, see 11004-11006)

Plain English Description

The physician makes a dorsal or lateral slit in the prepuce. The prepuce, also referred to as the foreskin, is the free fold of skin that covers the glans penis in uncircumcised males. If the prepuce is too tight, it is incised (slit) on the back (dorsum) or sides (lateral). Use 54000 when the procedure is performed on a newborn and 54001 when it is performed on a patient other than a newborn.

Slitting of prepuce, dorsal or lateral (separate procedure)

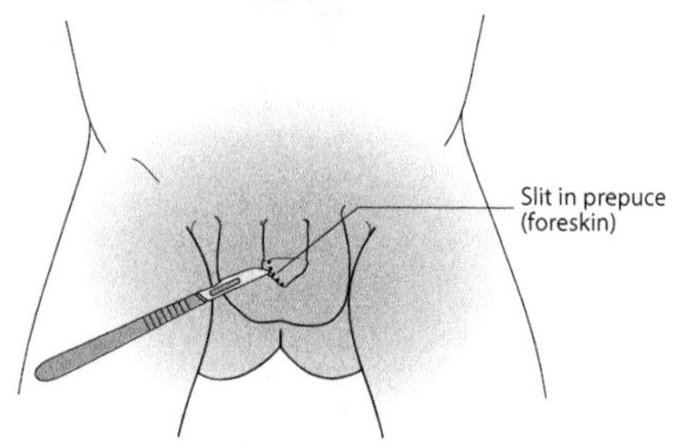

Newborn (54000); other than newborn (54001)

ICD-10-CM Diagnostic Codes

N47.0	Adherent prepuce, newborn ♂
N47.1	Phimosis ♂
N47.2	Paraphimosis ♂
N47.3	Deficient foreskin ♂
N47.4	Benign cyst of prepuce ♂
N47.5	Adhesions of prepuce and glans penis ♂
N47.6	Balanoposthitis ♂
N47.7	Other inflammatory diseases of prepuce ♂
N47.8	Other disorders of prepuce ♂
N48.1	Balanitis ♂

CCI Edits

Refer to Appendix A for CCI edits.

Facility RVUs ▯

Code	Work	PE Facility	MP	Total Facility
54000	1.59	1.45	0.20	3.24
54001	2.24	1.60	0.25	4.09

Non-facility RVUs ▯

Code	Work	PE Non-Facility	MP	Total Non-Facility
54000	1.59	3.06	0.20	4.85
54001	2.24	3.38	0.25	5.87

Modifiers (PAR) ▯

Code	Mod 50	Mod 51	Mod 62	Mod 66	Mod 80
54000	0	2	0	0	0
54001	0	2	0	0	1

Global Period

Code	Days
54000	010
54001	010

54015

54015 Incision and drainage of penis, deep

(For skin and subcutaneous abscess, see 10060-10160)

AMA Coding Notes

Incision Procedures on the Penis

(For abdominal perineal gangrene debridement, see 11004-11006)

Plain English Description

The patient is positioned supine and the penis is prepared with an antiseptic solution. The area is infiltrated with local anesthetic and an incision made through the skin and carried down to the corpus cavernosum and/or the corpus spongiosum until the infected area is opened and pus/fluid starts to drain. Infected or devitalized tissue is debrided including the epithelial cell lining. The wound is cleaned and irrigated with saline and/or antibacterial solution. A drain is placed and the wound closed with simple sutures. A sterile dressing is applied immediately following the procedure. The dressing and drain are removed 2-3 days later.

Incision and drainage of penis, deep

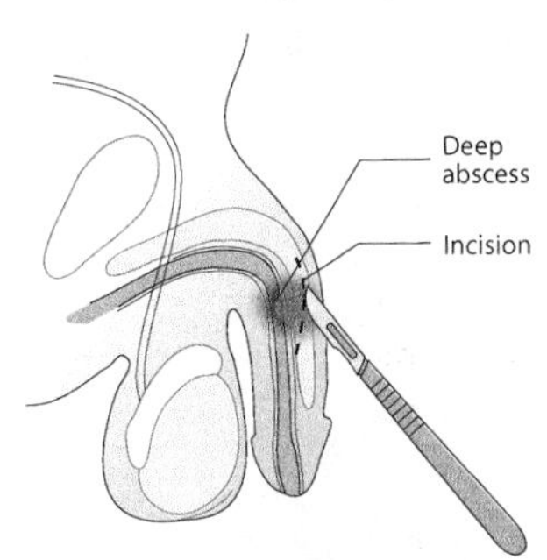

ICD-10-CM Diagnostic Codes

	A54.1	Gonococcal infection of lower genitourinary tract with periurethral and accessory gland abscess
	L98.495	Non-pressure chronic ulcer of skin of other sites with muscle involvement without evidence of necrosis
	L98.496	Non-pressure chronic ulcer of skin of other sites with bone involvement without evidence of necrosis
	N48.21	Abscess of corpus cavernosum and penis ♂
	N48.22	Cellulitis of corpus cavernosum and penis ♂
	N48.29	Other inflammatory disorders of penis ♂
	N48.5	Ulcer of penis ♂
	N48.89	Other specified disorders of penis ♂
❼	T79.8	Other early complications of trauma
❼	T81.42	Infection following a procedure, deep incisional surgical site

ICD-10-CM Coding Notes

For codes requiring a 7th character extension, refer to your ICD-10-CM book. Review the character descriptions and coding guidelines for proper selection. For some procedures, only certain characters will apply.

CCI Edits

Refer to Appendix A for CCI edits.

Facility RVUs ▯

Code	Work	PE Facility	MP	Total Facility
54015	5.36	2.92	0.64	8.92

Non-facility RVUs ▯

Code	Work	PE Non-Facility	MP	Total Non-Facility
54015	5.36	2.92	0.64	8.92

Modifiers (PAR) ▯

Code	Mod 50	Mod 51	Mod 62	Mod 66	Mod 80
54015	0	2	0	0	0

Global Period

Code	Days
54015	010

54050-54065

54050 Destruction of lesion(s), penis (eg, condyloma, papilloma, molluscum contagiosum, herpetic vesicle), simple; chemical

54055 Destruction of lesion(s), penis (eg, condyloma, papilloma, molluscum contagiosum, herpetic vesicle), simple; electrodesiccation

54056 Destruction of lesion(s), penis (eg, condyloma, papilloma, molluscum contagiosum, herpetic vesicle), simple; cryosurgery

54057 Destruction of lesion(s), penis (eg, condyloma, papilloma, molluscum contagiosum, herpetic vesicle), simple; laser surgery

54060 Destruction of lesion(s), penis (eg, condyloma, papilloma, molluscum contagiosum, herpetic vesicle), simple; surgical excision

54065 Destruction of lesion(s), penis (eg, condyloma, papilloma, molluscum contagiosum, herpetic vesicle), extensive (eg, laser surgery, electrosurgery, cryosurgery, chemosurgery)

(For destruction or excision of other lesions, see Integumentary System)

Plain English Description

The physician destroys one or more lesions on the penis using a method such as chemical destruction, electrodessication, cryosurgery, laser surgery, electrosurgery, or surgical excision. Common types of lesions treated include condylomata, papillomata, molluscum contagiosum, and herpetic vesicles. The lesion is examined and the most appropriate form of destruction determined. Local anesthesia is administered as needed. In 54050, a simple chemical destruction is performed with silver nitrate or other chemical compound. In 54055, a simple electrodessication is performed using a monopolar high-frequency electric current to destroy the lesion and control bleeding. In 54056, cryosurgery is performed using liquid nitrogen to freeze the lesion. A series of freeze-thaw cycles may be required to completely destroy the lesion. In 54057, a simple laser ablation is performed using a non-contact Nd-YAG laser or a contact laser probe with coaxial water to vaporize the lesion. In 54060, a simple excision is performed. A narrow margin of healthy tissue is identified and a full-thickness incision is made through the mucous and submucous tissue. The incision is carried around the lesion and the entire lesion is excised. The lesion is sent to the laboratory for separately reportable histologic evaluation. Bleeding is controlled by electrocautery or chemical cautery. The wound may be closed using simple single-layer suture technique or left open to granulate. In 54065, extensive destruction of a large lesion or multiple lesions is performed using laser surgery, electrosurgery, cryosurgery, or chemosurgery. Laser surgery, cryosurgery, or chemosurgery is performed as described above over an extensive area. Alternatively, electrosurgery may be performed. Electrosurgery uses heat applied to the lesion(s) with a high frequency current that passes through a metal probe or needle.

Destruction of lesion(s), penis

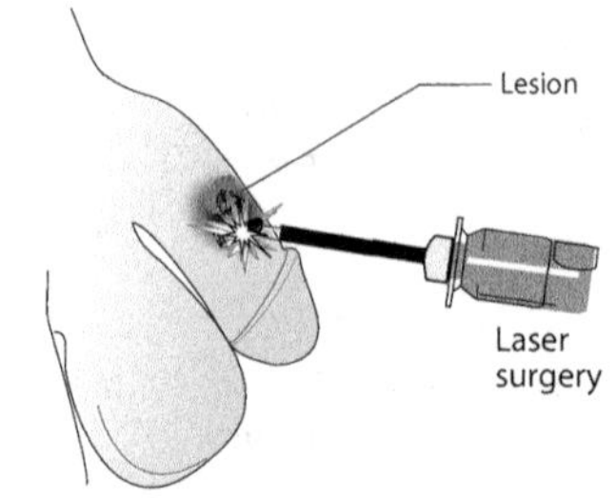

Simple, chemical (54050); simple, electrodesiccation (54055); simple, cryosurgery (54056); simple, laser surgery (54057); simple, surgical excision (54060); extensive (54065)

ICD-10-CM Diagnostic Codes

A60.01	Herpesviral infection of penis ♂
A63.0	Anogenital (venereal) warts
B07.8	Other viral warts
B07.9	Viral wart, unspecified
B08.1	Molluscum contagiosum
B97.7	Papillomavirus as the cause of diseases classified elsewhere
C60.0	Malignant neoplasm of prepuce ♂
C60.1	Malignant neoplasm of glans penis ♂
C60.2	Malignant neoplasm of body of penis ♂
C60.8	Malignant neoplasm of overlapping sites of penis ♂
C63.8	Malignant neoplasm of overlapping sites of male genital organs ♂
C79.82	Secondary malignant neoplasm of genital organs
D07.69	Carcinoma in situ of other male genital organs ♂
D29.0	Benign neoplasm of penis ♂
L82.1	Other seborrheic keratosis
N48.29	Other inflammatory disorders of penis ♂

CCI Edits

Refer to Appendix A for CCI edits.

Pub 100

54057: Pub 100-03, 1, 140.5
54065: Pub 100-03, 1, 140.5

Facility RVUs ▢

Code	Work	PE Facility	MP	Total Facility
54050	1.29	1.66	0.12	3.07
54055	1.25	1.38	0.12	2.75
54056	1.29	1.80	0.12	3.21
54057	1.29	1.40	0.14	2.83
54060	1.98	1.62	0.24	3.84
54065	2.47	2.27	0.25	4.99

Non-facility RVUs ▢

Code	Work	PE Non-Facility	MP	Total Non-Facility
54050	1.29	2.78	0.12	4.19
54055	1.25	2.64	0.12	4.01
54056	1.29	2.80	0.12	4.21
54057	1.29	2.75	0.14	4.18
54060	1.98	3.59	0.24	5.81
54065	2.47	3.83	0.25	6.55

Modifiers (PAR) ▢

Code	Mod 50	Mod 51	Mod 62	Mod 66	Mod 80
54050	0	2	0	0	1
54055	0	2	0	0	1
54056	0	2	0	0	1
54057	0	2	0	0	1
54060	0	2	0	0	1
54065	0	2	0	0	1

Global Period

Code	Days
54050	010
54055	010
54056	010
54057	010
54060	010
54065	010

54100-54105

54100 Biopsy of penis; (separate procedure)
54105 Biopsy of penis; deep structures

AMA *CPT® Assistant* ▢
54100: Nov 99: 26

Plain English Description
A biopsy of the penis is performed. In 54100, a simple biopsy is performed. The area to be biopsied is disinfected and a local anesthetic administered. An incision is made in the skin overlying the lesion. A tissue sample is obtained. The tissue is sent to the laboratory for separately reportable histological evaluation. In 54105, a biopsy of deeper tissue is performed, which may require use of a general anesthetic. Overlying tissues are dissected until the suspicious mass or lump is exposed. A tissue sample is obtained and sent for separately reportable histological evaluation.

Biopsy of penis

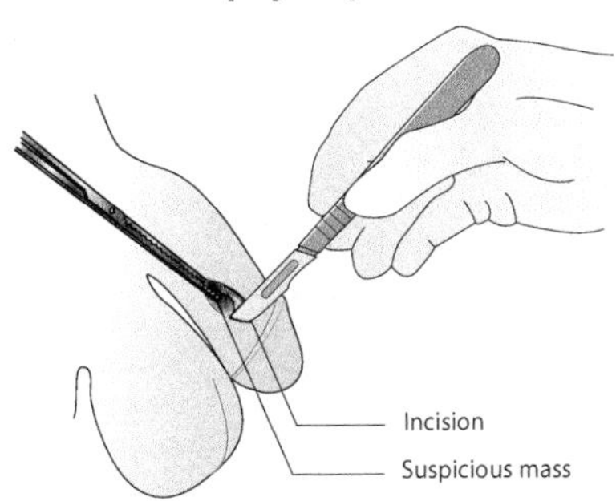

Separate procedure (54100); deep structures (54105)

ICD-10-CM Diagnostic Codes

A60.09	Herpesviral infection of other urogenital tract
A60.9	Anogenital herpesviral infection, unspecified
A63.0	Anogenital (venereal) warts
C60.0	Malignant neoplasm of prepuce ♂
C60.1	Malignant neoplasm of glans penis ♂
C60.2	Malignant neoplasm of body of penis ♂
C79.82	Secondary malignant neoplasm of genital organs
D07.4	Carcinoma in situ of penis ♂
D29.0	Benign neoplasm of penis ♂
D40.8	Neoplasm of uncertain behavior of other specified male genital organs ♂
D48.5	Neoplasm of uncertain behavior of skin
D49.59	Neoplasm of unspecified behavior of other genitourinary organ
L40.8	Other psoriasis
N47.6	Balanoposthitis ♂
N48.0	Leukoplakia of penis ♂
N48.1	Balanitis ♂
N48.29	Other inflammatory disorders of penis ♂
N48.5	Ulcer of penis ♂
N48.6	Induration penis plastica ♂
N48.83	Acquired buried penis ♂
N48.89	Other specified disorders of penis ♂
Z85.828	Personal history of other malignant neoplasm of skin

CCI Edits
Refer to Appendix A for CCI edits.

Facility RVUs ▢

Code	Work	PE Facility	MP	Total Facility
54100	1.90	1.41	0.20	3.51
54105	3.54	2.26	0.41	6.21

Non-facility RVUs ▢

Code	Work	PE Non-Facility	MP	Total Non-Facility
54100	1.90	3.92	0.20	6.02
54105	3.54	4.21	0.41	8.16

Modifiers (PAR) ▢

Code	Mod 50	Mod 51	Mod 62	Mod 66	Mod 80
54100	0	2	0	0	1
54105	0	2	0	0	1

Global Period

Code	Days
54100	000
54105	010

54110-54112

54110 Excision of penile plaque (Peyronie disease)

54111 Excision of penile plaque (Peyronie disease); with graft to 5 cm in length

54112 Excision of penile plaque (Peyronie disease); with graft greater than 5 cm in length

AMA *CPT® Assistant*

54111: Aug 99: 5

Plain English Description

Excision of penile plaque associated with Peyronie's disease is performed with or without graft repair. Peyronie's disease is characterized by the development of a hard, fibrous layer of scar tissue (plaque) under the skin in the spongy erectile tissue on the upper or lower side of the penis. The plaque causes the penis to curve when erect. The overlying tissue is incised and the plaque exposed. The plaque is then expanded by making several linear cuts in the plaque or excised. The areas of excision or expansion are covered as needed using a graft of skin, vein, or synthetic material. Use 54110, if the procedure is performed without a graft, 54111 if a graft of 5 cm or less is used, and 54112 if a graft of greater than 5 cm is required.

Excision of penile plaque

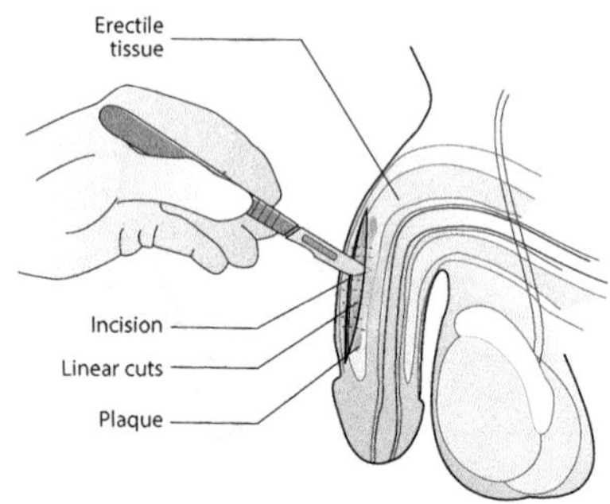

Excision (54110); with graft to 5 cm in length (54111); with graft greater than 5 cm in length (54112)

ICD-10-CM Diagnostic Codes

N48.6 Induration penis plastica ♂

CCI Edits

Refer to Appendix A for CCI edits.

Facility RVUs

Code	Work	PE Facility	MP	Total Facility
54110	10.92	6.14	1.32	18.38
54111	14.42	7.24	1.70	23.36
54112	16.98	8.40	2.01	27.39

Non-facility RVUs

Code	Work	PE Non-Facility	MP	Total Non-Facility
54110	10.92	6.14	1.32	18.38
54111	14.42	7.24	1.70	23.36
54112	16.98	8.40	2.01	27.39

Modifiers (PAR)

Code	Mod 50	Mod 51	Mod 62	Mod 66	Mod 80
54110	0	2	0	0	2
54111	0	2	1	0	2
54112	0	2	1	0	2

Global Period

Code	Days
54110	090
54111	090
54112	090

54115

54115 Removal foreign body from deep penile tissue (eg, plastic implant)

Plain English Description

To remove a foreign body, such as an implant, from deep penile tissue, the patient is positioned supine and the penis is prepared and draped. An incision is made along the shaft of the penis overlying the foreign body and carried down to the corpus cavernosum and/or corpus spongiosum until the object is visualized. Tissue surrounding the object is dissected free, including devitalized or infected tissue, and the wound irrigated with saline and/or antibacterial solution. A drain is placed and the wound closed with simple sutures. A sterile dressing is applied immediately following the procedure. The dressing and drain are removed 2-3 days later.

Removal of foreign body from deep penile tissue

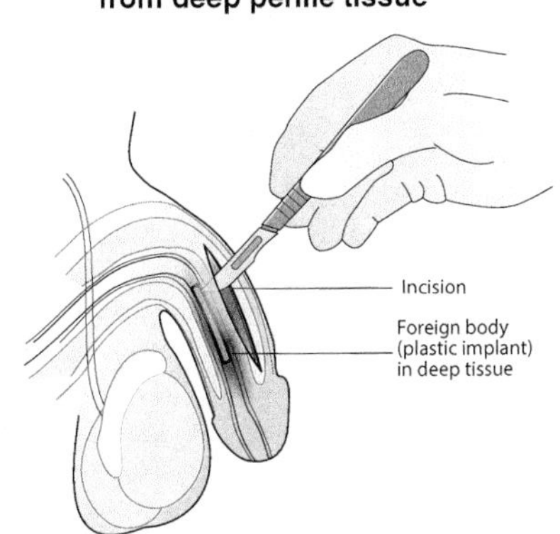

ICD-10-CM Diagnostic Codes

	M79.5	Residual foreign body in soft tissue
➐	T19.4	Foreign body in penis
➐	T83.410	Breakdown (mechanical) of implanted penile prosthesis
➐	T83.420	Displacement of implanted penile prosthesis
➐	T83.490	Other mechanical complication of implanted penile prosthesis
➐	T83.61	Infection and inflammatory reaction due to implanted penile prosthesis
➐	T83.82	Fibrosis due to genitourinary prosthetic devices, implants and grafts
➐	T83.83	Hemorrhage due to genitourinary prosthetic devices, implants and grafts
➐	T83.84	Pain due to genitourinary prosthetic devices, implants and grafts
➐	T83.85	Stenosis due to genitourinary prosthetic devices, implants and grafts
➐	T83.86	Thrombosis due to genitourinary prosthetic devices, implants and grafts
➐	T83.89	Other specified complication of genitourinary prosthetic devices, implants and grafts

ICD-10-CM Coding Notes

For codes requiring a 7th character extension, refer to your ICD-10-CM book. Review the character descriptions and coding guidelines for proper selection. For some procedures, only certain characters will apply.

CCI Edits

Refer to Appendix A for CCI edits.

Facility RVUs ▢

Code	Work	PE Facility	MP	Total Facility
54115	6.95	4.72	0.84	12.51

Non-facility RVUs ▢

Code	Work	PE Non-Facility	MP	Total Non-Facility
54115	6.95	5.65	0.84	13.44

Modifiers (PAR) ▢

Code	Mod 50	Mod 51	Mod 62	Mod 66	Mod 80
54115	0	2	0	0	2

Global Period

Code	Days
54115	090

CPT® Procedural Coding

54120

54120 Amputation of penis; partial

Plain English Description

Partial amputation of the penis, or penectomy, is performed with the patient in supine position under local, regional, or general anesthesia. The penis is prepared and draped and the tumor or lesion may be isolated by suturing a sterile condom or glove to the penile tip. A tourniquet is placed around the base of the penis and a circumferential incision is made in the skin 1.5 to 2.0 cm proximal to the tumor or lesion. Superficial and deep dorsal veins are identified, cut, and tied with sutures. Dissection continues through Buck's fascia and the tunica albuginea of the corpora. The corpora cavernosa is divided down to the urethra to identify the central cavernosal arteries, which are tied off with sutures. The urethra is now dissected free from the corpus spongiosum, leaving a 1 cm urethral stump distally to the transected corpora cavernosa and the specimen is removed. Tissue samples from the amputated penis are then prepared and examined by a pathologist in a separately reportable procedure to determine if margins are clear of cancer or other abnormal cells. The remaining urethral stump and transected corpora are washed off with an antiseptic or antibiotic solution and the closure begins by placing horizontal mattress sutures through the corpora, incorporating Buck's fascia, tunica albuginea, and intercavernous septum. The tourniquet is released from the base of the penis and bleeding controlled by fulguration. The urethra is spatulated and sutured to the skin. The skin is closed or, if a dorsal skin flap has been left, a button-hole incision is made in the flap, the flap is rotated ventrally anastomosing the dorsally spatulated urethra to the button-hole opening, and finally closing the skin flaps. One other option is to leave a slightly longer urethral stump, 1.5 to 2 cm, and spatulate ventrally, the dorsal flap is then rotated and sutured to the tunica albuginea of the corpora cavernosa and skin. A catheter is inserted transurethrally at the conclusion of the procedure.

Amputation of penis; partial

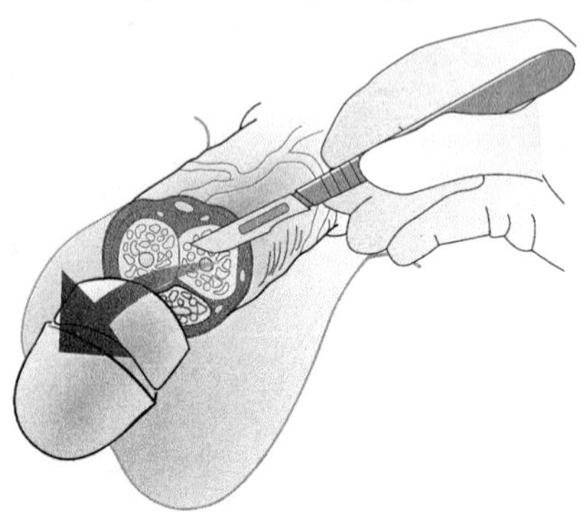

ICD-10-CM Diagnostic Codes

	C60.1	Malignant neoplasm of glans penis ♂
	C60.2	Malignant neoplasm of body of penis ♂
	C60.8	Malignant neoplasm of overlapping sites of penis ♂
	C60.9	Malignant neoplasm of penis, unspecified ♂
	C79.82	Secondary malignant neoplasm of genital organs
	D07.4	Carcinoma in situ of penis ♂
	I96	Gangrene, not elsewhere classified
	N48.0	Leukoplakia of penis ♂
	N48.21	Abscess of corpus cavernosum and penis ♂
	N48.22	Cellulitis of corpus cavernosum and penis ♂
	N48.29	Other inflammatory disorders of penis ♂
	N50.1	Vascular disorders of male genital organs ♂
❼	S31.21	Laceration without foreign body of penis
❼	S31.22	Laceration with foreign body of penis
❼	S31.23	Puncture wound without foreign body of penis
❼	S31.24	Puncture wound with foreign body of penis
❼	S31.25	Open bite of penis
❼	S38.222	Partial traumatic amputation of penis
❼	T21.36	Burn of third degree of male genital region
❼	T21.76	Corrosion of third degree of male genital region

ICD-10-CM Coding Notes

For codes requiring a 7th character extension, refer to your ICD-10-CM book. Review the character descriptions and coding guidelines for proper selection. For some procedures, only certain characters will apply.

CCI Edits

Refer to Appendix A for CCI edits.

Facility RVUs ▢

Code	Work	PE Facility	MP	Total Facility
54120	11.01	6.19	1.33	18.53

Non-facility RVUs ▢

Code	Work	PE Non-Facility	MP	Total Non-Facility
54120	11.01	6.19	1.33	18.53

Modifiers (PAR) ▢

Code	Mod 50	Mod 51	Mod 62	Mod 66	Mod 80
54120	0	2	1	0	2

Global Period

Code	Days
54120	090

54125

54125 Amputation of penis; complete

Plain English Description

Complete amputation of the penis may be necessary when a tumor or lesion is large or infiltrating. With the patient in dorsal lithotomy position, the penis, scrotum, and perineum are prepared and draped. The tumor or lesion is isolated with a sterile condom or glove sheathing the entire penis and sutured at the base. An elliptical skin incision is made at the base of the penis and carried through the subcutaneous tissue to the pubis. Blood vessels and lymphatic tissue are ligated or fulgurated. Penile suspensory ligaments are identified and isolated. The dorsal vein and penile arteries are identified, clamped, and ligated. Positioning the penis upward, Buck's fascia is opened and the urethra is dissected free from the corpora cavernosa. The urethra is divided at the distal bulbar region with adequate length to route to the perineum. Dissection of the corpora cavernosa continues to the ischiopubic rami where it is ligated and transected and the amputation is complete. Tissue samples from the amputated penis are then prepared and examined by a pathologist in a separately reportable procedure to determine if margins are clear of cancer or other abnormal cells. Dissection continues around the urethra to the urogenital diaphragm attempting a straight course to the perineal urethrostomy site. A 1 cm wedge of skin and subcutaneous tissue are removed from the perineum midline between the scrotum and the rectum. Using a curved clamp, a tunnel is created in the perineal subcutaneous tissue and the urethra is pulled through the perineal incision. After spatulating the urethra dorsally, a V-shaped skin inlay is created and anastomosed to the lining of the urethra. A catheter is inserted transurethrally. Penrose drains are placed on either side of the scrotum and the wound is closed transversely allowing elevation of the scrotum away from the perineal urethrostomy site.

Amputation of penis; complete

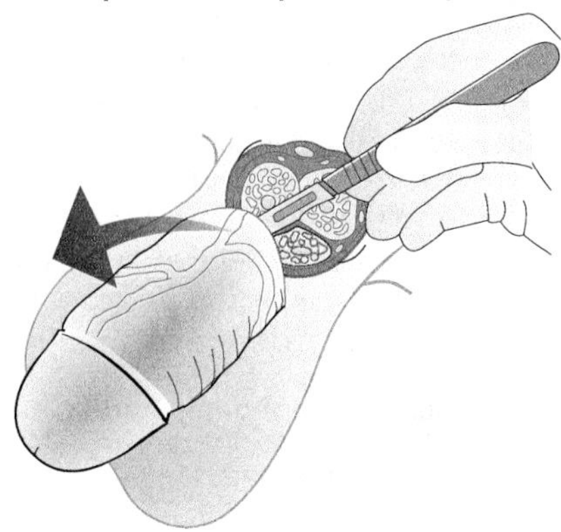

ICD-10-CM Diagnostic Codes

	C60.2	Malignant neoplasm of body of penis ♂
	C60.8	Malignant neoplasm of overlapping sites of penis ♂
	C60.9	Malignant neoplasm of penis, unspecified ♂
⇄	C63.11	Malignant neoplasm of right spermatic cord ♂
⇄	C63.12	Malignant neoplasm of left spermatic cord ♂
	C79.82	Secondary malignant neoplasm of genital organs
	D07.4	Carcinoma in situ of penis ♂
	D09.8	Carcinoma in situ of other specified sites
	I96	Gangrene, not elsewhere classified
	N48.0	Leukoplakia of penis ♂
	N49.8	Inflammatory disorders of other specified male genital organs ♂
	N50.1	Vascular disorders of male genital organs ♂
	N50.89	Other specified disorders of the male genital organs ♂
❼	S31.21	Laceration without foreign body of penis
❼	S31.22	Laceration with foreign body of penis
❼	S31.23	Puncture wound without foreign body of penis
❼	S31.24	Puncture wound with foreign body of penis
❼	S31.25	Open bite of penis
❼	S38.222	Partial traumatic amputation of penis
❼	T21.36	Burn of third degree of male genital region
❼	T21.76	Corrosion of third degree of male genital region

ICD-10-CM Coding Notes

For codes requiring a 7th character extension, refer to your ICD-10-CM book. Review the character descriptions and coding guidelines for proper selection. For some procedures, only certain characters will apply.

CCI Edits

Refer to Appendix A for CCI edits.

Facility RVUs ☐

Code	Work	PE Facility	MP	Total Facility
54125	14.56	7.64	1.83	24.03

Non-facility RVUs ☐

Code	Work	PE Non-Facility	MP	Total Non-Facility
54125	14.56	7.64	1.83	24.03

Modifiers (PAR) ☐

Code	Mod 50	Mod 51	Mod 62	Mod 66	Mod 80
54125	0	2	1	0	2

Global Period

Code	Days
54125	090

54130-54135

54130 Amputation of penis, radical; with bilateral inguinofemoral lymphadenectomy

54135 Amputation of penis, radical; in continuity with bilateral pelvic lymphadenectomy, including external iliac, hypogastric and obturator nodes

(For lymphadenectomy [separate procedure], see 38760-38770)

Plain English Description

The tumor or lesion in the penis is isolated with a sterile condom or glove sheathing the entire penis and sutured at the base. An elliptical skin incision is made at the base of the penis and carried through the subcutaneous tissue to the pubis. Blood vessels and lymphatic tissue are ligated or fulgurated. Penile suspensory ligaments are identified and isolated. The dorsal vein and penile arteries are identified, clamped, and ligated. Positioning the penis upward, Buck's fascia is opened and the urethra is dissected free from the corpora cavernosa. The urethra is divided at the distal bulbar region leaving adequate length to route to the perineum. The corpora cavernosa is dissected to the ischiopubic rami where it is ligated and transected and the amputation is complete. Dissection continues around the urethra to the urogenital diaphragm attempting a straight course to the perineal urethrostomy site. A wedge of skin and subcutaneous tissue are removed from the perineum midline between the scrotum and the rectum. Using a curved clamp, a tunnel is created in the perineal subcutaneous tissue and the urethra is pulled through the perineal incision. After spatulating the urethra dorsally, a V-shaped skin inlay is created and anastomosed to the lining of the urethra. A catheter is inserted. Penrose drains are placed on either side of the scrotum and the wound is closed transversely to elevate the scrotum away from the perineal urethrostomy site. In 54130, amputation of the penis is performed with bilateral inguinofemoral lymphadenectomy. An incision is made parallel to the inguinofemoral ligament and carried down to Camper's fascia. Skin flaps are elevated and separated from the underlying fat pad. Deep tissues at the superior aspect of the inguinal region are dissected. Cloquet's node is identified, excised, and frozen section performed. The fat pad containing nodal tissue is elevated and mobilized down to the inferior margin of the inguinal ligament. Dissection continues into the femoral triangle. The cribriform fascia is opened. Once the nodal tissue over the common femoral vein has been completely freed, the inguinofemoral nodal tissue is removed as a single specimen. In 54135, the amputation of the penis and inguinofemoral lymphadenectomy are performed as described above. If Cloquet's node is positive for malignancy, bilateral pelvic lymphadenectomy including excision of external iliac, hypogastric, and obturator nodes is performed. The abdomen is incised without opening the peritoneum, and the pelvic lymph nodes are explored. Fatty tissue is stripped from the mid-portion of the common iliac vessel and along the internal and external iliac vessels to the level of the circumflex iliac vein. Iliac, hypogastric, and obturator nodes are excised. The groin and abdominal incisions are closed in layers.

Amputation of penis, radical (bilateral inguinofemoral lymphadenectomy)

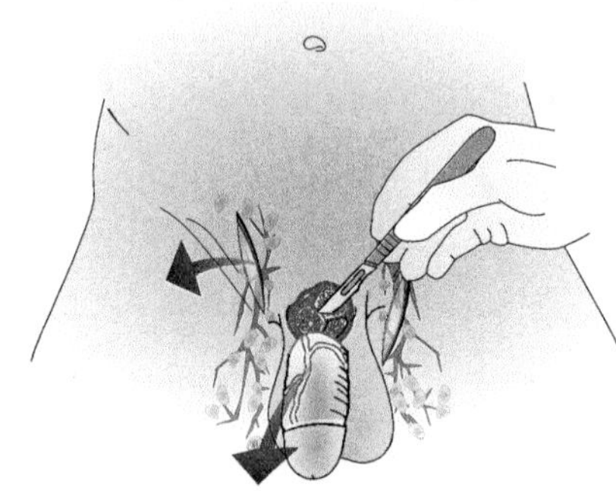

ICD-10-CM Diagnostic Codes

C60.0	Malignant neoplasm of prepuce ♂
C60.1	Malignant neoplasm of glans penis ♂
C60.2	Malignant neoplasm of body of penis ♂
C60.8	Malignant neoplasm of overlapping sites of penis ♂
C63.9	Malignant neoplasm of male genital organ, unspecified ♂
C77.2	Secondary and unspecified malignant neoplasm of intra-abdominal lymph nodes
C77.4	Secondary and unspecified malignant neoplasm of inguinal and lower limb lymph nodes
C77.5	Secondary and unspecified malignant neoplasm of intrapelvic lymph nodes
C79.82	Secondary malignant neoplasm of genital organs
D07.4	Carcinoma in situ of penis ♂
D40.8	Neoplasm of uncertain behavior of other specified male genital organs ♂
I96	Gangrene, not elsewhere classified
N48.0	Leukoplakia of penis ♂
N48.21	Abscess of corpus cavernosum and penis ♂
N48.22	Cellulitis of corpus cavernosum and penis ♂
N48.29	Other inflammatory disorders of penis ♂

CCI Edits

Refer to Appendix A for CCI edits.

Facility RVUs ▢

Code	Work	PE Facility	MP	Total Facility
54130	21.84	10.40	2.62	34.86
54135	28.17	12.54	3.36	44.07

Non-facility RVUs ▢

Code	Work	PE Non-Facility	MP	Total Non-Facility
54130	21.84	10.40	2.62	34.86
54135	28.17	12.54	3.36	44.07

Modifiers (PAR) ▢

Code	Mod 50	Mod 51	Mod 62	Mod 66	Mod 80
54130	2	2	1	0	2
54135	2	2	0	0	2

Global Period

Code	Days
54130	090
54135	090

54150

54150 Circumcision, using clamp or other device with regional dorsal penile or ring block

(Do not report modifier 63 in conjunction with 54150)

(Report 54150 with modifier 52 when performed without dorsal penile or ring block)

AMA *CPT® Assistant*

54150: Sep 96: 11, May 98: 11, Apr 03: 27, Aug 03: 6, May 07: 10, Jul 07: 5

Plain English Description

The foreskin on the head of the penis of a newborn is removed. The physician places a clamp or other device over the head of the penis to expose the foreskin, which is then removed. The clamp stays in place for a few days until all of the foreskin is gone. A regional block is included.

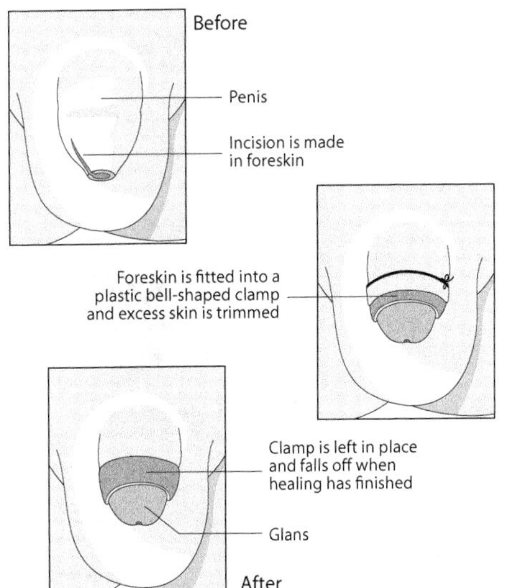
Circumcision
Using clamp or other device with regional dorsal penile or ring block
Before
Penis
Incision is made in foreskin
Foreskin is fitted into a plastic bell-shaped clamp and excess skin is trimmed
Clamp is left in place and falls off when healing has finished
Glans
After

ICD-10-CM Diagnostic Codes

N47.0	Adherent prepuce, newborn ♂
N47.1	Phimosis ♂
N47.2	Paraphimosis ♂
N47.3	Deficient foreskin ♂
N47.4	Benign cyst of prepuce ♂
N47.5	Adhesions of prepuce and glans penis ♂
N47.7	Other inflammatory diseases of prepuce ♂
N47.8	Other disorders of prepuce ♂
Z41.2	Encounter for routine and ritual male circumcision ♂

CCI Edits

Refer to Appendix A for CCI edits.

Facility RVUs

Code	Work	PE Facility	MP	Total Facility
54150	1.90	0.69	0.25	2.84

Non-facility RVUs

Code	Work	PE Non-Facility	MP	Total Non-Facility
54150	1.90	2.27	0.25	4.42

Modifiers (PAR)

Code	Mod 50	Mod 51	Mod 62	Mod 66	Mod 80
54150	0	2	0	0	0

Global Period

Code	Days
54150	000

54160-54161

54160 Circumcision, surgical excision other than clamp, device, or dorsal slit; neonate (28 days of age or less)

(Do not report modifier 63 in conjunction with 54160)

54161 Circumcision, surgical excision other than clamp, device, or dorsal slit; older than 28 days of age

AMA *CPT® Assistant*

54160: Sep 96: 11, May 98: 11, May 07: 10, Jul 07: 5

54161: Sep 96: 11, Dec 96: 10, May 98: 11, Jul 07: 5

Plain English Description

A male circumcision is performed using a method other than a clamp, device, or dorsal slit technique. Circumcision involves excision or removal of the prepuce, also referred to as the foreskin, which is the free fold of skin that covers the glans penis in uncircumcised males. A local anesthetic is injected. Alternatively, for older children and adults, a general anesthetic may be used. The physician then uses a freehand technique to excise of the prepuce. Use 54160 for a neonate defined as a patient aged 28 days or less. Use 54161 for a patient older than 28 days of age.

Circumcision, surgical excision (other than clamp, device, or dorsal slit)

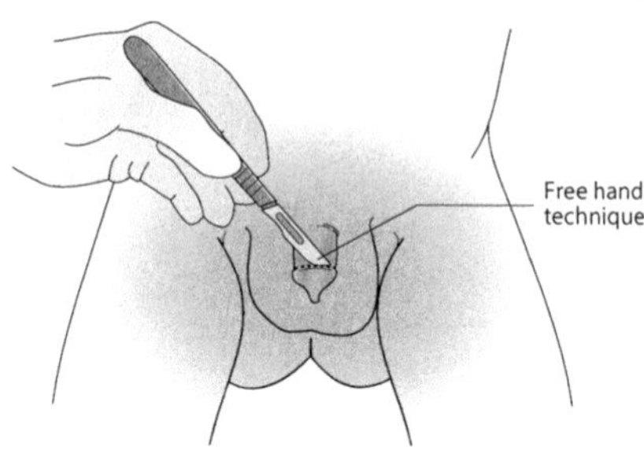

Neonate – 28 days of age or less (54160); older than 28 days of age (54161)

ICD-10-CM Diagnostic Codes

N47.0	Adherent prepuce, newborn ♂
N47.1	Phimosis ♂
N47.2	Paraphimosis ♂
N47.3	Deficient foreskin ♂
N47.4	Benign cyst of prepuce ♂
N47.5	Adhesions of prepuce and glans penis ♂
N47.7	Other inflammatory diseases of prepuce ♂
N47.8	Other disorders of prepuce ♂
Z41.2	Encounter for routine and ritual male circumcision ♂

CCI Edits

Refer to Appendix A for CCI edits.

Facility RVUs

Code	Work	PE Facility	MP	Total Facility
54160	2.53	1.43	0.29	4.25
54161	3.32	2.06	0.40	5.78

Non-facility RVUs

Code	Work	PE Non-Facility	MP	Total Non-Facility
54160	2.53	3.71	0.29	6.53
54161	3.32	2.06	0.40	5.78

Modifiers (PAR)

Code	Mod 50	Mod 51	Mod 62	Mod 66	Mod 80
54160	0	2	0	0	1
54161	0	2	0	0	1

Global Period

Code	Days
54160	010
54161	010

54162

54162 Lysis or excision of penile post-circumcision adhesions

Plain English Description

Adhesions sometimes form between the remaining prepuce (foreskin) and the glans penis following circumcision. While most adhesions resolve without surgical intervention, persistent adhesions may be cut (lysed) or excised. A general, regional, or local anesthetic is administered. A scalpel is then used to lyse or excise the adhesions.

Lysis or excision of penile post-circumcision adhesions

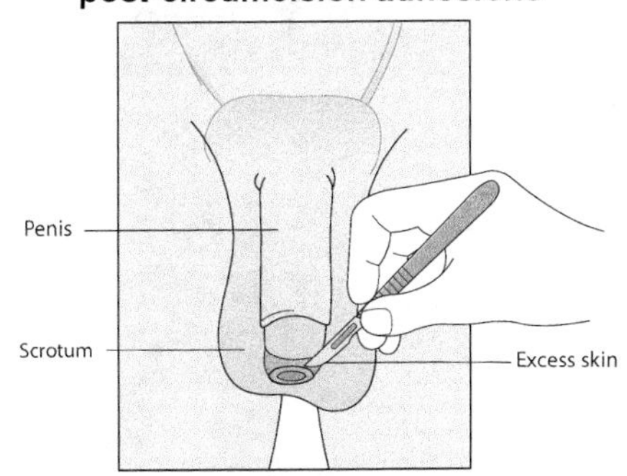

After a circumcision, the physician removes any leftover foreskin that has adhered to the end of the penis.

ICD-10-CM Diagnostic Codes

	N47.5	Adhesions of prepuce and glans penis ♂
	N48.21	Abscess of corpus cavernosum and penis ♂
	N48.22	Cellulitis of corpus cavernosum and penis ♂
	N48.29	Other inflammatory disorders of penis ♂
	N48.5	Ulcer of penis ♂
❼	T81.89	Other complications of procedures, not elsewhere classified

ICD-10-CM Coding Notes

For codes requiring a 7th character extension, refer to your ICD-10-CM book. Review the character descriptions and coding guidelines for proper selection. For some procedures, only certain characters will apply.

CCI Edits

Refer to Appendix A for CCI edits.

Facility RVUs ▢

Code	Work	PE Facility	MP	Total Facility
54162	3.32	2.15	0.40	5.87

Non-facility RVUs ▢

Code	Work	PE Non-Facility	MP	Total Non-Facility
54162	3.32	3.92	0.40	7.64

Modifiers (PAR) ▢

Code	Mod 50	Mod 51	Mod 62	Mod 66	Mod 80
54162	0	2	0	0	1

Global Period

Code	Days
54162	010

54163

54163 Repair incomplete circumcision

Plain English Description

This procedure is performed when there is excessive residual prepuce (foreskin) remaining following a previously performed circumcision. A general, regional, or local anesthetic is administered. If the head of the penis can be exposed, residual prepuce is then excised. If the head of the penis cannot be exposed due to the formation of adhesions between the glans penis and residual prepuce, the adhesions are first cut (lysed) and then the residual prepuce is excised.

Repair incomplete circumcision

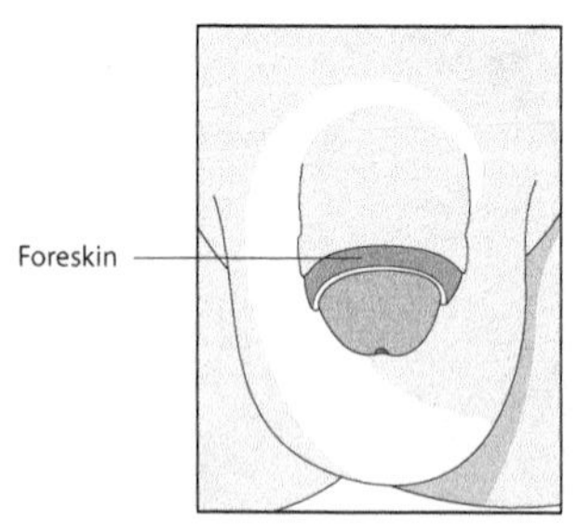

The physician finishes a circumcision that was not completed during the original procedure.

ICD-10-CM Diagnostic Codes

	L76.82	Other postprocedural complications of skin and subcutaneous tissue
	N47.0	Adherent prepuce, newborn ♂
	N47.1	Phimosis ♂
	N47.2	Paraphimosis ♂
	N47.3	Deficient foreskin ♂
	N47.5	Adhesions of prepuce and glans penis ♂
	N47.7	Other inflammatory diseases of prepuce ♂
	N47.8	Other disorders of prepuce ♂
	Q55.63	Congenital torsion of penis ♂
	Q55.69	Other congenital malformation of penis ♂
➐	T81.41	Infection following a procedure, superficial incisional surgical site
➐	T81.89	Other complications of procedures, not elsewhere classified
	Z41.1	Encounter for cosmetic surgery
	Z41.2	Encounter for routine and ritual male circumcision ♂

ICD-10-CM Coding Notes

For codes requiring a 7th character extension, refer to your ICD-10-CM book. Review the character descriptions and coding guidelines for proper selection. For some procedures, only certain characters will apply.

CCI Edits

Refer to Appendix A for CCI edits.

Facility RVUs ▯

Code	Work	PE Facility	MP	Total Facility
54163	3.32	2.67	0.40	6.39

Non-facility RVUs ▯

Code	Work	PE Non-Facility	MP	Total Non-Facility
54163	3.32	2.67	0.40	6.39

Modifiers (PAR) ▯

Code	Mod 50	Mod 51	Mod 62	Mod 66	Mod 80
54163	0	2	0	0	1

Global Period

Code	Days
54163	010

54164

54164 Frenulotomy of penis

(Do not report 54164 with circumcision codes 54150-54161, 54162, 54163)

Plain English Description

A frenulotomy of the penis may also be referred to as a frenuloplasty. With the patient positioned supine after a local anesthetic has been applied topically or injected, the penis is prepared and draped. A Z-shaped superficial skin incision is made with a slanting cut in the glans, followed by a vertical cut along the preputial fold and a second slanting cut in the prepuce. The incision is then straightened allowing the penis to elongate. Fine absorbable sutures are used to close the incision. A variation of this procedure may be performed using vascular clips. One clip is placed under the glans and the second parallel to the foreskin. A vertical incision is made between the two clips and they are pulled apart to stretch and elongate the frenulum. Sutures are not usually necessary and the clips fall off in a few days.

Frenulotomy of penis

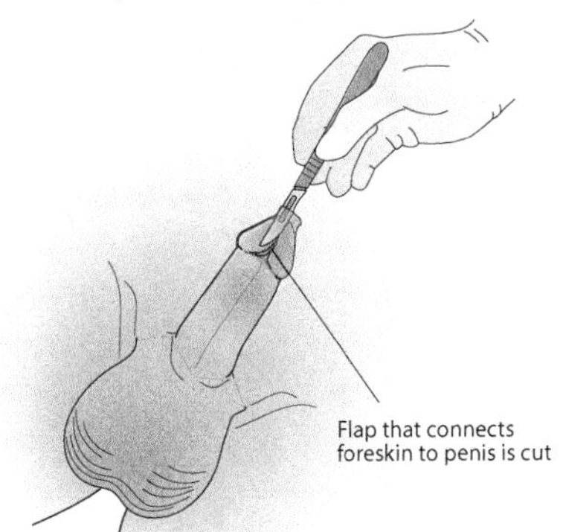
Flap that connects foreskin to penis is cut

ICD-10-CM Diagnostic Codes

N47.0	Adherent prepuce, newborn ♂
N47.1	Phimosis ♂
N47.2	Paraphimosis ♂
N47.3	Deficient foreskin ♂
N47.5	Adhesions of prepuce and glans penis ♂
N47.7	Other inflammatory diseases of prepuce ♂
N48.89	Other specified disorders of penis ♂

CCI Edits

Refer to Appendix A for CCI edits.

Facility RVUs ▯

Code	Work	PE Facility	MP	Total Facility
54164	2.82	2.52	0.34	5.68

Non-facility RVUs ▯

Code	Work	PE Non-Facility	MP	Total Non-Facility
54164	2.82	2.52	0.34	5.68

Modifiers (PAR) ▯

Code	Mod 50	Mod 51	Mod 62	Mod 66	Mod 80
54164	0	2	0	0	1

Global Period

Code	Days
54164	010

54200-54205

54200 Injection procedure for Peyronie disease

54205 Injection procedure for Peyronie disease; with surgical exposure of plaque

Plain English Description

Peyronie's disease is treated with an injection procedure with or without surgical exposure of plaque. Peyronie's disease is characterized by the development of a hard, fibrous layer of scar tissue (plaque) under the skin in the spongy erectile tissue on the upper or lower side of the penis. The plaque causes the penis to curve when erect. In 54200, the physician injects a drug that breaks down scar tissue and allows normal tissues to regenerate. Common drugs used include collagenase, calcium channel blockers such as verapamil, or interferons. The drugs are injected through the skin and into the plaque at multiple sites on the affected side of the penis. In 54205, the skin is incised and tissue dissected to expose the plaque. The drug is then injected at multiple sites directly into the plaque.

Injection procedure for Peyronie disease

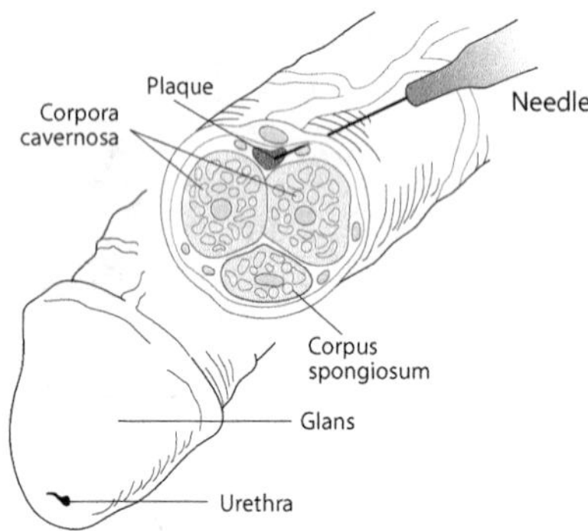

Medicine is injected into the penis to break down plaque in the spongy tissue (54200); with surgical access (54205).

ICD-10-CM Diagnostic Codes

N48.6 Induration penis plastica ♂

CCI Edits

Refer to Appendix A for CCI edits.

Facility RVUs

Code	Work	PE Facility	MP	Total Facility
54200	1.11	1.28	0.12	2.51
54205	8.97	5.57	1.06	15.60

Non-facility RVUs

Code	Work	PE Non-Facility	MP	Total Non-Facility
54200	1.11	2.17	0.12	3.40
54205	8.97	5.57	1.06	15.60

Modifiers (PAR)

Code	Mod 50	Mod 51	Mod 62	Mod 66	Mod 80
54200	0	2	0	0	1
54205	0	2	0	0	2

Global Period

Code	Days
54200	010
54205	090

54220

54220 Irrigation of corpora cavernosa for priapism

Plain English Description

Irrigation of the corpora cavernosa for priapism is accomplished with the patient awake. A penile ring block or local infiltration of anesthetic into the skin and tunica albuginea may be used for pain control. A 16 or 18 gauge needle is used to enter the lateral aspect of the corpus cavernosa. A 10 cc syringe is attached and an attempt made to aspirate blood from the tissue. If aspiration is unsuccessful, the syringe is removed from the needle and a 3-way stopcock attached. A liter of saline solution is connected via intravenous tubing to the stopcock opposite the needle and the syringe placed into the top port. Saline is drawn into the syringe and injected through the needle into the corpus cavernosa. The syringe is then used to aspirate thinned blood and the irrigation fluid back out of the tissue. The cycle continues until detumescence occurs. The needle can then be removed and firm pressure applied to the site for 5 minutes. Unilateral irrigation is usually successful in draining both sides of the corpora cavernosa. If saline alone does not relieve the priapism, epinephrine or phenylephrine may be added to the irrigation fluid.

Irrigation of corpora cavernosa for priapism

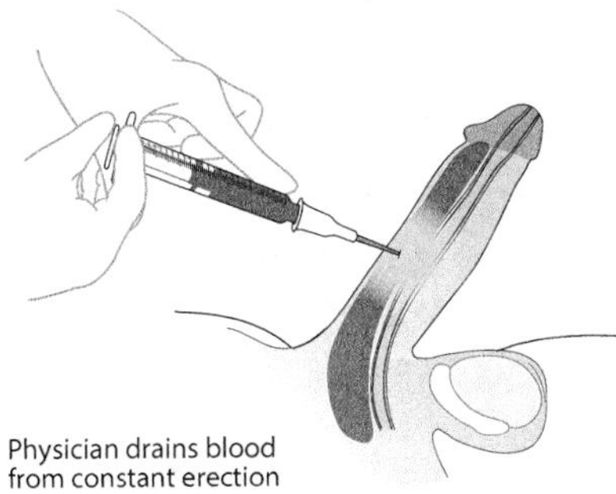
Physician drains blood from constant erection

ICD-10-CM Diagnostic Codes

N48.31	Priapism due to trauma ♂
N48.32	Priapism due to disease classified elsewhere ♂
N48.33	Priapism, drug-induced ♂
N48.39	Other priapism ♂

CCI Edits

Refer to Appendix A for CCI edits.

Facility RVUs ☐

Code	Work	PE Facility	MP	Total Facility
54220	2.42	1.11	0.37	3.90

Non-facility RVUs ☐

Code	Work	PE Non-Facility	MP	Total Non-Facility
54220	2.42	3.73	0.37	6.52

Modifiers (PAR) ☐

Code	Mod 50	Mod 51	Mod 62	Mod 66	Mod 80
54220	0	2	0	0	1

Global Period

Code	Days
54220	000

54230

54230 Injection procedure for corpora cavernosography

(For radiological supervision and interpretation, use 74445)

Plain English Description

Cavernosography involves the injection of contrast medium into the corpora cavernosa to examine radiographically the structure of the corpora cavernosa and the veins that drain blood from it. A 19-22 gauge needle is inserted into the tissue of the corpora cavernosa on the dorsal lateral aspect proximal to the glans penis. Contrast medium is injected and separately radiographic images are taken immediately from two angles, anterior/posterior and lateral/oblique. In less than a minute, the contrast medium should begin to flow through the channels between the two sides of the corpora cavernosa and drain down into the deep dorsal or crural veins. The needle is removed at the end of the procedure and pressure applied to the site. This code reports only the injection procedure. The radiologist's supervision and interpretation are reported separately.

Injection procedure for corpora cavernosography

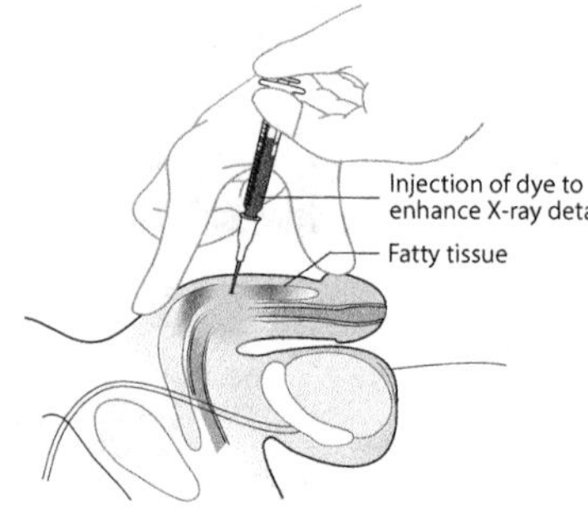

ICD-10-CM Diagnostic Codes

F52.21	Male erectile disorder ♂
N48.31	Priapism due to trauma ♂
N48.32	Priapism due to disease classified elsewhere ♂
N48.33	Priapism, drug-induced ♂
N48.39	Other priapism ♂
N48.6	Induration penis plastica ♂
N48.82	Acquired torsion of penis ♂
N48.89	Other specified disorders of penis ♂
N52.01	Erectile dysfunction due to arterial insufficiency ♂
N52.02	Corporo-venous occlusive erectile dysfunction ♂
N52.03	Combined arterial insufficiency and corporo-venous occlusive erectile dysfunction ♂
N52.1	Erectile dysfunction due to diseases classified elsewhere ♂
N52.31	Erectile dysfunction following radical prostatectomy ♂
N52.32	Erectile dysfunction following radical cystectomy ♂
N52.33	Erectile dysfunction following urethral surgery ♂
N52.34	Erectile dysfunction following simple prostatectomy ♂
N52.35	Erectile dysfunction following radiation therapy ♂
N52.36	Erectile dysfunction following interstitial seed therapy ♂
N52.37	Erectile dysfunction following prostate ablative therapy ♂
N52.39	Other and unspecified postprocedural erectile dysfunction ♂
N52.8	Other male erectile dysfunction ♂
Q55.69	Other congenital malformation of penis ♂
❼ S38.01	Crushing injury of penis

ICD-10-CM Coding Notes

For codes requiring a 7th character extension, refer to your ICD-10-CM book. Review the character descriptions and coding guidelines for proper selection. For some procedures, only certain characters will apply.

CCI Edits

Refer to Appendix A for CCI edits.

Facility RVUs ▯

Code	Work	PE Facility	MP	Total Facility
54230	1.34	0.81	0.17	2.32

Non-facility RVUs ▯

Code	Work	PE Non-Facility	MP	Total Non-Facility
54230	1.34	1.61	0.17	3.12

Modifiers (PAR) ▯

Code	Mod 50	Mod 51	Mod 62	Mod 66	Mod 80
54230	0	2	0	0	1

Global Period

Code	Days
54230	000

54231

54231 Dynamic cavernosometry, including intracavernosal injection of vasoactive drugs (eg, papaverine, phentolamine)

Plain English Description

Dynamic cavernosometry measures the vascular pressure in the corpus cavernosum during an erection. Using a 27-30 gauge needle, a vasodilatory drug such as Caverject or papaverine is injected into the corpora to produce arterial and sinusoidal relaxation. Following local injection of an anesthetic, a 19-gauge butterfly needle is inserted into the corpus cavernosum at a vertical angle to the penile axis to allow for movement during the erection. A perfusion pump with normal saline is attached to the needle and the fluid is pumped into the tissue until an erection is achieved. The pressure continues to be monitored and erectile activity observed until it reaches about 150 mm/Hg. The infusion is then stopped and the cavernosum pressure measured. Rapid fall in pressure and loss of an erection may indicate leakage into the vessels.

Dynamic cavernosometry; injection of vasoactive drugs

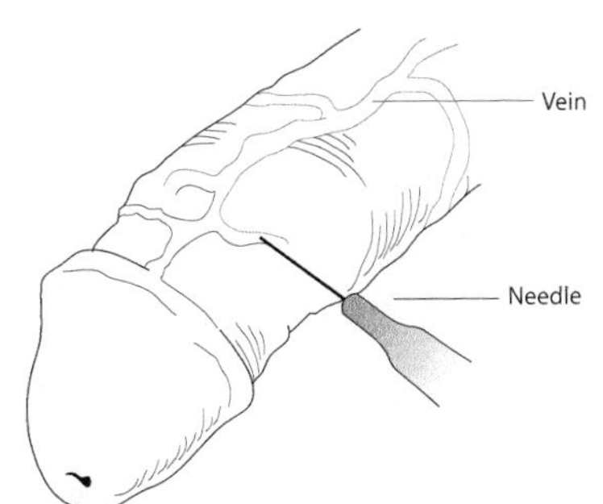

The physician injects drugs into the penis to measure the vascular pressure of the spongy tissue of the penis.

ICD-10-CM Diagnostic Codes

F52.21	Male erectile disorder ♂
N48.31	Priapism due to trauma ♂
N48.32	Priapism due to disease classified elsewhere ♂
N48.33	Priapism, drug-induced ♂
N48.39	Other priapism ♂
N48.6	Induration penis plastica ♂
N48.82	Acquired torsion of penis ♂
N48.89	Other specified disorders of penis ♂
N52.01	Erectile dysfunction due to arterial insufficiency ♂
N52.02	Corporo-venous occlusive erectile dysfunction ♂
N52.03	Combined arterial insufficiency and corporo-venous occlusive erectile dysfunction ♂
N52.1	Erectile dysfunction due to diseases classified elsewhere ♂
N52.2	Drug-induced erectile dysfunction ♂
N52.31	Erectile dysfunction following radical prostatectomy ♂
N52.32	Erectile dysfunction following radical cystectomy ♂
N52.33	Erectile dysfunction following urethral surgery ♂
N52.34	Erectile dysfunction following simple prostatectomy ♂
N52.35	Erectile dysfunction following radiation therapy ♂
N52.36	Erectile dysfunction following interstitial seed therapy ♂
N52.37	Erectile dysfunction following prostate ablative therapy ♂
N52.39	Other and unspecified postprocedural erectile dysfunction ♂
N52.8	Other male erectile dysfunction ♂
Q55.69	Other congenital malformation of penis ♂
❼ S38.1	Crushing injury of abdomen, lower back, and pelvis

ICD-10-CM Coding Notes

For codes requiring a 7th character extension, refer to your ICD-10-CM book. Review the character descriptions and coding guidelines for proper selection. For some procedures, only certain characters will apply.

CCI Edits

Refer to Appendix A for CCI edits.

Facility RVUs ▢

Code	Work	PE Facility	MP	Total Facility
54231	2.04	1.08	0.24	3.36

Non-facility RVUs ▢

Code	Work	PE Non-Facility	MP	Total Non-Facility
54231	2.04	1.90	0.24	4.18

Modifiers (PAR) ▢

Code	Mod 50	Mod 51	Mod 62	Mod 66	Mod 80
54231	0	2	0	0	1

Global Period

Code	Days
54231	000

CPT® Procedural Coding

54235

54235 Injection of corpora cavernosa with pharmacologic agent(s) (eg, papaverine, phentolamine)

AMA *CPT® Assistant* ☐

54235: Sep 96: 10

Plain English Description

The penis is laid across the thigh to stabilize and stretch it and the foreskin is retracted if the penis is uncircumcised. The injection site is selected and skin cleansed with alcohol. The site may be on either side of the penis, anywhere from the base to the glans. Care must be taken not to inject in the midline or underside of the penis or through visible veins. A needle is inserted at a 90-degree angle up to the needle hub and medication is injected over 1-2 minutes. The needle is removed and pressure applied to control bleeding. The corpora cavernosa is squeezed along one side and then the other and then pinched transversely at intervals to evenly distribute the medication along the entire length of the penis.

Injection of corpora cavernosa with pharmacologic agents

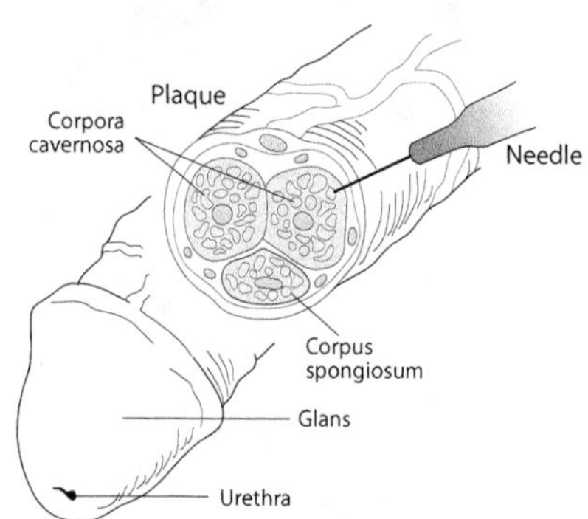

The physician injects drugs into the fatty tissue of the penis to treat erectile dysfunction.

ICD-10-CM Diagnostic Codes

F52.21 Male erectile disorder ♂
N48.31 Priapism due to trauma ♂
N48.32 Priapism due to disease classified elsewhere ♂
N48.33 Priapism, drug-induced ♂
N48.39 Other priapism ♂
N48.6 Induration penis plastica ♂
N48.82 Acquired torsion of penis ♂
N48.89 Other specified disorders of penis ♂
N50.1 Vascular disorders of male genital organs ♂
N52.01 Erectile dysfunction due to arterial insufficiency ♂
N52.02 Corporo-venous occlusive erectile dysfunction ♂
N52.03 Combined arterial insufficiency and corporo-venous occlusive erectile dysfunction ♂
N52.1 Erectile dysfunction due to diseases classified elsewhere ♂
N52.2 Drug-induced erectile dysfunction ♂
N52.31 Erectile dysfunction following radical prostatectomy ♂
N52.32 Erectile dysfunction following radical cystectomy ♂
N52.33 Erectile dysfunction following urethral surgery ♂
N52.34 Erectile dysfunction following simple prostatectomy ♂
N52.35 Erectile dysfunction following radiation therapy ♂
N52.36 Erectile dysfunction following interstitial seed therapy ♂
N52.37 Erectile dysfunction following prostate ablative therapy ♂
N52.39 Other and unspecified postprocedural erectile dysfunction ♂
N52.8 Other male erectile dysfunction ♂
Q55.69 Other congenital malformation of penis ♂
➐ S38.01 Crushing injury of penis

ICD-10-CM Coding Notes

For codes requiring a 7th character extension, refer to your ICD-10-CM book. Review the character descriptions and coding guidelines for proper selection. For some procedures, only certain characters will apply.

CCI Edits

Refer to Appendix A for CCI edits.

Facility RVUs ☐

Code	Work	PE Facility	MP	Total Facility
54235	1.19	0.80	0.12	2.11

Non-facility RVUs ☐

Code	Work	PE Non-Facility	MP	Total Non-Facility
54235	1.19	1.27	0.12	2.58

Modifiers (PAR) ☐

Code	Mod 50	Mod 51	Mod 62	Mod 66	Mod 80
54235	0	2	0	0	1

Global Period

Code	Days
54235	000

54240

54240 Penile plethysmography

Plain English Description

A plethysmograph is a device that measures blood flow in the various parts of the body. Penile plethysmography, also referred to as penile pulse volume recording, is used to diagnose erectile dysfunction. Either a volumetric air chamber type or a circumferential transducer type may be used. The volumetric air chamber type is placed over the patient's penis. As the penis becomes erect, air is displaced and the amount of air displacement is measured. The circumferential transducer type uses a rubber ring filled with mercury or indium/gallium that is placed around the shaft of the patient's penis. As the penis becomes erect, changes in diameter are measured. The physician reviews the results of the plethysmography and provides a written interpretation of the results.

Penile plethysmography

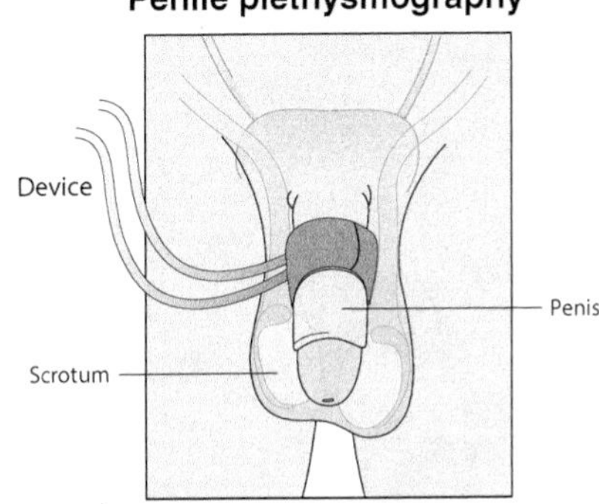

A device is placed around the penis to measure changes in diameter in response to stimulation.

ICD-10-CM Diagnostic Codes

E29.1	Testicular hypofunction ♂
F52.21	Male erectile disorder ♂
F52.32	Male orgasmic disorder ♂
F52.8	Other sexual dysfunction not due to a substance or known physiological condition
F52.9	Unspecified sexual dysfunction not due to a substance or known physiological condition
N48.29	Other inflammatory disorders of penis ♂
N48.6	Induration penis plastica ♂
N48.89	Other specified disorders of penis ♂
N50.1	Vascular disorders of male genital organs ♂
N52.01	Erectile dysfunction due to arterial insufficiency ♂
N52.02	Corporo-venous occlusive erectile dysfunction ♂
N52.03	Combined arterial insufficiency and corporo-venous occlusive erectile dysfunction ♂
N52.1	Erectile dysfunction due to diseases classified elsewhere ♂
N52.2	Drug-induced erectile dysfunction ♂
N52.31	Erectile dysfunction following radical prostatectomy ♂
N52.32	Erectile dysfunction following radical cystectomy ♂
N52.33	Erectile dysfunction following urethral surgery ♂
N52.34	Erectile dysfunction following simple prostatectomy ♂
N52.35	Erectile dysfunction following radiation therapy ♂
N52.36	Erectile dysfunction following interstitial seed therapy ♂
N52.37	Erectile dysfunction following prostate ablative therapy ♂
N52.39	Other and unspecified postprocedural erectile dysfunction ♂
N52.8	Other male erectile dysfunction ♂

CCI Edits

Refer to Appendix A for CCI edits.

Pub 100

54240: Pub 100-03, 1, 160.26

Facility RVUs

Code	Work	PE Facility	MP	Total Facility
54240	1.31	1.62	0.18	3.11

Non-facility RVUs

Code	Work	PE Non-Facility	MP	Total Non-Facility
54240	1.31	1.62	0.18	3.11

Modifiers (PAR)

Code	Mod 50	Mod 51	Mod 62	Mod 66	Mod 80
54240	0	0	0	0	0

Global Period

Code	Days
54240	000

54250

54250 Nocturnal penile tumescence and/or rigidity test

Plain English Description

This test is performed to determine whether the patient is having normal erections during sleep. The results are used to evaluate the cause of and/or level of erectile dysfunction. The test may be performed at home or in a sleep lab. An electronic monitoring device is used to record how many erections occur during sleep, how long the erections last, and how rigid the penis becomes during each erection. The physician reviews the recording and provides a written interpretation of the results.

Nocturnal penile tumescence and/or rigidity test

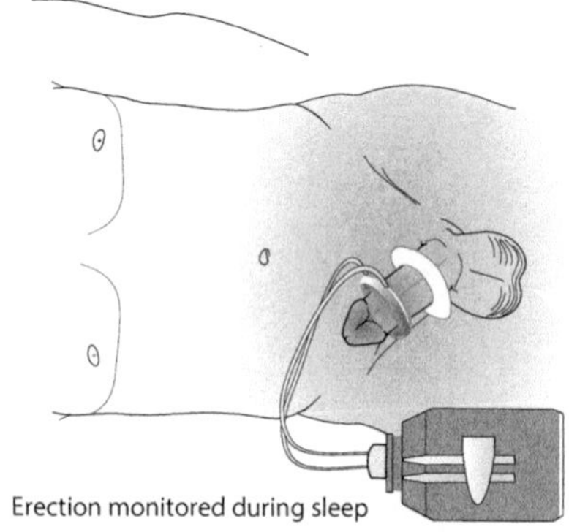

Erection monitored during sleep

ICD-10-CM Diagnostic Codes

E29.1	Testicular hypofunction ♂
F52.21	Male erectile disorder ♂
F52.32	Male orgasmic disorder ♂
F52.8	Other sexual dysfunction not due to a substance or known physiological condition
F52.9	Unspecified sexual dysfunction not due to a substance or known physiological condition
N48.29	Other inflammatory disorders of penis ♂
N48.6	Induration penis plastica ♂
N48.89	Other specified disorders of penis ♂
N50.1	Vascular disorders of male genital organs ♂
N52.01	Erectile dysfunction due to arterial insufficiency ♂
N52.02	Corporo-venous occlusive erectile dysfunction ♂
N52.03	Combined arterial insufficiency and corporo-venous occlusive erectile dysfunction ♂
N52.1	Erectile dysfunction due to diseases classified elsewhere ♂
N52.2	Drug-induced erectile dysfunction ♂
N52.31	Erectile dysfunction following radical prostatectomy ♂
N52.32	Erectile dysfunction following radical cystectomy ♂
N52.33	Erectile dysfunction following urethral surgery ♂
N52.34	Erectile dysfunction following simple prostatectomy ♂
N52.35	Erectile dysfunction following radiation therapy ♂
N52.36	Erectile dysfunction following interstitial seed therapy ♂
N52.37	Erectile dysfunction following prostate ablative therapy ♂
N52.39	Other and unspecified postprocedural erectile dysfunction ♂
N52.8	Other male erectile dysfunction ♂

CCI Edits

Refer to Appendix A for CCI edits.

Pub 100

54250: Pub 100-02, 15, 70

Facility RVUs ▯

Code	Work	PE Facility	MP	Total Facility
54250	2.22	1.16	0.20	3.58

Non-facility RVUs ▯

Code	Work	PE Non-Facility	MP	Total Non-Facility
54250	2.22	1.16	0.20	3.58

Modifiers (PAR) ▯

Code	Mod 50	Mod 51	Mod 62	Mod 66	Mod 80
54250	0	0	0	0	0

Global Period

Code	Days
54250	000

54300

54300 Plastic operation of penis for straightening of chordee (eg, hypospadias), with or without mobilization of urethra

AMA Coding Notes

Repair Procedures on the Penis

(For other urethroplasties, see 53400-53430)

(For penile revascularization, use 37788)

AMA *CPT® Assistant*

54300: Dec 14: 16

Plain English Description

There are several accepted techniques to straighten a penile curve or chordee. A longitudinal incision is made through the circumcision scar along the shaft of the penis, carried down to the superficial layer of Buck's fascia and the penile skin is degloved. A needle is inserted into the corpus cavernosum at a vertical angle to the penile axis to allow for movement during the erection. A perfusion pump with normal saline is attached to the needle and fluid pumped into the tissue until an erection is achieved and the location and degree of curvature observed. For a ventral curvature, the fibrous tissue in dartos fascia is mobilized for removal and the fibrous tissue in Buck's fascia is opened using scissors allowing mobilization of the urethra and corpus spongiosum between the glans and the penoscrotal junction. An erection is again induced with saline and if the penis is straight, the degloved skin is repositioned and the wound closed. An alternative approach when penile length does not need to be considered is excision and plication of the tunica albuginea. A circumferential skin incision is made at the glans and the penis degloved allowing the urethra to be mobilized by resection from the dartos and Buck's fascia. Erection is induced as described previously and if curvature remains, an ellipse of tissue opposite the concave curve is marked and excised from the tunica albuginea. The edges of the ellipse are sutured closed. If a penile curve remains, additional elliptical incisions are made until the penis is straight. The degloved skin is then mobilized back up the shaft of the penis and sutured around the glans. When only a lateral curve requires correction, erection is induced as previously described and a small vertical incision is made through Buck's fascia at the point of maximal curvature. A horizontal ellipse of tissue is removed from the tunica albuginea as previously described and the edges sutured. An erection is again induced and, if the penis is straight, Buck's fascia is sutured closed followed by closure of the skin.

Plastic operation of penis for straightening of chordee

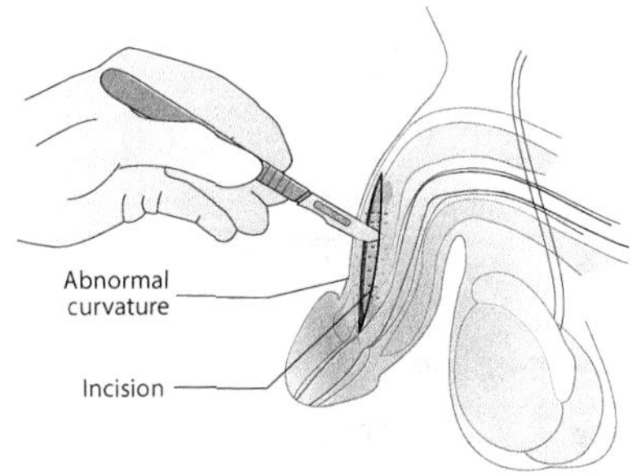

ICD-10-CM Diagnostic Codes

Q54.0	Hypospadias, balanic ♂
Q54.1	Hypospadias, penile ♂
Q54.2	Hypospadias, penoscrotal ♂
Q54.3	Hypospadias, perineal ♂
Q54.4	Congenital chordee ♂
Q54.8	Other hypospadias ♂
Q55.61	Curvature of penis (lateral) ♂

CCI Edits

Refer to Appendix A for CCI edits.

Facility RVUs

Code	Work	PE Facility	MP	Total Facility
54300	11.20	6.40	1.36	18.96

Non-facility RVUs

Code	Work	PE Non-Facility	MP	Total Non-Facility
54300	11.20	6.40	1.36	18.96

Modifiers (PAR)

Code	Mod 50	Mod 51	Mod 62	Mod 66	Mod 80
54300	0	2	1	0	2

Global Period

Code	Days
54300	090

54304

54304 Plastic operation on penis for correction of chordee or for first stage hypospadias repair with or without transplantation of prepuce and/or skin flaps

AMA Coding Notes

Repair Procedures on the Penis

(For other urethroplasties, see 53400-53430)

(For penile revascularization, use 37788)

Plain English Description

The penis may have a normal glans and urethral meatus but thin and poorly developed urethral mucosa and spongiosum tissue causing penile curvature. A staged repair is undertaken to correct the chordee and augment the urethra with an onlay island graft. The patient is positioned supine and the penis is prepared and draped. The repair begins with identification of the flat ventral glans surface as it begins to curve around the meatus. A vertical incision is made at the midline and widened along the glanular groove until an adequate meatal opening is formed. This incision will be left open to epithelialize. Next, an incision is made in the subcoronal tissue around the glans with extensions on either side of the urethral plate where it joins normal skin and on the side of the glandular groove to the apex of the glansplasty. The penile skin is then degloved exposing Buck's fascia but preserving the vascular connection to the preputial flap. The vascular pedicle is separated from the outer preputial skin maintaining blood supply to both layers. An onlay flap is created from the inner prepuce and running sutures are placed beginning under the pedicle to draw the glans together. The wing flaps are rotated medially around the neo-urethra and approximated in the midline with mattress sutures.

Plastic operation on penis for correction of chordee or for first stage hypospadias repair

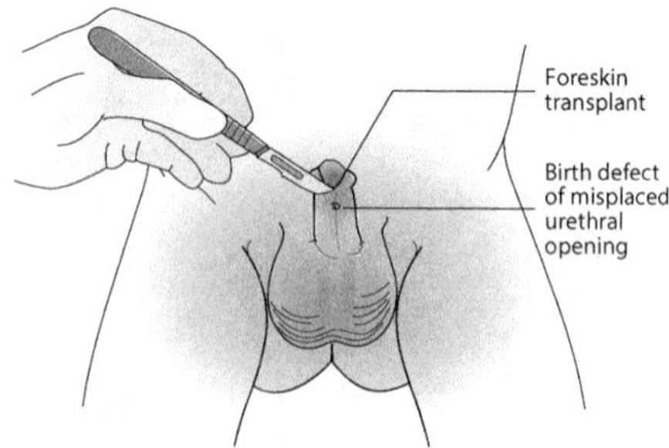

ICD-10-CM Diagnostic Codes

Q54.0	Hypospadias, balanic ♂
Q54.1	Hypospadias, penile ♂
Q54.2	Hypospadias, penoscrotal ♂
Q54.3	Hypospadias, perineal ♂
Q54.4	Congenital chordee ♂
Q54.8	Other hypospadias ♂
Q55.61	Curvature of penis (lateral) ♂

CCI Edits

Refer to Appendix A for CCI edits.

Facility RVUs ▯

Code	Work	PE Facility	MP	Total Facility
54304	13.28	7.03	1.59	21.90

Non-facility RVUs ▯

Code	Work	PE Non-Facility	MP	Total Non-Facility
54304	13.28	7.03	1.59	21.90

Modifiers (PAR) ▯

Code	Mod 50	Mod 51	Mod 62	Mod 66	Mod 80
54304	0	2	0	0	2

Global Period

Code	Days
54304	090

54308-54316

54308 Urethroplasty for second stage hypospadias repair (including urinary diversion); less than 3 cm

54312 Urethroplasty for second stage hypospadias repair (including urinary diversion); greater than 3 cm

54316 Urethroplasty for second stage hypospadias repair (including urinary diversion) with free skin graft obtained from site other than genitalia

AMA Coding Notes

Repair Procedures on the Penis

(For other urethroplasties, see 53400-53430)

(For penile revascularization, use 37788)

Plain English Description

The physician performs the second stage of a procedure to fix a birth defect in which the urethral opening is somewhere other than the tip of the penis. The urethra is moved less than 3 cm. Code 54312 if the urethra is moved more than 3 cm. Code 54316 if the physician uses a skin graft to complete the procedure. The graft is taken from somewhere other than the genitals.

Urethroplasty for second stage hypospadias repair

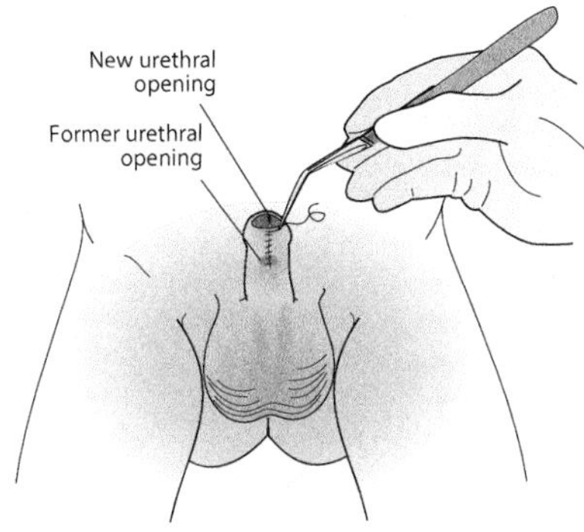

Less than 3 cm (54308); greater than 3 cm (54312); with free skin graft obtained from site other than genitalia (54316)

ICD-10-CM Diagnostic Codes

Q54.0	Hypospadias, balanic ♂
Q54.1	Hypospadias, penile ♂
Q54.2	Hypospadias, penoscrotal ♂
Q54.3	Hypospadias, perineal ♂
Q54.4	Congenital chordee ♂
Q54.8	Other hypospadias ♂

CCI Edits

Refer to Appendix A for CCI edits.

Facility RVUs

Code	Work	PE Facility	MP	Total Facility
54308	12.62	6.85	1.50	20.97
54312	14.51	7.71	1.71	23.93
54316	18.05	8.87	2.17	29.09

Non-facility RVUs

Code	Work	PE Non-Facility	MP	Total Non-Facility
54308	12.62	6.85	1.50	20.97
54312	14.51	7.71	1.71	23.93
54316	18.05	8.87	2.17	29.09

Modifiers (PAR)

Code	Mod 50	Mod 51	Mod 62	Mod 66	Mod 80
54308	0	2	1	0	2
54312	0	2	1	0	2
54316	0	2	1	0	2

Global Period

Code	Days
54308	090
54312	090
54316	090

CPT® Procedural Coding

54318

54318 Urethroplasty for third stage hypospadias repair to release penis from scrotum (eg, third stage Cecil repair)

AMA Coding Notes

Repair Procedures on the Penis

(For other urethroplasties, see 53400-53430)

(For penile revascularization, use 37788)

Plain English Description

The 3rd stage of a hypospadias repair to release the penis from the scrotum is performed a minimum of six weeks following the 2nd stage to allow for adequate epithelialization of the neo-urethra. The patient is positioned supine and the penis and scrotum are prepared and draped. A Foley catheter is placed transurethrally into the bladder. The approximated skin edges of the penis and scrotum are carefully excised to prevent any transfer of scrotal skin to the penile shaft. The soft tissue of the penile shaft is preserved and the edges of the penile skin from glans to scrotum are approximated and closed in the midline with absorbable sutures. The scrotal skin is then approximated and closed in the same fashion. The Foley catheter may be removed or left in place following the procedure.

Urethroplasty for third stage hypospadias repair to release penis from scrotum

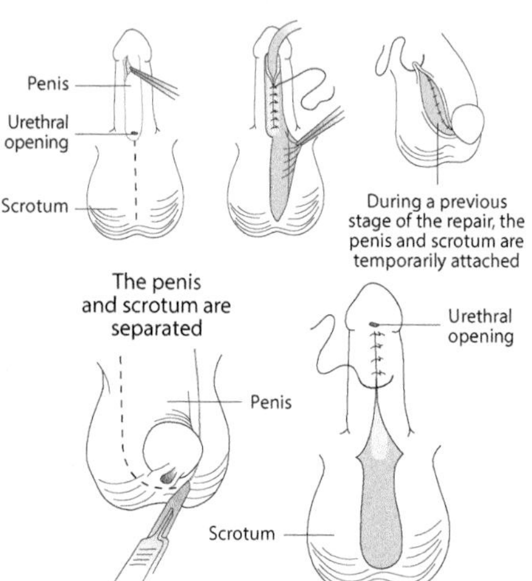
Penis
Urethral opening
Scrotum
During a previous stage of the repair, the penis and scrotum are temporarily attached
The penis and scrotum are separated
Penis
Scrotum
Urethral opening

ICD-10-CM Diagnostic Codes

Q54.2 Hypospadias, penoscrotal ♂

CCI Edits

Refer to Appendix A for CCI edits.

Facility RVUs

Code	Work	PE Facility	MP	Total Facility
54318	12.43	6.93	1.47	20.83

Non-facility RVUs

Code	Work	PE Non-Facility	MP	Total Non-Facility
54318	12.43	6.93	1.47	20.83

Modifiers (PAR)

Code	Mod 50	Mod 51	Mod 62	Mod 66	Mod 80
54318	0	2	1	0	2

Global Period

Code	Days
54318	090

54322-54326

54322 1-stage distal hypospadias repair (with or without chordee or circumcision); with simple meatal advancement (eg, Magpi, V-flap)

54324 1-stage distal hypospadias repair (with or without chordee or circumcision); with urethroplasty by local skin flaps (eg, flip-flap, prepucial flap)

54326 1-stage distal hypospadias repair (with or without chordee or circumcision); with urethroplasty by local skin flaps and mobilization of urethra

AMA Coding Notes

Repair Procedures on the Penis

(For other urethroplasties, see 53400-53430)

(For penile revascularization, use 37788)

Plain English Description

Hypospadias is a condition in which the urethral meatus is displaced from its normal position at the tip of the penis to the underside of the penis in males. Hypospadias is classified as distal or mild when the meatal opening is small and located in or near the glans. In 54322, mild hypospadias is repaired using simple metal advancement, also referred to as a meatal advancement and glanuloplasty (MAGPI), inverted Y-meatoglanuloplasty, or V-flap. To perform a MAGPI, a longitudinal circumcising incision is made in the glans followed by dorsal meatotomy to advance the edge of the meatus distally. The ventral edge of the meatus is elevated and brought forward. The flattened wings of the glans are rotated upwards and ventrally to form a cone shape after detaching the glans from the corpus spongiosum at the lateral margin and the corpora cavernosa at the side. The edges of the glans tissue are reapproximated in the midline around the excised urethral meatus in two layers, first incorporating the mesenchyme of the glans and finally the superficial glans epithelium. To perform an inverted Y-meatoglanuloplasty, a longitudinal incision is made midline from the meatus to the edge of the glans. Diverging limb incisions are made along the upper edge of the meatus creating space for the new urethra. The Y-incision is sutured as an inverted V and the glans flaps are wrapped around the urethra and sutured in the midline. In 54324, a single-stage repair with urethroplasty using local skin flaps is performed, such as a Mathieu or tubularized incised plate (TIP) urethroplasty, also known as a Snodgrass procedure. A U-shaped incision along the urethral plate is made and the penis is degloved. Longitudinal incisions are made along the urethral plate to create the glans wings. In the Mathieu procedure, a skin flap is developed proximal to the urethral meatus with sufficient length to reach the tip of the glans. The flap is elevated and sutured to each side of the distal urethra. In the Snodgrass procedure, a midline incision is made from the tip of the glans to the urethral meatus and carried down through the mucosal and submucosal tissue to the corporal bodies creating a tube over a catheter. Both procedures continue with dissection of dorsal subcutaneous tissue from the preputial and penile shaft skin, which is then rotated ventrally covering the neo-urethra. The wings of the glans form a second layer of support for the neo-urethra and are closed symmetrically in 2 layers. A urethral stent or catheter remains in place following the procedure. In 54326, a procedure similar to the Mathieu or Snodgrass procedure is performed except that the urethra is also mobilized. This involves detaching the entire urethra from the anterior aspect of the corpora cavernosa to increase ureteral length, also referred to as Koff's technique. If more length is required, the urethra is also freed proximally. This may be referred to as a Turner-Warwick procedure.

1-stage distal hypospadias repair; with simple meatal advancement

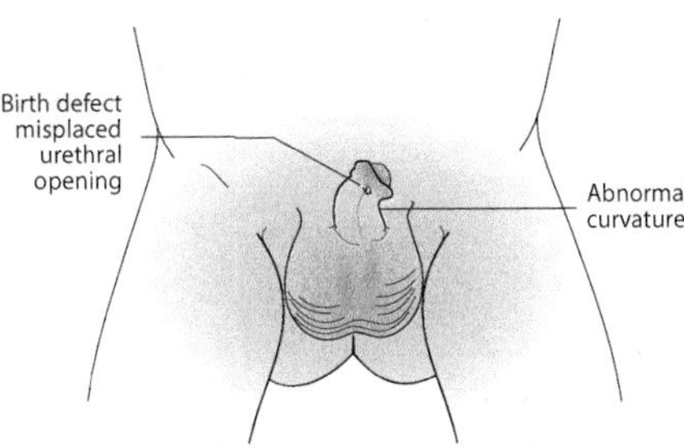

ICD-10-CM Diagnostic Codes

Q54.0	Hypospadias, balanic ♂
Q54.1	Hypospadias, penile ♂
Q54.2	Hypospadias, penoscrotal ♂
Q54.3	Hypospadias, perineal ♂
Q54.4	Congenital chordee ♂
Q54.8	Other hypospadias ♂

CCI Edits

Refer to Appendix A for CCI edits.

Facility RVUs

Code	Work	PE Facility	MP	Total Facility
54322	13.98	7.22	1.66	22.86
54324	17.55	8.67	2.08	28.30
54326	17.02	8.51	2.01	27.54

Non-facility RVUs

Code	Work	PE Non-Facility	MP	Total Non-Facility
54322	13.98	7.22	1.66	22.86
54324	17.55	8.67	2.08	28.30
54326	17.02	8.51	2.01	27.54

Modifiers (PAR)

Code	Mod 50	Mod 51	Mod 62	Mod 66	Mod 80
54322	0	2	0	0	2
54324	0	2	1	0	2
54326	0	2	1	0	2

Global Period

Code	Days
54322	090
54324	090
54326	090

54328

54328 1-stage distal hypospadias repair (with or without chordee or circumcision); with extensive dissection to correct chordee and urethroplasty with local skin flaps, skin graft patch, and/or island flap

(For urethroplasty and straightening of chordee, use 54308)

AMA Coding Notes

Repair Procedures on the Penis

(For other urethroplasties, see 53400-53430)

(For penile revascularization, use 37788)

AMA *CPT® Assistant*

54328: Oct 04: 15

Plain English Description

Hypospadias is a condition in which the urethral meatus is displaced from its normal position at the tip of the penis to the underside of the penis in males. Hypospadias is classified as distal or mild when the meatal opening is small and located in or near the glans. This procedure involves creation of a distal neo-urethra using grafts and/or flaps so that the urethral meatus can be relocated to the tip of the penis and also corrects chordee, which refers to curvature of the erect penis. An example of this type of hypospadias repair is a transverse preputial island flap (TPIF). A stent or catheter is placed in the urethra. A Y-shaped incision is made in the glans. The short limbs are approximately 0.5 cm long and the vertical limb extends to the coronal sulcus. Fibrotic tissue is identified and excised from the midline and laterally and the glans flaps elevated to allow the meatus to be enlarged and a core space made for the neo-urethra. A circumferential incision is made in the subcoronal tissue below the glans extending laterally to the area of excised fibrous tissue. The penile and preputial skin is degloved exposing Buck's fascia but preserving the vascular connection to the preputial flap. Once the penis has been degloved, an erection is induced and the degree of curvature evaluated. Due to the severity of the chordee, tissues are extensively dissected and the chordee corrected. The neo-urethra is then constructed. A rectangular flap is created and if necessary extended by using a horseshoe incision incorporating penile skin on either side. The flap is tubularized around a catheter with interrupted sutures beginning at the meatus under the vascular pedicle. The pedicle is separated from the preputial skin below the vascular bed of the outer prepuce. Next, the small upper median flap formed by the Y incision is anchored with sutures to the upper dorsal aspect of the tube. To create an aesthetic appearing meatus, a small V-shaped wedge of tissue is excised from the tip of the glans. The mobilized glans wings are then rotated medially around the neo-urethra and anchored with 3 mattress sutures placed transversely to approximate the wings in the midline which completes construction of the neo-urethra. Alternatively, a local skin flap or skin patch graft may be used to construct the neo-urethra. Following completion of the procedure, the urethral stent or catheter remains in place.

1-stage distal hypospadias repair; with extensive dissection to correct chordee and urethroplasty

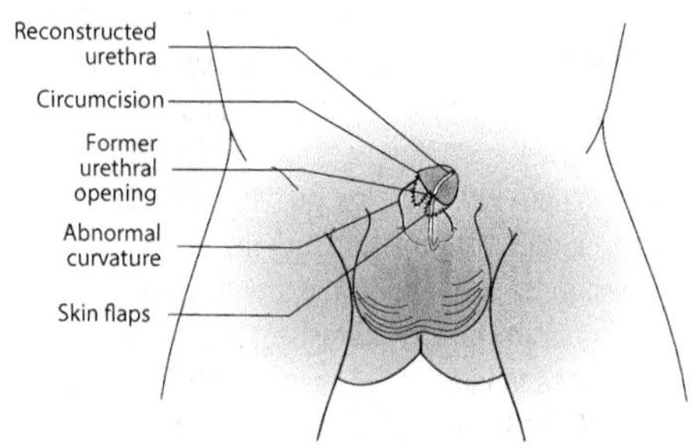

ICD-10-CM Diagnostic Codes

Q54.0	Hypospadias, balanic ♂
Q54.1	Hypospadias, penile ♂
Q54.4	Congenital chordee ♂
Q54.8	Other hypospadias ♂
Q55.3	Atresia of vas deferens ♂

CCI Edits

Refer to Appendix A for CCI edits.

Facility RVUs

Code	Work	PE Facility	MP	Total Facility
54328	16.89	8.48	2.01	27.38

Non-facility RVUs

Code	Work	PE Non-Facility	MP	Total Non-Facility
54328	16.89	8.48	2.01	27.38

Modifiers (PAR)

Code	Mod 50	Mod 51	Mod 62	Mod 66	Mod 80
54328	0	2	1	0	2

Global Period

Code	Days
54328	090

54332

54332 1-stage proximal penile or penoscrotal hypospadias repair requiring extensive dissection to correct chordee and urethroplasty by use of skin graft tube and/or island flap

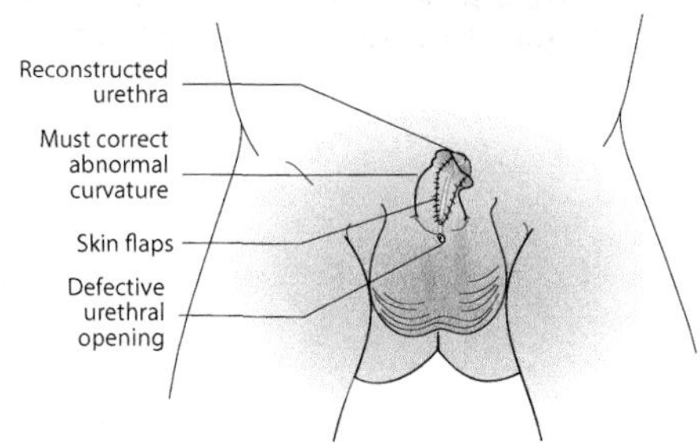

AMA Coding Notes

Repair Procedures on the Penis

(For other urethroplasties, see 53400-53430)

(For penile revascularization, use 37788)

AMA *CPT® Assistant* ◻

54332: Mar 04: 11, Sep 04: 12

Plain English Description

Hypospadias is a condition in which the urethral meatus is displaced from its normal position at the tip of the penis to the underside of the penis in males. In proximal hypospadias, the meatal opening is typically in the penoscrotal region and may range from a normal sized meatus to a long opening extending from the penoscrotal region to the midshaft. A lateral based flap can be used for proximal and penoscrotal hypospadias in a single-stage repair. A Y-shaped incision is made in the glans with the long vertical segment extending to the coronary sulcus. Fibrotic tissue is identified and excised from the midline and laterally to correct chordee followed by elevation of the three glans flaps to allow space for the neo-urethra. A long rectangular skin flap is created including a small cuff of skin containing the urethral meatus by incising proximally in the midline of the scrotum with distal and lateral extension to the prepuce if necessary. The penile skin is elevated and mobilized dorsally down to the root, carefully avoiding rotation of the flap. The flap is then tubularized over a catheter or stent, suturing distal to proximal using a continuous subcuticular stitch reinforced at intervals with interrupted sutures. The neo-meatus is created by suturing the terminal end of the neo-urethra to the ventral V-shaped incision in the glans. A slit-like opening and a conical glans can be accomplished by excising a small V-shaped tip in the neo-urethra. Next, the glanular wings wrap around the neo-urethra distally and are approximated in the midline. A layer of vascular areolar subcutaneous tissue is placed as reinforcement over the tubularized graft. The skin is approximated in the midline to simulate the normal penile raphae and closed with a continuous transverse mattress stitch.

ICD-10-CM Diagnostic Codes

Q54.0	Hypospadias, balanic ♂
Q54.1	Hypospadias, penile ♂
Q54.2	Hypospadias, penoscrotal ♂
Q54.4	Congenital chordee ♂
Q54.8	Other hypospadias ♂

CCI Edits

Refer to Appendix A for CCI edits.

Facility RVUs ◻

Code	Work	PE Facility	MP	Total Facility
54332	18.37	8.98	2.18	29.53

Non-facility RVUs ◻

Code	Work	PE Non-Facility	MP	Total Non-Facility
54332	18.37	8.98	2.18	29.53

Modifiers (PAR) ◻

Code	Mod 50	Mod 51	Mod 62	Mod 66	Mod 80
54332	0	2	1	0	2

Global Period

Code	Days
54332	090

54336

54336 1-stage perineal hypospadias repair requiring extensive dissection to correct chordee and urethroplasty by use of skin graft tube and/or island flap

AMA Coding Notes

Repair Procedures on the Penis

(For other urethroplasties, see 53400-53430)

(For penile revascularization, use 37788)

AMA *CPT® Assistant* ▢

54336: Oct 04: 15

Plain English Description

Perineal hypospadias is a condition in which the urethral meatus is displaced from its normal position at the tip of the penis to the perineal region near the anus in males. Often there is a cleft deformity of the scrotum as well. A single-stage repair of perineal hypospadias and chordee can be accomplished using a Koyanagi-Nonomura bucket release technique or a modified/augmented version of this repair. A catheter is placed transurethrally into the bladder. A circumferential incision is made just proximal to the coronal sulcus and carried down between dartos and Buck's fascia on the dorsal side. The urethral plate is exposed and fibrous bands on the ventral aspect proximal to the hypospadias meatus are excised down to the corpus spongiosum inside the scrotum to correct chordee. A U-shaped incision is made around the hypospadias meatus with extensions lateral and dorsal into the prepuce. The incisions in the prepuce are joined at the 12 o'clock position. The portion between the prepuce and dartos is dissected free on the dorsal side. The prepuce is fixed to the dartos as the neo-urethra without vascular compromise. A buttonhole incision is made through the pedicle of the dartos and the glans penis is passed through the hole. The parameatal skin flap and vascular pedicle are then mobilized to the ventral side maintaining a loop shape. The internal side of the loop is closed over the catheter with a running stitch beginning at the front wall and incorporating the full thickness. The external side of the loop is closed with a running subcuticular stitch beginning at the back wall of the neo-urethra. The neo-meatus is created by making a slit-like midline incision in the glans penis extending from the tip to the coronal sulcus and dissecting bilaterally to create a plane between the glans cap and the corpora. The neo-urethra fits into the created groove and the length is adjusted with the end of the neo-urethra finally sutured to the tip of the glans to complete the neo-meatus. The catheter now extends out the tip of the penis. The wings of the created flap are mobilized over the neo-urethra and sutured in the midline and Byer's flaps created from the dorsal foreskin are divided and sutured to cover the remaining ventral skin defects. The circumferential incision is closed around the corona creating the appearance of a circumcision. The catheter is left in place.

1-stage perineal hypospadias repair requiring extensive dissection

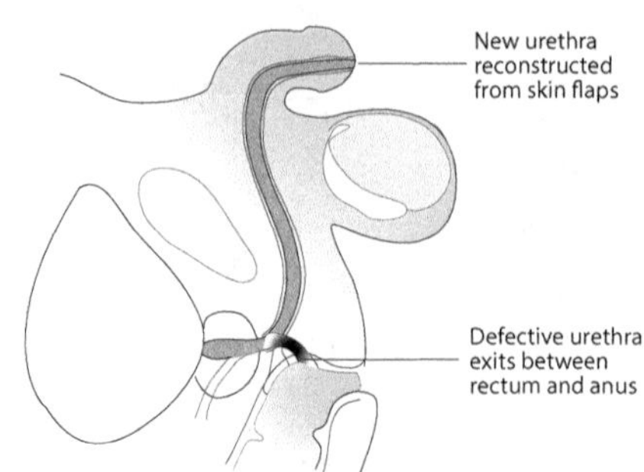
New urethra reconstructed from skin flaps
Defective urethra exits between rectum and anus

ICD-10-CM Diagnostic Codes

Q54.3	Hypospadias, perineal ♂
Q54.4	Congenital chordee ♂

CCI Edits

Refer to Appendix A for CCI edits.

Facility RVUs ▢

Code	Work	PE Facility	MP	Total Facility
54336	21.62	10.52	2.57	34.71

Non-facility RVUs ▢

Code	Work	PE Non-Facility	MP	Total Non-Facility
54336	21.62	10.52	2.57	34.71

Modifiers (PAR) ▢

Code	Mod 50	Mod 51	Mod 62	Mod 66	Mod 80
54336	0	2	1	0	2

Global Period

Code	Days
54336	090

54340-54348

▲ **54340 Repair of hypospadias complication(s) (ie, fistula, stricture, diverticula); by closure, incision, or excision, simple**

▲ **54344 Repair of hypospadias complication(s) (ie, fistula, stricture, diverticula); requiring mobilization of skin flaps and urethroplasty with flap or patch graft**

▲ **54348 Repair of hypospadias complication(s) (ie, fistula, stricture, diverticula); requiring extensive dissection, and urethroplasty with flap, patch or tubed graft (including urinary diversion, when performed)**

AMA Coding Notes

Repair Procedures on the Penis

(For other urethroplasties, see 53400-53430)

(For penile revascularization, use 37788)

Plain English Description

Complications of a previous hypospadias corrective procedure are repaired. Hypospadias is a birth defect in which the urethra opens somewhere besides the tip of the penis. Complications of a failed hypospadias repair include urethrocutaneous fistulas, strictures, diverticula and ventral penile curvature. Repairing complications can be challenging due to poor surrounding tissue from disruption of the normal vasculature. Stricture repairs, which can be the most challenging, will be described here. Use 54340 for simple repair of any of these defects that can be accomplished by closure, incision or excision. For a short stricture outside the area of previous hypospadias repair, simple excision with primary anastomosis is done. Use 54344 if skin flaps are mobilized and single-stage urethroplasty is done with flap or patch graft. This is appropriate for strictures that are proximal to, but separated from, the previous repair. Excision of the urethral stricture with anastomosis is done first, followed by the application of a small skin flap or, more often, grafting of a small patch of buccal mucosa onlay over the site. Report code 54348 if the physician must perform more extensive procedures to fix the defects, such as when a stricture is longer than 3 cm, requiring extensive dissection and repairing the urethra with a patch, flap or tubularization of a buccal graft.

Repair of hypospadias complications
(ie, fistula, stricture, diverticula)

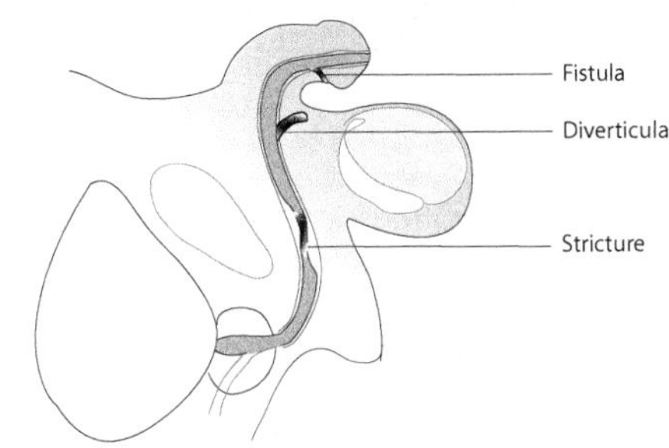

By closure, incision, or excision, simple (54340); requiring mobilization of skin flaps and urethroplasty with flap or patch graft (54344); requiring extensive dissection and urethroplasty with flap, patch, or tubed graft (includes urinary diversion) (54348)

ICD-10-CM Diagnostic Codes

	N36.1	Urethral diverticulum
	N99.110	Postprocedural urethral stricture, male, meatal ♂
	N99.111	Postprocedural bulbous urethral stricture, male ♂
	N99.112	Postprocedural membranous urethral stricture, male ♂
	N99.113	Postprocedural anterior bulbous urethral stricture, male ♂
	N99.114	Postprocedural urethral stricture, male, unspecified ♂
	N99.115	Postprocedural fossa navicularis urethral stricture ♂
	N99.116	Postprocedural urethral stricture, male, overlapping sites ♂
	N99.89	Other postprocedural complications and disorders of genitourinary system
➐	T81.83	Persistent postprocedural fistula
	Z87.710	Personal history of (corrected) hypospadias ♂

ICD-10-CM Coding Notes

For codes requiring a 7th character extension, refer to your ICD-10-CM book. Review the character descriptions and coding guidelines for proper selection. For some procedures, only certain characters will apply.

CCI Edits

Refer to Appendix A for CCI edits.

Facility RVUs 🗋

Code	Work	PE Facility	MP	Total Facility
54340	9.71	5.83	1.16	16.70
54344	17.06	8.53	2.03	27.62
54348	18.32	9.03	2.18	29.53

Non-facility RVUs 🗋

Code	Work	PE Non-Facility	MP	Total Non-Facility
54340	9.71	5.83	1.16	16.70
54344	17.06	8.53	2.03	27.62
54348	18.32	9.03	2.18	29.53

Modifiers (PAR) 🗋

Code	Mod 50	Mod 51	Mod 62	Mod 66	Mod 80
54340	0	2	1	0	2
54344	0	2	1	0	2
54348	0	2	1	0	2

Global Period

Code	Days
54340	090
54344	090
54348	090

54352

▲ **54352 Revision of prior hypospadias repair requiring extensive dissection and excision of previously constructed structures including re-release of chordee and reconstruction of urethra and penis by use of local skin as grafts and island flaps and skin brought in as flaps or grafts**

(Do not report 54352 in conjunction with 15275, 15574, 15740, 53235, 53410, 54300, 54336, 54340, 54344, 54348, 54360)

AMA Coding Notes

Repair Procedures on the Penis

(For other urethroplasties, see 53400-53430)

(For penile revascularization, use 37788)

Plain English Description

The physician revises a prior hypospadias repair that requires extensive dissection and excision of previously created structures done to repair a birth defect in which the urethra opens somewhere other than the tip of the penis. Some of the repairs that were performed during the original surgery must be reversed. The physician must perform extensive procedures to fix the defects, including re-releasing chordee and repairing the urethra or reconstructing the penis with local flaps or skin grafts as well as other skin patches or flaps.

Repair of hypospadias cripple requiring extensive dissection and excision of previously constructed structures

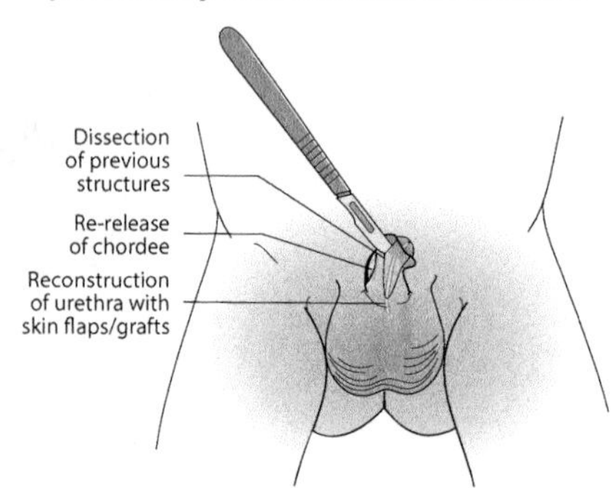

ICD-10-CM Diagnostic Codes

L76.82	Other postprocedural complications of skin and subcutaneous tissue
N99.110	Postprocedural urethral stricture, male, meatal ♂
N99.111	Postprocedural bulbous urethral stricture, male ♂
N99.112	Postprocedural membranous urethral stricture, male ♂
N99.113	Postprocedural anterior bulbous urethral stricture, male ♂
N99.115	Postprocedural fossa navicularis urethral stricture ♂
N99.116	Postprocedural urethral stricture, male, overlapping sites ♂
N99.89	Other postprocedural complications and disorders of genitourinary system
Q54.0	Hypospadias, balanic ♂
Q54.1	Hypospadias, penile ♂
Q54.2	Hypospadias, penoscrotal ♂
Q54.3	Hypospadias, perineal ♂
Q54.4	Congenital chordee ♂
Q54.8	Other hypospadias ♂
❼ T81.89	Other complications of procedures, not elsewhere classified
Z87.710	Personal history of (corrected) hypospadias ♂

ICD-10-CM Coding Notes

For codes requiring a 7th character extension, refer to your ICD-10-CM book. Review the character descriptions and coding guidelines for proper selection. For some procedures, only certain characters will apply.

CCI Edits

Refer to Appendix A for CCI edits.

Facility RVUs ▢

Code	Work	PE Facility	MP	Total Facility
54352	26.13	12.04	3.12	41.29

Non-facility RVUs ▢

Code	Work	PE Non-Facility	MP	Total Non-Facility
54352	26.13	12.04	3.12	41.29

Modifiers (PAR) ▢

Code	Mod 50	Mod 51	Mod 62	Mod 66	Mod 80
54352	0	2	1	0	2

Global Period

Code	Days
54352	090

54360

54360 Plastic operation on penis to correct angulation

AMA Coding Notes

Repair Procedures on the Penis

(For other urethroplasties, see 53400-53430)

(For penile revascularization, use 37788)

Plain English Description

Penile angulation, or curvature, may be a congenital or an acquired condition. Acquired angulation usually occurs when scar tissue replaces normal elastic penile tissue due to inflammation, infection, or injury. The angulation may be ventral (downward angle often associated with hypospadias), dorsal (upward angle associated with epispadias), or curve to the right or left side. Angulation may be present with a flaccid penis or only observed with penile erection. Severe angulation may impair penetration and cause discomfort to the patient and/or partner. Surgical correction of penile angulation may be performed through an infrapubic transverse dorsal incision or a subcoronal circumcising incision. The skin on the penis is then degloved to expose the tunica albuginea along the penile shaft. An artificial erection is induced using saline infusion and the exact location of the angle is identified. Plicating sutures are placed to mark the location and the erection is reduced. One or more small incision(s) are made in the tunica albuginea; tissue wedge(s) are removed to shorten the penis on the side opposite the angle; and the incision(s) is closed with absorbable sutures. Artificial erection is again induced to check for adequate angulation correction. The degloved skin is replaced over the penile shaft and the skin incision is closed.

Plastic operation on penis to correct angulation

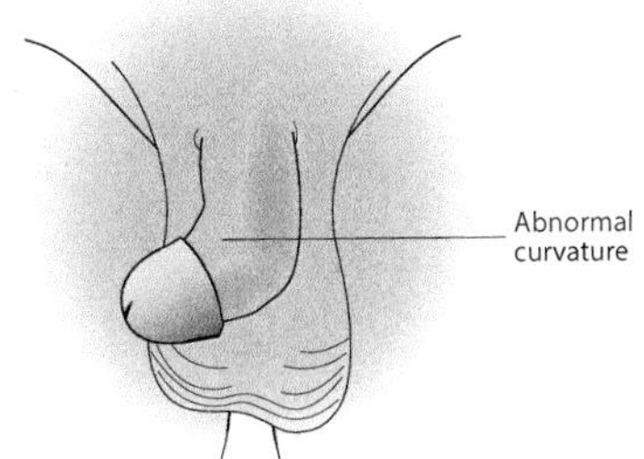

ICD-10-CM Diagnostic Codes

N48.0	Leukoplakia of penis ♂
N48.6	Induration penis plastica ♂
N48.82	Acquired torsion of penis ♂
Q55.61	Curvature of penis (lateral) ♂
Q55.63	Congenital torsion of penis ♂

CCI Edits

Refer to Appendix A for CCI edits.

Facility RVUs ▯

Code	Work	PE Facility	MP	Total Facility
54360	12.78	6.81	1.52	21.11

Non-facility RVUs ▯

Code	Work	PE Non-Facility	MP	Total Non-Facility
54360	12.78	6.81	1.52	21.11

Modifiers (PAR) ▯

Code	Mod 50	Mod 51	Mod 62	Mod 66	Mod 80
54360	0	2	1	0	2

Global Period

Code	Days
54360	090

54380-54390

54380 Plastic operation on penis for epispadias distal to external sphincter
54385 Plastic operation on penis for epispadias distal to external sphincter; with incontinence
54390 Plastic operation on penis for epispadias distal to external sphincter; with exstrophy of bladder

AMA Coding Notes

Repair Procedures on the Penis

(For other urethroplasties, see 53400-53430)

(For penile revascularization, use 37788)

Plain English Description

Epispadias is a congenital defect of the urinary tract in which the urethra does not fully develop causing urine to exit the body in an abnormal location. In males, the urethral opening is generally on the top or side of the penis rather than at the tip. The condition can be complicated by bladder neck and sphincter malformation and/or exstrophy of the bladder. These malformations may be treated in a single procedure or in a staged fashion.
In 54380, surgical correction of penile epispadias is performed. A circumferential incision is made below the glans and the penile skin is degloved exposing Buck's fascia. The urethral meatus is resected to the distal edge of the hypoplastic urethral tissue. An island flap is harvested from the penile preputial skin. A neourethra is then developed over a stent or catheter. The glans is split and flaps elevated to cover the distal neourethra, foreskin is trimmed, and excess tissue removed. The degloved penile skin is mobilized back up the penile shaft and the incision is sutured. In 54385, epispadias is complicated by absence of the bladder neck and sphincter resulting in incontinence. Epispadias repair and bladder neck reconstruction are typically performed in a staged fashion with the epispadias repair being performed around age 2 and bladder neck reconstruction at around age 4. To accomplish the bladder neck reconstruction, triangular lateral bladder mucosal wedges about 15 mm wide and 30 mm long are marked, developed, and demucosalized. The flaps are brought over the neourethra using a vest-over-pants technique to form the bladder neck. Suspension sutures are placed to suspend to the bladder neck. In 54390, bladder exstrophy, a condition where the bladder is turned inside out and protrudes through the abdominal wall, is also repaired. A skin incision is made above the umbilicus, carried around the sides of the bladder mucosa to approximately 1 cm from the midline, and continued parallel along the distal urethral plate to the lateral region of the male verumontanum. The incision is deepened around the umbilicus and a plane developed between the rectus muscle and the bladder wall. The peritoneum is dissected off the bladder and developed laterally until the trigone and the urogenital diaphragm are encountered. Ureteral stents are placed. The urogenital diaphragm is dissected completely off of the pubic bone parallel to the bladder and posterior urethra. Traction is placed on the pubic bone to bring the bladder neck deep into the pelvis. The bladder neck and posterior urethra are closed. An osteotomy is performed by bringing the pubic bone together in the midline with suture or wire and the abdominal wall defect is closed in layers. The pelvis may be immobilized with traction, cast, or external fixator.

Plastic operation on penis for epispadias distal to external sphincter

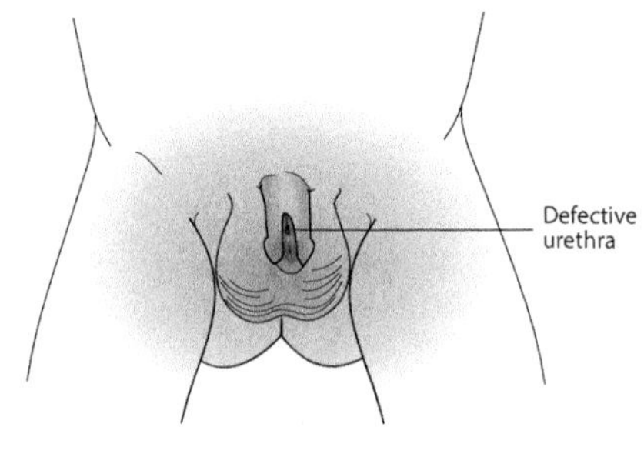

ICD-10-CM Diagnostic Codes

Q64.0 Epispadias

CCI Edits

Refer to Appendix A for CCI edits.

Facility RVUs

Code	Work	PE Facility	MP	Total Facility
54380	14.18	7.53	1.68	23.39
54385	16.56	8.70	1.98	27.24
54390	22.77	10.79	2.71	36.27

Non-facility RVUs

Code	Work	PE Non-Facility	MP	Total Non-Facility
54380	14.18	7.53	1.68	23.39
54385	16.56	8.70	1.98	27.24
54390	22.77	10.79	2.71	36.27

Modifiers (PAR)

Code	Mod 50	Mod 51	Mod 62	Mod 66	Mod 80
54380	0	2	1	0	2
54385	0	2	1	0	2
54390	0	2	1	0	2

Global Period

Code	Days
54380	090
54385	090
54390	090

54400-54401

54400 **Insertion of penile prosthesis; non-inflatable (semi-rigid)**

54401 **Insertion of penile prosthesis; inflatable (self-contained)**

(For removal or replacement of penile prosthesis, see 54415, 54416)

AMA Coding Notes

Repair Procedures on the Penis

(For other urethroplasties, see 53400-53430)

(For penile revascularization, use 37788)

Plain English Description

Placement of a penile prosthesis is performed to treat erectile dysfunction. In 54400, a non-inflatable/semi-rigid penile prosthesis is inserted. A catheter is placed transurethrally. A 180-degree skin incision is made along the subcoronal area of the penis and carried down to Buck's fascia. Stay sutures are then placed through the tunica albuginea lateral to the penile nerves securing each corpora cavernosa. Longitudinal incisions are made along the dorsal surface of the corpora cavernosa between the stay sutures. The incisions are extended and a space created on each side in the corporal tissue. The spaces are enlarged using a dilator. The tip of the dilator is positioned under the dorsolateral surface of the tunica albuginea and dilation proceeds at an angle away from the urethra and the penile septum. The spaces are measured and appropriately sized prosthetic cylinders are loaded into an inserter and placed into each of the corporal spaces. The inserting instrument is removed and the corporal incision is closed followed by closure of the tunica albuginea and skin. In 54401, an inflatable, self-contained penile prosthesis is inserted. A penoscrotal approach is most often used. A skin incision is made in the mid-raphe area of the penoscrotal junction and carried down to the dartos fascia. The fascia is carefully divided and a circular self-retaining hook retractor used as needed to facilitate exposure of the operative field. The corpus spongiosum is identified and dissection continues lateral to the urethra and spongiosum tissue until the corpora cavernosa is encountered. Stay sutures are placed through the tunica albuginea to secure each corpora cavernosa. A corporotomy is made between the sutures. The incisions are extended, spaces created, and the inflatable prosthesis placed as described above. A pouch is then created in the sub-dartos tissue of the scrotum. The pump is inserted and connected to the cylinders. The device is cycled to ensure that it is functioning properly and to check for leaks. Incisions are closed.

Insertion of penile prosthesis; non-inflatable (semi-rigid)

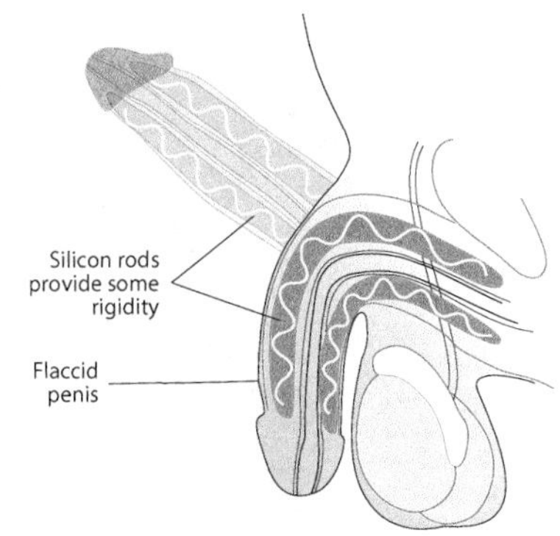

ICD-10-CM Diagnostic Codes

E10.59	Type 1 diabetes mellitus with other circulatory complications
E11.59	Type 2 diabetes mellitus with other circulatory complications
F52.21	Male erectile disorder ♂
F52.8	Other sexual dysfunction not due to a substance or known physiological condition
N48.6	Induration penis plastica ♂
N48.82	Acquired torsion of penis ♂
N48.89	Other specified disorders of penis ♂
N50.1	Vascular disorders of male genital organs ♂
N52.01	Erectile dysfunction due to arterial insufficiency ♂
N52.02	Corporo-venous occlusive erectile dysfunction ♂
N52.03	Combined arterial insufficiency and corporo-venous occlusive erectile dysfunction ♂
N52.1	Erectile dysfunction due to diseases classified elsewhere ♂
N52.2	Drug-induced erectile dysfunction ♂
N52.31	Erectile dysfunction following radical prostatectomy ♂
N52.32	Erectile dysfunction following radical cystectomy ♂
N52.33	Erectile dysfunction following urethral surgery ♂
N52.34	Erectile dysfunction following simple prostatectomy ♂
N52.35	Erectile dysfunction following radiation therapy ♂
N52.36	Erectile dysfunction following interstitial seed therapy ♂
N52.37	Erectile dysfunction following prostate ablative therapy ♂
N52.39	Other and unspecified postprocedural erectile dysfunction ♂
N52.8	Other male erectile dysfunction ♂

CCI Edits

Refer to Appendix A for CCI edits.

Pub 100

54400: Pub 100-03, 1, 230.4

54401: Pub 100-03, 1, 230.4

Facility RVUs ▯

Code	Work	PE Facility	MP	Total Facility
54400	9.17	5.35	1.09	15.61
54401	10.44	7.75	1.25	19.44

Non-facility RVUs ▯

Code	Work	PE Non-Facility	MP	Total Non-Facility
54400	9.17	5.35	1.09	15.61
54401	10.44	7.75	1.25	19.44

Modifiers (PAR) ▯

Code	Mod 50	Mod 51	Mod 62	Mod 66	Mod 80
54400	0	2	1	0	1
54401	0	2	1	0	1

Global Period

Code	Days
54400	090
54401	090

54405

54405 Insertion of multi-component, inflatable penile prosthesis, including placement of pump, cylinders, and reservoir

(For reduced services, report 54405 with modifier 52)

AMA Coding Notes

Repair Procedures on the Penis

(For other urethroplasties, see 53400-53430)

(For penile revascularization, use 37788)

Plain English Description

A multi-component, inflatable penile prosthesis allows the patient to maintain rigidity for intercourse. The device consists of two inflatable intracorporal cylinders, a scrotal pump, and a fluid reservoir placed in the abdomen. A Foley catheter is placed in the bladder. A transverse incision is made at the penoscrotal junction exposing the dartos fascia, which is then incised. The tunica albuginea of both corpora cavernosa are exposed. Small incisions are made in each corpus cavernosum and extended with scissors. The corpora cavernosa are dilated, taking care to avoid injury to the urethra, and the spaces are irrigated with antibiotic solution. The cylinders are inserted into the spaces and tested for patency. The incisions are closed with absorbable suture. A subdartos pouch is created in the center of the scrotum through a small incision in the dartos fascia and the pump is inserted into the pouch with the deflation button in an anteroinferior position. The pump tubing is passed through separate stab incisions in the dartos fascia to emerge from the posterior aspect of the pouch. The incision at the top of the pouch is closed. The cylinders and pump are checked for patency using a syringe and saline solution. The bladder is fully drained; the external inguinal ring is identified; and the spermatic cord is displaced medially for protection. The transversalis fascia is punctured for access to the retropubic space and the reservoir is inserted and filled with saline solution. The reservoir's position and the tubing exiting through the transversalis fascia are confirmed. The pump, reservoir, and cylinders are connected, and the device is checked again. The dartos fascia is closed with absorbable sutures followed by skin closure.

Insertion of a multi-component, inflatable penile prosthesis

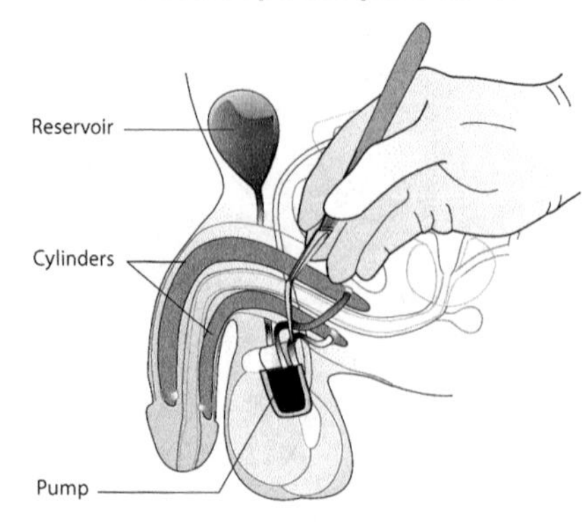

ICD-10-CM Diagnostic Codes

E10.59	Type 1 diabetes mellitus with other circulatory complications
E11.59	Type 2 diabetes mellitus with other circulatory complications
F52.21	Male erectile disorder ♂
F52.8	Other sexual dysfunction not due to a substance or known physiological condition
N48.6	Induration penis plastica ♂
N48.82	Acquired torsion of penis ♂
N48.89	Other specified disorders of penis ♂
N50.1	Vascular disorders of male genital organs ♂
N52.01	Erectile dysfunction due to arterial insufficiency ♂
N52.02	Corporo-venous occlusive erectile dysfunction ♂
N52.03	Combined arterial insufficiency and corporo-venous occlusive erectile dysfunction ♂
N52.1	Erectile dysfunction due to diseases classified elsewhere ♂
N52.2	Drug-induced erectile dysfunction ♂
N52.31	Erectile dysfunction following radical prostatectomy ♂
N52.32	Erectile dysfunction following radical cystectomy ♂
N52.34	Erectile dysfunction following simple prostatectomy ♂
N52.35	Erectile dysfunction following radiation therapy ♂
N52.36	Erectile dysfunction following interstitial seed therapy ♂
N52.39	Other and unspecified postprocedural erectile dysfunction ♂
N52.8	Other male erectile dysfunction ♂

CCI Edits

Refer to Appendix A for CCI edits.

Pub 100

54405: Pub 100-03, 1, 230.4

Facility RVUs ▯

Code	Work	PE Facility	MP	Total Facility
54405	14.52	7.41	1.72	23.65

Non-facility RVUs ▯

Code	Work	PE Non-Facility	MP	Total Non-Facility
54405	14.52	7.41	1.72	23.65

Modifiers (PAR) ▯

Code	Mod 50	Mod 51	Mod 62	Mod 66	Mod 80
54405	0	2	1	0	2

Global Period

Code	Days
54405	090

54406

54406 Removal of all components of a multi-component, inflatable penile prosthesis without replacement of prosthesis

(For reduced services, report 54406 with modifier 52)

AMA Coding Notes

Repair Procedures on the Penis

(For other urethroplasties, see 53400-53430)

(For penile revascularization, use 37788)

Plain English Description

A catheter is passed transurethrally. A midline skin incision is made in the lower abdomen and carried down through the subcutaneous tissue to the fascia. The dorsal venous complex and corporal bodies are identified and the incision is explored until tubing to the reservoir is encountered and tracked to its position under the rectus muscle. Using sharp and blunt dissection, the reservoir is freed. Tubing is tracked to the pump in the dartos pouch in the scrotum, dissected free, and brought out through the abdominal incision. Tubing is tracked to the two lateral cylinders in the corporal bodies and the cylinders are dissected free. All components are removed. Corporotomy incisions are closed. The tunica albuginea is closed followed by scrotal/dartos fascia. A drain may be placed in the abdominal incision. The rectus muscle, subcutaneous tissue, and skin are closed.

Removal of all components of a multi-component, inflatable penile prosthesis

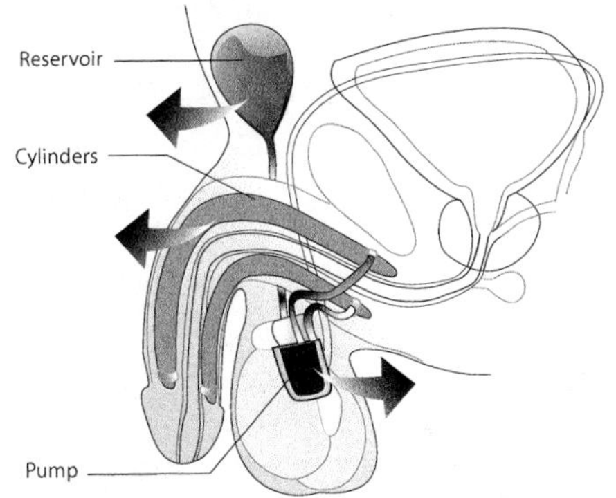

ICD-10-CM Diagnostic Codes

❼	T83.410	Breakdown (mechanical) of implanted penile prosthesis
❼	T83.420	Displacement of implanted penile prosthesis
❼	T83.490	Other mechanical complication of implanted penile prosthesis
❼	T83.61	Infection and inflammatory reaction due to implanted penile prosthesis
❼	T85.828	Fibrosis due to other internal prosthetic devices, implants and grafts
❼	T85.848	Pain due to other internal prosthetic devices, implants and grafts
❼	T85.868	Thrombosis due to other internal prosthetic devices, implants and grafts
❼	T85.898	Other specified complication of other internal prosthetic devices, implants and grafts

ICD-10-CM Coding Notes

For codes requiring a 7th character extension, refer to your ICD-10-CM book. Review the character descriptions and coding guidelines for proper selection. For some procedures, only certain characters will apply.

CCI Edits

Refer to Appendix A for CCI edits.

Pub 100

54406: Pub 100-03, 1, 230.4

Facility RVUs ▯

Code	Work	PE Facility	MP	Total Facility
54406	12.89	6.98	1.54	21.41

Non-facility RVUs ▯

Code	Work	PE Non-Facility	MP	Total Non-Facility
54406	12.89	6.98	1.54	21.41

Modifiers (PAR) ▯

Code	Mod 50	Mod 51	Mod 62	Mod 66	Mod 80
54406	0	2	1	0	2

Global Period

Code	Days
54406	090

54408

54408 Repair of component(s) of a multi-component, inflatable penile prosthesis

AMA Coding Notes

Repair Procedures on the Penis

(For other urethroplasties, see 53400-53430)

(For penile revascularization, use 37788)

Plain English Description

A catheter is inserted transurethrally. A midline skin incision is made in the lower abdomen and carried down through the subcutaneous tissue to the fascia. The dorsal venous complex and corporal bodies are identified and the incision is explored until tubing to the reservoir is encountered and tracked to its position under the rectus muscle. The tubing is checked for kinks and the reservoir for kinks/leaks. Tubing is then tracked to the pump in the dartos pouch in the scrotum, which is also examined for kinks/leaks. Finally, tubing is tracked to the cylinders in the corporal bodies and examined for kinks/leaks. Repair may include shortening of tubing if kinks are present, replacement of tubing, or replacement of connecters if leaks are occurring at the connection sites. The penile prosthesis is cycled to ensure that it is working properly and that there are no leaks. The tunica albuginea is closed followed by scrotal/dartos fascia. A drain may be placed in the abdominal incision. The rectus muscle, subcutaneous tissue, and skin are closed.

Repair of component(s) of a multicomponent, inflatable penile prosthesis

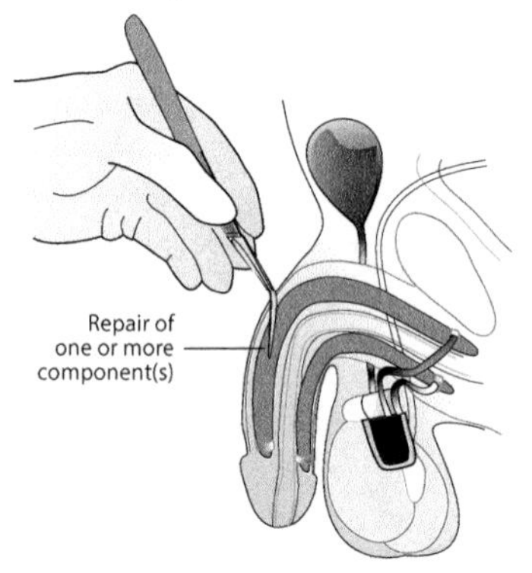

ICD-10-CM Diagnostic Codes

❼	T83.410	Breakdown (mechanical) of implanted penile prosthesis
❼	T83.420	Displacement of implanted penile prosthesis
❼	T83.490	Other mechanical complication of implanted penile prosthesis
❼	T85.828	Fibrosis due to other internal prosthetic devices, implants and grafts
❼	T85.838	Hemorrhage due to other internal prosthetic devices, implants and grafts
❼	T85.848	Pain due to other internal prosthetic devices, implants and grafts
❼	T85.898	Other specified complication of other internal prosthetic devices, implants and grafts
	Z44.8	Encounter for fitting and adjustment of other external prosthetic devices

ICD-10-CM Coding Notes

For codes requiring a 7th character extension, refer to your ICD-10-CM book. Review the character descriptions and coding guidelines for proper selection. For some procedures, only certain characters will apply.

CCI Edits

Refer to Appendix A for CCI edits.

Pub 100

54408: Pub 100-03, 1, 230.4

Facility RVUs ▯

Code	Work	PE Facility	MP	Total Facility
54408	13.91	7.58	1.66	23.15

Non-facility RVUs ▯

Code	Work	PE Non-Facility	MP	Total Non-Facility
54408	13.91	7.58	1.66	23.15

Modifiers (PAR) ▯

Code	Mod 50	Mod 51	Mod 62	Mod 66	Mod 80
54408	0	2	1	0	2

Global Period

Code	Days
54408	090

54410-54411

54410 Removal and replacement of all component(s) of a multi-component, inflatable penile prosthesis at the same operative session

54411 Removal and replacement of all components of a multi-component inflatable penile prosthesis through an infected field at the same operative session, including irrigation and debridement of infected tissue

(For reduced services, report 54411 with modifier 52)

(Do not report 11042, 11043 in addition to 54411)

AMA Coding Notes

Repair Procedures on the Penis

(For other urethroplasties, see 53400-53430)

(For penile revascularization, use 37788)

Plain English Description

A catheter is passed transurethrally. A midline skin incision is made in the lower abdomen and carried down through the subcutaneous tissue to the fascia. The dorsal venous complex and corporal bodies are identified and the incision is explored until tubing to the reservoir is encountered and tracked to its position under the rectus muscle. Using sharp and blunt dissection, the reservoir is freed. Tubing is tracked to the pump in the dartos pouch in the scrotum, dissected free, and brought out through the abdominal incision. Tubing is tracked to the two lateral cylinders in the corporal bodies and the cylinders are dissected free. All components are removed. If the removal is performed for infection, the wounds are copiously irrigated with antibiotic solution and any infected or necrotic tissue is debrided. The corporal bodies are resized and an appropriately sized replacement prosthetic device selected. The cylinders are filled with saline and cycled to check for leaks. The cylinders are then loaded into an inserter and placed into each of the corporal spaces. The inserting instrument is removed. The corporotomy incisions are closed. The pump is placed into the dartos pouch in the scrotum. The reservoir is placed in the rectus space in the lower abdomen. Tubing length is adjusted and connections secured. The device is cycled to ensure that it is functioning properly and to check for leaks. The tunica albuginea is closed followed by scrotal/dartos fascia. A drain may be placed in the abdominal incision. The rectus muscle, subcutaneous tissue, and skin are closed. Use 54410 for removal and replacement of all components for a reason other than infection. Use 54411 for removal and replacement through an infected field.

Removal and replacement of all component(s) of a multi-component, inflatable penile prosthesis

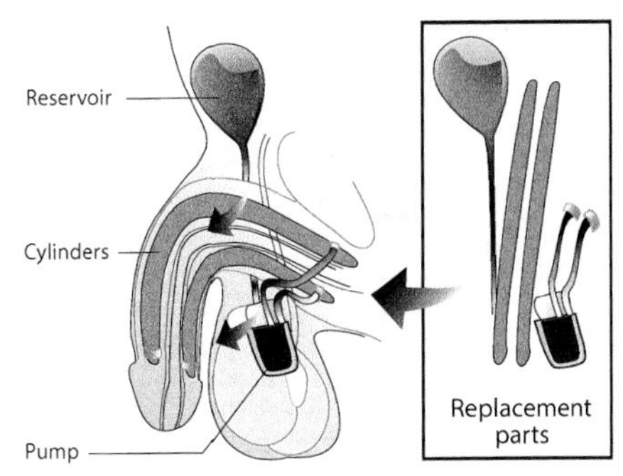

ICD-10-CM Diagnostic Codes

❼	T83.410	Breakdown (mechanical) of implanted penile prosthesis
❼	T83.420	Displacement of implanted penile prosthesis
❼	T83.490	Other mechanical complication of implanted penile prosthesis
❼	T83.61	Infection and inflammatory reaction due to implanted penile prosthesis
❼	T83.84	Pain due to genitourinary prosthetic devices, implants and grafts
❼	T83.89	Other specified complication of genitourinary prosthetic devices, implants and grafts
	Z44.8	Encounter for fitting and adjustment of other external prosthetic devices

ICD-10-CM Coding Notes

For codes requiring a 7th character extension, refer to your ICD-10-CM book. Review the character descriptions and coding guidelines for proper selection. For some procedures, only certain characters will apply.

CCI Edits

Refer to Appendix A for CCI edits.

Pub 100

54410: Pub 100-03, 1, 230.4
54411: Pub 100-03, 1, 230.4

Facility RVUs ☐

Code	Work	PE Facility	MP	Total Facility
54410	15.18	8.27	1.81	25.26
54411	18.35	9.57	2.17	30.09

Non-facility RVUs ☐

Code	Work	PE Non-Facility	MP	Total Non-Facility
54410	15.18	8.27	1.81	25.26
54411	18.35	9.57	2.17	30.09

Modifiers (PAR) ☐

Code	Mod 50	Mod 51	Mod 62	Mod 66	Mod 80
54410	0	2	1	0	2
54411	0	2	1	0	2

Global Period

Code	Days
54410	090
54411	090

54415

54415 Removal of non-inflatable (semi-rigid) or inflatable (self-contained) penile prosthesis, without replacement of prosthesis

AMA Coding Notes

Repair Procedures on the Penis

(For other urethroplasties, see 53400-53430)

(For penile revascularization, use 37788)

Plain English Description

Removal of a penile prosthesis is typically performed through the same incision used for placement. A catheter is placed transurethrally. To remove a non-inflatable, semi-rigid penile prosthesis, a 180-degree skin incision is made along the subcoronal area of the penis and carried down to Buck's fascia. Stay sutures are then placed through the tunica albuginea lateral to the penile nerves securing each corpora cavernosa. Longitudinal incisions are made along the dorsal surface of the corpora cavernosa between the stay sutures. Each implant (right and left) is dissected free of surrounding tissue. Hemostasis is achieved with electrocautery and the wound is irrigated with antibiotic solution. If infection is present, the wound may be left open to drain or a drain inserted. The incision is closed in layers. To remove an inflatable, self-contained penile prosthesis placed through a penoscrotal approach, a skin incision is made in the mid-raphe area of the penoscrotal junction and carried down to the dartos fascia. The fascia is divided and a self-retaining hook retractor placed to facilitate exposure of the operative field. The corpus spongiosum is identified. Dissection is performed lateral to the urethra and spongiosum tissue until the corpora cavernosa is encountered. Stay sutures are placed through the tunica albuginea to secure each corpora cavernosa. A corporotomy is made between the sutures. The cylinder implants are identified in the corporal bodies. The cylinder implants are identified within the corporal bodies. Each implant (right and left) is dissected free of surrounding tissue. Tubing is tracked to the pump in the sub-dartos pouch and the tubing and pump are dissected from surrounding tissue and removed. Incisions are closed as described above.

Removal of non-inflatable (semi-rigid) or inflatable penile prosthesis

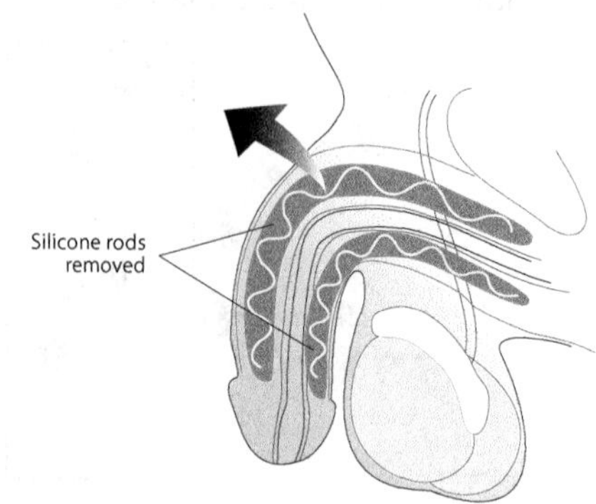

ICD-10-CM Diagnostic Codes

➐	T83.410	Breakdown (mechanical) of implanted penile prosthesis
➐	T83.420	Displacement of implanted penile prosthesis
➐	T83.490	Other mechanical complication of implanted penile prosthesis
➐	T83.61	Infection and inflammatory reaction due to implanted penile prosthesis
➐	T83.81	Embolism due to genitourinary prosthetic devices, implants and grafts
➐	T83.82	Fibrosis due to genitourinary prosthetic devices, implants and grafts
➐	T83.83	Hemorrhage due to genitourinary prosthetic devices, implants and grafts
➐	T83.84	Pain due to genitourinary prosthetic devices, implants and grafts
➐	T83.85	Stenosis due to genitourinary prosthetic devices, implants and grafts
➐	T83.86	Thrombosis due to genitourinary prosthetic devices, implants and grafts
➐	T83.89	Other specified complication of genitourinary prosthetic devices, implants and grafts

ICD-10-CM Coding Notes

For codes requiring a 7th character extension, refer to your ICD-10-CM book. Review the character descriptions and coding guidelines for proper selection. For some procedures, only certain characters will apply.

CCI Edits

Refer to Appendix A for CCI edits.

Pub 100

54415: Pub 100-03, 1, 230.4

Facility RVUs ▢

Code	Work	PE Facility	MP	Total Facility
54415	8.88	5.64	1.06	15.58

Non-facility RVUs ▢

Code	Work	PE Non-Facility	MP	Total Non-Facility
54415	8.88	5.64	1.06	15.58

Modifiers (PAR) ▢

Code	Mod 50	Mod 51	Mod 62	Mod 66	Mod 80
54415	0	2	1	0	2

Global Period

Code	Days
54415	090

54416-54417

54416 Removal and replacement of non-inflatable (semi-rigid) or inflatable (self-contained) penile prosthesis at the same operative session

54417 Removal and replacement of non-inflatable (semi-rigid) or inflatable (self-contained) penile prosthesis through an infected field at the same operative session, including irrigation and debridement of infected tissue

(Do not report 11042, 11043 in addition to 54417)

AMA Coding Notes

Repair Procedures on the Penis

(For other urethroplasties, see 53400-53430)

(For penile revascularization, use 37788)

Plain English Description

A penile prosthesis is removed and replaced at the same operative session. A catheter is placed transurethrally. The incision used for the insertion is reopened. The corpora cavernosa is exposed. Longitudinal incisions are made along the dorsal surface of the corpora cavernosa and the cylinder implants identified. Each prosthesis (right and left) is dissected free of surrounding tissue and removed. If the prosthesis is an inflatable semi-contained type, the tubing is tracked to the pump in the sub-dartos pouch and the tubing and pump are dissected from surrounding tissue and removed. Hemostasis is achieved with electrocautery and the wound is irrigated with antibiotic solution. If the procedure is performed through an infected surgical field, the wound is copiously irrigated and tissue debrided as needed. The penile prosthesis is then replaced. To replace a non-inflatable semi-rigid prosthesis, the length is measured and appropriately sized prosthetic cylinders are loaded into the insertion device. The cylinders are placed into each of the corporal spaces (right and left). The insertion device is removed and the incision is closed in layers. To replace a self-contained inflatable penile prosthesis, the cylinders are replaced as described above. The pump is inserted into the dartos pouch and connected to the cylinders. The device is cycled to evaluate function and to check for leaks. The corporal incisions are closed in layers. Use 54416 for removal and replacement for a reason other than infection. Use 54417 for removal and replacement through an infected field.

Removal and replacement of non-inflatable or inflatable penile prosthesis, same operative session

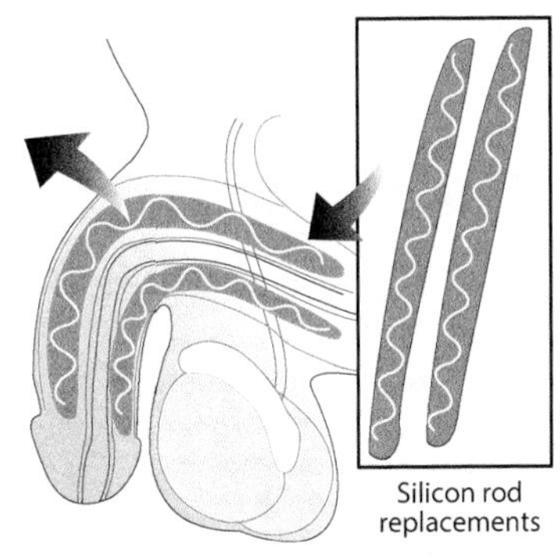

ICD-10-CM Diagnostic Codes

➐	T83.410	Breakdown (mechanical) of implanted penile prosthesis
➐	T83.420	Displacement of implanted penile prosthesis
➐	T83.490	Other mechanical complication of implanted penile prosthesis
➐	T83.61	Infection and inflammatory reaction due to implanted penile prosthesis
➐	T83.82	Fibrosis due to genitourinary prosthetic devices, implants and grafts
➐	T83.83	Hemorrhage due to genitourinary prosthetic devices, implants and grafts
➐	T83.84	Pain due to genitourinary prosthetic devices, implants and grafts
➐	T83.85	Stenosis due to genitourinary prosthetic devices, implants and grafts
➐	T83.86	Thrombosis due to genitourinary prosthetic devices, implants and grafts
➐	T83.89	Other specified complication of genitourinary prosthetic devices, implants and grafts
	Z44.8	Encounter for fitting and adjustment of other external prosthetic devices

ICD-10-CM Coding Notes

For codes requiring a 7th character extension, refer to your ICD-10-CM book. Review the character descriptions and coding guidelines for proper selection. For some procedures, only certain characters will apply.

CCI Edits

Refer to Appendix A for CCI edits.

Pub 100

54416: Pub 100-03, 1, 230.4

54417: Pub 100-03, 1, 230.4

Facility RVUs ▢

Code	Work	PE Facility	MP	Total Facility
54416	12.08	7.45	1.47	21.00
54417	16.10	8.27	1.93	26.30

Non-facility RVUs ▢

Code	Work	PE Non-Facility	MP	Total Non-Facility
54416	12.08	7.45	1.47	21.00
54417	16.10	8.27	1.93	26.30

Modifiers (PAR) ▢

Code	Mod 50	Mod 51	Mod 62	Mod 66	Mod 80
54416	0	2	1	0	2
54417	0	2	1	0	2

Global Period

Code	Days
54416	090
54417	090

54420-54430

54420 Corpora cavernosa-saphenous vein shunt (priapism operation), unilateral or bilateral

54430 Corpora cavernosa-corpus spongiosum shunt (priapism operation), unilateral or bilateral

AMA Coding Notes

Repair Procedures on the Penis

(For other urethroplasties, see 53400-53430)

(For penile revascularization, use 37788)

Plain English Description

A shunt procedure is performed to treat priapism. A Foley catheter is placed transurethrally. In 54420, a Grayhack procedure that creates a shunt between the corpora cavernosa and saphenous is perfomed. The first incision is made below the inguinal ligament at the saphenofemoral junction on either the right or left side and carried down until the saphenous vein is identified. An 8-10 cm length of vein is mobilized from surrounding tissue for harvesting. A lateral second incision is made in the skin at the base of the penis on the same side as the first incision and carried down to the corpora cavernosa/corpus spongiosum. An elliptical incision is then made in the tunica albuginea. The penis and glans may be irrigated using heparinized saline solution to remove accumulated blood and clots. A tunnel is created between the two incisions. The ligated saphenous vein is brought through to the penile incision. The end of the vein is spatulated open and sewn to the elliptical incision in the tunica albuginea. The skin of the penile incision is closed and then the inguinal/thigh incision is closed in layers. If a unilateral procedure fails to relieve pressure in the corpora cavernosa. an identical procedure may be performed on the opposite side. In 54430, a Quackles procedure that creates a shunt between the corpora cavernosa and corpus spongiosum is performed. A vertical skin incision is made in the perineum posterior to the scrotum. The incision is carried down to the bulbocavernosus muscle, which is reflected off the urethra. The junction of the cavernosa and spongiosum is identified and longitudinal or elliptical incisions are made through the tunica albuginea into one of the corpora cavernosa bodies and the tissue of the corpus spongiosum. The blood is evacuated from the corpora cavernosa by milking the penis. The posterior walls of the corpora cavernosa and corpus spongiosum are sutured together followed by the anterior walls. Pressure is measured for 10 minutes and if the intracavernosal pressure remains less than 40 mm Hg, the skin is closed. If the pressure is higher than 40 mm Hg an identical procedure is performed on the opposite side.

Corpora cavernosa-saphenous vein shunt, unilateral or bilateral

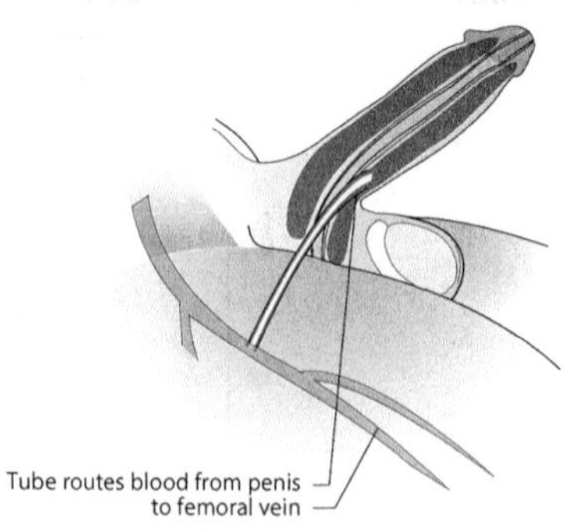
Tube routes blood from penis to femoral vein

ICD-10-CM Diagnostic Codes

N48.31	Priapism due to trauma ♂
N48.32	Priapism due to disease classified elsewhere ♂
N48.33	Priapism, drug-induced ♂
N48.39	Other priapism ♂

CCI Edits

Refer to Appendix A for CCI edits.

Facility RVUs ▯

Code	Work	PE Facility	MP	Total Facility
54420	12.39	6.72	1.47	20.58
54430	11.06	6.34	1.32	18.72

Non-facility RVUs ▯

Code	Work	PE Non-Facility	MP	Total Non-Facility
54420	12.39	6.72	1.47	20.58
54430	11.06	6.34	1.32	18.72

Modifiers (PAR) ▯

Code	Mod 50	Mod 51	Mod 62	Mod 66	Mod 80
54420	0	2	0	0	2
54430	2	2	0	0	2

Global Period

Code	Days
54420	090
54430	090

54435

54435 Corpora cavernosa-glans penis fistulization (eg, biopsy needle, Winter procedure, rongeur, or punch) for priapism

AMA Coding Notes

Repair Procedures on the Penis

(For other urethroplasties, see 53400-53430)

(For penile revascularization, use 37788)

Plain English Description

Creation of a fistula in the corpora cavernosa-glans penis to relieve priapism may also be referred to as an Ebbehoj or Winter procedure. These are minimally invasive surgical procedures and can often be performed using only a local anesthetic for pain control. With the patient positioned supine, the penis is prepared and draped. A large bore biopsy needle or scalpel tip is inserted through the glans penis into the corpora cavernosa and a core of tissue is removed, which allows accumulated blood to drain. Gentle pressure may be applied from the base of the penis toward the glans to milk blood out of the corporal tissue. The fistula is allowed to close spontaneously.

Corpora cavernosa-glans penis fistulization for priapism

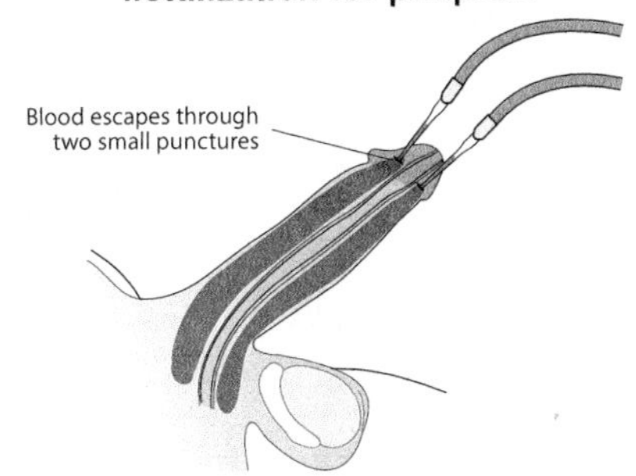
Blood escapes through two small punctures

ICD-10-CM Diagnostic Codes

N48.31	Priapism due to trauma ♂
N48.32	Priapism due to disease classified elsewhere ♂
N48.33	Priapism, drug-induced ♂
N48.39	Other priapism ♂

CCI Edits

Refer to Appendix A for CCI edits.

Facility RVUs

Code	Work	PE Facility	MP	Total Facility
54435	6.81	4.53	0.79	12.13

Non-facility RVUs

Code	Work	PE Non-Facility	MP	Total Non-Facility
54435	6.81	4.53	0.79	12.13

Modifiers (PAR)

Code	Mod 50	Mod 51	Mod 62	Mod 66	Mod 80
54435	0	2	0	0	1

Global Period

Code	Days
54435	090

54437

54437 Repair of traumatic corporeal tear(s)

(For repair of urethra, see 53410, 53415)

AMA Coding Notes

Repair Procedures on the Penis

(For other urethroplasties, see 53400-53430)

(For penile revascularization, use 37788)

Plain English Description

A procedure is performed to repair traumatic corporeal tear(s). The corpora cavernosa and corpus spongiosum are surrounded by a tough fibroelastic tissue called the tunica albuginea that stretches and thins during an erection. Traumatic corporeal injury occurs most often when the erect penile head strikes the pubic symphysis or perineum. Symptoms include a "popping" sound, rapid detumescence, pain, swelling, and abnormal penile curvature. Rarely, corporeal tears occur in the flaccid penis usually from sports injuries or other trauma. Tearing of the tunica albuginea and/or the corpora cavernosa causes a hematoma deep in Buck's fascia. Repair may be accomplished through a distal circumferential degloving incision or a lateral incision over the hematoma. For circumferential degloving, an incision is made in the skin between the glans and penile shaft, carried down to dartos fascia and Buck's fascia, and then degloved to the base of the penis. The right and left corpora cavernosa and the corpus spongiosum surrounding the urethra are carefully inspected. If a corporeal hematoma is present, Buck's fascia is incised and the hematoma is evacuated. The tunica albuginea is then inspected and lacerations are repaired. The fascia is closed with sutures; the skin is brought back up to cover the penile shaft (re-gloved); and the circumferential incision is closed. For a lateral incision over the hematoma, the skin is incised, carried down to dartos fascia and Buck's fascia, and the hematoma is evacuated. The tunica albuginea laceration is repaired with sutures and the incision is then closed in layers.

ICD-10-CM Diagnostic Codes

➐ S39.840 Fracture of corpus cavernosum penis

ICD-10-CM Coding Notes

For codes requiring a 7th character extension, refer to your ICD-10-CM book. Review the character descriptions and coding guidelines for proper selection. For some procedures, only certain characters will apply.

CCI Edits

Refer to Appendix A for CCI edits.

Facility RVUs ▯

Code	Work	PE Facility	MP	Total Facility
54437	11.50	6.98	1.37	19.85

Non-facility RVUs ▯

Code	Work	PE Non-Facility	MP	Total Non-Facility
54437	11.50	6.98	1.37	19.85

Modifiers (PAR) ▯

Code	Mod 50	Mod 51	Mod 62	Mod 66	Mod 80
54437	0	2	1	0	2

Global Period

Code	Days
54437	090

54438

54438 Replantation, penis, complete amputation including urethral repair

(To report replantation of incomplete penile amputation, see 54437 for repair of corporeal tear[s], and 53410, 53415 for repair of the urethra)

AMA Coding Notes

Repair Procedures on the Penis

(For other urethroplasties, see 53400-53430)

(For penile revascularization, use 37788)

Plain English Description

A procedure is performed to replant the penis following complete amputation. Bleeding from the penile stump may be controlled with a Penrose drain placed circumferentially and tightened with a hemostat. Necrotic tissue is debrided from the stump and penile remnant. Using a microscope, the skin is undermined from the stump and shaft to expose the dorsal veins, artery, and nerves and the urethra is spatulated. A Foley catheter is inserted into the urethra to bridge and stabilize the segments. The urethral mucosa is approximated and sutured 360° followed by a second layer of sutures through the corpus spongiosum. The deep cavernosal arteries may be reanastomosed if the amputation is proximal. The corporeal bodies are reattached and the tunica albuginea is approximated and sutured. Microvascular identification of the dorsal neurovascular bundles is performed and the dorsal arteries, vein, and nerves are reanastomosed. The dartos fascia is approximated and closed, followed by closure of the skin. Penrose drains may be placed as well as a suprapubic catheter.

ICD-10-CM Diagnostic Codes

❼ S38.221 Complete traumatic amputation of penis

ICD-10-CM Coding Notes

For codes requiring a 7th character extension, refer to your ICD-10-CM book. Review the character descriptions and coding guidelines for proper selection. For some procedures, only certain characters will apply.

CCI Edits

Refer to Appendix A for CCI edits.

Facility RVUs ▢

Code	Work	PE Facility	MP	Total Facility
54438	24.50	11.62	2.92	39.04

Non-facility RVUs ▢

Code	Work	PE Non-Facility	MP	Total Non-Facility
54438	24.50	11.62	2.92	39.04

Modifiers (PAR) ▢

Code	Mod 50	Mod 51	Mod 62	Mod 66	Mod 80
54438	0	2	1	0	2

Global Period

Code	Days
54438	090

54440

54440 Plastic operation of penis for injury

AMA Coding Notes

Repair Procedures on the Penis

(For other urethroplasties, see 53400-53430)

(For penile revascularization, use 37788)

Plain English Description

A plastic operation for penis injury called a phalloplasty is accomplished in stages. The first stage involves harvesting tissue from a donor site to create a neo-phallus with attachment of the neo-phallus to the genital area. The most common harvest site is a free transfer flap from the musculocutaneous latissimus dorsi (MLD). A skin incision is made and carried down to deep fascia to develop a plane between the latissimus dorsi and serratus cutaneous muscles. The flap is divided inferiorly and medially and then lifted to expose the neurovascular pedicle. After isolating a small strip of muscle to preserve the blood supply, dissection of the pedicle and subcutaneous fat continues proximally to the axillary vessels. The thoracodorsal nerve is identified and isolated, including the vascular blood supply for 3-4 cm proximally. Next, the neo-phallus is created while the graft is still attached to the blood supply of the vascular pedicle. The harvested flap is tubularized and a neo-glans is created by folding what will be the distal edge over and attaching it to the shaft. While the MLD is being harvested, a second surgical team is preparing the groin site. An inguinal skin incision is made and tissue gently dissected to locate and mobilize the superficial femoral artery, saphenous vein, and ilioinguinal nerve. A Y-incision is then made over the pubis and a tunnel created between the inguinal and Y incisions for the pedicle of the transfer graft. The neo-phallus is removed from the chest and transferred to the pubis. Using microsurgical technique, a lateral-to-terminal anastomosis is made between the subscapular and femoral arteries and a terminal-to-terminal anastomosis is made between the subscapular and saphenous veins. An epineural microneurorrhaphy is then completed between the ilioinguinal and thoracodorsal nerves. The next stage is a separately reportable urethroplasty, which may be combined with the first stage if a buccal mucosa graft is used or performed on its own after the neo-phallus has been implanted and is viable. The final stage is separately reportable penile prosthesis insertion. The penile implants are inserted 3-6 months after a successful urethroplasty has been accomplished.

Plastic repair of penis for injury

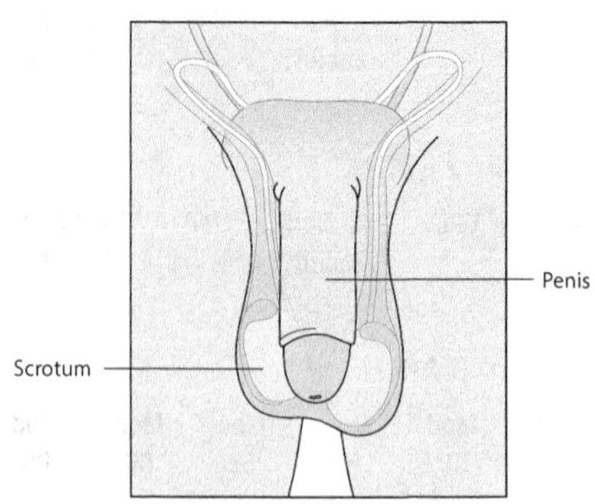

Injury of penis is repaired using one or more plastic surgery techniques.

ICD-10-CM Diagnostic Codes

- ❼ S31.21 Laceration without foreign body of penis
- ❼ S31.22 Laceration with foreign body of penis
- ❼ S31.23 Puncture wound without foreign body of penis
- ❼ S31.24 Puncture wound with foreign body of penis
- ❼ S31.25 Open bite of penis
- ❼ S38.01 Crushing injury of penis
- ❼ S38.222 Partial traumatic amputation of penis
- ❼ S39.840 Fracture of corpus cavernosum penis
- ❼ S39.848 Other specified injuries of external genitals

ICD-10-CM Coding Notes

For codes requiring a 7th character extension, refer to your ICD-10-CM book. Review the character descriptions and coding guidelines for proper selection. For some procedures, only certain characters will apply.

CCI Edits

Refer to Appendix A for CCI edits.

Facility RVUs ☐

Code	Work	PE Facility	MP	Total Facility
54440	0.00	0.00	0.00	0.00

Non-facility RVUs ☐

Code	Work	PE Non-Facility	MP	Total Non-Facility
54440	0.00	0.00	0.00	0.00

Modifiers (PAR) ☐

Code	Mod 50	Mod 51	Mod 62	Mod 66	Mod 80
54440	0	2	1	0	2

Global Period

Code	Days
54440	090

54450

54450 Foreskin manipulation including lysis of preputial adhesions and stretching

Plain English Description

This procedure may be performed for tight foreskin (phimosis) or adhesions in an uncircumcised male or adhesions between the remaining foreskin and glans pens in a circumcised male. In a circumscribed male, the remaining foreskin is manually manipulated by the physician to break up adhesions. In an uncircumcised male, the foreskin is pulled back to expose the glans penis and stretched, which also breaks up any adhesions.

Foreskin manipulation

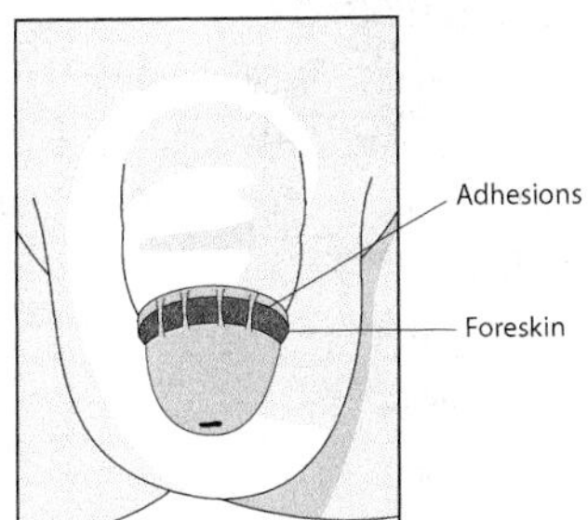

The foreskin is manually manipulated to break up adhesions.

ICD-10-CM Diagnostic Codes

N47.0	Adherent prepuce, newborn ♂
N47.1	Phimosis ♂
N47.2	Paraphimosis ♂
N47.3	Deficient foreskin ♂
N47.5	Adhesions of prepuce and glans penis ♂
N47.7	Other inflammatory diseases of prepuce ♂
N47.8	Other disorders of prepuce ♂

CCI Edits

Refer to Appendix A for CCI edits.

Facility RVUs ▯

Code	Work	PE Facility	MP	Total Facility
54450	1.12	0.41	0.12	1.65

Non-facility RVUs ▯

Code	Work	PE Non-Facility	MP	Total Non-Facility
54450	1.12	0.75	0.12	1.99

Modifiers (PAR) ▯

Code	Mod 50	Mod 51	Mod 62	Mod 66	Mod 80
54450	0	2	0	0	1

Global Period

Code	Days
54450	000

54500-54505

54500 Biopsy of testis, needle (separate procedure)

(For fine needle aspiration biopsy, see 10004, 10005, 10006, 10007, 10008, 10009, 10010, 10011, 10012, 10021)

(For evaluation of fine needle aspirate, see 88172, 88173)

54505 Biopsy of testis, incisional (separate procedure)

(For bilateral procedure, report 54505 with modifier 50)

(When combined with vasogram, seminal vesiculogram, or epididymogram, use 55300)

AMA Coding Notes

Excision Procedures on the Testis

(For abdominal perineal gangrene debridement, see 11004-11006)

AMA *CPT® Assistant* ☐

54505: Oct 01: 8

Plain English Description

A biopsy of the testis is performed. In 54500, a needle biopsy is performed. The skin over the planned puncture site is cleansed and a local anesthetic is administered as needed. A large bore needle is then inserted into the testis and a tissue sample obtained. In 54505, an incisional biopsy is performed. The skin is cleansed and a local anesthetic administered. If the biopsy is performed to evaluate a mass, the mass is exposed and a tissue sample obtained. The tissue sample is sent to the laboratory for separately reportable histological evaluation. If the biopsy is performed to evaluate the absence of living sperm in a semen sample (azoospermia), a sample of testis tissue is obtained. The tissue is placed in Bouin's fluid and sent to the infertility laboratory to determine whether sperm are present.

Biopsy of testis

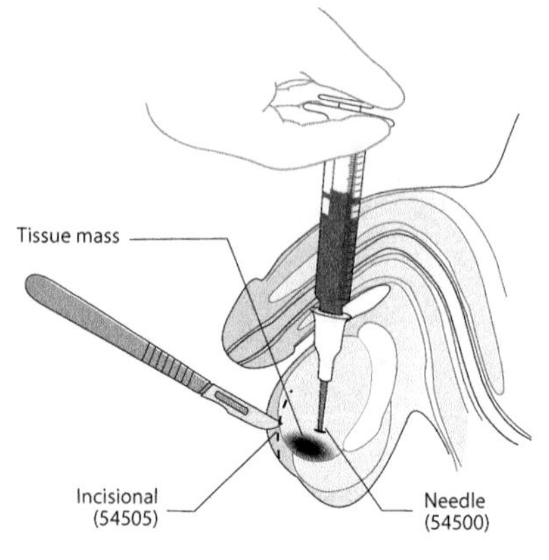

ICD-10-CM Diagnostic Codes

⇄	C62.01	Malignant neoplasm of undescended right testis ♂
⇄	C62.02	Malignant neoplasm of undescended left testis ♂
⇄	C62.11	Malignant neoplasm of descended right testis ♂
⇄	C62.12	Malignant neoplasm of descended left testis ♂
	C79.82	Secondary malignant neoplasm of genital organs
	D07.61	Carcinoma in situ of scrotum ♂
	D07.69	Carcinoma in situ of other male genital organs ♂
⇄	D29.21	Benign neoplasm of right testis ♂
⇄	D29.22	Benign neoplasm of left testis ♂
⇄	D40.11	Neoplasm of uncertain behavior of right testis ♂
⇄	D40.12	Neoplasm of uncertain behavior of left testis ♂
	D49.59	Neoplasm of unspecified behavior of other genitourinary organ
	E29.1	Testicular hypofunction ♂
	N44.1	Cyst of tunica albuginea testis ♂
	N44.2	Benign cyst of testis ♂
	N44.8	Other noninflammatory disorders of the testis ♂
	N46.01	Organic azoospermia ♂
	N46.021	Azoospermia due to drug therapy ♂
	N46.022	Azoospermia due to infection ♂
	N46.024	Azoospermia due to radiation ♂
	N46.025	Azoospermia due to systemic disease ♂
	N46.029	Azoospermia due to other extratesticular causes ♂
	N46.11	Organic oligospermia ♂
	N46.121	Oligospermia due to drug therapy ♂
	N46.122	Oligospermia due to infection ♂
	N46.124	Oligospermia due to radiation ♂
	N46.125	Oligospermia due to systemic disease ♂
	N46.129	Oligospermia due to other extratesticular causes ♂
	N46.8	Other male infertility ♂
	N50.0	Atrophy of testis ♂
	N50.3	Cyst of epididymis ♂
⇄	N50.811	Right testicular pain ♂
⇄	N50.812	Left testicular pain ♂
	N50.82	Scrotal pain ♂
	N50.89	Other specified disorders of the male genital organs ♂
	N53.12	Painful ejaculation ♂
	N53.8	Other male sexual dysfunction ♂
	Q53.111	Unilateral intraabdominal testis ♂
	Q53.112	Unilateral inguinal testis ♂
	Q53.13	Unilateral high scrotal testis ♂
	Q53.211	Bilateral intraabdominal testes ♂
	Q53.212	Bilateral inguinal testes ♂
	Q53.23	Bilateral high scrotal testes ♂
	R39.83	Unilateral non-palpable testicle ♂
	R39.84	Bilateral non-palpable testicles ♂

CCI Edits

Refer to Appendix A for CCI edits.

Facility RVUs ☐

Code	Work	PE Facility	MP	Total Facility
54500	1.31	0.69	0.17	2.17
54505	3.50	2.22	0.41	6.13

Non-facility RVUs ☐

Code	Work	PE Non-Facility	MP	Total Non-Facility
54500	1.31	0.69	0.17	2.17
54505	3.50	2.22	0.41	6.13

Modifiers (PAR) ☐

Code	Mod 50	Mod 51	Mod 62	Mod 66	Mod 80
54500	1	2	0	0	0
54505	1	2	0	0	0

Global Period

Code	Days
54500	000
54505	010

54512

54512 Excision of extraparenchymal lesion of testis

AMA Coding Notes

Excision Procedures on the Testis

(For abdominal perineal gangrene debridement, see 11004-11006)

AMA *CPT® Assistant*

54512: Oct 01: 8, Aug 05: 13

Plain English Description

An extraparenchymal lesion of the testis is excised. This type of lesion is located beneath the membranous covering (tunica vaginalis) of the testis and within the testicular capsule (tunica albuginea). Excision is performed for benign lesions such as fibroma, calcified pseudotumor, adenomatoid tumor, or testicular appendages. The scrotum is explored through a groin incision. The external oblique fascia is opened, taking care to protect the ilioinguinal nerve. The spermatic cord is mobilized and a tourniquet is placed around the cord. The testicle is delivered through the incision with the cord attached. The tunica vaginalis is incised and the testis and epididymis are inspected. The lesion is identified. Biopsies are obtained prior to excision and sent for separately reportable frozen section to confirm that the lesion is benign. The lesion is excised. The testis is replaced in the scrotal sac; the tourniquet around the cord is removed; the surgical wound irrigated; and the wound is closed.

Excision of extraparenchymal lesion of testis

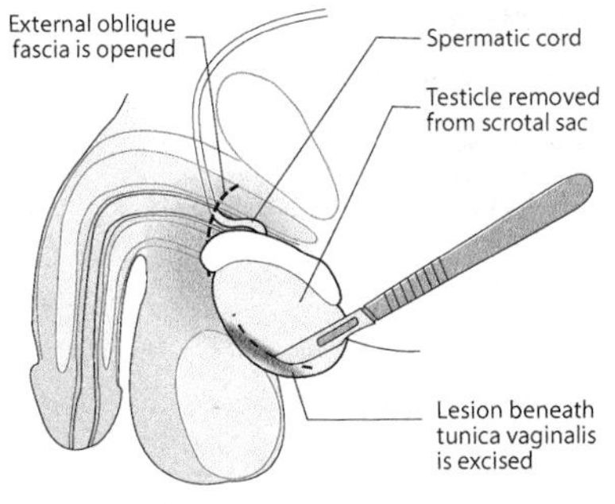
External oblique fascia is opened
Spermatic cord
Testicle removed from scrotal sac
Lesion beneath tunica vaginalis is excised

ICD-10-CM Diagnostic Codes

⇄	C62.01	Malignant neoplasm of undescended right testis ♂
⇄	C62.02	Malignant neoplasm of undescended left testis ♂
⇄	C62.11	Malignant neoplasm of descended right testis ♂
⇄	C62.12	Malignant neoplasm of descended left testis ♂
	C79.82	Secondary malignant neoplasm of genital organs
	D07.69	Carcinoma in situ of other male genital organs ♂
⇄	D29.21	Benign neoplasm of right testis ♂
⇄	D29.22	Benign neoplasm of left testis ♂
⇄	D40.10	Neoplasm of uncertain behavior of unspecified testis ♂
⇄	D40.11	Neoplasm of uncertain behavior of right testis ♂
⇄	D40.12	Neoplasm of uncertain behavior of left testis ♂
	N44.1	Cyst of tunica albuginea testis ♂
	N44.2	Benign cyst of testis ♂
	N44.8	Other noninflammatory disorders of the testis ♂
	N45.2	Orchitis ♂
	N45.3	Epididymo-orchitis ♂
	N49.1	Inflammatory disorders of spermatic cord, tunica vaginalis and vas deferens ♂
	N50.3	Cyst of epididymis ♂
	N50.89	Other specified disorders of the male genital organs ♂

CCI Edits

Refer to Appendix A for CCI edits.

Facility RVUs

Code	Work	PE Facility	MP	Total Facility
54512	9.33	5.29	1.12	15.74

Non-facility RVUs

Code	Work	PE Non-Facility	MP	Total Non-Facility
54512	9.33	5.29	1.12	15.74

Modifiers (PAR)

Code	Mod 50	Mod 51	Mod 62	Mod 66	Mod 80
54512	1	2	1	0	1

Global Period

Code	Days
54512	090

CPT® Procedural Coding

54520

54520 Orchiectomy, simple (including subcapsular), with or without testicular prosthesis, scrotal or inguinal approach

(For bilateral procedure, report 54520 with modifier 50)

AMA Coding Notes
Excision Procedures on the Testis

(For abdominal perineal gangrene debridement, see 11004-11006)

AMA *CPT® Assistant* ▢

54520: Winter 94: 13, Oct 01: 8, Mar 04: 3

Plain English Description

A simple orchiectomy or orchidectomy involves the removal of the testis. The surgical approach may be through the scrotum or inguinal area and testicular prosthesis may be implanted in the same operative session. In a scrotal approach, the skin incision is made at the median raphe and carried down through the subcutaneous tissue to the dartos fascia and cremasteric fibers to expose the tunica vaginalis. The gubernacular attachments are ligated and divided. The testis is removed through the scrotal incision. If an inguinal approach is used, a 4-6 cm skin incision is made superior to the pubic bone and parallel to the inguinal ligament on either the right or left side. The incision is carried down through the subcutaneous tissue to the aponeurosis of the external oblique muscle. Using a scalpel, an incision is made in the muscle between the internal and external rings following the direction of the fibers. The incision is widened preserving the ilioinguinal nerve and opening the inguinal canal to expose the spermatic cord. Using gentle pressure and traction on the spermatic cord, the testis is manipulated out of the scrotum through the open external inguinal ring and inguinal canal and delivered through the surgical wound to the operative field. If a gubernaculum is present at the inferior aspect of the testis, it is clamped, cut, and tied with absorbable suture. The surgical steps are the same at this point for scrotal and inguinal approach. The spermatic cord is clamped and divided above the epididymis, the vas deferens and vascular sections are ligated with sutures and then divided to facilitate removal of the testis. The scrotal structures are visually inspected, the wound is irrigated with saline solution, and hemostasis is achieved using electrocautery. A prosthetic testicular implant may be placed at this time into the empty scrotal sac. The hemiscrotum is closed. The surgical wound is closed in layers.

Orchiectomy, simple with/without testicular prosthesis, scrotal/inguinal approach

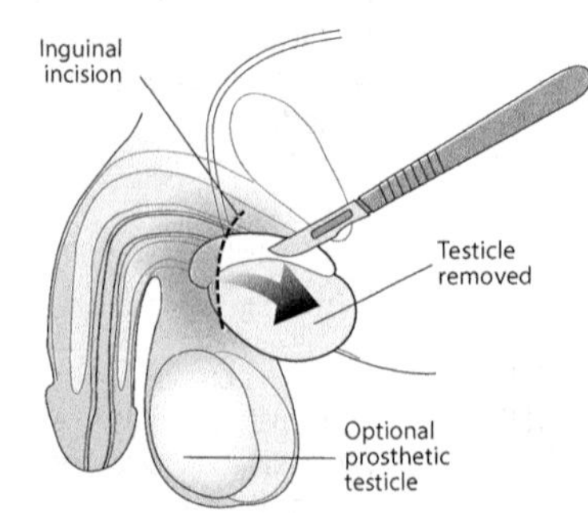

ICD-10-CM Diagnostic Codes

⇄	C62.01	Malignant neoplasm of undescended right testis ♂
⇄	C62.02	Malignant neoplasm of undescended left testis ♂
⇄	C62.11	Malignant neoplasm of descended right testis ♂
⇄	C62.12	Malignant neoplasm of descended left testis ♂
	C79.82	Secondary malignant neoplasm of genital organs
	D07.69	Carcinoma in situ of other male genital organs ♂
⇄	D29.21	Benign neoplasm of right testis ♂
⇄	D29.22	Benign neoplasm of left testis ♂
	N43.3	Hydrocele, unspecified ♂
	N44.01	Extravaginal torsion of spermatic cord ♂
	N44.02	Intravaginal torsion of spermatic cord ♂
	N44.03	Torsion of appendix testis ♂
	N44.04	Torsion of appendix epididymis ♂
	N45.2	Orchitis ♂
	N45.3	Epididymo-orchitis ♂
	N45.4	Abscess of epididymis or testis ♂
	N50.0	Atrophy of testis ♂
	Q53.111	Unilateral intraabdominal testis ♂
	Q53.112	Unilateral inguinal testis ♂
	Q53.13	Unilateral high scrotal testis ♂
	Q53.211	Bilateral intraabdominal testes ♂
	Q53.212	Bilateral inguinal testes ♂
	Q53.23	Bilateral high scrotal testes ♂
	Q55.22	Retractile testis ♂
	R39.83	Unilateral non-palpable testicle ♂
	R39.84	Bilateral non-palpable testicles ♂
❼	S31.31	Laceration without foreign body of scrotum and testes
❼	S31.32	Laceration with foreign body of scrotum and testes
❼	S31.33	Puncture wound without foreign body of scrotum and testes
❼	S31.34	Puncture wound with foreign body of scrotum and testes
❼	S31.35	Open bite of scrotum and testes
❼	S38.001	Crushing injury of unspecified external genital organs, male
❼	S38.02	Crushing injury of scrotum and testis
❼	S38.232	Partial traumatic amputation of scrotum and testis
	Z40.09	Encounter for prophylactic removal of other organ
	Z80.43	Family history of malignant neoplasm of testis

ICD-10-CM Coding Notes

For codes requiring a 7th character extension, refer to your ICD-10-CM book. Review the character descriptions and coding guidelines for proper selection. For some procedures, only certain characters will apply.

CCI Edits

Refer to Appendix A for CCI edits.

Pub 100

54520: Pub 100-03, 1, 230.3

Facility RVUs ▢

Code	Work	PE Facility	MP	Total Facility
54520	5.30	3.64	0.70	9.64

Non-facility RVUs ▢

Code	Work	PE Non-Facility	MP	Total Non-Facility
54520	5.30	3.64	0.70	9.64

Modifiers (PAR) ▢

Code	Mod 50	Mod 51	Mod 62	Mod 66	Mod 80
54520	1	2	0	0	1

Global Period

Code	Days
54520	090

54522

54522 Orchiectomy, partial

AMA Coding Notes

Excision Procedures on the Testis

(For abdominal perineal gangrene debridement, see 11004-11006)

AMA *CPT® Assistant*

54522: Oct 01: 8

Plain English Description

A partial orchiectomy is performed as a conservative intervention for benign intratesticular tumor or cyst, such as benign epidermoid cyst, hamartoma, or squamous epithelial cyst. Partial orchiectomy preserves the healthy testicular tissue. The scrotum is explored through a groin incision. The external oblique fascia is opened, taking care to protect the ilioinguinal nerve. The spermatic cord is mobilized and a tourniquet is placed around the cord. The testicle is delivered through the incision with the cord attached. The tunica vaginalis is incised and the testis and epididymis are inspected. The lesion is identified. Biopsies are obtained prior to excision and sent for separately reportable frozen section to confirm that the lesion is benign. The mass is carefully excised from the surrounding germinal testicular tissue. The testicular capsule (tunica albuginea) is closed. The testis is replaced in the scrotal sac; the tourniquet around the cord is removed; the surgical wound is irrigated; and the wound is closed.

Orchiectomy, partial

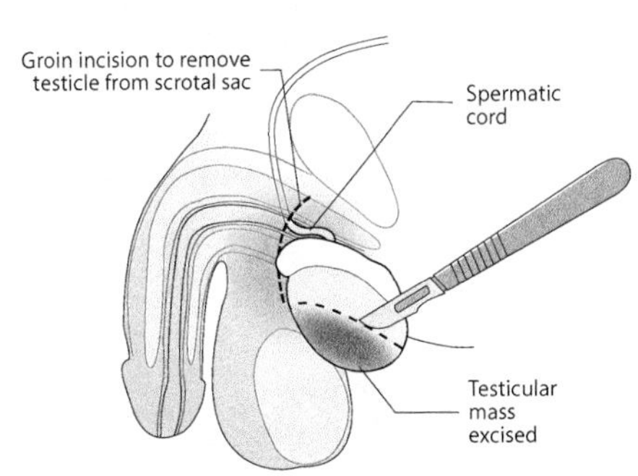

ICD-10-CM Diagnostic Codes

⇄	C62.01	Malignant neoplasm of undescended right testis ♂
⇄	C62.02	Malignant neoplasm of undescended left testis ♂
⇄	C62.11	Malignant neoplasm of descended right testis ♂
⇄	C62.12	Malignant neoplasm of descended left testis ♂
	C79.82	Secondary malignant neoplasm of genital organs
	N43.3	Hydrocele, unspecified ♂
	N44.01	Extravaginal torsion of spermatic cord ♂
	N44.02	Intravaginal torsion of spermatic cord ♂
	N44.03	Torsion of appendix testis ♂
	N44.04	Torsion of appendix epididymis ♂
	N44.1	Cyst of tunica albuginea testis ♂
	N44.2	Benign cyst of testis ♂
	N44.8	Other noninflammatory disorders of the testis ♂
	N45.1	Epididymitis ♂
	N45.3	Epididymo-orchitis ♂
	N45.4	Abscess of epididymis or testis ♂
	N50.0	Atrophy of testis ♂
	N50.1	Vascular disorders of male genital organs ♂
	N50.89	Other specified disorders of the male genital organs ♂
	Q53.111	Unilateral intraabdominal testis ♂
	Q53.112	Unilateral inguinal testis ♂
	Q53.13	Unilateral high scrotal testis ♂
	Q53.211	Bilateral intraabdominal testes ♂
	Q53.212	Bilateral inguinal testes ♂
	Q53.23	Bilateral high scrotal testes ♂
	Q55.22	Retractile testis ♂
	R39.83	Unilateral non-palpable testicle ♂
	R39.84	Bilateral non-palpable testicles ♂
❼	S31.31	Laceration without foreign body of scrotum and testes
❼	S31.32	Laceration with foreign body of scrotum and testes
❼	S31.33	Puncture wound without foreign body of scrotum and testes
❼	S31.34	Puncture wound with foreign body of scrotum and testes
❼	S31.35	Open bite of scrotum and testes
❼	S38.001	Crushing injury of unspecified external genital organs, male
❼	S38.02	Crushing injury of scrotum and testis
❼	S38.231	Complete traumatic amputation of scrotum and testis
❼	S38.232	Partial traumatic amputation of scrotum and testis
	Z85.47	Personal history of malignant neoplasm of testis ♂

ICD-10-CM Coding Notes

For codes requiring a 7th character extension, refer to your ICD-10-CM book. Review the character descriptions and coding guidelines for proper selection. For some procedures, only certain characters will apply.

CCI Edits

Refer to Appendix A for CCI edits.

Pub 100

54522: Pub 100-03, 1, 230.3

Facility RVUs

Code	Work	PE Facility	MP	Total Facility
54522	10.25	5.76	1.21	17.22

Non-facility RVUs

Code	Work	PE Non-Facility	MP	Total Non-Facility
54522	10.25	5.76	1.21	17.22

Modifiers (PAR)

Code	Mod 50	Mod 51	Mod 62	Mod 66	Mod 80
54522	1	2	1	0	2

Global Period

Code	Days
54522	090

CPT® Procedural Coding

54530-54535

54530 Orchiectomy, radical, for tumor; inguinal approach

54535 Orchiectomy, radical, for tumor; with abdominal exploration

(For orchiectomy with repair of hernia, see 49505 or 49507 and 54520)

(For radical retroperitoneal lymphadenectomy, use 38780)

AMA Coding Notes

Excision Procedures on the Testis

(For abdominal perineal gangrene debridement, see 11004-11006)

AMA *CPT® Assistant*

54530: Oct 01: 8

54535: Oct 01: 8

Plain English Description

Radical orchiectomy or orchidectomy for known or suspected testicular tumor is performed through an inguinal incision. In 54530, a 4-6 cm skin incision is made superior to the pubic bone and parallel to the inguinal ligament on the side correlating to the tumor. The incision is carried down through the subcutaneous tissue to the aponeurosis of the external oblique muscle. An incision is made in the muscle between the internal and external rings following the direction of the fibers. The incision is widened preserving the ilioinguinal nerve and opening the inguinal canal to expose the spermatic cord. The spermatic cord is bluntly dissected from the floor of the inguinal canal along its length to the pubic tubercle. A drain is then wrapped tightly around the spermatic cord and secured forming a tourniquet. With pressure and gentle traction on the spermatic cord, the testis is manipulated out of the scrotum through the open external inguinal ring and inguinal canal and delivered through the surgical wound to the operative field. If a gubernaculum is present at the inferior aspect of the testis, it is clamped, cut, and tied with absorbable suture. The vas deferens and vascular section of spermatic cord are then clamped, ligated, and divided as close to the inguinal ring as possible. A long silk or polypropylene suture is placed through the stump of the spermatic cord as a marker should later retroperitoneal lymph node dissection be necessary. Hemostasis is achieved using electrocautery and the wound irrigated. Closure begins at the inguinal floor, reinforcing with interrupted sutures if the area appears weak. Next, the ilioinguinal nerve is released and the external oblique muscle is closed with sutures beginning at the internal ring and terminating at the pubic tubercle. The wound may be irrigated again and the skin is then closed with skin sutures, staples, or clips. In 54535, following excision of the testis as described above, the abdomen is also explored. The incision is then extended cephalad and the peritoneum opened and explored for tumor. A separately reportable radical lymphadenectomy is performed as needed. Hemostasis is achieved using electrocautery and the wound irrigated. The peritoneum is closed with absorbable suture.

Orchiectomy, radical, for tumor

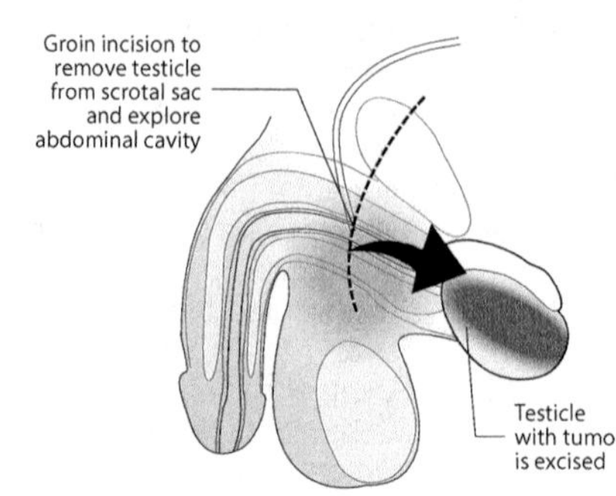

Inguinal approach (54530); with abdominal exploration (54535)

ICD-10-CM Diagnostic Codes

	C61	Malignant neoplasm of prostate ♂
⇄	C62.01	Malignant neoplasm of undescended right testis ♂
⇄	C62.02	Malignant neoplasm of undescended left testis ♂
⇄	C62.11	Malignant neoplasm of descended right testis ♂
⇄	C62.12	Malignant neoplasm of descended left testis ♂
	C79.82	Secondary malignant neoplasm of genital organs
	D07.69	Carcinoma in situ of other male genital organs ♂
⇄	D29.21	Benign neoplasm of right testis ♂
⇄	D29.22	Benign neoplasm of left testis ♂
⇄	D40.11	Neoplasm of uncertain behavior of right testis ♂
⇄	D40.12	Neoplasm of uncertain behavior of left testis ♂

CCI Edits

Refer to Appendix A for CCI edits.

Pub 100

54530: Pub 100-03, 1, 230.3

54535: Pub 100-03, 1, 230.3

Facility RVUs

Code	Work	PE Facility	MP	Total Facility
54530	8.46	5.41	1.04	14.91
54535	13.19	7.03	1.55	21.77

Non-facility RVUs

Code	Work	PE Non-Facility	MP	Total Non-Facility
54530	8.46	5.41	1.04	14.91
54535	13.19	7.03	1.55	21.77

Modifiers (PAR)

Code	Mod 50	Mod 51	Mod 62	Mod 66	Mod 80
54530	1	2	1	0	2
54535	1	2	0	0	2

Global Period

Code	Days
54530	090
54535	090

54550-54560

54550 Exploration for undescended testis (inguinal or scrotal area)

(For bilateral procedure, report 54550 with modifier 50)

54560 Exploration for undescended testis with abdominal exploration

(For bilateral procedure, report 54560 with modifier 50)

AMA *CPT® Assistant* ▯

54550: Oct 01: 8, Mar 17: 10
54560: Oct 01: 8

Plain English Description

Undescended testicle or cryptorchism occurs when one or both testes fail to descend into the scrotum before birth. Testes that have not descended by age 1 are typically treated surgically. The inguinal or scrotal area is explored for the undescended testis. Using an inguinal approach, the skin incision is made superior to the pubic bone and parallel to the inguinal ligament on either the right or left side. The incision is carried down through the subcutaneous tissue to the aponeurosis of the external oblique muscle. Using a scalpel, an incision is made in the muscle between the internal and external rings following the direction of the fibers. The incision is widened preserving the ilioinguinal nerve and opening the inguinal canal. If a spermatic cord is present, it is elevated and freed from the cremaster muscle with careful dissection and the undescended testis is repositioned in the scrotum. If spermatic cord structures and/or testicular remnants are present, they are removed and the surgery terminated at this point. If no cord structures or testicle can be identified, dissection moves to inside the internal ring, and if the results are still negative for cord structure or testis, an abdominal exploration may be performed. Abdominal exploration is performed through an incision in the lower abdomen. The abdominal muscles are separated and the peritoneum is entered and explored for spermatic cord and/or testis. If only remnants of spermatic cord structures and/or testis are present, they are removed and the surgery terminated at this point, closing the surgical incision in layers. If spermatic structures and testis are present, the spermatic vessels are dissected free from attachments and a broad flap shaped from the peritoneum with attachment to the vas deferens is brought down through a newly created external ring lateral to the pubic tubercle. The length of the spermatic cord is assessed, and if there is sufficient length, the testis is brought down into the scrotum. If there is not sufficient length or blood supply is compromised, a staged procedure may be required. Use 54550 for an inguinal or scrotal exploration. Use 54560 when abdominal exploration is required in addition to or instead of the inguinal or scrotal exploration.

ICD-10-CM Diagnostic Codes

Q53.00	Ectopic testis, unspecified ♂
Q53.01	Ectopic testis, unilateral ♂
Q53.02	Ectopic testes, bilateral ♂
Q53.111	Unilateral intraabdominal testis ♂
Q53.112	Unilateral inguinal testis ♂
Q53.12	Ectopic perineal testis, unilateral ♂
Q53.13	Unilateral high scrotal testis ♂
Q53.211	Bilateral intraabdominal testes ♂
Q53.212	Bilateral inguinal testes ♂
Q53.22	Ectopic perineal testis, bilateral ♂
Q53.23	Bilateral high scrotal testes ♂
Q55.0	Absence and aplasia of testis ♂
Q55.22	Retractile testis ♂
Q55.23	Scrotal transposition ♂
R39.83	Unilateral non-palpable testicle ♂
R39.84	Bilateral non-palpable testicles ♂

CCI Edits

Refer to Appendix A for CCI edits.

Facility RVUs ▯

Code	Work	PE Facility	MP	Total Facility
54550	8.41	5.00	1.00	14.41
54560	12.10	6.60	1.42	20.12

Non-facility RVUs ▯

Code	Work	PE Non-Facility	MP	Total Non-Facility
54550	8.41	5.00	1.00	14.41
54560	12.10	6.60	1.42	20.12

Modifiers (PAR) ▯

Code	Mod 50	Mod 51	Mod 62	Mod 66	Mod 80
54550	1	2	0	0	2
54560	1	2	1	0	2

Global Period

Code	Days
54550	090
54560	090

54600-54620

54600 Reduction of torsion of testis, surgical, with or without fixation of contralateral testis

54620 Fixation of contralateral testis (separate procedure)

AMA *CPT® Assistant*

54600: Aug 05: 13

Plain English Description

Testicular torsion is a condition in which the spermatic cord that is attached to the testicle becomes twisted, cutting off the blood supply to the testicle. The testis may be approached through single vertical midline incision in the scrotum, two separate hemiscrotal incisions, or a transverse incision. The incision is down to the dartos muscle. The testis is identified and the layers of the tunica albuginea are gently opened to expose the testis. The testis is inspected and gently manipulated to relieve the torsion. The testis may then be wrapped in warm moist gauze to recover while exploration of the contralateral testis is made. If the contralateral testis is normal, it may be fixed in place by everting the tunica vaginalis creating contact between the tunica albuginea and the dartos muscle and placing the testis in an extravaginal position. Two to three sutures are used to attach the peritesticular tissue to the dartos muscle anchoring the testis in place. The wrapped testis is then reexamined for viability. A dusty rose or pink color signifies adequate blood perfusion and the testis is fixed in the same manner as for the contralateral testis. The dartos layer is closed with sutures followed by closure of the skin. Use 54600 for reduction of torsion of testis with or without fixation of contralateral testis. Use 54620 for fixation of contralateral testis only, when performed as a separate procedure.

Reduction of torsion of testis, surgical, with/without fixation (contralateral)

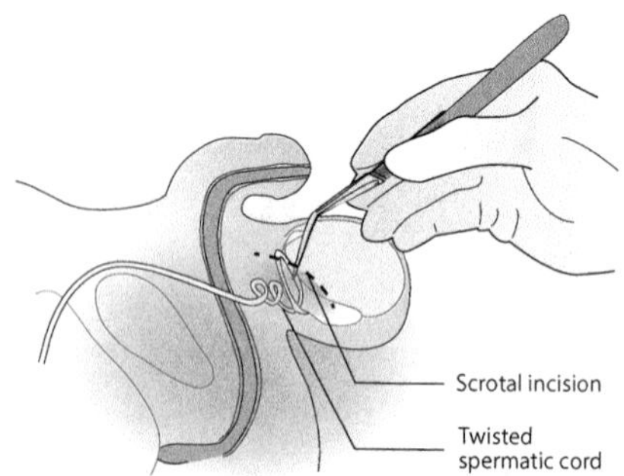

ICD-10-CM Diagnostic Codes

N44.00	Torsion of testis, unspecified ♂
N44.01	Extravaginal torsion of spermatic cord ♂
N44.02	Intravaginal torsion of spermatic cord ♂
N44.03	Torsion of appendix testis ♂
N44.04	Torsion of appendix epididymis ♂
N50.89	Other specified disorders of the male genital organs ♂

CCI Edits

Refer to Appendix A for CCI edits.

Facility RVUs

Code	Work	PE Facility	MP	Total Facility
54600	7.64	4.73	0.90	13.27
54620	5.21	2.91	0.61	8.73

Non-facility RVUs

Code	Work	PE Non-Facility	MP	Total Non-Facility
54600	7.64	4.73	0.90	13.27
54620	5.21	2.91	0.61	8.73

Modifiers (PAR)

Code	Mod 50	Mod 51	Mod 62	Mod 66	Mod 80
54600	1	2	0	0	1
54620	1	2	0	0	1

Global Period

Code	Days
54600	090
54620	010

54640

54640 Orchiopexy, inguinal or scrotal approach

(For bilateral procedure, report 54640 with modifier 50)

(For inguinal hernia repair performed in conjunction with inguinal orchiopexy, see 49495-49525)

AMA *CPT® Assistant*

54640: Oct 01: 8, Jan 04: 27, Mar 04: 10, Jun 08: 4, Mar 17: 11

Plain English Description

Orchiopexy is performed to reposition an undescended testis in the scrotum. A transverse inguinal incision is made in the skin and then carried down through the subcutaneous tissue to the external oblique aponeurosis. The inguinal canal is opened and the ilioinguinal nerve is identified and isolated. The spermatic cord and testicle are identified. If a fibrous cord called a gubernaculum is present, it is divided at the proximal end using a hemostat to allow for manipulation of the spermatic cord. Once the spermatic cord is free, it is elevated and blunt dissection continues off the anterior cremaster muscle fibers to the internal ring. If a hernia sac is present, it is dissected from the spermatic fascia and the cord structures are separated from the hernia sac. The sac can then be transected and dissected up to the internal inguinal ring where is it ligated with sutures. The testis and spermatic cord along with the distal hernia sac, if present, are delivered out of the inguinal incision. The hernia sac may be repositioned with absorbable suture behind the spermatic cord or testis to prevent formation of a hydrocele. A tunnel is made from the groin to the scrotum. A second transverse incision is made in the scrotum on the same side as the inguinal incision and a pouch is created by dissecting the scrotal skin from the underlying dartos muscle. A suture can be placed through the testicle and used to deliver the testis through the tunnel, or a clamp can be passed from the scrotum to the inguinal incision grasping the testis and pulling it through to the dartos pouch. The spermatic cord is carefully examined for torsion. To prevent the testis from migrating back to the inguinal area, the inlet to the pouch may be narrowed to a diameter smaller than the testis by placing a non-suture through the dartos muscle and incorporating the parietal tunica vaginalis in the stitch. Alternatively, the testis may be sutured to the scrotal septum to anchor it in the new location. The scrotal incision is closed. If a hernia sac was present, the transversalis fascia may require approximation to close the internal inguinal ring followed by closure of the external oblique aponeurosis and subcutaneous tissue and finally the skin edges.

Orchiopexy, inguinal approach

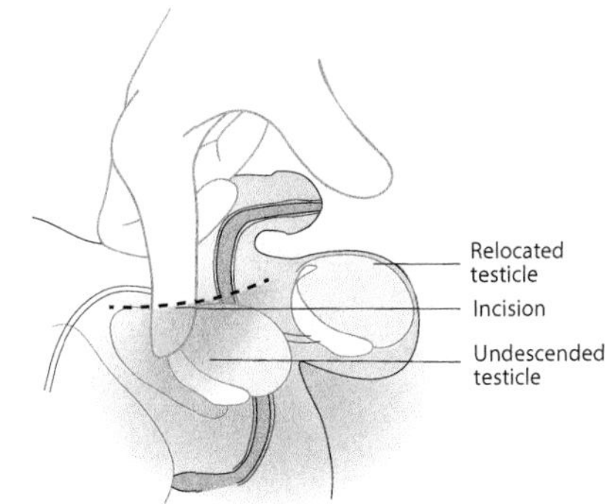

ICD-10-CM Diagnostic Codes

N44.0	Torsion of testis
N44.04	Torsion of appendix epididymis ♂
N44.1	Cyst of tunica albuginea testis ♂
N44.2	Benign cyst of testis ♂
Q53.01	Ectopic testis, unilateral ♂
Q53.02	Ectopic testes, bilateral ♂
Q53.112	Unilateral inguinal testis ♂
Q53.12	Ectopic perineal testis, unilateral ♂
Q53.13	Unilateral high scrotal testis ♂
Q53.212	Bilateral inguinal testes ♂
Q53.22	Ectopic perineal testis, bilateral ♂
Q53.23	Bilateral high scrotal testes ♂
Q55.20	Unspecified congenital malformations of testis and scrotum ♂
Q55.22	Retractile testis ♂
R39.83	Unilateral non-palpable testicle ♂
R39.84	Bilateral non-palpable testicles ♂

CCI Edits

Refer to Appendix A for CCI edits.

Facility RVUs

Code	Work	PE Facility	MP	Total Facility
54640	7.73	3.95	1.00	12.68

Non-facility RVUs

Code	Work	PE Non-Facility	MP	Total Non-Facility
54640	7.73	3.95	1.00	12.68

Modifiers (PAR)

Code	Mod 50	Mod 51	Mod 62	Mod 66	Mod 80
54640	1	2	0	0	0

Global Period

Code	Days
54640	090

54650

54650 Orchiopexy, abdominal approach, for intra-abdominal testis (eg, Fowler-Stephens)

(For laparoscopic approach, use 54692)

AMA *CPT® Assistant* ◻

54650: Nov 99: 26, May 00: 4, Oct 01: 8

Plain English Description

An orchiopexy performed through an open abdominal incision may be accomplished in a single-stage or a two-stage Fowler-Stephens technique. A midline skin incision is made from the pubis to just below the umbilicus, carried down through the rectus muscle, and the peritoneum opened. The intestines are moved aside to visualize the peritoneal cavity and the testis and spermatic cord located and inspected. The spermatic vessels are dissected free and vascular clips applied. The peritoneum is excised around the internal inguinal ring and the gubernaculum is transected distally leaving some testicular tissue attached. Grasping the freed gubernaculum, the peritoneum is incised laterally and medially over the spermatic vessels with the incisions joined proximally. Dissection continues until adequate length is obtained in the spermatic cord to allow mobilization of the testis to the scrotum. In a single-stage procedure, the spermatic vessels are divided between the previously applied vascular clips and the peritoneum incised lateral to the distal vessels with extension distally to the internal inguinal ring, superiorly to the vas deferens, and medially to the bladder. A skin incision is made in the scrotum on the same side as the testis. A pouch is developed in the dartos tissue and a neo-inguinal ring created using a clamp or forceps to open a tunnel from the dartos pouch, over the pubic tubercle, and through the peritoneum. The forceps are used to grasp the testis and gently mobilize it through the tunnel to the scrotum. The spermatic cord is inspected for tension or torsion. To prevent the testis from migrating back to the abdomen, it may be anchored to the scrotal septum with sutures. The scrotal incision is closed. The abdominal incision is checked for bleeding and hemostasis obtained with electrocautery. The intestines are moved back to their original position in the abdominal cavity. The incision is closed in layers. If a two-stage procedure is performed, the incision is closed following mobilization of the testis. The testes are given approximately 6 months to develop collateral vascular circulation from the cremasteric and vasal arteries. The abdomen is then reopened and the testis mobilized to the scrotum as described above.

Orchiopexy, abdominal approach, for intra-abdominal testis

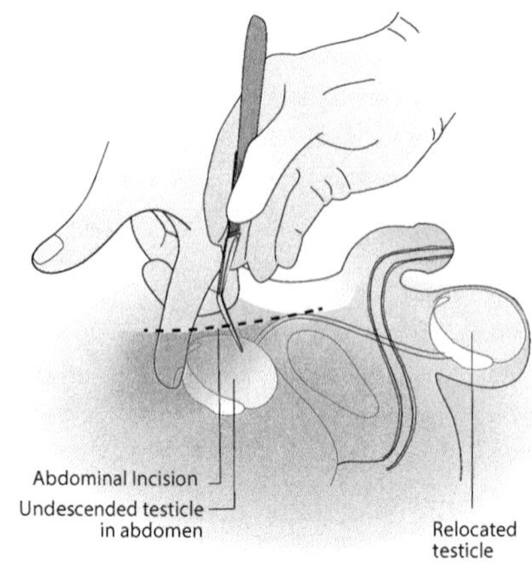

ICD-10-CM Diagnostic Codes

Q53.01	Ectopic testis, unilateral ♂
Q53.02	Ectopic testes, bilateral ♂
Q53.111	Unilateral intraabdominal testis ♂
Q53.211	Bilateral intraabdominal testes ♂
R39.83	Unilateral non-palpable testicle ♂
R39.84	Bilateral non-palpable testicles ♂

CCI Edits

Refer to Appendix A for CCI edits.

Facility RVUs ◻

Code	Work	PE Facility	MP	Total Facility
54650	12.39	6.99	1.47	20.85

Non-facility RVUs ◻

Code	Work	PE Non-Facility	MP	Total Non-Facility
54650	12.39	6.99	1.47	20.85

Modifiers (PAR) ◻

Code	Mod 50	Mod 51	Mod 62	Mod 66	Mod 80
54650	1	2	0	0	2

Global Period

Code	Days
54650	090

54660

54660 Insertion of testicular prosthesis (separate procedure)

(For bilateral procedure, report 54660 with modifier 50)

AMA *CPT® Assistant* □

54660: Oct 01: 8

Plain English Description

Insertion of a testicular prosthesis in a procedure separate from removal of testis can be accomplished through either an inguinal or a suprascrotal incision. Using an inguinal approach, the skin is incised over and carried down to the oblique muscle. The muscle is incised and the surgeon's finger used to probe and locate the scrotal neck and previous tunnel. Forceps are then used to dissect adhesions along the tunnel to the scrotum. The wound is irrigated and the prosthesis inserted through the incision. Using pressure on the outside skin, the prosthesis is gently manipulated through the tunnel into the scrotal space. Alternatively, Hegar dilators of increasing size may be used to expand the tunnel to the scrotum. Once the correct size dilator has been passed into the scrotum, an identical Hegar is placed on the outside of the scrotum and pushed up to invaginate the base of the scrotum through the inguinal incision. The prosthesis is placed into the invaginated scrotum, anchored with a suture, and manipulated back through the incision and tunnel to its original position. The wound is checked for bleeding and the incision closed in layers. Using a suprascrotal approach, the skin incision is made above the scrotum lateral to the penis and blunt dissection is used to form a pouch in the intrascrotal space. The prosthesis is inserted through the incision into the space and the incision is closed with absorbable suture.

Insertion of testicular prosthesis (separate procedure)

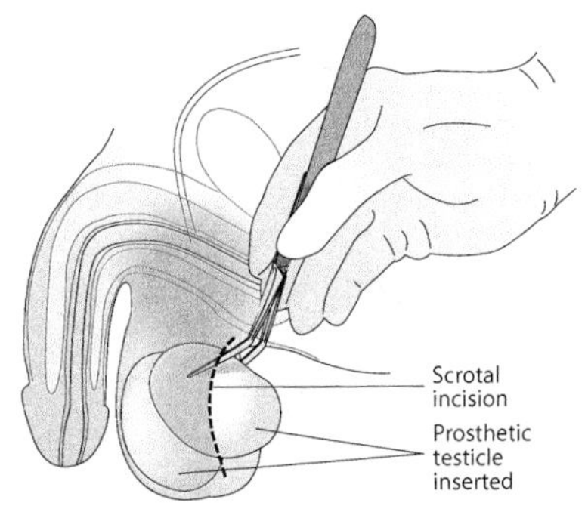

ICD-10-CM Diagnostic Codes

⇄	C62.01	Malignant neoplasm of undescended right testis ♂
⇄	C62.02	Malignant neoplasm of undescended left testis ♂
⇄	C62.11	Malignant neoplasm of descended right testis ♂
⇄	C62.12	Malignant neoplasm of descended left testis ♂
⇄	D29.21	Benign neoplasm of right testis ♂
⇄	D29.22	Benign neoplasm of left testis ♂
	E29.1	Testicular hypofunction ♂
	N50.0	Atrophy of testis ♂
	Q53.01	Ectopic testis, unilateral ♂
	Q53.02	Ectopic testes, bilateral ♂
	Q53.111	Unilateral intraabdominal testis ♂
	Q53.112	Unilateral inguinal testis ♂
	Q53.12	Ectopic perineal testis, unilateral ♂
	Q53.13	Unilateral high scrotal testis ♂
	Q53.211	Bilateral intraabdominal testes ♂
	Q53.212	Bilateral inguinal testes ♂
	Q53.22	Ectopic perineal testis, bilateral ♂
	Q53.23	Bilateral high scrotal testes ♂
	Q55.0	Absence and aplasia of testis ♂
	Q55.1	Hypoplasia of testis and scrotum ♂
	Q55.20	Unspecified congenital malformations of testis and scrotum ♂
	Q55.22	Retractile testis ♂
	Q55.29	Other congenital malformations of testis and scrotum ♂
	Q55.9	Congenital malformation of male genital organ, unspecified ♂
	R39.83	Unilateral non-palpable testicle ♂
	R39.84	Bilateral non-palpable testicles ♂
	Z85.47	Personal history of malignant neoplasm of testis ♂

CCI Edits

Refer to Appendix A for CCI edits.

Facility RVUs □

Code	Work	PE Facility	MP	Total Facility
54660	5.74	4.09	0.68	10.51

Non-facility RVUs □

Code	Work	PE Non-Facility	MP	Total Non-Facility
54660	5.74	4.09	0.68	10.51

Modifiers (PAR) □

Code	Mod 50	Mod 51	Mod 62	Mod 66	Mod 80
54660	1	2	0	0	0

Global Period

Code	Days
54660	090

54670

54670 Suture or repair of testicular injury

AMA *CPT® Assistant*

54670: Oct 01: 8

Plain English Description

If the injury is closed, the scrotum is incised. The tunica vaginalis is opened and the testis is exposed. If there is an open wound to the testis, the wound is explored and enlarged as needed to allow evaluation of the injury. The testis, spermatic cord, and tunica vaginalis are irrigated. Any foreign bodies are removed. The spermatic cord and testis are inspected for evidence of injury. If vascular injury is suspected, the tunica albuginea is incised and the blood flow to the testis evaluated. If the injury has resulted in extrusion of testicular contents, the contaminated seminiferous tubules are removed using sharp dissection and debridement. Following evaluation and repair of the testicular injury, the tunica albuginea is closed. The tunica vaginalis may be closed or left open and a drain placed. If the tunica vaginalis is closed, the scrotal fascia and skin are also closed.

Suture/repair of testicular injury

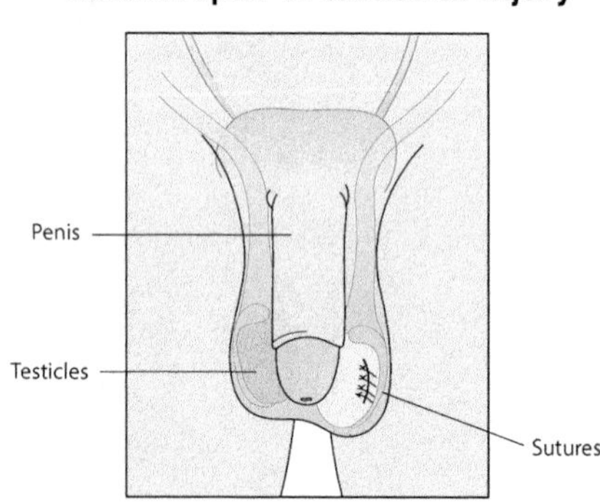

Sutures are placed after the wound is inspected for foreign matter/vascular injury/displacement.

ICD-10-CM Diagnostic Codes

❼	S31.31	Laceration without foreign body of scrotum and testes
❼	S31.32	Laceration with foreign body of scrotum and testes
❼	S31.33	Puncture wound without foreign body of scrotum and testes
❼	S31.34	Puncture wound with foreign body of scrotum and testes
❼	S31.35	Open bite of scrotum and testes
❼	S31.541	Puncture wound with foreign body of unspecified external genital organs, male
❼	S38.02	Crushing injury of scrotum and testis
❼	S38.231	Complete traumatic amputation of scrotum and testis
❼	S38.232	Partial traumatic amputation of scrotum and testis

ICD-10-CM Coding Notes

For codes requiring a 7th character extension, refer to your ICD-10-CM book. Review the character descriptions and coding guidelines for proper selection. For some procedures, only certain characters will apply.

CCI Edits

Refer to Appendix A for CCI edits.

Facility RVUs

Code	Work	PE Facility	MP	Total Facility
54670	6.65	4.57	0.78	12.00

Non-facility RVUs

Code	Work	PE Non-Facility	MP	Total Non-Facility
54670	6.65	4.57	0.78	12.00

Modifiers (PAR)

Code	Mod 50	Mod 51	Mod 62	Mod 66	Mod 80
54670	1	2	0	0	0

Global Period

Code	Days
54670	090

54680

54680 Transplantation of testis(es) to thigh (because of scrotal destruction)

AMA *CPT® Assistant*

54680: Oct 01: 8

Plain English Description

One or both testes can be preserved after scrotal destruction by surgical transplantation to the thigh. Small skin incisions are made in the thigh at the level of the scrotum. The skin is elevated with blunt dissection and a superficial subcutaneous pouch created. The dissection is extended to create a tunnel to the perineum to allow the spermatic cord to descend into the pouch without traction or torsion. The testis is gently manipulated through the tunnel to the subcutaneous pouch in the thigh and secured with absorbable suture. The skin incision in the thigh is closed. The procedure is repeated on the contralateral side as needed. The scrotal injury may be treated in a separately reportable procedure.

Transplantation of testis(es) to thigh (because of scrotal destruction)

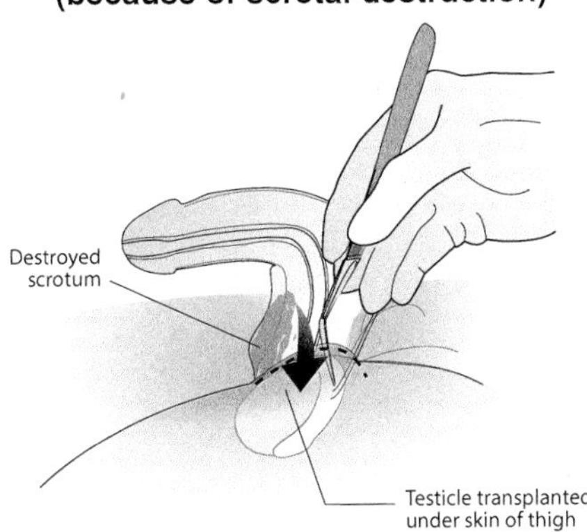

ICD-10-CM Diagnostic Codes

	C63.2	Malignant neoplasm of scrotum ♂
	C79.82	Secondary malignant neoplasm of genital organs
	D07.61	Carcinoma in situ of scrotum ♂
	D07.69	Carcinoma in situ of other male genital organs ♂
	L02.214	Cutaneous abscess of groin
	L02.215	Cutaneous abscess of perineum
	L03.314	Cellulitis of groin
	L03.315	Cellulitis of perineum
	L98.495	Non-pressure chronic ulcer of skin of other sites with muscle involvement without evidence of necrosis
	L98.496	Non-pressure chronic ulcer of skin of other sites with bone involvement without evidence of necrosis
➐	S31.31	Laceration without foreign body of scrotum and testes
➐	S31.32	Laceration with foreign body of scrotum and testes
➐	S31.33	Puncture wound without foreign body of scrotum and testes
➐	S31.34	Puncture wound with foreign body of scrotum and testes
➐	S31.35	Open bite of scrotum and testes
➐	S38.02	Crushing injury of scrotum and testis
➐	S38.232	Partial traumatic amputation of scrotum and testis
➐	S39.848	Other specified injuries of external genitals
➐	T21.36	Burn of third degree of male genital region
➐	T21.76	Corrosion of third degree of male genital region

ICD-10-CM Coding Notes

For codes requiring a 7th character extension, refer to your ICD-10-CM book. Review the character descriptions and coding guidelines for proper selection. For some procedures, only certain characters will apply.

CCI Edits

Refer to Appendix A for CCI edits.

Facility RVUs

Code	Work	PE Facility	MP	Total Facility
54680	14.04	7.34	1.68	23.06

Non-facility RVUs

Code	Work	PE Non-Facility	MP	Total Non-Facility
54680	14.04	7.34	1.68	23.06

Modifiers (PAR)

Code	Mod 50	Mod 51	Mod 62	Mod 66	Mod 80
54680	1	2	1	0	2

Global Period

Code	Days
54680	090

54690

54690 Laparoscopy, surgical; orchiectomy

AMA Coding Guideline

Laparoscopic Procedures on the Testis

Surgical laparoscopy always includes diagnostic laparoscopy. To report a diagnostic laparoscopy (peritoneoscopy) (separate procedure), use 49320.

AMA *CPT® Assistant* ▢

54690: Nov 99: 26, Mar 00: 5, Oct 01: 8

Plain English Description

Laparoscopic orchiectomy is performed with the patient in supine, Trendelenburg position. A Foley catheter is placed transurethrally. A small U-shaped skin incision is made at the umbilicus, and a clamp used to dissect down to the anterior rectus fascia, which is then opened a few millimeters to allow a Veress needle to be introduced into the peritoneal cavity. A pneumoperitoneum is created with insufflation of CO2. Using upward traction on the abdominal wall, the laparoscope is inserted through the umbilical incision and trocars placed into the abdomen along the mid-clavicular line. Abdominal organs are identified and inspected. The testis is grasped and dissected free from surrounding tissue, spermatic cord including the spermatic vessels and vas deferens are clipped and cut, and the testis is sealed and removed from the abdominal cavity through the ports. The laparoscopic instruments are withdrawn and CO2 removed from the cavity. The fascia is closed with suture followed by closure of the skin.

Laparoscopy, surgical; orchiectomy

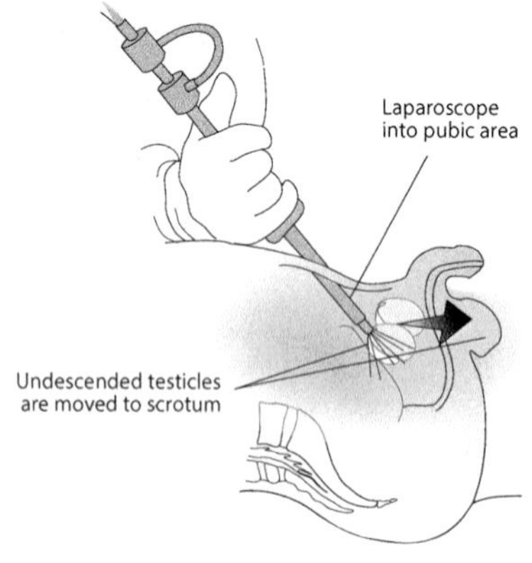

ICD-10-CM Diagnostic Codes

⇄ C62.01 Malignant neoplasm of undescended right testis ♂
⇄ C62.02 Malignant neoplasm of undescended left testis ♂
⇄ C62.11 Malignant neoplasm of descended right testis ♂
⇄ C62.12 Malignant neoplasm of descended left testis ♂
⇄ C62.91 Malignant neoplasm of right testis, unspecified whether descended or undescended ♂
⇄ C62.92 Malignant neoplasm of left testis, unspecified whether descended or undescended ♂
C79.82 Secondary malignant neoplasm of genital organs
D07.69 Carcinoma in situ of other male genital organs ♂
⇄ D29.21 Benign neoplasm of right testis ♂
⇄ D29.22 Benign neoplasm of left testis ♂
⇄ D40.11 Neoplasm of uncertain behavior of right testis ♂
⇄ D40.12 Neoplasm of uncertain behavior of left testis ♂
D49.59 Neoplasm of unspecified behavior of other genitourinary organ
N44.8 Other noninflammatory disorders of the testis ♂
N50.89 Other specified disorders of the male genital organs ♂
Q53.01 Ectopic testis, unilateral ♂
Q53.02 Ectopic testes, bilateral ♂
Q53.111 Unilateral intraabdominal testis ♂
Q53.112 Unilateral inguinal testis ♂
Q53.13 Unilateral high scrotal testis ♂
Q53.211 Bilateral intraabdominal testes ♂
Q53.212 Bilateral inguinal testes ♂
Q53.22 Ectopic perineal testis, bilateral ♂
Q53.23 Bilateral high scrotal testes ♂
R39.83 Unilateral non-palpable testicle ♂
R39.84 Bilateral non-palpable testicles ♂
➐ S31.31 Laceration without foreign body of scrotum and testes
➐ S31.32 Laceration with foreign body of scrotum and testes
➐ S31.33 Puncture wound without foreign body of scrotum and testes
➐ S31.34 Puncture wound with foreign body of scrotum and testes
➐ S31.35 Open bite of scrotum and testes
➐ S38.02 Crushing injury of scrotum and testis
➐ S38.232 Partial traumatic amputation of scrotum and testis
Z40.09 Encounter for prophylactic removal of other organ

ICD-10-CM Coding Notes

For codes requiring a 7th character extension, refer to your ICD-10-CM book. Review the character descriptions and coding guidelines for proper selection. For some procedures, only certain characters will apply.

CCI Edits

Refer to Appendix A for CCI edits.

Pub 100

54690: Pub 100-03, 1, 230.3

Facility RVUs ▢

Code	Work	PE Facility	MP	Total Facility
54690	11.70	6.10	1.40	19.20

Non-facility RVUs ▢

Code	Work	PE Non-Facility	MP	Total Non-Facility
54690	11.70	6.10	1.40	19.20

Modifiers (PAR) ▢

Code	Mod 50	Mod 51	Mod 62	Mod 66	Mod 80
54690	1	2	1	0	2

Global Period

Code	Days
54690	090

54692

54692 Laparoscopy, surgical; orchiopexy for intra-abdominal testis

AMA Coding Guideline

Laparoscopic Procedures on the Testis

Surgical laparoscopy always includes diagnostic laparoscopy. To report a diagnostic laparoscopy (peritoneoscopy) (separate procedure), use 49320.

AMA *CPT® Assistant* □

54692: Nov 99: 27, May 00: 4, Oct 01: 8

Plain English Description

Laparoscopic orchiopexy is performed with the patient in supine, Trendelenburg position. A Foley catheter is placed transurethrally. A small U-shaped skin incision is made at the umbilicus, and a clamp is used to dissect down to the anterior rectus fascia, which is then opened a few millimeters to allow a Veress needle to be introduced into the peritoneal cavity. A pneumoperitoneum is created with insufflation of CO2. With upward traction on the abdominal wall, the laparoscope is inserted through the umbilical incision and trocars are placed into the abdomen along the mid-clavicular line. Abdominal organs are identified and inspected. To free the testis and spermatic cord, dissection begins lateral to the structures at the gubernaculum near the internal inguinal ring. After dividing the gubernaculum, the peritoneum is incised and elevated off the spermatic vessels. The spermatic vessels are mobilized. The testis is grasped and stretched toward the contralateral inguinal ring to evaluate length. If necessary, additional mobility is achieved by incising a triangular section of peritoneum between the spermatic vessels and the vas deferens. Once adequate length of the spermatic cord has been obtained, a small transverse incision is made in the hemiscrotum ipsilateral to the testis and a subdartos pouch created by dissecting the scrotal skin from the underlying dartos muscle. A trocar is introduced through the scrotal incision and manipulated through the external inguinal ring lateral to the bladder and into the abdomen. The testis is grasped and delivered to the subdartos pouch where it is sutured to the scrotal septum anchoring it in the new location. The scrotal incision is closed. The laparoscopic instruments are withdrawn and CO2 removed from the cavity. The fascia is closed followed by closure of the skin.

Laparoscopy, surgical; orchiopexy for intra-abdominal testis

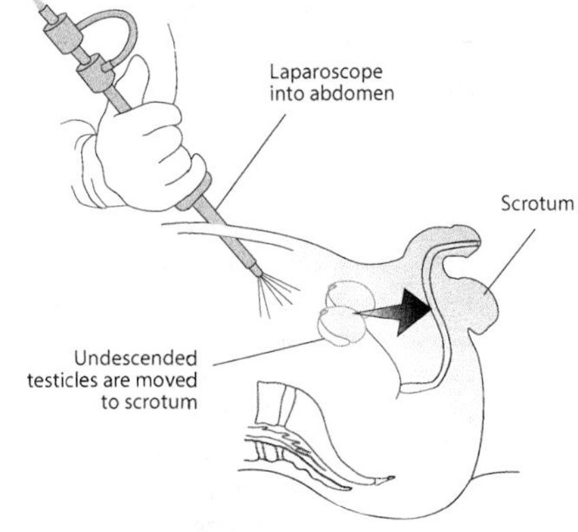

ICD-10-CM Diagnostic Codes

Q53.01	Ectopic testis, unilateral ♂
Q53.02	Ectopic testes, bilateral ♂
Q53.111	Unilateral intraabdominal testis ♂
Q53.211	Bilateral intraabdominal testes ♂
R39.83	Unilateral non-palpable testicle ♂
R39.84	Bilateral non-palpable testicles ♂

CCI Edits

Refer to Appendix A for CCI edits.

Facility RVUs □

Code	Work	PE Facility	MP	Total Facility
54692	13.74	6.74	1.64	22.12

Non-facility RVUs □

Code	Work	PE Non-Facility	MP	Total Non-Facility
54692	13.74	6.74	1.64	22.12

Modifiers (PAR) □

Code	Mod 50	Mod 51	Mod 62	Mod 66	Mod 80
54692	1	2	0	0	1

Global Period

Code	Days
54692	090

CPT® Procedural Coding

54700

54700 Incision and drainage of epididymis, testis and/or scrotal space (eg, abscess or hematoma)

(For debridement of necrotizing soft tissue infection of external genitalia, see 11004-11006)

AMA *CPT® Assistant* □

54700: Oct 01: 8

Plain English Description

The scrotum is examined and the location of the fluid collection determined. The scrotum is incised. If the abscess or hematoma is located in the scrotal space, the abscess pocket or hematoma is located and opened. If there is an abscess pocket, any loculations are broken up using blunt dissection and the pus drained. The abscess cavity is irrigated with sterile saline or antibiotic solution. If there is a hematoma, any blood clots are removed. If the abscess or hematoma is in the testis, the tunica vaginalis is opened and the abscess or hematoma drained as described above. If the abscess involves the epididymis, the epididymis is exposed and the abscess or hematoma drained. The incisions may be left open and packed with gauze or a drain placed. Alternatively, the incision may be closed.

Incision and drainage of epididymis, testis and/or scrotal space (eg, abscess or hematoma)

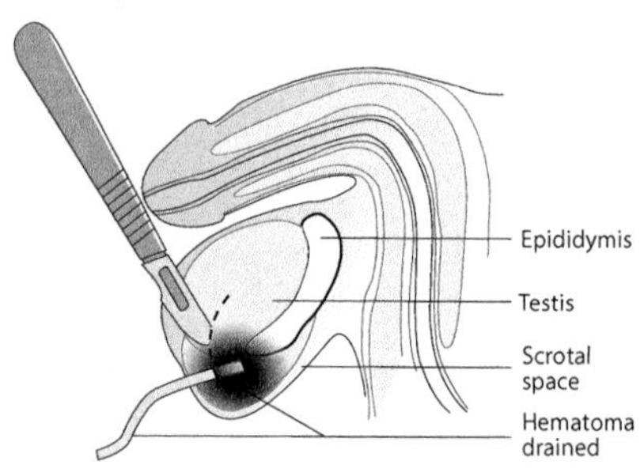

ICD-10-CM Diagnostic Codes

A54.23	Gonococcal infection of other male genital organs ♂
L02.214	Cutaneous abscess of groin
L02.215	Cutaneous abscess of perineum
L03.314	Cellulitis of groin
L03.315	Cellulitis of perineum
N45	Orchitis and epididymitis
N45.4	Abscess of epididymis or testis ♂
N49.1	Inflammatory disorders of spermatic cord, tunica vaginalis and vas deferens ♂
N49.2	Inflammatory disorders of scrotum ♂
N49.8	Inflammatory disorders of other specified male genital organs ♂
N99.820	Postprocedural hemorrhage of a genitourinary system organ or structure following a genitourinary system procedure
N99.821	Postprocedural hemorrhage of a genitourinary system organ or structure following other procedure
R36.1	Hematospermia ♂
R39.83	Unilateral non-palpable testicle ♂
R39.84	Bilateral non-palpable testicles ♂
❼ S30.21	Contusion of penis
❼ S30.22	Contusion of scrotum and testes
❼ T81.43	Infection following a procedure, organ and space surgical site

ICD-10-CM Coding Notes

For codes requiring a 7th character extension, refer to your ICD-10-CM book. Review the character descriptions and coding guidelines for proper selection. For some procedures, only certain characters will apply.

CCI Edits

Refer to Appendix A for CCI edits.

Facility RVUs □

Code	Work	PE Facility	MP	Total Facility
54700	3.47	2.33	0.45	6.25

Non-facility RVUs □

Code	Work	PE Non-Facility	MP	Total Non-Facility
54700	3.47	2.33	0.45	6.25

Modifiers (PAR) □

Code	Mod 50	Mod 51	Mod 62	Mod 66	Mod 80
54700	1	2	0	0	1

Global Period

Code	Days
54700	010

54800

54800 Biopsy of epididymis, needle

(For fine needle aspiration biopsy, see 10004, 10005, 10006, 10007, 10008, 10009, 10010, 10011, 10012, 10021)

(For evaluation of fine needle aspirate, see 88172, 88173)

AMA *CPT® Assistant* ☐

54800: Oct 01: 8

Plain English Description

A needle biopsy of the epididymis is performed under local anesthetic with the patient positioned supine and the scrotum prepared and draped. The testis is palpated in the scrotal sac and the epididymis located and stabilized between the surgeon's index finger and thumb. The scrotal skin is stretched tightly and a small skin incision made with the point of a scalpel. A spring-loaded needle is fired through the incision into the epididymal tissue to obtain tissue samples. The tissue samples are then prepared and examined by a pathologist in a separately reportable procedure to determine if cancer or other abnormal cells are present.

Biopsy of epididymis, needle

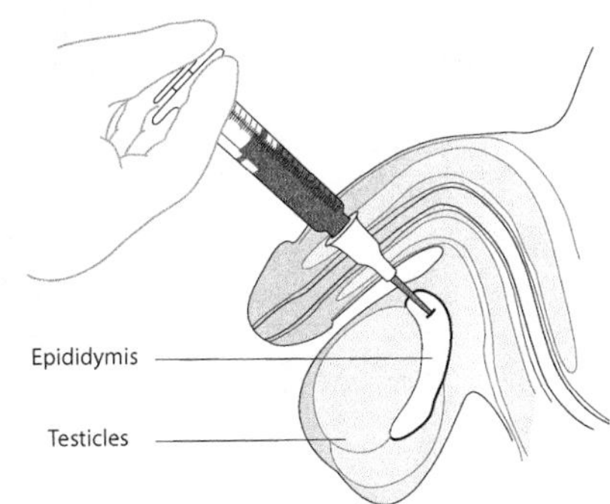

ICD-10-CM Diagnostic Codes

	A54.23	Gonococcal infection of other male genital organs ♂
⇄	C63.01	Malignant neoplasm of right epididymis ♂
⇄	C63.02	Malignant neoplasm of left epididymis ♂
	C79.82	Secondary malignant neoplasm of genital organs
	D07.69	Carcinoma in situ of other male genital organs ♂
⇄	D29.31	Benign neoplasm of right epididymis ♂
⇄	D29.32	Benign neoplasm of left epididymis ♂
	D40.8	Neoplasm of uncertain behavior of other specified male genital organs ♂
	D49.59	Neoplasm of unspecified behavior of other genitourinary organ
	N43.41	Spermatocele of epididymis, single ♂
	N43.42	Spermatocele of epididymis, multiple ♂
	N45.1	Epididymitis ♂
	N45.2	Orchitis ♂
	N45.3	Epididymo-orchitis ♂
	N45.4	Abscess of epididymis or testis ♂
	N50.3	Cyst of epididymis ♂
	N50.89	Other specified disorders of the male genital organs ♂
	N51	Disorders of male genital organs in diseases classified elsewhere ♂
	Z85.48	Personal history of malignant neoplasm of epididymis ♂

CCI Edits

Refer to Appendix A for CCI edits.

Facility RVUs ☐

Code	Work	PE Facility	MP	Total Facility
54800	2.33	1.04	0.27	3.64

Non-facility RVUs ☐

Code	Work	PE Non-Facility	MP	Total Non-Facility
54800	2.33	1.04	0.27	3.64

Modifiers (PAR) ☐

Code	Mod 50	Mod 51	Mod 62	Mod 66	Mod 80
54800	1	2	0	0	0

Global Period

Code	Days
54800	000

54830

54830 Excision of local lesion of epididymis

AMA *CPT® Assistant* ▢

54830: Oct 01: 8

Plain English Description

To excise a local lesion from the epididymis, the patient is positioned supine and the scrotum prepared and draped. The surgical approach may be through a vertical median raphe or a transverse hemiscrotal incision, which is then carried down to the tunica vaginalis. The testis and epididymis are brought out of the dartos fascia using blunt dissection or alternatively brought out through a completely incised tunica vaginalis. The lesion is then excised from the epididymal tissue. Bleeding is controlled with electrocautery. Tissue samples are prepared and examined by a pathologist in a separately reportable procedure to determine if cancer or other abnormal cells are present. If the lesion was large, the tunica vaginalis may be suture plicated in a radial fashion. The testis is returned to the scrotum and the tunica vaginalis or dartos layer closed followed by closure of the skin.

Excision of local lesion of epididymis

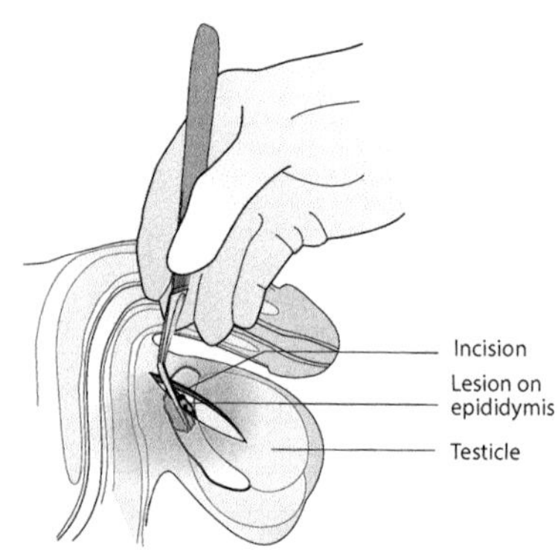

ICD-10-CM Diagnostic Codes

⇄	C63.01	Malignant neoplasm of right epididymis ♂
⇄	C63.02	Malignant neoplasm of left epididymis ♂
	C79.82	Secondary malignant neoplasm of genital organs
	D07.69	Carcinoma in situ of other male genital organs ♂
	D17.72	Benign lipomatous neoplasm of other genitourinary organ
⇄	D29.31	Benign neoplasm of right epididymis ♂
⇄	D29.32	Benign neoplasm of left epididymis ♂
	D40.8	Neoplasm of uncertain behavior of other specified male genital organs ♂
	D49.59	Neoplasm of unspecified behavior of other genitourinary organ
	N50.3	Cyst of epididymis ♂
	N50.89	Other specified disorders of the male genital organs ♂

CCI Edits

Refer to Appendix A for CCI edits.

Facility RVUs ▢

Code	Work	PE Facility	MP	Total Facility
54830	6.01	4.20	0.73	10.94

Non-facility RVUs ▢

Code	Work	PE Non-Facility	MP	Total Non-Facility
54830	6.01	4.20	0.73	10.94

Modifiers (PAR) ▢

Code	Mod 50	Mod 51	Mod 62	Mod 66	Mod 80
54830	1	2	0	0	0

Global Period

Code	Days
54830	090

54840

54840 Excision of spermatocele, with or without epididymectomy

AMA *CPT® Assistant*

54840: Oct 01: 8

Plain English Description

Excision of a spermatocele, with or without epididymectomy, is accomplished with the patient positioned supine and the scrotum prepared and draped. The surgical approach may be through a vertical median raphe or a transverse hemiscrotal incision, which is then carried down to the tunica vaginalis. The testis with epididymis are brought out of the dartos fascia using blunt dissection or alternatively brought out through a completely incised tunica vaginalis. Using sharp and blunt dissection, the spermatocele is isolated from the epididymis and the area explored for the connecting neck of the spermatocele to the epididymis. If located, the neck is suture ligated and divided. If the connecting neck cannot be located or the spermatocele is multiloculated, a partial epididymectomy is performed by excising a plane of normal epididymal tissue adjacent to the spermatocele. Bleeding in the epididymal bed is controlled by electrocautery. If the spermatocele was large in size, the tunica vaginalis may be suture plicated in a radial fashion. The testis is returned to the scrotum. The tunica vaginalis or dartos layer is closed followed by closure of the skin.

Excision of spermatocele, with or without epididymectomy

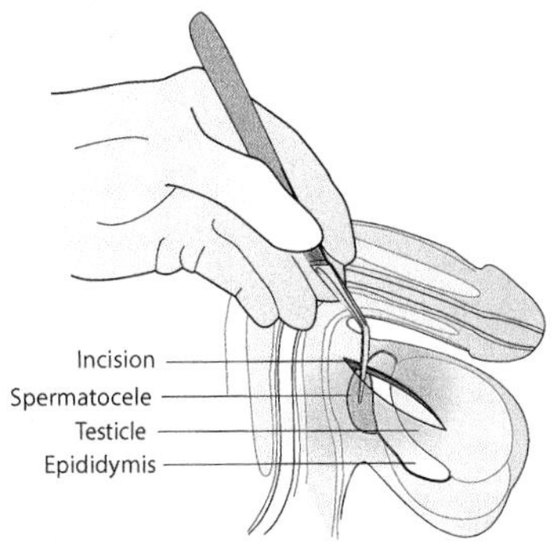

ICD-10-CM Diagnostic Codes

N43.41	Spermatocele of epididymis, single ♂
N43.42	Spermatocele of epididymis, multiple ♂

CCI Edits

Refer to Appendix A for CCI edits.

Facility RVUs

Code	Work	PE Facility	MP	Total Facility
54840	5.27	3.57	0.62	9.46

Non-facility RVUs

Code	Work	PE Non-Facility	MP	Total Non-Facility
54840	5.27	3.57	0.62	9.46

Modifiers (PAR)

Code	Mod 50	Mod 51	Mod 62	Mod 66	Mod 80
54840	1	2	0	0	1

Global Period

Code	Days
54840	090

54860-54861

54860 Epididymectomy; unilateral
54861 Epididymectomy; bilateral

Plain English Description

Epididymectomy is performed with the patient positioned supine and the penis and scrotum prepared and draped. A transverse incision is made in the skin of the hemiscrotum and carried down to the tunica vaginalis. Using sharp and blunt dissection in a plane between the tunica vaginalis and dartos fascia, the testis, epididymis and vas deferens are freed and delivered to the operative field. If a vasectomy was previously performed, dissection of the epididymis, and vas deferens continues to a level above the vasectomy site.
In the absence of a vasectomy, the vas deferens may be divided and ligated with absorbable suture at the junction of convoluted and straight vas deferens. After dividing the vas deferens, dissection continues to the vaso-epididymal junction creating a plane between the epididymis and testis. The epididymis is then grasped and lifted off the testis as the surgeon continues to dissect in an inferior to superior line, ligating the epididymal artery if encountered. When dissection reaches the testicular efferent ducts, they are ligated with absorbable suture or cauterized and the entire specimen is removed intact. The surgical site is irrigated and bleeding in the epididymal bed is controlled with electrocautery or fine absorbable sutures. The testis is then returned to the scrotal sac and the edges of the tunica vaginalis closed followed by layered closure of the dartos fascia and skin. Use 54860 for a unilateral epididymectomy. Use 54861 if the procedure is performed bilaterally.

Epididymectomy

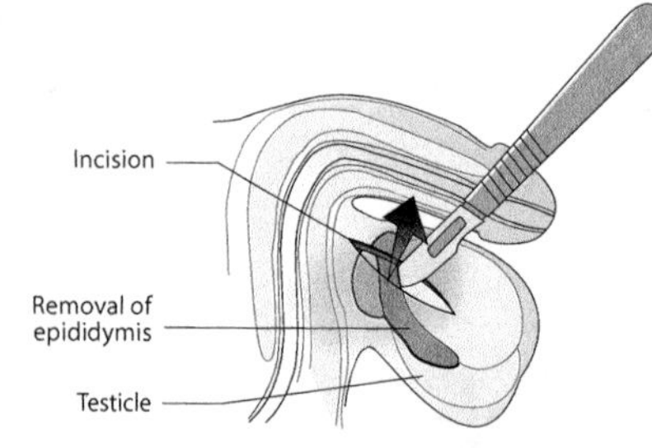

Unilateral (54860); bilateral (54861)

ICD-10-CM Diagnostic Codes

⇄	C63.01	Malignant neoplasm of right epididymis ♂
⇄	C63.02	Malignant neoplasm of left epididymis ♂
	C79.82	Secondary malignant neoplasm of genital organs
	D07.69	Carcinoma in situ of other male genital organs ♂
⇄	D29.31	Benign neoplasm of right epididymis ♂
⇄	D29.32	Benign neoplasm of left epididymis ♂
	D40.8	Neoplasm of uncertain behavior of other specified male genital organs ♂
	N44.04	Torsion of appendix epididymis ♂
	N44.2	Benign cyst of testis ♂
	N44.8	Other noninflammatory disorders of the testis ♂
	N45	Orchitis and epididymitis
	N45.1	Epididymitis ♂
	N45.4	Abscess of epididymis or testis ♂
	N50.3	Cyst of epididymis ♂
	N50.89	Other specified disorders of the male genital organs ♂
	N51	Disorders of male genital organs in diseases classified elsewhere ♂

CCI Edits

Refer to Appendix A for CCI edits.

Facility RVUs ▢

Code	Work	PE Facility	MP	Total Facility
54860	6.95	4.51	0.84	12.30
54861	9.70	5.81	1.16	16.67

Non-facility RVUs ▢

Code	Work	PE Non-Facility	MP	Total Non-Facility
54860	6.95	4.51	0.84	12.30
54861	9.70	5.81	1.16	16.67

Modifiers (PAR) ▢

Code	Mod 50	Mod 51	Mod 62	Mod 66	Mod 80
54860	0	2	0	0	1
54861	0	2	0	0	0

Global Period

Code	Days
54860	090
54861	090

54865

54865 Exploration of epididymis, with or without biopsy

Plain English Description

Epididymal exploration, with or without biopsy, is performed in cases of infertility in which the patient is suspected of having an obstructed epididymis with azoospermia. Exploration is performed through a midline scrotal incision. The testis is delivered from the scrotal sac and the tunica vaginalis is opened to access the epididymis. The operating microscope is used to examine the epididymis under magnification. An obstructed epididymis will have a characteristic appearance as the tail end will have dilated tubules of a yellowish color due to the presence of macrophages that phagocytize sperm remnants of degenerating and necrotic sperm, which has been blocked in its passage. The epididymal tunic may be punctured or opened to access the tubules and biopsies may be taken. Puncture sites or tunic incisions are closed, the tunica vaginalis is closed in a watertight way to avoid inflammation and later adhesions, the testicle is then returned to its position, and the incision is closed with sutures.

Exploration of epididymis, with or without biopsy

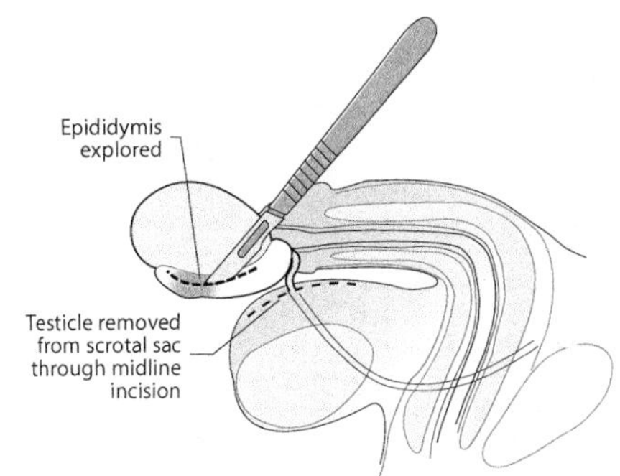

ICD-10-CM Diagnostic Codes

⇄	C63.01	Malignant neoplasm of right epididymis ♂
⇄	C63.02	Malignant neoplasm of left epididymis ♂
	C79.82	Secondary malignant neoplasm of genital organs
	D07.69	Carcinoma in situ of other male genital organs ♂
	D17.72	Benign lipomatous neoplasm of other genitourinary organ
⇄	D29.31	Benign neoplasm of right epididymis ♂
⇄	D29.32	Benign neoplasm of left epididymis ♂
	D40.8	Neoplasm of uncertain behavior of other specified male genital organs ♂
	D49.59	Neoplasm of unspecified behavior of other genitourinary organ
	N45.1	Epididymitis ♂
	N45.2	Orchitis ♂
	N45.3	Epididymo-orchitis ♂
	N45.4	Abscess of epididymis or testis ♂
	N46.02	Azoospermia due to extratesticular causes
	N46.023	Azoospermia due to obstruction of efferent ducts ♂
	N51	Disorders of male genital organs in diseases classified elsewhere ♂

CCI Edits

Refer to Appendix A for CCI edits.

Facility RVUs

Code	Work	PE Facility	MP	Total Facility
54865	5.77	4.10	0.68	10.55

Non-facility RVUs

Code	Work	PE Non-Facility	MP	Total Non-Facility
54865	5.77	4.10	0.68	10.55

Modifiers (PAR)

Code	Mod 50	Mod 51	Mod 62	Mod 66	Mod 80
54865	0	2	0	0	0

Global Period

Code	Days
54865	090

54900-54901

54900 Epididymovasostomy, anastomosis of epididymis to vas deferens; unilateral

54901 Epididymovasostomy, anastomosis of epididymis to vas deferens; bilateral

(For operating microscope, use 69990)

AMA *CPT® Assistant*

54900: Nov 98: 16, Jun 04: 11
54901: Nov 98: 16, Jun 04: 11

Plain English Description

The physician bypasses a blockage between the small organ that sits next to the testicle and stores sperm and the tube that carries sperm to the penis. The organ is reconnected to the tube at a different point, bypassing the blockage. Code 54900 if this procedure is only performed on one of the two sperm-storing organs. Code 54901 if this procedure is performing on both of the sperm-storing organs.

Epididymovasostomy, anastomosis of epididymis to vas deferens

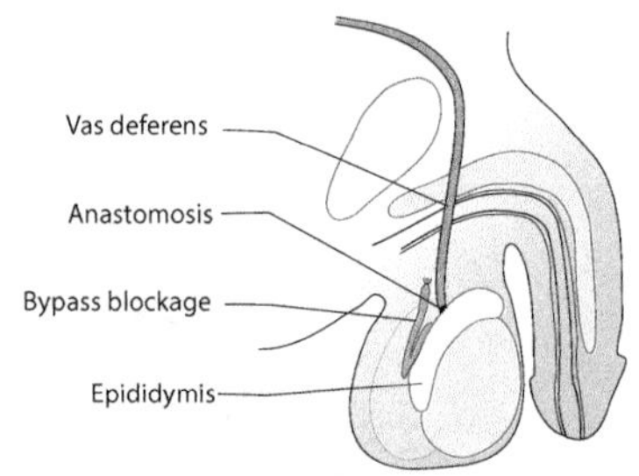

Unilateral (54900); bilateral (54901)

ICD-10-CM Diagnostic Codes

N46.023	Azoospermia due to obstruction of efferent ducts ♂
N46.029	Azoospermia due to other extratesticular causes ♂
N46.123	Oligospermia due to obstruction of efferent ducts ♂
Z31.0	Encounter for reversal of previous sterilization

CCI Edits

Refer to Appendix A for CCI edits.

Facility RVUs

Code	Work	PE Facility	MP	Total Facility
54900	14.20	7.54	1.69	23.43
54901	19.10	9.57	2.27	30.94

Non-facility RVUs

Code	Work	PE Non-Facility	MP	Total Non-Facility
54900	14.20	7.54	1.69	23.43
54901	19.10	9.57	2.27	30.94

Modifiers (PAR)

Code	Mod 50	Mod 51	Mod 62	Mod 66	Mod 80
54900	0	2	0	0	0
54901	2	2	0	0	0

Global Period

Code	Days
54900	090
54901	090

55000

55000 Puncture aspiration of hydrocele, tunica vaginalis, with or without injection of medication

Plain English Description

The tunica vaginalis is the serous sheath covering the testis and epididymis that consists of an outer parietal and inner visceral layer. A hydrocele is a collection of fluid between the parietal and visceral layers. The skin over the hydrocele is disinfected and a local anesthetic administered as needed. The skin is then punctured and the needle advanced into the fluid collection, which is aspirated. Following aspiration, a sclerosing medication may be injected to help prevent recurrence of the hydrocele.

Puncture aspiration of hydrocele, tunica vaginalis

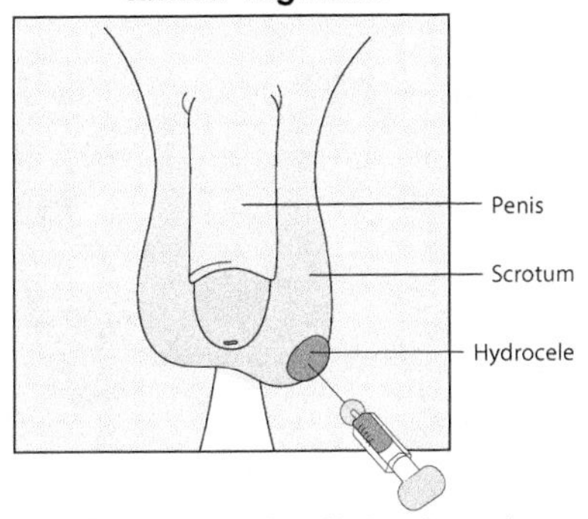

The physician drains a fluid-filled sac located on the membrane that surrounds the testicles.

ICD-10-CM Diagnostic Codes

N43.0	Encysted hydrocele ♂
N43.1	Infected hydrocele ♂
N43.2	Other hydrocele ♂
N50.89	Other specified disorders of the male genital organs ♂
P83.5	Congenital hydrocele ♂

CCI Edits

Refer to Appendix A for CCI edits.

Facility RVUs ☐

Code	Work	PE Facility	MP	Total Facility
55000	1.43	0.85	0.19	2.47

Non-facility RVUs ☐

Code	Work	PE Non-Facility	MP	Total Non-Facility
55000	1.43	1.96	0.19	3.58

Modifiers (PAR) ☐

Code	Mod 50	Mod 51	Mod 62	Mod 66	Mod 80
55000	1	2	0	0	1

Global Period

Code	Days
55000	000

55040-55041

55040 Excision of hydrocele; unilateral
55041 Excision of hydrocele; bilateral
(With hernia repair, see 49495-49501)

AMA *CPT® Assistant* ▯
55040: Jun 08: 4, Nov 17: 10

Plain English Description
The physician excises a hydrocele, also referred to as hydrocelectomy. The tunica vaginalis is the serous sheath covering the testis and epididymis that consists of an outer parietal and inner visceral layer. A hydrocele is a collection of fluid between the parietal and visceral layers. The scrotum is examined and the location of the fluid collection determined. An incision is made in the groin for children or in the scrotum for adults. The parietal layer of the tunica vaginalis is incised and the fluid drained. The wall of the hydrocele sac is closed or partially excised to prevent recurrence. Overlying tissues are closed in layers. Use 55040 for a unilateral procedure and 55041 for a bilateral hydrocele.

Excision of hydrocele

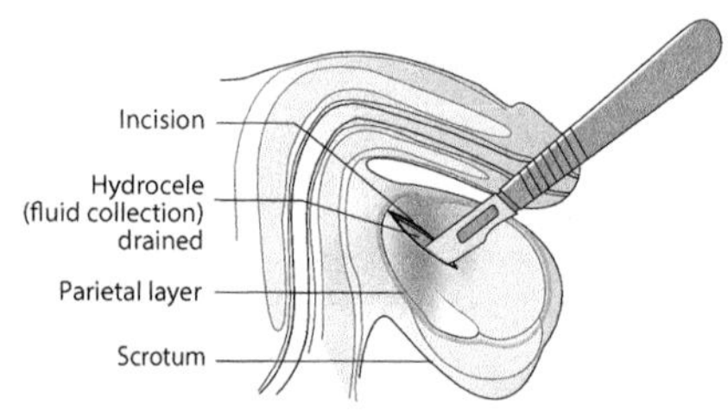

Unilateral (55040); bilateral (55041)

ICD-10-CM Diagnostic Codes

N43.0	Encysted hydrocele	♂
N43.1	Infected hydrocele	♂
N43.2	Other hydrocele	♂
P83.5	Congenital hydrocele	♂

CCI Edits
Refer to Appendix A for CCI edits.

Facility RVUs ▯

Code	Work	PE Facility	MP	Total Facility
55040	5.45	3.82	0.68	9.95
55041	8.54	5.45	1.04	15.03

Non-facility RVUs ▯

Code	Work	PE Non-Facility	MP	Total Non-Facility
55040	5.45	3.82	0.68	9.95
55041	8.54	5.45	1.04	15.03

Modifiers (PAR) ▯

Code	Mod 50	Mod 51	Mod 62	Mod 66	Mod 80
55040	0	2	0	0	1
55041	2	2	0	0	1

Global Period

Code	Days
55040	090
55041	090

55060

55060 Repair of tunica vaginalis hydrocele (Bottle type)

AMA *CPT® Assistant*

55060: Nov 14: 14

Plain English Description

A tunica vaginalis hydrocele is a collection of fluid within the tunica vaginalis of the scrotum. In a Bottle-type procedure, a transverse incision is made in the skin of the anterior scrotum and carried down through the dartos fascia to the tunica vaginalis exposing the fluid-filled sac surrounding the testis. The sac is incised vertically along the anterior border at the upper edge of the cord and the fluid drained. The hydrocele is everted around the testicle and secured with sutures. The scrotal incision is then closed in layers with absorbable suture starting with the dartos fascia followed by the skin.

Repair of tunica vaginalis (Bottle type)

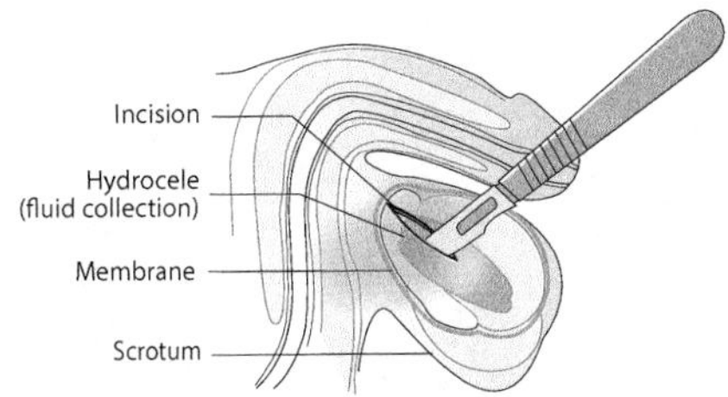

ICD-10-CM Diagnostic Codes

N43.0	Encysted hydrocele ♂
N43.1	Infected hydrocele ♂
N43.2	Other hydrocele ♂
P83.5	Congenital hydrocele ♂

CCI Edits

Refer to Appendix A for CCI edits.

Facility RVUs

Code	Work	PE Facility	MP	Total Facility
55060	6.15	4.25	0.76	11.16

Non-facility RVUs

Code	Work	PE Non-Facility	MP	Total Non-Facility
55060	6.15	4.25	0.76	11.16

Modifiers (PAR)

Code	Mod 50	Mod 51	Mod 62	Mod 66	Mod 80
55060	1	2	0	0	0

Global Period

Code	Days
55060	090

55100

55100 Drainage of scrotal wall abscess
(See also 54700)
(For debridement of necrotizing soft tissue infection of external genitalia, see 11004-11006)

Plain English Description

The scrotum is the sac that contains the testes. The scrotum is composed of skin that contains a network of nonstriated muscle fibers referred to as the dartos or scrotal fascia. An abscess of the scrotal wall involves the superficial layers of the scrotum. The skin of the scrotum is incised over the area of greatest fluctuance and the abscess pocket identified and opened. Any loculations are broken up using blunt dissection and the pus drained. The abscess cavity is irrigated with sterile saline or antibiotic solution. The incisions may be left open and packed with gauze or a drain placed. Alternatively, the incision may be closed.

Drainage of scrotal wall abscess

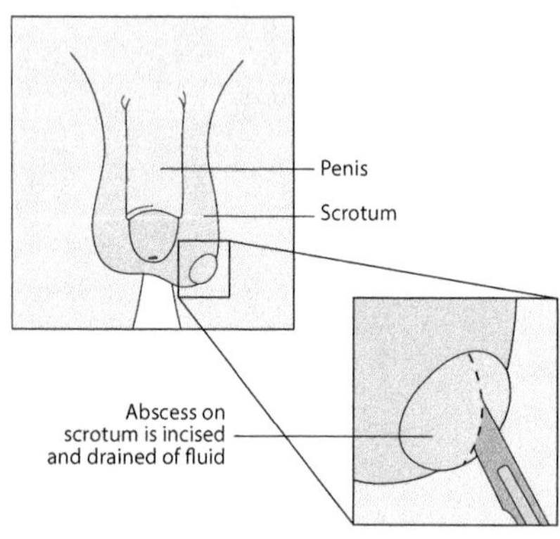
Penis
Scrotum
Abscess on scrotum is incised and drained of fluid

ICD-10-CM Diagnostic Codes

	N45.4	Abscess of epididymis or testis ♂
	N49.1	Inflammatory disorders of spermatic cord, tunica vaginalis and vas deferens ♂
	N49.2	Inflammatory disorders of scrotum ♂
	N49.8	Inflammatory disorders of other specified male genital organs ♂
❼	T81.41	Infection following a procedure, superficial incisional surgical site

ICD-10-CM Coding Notes

For codes requiring a 7th character extension, refer to your ICD-10-CM book. Review the character descriptions and coding guidelines for proper selection. For some procedures, only certain characters will apply.

CCI Edits

Refer to Appendix A for CCI edits.

Facility RVUs ▯

Code	Work	PE Facility	MP	Total Facility
55100	2.45	2.12	0.35	4.92

Non-facility RVUs ▯

Code	Work	PE Non-Facility	MP	Total Non-Facility
55100	2.45	4.07	0.35	6.87

Modifiers (PAR) ▯

Code	Mod 50	Mod 51	Mod 62	Mod 66	Mod 80
55100	0	2	0	0	1

Global Period

Code	Days
55100	010

55110

55110 Scrotal exploration

Plain English Description

A scrotal exploration may be performed after an injury, for acute symptoms indicating testicular pathology, or as part of a male infertility workup. The scrotal skin is incised transversely over the affected hemiscrotum or vertically along the median raphe and carried down through the dartos fascia to the tunica vaginalis and the testis/testes delivered out of the scrotum to the operative field. The structures are examined and any abnormalities noted. The incision is closed in layers starting with the dartos fascia and then the skin.

Scrotal exploration

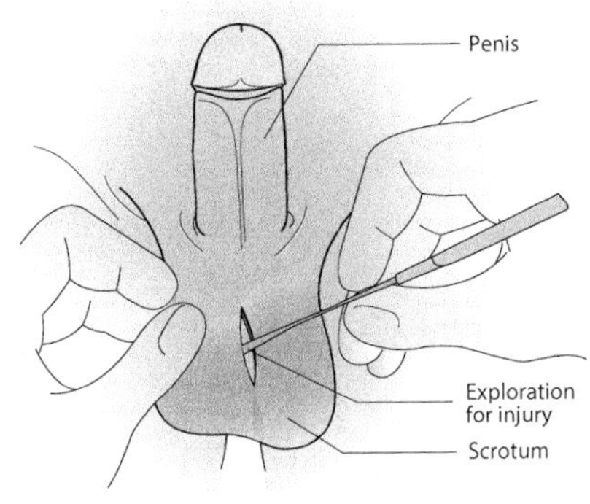

ICD-10-CM Diagnostic Codes

	C63.2	Malignant neoplasm of scrotum ♂
	C79.82	Secondary malignant neoplasm of genital organs
⇄	D29.21	Benign neoplasm of right testis ♂
⇄	D29.22	Benign neoplasm of left testis ♂
⇄	D29.31	Benign neoplasm of right epididymis ♂
⇄	D29.32	Benign neoplasm of left epididymis ♂
	D29.4	Benign neoplasm of scrotum ♂
	D29.8	Benign neoplasm of other specified male genital organs ♂
	D40.0	Neoplasm of uncertain behavior of prostate ♂
	D40.8	Neoplasm of uncertain behavior of other specified male genital organs ♂
	I86.1	Scrotal varices ♂
	N43.3	Hydrocele, unspecified ♂
	N44.01	Extravaginal torsion of spermatic cord ♂
	N44.02	Intravaginal torsion of spermatic cord ♂
	N44.03	Torsion of appendix testis ♂
	N44.04	Torsion of appendix epididymis ♂
	N44.1	Cyst of tunica albuginea testis ♂
	N44.2	Benign cyst of testis ♂
	N44.8	Other noninflammatory disorders of the testis ♂
	N45	Orchitis and epididymitis
	N45.1	Epididymitis ♂
	N45.2	Orchitis ♂
	N45.3	Epididymo-orchitis ♂
	N45.4	Abscess of epididymis or testis ♂
	N49.1	Inflammatory disorders of spermatic cord, tunica vaginalis and vas deferens ♂
	N49.2	Inflammatory disorders of scrotum ♂
	N49.8	Inflammatory disorders of other specified male genital organs ♂
	N50.3	Cyst of epididymis ♂
	N50.89	Other specified disorders of the male genital organs ♂
	N53.12	Painful ejaculation ♂
	N53.8	Other male sexual dysfunction ♂
	Q55.0	Absence and aplasia of testis ♂
	Q55.21	Polyorchism ♂
	Q55.8	Other specified congenital malformations of male genital organs ♂
	R10.2	Pelvic and perineal pain
❼	S39.848	Other specified injuries of external genitals
⇄	T81	Complications of procedures, not elsewhere classified

ICD-10-CM Coding Notes

For codes requiring a 7th character extension, refer to your ICD-10-CM book. Review the character descriptions and coding guidelines for proper selection. For some procedures, only certain characters will apply.

CCI Edits

Refer to Appendix A for CCI edits.

Facility RVUs ▯

Code	Work	PE Facility	MP	Total Facility
55110	6.33	4.27	0.83	11.43

Non-facility RVUs ▯

Code	Work	PE Non-Facility	MP	Total Non-Facility
55110	6.33	4.27	0.83	11.43

Modifiers (PAR) ▯

Code	Mod 50	Mod 51	Mod 62	Mod 66	Mod 80
55110	0	2	0	0	1

Global Period

Code	Days
55110	090

55120

55120 Removal of foreign body in scrotum

Plain English Description

The physician removes a foreign body from the scrotum following traumatic injury. The scrotum is the sac that contains the testes. The scrotum is composed of skin that contains a network of nonstriated muscle fibers referred to as the dartos or scrotal fascia. If there is a puncture wound, a straight or elliptical incision is made, the skin separated, and the scrotum explored. The foreign body is located. A hemostat or grasping forceps is then used to remove the foreign body. Alternatively, an open wound to the scrotum is explored and enlarged as needed to allow evaluation of the injury. The foreign body is located and removed. The wound is irrigated to remove any debris. The incision may be closed or packed open and a drain placed.

Removal of foreign body in scrotum

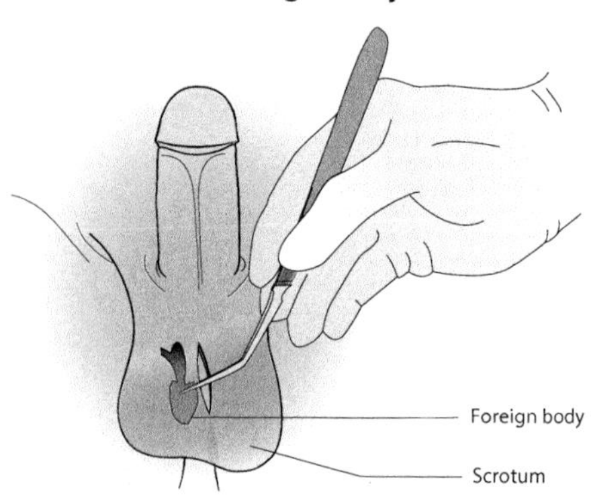

ICD-10-CM Diagnostic Codes

	L08.89	Other specified local infections of the skin and subcutaneous tissue
	L92.3	Foreign body granuloma of the skin and subcutaneous tissue
	M79.5	Residual foreign body in soft tissue
❼	S30.853	Superficial foreign body of scrotum and testes
❼	S31.32	Laceration with foreign body of scrotum and testes
❼	T81.500	Unspecified complication of foreign body accidentally left in body following surgical operation
❼	T81.508	Unspecified complication of foreign body accidentally left in body following other procedure
❼	T81.510	Adhesions due to foreign body accidentally left in body following surgical operation
❼	T81.518	Adhesions due to foreign body accidentally left in body following other procedure
❼	T81.520	Obstruction due to foreign body accidentally left in body following surgical operation
❼	T81.528	Obstruction due to foreign body accidentally left in body following other procedure
❼	T81.531	Perforation due to foreign body accidentally left in body following infusion or transfusion
❼	T81.538	Perforation due to foreign body accidentally left in body following other procedure

ICD-10-CM Coding Notes

For codes requiring a 7th character extension, refer to your ICD-10-CM book. Review the character descriptions and coding guidelines for proper selection. For some procedures, only certain characters will apply.

CCI Edits

Refer to Appendix A for CCI edits.

Facility RVUs ▢

Code	Work	PE Facility	MP	Total Facility
55120	5.72	4.02	0.67	10.41

Non-facility RVUs ▢

Code	Work	PE Non-Facility	MP	Total Non-Facility
55120	5.72	4.02	0.67	10.41

Modifiers (PAR) ▢

Code	Mod 50	Mod 51	Mod 62	Mod 66	Mod 80
55120	0	2	0	0	0

Global Period

Code	Days
55120	090

55150

55150 Resection of scrotum

AMA Coding Notes

Excision Procedures on the Scrotum

(For excision of local lesion of skin of scrotum, see Integumentary System)

Plain English Description

Scrotal resection may be necessary when skin lesions, soft tissue tumors, or excessive lymphatic tissue is present. An incision is made along the margin of healthy and affected skin and carried down to the dartos fascia in the inguinal, perineal, and crural areas. The testes and spermatic cords are dissected free and isolated. The abnormal skin and tissue are excised completely and sent to pathology where they may be prepared and examined by a pathologist in a separately reportable procedure. The tunica vaginalis is then inverted and the skin edges brought together to cover the scrotal structures. Bleeding is controlled with electrocautery, a drain is placed, and the edges of the incision are approximated and sutured in layers at the midline to simulate the scrotal raphe, starting with the dartos fascia followed by the skin.

Resection of scrotum

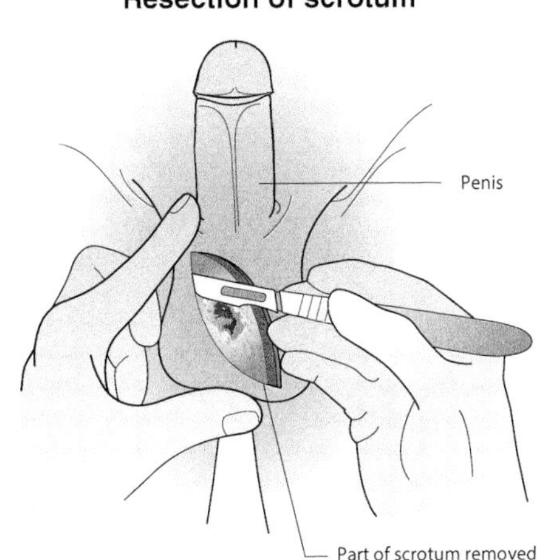

ICD-10-CM Diagnostic Codes

⇄	C62.11	Malignant neoplasm of descended right testis ♂
⇄	C62.12	Malignant neoplasm of descended left testis ♂
	C63.2	Malignant neoplasm of scrotum ♂
	C79.82	Secondary malignant neoplasm of genital organs
	D07.61	Carcinoma in situ of scrotum ♂
	D29.4	Benign neoplasm of scrotum ♂
	D40.8	Neoplasm of uncertain behavior of other specified male genital organs ♂
	D49.59	Neoplasm of unspecified behavior of other genitourinary organ
	N44.1	Cyst of tunica albuginea testis ♂
	N44.2	Benign cyst of testis ♂
	N44.8	Other noninflammatory disorders of the testis ♂
	N49.1	Inflammatory disorders of spermatic cord, tunica vaginalis and vas deferens ♂
	N49.2	Inflammatory disorders of scrotum ♂
	N49.3	Fournier gangrene ♂
	N49.8	Inflammatory disorders of other specified male genital organs ♂
	N50.1	Vascular disorders of male genital organs ♂
	N50.3	Cyst of epididymis ♂
	N50.89	Other specified disorders of the male genital organs ♂
	R10.2	Pelvic and perineal pain
❼	S31.30	Unspecified open wound of scrotum and testes
❼	S31.31	Laceration without foreign body of scrotum and testes
❼	S31.32	Laceration with foreign body of scrotum and testes
❼	S31.33	Puncture wound without foreign body of scrotum and testes
❼	S31.34	Puncture wound with foreign body of scrotum and testes
❼	S31.35	Open bite of scrotum and testes

ICD-10-CM Coding Notes

For codes requiring a 7th character extension, refer to your ICD-10-CM book. Review the character descriptions and coding guidelines for proper selection. For some procedures, only certain characters will apply.

CCI Edits

Refer to Appendix A for CCI edits.

Facility RVUs ▯

Code	Work	PE Facility	MP	Total Facility
55150	8.14	5.35	1.05	14.54

Non-facility RVUs ▯

Code	Work	PE Non-Facility	MP	Total Non-Facility
55150	8.14	5.35	1.05	14.54

Modifiers (PAR) ▯

Code	Mod 50	Mod 51	Mod 62	Mod 66	Mod 80
55150	0	2	1	0	2

Global Period

Code	Days
55150	090

55175-55180

55175 Scrotoplasty; simple
55180 Scrotoplasty; complicated

AMA *CPT® Assistant* ▢

55175: Dec 14: 16

Plain English Description

Scrotoplasty may be performed as a cosmetic procedure to remove excess skin due to aging, trauma, or injury; to repair congenital defects such as penoscrotal webbing; or for gender reassignment surgery. The scrotum is a thin, dual-chamber sac of skin and muscle that contains male reproductive organs including the testes, epididymis, vas deferens, and testicular artery and vein. The scrotal septum lies below the perineal raphe, a slightly raised, vertical ridge of skin running from the anus through the midline of the scrotum and up through the posterior midline of the penis. For simple scrotoplasty (55175), an incision is made along the perineal raphe, excess scrotal skin and muscle are removed, and the incision is sutured closed. For complicated scrotoplasty (55180) such as repair of congenital penoscrotal webbing, one or more incision(s) are made along the penoscrotal junction and the penis is dissected free of the attaching scrotal tissue. The excess scrotal tissue is then removed and the incision(s) is closed with suture. For female-to-male gender reassignment scrotoplasty, the labia majora are dissected to form two hollow cavities that are then unified to approximate a scrotum. Tissue expanders may be placed in preparation for silicon testicular prosthetic implants.

Scrotoplasty

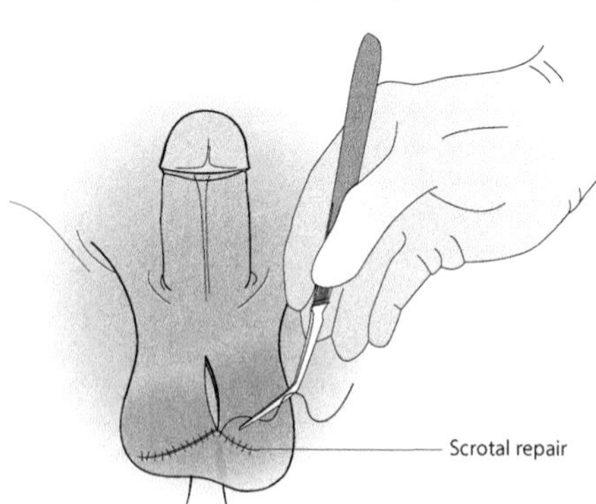

Simple (55175); complicated (55180)

ICD-10-CM Diagnostic Codes

C63.2	Malignant neoplasm of scrotum ♂
C79.82	Secondary malignant neoplasm of genital organs
D07.69	Carcinoma in situ of other male genital organs ♂
D29.4	Benign neoplasm of scrotum ♂
D40.8	Neoplasm of uncertain behavior of other specified male genital organs ♂
N43.0	Encysted hydrocele ♂
N43.1	Infected hydrocele ♂
N43.2	Other hydrocele ♂
N45	Orchitis and epididymitis
N45.4	Abscess of epididymis or testis ♂
N48.6	Induration penis plastica ♂
Q53.111	Unilateral intraabdominal testis ♂
Q53.112	Unilateral inguinal testis ♂
Q53.13	Unilateral high scrotal testis ♂
Q53.211	Bilateral intraabdominal testes ♂
Q53.212	Bilateral inguinal testes ♂
Q53.23	Bilateral high scrotal testes ♂
Q55.29	Other congenital malformations of testis and scrotum ♂
R39.83	Unilateral non-palpable testicle ♂
R39.84	Bilateral non-palpable testicles ♂
➐ S31.31	Laceration without foreign body of scrotum and testes
➐ S31.32	Laceration with foreign body of scrotum and testes
➐ S31.33	Puncture wound without foreign body of scrotum and testes
➐ S31.34	Puncture wound with foreign body of scrotum and testes
➐ S31.35	Open bite of scrotum and testes
➐ S38.232	Partial traumatic amputation of scrotum and testis

ICD-10-CM Coding Notes

For codes requiring a 7th character extension, refer to your ICD-10-CM book. Review the character descriptions and coding guidelines for proper selection. For some procedures, only certain characters will apply.

CCI Edits

Refer to Appendix A for CCI edits.

Facility RVUs ▢

Code	Work	PE Facility	MP	Total Facility
55175	5.87	4.12	0.73	10.72
55180	11.78	6.99	1.54	20.31

Non-facility RVUs ▢

Code	Work	PE Non-Facility	MP	Total Non-Facility
55175	5.87	4.12	0.73	10.72
55180	11.78	6.99	1.54	20.31

Modifiers (PAR) ▢

Code	Mod 50	Mod 51	Mod 62	Mod 66	Mod 80
55175	0	2	0	0	0
55180	0	2	0	0	0

Global Period

Code	Days
55175	090
55180	090

● New ▲ Revised ✚ Add On ⊘Modifier 51 Exempt ★Telemedicine ▢ CPT QuickRef ✗FDA Pending ⇄ Laterality ➐ Seventh Character ♂Male ♀Female

55200

55200 Vasotomy, cannulization with or without incision of vas, unilateral or bilateral (separate procedure)

Plain English Description

For a vasotomy with incision of the vas deferens, the scrotum is palpated to identify the vas, a small incision is made in the skin, and the vas is pulled up and delivered to the operative field. A straight clamp is placed under the vas and a hemi-vasotomy incision created utilizing an operative microscope and a micro-knife, with the clamp serving as a platform. Fluid is obtained from the opening of the vas and may be examined under a microscope in the operating room or sent to the laboratory for a separately reportable procedure. The vas deferens is then cannulized using an angiocath inserted into the distal end of the vasotomy and more fluid samples are obtained, examined, or sent to the laboratory for a separately reportable procedure. The angiocath is removed and the hemi-vasotomy closed in layers followed by closure of the skin. If both the right and left vas deferens are to be examined, the procedure is repeated on the opposite side. For a vasotomy without incision of the vas deferens, the scrotum is palpated to locate a straight portion of the structure. An angiocath or lymphangiogram needle with silastic tubing and a syringe attached is carefully threaded into the vasal lumen and fluid is aspirated and examined under a microscope in the operating room or sent to the laboratory for a separately reportable procedure. The needle is withdrawn from the vas deferens and removed from the scrotum. Firm pressure is applied to the puncture area to minimize bleeding. If both the right and left vas deferens are to be examined, the procedure is repeated on the opposite side.

Vasotomy

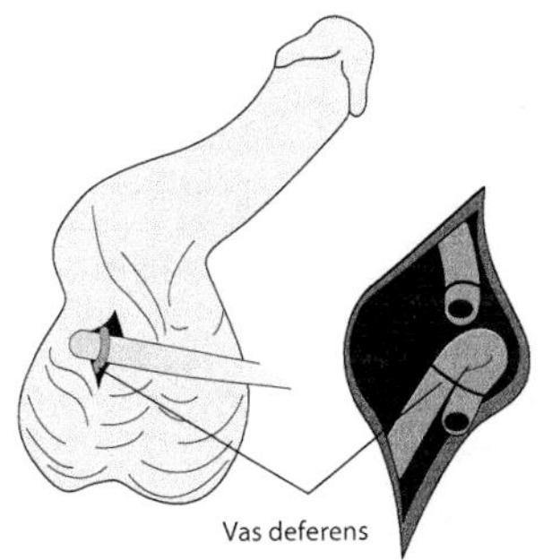

The vas is incised or punctured, a cannula is inserted, and fluid samples are obtained.

ICD-10-CM Diagnostic Codes

N46.023	Azoospermia due to obstruction of efferent ducts ♂
N46.12	Oligospermia due to extratesticular causes
N46.123	Oligospermia due to obstruction of efferent ducts ♂
N49.0	Inflammatory disorders of seminal vesicle ♂
N50.89	Other specified disorders of the male genital organs ♂
R36.1	Hematospermia ♂

CCI Edits

Refer to Appendix A for CCI edits.

Facility RVUs ☐

Code	Work	PE Facility	MP	Total Facility
55200	4.55	3.04	0.55	8.14

Non-facility RVUs ☐

Code	Work	PE Non-Facility	MP	Total Non-Facility
55200	4.55	6.36	0.55	11.46

Modifiers (PAR) ☐

Code	Mod 50	Mod 51	Mod 62	Mod 66	Mod 80
55200	2	2	0	0	0

Global Period

Code	Days
55200	090

55250

55250 Vasectomy, unilateral or bilateral (separate procedure), including postoperative semen examination(s)

AMA *CPT® Assistant*

55250: Jun 98: 10, Jul 98: 10, Apr 21: 13

Plain English Description

Vasectomy is considered a permanent form of birth control that involves interrupting the duct (vas deferens) that carries sperm from the testicles to the seminal vesicles. The vas deferens is located by palpation. A local anesthetic is injected. An incision is made in the scrotum and the vas deferens exposed. The vas deferens is cut and the ends tied, sutured, or closed using electrocautery. Scar tissue will develop over the cut ends to seal the duct and prevent release of sperm into the seminal vesicles. The vas deferens is replaced in the scrotum, which is closed with absorbable suture material. The procedure is repeated on the opposite side. Some physicians use a single incision of the scrotum to expose both vas deferens while others use two separate incisions, one on each side. It usually takes several months for all remaining sperm in the remaining vas deferens and seminal vesicles to be ejaculated or reabsorbed, so the patient must use an alternative form of birth control. The patient returns as instructed by the physician and postoperative semen examination is performed to ensure that the vas deferens has closed and that there are no sperm in the semen.

Vasectomy, unilateral or bilateral, including postoperative semen examination(s)

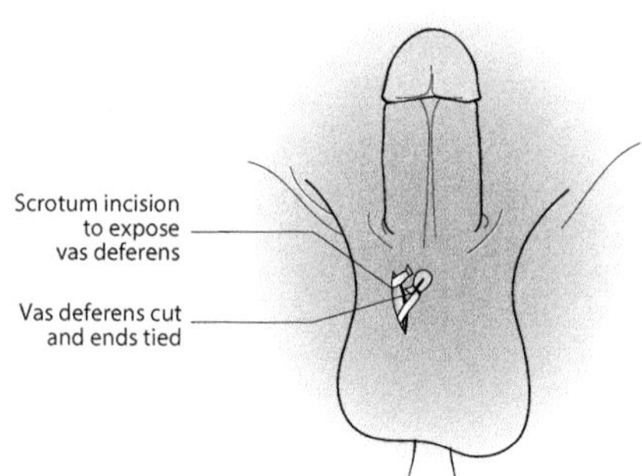

ICD-10-CM Diagnostic Codes

Z30.2 Encounter for sterilization

CCI Edits

Refer to Appendix A for CCI edits.

Pub 100

55250: Pub 100-03, 1, 230.3

Facility RVUs

Code	Work	PE Facility	MP	Total Facility
55250	3.37	2.93	0.40	6.70

Non-facility RVUs

Code	Work	PE Non-Facility	MP	Total Non-Facility
55250	3.37	6.24	0.40	10.01

Modifiers (PAR)

Code	Mod 50	Mod 51	Mod 62	Mod 66	Mod 80
55250	2	2	0	0	1

Global Period

Code	Days
55250	090

55300

55300 Vasotomy for vasograms, seminal vesiculograms, or epididymograms, unilateral or bilateral

(For radiological supervision and interpretation, use 74440)

(When combined with biopsy of testis, see 54505 and use modifier 51)

Plain English Description

A vasotomy is performed for injection of contrast for a unilateral or bilateral vasogram, seminal vesiculogram, or epididymogram. This code reports the vasotomy and injection procedure only. For vasotomy with incision of the vas, the scrotum is palpated to identify the vas, a small incision is made in the skin, and the vas is pulled up and delivered to the operative field. A straight clamp is placed under the vas and a hemi-vasotomy incision created utilizing an operative microscope and a micro-knife and the clamp serving as a platform. Fluid may be obtained from the opening of the vas and examined under a microscope in the operating room or sent to the laboratory for a separately reportable procedure. The vas deferens is then cannulized using an angiocath inserted into the distal end of the vasotomy and more fluid samples are obtained and examined or sent to the laboratory. A syringe containing 5-10 mL of contrast media is attached to the angiocath and the fluid is injected to examine the distal seminal duct under fluoroscopy. Proximal patency of the vas deferens and epididymal tubule may also be examined using the same technique by allowing passive flow contrast media into these structures. The angiocath is then removed and the hemi-vasotomy closed in layers followed by closure of the skin. If bilateral studies are performed, the procedure is repeated on the opposite side. For a procedure without incision of the vas, the scrotum is palpated to locate a straight portion of the structure. An angiocath or lymphangiogram needle with silastic tubing and a syringe attached is carefully threaded into the vasal lumen and the procedure continues as described for a vasotomy with incision. Upon completion of the procedure, the needle is removed from the scrotum and firm pressure applied to the puncture area to minimize bleeding. If bilateral studies are performed, the procedure is repeated on the opposite side.

Vasotomy for vasograms, seminal vesiculograms, or epididymograms, unilateral or bilateral

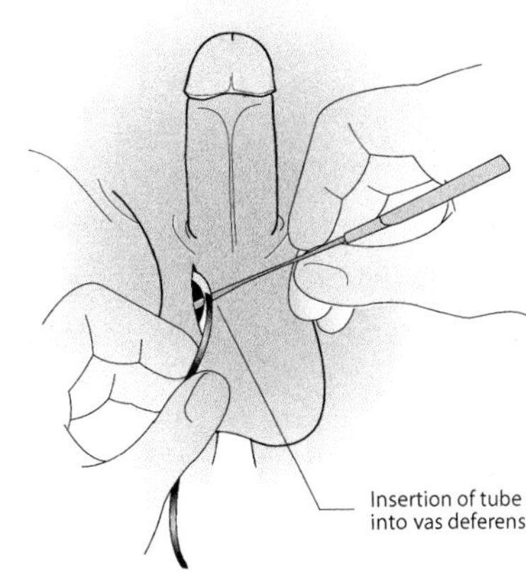

ICD-10-CM Diagnostic Codes

D17.6	Benign lipomatous neoplasm of spermatic cord ♂
N46.01	Organic azoospermia ♂
N46.021	Azoospermia due to drug therapy ♂
N46.022	Azoospermia due to infection ♂
N46.023	Azoospermia due to obstruction of efferent ducts ♂
N46.024	Azoospermia due to radiation ♂
N46.025	Azoospermia due to systemic disease ♂
N46.029	Azoospermia due to other extratesticular causes ♂
N46.11	Organic oligospermia ♂
N46.121	Oligospermia due to drug therapy ♂
N46.122	Oligospermia due to infection ♂
N46.123	Oligospermia due to obstruction of efferent ducts ♂
N46.124	Oligospermia due to radiation ♂
N46.125	Oligospermia due to systemic disease ♂
N46.129	Oligospermia due to other extratesticular causes ♂
N46.8	Other male infertility ♂
N50.0	Atrophy of testis ♂
N50.89	Other specified disorders of the male genital organs ♂
Q55.3	Atresia of vas deferens ♂
R36.1	Hematospermia ♂
Z31.41	Encounter for fertility testing

CCI Edits

Refer to Appendix A for CCI edits.

Facility RVUs

Code	Work	PE Facility	MP	Total Facility
55300	3.50	1.50	0.41	5.41

Non-facility RVUs

Code	Work	PE Non-Facility	MP	Total Non-Facility
55300	3.50	1.50	0.41	5.41

Modifiers (PAR)

Code	Mod 50	Mod 51	Mod 62	Mod 66	Mod 80
55300	2	2	0	0	0

Global Period

Code	Days
55300	000

CPT® Procedural Coding

55400

55400 Vasovasostomy, vasovasorrhaphy

(For bilateral procedure, report 55400 with modifier 50)

(For operating microscope, use 69990)

AMA *CPT® Assistant*

55400: Nov 98: 16, Oct 01: 8, Jun 04: 11

Plain English Description

A vasovasostomy or vasovasorrhaphy is performed to reconnect the ends of the vas deferens following a vasectomy or to repair an iatrogenic vasal injury that occurred during another surgical procedure. The scrotal skin is incised over the previous surgical scar and the vas deferens pulled up and delivered to the operative field. The ends of the vas deferens are incised and dilated using fine forceps, an angiocath is introduced into the vasal lumen, and the vas deferens is irrigated with saline to assess patency. The irrigation fluid is examined microscopically for spermatozoa or sperm fragments. The ends of the vas deferens are anastomosed using a single layer or multiple layer technique. The reconnected/repaired vas deferens is returned to the scrotum and the skin is then closed with absorbable suture.

Vasovasostomy, vasovasorrhaphy

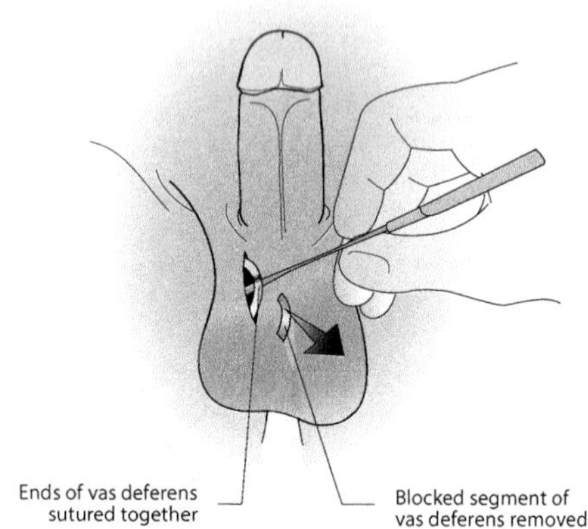

ICD-10-CM Diagnostic Codes

- N46.023 Azoospermia due to obstruction of efferent ducts ♂
- N46.123 Oligospermia due to obstruction of efferent ducts ♂
- N49.0 Inflammatory disorders of seminal vesicle ♂
- N50.89 Other specified disorders of the male genital organs ♂
- Q55.3 Atresia of vas deferens ♂
- Z31.0 Encounter for reversal of previous sterilization

CCI Edits

Refer to Appendix A for CCI edits.

Facility RVUs

Code	Work	PE Facility	MP	Total Facility
55400	8.61	5.01	1.02	14.64

Non-facility RVUs

Code	Work	PE Non-Facility	MP	Total Non-Facility
55400	8.61	5.01	1.02	14.64

Modifiers (PAR)

Code	Mod 50	Mod 51	Mod 62	Mod 66	Mod 80
55400	1	2	1	0	2

Global Period

Code	Days
55400	090

55500

55500 Excision of hydrocele of spermatic cord, unilateral (separate procedure)

AMA *CPT® Assistant* ☐

55500: Oct 01: 8

Plain English Description

Excision of a spermatic hydrocele is most often performed through an inguinal incision. A transverse inguinal incision is made in the skin and then carried down through the subcutaneous tissue to the external oblique aponeurosis. The inguinal canal is opened and the ilioinguinal nerve is identified and isolated. Next, the surgical wound is explored until the spermatic cord is identified and bluntly dissected off the anterior cremaster muscle fibers to the internal ring. After placement of a ligature suture near the base of the hydrocele sac, the sac is then carefully elevated off the spermatic cord, preserving the spermatic vessels and the vas deferens, and the sac dissected free from the spermatic fascia. The sac is then transected and dissected up to the internal inguinal ring where is it ligated with suture and bleeding controlled with electrocautery. The spermatic fascia is closed around the cord structures, and the external oblique muscle is closed followed by the skin.

Excision of hydrocele of spermatic cord, unilateral (separate procedure)

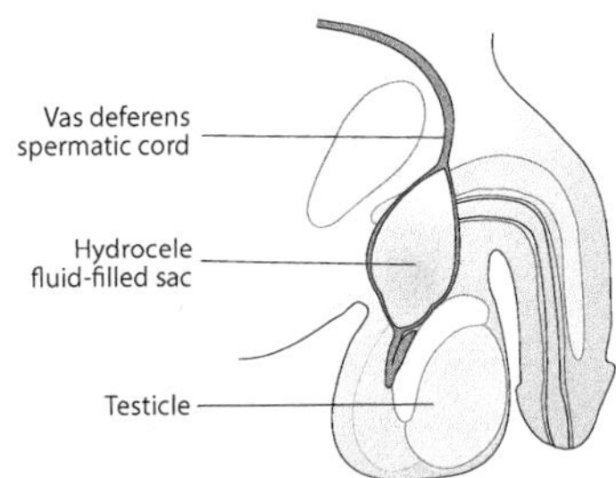

ICD-10-CM Diagnostic Codes

N43.0	Encysted hydrocele ♂
N43.1	Infected hydrocele ♂
N43.2	Other hydrocele ♂
P83.5	Congenital hydrocele ♂

CCI Edits

Refer to Appendix A for CCI edits.

Facility RVUs ☐

Code	Work	PE Facility	MP	Total Facility
55500	6.22	4.45	0.93	11.60

Non-facility RVUs ☐

Code	Work	PE Non-Facility	MP	Total Non-Facility
55500	6.22	4.45	0.93	11.60

Modifiers (PAR) ☐

Code	Mod 50	Mod 51	Mod 62	Mod 66	Mod 80
55500	1	2	0	0	0

Global Period

Code	Days
55500	090

CPT® Procedural Coding

55520

55520 Excision of lesion of spermatic cord (separate procedure)

AMA *CPT® Assistant*

55520: Sep 00: 10, Oct 01: 8

Plain English Description

The excision of a lesion from the spermatic cord is most often performed through an inguinal incision. A transverse inguinal incision is made in the skin and carried down through the subcutaneous tissue, Camper's fascia, and Scarpa's fascia to the external oblique aponeurosis. The inguinal canal is opened and the ilioinguinal nerve is identified and isolated. The surgical wound is explored until the spermatic cord is identified and bluntly dissected off the anterior cremaster muscle fibers to the internal ring. The cord is then stabilized using non-crushing clamps and ligated at the gubernaculum. The lesion is identified and excised. Bleeding is controlled with electrocautery and the spermatic fascia is closed with fine suture. The external oblique muscle, Scarpa's fascia, and Camper's fascia are closed in layers followed by the skin.

Excision of lesion of spermatic cord (separate procedure)

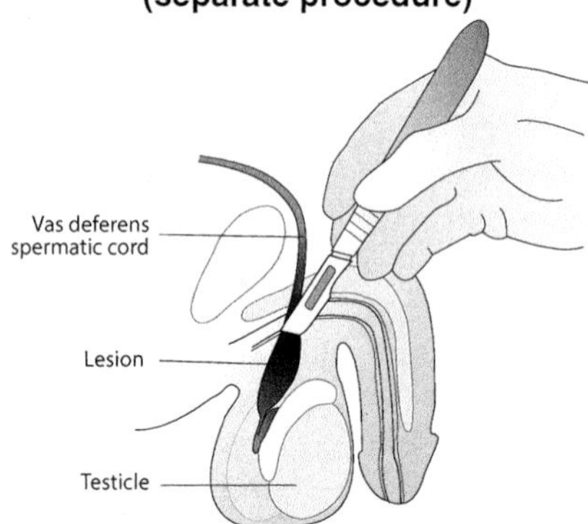

ICD-10-CM Diagnostic Codes

D17.6	Benign lipomatous neoplasm of spermatic cord ♂
D29.8	Benign neoplasm of other specified male genital organs ♂
D40.8	Neoplasm of uncertain behavior of other specified male genital organs ♂
N44.8	Other noninflammatory disorders of the testis ♂
N49.1	Inflammatory disorders of spermatic cord, tunica vaginalis and vas deferens ♂
N49.9	Inflammatory disorder of unspecified male genital organ ♂
N50.3	Cyst of epididymis ♂
N50.89	Other specified disorders of the male genital organs ♂
N53.12	Painful ejaculation ♂

CCI Edits

Refer to Appendix A for CCI edits.

Facility RVUs

Code	Work	PE Facility	MP	Total Facility
55520	6.66	5.43	1.61	13.70

Non-facility RVUs

Code	Work	PE Non-Facility	MP	Total Non-Facility
55520	6.66	5.43	1.61	13.70

Modifiers (PAR)

Code	Mod 50	Mod 51	Mod 62	Mod 66	Mod 80
55520	1	2	1	0	2

Global Period

Code	Days
55520	090

55530-55535

55530 Excision of varicocele or ligation of spermatic veins for varicocele; (separate procedure)

55535 Excision of varicocele or ligation of spermatic veins for varicocele; abdominal approach

AMA *CPT® Assistant*

55530: Oct 01: 8

55535: Oct 01: 8

Plain English Description

A varicocele is an enlargement of the veins in the scrotum. A varicocele may be treated by excision or ligation of the spermatic veins. In 55530, an inguinal or subinguinal approach is used. Using an inguinal approach, the external inguinal ring is located by invaginating the scrotal skin upwards. A transverse incision is made in the skin starting at the external inguinal ring and extending laterally along the line of Langer. The incision is carried down through the subcutaneous tissue, Camper's fascia, and Scarpa's fascia to the external oblique aponeurosis. The muscle fibers are incised and the ilioinguinal nerve identified and isolated. Alternatively, using a subinguinal approach, a skin incision is made in the groin above and to the side of the penis and then carried down through the subcutaneous tissue and fascia. Using blunt dissection, the spermatic cord is exposed to the level of the pubic tubercle. A ring clamp or Penrose drain is passed around the cord and the testis is delivered to the operative field. The external spermatic perforator scrotal and gubernacular collateral veins are identified, clamped, divided, and ligated and the testis is returned to the scrotal sac. The spermatic cord is elevated with a Penrose drain and the external and internal spermatic fascia opened to expose the varicocele. A solution of 1% Papaverine may be used to irrigate and induce dilation and pulsation of the arteries to facilitate identification. The testicular artery and lymphatic channels are identified and preserved. The spermatic veins are clamped, divided, and suture ligated. Alternatively, the varicocele may be excised. The vas deferens is examined and one set of vasal vessels may be ligated if enlarged. The Penrose drain is removed and the spermatic cord placed back into the incision. The incision is closed in layers. In 55535, a retroperitoneal approach is used. A skin incision is made along the line of Langer in the lower abdomen and carried down through the subcutaneous tissue to the external oblique aponeurosis. The muscle fibers are incised and the ilioinguinal nerve identified and isolated. The internal oblique muscle is exposed and blunt dissection used to expose the transverse abdominis muscle, which is then transected. The retroperitoneal space is entered just above the inguinal ligament. The peritoneum is displaced medially to expose the testicular artery and vein near the ureter and the femoral artery and inferior epigastric artery and vein near the vas deferens. The vessels are elevated using a loop and a solution of 1% Papaverine may be used for irrigation to induce dilation and pulsation to facilitate identification of the arteries. The veins, arteries, and lymphatic vessels are identified and the veins ligated using vascular clips or intracorporeal sutures. Alternatively, the varicocele may be excised. Hemostasis is obtained with electrocautery. The incision is closed in layers.

Excision of varicocele or ligation of spermatic veins for varicocele

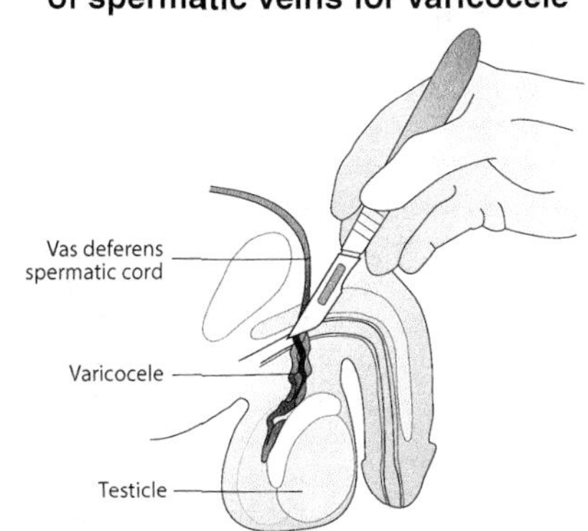

Transinguinal approach (55530); abdominal approach (55535)

ICD-10-CM Diagnostic Codes

I86.1 Scrotal varices ♂

CCI Edits

Refer to Appendix A for CCI edits.

Facility RVUs

Code	Work	PE Facility	MP	Total Facility
55530	5.75	3.90	0.73	10.38
55535	7.19	4.58	0.87	12.64

Non-facility RVUs

Code	Work	PE Non-Facility	MP	Total Non-Facility
55530	5.75	3.90	0.73	10.38
55535	7.19	4.58	0.87	12.64

Modifiers (PAR)

Code	Mod 50	Mod 51	Mod 62	Mod 66	Mod 80
55530	1	2	1	0	1
55535	1	2	1	0	2

Global Period

Code	Days
55530	090
55535	090

55540

55540 Excision of varicocele or ligation of spermatic veins for varicocele; with hernia repair

AMA *CPT® Assistant* ☐

55540: Oct 01: 8

Plain English Description

A varicocele is an enlargement of the veins in the scrotum. A varicocele may be treated by excision or ligation of the spermatic veins. A varicocelectomy or ligation of spermatic veins with concurrent hernia repair may be performed through a retroperitoneal incision in the lower abdomen. A skin incision is made along the line of Langer in the lower abdomen and carried down through the subcutaneous tissue to the external oblique aponeurosis. The muscle fibers are incised and the ilioinguinal nerve identified and isolated. The internal oblique muscle is exposed and blunt dissection used to expose the transverse abdominis muscle, which is then transected. The retroperitoneal space is entered just above the inguinal ligament. The peritoneum is displaced medially to expose the testicular artery and vein near the ureter and the femoral artery and inferior epigastric artery and vein near the vas deferens. The vessels are elevated using a loop and a solution of 1% Papaverine may be used for irrigation to induce dilation and pulsation to facilitate identification of the arteries. The veins, arteries, and lymphatic vessels are identified and the veins ligated using vascular clips or intracorporeal sutures. Alternatively, the varicocele may be excised. To repair an inguinal hernia from this approach, a mesh patch is most often used. The hernia sac is identified and dissected free of the surrounding tissue. The sac and contents are pulled into the abdominal cavity. The patch is laid over the opening in the inguinal canal and sutured in place. Hemostasis is obtained with electrocautery and the incision then closed in layers.

Excision of varicocele or ligation of spermatic veins for varicocele, with hernia repair

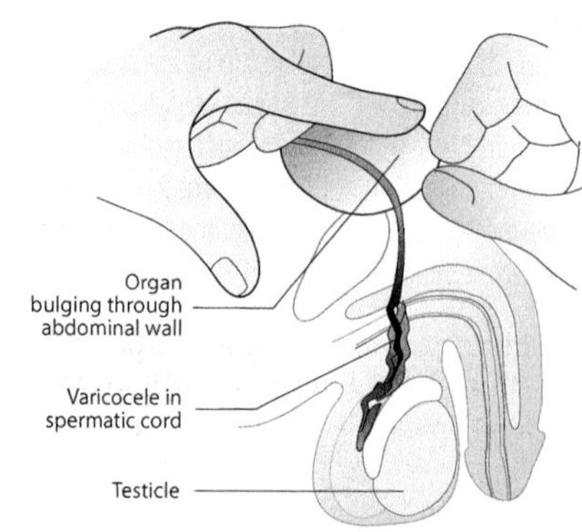

ICD-10-CM Diagnostic Codes

I86.1	Scrotal varices ♂
K40.00	Bilateral inguinal hernia, with obstruction, without gangrene, not specified as recurrent
K40.01	Bilateral inguinal hernia, with obstruction, without gangrene, recurrent
K40.10	Bilateral inguinal hernia, with gangrene, not specified as recurrent
K40.11	Bilateral inguinal hernia, with gangrene, recurrent
K40.20	Bilateral inguinal hernia, without obstruction or gangrene, not specified as recurrent
K40.21	Bilateral inguinal hernia, without obstruction or gangrene, recurrent
K40.30	Unilateral inguinal hernia, with obstruction, without gangrene, not specified as recurrent
K40.31	Unilateral inguinal hernia, with obstruction, without gangrene, recurrent
K40.40	Unilateral inguinal hernia, with gangrene, not specified as recurrent
K40.41	Unilateral inguinal hernia, with gangrene, recurrent
K40.90	Unilateral inguinal hernia, without obstruction or gangrene, not specified as recurrent
K40.91	Unilateral inguinal hernia, without obstruction or gangrene, recurrent
K42.9	Umbilical hernia without obstruction or gangrene
Q53.111	Unilateral intraabdominal testis ♂
Q53.112	Unilateral inguinal testis ♂
Q53.13	Unilateral high scrotal testis ♂
Q53.211	Bilateral intraabdominal testes ♂
Q53.212	Bilateral inguinal testes ♂
Q53.23	Bilateral high scrotal testes ♂
R39.83	Unilateral non-palpable testicle ♂
R39.84	Bilateral non-palpable testicles ♂

CCI Edits

Refer to Appendix A for CCI edits.

Facility RVUs ☐

Code	Work	PE Facility	MP	Total Facility
55540	8.30	6.22	2.09	16.61

Non-facility RVUs ☐

Code	Work	PE Non-Facility	MP	Total Non-Facility
55540	8.30	6.22	2.09	16.61

Modifiers (PAR) ☐

Code	Mod 50	Mod 51	Mod 62	Mod 66	Mod 80
55540	1	2	1	0	1

Global Period

Code	Days
55540	090

55550

55550 Laparoscopy, surgical, with ligation of spermatic veins for varicocele

AMA Coding Guideline

Laparoscopic Procedures on the Spermatic Cord

Surgical laparoscopy always includes diagnostic laparoscopy. To report a diagnostic laparoscopy (peritoneoscopy) (separate procedure), use 49320.

AMA *CPT® Assistant* ▯

55550: Nov 99: 27, Mar 00: 9, Oct 01: 8

Plain English Description

A varicocele is an enlargement of the veins in the scrotum. Using a laparoscopic approach, the spermatic veins are ligated. A small U-shaped skin incision is made at the umbilicus, and a clamp used to dissect down to the anterior rectus fascia, which is then opened a few millimeters to allow a Veress needle to be introduced into the peritoneal cavity. A pneumoperitoneum is created with insufflation of CO2. Using upward traction on the abdominal wall, the laparoscope is inserted through the umbilical incision and 3 ports are placed in a baseball diamond configuration in the lower abdomen. The intra-abdominal vas deferens is identified at the junction of the spermatic cord above the internal inguinal ring along with the gonadal vessels. The posterior peritoneum is then excised using cautery, laser, or endoscopic scissors. The gonadal artery is identified and preserved. The gonadal vein is isolated by blunt dissection using atraumatic graspers and ligated with vascular clips or intracorporeal sutures. The laparoscopic instruments are withdrawn and CO2 removed from the cavity. The fascia is closed with absorbable suture followed by closure of the skin with suture, skin clips, or surgical glue.

Laparoscopy, surgical, with ligation of spermatic veins for varicocele

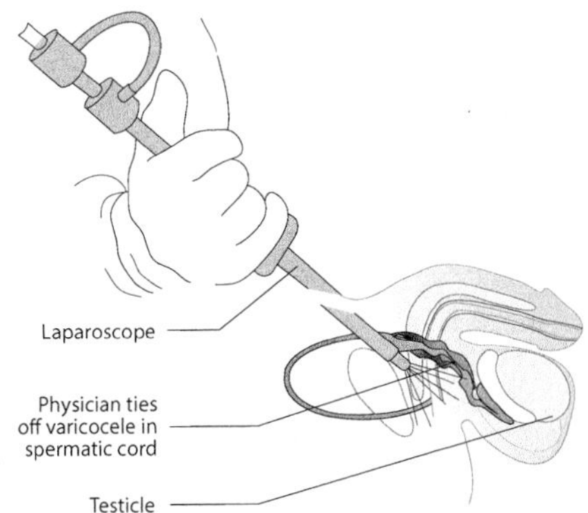

ICD-10-CM Diagnostic Codes

I86.1	Scrotal varices ♂

CCI Edits

Refer to Appendix A for CCI edits.

Facility RVUs ▯

Code	Work	PE Facility	MP	Total Facility
55550	7.20	4.54	0.87	12.61

Non-facility RVUs ▯

Code	Work	PE Non-Facility	MP	Total Non-Facility
55550	7.20	4.54	0.87	12.61

Modifiers (PAR) ▯

Code	Mod 50	Mod 51	Mod 62	Mod 66	Mod 80
55550	1	2	1	0	2

Global Period

Code	Days
55550	090

55600-55605

55600 Vesiculotomy

(For bilateral procedure, report 55600 with modifier 50)

55605 Vesiculotomy; complicated

Plain English Description

Vesiculotomy is the surgical exposure or opening of one or both seminal vesicles, a pair of tubular glands behind the bladder and above the prostate made up of an inner layer containing cells that produce components of seminal fluid, a middle layer of smooth muscle, and an outer layer of connective tissue. The seminal vesicles and vas deferens join to make the ejaculatory duct, which opens into the prostatic urethra. Symptoms of seminal vesicle disease may include abdominal, pelvic, or penile pain, pain with ejaculation and/or urination, low volume of semen, and blood in the semen and/or urine. Surgical approach for vesiculotomy may be through the retropubic space (between the pubic symphysis and bladder) or a perineal incision (between the anus and scrotum). For a retropubic incision in the lower abdomen, the bladder is retracted to gain access to the seminal vesicles and expose the glands. When more extensive dissection is required, report 55605. Code 55600 reports simple vesiculotomy.

Vesiculotomy

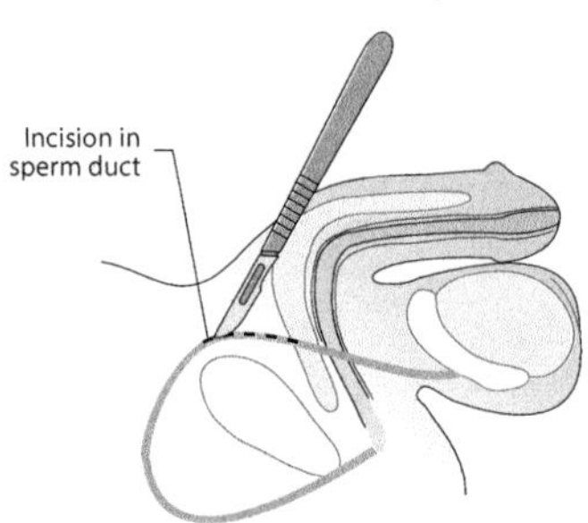

Vesiculotomy (55600); vesiculotomy, complicated (55605)

ICD-10-CM Diagnostic Codes

C63.7	Malignant neoplasm of other specified male genital organs ♂
C63.8	Malignant neoplasm of overlapping sites of male genital organs ♂
C79.82	Secondary malignant neoplasm of genital organs
D07.69	Carcinoma in situ of other male genital organs ♂
D29.8	Benign neoplasm of other specified male genital organs ♂
D40.8	Neoplasm of uncertain behavior of other specified male genital organs ♂
N49.0	Inflammatory disorders of seminal vesicle ♂
N50.1	Vascular disorders of male genital organs ♂
N50.89	Other specified disorders of the male genital organs ♂
R36.1	Hematospermia ♂

CCI Edits

Refer to Appendix A for CCI edits.

Facility RVUs

Code	Work	PE Facility	MP	Total Facility
55600	7.01	4.53	0.85	12.39
55605	8.76	5.56	1.04	15.36

Non-facility RVUs

Code	Work	PE Non-Facility	MP	Total Non-Facility
55600	7.01	4.53	0.85	12.39
55605	8.76	5.56	1.04	15.36

Modifiers (PAR)

Code	Mod 50	Mod 51	Mod 62	Mod 66	Mod 80
55600	1	2	0	0	0
55605	1	2	0	0	0

Global Period

Code	Days
55600	090
55605	090

55650

55650 Vesiculectomy, any approach

(For bilateral procedure, report 55650 with modifier 50)

Plain English Description

Vesiculectomy, removal of the seminal vesicle, is performed by any approach. Open surgical approaches to the seminal vesicles include: transperineal, transvesical through the posterior bladder wall, paravesical, retrovesical, or transcoccygeal. The procedure may also be performed laparoscopically. Using a transperineal approach, an inverted-U incision is made in the perineum and the central tendon is divided. A retractor is used to expose the anterior rectal fascial fibers. The rectourethralis is divided near the apex of the prostate. A weighted speculum is then used to expose the seminal vesicle. The rectum is dissected off the prostate and Denonvilliers fascia is incised. The seminal vesicle is dissected off the prostate, suture ligated at the base, and divided. Dissection is carried to the apex of the gland. The vascular pedicle is clamp ligated and the seminal vesicle is excised. To perform the procedure laparoscopically, a small U-shaped skin incision is made at the umbilicus, and a clamp used to dissect down to the anterior rectus fascia, which is then opened a few millimeters to allow a Veress needle to be introduced into the peritoneal cavity. A pneumoperitoneum is created with insufflation of CO2. Using upward traction on the abdominal wall, the laparoscope is inserted through the umbilical incision and 3-4 ports are placed in the lower abdomen. A transverse opening is made in the retrovesical peritoneum and the vas deferens is identified. The seminal vesicle is dissected from the vas deferens and the seminal artery is identified, ligated with vascular clips, and cut. Dissection of the seminal vesicle continues along the posterior trigone of the bladder and around the urethra. The seminal vesicle is then excised and removed from the abdomen. The laparoscopic instruments are withdrawn and CO2 removed from the cavity. The fascia is closed with absorbable suture followed by closure of the skin with suture, skin clips, or surgical glue.

Vesiculectomy, any approach

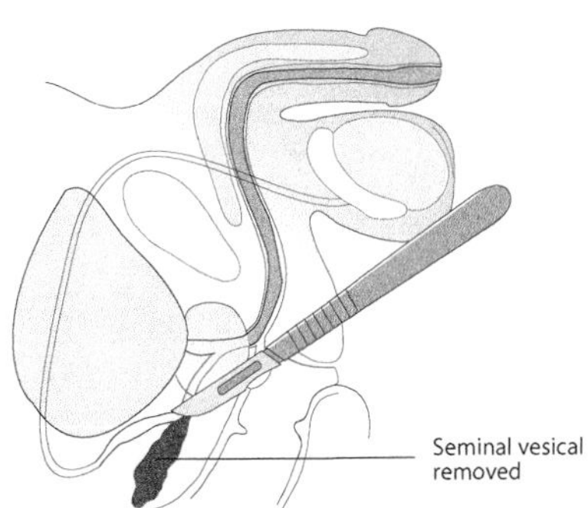

ICD-10-CM Diagnostic Codes

C63.7	Malignant neoplasm of other specified male genital organs ♂
C79.82	Secondary malignant neoplasm of genital organs
D07.69	Carcinoma in situ of other male genital organs ♂
D29.8	Benign neoplasm of other specified male genital organs ♂
D40.8	Neoplasm of uncertain behavior of other specified male genital organs ♂
D49.59	Neoplasm of unspecified behavior of other genitourinary organ
D49.8	Neoplasm of unspecified behavior of other specified sites
N49.0	Inflammatory disorders of seminal vesicle ♂
N50.89	Other specified disorders of the male genital organs ♂

CCI Edits

Refer to Appendix A for CCI edits.

Facility RVUs ☐

Code	Work	PE Facility	MP	Total Facility
55650	12.65	6.89	1.51	21.05

Non-facility RVUs ☐

Code	Work	PE Non-Facility	MP	Total Non-Facility
55650	12.65	6.89	1.51	21.05

Modifiers (PAR) ☐

Code	Mod 50	Mod 51	Mod 62	Mod 66	Mod 80
55650	1	2	1	0	2

Global Period

Code	Days
55650	090

CPT® Procedural Coding

55680

55680 Excision of Mullerian duct cyst

(For injection procedure, see 52010, 55300)

Plain English Description

A Mullerian duct cyst is a rare congenital anomaly in males that is a remnant of the caudal ends of the fused Mullerian duct that usually regresses before birth. These cysts are typically located in the midline, behind the bladder. They originate in the region of the verumontanum and are attached to the verumontanum with a stalk. They do not communicate with the urethra. Using a suprapubic approach, the abdomen is incised and the peritoneum is opened behind the bladder. The prostate gland and prostatic utricle are identified. The area is incised until the Mullerian duct and cyst are identified. The neck of the cyst is ligated and the cyst is excised. The peritoneum is closed and the abdominal incision is closed in layers.

Excision of Mullerian duct cyst

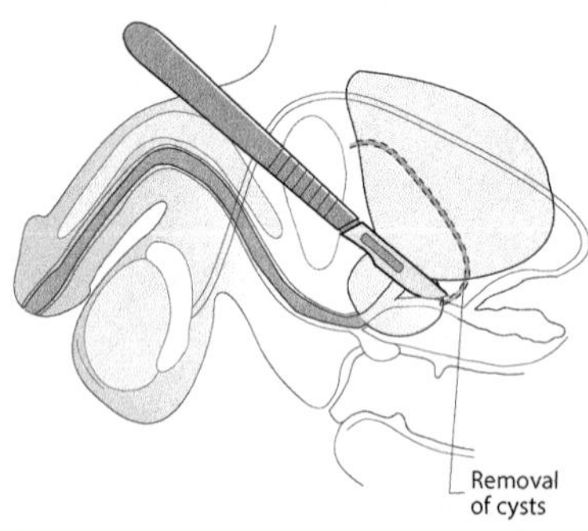

ICD-10-CM Diagnostic Codes

C63.7	Malignant neoplasm of other specified male genital organs ♂
D07.69	Carcinoma in situ of other male genital organs ♂
D29.8	Benign neoplasm of other specified male genital organs ♂
D40.8	Neoplasm of uncertain behavior of other specified male genital organs ♂
N49.0	Inflammatory disorders of seminal vesicle ♂
N50.89	Other specified disorders of the male genital organs ♂
Q55.29	Other congenital malformations of testis and scrotum ♂
Q55.4	Other congenital malformations of vas deferens, epididymis, seminal vesicles and prostate ♂

CCI Edits

Refer to Appendix A for CCI edits.

Facility RVUs

Code	Work	PE Facility	MP	Total Facility
55680	5.67	3.85	0.67	10.19

Non-facility RVUs

Code	Work	PE Non-Facility	MP	Total Non-Facility
55680	5.67	3.85	0.67	10.19

Modifiers (PAR)

Code	Mod 50	Mod 51	Mod 62	Mod 66	Mod 80
55680	1	2	0	0	0

Global Period

Code	Days
55680	090

55700-55705

55700 Biopsy, prostate; needle or punch, single or multiple, any approach

(If imaging guidance is performed, see 76942, 77002, 77012, 77021)

(For fine needle aspiration biopsy, see 10004, 10005, 10006, 10007, 10008, 10009, 10010, 10011, 10012, 10021)

(For evaluation of fine needle aspirate, see 88172, 88173)

(For transperineal stereotactic template guided saturation prostate biopsies, use 55706)

55705 Biopsy, prostate; incisional, any approach

AMA *CPT® Assistant* ▯

55700: May 96: 3, Nov 10: 5, Jul 18: 11

Plain English Description

A biopsy of the prostate is performed. Biopsy is performed when there is an enlargement or palpable mass of the prostate or when the patient has an elevated prostatic-specific antigen (PSA) blood test. In 55700, a needle or punch biopsy is performed by any approach. A large bore needle or spring-loaded (punch) needle is inserted through the rectum (transrectal biopsy) or through the urethra (transurethral biopsy), using a needle guide. The needle may be passed into a single site or multiple sites in the prostate may be punctured to obtain a tissue sample. If a transrectal approach is used, a separately reportable transrectal ultrasound (TRUS) may be used to guide placement of the needle. If a transurethral approach is used, the physician uses a cystoscope to visualize the prostate gland and obtain the biopsy. The tissue sample is sent to the laboratory for separately reportable histological evaluation. In 55705, an incisional biopsy is performed by any approach. Incisional biopsy is typically performed using a transperineal approach. The perineum between the anus and scrotum is incised and the prostate exposed. A tissue sample is obtained from one or more sites in the prostate.

Biopsy, prostate

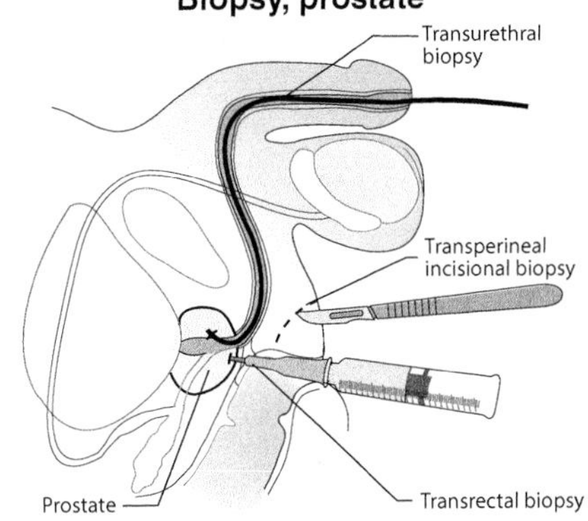

Needle or punch, single or multiple, any approach (55700); incisional, any approach (55705)

ICD-10-CM Diagnostic Codes

C61	Malignant neoplasm of prostate ♂
C79.82	Secondary malignant neoplasm of genital organs
D07.5	Carcinoma in situ of prostate ♂
D29.1	Benign neoplasm of prostate ♂
D40.0	Neoplasm of uncertain behavior of prostate ♂
D49.5	Neoplasm of unspecified behavior of other genitourinary organs
N40.0	Benign prostatic hyperplasia without lower urinary tract symptoms ♂
N40.1	Benign prostatic hyperplasia with lower urinary tract symptoms ♂
N40.2	Nodular prostate without lower urinary tract symptoms ♂
N40.3	Nodular prostate with lower urinary tract symptoms ♂
N41.1	Chronic prostatitis ♂
N41.2	Abscess of prostate ♂
N41.3	Prostatocystitis ♂
N41.4	Granulomatous prostatitis ♂
N41.8	Other inflammatory diseases of prostate ♂
N42.1	Congestion and hemorrhage of prostate ♂
N42.30	Unspecified dysplasia of prostate ♂
N42.31	Prostatic intraepithelial neoplasia ♂
N42.32	Atypical small acinar proliferation of prostate ♂
N42.39	Other dysplasia of prostate ♂
N42.81	Prostatodynia syndrome ♂
N42.82	Prostatosis syndrome ♂
N42.83	Cyst of prostate ♂
N42.89	Other specified disorders of prostate ♂
N44.1	Cyst of tunica albuginea testis ♂
N44.2	Benign cyst of testis ♂
N44.8	Other noninflammatory disorders of the testis ♂
N50.3	Cyst of epididymis ♂
N50.89	Other specified disorders of the male genital organs ♂
N53.12	Painful ejaculation ♂
N53.8	Other male sexual dysfunction ♂
N53.9	Unspecified male sexual dysfunction ♂
R97.20	Elevated prostate specific antigen [PSA] ♂
R97.21	Rising PSA following treatment for malignant neoplasm of prostate ♂

CCI Edits

Refer to Appendix A for CCI edits.

Facility RVUs ▯

Code	Work	PE Facility	MP	Total Facility
55700	2.50	0.99	0.29	3.78
55705	4.61	2.60	0.56	7.77

Non-facility RVUs ▯

Code	Work	PE Non-Facility	MP	Total Non-Facility
55700	2.50	4.43	0.29	7.22
55705	4.61	2.60	0.56	7.77

Modifiers (PAR) ▯

Code	Mod 50	Mod 51	Mod 62	Mod 66	Mod 80
55700	0	2	0	0	1
55705	0	2	1	0	1

Global Period

Code	Days
55700	000
55705	010

● New ▲ Revised ✚ Add On ⊘Modifier 51 Exempt ★Telemedicine ▯ CPT QuickRef ⁄FDA Pending ⇄ Laterality ❼ Seventh Character ♂Male ♀Female

55706

55706 Biopsies, prostate, needle, transperineal, stereotactic template guided saturation sampling, including imaging guidance

(Do not report 55706 in conjunction with 55700)

AMA *CPT® Assistant* □

55706: Nov 10: 5

Plain English Description

A transperineal needle biopsy of the prostate is performed by stereotactic template-guided saturation sampling, including imaging guidance. Using transrectal ultrasound (TRUS), a stereotactic template, and a stabilizing device, the prostate is positioned on the implant grid. The implant grid is divided into six or more sections. A linear probe with an attachment for needle guidance is used to obtain the tissue samples. Tissue cores are then obtained from each section and placed in separate specimen jars corresponding to the sections. As many as 60 tissue cores may be obtained and are sent to the laboratory for separately reportable pathology analysis.

Prostate biopsies, transperineal needle, stereotactic template

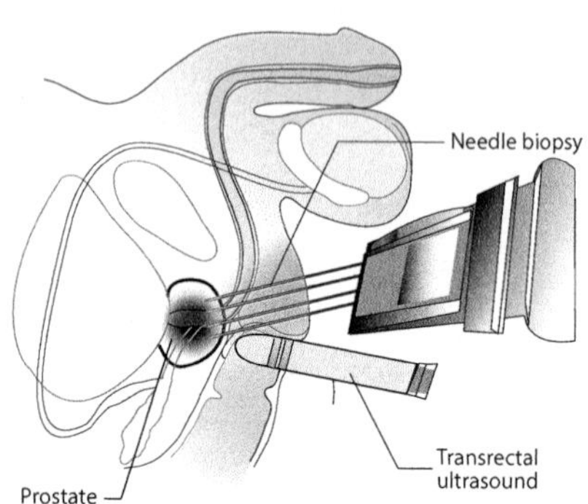

ICD-10-CM Diagnostic Codes

C61	Malignant neoplasm of prostate ♂
C79.82	Secondary malignant neoplasm of genital organs
D07.5	Carcinoma in situ of prostate ♂
D40.0	Neoplasm of uncertain behavior of prostate ♂

CCI Edits

Refer to Appendix A for CCI edits.

Facility RVUs □

Code	Work	PE Facility	MP	Total Facility
55706	6.28	4.00	0.73	11.01

Non-facility RVUs □

Code	Work	PE Non-Facility	MP	Total Non-Facility
55706	6.28	4.00	0.73	11.01

Modifiers (PAR) □

Code	Mod 50	Mod 51	Mod 62	Mod 66	Mod 80
55706	0	2	1	0	2

Global Period

Code	Days
55706	010

55720-55725

55720 Prostatotomy, external drainage of prostatic abscess, any approach; simple

55725 Prostatotomy, external drainage of prostatic abscess, any approach; complicated

(For transurethral drainage, use 52700)

Plain English Description

A prostatotomy by any approach is performed to drain an abscess in the prostate gland. In 55720, a simple prostatotomy with drainage is performed. The procedure may be performed using separately reportable transrectal ultrasound (TRUS) guidance. If TRUS guidance is used, the TRUS probe is inserted into the rectum. A small incision is made in the perineum and a biopsy needle and guide inserted and advanced under TRUS guidance into the abscess pocket in the prostate. Pus is aspirated. The needle is removed and a pigtail catheter is inserted into the abscess pocket to allow continued drainage. The catheter is secured and the perineum is dressed. In 55725, a complicated prostatotomy is performed. Using a perineal approach, an inverted-U incision is made in the mid-perineum above the anal opening. The incision is carried down to the ischiorectal fossa incising each side of the central tendon, which is then divided and cut. The fibrous confluence is exposed and dissected posterior to the raphe of the bulbospongiosus muscle, which is divided to expose the rectourethralis and levator ani muscles. With careful dissection around the rectum, the rectourethralis muscle is divided and the fibrous confluence elevated with forceps to expose the rectum and urethra at the apex of the prostate. The prostate is exposed and an incision is made in the prostate over the abscess pocket. The abscess pocket is opened and drained. Any loculations are broken up using blunt dissection. The abscess pocket is flushed with antibiotic solution, a drain is placed, and the incision is closed around the drain.

Prostatotomy, external drainage of prostatic abscess

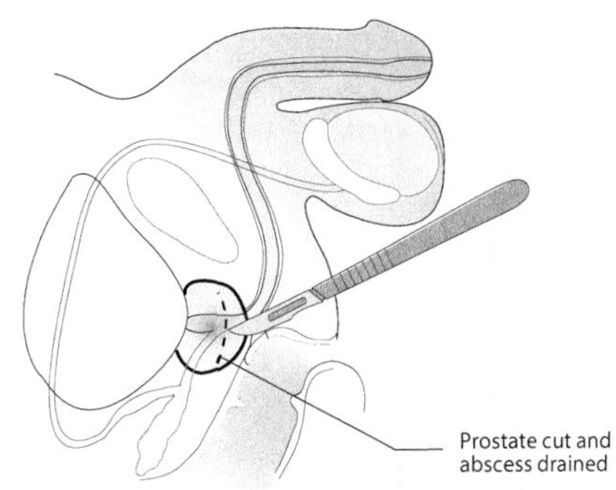

Any approach, simple (55720); any approach, complicated (55725)

ICD-10-CM Diagnostic Codes

A54.22	Gonococcal prostatitis ♂
A59.02	Trichomonal prostatitis ♂
N41.0	Acute prostatitis ♂
N41.1	Chronic prostatitis ♂
N41.2	Abscess of prostate ♂
N41.4	Granulomatous prostatitis ♂
N41.8	Other inflammatory diseases of prostate ♂
N41.9	Inflammatory disease of prostate, unspecified ♂

CCI Edits

Refer to Appendix A for CCI edits.

Facility RVUs ☐

Code	Work	PE Facility	MP	Total Facility
55720	7.73	4.61	0.93	13.27
55725	10.05	6.20	1.20	17.45

Non-facility RVUs ☐

Code	Work	PE Non-Facility	MP	Total Non-Facility
55720	7.73	4.61	0.93	13.27
55725	10.05	6.20	1.20	17.45

Modifiers (PAR) ☐

Code	Mod 50	Mod 51	Mod 62	Mod 66	Mod 80
55720	0	2	1	0	2
55725	0	2	1	0	2

Global Period

Code	Days
55720	090
55725	090

55801

55801 Prostatectomy, perineal, subtotal (including control of postoperative bleeding, vasectomy, meatotomy, urethral calibration and/or dilation, and internal urethrotomy)

AMA Coding Notes

Excision Procedures on the Prostate

(For transurethral removal of prostate, see 52601-52640)

(For transurethral destruction of prostate, see 53850-53852)

(For limited pelvic lymphadenectomy for staging [separate procedure], use 38562)

(For independent node dissection, see 38770-38780)

AMA *CPT® Assistant* ▯

55801: Jun 03: 6-7

Plain English Description

The physician enters the pubic cavity from the area between the rectum and the genitals and removes the prostate gland. The physician leaves in the seminal vesicles. During the procedure, the physician may control bleeding tissue, remove a section of the vas deferens, enlarge the opening of the urethra in the penis, increase or reduce the diameter of the urethra, and remove a section of the urethra.

Prostatectomy, perineal, subtotal

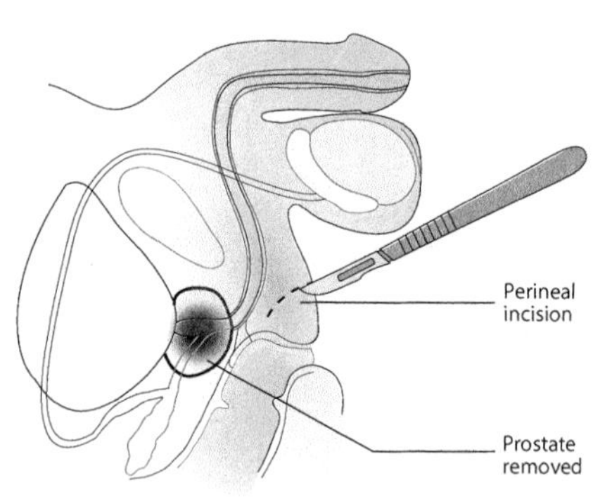

ICD-10-CM Diagnostic Codes

C61	Malignant neoplasm of prostate ♂
C79.82	Secondary malignant neoplasm of genital organs
D07.5	Carcinoma in situ of prostate ♂
D29.1	Benign neoplasm of prostate ♂
D40.0	Neoplasm of uncertain behavior of prostate ♂
N40.0	Benign prostatic hyperplasia without lower urinary tract symptoms ♂
N40.1	Benign prostatic hyperplasia with lower urinary tract symptoms ♂
N40.2	Nodular prostate without lower urinary tract symptoms ♂
N40.3	Nodular prostate with lower urinary tract symptoms ♂
N41.3	Prostatocystitis ♂
N41.4	Granulomatous prostatitis ♂
N41.8	Other inflammatory diseases of prostate ♂
N42.1	Congestion and hemorrhage of prostate ♂
N42.30	Unspecified dysplasia of prostate ♂
N42.31	Prostatic intraepithelial neoplasia ♂
N42.32	Atypical small acinar proliferation of prostate ♂
N42.39	Other dysplasia of prostate ♂
N42.8	Other specified disorders of prostate
N42.81	Prostatodynia syndrome ♂
N42.83	Cyst of prostate ♂
N42.89	Other specified disorders of prostate ♂
R97.21	Rising PSA following treatment for malignant neoplasm of prostate ♂
Z15.03	Genetic susceptibility to malignant neoplasm of prostate ♂
Z80.42	Family history of malignant neoplasm of prostate

CCI Edits

Refer to Appendix A for CCI edits.

Pub 100

55801: Pub 100-03, 1, 230.3

Facility RVUs ▯

Code	Work	PE Facility	MP	Total Facility
55801	19.80	9.85	2.34	31.99

Non-facility RVUs ▯

Code	Work	PE Non-Facility	MP	Total Non-Facility
55801	19.80	9.85	2.34	31.99

Modifiers (PAR) ▯

Code	Mod 50	Mod 51	Mod 62	Mod 66	Mod 80
55801	0	2	1	0	2

Global Period

Code	Days
55801	090

55810-55815

55810 Prostatectomy, perineal radical

55812 Prostatectomy, perineal radical; with lymph node biopsy(s) (limited pelvic lymphadenectomy)

55815 Prostatectomy, perineal radical; with bilateral pelvic lymphadenectomy, including external iliac, hypogastric and obturator nodes

(If 55815 is carried out on separate days, use 38770 with modifier 50 and 55810)

AMA Coding Notes

Excision Procedures on the Prostate

(For transurethral removal of prostate, see 52601-52640)

(For transurethral destruction of prostate, see 53850-53852)

(For limited pelvic lymphadenectomy for staging [separate procedure], use 38562)

(For independent node dissection, see 38770-38780)

AMA *CPT® Assistant*

55810: Jun 03: 7

Plain English Description

The prostate gland and seminal vesicles are removed through an incision in the perineum. If lymphadenectomy is needed, it is performed first. The lower abdomen is incised and, without opening the peritoneum, the pelvic lymph nodes on one side are explored. Taking care to preserve the genitofemoral nerve and psoas muscle, fatty tissue is stripped from the mid-portion of the common iliac vessel and along the external iliac vessel. Iliac, hypogastric, and obturator nodes are biopsied and sent for separately reportable frozen section. If the malignancy has spread to these lymph nodes, they are excised. The procedure may be repeated on the opposite side. Radical perineal prostatectomy is then performed. An inverted-U incision is made in the perineum above the anal opening. The incision is carried down to the ischiorectal fossa and each side of the central tendon divided. The fibrous confluence is exposed and dissected posterior to the raphe of the bulbospongiosus muscle, which is divided to expose the rectourethralis and levator ani muscles. The rectourethralis muscle is divided and the rectum and urethra exposed. The rectum is mobilized posteriorly from the prostatic apex and the Denonvilliers fascia is exposed. The prostate gland is mobilized toward the perineum. The rectum is mobilized away from the prostate. A transverse incision is made through the Denonvilliers fascia between the medial aspects of the vas deferens and seminal vesicles. Each vas deferens is freed from surrounding tissue, ligated, and divided. The seminal vesicles are retracted medially and the lateral aspects exposed, ligated, and divided. The base of the prostate is exposed. In a nerve sparing approach, the Denonvilliers aponeurosis is incised and the cavernosal nerve bundles separated from the prostate. In a non-nerve-sparing approach, the periprostatic tissue is dissected from the levator muscles and excised with the prostate. For both nerve-sparing and non-nerve-sparing procedures, the puboprostatic ligaments anterior to the prostate are divided. Prostate attachments anterior to the bladder neck are exposed and divided. A plane of dissection is created between the bladder neck and the base of the prostate. The urethra is exposed at its junction with the prostate. The urethra is dissected from the surrounding tissue and divided 1 cm below the bladder neck. The prostate is removed. The urethral ends are anastomosed. If the bladder neck cannot be preserved, it is excised and the bladder opening reduced in size to allow anastomosis of the urethra. A catheter is placed transurethrally into the bladder and the bladder is irrigated to remove clots. The perineal incision is closed. Use 55810 for radical perineal prostatectomy without lymph node biopsy or excision. Use 55812 when the procedure is performed with lymph node biopsy or limited pelvic lymphadenectomy. Use 55815 when the procedure is performed with bilateral excision of pelvic lymph nodes, including excision of the external iliac, hypogastric, and obturator nodes.

Radical perineal prostatectomy

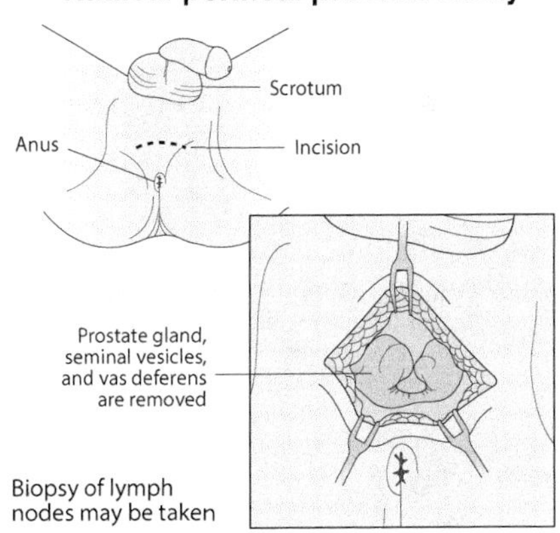

ICD-10-CM Diagnostic Codes

C61	Malignant neoplasm of prostate ♂
C77.5	Secondary and unspecified malignant neoplasm of intrapelvic lymph nodes
C79.82	Secondary malignant neoplasm of genital organs
D07.5	Carcinoma in situ of prostate ♂
D40.0	Neoplasm of uncertain behavior of prostate ♂
N40.1	Benign prostatic hyperplasia with lower urinary tract symptoms ♂
N40.3	Nodular prostate with lower urinary tract symptoms ♂
N42.1	Congestion and hemorrhage of prostate ♂
N42.30	Unspecified dysplasia of prostate ♂
N42.31	Prostatic intraepithelial neoplasia ♂
N42.32	Atypical small acinar proliferation of prostate ♂
N42.39	Other dysplasia of prostate ♂
N42.81	Prostatodynia syndrome ♂
N42.82	Prostatosis syndrome ♂
N42.89	Other specified disorders of prostate ♂

CCI Edits

Refer to Appendix A for CCI edits.

Facility RVUs

Code	Work	PE Facility	MP	Total Facility
55810	24.29	10.97	2.90	38.16
55812	29.89	13.45	3.56	46.90
55815	32.95	14.48	3.92	51.35

Non-facility RVUs

Code	Work	PE Non-Facility	MP	Total Non-Facility
55810	24.29	10.97	2.90	38.16
55812	29.89	13.45	3.56	46.90
55815	32.95	14.48	3.92	51.35

Modifiers (PAR)

Code	Mod 50	Mod 51	Mod 62	Mod 66	Mod 80
55810	0	2	1	0	2
55812	0	2	1	0	2
55815	2	2	1	0	2

Global Period

Code	Days
55810	090
55812	090
55815	090

55821

55821 Prostatectomy (including control of postoperative bleeding, vasectomy, meatotomy, urethral calibration and/or dilation, and internal urethrotomy); suprapubic, subtotal, 1 or 2 stages

AMA Coding Notes

Excision Procedures on the Prostate

(For transurethral removal of prostate, see 52601-52640)

(For transurethral destruction of prostate, see 53850-53852)

(For limited pelvic lymphadenectomy for staging [separate procedure], use 38562)

(For independent node dissection, see 38770-38780)

AMA *CPT® Assistant* ▢

55821: Jun 03: 6

Plain English Description

The physician enters the pubic cavity from above the lower abdomen and removes the prostate gland. The physician leaves in the seminal vesicles. During the procedure, the physician may control bleeding tissue, remove a section of the vas deferens, enlarge the opening of the urethra in the penis, increase or reduce the diameter of the urethra, and remove a section of the urethra. The procedure can be performed in one or two stages.

Prostatectomy, suprapubic, subtotal, 1 or 2 stages

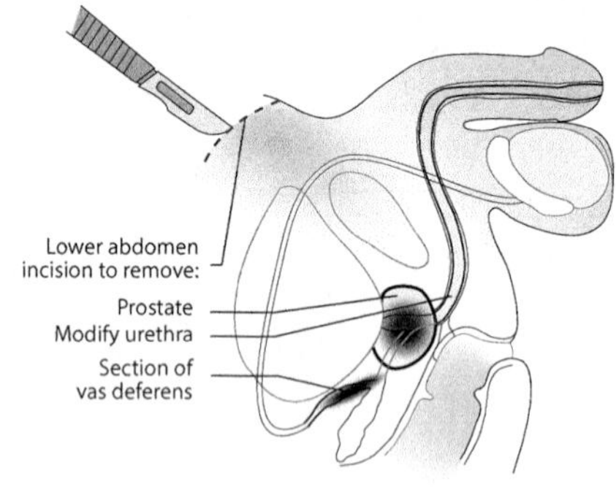

ICD-10-CM Diagnostic Codes

D07.5	Carcinoma in situ of prostate ♂
D29.1	Benign neoplasm of prostate ♂
D40.0	Neoplasm of uncertain behavior of prostate ♂
D49.5	Neoplasm of unspecified behavior of other genitourinary organs
N40.0	Benign prostatic hyperplasia without lower urinary tract symptoms ♂
N40.1	Benign prostatic hyperplasia with lower urinary tract symptoms ♂
N40.2	Nodular prostate without lower urinary tract symptoms ♂
N40.3	Nodular prostate with lower urinary tract symptoms ♂
N41.2	Abscess of prostate ♂
N41.3	Prostatocystitis ♂
N41.4	Granulomatous prostatitis ♂
N41.8	Other inflammatory diseases of prostate ♂
N42.1	Congestion and hemorrhage of prostate ♂
N42.30	Unspecified dysplasia of prostate ♂
N42.31	Prostatic intraepithelial neoplasia ♂
N42.32	Atypical small acinar proliferation of prostate ♂
N42.39	Other dysplasia of prostate ♂
N42.81	Prostatodynia syndrome ♂
N42.82	Prostatosis syndrome ♂
N42.83	Cyst of prostate ♂
N42.89	Other specified disorders of prostate ♂
Z80.42	Family history of malignant neoplasm of prostate

CCI Edits

Refer to Appendix A for CCI edits.

Pub 100

55821: Pub 100-03, 1, 230.3

Facility RVUs ▢

Code	Work	PE Facility	MP	Total Facility
55821	15.76	7.89	1.86	25.51

Non-facility RVUs ▢

Code	Work	PE Non-Facility	MP	Total Non-Facility
55821	15.76	7.89	1.86	25.51

Modifiers (PAR) ▢

Code	Mod 50	Mod 51	Mod 62	Mod 66	Mod 80
55821	0	2	1	0	2

Global Period

Code	Days
55821	090

55831

55831 Prostatectomy (including control of postoperative bleeding, vasectomy, meatotomy, urethral calibration and/or dilation, and internal urethrotomy); retropubic, subtotal

AMA Coding Notes

Excision Procedures on the Prostate

(For transurethral removal of prostate, see 52601-52640)

(For transurethral destruction of prostate, see 53850-53852)

(For limited pelvic lymphadenectomy for staging [separate procedure], use 38562)

(For independent node dissection, see 38770-38780)

AMA *CPT® Assistant* ☐

55831: Jun 03: 7

Plain English Description

The physician enters the pubic cavity from the lower abdomen and removes the prostate gland. The physician leaves in the seminal vesicles. During the procedure, the physician may control bleeding tissue, remove a section of the vas deferens, enlarge the opening of the urethra in the penis, increase or reduce the diameter of the urethra, and remove a section of the urethra.

Prostatectomy, retropubic, subtotal

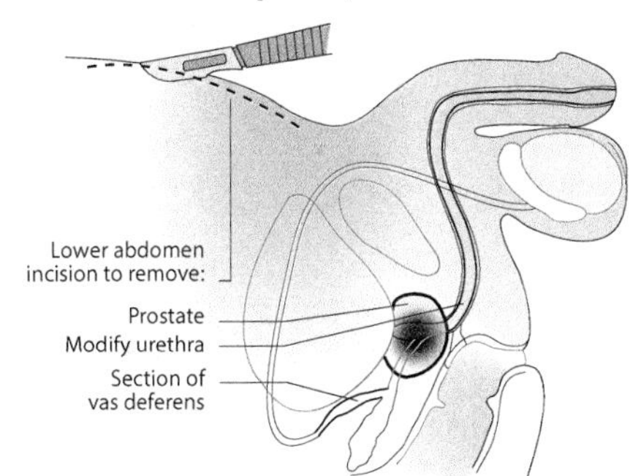

ICD-10-CM Diagnostic Codes

C61	Malignant neoplasm of prostate ♂
C79.82	Secondary malignant neoplasm of genital organs
D07.5	Carcinoma in situ of prostate ♂
D29.1	Benign neoplasm of prostate ♂
D40.0	Neoplasm of uncertain behavior of prostate ♂
N40.0	Benign prostatic hyperplasia without lower urinary tract symptoms ♂
N40.1	Benign prostatic hyperplasia with lower urinary tract symptoms ♂
N40.2	Nodular prostate without lower urinary tract symptoms ♂
N40.3	Nodular prostate with lower urinary tract symptoms ♂
N41.1	Chronic prostatitis ♂
N41.2	Abscess of prostate ♂
N41.3	Prostatocystitis ♂
N41.4	Granulomatous prostatitis ♂
N41.8	Other inflammatory diseases of prostate ♂
N42.1	Congestion and hemorrhage of prostate ♂
N42.30	Unspecified dysplasia of prostate ♂
N42.31	Prostatic intraepithelial neoplasia ♂
N42.32	Atypical small acinar proliferation of prostate ♂
N42.39	Other dysplasia of prostate ♂
N42.81	Prostatodynia syndrome ♂
N42.82	Prostatosis syndrome ♂
N42.83	Cyst of prostate ♂
N42.89	Other specified disorders of prostate ♂
Z80.42	Family history of malignant neoplasm of prostate

CCI Edits

Refer to Appendix A for CCI edits.

Pub 100

55831: Pub 100-03, 1, 230.3

Facility RVUs ☐

Code	Work	PE Facility	MP	Total Facility
55831	17.19	8.38	2.07	27.64

Non-facility RVUs ☐

Code	Work	PE Non-Facility	MP	Total Non-Facility
55831	17.19	8.38	2.07	27.64

Modifiers (PAR) ☐

Code	Mod 50	Mod 51	Mod 62	Mod 66	Mod 80
55831	0	2	1	0	2

Global Period

Code	Days
55831	090

55840-55845

55840 Prostatectomy, retropubic radical, with or without nerve sparing

55842 Prostatectomy, retropubic radical, with or without nerve sparing; with lymph node biopsy(s) (limited pelvic lymphadenectomy)

55845 Prostatectomy, retropubic radical, with or without nerve sparing; with bilateral pelvic lymphadenectomy, including external iliac, hypogastric, and obturator nodes

(If 55845 is carried out on separate days, use 38770 with modifier 50 and 55840)

(For laparoscopic retropubic radical prostatectomy, use 55866)

AMA Coding Notes

Excision Procedures on the Prostate

(For transurethral removal of prostate, see 52601-52640)

(For transurethral destruction of prostate, see 53850-53852)

(For limited pelvic lymphadenectomy for staging [separate procedure], use 38562)

(For independent node dissection, see 38770-38780)

AMA *CPT® Assistant*

55840: Jun 03: 8
55842: Jun 03: 8
55845: Jun 03: 8

Plain English Description

The lower abdomen is incised in the midline. If lymphadenectomy is needed, it is performed first. Without opening the peritoneum the pelvic lymph nodes on one side are explored. Taking care to preserve the genitofemoral nerve and psoas muscle, fatty tissue is stripped from the mid-portion of the common iliac vessel and along the external iliac vessel. Iliac, hypogastric, and obturator nodes are biopsied and sent for separately reportable pathology frozen section. If the malignancy has spread to these lymph nodes, they are excised. The procedure may be repeated on the opposite side. The prostate is approached by first removing retropubic fat. The superficial branch of the dorsal venous complex is isolated and cauterized. The prostatic fascia and dorsal venous complex are exposed. The dorsal venous complex is ligated and divided. The prostatic fascia is incised and the neurovascular bundles on either side of the prostate are identified, mobilized posteriorly, and protected. Alternatively, if the malignancy has spread to surrounding tissues, the neurovascular complex is excised. Using finger dissection the Denonvilliers fascia covering the posterior prostate and anterior rectum is separated. Finger dissection continues to the prostato-apical junction bilaterally. The lateral prostatic fascia on one side is incised. The membranous urethra is exposed and divided. The prostate is then completely mobilized while ligating vascular pedicles close to the prostate. The anterior layer of Denonvilliers fascia is divided and the ampullae of the vas deferens located, dissected off the medial aspect of the seminal vesicles and divided. The seminal vesicles are dissected free of the bladder base and posterior aspect of the bladder. The prostate is now free from all surrounding tissue and is removed en bloc. The bladder neck is repaired as needed. A sound is placed in the urethra and the bladder is anastomosed to the urethra. The surgical wound is closed in layers. Use 55840 for radical retropubic prostatectomy without lymph node biopsy or excision. Use 55842 when the procedure is performed with lymph node biopsy or limited pelvic lymphadenectomy. Use 55845 when the procedure is performed with bilateral pelvic lymphadenectomy, including the external iliac, hypogastric, and obturator nodes.

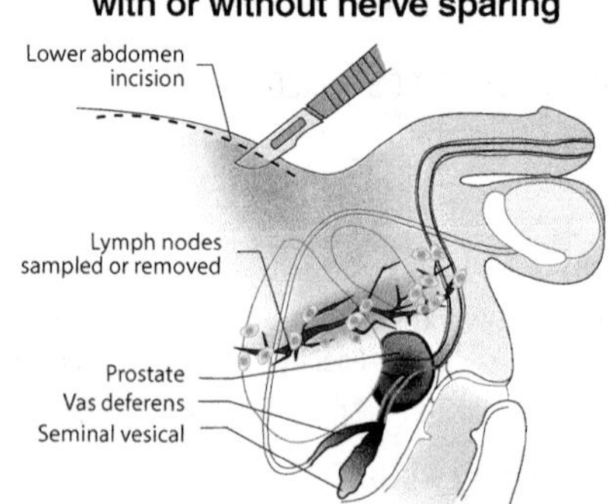

Prostatectomy (55840); with lymph node biopsy(ies) (55842); with bilateral pelvic lymphadenectomy (55845)

ICD-10-CM Diagnostic Codes

C61	Malignant neoplasm of prostate ♂
C79.82	Secondary malignant neoplasm of genital organs
D07.5	Carcinoma in situ of prostate ♂
D40.0	Neoplasm of uncertain behavior of prostate ♂
N41.1	Chronic prostatitis ♂
N41.4	Granulomatous prostatitis ♂
N41.8	Other inflammatory diseases of prostate ♂
N42.1	Congestion and hemorrhage of prostate ♂
N42.30	Unspecified dysplasia of prostate ♂
N42.31	Prostatic intraepithelial neoplasia ♂
N42.32	Atypical small acinar proliferation of prostate ♂
N42.39	Other dysplasia of prostate ♂
N42.81	Prostatodynia syndrome ♂
N42.82	Prostatosis syndrome ♂
N42.89	Other specified disorders of prostate ♂
Z80.42	Family history of malignant neoplasm of prostate

CCI Edits

Refer to Appendix A for CCI edits.

Facility RVUs

Code	Work	PE Facility	MP	Total Facility
55840	21.36	10.22	2.56	34.14
55842	21.36	10.23	2.56	34.15
55845	25.18	11.51	3.02	39.71

Non-facility RVUs

Code	Work	PE Non-Facility	MP	Total Non-Facility
55840	21.36	10.22	2.56	34.14
55842	21.36	10.23	2.56	34.15
55845	25.18	11.51	3.02	39.71

Modifiers (PAR)

Code	Mod 50	Mod 51	Mod 62	Mod 66	Mod 80
55840	0	2	1	0	2
55842	0	2	1	0	2
55845	2	2	1	0	2

Global Period

Code	Days
55840	090
55842	090
55845	090

● New ▲ Revised ✚ Add On ⊘Modifier 51 Exempt ★Telemedicine ▢ CPT QuickRef ⁄⁄FDA Pending ⇄ Laterality ➐ Seventh Character ♂Male ♀Female

55860-55865

55860 Exposure of prostate, any approach, for insertion of radioactive substance

(For application of interstitial radioelement, see 77770, 77771, 77772, 77778)

55862 Exposure of prostate, any approach, for insertion of radioactive substance; with lymph node biopsy(s) (limited pelvic lymphadenectomy)

55865 Exposure of prostate, any approach, for insertion of radioactive substance; with bilateral pelvic lymphadenectomy, including external iliac, hypogastric and obturator nodes

AMA Coding Notes

Excision Procedures on the Prostate

(For transurethral removal of prostate, see 52601-52640)

(For transurethral destruction of prostate, see 53850-53852)

(For limited pelvic lymphadenectomy for staging [separate procedure], use 38562)

(For independent node dissection, see 38770-38780)

Plain English Description

Surgical approach is used to expose the prostate for insertion of a radioactive substance for brachytherapy. This may include a retropubic or perineal incision. For a retropubic incision in the lower abdomen, the bladder is displaced to enter the space behind the pubic bone and reach the prostate. The physician may use a finger guide in the rectum to pass a hollow applicator needle into the prostate. When the needle is positioned in the target prostate tissue, radioactive seeds are introduced through the needle and implanted with the applicator. The needle is withdrawn and placed again in small millimeter increments and another seed is placed. The application process is repeated multiple times. In 55862, a limited pelvic lymphadenectomy is performed for lymph node biopsy, which usually removes unilateral obturator lymph node chain(s). In 55865, all lymph nodes on both sides are removed in an extended lymphadenectomy, which includes removal of all the nodes that run along the obturator fossa, external iliac vein, and hypogastric artery.

ICD-10-CM Diagnostic Codes

C61	Malignant neoplasm of prostate ♂
C77.5	Secondary and unspecified malignant neoplasm of intrapelvic lymph nodes
C79.82	Secondary malignant neoplasm of genital organs
D07.5	Carcinoma in situ of prostate ♂
D40.0	Neoplasm of uncertain behavior of prostate ♂
Z80.42	Family history of malignant neoplasm of prostate

CCI Edits

Refer to Appendix A for CCI edits.

Facility RVUs 🗆

Code	Work	PE Facility	MP	Total Facility
55860	15.84	7.86	1.87	25.57
55862	20.04	9.57	2.38	31.99
55865	24.57	11.48	2.93	38.98

Non-facility RVUs 🗆

Code	Work	PE Non-Facility	MP	Total Non-Facility
55860	15.84	7.86	1.87	25.57
55862	20.04	9.57	2.38	31.99
55865	24.57	11.48	2.93	38.98

Modifiers (PAR) 🗆

Code	Mod 50	Mod 51	Mod 62	Mod 66	Mod 80
55860	0	2	1	0	1
55862	0	2	1	0	2
55865	2	2	1	0	2

Global Period

Code	Days
55860	090
55862	090
55865	090

55866

55866 Laparoscopy, surgical prostatectomy, retropubic radical, including nerve sparing, includes robotic assistance, when performed

(For open procedure, use 55840)

AMA Coding Guideline

Laparoscopic Procedures on the Prostate

Surgical laparoscopy always includes diagnostic laparoscopy. To report a diagnostic laparoscopy (peritoneoscopy) (separate procedure), use 49320.

AMA *CPT® Assistant* ▢

55866: Jun 03: 8, Mar 12: 10

Plain English Description

Laparoscopic prostatectomy may be performed using either a transperitoneal or extraperitoneal approach. If a transperitoneal approach is used, a periumbilical incision is made for the initial laparoscopic port. Pneumoperitoneum is established. A conventional or robotic laparoscope is then inserted through the infraumbilical port into the peritoneum and the abdomen is inspected. Additional portal incisions are made for introduction of surgical instruments. An incision is made in the peritoneal fold between the rectum and bladder and the seminal vesicles are dissected and then retracted to allow exposure of Denonvilliers aponeurosis. The aponeurosis is incised and dissection continues to the rectourethral muscle, separating the prostate from the rectum. The peritoneum is incised and the space of Retzius is entered, resulting in the bladder falling posteriorly. The endopelvic fascia is incised and the levator muscle is pushed out of the way so that the prostate gland can be resected. The dorsal vein is ligated. The bladder neck is incised. The lateral pedicles are dissected. The urethra is transected and the prostate is removed along with the seminal vesicles. The urethra is re-anastomosed to the bladder neck. A drain is placed; the laparoscope and surgical instruments are removed; and portal incisions are closed. If an extraperitoneal approach is used, a small incision is made, the preperitoneum is insufflated, and the space of Retzius is developed using blunt dissection until the pubic symphysis is reached. The retropubic space is then further developed by placing a port in the midline above the symphysis and extraperitoneal robotic instruments through additional right and left ports. The procedure then continues as described above.

Laparoscopy, surgical prostatectomy, retropubic radical, including nerve sparing

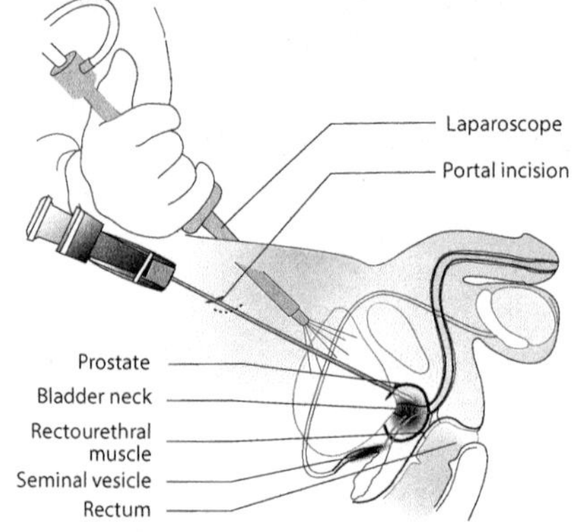

ICD-10-CM Diagnostic Codes

C61	Malignant neoplasm of prostate ♂
C79.82	Secondary malignant neoplasm of genital organs
D07	Carcinoma in situ of other and unspecified genital organs
D07.5	Carcinoma in situ of prostate ♂
D40.0	Neoplasm of uncertain behavior of prostate ♂
N40.1	Benign prostatic hyperplasia with lower urinary tract symptoms ♂
N40.3	Nodular prostate with lower urinary tract symptoms ♂
N41.1	Chronic prostatitis ♂
N41.4	Granulomatous prostatitis ♂
N41.8	Other inflammatory diseases of prostate ♂
N42.1	Congestion and hemorrhage of prostate ♂
N42.30	Unspecified dysplasia of prostate ♂
N42.31	Prostatic intraepithelial neoplasia ♂
N42.32	Atypical small acinar proliferation of prostate ♂
N42.39	Other dysplasia of prostate ♂
N42.8	Other specified disorders of prostate
N42.81	Prostatodynia syndrome ♂
N42.82	Prostatosis syndrome ♂
N42.89	Other specified disorders of prostate ♂
Z80.42	Family history of malignant neoplasm of prostate

CCI Edits

Refer to Appendix A for CCI edits.

Facility RVUs ▢

Code	Work	PE Facility	MP	Total Facility
55866	26.80	12.02	3.22	42.04

Non-facility RVUs ▢

Code	Work	PE Non-Facility	MP	Total Non-Facility
55866	26.80	12.02	3.22	42.04

Modifiers (PAR) ▢

Code	Mod 50	Mod 51	Mod 62	Mod 66	Mod 80
55866	0	2	1	0	2

Global Period

Code	Days
55866	090

● New ▲ Revised ✚ Add On ⊘Modifier 51 Exempt ★Telemedicine ▢ CPT QuickRef ✗FDA Pending ⇄ Laterality ❼ Seventh Character ♂Male ♀Female

55870

55870 Electroejaculation

AMA Coding Notes

Other Procedures on the Prostate

(For artificial insemination, see 58321, 58322)

Plain English Description

Electroejaculation may be used to obtain motile sperm from men with neurological impairments due to spinal cord injury, demyelinating neuropathies, diabetes, or pelvic/spinal surgeries. The bladder is emptied using a catheter and a lubricant such as simulated human tubal fluid/plasminate may be instilled. A digital rectal exam and/or anoscopy is performed to locate the prostate. A rectal probe is inserted and positioned against the prostate. Electrical energy is delivered through the probe at increasing frequency and amplitude until successful ejaculation is achieved. The ejaculate is collected into a specimen container and the bladder may be catheterized again to collect retrograde ejaculate. The probe is removed and the rectum may be examined again using anoscopy to detect any thermal or other injury from the procedure.

Electroejaculation

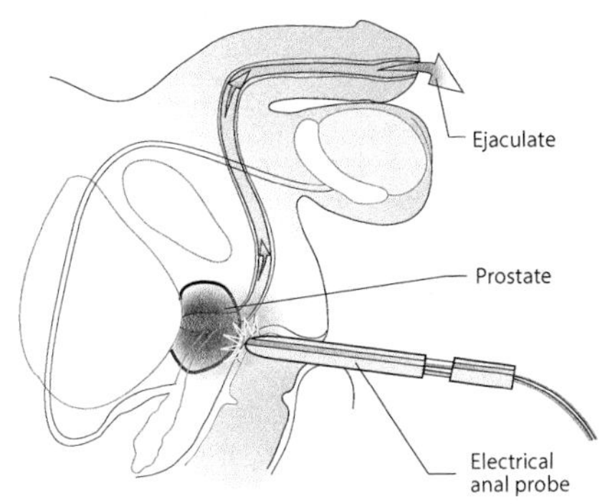

ICD-10-CM Diagnostic Codes

N53.11	Retarded ejaculation ♂
N53.13	Anejaculatory orgasm ♂
N53.19	Other ejaculatory dysfunction ♂
Z31.84	Encounter for fertility preservation procedure

CCI Edits

Refer to Appendix A for CCI edits.

Facility RVUs

Code	Work	PE Facility	MP	Total Facility
55870	2.58	1.23	0.31	4.12

Non-facility RVUs

Code	Work	PE Non-Facility	MP	Total Non-Facility
55870	2.58	2.27	0.31	5.16

Modifiers (PAR)

Code	Mod 50	Mod 51	Mod 62	Mod 66	Mod 80
55870	0	2	1	0	1

Global Period

Code	Days
55870	000

55873

55873 Cryosurgical ablation of the prostate (includes ultrasonic guidance and monitoring)

AMA Coding Notes

Other Procedures on the Prostate

(For artificial insemination, see 58321, 58322)

AMA *CPT® Assistant*

55873: Apr 01: 4, Sep 02: 9, Jun 03: 8, Feb 10: 7, Sep 15: 12, Sep 19: 11

Plain English Description

Cryosurgical ablation may be performed as an initial procedure to treat prostate cancer or it may be performed subsequent to a failed intervention such as failed radiation therapy. An ultrasound probe is placed in the rectum. Cryosurgical probes are then placed through the perineum into the prostate using real-time ultrasound imaging to monitor probe placement. The cryoprobes are then cooled to the appropriate temperature to create an ice ball. The growth of the ice ball is monitored with ultrasound. When it has reached the appropriate size, the cryoprobes are thawed. A second freeze/thaw cycle may be required. On occasion, a third freeze/thaw cycle is performed on a selected region such as the urethral diaphragm. This is accomplished by first removing posterior probes and then repeating the freeze/thaw cycle on the target region. The cryoprobes are thawed and removed. The cryoprobe sheath sites in the perineum are closed with sutures.

Cryosurgical ablation of the prostate (includes ultrasonic guidance and monitoring)

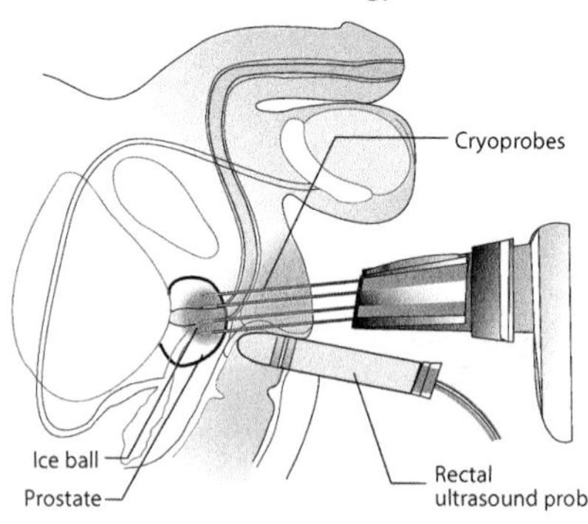

ICD-10-CM Diagnostic Codes

C61	Malignant neoplasm of prostate ♂
C79.82	Secondary malignant neoplasm of genital organs
D07.5	Carcinoma in situ of prostate ♂
D29.1	Benign neoplasm of prostate ♂
N40.1	Benign prostatic hyperplasia with lower urinary tract symptoms ♂
N40.3	Nodular prostate with lower urinary tract symptoms ♂
N41.1	Chronic prostatitis ♂
N41.4	Granulomatous prostatitis ♂
N41.8	Other inflammatory diseases of prostate ♂
N42.1	Congestion and hemorrhage of prostate ♂
N42.30	Unspecified dysplasia of prostate ♂
N42.31	Prostatic intraepithelial neoplasia ♂
N42.32	Atypical small acinar proliferation of prostate ♂
N42.39	Other dysplasia of prostate ♂
N42.8	Other specified disorders of prostate
N42.81	Prostatodynia syndrome ♂
N42.82	Prostatosis syndrome ♂
N42.83	Cyst of prostate ♂
N42.89	Other specified disorders of prostate ♂
R33.9	Retention of urine, unspecified
R39.14	Feeling of incomplete bladder emptying
R97.21	Rising PSA following treatment for malignant neoplasm of prostate ♂

CCI Edits

Refer to Appendix A for CCI edits.

Pub 100

55873: Pub 100-03, 1, 230.9, Pub 100-04, 32, 180-180.3

Facility RVUs

Code	Work	PE Facility	MP	Total Facility
55873	13.60	7.14	1.62	22.36

Non-facility RVUs

Code	Work	PE Non-Facility	MP	Total Non-Facility
55873	13.60	162.77	1.62	177.99

Modifiers (PAR)

Code	Mod 50	Mod 51	Mod 62	Mod 66	Mod 80
55873	0	2	0	0	1

Global Period

Code	Days
55873	090

55874

55874 Transperineal placement of biodegradable material, peri-prostatic, single or multiple injection(s), including image guidance, when performed

(Do not report 55874 in conjunction with 76942)

AMA Coding Notes

Other Procedures on the Prostate

(For artificial insemination, see 58321, 58322)

Plain English Description

Biodegradable spacer material may be placed between the anterior rectum and the prostate to protect healthy rectal tissue during radiotherapy for prostate cancer. The perineum is prepared and draped for injection. Using transrectal ultrasound for guidance, an 18-gauge needle is inserted through the perineum and advanced into the perirectal fat at the midgland of the prostate. Saline is injected to hydrodissect the space between Denonvilliers' fascia and the anterior wall of the rectum. The saline syringe is exchanged for a Y connector and syringe containing the biodegradable hydrogel liquid components. The needle position is verified and the biodegradable material is quickly injected solidifying into a hydrogel spacer within seconds. The biodegradable material will appear as a dark hypoechoic area on ultrasound. The needle is removed. The hydrogel begins decomposition back to a liquid form after approximately 3 months.

Transperineal placement of biodegradable material, peri-prostatic, single or multiple injection(s), including image guidance, when performed

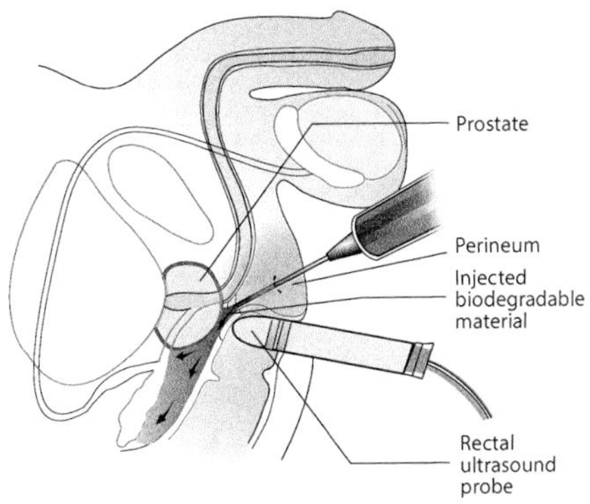

ICD-10-CM Diagnostic Codes

C61	Malignant neoplasm of prostate ♂
C79.82	Secondary malignant neoplasm of genital organs
D07.5	Carcinoma in situ of prostate ♂
D40.0	Neoplasm of uncertain behavior of prostate ♂
R97.20	Elevated prostate specific antigen [PSA] ♂
R97.21	Rising PSA following treatment for malignant neoplasm of prostate ♂

CCI Edits

Refer to Appendix A for CCI edits.

Facility RVUs

Code	Work	PE Facility	MP	Total Facility
55874	3.03	1.47	0.29	4.79

Non-facility RVUs

Code	Work	PE Non-Facility	MP	Total Non-Facility
55874	3.03	85.56	0.29	88.88

Modifiers (PAR)

Code	Mod 50	Mod 51	Mod 62	Mod 66	Mod 80
55874	0	2	1	1	1

Global Period

Code	Days
55874	000

CPT® Procedural Coding

55875

55875 Transperineal placement of needles or catheters into prostate for interstitial radioelement application, with or without cystoscopy

(For placement of needles or catheters into pelvic organs and/or genitalia [except prostate] for interstitial radioelement application, use 55920)

(For interstitial radioelement application, see 77770, 77771, 77772, 77778)

(For ultrasonic guidance for interstitial radioelement application, use 76965)

AMA Coding Notes

Other Procedures on the Prostate

(For artificial insemination, see 58321, 58322)

AMA *CPT® Assistant* ▯

55875: May 07: 1, Apr 09: 3

Plain English Description

Transperineal placement of needles or catheters into the prostate is performed for interstitial radioelement application, a form of brachytherapy. Radioactive isotopes are used for the slow delivery of internal radiation to the target tissue. Using fluoroscopy or ultrasonic guidance, encapsulated radioactive seeds are placed directly into prostate tissue through the perineum using applicators in the form of needles or tiny catheter tubes. The prostate will have been mapped out in a previous procedure to determine the exact locations and number of seeds to be placed. The tiny radioactive seeds contain isotopes such as iodine-125 or palladium-103 and are left in the prostate to deliver their dose of radiation steadily over a period of a few months before becoming inert. They do not need to be removed and cause no harm after becoming inert. By this method, the targeted tissue receives the radiation with minimal exposure to any surrounding tissue.

Transperineal placement of needles or catheters into prostate for interstitial radioelement application

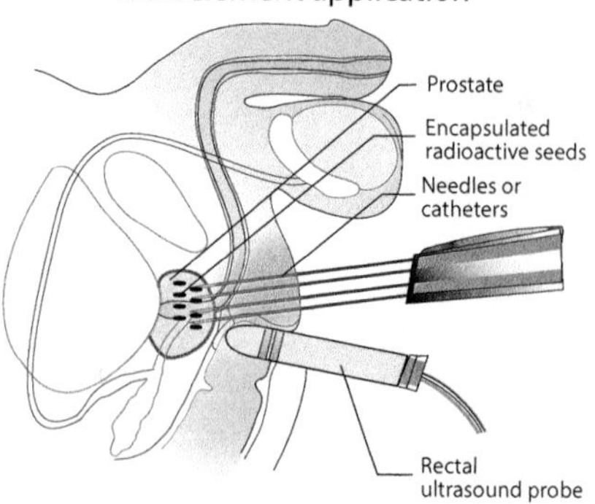

ICD-10-CM Diagnostic Codes

C61	Malignant neoplasm of prostate ♂
C79.82	Secondary malignant neoplasm of genital organs
D07.5	Carcinoma in situ of prostate ♂
D40.0	Neoplasm of uncertain behavior of prostate ♂

CCI Edits

Refer to Appendix A for CCI edits.

Facility RVUs ▯

Code	Work	PE Facility	MP	Total Facility
55875	13.46	7.83	1.40	22.69

Non-facility RVUs ▯

Code	Work	PE Non-Facility	MP	Total Non-Facility
55875	13.46	7.83	1.40	22.69

Modifiers (PAR) ▯

Code	Mod 50	Mod 51	Mod 62	Mod 66	Mod 80
55875	0	2	0	0	0

Global Period

Code	Days
55875	090

55876

55876 Placement of interstitial device(s) for radiation therapy guidance (eg, fiducial markers, dosimeter), prostate (via needle, any approach), single or multiple

(Report supply of device separately)

(For imaging guidance, see 76942, 77002, 77012, 77021)

AMA Coding Notes

Other Procedures on the Prostate

(For artificial insemination, see 58321, 58322)

AMA *CPT® Assistant* ☐

55876: May 07: 1, Oct 07: 1, Feb 10: 7, 12, Jun 16: 3

Plain English Description

Single or multiple interstitial devices for radiation therapy guidance, such as fiducial markers or dosimeter, are placed into the prostate using a needle by any approach. The prostate lies between the bladder and the rectum and its position changes in relation to the amount of rectal or bladder fullness. Since the rectum becomes less distended during a pelvic radiotherapy course, the prostate generally moves in a posterior, inferior direction. The change in position cannot be assessed with external landmarks. Since target motion is the major source of error in radiation treatment delivery, a safety margin is applied to ensure accurate, daily target localization for correct radiation. Radiopaque fiducial markers are one type of interstitial device placed in the prostate prior to starting therapy to be used with X-ray imaging to monitor and guide accuracy of the beam isocenter before delivery. Interstitial devices, such as fiducial markers, are placed prior to radiation therapy and are used to precisely locate the tumor or mass in the prostate. This allows radiation to be directed at the malignant tissue and helps prevent extensive radiation damage to surrounding tissues and structures. Fiducial markers are gold seeds that are implanted in or around a malignant tumor or the prostate. The procedure is performed using separately reportable ultrasound, fluoroscopic, CT, or MR guidance. A digital rectal exam is performed. If ultrasound guidance is used, the anus is dilated and a transrectal ultrasound probe inserted. The prostate is visualized and measured. A local anesthetic is administered to numb tissue along the planned insertion sites. Using radiological guidance, one or more gold seeds are passed through a needle that is passed through the ultrasound probe. The gold seeds are placed at strategic locations in and around the prostate or the prostate tumor. The positions of the gold seeds are checked radiographically to ensure that they are properly placed. The transrectal ultrasound probe is removed.

Placement of interstitial device(s) into the prostate for radiation therapy guidance

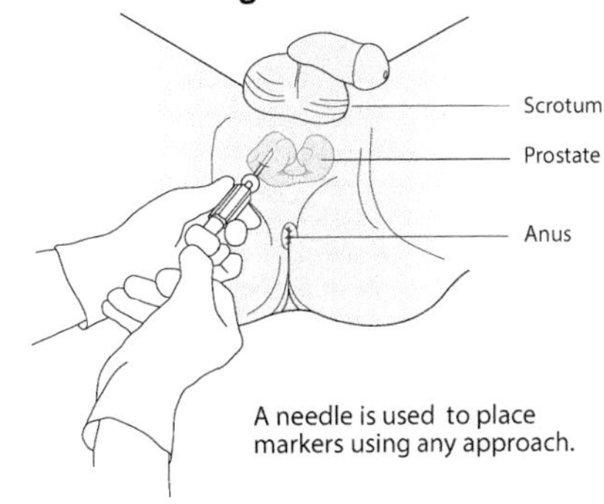
Scrotum
Prostate
Anus
A needle is used to place markers using any approach.

ICD-10-CM Diagnostic Codes

C61	Malignant neoplasm of prostate ♂
C79.82	Secondary malignant neoplasm of genital organs
D07.5	Carcinoma in situ of prostate ♂
D40.0	Neoplasm of uncertain behavior of prostate ♂

CCI Edits

Refer to Appendix A for CCI edits.

Facility RVUs ☐

Code	Work	PE Facility	MP	Total Facility
55876	1.73	1.04	0.19	2.96

Non-facility RVUs ☐

Code	Work	PE Non-Facility	MP	Total Non-Facility
55876	1.73	2.56	0.19	4.48

Modifiers (PAR) ☐

Code	Mod 50	Mod 51	Mod 62	Mod 66	Mod 80
55876	0	2	1	1	1

Global Period

Code	Days
55876	000

55880

55880 Ablation of malignant prostate tissue, transrectal, with high intensity-focused ultrasound (HIFU), including ultrasound guidance

AMA Coding Notes

Other Procedures on the Prostate

(For artificial insemination, see 58321, 58322)

Plain English Description

High intensity–focused ultrasound (HIFU) is a minimally invasive procedure that uses precisely focused sound wave energy to heat and destroy malignant prostate tissue. This procedure provides personalized, radiation-free treatment with minimal side effects and is appropriate for low to intermediate risk prostate cancer when the prostate is not too enlarged. Sound wave energy is delivered across the rectal wall using a transducer and focused at the target tissue within the prostate, which is often identified by MRI and confirmed with real time imaging guidance. With the sound waves aimed at the tissue, the temperature of the tissue at the target site is rapidly increased, destroying the cancerous cells within seconds and leaving healthy, surrounding tissue untouched, similar to focusing light through a magnifying glass. The process is repeated until the entire selected area, or even the entire gland, is destroyed. This is usually accomplished in a single therapy session.

ICD-10-CM Diagnostic Codes

C61	Malignant neoplasm of prostate ♂
D07.5	Carcinoma in situ of prostate ♂

CCI Edits

Refer to Appendix A for CCI edits.

Facility RVUs ▯

Code	Work	PE Facility	MP	Total Facility
55880	17.73	8.78	2.16	28.67

Non-facility RVUs ▯

Code	Work	PE Non-Facility	MP	Total Non-Facility
55880	17.73	8.78	2.16	28.67

Modifiers (PAR) ▯

Code	Mod 50	Mod 51	Mod 62	Mod 66	Mod 80
55880	0	2	0	0	1

Global Period

Code	Days
55880	090

55920

55920 Placement of needles or catheters into pelvic organs and/or genitalia (except prostate) for subsequent interstitial radioelement application

(For placement of needles or catheters into prostate, use 55875)

(For insertion of uterine tandems and/or vaginal ovoids for clinical brachytherapy, use 57155)

(For insertion of Heyman capsules for clinical brachytherapy, use 58346)

AMA *CPT® Assistant*

55920: Apr 09: 10

Plain English Description

Needles or catheters are placed in the pelvic organs and/or genitalia, excluding the prostate, for interstitial radioelement application. This code reports the placement of the needles or catheters only. The interstitial radioelement application (brachytherapy) is reported separately. This procedure varies depending on the exact site of the malignant neoplasm and male or female anatomy. A radiopaque urinary tract catheter with a steel ring to mark the urethral meatus may be inserted into the bladder. Tumor volume is assessed. The relationship of the tumor to normal structures is evaluated. A template device may be selected and prepared to orient the brachytherapy needles or catheters, and then sutured into place. Needles, catheters, and other devices, such as guide probes, guidewires, or a vaginal cylinder in females, are selected and prepared for placement. The number of needles or catheters and depth of insertion are adjusted depending on the extent and anatomic distribution of the tumor. The skin over the first insertion site is punctured and the brachytherapy needle or catheter is advanced to the selected site. Digital rectal palpation may be used to guide placement of needles and catheters in the posterior aspect of the genital region. This is repeated until all catheter tubes are in place.

Placement of needles or catheters into pelvic organs and/or genitalia (except prostate)

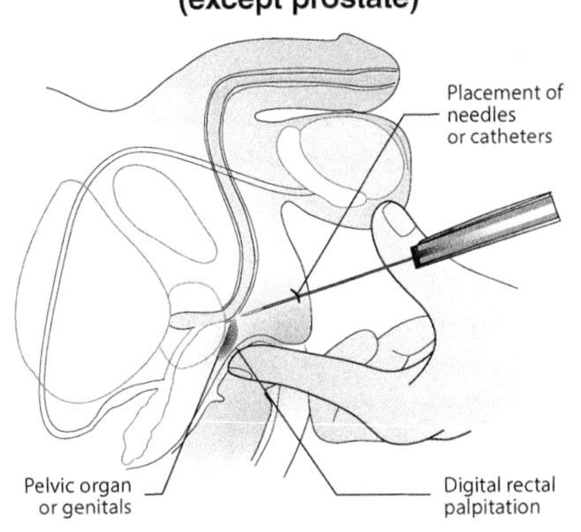

ICD-10-CM Diagnostic Codes

	C51.0	Malignant neoplasm of labium majus ♀
	C51.1	Malignant neoplasm of labium minus ♀
	C51.2	Malignant neoplasm of clitoris ♀
	C51.8	Malignant neoplasm of overlapping sites of vulva ♀
	C51.9	Malignant neoplasm of vulva, unspecified ♀
	C57.3	Malignant neoplasm of parametrium ♀
	C57.7	Malignant neoplasm of other specified female genital organs ♀
	C57.8	Malignant neoplasm of overlapping sites of female genital organs ♀
⇄	C62.01	Malignant neoplasm of undescended right testis ♂
⇄	C62.02	Malignant neoplasm of undescended left testis ♂
⇄	C62.11	Malignant neoplasm of descended right testis ♂
⇄	C62.12	Malignant neoplasm of descended left testis ♂
⇄	C62.91	Malignant neoplasm of right testis, unspecified whether descended or undescended ♂
⇄	C62.92	Malignant neoplasm of left testis, unspecified whether descended or undescended ♂
	C63.2	Malignant neoplasm of scrotum ♂
	C63.7	Malignant neoplasm of other specified male genital organs ♂
	C63.8	Malignant neoplasm of overlapping sites of male genital organs ♂
⇄	C64.1	Malignant neoplasm of right kidney, except renal pelvis
⇄	C64.2	Malignant neoplasm of left kidney, except renal pelvis
⇄	C65.1	Malignant neoplasm of right renal pelvis
⇄	C65.2	Malignant neoplasm of left renal pelvis
⇄	C66.1	Malignant neoplasm of right ureter
⇄	C66.2	Malignant neoplasm of left ureter
	C67.0	Malignant neoplasm of trigone of bladder
	C67.1	Malignant neoplasm of dome of bladder
	C67.2	Malignant neoplasm of lateral wall of bladder
	C67.3	Malignant neoplasm of anterior wall of bladder
	C67.4	Malignant neoplasm of posterior wall of bladder
	C67.5	Malignant neoplasm of bladder neck
	C67.6	Malignant neoplasm of ureteric orifice
	C67.7	Malignant neoplasm of urachus
	C67.8	Malignant neoplasm of overlapping sites of bladder
	C67.9	Malignant neoplasm of bladder, unspecified
	C68.0	Malignant neoplasm of urethra
	C68.1	Malignant neoplasm of paraurethral glands
	C68.8	Malignant neoplasm of overlapping sites of urinary organs
	C79.82	Secondary malignant neoplasm of genital organs

CCI Edits

Refer to Appendix A for CCI edits.

Facility RVUs

Code	Work	PE Facility	MP	Total Facility
55920	8.31	4.42	0.65	13.38

Non-facility RVUs

Code	Work	PE Non-Facility	MP	Total Non-Facility
55920	8.31	4.42	0.65	13.38

Modifiers (PAR)

Code	Mod 50	Mod 51	Mod 62	Mod 66	Mod 80
55920	0	2	0	0	0

Global Period

Code	Days
55920	000

57220

57220 Plastic operation on urethral sphincter, vaginal approach (eg, Kelly urethral plication)

AMA Coding Notes

Repair Procedures on the Vagina

(For urethral suspension, Marshall-Marchetti-Krantz type, abdominal approach, see 51840, 51841)

(For laparoscopic suspension, use 51990)

Surgical Procedures on the Female Genital System

(For pelvic laparotomy, use 49000)

(For excision or destruction of endometriomas, open method, see 49203-49205, 58957, 58958)

(For paracentesis, see 49082, 49083, 49084)

(For secondary closure of abdominal wall evisceration or disruption, use 49900)

(For fulguration or excision of lesions, laparoscopic approach, use 58662)

(For chemotherapy, see 96401-96549)

AMA *CPT® Assistant* ▢

57220: Winter 90: 7

Plain English Description

The physician performs a plastic operation on the urethral sphincter via a vaginal approach, such as a Kelly plication or urethral plication. This procedure is performed to treat stress incontinence and is accomplished using a plication procedure to reduce the diameter of the urethra. Using a vaginal approach, a tenaculum is placed on the cervix and a transverse incision made at the junction of the vaginal mucosa and cervix and carried down to the pubovesical cervical fascia. The vaginal mucosa is dissected off the pubovesical cervical fascia. The vaginal mucosa is opened in the midline to approximately 1 cm from the urethral meatus. Dissection continues until the bladder and urethra are separated from the vaginal mucosa and the urethral vesical angle has been identified. A mattress suture is placed in the wall of the urethra along the lateral margin approximately 1 cm below the urethral meatus. The urethral tissue is then inverted and plicated, and the suture tied. Additional plication sutures are placed along the urethra to a point approximately 2 cm beyond the urethral vesical angle. Overlying tissues are reapproximated and a Foley or suprapubic catheter placed.

Plastic operation on urethral sphincter, vaginal approach

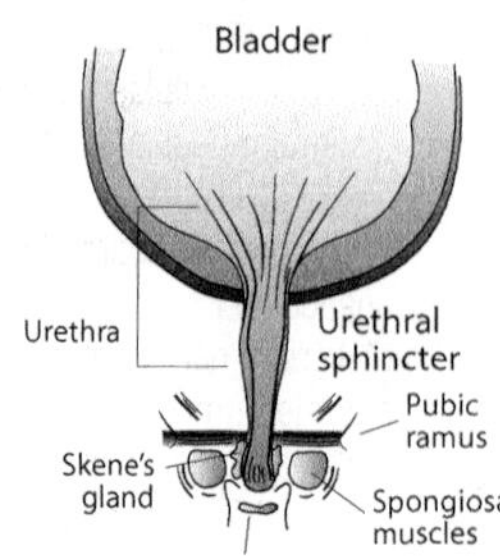

ICD-10-CM Diagnostic Codes

N36.41	Hypermobility of urethra
N36.42	Intrinsic sphincter deficiency (ISD)
N36.43	Combined hypermobility of urethra and intrinsic sphincter deficiency
N36.8	Other specified disorders of urethra
N39.3	Stress incontinence (female) (male)
N39.8	Other specified disorders of urinary system
N94.89	Other specified conditions associated with female genital organs and menstrual cycle ♀
R10.2	Pelvic and perineal pain
R33.8	Other retention of urine

CCI Edits

Refer to Appendix A for CCI edits.

Facility RVUs ▢

Code	Work	PE Facility	MP	Total Facility
57220	4.85	4.76	0.77	10.38

Non-facility RVUs ▢

Code	Work	PE Non-Facility	MP	Total Non-Facility
57220	4.85	4.76	0.77	10.38

Modifiers (PAR) ▢

Code	Mod 50	Mod 51	Mod 62	Mod 66	Mod 80
57220	0	2	1	0	2

Global Period

Code	Days
57220	090

57230

57230 Plastic repair of urethrocele

AMA Coding Notes

Repair Procedures on the Vagina

(For urethral suspension, Marshall-Marchetti-Krantz type, abdominal approach, see 51840, 51841)

(For laparoscopic suspension, use 51990)

Surgical Procedures on the Female Genital System

(For pelvic laparotomy, use 49000)

(For excision or destruction of endometriomas, open method, see 49203-49205, 58957, 58958)

(For paracentesis, see 49082, 49083, 49084)

(For secondary closure of abdominal wall evisceration or disruption, use 49900)

(For fulguration or excision of lesions, laparoscopic approach, use 58662)

(For chemotherapy, see 96401-96549)

AMA *CPT® Assistant* ◻

57230: Winter 90: 7

Plain English Description

The physician performs a plastic repair of a prolapsed urethra. Using a vaginal approach, a tenaculum is placed on the cervix and a transverse incision is made at the junction of the vaginal mucosa and cervix and carried down to the cervical fascia. The vaginal mucosa is dissected off the cervical fascia down to the level of the pubic bone and bladder. The vaginal mucosa is opened in the midline to approximately 1 cm from the urethral opening (meatus). Dissection continues until the urethra is separated from the vaginal mucosa and the junction between the urethra and bladder (urethrovesical angle) has been identified. Beginning immediately below the urethral meatus, plication sutures are placed in the fascia. By folding (plicating) the fascia, the prolapsed urethra is returned to normal position (reduced). The vaginal mucosa is then closed. A Foley or suprapubic catheter is placed.

Plastic repair of urethrocele

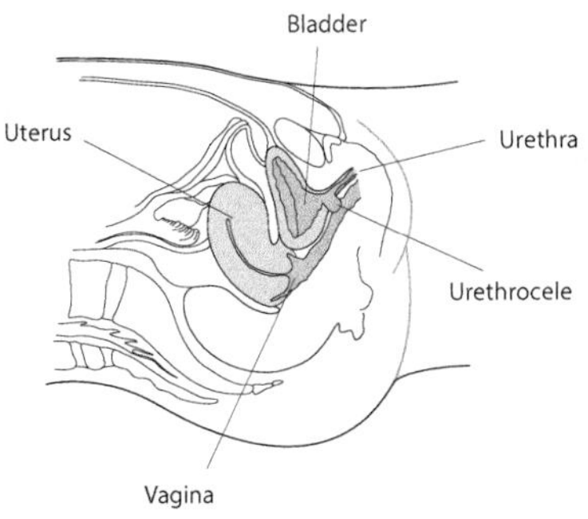

The urethra bulges into the vaginal canal.

ICD-10-CM Diagnostic Codes

N36.8	Other specified disorders of urethra
N81.0	Urethrocele ♀
Q64.71	Congenital prolapse of urethra

CCI Edits

Refer to Appendix A for CCI edits.

Facility RVUs ◻

Code	Work	PE Facility	MP	Total Facility
57230	6.30	5.21	1.02	12.53

Non-facility RVUs ◻

Code	Work	PE Non-Facility	MP	Total Non-Facility
57230	6.30	5.21	1.02	12.53

Modifiers (PAR) ◻

Code	Mod 50	Mod 51	Mod 62	Mod 66	Mod 80
57230	0	2	1	0	2

Global Period

Code	Days
57230	090

57240

57240 Anterior colporrhaphy, repair of cystocele with or without repair of urethrocele, including cystourethroscopy, when performed

(Do not report 57240 in conjunction with 52000)

AMA Coding Notes

Repair Procedures on the Vagina

(For urethral suspension, Marshall-Marchetti-Krantz type, abdominal approach, see 51840, 51841)

(For laparoscopic suspension, use 51990)

Surgical Procedures on the Female Genital System

(For pelvic laparotomy, use 49000)

(For excision or destruction of endometriomas, open method, see 49203-49205, 58957, 58958)

(For paracentesis, see 49082, 49083, 49084)

(For secondary closure of abdominal wall evisceration or disruption, use 49900)

(For fulguration or excision of lesions, laparoscopic approach, use 58662)

(For chemotherapy, see 96401-96549)

AMA *CPT® Assistant* ▫

57240: Winter 90: 7, Jan 97: 3, Jun 02: 5, Jun 10: 6

Plain English Description

This procedure is performed on the anterior aspect (front) of the vaginal wall to treat prolapse of the bladder (cystocele) with prolapse of the urethra (urethrocele), if present. Cystourethroscopy is included, if performed. Using a vaginal approach, a tenaculum is placed on the cervix and a transverse incision is made at the junction of the vaginal mucosa and cervix and carried down to the cervical fascia. The vaginal mucosa is dissected off underlying fascia. Dissection continues until the urethra is separated from the vaginal mucosa and the junction between the urethra and bladder (urethrovesical angle) has been exposed. The defect in the underlying fascia is repaired using plication sutures. By folding (plicating) the fascia, the prolapsed bladder and urethra are returned to normal position (reduced). Excessive vaginal mucosa is excised. The vaginal mucosa is then closed in the midline and the vaginal cuff is repaired with sutures. A Foley or suprapubic catheter is placed.

Anterior colporrhaphy, repair of cystocele with or without repair of urethrocele

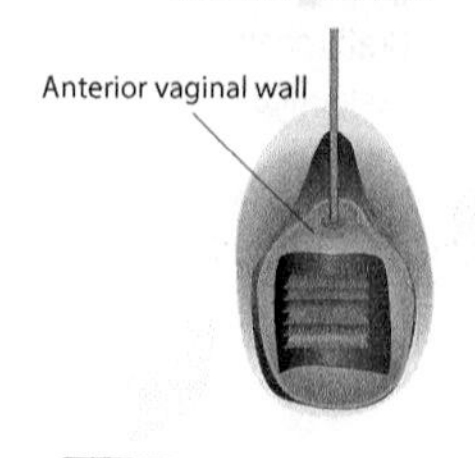

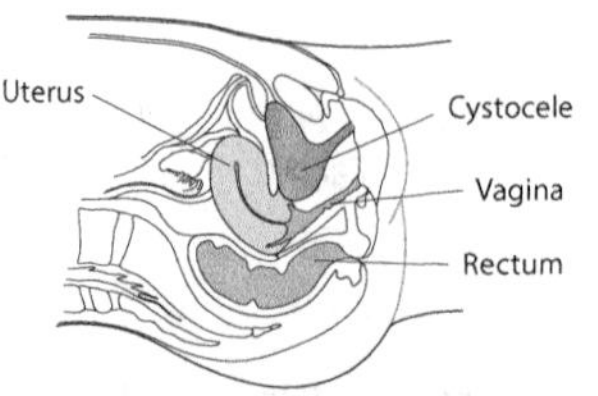

The physician repairs a condition in which the bladder protrudes through its support tissue and into the vagina, and may also repair the urethra if it is bulging into the vagina.

ICD-10-CM Diagnostic Codes

N36.1	Urethral diverticulum
N36.2	Urethral caruncle
N36.41	Hypermobility of urethra
N36.42	Intrinsic sphincter deficiency (ISD)
N36.43	Combined hypermobility of urethra and intrinsic sphincter deficiency
N36.8	Other specified disorders of urethra
N39.3	Stress incontinence (female) (male)
N81.0	Urethrocele ♀
N81.10	Cystocele, unspecified ♀
N81.11	Cystocele, midline ♀
N81.12	Cystocele, lateral ♀
N81.2	Incomplete uterovaginal prolapse ♀
N81.3	Complete uterovaginal prolapse ♀
N81.4	Uterovaginal prolapse, unspecified ♀
N81.5	Vaginal enterocele ♀
N81.6	Rectocele ♀
N81.81	Perineocele ♀
N81.82	Incompetence or weakening of pubocervical tissue ♀
N81.83	Incompetence or weakening of rectovaginal tissue ♀
N81.89	Other female genital prolapse ♀
N99.3	Prolapse of vaginal vault after hysterectomy ♀
Q64.71	Congenital prolapse of urethra

CCI Edits

Refer to Appendix A for CCI edits.

Facility RVUs ▫

Code	Work	PE Facility	MP	Total Facility
57240	10.08	6.66	1.51	18.25

Non-facility RVUs ▫

Code	Work	PE Non-Facility	MP	Total Non-Facility
57240	10.08	6.66	1.51	18.25

Modifiers (PAR) ▫

Code	Mod 50	Mod 51	Mod 62	Mod 66	Mod 80
57240	0	2	1	0	2

Global Period

Code	Days
57240	090

57284

57284 Paravaginal defect repair (including repair of cystocele, if performed); open abdominal approach

(Do not report 57284 in conjunction with 51840, 51841, 51990, 57240, 57260, 57265, 58152, 58267)

AMA Coding Notes

Repair Procedures on the Vagina

(For urethral suspension, Marshall-Marchetti-Krantz type, abdominal approach, see 51840, 51841)

(For laparoscopic suspension, use 51990)

Surgical Procedures on the Female Genital System

(For pelvic laparotomy, use 49000)

(For excision or destruction of endometriomas, open method, see 49203-49205, 58957, 58958)

(For paracentesis, see 49082, 49083, 49084)

(For secondary closure of abdominal wall evisceration or disruption, use 49900)

(For fulguration or excision of lesions, laparoscopic approach, use 58662)

(For chemotherapy, see 96401-96549)

AMA *CPT® Assistant* ▯

57284: Jan 97: 1, Jun 02: 7, Jul 05: 16, Jun 10: 6

Plain English Description

A paravaginal defect is repaired using an open abdominal approach. Any repair of cystocele is included. A paravaginal defect results from loss of support of the arcus tendineus fascia pelvis (ATFP), which forms the lateral attachments of the vagina. Without the support of the ATFP, the bladder and urethra drop from their normal position (prolapse), resulting in a cystocele or cystourethrocele. The defect may affect only one side (unilateral) or both sides (bilateral) of the ATFP. Using an open abdominal approach, the retropubic space of Retzius is accessed, taking care to protect vascular structures. The bladder is mobilized and the lateral retropubic spaces are exposed. The ischial spine is identified by palpation. The entire length of the ATFP is visualized as a white ligamentous band extending from the ischial spine toward the ipsilateral posterior pubic symphysis. The paravaginal defect is visualized, which may present as a unilateral or bilateral defect with avulsion of the vagina off the ATFP or as avulsion of the ATFP off the obturator internus muscle. The bladder is deflected. A few fingers of the nondominant hand are inserted into the vagina and the ipsilateral anterolateral vaginal sulcus is elevated. A suture is placed through the fibromuscular tissue of the lateral vaginal apex and into the ATFP or obturator internus fascia just distal to the ischial spine. Additional sutures are placed in a similar fashion with the last suture placed into the pubourethral ligament as close as possible to the pubic ramus. The sutures are tied sequentially and the defect is obliterated. If a bilateral defect is present, the procedure is repeated on the contralateral side.

Paravaginal defect repair; open abdominal approach

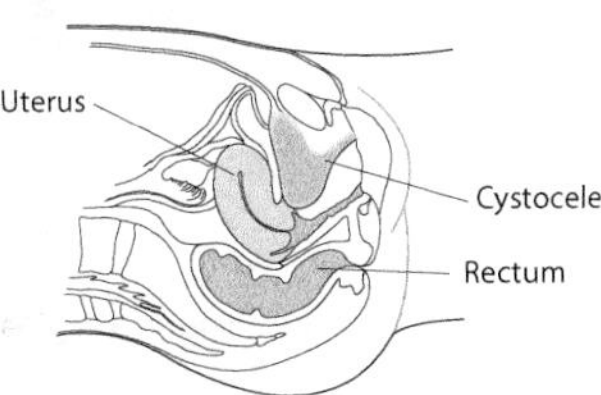

A paravaginal defect is repaired using an open abdominal approach.

ICD-10-CM Diagnostic Codes

N39.3	Stress incontinence (female) (male)
N39.46	Mixed incontinence
N81.0	Urethrocele ♀
N81.12	Cystocele, lateral ♀
N81.2	Incomplete uterovaginal prolapse ♀
N81.3	Complete uterovaginal prolapse ♀
N81.6	Rectocele ♀
N81.81	Perineocele ♀
N81.82	Incompetence or weakening of pubocervical tissue ♀
N81.83	Incompetence or weakening of rectovaginal tissue ♀
N81.84	Pelvic muscle wasting ♀
N81.85	Cervical stump prolapse ♀
N81.89	Other female genital prolapse ♀
N99.3	Prolapse of vaginal vault after hysterectomy ♀

CCI Edits

Refer to Appendix A for CCI edits.

Facility RVUs ▯

Code	Work	PE Facility	MP	Total Facility
57284	14.33	8.28	2.17	24.78

Non-facility RVUs ▯

Code	Work	PE Non-Facility	MP	Total Non-Facility
57284	14.33	8.28	2.17	24.78

Modifiers (PAR) ▯

Code	Mod 50	Mod 51	Mod 62	Mod 66	Mod 80
57284	0	2	2	0	2

Global Period

Code	Days
57284	090

57285

57285 Paravaginal defect repair (including repair of cystocele, if performed); vaginal approach

(Do not report 57285 in conjunction with 51990, 57240, 57260, 57265, 58267)

AMA Coding Notes

Repair Procedures on the Vagina

(For urethral suspension, Marshall-Marchetti-Krantz type, abdominal approach, see 51840, 51841)

(For laparoscopic suspension, use 51990)

Surgical Procedures on the Female Genital System

(For pelvic laparotomy, use 49000)

(For excision or destruction of endometriomas, open method, see 49203-49205, 58957, 58958)

(For paracentesis, see 49082, 49083, 49084)

(For secondary closure of abdominal wall evisceration or disruption, use 49900)

(For fulguration or excision of lesions, laparoscopic approach, use 58662)

(For chemotherapy, see 96401-96549)

AMA *CPT® Assistant* ▢

57285: Jun 10: 6

Plain English Description

A paravaginal defect is repaired using a vaginal approach. Any cystocele repair is included, when performed. A paravaginal defect results from loss of support of the arcus tendineus fascia pelvis (ATFP), which forms the lateral attachments of the vagina. Without the support of the ATFP, the bladder and urethra drop out of their normal position (prolapse), resulting in a cystocele or cystourethrocele. Using a vaginal approach, the anterior vaginal wall is incised and the bladder is dissected free of the vaginal epithelium to gain access to the retropubic space (space of Retzius). The ATFP is exposed. Sutures are placed along the anterior lateral vaginal sulcus at the site of the defect, which may be either unilateral or bilateral, and carried through the pubocervical fascia. The sutures are then brought through the internal obturator muscle immediately above the ATFP and placed from the underside along the full length of the pubic synthesis to the ischial spine. The sutures are tied sequentially and the defect is obliterated. The incisions in the vaginal wall are repaired.

Paravaginal defect repair; vaginal approach

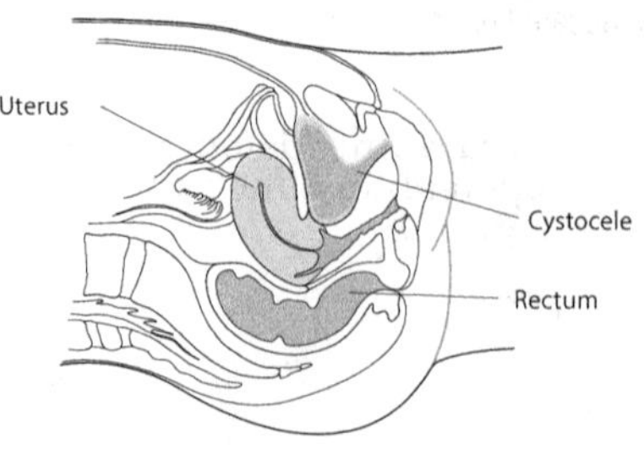

A paravaginal defect is repaired using a vaginal approach.

ICD-10-CM Diagnostic Codes

N81.0	Urethrocele ♀
N81.11	Cystocele, midline ♀
N81.12	Cystocele, lateral ♀
N81.2	Incomplete uterovaginal prolapse ♀
N81.3	Complete uterovaginal prolapse ♀
N81.6	Rectocele ♀
N81.81	Perineocele ♀
N81.83	Incompetence or weakening of rectovaginal tissue ♀
N81.84	Pelvic muscle wasting ♀
N81.85	Cervical stump prolapse ♀
N81.89	Other female genital prolapse ♀
N99.3	Prolapse of vaginal vault after hysterectomy ♀

CCI Edits

Refer to Appendix A for CCI edits.

Facility RVUs ▢

Code	Work	PE Facility	MP	Total Facility
57285	11.60	7.28	1.76	20.64

Non-facility RVUs ▢

Code	Work	PE Non-Facility	MP	Total Non-Facility
57285	11.60	7.28	1.76	20.64

Modifiers (PAR) ▢

Code	Mod 50	Mod 51	Mod 62	Mod 66	Mod 80
57285	0	2	2	0	2

Global Period

Code	Days
57285	090

57287

57287 Removal or revision of sling for stress incontinence (eg, fascia or synthetic)

AMA Coding Notes

Repair Procedures on the Vagina

(For urethral suspension, Marshall-Marchetti-Krantz type, abdominal approach, see 51840, 51841)

(For laparoscopic suspension, use 51990)

Surgical Procedures on the Female Genital System

(For pelvic laparotomy, use 49000)

(For excision or destruction of endometriomas, open method, see 49203-49205, 58957, 58958)

(For paracentesis, see 49082, 49083, 49084)

(For secondary closure of abdominal wall evisceration or disruption, use 49900)

(For fulguration or excision of lesions, laparoscopic approach, use 58662)

(For chemotherapy, see 96401-96549)

AMA CPT® Assistant ☐

57287: Jun 02: 7, Nov 07: 9

Plain English Description

A previously placed fascial or synthetic sling used to treat stress incontinence is removed or revised. Removal of the sling is usually performed for complications such as urethral erosion and may also be performed for vaginal extrusion of the sling. Revision may be performed for recurrent stress incontinence or vaginal extrusion of the sling. A Foley catheter is placed through the urethra and into the bladder. Removal is performed using a vaginal approach. The sling is dissected free of surrounding tissue and removed along with any permanent suture material. If urethral erosion is present, the urethral defect is repaired over the catheter by suture repair of the periurethral fascia. A labial fat graft may be used to strengthen the repair. If the sling has extruded through the vagina, the sling may be removed or revised. Removal is performed as described above and the vaginal defect is then repaired. Revision following vaginal extrusion of the sling consists of trimming the mesh, excising granulation tissue, and performing a two-layer repair of the vaginal defect. If revision is performed for recurrent stress incontinence, the sling may be shortened. An incision is made in the vagina and the sling is dissected free of surrounding tissue, then shortened and reattached to the pelvic fascia or abdominal wall.

Removal or revision of sling for stress incontinence (eg, fascia or synthetic)

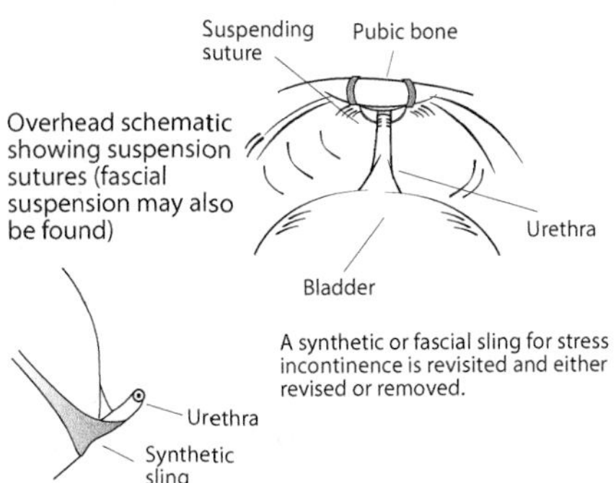

The physician removes or performs a revision to a device that supports the bladder or urethra to fix a condition in which the patient cannot control the release of urine.

ICD-10-CM Diagnostic Codes

	N39.3	Stress incontinence (female) (male)
	N99.89	Other postprocedural complications and disorders of genitourinary system
➐	T83.118	Breakdown (mechanical) of other urinary devices and implants
➐	T83.128	Displacement of other urinary devices and implants
➐	T83.198	Other mechanical complication of other urinary devices and implants
➐	T83.21	Breakdown (mechanical) of graft of urinary organ
➐	T83.22	Displacement of graft of urinary organ
➐	T83.23	Leakage of graft of urinary organ
➐	T83.29	Other mechanical complication of graft of urinary organ
➐	T83.498	Other mechanical complication of other prosthetic devices, implants and grafts of genital tract
➐	T83.598	Infection and inflammatory reaction due to other prosthetic device, implant and graft in urinary system
➐	T83.81	Embolism due to genitourinary prosthetic devices, implants and grafts
➐	T83.82	Fibrosis due to genitourinary prosthetic devices, implants and grafts
➐	T83.83	Hemorrhage due to genitourinary prosthetic devices, implants and grafts
➐	T83.84	Pain due to genitourinary prosthetic devices, implants and grafts
➐	T83.85	Stenosis due to genitourinary prosthetic devices, implants and grafts
➐	T83.86	Thrombosis due to genitourinary prosthetic devices, implants and grafts
➐	T83.89	Other specified complication of genitourinary prosthetic devices, implants and grafts
➐	T85.692	Other mechanical complication of permanent sutures
➐	T85.698	Other mechanical complication of other specified internal prosthetic devices, implants and grafts
	Z46.6	Encounter for fitting and adjustment of urinary device

ICD-10-CM Coding Notes

For codes requiring a 7th character extension, refer to your ICD-10-CM book. Review the character descriptions and coding guidelines for proper selection. For some procedures, only certain characters will apply.

CCI Edits

Refer to Appendix A for CCI edits.

Facility RVUs ☐

Code	Work	PE Facility	MP	Total Facility
57287	11.15	9.37	1.62	22.14

Non-facility RVUs ☐

Code	Work	PE Non-Facility	MP	Total Non-Facility
57287	11.15	9.37	1.62	22.14

Modifiers (PAR) ☐

Code	Mod 50	Mod 51	Mod 62	Mod 66	Mod 80
57287	0	2	1	0	2

Global Period

Code	Days
57287	090

57288

57288 Sling operation for stress incontinence (eg, fascia or synthetic)

(For laparoscopic approach, use 51992)

AMA Coding Notes

Repair Procedures on the Vagina

(For urethral suspension, Marshall-Marchetti-Krantz type, abdominal approach, see 51840, 51841)

(For laparoscopic suspension, use 51990)

Surgical Procedures on the Female Genital System

(For pelvic laparotomy, use 49000)

(For excision or destruction of endometriomas, open method, see 49203-49205, 58957, 58958)

(For paracentesis, see 49082, 49083, 49084)

(For secondary closure of abdominal wall evisceration or disruption, use 49900)

(For fulguration or excision of lesions, laparoscopic approach, use 58662)

(For chemotherapy, see 96401-96549)

AMA *CPT® Assistant* ▢

57288: Nov 99: 28, May 00: 4, Oct 00: 7, Apr 02: 18, Jun 02: 7

Plain English Description

A sling operation is performed to treat stress incontinence using a fascial or synthetic graft. If a fascial autograft is being used, an incision is made in the lower abdomen and a strip of abdominal fascia is removed. A second incision is then made in the vaginal wall just below the urethra. Two small tunnels are created on either side of the urethra and extended into the space below the pubic bone. The fascial or synthetic sling is placed under the urethra and around the bladder neck. The ends of the sling are then brought up through the tunnels and sutured to the pelvic fascia or the abdominal wall. The incisions in the abdomen and vaginal wall are closed.

Sling operation for stress incontinence

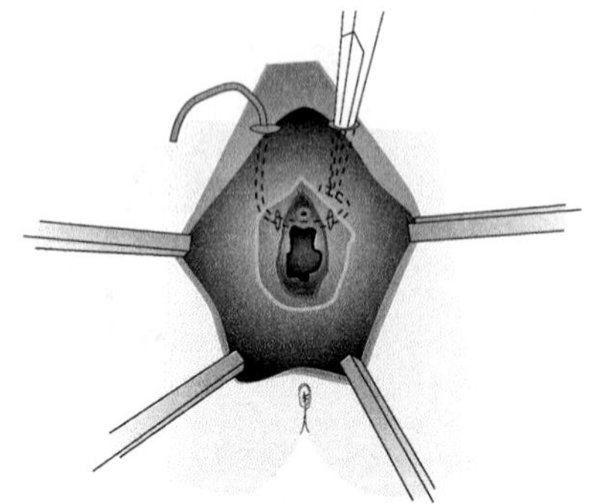

The physician places a device under the urethra and/or bladder to fix a condition in which the patient cannot control the release of urine.

ICD-10-CM Diagnostic Codes

N36.42	Intrinsic sphincter deficiency (ISD)
N39.3	Stress incontinence (female) (male)
N39.46	Mixed incontinence

CCI Edits

Refer to Appendix A for CCI edits.

Facility RVUs ▢

Code	Work	PE Facility	MP	Total Facility
57288	12.13	8.17	1.78	22.08

Non-facility RVUs ▢

Code	Work	PE Non-Facility	MP	Total Non-Facility
57288	12.13	8.17	1.78	22.08

Modifiers (PAR) ▢

Code	Mod 50	Mod 51	Mod 62	Mod 66	Mod 80
57288	0	2	1	0	2

Global Period

Code	Days
57288	090

57289

57289 Pereyra procedure, including anterior colporrhaphy

AMA Coding Notes

Repair Procedures on the Vagina

(For urethral suspension, Marshall-Marchetti-Krantz type, abdominal approach, see 51840, 51841)

(For laparoscopic suspension, use 51990)

Surgical Procedures on the Female Genital System

(For pelvic laparotomy, use 49000)

(For excision or destruction of endometriomas, open method, see 49203-49205, 58957, 58958)

(For paracentesis, see 49082, 49083, 49084)

(For secondary closure of abdominal wall evisceration or disruption, use 49900)

(For fulguration or excision of lesions, laparoscopic approach, use 58662)

(For chemotherapy, see 96401-96549)

AMA *CPT® Assistant*

57289: Jan 97: 3, Jun 02: 7

Plain English Description

The physician performs an operation to fix a condition in which the patient is unable to control the release of urine. The physician performs a procedure to tie the urethrovesical junction to the rectus abdominis muscles and also repairs a protrusion of the bladder through its supporting tissue, pushing against the vaginal wall. A U-shaped incision is made up and around the vaginal opening between the urethra and the vagina. The space on either side of the urethra is opened up where it joins with the bladder. The fascial tissues along each side of the urethra are sutured to the urethrovesical junction. An incision is then made in the abdomen above the pubis and a Pereyra ligature instrument is placed down through the tissues on either side of the midline until it reaches the sutured tissue. Sutures are then threaded into the instrument and brought back out through the abdominal incision. The urethrovesical junction is next elevated by pulling on the sutures and securing them around the rectus abdominis muscle. Anterior colporrhaphy is performed to repair the cystocele bulging the vaginal wall.

Pereyra procedure (including anterior colporrhaphy)

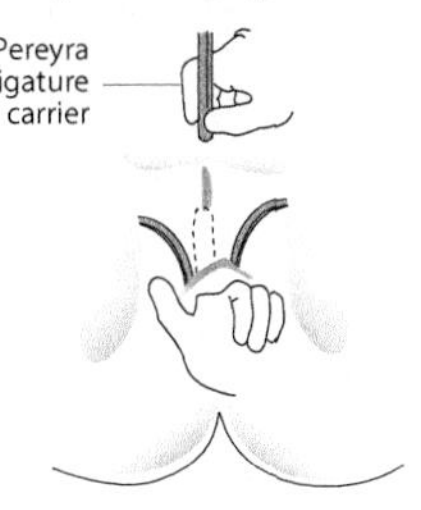

The physician guides the ligature with a finger inserted in the vagina.

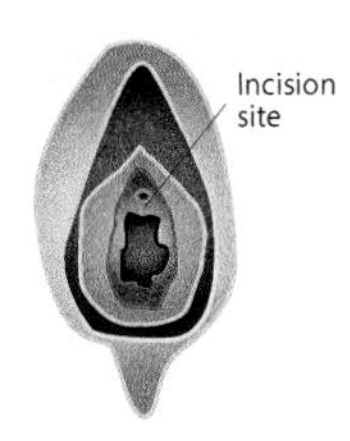

A cystocele is also repaired.

The physician performs an operation to fix a condition in which the patient is unable to control the release of urine.

ICD-10-CM Diagnostic Codes

N36.42	Intrinsic sphincter deficiency (ISD)
N39.3	Stress incontinence (female) (male)
N39.46	Mixed incontinence
N81.0	Urethrocele ♀
N81.11	Cystocele, midline ♀
N81.12	Cystocele, lateral ♀
N81.2	Incomplete uterovaginal prolapse ♀
N81.5	Vaginal enterocele ♀
N81.82	Incompetence or weakening of pubocervical tissue ♀
N81.83	Incompetence or weakening of rectovaginal tissue ♀
N81.85	Cervical stump prolapse ♀
N81.89	Other female genital prolapse ♀

CCI Edits

Refer to Appendix A for CCI edits.

Facility RVUs

Code	Work	PE Facility	MP	Total Facility
57289	12.80	8.83	2.09	23.72

Non-facility RVUs

Code	Work	PE Non-Facility	MP	Total Non-Facility
57289	12.80	8.83	2.09	23.72

Modifiers (PAR)

Code	Mod 50	Mod 51	Mod 62	Mod 66	Mod 80
57289	0	2	1	0	2

Global Period

Code	Days
57289	090

57423

57423 Paravaginal defect repair (including repair of cystocele, if performed), laparoscopic approach

(Do not report 57423 in conjunction with 49320, 51840, 51841, 51990, 57240, 57260, 58152, 58267)

AMA Coding Notes

Surgical Procedures on the Female Genital System

(For pelvic laparotomy, use 49000)

(For excision or destruction of endometriomas, open method, see 49203-49205, 58957, 58958)

(For paracentesis, see 49082, 49083, 49084)

(For secondary closure of abdominal wall evisceration or disruption, use 49900)

(For fulguration or excision of lesions, laparoscopic approach, use 58662)

(For chemotherapy, see 96401-96549)

AMA *CPT® Assistant* ▯

57423: Jun 10: 6

Plain English Description

A paravaginal defect is repaired using a laparoscopic approach. Any repair of a cystocele is included, when performed. A paravaginal defect results from loss of support of the arcus tendineus fascia pelvis (ATFP), which forms the lateral attachments of the vagina. Without the support of the ATFP, the bladder and urethra drop out of their normal position (prolapse), resulting in a cystocele or cystourethrocele. Using a laparoscopic approach, a small incision is made below the umbilicus and the laparoscope is inserted. Additional small incisions are made and trocars are placed, including a small incision into the peritoneum above the bladder and behind the pubic bone. The retropubic space (space of Retzius) is entered and dissected. Using the laparoscope, the paravaginal defect is identified and the location is confirmed with digital vaginal exam. Sutures are placed along the anterior lateral vaginal sulcus at the site of the defect, which may be either unilateral or bilateral, and carried through the pubocervical fascia. The sutures are then brought through the internal obturator muscle immediately above the ATFP and placed from the underside along the full length of the pubic synthesis to the ischial spine. A retractor is placed in the vaginal vault and the sutures are tied sequentially using intracorporeal or extracorporeal knot tying technique. Repair of the defect is confirmed by digital vaginal exam and direct laparoscopic view.

Paravaginal defect repair, laparoscopic approach

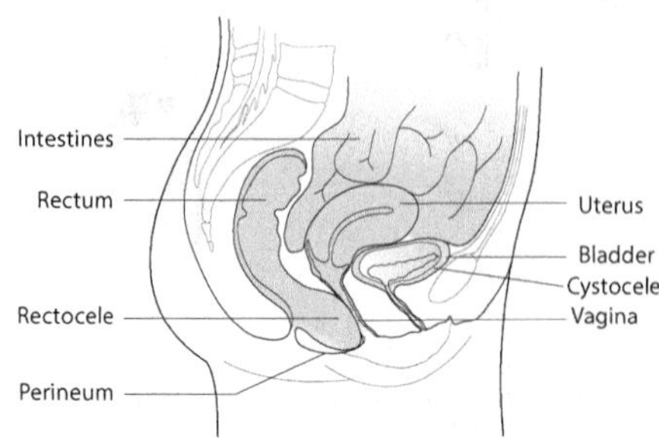

A paravaginal defect is repaired using a laparoscopic approach. Any repair of a cystocele is included, when performed.

ICD-10-CM Diagnostic Codes

N81.0	Urethrocele ♀
N81.11	Cystocele, midline ♀
N81.12	Cystocele, lateral ♀
N81.2	Incomplete uterovaginal prolapse ♀
N81.3	Complete uterovaginal prolapse ♀
N81.6	Rectocele ♀
N81.81	Perineocele ♀
N81.83	Incompetence or weakening of rectovaginal tissue ♀
N81.85	Cervical stump prolapse ♀
N81.89	Other female genital prolapse ♀
N99.3	Prolapse of vaginal vault after hysterectomy ♀

CCI Edits

Refer to Appendix A for CCI edits.

Facility RVUs ▯

Code	Work	PE Facility	MP	Total Facility
57423	16.08	9.04	2.50	27.62

Non-facility RVUs ▯

Code	Work	PE Non-Facility	MP	Total Non-Facility
57423	16.08	9.04	2.50	27.62

Modifiers (PAR) ▯

Code	Mod 50	Mod 51	Mod 62	Mod 66	Mod 80
57423	0	2	2	0	2

Global Period

Code	Days
57423	090

60540-60545

60540 Adrenalectomy, partial or complete, or exploration of adrenal gland with or without biopsy, transabdominal, lumbar or dorsal (separate procedure)

60545 Adrenalectomy, partial or complete, or exploration of adrenal gland with or without biopsy, transabdominal, lumbar or dorsal (separate procedure); with excision of adjacent retroperitoneal tumor

(Do not report 60540, 60545 in conjunction with 50323)

(For bilateral procedure, report 60540 with modifier 50)

(For excision of remote or disseminated pheochromocytoma, see 49203-49205)

(For laparoscopic approach, use 60650)

AMA Coding Notes

Excision Procedures on the Parathyroid, Thymus, Adrenal Glands, Pancreas, and Carotid Body

(For pituitary and pineal surgery, see Nervous System)

Surgical Procedures on the Endocrine System

(For pituitary and pineal surgery, see Nervous System)

AMA *CPT® Assistant* ▯

60540: Nov 98: 17

60545: Nov 98: 17

Plain English Description

The adrenal glands are paired endocrine glands located above each kidney. The adrenal glands excrete hormones including epinephrine, norepinephrine, androgens, estrogens, aldosterone, and cortisol. Exploration, biopsy, and/or excision are typically performed for enlargement or tumors of these glands. Tumors often excrete excessive amounts of hormones causing severe hormonal imbalances. The adrenal gland is typically approached through an anterior or posterior subcostal incision, a midline abdominal incision, or a flank incision. Overlying tissues are dissected and the adrenal gland exposed. If exploration and biopsy are performed, the adrenal gland is carefully inspected and a tissue sample obtained. If the adrenal gland is excised, blood vessels supplying the adrenal gland are ligated and divided. The adrenal gland is dissected free of surrounding tissue and removed. The wound is irrigated with sterile saline and the wound closed in layers. Use 60540 when exploration and excision of the adrenal gland are performed without excision of an adjacent retroperitoneal tumor and 60545 when an adjacent retroperitoneal tumor is also excised. The most common approach is an abdominal transperitoneal route. The tumor is typically excised along with a wide margin of normal tissue to ensure that all tumor tissue is removed.

Adrenalectomy

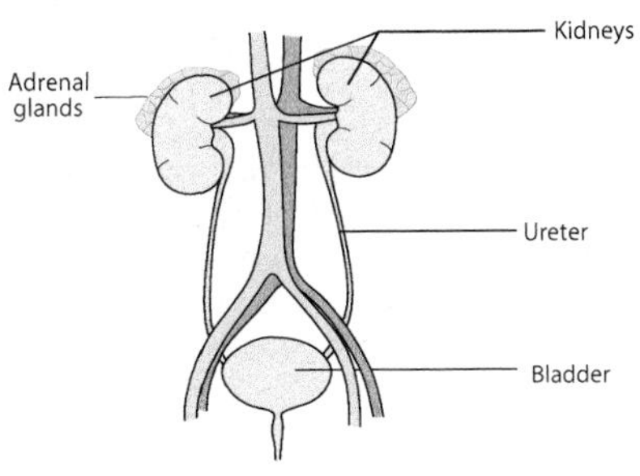

All or part of the adrenal gland is removed or explored (60540); with adjacent retroperitoneal tumor excision (60545).

ICD-10-CM Diagnostic Codes

⇄	C74.01	Malignant neoplasm of cortex of right adrenal gland
⇄	C74.11	Malignant neoplasm of medulla of right adrenal gland
⇄	C74.12	Malignant neoplasm of medulla of left adrenal gland
⇄	C79.71	Secondary malignant neoplasm of right adrenal gland
⇄	C79.72	Secondary malignant neoplasm of left adrenal gland
	D09.3	Carcinoma in situ of thyroid and other endocrine glands
⇄	D35.01	Benign neoplasm of right adrenal gland
⇄	D35.02	Benign neoplasm of left adrenal gland
⇄	D44.11	Neoplasm of uncertain behavior of right adrenal gland
⇄	D44.12	Neoplasm of uncertain behavior of left adrenal gland
	E24.3	Ectopic ACTH syndrome
	E25.0	Congenital adrenogenital disorders associated with enzyme deficiency
	E26.01	Conn's syndrome
	E26.02	Glucocorticoid-remediable aldosteronism
	E26.09	Other primary hyperaldosteronism
	E26.1	Secondary hyperaldosteronism
	E26.89	Other hyperaldosteronism
	E27.0	Other adrenocortical overactivity
	E27.1	Primary adrenocortical insufficiency
	E27.2	Addisonian crisis
	E27.3	Drug-induced adrenocortical insufficiency
	E27.49	Other adrenocortical insufficiency
	E27.5	Adrenomedullary hyperfunction
	E27.8	Other specified disorders of adrenal gland

CCI Edits

Refer to Appendix A for CCI edits.

Facility RVUs ▯

Code	Work	PE Facility	MP	Total Facility
60540	18.02	10.16	3.65	31.83
60545	20.93	11.45	4.55	36.93

Non-facility RVUs ▯

Code	Work	PE Non-Facility	MP	Total Non-Facility
60540	18.02	10.16	3.65	31.83
60545	20.93	11.45	4.55	36.93

Modifiers (PAR) ▯

Code	Mod 50	Mod 51	Mod 62	Mod 66	Mod 80
60540	1	2	1	0	2
60545	1	2	1	0	2

Global Period

Code	Days
60540	090
60545	090

CPT® Procedural Coding

60650

60650 Laparoscopy, surgical, with adrenalectomy, partial or complete, or exploration of adrenal gland with or without biopsy, transabdominal, lumbar or dorsal

AMA Coding Guideline

Laparoscopic Procedures on the Parathyroid, Thymus, Adrenal Glands, Pancreas, and Carotid Body

Surgical laparoscopy always includes diagnostic laparoscopy. To report a diagnostic laparoscopy (peritoneoscopy) (separate procedure), use 49320.

AMA Coding Notes

Surgical Procedures on the Endocrine System

(For pituitary and pineal surgery, see Nervous System)

AMA *CPT® Assistant* ▢

60650: Nov 99: 30, Mar 00: 10, Nov 01: 8

Plain English Description

The adrenal glands are paired endocrine glands located above each kidney. The adrenal glands excrete hormones including epinephrine, norepinephrine, androgens, estrogens, aldosterone, and cortisol. Exploration, biopsy, and/or excision are typically performed for enlargement or tumors of these glands. Tumors often excrete excessive amounts of hormones causing severe hormonal imbalances. Laparoscopic surgery is typically performed using an abdominal transperitoneal approach, although a retroperitoneal approach is sometimes used instead. A small incision is made in the upper abdomen on the affected side. A trocar is placed and the laparoscope introduced into the abdomen. Pneumoperitoneum is established. If the affected adrenal gland is on the right, the right lobe of the liver is mobilized. The triangular ligament is incised up to the diaphragm. The retroperitoneum is opened. The inferior vena cava is identified and a plane of dissection developed between the vena cava and the adrenal gland. If the affected adrenal gland is on the left, the splenic flexure and pancreas are mobilized and the retroperitoneum opened. Surrounding tissues are dissected and the adrenal gland exposed. If exploration and biopsy are performed, the adrenal gland is carefully inspected and a tissue sample obtained. If the adrenal gland is excised, the adrenal vein and other blood vessels supplying the adrenal gland are ligated and divided. The adrenal gland is dissected free of surrounding tissue, placed in an endobag, and removed. The surgical instruments are removed, gas released from the abdomen, and the laparoscope and trocars are removed. Portal incisions are closed.

ICD-10-CM Diagnostic Codes

⇄	C74.01	Malignant neoplasm of cortex of right adrenal gland
⇄	C74.02	Malignant neoplasm of cortex of left adrenal gland
⇄	C74.11	Malignant neoplasm of medulla of right adrenal gland
⇄	C74.12	Malignant neoplasm of medulla of left adrenal gland
⇄	C79.71	Secondary malignant neoplasm of right adrenal gland
⇄	C79.72	Secondary malignant neoplasm of left adrenal gland
	D09.3	Carcinoma in situ of thyroid and other endocrine glands
⇄	D35.01	Benign neoplasm of right adrenal gland
⇄	D35.02	Benign neoplasm of left adrenal gland
⇄	D44.11	Neoplasm of uncertain behavior of right adrenal gland
⇄	D44.12	Neoplasm of uncertain behavior of left adrenal gland
	E24.3	Ectopic ACTH syndrome
	E25.0	Congenital adrenogenital disorders associated with enzyme deficiency
	E25.8	Other adrenogenital disorders
	E26.01	Conn's syndrome
	E26.02	Glucocorticoid-remediable aldosteronism
	E26.09	Other primary hyperaldosteronism
	E27.0	Other adrenocortical overactivity
	E27.1	Primary adrenocortical insufficiency
	E27.2	Addisonian crisis
	E27.3	Drug-induced adrenocortical insufficiency
	E27.49	Other adrenocortical insufficiency
	E27.5	Adrenomedullary hyperfunction
	E27.8	Other specified disorders of adrenal gland

CCI Edits

Refer to Appendix A for CCI edits.

Facility RVUs ▢

Code	Work	PE Facility	MP	Total Facility
60650	20.73	10.19	4.30	35.22

Non-facility RVUs ▢

Code	Work	PE Non-Facility	MP	Total Non-Facility
60650	20.73	10.19	4.30	35.22

Modifiers (PAR) ▢

Code	Mod 50	Mod 51	Mod 62	Mod 66	Mod 80
60650	1	2	1	0	2

Global Period

Code	Days
60650	090

64566

64566 Posterior tibial neurostimulation, percutaneous needle electrode, single treatment, includes programming

(Do not report 64566 in conjunction with 64555, 95970-95972)

AMA Coding Guideline

Neurostimulator Procedures on the Peripheral Nerves

For electronic analysis with programming, when performed, of peripheral nerve neurostimulator pulse generator/transmitters, see codes 95970, 95971, 95972. An electrode array is a catheter or other device with more than one contact. The function of each contact may be capable of being adjusted during programming services. Test stimulation to confirm correct target site placement of the electrode array(s) and/or to confirm the functional status of the system is inherent to placement, and is not separately reported as electronic analysis or programming of the neurostimulator system. Electronic analysis (95970) at the time of implantation is not separately reported.

Codes 64553, 64555, and 64561 may be used to report both temporary and permanent placement of percutaneous electrode arrays.

AMA Coding Notes

Neurostimulator Procedures on the Peripheral Nerves

(For transcutaneous nerve stimulation [TENS], use 97014 for electrical stimulation requiring supervision only or use 97032 for electrical stimulation requiring constant attendance)

(For percutaneous implantation or replacement of integrated neurostimulation system, posterior tibial nerve, use 0587T)

Surgical Procedures on the Extracranial Nerves, Peripheral Nerves, and Autonomic Nervous System

(For intracranial surgery on cranial nerves, see 61450, 61460, 61790)

AMA *CPT® Assistant* ▢

64566: Feb 11: 5, Sep 11: 8

Plain English Description

Posterior tibial neurostimulation is used to treat overactive bladder, urge incontinence, and the symptom of frequent urination in patients who have failed other treatment modalities. The posterior tibial nerve located near the ankle is a branch derived from the sacral nerve plexus, the nerves responsible for bladder and pelvic floor function. Neuromodulation of the posterior tibial nerve sends mild electrical impulses to stimulate the sacral nerve plexus, thereby improving voiding function and control. The patient's foot is comfortably elevated and supported. The skin just above the ankle over the tibial nerve is cleansed. The neurostimulator is programmed. A fine-needle electrode is inserted adjacent to the nerve and low-voltage electrical stimulation is delivered using the prescribed voltage for the prescribed amount of time. This code reports a single treatment session. Most patients receive once-a-week sessions over a 10- to 12-week period.

ICD-10-CM Diagnostic Codes

N32.81	Overactive bladder
N39.41	Urge incontinence
R35.0	Frequency of micturition
R39.15	Urgency of urination

CCI Edits

Refer to Appendix A for CCI edits.

Facility RVUs ▢

Code	Work	PE Facility	MP	Total Facility
64566	0.60	0.21	0.09	0.90

Non-facility RVUs ▢

Code	Work	PE Non-Facility	MP	Total Non-Facility
64566	0.60	2.89	0.09	3.58

Modifiers (PAR) ▢

Code	Mod 50	Mod 51	Mod 62	Mod 66	Mod 80
64566	0	2	0	0	0

Global Period

Code	Days
64566	000

64581

▲ **64581 Open implantation of neurostimulator electrode array; sacral nerve (transforaminal placement)**

AMA Coding Guideline

Neurostimulator Procedures on the Peripheral Nerves

For electronic analysis with programming, when performed, of peripheral nerve neurostimulator pulse generator/transmitters, see codes 95970, 95971, 95972. An electrode array is a catheter or other device with more than one contact. The function of each contact may be capable of being adjusted during programming services. Test stimulation to confirm correct target site placement of the electrode array(s) and/or to confirm the functional status of the system is inherent to placement, and is not separately reported as electronic analysis or programming of the neurostimulator system. Electronic analysis (95970) at the time of implantation is not separately reported.

Codes 64553, 64555, and 64561 may be used to report both temporary and permanent placement of percutaneous electrode arrays.

AMA Coding Notes

Neurostimulator Procedures on the Peripheral Nerves

(For transcutaneous nerve stimulation [TENS], use 97014 for electrical stimulation requiring supervision only or use 97032 for electrical stimulation requiring constant attendance)

(For percutaneous implantation or replacement of integrated neurostimulation system, posterior tibial nerve, use 0587T)

Surgical Procedures on the Extracranial Nerves, Peripheral Nerves, and Autonomic Nervous System

(For intracranial surgery on cranial nerves, see 61450, 61460, 61790)

AMA *CPT® Assistant* ▯

64581: Dec 12: 14, Sep 14: 5

Plain English Description

Direct transforaminal sacral nerve stimulation is used to treat voiding dysfunction, including urge incontinence, urgency, frequency, and nonobstructive urinary retention. For open transforaminal implantation of a sacral nerve neurostimulator electrode array, the skin is prepared and a local anesthetic is injected into the skin and periosteum of the sacrum. The skin over the sacrum is incised in the midline. Overlying tissue is dissected and the sacrum is exposed. A foramen needle is inserted into the selected sacral foramen. A power source is connected to the needle; stimulation is applied; and the motor responses are evaluated as the position of the needle is changed until the desired response is achieved. The needle is disconnected from the power source and removed. An electrode array is then passed through the foramen and positioned in the desired location next to the sacral nerve. Correct placement is verified by testing motor response to stimulation. The electrode array is tunneled to the site of the generator/receiver, which is implanted in a separately reportable procedure. The presacral fascia is closed over the electrode array, followed by closure of the subcutaneous tissue and skin.

ICD-10-CM Diagnostic Codes

	G83.4	Cauda equina syndrome
	G95.89	Other specified diseases of spinal cord
	N31.0	Uninhibited neuropathic bladder, not elsewhere classified
	N31.1	Reflex neuropathic bladder, not elsewhere classified
	N31.2	Flaccid neuropathic bladder, not elsewhere classified
	N31.8	Other neuromuscular dysfunction of bladder
	N31.9	Neuromuscular dysfunction of bladder, unspecified
	N39.41	Urge incontinence
	N39.42	Incontinence without sensory awareness
	N39.43	Post-void dribbling
	N39.44	Nocturnal enuresis
	N39.45	Continuous leakage
	N39.46	Mixed incontinence
	N39.490	Overflow incontinence
	N39.498	Other specified urinary incontinence
	N39.8	Other specified disorders of urinary system
	R32	Unspecified urinary incontinence
	R33.8	Other retention of urine
	R33.9	Retention of urine, unspecified
	R35.0	Frequency of micturition
	R35.1	Nocturia
	R35.81	Nocturnal polyuria
	R35.89	Other polyuria
❼	S34.3	Injury of cauda equina

ICD-10-CM Coding Notes

For codes requiring a 7th character extension, refer to your ICD-10-CM book. Review the character descriptions and coding guidelines for proper selection. For some procedures, only certain characters will apply.

CCI Edits

Refer to Appendix A for CCI edits.

Pub 100

64581: Pub 100-04, 32, 40.2.1

Facility RVUs ▯

Code	Work	PE Facility	MP	Total Facility
64581	12.20	5.49	1.63	19.32

Non-facility RVUs ▯

Code	Work	PE Non-Facility	MP	Total Non-Facility
64581	12.20	5.49	1.63	19.32

Modifiers (PAR) ▯

Code	Mod 50	Mod 51	Mod 62	Mod 66	Mod 80
64581	0	2	0	0	1

Global Period

Code	Days
64581	090

72191

72191 Computed tomographic angiography, pelvis, with contrast material(s), including noncontrast images, if performed, and image postprocessing

(Do not report 72191 in conjunction with 73706 or 75635. For CTA aorto-iliofemoral runoff, use 75635)

(Do not report 72191 in conjunction with 74175. For a combined computed tomographic angiography abdomen and pelvis study, use 74174)

(For noninvasive arterial plaque analysis using software processing of data from computerized tomography angiography to quantify structure and composition of the vessel wall, including assessment for lipid-rich necrotic core plaque, see 0710T, 0711T, 0712T, 0713T)

Plain English Description

A computed tomographic angiography (CTA) of the pelvis is performed with contrast material including image postprocessing. Noncontrast images may also be obtained and are included when performed. CTA provides images of the blood vessels using a combination of computed tomography (CT) and angiography with contrast material. When angiography is performed using CT, multiple images are obtained and processed on a computer to create detailed, two-dimensional, cross-sectional views of the blood vessels. These images are then displayed on a computer monitor. The patient is positioned on the CT table. An intravenous line is inserted into a blood vessel, usually in the arm or hand. Non-contrast images may be obtained. A small dose of contrast is injected and test images are obtained to verify correct positioning. The CTA is then performed. Contrast is injected at a controlled rate and the CT table moves through the CT machine as the scanning is performed. After completion of the CTA, the radiologist reviews and interprets the CTA images of the pelvis.

RVUs

Code	Work	PE	PE Non-Facility	MP	Total Non-Facility	Total Facility	Global
72191	1.81	7.65	7.65	0.11	9.57	9.57	XXX

72192-72194

72192 Computed tomography, pelvis; without contrast material

72193 Computed tomography, pelvis; with contrast material(s)

72194 Computed tomography, pelvis; without contrast material, followed by contrast material(s) and further sections

(For a combined CT abdomen and pelvis study, see 74176-74178)

(To report 3D rendering, see 76376, 76377)

(For computed tomographic colonography, diagnostic, see 74261-74262. For computed tomographic colonography, screening, use 74263)

(Do not report 72192-72194 in conjunction with 74261-74263)

Plain English Description

Diagnostic computed tomography (CT) is performed on the pelvis to provide detailed visualization of the organs and structures within or near the pelvis, such as kidneys, bladder, prostate, uterus, cervix, vagina, lymph nodes, and pelvic bones. CT uses multiple, narrow X-ray beams aimed around a single rotational axis, taking a series of two-dimensional (2D) images of the target structure from multiple angles. Contrast material is used to enhance the images. Computer software processes the data and produces several images of thin, cross-sectional 2D slices of the targeted organ or area. Three-dimensional (3D) models of organs within the pelvis can be created by stacking multiple, individual 2D slices together. The patient is placed inside the CT scanner on the table and images are obtained of the pelvis area. In 72192, no contrast medium is used. In 72193, an iodine contrast dye is administered intravenously to see the target area better before images are taken. In 72194, images are taken without contrast and again after the administration of the contrast. The physician reviews the images to gather information for specified purposes, such as diagnosing or monitoring cancer, evaluating the pelvic bones for fractures or other injury following trauma, locating abscesses or masses found during physical exam, finding the cause of pelvic pain, providing more detailed information before surgery, and evaluating the patient after surgery.

RVUs

Code	Work	PE	PE Non-Facility	MP	Total Non-Facility	Total Facility	Global
72192	1.09	2.97	2.97	0.06	4.12	4.12	XXX
72193	1.16	6.05	6.05	0.06	7.27	7.27	XXX
72194	1.22	6.71	6.71	0.09	8.02	8.02	XXX

72195-72197

72195 Magnetic resonance (eg, proton) imaging, pelvis; without contrast material(s)

72196 Magnetic resonance (eg, proton) imaging, pelvis; with contrast material(s)

72197 Magnetic resonance (eg, proton) imaging, pelvis; without contrast material(s), followed by contrast material(s) and further sequences

(Do not report 72195, 72196, 72197 in conjunction with 74712, 74713)

(For magnetic resonance imaging of a fetus[es], see 74712, 74713)

Plain English Description

Magnetic resonance imaging (MRI) is performed on the pelvis and organs within the pelvic area. MRI is a noninvasive, non-radiating imaging technique that uses the magnetic properties of nuclei within hydrogen atoms of the body. The powerful magnetic field forces the hydrogen atoms to line up. Radio waves are then transmitted within the strong magnetic field. Protons in the nuclei of different types of tissues emit a specific radiofrequency signal that bounces back to the computer, which records the images. The computer processes the signals and converts the data into tomographic, 3D, sectional images in slices with very high resolution. The patient is placed on a motorized table within a large MRI tunnel scanner that contains the magnet. Small coils that help transmit and receive the radio waves may be placed around the hip area. MRI scans of the pelvis are often performed for injury, trauma, birth defects, or unexplained hip or pelvic pain. In 72195, no contrast medium is used. In 72196, an iodine contrast dye is administered intravenously to see the target area better before images are taken. In 72197, images are taken without contrast and again after the administration of contrast. The physician reviews the images to look for information that may correlate to the patient's signs or symptoms. Pelvic MRI may be performed on males to evaluate lumps or swelling of the testicles or scrotum and locate an undescended testicle that does not appear on ultrasound. For females, an MRI scan may be used to evaluate abnormal vaginal bleeding, endometriosis, a pelvic mass, or unexplained infertility.

RVUs

Code	Work	PE	PE Non-Facility	MP	Total Non-Facility	Total Facility	Global
72195	1.46	5.70	5.70	0.10	7.26	7.26	XXX
72196	1.73	6.66	6.66	0.11	8.50	8.50	XXX
72197	2.20	8.34	8.34	0.14	10.68	10.68	XXX

74018-74022

74018 Radiologic examination, abdomen; 1 view

74019 Radiologic examination, abdomen; 2 views

74021 Radiologic examination, abdomen; 3 or more views

74022 Radiologic examination, complete acute abdomen series, including 2 or more views of the abdomen (eg, supine, erect, decubitus), and a single view chest

Plain English Description

A radiologic examination of the abdomen images the internal organs, soft tissue (muscle, fat), and supporting skeleton. X-ray imaging uses indirect ionizing radiation to take pictures of non-uniform material, such as human tissue, because of its different density and composition, which allows some of the x-rays to be absorbed and some to pass through and be captured. This produces a 2D image of the structures. The radiographs may be taken to look for size, shape, and position of organs, pattern of air (bowel gas), obstruction, foreign objects, and calcification in the gallbladder, urinary tract, and aorta. A radiologic examination of the abdomen may be ordered to diagnose abdominal distention and pain, vomiting, diarrhea or constipation, and traumatic injury; it may also be obtained as a screening exam or scout film prior to other imagining procedures. Code 74018 is used to report a single view; code 74019 reports 2 views; 74021 reports 3 or more views. Code 74022 is used to report a complete acute abdomen series which includes at least 2 views of the abdomen in supine, erect, and/or decubitus views and a single view of the chest. Common views of the abdomen include front-to-back anteroposterior (AP) with the patient lying supine or standing erect, back-to-front posteroanterior (PA) with the patient lying prone, lateral with the patient lying on the side, lateral decubitus anteroposterior (side lying, front-to-back view), lateral dorsal decubitus (lying supine, side view), oblique (anterior or posterior rotation), and coned (small collimated) views, which may be used to localize and differentiate lesions, calcifications, or herniations.

RVUs

Code	Work	PE	PE Non-Facility	MP	Total Non-Facility	Total Facility	Global
74018	0.18	0.70	0.70	0.02	0.90	0.90	XXX
74019	0.23	0.85	0.85	0.02	1.10	1.10	XXX
74021	0.27	1.00	1.00	0.02	1.29	1.29	XXX
74022	0.32	1.15	1.15	0.02	1.49	1.49	XXX

74150-74170

74150 Computed tomography, abdomen; without contrast material

74160 Computed tomography, abdomen; with contrast material(s)

74170 Computed tomography, abdomen; without contrast material, followed by contrast material(s) and further sections

(For a combined CT abdomen and pelvis study, see 74176-74178)

(To report 3D rendering, see 76376, 76377)

(For computed tomographic colonography, diagnostic, see 74261-74262. For computed tomographic colonography, screening, use 74263)

(Do not report 74150-74170 in conjunction with 74261-74263)

Plain English Description

Diagnostic computed tomography (CT) is performed on the abdomen to provide detailed visualization of the tissues and organs within the abdominal area. CT uses multiple, narrow X-ray beams aimed around a single rotational axis, taking a series of 2D images of the target structure from multiple angles. Contrast material is used to enhance the images. Computer software processes the data and produces several images of thin, cross-sectional 2D slices of the targeted organ or area. Three-dimensional (3D) models can be created by stacking multiple, individual 2D slices together. The patient is placed inside the CT scanner on the table and images are obtained of the abdomen. In 74150, no contrast medium is used. In 74160, an iodine contrast dye is administered intravenously to see the target area better before images are taken. In 74170, CT is first performed without contrast followed by the administration of contrast and acquisition of additional sections. The physician reviews the images for the cause of abdominal pain, swelling, and fever; for other suspected problems such as appendicitis and kidney stones; for locating tumors, abscesses, or masses; or for evaluating the abdominal area for hernias, infections, or internal injury. The physician reviews the CT scan, notes any abnormalities, and provides a written interpretation of the findings.

RVUs

Code	Work	PE	PE Non-Facility	MP	Total Non-Facility	Total Facility	Global
74150	1.19	2.98	2.98	0.08	4.25	4.25	XXX
74160	1.27	6.07	6.07	0.08	7.42	7.42	XXX
74170	1.40	6.81	6.81	0.10	8.31	8.31	XXX

74174

74174 Computed tomographic angiography, abdomen and pelvis, with contrast material(s), including noncontrast images, if performed, and image postprocessing

(Do not report 74174 in conjunction with 72191, 73706, 74175, 75635, 76376, 76377)

(For CTA aorto-iliofemoral runoff, use 75635)

Plain English Description

Computed tomographic angiography (CTA) provides images of the blood vessels using a combination of computed tomography (CT) and angiography with contrast material. When angiography is performed using CT, multiple images are obtained and processed on a computer to create detailed, two-dimensional, cross-sectional views of the blood vessels. These images are then displayed on a computer monitor. The patient is positioned on the CT table. An intravenous line is inserted into a blood vessel, usually in the arm or hand. Non-contrast images of the abdomen and pelvis are obtained as needed. A small dose of contrast is injected and test images are obtained to verify correct positioning. The CTA of the abdomen and pelvis is then performed. Contrast is injected at a controlled rate and the CT table moves through the CT machine as the scanning is performed. After completion of the CTA, the radiologist reviews and interprets the CTA images of the blood vessels of the abdomen and pelvis.

RVUs

Code	Work	PE	PE Non-Facility	MP	Total Non-Facility	Total Facility	Global
74174	2.20	9.58	9.58	0.15	11.93	11.93	XXX

74175

74175 Computed tomographic angiography, abdomen, with contrast material(s), including noncontrast images, if performed, and image postprocessing

(Do not report 74175 in conjunction with 73706 or 75635. For CTA aorto-iliofemoral runoff, use 75635)

(Do not report 74175 in conjunction with 72191. For a combined computed tomographic angiography abdomen and pelvis study, use 74174)

(For noninvasive arterial plaque analysis using software processing of data from computerized tomography angiography to quantify structure and composition of the vessel wall, including assessment for lipid-rich necrotic core plaque, see 0710T, 0711T, 0712T, 0713T)

Plain English Description

A computed tomographic angiography (CTA) of the abdomen is performed with contrast material including image postprocessing. Non-contrast images may also be obtained and are included when performed. CTA provides images of the blood vessels using a combination of computed tomography (CT) and angiography with contrast material. When angiography is performed using CT, multiple images are obtained and processed on a computer to create detailed, two-dimensional, cross-sectional views of the blood vessels. These images are then displayed on a computer monitor. The patient is positioned on the CT table. An intravenous line is inserted into a blood vessel, usually in the arm or hand. Non-contrast images may be obtained. A small dose of contrast is injected and test images are obtained to verify correct positioning. The CTA is then performed. Contrast is injected at a controlled rate and the CT table moves through the CT machine as the scanning is performed. After completion of the CTA, the radiologist reviews and interprets the CTA images of the blood vessels of the abdomen.

RVUs

Code	Work	PE	PE Non-Facility	MP	Total Non-Facility	Total Facility	Global
74175	1.82	7.65	7.65	0.11	9.58	9.58	XXX

74176-74178

74176 Computed tomography, abdomen and pelvis; without contrast material

74177 Computed tomography, abdomen and pelvis; with contrast material(s)

74178 Computed tomography, abdomen and pelvis; without contrast material in one or both body regions, followed by contrast material(s) and further sections in one or both body regions

(Do not report 74176-74178 in conjunction with 72192-72194, 74150-74170)

(Report 74176, 74177, or 74178 only once per CT abdomen and pelvis examination)

Plain English Description

Computed tomography, also referred to as a CT scan, uses special X-ray equipment and computer technology to produce multiple cross-sectional images of the abdomen and pelvis. The patient is positioned on the CT examination table. An initial pass is made through the CT scanner to determine the starting position of the scans. The CT scan is then performed. As the table moves slowly through the scanner, numerous X-ray beams and electronic X-ray detectors rotate around the abdomen and pelvis. The amount of radiation being absorbed is measured. As the beams and detectors rotate around the body, the table is moved through the scanner. A computer program processes the data that are then displayed on the monitor as two-dimensional cross-sectional images of the abdomen or pelvis. The physician reviews the data and images as they are obtained and may request additional sections to provide more detail on areas of interest. Use 74176 for CT scan of the abdomen and pelvis without intravenous contrast material. Use 74177 for CT scan of the abdomen and pelvis in which intravenous contrast material is administered before CT scanning begins and contrast enhanced images are obtained. Use 74178 when CT is first performed without intravenous contrast followed by the administration of intravenous contrast and acquisition of additional sections. The physician reviews the CT scan, notes any abnormalities, and provides a written interpretation of the findings.

RVUs

Code	Work	PE	PE Non-Facility	MP	Total Non-Facility	Total Facility	Global
74176	1.74	3.82	3.82	0.10	5.66	5.66	XXX
74177	1.82	7.70	7.70	0.11	9.63	9.63	XXX
74178	2.01	8.66	8.66	0.11	10.78	10.78	XXX

74181-74183

74181 Magnetic resonance (eg, proton) imaging, abdomen; without contrast material(s)

74182 Magnetic resonance (eg, proton) imaging, abdomen; with contrast material(s)

74183 Magnetic resonance (eg, proton) imaging, abdomen; without contrast material(s), followed by with contrast material(s) and further sequences

Plain English Description

Magnetic resonance imaging (MRI) is performed on the abdomen. Magnetic resonance is a noninvasive, non-radiating imaging technique that uses the magnetic properties of hydrogen atoms in the body. The patient is placed on a motorized table within a large MRI tunnel scanner that contains the magnet. The powerful magnetic field forces the hydrogen atoms to line up. Radio waves are then transmitted within the strong magnetic field. Protons in the nuclei of different types of tissues emit a specific radiofrequency signal that bounces back to the computer, which processes the signals and converts the data into tomographic, 3D images with very high resolution. The patient is placed on a motorized table within a large MRI tunnel scanner that contains the magnet. Small coils that help transmit and receive the radio waves may be placed around the abdomen. MRI is often performed for trauma and suspected internal injury, and unexplained abdominal pain, swelling, and fever. MRI scans provide clear images of areas that may be difficult to see on CT. In 74181, no contrast medium is used. In 74182, an iodine contrast dye is administered to see the target area better before images are taken. In 74183, images are taken without contrast and again after the administration of contrast. The physician reviews the images to look for information that may correlate to the patient's signs or symptoms, such as the location of tumors, abscesses, or masses; the presence of kidney stones, hernias, appendicitis or other infections, and internal injury.

RVUs

Code	Work	PE	PE Non-Facility	MP	Total Non-Facility	Total Facility	Global
74181	1.46	4.60	4.60	0.09	6.15	6.15	XXX
74182	1.73	7.73	7.73	0.11	9.57	9.57	XXX
74183	2.20	8.36	8.36	0.14	10.70	10.70	XXX

74190

74190 Peritoneogram (eg, after injection of air or contrast), radiological supervision and interpretation

(For procedure, use 49400)

(For computed tomography, see 72192 or 74150)

Plain English Description

Peritoneogram is used to visualize the contours and external surfaces of the abdominal viscera and peritoneum, measure the wall thickness of portions of the digestive organs, and detect the presence and extent of extra-abdominal tumors or disease. An appropriate site is selected in the abdominal area and the skin and subcutaneous tissue are infiltrated with local anesthesia to the level of the peritoneum. Under fluoroscopy (X-ray guidance), a needle is inserted into the peritoneum and a flexible catheter is threaded into place. Contrast dye and/or air are injected into the peritoneal space and further X-rays are obtained with the patient in varying positions. The catheter is removed at the end of the procedure. Code 74190 is used to report the radiologist's supervision of the procedure and interpretation of the findings.

RVUs

Code	Work	PE	PE Non-Facility	MP	Total Non-Facility	Total Facility	Global
74190	0.00	0.00	0.00	0.00	0.00	0.00	XXX

74400

74400 Urography (pyelography), intravenous, with or without KUB, with or without tomography

Plain English Description

A procedure is performed to visualize and study the kidneys (calyces and renal pelvis), ureters, bladder, and urethra by injecting contrast into a vein causing opacification of the urinary tract. This study may be used to assess normal functioning of the urinary system, determine anatomical variants or congenital anomalies, or detect and localize obstructions and tumors. Intravenous access is established and scout films of the kidneys, ureters, bladder (KUB) may be obtained. Contrast is injected and fluoroscopic films are obtained at intervals with the patient positioned supine, prone, and/or oblique. If tomography is performed, the urinary system is imaged by sections to produce a 3-dimensional picture. Once the contrast has filtered through the kidneys and descended through the ureters to collect in the bladder, the patient voids and additional films may be obtained to monitor the function of the urethra. One or more post void film(s) may be obtained to ensure that the bladder is completely empty.

RVUs

Code	Work	PE	PE Non-Facility	MP	Total Non-Facility	Total Facility	Global
74400	0.49	3.61	3.61	0.03	4.13	4.13	XXX

74410

74410 Urography, infusion, drip technique and/or bolus technique

Plain English Description

A procedure is performed to visualize and study the kidneys (calyces and renal pelvis), ureters, bladder, and urethra by injecting contrast into a vein causing opacification of the urinary tract. This study may be used to assess normal functioning of the urinary system, determine anatomical variants or congenital anomalies, or detect and localize obstructions and tumors. Intravenous access is established and scout films of the kidneys, ureters, bladder (KUB) may be obtained. Contrast is infused by bolus or drip technique and fluoroscopic films are obtained at intervals with the patient positioned supine, prone, and/or oblique. A bolus infusion provides greater renal opacification for a shorter period of time requiring more images (fluoroscopic films) to be taken, thus increasing the amount of radiation exposure to the patient. A drip infusion delivers a greater volume of contrast over a longer period of time so fewer images (fluoroscopic films) are required, decreasing the radiation exposure to the patient. When nephrotomography is performed, the urinary system is imaged by sections to produce a 3-dimensional picture. Once the contrast has filtered through the kidneys and descended through the ureters to collect in the bladder, the patient voids and additional films may be obtained to monitor the function of the urethra. One or more post void film(s) may be obtained to ensure that the bladder is completely empty. Code 74410 includes urography by infusion of contrast using drip or bolus technique. Code 74415 includes the addition of nephrotomography.

RVUs

Code	Work	PE	PE Non-Facility	MP	Total Non-Facility	Total Facility	Global
74410	0.49	3.75	3.75	0.03	4.27	4.27	XXX

74415

74415 Urography, infusion, drip technique and/or bolus technique; with nephrotomography

Plain English Description

A procedure is performed to visualize and study the kidneys (calyces and renal pelvis), ureters, bladder, and urethra by injecting contrast into a vein causing opacification of the urinary tract. This study may be used to assess normal functioning of the urinary system, determine anatomical variants or congenital anomalies, or detect and localize obstructions and tumors. Intravenous access is established and scout films of the kidneys, ureters, bladder (KUB) may be obtained. Contrast is infused by bolus or drip technique and fluoroscopic films are obtained at intervals with the patient positioned supine, prone, and/or oblique. A bolus infusion provides greater renal opacification for a shorter period of time requiring more images (fluoroscopic films) to be taken, thus increasing the amount of radiation exposure to the patient. A drip infusion delivers a greater volume of contrast over a longer period of time so fewer images (fluoroscopic films) are required, decreasing the radiation exposure to the patient. When nephrotomography is performed, the urinary system is imaged by sections to produce a 3-dimensional picture. Once the contrast has filtered through the kidneys and descended through the ureters to collect in the bladder, the patient voids and additional films may be obtained to monitor the function of the urethra. One or more post void film(s) may be obtained to ensure that the bladder is completely empty. Code 74410 includes urography by infusion of contrast using drip or bolus technique. Code 74415 includes the addition of nephrotomography.

RVUs

Code	Work	PE	PE Non-Facility	MP	Total Non-Facility	Total Facility	Global
74415	0.49	4.20	4.20	0.03	4.72	4.72	XXX

74420

74420 Urography, retrograde, with or without KUB

Plain English Description

The physician introduces a special dye into the kidneys and the tubes that carry urine from the kidneys to the bladder (ureters). The dye is inserted so it enters the kidneys and ureters against the normal flow of liquid through these structures. The physician then takes and examines an X-ray image of these structures. The physician may also take a general X-ray image of the abdomen during the procedure.

RVUs

Code	Work	PE	PE Non-Facility	MP	Total Non-Facility	Total Facility	Global
74420	0.52	1.74	1.74	0.03	2.29	2.29	XXX

74425

74425 Urography, antegrade, radiological supervision and interpretation

(Use 74425 in conjunction with 50390, 50396, 50684, 50690)

(Do not report 74425 in conjunction with 50430, 50431, 50432, 50433, 50434, 50435, 50693, 50694, 50695)

Plain English Description

A procedure is performed to visualize the condition of the kidney and/or ureter, assess urinary drainage, aspirate a cyst, or perform pressure studies by injecting radiopaque contrast medium either through a percutaneously placed needle or tube, or an indwelling catheter. Antegrade urography, which may include procedures such as a pyelostogram, nephrostogram, or ureteropyelogram, is also used to diagnose strictures, stones, and tumors, check previously placed nephrostomy, pyelostomy, or ureterostomy catheters and the flow of urine, or view the implanted ureters in an ileal conduit. For percutaneous antegrade urography, a local anesthetic is injected into the skin and muscle over the kidney. Using fluoroscopic guidance, a needle is inserted through the skin and advanced to the target site, such as the renal pelvis of the kidney. Contrast medium is then injected through the needle and radiologic images of the upper collection system and ureter are obtained as urine drains to the bladder. For antegrade urography through a previously placed indwelling catheter in the kidney, renal pelvis, or ureter, a syringe filled with contrast dye is connected to the catheter. Contrast is injected and X-ray images are taken of the catheter, the kidney, and ureter as urine drains. A similar injection procedure may be performed through an existing stoma for ureteropyelography or to visualize implanted ureters and section of small bowel (ileal conduit) that has been repositioned to function as a bladder and allow urine to drain. Code 74425 reports only the radiological supervision and interpretation portion of an antegrade urography procedure, including the review of images obtained and a written report of the findings.

RVUs

Code	Work	PE	PE Non-Facility	MP	Total Non-Facility	Total Facility	Global
74425	0.51	3.62	3.62	0.03	4.16	4.16	XXX

74430

74430 Cystography, minimum of 3 views, radiological supervision and interpretation

Plain English Description

Radiological supervision is provided for a procedure to examine the bladder using fluoroscopy and radiopaque contrast medium. Cystography may be used to diagnose vesicoureteral reflux, bladder tumors, polyps, or injury. An X-ray of the bladder/urinary tract without contrast may be obtained prior to beginning the cystogram. A catheter is inserted through the urethra into the bladder. Contrast is instilled through the catheter until the bladder is distended. X-rays are obtained of the bladder/ureters from one or more angles. The catheter is removed and the patient allowed to void. An X-ray is obtained after the patient voids to determine if all contrast has been expelled from the bladder. Code 74430 reports the radiological supervision of the cystography procedure with a minimum of 3 views taken, review of records obtained, interpretation of the findings, and a written report.

RVUs

Code	Work	PE	PE Non-Facility	MP	Total Non-Facility	Total Facility	Global
74430	0.32	0.87	0.87	0.02	1.21	1.21	XXX

74440

74440 Vasography, vesiculography, or epididymography, radiological supervision and interpretation

Plain English Description

Radiological supervision is provided for a procedure to examine the male reproductive system for tumors, cysts, abscesses, inflammation, or obstruction using fluoroscopy and a radiopaque contrast medium. Small bilateral incisions are made in the upper scrotum to expose and identify the vas deferens. A needle or small catheter is inserted into the vas deferens, contrast medium is injected, and the flow of contrast through the vas deferens, seminal vesicles, or ejaculatory ducts is observed and recorded. At the conclusion of the procedure, the needles or catheters are removed and the incisions are closed. Code 74440 reports the radiological supervision of the vasography, vesiculography, or epididymography procedure, review of records obtained, and interpretation of the findings, with a written report provided.

RVUs

Code	Work	PE	PE Non-Facility	MP	Total Non-Facility	Total Facility	Global
74440	0.38	2.56	2.56	0.02	2.96	2.96	XXX

74445

74445 Corpora cavernosography, radiological supervision and interpretation

Plain English Description

Cavernosography involves the injection of contrast medium into the corpora cavernosa to examine radiographically the structure of the corpora cavernosa and the veins that drain blood from it. During a separately reportable injection procedure, a 19-22 gauge needle is inserted into the tissue of the corpora cavernosa on the dorsal lateral aspect proximal to the glans penis and contrast medium injected. Radiographic images are taken immediately from two angles, anterior/posterior and lateral/oblique. The radiologist supervises the injection procedure and provides a written interpretation of the procedure.

RVUs

Code	Work	PE	PE Non-Facility	MP	Total Non-Facility	Total Facility	Global
74445	0.00	0.00	0.00	0.00	0.00	0.00	XXX

74450

74450 Urethrocystography, retrograde, radiological supervision and interpretation

Plain English Description

Radiological supervision is provided for a procedure to examine the urethra and bladder using fluoroscopy and radiopaque contrast medium. Urethrocystography may be used to diagnose injury, congenital anomalies, tumors, diverticula, stones, fistulas, strictures, or obstruction. Contrast is instilled through the external urethral orifice, distending and filling the urethra and bladder. X-rays are obtained of the urethra and bladder from one or more angles. The patient is then allowed to void and an X-ray is obtained after voiding to determine if all contrast has been expelled. Code 74450 reports the radiological supervision of the urethrocystography procedure, review of records obtained, and interpretation of the findings, with a written report provided.

RVUs

Code	Work	PE	PE Non-Facility	MP	Total Non-Facility	Total Facility	Global
74450	0.00	0.00	0.00	0.00	0.00	0.00	XXX

74455

74455 Urethrocystography, voiding, radiological supervision and interpretation

Plain English Description

Radiological supervision is provided for a procedure to examine the urethra and bladder using fluoroscopy and radiopaque contrast medium. Voiding urethrocystography may be used to diagnose injury, congenital anomalies, tumors, diverticula, stones, fistulas, strictures, or obstruction. Contrast is instilled through the external urethral orifice, distending and filling the urethra and bladder. X-rays are obtained of the urethra and bladder from one or more angles. The patient then voids on the table while additional X-rays are obtained to monitor the flow of contrast out of the bladder and through the urethra until all contrast has been expelled. Code 74455 reports the radiological supervision of the voiding urethrocystography procedure, review of records obtained, and interpretation of the findings, with a written report provided.

RVUs

Code	Work	PE	PE Non-Facility	MP	Total Non-Facility	Total Facility	Global
74455	0.33	2.83	2.83	0.02	3.18	3.18	XXX

74470

74470 Radiologic examination, renal cyst study, translumbar, contrast visualization, radiological supervision and interpretation

Plain English Description

A procedure is performed for radiologic study of a renal cyst using a translumbar approach. Under fluoroscopic guidance, a needle is placed through the skin in the lower back and into the renal cyst. A radiopaque contrast medium is injected and X-ray images are obtained. The radiologist will examine the images for characteristics in the cyst that might indicate malignancy, including shape, margination of the walls, enhancement properties, and the presence of septa and nodular protuberances. Code 74470 reports the radiological supervision of the translumbar injection of contrast medium to visualize and study a renal cyst, review of records obtained, and interpretation of the findings, and a written report.

RVUs

Code	Work	PE	PE Non-Facility	MP	Total Non-Facility	Total Facility	Global
74470	0.00	0.00	0.00	0.00	0.00	0.00	XXX

74485

74485 Dilation of ureter(s) or urethra, radiological supervision and interpretation

(Do not report 74485 in conjunction with 50436, 50437)

(For dilation of ureter without radiologic guidance, use 52341, 52344)

(For change of nephrostomy or pyelostomy tube, use 50435)

(For dilation of a nephrostomy tract for endourologic procedure, see 50436, 50437)

Plain English Description

Radiological supervision is provided for a procedure to dilate the ureter(s) or urethra. This procedure may be required when stenosis or obstruction of one or more of these structures is documented or suspected. To dilate the ureter(s), a cystourethroscope is inserted into the urethra, advanced through the bladder into the ureter, and a guidewire passed through the area of the stricture. A semi-rigid or flexible ureteroscope is passed over the guidewire to the area of the stricture. Contrast medium is injected and X-ray images are obtained. A balloon dilator may then be advanced and inflated to dilate the stricture. To dilate the urethra, radiopaque contrast medium is injected through the external urethral orifice and X-ray images are obtained. The urethra is then dilated using progressively larger dilators or a balloon catheter. Code 74485 reports the radiological supervision of a ureteral or urethral dilation procedure, review of records obtained, interpretation of the findings, and provision of a written report.

RVUs

Code	Work	PE	PE Non-Facility	MP	Total Non-Facility	Total Facility	Global
74485	0.83	2.72	2.72	0.03	3.58	3.58	XXX

75831

75831 Venography, renal, unilateral, selective, radiological supervision and interpretation

Plain English Description

Radiological supervision is provided for a procedure to evaluate the renal veins using radiopaque contrast medium and fluoroscopy. The study may be performed to diagnose blood clots, tumors, retroperitoneal fibrosis, renal agenesis, venous anomalies, and renovascular hypertension. Normally, the femoral vein is used and accessed with a large bore needle in the right or left groin. A guidewire is threaded through the needle and advanced into the vena cava and into the renal veins. A catheter is then threaded over the guidewire to the selected location and the guidewire is removed. Blood samples may be obtained and tested for renin levels if renovascular hypertension is suspected. Contrast medium is injected through the catheter and X-rays are taken as the dye moves through the right and/or left renal veins. At the conclusion of the study, the catheter is removed. These codes report the radiological supervision of the unilateral (75831) or bilateral (75833) selective renal venography procedure, review and interpretation of the images obtained, and written report of the findings.

RVUs

Code	Work	PE	PE Non-Facility	MP	Total Non-Facility	Total Facility	Global
75831	1.14	2.32	2.32	0.10	3.56	3.56	XXX

75833

75833 Venography, renal, bilateral, selective, radiological supervision and interpretation

Plain English Description

Radiological supervision is provided for a procedure to evaluate the renal veins using radiopaque contrast medium and fluoroscopy. The study may be performed to diagnose blood clots, tumors, retroperitoneal fibrosis, renal agenesis, venous anomalies, and renovascular hypertension. Normally, the femoral vein is used and accessed with a large bore needle in the right or left groin. A guidewire is threaded through the needle and advanced into the vena cava and into the renal veins. A catheter is then threaded over the guidewire to the selected location and the guidewire is removed. Blood samples may be obtained and tested for renin levels if renovascular hypertension is suspected. Contrast medium is injected through the catheter and X-rays are taken as the dye moves through the right and/or left renal veins. At the conclusion of the study, the catheter is removed. These codes report the radiological supervision of the unilateral (75831) or bilateral (75833) selective renal venography procedure, review and interpretation of the images obtained, and written report of the findings.

RVUs

Code	Work	PE	PE Non-Facility	MP	Total Non-Facility	Total Facility	Global
75833	1.49	2.72	2.72	0.20	4.41	4.41	XXX

75984

75984 Change of percutaneous tube or drainage catheter with contrast monitoring (eg, genitourinary system, abscess), radiological supervision and interpretation

(For percutaneous replacement of gastrostomy, duodenostomy, jejunostomy, gastro-jejunostomy, or cecostomy [or other colonic] tube including fluoroscopic imaging guidance, see 49450-49452)

(To report exchange of a percutaneous nephrostomy catheter, use 50435)

(For percutaneous cholecystostomy, use 47490)

(For percutaneous biliary procedures, including radiological supervision and interpretation, see 47531-47544)

(For percutaneous nephrostolithotomy or pyelostolithotomy, see 50080, 50081)

(For removal and/or replacement of an internally dwelling ureteral stent via a transurethral approach, see 50385-50386)

Plain English Description

Radiological supervision and interpretation is performed during a separately reportable change of a percutaneous tube or drainage catheter with the use of contrast monitoring. A tube of the genitourinary system, an abscess, or other type drainage catheter is visualized and changed using ultrasound, fluoroscopy, or CT. Contrast media is injected into the existing tube or drainage catheter to identify the current location and any malfunction. The existing tube or drainage catheter is visualized as it is removed. A replacement tube or drainage catheter is then placed under radiographic guidance through the existing tract. Contrast media is injected to verify correct placement of the replacement tube or drainage catheter.

RVUs

Code	Work	PE	PE Non-Facility	MP	Total Non-Facility	Total Facility	Global
75984	0.83	2.03	2.03	0.05	2.91	2.91	XXX

75989

75989 Radiological guidance (ie, fluoroscopy, ultrasound, or computed tomography), for percutaneous drainage (eg, abscess, specimen collection), with placement of catheter, radiological supervision and interpretation

(Do not report 75989 in conjunction with 10030, 32554, 32555, 32556, 32557, 33017, 33018, 33019, 47490, 49405, 49406, 49407)

Plain English Description

Radiological guidance for placement of a minimally invasive percutaneous drainage catheter may be accomplished using fluoroscopy, ultrasound, or computed tomography (CT). The drainage catheter is a thin, flexible, hollow tube that can be inserted through the skin into an area of collected fluid in order to drain the serum, blood, pus, and cellular debris and/or obtain a specimen sample for testing. The most common areas in which fluid accumulates are the chest, abdomen, and pelvic cavities. Code 75989 reports the radiologist's supervision of the percutaneous drainage procedure, review and interpretation of the findings, and the written report.

RVUs

Code	Work	PE	PE Non-Facility	MP	Total Non-Facility	Total Facility	Global
75989	1.19	2.14	2.14	0.09	3.42	3.42	XXX

76000

76000 Fluoroscopy (separate procedure), up to 1 hour physician or other qualified health care professional time

(Do not report 76000 in conjunction with 33274, 33275, 33957, 33958, 33959, 33962, 33963, 33964, 0515T, 0516T, 0517T, 0518T, 0519T, 0520T)

Plain English Description

Fluoroscopic monitoring of a separately reportable procedure is performed. Fluoroscopy is an imaging technique used to obtain real-time moving images of internal structures using a device that consists of an X-ray source and a fluorescent screen. These devices include image intensifiers and video cameras that allow images to be recorded and displayed on a monitor. In 76000, the physician or other qualified health care professional provides fluoroscopic monitoring for up to 1 hour for a service or procedure that does not include the fluoroscopy service as part of the procedure.

RVUs

Code	Work	PE	PE Non-Facility	MP	Total Non-Facility	Total Facility	Global
76000	0.30	0.93	0.93	0.05	1.28	1.28	XXX

76700-76705

76700 Ultrasound, abdominal, real time with image documentation; complete

76705 Ultrasound, abdominal, real time with image documentation; limited (eg, single organ, quadrant, follow-up)

Plain English Description

A real-time abdominal ultrasound is performed with image documentation. The patient is placed supine. Acoustic coupling gel is applied to the skin of the abdomen. The transducer is pressed firmly against the skin and swept back and forth over the abdomen and images obtained. The ultrasonic wave pulses directed at the abdomen are imaged by recording the ultrasound echoes. Any abnormalities are evaluated to identify characteristics that might provide a definitive diagnosis. The physician reviews the ultrasound images of the abdomen and provides a written interpretation. Code 76700 is used for a complete abdominal ultrasound, which includes real-time scanning of the liver, gallbladder, common bile duct, pancreas, spleen, kidneys, upper abdominal aorta, and inferior vena cava. Code 76705 is used when a limited ultrasound examination is performed such as a single organ, single quadrant, or a follow-up scan.

RVUs

Code	Work	PE	PE Non-Facility	MP	Total Non-Facility	Total Facility	Global
76700	0.81	2.67	2.67	0.05	3.53	3.53	XXX
76705	0.59	2.00	2.00	0.05	2.64	2.64	XXX

76770-76775

76770 Ultrasound, retroperitoneal (eg, renal, aorta, nodes), real time with image documentation; complete

76775 Ultrasound, retroperitoneal (eg, renal, aorta, nodes), real time with image documentation; limited

Plain English Description

A real-time retroperitoneal ultrasound is performed with image documentation. The patient is placed supine. Acoustic coupling gel is applied to the skin of the abdomen. The transducer is pressed firmly against the skin and swept back and forth over the abdomen and images obtained of the retroperitoneal area. The ultrasonic wave pulses directed at the retroperitoneum are imaged by recording the ultrasound echoes. Any abnormalities are evaluated to identify characteristics that might provide a definitive diagnosis. The physician reviews the ultrasound images of the retroperitoneum and provides a written interpretation. Code 76770 is used for a complete retroperitoneal ultrasound, which includes real-time scanning of the kidneys, abdominal aorta, common iliac artery origins, and inferior vena cava. Alternatively, if ultrasonography is being performed to evaluate the urinary tract, examination of the kidneys and urinary bladder constitutes a complete exam. Code 76775 is used when a limited retroperitoneal ultrasound examination is performed.

RVUs

Code	Work	PE	PE Non-Facility	MP	Total Non-Facility	Total Facility	Global
76770	0.74	2.48	2.48	0.05	3.27	3.27	XXX
76775	0.58	1.10	1.10	0.05	1.73	1.73	XXX

76776

76776 Ultrasound, transplanted kidney, real time and duplex Doppler with image documentation

(For ultrasound of transplanted kidney without duplex Doppler, use 76775)

(For ultrasound and duplex Doppler of a transplanted kidney, do not report 76776 in conjunction with 93975, 93976)

Plain English Description

An ultrasound (US) study of the transplanted kidney in real time and duplex Doppler may be performed in the early perioperative period or later for routine follow-up. US studies are used to evaluate renal function and monitor the patient for complications. There are two elements to renal US gray scale to evaluate structures without assessing motion, and Doppler to visualize blood flow. They are displayed on the same screen as overlapping images to provide a real-time picture for documentation and interpretation by the radiologist. A transplanted kidney is most often positioned in the extraperitoneal area of the right or left iliac fossa, which allows for excellent visualization of the organ during US examination. The patient history should be reviewed including the exact renal transplant procedure used to ensure accurate documentation of abnormal or normal findings. The perinephric space is examined for fluid collection of urine, blood, lymph, or pus. Urinomas and hematomas are common in the first 2 weeks of the postoperative period. Lymphoceles are a later complication, typically appearing 4-8 weeks postoperatively. The renal parenchyma is then examined for cortical thickening or enlargement, changes in echogenicity, loss of corticomedullary differentiation, prominent pyramids, or thickened collecting systems. All can be signs of decreased renal function and possible rejection of the transplanted organ. The urinary collecting system is assessed for urine leak or urinoma, obstruction, or calculi. Finally, the vasculature is examined for renal artery occlusion, renal vein thrombosis, or stenosis of either vessel.

RVUs

Code	Work	PE	PE Non-Facility	MP	Total Non-Facility	Total Facility	Global
76776	0.76	3.67	3.67	0.06	4.49	4.49	XXX

76870

76870 Ultrasound, scrotum and contents

Plain English Description

An ultrasound examination of the scrotum and its contents is a non-invasive procedure that uses a transducer probe placed firmly against the skin to deliver high-frequency sound waves and create a gray scale and/or color (Doppler) image of the internal anatomy. Ultrasound may be used to detect scrotal masses/tumors and undescended testicle(s), as well as to evaluate testicular torsion, scrotal injury or trauma, hydrocele(s), varicocele(s), and male infertility. Ultrasonic conduction gel is applied to the scrotum and the transducer probe is held against the skin and swept over the area. The images produced are captured on a screen and viewed in real-time and/or saved for later analysis.

RVUs

Code	Work	PE	PE Non-Facility	MP	Total Non-Facility	Total Facility	Global
76870	0.64	2.35	2.35	0.05	3.04	3.04	XXX

76872-76873

76872 Ultrasound, transrectal

(Do not report 76872 in conjunction with 45341, 45342, 45391, 45392, 46948, 0421T, 0619T)

76873 Ultrasound, transrectal; prostate volume study for brachytherapy treatment planning (separate procedure)

Plain English Description

The physician inserts an ultrasound probe through the rectum to view an ultrasound image of tissue inside the digestive tract. This imaging technique bounces waves through tissue in the body and a response is given to a receiving unit. The unit converts what is received into electrical pulses that are displayed on a screen. Code 76873 if the physician measures the size of the prostate, allowing the physician to determine the best course of brachytherapy, the implantation of radioactive beads for prostate cancer.

RVUs

Code	Work	PE	PE Non-Facility	MP	Total Non-Facility	Total Facility	Global
76872	0.69	5.38	5.38	0.04	6.11	6.11	XXX
76873	1.55	3.57	3.57	0.06	5.18	5.18	XXX

76940

76940 Ultrasound guidance for, and monitoring of, parenchymal tissue ablation

(Do not report 76940 in conjunction with 20982, 20983, 32994, 32998, 50250, 50542, 76942, 76998, 0582T, 0600T, 0601T)

(For ablation, see 47370-47382, 47383, 50592, 50593)

Plain English Description

Ultrasound (US) may be used to guide and monitor parenchymal tissue ablation procedures in a patient undergoing microwave ablation (MVA) or radiofrequency ablation (RVA) of a tumor or abnormal tissue in an organ or gland. US may be used to map the area of treatment and guide the needle(s) to the correct site. It can then be used to monitor the treatment and aid the physician in determining when adequate ablation of the tumor or abnormal tissue has been achieved. Code 76940 reports the ultrasound used during the separately reportable tissue ablation procedure.

RVUs

Code	Work	PE	PE Non-Facility	MP	Total Non-Facility	Total Facility	Global
76940	0.00	0.00	0.00	0.00	0.00	0.00	YYY

76942

76942 Ultrasonic guidance for needle placement (eg, biopsy, aspiration, injection, localization device), imaging supervision and interpretation

(Do not report 76942 in conjunction with 10004, 10005, 10006, 10021, 10030, 19083, 19285, 20604, 20606, 20611, 27096, 32408, 32554, 32555, 32556, 32557, 37760, 37761, 43232, 43237, 43242, 45341, 45342, 46948, 55874, 64479, 64480, 64483, 64484, 64490, 64491, 64493, 64494, 64495, 76975, 0213T, 0214T, 0215T, 0216T, 0217T, 0218T, 0232T, 0481T, 0582T)

(For harvesting, preparation, and injection[s] of platelet rich plasma, use 0232T)

Plain English Description

Ultrasound (US) guidance including imaging supervision and interpretation is performed for needle placement during a separately reportable biopsy, aspiration, injection, or placement of a localization device. A local anesthetic is injected at the site of the planned needle or localization device placement. A transducer is then used to locate the lesion, site of the planned injection, or site of the planned placement of the localization device. The radiologist constantly monitors needle placement with the US probe to ensure the needle is properly placed. The radiologist also uses US imaging to monitor separately reportable biopsy, aspiration, injection, or device localization procedures. Upon completion of the procedure, the needle is withdrawn and pressure applied to control bleeding. A dressing is applied as needed. The radiologist then provides a written report of the US imaging component of the procedure.

RVUs

Code	Work	PE	PE Non-Facility	MP	Total Non-Facility	Total Facility	Global
76942	0.67	1.00	1.00	0.05	1.72	1.72	XXX

77002

✚ **77002 Fluoroscopic guidance for needle placement (eg, biopsy, aspiration, injection, localization device) (List separately in addition to code for primary procedure)**

(Use 77002 in conjunction with 10160, 20206, 20220, 20225, 20520, 20525, 20526, 20550, 20551, 20552, 20553, 20555, 20600, 20605, 20610, 20612, 20615, 21116, 21550, 23350, 24220, 25246, 27093, 27095, 27369, 27648, 32400, 32553, 36002, 38220, 38221, 38222, 38505, 38794, 41019, 42400, 42405, 47000, 47001, 48102, 49180, 49411, 50200, 50390, 51100, 51101, 51102, 55700, 55876, 60100, 62268, 62269, 64400-64448, 64450, 64455, 64505, 64600, 64605)

(77002 is included in all arthrography radiological supervision and interpretation codes. See Administration of Contrast Material[s] introductory guidelines for reporting of arthrography procedures)

Plain English Description

This code reports the radiological portion of fluoroscopic guidance used in needle placement for biopsy, aspiration, injection, or localization type procedures. Fluoroscopy is a continuous, X-ray beam passed through the body part being examined and projected onto a TV-like monitor to create a kind of X-ray movie. This uses more radiation than standard X-rays and can image many different body systems to study a specific structure or organ, localize a tumor or foreign body, and also study movement within the body. The area is identified with fluoroscopy and anesthetized. The appropriate type of needle is inserted under fluoroscopic guidance to perform the specified procedure such as removing aspirate or tissue samples for biopsy, injecting a therapeutic or diagnostic substance, or localizing a tumor or mass for further study. The primary procedural code reports the type of procedure and anatomic location.

RVUs

Code	Work	PE	PE Non-Facility	MP	Total Non-Facility	Total Facility	Global
77002	0.54	2.90	2.90	0.05	3.49	3.49	ZZZ

77012

77012 Computed tomography guidance for needle placement (eg, biopsy, aspiration, injection, localization device), radiological supervision and interpretation

(Do not report 77011, 77012 in conjunction with 22586)

(Do not report 77012 in conjunction with 10009, 10010, 10030, 27096, 32408, 32554, 32555, 32556, 32557, 62270, 62272, 62328, 62329, 64479, 64480, 64483, 64484, 64490, 64491, 64492, 64493, 64494, 64495, 64633, 64634, 64635, 64636, 0232T, 0481T, 0629T, 0630T)

(For harvesting, preparation, and injection[s] of platelet-rich plasma, use 0232T)

Plain English Description

This code reports the radiological supervision and interpretation portion of computed tomography (CT) guidance used in needle placement for biopsy, aspiration, injection, or localization procedures. The target area is localized using CT and then anesthetized. The appropriate type of needle is inserted under CT guidance to perform the specified procedure, such as removing aspirate or tissue samples for biopsy, injecting a therapeutic or diagnostic substance, or localizing a tumor or mass for further study. The surgical code reports the procedure and anatomic location. CT aims multiple, narrow X-ray beams around a single rotational axis, taking a large series of two-dimensional images of the target structure from multiple angles. The computer can digitally reconstruct the data into a 3D image and produce thin, cross-sectional 2D or 3D images (slices) of the test object.

RVUs

Code	Work	PE	PE Non-Facility	MP	Total Non-Facility	Total Facility	Global
77012	1.50	2.65	2.65	0.10	4.25	4.25	XXX

77013

77013 Computed tomography guidance for, and monitoring of, parenchymal tissue ablation

(Do not report 77013 in conjunction with 20982, 20983, 32994, 32998, 0600T)

(For percutaneous ablation, see 47382, 47383, 50592, 50593)

Plain English Description

This code reports the radiological supervision and interpretation portion of computed tomography (CT) guidance used in tissue ablation procedures. The target area is localized using CT and then anesthetized. The appropriate type of needle is inserted under CT guidance to perform the specified procedure, such as removing aspirate or tissue samples for biopsy, injecting a therapeutic or diagnostic substance, or localizing a tumor or mass for further study. The surgical code reports the procedure and anatomic location. CT aims multiple, narrow X-ray beams around a single rotational axis, taking a large series of 2D images of the target structure from multiple angles. The computer can digitally reconstruct the data into a 3D image and produce thin, cross-sectional 2D or 3D images (slices) of the test object.

RVUs

Code	Work	PE	PE Non-Facility	MP	Total Non-Facility	Total Facility	Global
77013	0.00	0.00	0.00	0.00	0.00	0.00	XXX

77021

77021 Magnetic resonance imaging guidance for needle placement (eg, for biopsy, needle aspiration, injection, or placement of localization device) radiological supervision and interpretation

(For procedure, see appropriate organ or site)

(Do not report 77021 in conjunction with 10011, 10012, 10030, 19085, 19287, 32408, 32554, 32555, 32556, 32557, 0232T, 0481T)

(For harvesting, preparation, and injection[s] of platelet-rich plasma, use 0232T)

Plain English Description

This code reports the radiological supervision and interpretation portion of magnetic resonance imaging (MRI) guidance used in needle placement for biopsy, aspiration, injection, or localization procedures. The target area is localized using MRI and then anesthetized. The appropriate type of needle is inserted under MRI guidance to perform the specified procedure, such as removing aspirate or tissue samples for biopsy, injecting a therapeutic or diagnostic substance, or localizing a tumor or mass for further study. The surgical code reports the procedure and anatomic location. MRI is a noninvasive, non-radiating imaging technique that uses the magnetic properties of hydrogen atoms in the body. The nuclei of hydrogen atoms emit radiofrequency signals when the body is exposed to radio waves transmitted within a strong magnetic field. The computer processes the signals and converts the data into tomographic, 3D images with very high resolution. The needle being used with MRI guidance may have special metallic ringlets around it, be coated with contrast material, or have a signal-receiving coil in its tip.

RVUs

Code	Work	PE	PE Non-Facility	MP	Total Non-Facility	Total Facility	Global
77021	1.50	11.26	11.26	0.07	12.83	12.83	XXX

77022

77022 Magnetic resonance imaging guidance for, and monitoring of, parenchymal tissue ablation

(Do not report 77022 in conjunction with 20982, 20983, 32994, 32998, 0071T, 0072T, 0600T)

(For percutaneous ablation, see 47382, 47383, 50592, 50593)

(For focused ultrasound ablation treatment of uterine leiomyomata, see Category III codes 0071T, 0072T)

(To report stereotactic localization guidance for breast biopsy or for placement of breast localization device[s], see 19081, 19283)

(To report mammographic guidance for placement of breast localization device[s], use 19281)

Plain English Description

This code reports magnetic resonance imaging (MRI) guidance used in monitoring parenchymal tissue ablation procedures. Parenchymal tissue is the bulk of functional cells within an organ, such as the liver, kidneys, or glands as opposed to the structural stroma cells, such as blood vessels and connective tissue. Ablation causes cell death by the targeted application of destructive energy, inducing localized necrosis and scar tissue that eventually shrinks. The target area is localized using MRI. The appropriate type of needle, catheter, or other energy application device is inserted under MRI guidance to perform the specified ablation procedure, such as tumor or mass destruction. The surgical code reports the procedure and anatomic location. Magnetic resonance is a noninvasive, non-radiating imaging technique that uses the magnetic properties of hydrogen atoms in the body. The nuclei of hydrogen atoms emit radiofrequency signals when the body is exposed to radio waves transmitted within a strong magnetic field. The computer processes the signals and converts the data into tomographic, 3D images with very high resolution. The device being used with MRI guidance may have special metallic ringlets around it, be coated with contrast material, or have a signal-receiving coil in its tip.

RVUs

Code	Work	PE	PE Non-Facility	MP	Total Non-Facility	Total Facility	Global
77022	0.00	0.00	0.00	0.00	0.00	0.00	XXX

78700-78701

78700 Kidney imaging morphology

78701 Kidney imaging morphology; with vascular flow

Plain English Description

The size, shape, and structure (morphology) of the kidney and its function, including vascular flow, is assessed using scintigraphy and a radiolabeled isotope tracer. The kidneys filter waste from the blood; maintain a balance of certain chemicals; and produce erythropoietin for red blood cell growth, renin for blood pressure control, and calcitriol for calcium uptake by the bones. This procedure may be used to evaluate renal blood flow, renovascular hypertension, renal cysts, tumors, abscesses, and kidney disease, as well as monitoring kidney transplants. An intravenous line is established and the radiolabeled isotope tracer is injected directly into the circulatory system. The patient is positioned on the imaging table with the gamma camera focused on the kidneys. Scanning is performed at specific intervals and the radioactive energy emitted is converted into an image. Code 78700 is used when only the morphology of the kidney is being studied. Code 78701 is used when morphology and vascular flow are studied. The physician interprets the study and provides a written report of the findings.

RVUs

Code	Work	PE	PE Non-Facility	MP	Total Non-Facility	Total Facility	Global
78700	0.45	4.34	4.34	0.06	4.85	4.85	XXX
78701	0.49	5.72	5.72	0.06	6.27	6.27	XXX

78707-78709

78707 Kidney imaging morphology; with vascular flow and function, single study without pharmacological intervention

78708 Kidney imaging morphology; with vascular flow and function, single study, with pharmacological intervention (eg, angiotensin converting enzyme inhibitor and/or diuretic)

78709 Kidney imaging morphology; with vascular flow and function, multiple studies, with and without pharmacological intervention (eg, angiotensin converting enzyme inhibitor and/or diuretic)

(For introduction of radioactive substance in association with renal endoscopy, use 77778)

Plain English Description

The size, shape, and structure (morphology) of the kidney and its function, including vascular flow, is assessed using scintigraphy and a radiolabeled isotope tracer. The kidneys filter waste from the blood; maintain a balance of certain chemicals; and produce erythropoietin for red blood cell growth, renin for blood pressure control, and calcitriol for calcium uptake by the bones. This procedure may be used to evaluate renal blood flow, renovascular hypertension, renal cysts, tumors, abscesses, and kidney disease, as well as monitor kidney transplants. An intravenous line is established and the radiolabeled isotope tracer is injected directly into the circulatory system. The patient is positioned on the imaging table with the gamma camera focused on the kidneys. Scanning is performed at specific intervals and the radioactive energy emitted is converted into an image. A diuretic may be administered during the procedure for more detailed images of kidney obstruction. An angiotensin converting enzyme (ACE-inhibitor) medication may be administered to help determine if hypertension is associated with renal vascular flow. Code 78707 is used when kidney morphology, vascular flow, and function are assessed in a single study without the use of diuretics or ACE-inhibitor medications. Code 78708 is used when kidney morphology, vascular flow, and function are assessed in a single study with the use of diuretics and/or ACE-inhibitors. Code 78709 is used when morphology, vascular flow, and function are assessed in multiple studies both with and without the use of diuretics and/or ACE-inhibiting medications. The physician interprets the study and provides a written report of the findings.

RVUs

Code	Work	PE	PE Non-Facility	MP	Total Non-Facility	Total Facility	Global
78707	0.96	5.54	5.54	0.08	6.58	6.58	XXX
78708	1.21	3.87	3.87	0.10	5.18	5.18	XXX
78709	1.41	8.94	8.94	0.12	10.47	10.47	XXX

78725

78725 Kidney function study, non-imaging radioisotopic study

Plain English Description

A study of kidney function is performed using a scintillation counter and a radiolabeled isotope tracer. The kidneys filter waste from the blood; maintain a balance of certain chemicals; and produce erythropoietin for red blood cell growth, renin for blood pressure control, and calcitriol for calcium uptake by the bones. An intravenous line is established and the radiolabeled isotope tracer is injected directly into the circulatory system. The patient is positioned on the procedure table with the scintillation counter focused on the kidneys. The counter records the amount of radiolabeled isotope tracer that is filtered by the kidneys and excreted in urine via the bladder. The physician interprets the study and provides a written report of the findings.

RVUs

Code	Work	PE	PE Non-Facility	MP	Total Non-Facility	Total Facility	Global
78725	0.38	2.90	2.90	0.05	3.33	3.33	XXX

78730

+ **78730 Urinary bladder residual study (List separately in addition to code for primary procedure)**

(Use 78730 in conjunction with 78740)

(For measurement of postvoid residual urine and/or bladder capacity by ultrasound, nonimaging, use 51798)

(For ultrasound imaging of the bladder only, with measurement of postvoid residual urine when performed, use 76857)

Plain English Description

A urinary bladder residual study is performed using scintigraphy and a radiolabeled isotope tracer. This procedure is used to examine how well the bladder empties and to assess for obstruction or dysfunction. The bladder may be catheterized with direct radionucleotide cystography (DRC) and the radiolabeled isotope tracer instilled with fluid to distend the bladder, after which the patient voids and the urine remaining in the bladder is measured or calculated; or, the radiolabeled isotope tracer can be injected directly into the circulatory system with indirect radionucleotide cystography (IRC) and images obtained of the kidney, ureters, and bladder, including post void to detect residual urine. The patient is prepared appropriately for either approach, bladder catheterization or intravenous line insertion, and the gamma camera is positioned to capture images of the bladder. Scanning is performed at specific intervals and the radioactive energy emitted is converted into an image. The physician interprets the study and provides a written report of the findings.

RVUs

Code	Work	PE	PE Non-Facility	MP	Total Non-Facility	Total Facility	Global
78730	0.15	1.98	1.98	0.01	2.14	2.14	ZZZ

78740

78740 Ureteral reflux study (radiopharmaceutical voiding cystogram)

(Use 78740 in conjunction with 78730 for urinary bladder residual study)

(For catheterization, see 51701, 51702, 51703)

Plain English Description

A ureteral reflux study is performed using scintigraphy and a radiolabeled isotope tracer. This procedure is used to assess backflow of urine from the bladder to the kidneys. The bladder may be catheterized with direct radionucleotide cystography (DRC) and the radiolabeled isotope tracer instilled with fluid to distend the bladder, which is observed for retrograde movement of urine through the vesicoureteral valves. The radiolabeled isotope tracer can also be injected directly into the circulatory system with indirect radionucleotide cystography (IRC) and images obtained of the kidney, ureters, and bladder, including retrograde movement of urine from the bladder to the kidneys and bladder emptying. The patient is prepared appropriately for either approach, bladder catheterization for DRC or intravenous line insertion for IRC, and the gamma camera is positioned to capture images of the urinary system. Scanning is performed at specific intervals and the radioactive energy emitted is converted into an image. The physician interprets the study and provides a written report of the findings.

RVUs

Code	Work	PE	PE Non-Facility	MP	Total Non-Facility	Total Facility	Global
78740	0.57	5.55	5.55	0.05	6.17	6.17	XXX

78761

78761 Testicular imaging with vascular flow

Plain English Description

Testicular imaging with vascular flow is performed using scintigraphy and a radiolabeled isotope tracer. This procedure may be used to diagnose spermatic cord torsion, epididymitis, or orchitis. An intravenous line is established and the radiolabeled isotope tracer is injected directly into the circulatory system. The patient is positioned on the procedure table with the gamma camera positioned for scrotal imaging. Flow studies are obtained to document vascular perfusion of the testis, which may be displayed in cinematic mode followed by static images of the testis, spermatic cords, and other structures. The radioactive energy emitted is converted into an image and the physician interprets the study and provides a written report of the findings.

RVUs

Code	Work	PE	PE Non-Facility	MP	Total Non-Facility	Total Facility	Global
78761	0.71	5.24	5.24	0.08	6.03	6.03	XXX

80047-80048

80047 Basic metabolic panel (Calcium, ionized)

This panel must include the following:

Calcium, ionized (82330); Carbon dioxide (bicarbonate) (82374); Chloride (82435); Creatinine (82565); Glucose (82947); Potassium (84132); Sodium (84295); Urea Nitrogen (BUN) (84520)

80048 Basic metabolic panel (Calcium, total)

This panel must include the following:

Calcium, total (82310); Carbon dioxide (bicarbonate) (82374); Chloride (82435); Creatinine (82565); Glucose (82947); Potassium (84132); Sodium (84295); Urea nitrogen (BUN) (84520)

Plain English Description

A basic metabolic blood panel is obtained that includes ionized calcium levels along with carbon dioxide (bicarbonate) (CO_2), chloride, creatinine, glucose, potassium, sodium, and urea nitrogen (BUN). A basic metabolic panel with measurement of ionized calcium may be used to screen for or monitor overall metabolic function or identify imbalances. Ionized or free calcium flows freely in the blood, is not attached to any proteins, and represents the amount of calcium available to support metabolic processes, such as heart function, muscle contraction, nerve function, and blood clotting. Total carbon dioxide (bicarbonate) (CO_2) level is composed of CO_2, bicarbonate (HCO_3), and carbonic acid (HCO_3) with the primary constituent being bicarbonate, a negatively charged electrolyte that works in conjunction with other electrolytes, such as potassium, sodium, and chloride, to maintain proper acid-base balance and electrical neutrality at the cellular level. Chloride is also a negatively charged electrolyte that helps regulate body fluid and maintain proper acid-base balance. Creatinine is a waste product excreted by the kidneys that is produced in the muscles while breaking down creatine, a compound used by the muscles to create energy. Blood levels of creatinine provide a good measurement of renal function. Glucose is a simple sugar and the main source of energy for the body, regulated by insulin. When more glucose is available than is required, it is stored in the liver as glycogen or stored in adipose tissue as fat. Glucose measurement determines whether the glucose/insulin metabolic process is functioning properly. Both potassium and sodium are positively charged electrolytes that work in conjunction with other electrolytes to regulate body fluid, stimulate muscle contraction, and maintain proper acid-base balance, and both are essential for maintaining normal metabolic processes. Urea is a waste product produced in the liver by the breakdown of protein from a sequence of chemical reactions referred to as the urea or Krebs-Henseleit cycle. Urea is taken up by the kidneys and excreted in the urine. Blood urea nitrogen, BUN, is a measure of renal function, and helps monitor renal disease and the effectiveness of dialysis. Report 80048 for the same basic metabolic panel, but with total calcium measured instead of ionized calcium. Total calcium is a measurement of the total amount of both ionized (free) calcium and calcium attached (bound) to proteins circulating in the blood. The measurement can screen for or monitor a number of conditions, including those affecting the bones, heart, nerves, kidneys, and teeth.

RVUs

Code	Work	PE	PE Non-Facility	MP	Total Non-Facility	Total Facility	Global
80047	0.00	0.00	0.00	0.00	0.00	0.00	XXX
80048	0.00	0.00	0.00	0.00	0.00	0.00	XXX

80050

80050 General health panel
This panel must include the following:
Comprehensive metabolic panel (80053); Blood count, complete (CBC), automated and automated differential WBC count (85025 or 85027 and 85004); OR Blood count, complete (CBC), automated (85027); and appropriate manual differential WBC count (85007 or 85009); Thyroid stimulating hormone (TSH) (84443)

Plain English Description

A general health panel is obtained that includes a comprehensive metabolic panel with albumin, bilirubin, total calcium, carbon dioxide, chloride, creatinine, glucose, alkaline phosphatase, potassium, total protein, sodium, alanine amino transferase (ALT) (SGPT), aspartate amino transferase (AST) (SGOT), urea nitrogen (BUN); a complete blood count with differential white blood cell count; and thyroid stimulating hormone (TSH). This test is used to evaluate electrolytes and fluid balance, as well as liver and kidney function, and is used to help rule out conditions such as diabetes, thyroid disease, and anemia. Tests related to electrolytes and fluid balance include carbon dioxide, chloride, potassium, and sodium. Tests specific to liver function include albumin, bilirubin, alkaline phosphatase, ALT, AST, and total protein. Tests specific to kidney function include BUN and creatinine. Calcium is needed to support metabolic processes such as heart function, muscle contraction, nerve function, and blood clotting. Glucose is the main source of energy for the body and is regulated by insulin. Glucose measurement determines whether the glucose/insulin metabolic process is functioning properly. A CBC is performed to test for anemia, infection, blood clotting disorders, as well as many other diseases. TSH is produced in the pituitary and helps to regulate two other thyroid hormones, T3 and T4, which in turn help regulate the body's metabolic processes.

RVUs

Code	Work	PE	PE Non-Facility	MP	Total Non-Facility	Total Facility	Global
80050	0.00	0.00	0.00	0.00	0.00	0.00	XXX

80051

80051 Electrolyte panel
This panel must include the following:
Carbon dioxide (bicarbonate) (82374); Chloride (82435); Potassium (84132); Sodium (84295)

Plain English Description

An electrolyte panel is obtained to detect problems with fluid and electrolyte balance and monitor the health status of persons with acute or chronic medical conditions including high blood pressure, heart failure, and kidney or liver disease. The test measures electrically charged minerals such as sodium, potassium, and chloride found in body tissues and blood. Sodium is primarily found outside cells and maintains water balance in the tissues, as well as nerve and muscle function. Potassium is primarily found inside cells and affects heart rhythm, cell metabolism, and muscle function. Chloride moves freely in and out of cells to regulate fluid levels and help maintain electrical neutrality. Carbon dioxide, or bicarbonate, maintains body pH and the acid-base balance of the blood. A test called an "anion gap" may be included in the electrolyte panel. Anion gap is a calculated value of the test components that measures the difference between the negatively charged ions (anions) and the positivity charged ions (cations). Anion-gap values can be affected by many conditions, such as metabolic disorders, starvation, and diabetes or exposure to toxins. A blood sample is obtained by separately reportable venipuncture, or heel or finger stick. Serum and/or plasma is tested using quantitative ion-selective electrode/enzymatic method.

RVUs

Code	Work	PE	PE Non-Facility	MP	Total Non-Facility	Total Facility	Global
80051	0.00	0.00	0.00	0.00	0.00	0.00	XXX

80053

80053 Comprehensive metabolic panel
This panel must include the following:
Albumin (82040); Bilirubin, total (82247); Calcium, total (82310); Carbon dioxide (bicarbonate) (82374); Chloride (82435); Creatinine (82565); Glucose (82947); Phosphatase, alkaline (84075); Potassium (84132); Protein, total (84155); Sodium (84295); Transferase, alanine amino (ALT) (SGPT) (84460); Transferase, aspartate amino (AST) (SGOT) (84450); Urea nitrogen (BUN) (84520)

Plain English Description

A comprehensive metabolic panel that includes albumin, bilirubin, total calcium, carbon dioxide, chloride, creatinine, glucose, alkaline phosphatase, potassium, total protein, sodium, alanine amino transferase (ALT) (SGPT), aspartate amino transferase (AST) (SGOT), and urea nitrogen (BUN) is obtained. This test is used to evaluate electrolytes and fluid balance as well as liver and kidney function. It is also used to help rule out conditions such as diabetes. Tests related to electrolytes and fluid balance include carbon dioxide, chloride, potassium, and sodium. Tests specific to liver function include albumin, bilirubin, alkaline phosphatase, ALT, AST, and total protein. Tests specific to kidney function include BUN and creatinine. Calcium is needed to support metabolic processes such as heart function, muscle contraction, nerve function, and blood clotting. Glucose is the main source of energy for the body and is regulated by insulin. Glucose measurement determines whether the glucose/insulin metabolic process is functioning properly.

RVUs

Code	Work	PE	PE Non-Facility	MP	Total Non-Facility	Total Facility	Global
80053	0.00	0.00	0.00	0.00	0.00	0.00	XXX

80069

80069 Renal function panel
This panel must include the following:
Albumin (82040); Calcium, total (82310); Carbon dioxide (bicarbonate) (82374); Chloride (82435); Creatinine (82565); Glucose (82947); Phosphorus inorganic (phosphate) (84100); Potassium (84132); Sodium (84295); Urea nitrogen (BUN) (84520)

Plain English Description

A renal panel is obtained for routine health screening and to monitor conditions such as diabetes, renal disease, liver disease, nutritional disorders, thyroid and parathyroid function, and interventional drug therapies. Tests in a renal panel include glucose or blood sugar; electrolytes and minerals as sodium, potassium, chloride, total calcium, and phosphorus; the waste products blood urea nitrogen (BUN) and creatinine; a protein called albumin; and bicarbonate (carbon dioxide, CO_2) responsible for acid/base balance. Glucose is the main source of energy for the body and is regulated by insulin. High levels may indicate diabetes or impaired kidney function. Sodium is found primarily outside cells and maintains water balance in the tissues, as well as nerve and muscle function. Potassium is primarily found inside cells and affects heart rhythm, cell metabolism, and muscle function. Chloride moves freely in and out of cells to regulate fluid levels and help maintain electrical neutrality. Calcium is needed to support metabolic processes, heart and nerve function, muscle contraction, and blood clotting. Phosphorus is essential for energy production, nerve and muscle function, and bone growth. Blood urea nitrogen (BUN) and creatinine are waste products from tissue breakdown that circulate in the blood and are filtered out by the kidneys. Albumin, a protein made by the liver, helps to nourish tissue and transport hormones, vitamins, drugs, and calcium throughout the body. Bicarbonate (HCO3) may also be referred to as carbon dioxide (CO2) and maintains body pH or the acid/base balance. A specimen is obtained by separately reportable venipuncture. Serum/plasma is tested using quantitative chemiluminescent immunoassay or quantitative enzyme-linked immunosorbent assay.

RVUs

Code	Work	PE	PE Non-Facility	MP	Total Non-Facility	Total Facility	Global
80069	0.00	0.00	0.00	0.00	0.00	0.00	XXX

80169

80169 Everolimus

Plain English Description

A blood test is performed to measure everolimus levels. Everolimus (Zortress, Certican, Afinitor) is an immunosuppressive agent that is used to prevent organ rejection (Zortress, Certican) in patients with kidney or liver transplants and to treat certain cancers (Afinitor) including advanced renal cell carcinoma (aRCC), subependymal giant cell astrocytoma (SEGA) associated with tuberous sclerosis complex (TSC) when the patient cannot undergo curative surgical resection, progressive or metastatic pancreatic neuroendocrine tumors (PNET) not surgically removable, and advanced hormone-receptor positive HER2-negative breast cancer in post-menopausal women. Everolimus levels should be monitored by pre-dose (trough) blood draws. A blood sample is obtained by separately reportable venipuncture. Whole blood is tested using quantitative liquid chromatography-tandem mass spectrometry.

RVUs

Code	Work	PE	PE Non-Facility	MP	Total Non-Facility	Total Facility	Global
80169	0.00	0.00	0.00	0.00	0.00	0.00	XXX

80197

80197 Tacrolimus

Plain English Description

A blood test is performed to measure tacrolimus levels. Tacrolimus, also known as Prograf, is an immunosuppressant drug that affects the ability of certain white blood cells in the body to recognize and respond to transplanted body organs such as kidney, liver, heart, and lung. The drug is administered intravenously, either alone or in combination with other immunosuppressant drugs. Tacrolimus has a narrow therapeutic range and blood levels may be assessed daily at the start of therapy, taper to 1-2 times per week, and finally to once every 1-2 months. For routine monitoring, the specimen is collected as a trough level, immediately prior to a scheduled dose and at least 12 hours after the previous dose. A blood sample is obtained by a separately reportable venipuncture. Whole blood is then tested using liquid chromatography-tandem mass spectrometry. Prograf may be tested with chromatographic or immunoassay technique and the results will be somewhat different. Make note of the technique used when comparing results with previous levels.

RVUs

Code	Work	PE	PE Non-Facility	MP	Total Non-Facility	Total Facility	Global
80197	0.00	0.00	0.00	0.00	0.00	0.00	XXX

80200

80200 Tobramycin

Plain English Description

A blood test is performed to measure tobramycin levels. The levels may be measured at random, peak, and trough times. Tobramycin is an injectable aminoglycoside prescribed to treat severe or serious bacterial infections. Blood level monitoring is necessary because the drug has the potential to cause auditory, vestibular, and renal toxicity. A random sample may be drawn any time. Peak and trough levels are time dependent and are usually drawn 24 hours after initiating therapy and every 2-3 days thereafter. A trough level is drawn 5-90 minutes prior to intravenous infusion or intramuscular injection. A peak level is drawn 30 minutes after intravenous infusion is complete and 30-90 minutes after an intramuscular injection. A blood sample is obtained by separately reportable venipuncture. Blood serum is then tested using fluorescence polarization immunoassay.

RVUs

Code	Work	PE	PE Non-Facility	MP	Total Non-Facility	Total Facility	Global
80200	0.00	0.00	0.00	0.00	0.00	0.00	XXX

80408

80408 Aldosterone suppression evaluation panel (eg, saline infusion)
This panel must include the following:
Aldosterone (82088 x 2); Renin (84244 x 2)

Plain English Description

A laboratory test is performed to assess aldosterone and renin levels in patients with suspected primary and/or secondary hyperaldosteronism. Primary hyperaldosteronism causes elevated aldosterone levels, sodium retention, potassium depletion, and elevated blood pressure. It can result from benign adrenal tumors, bilateral adrenal hyperplasia, or an unknown etiology. Secondary hyperaldosteronism is more common and renin levels will be elevated along with aldosterone. Causes of secondary hyperaldosteronism include renal artery stenosis, congestive heart failure, cirrhosis, kidney disease, and preeclampsia. Symptoms include urinary frequency, increased thirst, fatigue, muscle weakness or cramping, palpitations, and headache. The aldosterone suppression evaluation test measures aldosterone and renin at baseline and the changes that occur following an intravenous infusion of isotonic (0.9%) sodium chloride (NaCl) solution. Patient preparation includes a normal sodium diet (100-200 mEq/day) x 3 days and no medication known to affect the renin/aldosterone system. If the physician has specified a supine test, the baseline blood draw should be performed between 8 and 10 a.m. with the patient supine for a minimum of 2 hours before the blood draw and remaining supine until the test is over. If the test is ordered in the upright position, the baseline blood draw must be performed before noon with the patient sitting or standing upright for at least 2 hours prior to the blood draw and remaining sitting or standing for the duration of the test. An IV line is established in a separately reportable procedure. A blood sample may be obtained from this IV line or by separately reportable venipuncture and used to measure the baseline aldosterone and renin levels. The IV infusion of sodium chloride is started at a rate of 500 mL/h x 4 hours for a total of 2L. At the end of the infusion, a second blood sample is obtained and used to measure the post infusion levels of aldosterone and renin. Serum/plasma is tested using quantitative radioimmunoassay or quantitative immunoradiometry.

RVUs

Code	Work	PE	PE Non-Facility	MP	Total Non-Facility	Total Facility	Global
80408	0.00	0.00	0.00	0.00	0.00	0.00	XXX

80416

80416 Renal vein renin stimulation panel (eg, captopril)
This panel must include the following:
Renin (84244 x 6)

Plain English Description

A laboratory test is performed to diagnose renovascular hypertension, which may be caused by renal artery stenosis (RAS), a narrowing of the renovascular bed often due to atherosclerotic plaque formation, or fibromuscular hyperplasia. When hypertension is caused by RAS it can be treated using angiotensin converting enzyme (ACE) inhibitors. Plasma renin activity will be increased in patients with renovascular hypertension. The renal vein renin stimulation test is performed to determine the baseline renin level in the kidneys and the changes that occur following administration of an ACE inhibiting medication, captopril. The patient discontinues diuretics and ACE inhibiting medications at least 14 days prior to the test and eats a normal sodium diet (100-200 mEq/day) x 3 days. Angiography is performed as a separately reportable procedure. The patient is positioned supine on the table, prepared and draped in the usual sterile manner. The renal veins are catheterized from a transfemoral or jugular approach using a 4 or 5 F cobra or shepard catheter with side hole. Small injections of contrast are given to confirm catheter location. A baseline blood sample is obtained from the right and left renal veins to determine renin levels. Captopril 25-50 mg is administered and additional blood samples are then taken at timed intervals from the right and left veins to determine renin levels. Serum/plasma is tested using quantitative immunoradiometry.

RVUs

Code	Work	PE	PE Non-Facility	MP	Total Non-Facility	Total Facility	Global
80416	0.00	0.00	0.00	0.00	0.00	0.00	XXX

80417

80417 Peripheral vein renin stimulation panel (eg, captopril)
This panel must include the following:
Renin (84244 x 2)

Plain English Description

A laboratory test is performed to diagnose renovascular hypertension, which may be caused by renal artery stenosis (RAS), a narrowing of the renovascular bed often due to atherosclerotic plaque formation, or fibromuscular hyperplasia. When hypertension is caused by RAS, it can be treated using angiotensin converting enzyme (ACE) inhibitors. Plasma renin activity will be increased in patients with renovascular hypertension. The peripheral vein renin stimulation test is performed to determine the baseline renin level in the peripheral circulating blood and the changes that occur following ingestion of an ACE inhibiting medication, captopril. The patient discontinues diuretics and ACE inhibiting medications at least 14 days prior to the test and eats a normal sodium diet (100-200 mEq/day) x 3 days. If the physician has specified a supine test, the baseline blood draw should be performed between 8 and 10 a.m. with the patient supine for a minimum of 2 hours before the blood draw and remaining supine until the test is over. If the test is ordered in the upright position, the baseline blood draw must be performed before noon with the patient sitting or standing upright for at least 2 hours prior to the blood draw and remaining sitting or standing for the duration of the test. The baseline blood sample is obtained by separately reportable venipuncture. Captopril 25-50 mg is administered orally and the second blood sample is obtained 30 minutes later. Serum/plasma is tested using quantitative immunoradiometry.

RVUs

Code	Work	PE	PE Non-Facility	MP	Total Non-Facility	Total Facility	Global
80417	0.00	0.00	0.00	0.00	0.00	0.00	XXX

81000-81003

81000 Urinalysis, by dip stick or tablet reagent for bilirubin, glucose, hemoglobin, ketones, leukocytes, nitrite, pH, protein, specific gravity, urobilinogen, any number of these constituents; non-automated, with microscopy

81001 Urinalysis, by dip stick or tablet reagent for bilirubin, glucose, hemoglobin, ketones, leukocytes, nitrite, pH, protein, specific gravity, urobilinogen, any number of these constituents; automated, with microscopy

81002 Urinalysis, by dip stick or tablet reagent for bilirubin, glucose, hemoglobin, ketones, leukocytes, nitrite, pH, protein, specific gravity, urobilinogen, any number of these constituents; non-automated, without microscopy

81003 Urinalysis, by dip stick or tablet reagent for bilirubin, glucose, hemoglobin, ketones, leukocytes, nitrite, pH, protein, specific gravity, urobilinogen, any number of these constituents; automated, without microscopy

Plain English Description

A urinalysis is performed with dip stick or tablet reagent for bilirubin, glucose, hemoglobin, ketones, leukocytes, nitrite, pH, protein, specific gravity, and/or urobilinogen. Urinalysis can quickly screen for conditions that do not immediately produce symptoms, such as diabetes mellitus, kidney disease, or urinary tract infection. A dip stick allows qualitative and semi-quantitative analysis using a paper or plastic stick with color strips for each agent being tested. The stick is dipped in the urine specimen and the color strips are then compared to a color chart to determine the presence or absence and/or a rough estimate of the concentration of each agent tested. Reagent tablets use an absorbent mat with a few drops of urine placed on the mat followed by a reagent tablet. A drop of distilled, deionized water is then placed on the tablet and the color change is observed. Bilirubin is a byproduct of the breakdown of red blood cells by the liver. Normally bilirubin is excreted through the bowel, but in patients with liver disease, bilirubin is filtered by the kidneys and excreted in the urine. Glucose is a sugar that is normally filtered by the glomerulus and excreted only in small quantities in the urine. Excess sugar in the urine (glycosuria) is indicative of diabetes mellitus. The peroxidase activity of erythrocytes is used to detect hemoglobin in the urine, which may be indicative of hematuria, myoglobinuria, or hemoglobinuria. Ketones in the urine are the result of diabetic ketoacidosis or calorie deprivation (starvation). A leukocyte esterase test identifies the presence of white blood cells in the urine. The presence of nitrites in the urine is indicative of bacteria. The pH identifies the acid-base levels in the urine. The presence of excessive amounts of protein (proteinuria) may be indicative of nephrotic syndrome. Specific gravity measures urine density and is indicative of the kidneys' ability to concentrate and dilute urine. Following dip stick or reagent testing, the urine sample may be examined under a microscope. The urine sample is placed in a test tube and centrifuged. The sediment is resuspended. A drop of the resuspended sediment is then placed on a glass slide, cover-slipped, and examined under a microscope for crystals, casts, squamous cells, blood (white, red) cells, and bacteria. Use 81000 for a non-automated test with microscopy and 81001 for an automated test with microscopy. Use 81002 for a non-automated test without microscopy and 81003 for an automated test without microscopy.

RVUs

Code	Work	PE	PE Non-Facility	MP	Total Non-Facility	Total Facility	Global
81000	0.00	0.00	0.00	0.00	0.00	0.00	XXX
81001	0.00	0.00	0.00	0.00	0.00	0.00	XXX
81002	0.00	0.00	0.00	0.00	0.00	0.00	XXX
81003	0.00	0.00	0.00	0.00	0.00	0.00	XXX

81005

81005 Urinalysis; qualitative or semiquantitative, except immunoassays

(For non-immunoassay reagent strip urinalysis, see 81000, 81002)

(For immunoassay, qualitative or semiquantitative, use 83518)

(For microalbumin, see 82043, 82044)

Plain English Description

A laboratory test is performed to detect abnormal cellular material or substances in urine. Qualitative or semiquantitative urinalysis may be used as a routine screening tool to detect substances such as protein, glucose, bacteria, and red or white blood cells in urine that may require follow up; it may also be performed to monitor organ function and response to treatment in patients with a known disease. Urinalysis usually includes a visual examination and chemical analysis and may also include a microscopic study. A urine sample is obtained by clean catch, mid-stream void, or catheterization. The sample is observed visually for color, odor, and clarity. Drops of urine are then applied to a plastic test strip affixed with several reagent areas impregnated with chemicals and the color changes, of the reagent areas are compared to a standardized chart to determine pH level, specific gravity, and the absence or presence of glucose, bilirubin, ketones, blood, protein, urobilinogen, nitrate, leukocytes, and ascorbic acid. The sample may then be centrifuged to separate the fluid and sediment. The sediment is examined microscopically for crystals, casts, squamous cells, red or white blood cells, epithelial cells, bacteria, or yeast cells. Any cells present are counted and reported.

RVUs

Code	Work	PE	PE Non-Facility	MP	Total Non-Facility	Total Facility	Global
81005	0.00	0.00	0.00	0.00	0.00	0.00	XXX

81007

81007 Urinalysis; bacteriuria screen, except by culture or dipstick

(For culture, see 87086-87088)

(For dipstick, use 81000 or 81002)

Plain English Description

A laboratory test is performed to measure bacteria in urine. Bacteriuria may be associated with acute or chronic urinary tract infection. A urine sample is obtained by clean catch, mid-stream void, or catheterization. The sample is mixed well and diluted with fluorescent staining dyes. Using automated flow cytometry, the sample is passed through a sheath and illuminated with an argon laser beam. Red blood cells, white blood cells, epithelial cells, casts, and bacteria are counted and recorded. The qualitative results may be used to determine bacterial concentrations and aid in the diagnosis of urinary tract infection.

RVUs

Code	Work	PE	PE Non-Facility	MP	Total Non-Facility	Total Facility	Global
81007	0.00	0.00	0.00	0.00	0.00	0.00	XXX

81015

81015 Urinalysis; microscopic only

(For sperm evaluation for retrograde ejaculation, use 89331)

Plain English Description

Microscopic analysis is performed to determine if sediment in the urine specimen is normal or indicative of an abnormality such as infection. Microscopy can be performed using a standard glass counting chamber and coverslips or a disposable system. Most laboratories use disposable systems. Urine from the sample is centrifuged to concentrate the sediment in a button at the bottom of the tube. The specimen is decanted leaving only 0.2-0.5 mL liquid. The sediment is resuspended. The sediment is placed in a test well and examined under a microscope at low power to identify crystals, casts, squamous cells, and other debris. The test well is 0.1 mm deep and contains a grid that measures 3x3 mm with 90 small squares in the grid. Each of the 90 small squares are grouped together in 1x1 mm squares, which are the medium squares, and each contains 9 small squares. Casts are usually counted at low power. The urine is then examined under high power for the presence of red blood cells (RBCs), white blood cells (WBCs), epithelial cells, bacteria, yeast, and crystals and each of the constituents is characterized and counted. Counts may be performed on a single small cell or all 90 cells may be counted depending on the concentration of each of the constituents in the specimen. For example, WBCs may be counted in only a single small square when high numbers of cells are present, 9 medium squares when moderate levels of cells are present, or the entire 90 cells when low cell counts are present. If a single small square is counted, the results are multiplied by 90 to obtain the WBC count. If a medium square is counted (9 small cells), the results are multiplied by 10. If all 90 cells are counted, the total count is reported.

RVUs

Code	Work	PE	PE Non-Facility	MP	Total Non-Facility	Total Facility	Global
81015	0.00	0.00	0.00	0.00	0.00	0.00	XXX

81020

81020 Urinalysis; 2 or 3 glass test

Plain English Description

This test is performed to help diagnose the site and cause of inflammation of the urethra, particularly in males. First morning urine is collected in two or three glasses. Each glass is then tested for the presence of white blood cells (WBCs) as indicated by turbidity (cloudiness) of the specimen and red blood cells (RBCs). If the first glass is turbid and the second glass and third glass clear, urethritis is present in the anterior segment only. If all two or three glasses are turbid, both anterior and posterior urethritis is present. If only the anterior urethra is inflamed, the first glass will contain blood while the other two will not. If both anterior and posterior urethritis is present, all two or three glasses will contain blood.

RVUs

Code	Work	PE	PE Non-Facility	MP	Total Non-Facility	Total Facility	Global
81020	0.00	0.00	0.00	0.00	0.00	0.00	XXX

81050

81050 Volume measurement for timed collection, each

Plain English Description

A procedure is performed to collect urine and measure volume over a specific period of time. The volumetric measurement of urine may be required to report certain biomarkers and variations in the concentration over a specific length of time. The timed collection begins by discarding the first sample of urine and noting the time. All subsequent urine is then collected and pooled in the collection container for the designated period of time. When the last sample is collected, the end time is noted and the collected specimen is sent to the laboratory for processing and analysis.

RVUs

Code	Work	PE	PE Non-Facility	MP	Total Non-Facility	Total Facility	Global
81050	0.00	0.00	0.00	0.00	0.00	0.00	XXX

81224

81224 *CFTR (cystic fibrosis transmembrane conductance regulator)* (eg, cystic fibrosis) gene analysis; intron 8 poly-T analysis (eg, male infertility)

Plain English Description

Molecular genetic testing is performed to identify a specific mutation of the CFTR gene found on chromosome 7 and responsible for encoding the protein, cystic fibrosis transmembrane conductance regulator, which causes cystic fibrosis (CF) and congenital bilateral absence of the vas deferens (CBAVD). Males who present with azoospermia, low semen ejaculatory volume, and absence of vas deferens on clinical exam or ultrasound are candidates for molecular genetic testing to determine if they are carriers of a CFTR gene mutation. An intron 8 poly-T analysis is a reflex test performed when a R117H mutation (or other disease-causing mutation) is identified. The poly-T tract is a string of thymidine bases located on intron 8, with 3 common variants, 5T, a penetrant mutation variable, and 7T and 9T, both polymorphic variants.

RVUs

Code	Work	PE	PE Non-Facility	MP	Total Non-Facility	Total Facility	Global
81224	0.00	0.00	0.00	0.00	0.00	0.00	XXX

81225

81225 *CYP2C19 (cytochrome P450, family 2, subfamily C, polypeptide 19)* (eg, drug metabolism), gene analysis, common variants (eg, *2, *3, *4, *8, *17)

Plain English Description

Molecular genetic testing is performed to identify a specific mutation of the CYP2C19 gene located on chromosome 10, responsible for encoding the cytochrome P450, family 2, subfamily C, polypeptide 19. This complex polypeptide is part of a mixed function oxidase system that metabolizes xenobiotics (compounds foreign to the body such as drugs and toxins) and also bioactivates and synthesizes substances such as cholesterol, steroids, and other lipids. A large phenotypical variability factor is present due to genetic polymorphism. The common variants are categorized as normal-fully functional (*1), decreased or non-functioning (*2, *3), decreased or partial-functioning (*4, *5, *6, *7, *8), or increased-partial functioning (*17). Genetic testing may be ordered for individuals undergoing certain drug therapy (antiepileptics, proton pump inhibitors, antidepressants) to identify gene mutations that alter the metabolism of the compound-leading to an adverse drug response or effect.

RVUs

Code	Work	PE	PE Non-Facility	MP	Total Non-Facility	Total Facility	Global
81225	0.00	0.00	0.00	0.00	0.00	0.00	XXX

81226

81226 *CYP2D6 (cytochrome P450, family 2, subfamily D, polypeptide 6)* (eg, drug metabolism), gene analysis, common variants (eg, *2, *3, *4, *5, *6, *9, *10, *17, *19, *29, *35, *41, *1XN, *2XN, *4XN)

Plain English Description

Molecular genetic testing is performed to identify a specific mutation of the CYP2D6 gene located on chromosome 22, responsible for encoding the cytochrome P450, family 2, subfamily D, polypeptide 6. This complex polypeptide is part of a mixed function oxidase system that metabolizes xenobiotics (compounds foreign to the body such as drugs and toxins) and also bioactivates and synthesizes substances such as cholesterol, steroids, and other lipids. A large phenotypical variability factor is present due to genetic polymorphism. The common variants are categorized as: normal-fully functional (*1, *2 [except for *1xN and *2xN]), partial functioning-decreased (*9, *10, *17, *29, *41), partial functioning-increased (*1xN, *2xN), non-functioning (*3, *4, *5, *6, *19, *4xN). Genetic testing may be ordered for individuals undergoing certain types of drug therapy (such as Tamoxifen for breast cancer) to identify gene mutations that alter the metabolism of the compound leading to an adverse drug response or effect.

RVUs

Code	Work	PE	PE Non-Facility	MP	Total Non-Facility	Total Facility	Global
81226	0.00	0.00	0.00	0.00	0.00	0.00	XXX

81227

81227 *CYP2C9 (cytochrome P450, family 2, subfamily C, polypeptide 9)* (eg, drug metabolism), gene analysis, common variants (eg, *2, *3, *5, *6)

Plain English Description

Molecular genetic testing is performed to identify a specific mutation of the CYP2C9 gene located on chromosome 10, responsible for encoding the cytochrome P450, family 2, subfamily C, polypeptide 9. This complex protein of monooxygenases catalyzes the metabolism of xenobiotics (compounds foreign to the body such as drugs and toxins) and also bioactivates and synthesizes substances such as cholesterol, steroids, and other lipids. At least 50 single nucleotide polymorphisms (SNP) have been identified in coding regions associated with decreased enzyme activity. Adverse drug reactions are often a result of unexpected enzymatic alteration due to polymorphism. The common variants *2, *3 are associated with reduced warfarin metabolism. Individuals with this mutation require a lower dose of warfarin during anti-coagulation therapy and are at increased risk for bleeding. Low-frequency variants *5, *6 have been identified in African-American populations and are associated with decreased activity for *5 and no activity for *6. Genetic testing may be ordered for individuals undergoing certain types of drug therapy (such as warfarin and phenytoin) to identify gene mutations that alter the metabolism of the compound, leading to toxicity at normal therapeutic dosages.

RVUs

Code	Work	PE	PE Non-Facility	MP	Total Non-Facility	Total Facility	Global
81227	0.00	0.00	0.00	0.00	0.00	0.00	XXX

81250

81250 *G6PC (glucose-6-phosphatase, catalytic subunit)* (eg, Glycogen storage disease, type 1a, von Gierke disease) gene analysis, common variants (eg, R83C, Q347X)

Plain English Description

Molecular genetic testing is performed to identify a specific mutation of the G6PC (glucose-6-phosphatase, catalytic subunit) gene. Located on chromosome 17, as many as 85 mutations of the G6PC gene have been identified for the glycogen storage disease, type 1a, also known as von Gierke disease. Most change a single amino acid in the enzyme, glucose-6-phosphatase on the membrane of the endoplasmic reticulum. This membrane, located inside of cells, involves protein transport and processing along with the glucose-6-phosphate translocase protein (produced from the 5LC37A4 gene) to break down the glucose 6 phosphate sugar molecule forming a simple glucose sugar for energy use by the cell. This enzyme is the main regulator of glucose produced by the liver and is also active in the kidneys and intestine. Mutation impairs the glucose-6-phosphatase enzyme, which then impairs the glucose 6 phosphate sugar molecule from breaking down into glucose, instead converting it into fat and glycogen. Fat and glycogen accumulation in the cell leads to tissue and organ damage, particularly in the kidneys and liver. The disease is autosomal recessive. Individuals with mutation of the G6PC gene from both parents develop von Gierke disease. Individuals who receive the G6PC mutation from only one parent are carriers of the disease. Symptoms of this inherited disorder include severe hypoglycemia, constant hunger, irritability, excess bleeding/bruising, fatigue, abdominal distention with thin extremities and puffy cheeks, inflammatory bowel disease, stunted growth, and delayed puberty. The disease is treated by restricting fructose (fruits) and galactose (dairy products), avoiding low blood glucose levels by eating starches such as uncooked cornstarch, and taking allopurinol to decrease uric acid levels. Molecular genetic testing is indicated in individuals with symptoms associated with von Gierke disease or when there is a family history of the disorder.

RVUs

Code	Work	PE	PE Non-Facility	MP	Total Non-Facility	Total Facility	Global
81250	0.00	0.00	0.00	0.00	0.00	0.00	XXX

81539

81539 Oncology (high-grade prostate cancer), biochemical assay of four proteins (Total PSA, Free PSA, Intact PSA, and human kallikrein-2 [hK2]), utilizing plasma or serum, prognostic algorithm reported as a probability score

Plain English Description

Total PSA (tPSA), Free PSA (fPSA), Intact PSA (iPSA), and human kallikrein-2 (hK2) in plasma or serum are assayed. Prostate specific antigen (PSA) is a glycoprotein enzyme belonging to the kallikrein family and secreted in the prostate gland by epithelial cells. Elevated PSA levels in plasma/serum may indicate benign prostatic hypertrophy, prostatitis, and possible malignancy. Human kallidrein-2 (hK2) is also secreted in the prostate gland by epithelial cells and elevated levels are more likely to be associated with malignant prostate tumors, which may be aggressive and metastasize quickly or never progress or cause no harm. A blood sample is obtained by separately reportable venipuncture. Serum/plasma is tested using electrochemiluminescence immunoassay. The results of the blood test are combined in an algorithm using the patient's age, absence or presence of prostate nodules on digital rectal exam (DRE), and prior negative biopsy results to generate a risk score for the probability of high-grade prostate cancer (a Gleason score of ≥ 7) being found on biopsy. The probability score that is reported can assist the physician and patient in the decision to proceed with a prostate biopsy. This test is contraindicated in patients with a previous diagnosis of prostate cancer, DRE within 4 days, 5-alpha reductase inhibitor therapy, or treatment for symptomatic benign prostatic hypertrophy within 6 months.

RVUs

Code	Work	PE	PE Non-Facility	MP	Total Non-Facility	Total Facility	Global
81539	0.00	0.00	0.00	0.00	0.00	0.00	XXX

81541

81541 Oncology (prostate), mRNA gene expression profiling by real-time RT-PCR of 46 genes (31 content and 15 housekeeping), utilizing formalin-fixed paraffin-embedded tissue, algorithm reported as a disease-specific mortality risk score

Plain English Description

Molecular genomic testing is performed using real-time RT-PCR for mRNA gene expression profiling of 31 content (signature) and 15 control (housekeeping) genes utilizing formalin-fixed paraffin-embedded prostate tumor tissue. The test examines tumor cells for cell cycle progression (CCP) genes to stratify the risk of prostate cancer progression. The algorithm reports a score of -3 to +3 for CCP gene expression levels. A higher score indicates a greater possibility of tumor growth or other adverse event. The test can aid in developing a treatment plan such as active surveillance vs. aggressive surgery.

RVUs

Code	Work	PE	PE Non-Facility	MP	Total Non-Facility	Total Facility	Global
81541	0.00	0.00	0.00	0.00	0.00	0.00	XXX

81542

81542 Oncology (prostate), mRNA, microarray gene expression profiling of 22 content genes, utilizing formalin-fixed paraffin-embedded tissue, algorithm reported as metastasis risk score

Plain English Description

Molecular genetic testing is performed on formalin-fixed paraffin-embedded (FFPE) prostate tissue to identify messenger RNA (mRNA) in 22 content genes and predict the likelihood of metastasis following radical prostatectomy. This test is most often used on patients with Stage 2 disease and positive margins, Stage 3 disease, or any patient with rising PSA levels following surgery. Using microarray gene expression profiling, the test measures mRNA at a given point in time to identify current disease status and assist in making a prediction for response to treatment. An algorithm is created from the genetic information in mRNA and a risk score of 0-1 is assigned for predicting clinical metastasis in patients with biochemical recurrence after surgery, and can also help determine the timing of postoperative radiotherapy.

RVUs

Code	Work	PE	PE Non-Facility	MP	Total Non-Facility	Total Facility	Global
81542	0.00	0.00	0.00	0.00	0.00	0.00	XXX

81551

81551 Oncology (prostate), promoter methylation profiling by real-time PCR of 3 genes (*GSTP1, APC, RASSF1*), utilizing formalin-fixed paraffin-embedded tissue, algorithm reported as a likelihood of prostate cancer detection on repeat biopsy

Plain English Description

Molecular genomic testing is performed using promoter methylation profiling by real-time PCR of 3 genes (*GSTP1, APC, RASSF1*) utilizing formalin-fixed paraffin-embedded prostate tumor tissue. The test examines cells in tissue surrounding the tumor for molecular changes related to DNA methylation. Cells that are positive for methylation changes indicate a high probability that prostate cancer is present. The 3 gene test can aide in the identification of false-negative histopathology biopsy specimens and the algorithm score reports the likelihood of prostate cancer detection on repeat biopsy.

RVUs

Code	Work	PE	PE Non-Facility	MP	Total Non-Facility	Total Facility	Global
81551	0.00	0.00	0.00	0.00	0.00	0.00	XXX

82009-82010

82009 Ketone body(s) (eg, acetone, acetoacetic acid, beta-hydroxybutyrate); qualitative

82010 Ketone body(s) (eg, acetone, acetoacetic acid, beta-hydroxybutyrate); quantitative

Plain English Description

A blood test is performed for acetone, acetoacetic acid, beta-hydroxybutyrate, or other ketone bodies. The qualitative test (82009) evaluates blood serum for the presence or absence of ketone bodies. A visual test is performed. Because visual tests show a spectrum of low to high levels, which are based on color changes, they are sometimes also referred to as semi-quantitative tests. The presence of ketone bodies in the blood are indicative of decreased carbohydrate utilization, which is found in patients with diabetes mellitus; malnutrition, anorexia, or other inadequate calorie intake; vomiting; and glycogen storage disease. The quantitative test (82010) measures the level of ketone bodies in blood serum. Quantitative testing is used to evaluate and manage diseases such as diabetic and alcoholic ketoacidosis either emergently or as a routine test. A blood sample is obtained by separately reportable venipuncture. Blood serum is then tested using gas chromatography.

RVUs

Code	Work	PE	PE Non-Facility	MP	Total Non-Facility	Total Facility	Global
82009	0.00	0.00	0.00	0.00	0.00	0.00	XXX
82010	0.00	0.00	0.00	0.00	0.00	0.00	XXX

82040

82040 Albumin; serum, plasma or whole blood

Plain English Description

A blood test is performed to measure albumin levels in serum, plasma, or whole blood. Albumin is a plasma protein responsible for regulating the colloidal osmotic pressure of blood. It is capable of binding water, electrolytes (sodium, potassium, calcium), fatty acids, hormones, bilirubin, and drugs/medications. Albumin levels are used to assess nutritional status. A blood sample is obtained by separately reportable venipuncture. The plasma, serum, or whole blood is tested using spectrophotometry or quantitative nephelometry.

RVUs

Code	Work	PE	PE Non-Facility	MP	Total Non-Facility	Total Facility	Global
82040	0.00	0.00	0.00	0.00	0.00	0.00	XXX

82042

82042 Albumin; other source, quantitative, each specimen

(For total protein, see 84155, 84156, 84157, 84160)

Plain English Description

A test on other body fluids, other than blood or urine, is performed to measure the amount of albumin present. Albumin is a plasma protein responsible for regulating the colloidal osmotic pressure of blood. It is capable of binding water, electrolytes (sodium, potassium, calcium), fatty acids, hormones, bilirubin, and drugs/medications. Albumin levels are used to assess nutritional status and renal function. A sample of body fluid to be tested is obtained and tested using quantitative nephelometry or spectrophotometry.

RVUs

Code	Work	PE	PE Non-Facility	MP	Total Non-Facility	Total Facility	Global
82042	0.00	0.00	0.00	0.00	0.00	0.00	XXX

82043-82044

82043 Albumin; urine (eg, microalbumin), quantitative

82044 Albumin; urine (eg, microalbumin), semiquantitative (eg, reagent strip assay)

(For prealbumin, use 84134)

Plain English Description

A test on urine is used to measure microalbumin levels and is routinely performed annually on diabetic patients with stable blood glucose levels to assess for early onset nephropathy. The quantitative test (82043), which measures the actual amount of microalbumin present in the urine, may be performed on a random urine sample, with a notation of total volume and voiding time, or a 24-hour urine sample using immunoturbidimetric technique. The semi-quantitative test (82044) identifies the presence of elevated microalbumin levels in the urine within a general range and involves a chemical dipstick placed into the urine sample which reacts and changes color when albumin is present.

RVUs

Code	Work	PE	PE Non-Facility	MP	Total Non-Facility	Total Facility	Global
82043	0.00	0.00	0.00	0.00	0.00	0.00	XXX
82044	0.00	0.00	0.00	0.00	0.00	0.00	XXX

82108

82108 Aluminum

Plain English Description

A blood test is performed to measure aluminum levels and monitor patients at risk for aluminum toxicity. Certain diseases or environmental exposure can result in toxic levels of aluminum accumulating in the body, such as with chronic kidney disease. Aluminum is a member of the boron group of chemical elements and may be ingested orally in foods, nutritional supplements, and medications. Symptoms of toxicity can include encephalopathy, osteomalacia, aplastic bone disease, cardiac changes or arrhythmias, and microcytic anemia. A blood sample is obtained by a separately reportable venipuncture. Blood serum is then tested using quantitative inductively coupled plasma mass spectrometry.

RVUs

Code	Work	PE	PE Non-Facility	MP	Total Non-Facility	Total Facility	Global
82108	0.00	0.00	0.00	0.00	0.00	0.00	XXX

82127-82131

82127 Amino acids; single, qualitative, each specimen

82128 Amino acids; multiple, qualitative, each specimen

82131 Amino acids; single, quantitative, each specimen

Plain English Description

A laboratory test is performed to identify the presence of a single amino acid (82127) or multiple amino acids (82128) in the blood or urine of an individual with a suspected inborn error of metabolism. Amino acids are the building blocks of proteins and an intermediate in metabolism, possessing a vast chemical versatility to catalyze reactions and control cellular activity. The clinical presentation of metabolic error disorders usually manifests in infancy or early childhood and depends on the specific amino acid involved. Common symptoms can include feeding problems, poor growth or failure to thrive, seizures, muscle weakness, renal or liver failure, developmental delays, and cognitive deficits. A blood sample is obtained by separately reportable venipuncture. A urine sample is obtained by voided specimen or catheterization. Serum/plasma and urine are tested using liquid chromatography-tandem mass spectrometry. Report code 82131 if the test measures the quantitative amount of a single amino acid in a specimen. Quantitative amino acid testing can be used to monitor treatment and dietary compliance in patients with phenylketonuria (PKU), a disorder of phenylalanine metabolism; cystinuria, a disorder of cystine metabolism that causes stones to form in the kidney and bladder; and Hartnup disease, a genetic disorder that inhibits the protein tryptophan from being absorbed by the intestines and then reabsorbed in the kidneys.

RVUs

Code	Work	PE	PE Non-Facility	MP	Total Non-Facility	Total Facility	Global
82127	0.00	0.00	0.00	0.00	0.00	0.00	XXX
82128	0.00	0.00	0.00	0.00	0.00	0.00	XXX
82131	0.00	0.00	0.00	0.00	0.00	0.00	XXX

82136-82139

82136 Amino acids, 2 to 5 amino acids, quantitative, each specimen

82139 Amino acids, 6 or more amino acids, quantitative, each specimen

Plain English Description

A blood, urine, or cerebral spinal fluid (CSF) sample is obtained to measure amino acid levels. Amino acids (AA) are molecules that contain an amine group, a carboxylic acid group, and a side chain that varies to differentiate each molecule. Amino acids are the building blocks of protein (linear chains of amino acids) and are critical to metabolism and sustaining life. Symptoms that may indicate a problem with amino acid levels include: failure to thrive, persistent vomiting, neurological deterioration, hyperammonemia, extreme lethargy, and metabolic acidosis. Medical conditions, that warrant amino acid analysis include acute life-threatening episodes and inborn errors of metabolism. The blood, urine, or CSF specimen is then tested using ion exchange chromatography. A quantitative analysis measures the amount, level, or concentration of each specific amino acid being tested. The specific amino acids tested for are dependent on the condition being evaluated. For example, a cystinuria panel measures four amino acids, arginine, cystine, lysine, and ornithine. Use 82136 for quantitative analysis of 2-5 amino acids. Use 82139 for quantitative analysis of 6 or more amino acids. These codes are reported for each separate specimen tested.

RVUs

Code	Work	PE	PE Non-Facility	MP	Total Non-Facility	Total Facility	Global
82136	0.00	0.00	0.00	0.00	0.00	0.00	XXX
82139	0.00	0.00	0.00	0.00	0.00	0.00	XXX

82140

82140 Ammonia

Plain English Description

A blood test is performed to measure ammonia levels. Ammonia is a byproduct of protein metabolism and is normally converted to urea by the liver and excreted via the kidney. Elevated ammonia levels may result from cirrhosis or hepatitis. Symptoms of elevated ammonia levels are confusion, tremors, excessive sleepiness, or coma. Testing may be performed in disease states such as Reyes syndrome or liver failure. A blood sample is obtained by a separately reportable venipuncture or arterial access line. The specimen is then tested using colorimetry.

RVUs

Code	Work	PE	PE Non-Facility	MP	Total Non-Facility	Total Facility	Global
82140	0.00	0.00	0.00	0.00	0.00	0.00	XXX

82163

82163 Angiotensin II

Plain English Description

A blood test is performed to measure angiotensin II. Angiotensin II is converted from angiotensin I by angiotensin I-converting enzyme (ACE). Angiotensin II functions as a hormone, primarily acting on smooth muscle, and stimulating aldosterone secretion. It is a strong vasopressor responsible for raising blood pressure and reducing fluid loss in the kidneys by restricting blood flow. A blood sample is obtained by separately reportable venipuncture. The plasma is then tested using immunoassay.

RVUs

Code	Work	PE	PE Non-Facility	MP	Total Non-Facility	Total Facility	Global
82163	0.00	0.00	0.00	0.00	0.00	0.00	XXX

82340

82340 Calcium; urine quantitative, timed specimen

Plain English Description

A laboratory test is performed to measure urine calcium levels. Calcium is a mineral essential to bone health, heart function, muscle contraction, nerve signaling, and blood clotting. Most of the body's calcium is found in the bones. A very small percentage (1%) circulates in the blood with half that amount metabolically active, and the rest bound to albumin or complexed with phosphate. Small amounts of calcium are normally excreted in urine. Urine calcium levels may be evaluated when a patient presents with abnormal serum calcium levels. Elevated urine calcium can differentially diagnose parathyroid disorders and familial hypocalciuric hypercalcemia (FHH). Intermittent monitoring of urine calcium levels may help direct treatment of these diseases. A random, timed, or 24-hour urine sample is obtained by voided specimen or catheterization. Urine is tested using quantitative spectrophotometry.

RVUs

Code	Work	PE	PE Non-Facility	MP	Total Non-Facility	Total Facility	Global
82340	0.00	0.00	0.00	0.00	0.00	0.00	XXX

82355-82360

82355 Calculus; qualitative analysis
82360 Calculus; quantitative analysis, chemical

Plain English Description

A laboratory test is performed to analyze and record the characteristics of renal calculi. As the kidney filters blood and makes urine, chemicals can precipitate and form crystals. These crystals typically contain minerals, cysteine, or both. Kidney stones can obstruct urine and blood flow in the kidneys or dislodge and travel down the ureters, stretching, irritating, and damaging the ureteral walls. To analyze calculi, urine is caught in a clean container and strained through fine mesh. Calculi are collected in a container and brought to the lab. The collected calculi are washed and dried, then weighed and measured. Observations are made regarding the qualitative (82355) characteristics of the stones, rough, smooth, horned, or waxy, and the stones are cut in half to check for a nucleus. If a nucleus is present, the nucleus and shell are divided and analyzed separately. After qualitative analysis of the stone(s) has been performed and recorded, if the stone does not appear to have a nucleus, the whole stone may be pulverized and a chemical analysis performed to determine the composition of the calculi (82360). Calcium, magnesium, inorganic phosphate, and oxalate are each measured and their levels are used to calculate the stone's composition in terms of calcium, oxalate, apatite, and magnesium ammonium phosphate.

RVUs

Code	Work	PE	PE Non-Facility	MP	Total Non-Facility	Total Facility	Global
82355	0.00	0.00	0.00	0.00	0.00	0.00	XXX
82360	0.00	0.00	0.00	0.00	0.00	0.00	XXX

82365-82370

82365 Calculus; infrared spectroscopy
82370 Calculus; X-ray diffraction
(Carbamates, see individual listings)

Plain English Description

A laboratory test is performed to analyze the composition of renal calculi. As the kidney filters blood and makes urine, chemicals can precipitate and form crystals. These crystals typically contain minerals, cysteine, or both. Kidney stones can obstruct urine and blood flow in the kidneys or dislodge and travel down the ureters, stretching, irritating, and damaging the ureteral walls. To analyze calculi, urine is caught in a clean container and strained through fine mesh. Calculi are collected in a container and brought to the lab. Usually after qualitative analysis of the stone(s) has been performed and recorded separately, samples of the stones' surface, core, and cross section are taken and analyzed using infrared spectrometry in 82365 or the stone(s) are analyzed using roentgenogram (X-ray) diffraction to create a diffractogram in 82370. The sample is compared to a known database of possible stone composition materials and a determination of the calculi composition is then made.

RVUs

Code	Work	PE	PE Non-Facility	MP	Total Non-Facility	Total Facility	Global
82365	0.00	0.00	0.00	0.00	0.00	0.00	XXX
82370	0.00	0.00	0.00	0.00	0.00	0.00	XXX

82379

82379 Carnitine (total and free), quantitative, each specimen
(For acylcarnitine, see 82016, 82017)

Plain English Description

A laboratory test is obtained to measure free and total carnitine. Carnitine is a hydrophilic amino acid derivative produced in the liver and kidneys and absorbed from ingested meats and dairy. Carnitine is required for energy metabolism, specifically the breakdown of long chain fatty acids for use by the mitochondria. If long chain fatty acids are not available to the body for beta oxidation and energy production, ketones will not be available for use by the brain. Symptoms of carnitine deficiency include hypoglycemia (all available glucose is being used for energy by the cells), muscle weakness, anemia, and heart and kidney problems. Newborns are screened for primary carnitine deficiency soon after birth. Secondary or acquired carnitine deficiency can develop as a result of type 2 diabetes, gastrointestinal disorders, familial cardiomyopathy, renal tubule disease, chronic renal failure, and prolonged treatment with steroids, antibiotics, anticonvulsants, and total parenteral nutrition (TPN). A blood sample is obtained by separately reportable venipuncture or heel stick. A urine sample is obtained by voided specimen or catheterization. Serum/plasma and urine are tested using tandem mass spectrometry.

RVUs

Code	Work	PE	PE Non-Facility	MP	Total Non-Facility	Total Facility	Global
82379	0.00	0.00	0.00	0.00	0.00	0.00	XXX

82435

82435 Chloride; blood

Plain English Description

A blood sample is taken to measure chloride level. Chloride is a negatively charged electrolyte that works in conjunction with other electrolytes, such as potassium, sodium, and carbon dioxide (CO2), to regulate fluid in the body and maintain proper acid-base balance. Chloride is found in all body fluids, but is concentrated in the blood. Chloride levels mirror sodium levels, increasing and decreasing in direct relationship to sodium, except when there is an acid-base imbalance. When an acid-base imbalance occurs, chloride acts as a buffer and chloride levels move independently of sodium. Chloride is measured to screen for or monitor electrolyte or acid-base balance. Chloride is measured by ion-selective electrode (ISE) methodology.

RVUs

Code	Work	PE	PE Non-Facility	MP	Total Non-Facility	Total Facility	Global
82435	0.00	0.00	0.00	0.00	0.00	0.00	XXX

82436

82436 Chloride; urine

Plain English Description

Chloride is a negatively charged molecule known as an electrolyte. It works with other electrolytes, such as potassium, salt (sodium), and carbon dioxide (CO2), to help keep the proper balance of body fluids and maintain the body's acid-base balance. This test may be used to help determine the causes of hypokalemia and to aid in the diagnosis of renal tubular acidosis. This test is performed by measuring the amount of chloride in a urine sample.

RVUs

Code	Work	PE	PE Non-Facility	MP	Total Non-Facility	Total Facility	Global
82436	0.00	0.00	0.00	0.00	0.00	0.00	XXX

82441

82441 Chlorinated hydrocarbons, screen

(Cholecalciferol [Vitamin D], use 82306)

Plain English Description

A screening test for toxic exposure levels to chlorinated hydrocarbons is performed on blood, urine, or exhaled air from the lungs. Chlorinated hydrocarbons are chemical compounds made up of carbon, chlorine, and hydrogen most often used as an insecticide to control vectors (disease carrying insects) or in solvents and include substances such as chloroform, carbon tetrachloride, dichloromethane, and tri- or tetrachloroethylene. Exposure usually occurs in occupational settings via inhalation of vaporous fumes or direct contact with skin. Prolonged or excessive exposure can cause liver and kidney damage.

RVUs

Code	Work	PE	PE Non-Facility	MP	Total Non-Facility	Total Facility	Global
82441	0.00	0.00	0.00	0.00	0.00	0.00	XXX

82507

82507 Citrate

(Cocaine, qualitative analysis, use 80353)

(Codeine, qualitative analysis, use 80361)

(Complement, see 86160-86162)

Plain English Description

A blood or urine test is performed to measure citrate (citric acid) levels. Citrate plays an important role in metabolism. Citrate levels in urine are also useful in evaluating nephrolithiasis. A blood sample is obtained by separately reportable venipuncture. Urine may be collected over a 24-hour period or submitted as a single random sample. Serum is tested using spectrophotometry or enzymatic methodology. Urine is tested using quantitative enzymatic methodology.

RVUs

Code	Work	PE	PE Non-Facility	MP	Total Non-Facility	Total Facility	Global
82507	0.00	0.00	0.00	0.00	0.00	0.00	XXX

82565-82575

82565 Creatinine; blood

82570 Creatinine; other source

82575 Creatinine; clearance

Plain English Description

A blood sample is taken to measure creatinine levels in 82565 and a sample other than blood is taken to measure creatinine levels in 82570. Creatinine is a waste product produced by the muscles in the breakdown of creatine, which is a compound used by the muscles to create energy for contraction. The waste product, creatinine, is excreted by the kidneys and blood levels provide a good measurement of renal function. Creatinine may be checked to screen for or monitor treatment of renal disease. Creatinine levels may also be monitored in patients with acute or chronic illnesses that may impair renal function and in patients on medications that affect renal function. Creatinine is measured using spectrophotometry. Creatinine clearance (82575), also known as urea or urea nitrogen clearance, tests both blood and urine samples for a calculation of creatinine content adjusted for urine volume and physical size as a general indicator of glomerular filtration function.

RVUs

Code	Work	PE	PE Non-Facility	MP	Total Non-Facility	Total Facility	Global
82565	0.00	0.00	0.00	0.00	0.00	0.00	XXX
82570	0.00	0.00	0.00	0.00	0.00	0.00	XXX
82575	0.00	0.00	0.00	0.00	0.00	0.00	XXX

82610

82610 Cystatin C

Plain English Description

A blood sample is obtained to measure the cystatin C level. Cystatin C, also referred to as cystatin 3 or CST 3, is a serum protein produced by all nucleated cells in the body, and has a low molecular mass that allows it to be filtered by the glomerular membrane in the kidneys. Cystatin C contained in the filtrate is then reabsorbed by the body and broken down. It is not returned to the blood. When glomerular filtration rate is impaired, cystatin C levels in the blood increase, indicating decreased kidney function. Cystatin C measurement is used to evaluate glomerular filtration rate, screen for and monitor renal disease, and monitor treatment in patients with known renal disease. Cystatin C levels may also be used to predict survival following a heart attack, with elevated levels indicating a poorer prognosis. Cystatin C is measured by nephelometry.

RVUs

Code	Work	PE	PE Non-Facility	MP	Total Non-Facility	Total Facility	Global
82610	0.00	0.00	0.00	0.00	0.00	0.00	XXX

82615

82615 Cystine and homocystine, urine, qualitative

Plain English Description

A laboratory test is performed to determine the presence of cystine and homocystine in urine. The amino acids lysine, ornithine, and arginine break down into cystine. When cystine fails to be reabsorbed in the kidney, it can precipitate in the urine and form stones. Cystinuria is usually caused by an inherited genetic disorder. Homocystinuria may result from an inherited metabolic disorder of the amino acid methionine (cystathionine beta synthase deficiency), re-methylation defects, or vitamin B deficiencies (B2, B6, B9, B12). Symptoms of elevated homocystine can be multisystemic and include connective tissue and muscle disorders, central nervous system disorders, and cardiovascular problems. A urine sample is obtained by voided specimen or catheterization. Urine is tested for cystine and homocystine using spectrometry.

RVUs

Code	Work	PE	PE Non-Facility	MP	Total Non-Facility	Total Facility	Global
82615	0.00	0.00	0.00	0.00	0.00	0.00	XXX

82642

82642 Dihydrotestosterone (DHT)

(For dihydrotestosterone analysis for anabolic drug testing, see 80327, 80328)

(Dipropylacetic acid, use 80164)

(Dopamine, see 82382-82384)

(Duodenal contents, see individual enzymes; for intubation and collection, see 43756, 43757)

Plain English Description

A laboratory test is performed to measure dihydrotesterone (DHT) level. DHT has a role in male pattern baldness and prostate disease and is necessary for male virilization to mitigate the effects of estrogen. DHT is a biologically active metabolite of testosterone belonging to the androgen class of hormones. DHT is generated from the reduction of testosterone by the enzyme 5-alpha-reductase to form 2 isoenzymes. DHT Type 1 can be found in most body tissue and is the dominant form found in sebaceous glands. DHT Type 2 is the dominant isoenzyme in genital tissue including the prostate gland. Serum levels of DHT are not affected by aging despite lower levels of serum testosterone and do not increase when benign prostatic hyperplasia (BPH) is present. A serum DHT measurement may be used to evaluate and diagnose DHT deficiency and to monitor patients receiving 5-alpha-reductase therapy/chemotherapy such as finasteride or saw palmetto. A blood sample is obtained by separately reported procedure. Serum is tested using liquid chromatography-tandem mass spectrometry (LC-MS/MS).

RVUs

Code	Work	PE	PE Non-Facility	MP	Total Non-Facility	Total Facility	Global
82642	0.00	0.00	0.00	0.00	0.00	0.00	XXX

82947-82948

82947 Glucose; quantitative, blood (except reagent strip)
82948 Glucose; blood, reagent strip

Plain English Description

A blood sample is obtained to measure total (quantitative) blood glucose level. Glucose is a simple sugar that is the main source of energy for the body. Carbohydrates are broken down into simple sugars, primarily glucose, absorbed by the intestine, and circulated in the blood. Insulin, a hormone produced by the pancreas, regulates glucose level in the blood and transports glucose to cells in other tissues and organs. When more glucose is available in the blood than is required, it is converted to glycogen and stored in the liver or converted to fat and stored in adipose (fat) tissue. If the glucose/insulin metabolic process is working properly, blood glucose will remain at a fairly constant, healthy level. Glucose is measured to determine whether the glucose/insulin metabolic process is functioning properly. It is used to monitor glucose levels and determine whether they are too low (hypoglycemia) or too high (hyperglycemia) as well as test for diabetes and to monitor blood sugar control in diabetics. Use 82947 for quantitative blood glucose determination by enzymatic methodology or any method other than reagent strip. Use 82948 for blood glucose determination by reagent strip. A drop of blood is placed on a reagent strip, which is then compared to a calibrated color scale, and a visual determination is made as to the amount of glucose present in the specimen.

RVUs

Code	Work	PE	PE Non-Facility	MP	Total Non-Facility	Total Facility	Global
82947	0.00	0.00	0.00	0.00	0.00	0.00	XXX
82948	0.00	0.00	0.00	0.00	0.00	0.00	XXX

82950

82950 Glucose; post glucose dose (includes glucose)

Plain English Description

A laboratory test is performed to measure the level of glucose, a simple sugar molecule that provides energy to cells. Glucose is ingested in many different foods and can also be synthesized from glycogen stores in the liver and muscle tissue. The pancreatic hormones insulin and glucagon help to regulate blood glucose levels (BGL). A post-load BGL is routinely monitored during pregnancy, usually between 24 and 28 weeks gestation. Hormones produced by the placenta can cause impaired glucose metabolism in the mother, leading to elevated maternal BGL and overnutrition/excess growth of the baby. The patient does not need to be fasting for this test. A 50 g oral dose of concentrated glucose (Glucola) is given to the patient. A blood sample is obtained by separately reportable venipuncture 60 minutes post ingestion. Plasma is tested using quantitative enzymatic method.

RVUs

Code	Work	PE	PE Non-Facility	MP	Total Non-Facility	Total Facility	Global
82950	0.00	0.00	0.00	0.00	0.00	0.00	XXX

82951-82952

82951 Glucose; tolerance test (GTT), 3 specimens (includes glucose)

✚ **82952 Glucose; tolerance test, each additional beyond 3 specimens (List separately in addition to code for primary procedure)**

(Use 82952 in conjunction with 82951)

(For insulin tolerance test, see 80434, 80435)

(For leucine tolerance test, use 80428)

(For semiquantitative urine glucose, see 81000, 81002, 81005, 81099)

Plain English Description

A laboratory test is performed to measure glucose, a simple sugar molecule that provides energy to cells. Glucose is ingested in many different foods and can also be synthesized from glycogen stores in the liver and muscle tissue. The pancreatic hormones insulin and glucagon help to regulate blood glucose levels (BGL). A glucose tolerance test (GTT) may be ordered when a patient has a positive glucose screening test to diagnose gestational diabetes, diabetes mellitus, or impaired glucose tolerance and may also be used to test for lactose intolerance and malabsorption disorders. The patient should fast for a minimum of 8 hours prior to the test. A blood sample is obtained by separately reportable venipuncture for a baseline blood glucose level. A 75 g (100 g if the patient is pregnant) oral dose of concentrated glucose (Glucola) is given to the patient. A blood sample is obtained by separately reportable venipuncture at 60, 120, and 180 minutes post ingestion. Plasma is tested using quantitative enzymatic method. When testing for lactose intolerance and malabsorption disorders, a baseline blood glucose level is obtained followed by a 50 g oral dose of concentrated glucose (Glucola). Blood samples are obtained at 30, 60, 120, and 180 minutes post ingestion and plasma is tested for glucose levels using quantitative enzymatic method. The first 3 blood samples are reported using code 82951; additional samples are reported using code 82952.

RVUs

Code	Work	PE	PE Non-Facility	MP	Total Non-Facility	Total Facility	Global
82951	0.00	0.00	0.00	0.00	0.00	0.00	XXX
82952	0.00	0.00	0.00	0.00	0.00	0.00	XXX

83735

83735 Magnesium

Plain English Description

A blood, urine, or fecal test is performed to measure magnesium levels. Magnesium is an essential dietary mineral responsible for enzyme function, energy production, and contraction and relaxation of muscle fibers. Decreased levels may result from severe burns, metabolic disorders, certain medications, and low blood calcium levels. A blood sample is obtained by separately reportable venipuncture. Red blood cells (RBCs) are tested using quantitative inductively coupled plasma-mass spectrometry. Serum/plasma is tested using quantitative spectrophotometry. A 24-hour voided urine specimen is tested using quantitative spectrophotometry. A random or 24-hour fecal sample is tested using quantitative spectrophotometry.

RVUs

Code	Work	PE	PE Non-Facility	MP	Total Non-Facility	Total Facility	Global
83735	0.00	0.00	0.00	0.00	0.00	0.00	XXX

84066

84066 Phosphatase, acid; prostatic

Plain English Description

A blood test is performed to measure prostatic acid phosphatase (PAP) levels. PAP is an enzyme specific to the prostate and is present in seminal fluid. The enzyme fuses endosomes to create an acidic pH environment. Levels may be elevated in patients with benign prostatic hyperplasia (BPH), prostate cancer, infection, or infarction and in Paget's or Gaucher's disease. Prostate manipulation such as biopsy or massage may elevate PAP levels for 24-48 hours following the procedure. The test for PAP is not useful in screening but may be helpful in predicting disease recurrence and to monitor response to treatment. A blood sample is obtained by separately reportable venipuncture. Serum is tested using quantitative chemiluminescent immunoassay.

RVUs

Code	Work	PE	PE Non-Facility	MP	Total Non-Facility	Total Facility	Global
84066	0.00	0.00	0.00	0.00	0.00	0.00	XXX

84100-84105

84100 Phosphorus inorganic (phosphate)

84105 Phosphorus inorganic (phosphate); urine

(Pituitary gonadotropins, see 83001-83002)

(PKU, see 84030, 84035)

Plain English Description

A blood or urine test is performed to measure inorganic phosphorus (phosphate) levels. Phosphate is an intracellular anion, found primarily in bone and soft tissue. It plays an important role in cellular energy (nerve and muscle function) and the building/repair of bone and teeth. Decreased levels are most often caused by malnutrition and lead to muscle and neurological dysfunction. Elevated levels may be due to kidney or parathyroid gland problems. In 84100, a blood sample is obtained by separately reportable venipuncture. Serum/plasma is tested using quantitative spectrophotometry. In 84105, a 24-hour or random urine sample is obtained. Urine is tested using quantitative spectrophotometry.

RVUs

Code	Work	PE	PE Non-Facility	MP	Total Non-Facility	Total Facility	Global
84100	0.00	0.00	0.00	0.00	0.00	0.00	XXX
84105	0.00	0.00	0.00	0.00	0.00	0.00	XXX

84119-84120

84119 Porphyrins, urine; qualitative

84120 Porphyrins, urine; quantitation and fractionation

Plain English Description

A urine test is performed to determine the presence of porphyrin in 84119 and to measure porphyrin levels in 84120. Elevated levels may be diagnostic for lead poisoning, liver disease, or porphyria, an inherited metabolic disorder involving a deficiency of enzymes in the heme synthesis pathway. Heme is a component of red blood cells and muscle cells. Porphyrins help form many important substances for the body, including hemoglobin. A quantitation and fractionation test (84120) is often ordered in conjunction with urine porphobilinogen (84106). A 24-hour urine sample is obtained. A random sample may also be used during acute symptomatic periods. Urine is tested using quantitative high-performance liquid chromatography.

RVUs

Code	Work	PE	PE Non-Facility	MP	Total Non-Facility	Total Facility	Global
84119	0.00	0.00	0.00	0.00	0.00	0.00	XXX
84120	0.00	0.00	0.00	0.00	0.00	0.00	XXX

84132

84132 Potassium; serum, plasma or whole blood

Plain English Description

A blood sample is obtained to measure potassium level. Potassium is a positively charged electrolyte that works in conjunction with other electrolytes, such as sodium, chloride, and carbon dioxide (CO2), to regulate body fluid, stimulate muscle contraction, and maintain proper acid-base balance. Potassium is found in all body fluids but mostly stored within cells, not in extracellular fluids, blood serum, or plasma. Small fluctuations in blood potassium, either too high (hyperkalemia) or too low (hypokalemia), can have serious, even life-threatening consequences. Potassium level is used to screen for and monitor renal disease; monitor patients on certain medications, such as diuretics; and patients with acute and chronic conditions, such as dehydration or endocrine disorders. Because blood potassium affects heart rhythm and respiratory rate, it is routinely checked prior to major surgical procedures. Potassium is measured by ion-selective electrode (ISE) methodology.

RVUs

Code	Work	PE	PE Non-Facility	MP	Total Non-Facility	Total Facility	Global
84132	0.00	0.00	0.00	0.00	0.00	0.00	XXX

84133

84133 Potassium; urine

Plain English Description

A urine test is performed to measure potassium levels. Potassium is a chemical element essential for proper functioning of the heart, kidneys, intestine, muscles, and nerves. Levels may be elevated in kidney disease, Cushing's syndrome, hyperaldosteronism, eating disorders, diabetic/metabolic acidosis, hypomagnesemia, and with the use of certain diuretics. Decreased levels may be caused by adrenal gland insufficiency, hypoaldosteronism, and medications such as beta blockers, lithium, and NSAIDs. A 24-hour or random urine sample is obtained. Urine is tested using quantitative ion-selective electrode.

RVUs

Code	Work	PE	PE Non-Facility	MP	Total Non-Facility	Total Facility	Global
84133	0.00	0.00	0.00	0.00	0.00	0.00	XXX

84134

84134 Prealbumin

(For microalbumin, see 82043, 82044)

Plain English Description

A blood test is performed to measure prealbumin levels. Prealbumin, also referred to as transthyretin (TTR), is found in serum and cerebral spinal fluid (CSF). It is responsible for transporting thyroxin and retinol binding protein carried on retinol. The test may be ordered to detect protein-calorie malnutrition in chronically or critically ill individuals. Levels may be elevated with the use of high dose corticosteroids or non-steroidal anti-inflammatory drugs (NSAIDs), adrenal gland disorders, Hodgkin's disease, and kidney failure. Decreased levels may be caused by hyperthyroidism, liver disease, severe infection, inflammatory diseases, and certain digestive disorders. A blood sample is obtained by separately reportable venipuncture. Serum and/or plasma is tested using immunoturbidimetric method.

RVUs

Code	Work	PE	PE Non-Facility	MP	Total Non-Facility	Total Facility	Global
84134	0.00	0.00	0.00	0.00	0.00	0.00	XXX

84152-84154

84152 Prostate specific antigen (PSA); complexed (direct measurement)

84153 Prostate specific antigen (PSA); total

84154 Prostate specific antigen (PSA); free

Plain English Description

Prostate specific antigen (PSA) is measured. PSA is a protein produced by normal prostate cells found in serum and exists in both free form and complexed with other proteins. In 84152, complexed PSA is measured by direct measurement. A higher level of complexed PSA is suggestive of prostate cancer and is a better indicator of malignancy than total PSA. In 84153, total PSA is measured as the total amount of both free and complexed forms. Total PSA levels are higher in men with benign prostatic hyperplasia (BPH), acute bacterial prostatitis, or prostate cancer. Total PSA is used to screen for prostate cancer and evaluate the response to treatment in those with prostate cancer, but cannot be used by itself to definitively diagnose prostate cancer. In 84154, free PSA is measured, often in conjunction with total PSA, to provide an indirect measurement of complexed PSA.

RVUs

Code	Work	PE	PE Non-Facility	MP	Total Non-Facility	Total Facility	Global
84152	0.00	0.00	0.00	0.00	0.00	0.00	XXX
84153	0.00	0.00	0.00	0.00	0.00	0.00	XXX
84154	0.00	0.00	0.00	0.00	0.00	0.00	XXX

84155

84155 Protein, total, except by refractometry; serum, plasma or whole blood

Plain English Description

A blood test is performed to measure total protein levels. Total protein is often reported as a ratio of albumin to globulin (A/G ratio), and normal results will show albumin slightly greater than globulin. The test may be used to monitor nutritional status or diagnose kidney and liver disease. Elevated levels can indicate chronic inflammation, viral hepatitis, HIV infection, and multiple myeloma. Levels that are decreased may result from malnutrition or malabsorption syndromes such as celiac disease or inflammatory bowel disease. A blood sample is obtained by separately reportable venipuncture. Serum, plasma, or whole blood may be tested using quantitative spectrophotometry.

RVUs

Code	Work	PE	PE Non-Facility	MP	Total Non-Facility	Total Facility	Global
84155	0.00	0.00	0.00	0.00	0.00	0.00	XXX

84156

84156 Protein, total, except by refractometry; urine

Plain English Description

A urine test is performed to measure total protein levels. Protein is not normally found in urine and usually indicates damage or disease in the kidneys. Elevated levels are often present in patients with diabetes, hypertension, and multiple myeloma. A 24-hour or random urine sample is obtained and tested using quantitative spectrophotometry.

RVUs

Code	Work	PE	PE Non-Facility	MP	Total Non-Facility	Total Facility	Global
84156	0.00	0.00	0.00	0.00	0.00	0.00	XXX

84160

84160 Protein, total, by refractometry, any source

(For urine total protein by dipstick method, use 81000-81003)

Plain English Description

Total protein levels may be measured in any fluid or liquid substances of the body including urine, serum, cerebral spinal fluid, and synovial fluid using refractometry. A sample of blood, urine, amniotic fluid, or serum is obtained and the patient's level of protein is measured. The total protein level determines the overall nutritional level of the patient.

RVUs

Code	Work	PE	PE Non-Facility	MP	Total Non-Facility	Total Facility	Global
84160	0.00	0.00	0.00	0.00	0.00	0.00	XXX

84165

84165 Protein; electrophoretic fractionation and quantitation, serum

Plain English Description

A blood test is performed to measure protein levels in serum. This test is often performed in conjunction with total protein (84155) to detect pathophysiologic states such as inflammation, gammopathies, and dysproteinemias. There are more sensitive tests available to detect these and similar disorders. A blood sample is obtained by separately reportable venipuncture. Serum is tested using electrophoretic fractionation and quantitation.

RVUs

Code	Work	PE	PE Non-Facility	MP	Total Non-Facility	Total Facility	Global
84165	0.00	0.00	0.00	0.00	0.00	0.00	XXX

84166

84166 Protein; electrophoretic fractionation and quantitation, other fluids with concentration (eg, urine, CSF)

Plain English Description

A test is performed on body fluids with concentration, such as cerebral spinal fluid (CSF) or urine, to measure protein levels. Elevated protein levels in CSF may be caused by central nervous system tumors or neurological illness. Elevated protein levels in urine may indicate kidney disease or damage. There are more sensitive tests available to detect these and similar disorders. CSF is obtained by separately reportable lumbar puncture (spinal tap), while urine is obtained from a 24-hour specimen. Body fluids are tested for fractionation and quantitation using quantitative electrophoresis.

RVUs

Code	Work	PE	PE Non-Facility	MP	Total Non-Facility	Total Facility	Global
84166	0.00	0.00	0.00	0.00	0.00	0.00	XXX

84206

84206 Proinsulin

(Pseudocholinesterase, use 82480)

Plain English Description

A blood test is performed to measure proinsulin levels. Proinsulin is a hormone precursor to insulin produced by beta cells in the pancreas, specifically in an area called the islets of Langerhans. A blood sample is obtained by separately reportable venipuncture. Serum is tested using qualitative enzyme-linked immunosorbent assay. This test is often performed to measure stages of pre-diabetes and progression toward type 2 diabetes mellitus. Elevated proinsulin levels may also be present in patients with benign or malignant B-cell tumors of the pancreas, renal failure, cirrhosis, or hyperthyroidism.

RVUs

Code	Work	PE	PE Non-Facility	MP	Total Non-Facility	Total Facility	Global
84206	0.00	0.00	0.00	0.00	0.00	0.00	XXX

84244

84244 Renin

Plain English Description

A blood test is performed to measure renin levels. Renin is an enzyme released by the kidney in response to decreased sodium levels or blood volume, working with angiotensin and aldosterone to regulate mean arterial pressure. Levels may be elevated in Addison's disease, cirrhosis, congestive heart failure, dehydration, hemorrhage, hypertension, hypokalemia, nephrotic syndrome, and renal tumors. Decreased levels may be caused by ADH therapy, hyperaldosteronism, steroid use, or sodium sensitive hypertension. This test is often ordered in conjunction with Aldosterone (82088). A blood sample is obtained by separately reportable venipuncture. Plasma is tested for direct renin using quantitative immunoradiometric assay and for plasma renin activity using quantitative radioimmunoassay.

RVUs

Code	Work	PE	PE Non-Facility	MP	Total Non-Facility	Total Facility	Global
84244	0.00	0.00	0.00	0.00	0.00	0.00	XXX

84295-84302

84295 Sodium; serum, plasma or whole blood

84300 Sodium; urine

84302 Sodium; other source

(Somatomammotropin, use 83632)

(Somatotropin, use 83003)

Plain English Description

A blood sample is obtained to measure sodium level in 84295. A urine sample is obtained to measure sodium level in 84300. A sample other than urine, blood, plasma, or serum is obtained to measure sodium level in 84302. Sodium is a positively charged electrolyte that works in conjunction with other electrolytes, such as potassium, chloride, and carbon dioxide (CO2), to regulate fluid in the body and maintain proper acid-base balance. Sodium is an essential mineral in the body, necessary for maintaining normal metabolic processes, fluid levels, and vascular pressure. Sodium level is used to screen for and monitor elevated blood sodium (hypernatremia), low blood sodium (hyponatremia), and electrolyte imbalances. Sodium may be monitored in patients on certain medications, such as diuretics, which can cause electrolyte imbalance. Sodium is measured by ion-selective electrode (ISE) methodology.

RVUs

Code	Work	PE	PE Non-Facility	MP	Total Non-Facility	Total Facility	Global
84295	0.00	0.00	0.00	0.00	0.00	0.00	XXX
84300	0.00	0.00	0.00	0.00	0.00	0.00	XXX
84302	0.00	0.00	0.00	0.00	0.00	0.00	XXX

84402-84403

84402 Testosterone; free

84403 Testosterone; total

Plain English Description

A blood test is performed to measure free testosterone levels in 84402 or a blood and urine test is performed to measure total testosterone level in 84403. Testosterone is an androgen hormone secreted in the testes of men, ovaries of women, and the adrenal glands of both sexes. Testosterone helps promote protein synthesis and supports the growth of cells and tissue. This test is often performed in conjunction with sex hormone binding globulin (84270). A blood sample is obtained by separately reportable venipuncture. Serum/plasma of adult males is tested using quantitative electrochemiluminescent immunoassay with the value derived from a mathematical expression using sex hormone binding globulin (SHBG). Serum/plasma of adult males may also be tested using quantitative equilibrium dialysis/high-performance liquid chromatography-tandem mass spectrometry. Serum/plasma of children and adult females is tested using quantitative high-performance liquid chromatography-tandem mass spectrometry/electrochemiluminescent immunoassay with the value also derived from a mathematical expression using SHBG.

RVUs

Code	Work	PE	PE Non-Facility	MP	Total Non-Facility	Total Facility	Global
84402	0.00	0.00	0.00	0.00	0.00	0.00	XXX
84403	0.00	0.00	0.00	0.00	0.00	0.00	XXX

84410

84410 Testosterone; bioavailable, direct measurement (eg, differential precipitation)

(Do not report 84402, 84403 in conjunction with 80327, 80328 to identify anabolic steroid testing for testosterone)

Plain English Description

A laboratory test is performed to measure bioavailable testosterone in serum. Testosterone is an androgen hormone secreted by both males and females. The majority of circulating testosterone is tightly bound to sex hormone binding globulin (SHBG) and biologically inactive. Free and albumin bound testosterone are active, bioavailable compounds. This test may be used to diagnose androgen deficiency in males when total testosterone is at the lower limits of normal and/or for suspected alteration of SHBG due to aging, obesity, or ingestion of certain medications. The test may also be used to diagnose hyperandrogenism in women who present with amenorrhea, hirsutism, polycystic ovarian syndrome (PCOS), and/or virilization. A blood sample is obtained by separately reportable venipuncture. The serum concentration of free testosterone is measured by differential precipitation of SHBG and ammonium sulfate following equilibration of the serum specimen tracer amounts of tritium-labeled testosterone.

RVUs

Code	Work	PE	PE Non-Facility	MP	Total Non-Facility	Total Facility	Global
84410	0.00	0.00	0.00	0.00	0.00	0.00	XXX

84520

84520 Urea nitrogen; quantitative

Plain English Description

A blood sample is obtained to measure total (quantitative) urea nitrogen (BUN) level. Urea is a waste product produced in the liver by the breakdown of protein from a sequence of chemical reactions referred to as the urea or Krebs-Henseleit cycle. Urea then enters the bloodstream, is taken up by the kidneys, and excreted in the urine. Blood BUN is measured to evaluate renal function, to monitor patients with renal disease, and to evaluate effectiveness of dialysis. BUN may also be measured in patients with acute or chronic illnesses that affect renal function. BUN is measured using spectrophotometry.

RVUs

Code	Work	PE	PE Non-Facility	MP	Total Non-Facility	Total Facility	Global
84520	0.00	0.00	0.00	0.00	0.00	0.00	XXX

84525-84545

84525 Urea nitrogen; semiquantitative (eg, reagent strip test)

84540 Urea nitrogen, urine

84545 Urea nitrogen, clearance

Plain English Description

A blood sample is obtained to measure total (quantitative) blood urea nitrogen (BUN) level. Urea is a waste product made in the liver by the breakdown of protein through a sequence of chemical reactions referred to as the urea or Krebs-Henseleit cycle. Urea enters the bloodstream, is taken up by the kidneys, and excreted in the urine. BUN is measured to evaluate renal function, monitor current renal disease, and evaluate the effectiveness of dialysis. BUN may also be measured in patients with acute or chronic illnesses that affect renal function. In 84525, the test is performed with a reagent strip, which reacts with a urine sample. In 84540, only the BUN is performed. In 84545, a urine sample is collected over a 24-hour period.

RVUs

Code	Work	PE	PE Non-Facility	MP	Total Non-Facility	Total Facility	Global
84525	0.00	0.00	0.00	0.00	0.00	0.00	XXX
84540	0.00	0.00	0.00	0.00	0.00	0.00	XXX
84545	0.00	0.00	0.00	0.00	0.00	0.00	XXX

84550

84550 Uric acid; blood

Plain English Description

A blood test is performed to measure uric acid levels. Uric acid forms from the natural breakdown of body cells and the food we ingest. Uric acid is normally filtered by the kidneys and excreted in urine. Elevated blood levels may result from kidney disease, certain cancers and/or cancer therapies, hemolytic or sickle cell anemia, heart failure, cirrhosis, lead poisoning, and low levels of thyroid or parathyroid hormones. Levels may be decreased in Wilson's disease, with poor dietary intake of protein, and with the use of certain drugs. A blood sample is obtained by separately reportable venipuncture. Serum/plasma is tested using quantitative spectrophotometry.

RVUs

Code	Work	PE	PE Non-Facility	MP	Total Non-Facility	Total Facility	Global
84550	0.00	0.00	0.00	0.00	0.00	0.00	XXX

84560

84560 Uric acid; other source

Plain English Description

A test is performed on urine or synovial (joint) fluid to measure uric acid levels. Uric acid forms from the natural breakdown of body cells and the food we ingest. It is normally filtered by the kidneys and excreted in urine. Elevated levels may result from kidney disease, certain cancers and/or cancer therapies, hemolytic or sickle cell anemia, heart failure, cirrhosis, a diet high in purine, lead poisoning, and low levels of thyroid or parathyroid hormones. Levels may be decreased with gout, folic acid deficiency, and certain medications. A 24-hour or random urine specimen is obtained and tested using quantitative spectrophotometry. Uric acid found in synovial fluid is usually in the form of monosodium urate crystals. The joints most commonly affected are in the feet and legs. Synovial fluid is aspirated from the affected joint(s) by separately reportable arthrocentesis and tested using quantitative spectrophotometry.

RVUs

Code	Work	PE	PE Non-Facility	MP	Total Non-Facility	Total Facility	Global
84560	0.00	0.00	0.00	0.00	0.00	0.00	XXX

84578-84583

84578 Urobilinogen, urine; qualitative

84580 Urobilinogen, urine; quantitative, timed specimen

84583 Urobilinogen, urine; semiquantitative

(Uroporphyrins, use 84120)

(Valproic acid [dipropylacetic acid], use 80164)

Plain English Description

Urobilinogen is a product of bilirubin reduction, which takes place in the intestine. A small amount is reabsorbed from the intestine and circulated via blood to the kidneys for filtration. This is called the enterohepatic urobilinogen cycle. Elevated levels in urine may result from biliary obstruction; hepatic infection, poisoning, or inflammation; and from hemolytic anemia. Elevated levels may also occur in the presence of a large hematoma that the body must absorb. Levels may be deceased with congenital enzymatic jaundice and in the presence of urine acidifying drugs. Use 84578 for qualitative evaluation; 84580 for quantitative, timed specimen urobilinogen evaluation; and 84583 for a semiquantitative evaluation.

RVUs

Code	Work	PE	PE Non-Facility	MP	Total Non-Facility	Total Facility	Global
84578	0.00	0.00	0.00	0.00	0.00	0.00	XXX
84580	0.00	0.00	0.00	0.00	0.00	0.00	XXX
84583	0.00	0.00	0.00	0.00	0.00	0.00	XXX

84588

84588 Vasopressin (antidiuretic hormone, ADH)

Plain English Description

A blood test is performed to measure arginine vasopressin hormone (antidiuretic hormone, ADH) levels. ADH is a neurohypophyseal hormone that regulates water, glucose, and sodium levels in the blood. It is synthesized by the hypothalamus and stored in the posterior pituitary gland. ADH is released in response to dehydration causing the kidney to conserve water and concentrate urine volume. The hormone also increases peripheral vascular resistance, which causes an elevation in blood pressure from vasoconstriction. A blood sample is obtained by separately reportable venipuncture. Plasma is tested using quantitative radioimmunoassay.

RVUs

Code	Work	PE	PE Non-Facility	MP	Total Non-Facility	Total Facility	Global
84588	0.00	0.00	0.00	0.00	0.00	0.00	XXX

85004

85004 Blood count; automated differential WBC count

Plain English Description

A WBC count is a count of the number of white blood cells (leukocytes) in a specific volume of blood. This test is performed to evaluate overall health and can help the physician evaluate conditions such as infection, allergy, systemic illness, inflammation, and leukemia. There are five types of WBCs: neutrophils, eosinophils, basophils, monocytes, and lymphocytes. In an automated WBC count, each of the five types is counted separately using an electronic cell counter or an image analysis instrument.

RVUs

Code	Work	PE	PE Non-Facility	MP	Total Non-Facility	Total Facility	Global
85004	0.00	0.00	0.00	0.00	0.00	0.00	XXX

85007-85008

85007 Blood count; blood smear, microscopic examination with manual differential WBC count

85008 Blood count; blood smear, microscopic examination without manual differential WBC count

(For other fluids [eg, CSF], see 89050, 89051)

Plain English Description

A blood smear is performed with microscopic examination with or without a manual differential WBC count. A blood smear is typically performed following an automated test that indicates the presence of abnormal or immature blood cells. It may also be performed when the physician suspects a condition that affects blood cell production, such as anemia. A blood sample is obtained by separately reportable venipuncture. A blood smear is prepared and examined under a microscope by a technician for immature or abnormal cells. In 85007, the test is performed with a manual differential white blood cell (WBC) count. The technician examines and counts each of the five types of WBCs separately. Neutrophils comprise the majority of WBCs in healthy adults and are differentiated by cytoplasm with pink or purple granules. Eosinophils normally comprise 1-3% of total WBCs and are differentiated in stained smears by their large, red-orange granules. Elevated levels of eosinophils may indicate allergy or parasitic infection. Basophils normally comprise only 1% of total WBCs and are differentiated by their large, black granules. Elevated levels of basophils may be indicative of certain leukemias, varicella (chicken pox) infection, or ulcerative colitis. Monocytes are the largest WBCs and act as scavengers to ingest (phagocytize) cellular debris, bacteria, and other particles. Lymphocytes produce antibodies (immunoglobulins) and are differentiated by their homogenous cytoplasm and smooth, round nucleus. In 85008, the blood smear is performed without manual differential WBC count.

RVUs

Code	Work	PE	PE Non-Facility	MP	Total Non-Facility	Total Facility	Global
85007	0.00	0.00	0.00	0.00	0.00	0.00	XXX
85008	0.00	0.00	0.00	0.00	0.00	0.00	XXX

85009

85009 Blood count; manual differential WBC count, buffy coat

(Eosinophils, nasal smear, use 89190)

Plain English Description

A manual white blood cell (WBC) count is estimated using a rapid technique referred to as buffy coat. A blood sample is obtained by separately reportable venipuncture. The blood specimen is placed in a microhematocrit tube and centrifuged (spun) to separate the WBCs, which appear as a thin layer of white cells between the RBCs and plasma. This thin layer is called the buffy coat and is used to estimate whether WBC count is higher than normal. The technician then performs a manual differential WBC count, which involves identifying and counting each of the five types of WBCs separately. Neutrophils comprise the majority of WBCs in healthy adults and are differentiated by cytoplasm with pink or purple granules. Eosinophils normally comprise 1-3% of total WBCs and are differentiated in stained smears by their large, red-orange granules. Elevated levels of eosinophils may indicate allergy or parasitic infection. Basophils normally comprise only 1% of total WBCs and are differentiated by their large, black granules. Elevated levels of basophils may be indicative of certain leukemias, varicella (chicken pox) infection, or ulcerative colitis. Monocytes are the largest WBCs and act as scavengers to ingest (phagocytize) cellular debris, bacteria, and other particles. Lymphocytes produce antibodies (immunoglobulins) and are differentiated by their homogenous cytoplasm and smooth, round nucleus.

RVUs

Code	Work	PE	PE Non-Facility	MP	Total Non-Facility	Total Facility	Global
85009	0.00	0.00	0.00	0.00	0.00	0.00	XXX

85013-85014

85013 Blood count; spun microhematocrit

85014 Blood count; hematocrit (Hct)

Plain English Description

A blood test is performed to determine hematocrit (Hct). Hematocrit refers to the volume of red blood cells (erythrocytes) in a given volume of blood and is usually expressed as a percentage of total blood volume. A blood sample is obtained by separately reportable venipuncture or finger, heel, or ear stick. In 85013, the blood sample is collected in a microhematocrit tube that is centrifuged (spun) to separate the WBCs and plasma from the RBCs. The Hct (volume of RBCs) is then calculated and expressed as a percentage of total blood volume (RBCs + WBCs + plasma). In 85014, Hct is calculated using an electronic cell counter.

RVUs

Code	Work	PE	PE Non-Facility	MP	Total Non-Facility	Total Facility	Global
85013	0.00	0.00	0.00	0.00	0.00	0.00	XXX
85014	0.00	0.00	0.00	0.00	0.00	0.00	XXX

85018

85018 Blood count; hemoglobin (Hgb)

(For other hemoglobin determination, see 83020-83069)

(For immunoassay, hemoglobin, fecal, use 82274)

(For transcutaneous hemoglobin measurement, use 88738)

Plain English Description

A blood test is performed to determine hemoglobin (Hgb), which is a measurement of the amount of oxygen-carrying protein in the blood. Hgb is measured to determine the severity of anemia or polycythemia, monitor response to treatment for these conditions, or determine the need for blood transfusion. A blood sample is collected by separately reportable venipuncture or finger, heel, or ear stick. The sample may be sent to the lab or a rapid testing system may be used in the physician's office. Systems consist of a portable photometer and pipettes that contain reagent. The pipette is used to collect the blood sample from a capillary stick and the blood is automatically mixed with the reagent in the pipette. The photometer is then used to read the result, which is displayed on the photometer device.

RVUs

Code	Work	PE	PE Non-Facility	MP	Total Non-Facility	Total Facility	Global
85018	0.00	0.00	0.00	0.00	0.00	0.00	XXX

85025-85027

85025 Blood count; complete (CBC), automated (Hgb, Hct, RBC, WBC and platelet count) and automated differential WBC count

85027 Blood count; complete (CBC), automated (Hgb, Hct, RBC, WBC and platelet count)

Plain English Description

An automated complete blood count (CBC) is performed with or without automated differential white blood cell (WBC) count. A CBC is used as a screening test to evaluate overall health and symptoms such as fatigue, bruising, bleeding, and inflammation, or to help diagnose infection. A CBC includes measurement of Hgb and Hct, RBC count, WBC count with or without differential, and platelet count. Hgb measures the amount of oxygen-carrying protein in the blood. Hct refers to the volume of red blood cells (erythrocytes) in a given volume of blood and is usually expressed as a percentage of total blood volume. RBC count is the number of red blood cells (erythrocytes) in a specific volume of blood. WBC count is the number of white blood cells (leukocytes) in a specific volume of blood. There are five types of WBCs: neutrophils, eosinophils, basophils, monocytes, and lymphocytes. If a differential is performed, each of the five types is counted separately. Platelet count is the number of platelets (thrombocytes) in the blood. Platelets are responsible for blood clotting. The CBC is performed with an automated blood cell counting instrument that can also be programmed to provide an automated WBC differential count. Use 85025 for CBC with automated differential WBC count or 85027 for CBC without differential WBC count.

RVUs

Code	Work	PE	PE Non-Facility	MP	Total Non-Facility	Total Facility	Global
85025	0.00	0.00	0.00	0.00	0.00	0.00	XXX
85027	0.00	0.00	0.00	0.00	0.00	0.00	XXX

85032

85032 Blood count; manual cell count (erythrocyte, leukocyte, or platelet) each

Plain English Description

A manual blood cell count of red blood cells (RBCs/erythrocytes), white blood cells (WBCs/leukocytes), or platelets (thrombocytes) is performed. A blood sample is obtained. A capillary pipette and hemocytometer may be used to obtain the sample. Manual erythrocyte count is performed by placing the hemocytometer on the microscope stage. The central area is ruled off into 25 squares. Erythrocytes in the four corner squares and the middle square are then counted. The number of erythrocytes in each square should not vary by more than 10 cells. The erythrocyte count is calculated by averaging the number of erythrocytes in the squares counted. Leukocytes and platelets are counted in the same manner except that the hemocytometer is divided into nine squares, and cells in all nine squares are counted and then averaged. Report 85032 for each type of blood cell (erythrocyte, leukocyte, or platelet) counted.

RVUs

Code	Work	PE	PE Non-Facility	MP	Total Non-Facility	Total Facility	Global
85032	0.00	0.00	0.00	0.00	0.00	0.00	XXX

85041

85041 Blood count; red blood cell (RBC), automated

(Do not report code 85041 in conjunction with 85025 or 85027)

Plain English Description

An automated red blood cell (RBC) count is performed to evaluate any decrease or increase in the number of RBCs in a specific volume of blood. RBC count may be performed as part of a general health screen or prior to a surgical procedure. It may also be performed to monitor patients undergoing chemotherapy or radiation therapy, or to monitor and evaluate response to treatment in patients with bleeding disorders, chronic anemia, or polycythemia. The RBC count is performed with an automated blood cell counting instrument.

RVUs

Code	Work	PE	PE Non-Facility	MP	Total Non-Facility	Total Facility	Global
85041	0.00	0.00	0.00	0.00	0.00	0.00	XXX

85048

85048 Blood count; leukocyte (WBC), automated

Plain English Description

An automated white blood cell (WBC/leukocyte) count is performed to evaluate any decrease or increase in the number of leukocytes in a specific volume of blood. Leukocyte count may be performed to monitor conditions such as HIV and AIDS, or to monitor medical therapies such as chemotherapy or radiation therapy that weaken the immune system and cause a decrease in WBCs. It may also be performed to screen for elevated levels found with bacterial infections, inflammation, leukemia, or trauma. The leukocyte count is performed with an automated blood cell counting instrument.

RVUs

Code	Work	PE	PE Non-Facility	MP	Total Non-Facility	Total Facility	Global
85048	0.00	0.00	0.00	0.00	0.00	0.00	XXX

85049

85049 Blood count; platelet, automated

Plain English Description

An automated platelet count is performed. Platelets, also referred to as thrombocytes, are responsible for blood clotting. A platelet count is performed to diagnose bleeding disorders such as von Willebrand disease, or bone marrow diseases such as leukemia, or other blood cancers. Platelet levels may also be monitored in patients who have undergone bone marrow transplant, who are receiving chemotherapy, or who have chronic kidney disease or autoimmune disorders. Platelets are counted electronically using an automated device.

RVUs

Code	Work	PE	PE Non-Facility	MP	Total Non-Facility	Total Facility	Global
85049	0.00	0.00	0.00	0.00	0.00	0.00	XXX

85060

85060 Blood smear, peripheral, interpretation by physician with written report

Plain English Description

A laboratory test is performed by a physician to examine, interpret, and submit a written report of a peripheral blood smear. This test is usually ordered when an automated complete blood count (CBC) is abnormal. A drop of blood is placed on a glass slide, spread thinly, and fixed in place with a special stain. The slide is then placed under a microscope and the cells are counted and examined for size, shape, and appearance. Characteristics of red blood cells (RBC, erythrocytes), white blood cells (WBC, leukocytes) and platelets (thrombocytes) can diagnose a number of diseases and deficiencies involving blood production, function, and cell destruction. Cell production and maturity may be monitored using a blood smear in patients with anemia, myeloproliferative disorders, bone marrow disease, leukemia, and hemoglobin variant conditions such as sickle cell disease and thalassemia, and during cancer treatment with chemotherapy or radiation. A blood sample is obtained by separately reportable venipuncture, finger, ear, or heel stick. Whole blood is examined using stain and microscope.

RVUs

Code	Work	PE	PE Non-Facility	MP	Total Non-Facility	Total Facility	Global
85060	0.45	0.22	0.22	0.04	0.71	0.71	XXX

86294

86294 Immunoassay for tumor antigen, qualitative or semiquantitative (eg, bladder tumor antigen)

(For qualitative NMP22 protein, use 86386)

Plain English Description

A qualitative or semi-quantitative immunoassay for tumor antigen, such as bladder tumor antigen, is performed. Tumor antigens, also referred to as tumor markers, are indicators that a malignant neoplasm may be present. Significant circulating levels found in serum are associated with malignancy. In the case of bladder tumor antigen (BTA), a latex agglutination assay is used to determine the presence or absence of BTA in urine. The presence of BTA in the urine is not a definitive test for bladder tumor since other conditions, such as renal stones, nephritis, renal cancer, urinary tract infection, cystitis, or recent trauma to the bladder or kidneys, can cause a positive result. A positive test for BTA indicates the need for further testing to determine whether a bladder tumor is present.

RVUs

Code	Work	PE	PE Non-Facility	MP	Total Non-Facility	Total Facility	Global
86294	0.00	0.00	0.00	0.00	0.00	0.00	XXX

86328

86328 Immunoassay for infectious agent antibody(ies), qualitative or semiquantitative, single-step method (eg, reagent strip); severe acute respiratory syndrome coronavirus 2 (SARS-CoV-2) (coronavirus disease [COVID-19])

(For severe acute respiratory syndrome coronavirus 2 [SARS-CoV-2] [coronavirus disease {COVID-19}] antibody testing using multiple-step method, use 86769)

Plain English Description

The rapid reagent test strip method for diagnosing COVID-19 can provide a diagnosis in one step within about 10-15 minutes by detecting antibodies produced against SARS-CoV-2 between 3 and 7 days after initial infection. The reagent strip cartridge, or rapid test cassette, is a qualitative or semiquantitative membrane-based immunoassay test used to detect SARS-CoV-2 antibodies, both IgG and IgM class, in serum, plasma, or whole blood. The test strip is composed of the IgG component, or test region, coated with anti-human IgG; an IgM test region coated with anti-human IgM; and a control test area of the reagent strip. A sample of the patient's blood is added to the specimen well of the cassette along with diluent. The specimen then reacts with the SARS-CoV-2 antigen-coated particles in the cassette and the mixture moves along the test membrane by capillary action. A colored band should appear in the control line region to verify that the specimen volume is sufficient and that the membrane is wicking. If IgG antibodies to SARS-CoV-2 are present in the sample, it reacts with the anti-human IgG in that test region of the strip, forming a complex. A colored line then appears in the band for the IgG test region, and the same for IgM antibodies to SARS-CoV-2, if present. If the test sample does not contain any antibodies to SARS-CoV-2, no colored line will appear in either of the test line regions. The results are read and reported.

RVUs

Code	Work	PE	PE Non-Facility	MP	Total Non-Facility	Total Facility	Global
86328	0.00	0.00	0.00	0.00	0.00	0.00	XXX

86386

86386 Nuclear Matrix Protein 22 (NMP22), qualitative

(Ouchterlony diffusion, use 86331)

(Platelet antibodies, see 86022, 86023)

Plain English Description

A screening test for Nuclear Matrix Protein 22 (NMP22) is performed in a patient with hematuria to help differentiate hematuria due to bladder cancer from hematuria due to other causes. NMP22 is a protein found in the cell nucleus. Malignant neoplasms of the bladder increase the intracellular levels of NMP22 and cause shedding of the protein into the urine. A urine sample is obtained. A test kit specific to NMP22 is then used to identify the presence or absence of NMP22 in the urine and to estimate the concentration of the protein. A level of NMP22 greater than 7 is suggestive of bladder malignancy.

RVUs

Code	Work	PE	PE Non-Facility	MP	Total Non-Facility	Total Facility	Global
86386	0.00	0.00	0.00	0.00	0.00	0.00	XXX

86609

86609 Antibody; bacterium, not elsewhere specified

Plain English Description

A blood sample is tested for antibodies to bacteria not specified in any other code. Some of the commonly tested antibodies reported with this code include listeria, mycobacterium tuberculosis, and toxic shock syndrome antibody. A humoral immunity panel, which tests for multiple organisms in patients with chronic and recurrent infections also includes tests for bacteria not listed in other codes. Methodology depends on the antibody being tested. Listeria uses complement fixation. Mycobacterium tuberculosis uses enzyme-linked immunosorbent assay (ELISA). Toxic shock syndrome uses multi-analyte immunodetection (MAID). IgG antibody is the most common antibody class tested. This code may be reported multiple times depending on how many organisms are tested, the number of antibody classes (IgG, IgM), and the different methodologies used for each organism.

RVUs

Code	Work	PE	PE Non-Facility	MP	Total Non-Facility	Total Facility	Global
86609	0.00	0.00	0.00	0.00	0.00	0.00	XXX

86631-86632

86631 Antibody; Chlamydia

86632 Antibody; Chlamydia, IgM

(For chlamydia antigen, see 87270, 87320. For fluorescent antibody technique, see 86255, 86256)

Plain English Description

A blood sample is tested for antibodies to Chlamydia, a group of bacteria that cause a variety of infections. The most common infection is C. trachomatis, a sexually transmitted disease (STD) that often produces no symptoms, but can cause irreversible damage to the female reproductive tract, resulting in infertility. In men, symptoms include burning and itching of the urethra, but men rarely suffer reproductive damage from the infection. Another species, C. pneumoniae, causes upper respiratory infection, including pneumonia, bronchitis, rhinitis, and pharyngitis. A third species, C. psittaci, primarily affects birds but humans can acquire the disease by handling or being exposed to infected birds. C. psittaci causes flu-like symptoms. There are several methods available to test for Chlamydia antibodies including indirect fluorescent antibody and enzyme-linked immunosorbent assay (ELISA). Use 86631 for screening tests for all chlamydial species and tests for IgG antibodies. Use 86632 for IgM antibodies. Each species and each immunoglobulin class (IgG, IgM) tested is reported separately.

RVUs

Code	Work	PE	PE Non-Facility	MP	Total Non-Facility	Total Facility	Global
86631	0.00	0.00	0.00	0.00	0.00	0.00	XXX
86632	0.00	0.00	0.00	0.00	0.00	0.00	XXX

86694-86696

86694 Antibody; herpes simplex, non-specific type test

86695 Antibody; herpes simplex, type 1

86696 Antibody; herpes simplex, type 2

Plain English Description

A blood or cerebrospinal fluid sample is tested for antibodies to the herpes simplex virus (HSV). HSV is spread by direct contact. The primary infection typically presents with an area of ulceration in the skin or mucous membrane. Following the primary infection, the virus enters a latent phase and is reactivated in response to other illnesses, infection, and stress. Neonates and immunocompromised individuals are at risk for developing ocular or central nervous system infection. There are several methods available to test for HSV infection including indirect hemagglutination (IHA), chemiluminescent immunoassay, or enzyme-linked immunosorbent assay (ELISA). IgG and IgM testing is performed to diagnose HSV infection. If both IgG and IgM testing is performed, the test for each immunoglobulin class should be reported separately. Use 86694 when a non-specific type HSV test is performed. Use 86695 when the test is specific for HSV type 1 or 86696 when the test is specific for HSV type 2. These codes are also used to report HSV type 1 and/or type 2 glycoprotein G-specific antibody IgG and/or IgM.

RVUs

Code	Work	PE	PE Non-Facility	MP	Total Non-Facility	Total Facility	Global
86694	0.00	0.00	0.00	0.00	0.00	0.00	XXX
86695	0.00	0.00	0.00	0.00	0.00	0.00	XXX
86696	0.00	0.00	0.00	0.00	0.00	0.00	XXX

86769

86769 Antibody; severe acute respiratory syndrome coronavirus 2 (SARS-CoV-2) (coronavirus disease [COVID-19])

(For severe acute respiratory syndrome coronavirus 2 [SARS-CoV-2] [coronavirus disease {COVID-19}] antibody testing using single-step method, use 86328)

Plain English Description

Enzyme-linked immunosorbent assays are multiple-step methods used to detect IgG and/or IgM antibodies to the novel coronavirus 2 (SARS-CoV-2) and diagnose acute COVID-19 disease or a convalescent phase of COVID-19. IgG testing is performed to diagnose a current or past infection, as it is the most abundant immunoglobulin produced against an antigen and is maintained for long-term response. IgM testing is performed to identify a current infection in the early onset as IgM is the first immunoglobulin produced and primarily detected at disease onset. Assay protocols differ depending on the specific type of test performed and antigen-antibody combinations used. A sample of the patient's serum or plasma is diluted. Aliquots of diluted sample and control samples are placed in designated microplate wells coated with the SARS-CoV-2 recombinant antigen. The samples are incubated and washed. An enzyme-labeled antibody to the target protein, such as labeled anti-human IgG and/or IgM tracer antibody, is added and incubated. If the patient's sample contains antibodies against SARS-CoV-2, a complex will form. The enzyme activity is measured colorimetrically by adding a chromogenic substrate that changes color when modified by the enzyme, and the samples are again incubated. Color indicates that the patient's blood contains antibodies against the novel coronavirus 2. The higher the concentration, the higher the degree of color. A stop solution is added and light absorption of the product formed is read using a 450 nm microtiter plate reader and converted to numeric values.

RVUs

Code	Work	PE	PE Non-Facility	MP	Total Non-Facility	Total Facility	Global
86769	0.00	0.00	0.00	0.00	0.00	0.00	XXX

86780

86780 Antibody; Treponema pallidum

(For syphilis testing by non-treponemal antibody analysis, see 86592-86593)

Plain English Description

An antibody test for Treponema pallidum, the causative agent of syphilis, is performed using a technique such as fluorescent treponemal antibody absorption (FTA-ABS), T. pallidum particle agglutination (TP-PA), or indirect fluorescent antibody (IFA). Syphilis is a sexually transmitted disease (STD). During the primary stage of syphilis, a sore called a chancre appears at the site where the syphilis bacterium entered the body. The chancre resolves without treatment in three to six weeks but the patient remains infected and without treatment the infection will progress to a secondary stage. During the second stage, a skin rash and mucous membrane lesions appear. The most common sites of the rash are the palms of the hands and soles of the feet. Other symptoms during the secondary stage include fever, swollen lymph nodes, sore throat, hair loss, headaches, weight loss, muscle aches, and fatigue. Symptoms of secondary syphilis also resolve spontaneously but the patient remains infected. The patient then enters the late or latent stage of the disease and symptoms of this stage may not appear for 10-20 years. Symptoms of late stage syphilis include difficulty coordinating muscle movements, paralysis, numbness, gradual blindness, and dementia. These symptoms occur as the disease damages internal organs including the brain, nerves, eyes, heart, blood vessels, liver, bones, and joints. Of particular concern is undiagnosed syphilis infection during pregnancy as the infection can be passed to the baby in utero. This increases the risk of stillbirth or of a live born infant dying shortly after birth. Untreated infants who survive often experience developmental delays or seizures. The FTA-ABS and IFA tests can be performed on blood or cerebrospinal fluid (CSF) samples. TP-PA is used only on blood samples.

RVUs

Code	Work	PE	PE Non-Facility	MP	Total Non-Facility	Total Facility	Global
86780	0.00	0.00	0.00	0.00	0.00	0.00	XXX

87086

87086 Culture, bacterial; quantitative colony count, urine

Plain English Description

A laboratory test is performed to determine the presence or absence of bacterial colonies in urine and provide a colony count. Bacteria in urine may indicate an acute or chronic urinary tract infection (UTI) including pyelonephritis, cystitis, urethritis, or acute urethral syndrome. A urine sample is obtained by clean catch, mid-stream void, or catheterization. Using a calibrated loop, the urine specimen is inoculated onto agar plates and incubated. Quantitative colony counts are determined and potential pathogens are identified. A colony count of 10,000 cfu/mL is reported as "organism present" and may indicate an infection. Comingled flora of the urethra and mixed organisms in the colony counts are reported as "mixed flora" and most often represent contamination.

RVUs

Code	Work	PE	PE Non-Facility	MP	Total Non-Facility	Total Facility	Global
87086	0.00	0.00	0.00	0.00	0.00	0.00	XXX

87088

87088 Culture, bacterial; with isolation and presumptive identification of each isolate, urine

Plain English Description

A laboratory test is performed to isolate and identify bacteria colonizing in urine. Bacteria in urine may indicate an acute or chronic urinary tract infection (UTI) including pyelonephritis, cystitis, urethritis, or acute urethral syndrome (infection of the urethra). A urine sample is obtained by clean catch, mid-stream void, or catheterization. Using a calibrated loop, the urine specimen is inoculated onto agar plates and incubated. Semi-quantitative colony counts are determined and potential pathogens are identified. A colony count of 10,000 cfu/mL usually indicates a pathogen is present. A colony count of 100,000 cfu/mL is significant for urinary tract infection. Each isolated bacterial colony is then examined using conventional or rapid identification technique to determine what pathogen is present. Code 87088 is reported for each isolate.

RVUs

Code	Work	PE	PE Non-Facility	MP	Total Non-Facility	Total Facility	Global
87088	0.00	0.00	0.00	0.00	0.00	0.00	XXX

87110

87110 Culture, chlamydia, any source

(For immunofluorescence staining of shell vials, use 87140)

Plain English Description

A Chlamydia culture is performed on a tissue or cell sample from any source. Chlamydia is a group of bacteria that cause a variety of infections. The most common infection is C. trachomatis, which is a sexually transmitted disease (STD) that often produces no symptoms, but can cause irreversible damage to the female reproductive tract, resulting in infertility. In men, symptoms include burning and itching of the urethra, but men rarely suffer reproductive damage from the infection. The specimen may be obtained from the cervix, urethra, rectum, eye, nose, or throat. Excess mucous or secretions are removed from the infected site using a swab. A second swab is then used to obtain the specimen culture, taking care to obtain adequate numbers of columnar epithelial cells. The swabs are placed in viral chlamydial transport medium. Specimens are then inoculated onto tissue culture cells with trachomatis-specific antibodies and incubated. Immunofluorescence is then used to identify whether the patient has a Chlamydia infection.

RVUs

Code	Work	PE	PE Non-Facility	MP	Total Non-Facility	Total Facility	Global
87110	0.00	0.00	0.00	0.00	0.00	0.00	XXX

87164-87166

87164 Dark field examination, any source (eg, penile, vaginal, oral, skin); includes specimen collection

87166 Dark field examination, any source (eg, penile, vaginal, oral, skin); without collection

Plain English Description

A dark field examination, also called dark field microscopy, is performed on a specimen from any source including penile, vaginal, oral, skin, or lymph node. This test is performed to identify microorganisms that are easily visible against a dark background, such as Treponema pallidum spirochetes that cause syphilis. If the sample is from a lymph node, lymph node aspiration biopsy is first performed. If the sample is obtained from an ulcerative lesion on the skin or mucous membrane, the lesion is first cleaned and abraded with gauze, then squeezed to obtain a drop of serous transudate that is placed on a glass slide and covered with a cover slip. The slide is then examined using a microscope with a dark-field condenser or with a phase contrast microscope for the presence or absence of motile spirochetes. Use 87164 for the dark field examination including specimen collection. Use 87166 when the laboratory that performs the test is not responsible for collecting the specimen.

RVUs

Code	Work	PE	PE Non-Facility	MP	Total Non-Facility	Total Facility	Global
87164	0.00	0.00	0.00	0.00	0.00	0.00	XXX
87166	0.00	0.00	0.00	0.00	0.00	0.00	XXX

87270

87270 Infectious agent antigen detection by immunofluorescent technique; Chlamydia trachomatis

Plain English Description

A specimen is tested for Chlamydia trachomatis using C. trachomatis antigen detection by immunofluorescent technique. C. trachomatis is a sexually transmitted disease (STD) that often produces no symptoms, but can cause irreversible damage to the female reproductive tract, resulting in infertility. In men, symptoms include burning and itching of the urethra, but men rarely suffer reproductive damage from the infection. Immunofluorescent antigen detection for C. trachomatis is performed by direct fluorescent antibody (DFA) technique. A genital, rectal, ocular, or nasopharyngeal swab is obtained. Reagent for C. trachomatis is then applied to the specimen and incubated for 15-30 min at body temperature in a humid environment to allow the antigen-antibody reaction to occur. The specimen is washed to remove unbound conjugate and then dried and mounted. A fluorescence microscope fitted with the appropriate fluorescent light source and barrier filters is then used to examine the specimen for antigen-antibody binding. Binding appears as bright green or orange-yellow objects when viewed under the microscope, which indicates a positive test result.

RVUs

Code	Work	PE	PE Non-Facility	MP	Total Non-Facility	Total Facility	Global
87270	0.00	0.00	0.00	0.00	0.00	0.00	XXX

87273-87274

87273 Infectious agent antigen detection by immunofluorescent technique; Herpes simplex virus type 2

87274 Infectious agent antigen detection by immunofluorescent technique; Herpes simplex virus type 1

Plain English Description

A blood sample is tested for Herpes simplex virus (HSV) using HSV antigen detection by immunofluorescent technique. HSV is spread by direct contact and the primary infection typically presents with an area of ulceration in the skin or mucous membrane. Following the primary infection, the virus enters a latent phase and is reactivated in response to other illnesses, infection, or stress. Neonates and immunocompromised individuals are at risk for developing ocular or central nervous system infection. There are two types of HSV referred to as type 1 and type 2. Type 1 typically causes oral herpes, also referred to as cold sores, but can also cause genital infections. Type 2 typically causes genital herpes. Immunofluorescent antigen detection for HSV is performed by direct fluorescent antibody (DFA) technique. A blood sample is obtained. Reagent for HSV is then applied to the specimen and incubated for 15-30 min at body temperature in a humid environment to allow the antigen-antibody reaction to occur. The specimen is washed to remove unbound conjugate and then dried and mounted. A fluorescence microscope fitted with the appropriate fluorescent light source and barrier filters is then used to examine the specimen for antigen-antibody binding. Binding appears as bright green or orange-yellow objects when viewed under the microscope and indicates a positive test result. Use 87273 for HSV type 2 and 87274 for HSV type 1.

RVUs

Code	Work	PE	PE Non-Facility	MP	Total Non-Facility	Total Facility	Global
87273	0.00	0.00	0.00	0.00	0.00	0.00	XXX
87274	0.00	0.00	0.00	0.00	0.00	0.00	XXX

87285

87285 Infectious agent antigen detection by immunofluorescent technique; Treponema pallidum

Plain English Description

A test for Treponema pallidum, the causative agent of syphilis, is performed using T. pallidum antigen detection by immunofluorescent technique. Syphilis is a sexually transmitted disease (STD). This test uses cells or tissues from a suspicious lesion to test for primary syphilis, or less commonly, tissue from the umbilical cord is used if there is concern about congenital syphilis. During the primary stage of syphilis, a sore called a chancre appears at the site where the syphilis bacteria entered the body. Undiagnosed syphilis infection during pregnancy can be passed to the baby in utero, increasing the risk of stillbirth or death shortly after birth. Untreated infants who survive often experience developmental delays or seizures. Immunofluorescent antigen detection for T. pallidum is performed by direct fluorescent antibody (DFA) technique. The suspicious lesion (chancre) is scraped to obtain a specimen. Reagent for T. pallidum is then applied to the specimen and incubated for 15-30 min at body temperature in a humid environment to allow the antigen-antibody reaction to occur. The specimen is washed to remove unbound conjugate and then dried and mounted. A fluorescence microscope fitted with the appropriate fluorescent light source and barrier filters is then used to examine the specimen for antigen-antibody binding. Binding appears as bright green or orange-yellow objects when viewed under the microscope and indicates a positive test result.

RVUs

Code	Work	PE	PE Non-Facility	MP	Total Non-Facility	Total Facility	Global
87285	0.00	0.00	0.00	0.00	0.00	0.00	XXX

87320

▲ **87320 Infectious agent antigen detection by immunoassay technique (eg, enzyme immunoassay [EIA], enzyme-linked immunosorbent assay [ELISA], fluorescence immunoassay [FIA], immunochemiluminometric assay [IMCA]), qualitative or semiquantitative; Chlamydia trachomatis**

Plain English Description

A specimen is tested for Chlamydia trachomatis using antigen detection by any immunoassay technique such as enzyme immunoassay (EIA), enzyme-linked immunosorbent assay (ELISA), fluorescence immunoassay (FIA), and immunochemiluminometric assay (IMCA). Chlamydia is a sexually transmitted disease that often produces no symptoms, but can cause irreversible damage to the female reproductive tract, resulting in infertility. In men, symptoms include burning and itching of the urethra, although men rarely suffer reproductive damage. A cervical, urethral, or rectal swab is obtained and the sample is tested. Both EIA and ELISA detect very small quantities of the antigen when bound to its specific antibody in a sample by adding a secondary, enzyme-labeled antibody to detect its presence. A chromogenic reaction of the enzyme produces a visible color change or fluorescence. Qualitative and semi-quantitative measures are assessed by the colorimetric reading. FIA detects binding of the "detection" antibody with the analyte molecule by using a fluorescent compound as the detecting reagent that absorbs light at a different wavelength than it emits. IMCA uses the reaction of antibodies labeled with a chemiluminescent substance to identify and quantify the bound antigen-antibody complex by light emission.

RVUs

Code	Work	PE	PE Non-Facility	MP	Total Non-Facility	Total Facility	Global
87320	0.00	0.00	0.00	0.00	0.00	0.00	XXX

87389-87391

▲ **87389 Infectious agent antigen detection by immunoassay technique (eg, enzyme immunoassay [EIA], enzyme-linked immunosorbent assay [ELISA], fluorescence immunoassay [FIA], immunochemiluminometric assay [IMCA]), qualitative or semiquantitative; HIV-1 antigen(s), with HIV-1 and HIV-2 antibodies, single result**

▲ **87390 Infectious agent antigen detection by immunoassay technique (eg, enzyme immunoassay [EIA], enzyme-linked immunosorbent assay [ELISA], fluorescence immunoassay [FIA], immunochemiluminometric assay [IMCA]), qualitative or semiquantitative; HIV-1**

▲ **87391 Infectious agent antigen detection by immunoassay technique (eg, enzyme immunoassay [EIA], enzyme-linked immunosorbent assay [ELISA], fluorescence immunoassay [FIA], immunochemiluminometric assay [IMCA]), qualitative or semiquantitative; HIV-2**

Plain English Description

A blood or saliva sample is tested for human immunodeficiency virus (HIV) antigen by any immunoassay technique test such as enzyme immunoassay (EIA), enzyme-linked immunosorbent assay (ELISA), fluorescence immunoassay (FIA) and immunochemiluminometric assay (IMCA). HIV virus infections are sexually transmitted diseases that can also be transmitted from unscreened blood and shared needles, from mother to child in utero, or by breast feeding. HIV attacks the immune system by destroying T cells or CD4 cells, types of white blood cells. This hampers the body's ability to fight infection. AIDS is the final stage of HIV infection. A blood or saliva sample is obtained and placed in a fixative or sent fresh to the laboratory for processing. Both EIA and ELISA detect very small quantities of the antigen when bound to its specific antibody in a sample by adding a secondary, enzyme-labeled antibody to detect its presence. A chromogenic reaction of the enzyme produces a visible color change or fluorescence. Qualitative and semi-quantitative measures are assessed by the colorimetric reading. FIA detects the binding of the "detection" antibody with the analyte molecule by using a fluorescent compound as the detecting reagent that absorbs light at a different wavelength than it emits. IMCA uses the reaction of antibodies labeled with a chemiluminescent substance to identify and quantify the bound antigen-antibody complex by light emission. Use 87389 when testing for HIV-1 antigen(s), with HIV-1 and HIV-2 antibodies, single result. Use 87390 when testing for HIV-I alone. Use 87391 for HIV-II alone.

RVUs

Code	Work	PE	PE Non-Facility	MP	Total Non-Facility	Total Facility	Global
87389	0.00	0.00	0.00	0.00	0.00	0.00	XXX
87390	0.00	0.00	0.00	0.00	0.00	0.00	XXX
87391	0.00	0.00	0.00	0.00	0.00	0.00	XXX

87490-87492

87490 Infectious agent detection by nucleic acid (DNA or RNA); Chlamydia trachomatis, direct probe technique

87491 Infectious agent detection by nucleic acid (DNA or RNA); Chlamydia trachomatis, amplified probe technique

87492 Infectious agent detection by nucleic acid (DNA or RNA); Chlamydia trachomatis, quantification

Plain English Description

Infectious agent antibody detection by nucleic acid technique (DNA or RNA) is used to identify Chlamydia trachomatis infection using direct probe (87490), amplified probe (87491), or quantification (87492) of the amplified probe. C. trachomatis infection is a sexually transmitted disease (STD) that often produces no symptoms, but can cause irreversible damage to the female reproductive tract, resulting in infertility. In men, symptoms include burning and itching of the urethra, but men rarely suffer reproductive damage from the infection. Some types of nucleic acid tests are rapid tests that may be performed in the physician office using a test kit. A swab is used to obtain a specimen from the cervix, male urethra, or eye. In 87490, the exact methodology is dependent on the test kit used as there are several manufacturers. One test kit uses a nucleic acid hybridization method. A single stranded chemiluminescent DNA probe is used that is complementary to the ribosomal RNA of the Chlamydia organism. Lysate is used to rupture cells and release nucleic acids. The ribosomal RNA from the Chlamydia organism then combines with the labeled DNA probe to form a stable DNA:RNA hybrid. The presence of DNA:RNA hybrids is then detected using a luminometer. In 87491, an amplification technique, such as polymerase chain reaction (PCR), is used to create copies of the Chlamydia nucleic acids. Amplification is used when it is suspected that there are low levels of the targeted microorganism in the specimen that would not be detected using a direct probe. The Chlamydia nucleic acid is then detected using a variety of techniques. In 87492, the amplified product is quantified to provide an assessment of how many Chlamydia organisms are present. Quantification may be used to evaluate the severity of the infection and response to treatment.

RVUs

Code	Work	PE	PE Non-Facility	MP	Total Non-Facility	Total Facility	Global
87490	0.00	0.00	0.00	0.00	0.00	0.00	XXX
87491	0.00	0.00	0.00	0.00	0.00	0.00	XXX
87492	0.00	0.00	0.00	0.00	0.00	0.00	XXX

87500

87500 Infectious agent detection by nucleic acid (DNA or RNA); vancomycin resistance (eg, enterococcus species van A, van B), amplified probe technique

Plain English Description

An amplified probe technique is used to identify vancomycin-resistant infectious agents, such as enterococcus species van A and van B. Vancomycin is a strong antibiotic used to treat gram-positive bacterial infections. However, vancomycin-resistant enterococci are becoming increasingly common. Vancomycin-resistant enterococci can be detected by nucleic acid (DNA or RNA) amplified probe technique that identifies the presence of the vancomycin-resistant gene in the bacteria. A specimen is obtained and the bacteria isolated. Cells contained in the specimen are treated to expose single-stranded target nucleic acid molecules that react with a probe nucleic acid sequence that allows the target and the probe strands to hybridize to each other. The target and the probe form a double-stranded, target-probe complex. Then, an enzyme molecule cleaves the link of the target-probe complex and one or more fragments of the nucleic acid probe are released. If cleaved portions of the nucleic acid probe are produced, the bacterium causing the infection is vancomycin resistant. Nucleic acid probes also identify the genotype A or B.

RVUs

Code	Work	PE	PE Non-Facility	MP	Total Non-Facility	Total Facility	Global
87500	0.00	0.00	0.00	0.00	0.00	0.00	XXX

87528-87530

87528 Infectious agent detection by nucleic acid (DNA or RNA); Herpes simplex virus, direct probe technique

87529 Infectious agent detection by nucleic acid (DNA or RNA); Herpes simplex virus, amplified probe technique

87530 Infectious agent detection by nucleic acid (DNA or RNA); Herpes simplex virus, quantification

Plain English Description

Infectious agent antibody detection by nucleic acid technique (RNA or DNA) is used to identify Herpes simplex virus (HSV) using direct probe (87528), amplified probe (87529), or quantification (87530) of the amplified probe. HSV is spread by direct contact and the primary infection typically presents with an area of ulceration in the skin or mucous membrane. Following the primary infection, the virus enters a latent phase and is reactivated in response to other illnesses, infection, or stress. Neonates and immunocompromised individuals are at risk for developing ocular or central nervous system infection. There are two types of HSV: type 1 and type 2. Type 1 typically causes oral herpes, also referred to as cold sores, but can also cause genital infections. Type 2 typically causes genital herpes. A specimen is obtained from an oral or genital lesion, from vitreous of the eye, or from a blood sample. In 87528, the specimen is incubated with lysate to rupture all cells and release nucleic acids. The lysate is placed in the sample well and the test slide is dipped and incubated. Probes specific for HSV-1 and/or HSV-2 are introduced. The slide is washed to remove cellular debris and unbound nucleic acids. A second probe

containing a color development substrate is added. The slide is again washed and an enzyme is added to catalyze the color substrate. A luminometer is used to determine whether HSV-1 or HSV-2 is present. In 87529, an amplification technique, such as polymerase chain reaction (PCR), is used to create copies of the HSV-1 and/or HSV-2 nucleic acids. Amplification is used when it is suspected that there are low levels of the targeted microorganism in the specimen that would not be detected using a direct probe. The HSV-1 and/or HSV-2 nucleic acids are then detected using a variety of techniques.
In 87530, the amplified product is quantified to provide an assessment of how many HSV-1 and/or HSV-2 organisms are present. Quantification may be used to evaluate the severity of the infection and response to treatment. If the specimen is tested for both HSV-1 and HSV-2, the code for the direct or amplified probe is reported for each serotype as is the quantification procedure if quantification is also performed.

RVUs

Code	Work	PE	PE Non-Facility	MP	Total Non-Facility	Total Facility	Global
87528	0.00	0.00	0.00	0.00	0.00	0.00	XXX
87529	0.00	0.00	0.00	0.00	0.00	0.00	XXX
87530	0.00	0.00	0.00	0.00	0.00	0.00	XXX

87534-87536

87534 Infectious agent detection by nucleic acid (DNA or RNA); HIV-1, direct probe technique

87535 Infectious agent detection by nucleic acid (DNA or RNA); HIV-1, amplified probe technique, includes reverse transcription when performed

87536 Infectious agent detection by nucleic acid (DNA or RNA); HIV-1, quantification, includes reverse transcription when performed

Plain English Description

Infectious agent antibody detection by nucleic acid technique (RNA or DNA) is used to identify HIV-1 using direct probe (87534), amplified probe (87535), or quantification (87536) of the amplified probe. HIV virus infections are sexually transmitted diseases that can also be transmitted from unscreened blood, shared needles, from mother to child in utero, or by breast feeding. HIV attacks the immune system by destroying T-cells or CD4 cells, which are types of white blood cell. This hampers the body's ability to fight infection. Acquired immunodeficiency syndrome (AIDS) is the final stage of HIV infection. There are two HIV serotypes (HIV-1, HIV-2). These tests are performed to identify HIV-1. A blood sample is obtained. In 87534, a direct probe is performed. Direct probes are rarely used as they require culture of the specimen.
In 87535, an amplification technique such as reverse transcription polymerase chain reaction (RT-PCR) is used to create copies of the HIV-1 nucleic acids. Amplification is used when there may be such low levels of the suspected microorganism in the specimen that it would not be detected using a direct probe. The HIV-1 nucleic acids are then detected using a variety of techniques. Test kits that may be used have three components: the specimen collection and preparation component, an amplification component, and a detection component. Red blood cells are selectively lysed leaving leukocytes intact. The leukocytes are pelleted and then washed several times. DNA is extracted from the pellet. Proviral HIV-1 DNA is then amplified. The detection component is then used to determine whether HIV-1 DNA is present in the specimen.
In 87536, the amount of the infectious agent in the sample is evaluated following amplification. Using reverse transcription and quantification techniques, the HIV-1 viral load is determined. Quantification of HIV-1 is typically performed to evaluate response to treatment.

RVUs

Code	Work	PE	PE Non-Facility	MP	Total Non-Facility	Total Facility	Global
87534	0.00	0.00	0.00	0.00	0.00	0.00	XXX
87535	0.00	0.00	0.00	0.00	0.00	0.00	XXX
87536	0.00	0.00	0.00	0.00	0.00	0.00	XXX

87537-87539

87537 Infectious agent detection by nucleic acid (DNA or RNA); HIV-2, direct probe technique

87538 Infectious agent detection by nucleic acid (DNA or RNA); HIV-2, amplified probe technique, includes reverse transcription when performed

87539 Infectious agent detection by nucleic acid (DNA or RNA); HIV-2, quantification, includes reverse transcription when performed

Plain English Description

Infectious agent antibody detection by nucleic acid technique (RNA or DNA) is used to identify HIV-2 using direct probe (87537), amplified probe (87538), or quantification (87539) of the amplified probe. HIV virus infections are sexually transmitted diseases that can also be transmitted from unscreened blood, shared needles, from mother to child in utero, or by breast feeding. HIV attacks the immune system by destroying T-cells or CD4 cells, which are types of white blood cell. This hampers the body's ability to fight infection. Acquired immunodeficiency syndrome (AIDS) is the final stage of HIV infection. There are two HIV serotypes (HIV-1, HIV-2). These tests are performed to identify HIV-2. A blood sample is obtained. In 87537, a direct probe is performed. Direct probes are rarely used as they require culture of the specimen.
In 87538, an amplification technique such as reverse transcription polymerase chain reaction (RT-PCR) is used to create copies of the HIV-2 nucleic acids. Amplification is used when there may be such low levels of the suspected microorganism in the specimen that it would not be detected using a direct probe. The HIV-2 nucleic acids are then detected using a variety of techniques. Test kits that may be used have three components: the specimen collection and preparation component, an amplification component, and a detection component. Red blood cells are selectively lysed leaving leukocytes intact. The leukocytes are pelleted and then washed several times. DNA is extracted from the pellet. Proviral HIV-2 DNA is then amplified. The detection component is then used to determine whether HIV-2 DNA is present in the specimen.
In 87539, the amount of the infectious agent in the sample is evaluated following amplification. Using reverse transcription and quantification techniques, the HIV-2 viral load is determined. Quantification of HIV-2 is typically performed to evaluate response to treatment.

RVUs

Code	Work	PE	PE Non-Facility	MP	Total Non-Facility	Total Facility	Global
87537	0.00	0.00	0.00	0.00	0.00	0.00	XXX
87538	0.00	0.00	0.00	0.00	0.00	0.00	XXX
87539	0.00	0.00	0.00	0.00	0.00	0.00	XXX

87563

87563 Infectious agent detection by nucleic acid (DNA or RNA); Mycoplasma genitalium, amplified probe technique

Plain English Description

A laboratory test is performed to identify the presence of Mycobacterium genitalium (M. genitalium), a tiny gram-negative bacterium in epithelial cells lining the male or female genital tract. M. genitalium causes inflammation of the urethra (urethritis) and cervix (cervicitis) and has also been identified in female pelvic inflammatory disease (PID). Using a swab, the clinician collects a specimen from the penile urethra or meatus, the endo-cervix, or the vagina. The patient may self-collect a specimen from the penile meatus or from first catch urine in either males and females. The collected specimen is placed into an appropriate transport tube containing target rRNA which isolates the M. genitalium, if present, using a capture oligomer and magnetic microparticles. The sample is hybridized to allow the capture oligomer to bind to the target molecule forming a complex that can then be removed by covalent attachment to the magnetic particles. The rRNA is amplified along specific regions and a single stranded chemiluminescent labeled, complimentary DNA probe is added, forming a DNA/RNA hybrid. Light emitted from the labeled DNA/RNA hybrid can then be measured as a photon signal by an illuminator reading device.

RVUs

Code	Work	PE	PE Non-Facility	MP	Total Non-Facility	Total Facility	Global
87563	0.00	0.00	0.00	0.00	0.00	0.00	XXX

87590-87592

87590 Infectious agent detection by nucleic acid (DNA or RNA); Neisseria gonorrhoeae, direct probe technique

87591 Infectious agent detection by nucleic acid (DNA or RNA); Neisseria gonorrhoeae, amplified probe technique

87592 Infectious agent detection by nucleic acid (DNA or RNA); Neisseria gonorrhoeae, quantification

Plain English Description

Neisseria gonorrhoeae (N. gonorrhoeae) causes gonorrhea, a sexually transmitted disease (STD) that is spread through direct contact and can infect the reproductive tract, mouth, throat, eyes, and anus. N. gonorrhoeae often causes no symptoms in women, but can cause irreversible damage to the reproductive tract of women, which can result in infertility. In men, symptoms include burning, itching, and discharge of the urethra, but men rarely suffer reproductive damage from the infection. Some types of nucleic acid tests are rapid tests that may be performed in the physician office using a test kit. A swab is used to obtain a specimen from the cervix, male urethra, mouth, throat, or eye. In 87590, the exact methodology is dependent on the test kit used as there are several manufacturers. One test kit uses a nucleic acid hybridization method. A single stranded chemiluminescent DNA probe is used that is complementary to the ribosomal RNA of the N. gonorrhoeae organism. Lysate is used to rupture cells and release nucleic acids. The ribosomal RNA from the organism then combines with the labeled DNA probe to form a stable DNA:RNA hybrid. The presence of DNA:RNA hybrids is then detected using a luminometer. In 87591, an amplification technique, such as polymerase chain reaction (PCR) or transcription mediated amplification (TMA), is used to create copies of the N. gonorrhoeae nucleic acids. Amplification is used when there may be low levels of the suspected microorganism in the specimen that would not be detected using a direct probe. The N. gonorrhoeae nucleic acid is then detected using a variety of techniques. In 87592, the amplified product is quantified to provide an assessment of how many N. gonorrhoeae organisms are present. Quantification may be used to evaluate severity of infection and response to treatment.

RVUs

Code	Work	PE	PE Non-Facility	MP	Total Non-Facility	Total Facility	Global
87590	0.00	0.00	0.00	0.00	0.00	0.00	XXX
87591	0.00	0.00	0.00	0.00	0.00	0.00	XXX
87592	0.00	0.00	0.00	0.00	0.00	0.00	XXX

87623-87625

87623 Infectious agent detection by nucleic acid (DNA or RNA); Human Papillomavirus (HPV), low-risk types (eg, 6, 11, 42, 43, 44)

87624 Infectious agent detection by nucleic acid (DNA or RNA); Human Papillomavirus (HPV), high-risk types (eg, 16, 18, 31, 33, 35, 39, 45, 51, 52, 56, 58, 59, 68)

(When both low-risk and high-risk HPV types are performed in a single assay, use only 87624)

87625 Infectious agent detection by nucleic acid (DNA or RNA); Human Papillomavirus (HPV), types 16 and 18 only, includes type 45, if performed

(For Human Papillomavirus [HPV] detection of five or greater separately reported high-risk HPV types [ie, genotyping], use 0500T)

Plain English Description

Human papillomavirus (HPV) invades skin and mucosal epithelia causing site-specific clinical and subclinical infection. There are more than 100 types of HPV known to cause infection in humans, and 40 types can be found predominately in the anogenital tract. High-risk oncogenic HPV types are frequently detected in high-grade squamous intraepithelial lesions (HSIL) and invasive cancers. Low-risk HPV types are associated with acuminate condylomas of the genitals and low-grade squamous intraepithelial lesions (LSIL) of the cervix. Infectious agent detection by nucleic acid (DNA or RNA) for HPV is now considered routine in the management of cervical disease in women. Exfoliated cervical cells are collected using a cytobrush, swab, or plastic spatula and re-suspended in a liquid transport medium. The cell sample is treated with sodium hydroxide to denature the DNA and then hybridized in a solution with two mixtures of non-isotope single-stranded RNA probes. One probe detects 5 low-risk HPV types and the other probe detects 13 high-risk HPV types. The hybridized products are transferred to a microplate with antibody-coated wells that will specifically recognize the HPV DNA/RNA hybrids. An alkaline phosphatase-labeled monoclonal antibody against the DNA/RNA hybrids is added along with a chemiluminescent substrate and the light produced is measured with a luminometer to give the ratio of reactivity. Code 87623 is used when testing for low-risk HPV types (6, 11, 42, 43, and 44). Code 87624 is used when testing for high-risk HPV types (16, 18, 31, 33, 35, 39, 45, 51, 52, 56, 58, 59, and 68). Code 87624 is also the default code used when both low- and high-risk types are tested within a single assay. Code 87625 is used when testing for HPV types 16 and 18 only, and includes type 45 also, if performed.

RVUs

Code	Work	PE	PE Non-Facility	MP	Total Non-Facility	Total Facility	Global
87623	0.00	0.00	0.00	0.00	0.00	0.00	XXX
87624	0.00	0.00	0.00	0.00	0.00	0.00	XXX
87625	0.00	0.00	0.00	0.00	0.00	0.00	XXX

87635

87635 Infectious agent detection by nucleic acid (DNA or RNA); severe acute respiratory syndrome coronavirus 2 (SARS-CoV-2) (coronavirus disease [COVID-19]), amplified probe technique

Plain English Description

Nucleic acid amplification tests can identify very small amounts of DNA and detect the presence of viruses and other pathogens in a sample, even with very little genetic material available. This is done by copying (amplifying) one specific target section of the viral DNA hundreds of thousands of times to confirm its presence accurately. One of the most common and accurate tests for detecting SARS-CoV-2 is real time reverse transcription-polymerase chain reaction (RT-PCR). The SARS-CoV-2 contains only RNA; however, only DNA can be amplified so the RNA must be converted to DNA through a reverse transcription process in order to detect it. Sputum or other sample is taken from the patient's nose, throat, bronchus, or lungs via swabbing, washing, aspirate, or bronchoalveolar lavage. The sample is treated with different chemical solutions to remove fats and proteins, and RNA is extracted, both the person's own and that of the virus, if present. A specific enzyme is added to reverse transcribe RNA to DNA. Oligonucleotide probes and primers containing special markers with fluorescent dyes are added, which attach to the nucleic acid target sequence and demarcate the segment to be amplified. The target DNA is then isolated and purified. The sample is placed in the RT-PCR machine and cycled through chemical reactions that create identical copies of the viral target DNA sections, doubling the amount with each cycle. As the new copies are made, the fluorescent marker attaches to them and is measured by the computer in real time with each cycle. When a certain level of fluorescence is reached, the virus is confirmed to be present. The number of cycles it takes to reach confirmation level also helps diagnose the disease severity.

RVUs

Code	Work	PE	PE Non-Facility	MP	Total Non-Facility	Total Facility	Global
87635	0.00	0.00	0.00	0.00	0.00	0.00	XXX

87850

▲ **87850 Infectious agent antigen detection by immunoassay with direct optical (ie, visual) observation; Neisseria gonorrhoeae**

Plain English Description

Neisseria gonorrhoeae causes gonorrhea, a sexually transmitted disease spread through direct contact that can infect the reproductive tract, mouth, throat, eyes, and anus. Neisseria gonorrhoeae often causes no symptoms in women, but can cause irreversible damage to the female reproductive tract, which can result in infertility. In men, symptoms include urethral burning, itching, and discharge, but men rarely suffer reproductive damage from the infection. A swab is used to obtain a specimen from the cervix, male urethra, mouth, throat, or eye. Alternatively, a urine sample may be obtained. This test is a rapid, qualitative sandwich immunoassay that detects gonorrhea antigen in the specimen. The specimen is placed in a tube containing a reagent that extracts the gonorrhea antigen. Monoclonal and polyclonal antibodies are then used to identify Neisseria gonorrhoeae. If the sample contains the antigen, the test strip, line, or dot will change color as will a second control strip, line, or dot, indicating a positive result.

RVUs

Code	Work	PE	PE Non-Facility	MP	Total Non-Facility	Total Facility	Global
87850	0.00	0.00	0.00	0.00	0.00	0.00	XXX

87901

87901 Infectious agent genotype analysis by nucleic acid (DNA or RNA); HIV-1, reverse transcriptase and protease regions

Plain English Description

This test is used to analyze and identify mutations in HIV-1 genes that cause resistance to 19 commonly prescribed reverse transcriptase and protease inhibitors, which are types of medications used to treat HIV-1. Human immunodeficiency virus (HIV) attacks the immune system by destroying T cells or CD4 cells, which are types of white blood cells. This hampers the ability of the body to fight infection. HIV is the virus that causes acquired immunodeficiency syndrome (AIDS) and AIDS is the final stage of HIV infection. HIV is an RNA virus with a high replication rate. The reverse transcription enzyme required for replication can cause mutations and some of these mutations result in resistance to anti-viral drugs. Initial drug therapy for HIV typically uses a combination of anti-retrovirals with different mechanisms of action to reduce the viral load and help prevent mutations that cause drug resistance. This is referred to as highly active anti-retroviral therapy (HAART). When initial drug therapy fails, a genotype analysis is performed using reverse transcriptase and protease genes to detect known mutations that cause drug resistance. Genotyping is a very complex test that uses a blood sample to evaluate HIV-1 for the presence of specific nucleic acid sequences. Three steps are required. First, one or more very specific nucleic acid sequences are amplified using a technique such as polymerase chain reaction (PCR). Next, the amplified product is purified and further molecular analysis is performed. Then, the amplified sequence is compared to known sequences that confer known drug resistance. This information is used to develop a drug regimen that will better control the HIV infection.

RVUs

Code	Work	PE	PE Non-Facility	MP	Total Non-Facility	Total Facility	Global
87901	0.00	0.00	0.00	0.00	0.00	0.00	XXX

87905

87905 Infectious agent enzymatic activity other than virus (eg, sialidase activity in vaginal fluid)

(For virus isolation including identification by non-immunologic method, other than by cytopathic effect, use 87255)

Plain English Description

A body fluid specimen is obtained, such as a vaginal swab for vaginal fluid, to test for infectious agent enzymatic activity other than that due to viral infection, such as sialidase activity. Sialidases are enzymes that enhance the ability of microorganisms to invade and destroy tissue. Elevated levels of sialidase activity in vaginal fluid may be an indication of bacterial vaginosis. To test for sialidase, the lower third of the vaginal wall is swabbed. The swab is rotated for 10 to 20 seconds to collect a sufficient amount of fluid and then placed in a tube, which is capped. A chromogenic enzyme activity test is performed to identify the presence of sialidase activity. Code 87905 may be used to report other enzymatic activity tests for infectious agents other than viruses in other body fluids.

RVUs

Code	Work	PE	PE Non-Facility	MP	Total Non-Facility	Total Facility	Global
87905	0.00	0.00	0.00	0.00	0.00	0.00	XXX

88104-88106

88104 Cytopathology, fluids, washings or brushings, except cervical or vaginal; smears with interpretation

88106 Cytopathology, fluids, washings or brushings, except cervical or vaginal; simple filter method with interpretation

(Do not report 88106 in conjunction with 88104)

(For nongynecological selective cellular enhancement including filter transfer techniques, use 88112)

Plain English Description

A laboratory test is performed on fluid or washing or brushing samples to diagnose malignant, premalignant, infectious, or autoimmune disease, inflammation, immune reactions, cell aging, or amyloidosis. Cytopathology is the microscopic study of cells that spontaneously exfoliate or can be removed from a body surface by washing or brushing. This technique can be used on samples from sputum, urine, breast (nipple) discharge, cerebrospinal fluid, pleural, peritoneal, pericardial, or joint effusions, vitreous of the eye, skin, and the gastrointestinal tract. A sample is obtained by separately reportable procedure. When testing by smear technique (88104), the sample is placed on a glass slide and fixed in place. To test for cells in fluid, the simple filter method (88106) is used. The fluid is filtered to separate cells and the sediment collected is fixed on a glass slide. The pathologist examines the slide under a microscope and provides a written report of the findings.

RVUs

Code	Work	PE	PE Non-Facility	MP	Total Non-Facility	Total Facility	Global
88104	0.56	1.39	1.39	0.02	1.97	1.97	XXX
88106	0.37	1.58	1.58	0.02	1.97	1.97	XXX

88120-88121

88120 Cytopathology, in situ hybridization (eg, FISH), urinary tract specimen with morphometric analysis, 3-5 molecular probes, each specimen; manual

88121 Cytopathology, in situ hybridization (eg, FISH), urinary tract specimen with morphometric analysis, 3-5 molecular probes, each specimen; using computer-assisted technology

(For morphometric in situ hybridization on cytologic specimens other than urinary tract, see 88367, 88368)

(For more than 5 probes, use 88399)

Plain English Description

A specimen containing cells from the urinary tract, such as a urine sample or bladder irrigation (washing) specimen, is tested for the presence of abnormal cells using an in situ hybridization technique such as fluorescence in situ hybridization (FISH). This test evaluates exfoliated urothelial cells for genetic alterations indicative of urinary tract cancer. The test involves the use of multiple (3-5) DNA probes that identify chromosome changes in specific regions of specific chromosomes that are indicative of a urinary tract cancer. A DNA probe is labeled with fluorescent dye and applied to cells in which the nuclei are in interphase. The probe binds to its complementary sequence and labels a specific chromosome that is then visualized under fluorescent microscope. Nuclei exhibiting chromosomal changes indicative of urothelial cancer fluoresce when viewed under the fluorescent microscope. Use 88120 for a manual test. Use 88121 when computer-assisted technology is used to evaluate the specimen. Report these codes for each specimen tested using manual or computer-assisted technology.

RVUs

Code	Work	PE	PE Non-Facility	MP	Total Non-Facility	Total Facility	Global
88120	1.20	16.96	16.96	0.06	18.22	18.22	XXX
88121	1.00	11.80	11.80	0.03	12.83	12.83	XXX

88160-88162

88160 Cytopathology, smears, any other source; screening and interpretation

88161 Cytopathology, smears, any other source; preparation, screening and interpretation

88162 Cytopathology, smears, any other source; extended study involving over 5 slides and/or multiple stains

(For aerosol collection of sputum, use 89220)

(For special stains, see 88312-88314)

Plain English Description

A laboratory test is performed on fluid or washing or brushing samples to diagnose malignant, premalignant, infectious or autoimmune disease, inflammation, immune reactions, cell aging, or amyloidosis. Cytopathology is the microscopic study of cells that spontaneously exfoliate or can be removed from a body surface by washing or brushing. Codes 88160-88162 may be used for herpetic lesions (Tzanck smear), conjunctival scrapings, and anal cell analysis. A sample is obtained by separately reportable procedure. The slide(s) is prepared by a technician or the pathologist. The pathologist examines the slide(s) under a microscope and provides a written report of the findings. Code 88160 is used for screening and interpretation. Code 88161 is used when the sample requires preparation before the screening and interpretation. Code 88162 is used when the sample involves extended study of more than 5 slides and/or multiple stains.

RVUs

Code	Work	PE	PE Non-Facility	MP	Total Non-Facility	Total Facility	Global
88160	0.50	1.58	1.58	0.02	2.10	2.10	XXX
88161	0.50	1.64	1.64	0.02	2.16	2.16	XXX
88162	0.76	2.54	2.54	0.03	3.33	3.33	XXX

88172-88173

88172 Cytopathology, evaluation of fine needle aspirate; immediate cytohistologic study to determine adequacy for diagnosis, first evaluation episode, each site

(The evaluation episode represents a complete set of cytologic material submitted for evaluation and is independent of the number of needle passes or slides prepared. A separate evaluation episode occurs if the proceduralist provider obtains additional material from the same site, based on the prior immediate adequacy assessment, or a separate lesion is aspirated)

88173 Cytopathology, evaluation of fine needle aspirate; interpretation and report

(Report one unit of 88173 for the interpretation and report from each anatomic site, regardless of the number of passes or evaluation episodes performed during the aspiration procedure)

(For fine needle aspirate biopsy, see 10004, 10005, 10006, 10007, 10008, 10009, 10010, 10011, 10012, 10021)

(Do not report 88172, 88173 in conjunction with 88333 and 88334 for the same specimen)

Plain English Description

A separately reportable fine needle aspiration is performed to obtain fluid or tissue. The cells are placed on a slide at which time the cells form clusters of approximately 10 cells each. A smear is then created by laying another slide on top. Stains are used to enhance cellular detail as needed. The cells are then examined for evidence of disease, such as malignancy. In 88172, an immediate cytohistologic study is performed to determine the adequacy of the specimen. The physician examines the specimen under a microscope to determine whether the cell sample contains a sufficient number of cells for evaluation and diagnosis. Diagnostic accuracy increases when there are six or more cell clusters available for review. If an inadequate number of cells are present, the aspiration procedure may be repeated. Report this for the first evaluation episode for each site from which separate specimens are obtained. In 88173, a cell sample with an adequate number of cells is examined for definitive diagnosis. The cells are examined under a microscope for evidence of malignancy or other disease. The physician provides an interpretation that describes the characteristics of the cells in the sample and will typically indicate whether the cells are clearly benign, clearly malignant, or indeterminate—meaning no definitive diagnosis can be made. A written report is provided.

RVUs

Code	Work	PE	PE Non-Facility	MP	Total Non-Facility	Total Facility	Global
88172	0.69	0.88	0.88	0.02	1.59	1.59	XXX
88173	1.39	3.14	3.14	0.08	4.61	4.61	XXX

88177

✚ **88177 Cytopathology, evaluation of fine needle aspirate; immediate cytohistologic study to determine adequacy for diagnosis, each separate additional evaluation episode, same site (List separately in addition to code for primary procedure)**

(When repeat immediate evaluation episode(s) is required on subsequent cytologic material from the same site, eg, following determination the prior sampling that was not adequate for diagnosis, use 1 unit of 88177 for each additional evaluation episode)

(Use 88177 in conjunction with 88172)

Plain English Description

A separately reportable fine needle aspiration is performed to obtain fluid or tissue. Following a separately reportable initial evaluation episode, one or more additional cytohistologic studies are performed on a specimen from the same site to determine the adequacy of the specimen. The cells are placed on a slide at which time the cells form clusters of approximately 10 cells each. A smear is then created by laying another slide on top. Stains are used to enhance cellular detail as needed. The cells are then examined for evidence of disease, such as malignancy. The physician examines the specimen under a microscope to determine whether the cell sample contains a sufficient number of cells for evaluation and diagnosis. Diagnostic accuracy increases when there are six or more cell clusters available for review. If an inadequate number of cells are present, the aspiration procedure may be repeated. Report 88177 for each additional separate evaluation episode performed on a specimen from the same site following the initial evaluation episode.

RVUs

Code	Work	PE	PE Non-Facility	MP	Total Non-Facility	Total Facility	Global
88177	0.42	0.41	0.41	0.01	0.84	0.84	ZZZ

88302-88309

88302 Level II - Surgical pathology, gross and microscopic examination

Appendix, incidental; Fallopian tube, sterilization; Fingers/toes, amputation, traumatic; Foreskin, newborn; Hernia sac, any location; Hydrocele sac; Nerve; Skin, plastic repair; Sympathetic ganglion; Testis, castration; Vaginal mucosa, incidental; Vas deferens, sterilization

88304 Level III - Surgical pathology, gross and microscopic examination

Abortion, induced; Abscess; Aneurysm - arterial/ventricular; Anus, tag; Appendix, other than incidental; Artery, atheromatous plaque; Bartholin's gland cyst; Bone fragment(s), other than pathologic fracture; Bursa/synovial cyst; Carpal tunnel tissue; Cartilage, shavings; Cholesteatoma; Colon, colostomy stoma; Conjunctiva - biopsy/pterygium; Cornea; Diverticulum - esophagus/small intestine; Dupuytren's contracture tissue; Femoral head, other than fracture; Fissure/fistula; Foreskin, other than newborn; Gallbladder; Ganglion cyst; Hematoma; Hemorrhoids; Hydatid of Morgagni; Intervertebral disc; Joint, loose body; Meniscus; Mucocele, salivary; Neuroma - Morton's/traumatic; Pilonidal cyst/sinus; Polyps, inflammatory - nasal/sinusoidal; Skin - cyst/tag/debridement; Soft tissue, debridement; Soft tissue, lipoma; Spermatocele; Tendon/tendon sheath; Testicular appendage; Thrombus or embolus; Tonsil and/or adenoids; Varicocele; Vas deferens, other than sterilization; Vein, varicosity

88305 Level IV - Surgical pathology, gross and microscopic examination

Abortion - spontaneous/missed; Artery, biopsy; Bone marrow, biopsy; Bone exostosis; Brain/meninges, other than for tumor resection; Breast, biopsy, not requiring microscopic evaluation of surgical margins; Breast, reduction mammoplasty; Bronchus, biopsy; Cell block, any source; Cervix, biopsy; Colon, biopsy; Duodenum, biopsy; Endocervix, curettings/biopsy; Endometrium, curettings/biopsy; Esophagus, biopsy; Extremity, amputation, traumatic; Fallopian tube, biopsy; Fallopian tube, ectopic pregnancy; Femoral head, fracture; Fingers/toes, amputation, non-traumatic; Gingiva/oral mucosa, biopsy; Heart valve; Joint, resection; Kidney, biopsy; Larynx, biopsy; Leiomyoma(s), uterine myomectomy - without uterus; Lip, biopsy/wedge resection; Lung, transbronchial biopsy; Lymph node, biopsy; Muscle, biopsy; Nasal mucosa, biopsy; Nasopharynx/oropharynx, biopsy; Nerve, biopsy; Odontogenic/dental cyst; Omentum, biopsy; Ovary with or without tube, non-neoplastic; Ovary, biopsy/wedge resection; Parathyroid gland; Peritoneum, biopsy; Pituitary tumor; Placenta, other than third trimester; Pleura/pericardium - biopsy/tissue; Polyp, cervical/endometrial; Polyp, colorectal; Polyp, stomach/small intestine; Prostate, needle biopsy Prostate, TUR; Salivary gland, biopsy; Sinus, paranasal biopsy; Skin, other than cyst/tag/debridement/plastic repair; Small intestine, biopsy; Soft tissue, other than tumor/mass/lipoma/debridement; Spleen; Stomach, biopsy; Synovium; Testis, other than tumor/biopsy/castration; Thyroglossal duct/brachial cleft cyst; Tongue, biopsy; Tonsil, biopsy; Trachea, biopsy; Ureter, biopsy; Urethra, biopsy; Urinary bladder, biopsy; Uterus, with or without tubes and ovaries, for prolapse; Vagina, biopsy; Vulva/labia, biopsy

88307 Level V - Surgical pathology, gross and microscopic examination

Adrenal, resection; Bone - biopsy/curettings; Bone fragment(s), pathologic fracture; Brain, biopsy; Brain/meninges, tumor resection; Breast, excision of lesion, requiring microscopic evaluation of surgical margins; Breast, mastectomy - partial/simple; Cervix, conization; Colon, segmental resection, other than for tumor; Extremity, amputation, non-traumatic; Eye, enucleation; Kidney, partial/total nephrectomy; Larynx, partial/total resection; Liver, biopsy - needle/wedge; Liver, partial resection; Lung, wedge biopsy; Lymph nodes, regional resection; Mediastinum, mass; Myocardium, biopsy; Odontogenic tumor; Ovary with or without tube, neoplastic; Pancreas, biopsy; Placenta, third trimester; Prostate, except radical resection; Salivary gland; Sentinel lymph node; Small intestine, resection, other than for tumor; Soft tissue mass (except lipoma) - biopsy/simple excision; Stomach - subtotal/total resection, other than for tumor; Testis, biopsy; Thymus, tumor; Thyroid, total/lobe; Ureter, resection; Urinary bladder, TUR; Uterus, with or without tubes and ovaries, other than neoplastic/prolapse

88309 Level VI - Surgical pathology, gross and microscopic examination

Bone resection; Breast, mastectomy - with regional lymph nodes; Colon, segmental resection for tumor; Colon, total resection; Esophagus, partial/total resection; Extremity, disarticulation; Fetus, with dissection; Larynx, partial/total resection - with regional lymph nodes; Lung - total/lobe/segment resection; Pancreas, total/subtotal resection; Prostate, radical resection; Small intestine, resection for tumor; Soft tissue tumor, extensive resection; Stomach - subtotal/total resection for tumor; Testis, tumor; Tongue/tonsil -resection for tumor; Urinary bladder, partial/total resection; Uterus, with or without tubes and ovaries, neoplastic; Vulva, total/subtotal resection

(For fine needle aspiration biopsy, see 10004, 10005, 10006, 10007, 10008, 10009, 10010, 10011, 10012, 10021)

(For evaluation of fine needle aspirate, see 88172-88173)

(Do not report 88302-88309 on the same specimen as part of Mohs surgery)

Plain English Description

Tissue removed during a surgical procedure, such as a biopsy, excision, or resection, is examined macroscopically (gross or visual examination) and then under a microscope. The cells, tissues, or organ are transported from the surgical suite to the pathologist. The pathologist first visually examines the specimen and notes any defining characteristics. The specimen is then prepared for microscopic evaluation. The physician carefully analyzes the specimen to help establish a diagnosis, identify the presence or absence of malignant neoplasm, identify the exact type of malignancy if present, and examine the margins of the specimen to determine whether or not the entire diseased area was removed. A written report of findings is then prepared and a copy sent to the treating physician. Pathology services are reported based on the type of tissue examined, whether or not the tissue is expected to be normal or diseased, the difficulty of the pathology exam, and the time required to complete the exam. Use 88302 for a Level II pathology examination; 88304 for a Level III exam; 88305 for a Level IV exam; 88307 for a Level V exam; and 88309 for a Level VI exam.

RVUs

Code	Work	PE	PE Non-Facility	MP	Total Non-Facility	Total Facility	Global
88302	0.13	0.78	0.78	0.02	0.93	0.93	XXX
88304	0.22	0.98	0.98	0.02	1.22	1.22	XXX
88305	0.75	1.31	1.31	0.02	2.08	2.08	XXX
88307	1.59	6.73	6.73	0.08	8.40	8.40	XXX
88309	2.80	9.87	9.87	0.09	12.76	12.76	XXX

88311

✚ **88311 Decalcification procedure (List separately in addition to code for surgical pathology examination)**

Plain English Description

A surgical or other specimen containing calcium, such as bone, bone marrow, or other calcified tissue, is treated to remove the calcium. The specimen is first placed in an acid solution to remove the calcium. Ion exchange is then performed by bathing the specimen in another solution that removes calcium ions. The decalcified specimen is then prepared for examination.

RVUs

Code	Work	PE	PE Non-Facility	MP	Total Non-Facility	Total Facility	Global
88311	0.24	0.35	0.35	0.02	0.61	0.61	XXX

89260-89261

89260 Sperm isolation; simple prep (eg, sperm wash and swim-up) for insemination or diagnosis with semen analysis

89261 Sperm isolation; complex prep (eg, Percoll gradient, albumin gradient) for insemination or diagnosis with semen analysis

(For semen analysis without sperm wash or swim-up, use 89320)

Plain English Description

Sperm are isolated for use in an assisted reproductive procedure or for diagnostic purposes. A semen analysis is performed first. Semen analysis includes an evaluation for the presence and motility of sperm. The total density of sperm per millimeter of semen is calculated and then the motile density is calculated. Motile density evaluates the number of sperm showing good forward motion. Semen analysis may also include an evaluation of volume and differential. Volume refers to the total volume of semen in a single ejaculation. Differential is an evaluation of the number of sperm that appear normal when examined under a microscope. Following semen analysis, the sperm are isolated. In 89260, a sample of unsorted spermatozoa is placed in the bottom of a laboratory test tube containing sperm wash medium. The tube is then placed in an upright position and allowed to stand for 30-60 minutes while maintaining a constant temperature of 37 degrees C. During this 30-60 minute period, viable, motile sperm will swim up to the top of the tube. In 89261, a test tube is prepared with a solution of 90% Percoll or albumin gradient on the bottom half of the tube and a second solution on the top half containing a 45% Percoll or albumin gradient solution. Unsorted spermatozoa are then placed on top of the 45% solution. The test tube is centrifuged for 30 minutes while maintaining a temperature of 25 degrees C. Following the centrifugation process, nonviable sperm remain suspended in the 45% solution while viable sperm fall to the bottom of the tube. Following sperm wash and swim up or Percoll gradient sperm isolation, the viable sperm are removed for further diagnostic analysis or prepared for a separately reportable artificial insemination procedure.

RVUs

Code	Work	PE	PE Non-Facility	MP	Total Non-Facility	Total Facility	Global
89260	0.00	0.00	0.00	0.00	0.00	0.00	XXX
89261	0.00	0.00	0.00	0.00	0.00	0.00	XXX

89264

89264 Sperm identification from testis tissue, fresh or cryopreserved

(For biopsy of testis, see 54500, 54505)

(For sperm identification from aspiration, use 89257)

(For semen analysis, see 89300-89320)

Plain English Description

Fresh or frozen sperm retrieved from testis tissue by a separately reportable aspiration or biopsy procedure are identified in the embryology lab. Prior to transport to the lab, the tissue is minced into very small segments and placed in a tube containing yolk test buffer. At the embryology lab the tissue samples are carefully examined under a microscope for the presence of viable sperm. Identification of sperm in testis tissue can be a time-consuming and tedious procedure. Once sperm are identified, they are prepared for use in a separately reportable assisted reproduction procedure. Frozen testis tissue is thawed and then examined in the embryology lab to identify viable sperm using the same techniques as those described for fresh testicular tissue.

RVUs

Code	Work	PE	PE Non-Facility	MP	Total Non-Facility	Total Facility	Global
89264	0.00	0.00	0.00	0.00	0.00	0.00	XXX

89310-89320

89310 Semen analysis; motility and count (not including Huhner test)

89320 Semen analysis; volume, count, motility, and differential

(Skin tests, see 86485-86580 and 95012-95199)

Plain English Description

A semen analysis to evaluate the presence and/or motility of sperm is performed. The total density of sperm per milliliter of semen is calculated, with a normal sperm count being 20 million per milliliter or above. The motile density is then evaluated. Motile density evaluates the number of active sperm showing good forward motion that would be capable of moving from the site of sperm deposition to the site of fertilization. A normal motility count is 8 million per milliliter or higher. Use 89320 when motility and count as described above are performed with an evaluation of volume and differential. Volume evaluates the total volume of semen in a single ejaculation. Differential is an evaluation of the number of sperm that appear normal when viewed under the microscope.

RVUs

Code	Work	PE	PE Non-Facility	MP	Total Non-Facility	Total Facility	Global
89310	0.00	0.00	0.00	0.00	0.00	0.00	XXX
89320	0.00	0.00	0.00	0.00	0.00	0.00	XXX

89321

89321 Semen analysis; sperm presence and motility of sperm, if performed

(To report Hyaluronan binding assay [HBA], use 89398)

Plain English Description

A semen analysis is performed to identify the presence of sperm. This test is typically performed following vasectomy to verify that the sterilization procedure was successful. A successful vasectomy result shows no sperm present in the semen. If sperm are present, the motility (movement) of sperm may be evaluated.

RVUs

Code	Work	PE	PE Non-Facility	MP	Total Non-Facility	Total Facility	Global
89321	0.00	0.00	0.00	0.00	0.00	0.00	XXX

89322

89322 Semen analysis; volume, count, motility, and differential using strict morphologic criteria (eg, Kruger)

Plain English Description

A semen analysis is performed to evaluate the volume of semen in a single ejaculation, the number of sperm present per milliliter, the motility (movement) of sperm, and the differential number of sperm that are normal using strict morphologic criteria. The total volume of semen in a single ejaculation is measured. The total density of sperm per milliliter of semen is calculated with a normal sperm count being 20 million per milliliter or above. The motile density is then evaluated for the number of active sperm, showing good forward motion, capable of moving from the site of sperm deposition to the site of fertilization. A normal motility count is 8 million per milliliter or higher. Next, a differential using strict morphologic criteria is performed. A stained slide is prepared and several hundred individual sperm are evaluated. Each sperm is carefully inspected and any abnormalities in structure of the head, neck, or tail are noted. This detailed morphologic exam allows greater accuracy in the determination of the number of normal versus abnormal sperm present.

RVUs

Code	Work	PE	PE Non-Facility	MP	Total Non-Facility	Total Facility	Global
89322	0.00	0.00	0.00	0.00	0.00	0.00	XXX

89331

89331 Sperm evaluation, for retrograde ejaculation, urine (sperm concentration, motility, and morphology, as indicated)

(For semen analysis on concurrent semen specimen, see 89300-89322 in conjunction with 89331)

(For detection of sperm in urine, use 81015)

Plain English Description

A urine specimen is obtained to evaluate sperm concentration, motility, and morphology in a patient with suspected retrograde ejaculation. Retrograde ejaculation is a condition in which semen enters the bladder during ejaculation rather than being discharged through the urethra and is relatively uncommon. Diabetes, some medications, or previous urinary tract procedures increase the risk of developing retrograde ejaculation. Medication is administered to increase the alkalinity of the urine. Following sexual climax, a urine specimen is obtained. The number, or concentration, of sperm in the urine is evaluated. Motility is then evaluated to determine the number of active sperm showing good forward motion. A morphological examination of the sperm may also be performed to determine the number of normal to abnormal sperm.

RVUs

Code	Work	PE	PE Non-Facility	MP	Total Non-Facility	Total Facility	Global
89331	0.00	0.00	0.00	0.00	0.00	0.00	XXX

90935-90937

90935 Hemodialysis procedure with single evaluation by a physician or other qualified health care professional

90937 Hemodialysis procedure requiring repeated evaluation(s) with or without substantial revision of dialysis prescription

Plain English Description

A nurse or technician inserts two needles into a previously created vascular access site. The vascular access site may be a surgically created internal fistula or shunt, an internal graft, or less commonly a central venous catheter. Each needle is attached to a separate piece of flexible plastic tubing that is connected to the dialysis machine. One tube removes blood from the body. The blood is circulated through the dialysis machine and then returned to the body through the second tube. The blood circulating through the dialysis machine passes on one side of a membrane and dialysis fluid passes on the other. The wastes and excess fluid pass from the blood through the membrane and into the dialysis fluid. These wastes are discarded with the dialysis fluid. The cleansed blood is returned to the bloodstream through the second tube. The hemodialysis procedure includes all evaluation and management services performed on the date of the dialysis procedure that are related to the patient's renal disease. Code 90935 is used when a single evaluation and management service is performed on the date of the hemodialysis procedure. Code 90937 is used when repeated evaluation and management services are required during the course of the hemodialysis procedure.

RVUs

Code	Work	PE	PE Non-Facility	MP	Total Non-Facility	Total Facility	Global
90935	1.48	0.54	0.54	0.09	2.11	2.11	000
90937	2.11	0.79	0.79	0.12	3.02	3.02	000

90940

90940 Hemodialysis access flow study to determine blood flow in grafts and arteriovenous fistulae by an indicator method

(For duplex scan of hemodialysis access, use 93990)

Plain English Description

A hemodialysis access flow study is performed to determine blood flow in grafts and arteriovenous (AV) fistulae using an indicator method. Monitoring of AV graft patency using an indicator method provides early detection of stenosis, reduces graft thrombosis, and can extend the life of the graft. The physician or other trained staff member performs the procedure during a regularly scheduled hemodialysis session. Two ultrasound sensors are clipped onto hemodialysis tubing blood lines, one sensor on the tube receiving the blood from the body and another one on the tube returning the cleansed blood from the dialyzer. These sensors transmit minute levels of ultrasound through the tubing wall into the blood stream. An isotonic saline solution is injected into the blood to dilute it and reduce the ultrasound velocity. As the saline bolus passes through the tubing, two sensors measure changes in the ultrasound characteristics of the blood in the tubes of the extracorporeal circuit. These measurements are evaluated and used to identify any blood flow problems. Hook-up, measurement, and disconnection from the monitoring device are included.

RVUs

Code	Work	PE	PE Non-Facility	MP	Total Non-Facility	Total Facility	Global
90940	0.00	0.00	0.00	0.00	0.00	0.00	XXX

90945-90947

90945 Dialysis procedure other than hemodialysis (eg, peritoneal dialysis, hemofiltration, or other continuous renal replacement therapies), with single evaluation by a physician or other qualified health care professional

(For home infusion of peritoneal dialysis, use 99601, 99602)

90947 Dialysis procedure other than hemodialysis (eg, peritoneal dialysis, hemofiltration, or other continuous renal replacement therapies) requiring repeated evaluations by a physician or other qualified health care professional, with or without substantial revision of dialysis prescription

Plain English Description

A dialysis procedure other than hemodialysis with related evaluation services is performed. Types of dialysis procedures performed include peritoneal dialysis, hemofiltration, or other continuous renal replacement therapies. Peritoneal dialysis, hemofiltration, and other continuous renal replacement therapies filter blood continuously without interruption. If peritoneal dialysis is performed, a nurse or technician instills dialysis fluid through a previously placed abdominal catheter. The dialysis solution contains the sugar dextrose, which pulls wastes and extra fluid out of the blood through the peritoneal membrane and into the abdominal cavity. The dialysis fluid remains in the abdominal cavity for a period of four to six hours after which the dialysis solution along with the wastes and excess fluid is removed from the abdomen through the catheter. This process of filling and draining the abdomen may be repeated several times during the day. Hemofiltration may be performed by an arteriovenous or venovenous procedure. In an arteriovenous procedure, the femoral artery is cannulated. Arterial pressure forces blood through a filter into the femoral vein. Water and soluble waste products filter from the blood through a permeable membrane and are discarded. The cleansed blood is returned to the body with replacement fluid of physiologically balanced water and electrolytes. The procedure for venovenous filtration is similar. A double lumen catheter is placed in the femoral, subclavian, or internal jugular vein. A pump is used to push blood from the vein through the dialysis circuit. The cleansed blood is then pushed back into the same vein. Code 90945 is used when a single evaluation and management service is performed on the date of the peritoneal dialysis, hemofiltration, or other continuous renal replacement therapy. Code 90947 is used when repeated evaluation and management services are required during the course of the peritoneal dialysis procedure, hemofiltration procedure, or other continuous renal replacement therapy procedure.

RVUs

Code	Work	PE	PE Non-Facility	MP	Total Non-Facility	Total Facility	Global
90945	1.56	0.85	0.85	0.10	2.51	2.51	000
90947	2.52	0.93	0.93	0.18	3.63	3.63	000

90951-90953

★ **90951 End-stage renal disease (ESRD) related services monthly, for patients younger than 2 years of age to include monitoring for the adequacy of nutrition, assessment of growth and development, and counseling of parents; with 4 or more face-to-face visits by a physician or other qualified health care professional per month**

★ **90952 End-stage renal disease (ESRD) related services monthly, for patients younger than 2 years of age to include monitoring for the adequacy of nutrition, assessment of growth and development, and counseling of parents; with 2-3 face-to-face visits by a physician or other qualified health care professional per month**

90953 End-stage renal disease (ESRD) related services monthly, for patients younger than 2 years of age to include monitoring for the adequacy of nutrition, assessment of growth and development, and counseling of parents; with 1 face-to-face visit by a physician or other qualified health care professional per month

Plain English Description

End-stage renal disease (ESRD) related services are provided per 1 full month in an outpatient setting, including monitoring of the adequacy of nutrition, assessment of growth and development, and counseling of parents for services provided to a child younger than 2 years of age. The physician or other qualified health care professional establishes the dialyzing cycle, performs outpatient evaluation and management services related to the dialysis services, and provides oversight and management of the patient during the dialysis services as well as telephone follow-up as needed for the entire month. The patient is examined on a routine basis for existing and potential medical problems. The patient is seen as needed when new symptoms or problems develop. The physician or other qualified health care professional ensures that dialysis services are being provided as prescribed and makes adjustments to the dialysis prescription as needed, including monitoring the patient's weight, making recommendations regarding diet and fluid intake, and prescribing special renal supplement formula as needed. Laboratory data are reviewed. Medications and nutritional supplements are monitored, and changes are made as needed. Interventions for delays in growth or development are initiated as needed, which may include injection of growth hormones. Social development is monitored and any behavioral or school problems are also addressed. The physician or other health care professional counsels the parents and caregivers and responds to their questions and concerns. These ESRD services are included in one code, which is reported only once per month based on the number of face-to-face visits provided each month. Code 90951 is for 4 or more face-to-face visits per month; code 90952 is for 2 to 3 face-to-face visits per month; and code 90953 reports 1 face-to-face visit per month.

RVUs

Code	Work	PE	PE Non-Facility	MP	Total Non-Facility	Total Facility	Global
90951	23.92	9.21	9.21	1.60	34.73	34.73	XXX
90952	0.00	0.00	0.00	0.00	0.00	0.00	XXX
90953	0.00	0.00	0.00	0.00	0.00	0.00	XXX

90954-90956

★ 90954 End-stage renal disease (ESRD) related services monthly, for patients 2-11 years of age to include monitoring for the adequacy of nutrition, assessment of growth and development, and counseling of parents; with 4 or more face-to-face visits by a physician or other qualified health care professional per month

★ 90955 End-stage renal disease (ESRD) related services monthly, for patients 2-11 years of age to include monitoring for the adequacy of nutrition, assessment of growth and development, and counseling of parents; with 2-3 face-to-face visits by a physician or other qualified health care professional per month

90956 End-stage renal disease (ESRD) related services monthly, for patients 2-11 years of age to include monitoring for the adequacy of nutrition, assessment of growth and development, and counseling of parents; with 1 face-to-face visit by a physician or other qualified health care professional per month

Plain English Description

End-stage renal disease (ESRD) related services are provided per 1 full month in an outpatient setting, including monitoring of the adequacy of nutrition, assessment of growth and development, and counseling of parents for services provided to children aged 2 through 11 years. The physician or other qualified health care professional establishes the dialyzing cycle, performs outpatient evaluation and management services related to the dialysis services, and provides oversight and management of the patient during the dialysis service as well as telephone follow-up as needed for the entire month. The patient is examined on a routine basis for existing and potential medical problems. The patient is seen as needed when new symptoms or problems develop. The physician or other qualified health care professional ensures that dialysis services are being provided as prescribed and makes adjustments to the dialysis prescription as needed, including monitoring the patient's weight, making recommendations regarding diet and fluid intake, and prescribing special renal supplement formula as needed. Laboratory data are reviewed. Medications and nutritional supplements are monitored, and changes are made as needed. Interventions for delays in growth or development are initiated as needed, which may include injection of growth hormones. Social development is monitored and any behavioral or school problems are also addressed. The physician or other qualified health care professional counsels the parents and caregivers and responds to their questions and concerns. These ESRD services are included in one code, which is reported only once per month based on the number of face-to-face visits provided each month. Code 90954 is for 4 or more face-to-face visits per month; code 90955 is for 2 to 3 face-to-face visits per month; and code 90956 reports 1 face-to-face visit per month.

RVUs

Code	Work	PE	PE Non-Facility	MP	Total Non-Facility	Total Facility	Global
90954	20.86	7.62	7.62	1.36	29.84	29.84	XXX
90955	10.32	4.46	4.46	0.64	15.42	15.42	XXX
90956	6.64	3.16	3.16	0.41	10.21	10.21	XXX

90957-90959

★ 90957 End-stage renal disease (ESRD) related services monthly, for patients 12-19 years of age to include monitoring for the adequacy of nutrition, assessment of growth and development, and counseling of parents; with 4 or more face-to-face visits by a physician or other qualified health care professional per month

★ 90958 End-stage renal disease (ESRD) related services monthly, for patients 12-19 years of age to include monitoring for the adequacy of nutrition, assessment of growth and development, and counseling of parents; with 2-3 face-to-face visits by a physician or other qualified health care professional per month

90959 End-stage renal disease (ESRD) related services monthly, for patients 12-19 years of age to include monitoring for the adequacy of nutrition, assessment of growth and development, and counseling of parents; with 1 face-to-face visit by a physician or other qualified health care professional per month

Plain English Description

End-stage renal disease (ESRD) related services are provided per 1 full month in an outpatient setting, including monitoring of the adequacy of nutrition, assessment of growth and development, and counseling of parents for services provided to a child aged 12-19 years. The physician or other qualified health care professional establishes the dialyzing cycle, performs outpatient evaluation and management services related to the dialysis services, and provides oversight and management of the patient during the dialysis services as well as telephone follow-up as needed for the entire month. The patient is examined on a routine basis for existing and potential medical problems, and is seen as needed when new symptoms or problems develop. The physician or other qualified health care professional ensures that dialysis services are being provided as prescribed and makes adjustments to the dialysis prescription as needed, including monitoring the patient's weight, making recommendations regarding diet and fluid intake, and prescribing special renal supplement formula as needed. Laboratory data are reviewed. Medications and nutritional supplements are monitored, and changes are made as needed. Interventions for delays in growth or development are initiated as needed, which may include injection of growth hormones. Social development is monitored and any behavioral or school problems are also addressed. The physician or other qualified health care professional counsels the parents and caregivers and responds to their questions and concerns. These ESRD services are included in one code, and reported only once per month based on the number of face-to-face visits. Code 90957 is for 4 or more face-to-face visits per month; code 90958 is for 2-3 face-to-face visits per month; and code 90959 reports 1 face-to-face visit per month.

RVUs

Code	Work	PE	PE Non-Facility	MP	Total Non-Facility	Total Facility	Global
90957	15.46	6.35	6.35	1.00	22.81	22.81	XXX
90958	9.87	4.35	4.35	0.62	14.84	14.84	XXX
90959	6.19	3.01	3.01	0.39	9.59	9.59	XXX

90960-90962

★ **90960 End-stage renal disease (ESRD) related services monthly, for patients 20 years of age and older; with 4 or more face-to-face visits by a physician or other qualified health care professional per month**

★ **90961 End-stage renal disease (ESRD) related services monthly, for patients 20 years of age and older; with 2-3 face-to-face visits by a physician or other qualified health care professional per month**

90962 End-stage renal disease (ESRD) related services monthly, for patients 20 years of age and older; with 1 face-to-face visit by a physician or other qualified health care professional per month

Plain English Description

End-stage renal disease (ESRD) related services are provided per 1 full month in an outpatient setting to a patient 20 years of age and older. The physician or other qualified health care professional establishes the dialyzing cycle, performs outpatient evaluation and management services related to the dialysis services, and provides oversight and management of the patient during the dialysis service as well as telephone follow-up as needed for the entire month. The patient is examined on a routine basis for existing and potential medical problems, and is seen as needed when new symptoms or problems develop. The physician or other qualified health care professional ensures that dialysis services are being provided as prescribed and makes adjustments to the dialysis prescription as needed. Laboratory data are reviewed. Medications and nutritional supplements are monitored, and changes are made as needed. The physician or other qualified health care professional also establishes, monitors, and coordinates care, which may include social service interventions, nutritional support, kidney transplant planning, and services provided by other medical and/or surgical specialists. These ESRD services are included in one code, which is reported only once per month based on the number of face-to-face visits. Code 90960 is for 4 or more face-to-face visits per month; code 90961 is for 2-3 face-to-face visits per month; and code 90962 reports 1 face-to-face visit per month.

RVUs

Code	Work	PE	PE Non-Facility	MP	Total Non-Facility	Total Facility	Global
90960	6.77	3.26	3.26	0.41	10.44	10.44	XXX
90961	5.52	2.80	2.80	0.34	8.66	8.66	XXX
90962	3.57	2.16	2.16	0.22	5.95	5.95	XXX

90963-90965

★ **90963 End-stage renal disease (ESRD) related services for home dialysis per full month, for patients younger than 2 years of age to include monitoring for the adequacy of nutrition, assessment of growth and development, and counseling of parents**

★ **90964 End-stage renal disease (ESRD) related services for home dialysis per full month, for patients 2-11 years of age to include monitoring for the adequacy of nutrition, assessment of growth and development, and counseling of parents**

★ **90965 End-stage renal disease (ESRD) related services for home dialysis per full month, for patients 12-19 years of age to include monitoring for the adequacy of nutrition, assessment of growth and development, and counseling of parents**

Plain English Description

End-stage renal disease (ESRD) related services are provided for 1 full month for home dialysis, including monitoring of the adequacy of nutrition, assessment of growth and development, and counseling of parents for services provided to a child. The physician establishes the dialyzing cycle, performs outpatient evaluation and management services related to the home dialysis services, and provides oversight and management of the patient during the dialysis as well as telephone follow-up as needed for the entire month. The physician examines the patient on a routine basis for existing and potential medical problems. The patient is seen as needed when new symptoms or problems develop. The physician ensures that dialysis services are being provided in the home as prescribed and makes adjustments to the dialysis prescription as needed. The physician monitors the patient's weight and makes recommendations regarding the patient's diet and fluid intake and prescribes special renal supplement formula as needed. Laboratory data are reviewed. Medications and nutritional supplements are monitored, and changes are made as needed. The physician initiates the necessary interventions for delays in growth or development, which may include injection of growth hormones. The physician reviews social development and monitors any behavioral or school problems, making referrals and intervening as needed. The physician counsels the parents and caregivers and responds to their questions and concerns. These ESRD-related services for home dialysis are included in one code, which is reported only once per month and are age-specific. Code 90963 is reported for patients younger than 2 years of age; code 90964 is for patients 2-11 years old; and code 90965 is for patients aged 12-19.

RVUs

Code	Work	PE	PE Non-Facility	MP	Total Non-Facility	Total Facility	Global
90963	12.09	5.06	5.06	0.77	17.92	17.92	XXX
90964	10.25	4.47	4.47	0.65	15.37	15.37	XXX
90965	9.80	4.35	4.35	0.62	14.77	14.77	XXX

90966

★ **90966 End-stage renal disease (ESRD) related services for home dialysis per full month, for patients 20 years of age and older**

Plain English Description

End-stage renal disease (ESRD) related services are provided for 1 full month for home dialysis for patients 20 years of age and older. The physician establishes the dialyzing cycle, performs outpatient evaluation and management services related to the home dialysis services, and provides oversight and management of the patient during the dialysis as well as telephone follow-up as needed for the entire month. The physician examines the patient on a routine basis for existing and potential medical problems. The patient is seen as needed when new symptoms or problems develop. The physician ensures that dialysis services are being provided as prescribed and makes adjustments to the dialysis prescription as needed. Laboratory data are reviewed. Medications and nutritional supplements are monitored, and changes are made as needed. The physician also establishes, monitors, and coordinates care, which may include social service interventions, nutritional support, kidney transplant planning, and services provided by other medical and/or surgical specialists.

RVUs

Code	Work	PE	PE Non-Facility	MP	Total Non-Facility	Total Facility	Global
90966	5.52	2.80	2.80	0.34	8.66	8.66	XXX

90967-90970

★ **90967 End-stage renal disease (ESRD) related services for dialysis less than a full month of service, per day; for patients younger than 2 years of age**

★ **90968 End-stage renal disease (ESRD) related services for dialysis less than a full month of service, per day; for patients 2-11 years of age**

★ **90969 End-stage renal disease (ESRD) related services for dialysis less than a full month of service, per day; for patients 12-19 years of age**

★ **90970 End-stage renal disease (ESRD) related services for dialysis less than a full month of service, per day; for patients 20 years of age and older**

Plain English Description

End-stage renal disease (ESRD) services are provided per day in an outpatient setting when less than a full month of service is required. Outpatient ESRD services may be provided for only part of a month due to inpatient hospitalization or initiation of the services after the first of the month. The physician establishes the dialyzing cycle, performs outpatient evaluation and management services related to the dialysis services, and provides oversight and management of the patient during the dialysis as well as telephone follow-up as needed. The physician examines the patient on a routine basis for existing and potential medical problems. The patient is seen as needed when new symptoms or problems develop. The physician ensures that dialysis services are being provided as prescribed and makes adjustments to the dialysis prescription as needed. The physician monitors the patient's weight, makes recommendations regarding the patient's diet and fluid intake, and prescribes special renal supplement formula as needed. Laboratory data are reviewed. Medications and nutritional supplements are monitored and changes are made as needed. The physician also establishes, monitors, and coordinates care, which may include social service interventions, nutritional support, kidney transplant planning, and services provided by other medical and/or surgical specialists. For younger patients, the physician initiates the necessary interventions for delays in growth or development, which may include injection of growth hormones. Social development is monitored and any behavioral or school problems are addressed by making referrals and intervening as needed. The physician counsels the parents and/or caregivers and responds to questions and concerns. These ESRD services are age-specific and reported on a daily basis. Code 90967 is for patients younger than 2; code 90968 is for patients aged 2-11; code 90969 is for patients 12-19 years of age; and code 90970 is for patients aged 20 or older.

RVUs

Code	Work	PE	PE Non-Facility	MP	Total Non-Facility	Total Facility	Global
90967	0.35	0.15	0.15	0.02	0.52	0.52	XXX
90968	0.34	0.15	0.15	0.02	0.51	0.51	XXX
90969	0.33	0.15	0.15	0.02	0.50	0.50	XXX
90970	0.18	0.09	0.09	0.01	0.28	0.28	XXX

90989-90993

90989 Dialysis training, patient, including helper where applicable, any mode, completed course

90993 Dialysis training, patient, including helper where applicable, any mode, course not completed, per training session

Plain English Description

The physician performs administrative, routine professional services, and supervision or direction of a dialysis patient, including a helper where applicable, during self-dialysis training. During self-dialysis training, the physician provides the following administrative services: training and supervision of staff, participation in staff conferences and management of the facility, advising staff on procurement of supplies, and medical direction of staff delivering the self-training services to the patient. The physician's routine professional services may include such things as direction of and participation in training of dialysis patients; review of family, home status, and environment of the patient; counseling and training of family members; review of the training process; review of laboratory results, nurses' notes, and any other medical documentation; adjustment of patient's medication, diet, or the dialysis procedure; prescription of medical supplies; evaluation of the patient's psychosocial status; evaluation of the appropriateness of the treatment; pre-dialysis and post-dialysis patient examinations; and observation of a complete successful self-dialysis procedure by the patient. Code 90989 is used for a completed self-dialysis training course, which typically includes at least 25 training sessions. Code 90993 is used when the course is not completed and is reported for each training session performed.

RVUs

Code	Work	PE	PE Non-Facility	MP	Total Non-Facility	Total Facility	Global
90989	0.00	0.00	0.00	0.00	0.00	0.00	XXX
90993	0.00	0.00	0.00	0.00	0.00	0.00	XXX

90997

90997 Hemoperfusion (eg, with activated charcoal or resin)

Plain English Description

A hemoperfusion procedure is performed using activated charcoal or resin. Hemoperfusion is used to remove drugs, poisons, or other toxic substances from the blood that are harmful to the kidneys, to remove waste products from the blood in patients with kidney disease, or to provide supportive treatment to patients with liver failure before and after liver transplant. Hemoperfusion can clear toxins from a larger volume of blood than other filtration methods, such as hemodialysis, and can process over 300 mL of blood per minute. Two catheters are placed in the arm, one in an artery and one in a nearby vein, and connected to plastic tubing. The tubing from the arterial access site removes blood from the body and passes it through a hemoperfusion system. In the hemoperfusion system, the blood is passed over a column or cartridge containing the activated charcoal or resin, and the toxic molecules or particles are trapped within the column or cartridge. The cleansed blood flows out of the hemoperfusion system through the second tube and is returned to the body through the venous access site.

RVUs

Code	Work	PE	PE Non-Facility	MP	Total Non-Facility	Total Facility	Global
90997	1.84	0.65	0.65	0.11	2.60	2.60	000

93975-93976

93975 Duplex scan of arterial inflow and venous outflow of abdominal, pelvic, scrotal contents and/or retroperitoneal organs; complete study

93976 Duplex scan of arterial inflow and venous outflow of abdominal, pelvic, scrotal contents and/or retroperitoneal organs; limited study

Plain English Description

A vascular ultrasound study is performed to evaluate the arterial inflow and venous outflow of abdominal, pelvic, and scrotal contents and/or retroperitoneal organs. A duplex scan uses both B-mode and Doppler studies. A clear gel is placed on the skin over the region to be studied. A B-mode transducer is placed on the skin and real-time images of the arteries and veins are obtained. A Doppler probe within the B-mode transducer provides information on the pattern and direction of blood flow in the arteries and veins. The B-mode transducer produces ultrasonic sound waves that move through the skin and bounce off the arteries and veins when the probe is moved over the region being studied. The Doppler probe produces sound waves that bounce off blood cells moving within the arteries and veins. The reflected sound waves are sent to an amplifier that makes the sound waves audible. The pitch of the sound waves changes if there is reduced blood flow, or ceases altogether if a vessel is completely obstructed. A computer converts the sound waves to images that are overlaid with colors to produce video images showing the speed and direction of blood flow as well as any obstruction. Spectral Doppler analysis is performed to provide information on anatomy and hemodynamic function, including information on the presence of narrowing and plaque formation within the blood vessels. The physician reviews the duplex scan and provides a written interpretation of findings. Use code 93975 for a complete study. Use code 93976 for a limited study.

RVUs

Code	Work	PE	PE Non-Facility	MP	Total Non-Facility	Total Facility	Global
93975	1.16	6.71	6.71	0.13	8.00	8.00	XXX
93976	0.80	3.89	3.89	0.06	4.75	4.75	XXX

93980-93981

93980 Duplex scan of arterial inflow and venous outflow of penile vessels; complete study

93981 Duplex scan of arterial inflow and venous outflow of penile vessels; follow-up or limited study

Plain English Description

A vascular ultrasound study is performed to evaluate the arterial inflow and venous outflow of the penile vessels. A duplex scan uses both B-mode and Doppler studies. A clear gel is placed on the skin. The B-mode transducer is then placed on the skin and real-time images of the arteries and veins are obtained. A Doppler probe within the B-mode transducer provides information on the pattern and direction of blood flow in the penile blood vessels. The B-mode transducer produces ultrasonic sound waves that move through the skin and bounce off the blood vessels when the probe is moved over the penis. The Doppler probe produces sound waves that bounce off blood cells moving within the penile vessels. The reflected sound waves are sent to an amplifier that makes the sound waves audible. The pitch of the sound waves changes if there is reduced blood flow, or ceases altogether if a vessel is completely obstructed. A computer converts the sound waves to images that are overlaid with colors to produce video images showing the speed and direction of blood flow as well as any obstruction. Spectral Doppler analysis is performed to provide information on anatomy and hemodynamic function, including information on the presence of narrowing and plaque formation within the blood vessels. The physician reviews the duplex scan and provides a written interpretation of findings. Use code 93980 for a complete study. Use code 93981 for a follow-up or limited study.

RVUs

Code	Work	PE	PE Non-Facility	MP	Total Non-Facility	Total Facility	Global
93980	1.25	2.13	2.13	0.05	3.43	3.43	XXX
93981	0.44	1.60	1.60	0.03	2.07	2.07	XXX

93985-93986

93985 Duplex scan of arterial inflow and venous outflow for preoperative vessel assessment prior to creation of hemodialysis access; complete bilateral study

(Do not report 93985 in conjunction with 93925, 93930, 93970 for the same extremity[ies])

(Do not report 93985 in conjunction with 93990 for the same extremity)

93986 Duplex scan of arterial inflow and venous outflow for preoperative vessel assessment prior to creation of hemodialysis access; complete unilateral study

(Do not report 93986 in conjunction with 93926, 93931, 93971, 93990 for the same extremity)

Plain English Description

Ultrasound duplex scanning is a technique that images how blood flows through arteries and veins and its speed, as well as the blood vessel tissue structure. Duplex ultrasonography combines traditional ultrasound with pulsed wave color flow Doppler imaging to provide a color picture detecting blood flow as well as a 2D black-and-white ultrasound image of surrounding tissues. Pre-operative duplex scans are performed to evaluate upper extremity vessels in patients with kidney failure for arteriovenous fistula (AVF) access for hemodialysis. An AVF is formed by connecting a vein to an artery or placing a synthetic conduit between the two vessels. Obese patients, those with multiple previous access surgeries or suspected arterial or venous disease may undergo duplex ultrasound in addition to physical examination. The transducer wand is moved over the area being examined and sends out sound waves that are reflected back to the computer after bouncing off different tissues. Doppler imaging records waves that bounce off blood as it flows through the arteries and veins, while traditional ultrasound bounces off nonmoving structures to view the blood vessels themselves. The computer changes the waves that bounce back at different frequencies into duplex ultrasound images. Blood flow and vessel integrity can then be assessed and any abnormalities identified before surgical creation an AVF access. Use 93985 for a complete bilateral study, and 93986 for a complete unilateral study.

RVUs

Code	Work	PE	PE Non-Facility	MP	Total Non-Facility	Total Facility	Global
93985	0.80	6.60	6.60	0.15	7.55	7.55	XXX
93986	0.50	3.89	3.89	0.10	4.49	4.49	XXX

93990

93990 Duplex scan of hemodialysis access (including arterial inflow, body of access and venous outflow)

(For measurement of hemodialysis access flow using indicator dilution methods, use 90940)

Plain English Description

A vascular ultrasound study is performed to evaluate a hemodialysis graft or fistula. Periodic evaluation of the hemodialysis access site is performed to identify abnormalities such as reduced flow and stenosis that may threaten the function of hemodialysis access if left untreated. A duplex scan uses both B-mode and Doppler studies. A clear gel is placed on the skin over the hemodialysis access site. A B-mode transducer is placed on the skin and real-time images of the arterial inflow and venous outflow are obtained. A Doppler probe within the B-mode transducer provides information on the pattern and direction of blood within the hemodialysis access. The B-mode transducer produces ultrasonic sound waves that move through the skin and bounce off the hemodialysis graft/fistula when the probe is moved over the site. The Doppler probe produces sound waves that bounce off blood cells moving within the graft/fistula. The reflected sound waves are sent to an amplifier that makes the sound waves audible. The pitch of the sound waves changes if there is reduced blood flow, or ceases altogether if the graft/fistula is completely obstructed. A computer converts the sound waves to images that are overlaid with colors to produce video images showing the speed and direction of blood flow as well as any obstruction. Spectral Doppler analysis is performed to provide information on anatomy and hemodynamic function including information on the presence of narrowing and plaque formation within the blood vessels. The physician reviews the duplex scan and provides a written interpretation of findings.

RVUs

Code	Work	PE	PE Non-Facility	MP	Total Non-Facility	Total Facility	Global
93990	0.50	3.83	3.83	0.11	4.44	4.44	XXX

96360-96361

96360 Intravenous infusion, hydration; initial, 31 minutes to 1 hour

(Do not report 96360 if performed as a concurrent infusion service)

(Do not report intravenous infusion for hydration of 30 minutes or less)

✚ **96361 Intravenous infusion, hydration; each additional hour (List separately in addition to code for primary procedure)**

(Use 96361 in conjunction with 96360)

(Report 96361 for hydration infusion intervals of greater than 30 minutes beyond 1 hour increments)

(Report 96361 to identify hydration if provided as a secondary or subsequent service after a different initial service [96360, 96365, 96374, 96409, 96413] is administered through the same IV access)

Plain English Description

An intravenous infusion is administered for hydration. An intravenous line is placed into a vein, usually in the arm, and fluid is administered to provide additional fluid levels and electrolytes to counteract the effects of dehydration or supplement deficient oral fluid intake. The physician provides direct supervision of the fluid administration and is immediately available to intervene should complications arise. The physician provides periodic assessments of the patient and documentation of the patient's response to treatment. Use 96360 for the initial 31 minutes to 1 hour of hydration. Use 96361 for each additional hour.

RVUs

Code	Work	PE	PE Non-Facility	MP	Total Non-Facility	Total Facility	Global
96360	0.17	0.82	0.82	0.02	1.01	1.01	XXX
96361	0.09	0.28	0.28	0.01	0.38	0.38	ZZZ

96365-96368

96365 Intravenous infusion, for therapy, prophylaxis, or diagnosis (specify substance or drug); initial, up to 1 hour

✚ **96366 Intravenous infusion, for therapy, prophylaxis, or diagnosis (specify substance or drug); each additional hour (List separately in addition to code for primary procedure)**

(Report 96366 in conjunction with 96365, 96367)

(Report 96366 for additional hour[s] of sequential infusion)

(Report 96366 for infusion intervals of greater than 30 minutes beyond 1 hour increments)

(Report 96366 in conjunction with 96365 to identify each second and subsequent infusions of the same drug/substance)

✚ **96367 Intravenous infusion, for therapy, prophylaxis, or diagnosis (specify substance or drug); additional sequential infusion of a new drug/substance, up to 1 hour (List separately in addition to code for primary procedure)**

(Report 96367 in conjunction with 96365, 96374, 96409, 96413 to identify the infusion of a new drug/substance provided as a secondary or subsequent service after a different initial service is administered through the same IV access. Report 96367 only once per sequential infusion of same infusate mix)

✚ **96368 Intravenous infusion, for therapy, prophylaxis, or diagnosis (specify substance or drug); concurrent infusion (List separately in addition to code for primary procedure)**

(Report 96368 only once per date of service)

(Report 96368 in conjunction with 96365, 96366, 96413, 96415, 96416)

Plain English Description

An intravenous infusion of a specified substance or drug is administered for therapy, prophylaxis, or diagnosis. An intravenous line is placed into a vein, usually in the arm, and the specified substance or drug is administered. The physician provides direct supervision of the administration and is immediately available to intervene should complications arise. The physician provides periodic assessments of the patient and documentation of the patient's response to treatment. Use code 96365 for an intravenous infusion up to 1 hour. Use add-on code 96366 for each additional hour of the same infusion. Use add-on code 96367 for another, sequential infusion of a different substance or drug for up to 1 hour. Use add-on code 96368 when a different substance or drug is administered at the same time as another drug in a concurrent infusion.

RVUs

Code	Work	PE	PE Non-Facility	MP	Total Non-Facility	Total Facility	Global
96365	0.21	1.75	1.75	0.04	2.00	2.00	XXX
96366	0.18	0.43	0.43	0.01	0.62	0.62	ZZZ
96367	0.19	0.68	0.68	0.02	0.89	0.89	ZZZ
96368	0.17	0.42	0.42	0.01	0.60	0.60	ZZZ

96372

96372 Therapeutic, prophylactic, or diagnostic injection (specify substance or drug); subcutaneous or intramuscular

(For administration of vaccines/toxoids, see 90460, 90461, 90471, 90472, 0001A, 0002A, 0003A, 0011A, 0012A, 0013A, 0021A, 0022A, 0031A, 0041A, 0042A)

(Report 96372 for non-antineoplastic hormonal therapy injections)

(Report 96401 for anti-neoplastic nonhormonal injection therapy)

(Report 96402 for anti-neoplastic hormonal injection therapy)

(For intradermal cancer immunotherapy injection, see 0708T, 0709T)

(Do not report 96372 for injections given without direct physician or other qualified health care professional supervision. To report, use 99211. Hospitals may report 96372 when the physician or other qualified health care professional is not present)

(96372 does not include injections for allergen immunotherapy. For allergen immunotherapy injections, see 95115-95117)

Plain English Description

A subcutaneous or intramuscular injection of a therapeutic, prophylactic, or diagnostic substance or drug is given. A subcutaneous injection is administered just under the skin in the fatty tissue of the abdomen, upper arm, upper leg, or buttocks. The skin is cleansed. A 2-inch fold of skin is pinched between the thumb and forefinger. The needle is inserted completely under the skin at a 45- to 90-degree angle using a quick, sharp thrust. The plunger is retracted to check for blood. If blood is present, a new site is selected. If no blood is present, the medication is injected slowly into the tissue. The needle is withdrawn and mild pressure is applied. An intramuscular injection is administered in a similar fashion deep into muscle tissue, differing only in the sites of administration and the angle of needle insertion. Common sites include the gluteal muscles of the buttocks, the vastus lateralis muscle of the thigh, or the deltoid muscle of the upper arm. The angle of insertion is 90 degrees. Intramuscular administration provides rapid systemic absorption and can be used for administration of relatively large doses of medication.

RVUs

Code	Work	PE	PE Non-Facility	MP	Total Non-Facility	Total Facility	Global
96372	0.17	0.24	0.24	0.01	0.42	0.42	XXX

96373

96373 Therapeutic, prophylactic, or diagnostic injection (specify substance or drug); intra-arterial

Plain English Description

An intra-arterial injection of a therapeutic, prophylactic, or diagnostic substance or drug is given. Intra-arterial injection delivers medication directly to an artery or organ. Very few medications are delivered into an artery. The arterial site is identified and the skin is cleansed. The artery is punctured and the specified substance or drug is injected.

RVUs

Code	Work	PE	PE Non-Facility	MP	Total Non-Facility	Total Facility	Global
96373	0.17	0.35	0.35	0.01	0.53	0.53	XXX

96374-96376

96374 **Therapeutic, prophylactic, or diagnostic injection (specify substance or drug); intravenous push, single or initial substance/drug**

✚ 96375 **Therapeutic, prophylactic, or diagnostic injection (specify substance or drug); each additional sequential intravenous push of a new substance/drug (List separately in addition to code for primary procedure)**

(Use 96375 in conjunction with 96365, 96374, 96409, 96413)

(Report 96375 to identify intravenous push of a new substance/drug if provided as a secondary or subsequent service after a different initial service is administered through the same IV access)

✚ 96376 **Therapeutic, prophylactic, or diagnostic injection (specify substance or drug); each additional sequential intravenous push of the same substance/drug provided in a facility (List separately in addition to code for primary procedure)**

(Do not report 96376 for a push performed within 30 minutes of a reported push of the same substance or drug)

(96376 may be reported by facilities only)

(Report 96376 in conjunction with 96365, 96374, 96409, 96413)

Plain English Description

A therapeutic, prophylactic, or diagnostic injection is administered by intravenous push (IVP) technique. The specified substance or drug is injected using a syringe directly into an injection site of an existing intravenous line or intermittent infusion set (saline lock). The injection is given over a short period of time, usually less than 15 minutes. Use 96374 for a single or initial substance or drug. Use 96375 as an add-on code for each additional sequential push of a new substance or drug provided through the same venous access site. Use 96376 for the facility component for each additional sequential intravenous push of the same substance/drug when the interval between each administration is 30 minutes or more.

RVUs

Code	Work	PE	PE Non-Facility	MP	Total Non-Facility	Total Facility	Global
96374	0.18	0.96	0.96	0.02	1.16	1.16	XXX
96375	0.10	0.36	0.36	0.01	0.47	0.47	ZZZ
96376	0.00	0.00	0.00	0.00	0.00	0.00	ZZZ

97802

★ 97802 **Medical nutrition therapy; initial assessment and intervention, individual, face-to-face with the patient, each 15 minutes**

Plain English Description

A registered dietician (RD) provides medical nutrition therapy (MNT) to an individual. In 97802, initial assessment and intervention is provided to an individual in a face-to-face encounter. During the initial assessment, the RD determines the need for therapy, develops a plan, and determines how the therapy will be provided. A detailed medical history is obtained of all acute and chronic illnesses and other conditions. A psychosocial assessment is also performed including economic status, ethnic and cultural background, education level, occupation, and mental status. The RD determines whether the patient has access to the foods required to maintain health. Handicaps are noted, specifically those affecting the ability to obtain and/or prepare food. A list of current medications, including all vitamin, mineral, and herbal supplements, is obtained and reviewed for interactions between food and medications, particularly adverse reactions related to nutrient absorption and excretion. Vitamin and mineral supplements are also evaluated to determine whether they are adequate or if toxic levels of supplements are being used. A diet history is obtained including number of meals per day and what the patient eats in a typical 24-hour period. Food preparation techniques may also be evaluated to determine the amount of sodium or fat consumed each day. The patient may be asked to rate appetite from poor to good. Any taste alterations, food allergies, or religious restrictions are noted as are chewing or swallowing difficulties and bowel habits. A physical examination is performed including height, weight, body mass index, and arm or wrist circumference. Any recent weight changes are noted. The appearance of hair, skin, and nails is also evaluated for evidence of nutritional deficiencies. The RD then develops a nutrition therapy plan that addresses the patient's needs. Initial MNT is reported per 15-min interval.

RVUs

Code	Work	PE	PE Non-Facility	MP	Total Non-Facility	Total Facility	Global
97802	0.53	0.40	0.53	0.02	1.08	0.95	XXX

97803-97804

★ 97803 **Medical nutrition therapy; re-assessment and intervention, individual, face-to-face with the patient, each 15 minutes**

★ 97804 **Medical nutrition therapy; group (2 or more individual(s)), each 30 minutes**

(Physicians and other qualified health care professionals who may report evaluation and management services should use the appropriate evaluation and management codes)

Plain English Description

In 97803, a registered dietician (RD) provides medical nutrition therapy (MNT) re-assessment and intervention to an individual in a face-to-face encounter. The RD evaluates the effectiveness of the previously developed nutrition therapy plan. The patient is weighed. If the patient has been keeping a daily food diary, it is reviewed. Changes to the diet are suggested. The RD may provide food and recipe suggestions to help the patient meet nutritional needs. Re-assessment is reported per 15-min interval. In 97804, MNT is provided in a group setting of two or more individuals, usually for patients with similar health problems, such as diabetes or renal disease. Nutrition and lifestyle of each individual is evaluated. Ongoing nutrition counseling is provided along with counseling related to managing lifestyle factors affecting diet and exercise. The patient's progress in managing specific dietary needs is monitored. Group MNT is reported per patient per 30-min interval.

RVUs

Code	Work	PE	PE Non-Facility	MP	Total Non-Facility	Total Facility	Global
97803	0.45	0.34	0.47	0.02	0.94	0.81	XXX
97804	0.25	0.19	0.24	0.01	0.50	0.45	XXX

98960-98962

- ★ **98960 Education and training for patient self-management by a qualified, nonphysician health care professional using a standardized curriculum, face-to-face with the patient (could include caregiver/family) each 30 minutes; individual patient**
- ★ **98961 Education and training for patient self-management by a qualified, nonphysician health care professional using a standardized curriculum, face-to-face with the patient (could include caregiver/family) each 30 minutes; 2-4 patients**
- ★ **98962 Education and training for patient self-management by a qualified, nonphysician health care professional using a standardized curriculum, face-to-face with the patient (could include caregiver/family) each 30 minutes; 5-8 patients**

Plain English Description

A physician or other health care professional provides education and training to a patient on how to manage a disease, injury, or other health problem. Family members of the patient or other caregivers may also be present. The instruction is based on a standard curriculum, though it may be modified slightly as circumstances dictate. Code 98961 if the education session is given to 2-4 patients at the same time, and 98962 if 5-8 patients are present.

RVUs

Code	Work	PE	PE Non-Facility	MP	Total Non-Facility	Total Facility	Global
98960	0.00	0.81	0.81	0.04	0.85	0.85	XXX
98961	0.00	0.39	0.39	0.01	0.40	0.40	XXX
98962	0.00	0.29	0.29	0.01	0.30	0.30	XXX

98966-98968

- **98966 Telephone assessment and management service provided by a qualified nonphysician health care professional to an established patient, parent, or guardian not originating from a related assessment and management service provided within the previous 7 days nor leading to an assessment and management service or procedure within the next 24 hours or soonest available appointment; 5-10 minutes of medical discussion**
- **98967 Telephone assessment and management service provided by a qualified nonphysician health care professional to an established patient, parent, or guardian not originating from a related assessment and management service provided within the previous 7 days nor leading to an assessment and management service or procedure within the next 24 hours or soonest available appointment; 11-20 minutes of medical discussion**
- **98968 Telephone assessment and management service provided by a qualified nonphysician health care professional to an established patient, parent, or guardian not originating from a related assessment and management service provided within the previous 7 days nor leading to an assessment and management service or procedure within the next 24 hours or soonest available appointment; 21-30 minutes of medical discussion**

(Do not report 98966-98968 during the same month with 99426, 99427, 99439, 99487, 99489, 99490, 99491)

(Do not report 98966, 98967, 98968 in conjunction with 93792, 93793)

Plain English Description

An established patient, parent, or guardian initiates a telephone conversation that results in a telephone assessment and management service provided by a qualified nonphysician health care professional, such as a registered dietician, physical therapist, occupational therapist, or speech-language pathologist. The phone call is not related to any previous face-to-face assessment and management service within the last 7 days prior to the telephone service nor does it lead to a subsequent face-to-face assessment and management service within the following 24 hours or the soonest available urgent care appointment. The telephone assessment and management service are also not performed during the post-operative period of a related surgical procedure. During the telephone conversation, the qualified nonphysician health care professional listens to the patient's complaints and concerns, answers questions, requests additional related information, provides counseling and instruction as needed, and modifies the treatment plan, if necessary. The conversation is documented in the medical record and the amount of time spent conversing with the patient is noted. Use 98966 for a medical discussion lasting 5-10 minutes, 98967 for 11-20 minutes, and 98968 for 21-30 minutes.

RVUs

Code	Work	PE	PE Non-Facility	MP	Total Non-Facility	Total Facility	Global
98966	0.25	0.07	0.12	0.01	0.38	0.33	XXX
98967	0.50	0.12	0.18	0.02	0.70	0.64	XXX
98968	0.75	0.14	0.20	0.04	0.99	0.93	XXX

98970-98972

98970 Qualified nonphysician health care professional online digital assessment and management, for an established patient, for up to 7 days, cumulative time during the 7 days; 5-10 minutes

98971 Qualified nonphysician health care professional online digital assessment and management, for an established patient, for up to 7 days, cumulative time during the 7 days; 11-20 minutes

98972 Qualified nonphysician health care professional online digital assessment and management, for an established patient, for up to 7 days, cumulative time during the 7 days; 21 or more minutes

(Report 98970, 98971, 98972 once per 7-day period)

(Do not report online digital E/M services for cumulative visit time less than 5 minutes)

(Do not count 98970, 98971, 98972 time otherwise reported with other services)

(Do not report 98970, 98971, 98972 for home and outpatient INR monitoring when reporting 93792, 93793)

(Do not report 98970, 98971, 98972 when using 99091, 99339, 99340, 99374, 99375, 99377, 99378, 99379, 99380, 99426, 99427, 99437, 99439, 99487, 99489, 99490, 99491, for the same communication[s])

Plain English Description

An established patient initiates an online (e-mail, EHR portal, or similar) electronic communication encounter that results in digital evaluation and management services that require decision making provided by a qualified nonphysician health care professional. Examples of qualified nonphysician health care professionals include registered dietician, physical therapist, occupational therapist, and speech-language pathologist. During the digital service the qualified nonphysician professional reviews the patient's initial inquiry with complaints and concerns, answers questions, reviews the patient's record and any other pertinent data, requests additional related information, may collaborate with clinical staff over the patient problem, develops a management or treatment plan, writes prescriptions or orders tests, and provides patient counseling and instruction as needed through communication online, via telephone, email or other digital mode. The online service is documented and stored in the medical record. The digital encounter begins with review of the patient's new inquiry unrelated to any postoperative or previous assessment and management service within the last seven days and is reported by cumulative time spent on the problem in a 7 day period. Report 98970 for 5-10 minutes; 98971 for 11-20 minutes; and 98972 for 21 or more minutes.

RVUs

Code	Work	PE	PE Non-Facility	MP	Total Non-Facility	Total Facility	Global
98970	0.25	0.08	0.08	0.01	0.34	0.34	XXX
98971	0.44	0.13	0.14	0.02	0.60	0.59	XXX
98972	0.69	0.19	0.20	0.04	0.93	0.92	XXX

99000-99001

99000 Handling and/or conveyance of specimen for transfer from the office to a laboratory

99001 Handling and/or conveyance of specimen for transfer from the patient in other than an office to a laboratory (distance may be indicated)

Plain English Description

A specimen is transported from the office (99000) or from another setting (99001) where it was obtained to the laboratory where the requested laboratory study will be performed. Prior to transport, the specimen is stored in the office or other location where it was obtained following the specific protocol for handling of the specimen. The specimen is transported as required by the laboratory protocol designed for the specific specimen, which may include keeping the specimen at a specific temperature (frozen or refrigerated). All safety precautions are adhered to when handling and transporting the specimen.

RVUs

Code	Work	PE	PE Non-Facility	MP	Total Non-Facility	Total Facility	Global
99000	0.00	0.00	0.00	0.00	0.00	0.00	XXX
99001	0.00	0.00	0.00	0.00	0.00	0.00	XXX

99058-99060

99058 Service(s) provided on an emergency basis in the office, which disrupts other scheduled office services, in addition to basic service

99060 Service(s) provided on an emergency basis, out of the office, which disrupts other scheduled office services, in addition to basic service

Plain English Description

The physician or other qualified health care professional provides needed basic procedures or services in an emergency-type situation either within the office (99058) or outside of the office (99060), which causes consequential disruption in the regularly scheduled office routine.

RVUs

Code	Work	PE	PE Non-Facility	MP	Total Non-Facility	Total Facility	Global
99058	0.00	0.00	0.00	0.00	0.00	0.00	XXX
99060	0.00	0.00	0.00	0.00	0.00	0.00	XXX

99151-99153

⊘ **99151 Moderate sedation services provided by the same physician or other qualified health care professional performing the diagnostic or therapeutic service that the sedation supports, requiring the presence of an independent trained observer to assist in the monitoring of the patient's level of consciousness and physiological status; initial 15 minutes of intraservice time, patient younger than 5 years of age**

⊘ **99152 Moderate sedation services provided by the same physician or other qualified health care professional performing the diagnostic or therapeutic service that the sedation supports, requiring the presence of an independent trained observer to assist in the monitoring of the patient's level of consciousness and physiological status; initial 15 minutes of intraservice time, patient age 5 years or older**

✚ **99153 Moderate sedation services provided by the same physician or other qualified health care professional performing the diagnostic or therapeutic service that the sedation supports, requiring the presence of an independent trained observer to assist in the monitoring of the patient's level of consciousness and physiological status; each additional 15 minutes intraservice time (List separately in addition to code for primary service)**

(Use 99153 in conjunction with 99151, 99152)

(Do not report 99153 in conjunction with 99155, 99156)

Plain English Description

Moderate sedation services are provided by the same physician or other qualified health care professional who is performing the diagnostic or therapeutic service requiring the sedation with an independent trained observer to assist in monitoring the patient. A patient assessment is performed. An intravenous line is inserted and fluids are administered as needed. A sedative agent is then administered. The patient is maintained under moderate sedation, with monitoring of the patient's consciousness level and physiological status that includes oxygen saturation, heart rate, and blood pressure. Following completion of the procedure, the physician or other qualified health care professional continues to monitor the patient until the patient has recovered from the sedation and can be turned over to nursing staff for continued care. Use 99151 for the first 15 minutes of intraservice time for a patient younger than 5 years old; 99152 for the first 15 minutes of intraservice time for a patient age 5 years or older; and 99153 for each additional 15 minutes.

RVUs

Code	Work	PE	PE Non-Facility	MP	Total Non-Facility	Total Facility	Global
99151	0.50	0.19	1.52	0.04	2.06	0.73	XXX
99152	0.25	0.08	1.22	0.04	1.51	0.37	XXX
99153	0.00	0.30	0.30	0.02	0.32	0.32	ZZZ

99155-99157

99155 Moderate sedation services provided by a physician or other qualified health care professional other than the physician or other qualified health care professional performing the diagnostic or therapeutic service that the sedation supports; initial 15 minutes of intraservice time, patient younger than 5 years of age

99156 Moderate sedation services provided by a physician or other qualified health care professional other than the physician or other qualified health care professional performing the diagnostic or therapeutic service that the sedation supports; initial 15 minutes of intraservice time, patient age 5 years or older

✚ **99157 Moderate sedation services provided by a physician or other qualified health care professional other than the physician or other qualified health care professional performing the diagnostic or therapeutic service that the sedation supports; each additional 15 minutes intraservice time (List separately in addition to code for primary service)**

(Use 99157 in conjunction with 99155, 99156)

(Do not report 99157 in conjunction with 99151, 99152)

Plain English Description

Moderate sedation services are provided by a physician or other qualified health care professional other than the one performing the diagnostic or therapeutic service requiring the sedation. A patient assessment is performed. An intravenous line is inserted and fluids are administered as needed. A sedative agent is then administered. The patient is maintained under moderate sedation, with monitoring of the patient's consciousness level and physiological status that includes oxygen saturation, heart rate, and blood pressure. Following completion of the procedure, the physician or other qualified health care professional continues to monitor the patient until the patient has recovered from the sedation and can be turned over to nursing staff for continued care. Use 99155 for the first 15 minutes of intraservice time for a patient younger than 5 years old; 99156 for the first 15 minutes of intraservice time for a patient age 5 years or older; and 99157 for each additional 15 minutes.

RVUs

Code	Work	PE	PE Non-Facility	MP	Total Non-Facility	Total Facility	Global
99155	1.90	0.32	0.32	0.21	2.43	2.43	XXX
99156	1.65	0.40	0.40	0.18	2.23	2.23	XXX
99157	1.25	0.46	0.46	0.11	1.82	1.82	ZZZ

0421T

0421T Transurethral waterjet ablation of prostate, including control of post-operative bleeding, including ultrasound guidance, complete (vasectomy, meatotomy, cystourethroscopy, urethral calibration and/or dilation, and internal urethrotomy are included when performed)

(Do not report 0421T in conjunction with 52500, 52630, 76872)

Plain English Description

A procedure is performed using water-jet hydrodissection (aqua ablation) to treat benign prostatic hypertrophy (BPH) with lower urinary tract symptoms (LUTS) of bladder outlet obstruction. Transrectal ultrasound imaging is used to map the target area and the surgeon programs a robotic system with precise tissue contours/depth. Using electromechanical control and real-time ultrasound guidance, a high-velocity stream of saline is delivered to the prostate via the urethra, which may require meatotomy, internal urethrotomy, and urethral calibration or dilation for access and successful ablation. The water jet selectively ablates the glandular tissue, which is simultaneously collected for post procedural laboratory analysis. A laser beam captured by a low-pressure water jet may be employed to obtain surface coagulation and hemostasis. Ultrasound guidance and control of post procedural bleeding are included as well as vasectomy and cystourethroscopy, when performed.

RVUs

Code	Work	PE	PE Non-Facility	MP	Total Non-Facility	Total Facility	Global
0421T	0.00	0.00	0.00	0.00	0.00	0.00	XXX

0443T

✚ **0443T Real-time spectral analysis of prostate tissue by fluorescence spectroscopy, including imaging guidance (List separately in addition to code for primary procedure)**

(Use 0443T in conjunction with 55700)

(Report 0443T only once per session)

Plain English Description

A procedure is performed to identify malignant prostate tissue using real-time spectral analysis during separately reportable needle or punch prostate biopsy. Fluorescence spectroscopy (FS) analyzes naturally fluorescing endogenous proteins and enzymes in body tissue that scatter signals after undergoing photon-electron stimulation. Since the amount of endogenous fluorophores in prostate tissue differs with disease states, FS is used to help quantify the variation and identify malignant lesions. The FS signals are read by a custom fluorometer interfaced with software to differentiate benign from malignant tissue and provide a histopathological grade to suspected malignant tumors. An optical biopsy needle containing a built-in light sensitive optical probe/sensor with fibers for tissue excitation and collection of the spectral data is advanced into the prostate under FS guidance. The custom fluorometer has light-emitting diodes and spectrometer and reads the acquired spectral data acquired for real-time in vivo prostate cancer diagnosis or recognition of suspicious target areas within the prostate gland, thereby increasing the yield of diagnostic information attained with the biopsy sample.

RVUs

Code	Work	PE	PE Non-Facility	MP	Total Non-Facility	Total Facility	Global
0443T	0.00	0.00	0.00	0.00	0.00	0.00	ZZZ

0487T

0487T Biomechanical mapping, transvaginal, with report

Plain English Description

Transvaginal biomechanical mapping can be used to evaluate soft tissue elasticity and weak or damaged muscles and ligaments that may disrupt pelvic floor support and function. Changes in the pelvic floor structure and function can be caused by advanced age, childbirth, genetics, and neurologic conditions. Changes include muscle weakness, avulsion, connective tissue laxity, and disruption in tissue structure. With the patient in dorsal lithotomy position and bladder and rectum empty, a probe with tactile sensors is inserted into the vagina. The initial insertion provides pressure responses of the anterior and posterior vagina along the entire vaginal length and a computer software program calculates the pressure gradient and anatomical dimensions. The probe is then elevated to capture the pressure responses for the apical, anterior, and posterior compartments that relate to the pelvic floor support structures, and the pressure gradients and anatomical dimensions are calculated and stored. Next, the probe is rotated to obtain pressure readings from the left and right sides of the vagina. The circumferential tactile image of the vaginal walls detects underlying muscle or tissue irregularities, presence of foreign bodies, scar tissue, and hypertonic muscle movement. The pelvic floor muscles are then stimulated with pressure on the lower abdomen by the technician or Valsalva maneuver by the patient to measure dynamic muscle response of the pelvic floor structures. The probe is removed and the data are integrated and analyzed into a mapped report of the vagina and surrounding pelvic floor structures.

RVUs

Code	Work	PE	PE Non-Facility	MP	Total Non-Facility	Total Facility	Global
0487T	0.00	0.00	0.00	0.00	0.00	0.00	XXX

0499T

0499T Cystourethroscopy, with mechanical dilation and urethral therapeutic drug delivery for urethral stricture or stenosis, including fluoroscopy, when performed

(Do not report 0499T in conjunction with 52281, 52283)

Plain English Description

Cystourethroscopy including mechanical dilation and therapeutic urethral drug injection is performed for urethral stricture or stenosis, characterized by narrowing of the urethral lumen due to injury, inflammation, infection, previous interventions (surgery, catheterization, instrumentation, prostate cancer treatment), and congenital or idiopathic etiologies. With the patient prepared and draped in dorsolithotomy position, the cystourethroscope is passed through the urethra into the bladder. Fluoroscopy may also be used to enhance the examination and capture and save images. The bladder is inspected and the scope is then slowly withdrawn, allowing inspection along the length of the urethra. A thin wire is inserted into the urethra and progressively larger dilators are passed over the wire gradually increasing the diameter of the urethral lumen for mechanical dilation. The cystourethroscope is again inserted and the urethra is inspected to identify the targeted tissue for injection. The most common pharmacological agent injected for stricture or stenosis is an anti-proliferative, anti-scar drug. The injection is accomplished through the working port of the cystourethroscope, which is removed at the completion of the procedure.

RVUs

Code	Work	PE	PE Non-Facility	MP	Total Non-Facility	Total Facility	Global
0499T	0.00	0.00	0.00	0.00	0.00	0.00	000

0582T

0582T Transurethral ablation of malignant prostate tissue by high-energy water vapor thermotherapy, including intraoperative imaging and needle guidance

(Do not report 0582T in conjunction with 52000, 72195, 72196, 72197, 76376, 76377, 76872, 76940, 76942, 77021, 77022)

(For transurethral destruction of prostate tissue by radiofrequency-generated water vapor thermotherapy for benign prostatic hypertrophy [BPH], use 53854)

Plain English Description

Transurethral water vapor thermotherapy uses the thermal energy in steam to ablate malignant prostate tissue and help improve accompanying lower urinary tract symptoms. Tissue is ablated in a minimally invasive way using radiofrequency to generate wet thermal energy and employ convective vs.

conductive heat transfer. Most patients are given an oral pain medication/anxiolytic or conscious sedation. A prostate block may also be used. With the patient in the lithotomy position, the hand-held delivery device containing a lens allowing for direct cystoscopic visualization is inserted into the urethra. The needle is positioned within the malignant prostatic tissue of the lateral or median lobes. A generator applies radiofrequency current to the inductive coil within the device and converts a few drops of water into steam. The water vapor is injected into the prostate tissue through the retractable needle that has small emitter holes spaced circumferentially around the tip. The vapor immediately turns back into water, releasing the energy stored in the vapor into the cell membranes, causing instant cell death. The needle is retracted and repositioned after each treatment until the target prostate tissue is ablated. Over time, this ablated tissue is reabsorbed by the body, reducing the volume of tissue and allowing the urethra to open.

RVUs

Code	Work	PE	PE Non-Facility	MP	Total Non-Facility	Total Facility	Global
0582T	0.00	0.00	0.00	0.00	0.00	0.00	YYY

0587T-0588T

0587T Percutaneous implantation or replacement of integrated single device neurostimulation system including electrode array and receiver or pulse generator, including analysis, programming, and imaging guidance when performed, posterior tibial nerve

(Do not report 0587T in conjunction with 64555, 64566, 64575, 64590, 95970, 95971, 95972, 0588T, 0589T, 0590T)

0588T Revision or removal of integrated single device neurostimulation system including electrode array and receiver or pulse generator, including analysis, programming, and imaging guidance when performed, posterior tibial nerve

(Do not report 0588T in conjunction with 64555, 64566, 64575, 64590, 95970, 95971, 95972, 0587T, 0589T, 0590T)

Plain English Description

A percutaneous implanted posterior tibial nerve stimulating device may be used to treat overactive bladder (OAB). OAB is a chronic medical condition affecting the storage of urine and the urge to urinate which may lead to urinary frequency and/or involuntary loss of urine (incontinence). Electrical signals from the nerve stimulator alter the messaging between sympathetic and parasympathetic post-ganglionic nerve terminals and synapses involved with the voiding reflex to facilitate better bladder storage and reduced frequency, urgency, and incontinence. The device consists of an implanted lead/electrode, an external pulse transmitter (EPT) worn externally over the electrode, and a hand held wireless remote control programmed by the physician or other qualified health care professional. Under local anesthesia, the lead/electrode is implanted through a small incision or injected via a delivery system close to the tibial neurovascular bundle just above the ankle. If the injection method is used, ultrasound or active stimulation guidance may be performed to ensure correct positioning. The external pulse transmitter is placed over the lead/electrode to stimulate the target nerve wirelessly from the hand held remote. The physician analyzes and programs the pulse transmitter and remote device to appropriate stimulation settings (0587T). To revise or remove the posterior tibial nerve stimulating device, a small incision is made in the skin over the implanted electrode and the lead is repositioned or removed entirely. Ultrasound or active stimulation guidance may be used to ensure correct repositioning and the transmitter and remote device may then be re-analyzed and programmed by the physician to attain appropriate stimulation settings. (0588T).

RVUs

Code	Work	PE	PE Non-Facility	MP	Total Non-Facility	Total Facility	Global
0587T	0.00	0.00	0.00	0.00	0.00	0.00	YYY
0588T	0.00	0.00	0.00	0.00	0.00	0.00	YYY

0589T-0590T

0589T Electronic analysis with simple programming of implanted integrated neurostimulation system (eg, electrode array and receiver), including contact group(s), amplitude, pulse width, frequency (Hz), on/off cycling, burst, dose lockout, patient-selectable parameters, responsive neurostimulation, detection algorithms, closed-loop parameters, and passive parameters, when performed by physician or other qualified health care professional, posterior tibial nerve, 1-3 parameters

(Do not report 0589T in conjunction with 43647, 43648, 43881, 43882, 61850-61888, 63650, 63655, 63661, 63662, 63663, 63664, 63685, 63688, 64553-64595, 95970, 95971, 95972, 95976, 95977, 95983, 95984, 0587T, 0588T, 0590T)

0590T Electronic analysis with complex programming of implanted integrated neurostimulation system (eg, electrode array and receiver), including contact group(s), amplitude, pulse width, frequency (Hz), on/off cycling, burst, dose lockout, patient-selectable parameters, responsive neurostimulation, detection algorithms, closed-loop parameters, and passive parameters, when performed by physician or other qualified health care professional, posterior tibial nerve, 4 or more parameters

(Do not report 0590T in conjunction with 43647, 43648, 43881, 43882, 61850-61888, 63650, 63655, 63661, 63662, 63663, 63664, 63685, 63688, 64553-64595, 95970, 95971, 95972, 95976, 95977, 95983, 95984, 0587T, 0588T, 0589T)

Plain English Description

An implanted posterior tibial nerve stimulating system is used to treat overactive bladder (OAB). OAB is a chronic medical condition affecting the storage of urine and the urge to urinate which may lead to urinary frequency and/or involuntary loss of urine (incontinence). Electrical signals from the nerve stimulator alter the messaging between sympathetic and parasympathetic post-ganglionic nerve terminals and synapses involved with the voiding reflex to facilitate better bladder storage and reduced frequency, urgency, and incontinence. The device consists of an implanted lead/electrode, an external pulse transmitter (EPT) worn externally over the electrode, and a hand held wireless remote control programmed by the physician or other qualified health care professional. Following implantation, the posterior tibial neurostimulation system is monitored and programmed at regular intervals to find optimal settings for the patient. Monitoring and programming may include contact group(s), amplitude, pulse width, frequency (Hz), on/off cycling, burst, dose lockout, patient-selectable parameters, responsive neurostimulation, algorithm detection, closed loop parameters, and passive parameters. Code 0589T reports electronic analysis with simple (1-3 parameters) programming of the neurostimulation system; code 0590T reports complex programming of 4 or more parameters.

RVUs

Code	Work	PE	PE Non-Facility	MP	Total Non-Facility	Total Facility	Global
0589T	0.00	0.00	0.00	0.00	0.00	0.00	YYY
0590T	0.00	0.00	0.00	0.00	0.00	0.00	YYY

0596T-0597T

0596T Temporary female intraurethral valve-pump (ie, voiding prosthesis); initial insertion, including urethral measurement

0597T Temporary female intraurethral valve-pump (ie, voiding prosthesis); replacement

(Do not report 0596T, 0597T in conjunction with 51610, 51700, 51701, 51702, 51703, 51705)

Plain English Description

The inFlow™ intraurethral valve pump with activator is a temporary urinary prosthesis for use in females 18 years and older who suffer permanent urinary retention due to neurologic impairment of the detrusor muscle. Insufficient detrusor muscle contractility results in the inability to urinate as needed on one's own and leads to other serious urinary complications. The condition is generally incurable, caused by spinal cord injury or disease, and neurologic conditions. The inFlow™ system allows for near normal voiding without assistance, without tubes or urinary bags. The device is replaced every 29 days or less. The physician performs initial insertion with prior device sizing (0596T). The plastic sizing device with gradient markings corresponding to urethral length is inserted and the adjustable tab is moved back until it touches the meatus to determine urethral length. The intraurethral device is 3-7 cm long in a silicone housing with flexible petal-like fins that open to fix the device at the bladder neck and hold it in the urethra. Inside the housing tube is the internal, magnetically activated miniature valve-pump. The device comes with a disposable introducer and insertion of the device is similar to a urinary catheter. The other component of the system is a hand held remote control activator that operates the valve pump and is placed on a charger. The user holds the remote control activator over her pelvis and presses the button down to activate the small magnetic pump and empty the bladder. When the button is released, urine flow is stopped. When it's time for replacement, the device is removed by simply grasping the external tab and pulling it out. Report 0597T for replacement of the device (which may also be done by a trained caregiver at home).

RVUs

Code	Work	PE	PE Non-Facility	MP	Total Non-Facility	Total Facility	Global
0596T	0.00	0.00	0.00	0.00	0.00	0.00	YYY
0597T	0.00	0.00	0.00	0.00	0.00	0.00	YYY

0602T-0603T

0602T Glomerular filtration rate (GFR) measurement(s), transdermal, including sensor placement and administration of a single dose of fluorescent pyrazine agent

0603T Glomerular filtration rate (GFR) monitoring, transdermal, including sensor placement and administration of more than one dose of fluorescent pyrazine agent, each 24 hours

(Do not report 0603T in conjunction with 0602T)

Plain English Description

Glomerular filtration rate (GFR) measurement (0602T) or monitoring (0603T) is done in a noninvasive way through a transdermal sensor device to check kidney function, monitor kidney disease, or prevent a staging misdiagnosis of kidney disease. The estimated GFR rate is current clinical practice for monitoring renal function, but calculation of eGFR requires a blood draw and is dependent on serum creatinine concentration, which can be affected by many different factors or may not reflect abnormally in a timely manner, making the calculation less than optimal or even unusable. Point of care measurement (not estimation) of GFR is a valuable tool, particularly as real time measurements can be made as the tracer is cleared by glomerular filtration. The sensor site is prepared by cleansing and shaving, and the sensor is attached to the skin surface with medical grade two-sided adhesive. The fluorescent pyrazine tracer agent is administered in a single dose (0602T) for GFR measurement as an intravenous bolus injection, or multiple doses, each 24 hours (0603T) for longer monitoring. The tracer then distributes into the extracellular space before being cleared by the kidneys. The length of time that monitoring can be done after tracer administration depends on kidney health. The transdermal sensor contains a fiber optic bundle consisting of closely packed arrays of light source and detection fibers with a prism used to collect the backscattered light source and the fluorescent light emitted from the tracer, which is detected, amplified, and converted from analog to digital readout with custom software as the tracer is cleared.

RVUs

Code	Work	PE	PE Non-Facility	MP	Total Non-Facility	Total Facility	Global
0602T	0.00	0.00	0.00	0.00	0.00	0.00	YYY
0603T	0.00	0.00	0.00	0.00	0.00	0.00	YYY

0619T

0619T Cystourethroscopy with transurethral anterior prostate commissurotomy and drug delivery, including transrectal ultrasound and fluoroscopy, when performed

(Do not report 0619T in conjunction with 52000, 52441, 52442, 52450, 52500, 52601, 52630, 52640, 52647, 52648, 52649, 53850, 53852, 53854, 76872, 0499T)

Plain English Description

Transurethral anterior prostatic commissurotomy (TUAP) is a minimally invasive technique used to treat urinary symptoms caused by benign prostatic hypertrophy (BPH). A scope that combines visual and surgical capabilities is threaded up the urethra to the bladder and the area where the prostate surrounds the urethra is visualized. The instrument may generate electrical current or laser energy and one or two small grooves are cut into the area where the prostate and the bladder are connected, dividing the anterior prostatic commissure and the bladder neck while sparing mucosa. Cutting the musculature relaxes the bladder opening and decompresses the urethra. Resistance is decreased and the urinary channel is opened, which allows urine to pass more easily. A drug to keep the urinary channel open is then delivered to the prostatic urethra through the catheter. A new system known as the Optilume ™ BPH catheter system makes it possible to achieve prostate resection-type results and perform the commissurotomy without cutting, burning, vaporizing, or lasering. A predilation balloon catheter is passed through the urethra and performs TUAP by exerting radial force to dilate the prostatic urethra, resulting in a commissurotomy that alleviates obstruction. A drug-coated balloon tipped catheter is introduced with a proprietary coating of paclitaxel, a drug used to maintain the newly divided tissue open. When the balloon is inflated, the drug gets transferred onto the lining of the urethra.

RVUs

Code	Work	PE	PE Non-Facility	MP	Total Non-Facility	Total Facility	Global
0619T	0.00	0.00	0.00	0.00	0.00	0.00	YYY

0655T

● **0655T Transperineal focal laser ablation of malignant prostate tissue, including transrectal imaging guidance, with MR-fused images or other enhanced ultrasound imaging**

(Do not report 0655T in conjunction with 52000, 76376, 76377, 76872, 76940, 76942, 76998)

Plain English Description

Focal laser ablation (FLA) delivers targeted laser energy for thermal destruction of malignant prostate tissue while sparing the rest of the gland. FLA is a minimally invasive, outpatient procedure with a lower risk of side effects that can be repeated in the future. The tissue absorbs the light energy, inducing heat within a few seconds. Temperature, heat transfer duration, and the depth of light distribution help determine the wavelength of the laser. A Foley catheter is placed. An ultrasound probe is inserted into the rectum, generally under IV sedation with a local anesthetic. A catheter is inserted percutaneously through the perineum to deliver an optical fiber with diffusing tip and diode laser surrounded by a cooling system, which is attached to a flow circuit of room-temperature sterile saline. Using contrast enhanced ultrasonography or 3D ultrasound guided by MRI-fused images, the laser fiber is guided to the exact location of the cancerous area. The laser is first activated at a reduced power level to verify proper placement and then treatment is initiated. Tissue necrosis is montored closely in real time as well as temperature around the treatment region. The system terminates laser delivery if temperatures at critical structures reaches the assigned limit. At the conclusion, the Foley catheter is removed and the patient is monitored before being discharged.

RVUs

Code	Work	PE	PE Non-Facility	MP	Total Non-Facility	Total Facility	Global
0655T	0.00	0.00	0.00	0.00	0.00	0.00	YYY

0672T

● **0672T Endovaginal cryogen-cooled, monopolar radiofrequency remodeling of the tissues surrounding the female bladder neck and proximal urethra for urinary incontinence**

Plain English Description

Endovaginal cryogen-cooled, monopolar radiofrequency tissue remodeling is a non-invasive, dual-energy treatment for urethral hypermobility and stress urinary incontinency in females. The Viveve System applies uniform heat to deeper tissues while simultaneously cooling and protecting surface tissue to stimulate new collagen formation in just one office session. Rebuilding natural collagen restores tissue support for the urethra and improves incontinence. The system consists of the main console, sterile single-use treatment tips and special coupling gel used only with the Viveve system, and a return pad with electrode for grounding. The pad is placed in direct contact with a clean, dry area of skin appropriate for grounding the treatment area, such as the upper outer thigh for treating the pelvic floor. The coupling fluid is applied to the treatment area and the tip regularly throughout treatment for good electrical contact to deliver the radiofrequency (RF) energy safely. The treatment tip is placed in good contact with the treatment surface area and RF energy is delivered to the target area for a total of 5 passes along with an overlapping area of about 50% more or 0.5 cm to ensure good coverage. The patient can then resume normal activities per her health care provider and personal tolerance of the procedure.

RVUs

Code	Work	PE	PE Non-Facility	MP	Total Non-Facility	Total Facility	Global
0672T	0.00	0.00	0.00	0.00	0.00	0.00	YYY

A4311

ⓘ⚕A4311 Insertion tray without drainage bag with indwelling catheter, foley type, two-way latex with coating (teflon, silicone, silicone elastomer or hydrophilic, etc.)

RVUs

Global: XXX

	Work	PE	MP	Total
Facility	0.00	0.00	0.00	0.00
Non-facility	0.00	0.00	0.00	0.00

Modifiers (PAR)

Mod 50	Mod 51	Mod 62	Mod 80
9	9	9	9

CCI Edits

Refer to Appendix A for CCI edits.

A4312

ⓘ⚕A4312 Insertion tray without drainage bag with indwelling catheter, foley type, two-way, all silicone

RVUs

Global: XXX

	Work	PE	MP	Total
Facility	0.00	0.00	0.00	0.00
Non-facility	0.00	0.00	0.00	0.00

Modifiers (PAR)

Mod 50	Mod 51	Mod 62	Mod 80
9	9	9	9

CCI Edits

Refer to Appendix A for CCI edits.

A4313

ⓘ⚕A4313 Insertion tray without drainage bag with indwelling catheter, foley type, three-way, for continuous irrigation

RVUs

Global: XXX

	Work	PE	MP	Total
Facility	0.00	0.00	0.00	0.00
Non-facility	0.00	0.00	0.00	0.00

Modifiers (PAR)

Mod 50	Mod 51	Mod 62	Mod 80
9	9	9	9

CCI Edits

Refer to Appendix A for CCI edits.

A4314

ⓘ⚕A4314 Insertion tray with drainage bag with indwelling catheter, foley type, two-way latex with coating (teflon, silicone, silicone elastomer or hydrophilic, etc.)

RVUs

Global: XXX

	Work	PE	MP	Total
Facility	0.00	0.00	0.00	0.00
Non-facility	0.00	0.00	0.00	0.00

Modifiers (PAR)

Mod 50	Mod 51	Mod 62	Mod 80
9	9	9	9

CCI Edits

Refer to Appendix A for CCI edits.

A4315

ⓘ⚕A4315 Insertion tray with drainage bag with indwelling catheter, foley type, two-way, all silicone

RVUs

Global: XXX

	Work	PE	MP	Total
Facility	0.00	0.00	0.00	0.00
Non-facility	0.00	0.00	0.00	0.00

Modifiers (PAR)

Mod 50	Mod 51	Mod 62	Mod 80
9	9	9	9

CCI Edits

Refer to Appendix A for CCI edits.

A4316

ⓘ⚕A4316 Insertion tray with drainage bag with indwelling catheter, foley type, three-way, for continuous irrigation

RVUs

Global: XXX

	Work	PE	MP	Total
Facility	0.00	0.00	0.00	0.00
Non-facility	0.00	0.00	0.00	0.00

Modifiers (PAR)

Mod 50	Mod 51	Mod 62	Mod 80
9	9	9	9

CCI Edits

Refer to Appendix A for CCI edits.

A4338

ⓘ⚲A4338 Indwelling catheter; foley type, two-way latex with coating (teflon, silicone, silicone elastomer, or hydrophilic, etc.), each

RVUs

Global: XXX

	Work	PE	MP	Total
Facility	0.00	0.00	0.00	0.00
Non-facility	0.00	0.00	0.00	0.00

Modifiers (PAR)

Mod 50	Mod 51	Mod 62	Mod 80
9	9	9	9

Pub 100

A4338: Pub 100-04, 20, 110.2, 130.1 ; Pub 100-04, 20, 130.1

CCI Edits

Refer to Appendix A for CCI edits.

A4340

ⓘ⚲A4340 Indwelling catheter; specialty type, (e.g., coude, mushroom, wing, etc.), each

RVUs

Global: XXX

	Work	PE	MP	Total
Facility	0.00	0.00	0.00	0.00
Non-facility	0.00	0.00	0.00	0.00

Modifiers (PAR)

Mod 50	Mod 51	Mod 62	Mod 80
9	9	9	9

CCI Edits

Refer to Appendix A for CCI edits.

A4344

ⓘ⚲A4344 Indwelling catheter, foley type, two-way, all silicone, each

RVUs

Global: XXX

	Work	PE	MP	Total
Facility	0.00	0.00	0.00	0.00
Non-facility	0.00	0.00	0.00	0.00

Modifiers (PAR)

Mod 50	Mod 51	Mod 62	Mod 80
9	9	9	9

CCI Edits

Refer to Appendix A for CCI edits.

A4351

ⓘ⚲A4351 Intermittent urinary catheter; straight tip, with or without coating (teflon, silicone, silicone elastomer, or hydrophilic, etc.), each

RVUs

Global: XXX

	Work	PE	MP	Total
Facility	0.00	0.00	0.00	0.00
Non-facility	0.00	0.00	0.00	0.00

Modifiers (PAR)

Mod 50	Mod 51	Mod 62	Mod 80
9	9	9	9

CCI Edits

Refer to Appendix A for CCI edits.

A4352

ⓘ⚲A4352 Intermittent urinary catheter; coude (curved) tip, with or without coating (teflon, silicone, silicone elastomeric, or hydrophilic, etc.), each

RVUs

Global: XXX

	Work	PE	MP	Total
Facility	0.00	0.00	0.00	0.00
Non-facility	0.00	0.00	0.00	0.00

Modifiers (PAR)

Mod 50	Mod 51	Mod 62	Mod 80
9	9	9	9

CCI Edits

Refer to Appendix A for CCI edits.

A4358

ⓘ⚲A4358 Urinary drainage bag, leg or abdomen, vinyl, with or without tube, with straps, each

RVUs

Global: XXX

	Work	PE	MP	Total
Facility	0.00	0.00	0.00	0.00
Non-facility	0.00	0.00	0.00	0.00

Modifiers (PAR)

Mod 50	Mod 51	Mod 62	Mod 80
9	9	9	9

CCI Edits

Refer to Appendix A for CCI edits.

G0102

ⓘ♂G0102 Prostate cancer screening; digital rectal examination

RVUs

Global: XXX

	Work	PE	MP	Total
Facility	0.18	0.07	0.01	0.26
Non-facility	0.18	0.49	0.01	0.68

Modifiers (PAR)

Mod 50	Mod 51	Mod 62	Mod 80
9	9	9	9

Pub 100

G0102: Pub 100-04, 18, 1.2, 50.3, 50.3.1, 50.4

CCI Edits

Refer to Appendix A for CCI edits.

G0103

ⓘ♂G0103 Prostate cancer screening; prostate specific antigen test (psa)

RVUs

Global: XXX

	Work	PE	MP	Total
Facility	0.00	0.00	0.00	0.00
Non-facility	0.00	0.00	0.00	0.00

Modifiers (PAR)

Mod 50	Mod 51	Mod 62	Mod 80
9	9	9	9

Pub 100

G0103: Pub 100-04, 18, 1.2, 50.3, 50.4

CCI Edits

Refer to Appendix A for CCI edits.

G0491

G0491 Dialysis procedure at a medicare certified esrd facility for acute kidney injury without esrd

RVUs

Global: XXX

	Work	PE	MP	Total
Facility	0.00	0.00	0.00	0.00
Non-facility	0.00	0.00	0.00	0.00

Modifiers (PAR)

Mod 50	Mod 51	Mod 62	Mod 80
9	9	9	9

CCI Edits

Refer to Appendix A for CCI edits.

G0492

G0492 Dialysis procedure with single evaluation by a physician or other qualified health care professional for acute kidney injury without esrd

RVUs

Global: XXX

	Work	PE	MP	Total
Facility	0.00	0.00	0.00	0.00
Non-facility	0.00	0.00	0.00	0.00

Modifiers (PAR)

Mod 50	Mod 51	Mod 62	Mod 80
9	9	9	9

CCI Edits

Refer to Appendix A for CCI edits.

Modifiers

The CPT® code selected must be the one that most closely describes the service(s) and/or procedure(s) documented by the physician. However, sometimes certain services or procedures go above and beyond the definition of the assigned CPT code definition and require further clarification. For these and other reasons, modifiers were developed and implemented by the American Medical Association (AMA), the Centers for Medicare & Medicaid Services (CMS), and local Part B Medicare Administrative Contractors (MACs). These modifiers give health care providers a way to indicate that a service or procedure has been modified by some circumstance but still meets the code definition. Modifiers were designed to expand on the information already provided by the current CPT coding system and to assist in the prompt processing of claims. A CPT modifier is a two-digit numeric character reported with the appropriate CPT code, and is intended to transfer specific information regarding a certain procedure or service.

Modifiers are used to ensure payment accuracy, coding consistency, and editing under the outpatient prospective payment system (OPPS), and are also mandated for private practitioners (solo and multiple), ambulatory surgery centers (ASCs), and other outpatient hospital services.

Modifier Usage

Modifiers are indicated when:

- A service/procedure contains a professional and technical component but only one is applicable
- A service/procedure was performed by more than one physician and/or in more than one location
- The service reported was increased or decreased from that of the original definition
- Unusual events occurred during the service/procedure
- A service/procedure was performed more than once
- A bilateral procedure was performed
- Only part of a service was performed
- An adjunctive service was performed

If a modifier is to be utilized, the following must be documented in the patient's medical record:

- The special circumstances indicating the need to add that modifier
- All pertinent information and an adequate definition of the service/procedure performed supporting the use of the assigned modifier

CPT Modifiers

CPT modifiers are attached to the end of the appropriate CPT code. For professional services, modifiers will be reported as an attachment to the CPT code as reported on the CMS-1500 form, and for outpatient services, modifiers will be reported as an attachment to the CPT code as reported in the UB-04 form locator FL 44.

Some modifiers are strictly informational:

- Modifier 57, identifying a decision for surgery at the time of an evaluation and management service

Other modifiers are informational and indicate additional reimbursement may be warranted:

- Modifier 22, identifying an unusual service that is greater than what is typical for that code

Placement of a modifier after a CPT code does not always ensure additional reimbursement. A special report may be required if the service is rarely provided, unusual, variable, or new. The report should include pertinent information and an adequate definition or description of the nature, extent, and need for the service/procedure. It should also describe the complexity of the patient's symptoms, pertinent history and physical findings, diagnostic and therapeutic procedures, final diagnosis and associated conditions, and follow-up care.

Like CPT codes, the use of modifiers requires understanding of the purpose of each modifier. It is also important to identify when a modifier has been expanded or restricted by a payer prior to submission of a claim. There will also be times when the coding and modifier information issued by the CMS differs from that of CPT's coding guidelines on the usage of modifiers.

Note: For the purposes of this Modifier chapter, payer-specific information is indicated with the symbol ⓘ. It is good to check with individual payers to determine modifier acceptance.

The following is a list of CPT modifiers:

22 Increased Procedural Services

When the work required to provide a service is substantially greater than typically required, it may be identified by adding modifier 22 to the usual procedure code. Documentation must support the substantial additional work and the reason for the additional work (i.e., increased intensity, time, technical difficulty of procedure, severity of patient's condition, physical and mental effort required).

Note: This modifier should not be appended to an E/M service.

ⓘ Claims submitted to Medicare, Medicaid, and other payers containing modifier 22 for unusual procedural services that do not have attached supporting documentation that illustrates the unusual distinction of the services will be processed as if the procedure codes were not appended with this modifier. Some payers might suspend the claims and request additional information from the provider, but this is the exception rather than the rule. For most payers, this modifier includes additional reimbursement to the provider for the additional work.

23 Unusual Anesthesia

Occasionally, a procedure, which usually requires either no anesthesia or local anesthesia, because of unusual circumstances must be done under general anesthesia. This circumstance may be reported by adding modifier 23 to the procedure code of the basic service.

24 Unrelated Evaluation and Management Service by the Same Physician or Other Qualified Health Care Professional During a Postoperative Period

The physician or other qualified health care professional may need to indicate that an evaluation and management service was performed during a postoperative period for a reason(s) unrelated to the original procedure. This circumstance may be reported by adding modifier 24 to the appropriate level of E/M service.

ⓘ By payer definition, a postoperative period is one that has been determined to be included in the payment for the procedure that was performed. During this time, the provider offers treatment for the procedure in follow-up visits, which is not reimbursed. Medicare has postoperative periods for procedures of 0, 10, or 90 days (number of days applicable for each procedure can be found in the Federal Register or Physician Fee Schedule (RBRVS) put out by CMS.) Commercial payers may vary the postoperative days; check with each to determine the appropriate number of days for a given procedure.

25 Significant, Separately Identifiable Evaluation and Management Service by the Same Physician or Other Qualified Health Care Professional on the Same Day of the Procedure or Other Service

It may be necessary to indicate that on the day a procedure or service identified by a CPT code was performed, the patient's condition required a significant, separately identifiable E/M service above and beyond the other service provided or beyond the usual preoperative or postoperative care associated with the procedure that was performed. A significant, separately identifiable E/M service is defined or substantiated by documentation that satisfies the relevant criteria for the respective E/M service to be reported (see **Evaluation and Management Services Guidelines** for instructions on determining level of E/M service). The E/M service may be prompted by the symptom or condition for which the procedure and/or service was provided. As such, different diagnoses are not required for reporting of the E/M service on the same date. This circumstance may be reported by adding modifier 25 to the appropriate level of E/M service.

Note: This modifier is not used to report an E/M service that resulted in a decision to perform surgery. See modifier 57. For significant, separately identifiable non-E/M services, see modifier 59.

ⓘ Modifier 25 Guidelines

1. Modifier 25 should be used only when a visit is separately payable when billed in addition to a minor surgical procedure (any surgery with a 0- or 10-day postoperative period per Medicare). Payment for pre- and postoperative work in minor procedures is included in the payment for the procedure. Where the decision to perform the minor procedure is typically made immediately before the service (e.g., sutures are needed to close a wound), it is considered to be a routine preoperative service and an E/M service should not be billed in addition to the minor procedure. In circumstances in which the physician provides an E/M service that is beyond the usual pre- and postoperative work for the service, the visit may be billed with a modifier 25. A modifier is not needed if the visit was performed the day before a minor surgery because the global period for minor procedures does not include the day prior to the surgery.
2. The global surgery policy does not apply to services of other physicians who may be rendering services during the pre- or postoperative period unless the physician is a member of the same group as the operating physician.
3. The provider must determine if the E/M service for which they are billing is clearly distinct from the surgical service. When the decision to perform the minor procedure is typically done immediately before the procedure is rendered, the visit should not be billed separately.

26 Professional Component

Certain procedures are a combination of a physician or other qualified health care professional component and a technical component. When the physician or other qualified health care professional component is reported separately, the service may be identified by adding modifier 26 to the usual procedure number.

ⓘ To determine which codes have both a professional and technical component for CMS, review the Federal Register and/or the Physician Fee Schedule for a breakdown. Usually commercial payers go along with CMS determinations of professional and technical components. Some CPT codes are already broken down into professional and technical components. Examples of these are:

93005 Electrocardiography, routine ECG with at least 12 leads; tracing only, without interpretation and report (technical component)

93010 Electrocardiography, routine ECG with at least 12 leads; interpretation and report only

Modifier 26 should not be appended to either of the codes because the nomenclature itself has determined that they are already technical or professional components.

32 Mandated Services

Services related to *mandated* consultation and/or related services (e.g., third-party payer, governmental, legislative, or regulatory requirement) may be identified by adding modifier 32 to the basic procedure.

33 Preventive Services

When the primary purpose of the service is the delivery of an evidence based service in accordance with the US Preventive Services Task Force A or B rating in effect and other preventive services identified in preventive services mandates (legislative or regulatory), the service may be identified by adding 33 to the procedure. For separately reported services specifically identified as preventive, the modifier should not be used.

47 Anesthesia by Surgeon

Regional or general anesthesia provided by the surgeon may be reported by adding modifier 47 to the basic service. (This does not include local anesthesia.)

Note: Modifier 47 would not be used as a modifier for the anesthesia procedures.

ⓘ This service is not covered by Medicare and many state Medicaid programs. Commercial payers and managed care organizations may cover this additional service.

50 Bilateral Procedure

Unless otherwise identified in the listings, bilateral procedures that are performed at the same session should be identified by adding modifier 50 to the appropriate 5-digit code.

Note: This modifier should not be appended to designated "add-on" codes (see Appendix D*).

ⓘ Reported as a one-line item for Medicare claims with modifier 50 appended to the end of the code. Some carriers or payers may request that bilateral procedures be reported with the LT and RT HCPCS Level II modifiers as two-line items.

51 Multiple Procedures

When multiple procedures, other than E/M Services, Physical Medicine and Rehabilitation services, or provision of supplies (e.g., vaccines), are performed at the same session by the same individual, the primary procedure or service may be reported as listed. The additional procedure(s) or service(s) may be identified by appending modifier 51 to the additional procedure or service code(s).

Note: This modifier should not be appended to designated "add-on" codes (see Appendix D*).

52 Reduced Services

Under certain circumstances a service or procedure is partially reduced or eliminated at the discretion of the physician or other qualified health care professional. Under these circumstances the service provided can be identified by its usual procedure number and the addition of modifier 52, signifying that the service is reduced. This provides a means of reporting reduced services without disturbing the identification of the basic service.

Note: For hospital outpatient reporting of a previously scheduled procedure/service that is partially reduced or cancelled as a result of extenuating circumstances or those that threaten the well-being of the patient prior to or after administration of anesthesia, see modifiers 73 and 74 (see modifiers approved for ASC hospital outpatient use).

ⓘ Procedures reported with modifier 52 are typically billed at a reduced amount. Most payers do not require documentation to support the use of modifier 52 and will reimburse the procedure at a reduced level.

53 Discontinued Procedure

Under certain circumstances, the physician or other qualified health care professional may elect to terminate a surgical or diagnostic procedure. Due to extenuating circumstances or those that threaten the well being of the patient, it may be necessary to indicate that a surgical or diagnostic procedure was started but discontinued. This circumstance may be reported by adding modifier 53 to the code reported by the individual for the discontinued procedure.

Note: This modifier is not used to report the elective cancellation of a procedure prior to the patient's anesthesia induction and/or surgical preparation in the operating suite. For outpatient hospital/ambulatory surgery center (ASC) reporting of a previously scheduled procedure/service that is partially reduced or cancelled as a result of extenuating circumstances or those that threaten the well being of the patient prior to or after administration of anesthesia, see modifiers 73 and 74 (see modifiers approved for ASC hospital outpatient use).

54 Surgical Care Only

When 1 physician or other qualified health care professional performs a surgical procedure and another provides preoperative and/or postoperative management, surgical services may be identified by adding modifier 54 to the usual procedure number.

ⓘ Both claims submitted by the surgeon and the other provider must report the date patient care was assumed and relinquished in block 19 of the CMS-1500 or electronic equivalent. Both the surgeon and the other provider must keep a copy of the written transfer agreement in the patient's medical record. Both providers will use the same CPT code, but they will use different modifiers that identify which portion of care they provided.

55 Postoperative Management Only

When 1 physician or other qualified health care professional performed the postoperative management and another performed the surgical procedure, the postoperative component may be identified by adding modifier 55 to the usual procedure number.

ⓘ Both providers will use the same CPT code, but they will use different modifiers that identify which portion of care they provided.

56 Preoperative Management Only

When 1 physician or other qualified health care professional performed the preoperative care and evaluation and another performed the surgical procedure, the preoperative component may be identified by adding modifier 56 to the usual procedure number.

ⓘ Both providers will use the same CPT code, but will they will use different modifiers that identify which portion of care they provided. Some payers do not allow modifier 56 as by their definition the pre-operative care is included in the surgical component.

57 Decision for Surgery

An evaluation and management service that resulted in the initial decision to perform the surgery may be identified by adding modifier 57 to the appropriate level of E/M service.

ⓘ Major Surgical Procedures

Major Surgery with a global period of 90 days (as defined by Medicare) include the day before and the day of surgery. For example, a visit the day before or the same day could be properly billed in addition to a cholecystotomy if the need for the surgery was found during the encounter. Modifier 57 should be added to the E/M code. Billing for a visit would not be appropriate if the physician was only discussing the upcoming surgical procedure.

Procedures with a 90 day global period are considered to be major surgery, as categorized by CMS. The RBRVS (Resource-Based Relative Value Scale) manual or Federal Register lists the global period for all procedure codes eligible for payment by Medicare.

ⓘ Minor Surgical Procedures

Procedures with a 0 or 10 day global period are considered to be minor or endoscopic surgeries, as categorized by CMS. E/M visits by the same physician on the same day as a minor surgery or endoscopy are included in the payment for the procedure, unless a significant, separately identifiable service is also performed.

58 Staged or Related Procedure or Service by the Same Physician or Other Qualified Health Care Professional During the Postoperative Period

It may be necessary to indicate that the performance of a procedure or service during the postoperative period was: (a) planned or anticipated (staged); (b) more extensive than the original procedure; or (c) for therapy following a diagnostic surgical procedure. This circumstance may be reported by adding modifier 58 to the staged or related procedure.

Note: For treatment of a problem that requires a return to the operating/procedure room (eg, unanticipated clinical condition), see modifier 78.

ⓘ Modifier 58 must be used for purposes of identifying procedures performed by the original physician during the postoperative period of the original procedure, within the constraints of the modifier's definition. These procedures cannot be repeat operations (unless the procedures are more extensive than the original procedure) and cannot be for the treatment of complications requiring a return trip to the operating room.

Modifiers

*Pages in this section refer to the AMA *CPT® 2022 Professional Edition*

The existence of modifier 58 does not negate the global fee concept. Services that are included in CPT as multiple sessions or are defined as including multiple services or events may not be billed with this modifier. This modifier is designed to allow a method of reporting additional, related surgeries that are due to a progression of the disease and are not to be used to avoid global surgery edits applicable to staged procedures.

Modifier 58 should be used on surgical codes only and has no effect on the payment amount. It should not be used with the following codes because the codes are defined as "one or more sessions or stages":

66762	67031	67218
66821	67208	67220
66840	67210	67229

59 Distinct Procedural Service

Under certain circumstances, it may be necessary to indicate that a procedure or service was distinct or independent from other non-E/M services performed on the same day. Modifier 59 is used to identify procedures/services, other than E/M services, that are not normally reported together, but are appropriate under the circumstances. Documentation must support a different session, different procedure or surgery, different site or organ system, separate incision/excision, separate lesions, or separate injury (or area of injury in extensive injuries) not ordinarily encountered or performed on the same day by the same individual. However, when another already established modifier is more appropriate, it should be used rather than modifier 59. Only if no more descriptive modifier is available, and the use of modifier 59 best explains the circumstances, should modifier 59 be used.

Note: Modifier 59 should not be appended to an E/M service. To report a separate and distinct E/M service with a non-E/M service performed on the same date, see modifier 25.

ⓘ Modifier 59 was established to demonstrate that multiple, yet distinct, services were provided to a patient on the same date of service by the same provider. Because distinct procedures or services rendered on the same day by the same physician cannot be easily identified and properly adjudicated by simply listing the CPT procedure codes, modifier 59 assists the payer or Medicare carrier in applying the appropriate reimbursement protocol. If the modifier is not used in these circumstances, services may be denied, with the explanation of benefits stating that the payer does not reimburse for this service because it is part of another service that was performed at the same time.

62 Two Surgeons

When 2 surgeons work together as primary surgeons performing distinct part(s) of a procedure, each surgeon should report his/her distinct operative work by adding modifier 62 to the procedure code and any associated add-on code(s) for that procedure as long as both surgeons continue to work together as primary surgeons. Each surgeon should report the co-surgery once using the same procedure code. If additional procedure(s) (including add-on procedures[s]) are performed during the same surgical session, separate code(s) may also be reported with modifier 62 added.

Note: If a co-surgeon acts as an assistant in the performance of additional procedure(s), other than those reported with the modifier 62, during the same surgical session, those services may be reported using separate procedure code(s) with modifier 80 or modifier 82 added, as appropriate.

ⓘ According to Medicare, payment for the two physicians is based on the two physicians splitting 125% of the allowed charge(s). Check with other payers to determine payment based on this modifier. This modifier should not be confused with modifier 80 (assistant surgeon).

63 Procedure Performed on Infants Less Than 4 kg

Procedures performed on neonates and infants up to a present body weight of 4 kg may involve significantly increased complexity and physician or other qualified health care professional work commonly associated with these patients. This circumstance may be reported by adding modifier 63 to the procedure number.

Note: Unless otherwise designated, this modifier may only be appended to procedures/services listed in the 20100-69990 code series and 92920, 92928, 92953, 92960, 92986, 92987, 92990, 92997, 92998, 93312, 93313, 93314, 93315, 93316, 93317, 93318, 93452, 93505, 93563, 93564, 93568, 93580, 93582, 93590, 93591, 93592, 93593, 93594, 93595, 93596, 93597, 93598, 93615, 93616 from the Medicine/Cardiovascular section. Modifier 63 should not be appended to any CPT codes listed in the **Evaluation and Management Services, Anesthesia, Radiology, Pathology/Laboratory,** or **Medicine** sections (other than those identified above from the Medicine/Cardiovascular section).

66 Surgical Team

Under some circumstances, highly complex procedures (requiring the concomitant services of several physicians or other qualified health care professionals, often of different specialties, plus other highly skilled, specially trained personnel, various types of complex equipment) are carried out under the "surgical team" concept. Such circumstances may be identified by each participating individual with the addition of modifier 66 to the basic procedure number used for reporting services.

ⓘ Each surgeon that participates in the procedure would report the same CPT code with modifier 66. Only surgical CPT codes (10021-69990) should be used with modifier 66 unless otherwise stated by the payer.

76 Repeat Procedure or Service by Same Physician or Other Qualified Health Care Professional

It may be necessary to indicate that a procedure or service was repeated by the same physician or other qualified health care professional subsequent to the original procedure or service. This circumstance may be reported by adding modifier 76 to the repeated procedure or service.

Note: This modifier should not be appended to an E/M service.

77 Repeat Procedure or Service by Another Physician or Other Qualified Health Care Professional

It may be necessary to indicate that a basic procedure or service was repeated by another physician or other qualified health care professional subsequent to the original procedure or service. This circumstance may be reported by adding modifier 77 to the repeated procedure or service.

Note: This modifier should not be appended to an E/M service.

ⓘ Appending this modifier does not guarantee payment of the repeat procedure, but will assist in determining duplicate billings for the procedure.

78 Unplanned Return to the Operating/Procedure Room by the Same Physician or Other Qualified Health Care Professional Following Initial Procedure for a Related Procedure During the Postoperative Period

It may be necessary to indicate that another procedure was performed during the postoperative period of the initial procedure (unplanned procedure following initial procedure). When this procedure is related to the first, and requires the use of an operating/procedure room, it may be reported by adding modifier 78 to the related procedure. (For repeat procedures, see modifier 76.)

ⓘ Medicare includes specific medical and/or surgical care for postoperative complications within the global surgical package and does not allow additional payment. Included in the global surgical package are "additional medical and surgical services required of the surgeon during the postoperative period of the surgery because of complications which do not require additional trips to the operating room."

79 Unrelated Procedure or Service by the Same Physician or Other Qualified Health Care Professional During the Postoperative Period

The individual may need to indicate that the performance of a procedure or service during the postoperative period was unrelated to the original procedure. This circumstance may be reported by using modifier 79. (For repeat procedures on the same day, see modifier 76.)

ⓘ When billing for an unrelated procedure by the same physician during the postoperative period of an original procedure, a new postoperative period will begin with the subsequent procedure. A different ICD-10-CM diagnosis should be indicated on the claim.

80 Assistant Surgeon

Surgical assistant services may be identified by adding modifier 80 to the usual procedure number(s).

ⓘ Some surgical procedures are not eligible for this modifier; check the Medicare physician fee schedule or with other payers to determine payment eligibility

81 Minimum Assistant Surgeon

Minimum surgical assistant services are identified by adding modifier 81 to the usual procedure number.

ⓘ Check with payers to determine if payment is allowed for this modifier.

82 Assistant Surgeon (When Qualified Resident Surgeon Not Available)

The unavailability of a qualified resident surgeon is a prerequisite for use of modifier 82 appended to the usual procedure code number(s).

ⓘ In some hospitals with residency programs, Medicare pays through the medical program or graduate medical education (GME) program. Because of this, they will not reimburse for a resident when they are used as an assistant surgeon. Although under special circumstances, payment may be made if there is a emergent situation that is life-threatening.

90 Reference (Outside) Laboratory

When laboratory procedures are performed by a party other than the treating or reporting physician or other qualified health care professional, the procedure may be identified by adding modifier 90 to the usual procedure number.

ⓘ Check with payers to determine if the provider may bill for the laboratory procedure if not performed by the provider.

91 Repeat Clinical Diagnostic Laboratory Test

In the course of treatment of the patient, it may be necessary to repeat the same laboratory test on the same day to obtain subsequent (multiple) test results. Under these circumstances, the laboratory test performed can be identified by its usual procedure number and the addition of modifier 91.

Note: This modifier may not be used when tests are rerun to confirm initial results; due to testing problems with specimens or equipment; or for any other reason when a normal, one-time, reportable result is all that is required. This modifier may not be used when other code(s) describe a series of test results (eg, glucose tolerance tests, evocative/suppression testing). This modifier may only be used for laboratory test(s) performed more than once on the same day on the same patient.

92 Alternative Laboratory Platform Testing

When laboratory testing is performed using a kit or transportable instrument that wholly or in part consists of a single use, disposable analytical chamber, the service may be identified by adding modifier 92 to the usual laboratory procedure code (HIV testing 86701-86703, and 87389). The test does not require permanent dedicated space, hence by its design may be hand carried or transported to the vicinity of the patient for immediate testing at that site, although location of testing is not in itself determinative of the use of this modifier.

95 Synchronous Telemedicine Service Rendered Via a Real-Time Interactive Audio and Video Telecommunications System

Synchronous telemedicine service is defined as a real-time interaction between a physician or other qualified health care professional and a patient who is located at a distant site from the physician or other qualified health care professional. The totality of the communication of information exchanged between the physician or other qualified health care professional and the patient during the course of the synchronous telemedicine service must be of an amount and nature that would be sufficient to meet the key components and/or requirements of the same services when rendered via a face-to-face interaction. Modifier 95 may only be appended to the services listed in Appendix P*. Appendix P is the list of the CPT codes for services that are typically performed face-to-face, but may be rendered via a real-time (synchronous) interactive audio and video telecommunications system.

96 Habilitative Services

When a service or procedure that may be either habilitative or rehabilitative in nature is provided for habilitative purposes, the physician or other qualified health care professional may add modifier 96 to the service or procedure code to indicate that the service or procedure provided was a habilitative service. Habilitative services help an individual learn skills and functioning for daily living that the individual has not yet developed, and then keep and/or improve those learned skills. Habilitative services also help an individual keep, learn, or improve skills and functioning for daily living.

97 Rehabilitative Services

When a service or procedure that may be either habilitative or rehabilitative in nature is provided for rehabilitative purposes, the physician or other qualified health care professional may add modifier 97 to the service or procedure code to indicate that the service or procedure provided was a rehabilitative service. Rehabilitative services help an individual keep, get back, or improve skills and functioning for daily living that have been lost or impaired because the individual was sick, hurt, or disabled.

99 Multiple Modifiers

Under certain circumstances 2 or more modifiers may be necessary to completely delineate a service. In such situations modifier 99 should be added to the basic procedure, and other applicable modifiers may be listed as part of the description of the service.

ⓘ Check with payers to determine if this modifier is necessary when reporting multiple modifiers.

Modifiers Approved for Ambulatory Surgery Center (ASC) Hospital Outpatient Use

There are some differences in modifiers for professional and ASC hospital use. The following list consists of the only approved modifiers that can be used in an ASC/hospital setting:

Modifiers

*Pages in this section refer to the AMA *CPT® 2022 Professional Edition*

25 Significant, Separately Identifiable Evaluation and Management Service by the Same Physician or Other Qualified Health Care Professional on the Same Day of the Procedure or Other Service

It may be necessary to indicate that on the day a procedure or service identified by a CPT code was performed, the patient's condition required a significant, separately identifiable E/M service above and beyond the other service provided or beyond the usual preoperative and postoperative care associated with the procedure that was performed. A significant, separately identifiable E/M service is defined or substantiated by documentation that satisfies the relevant criteria for the respective E/M service to be reported (see **Evaluation and Management Services Guidelines** for instructions on determining level of E/M service). The E/M service may be prompted by the symptom or condition for which the procedure and/or service was provided. As such, different diagnoses are not required for reporting of the E/M services on the same date. This circumstance may be reported by adding modifier 25 to the appropriate level of E/M service.

Note: This modifier is not used to report an E/M service that resulted in a decision to perform surgery. See modifier 57. For significant, separately identifiable non-E/M services, see modifier 59.

ⓘ According to Medicare, modifier 25 may be appended to an Emergency Department Services E/M code (99281-99285) if provided on the same day as a diagnostic or therapeutic procedure.

27 Multiple Outpatient Hospital E/M Encounters on the Same Date

For hospital outpatient reporting purposes, utilization of hospital resources related to separate and distinct E/M encounters performed in multiple outpatient hospital settings on the same date may be reported by adding modifier 27 to each appropriate level outpatient and/or emergency department E/M code(s). This modifier provides a means of reporting circumstances involving evaluation and management services provided by physician(s) in more than one (multiple) outpatient hospital setting(s) (e.g., hospital emergency department, clinic).

Note: This modifier is not to be used for physician reporting of multiple E/M services performed by the same physician on the same date. For physician reporting of all outpatient E/M services provided by the same physician on the same date and performed in multiple outpatient setting(s) (eg, hospital emergency department, clinic), see **Evaluation and Management, Emergency Department**, or **Preventive Medicine Services** codes.

33 Preventive Services

When the primary purpose of the service is the delivery of an evidence based service in accordance with a US Preventive Services Task Force A or B rating in effect and other preventive services identified in preventive services mandates (legislative or regulatory), the services may be identified by adding 33 to the procedure. For separately reported services specifically identified as preventive, the modifier should not be used.

50 Bilateral Procedure

Unless otherwise identified in the listings, bilateral procedures that are performed at the same session should be identified by adding modifier 50 to the appropriate 5-digit code.

Note: This modifier should not be appended to designated "add-on" codes (see Appendix D*)

ⓘ Reported on procedures performed at the same operative session, this modifier should be reported only once as a one-line item for Medicare, with the modifier appended to the end of the code.

ⓘ Some payers may accept the bilateral procedures as two-line items, with HCPCS Level II modifiers LT and RT appended to the end of the codes.

52 Reduced Services

Under certain circumstances a service or procedure is partially reduced or eliminated at the discretion of the physician or other qualified health care professional. Under these circumstances the service provided can be identified by its usual procedure number and the addition of modifier 52, signifying that the service is reduced. This provides a means of reporting reduced services without disturbing the identification of the basic service.

Note: For hospital outpatient reporting of a previously scheduled procedure/ service that is partially reduced or cancelled as a result of extenuating circumstances or those that threaten the well-being of the patient prior to or after administration of anesthesia, see modifiers 73 and 74. (see modifiers approved for ASC hospital outpatient use)

ⓘ Procedures reported with modifier 52 are typically billed at a reduced amount. Most payers do not require documentation to support the use of modifier 52 and will reimburse the procedure at a reduced level.

58 Staged or Related Procedure or Service by the Same Physician or Other Qualified Health Care Professional During the Postoperative Period

It may be necessary to indicate that the performance of a procedure or service during the postoperative period was: (a) planned or anticipated (staged); (b) more extensive than the original procedure; or (c) for therapy following a diagnostic surgical procedure. This circumstance may be reported by adding modifier 58 to the staged or related procedure.

Note: For treatment of a problem that requires a return to the operating/ procedure room (e.g., unanticipated clinical condition), see modifier 78.

ⓘ Modifier 58 must be used for purposes of identifying procedures performed by the original physician during the postoperative period of the original procedure, within the constraints of the modifier's definition. These procedures cannot be repeat operations (unless the procedures are more extensive than the original procedure) and cannot be for the treatment of complications requiring a return trip to the operating room.

The existence of modifier 58 does not negate the global fee concept. Services that are included in CPT as multiple sessions or are defined as including multiple services or events may not be billed with this modifier. This modifier is designed to allow a method of reporting additional, related surgeries that are due to a progression of the disease and are not to be used to avoid global surgery edits applicable to staged procedures.

Modifier 58 should be used on surgical codes only and has no effect on the payment amount.

59 Distinct Procedural Service

Under certain circumstances, it may be necessary to indicate that a procedure or service was distinct or independent from other non-E/M services performed on the same day. Modifier 59 is used to identify procedures/services, other than E/M services, that are not normally reported together, but are appropriate under the circumstances. Documentation must support a different session, different procedure or surgery, different site or organ system, separate incision/excision, separate lesion, or separate injury (or area of injury in extensive injuries) not ordinarily encountered or performed on the same day by the same individual. However, when another already established modifier is appropriate it should be used rather than modifier 59. Only if no more descriptive modifier is available, and the use of modifier 59 best explains the circumstances, should modifier 59 be used.

*Pages in this section refer to the AMA *CPT® 2022 Professional Edition*

Note: Modifier 59 should not be appended to an E/M service. To report a separate and distinct E/M service with a non-E/M service performed on the same date, see modifier 25.

ⓘ Modifier 59 was established to demonstrate that multiple, yet distinct, services were provided to a patient on the same date of service by the same provider. Because distinct procedures or services rendered on the same day by the same physician cannot be easily identified and properly adjudicated by simply listing the CPT procedure codes, modifier 59 assists the payer or Medicare carrier in applying the appropriate reimbursement protocol. If the modifier is not used in these circumstances, services may be denied, with the explanation of benefits stating that the payer does not reimburse for this service because it is part of another service that was performed at the same time.

73 Discontinued Out-Patient Hospital/Ambulatory Surgery Center (ASC) Procedure Prior to Administration of Anesthesia

Due to extenuating circumstances or those that threaten the well being of the patient, the physician may cancel a surgical or diagnostic procedure subsequent to the patient's surgical preparation (including sedation when provided, and being taken to the room where the procedure is to be performed), but prior to the administration of anesthesia (local, regional block(s), or general). Under these circumstances, the intended service that is prepared for but cancelled can be reported by its usual procedure number and the addition of modifier 73.

Note: The elective cancellation of a service prior to the administration of anesthesia and/or surgical preparation of the patient should not be reported. For physician reporting of a discontinued procedure, see modifier 53.

74 Discontinued Out-Patient Hospital/Ambulatory Surgery Center (ASC) Procedure After Administration of Anesthesia

Due to extenuating circumstances or those that threaten the well being of the patient, the physician may terminate a surgical or diagnostic procedure after the administration of anesthesia (local, regional block(s), or general) or after the procedure was started (e.g., incision made, intubation started, scope inserted, etc.). Under these circumstances, the intended service that is prepared for but cancelled can be reported by its usual procedure number and the addition of modifier 74.

Note: The elective cancellation of a service prior to the administration of anesthesia and/or surgical preparation of the patient should not be reported. For physician reporting of a discontinued procedure, see modifier 53.

76 Repeat Procedure or Service by Same Physician or Other Qualified Health Care Professional

It may be necessary to indicate that a procedure or service was repeated subsequent to the original procedure or service. This circumstance may be reported by adding modifier 76 to the repeated procedure or service.

Note: This modifier should not be appended to an E/M service.

77 Repeat Procedure by Another Physician or Other Qualified Health Care Professional

It may be necessary to indicate that a basic procedure or service was repeated by another physician or other qualified health care professional subsequent to the original procedure or service. This circumstance may be reported by adding modifier 77 to the repeated procedure or service.

Note: This modifier should not be appended to an E/M service.

ⓘ Appending this modifier does not guarantee payment of the repeat procedure, but will assist in determining duplicate billings for the procedure.

78 Unplanned Return to the Operating/Procedure Room by the Same Physician or Other Qualified Health Care Professional Following Initial Procedure for a Related Procedure During the Postoperative Period

It may be necessary to indicate that another procedure was performed during the postoperative period of the initial procedure (unplanned procedure following initial procedure). When this procedure is related to the first, and requires the use of an operating/procedure room, it may be reported by adding modifier 78 to the related procedure. (For repeat procedures, see modifier 76.)

ⓘ Medicare includes specific medical and/or surgical care for postoperative complications within the global surgical package and does not allow additional payment. Included in the global surgical package are "additional medical and surgical services required of the surgeon during the postoperative period of the surgery because of complications which do not require additional trips to the operating room."

79 Unrelated Procedure or Service by the Same Physician or Other Qualified Health Care Professional During the Postoperative Period

The individual may need to indicate that the performance of a procedure or service during the postoperative period was unrelated to the original procedure. This circumstance may be reported by using modifier 79. (For repeat procedures on the same day, see modifier 76.)

ⓘ When billing for an unrelated procedure by the same physician during the postoperative period of an original procedure, a new postoperative period will begin with the subsequent procedure. A different diagnosis should be indicated on the claim to identify the unrelated procedure.

91 Repeat Clinical Diagnostic Laboratory Test

In the course of treatment of the patient, it may be necessary to repeat the same laboratory test on the same day to obtain subsequent (multiple) test results. Under these circumstances, the laboratory test performed can be identified by its usual procedure number and the addition of modifier 91.

Note: This modifier may not be used when tests are rerun to confirm initial results; due to testing problems with specimens or equipment; or for any other reason when a normal, one-time, reportable result is all that is required. This modifier may not be used when other code(s) describe a series of test results (e.g., glucose tolerance tests, evocative/suppression testing). This modifier may only be used for laboratory test(s) performed more than once on the same day on the same patient.

Category II Modifiers

The following performance measurement modifiers may be used for Category II codes to indicate that a service specified in the associated measure(s) was considered but, due to either medical, patient, or system circumstance(s) documented in the medical record, the service was not provided. These modifiers serve as denominator exclusions from the performance measure. The user should note that not all listed measures provide for exclusions (see Alphabetical Clinical Topics Listing for more discussion regarding exclusion criteria).

Category II modifiers should only be reported with Category II codes—they should not be reported with Category I or Category III codes. In addition, the modifiers in the Category II section should only be used where specified in the guidelines, reporting instructions, parenthetic notes, or code descriptor language listed in the Category II section (code listing and the Alphabetical Clinical Topics Listing).

1P Performance Measure Exclusion Modifier due to Medical Reasons

Reasons include:

- Not indicated (absence of organ/limb, already received/performed, other)
- Contraindicated (patient allergic history, potential adverse drug interaction, other)
- Other medical reasons

2P Performance Measure Exclusion Modifier due to Patient Reasons

Reasons include:

- Patient declined
- Economic, social, or religious reasons
- Other patient reasons

3P Performance Measure Exclusion Modifier due to System Reasons

Reasons include:

- Resources to perform the services not available
- Insurance coverage/payor-related limitations
- Other reasons attributable to health care delivery system

Modifier 8P is intended to be used as a "reporting modifier" to allow the reporting of circumstances when an action described in a measure's numerator is not performed and the reason is not otherwise specified.

8P Performance measure reporting modifier–action not performed, reason not otherwise specified

Level II (HCPCS/National) Modifiers

E1 Upper left, eyelid
E2 Lower left, eyelid
E3 Upper right, eyelid
E4 Lower right, eyelid
F1 Left hand, second digit
F2 Left hand, third digit
F3 Left hand, fourth digit
F4 Left hand, fifth digit
F5 Right hand, thumb
F6 Right hand, second digit
F7 Right hand, third digit
F8 Right hand, fourth digit
F9 Right hand, fifth digit
FA Left hand, thumb
GG Performance and payment of a screening mammogram and diagnostic mammogram on the same patient, same day
GH Diagnostic mammogram converted from screening mammogram on same day
LC Left circumflex coronary artery
LD Left anterior descending coronary artery
LM Left main coronary artery
LT Left side (used to identify procedures performed on the left side of the body)
QM Ambulance service provided under arrangement by a provider of services
QN Ambulance service furnished directly by a provider of services
RC Right coronary artery
RI Ramus intermedius coronary artery
RT Right side (used to identify procedures performed on the right side of the body)
T1 Left foot, second digit
T2 Left foot, third digit
T3 Left foot, fourth digit
T4 Left foot, fifth digit
T5 Right foot, great toe
T6 Right foot, second digit
T7 Right foot, third digit
T8 Right foot, fourth digit
T9 Right foot, fifth digit
TA Left foot, great toe
XE Separate Encounter *
XS Separate Structure *
XP Separate Practitioner *
XU Unusual Non-Overlapping Service *

(*HCPCS modifiers for selective identification of subsets of Distinct Procedural Services [59 modifier])

Modifier Rules

Mult Proc = Multiple Procedure (Modifier 51)

Indicates applicable payment-adjustment rule for multiple procedures:

0 No payment-adjustment rules for multiple procedures apply. If procedure is reported on the same day as another procedure, base the payment on the lower of (a) the actual charge, or (b) the fee-schedule amount for the procedure.

1 Standard payment-adjustment rules in effect before January 1, 1995 for multiple procedures apply. In the 1995 file, this indicator only applies to codes with a status code of "D." If procedure is reported on the same day as another procedure that has an indicator of 1, 2, or 3, rank the procedures by fee-schedule amount and apply the appropriate reduction to this code (100%, 50%, 25%, 25%, 25%, and by report). Base the payment on the lower of (a) the actual charge, or (b) the fee-schedule amount reduced by the appropriate percentage.

2 Standard payment-adjustment rules for multiple procedures apply. If procedure is reported on the same day as another procedure with an indicator of 1, 2, or 3, rank the procedures by fee-schedule amount and apply the appropriate reduction to this code (100%, 50%, 50%, 50%, 50% and by report). Base the payment on the lower of (a) the actual charge, or (b) the fee-schedule amount reduced by the appropriate percentage.

3 Special rules for multiple endoscopic procedures apply if procedure is billed with another endoscopy in the same family (i.e., another endoscopy that has the same base procedure). The base procedure for each code with this indicator is identified in the ENDO BASE field of this file. Apply the multiple endoscopy rules to a family before ranking the family

with the other procedures performed on the same day (for example, if multiple endoscopies in the same family are reported on the same day as endoscopies in another family or on the same day as a non-endoscopic procedure). If an endoscopic procedure is reported with only its base procedure, do not pay separately for the base procedure. Payment for the base procedure is included in the payment for the other endoscopy.

5 Subject to 20% of the practice expense component for certain therapy services (25% reduction for services rendered in an institutional setting - effective for services January 1, 2012 and after).

9 Concept does not apply.

Bilat Surg = Bilateral Surgery (Modifier 50)

Indicates services subject to payment adjustment.

0 150% payment adjustment for bilateral procedures does not apply. If procedure is reported with modifier 50 or with modifiers RT and LT, base the payment for the two sides on the lower of: (a) the total actual charge for both sides or (b) 100% of the fee-schedule amount for a single code. Example: The fee-schedule amount for code XXXXX is $125. The physician reports code XXXXX-LT with an actual charge of $100 and XXXXX-RT with an actual charge of $100. Payment should be based on the fee-schedule amount ($125) since it is lower than the total actual charges for the left and right sides ($200). The bilateral adjustment is inappropriate for codes in this category (a) because of physiology or anatomy, or (b) because the code description specifically states that it is a unilateral procedure and there is an existing code for the bilateral procedure.

1 150% payment adjustment for bilateral procedures applies. If the code is billed with the bilateral modifier or is reported twice on the same day by any other means (e.g., with RT and LT modifiers, or with a "2" in the units field), base the payment for these codes when reported as bilateral procedures on the lower of: (a) the total actual charge for both sides or (b) 150% of the fee-schedule amount for a single code. If the code is reported as a bilateral procedure and is reported with other procedure codes on the same day, apply the bilateral adjustment before applying any multiple procedure rules.

2 150% payment adjustment does not apply. RVUs are already based on the procedure being performed as a bilateral procedure. If the procedure is reported with modifier 50 or is reported twice on the same day by any other means (e.g., with RT and LT modifiers or with a "2" in the units field), base the payment for both sides on the lower of (a) the total actual charge by the physician for both sides, or (b) 100% of the fee-schedule for a single code. Example: The fee-schedule amount for code YYYYY is $125. The physician reports code YYYYY-LT with an actual charge of $100 and YYYYY-RT with an actual charge of $100. Payment should be based on the fee-schedule amount ($125) since it is lower than the total actual charges for the left and right sides ($200). The RVUs are based on a bilateral procedure because (a) the code descriptor specifically states that the procedure is bilateral, (b) the code descriptor states that the procedure may be performed either unilaterally or bilaterally, or (c) the procedure is usually performed as a bilateral procedure.

3 The usual payment adjustment for bilateral procedures does not apply. If the procedure is reported with modifier 50 or is reported for both sides on the same day by any other means (e.g., with RT and LT modifiers or with a "2" in the units field), base the payment for each side or organ or site of a paired organ on the lower of (a) the actual charge for each side or (b) 100% of the fee-schedule amount for each side. If the procedure is reported as a bilateral procedure and with other procedure codes on the same day, determine the fee-schedule amount for a bilateral procedure before applying any multiple procedure rules. Services in this category are generally radiology procedures or other diagnostic tests, which are not subject to the special payment rules for other bilateral surgeries.

9 Concept does not apply.

Asst Surg = Assistant at Surgery (Modifier 80)

Indicates services where an assistant at surgery is never paid for per Medicare Claims Manual.

0 Payment restriction for assistants at surgery applies to this procedure unless supporting documentation is submitted to establish medical necessity.

1 Statutory payment restriction for assistants at surgery applies to this procedure. Assistant at surgery may not be paid.

2 Payment restriction for assistants at surgery does not apply to this procedure. Assistant at surgery may be paid.

9 Concept does not apply.

Co Surg = Co-surgeons (Modifier 62)

Indicates services for which two surgeons, each in a different specialty, may be paid.

0 Co-surgeons not permitted for this procedure.

1 Co-surgeons could be paid, though supporting documentation is required to establish the medical necessity of two surgeons for the procedure.

2 Co-surgeons permitted and no documentation required if the two-specialty requirement is met.

9 Concept does not apply.

Team Surg = Team Surgery (Modifier 66)

Indicates services for which team surgeons may be paid.

0 Team surgeons not permitted for this procedure.

1 Team surgeons could be paid, though supporting documentation required to establish medical necessity of a team; pay by report.

2 Team surgeons permitted; pay by report.

9 Concept does not apply.

National Correct Coding Initiative

A. Introduction

The principles of correct coding apply to the CPT codes in the range 50010-59897. Several general guidelines are repeated in this Chapter.

Physicians should report the HCPCS/CPT code that describes the procedure performed to the greatest specificity possible. A HCPCS/CPT code should be reported only if all services described by the code are performed. A physician should not report multiple HCPCS/CPT codes if a single HCPCS/CPT code exists that describes the services. This type of unbundling is incorrect coding.

HCPCS/CPT codes include all services usually performed as part of the procedure as a standard of medical/surgical practice. A physician should not separately report these services simply because HCPCS/CPT codes exist for them. Specific issues unique to this section of CPT are clarified in this Chapter.

B. Evaluation and Management (E/M) Services

Medicare Global Surgery Rules define the rules for reporting evaluation and management (E/M) services with procedures covered by these rules. This section summarizes some of the rules.

All procedures on the Medicare Physician Fee Schedule are assigned a global period of 000, 010, 090, XXX, YYY, ZZZ, or MMM. The global concept does not apply to XXX procedures. The global period for YYY procedures is defined by the Carrier. All procedures with a global period of ZZZ are related to another procedure, and the applicable global period for the ZZZ code is determined by the related procedure. Procedures with a global period of MMM are maternity procedures.

Since NCCI PTP edits are applied to same day services by the same provider to the same beneficiary, certain Global Surgery Rules are applicable to NCCI. An E/M service is separately reportable on the same date of service as a procedure with a global period of 000, 010, or 090 under limited circumstances.

If a procedure has a global period of 090 days, it is defined as a major surgical procedure. If an E/M is performed on the same date of service as a major surgical procedure for the purpose of deciding whether to perform this surgical procedure, the E/M service is separately reportable with modifier 57. Other preoperative E/M services on the same date of service as a major surgical procedure are included in the global payment for the procedure and are not separately reportable. NCCI does not contain edits based on this rule because Medicare Carriers have separate edits.

If a procedure has a global period of 000 or 010 days, it is defined as a minor surgical procedure. In general E/M services on the same date of service as the minor surgical procedure are included in the payment for the procedure. The decision to perform a minor surgical procedure is included in the payment for the minor surgical procedure and should not be reported separately as an E/M service. However, a significant and separately identifiable E/M service unrelated to the decision to perform the minor surgical procedure is separately reportable with modifier 25.The E/M service and minor surgical procedure do not require different diagnoses. If a minor surgical procedure is performed on anew patient, the same rules for reporting E/M services apply. The fact that the patient is "new" to the provider is not sufficient alone to justify reporting an E/M service on the same date of service as a minor surgical procedure. NCCI contains many, but not all, possible edits based on these principles.

Example: If a physician determines that a new patient with head trauma requires sutures, confirms the allergy and immunization status, obtains informed consent, and performs the repair, an E/M service is not separately reportable. However, if the physician also performs a medically reasonable and necessary full neurological examination, an E/M service may be separately reportable.

For major and minor surgical procedures, postoperative E/M services related to recovery from the surgical procedure during the postoperative period are included in the global surgical packages are E/M services related to complications of the surgery. Postoperative visits unrelated to the diagnosis for which the surgical procedure was performed unless related to a complication of surgery may be reported separately on the same day as surgical procedure with modifier 24 ("Unrelated Evaluation and Management Service by the Same Physician or Other Qualified Health Care Professional During a Postoperative Period").

Procedures with a global surgery indicator of "XXX" are not covered by these rules. Many of these "XXX" procedures are performed by physicians and have inherent pre-procedure, intraprocedure, and post-procedure work usually performed each time the procedure is completed. This work should never be reported as a separate E/M code. Other "XXX" procedures are not usually performed by a physician and have no physician work relative value units associated with them. A physician should never report a separate E/M code with these procedures for the supervision of others performing the procedure or for the interpretation of the procedure. With most "XXX" procedures, the physician may, however, perform a significant and separately identifiable E/M service on the same date of service which may be reported by appending modifier 25 to the E/M code. This E/M service may be related to the same diagnosis necessitating performance of the "XXX" procedure but cannot include any work inherent in the "XXX" procedure, supervision of others performing the "XXX" procedure, or time for interpreting the result of the "XXX" procedure. Appending modifier 25 to a significant, separately identifiable E/M service when performed on the same date of service as an "XXX" procedure is correct coding.

C. Urinary System

1. Insertion of a urinary bladder catheter is a component of the global surgical package. Urinary bladder catheterization (CPT codes 51701, 51702, and 51703) is not separately reportable with a surgical procedure when performed at the time of or just prior to the procedure.
   Additionally, many procedures involving the urinary tract include the placement of a urethral/bladder catheter for post-operative drainage. Because this is integral to the procedure, placement of a urinary catheter is not separately reportable.
2. Cystourethroscopy, with biopsy(s) (CPT code 52204) includes all biopsies during the procedure and should be reported with one unit of service.
3. Some lesions of the genitourinary tract occur at mucocutaneous borders. The CPT Manual contains integumentary system (CPT codes 10000-19999) and genitourinary system (CPT codes 50000-59899) codes to describe various procedures such as biopsy, excision, or destruction. A single code from one of these two sections of the CPT Manual that best describes the biopsy, excision, destruction, or other procedure performed on one or multiple similar lesions at a mucocutaneous border should be reported. Separate codes from the integumentary system and genitourinary system sections of the CPT Manual may only be reported if separate procedures are performed on completely separate lesions on the skin and genitourinary tract. Modifier 59 should be utilized to indicate that the procedures are on separate lesions. The medical record should accurately describe the precise locations of the lesions.
4. If an irrigation or drainage procedure is necessary and integral to complete a genitourinary or other procedure, only the more extensive procedure should be reported. The irrigation or drainage procedure is not separately reportable.
5. The CPT code descriptor for some genitourinary procedures includes a hernia repair. A HCPCS/CPT code for a hernia repair is not separately reportable unless the hernia repair is performed at a different site through a separate incision. In the latter case, the hernia repair may be reported with modifier 59.
6. In general, multiple methods of performing a procedure (e.g., prostatectomy) cannot be performed at the same patient encounter. (See general policy on mutually exclusive services.) Therefore, only one method of accomplishing a given procedure may be reported. If an initial approach fails and is followed by an alternative approach, only the completed or last uncompleted approach may be reported.
7. If a diagnostic endoscopy leads to the performance of a laparoscopic or open procedure, the diagnostic endoscopy may be separately reportable. Modifier 58 may be reported to indicate that the diagnostic endoscopy and non-endoscopic therapeutic procedures were staged or planned procedures. The medical record must indicate the medical necessity for the diagnostic endoscopy. However, if an endoscopic procedure is performed as an integral part of an open procedure, only the open procedure is reportable. If the endoscopy is confirmatory or is performed to assess the surgical field ("scout endoscopy"), the endoscopy does not represent a separate diagnostic or surgical endoscopy. The endoscopy represents exploration of the surgical field, and should not be reported separately with a diagnostic or surgical endoscopy code.
   If an endoscopic procedure is performed at the same patient encounter as a non-endoscopic procedure to ensure no intra-operative injury occurred or verify the procedure was performed correctly, the endoscopic procedure is not separately reportable with the non-endoscopic procedure.
8. If an endoscopic procedure is converted to an open procedure, only the open procedure may be reported. Neither a surgical endoscopy nor a diagnostic endoscopy code should be reported with the open procedure code when an endoscopic procedure is converted to an open procedure.
9. Surgical endoscopy includes diagnostic endoscopy which is not separately reportable. If a diagnostic endoscopy leads to a surgical endoscopy at the same patient encounter, only the surgical endoscopy may be reported.
10. When multiple endoscopic procedures are performed at the same patient encounter, the most comprehensive code accurately describing the service(s) performed should be reported. If several procedures not included in a more comprehensive code are performed at the same endoscopic session, multiple HCPCS/CPT codes may be reported with modifier 51. (For example, if renal endoscopy is performed through an established nephrostomy with biopsy, fulguration of a lesion, and foreign body (calculus) removal, the appropriate CPT coding would be CPT codes 50557 and 50561-51, not CPT codes 50551, 50555, 50557, and 50561.) This policy applies to all endoscopic procedures, not only those of the genitourinary system.
11. CPT code 51700 (bladder irrigation, simple, lavage and/or instillation) is used to report irrigation with therapeutic agents or as an independent therapeutic procedure. It is not separately reportable if bladder irrigation is part of a more comprehensive service such as to gain access to or visualize the urinary system. Irrigation of a urinary catheter is included in the global surgical package. CPT code 51700 should not be misused to report irrigation of a urinary catheter.
12. CPT codes 51784 and 51785 describe diagnostic electromyography (EMG). When EMG is performed as part of a biofeedback session, neither CPT code 51784 nor 51785 should be reported unless a significant, separately identifiable diagnostic EM service is provided. If either CPT code 51784 or CPT code 51785 is reported for a diagnostic electromyogram, a separate report must be available in the medical record to indicate this service was performed for diagnostic purposes.
13. When endoscopic visualization of the urinary system involves several regions (e.g., kidney, renal pelvis, calyx, and ureter), the appropriate CPT code is defined by the approach (e.g., nephrostomy, pyelostomy, ureterostomy, etc.) as indicated in the CPT descriptor. When multiple endoscopic approaches at the same patient encounter are medically reasonable and

necessary (e.g., renal endoscopy through a nephrostomy and cystourethroscopy) to perform different procedures, they may be separately reported appending modifier 51 to the less extensive procedure codes. However, when multiple endoscopic approaches are utilized to attempt the same procedure, only the completed approach should be reported.

14. Endoscopic procedures include all minor related functions performed at the same encounter. Although CPT codes may exist to describe these functions, they should not be reported separately. For example, transurethral resection of the prostate includes meatotomy, urethral calibration and/or dilation, urethroscopy, and cystoscopy. Codes for the included procedures should not be reported separately.
15. When urethral catheterization or urethral dilation (e.g., CPT codes 51701-51703) is necessary to complete a more extensive procedure, the urethral catheterization/dilation is not separately reportable.
16. Ureteral anastomosis procedures are described by CPT codes 50740-50825, and 50860. In general, they represent mutually exclusive procedures that are not reported together. If one type of anastomosis is performed on one ureter, and a different type of anastomosis is performed on the contralateral ureter, the appropriate modifier (e.g., LT, RT) should be reported with the CPT code to describe the service performed on each ureter.
    For example, the procedure described by CPT code 50860 (ureterostomy, transplantation of ureter to skin) is mutually exclusive with the procedures described by CPT codes 50800- 50830 (e.g., ureteroenterostomy, ureterocolon conduit, urinary undiversion) unless performed on contralateral ureters in which case anatomic modifiers should be reported.
17. CPT codes 53502-53515 describe urethral repair codes for urethral wounds or injuries (urethrorrhaphy). When an urethroplasty is performed, codes for urethrorrhaphy should not be reported in addition since "suture to repair wound or injury" is included in the urethroplasty service.
18. CPT code 78730 (Urinary bladder, residual study) is a nuclear medicine procedure requiring use of a radio- pharmaceutical. This CPT code should not be utilized to report measurement of residual urine in the urinary bladder determined by other methods.
19. CPT code 52332 (Cystourethroscopy, with insertion of indwelling ureteral stent) describes insertion of a self-retaining indwelling stent during cystourethroscopy with ureteroscopy and/or pyeloscopy and should not be reported to describe insertion and removal of a temporary ureteral stent during diagnostic or therapeutic cystourethroscopy with ureteroscopy and/or pyeloscopy (e.g., CPT codes 52320-52330, 52334- 52355). The insertion and removal of a temporary ureteral catheter (stent) during these procedures is not separately reportable and should not be reported with CPT codes 52005 (Cystourethroscopy, with ureteral catheterization, with or without irrigation, instillation, or ureteropyelography, exclusive of radiologic service;) or 52007 (Cystourethroscopy, with ureteral catheterization, with or without irrigation, instillation, or ureteropyelography, exclusive of radiologic service; with brush biopsy of ureter and/or renal pelvis). CPT codes 52332 and 52005 are not separately reportable for the same ureter for the same patient encounter.
20. Prostatectomy procedures (CPT codes 55801-55845) include cystoplasty or cystourethroplasty as a standard of surgical practice. CPT code 51800 (cystoplasty or cystourethroplasty...) should not be reported separately with prostatectomy procedures.
21. CPT code 50650 (ureterectomy, with bladder cuff (separate procedure)) should not be reported with other procedures on the ipsilateral ureter. Since CPT code 50650 includes the "separate procedure" designation, CMS does not allow additional payment for the procedure when it is performed with other procedures in an anatomically related area.
22. The code descriptors for CPT codes 52310 and 52315 (cystourethroscopy, with removal of foreign body, calculus, or ureteral stent from urethra or bladder (separate procedure)...) include the "separate procedure" designation. Per CMS payment policy for procedures with the "separate procedure" designation, these codes should not be reported with other cystourethroscopy CPT codes for the same patient encounter.
23. Fluoroscopy (CPT codes 76000 and 76001) is an integral component of all endoscopic procedures when performed. CPT codes 76000 and/or 76001 should not be reported separately with an endoscopic procedure.
24. Cystourethroscopy and transurethral procedures include fluoroscopy when performed. CPT codes describing fluoroscopy or fluoroscopic guidance (e.g. 76000, 76001, 77002) should not be reported separately with a cystourethroscopy or transurethral procedure CPT code.
25. A ureteral stent is commonly inserted at the site of an anastomosis of a ureter and another structure in order to maintain patency of the ureter. A ureteral stent is also often inserted into a ureter if the ureter is incised during a procedure (e.g., nephrectomy, cystectomy, ureteral anastomosis). With these procedures, insertion of the ureteral stent is integral to the procedure and is not separately reportable. For example, CPT code 50605 (Ureterotomy for insertion of indwelling stent, all types) should not be reported with CPT codes describing cystectomy, urinary diversion, or ureteral anastomosis for insertion of a ureteral stent to maintain patency at the site of a ureteral anastomosis.
26. Pelvic exenteration procedures (CPT codes 45126, 51597, 58240) include extensive removal of structures from the pelvis. Physicians should not separately report codes for the removal of pelvic structures (e.g., colon, rectum, urinary bladder, uterine body and/or cervix, fallopian tubes, ovaries, lymph nodes, prostate gland).
27. CPT code 50398 describes change of a nephrostomy or pyelostomy tube. If the tube change occurs in a patient without new symptoms related to the tube, CPT code 50394 (injection procedure for pyelography through a nephrostomy or pyelostomy tube) should not be reported separately for the tube check. However, if the patient has new symptoms related to the tube, the provider may separately report CPT code 50394 with an NCCI-associated modifier for the tube

check. (CPT codes 50394 and 50398 were deleted January 1, 2016.)

28. CPT codes 52317 and 52318 describe litholapaxy (crushing/fragmentation and removal) of calculus in the urinary bladder. These codes may be reported for crushing/fragmentation with removal of calculi originating de novo in the urinary bladder. These codes should not be reported for crushing/fragmentation and removal of calculi in the urinary bladder that result from a procedure to remove, manipulate, and/or fragment calculi higher up in the urinary tract.

D. Male Genital System

1. Transurethral drainage of a prostatic abscess (e.g., CPT code 52700) is included in male transurethral prostatic procedures and should not be reported separately.
2. The puncture aspiration of a hydrocele (e.g., CPT code 55000) is included in services involving the tunica vaginalis and proximate anatomy (e.g., scrotum, vas deferens) and in inguinal hernia repairs and should not be reported separately.
3. The CPT Manual contains many codes (CPT codes 52601-52649, 53850-53853, 55801-55845, 55866) which describe various methods of removing or destroying prostate tissue. These procedures are mutually exclusive, and two codes from these code ranges should not be reported together.
4. Scrotal exploration (CPT code 55110) is not separately reportable with procedures of the scrotum, scrotal sac, or its contents including the testes and epididymis. Exploration of the surgical field is not separately reportable.
5. If a prostatectomy procedure necessitates reconstruction of the bladder neck, the bladder neck reconstruction is not separately reportable. For example, CPT code 51800 (cystoplasty or cystourethroplasty, plastic operation on bladder and/or vesical neck...) should not be reported with a prostatectomy CPT code where the cystoplasty or cystourethroplasty is necessitated by the prostatectomy procedure.

E. Female Genital System

1. When a pelvic examination is performed in conjunction with a gynecologic procedure, either as a necessary part of the procedure or as a confirmatory examination, the pelvic examination is not separately reportable. A diagnostic pelvic examination may be performed for the purpose of deciding to perform a procedure. This examination is included in the evaluation and management service at the time the decision to perform the procedure is made.
2. All surgical laparoscopic, hysteroscopic or peritoneoscopic procedures include diagnostic procedures. Therefore, CPT code 49320 is included in CPT codes 38120, 38570-38572, 43280, 43651-43653, 44180-44227, 44970, 47562-47570, 49321-49323, 49650-49651, 54690-54692, 55550, 58545-58554, 58660-58673, and 60650. CPT code 58555 is included in CPT codes 58558-58565.
3. Pelvic examination under anesthesia (CPT code 57410) is included in all major and most minor gynecological procedures and is not separately reportable. This procedure represents routine evaluation of the surgical field.
4. Dilation of vagina or cervix (CPT codes 57400 or 57800) in conjunction with vaginal approach procedures is not separately reportable unless the CPT code descriptor states "without cervical dilation."
5. Colposcopy (CPT codes 56820, 57420, 57452) should not be reported separately when performed as a "scout" procedure to confirm a lesion or to assess the surgical field prior to a surgical procedure. A diagnostic colposcopy resulting in the decision to perform a non-colposcopic procedure may be reported separately with modifier 58 appended to the non-colposcopic procedure code. Diagnostic colposcopies (CPT codes 56820, 57420, 57452) are not separately reportable with other colposcopic procedures.
6. Pelvic exenteration procedures (CPT codes 45126, 51597, 58240) include extensive removal of structures from the pelvis. Physicians should not separately report codes for the removal of pelvic structures (e.g., colon, rectum, urinary bladder, uterine body and/or cervix, fallopian tubes, ovaries, lymph nodes, prostate gland).
7. CPT code 57250 describes posterior colporrhaphy for repair of rectocele including perineorrhaphy if performed. If a vaginal hysterectomy is accompanied by additional dissection to repair a rectocele (with perineorrhaphy if performed), both the vaginal hysterectomy CPT code and CPT code 57250 may be reported together with an NCCI-associated modifier.
8. CPT code 57240 describes anterior colporrhaphy for repair of cystocele including repair of urethrocele if performed. If a vaginal hysterectomy is accompanied by additional dissection to repair a cystocele (with repair of urethrocele if performed), both the vaginal hysterectomy CPT code and CPT code 57240 may be reported together with an NCCI-associated modifier.
9. CPT code 57260 describes a combined anteroposterior colporrhaphy. If a vaginal hysterectomy is accompanied by additional dissection to repair a rectocele (with perineorrhaphy if performed) and repair a cystocele (with repair of urethrocele if performed), both the vaginal hysterectomy CPT code and CPT code 57260 may be reported together with an NCCI associated modifier.
10. A vaginal hysterectomy normally includes fixation of the vagina to surrounding tissues. It is a misuse of CPT code 57282 (Colpopexy, vaginal; extra-peritoneal approach (sacrospinous, iliococcygeus)) or 57283 (Colpopexy, vaginal; intra-peritoneal approach (uterosacral, levator myorrhaphy)) to report this fixation of the vagina to describe the fixation that routinely occurs during a vaginal hysterectomy. If a more extensive colpopexy consistent with the requirements of CPT code 57282 or 57283 is performed, CPT codes 57282 or 57283 may be reported with the vaginal hysterectomy CPT code utilizing an NCCI-associated modifier.

F. Laparoscopy

1. Surgical laparoscopy includes diagnostic laparoscopy which is not separately reportable. If a diagnostic laparoscopy leads to a surgical laparoscopy at the same patient encounter, only the surgical laparoscopy may be reported.

2. If a laparoscopy is performed as a "scout" procedure to assess the surgical field or extent of disease, it is not separately reportable. If the findings of a diagnostic laparoscopy lead to the decision to perform an open procedure, the diagnostic laparoscopy may be separately reportable.
   Modifier 58 may be reported to indicate that the diagnostic laparoscopy and non-laparoscopic therapeutic procedures were staged or planned procedures. The medical record must indicate the medical necessity for the diagnostic laparoscopy.
3. CPT code 49321 describes a laparoscopic biopsy. If this procedure is performed for diagnostic purposes and the decision to proceed with an open or laparoscopic -ectomy procedure is based on this biopsy, CPT code 49321 may be reported in addition to the CPT code for the -ectomy procedure. However, if the laparoscopic biopsy is performed for a different purpose such as assessing the margins of resection, CPT code 49321 is not separately reportable.
4. If a laparoscopic procedure is converted to an open procedure, only the open procedure may be reported. Neither a surgical laparoscopy nor a diagnostic laparoscopy code should be reported with the open procedure code when a laparoscopic procedure is converted to an open procedure.
5. Laparoscopic lysis of adhesions (CPT codes 44180 or 58660) is not separately reportable with other surgical laparoscopic procedures.
6. CPT code 44970 describes a laparoscopic appendectomy and may be reported separately with another laparoscopic procedure code when a diseased appendix is removed. Since removal of a normal appendix with another laparoscopic procedure is not separately reportable, this code should not be reported for an incidental laparoscopic appendectomy.
7. Fluoroscopy (CPT codes 76000 and 76001) is an integral component of all laparoscopic procedures when performed. CPT codes 76000 and/or 76001 should not be reported separately with a laparoscopic procedure.

G. Medically Unlikely Edits (MUEs)

1. MUEs are described in Chapter I, Section V.
2. Providers/suppliers should be cautious about reporting services on multiple lines of a claim utilizing modifiers to bypass MUEs. MUEs were set so that such occurrences should be uncommon. If a provider/supplier does this frequently for any HCPCS/CPT code, the provider/supplier may be coding units of service incorrectly. The provider/supplier should consider contacting his/her national healthcare organization or the national medical/surgical society whose members commonly perform the procedure to clarify the correct reporting of units of service. A national healthcare organization, provider/ supplier, or other interested third party may request a reconsideration of the MUE value of a HCPCS/CPT code by CMS by writing the MUE contractor, Correct Coding Solutions, LLC, at the address indicated in Chapter I, Section V.
3. The unit of service (UOS) for a procedure describing destruction or removal of renal system calculus(i) is one (1). The UOS is not each calculus. If a procedure for destruction or removal of renal system calculi is performed bilaterally, the CPT code may be reported with modifier 50 and one (1) UOS. For example, CPT code 52353 (cystourethroscopy, with ureteroscopy and/or pyeloscopy; with lithotripsy (ureteral catheterization is included)) should be reported with only one unit of service (UOS) per ureter regardless of the number of calculi in the ureter. If the procedure is performed on bilateral ureters, it may be reported with modifier 50 and one UOS. This code should not be reported with a separate UOS for each calculus.
4. The CMS Internet-Only Manual (Publication 100-04 Medicare Claims Processing Manual, Chapter 12 (Physicians/ Nonphysician Practitioners), Section 40.7.B. and Chapter 4 (Part B Hospital (Including Inpatient Hospital Part B and OPPS)), Section 20.6.2 requires that practitioners and outpatient hospitals report bilateral surgical procedures with modifier 50 and one (1) UOS on a single claim line. MUE values for surgical procedures that may be performed bilaterally are based on this reporting requirement. Since this reporting requirement does not apply to an ambulatory surgical center (ASC), an ASC should report a bilateral surgical procedure on two claim lines, each with one (1) UOS using modifiers LT and RT on different claim lines. This reporting requirement does not apply to non-surgical diagnostic procedures.

H. General Policy Statements

1. MUE and NCCI PTP edits are based on services provided by the same physician to the same beneficiary on the same date of service. Physicians should not inconvenience beneficiaries nor increase risks to beneficiaries by performing services on different dates of service to avoid MUE or NCCI PTP edits.
2. In this Manual many policies are described utilizing the term "physician." Unless indicated differently the usage of this term does not restrict the policies to physicians only but applies to all practitioners, hospitals, providers, or suppliers eligible to bill the relevant HCPCS/CPT codes pursuant to applicable portions of the Social Security Act (SSA) of 1965, the Code of Federal Regulations (CFR), and Medicare rules. In some sections of this Manual, the term "physician" would not include some of these entities because specific rules do not apply to them. For example, Anesthesia Rules [e.g., CMS Internet-Only Manual, Publication 100-04 (Medicare Claims Processing Manual), Chapter 12 (Physician/Nonphysician Practitioners), Section 50(Payment for Anesthesiology Services)] and Global Surgery Rules [e.g., CMS Internet-Only Manual, Publication 100-04 (Medicare Claims Processing Manual), Chapter 12 (Physician/Nonphysician Practitioners), Section 40 (Surgeons and Global Surgery)] do not apply to hospitals.
3. Providers reporting services under Medicare's hospital outpatient prospective payment system (OPPS) should report all services in accordance with appropriate Medicare Internet- Only Manual (IOM) instructions.
4. In 2010 the CPT Manual modified the numbering of codes so that the sequence of codes as they appear in the CPT Manual does not necessarily correspond to a sequential numbering

of codes. In the National Correct Coding Initiative Policy Manual for Medicare Services, use of a numerical range of codes reflects all codes that numerically fall within the range regardless of their sequential order in the CPT Manual.

5. With few exceptions the payment for a surgical procedure includes payment for dressings, supplies, and local anesthesia. These items are not separately reportable under their own HCPCS/CPT codes. Wound closures utilizing adhesive strips or tape alone are not separately reportable. In the absence of an operative procedure, these types of wound closures are included in an E/M service. Under limited circumstances wound closure utilizing tissue adhesive may be reported separately. If a practitioner utilizes a tissue adhesive alone for a wound closure, it may be reported separately with HCPCS code G0168 (wound closure utilizing tissue adhesive(s) only). If a practitioner utilizes tissue adhesive in addition to staples or sutures to close a wound, HCPCS code G0168 is not separately reportable but is included in the tissue repair. Under OPPS HCPCS code G0168 is not recognized and paid. Facilities may report wound closure utilizing sutures, staples, or tissue adhesives, either singly or in combination with each other, with the appropriate CPT code in the "Repair (Closure)" section of the CPT Manual.
6. With limited exceptions Medicare Anesthesia Rules prevent separate payment for anesthesia for a medical or surgical procedure when provided by the physician performing the procedure. The physician should not report CPT codes 00100-01999, 62320-62327, or 64400-64530 for anesthesia for a procedure. Additionally, the physician should not unbundle the anesthesia procedure and report component codes individually. For example, introduction of a needle or intracatheter into a vein (CPT code 36000), venipuncture (CPT code 36410), drug administration (CPT codes 96360-96377) or cardiac assessment (e.g., CPT codes 93000-93010, 93040-93042) should not be reported when these procedures are related to the delivery of an anesthetic agent.
7. Medicare allows separate reporting for moderate conscious sedation services (CPT codes 99151-99153) when provided by the same physician performing a medical or surgical procedure.
8. Under Medicare Global Surgery Rules, drug administration services (CPT codes 96360-96377) are not separately reportable by the physician performing a procedure for drug administration services related to the procedure.
9. Under the OPPS drug administration services related to operative procedures are included in the associated procedural HCPCS/CPT codes. Examples of such drug administration services include, but are not limited to, anesthesia (local or other), hydration, and medications such as anxiolytics or antibiotics. Providers should not report CPT codes 96360-96377 for these services.
10. Medicare Global Surgery Rules prevent separate payment for postoperative pain management when provided by the physician performing an operative procedure. CPT codes 36000, 36410, 62320-62327, 64400-64489, and 96360-96377 describe some services that may be utilized for postoperative pain management. The services described by these codes may be reported by the physician performing the operative procedure only if provided for purposes unrelated to the postoperative pain management, the operative procedure, or anesthesia for the procedure.
11. If a physician performing an operative procedure provides a drug administration service (CPT codes 96360-96375) for a purpose unrelated to anesthesia, intra-operative care, or post-procedure pain management, the drug administration service (CPT codes 96360-96375) may be reported with an NCCI-associated modifier if performed in a non-facility site of service.
12. The Medicare global surgery package includes insertion of urinary catheters. CPT codes 51701-51703 (insertion of bladder catheters) should not be reported with any procedure with a global period of 000, 010, or 090 days nor with some procedures with a global period of MMM.
13. Closure/repair of a surgical incision is included in the global surgical package. Wound repair CPT codes 12001-13153 should not be reported separately to describe closure of surgical incisions for procedures with global surgery indicators of 000, 010, 090, or MMM.
14. Control of bleeding during an operative procedure is an integral component of a surgical procedure and is not separately reportable. Postoperative control of bleeding not requiring return to the operating room is included in the global surgical package and is not separately reportable. However, control of bleeding requiring return to the operating room in the postoperative period is separately reportable utilizing modifier 78.
15. A biopsy performed at the time of another more extensive procedure (e.g., excision, destruction, removal) is separately reportable under specific circumstances. If the biopsy is performed on a separate lesion, it is separately reportable. This situation may be reported with anatomic modifiers or modifier 59. If the biopsy is performed on the same lesion on which a more extensive procedure is performed, it is separately reportable only if the biopsy is utilized for immediate pathologic diagnosis prior to the more extensive procedure, and the decision to proceed with the more extensive procedure is based on the diagnosis established by the pathologic examination. The biopsy is not separately reportable if the pathologic examination at the time of surgery is for the purpose of assessing margins of resection or verifying resectability. When separately reportable modifier 58 may be reported to indicate that the biopsy and the more extensive procedure were planned or staged procedures. If a biopsy is performed and submitted for pathologic evaluation that will be completed after the more extensive procedure is performed, the biopsy is not separately reportable with the more extensive procedure.
16. Fine needle aspiration (FNA) (CPT codes 10021, 10022) should not be reported with another biopsy procedure code for the same lesion unless one specimen is inadequate for diagnosis. For example, an FNA specimen is usually examined for adequacy when the specimen is aspirated. If the specimen is adequate for diagnosis, it is not necessary to obtain an additional biopsy specimen. However, if the specimen is not

adequate and another type of biopsy (e.g., needle, open) is subsequently performed at the same patient encounter, the other biopsy procedure code may also be reported with an NCCI-associated modifier.

17. If the code descriptor of a HCPCS/CPT code includes the phrase, "separate procedure", the procedure is subject to NCCI PTP edits based on this designation. CMS does not allow separate reporting of a procedure designated as a "separate procedure" when it is performed at the same patient encounter as another procedure in an anatomically related area through the same skin incision, orifice, or surgical approach.
18. Most NCCI PTP edits for codes describing procedures that may be performed on bilateral organs or structures (e.g., arms, eyes, kidneys, lungs) allow use of NCCI-associated modifiers (modifier indicator of "1") because the two codes of the code pair edit may be reported if the two procedures are performed on contralateral organs or structures. Most of these code pairs should not be reported with NCCI-associated modifiers when the corresponding procedures are performed on the ipsilateral organ or structure unless there is a specific coding rationale to bypass the edit. The existence of the NCCI PTP edit indicates that the two codes generally should not be reported together unless the two corresponding procedures are performed at two separate patient encounters or two separate anatomic sites. However, if the corresponding procedures are performed at the same patient encounter and in contiguous structures, NCCI- associated modifiers should generally not be utilized.
19. If fluoroscopy is performed during an endoscopic procedure, it is integral to the procedure. This principle applies to all endoscopic procedures including, but not limited to, laparoscopy, hysteroscopy, thoracoscopy, arthroscopy, esophagoscopy, colonoscopy, other GI endoscopy, laryngoscopy, bronchoscopy, and cystourethroscopy.
20. If the code descriptor for a HCPCS/CPT code, CPT Manual instruction for a code, or CMS instruction for a code indicates that the procedure includes radiologic guidance, a physician should not separately report a HCPCS/CPT code for radiologic guidance including, but not limited to, fluoroscopy, ultrasound, computed tomography, or magnetic resonance imaging codes. If the physician performs an additional procedure on the same date of service for which a radiologic guidance or imaging code may be separately reported, the radiologic guidance or imaging code appropriate for that additional procedure may be reported separately with an NCCI-associated modifier if appropriate.
21. A cystourethroscopy (e.g., CPT code 52000) or cystourethroscopy with ureteroscopy (e.g., CPT code 52351) performed near the termination of an intra-abdominal, intra-pelvic, or retroperitoneal surgical procedure to assure that there was no intraoperative injury to the ureters or urinary bladder and that they are functioning properly is not separately reportable with the surgical procedure.

CCI Table Information

The CCI Modification indicator is noted with superscript letters and is also located in the footer of each page for reference purposes The codes are suffixed as **0** or **1**.

- **0** indicates there is no circumstance in which a modifier would be allowed or appropriate, meaning services represented by the code combination will not be paid separately.
- **1** signifies a modifier is allowed in order to differentiate between the services provided.

Note: The responsibility for the content of this product is the Centers for Medicare and Medicaid Services (CMS) and no endorsement by the American Medical Association (AMA) is intended or should be implied. The AMA disclaims responsibility for any consequences or liability attributable to or related to any uses, non-use, or interpretation of information contained or not contained in this product.

The NCCI edits on the following tables represent only the codes contained in this book. There are NCCI edits for CPT codes not found in this guide. The edits herein represent all active edits as of 1/1/2022. NCCI edits are updated quarterly. To view all NCCI edits, as well as quarterly updates, visit www.cms.gov/nationalcorrectcodeinited/.

Code 1	Code 2
10004	0213T[1], 0216T[1], 10012[1], 10035[1], 19281[1], 19283[1], 19285[1], 19287[1], 36000[1], 36410[1], 36591[0], 36592[0], 61650[1], 62324[1], 62325[1], 62326[1], 62327[1], 64415[1], 64416[1], 64417[1], 64450[1], 64454[1], 64486[1], 64487[1], 64488[1], 64489[1], 64490[1], 64493[1], 76000[1], 76380[1], 76942[1], 76998[1], 77001[1], 77002[1], 77012[1], 77021[1], 96360[1], 96365[1], 96372[1], 96374[1], 96375[1], 96376[1], 96377[1], 96523[0], J2001[1]
10005	0213T[1], 0216T[1], 10004[1], 10008[1], 10010[1], 10011[1], 10012[1], 10021[1], 10035[1], 11102[1], 11103[1], 11104[1], 11105[1], 11106[1], 11107[1], 19281[1], 19283[1], 19285[1], 19287[1], 36000[1], 36410[1], 36591[0], 36592[0], 61650[1], 62324[1], 62325[1], 62326[1], 62327[1], 64415[1], 64416[1], 64417[1], 64450[1], 64454[1], 64486[1], 64487[1], 64488[1], 64489[1], 64490[1], 64493[1], 76000[1], 76380[1], 76942[1], 76998[1], 77001[1], 77002[1], 77012[1], 77021[1], 96360[1], 96365[1], 96372[1], 96374[1], 96375[1], 96376[1], 96377[1], 96523[0], J2001[1]
10006	0213T[1], 0216T[1], 10004[1], 10035[1], 19281[1], 19283[1], 19285[1], 19287[1], 36000[1], 36410[1], 36591[0], 36592[0], 61650[1], 62324[1], 62325[1], 62326[1], 62327[1], 64415[1], 64416[1], 64417[1], 64450[1], 64454[1], 64486[1], 64487[1], 64488[1], 64489[1], 64490[1], 64493[1], 76000[1], 76380[1], 76942[1], 76998[1], 77001[1], 77002[1], 77012[1], 77021[1], 96360[1], 96365[1], 96372[1], 96374[1], 96375[1], 96376[1], 96377[1], 96523[0], J2001[1]
10007	0213T[1], 0216T[1], 10004[1], 10005[1], 10006[1], 10010[1], 10011[1], 10012[1], 10021[1], 10035[1], 11102[1], 11103[1], 11104[1], 11105[1], 11106[1], 11107[1], 19281[1], 19283[1], 19285[1], 19287[1], 36000[1], 36410[1], 36591[0], 36592[0], 61650[1], 62324[1], 62325[1], 62326[1], 62327[1], 64415[1], 64416[1], 64417[1], 64450[1], 64454[1], 64486[1], 64487[1], 64488[1], 64489[1], 64490[1], 64493[1], 76000[1], 76380[1], 76942[1], 76998[1], 77001[1], 77002[1], 77012[1], 77021[1], 96360[1], 96365[1], 96372[1], 96374[1], 96375[1], 96376[1], 96377[1], 96523[0], J2001[1]
10008	0213T[1], 0216T[1], 10004[1], 10021[1], 10035[1], 19281[1], 19283[1], 19285[1], 19287[1], 36000[1], 36410[1], 36591[0], 36592[0], 61650[1], 62324[1], 62325[1], 62326[1], 62327[1], 64415[1], 64416[1], 64417[1], 64450[1], 64454[1], 64486[1], 64487[1], 64488[1], 64489[1], 64490[1], 64493[1], 76000[1], 76380[1], 76942[1], 76998[1], 77001[1], 77002[1], 77012[1], 77021[1], 96360[1], 96365[1], 96372[1], 96374[1], 96375[1], 96376[1], 96377[1], 96523[0], J2001[1]
10009	0213T[1], 0216T[1], 10004[1], 10005[1], 10006[1], 10007[1], 10008[1], 10011[1], 10012[1], 10021[1], 10035[1], 11102[1], 11103[1], 11104[1], 11105[1], 11106[1], 19281[1], 19283[1], 19285[1], 19287[1], 36000[1], 36410[1], 36591[0], 36592[0], 61650[1], 62324[1], 62325[1], 62326[1], 62327[1], 64415[1], 64416[1], 64417[1], 64450[1], 64454[1], 64486[1], 64487[1], 64488[1], 64489[1], 64490[1], 64493[1], 76000[1], 76380[1], 76942[1], 76998[1], 77001[1], 77002[1], 77012[1], 77021[1], 96360[1], 96365[1], 96372[1], 96374[1], 96375[1], 96376[1], 96377[1], 96523[0], J2001[1]
10010	0213T[1], 0216T[1], 10004[1], 10021[1], 10035[1], 19281[1], 19283[1], 19285[1], 19287[1], 36000[1], 36410[1], 36591[0], 36592[0], 61650[1], 62324[1], 62325[1], 62326[1], 62327[1], 64415[1], 64416[1], 64417[1], 64450[1], 64454[1], 64486[1], 64487[1], 64488[1], 64489[1], 64490[1], 64493[1], 76000[1], 76380[1], 76942[1], 76998[1], 77001[1], 77002[1], 77012[1], 77021[1], 96360[1], 96365[1], 96372[1], 96374[1], 96375[1], 96376[1], 96377[1], 96523[0], J2001[1]
10011	0213T[1], 0216T[1], 10004[1], 10006[1], 10008[1], 10010[1], 10035[1], 19281[1], 19283[1], 19285[1], 19287[1], 36000[1], 36410[1], 36591[0], 36592[0], 61650[1], 62324[1], 62325[1], 62326[1], 62327[1], 64415[1], 64416[1], 64417[1], 64450[1], 64454[1], 64486[1], 64487[1], 64488[1], 64489[1], 64490[1], 64493[1], 76000[1], 76380[1], 76942[1], 76998[1], 77001[1], 77002[1], 77012[1], 77021[1], 96360[1], 96365[1], 96372[1], 96374[1], 96375[1], 96376[1], 96377[1], 96523[0], J2001[1]
10012	0213T[1], 0216T[1], 10035[1], 19281[1], 19283[1], 19285[1], 19287[1], 36000[1], 36410[1], 36591[0], 36592[0], 61650[1], 62324[1], 62325[1], 62326[1], 62327[1], 64415[1], 64416[1], 64417[1], 64450[1], 64454[1], 64486[1], 64487[1], 64488[1], 64489[1], 64490[1], 64493[1], 76000[1], 76380[1], 76942[1], 76998[1], 77001[1], 77002[1], 77012[1], 77021[1], 96360[1], 96365[1], 96372[1], 96374[1], 96375[1], 96376[1], 96377[1], 96523[0], J2001[1]
10021	0213T[1], 0216T[1], 10006[1], 10011[1], 10012[1], 10035[1], 11102[1], 11103[1], 11104[1], 11105[1], 11107[1], 19281[1], 19283[1], 19285[1], 19287[1], 36000[1], 36410[1], 36591[0], 36592[0], 61650[1], 62324[1], 62325[1], 62326[1], 62327[1], 64415[1], 64416[1], 64417[1], 64450[1], 64454[1], 64486[1], 64487[1], 64488[1], 64489[1], 64490[1], 64493[1], 76000[1], 76380[1], 76942[1], 76998[1], 77001[1], 77002[1], 77012[1], 77021[1], 96360[1], 96365[1], 96372[1], 96374[1], 96375[1], 96376[1], 96377[1], 96523[0], J2001[1]
10030	0213T[0], 0216T[0], 0596T[1], 0597T[1], 10060[1], 10061[1], 10080[1], 10081[1], 10140[1], 10160[1], 11055[1], 11056[1], 11057[1], 11401[1], 11402[1], 11403[1], 11404[1], 11406[1], 11421[1], 11422[1], 11423[1], 11424[1], 11426[1], 11441[1], 11442[1], 11443[1], 11444[1], 11446[1], 11450[1], 11451[1], 11462[1], 11463[1], 11470[1], 11471[1], 11600[1], 11601[1], 11602[1], 11603[1], 11604[1], 11606[1], 11620[1], 11621[1], 11622[1], 11623[1], 11624[1], 11626[1], 11640[1], 11641[1], 11642[1], 11643[1], 11644[1], 11646[1], 11719[1], 11720[1], 11721[1], 11765[1], 12001[1], 12002[1], 12004[1], 12005[1], 12006[1], 12007[1], 12011[1], 12013[1], 12014[1], 12015[1], 12016[1], 12017[1], 12018[1], 12020[1], 12021[1], 12031[1], 12032[1], 12034[1], 12035[1], 12036[1], 12037[1], 12041[1], 12042[1], 12044[1], 12045[1], 12046[1], 12047[1], 12051[1], 12052[1], 12053[1], 12054[1], 12055[1], 12056[1], 12057[1], 13100[1], 13101[1], 13102[1], 13120[1], 13121[1], 13122[1], 13131[1], 13132[1], 13133[1], 13151[1], 13152[1], 13153[1], 20500[1], 29580[1], 29581[1], 36000[1], 36400[1], 36405[1], 36406[1], 36410[1], 36420[1], 36425[1], 36430[1], 36440[1], 36591[0], 36592[0], 36600[1], 36640[1], 43752[1], 51701[1], 51702[1], 51703[1], 61650[1], 62320[0], 62321[0], 62322[0], 62323[0], 62324[0], 62325[0], 62326[0], 62327[0], 64400[0], 64405[0], 64408[0], 64415[0], 64416[0], 64417[0], 64418[0], 64420[0], 64421[0], 64425[0], 64430[0], 64435[0], 64445[0], 64446[0], 64447[0], 64448[0], 64449[0], 64450[1], 64451[0], 64454[1], 64461[0], 64462[0], 64463[0], 64479[0], 64480[0], 64483[0], 64484[0], 64486[0], 64487[0], 64488[0], 64489[0], 64490[0], 64491[0], 64492[0], 64493[0], 64494[0], 64495[0], 64505[0], 64510[0], 64517[0], 64520[0], 64530[0], 69990[0], 75989[1], 76000[1], 76380[1], 76942[1], 76998[1], 77002[1], 77003[1], 77012[1], 77021[1], 92012[1], 92014[1], 93000[1], 93005[1], 93010[1], 93040[1], 93041[1], 93042[1], 93318[1], 93355[1], 94002[1], 94200[1], 94680[1], 94681[1], 94690[1], 95812[1], 95813[1], 95816[1], 95819[1], 95822[1], 95829[1], 95955[1], 96360[1], 96361[1], 96365[1], 96366[1], 96367[1], 96368[1], 96372[1], 96374[1], 96375[1], 96376[1], 96377[1], 96523[0], 97597[1], 97598[1], 97602[1], 97605[1], 97606[1], 97607[1], 97608[1], 99155[0], 99156[0], 99157[0], 99211[1], 99212[1], 99213[1], 99214[1], 99215[1], 99217[1], 99218[1], 99219[1], 99220[1], 99221[1], 99222[1], 99223[1], 99231[1], 99232[1], 99233[1], 99234[1], 99235[1], 99236[1], 99238[1], 99239[1], 99241[1], 99242[1], 99243[1], 99244[1], 99245[1], 99251[1], 99252[1], 99253[1], 99254[1], 99255[1], 99291[1], 99292[1], 99304[1], 99305[1], 99306[1], 99307[1], 99308[1], 99309[1], 99310[1], 99315[1], 99316[1], 99334[1], 99335[1], 99336[1], 99337[1], 99347[1], 99348[1], 99349[1], 99350[1], 99374[1], 99375[1], 99377[1], 99378[1], 99446[0], 99447[0], 99448[0], 99449[0], 99451[0], 99452[0], G0127[1], G0463[1], G0471[1], J0670[1], J2001[1]
10180	0213T[0], 0216T[0], 0596T[1], 0597T[1], 11720[1], 11721[1], 12001[1], 12002[1], 12004[1], 12005[1], 12006[1], 12007[1], 12011[1], 12013[1], 12014[1], 12015[1], 12016[1], 12017[1], 12018[1], 12020[1], 12021[1], 12031[1], 12032[1], 12034[1], 12035[1], 12036[1], 12037[1], 12041[1], 12042[1], 12044[1], 12045[1], 12046[1], 12047[1], 12051[1], 12052[1], 12053[1], 12054[1], 12055[1], 12056[1], 12057[1], 13100[1], 13101[1], 13102[1], 13120[1], 13121[1], 13122[1], 13131[1], 13132[1], 13133[1], 13151[1], 13152[1], 13153[1], 20500[1], 36000[1], 36400[1], 36405[1], 36406[1], 36410[1], 36420[1], 36425[1], 36430[1], 36440[1], 36591[0], 36592[0], 36600[1], 36640[1], 43752[1], 51701[1], 51702[1], 51703[1], 62320[0], 62321[0], 62322[0], 62323[0], 62324[0], 62325[0], 62326[0], 62327[0], 64400[0], 64405[0], 64408[0], 64415[0], 64416[0], 64417[0], 64418[0], 64420[0], 64421[0], 64425[0], 64430[0], 64435[0], 64445[0], 64446[0], 64447[0], 64448[0], 64449[0], 64450[1], 64451[0], 64454[1], 64461[0], 64462[0], 64463[0], 64479[0], 64480[0], 64483[0], 64484[0], 64486[0], 64487[0], 64488[0], 64489[0], 64490[0], 64491[0], 64492[0], 64493[0], 64494[0], 64495[0], 64505[0], 64510[0], 64517[0], 64520[0], 64530[0], 69990[0], 92012[1], 92014[1], 93000[1], 93005[1], 93010[1], 93040[1], 93041[1], 93042[1], 93318[1], 93355[1], 94002[1], 94200[1], 94680[1], 94681[1], 94690[1], 95812[1], 95813[1], 95816[1], 95819[1], 95822[1], 95829[1], 95955[1], 96360[1], 96361[1], 96365[1], 96366[1], 96367[1], 96368[1], 96372[1], 96374[1], 96375[1], 96376[1], 96377[1], 96523[0], 99155[0], 99156[0], 99157[0], 99211[1], 99212[1], 99213[1], 99214[1], 99215[1], 99217[1], 99218[1], 99219[1], 99220[1], 99221[1], 99222[1], 99223[1], 99231[1], 99232[1], 99233[1], 99234[1], 99235[1], 99236[1], 99238[1], 99239[1], 99241[1], 99242[1], 99243[1], 99244[1], 99245[1], 99251[1], 99252[1], 99253[1], 99254[1], 99255[1], 99291[1], 99292[1], 99304[1], 99305[1], 99306[1], 99307[1], 99308[1], 99309[1], 99310[1], 99315[1], 99316[1], 99334[1], 99335[1], 99336[1], 99337[1], 99347[1], 99348[1], 99349[1], 99350[1], 99374[1], 99375[1], 99377[1], 99378[1], 99446[0], 99447[0], 99448[0], 99449[0], 99451[0], 99452[0], 99495[0], 99496[0], G0463[1], G0471[1], J0670[1], J2001[1]
11004	0213T[0], 0216T[0], 0437T[1], 0552T[1], 10030[1], 10060[1], 10061[1], 11000[1], 11010[1], 11011[1], 11012[1], 11042[1], 11043[1], 11044[1], 11102[1], 11103[1], 11104[1], 11105[1], 11106[1], 11107[1], 12001[1], 12002[1], 12004[1], 12005[1], 12006[1], 12007[1], 12011[1], 12013[1], 12014[1], 12015[1], 12016[1], 12017[1], 12018[1], 12021[1], 12031[1], 12032[1], 12034[1], 12035[1], 12036[1], 12037[1], 12041[1], 12042[1], 12044[1], 12045[1], 12046[1], 12047[1], 12051[1], 12052[1], 12053[1], 12054[1], 12055[1], 12056[1], 12057[1], 13100[1], 13101[1], 13102[1], 13120[1], 13121[1], 13122[1], 13131[1], 13132[1], 13133[1], 13151[1], 13152[1], 13153[1], 15769[1], 15777[1], 20552[1], 20553[1], 20560[1], 20561[1], 20700[1], 20701[1], 36000[1], 36400[1], 36405[1], 36406[1], 36410[1], 36420[1], 36425[1], 36430[1], 36440[1], 36591[0], 36592[0], 36600[1], 36640[1], 43752[1], 57267[1], 62320[0], 62321[0], 62322[0], 62323[0], 62324[0], 62325[0], 62326[0], 62327[0], 64400[0], 64405[0], 64408[0], 64415[0], 64416[0], 64417[0], 64418[0], 64420[0], 64421[0], 64425[0], 64430[0], 64435[0], 64445[0], 64446[0], 64447[0], 64448[0], 64449[0], 64450[1], 64451[0], 64454[1], 64461[0], 64462[0], 64463[0], 64479[0], 64480[0], 64483[0], 64484[0], 64486[0], 64487[0], 64488[0], 64489[0], 64490[0], 64491[0], 64492[0], 64493[0], 64494[0], 64495[0], 64505[0], 64510[0], 64517[0], 64520[0], 64530[0], 66987[1], 66988[1], 69990[0], 92012[1], 92014[1], 93000[1], 93005[1], 93010[1], 93040[1], 93041[1], 93042[1], 93318[1], 93355[1], 94002[1], 94200[1], 94680[1], 94681[1], 94690[1], 95812[1], 95813[1], 95816[1], 95819[1], 95822[1], 95829[1], 95955[1], 96360[1], 96361[1], 96365[1], 96366[1], 96367[1], 96368[1], 96372[1], 96374[1], 96375[1], 96376[1], 96377[1], 96523[0], 97597[1], 97598[1], 97610[1], 99155[0], 99156[0], 99157[0], 99211[1], 99212[1], 99213[1], 99214[1], 99215[1], 99217[1], 99218[1], 99219[1], 99220[1], 99221[1], 99222[1], 99223[1], 99231[1], 99232[1], 99233[1], 99234[1], 99235[1], 99236[1], 99238[1], 99239[1], 99241[1], 99242[1], 99243[1], 99244[1], 99245[1], 99251[1], 99252[1], 99253[1], 99254[1], 99255[1], 99291[1], 99292[1], 99304[1], 99305[1], 99306[1], 99307[1], 99308[1], 99309[1], 99310[1], 99315[1], 99316[1], 99334[1], 99335[1], 99336[1], 99337[1], 99347[1], 99348[1], 99349[1], 99350[1],

0 = Modifier usage not allowed or inappropriate 1 = Modifier usage allowed

Code 1	Code 2
	99374[1], 99375[1], 99377[1], 99378[1], 99446[0], 99447[0], 99448[0], 99449[0], 99451[0], 99452[0], 99495[1], 99496[1], G0463[1], G0471[1]
11005	0213T[0], 0216T[0], 0437T[1], 0552T[1], 10030[1], 10060[1], 10061[1], 11000[1], 11004[0], 11010[1], 11011[1], 11012[1], 11042[1], 11043[1], 11044[1], 11102[1], 11103[1], 11104[1], 11105[1], 11106[1], 11107[1], 12001[1], 12002[1], 12004[1], 12005[1], 12006[1], 12007[1], 12011[1], 12013[1], 12014[1], 12015[1], 12016[1], 12017[1], 12018[1], 12021[1], 12031[1], 12032[1], 12034[1], 12035[1], 12036[1], 12037[1], 12041[1], 12042[1], 12044[1], 12045[1], 12046[1], 12047[1], 12051[1], 12052[1], 12053[1], 12054[1], 12055[1], 12056[1], 12057[1], 13100[1], 13101[1], 13102[1], 13120[1], 13121[1], 13122[1], 13131[1], 13132[1], 13133[1], 13151[1], 13152[1], 13153[1], 15769[1], 15777[1], 20552[1], 20553[1], 20560[1], 20561[1], 20700[1], 20701[1], 36000[1], 36400[1], 36405[1], 36406[1], 36410[1], 36420[1], 36425[1], 36430[1], 36440[1], 36591[0], 36592[0], 36600[1], 36640[1], 43752[1], 57267[1], 62320[0], 62321[0], 62322[0], 62323[0], 62324[0], 62325[0], 62326[0], 62327[0], 64400[0], 64405[0], 64408[0], 64415[0], 64416[0], 64417[0], 64418[0], 64420[0], 64421[0], 64425[0], 64430[0], 64435[0], 64445[0], 64446[0], 64447[0], 64448[0], 64449[0], 64450[1], 64451[0], 64454[1], 64461[0], 64462[0], 64463[0], 64479[0], 64480[0], 64483[0], 64484[0], 64486[0], 64487[0], 64488[0], 64489[0], 64490[0], 64491[0], 64492[0], 64493[0], 64494[0], 64495[0], 64505[0], 64510[0], 64517[0], 64520[0], 64530[0], 66987[1], 66988[1], 69990[0], 92012[1], 92014[1], 93000[1], 93005[1], 93010[1], 93040[1], 93041[1], 93042[1], 93318[1], 93355[1], 94002[1], 94200[1], 94680[1], 94681[1], 94690[1], 95812[1], 95813[1], 95816[1], 95819[1], 95822[1], 95829[1], 95955[1], 96360[1], 96361[1], 96365[1], 96366[1], 96367[1], 96368[1], 96372[1], 96374[1], 96375[1], 96376[1], 96377[1], 96523[0], 97597[1], 97598[1], 97610[1], 99155[0], 99156[0], 99157[0], 99211[1], 99212[1], 99213[1], 99214[1], 99215[1], 99217[1], 99218[1], 99219[1], 99220[1], 99221[1], 99222[1], 99223[1], 99231[1], 99232[1], 99233[1], 99234[1], 99235[1], 99236[1], 99238[1], 99239[1], 99241[1], 99242[1], 99243[1], 99244[1], 99245[1], 99251[1], 99252[1], 99253[1], 99254[1], 99255[1], 99291[1], 99292[1], 99304[1], 99305[1], 99306[1], 99307[1], 99308[1], 99309[1], 99310[1], 99315[1], 99316[1], 99334[1], 99335[1], 99336[1], 99337[1], 99347[1], 99348[1], 99349[1], 99350[1], 99374[1], 99375[1], 99377[1], 99378[1], 99446[0], 99447[0], 99448[0], 99449[0], 99451[0], 99452[0], 99495[1], 99496[1], G0463[1], G0471[1]
11006	0213T[0], 0216T[0], 0437T[1], 0552T[1], 10030[1], 10060[1], 10061[1], 11000[1], 11004[0], 11005[0], 11010[1], 11011[1], 11012[1], 11042[1], 11043[1], 11044[1], 11102[1], 11103[1], 11104[1], 11105[1], 11106[1], 11107[1], 12001[1], 12002[1], 12004[1], 12005[1], 12006[1], 12007[1], 12011[1], 12013[1], 12014[1], 12015[1], 12016[1], 12017[1], 12018[1], 12021[1], 12031[1], 12032[1], 12034[1], 12035[1], 12036[1], 12037[1], 12041[1], 12042[1], 12044[1], 12045[1], 12046[1], 12047[1], 12051[1], 12052[1], 12053[1], 12054[1], 12055[1], 12056[1], 12057[1], 13100[1], 13101[1], 13102[1], 13120[1], 13121[1], 13122[1], 13131[1], 13132[1], 13133[1], 13151[1], 13152[1], 13153[1], 15769[1], 15777[1], 20552[1], 20553[1], 20560[1], 20561[1], 20700[1], 20701[1], 36000[1], 36400[1], 36405[1], 36406[1], 36410[1], 36420[1], 36425[1], 36430[1], 36440[1], 36591[0], 36592[0], 36600[1], 36640[1], 43752[1], 57267[1], 62320[0], 62321[0], 62322[0], 62323[0], 62324[0], 62325[0], 62326[0], 62327[0], 64400[0], 64405[0], 64408[0], 64415[0], 64416[0], 64417[0], 64418[0], 64420[0], 64421[0], 64425[0], 64430[0], 64435[0], 64445[0], 64446[0], 64447[0], 64448[0], 64449[0], 64450[1], 64451[0], 64454[1], 64461[0], 64462[0], 64463[0], 64479[0], 64480[0], 64483[0], 64484[0], 64486[0], 64487[0], 64488[0], 64489[0], 64490[0], 64491[0], 64492[0], 64493[0], 64494[0], 64495[0], 64505[0], 64510[0], 64517[0], 64520[0], 64530[0], 66987[1], 66988[1], 69990[0], 92012[1], 92014[1], 93000[1], 93005[1], 93010[1], 93040[1], 93041[1], 93042[1], 93318[1], 93355[1], 94002[1], 94200[1], 94680[1], 94681[1], 94690[1], 95812[1], 95813[1], 95816[1], 95819[1], 95822[1], 95829[1], 95955[1], 96360[1], 96361[1], 96365[1], 96366[1], 96367[1], 96368[1], 96372[1], 96374[1], 96375[1], 96376[1], 96377[1], 96523[0], 97597[1], 97598[1], 97610[1], 99155[0], 99156[0], 99157[0], 99211[1], 99212[1], 99213[1], 99214[1], 99215[1], 99217[1], 99218[1], 99219[1], 99220[1], 99221[1], 99222[1], 99223[1], 99231[1], 99232[1], 99233[1], 99234[1], 99235[1], 99236[1], 99238[1], 99239[1], 99241[1], 99242[1], 99243[1], 99244[1], 99245[1], 99251[1], 99252[1], 99253[1], 99254[1], 99255[1], 99291[1], 99292[1], 99304[1], 99305[1], 99306[1], 99307[1], 99308[1], 99309[1], 99310[1], 99315[1], 99316[1], 99334[1], 99335[1], 99336[1], 99337[1], 99347[1], 99348[1], 99349[1], 99350[1], 99374[1], 99375[1], 99377[1], 99378[1], 99446[0], 99447[0], 99448[0], 99449[0], 99451[0], 99452[0], 99495[1], 99496[1], G0463[1], G0471[1]
11420	00400[0], 0213T[0], 0216T[0], 0470T[1], 0471T[1], 0596T[1], 0597T[1], 0700T[1], 0701T[1], 0708T[1], 0709T[1], 10030[1], 10060[1], 10061[1], 11000[1], 11001[1], 11004[1], 11005[1], 11006[1], 11042[1], 11043[1], 11044[1], 11045[1], 11046[1], 11047[1], 11102[1], 11104[1], 11106[1], 11719[1], 11900[1], 11901[1], 12001[1], 12002[1], 12004[1], 12005[1], 12006[1], 12007[1], 12011[1], 12013[1], 12014[1], 12015[1], 12016[1], 12017[1], 12018[1], 12020[1], 12021[1], 12031[1], 12032[1], 12034[1], 12035[1], 12036[1], 12037[1], 12041[1], 12042[1], 12044[1], 12045[1], 12046[1], 12047[1], 12051[1], 12052[1], 12053[1], 12054[1], 12055[1], 12056[1], 12057[1], 13100[1], 13101[1], 13102[1], 13120[1], 13121[1], 13122[1], 13131[1], 13132[1], 13133[1], 13151[1], 13152[1], 13153[1], 17000[1], 17250[1], 36000[1], 36400[1], 36405[1], 36406[1], 36410[1], 36420[1], 36425[1], 36430[1], 36440[1], 36591[0], 36592[0], 36600[1], 36640[1], 43752[1], 51701[1], 51702[1], 51703[1], 62320[0], 62321[0], 62322[0], 62323[0], 62324[0], 62325[0], 62326[0], 62327[0], 64400[0], 64405[0], 64408[0], 64415[0], 64416[0], 64417[0], 64418[0], 64420[0], 64421[0], 64425[0], 64430[0], 64435[0], 64445[0], 64446[0], 64447[0], 64448[0], 64449[0], 64450[1], 64451[0], 64454[1], 64461[0], 64462[0], 64463[0], 64479[0], 64480[0], 64483[0], 64484[0], 64486[0], 64487[0], 64488[0], 64489[0], 64490[0], 64491[0], 64492[0], 64493[0], 64494[0], 64495[0], 64505[0], 64510[0], 64517[0], 64520[0], 64530[0], 69990[0], 92012[1], 92014[1], 93000[1], 93005[1], 93010[1], 93040[1], 93041[1], 93042[1], 93318[1], 93355[1], 94002[1], 94200[1], 94680[1], 94681[1], 94690[1], 95812[1], 95813[1], 95816[1], 95819[1], 95822[1], 95829[1], 95955[1], 96360[1], 96361[1], 96365[1], 96366[1], 96367[1], 96368[1], 96372[1], 96374[1], 96375[1], 96376[1], 96377[1], 96405[1], 96406[1], 96523[0], 96931[1], 96932[1], 96933[1], 96934[1], 96935[1], 96936[1], 97597[1], 97598[1], 97602[1], 99155[0], 99156[0], 99157[0], 99211[1], 99212[1], 99213[1], 99214[1], 99215[1], 99217[1], 99218[1], 99219[1], 99220[1], 99221[1], 99222[1], 99223[1], 99231[1], 99232[1], 99233[1], 99234[1], 99235[1], 99236[1], 99238[1], 99239[1], 99241[1], 99242[1], 99243[1], 99244[1], 99245[1], 99251[1], 99252[1], 99253[1], 99254[1], 99255[1], 99291[1], 99292[1], 99304[1], 99305[1], 99306[1], 99307[1], 99308[1], 99309[1], 99310[1], 99315[1], 99316[1], 99334[1], 99335[1], 99336[1], 99337[1], 99347[1], 99348[1], 99349[1], 99350[1], 99374[1], 99375[1], 99377[1], 99378[1], 99446[0], 99447[0], 99448[0], 99449[0], 99451[0], 99452[0], 99495[0], 99496[0], G0168[1], G0463[1], G0471[1], J0670[1], J2001[1]
11421	00400[0], 0213T[0], 0216T[0], 0470T[1], 0471T[1], 0596T[1], 0597T[1], 0700T[1], 0701T[1], 0708T[1], 0709T[1], 10061[1], 11000[1], 11001[1], 11004[1], 11005[1], 11006[1], 11042[1], 11043[1], 11044[1], 11045[1], 11046[1], 11047[1], 11102[1], 11104[1], 11106[1], 11719[1], 11900[1], 11901[1], 12001[1], 12002[1], 12004[1], 12005[1], 12006[1], 12007[1], 12011[1], 12013[1], 12014[1], 12015[1], 12016[1], 12017[1], 12018[1], 17000[1], 17004[1], 17250[1], 36000[1], 36400[1], 36405[1], 36406[1], 36410[1], 36420[1], 36425[1], 36430[1], 36440[1], 36591[0], 36592[0], 36600[1], 36640[1], 43752[1], 51701[1], 51702[1], 51703[1], 62320[0], 62321[0], 62322[0], 62323[0], 62324[0], 62325[0], 62326[0], 62327[0], 64400[0], 64405[0], 64408[0], 64415[0], 64416[0], 64417[0], 64418[0], 64420[0], 64421[0], 64425[0], 64430[0], 64435[0], 64445[0], 64446[0], 64447[0], 64448[0], 64449[0], 64450[1], 64451[0], 64454[1], 64461[0], 64462[0], 64463[0], 64479[0], 64480[0], 64483[0], 64484[0], 64486[0], 64487[0], 64488[0], 64489[0], 64490[0], 64491[0], 64492[0], 64493[0], 64494[0], 64495[0], 64505[0], 64510[0], 64517[0], 64520[0], 64530[0], 69990[0], 92012[1], 92014[1], 93000[1], 93005[1], 93010[1], 93040[1], 93041[1], 93042[1], 93318[1], 93355[1], 94002[1], 94200[1], 94680[1], 94681[1], 94690[1], 95812[1], 95813[1], 95816[1], 95819[1], 95822[1], 95829[1], 95955[1], 96360[1], 96361[1], 96365[1], 96366[1], 96367[1], 96368[1], 96372[1], 96374[1], 96375[1], 96376[1], 96377[1], 96405[1], 96406[1], 96523[0], 96931[1], 96932[1], 96933[1], 96934[1], 96935[1], 96936[1], 97597[1], 97598[1], 97602[1], 99155[0], 99156[0], 99157[0], 99211[1], 99212[1], 99213[1], 99214[1], 99215[1], 99217[1], 99218[1], 99219[1], 99220[1], 99221[1], 99222[1], 99223[1], 99231[1], 99232[1], 99233[1], 99234[1], 99235[1], 99236[1], 99238[1], 99239[1], 99241[1], 99242[1], 99243[1], 99244[1], 99245[1], 99251[1], 99252[1], 99253[1], 99254[1], 99255[1], 99291[1], 99292[1], 99304[1], 99305[1], 99306[1], 99307[1], 99308[1], 99309[1], 99310[1], 99315[1], 99316[1], 99334[1], 99335[1], 99336[1], 99337[1], 99347[1], 99348[1], 99349[1], 99350[1], 99374[1], 99375[1], 99377[1], 99378[1], 99446[0], 99447[0], 99448[0], 99449[0], 99451[0], 99452[0], 99495[0], 99496[0], G0168[1], G0463[1], G0471[1], J0670[1], J2001[1]
11422	00400[0], 0213T[0], 0216T[0], 0470T[1], 0471T[1], 0596T[1], 0597T[1], 0700T[1], 0701T[1], 0708T[1], 0709T[1], 10061[1], 11000[1], 11001[1], 11004[1], 11005[1], 11006[1], 11042[1], 11043[1], 11044[1], 11045[1], 11046[1], 11047[1], 11102[1], 11104[1], 11106[1], 11900[1], 11901[1], 12001[1], 12002[1], 12004[1], 12005[1], 12006[1], 12007[1], 12011[1], 12013[1], 12014[1], 12015[1], 12016[1], 12017[1], 12018[1], 17000[1], 17004[1], 17250[1], 36000[1], 36400[1], 36405[1], 36406[1], 36410[1], 36420[1], 36425[1], 36430[1], 36440[1], 36591[0], 36592[0], 36600[1], 36640[1], 43752[1], 51701[1], 51702[1], 51703[1], 62320[0], 62321[0], 62322[0], 62323[0], 62324[0], 62325[0], 62326[0], 62327[0], 64400[0], 64405[0], 64408[0], 64415[0], 64416[0], 64417[0], 64418[0], 64420[0], 64421[0], 64425[0], 64430[0], 64435[0], 64445[0], 64446[0], 64447[0], 64448[0], 64449[0], 64450[1], 64451[0], 64454[1], 64461[0], 64462[0], 64463[0], 64479[0], 64480[0], 64483[0], 64484[0], 64486[0], 64487[0], 64488[0], 64489[0], 64490[0], 64491[0], 64492[0], 64493[0], 64494[0], 64495[0], 64505[0], 64510[0], 64517[0], 64520[0], 64530[0], 69990[0], 92012[1], 92014[1], 93000[1], 93005[1], 93010[1], 93040[1], 93041[1], 93042[1], 93318[1], 93355[1], 94002[1], 94200[1], 94680[1], 94681[1], 94690[1], 95812[1], 95813[1], 95816[1], 95819[1], 95822[1], 95829[1], 95955[1], 96360[1], 96361[1], 96365[1], 96366[1], 96367[1], 96368[1], 96372[1], 96374[1], 96375[1], 96376[1], 96377[1], 96405[1], 96406[1], 96523[0], 96931[1], 96932[1], 96933[1], 96934[1], 96935[1], 96936[1], 97597[1], 97598[1], 97602[1], 99155[0], 99156[0], 99157[0], 99211[1], 99212[1], 99213[1], 99214[1], 99215[1], 99217[1], 99218[1], 99219[1], 99220[1], 99221[1], 99222[1], 99223[1], 99231[1], 99232[1], 99233[1], 99234[1], 99235[1], 99236[1], 99238[1], 99239[1], 99241[1], 99242[1], 99243[1], 99244[1], 99245[1], 99251[1], 99252[1], 99253[1], 99254[1], 99255[1], 99291[1], 99292[1], 99304[1], 99305[1], 99306[1], 99307[1], 99308[1], 99309[1], 99310[1], 99315[1], 99316[1], 99334[1], 99335[1], 99336[1], 99337[1], 99347[1], 99348[1], 99349[1], 99350[1], 99374[1], 99375[1], 99377[1], 99378[1], 99446[0], 99447[0], 99448[0], 99449[0], 99451[0], 99452[0], 99495[0], 99496[0], G0168[1], G0463[1], G0471[1], J0670[1], J2001[1]
11423	00400[0], 0213T[0], 0216T[0], 0470T[1], 0471T[1], 0596T[1], 0597T[1], 0700T[1], 0701T[1], 0708T[1], 0709T[1], 10061[1], 11000[1], 11001[1], 11004[1], 11005[1], 11006[1], 11042[1], 11043[1], 11044[1], 11045[1], 11046[1], 11047[1], 11102[1], 11104[1], 11106[1], 11900[1], 11901[1], 12001[1], 12002[1], 12004[1], 12005[1], 12006[1], 12007[1], 12011[1], 12013[1], 12014[1], 12015[1], 12016[1], 12017[1], 12018[1], 17000[1], 17004[1], 17250[1], 36000[1], 36400[1], 36405[1], 36406[1], 36410[1], 36420[1],

0 = Modifier usage not allowed or inappropriate 1 = Modifier usage allowed

Appendix A: NCCI - CPT Codes

Code 1	Code 2
	36425[1], 36430[1], 36440[1], 36591[0], 36592[0], 36600[1], 36640[1], 43752[1], 51701[1], 51702[1], 51703[1], 62320[0], 62321[0], 62322[0], 62323[0], 62324[0], 62325[0], 62326[0], 62327[0], 64400[0], 64405[0], 64408[0], 64415[0], 64416[0], 64417[0], 64418[0], 64420[0], 64421[0], 64425[0], 64430[0], 64435[0], 64445[0], 64446[0], 64447[0], 64448[0], 64449[0], 64450[1], 64451[0], 64454[1], 64461[0], 64462[0], 64463[0], 64479[0], 64480[0], 64483[0], 64484[0], 64486[0], 64487[0], 64488[0], 64489[0], 64490[0], 64491[0], 64492[0], 64493[0], 64494[0], 64495[0], 64505[0], 64510[0], 64517[0], 64520[0], 64530[0], 69990[0], 92012[1], 92014[1], 93000[1], 93005[1], 93010[1], 93040[1], 93041[1], 93042[1], 93318[1], 93355[1], 94002[1], 94200[1], 94680[1], 94681[1], 94690[1], 95812[1], 95813[1], 95816[1], 95819[1], 95822[1], 95829[1], 95955[1], 96360[1], 96361[1], 96365[1], 96366[1], 96367[1], 96368[1], 96372[1], 96374[1], 96375[1], 96376[1], 96377[1], 96405[1], 96406[1], 96523[0], 96931[1], 96932[1], 96933[1], 96934[1], 96935[1], 96936[1], 97597[1], 97598[1], 97602[1], 99155[0], 99156[0], 99157[0], 99211[1], 99212[1], 99213[1], 99214[1], 99215[1], 99217[1], 99218[1], 99219[1], 99220[1], 99221[1], 99222[1], 99223[1], 99231[1], 99232[1], 99233[1], 99234[1], 99235[1], 99236[1], 99238[1], 99239[1], 99241[1], 99242[1], 99243[1], 99244[1], 99245[1], 99251[1], 99252[1], 99253[1], 99254[1], 99255[1], 99291[1], 99292[1], 99304[1], 99305[1], 99306[1], 99307[1], 99308[1], 99309[1], 99310[1], 99315[1], 99316[1], 99334[1], 99335[1], 99336[1], 99337[1], 99347[1], 99348[1], 99349[1], 99350[1], 99374[1], 99375[1], 99377[1], 99378[1], 99446[0], 99447[0], 99448[0], 99449[0], 99451[0], 99452[0], 99495[0], 99496[0], G0168[1], G0463[1], G0471[1], J0670[1], J2001[1]
11424	00400[0], 0213T[0], 0216T[0], 0470T[1], 0471T[1], 0596T[1], 0597T[1], 0700T[1], 0701T[1], 0708T[1], 0709T[1], 11000[1], 11001[1], 11004[1], 11005[1], 11006[1], 11042[1], 11043[1], 11044[1], 11045[1], 11046[1], 11047[1], 11102[1], 11104[1], 11106[1], 11900[1], 11901[1], 12001[1], 12002[1], 12004[1], 12005[1], 12006[1], 12007[1], 12011[1], 12013[1], 12014[1], 12015[1], 12016[1], 12017[1], 12018[1], 17000[1], 17004[1], 17250[1], 36000[1], 36400[1], 36405[1], 36406[1], 36410[1], 36420[1], 36425[1], 36430[1], 36440[1], 36591[0], 36592[0], 36600[1], 36640[1], 43752[1], 51701[1], 51702[1], 51703[1], 62320[0], 62321[0], 62322[0], 62323[0], 62324[0], 62325[0], 62326[0], 62327[0], 64400[0], 64405[0], 64408[0], 64415[0], 64416[0], 64417[0], 64418[0], 64420[0], 64421[0], 64425[0], 64430[0], 64435[0], 64445[0], 64446[0], 64447[0], 64448[0], 64449[0], 64450[1], 64451[0], 64454[1], 64461[0], 64462[0], 64463[0], 64479[0], 64480[0], 64483[0], 64484[0], 64486[0], 64487[0], 64488[0], 64489[0], 64490[0], 64491[0], 64492[0], 64493[0], 64494[0], 64495[0], 64505[0], 64510[0], 64517[0], 64520[0], 64530[0], 69990[0], 92012[1], 92014[1], 93000[1], 93005[1], 93010[1], 93040[1], 93041[1], 93042[1], 93318[1], 93355[1], 94002[1], 94200[1], 94680[1], 94681[1], 94690[1], 95812[1], 95813[1], 95816[1], 95819[1], 95822[1], 95829[1], 95955[1], 96360[1], 96361[1], 96365[1], 96366[1], 96367[1], 96368[1], 96372[1], 96374[1], 96375[1], 96376[1], 96377[1], 96405[1], 96406[1], 96523[0], 96931[1], 96932[1], 96933[1], 96934[1], 96935[1], 96936[1], 97597[1], 97598[1], 97602[1], 99155[0], 99156[0], 99157[0], 99211[1], 99212[1], 99213[1], 99214[1], 99215[1], 99217[1], 99218[1], 99219[1], 99220[1], 99221[1], 99222[1], 99223[1], 99231[1], 99232[1], 99233[1], 99234[1], 99235[1], 99236[1], 99238[1], 99239[1], 99241[1], 99242[1], 99243[1], 99244[1], 99245[1], 99251[1], 99252[1], 99253[1], 99254[1], 99255[1], 99291[1], 99292[1], 99304[1], 99305[1], 99306[1], 99307[1], 99308[1], 99309[1], 99310[1], 99315[1], 99316[1], 99334[1], 99335[1], 99336[1], 99337[1], 99347[1], 99348[1], 99349[1], 99350[1], 99374[1], 99375[1], 99377[1], 99378[1], 99446[0], 99447[0], 99448[0], 99449[0], 99451[0], 99452[0], 99495[0], 99496[0], G0168[1], G0463[1], G0471[1], J0670[1], J2001[1]
11426	00400[0], 0213T[0], 0216T[0], 0470T[1], 0471T[1], 0596T[1], 0597T[1], 0700T[1], 0701T[1], 0708T[1], 0709T[1], 11000[1], 11001[1], 11004[1], 11005[1], 11006[1], 11042[1], 11043[1], 11044[1], 11045[1], 11046[1], 11047[1], 11102[1], 11104[1], 11106[1], 11900[1], 11901[1], 12001[1], 12002[1], 12004[1], 12005[1], 12006[1], 12007[1], 12011[1], 12013[1], 12014[1], 12015[1], 12016[1], 12017[1], 12018[1], 17000[1], 17004[1], 17250[1], 36000[1], 36400[1], 36405[1], 36406[1], 36410[1], 36420[1], 36425[1], 36430[1], 36440[1], 36591[0], 36592[0], 36600[1], 36640[1], 43752[1], 51701[1], 51702[1], 51703[1], 62320[0], 62321[0], 62322[0], 62323[0], 62324[0], 62325[0], 62326[0], 62327[0], 64400[0], 64405[0], 64408[0], 64415[0], 64416[0], 64417[0], 64418[0], 64420[0], 64421[0], 64425[0], 64430[0], 64435[0], 64445[0], 64446[0], 64447[0], 64448[0], 64449[0], 64450[1], 64451[0], 64454[1], 64461[0], 64462[0], 64463[0], 64479[0], 64480[0], 64483[0], 64484[0], 64486[0], 64487[0], 64488[0], 64489[0], 64490[0], 64491[0], 64492[0], 64493[0], 64494[0], 64495[0], 64505[0], 64510[0], 64517[0], 64520[0], 64530[0], 69990[0], 92012[1], 92014[1], 93000[1], 93005[1], 93010[1], 93040[1], 93041[1], 93042[1], 93318[1], 93355[1], 94002[1], 94200[1], 94680[1], 94681[1], 94690[1], 95812[1], 95813[1], 95816[1], 95819[1], 95822[1], 95829[1], 95955[1], 96360[1], 96361[1], 96365[1], 96366[1], 96367[1], 96368[1], 96372[1], 96374[1], 96375[1], 96376[1], 96377[1], 96405[1], 96406[1], 96523[0], 96931[1], 96932[1], 96933[1], 96934[1], 96935[1], 96936[1], 97597[1], 97598[1], 97602[1], 99155[0], 99156[0], 99157[0], 99211[1], 99212[1], 99213[1], 99214[1], 99215[1], 99217[1], 99218[1], 99219[1], 99220[1], 99221[1], 99222[1], 99223[1], 99231[1], 99232[1], 99233[1], 99234[1], 99235[1], 99236[1], 99238[1], 99239[1], 99241[1], 99242[1], 99243[1], 99244[1], 99245[1], 99251[1], 99252[1], 99253[1], 99254[1], 99255[1], 99291[1], 99292[1], 99304[1], 99305[1], 99306[1], 99307[1], 99308[1], 99309[1], 99310[1], 99315[1], 99316[1], 99334[1], 99335[1], 99336[1], 99337[1], 99347[1], 99348[1], 99349[1], 99350[1], 99374[1], 99375[1], 99377[1], 99378[1], 99446[0], 99447[0], 99448[0], 99449[0], 99451[0], 99452[0], 99495[0], 99496[0], G0168[1], G0463[1], G0471[1], J0670[1], J2001[1]
11620	00400[0], 0213T[0], 0216T[0], 0596T[1], 0597T[1], 10061[1], 11000[1], 11001[1], 11004[1], 11005[1], 11006[1], 11042[1], 11043[1], 11044[1], 11045[1], 11046[1], 11047[1], 11102[1], 11104[1], 11106[1], 11900[1], 11901[1], 12001[1], 12002[1], 12004[1], 12005[1], 12006[1], 12007[1], 12011[1], 12013[1], 12014[1], 12015[1], 12016[1], 12017[1], 12018[1], 17000[1], 17004[1], 17250[1], 17262[1], 17263[1], 17264[1], 17266[1], 17271[1], 17272[1], 17273[1], 17274[1], 17276[1], 17281[1], 17282[1], 17283[1], 17284[1], 17286[1], 36000[1], 36400[1], 36405[1], 36406[1], 36410[1], 36420[1], 36425[1], 36430[1], 36440[1], 36591[0], 36592[0], 36600[1], 36640[1], 43752[1], 51701[1], 51702[1], 51703[1], 62320[0], 62321[0], 62322[0], 62323[0], 62324[0], 62325[0], 62326[0], 62327[0], 64400[0], 64405[0], 64408[0], 64415[0], 64416[0], 64417[0], 64418[0], 64420[0], 64421[0], 64425[0], 64430[0], 64435[0], 64445[0], 64446[0], 64447[0], 64448[0], 64449[0], 64450[1], 64451[0], 64454[1], 64461[0], 64462[0], 64463[0], 64479[0], 64480[0], 64483[0], 64484[0], 64486[0], 64487[0], 64488[0], 64489[0], 64490[0], 64491[0], 64492[0], 64493[0], 64494[0], 64495[0], 64505[0], 64510[0], 64517[0], 64520[0], 64530[0], 69990[0], 92012[1], 92014[1], 93000[1], 93005[1], 93010[1], 93040[1], 93041[1], 93042[1], 93318[1], 93355[1], 94002[1], 94200[1], 94680[1], 94681[1], 94690[1], 95812[1], 95813[1], 95816[1], 95819[1], 95822[1], 95829[1], 95955[1], 96360[1], 96361[1], 96365[1], 96366[1], 96367[1], 96368[1], 96372[1], 96374[1], 96375[1], 96376[1], 96377[1], 96523[0], 97597[1], 97598[1], 97602[1], 99155[0], 99156[0], 99157[0], 99211[1], 99212[1], 99213[1], 99214[1], 99215[1], 99217[1], 99218[1], 99219[1], 99220[1], 99221[1], 99222[1], 99223[1], 99231[1], 99232[1], 99233[1], 99234[1], 99235[1], 99236[1], 99238[1], 99239[1], 99241[1], 99242[1], 99243[1], 99244[1], 99245[1], 99251[1], 99252[1], 99253[1], 99254[1], 99255[1], 99291[1], 99292[1], 99304[1], 99305[1], 99306[1], 99307[1], 99308[1], 99309[1], 99310[1], 99315[1], 99316[1], 99334[1], 99335[1], 99336[1], 99337[1], 99347[1], 99348[1], 99349[1], 99350[1], 99374[1], 99375[1], 99377[1], 99378[1], 99446[0], 99447[0], 99448[0], 99449[0], 99451[0], 99452[0], 99495[0], 99496[0], G0168[1], G0463[1], G0471[1], J0670[1], J2001[1]
11621	00400[0], 0213T[0], 0216T[0], 0596T[1], 0597T[1], 10061[1], 11000[1], 11001[1], 11004[1], 11005[1], 11006[1], 11042[1], 11043[1], 11044[1], 11045[1], 11046[1], 11047[1], 11102[1], 11104[1], 11106[1], 11900[1], 11901[1], 12001[1], 12002[1], 12004[1], 12005[1], 12006[1], 12007[1], 12011[1], 12013[1], 12014[1], 12015[1], 12016[1], 12017[1], 12018[1], 17000[1], 17004[1], 17250[1], 17266[1], 17273[1], 17274[1], 17276[1], 17282[1], 17283[1], 17284[1], 17286[1], 36000[1], 36400[1], 36405[1], 36406[1], 36410[1], 36420[1], 36425[1], 36430[1], 36440[1], 36591[0], 36592[0], 36600[1], 36640[1], 43752[1], 51701[1], 51702[1], 51703[1], 62320[0], 62321[0], 62322[0], 62323[0], 62324[0], 62325[0], 62326[0], 62327[0], 64400[0], 64405[0], 64408[0], 64415[0], 64416[0], 64417[0], 64418[0], 64420[0], 64421[0], 64425[0], 64430[0], 64435[0], 64445[0], 64446[0], 64447[0], 64448[0], 64449[0], 64450[1], 64451[0], 64454[1], 64461[0], 64462[0], 64463[0], 64479[0], 64480[0], 64483[0], 64484[0], 64486[0], 64487[0], 64488[0], 64489[0], 64490[0], 64491[0], 64492[0], 64493[0], 64494[0], 64495[0], 64505[0], 64510[0], 64517[0], 64520[0], 64530[0], 69990[0], 92012[1], 92014[1], 93000[1], 93005[1], 93010[1], 93040[1], 93041[1], 93042[1], 93318[1], 93355[1], 94002[1], 94200[1], 94680[1], 94681[1], 94690[1], 95812[1], 95813[1], 95816[1], 95819[1], 95822[1], 95829[1], 95955[1], 96360[1], 96361[1], 96365[1], 96366[1], 96367[1], 96368[1], 96372[1], 96374[1], 96375[1], 96376[1], 96377[1], 96523[0], 97597[1], 97598[1], 97602[1], 99155[0], 99156[0], 99157[0], 99211[1], 99212[1], 99213[1], 99214[1], 99215[1], 99217[1], 99218[1], 99219[1], 99220[1], 99221[1], 99222[1], 99223[1], 99231[1], 99232[1], 99233[1], 99234[1], 99235[1], 99236[1], 99238[1], 99239[1], 99241[1], 99242[1], 99243[1], 99244[1], 99245[1], 99251[1], 99252[1], 99253[1], 99254[1], 99255[1], 99291[1], 99292[1], 99304[1], 99305[1], 99306[1], 99307[1], 99308[1], 99309[1], 99310[1], 99315[1], 99316[1], 99334[1], 99335[1], 99336[1], 99337[1], 99347[1], 99348[1], 99349[1], 99350[1], 99374[1], 99375[1], 99377[1], 99378[1], 99446[0], 99447[0], 99448[0], 99449[0], 99451[0], 99452[0], 99495[0], 99496[0], G0168[1], G0463[1], G0471[1], J0670[1], J2001[1]
11622	00400[0], 0213T[0], 0216T[0], 0596T[1], 0597T[1], 10061[1], 11000[1], 11001[1], 11004[1], 11005[1], 11006[1], 11042[1], 11043[1], 11044[1], 11045[1], 11046[1], 11047[1], 11102[1], 11104[1], 11106[1], 11900[1], 11901[1], 12001[1], 12002[1], 12004[1], 12005[1], 12006[1], 12007[1], 12011[1], 12013[1], 12014[1], 12015[1], 12016[1], 12017[1], 12018[1], 17000[1], 17004[1], 17250[1], 17274[1], 17276[1], 17283[1], 17284[1], 17286[1], 36000[1], 36400[1], 36405[1], 36406[1], 36410[1], 36420[1], 36425[1], 36430[1], 36440[1], 36591[0], 36592[0], 36600[1], 36640[1], 43752[1], 51701[1], 51702[1], 51703[1], 62320[0], 62321[0], 62322[0], 62323[0], 62324[0], 62325[0], 62326[0], 62327[0], 64400[0], 64405[0], 64408[0], 64415[0], 64416[0], 64417[0], 64418[0], 64420[0], 64421[0], 64425[0], 64430[0], 64435[0], 64445[0], 64446[0], 64447[0], 64448[0], 64449[0], 64450[1], 64451[0], 64454[1], 64461[0], 64462[0], 64463[0], 64479[0], 64480[0], 64483[0], 64484[0], 64486[0], 64487[0], 64488[0], 64489[0], 64490[0], 64491[0], 64492[0], 64493[0], 64494[0], 64495[0], 64505[0], 64510[0], 64517[0], 64520[0], 64530[0], 69990[0], 92012[1], 92014[1], 93000[1], 93005[1], 93010[1], 93040[1], 93041[1], 93042[1], 93318[1], 93355[1], 94002[1], 94200[1], 94680[1], 94681[1], 94690[1], 95812[1], 95813[1], 95816[1], 95819[1], 95822[1], 95829[1], 95955[1], 96360[1], 96361[1], 96365[1], 96366[1], 96367[1], 96368[1], 96372[1], 96374[1], 96375[1], 96376[1], 96377[1], 96523[0], 97597[1], 97598[1], 97602[1], 99155[0], 99156[0], 99157[0], 99211[1], 99212[1], 99213[1], 99214[1], 99215[1], 99217[1], 99218[1], 99219[1], 99220[1], 99221[1], 99222[1], 99223[1], 99231[1], 99232[1], 99233[1], 99234[1], 99235[1], 99236[1], 99238[1], 99239[1], 99241[1], 99242[1], 99243[1], 99244[1], 99245[1], 99251[1], 99252[1], 99253[1], 99254[1], 99255[1], 99291[1], 99292[1], 99304[1], 99305[1], 99306[1], 99307[1], 99308[1], 99309[1], 99310[1], 99315[1], 99316[1], 99334[1], 99335[1], 99336[1], 99337[1], 99347[1], 99348[1], 99349[1], 99350[1],

0 = Modifier usage not allowed or inappropriate 1 = Modifier usage allowed

Code 1	Code 2
	99374[1], 99375[1], 99377[1], 99378[1], 99446[0], 99447[0], 99448[0], 99449[0], 99451[0], 99452[0], 99495[0], 99496[0], G0168[1], G0463[1], G0471[1], J0670[1], J2001[1]
11623	00400[0], 0213T[0], 0216T[0], 0596T[1], 0597T[1], 11000[1], 11001[1], 11004[1], 11005[1], 11006[1], 11042[1], 11043[1], 11044[1], 11045[1], 11046[1], 11047[1], 11102[1], 11104[1], 11106[1], 11900[1], 11901[1], 12001[1], 12002[1], 12004[1], 12005[1], 12006[1], 12007[1], 12011[1], 12013[1], 12014[1], 12015[1], 12016[1], 12017[1], 12018[1], 17000[1], 17004[1], 17250[1], 17276[1], 17284[1], 17286[1], 36000[1], 36400[1], 36405[1], 36406[1], 36410[1], 36420[1], 36425[1], 36430[1], 36440[1], 36591[0], 36592[0], 36600[1], 36640[1], 43752[1], 51701[1], 51702[1], 51703[1], 62320[0], 62321[0], 62322[0], 62323[0], 62324[0], 62325[0], 62326[0], 62327[0], 64400[0], 64405[0], 64408[0], 64415[0], 64416[0], 64417[0], 64418[0], 64420[0], 64421[0], 64425[0], 64430[0], 64435[0], 64445[0], 64446[0], 64447[0], 64448[0], 64449[0], 64450[1], 64451[0], 64454[1], 64461[0], 64462[0], 64463[0], 64479[0], 64480[0], 64483[0], 64484[0], 64486[0], 64487[0], 64488[0], 64489[0], 64490[0], 64491[0], 64492[0], 64493[0], 64494[0], 64495[0], 64505[0], 64510[0], 64517[0], 64520[0], 64530[0], 69990[0], 92012[1], 92014[1], 93000[1], 93005[1], 93010[1], 93040[1], 93041[1], 93042[1], 93318[1], 93355[1], 94002[1], 94200[1], 94680[1], 94681[1], 94690[1], 95812[1], 95813[1], 95816[1], 95819[1], 95822[1], 95829[1], 95955[1], 96360[1], 96361[1], 96365[1], 96366[1], 96367[1], 96368[1], 96372[1], 96374[1], 96375[1], 96376[1], 96377[1], 96523[0], 97597[1], 97598[1], 97602[1], 99155[0], 99156[0], 99157[0], 99211[1], 99212[1], 99213[1], 99214[1], 99215[1], 99217[1], 99218[1], 99219[1], 99220[1], 99221[1], 99222[1], 99223[1], 99231[1], 99232[1], 99233[1], 99234[1], 99235[1], 99236[1], 99238[1], 99239[1], 99241[1], 99242[1], 99243[1], 99244[1], 99245[1], 99251[1], 99252[1], 99253[1], 99254[1], 99255[1], 99291[1], 99292[1], 99304[1], 99305[1], 99306[1], 99307[1], 99308[1], 99309[1], 99310[1], 99315[1], 99316[1], 99334[1], 99335[1], 99336[1], 99337[1], 99347[1], 99348[1], 99349[1], 99350[1], 99374[1], 99375[1], 99377[1], 99378[1], 99446[0], 99447[0], 99448[0], 99449[0], 99451[0], 99452[0], 99495[0], 99496[0], G0168[1], G0463[1], G0471[1], J0670[1], J2001[1]
11624	00400[0], 0213T[0], 0216T[0], 0596T[1], 0597T[1], 11000[1], 11001[1], 11004[1], 11005[1], 11006[1], 11042[1], 11043[1], 11044[1], 11045[1], 11046[1], 11047[1], 11102[1], 11104[1], 11106[1], 11900[1], 11901[1], 12001[1], 12002[1], 12004[1], 12005[1], 12006[1], 12007[1], 12011[1], 12013[1], 12014[1], 12015[1], 12016[1], 12017[1], 12018[1], 17000[1], 17004[1], 17250[1], 17286[1], 36000[1], 36400[1], 36405[1], 36406[1], 36410[1], 36420[1], 36425[1], 36430[1], 36440[1], 36591[0], 36592[0], 36600[1], 36640[1], 43752[1], 51701[1], 51702[1], 51703[1], 62320[0], 62321[0], 62322[0], 62323[0], 62324[0], 62325[0], 62326[0], 62327[0], 64400[0], 64405[0], 64408[0], 64415[0], 64416[0], 64417[0], 64418[0], 64420[0], 64421[0], 64425[0], 64430[0], 64435[0], 64445[0], 64446[0], 64447[0], 64448[0], 64449[0], 64450[1], 64451[0], 64454[1], 64461[0], 64462[0], 64463[0], 64479[0], 64480[0], 64483[0], 64484[0], 64486[0], 64487[0], 64488[0], 64489[0], 64490[0], 64491[0], 64492[0], 64493[0], 64494[0], 64495[0], 64505[0], 64510[0], 64517[0], 64520[0], 64530[0], 69990[0], 92012[1], 92014[1], 93000[1], 93005[1], 93010[1], 93040[1], 93041[1], 93042[1], 93318[1], 93355[1], 94002[1], 94200[1], 94680[1], 94681[1], 94690[1], 95812[1], 95813[1], 95816[1], 95819[1], 95822[1], 95829[1], 95955[1], 96360[1], 96361[1], 96365[1], 96366[1], 96367[1], 96368[1], 96372[1], 96374[1], 96375[1], 96376[1], 96377[1], 96523[0], 97597[1], 97598[1], 97602[1], 99155[0], 99156[0], 99157[0], 99211[1], 99212[1], 99213[1], 99214[1], 99215[1], 99217[1], 99218[1], 99219[1], 99220[1], 99221[1], 99222[1], 99223[1], 99231[1], 99232[1], 99233[1], 99234[1], 99235[1], 99236[1], 99238[1], 99239[1], 99241[1], 99242[1], 99243[1], 99244[1], 99245[1], 99251[1], 99252[1], 99253[1], 99254[1], 99255[1], 99291[1], 99292[1], 99304[1], 99305[1], 99306[1], 99307[1], 99308[1], 99309[1], 99310[1], 99315[1], 99316[1], 99334[1], 99335[1], 99336[1], 99337[1], 99347[1], 99348[1], 99349[1], 99350[1], 99374[1], 99375[1], 99377[1], 99378[1], 99446[0], 99447[0], 99448[0], 99449[0], 99451[0], 99452[0], 99495[0], 99496[0], G0168[1], G0463[1], G0471[1], J0670[1], J2001[1]
11626	00400[0], 0213T[0], 0216T[0], 0596T[1], 0597T[1], 11000[1], 11001[1], 11004[1], 11005[1], 11006[1], 11042[1], 11043[1], 11044[1], 11045[1], 11046[1], 11047[1], 11102[1], 11104[1], 11106[1], 11900[1], 11901[1], 12001[1], 12002[1], 12004[1], 12005[1], 12006[1], 12007[1], 12011[1], 12013[1], 12014[1], 12015[1], 12016[1], 12017[1], 12018[1], 15002[1], 17000[1], 17004[1], 17250[1], 17286[1], 36000[1], 36400[1], 36405[1], 36406[1], 36410[1], 36420[1], 36425[1], 36430[1], 36440[1], 36591[0], 36592[0], 36600[1], 36640[1], 43752[1], 51701[1], 51702[1], 51703[1], 62320[0], 62321[0], 62322[0], 62323[0], 62324[0], 62325[0], 62326[0], 62327[0], 64400[0], 64405[0], 64408[0], 64415[0], 64416[0], 64417[0], 64418[0], 64420[0], 64421[0], 64425[0], 64430[0], 64435[0], 64445[0], 64446[0], 64447[0], 64448[0], 64449[0], 64450[1], 64451[0], 64454[1], 64461[0], 64462[0], 64463[0], 64479[0], 64480[0], 64483[0], 64484[0], 64486[0], 64487[0], 64488[0], 64489[0], 64490[0], 64491[0], 64492[0], 64493[0], 64494[0], 64495[0], 64505[0], 64510[0], 64517[0], 64520[0], 64530[0], 69990[0], 92012[1], 92014[1], 93000[1], 93005[1], 93010[1], 93040[1], 93041[1], 93042[1], 93318[1], 93355[1], 94002[1], 94200[1], 94680[1], 94681[1], 94690[1], 95812[1], 95813[1], 95816[1], 95819[1], 95822[1], 95829[1], 95955[1], 96360[1], 96361[1], 96365[1], 96366[1], 96367[1], 96368[1], 96372[1], 96374[1], 96375[1], 96376[1], 96377[1], 96523[0], 97597[1], 97598[1], 97602[1], 99155[0], 99156[0], 99157[0], 99211[1], 99212[1], 99213[1], 99214[1], 99215[1], 99217[1], 99218[1], 99219[1], 99220[1], 99221[1], 99222[1], 99223[1], 99231[1], 99232[1], 99233[1], 99234[1], 99235[1], 99236[1], 99238[1], 99239[1], 99241[1], 99242[1], 99243[1], 99244[1], 99245[1], 99251[1], 99252[1], 99253[1], 99254[1], 99255[1], 99291[1], 99292[1], 99304[1], 99305[1], 99306[1], 99307[1], 99308[1], 99309[1], 99310[1], 99315[1], 99316[1], 99334[1], 99335[1], 99336[1], 99337[1], 99347[1], 99348[1], 99349[1], 99350[1], 99374[1], 99375[1], 99377[1], 99378[1], 99446[0], 99447[0], 99448[0], 99449[0], 99451[0], 99452[0], 99495[0], 99496[0], G0168[1], G0463[1], G0471[1], J0670[1], J2001[1]
12001	0213T[0], 0216T[0], 0543T[1], 0544T[1], 0545T[1], 0567T[1], 0568T[1], 0569T[1], 0570T[1], 0571T[1], 0572T[1], 0573T[1], 0574T[1], 0580T[1], 0581T[1], 0582T[1], 0655T[1], 11042[1], 11055[1], 11056[1], 11719[1], 11740[1], 11750[1], 11900[1], 11901[1], 20560[1], 20561[1], 36000[1], 36400[1], 36405[1], 36406[1], 36410[1], 36420[1], 36425[1], 36430[1], 36440[1], 36591[0], 36592[0], 36600[1], 36640[1], 43752[1], 51701[1], 51702[1], 51703[1], 64400[0], 64405[0], 64408[0], 64415[0], 64416[0], 64417[0], 64418[0], 64420[0], 64421[0], 64425[0], 64430[0], 64435[0], 64445[0], 64446[0], 64447[0], 64448[0], 64449[0], 64450[1], 64479[0], 64480[0], 64483[0], 64484[0], 64490[0], 64491[0], 64492[0], 64493[0], 64494[0], 64495[0], 64505[0], 64510[0], 64517[0], 64520[0], 64530[0], 66987[1], 66988[1], 69990[0], 92012[1], 92014[1], 93000[1], 93005[1], 93010[1], 93040[1], 93041[1], 93042[1], 93318[1], 93355[1], 94002[1], 94200[1], 94680[1], 94681[1], 94690[1], 95812[1], 95813[1], 95816[1], 95819[1], 95822[1], 95829[1], 95955[1], 96360[1], 96361[1], 96365[1], 96366[1], 96367[1], 96368[1], 96372[1], 96374[1], 96375[1], 96376[1], 96377[1], 96523[0], 97597[1], 97598[1], 97602[1], 97605[1], 97606[1], 97607[1], 97608[1], 99155[0], 99156[0], 99157[0], 99211[1], 99212[1], 99213[1], 99214[1], 99215[1], 99217[1], 99218[1], 99219[1], 99220[1], 99221[1], 99222[1], 99223[1], 99231[1], 99232[1], 99233[1], 99234[1], 99235[1], 99236[1], 99238[1], 99239[1], 99241[1], 99242[1], 99243[1], 99244[1], 99245[1], 99251[1], 99252[1], 99253[1], 99254[1], 99255[1], 99291[1], 99292[1], 99304[1], 99305[1], 99306[1], 99307[1], 99308[1], 99309[1], 99310[1], 99315[1], 99316[1], 99334[1], 99335[1], 99336[1], 99337[1], 99347[1], 99348[1], 99349[1], 99350[1], 99374[1], 99375[1], 99377[1], 99378[1], 99446[0], 99447[0], 99448[0], 99449[0], 99451[0], 99452[0], 99495[1], 99496[1], G0168[1], G0463[1], G0471[1], J0670[1], J2001[1]
12002	0213T[0], 0216T[0], 0543T[1], 0544T[1], 0545T[1], 0567T[1], 0568T[1], 0569T[1], 0570T[1], 0571T[1], 0572T[1], 0573T[1], 0574T[1], 0580T[1], 0581T[1], 0582T[1], 0655T[1], 11042[1], 11740[1], 11900[1], 11901[1], 12001[0], 12013[1], 12014[1], 20560[1], 20561[1], 20701[1], 36000[1], 36400[1], 36405[1], 36406[1], 36410[1], 36420[1], 36425[1], 36430[1], 36440[1], 36591[0], 36592[0], 36600[1], 36640[1], 43752[1], 51701[1], 51702[1], 51703[1], 64400[0], 64405[0], 64408[0], 64415[0], 64416[0], 64417[0], 64418[0], 64420[0], 64421[0], 64425[0], 64430[0], 64435[0], 64445[0], 64446[0], 64447[0], 64448[0], 64449[0], 64450[1], 64479[0], 64480[0], 64483[0], 64484[0], 64490[0], 64491[0], 64492[0], 64493[0], 64494[0], 64495[0], 64505[0], 64510[0], 64517[0], 64520[0], 64530[0], 66987[1], 66988[1], 69990[0], 92012[1], 92014[1], 93000[1], 93005[1], 93010[1], 93040[1], 93041[1], 93042[1], 93318[1], 93355[1], 94002[1], 94200[1], 94680[1], 94681[1], 94690[1], 95812[1], 95813[1], 95816[1], 95819[1], 95822[1], 95829[1], 95955[1], 96360[1], 96361[1], 96365[1], 96366[1], 96367[1], 96368[1], 96372[1], 96374[1], 96375[1], 96376[1], 96377[1], 96523[0], 97597[1], 97598[1], 97602[1], 97605[1], 97606[1], 97607[1], 97608[1], 99155[0], 99156[0], 99157[0], 99211[1], 99212[1], 99213[1], 99214[1], 99215[1], 99217[1], 99218[1], 99219[1], 99220[1], 99221[1], 99222[1], 99223[1], 99231[1], 99232[1], 99233[1], 99234[1], 99235[1], 99236[1], 99238[1], 99239[1], 99241[1], 99242[1], 99243[1], 99244[1], 99245[1], 99251[1], 99252[1], 99253[1], 99254[1], 99255[1], 99291[1], 99292[1], 99304[1], 99305[1], 99306[1], 99307[1], 99308[1], 99309[1], 99310[1], 99315[1], 99316[1], 99334[1], 99335[1], 99336[1], 99337[1], 99347[1], 99348[1], 99349[1], 99350[1], 99374[1], 99375[1], 99377[1], 99378[1], 99446[0], 99447[0], 99448[0], 99449[0], 99451[0], 99452[0], 99495[1], 99496[1], G0168[1], G0463[1], G0471[1], J0670[1], J2001[1]
12004	0213T[0], 0216T[0], 0543T[1], 0544T[1], 0545T[1], 0567T[1], 0568T[1], 0569T[1], 0570T[1], 0571T[1], 0572T[1], 0573T[1], 0574T[1], 0580T[1], 0581T[1], 0582T[1], 0655T[1], 11042[1], 11900[1], 11901[1], 12001[0], 12002[0], 12015[1], 20560[1], 20561[1], 20701[1], 36000[1], 36400[1], 36405[1], 36406[1], 36410[1], 36420[1], 36425[1], 36430[1], 36440[1], 36591[0], 36592[0], 36600[1], 36640[1], 43752[1], 51701[1], 51702[1], 51703[1], 64400[0], 64405[0], 64408[0], 64415[0], 64416[0], 64417[0], 64418[0], 64420[0], 64421[0], 64425[0], 64430[0], 64435[0], 64445[0], 64446[0], 64447[0], 64448[0], 64449[0], 64450[1], 64479[0], 64480[0], 64483[0], 64484[0], 64490[0], 64491[0], 64492[0], 64493[0], 64494[0], 64495[0], 64505[0], 64510[0], 64517[0], 64520[0], 64530[0], 66987[1], 66988[1], 69990[0], 92012[1], 92014[1], 93000[1], 93005[1], 93010[1], 93040[1], 93041[1], 93042[1], 93318[1], 93355[1], 94002[1], 94200[1], 94680[1], 94681[1], 94690[1], 95812[1], 95813[1], 95816[1], 95819[1], 95822[1], 95829[1], 95955[1], 96360[1], 96361[1], 96365[1], 96366[1], 96367[1], 96368[1], 96372[1], 96374[1], 96375[1], 96376[1], 96377[1], 96523[0], 97597[1], 97598[1], 97602[1], 97605[1], 97606[1], 97607[1], 97608[1], 99155[0], 99156[0], 99157[0], 99211[1], 99212[1], 99213[1], 99214[1], 99215[1], 99217[1], 99218[1], 99219[1], 99220[1], 99221[1], 99222[1], 99223[1], 99231[1], 99232[1], 99233[1], 99234[1], 99235[1], 99236[1], 99238[1], 99239[1], 99241[1], 99242[1], 99243[1], 99244[1], 99245[1], 99251[1], 99252[1], 99253[1], 99254[1], 99255[1], 99291[1], 99292[1], 99304[1], 99305[1], 99306[1], 99307[1], 99308[1], 99309[1], 99310[1], 99315[1], 99316[1], 99334[1], 99335[1], 99336[1], 99337[1], 99347[1], 99348[1], 99349[1], 99350[1], 99374[1], 99375[1], 99377[1], 99378[1], 99446[0], 99447[0], 99448[0], 99449[0], 99451[0], 99452[0], 99495[1], 99496[1], G0168[1], G0463[1], G0471[1], J0670[1], J2001[1]
12005	0213T[0], 0216T[0], 0543T[1], 0544T[1], 0545T[1], 0567T[1], 0568T[1], 0569T[1], 0570T[1], 0571T[1], 0572T[1], 0573T[1], 0574T[1], 0580T[1], 0581T[1], 0582T[1], 0655T[1], 11042[1], 11043[1], 11900[1], 11901[1], 12001[0], 12002[0], 12004[0], 12016[1], 20560[1], 20561[1], 20700[1], 20701[1], 36000[1], 36400[1], 36405[1], 36406[1], 36410[1], 36420[1], 36425[1], 36430[1], 36440[1], 36591[0], 36592[0], 36600[1], 36640[1], 43752[1], 51701[1], 51702[1], 51703[1], 64400[0], 64405[0], 64408[0], 64415[0],

0 = Modifier usage not allowed or inappropriate 1 = Modifier usage allowed

Appendix A: NCCI - CPT Codes

Code 1	Code 2
	64416[0], 64417[0], 64418[0], 64420[0], 64421[0], 64425[0], 64430[0], 64435[0], 64445[0], 64446[0], 64447[0], 64448[0], 64449[0], 64450[1], 64451[1], 64479[0], 64480[0], 64483[0], 64484[0], 64490[0], 64491[0], 64492[0], 64493[0], 64494[0], 64495[0], 64505[0], 64510[0], 64517[0], 64520[0], 64530[0], 66987[1], 66988[1], 69990[0], 92012[1], 92014[1], 93000[1], 93005[1], 93010[1], 93040[1], 93041[1], 93042[1], 93318[1], 93355[1], 94002[1], 94200[1], 94680[1], 94681[1], 94690[1], 95812[1], 95813[1], 95816[1], 95819[1], 95822[1], 95829[1], 95955[1], 96360[1], 96361[1], 96365[1], 96366[1], 96367[1], 96368[1], 96372[1], 96374[1], 96375[1], 96376[1], 96377[1], 96523[0], 97597[1], 97598[1], 97602[1], 97605[1], 97606[1], 97607[1], 97608[1], 99155[0], 99156[0], 99157[0], 99211[1], 99212[1], 99213[1], 99214[1], 99215[1], 99217[1], 99218[1], 99219[1], 99220[1], 99221[1], 99222[1], 99223[1], 99231[1], 99232[1], 99233[1], 99234[1], 99235[1], 99236[1], 99238[1], 99239[1], 99241[1], 99242[1], 99243[1], 99244[1], 99245[1], 99251[1], 99252[1], 99253[1], 99254[1], 99255[1], 99291[1], 99292[1], 99304[1], 99305[1], 99306[1], 99307[1], 99308[1], 99309[1], 99310[1], 99315[1], 99316[1], 99334[1], 99335[1], 99336[1], 99337[1], 99347[1], 99348[1], 99349[1], 99350[1], 99374[1], 99375[1], 99377[1], 99378[1], 99446[0], 99447[0], 99448[0], 99449[0], 99451[0], 99452[0], 99495[1], 99496[1], G0168[1], G0463[1], G0471[1], J0670[1], J2001[1]
12006	0213T[0], 0216T[0], 0543T[1], 0544T[1], 0545T[1], 0567T[1], 0568T[1], 0569T[1], 0570T[1], 0571T[1], 0572T[1], 0573T[1], 0574T[1], 0580T[1], 0581T[1], 0582T[1], 0655T[1], 11042[1], 11043[1], 11900[1], 11901[1], 12001[0], 12002[0], 12004[0], 12005[0], 12017[1], 20560[1], 20561[1], 20700[1], 20701[1], 36000[1], 36400[1], 36405[1], 36406[1], 36410[1], 36420[1], 36425[1], 36430[1], 36440[1], 36591[0], 36592[0], 36600[1], 36640[1], 43752[1], 51701[1], 51702[1], 51703[1], 64400[0], 64405[0], 64408[0], 64415[0], 64416[0], 64417[0], 64418[0], 64420[0], 64421[0], 64425[0], 64430[0], 64435[0], 64445[0], 64446[0], 64447[0], 64448[0], 64449[0], 64450[1], 64451[1], 64479[0], 64480[0], 64483[0], 64484[0], 64490[0], 64491[0], 64492[0], 64493[0], 64494[0], 64495[0], 64505[0], 64510[0], 64517[0], 64520[0], 64530[0], 66987[1], 66988[1], 69990[0], 92012[1], 92014[1], 93000[1], 93005[1], 93010[1], 93040[1], 93041[1], 93042[1], 93318[1], 93355[1], 94002[1], 94200[1], 94680[1], 94681[1], 94690[1], 95812[1], 95813[1], 95816[1], 95819[1], 95822[1], 95829[1], 95955[1], 96360[1], 96361[1], 96365[1], 96366[1], 96367[1], 96368[1], 96372[1], 96374[1], 96375[1], 96376[1], 96377[1], 96523[0], 97597[1], 97598[1], 97602[1], 97605[1], 97606[1], 97607[1], 97608[1], 99155[0], 99156[0], 99157[0], 99211[1], 99212[1], 99213[1], 99214[1], 99215[1], 99217[1], 99218[1], 99219[1], 99220[1], 99221[1], 99222[1], 99223[1], 99231[1], 99232[1], 99233[1], 99234[1], 99235[1], 99236[1], 99238[1], 99239[1], 99241[1], 99242[1], 99243[1], 99244[1], 99245[1], 99251[1], 99252[1], 99253[1], 99254[1], 99255[1], 99291[1], 99292[1], 99304[1], 99305[1], 99306[1], 99307[1], 99308[1], 99309[1], 99310[1], 99315[1], 99316[1], 99334[1], 99335[1], 99336[1], 99337[1], 99347[1], 99348[1], 99349[1], 99350[1], 99374[1], 99375[1], 99377[1], 99378[1], 99446[0], 99447[0], 99448[0], 99449[0], 99451[0], 99452[0], 99495[1], 99496[1], G0168[1], G0463[1], G0471[1], J0670[1], J2001[1]
12007	0213T[0], 0216T[0], 0543T[1], 0544T[1], 0545T[1], 0567T[1], 0568T[1], 0569T[1], 0570T[1], 0571T[1], 0572T[1], 0573T[1], 0574T[1], 0580T[1], 0581T[1], 0582T[1], 0655T[1], 11900[1], 11901[1], 12001[0], 12002[0], 12004[0], 12005[0], 12006[0], 12018[1], 15772[1], 15774[1], 20560[1], 20561[1], 20700[1], 20701[1], 36000[1], 36400[1], 36405[1], 36406[1], 36410[1], 36420[1], 36425[1], 36430[1], 36440[1], 36591[0], 36592[0], 36600[1], 36640[1], 43752[1], 51701[1], 51702[1], 51703[1], 64400[0], 64405[0], 64408[0], 64415[0], 64416[0], 64417[0], 64418[0], 64420[0], 64421[0], 64425[0], 64430[0], 64435[0], 64445[0], 64446[0], 64447[0], 64448[0], 64449[0], 64450[1], 64451[1], 64479[0], 64480[0], 64483[0], 64484[0], 64490[0], 64491[0], 64492[0], 64493[0], 64494[0], 64495[0], 64505[0], 64510[0], 64517[0], 64520[0], 64530[0], 66987[1], 66988[1], 69990[0], 92012[1], 92014[1], 93000[1], 93005[1], 93010[1], 93040[1], 93041[1], 93042[1], 93318[1], 93355[1], 94002[1], 94200[1], 94680[1], 94681[1], 94690[1], 95812[1], 95813[1], 95816[1], 95819[1], 95822[1], 95829[1], 95955[1], 96360[1], 96361[1], 96365[1], 96366[1], 96367[1], 96368[1], 96372[1], 96374[1], 96375[1], 96376[1], 96377[1], 96523[0], 97597[1], 97598[1], 97602[1], 97605[1], 97606[1], 97607[1], 97608[1], 99155[0], 99156[0], 99157[0], 99211[1], 99212[1], 99213[1], 99214[1], 99215[1], 99217[1], 99218[1], 99219[1], 99220[1], 99221[1], 99222[1], 99223[1], 99231[1], 99232[1], 99233[1], 99234[1], 99235[1], 99236[1], 99238[1], 99239[1], 99241[1], 99242[1], 99243[1], 99244[1], 99245[1], 99251[1], 99252[1], 99253[1], 99254[1], 99255[1], 99291[1], 99292[1], 99304[1], 99305[1], 99306[1], 99307[1], 99308[1], 99309[1], 99310[1], 99315[1], 99316[1], 99334[1], 99335[1], 99336[1], 99337[1], 99347[1], 99348[1], 99349[1], 99350[1], 99374[1], 99375[1], 99377[1], 99378[1], 99446[0], 99447[0], 99448[0], 99449[0], 99451[0], 99452[0], 99495[1], 99496[1], G0168[1], G0463[1], G0471[1], J0670[1], J2001[1]
12020	0213T[0], 0216T[0], 0543T[1], 0544T[1], 0545T[1], 0567T[1], 0568T[1], 0569T[1], 0570T[1], 0571T[1], 0572T[1], 0573T[1], 0574T[1], 0580T[1], 0581T[1], 0582T[1], 0655T[1], 11000[1], 11001[1], 11004[1], 11005[1], 11006[1], 11042[1], 11043[1], 11044[1], 11045[1], 11046[1], 11047[1], 11900[1], 11901[1], 12021[1], 15772[1], 15774[1], 20560[1], 20561[1], 20700[1], 20701[1], 36000[1], 36400[1], 36405[1], 36406[1], 36410[1], 36420[1], 36425[1], 36430[1], 36440[1], 36591[0], 36592[0], 36600[1], 36640[1], 43752[1], 51701[1], 51702[1], 51703[1], 64400[0], 64405[0], 64408[0], 64415[0], 64416[0], 64417[0], 64418[0], 64420[0], 64421[0], 64425[0], 64430[0], 64435[0], 64445[0], 64446[0], 64447[0], 64448[0], 64449[0], 64450[1], 64451[1], 64479[0], 64480[0], 64483[0], 64484[0], 64490[0], 64491[0], 64492[0], 64493[0], 64494[0], 64495[0], 64505[0], 64510[0], 64517[0], 64520[0], 64530[0], 66987[1], 66988[1], 69990[0], 92012[1], 92014[1], 93000[1], 93005[1], 93010[1], 93040[1], 93041[1], 93042[1], 93318[1], 93355[1], 94002[1], 94200[1], 94680[1], 94681[1], 94690[1], 95812[1], 95813[1], 95816[1], 95819[1], 95822[1], 95829[1], 95955[1], 96360[1], 96361[1], 96365[1], 96366[1], 96367[1], 96368[1], 96372[1], 96374[1], 96375[1], 96376[1], 96377[1], 96523[0], 97597[1], 97598[1], 97602[1], 97605[1], 97606[1], 97607[1], 97608[1], 99155[0], 99156[0], 99157[0], 99211[1], 99212[1], 99213[1], 99214[1], 99215[1], 99217[1], 99218[1], 99219[1], 99220[1], 99221[1], 99222[1], 99223[1], 99231[1], 99232[1], 99233[1], 99234[1], 99235[1], 99236[1], 99238[1], 99239[1], 99241[1], 99242[1], 99243[1], 99244[1], 99245[1], 99251[1], 99252[1], 99253[1], 99254[1], 99255[1], 99291[1], 99292[1], 99304[1], 99305[1], 99306[1], 99307[1], 99308[1], 99309[1], 99310[1], 99315[1], 99316[1], 99334[1], 99335[1], 99336[1], 99337[1], 99347[1], 99348[1], 99349[1], 99350[1], 99374[1], 99375[1], 99377[1], 99378[1], 99446[0], 99447[0], 99448[0], 99449[0], 99451[0], 99452[0], 99495[0], 99496[0], G0168[1], G0463[1], G0471[1], J0670[1], J2001[1]
12021	0213T[0], 0216T[0], 0543T[1], 0544T[1], 0567T[1], 0568T[1], 0569T[1], 0570T[1], 0571T[1], 0572T[1], 0573T[1], 0574T[1], 0580T[1], 0581T[1], 0582T[1], 0655T[1], 11042[1], 11900[1], 11901[1], 20560[1], 20561[1], 20700[1], 20701[1], 36000[1], 36400[1], 36405[1], 36406[1], 36410[1], 36420[1], 36425[1], 36430[1], 36440[1], 36591[0], 36592[0], 36600[1], 36640[1], 43752[1], 51701[1], 51702[1], 51703[1], 64400[0], 64405[0], 64408[0], 64415[0], 64416[0], 64417[0], 64418[0], 64420[0], 64421[0], 64425[0], 64430[0], 64435[0], 64445[0], 64446[0], 64447[0], 64448[0], 64449[0], 64450[1], 64451[1], 64479[0], 64480[0], 64483[0], 64484[0], 64490[0], 64491[0], 64492[0], 64493[0], 64494[0], 64495[0], 64505[0], 64510[0], 64517[0], 64520[0], 64530[0], 66987[1], 66988[1], 69990[0], 92012[1], 92014[1], 93000[1], 93005[1], 93010[1], 93040[1], 93041[1], 93042[1], 93318[1], 93355[1], 94002[1], 94200[1], 94680[1], 94681[1], 94690[1], 95812[1], 95813[1], 95816[1], 95819[1], 95822[1], 95829[1], 95955[1], 96360[1], 96361[1], 96365[1], 96366[1], 96367[1], 96368[1], 96372[1], 96374[1], 96375[1], 96376[1], 96377[1], 96523[0], 97597[1], 97598[1], 97602[1], 97605[1], 97606[1], 97607[1], 97608[1], 99155[0], 99156[0], 99157[0], 99211[1], 99212[1], 99213[1], 99214[1], 99215[1], 99217[1], 99218[1], 99219[1], 99220[1], 99221[1], 99222[1], 99223[1], 99231[1], 99232[1], 99233[1], 99234[1], 99235[1], 99236[1], 99238[1], 99239[1], 99241[1], 99242[1], 99243[1], 99244[1], 99245[1], 99251[1], 99252[1], 99253[1], 99254[1], 99255[1], 99291[1], 99292[1], 99304[1], 99305[1], 99306[1], 99307[1], 99308[1], 99309[1], 99310[1], 99315[1], 99316[1], 99334[1], 99335[1], 99336[1], 99337[1], 99347[1], 99348[1], 99349[1], 99350[1], 99374[1], 99375[1], 99377[1], 99378[1], 99446[0], 99447[0], 99448[0], 99449[0], 99451[0], 99452[0], 99495[0], 99496[0], G0168[1], G0463[1], G0471[1], J2001[1]
12041	0213T[0], 0216T[0], 0543T[1], 0544T[1], 0567T[1], 0568T[1], 0569T[1], 0570T[1], 0571T[1], 0572T[1], 0573T[1], 0574T[1], 0580T[1], 0581T[1], 0582T[1], 0655T[1], 11055[1], 11056[1], 11740[1], 11900[1], 11901[1], 12031[1], 20560[1], 20561[1], 20700[1], 20701[1], 36000[1], 36400[1], 36405[1], 36406[1], 36410[1], 36420[1], 36425[1], 36430[1], 36440[1], 36591[0], 36592[0], 36600[1], 36640[1], 43752[1], 51701[1], 51702[1], 51703[1], 64400[0], 64405[0], 64408[0], 64415[0], 64416[0], 64417[0], 64418[0], 64420[0], 64421[0], 64425[0], 64430[0], 64435[0], 64445[0], 64446[0], 64447[0], 64448[0], 64449[0], 64450[1], 64451[1], 64479[0], 64480[0], 64483[0], 64484[0], 64490[0], 64491[0], 64492[0], 64493[0], 64494[0], 64495[0], 64505[0], 64510[0], 64517[0], 64520[0], 64530[0], 66987[1], 66988[1], 69990[0], 92012[1], 92014[1], 93000[1], 93005[1], 93010[1], 93040[1], 93041[1], 93042[1], 93318[1], 93355[1], 94002[1], 94200[1], 94680[1], 94681[1], 94690[1], 95812[1], 95813[1], 95816[1], 95819[1], 95822[1], 95829[1], 95955[1], 96360[1], 96361[1], 96365[1], 96366[1], 96367[1], 96368[1], 96372[1], 96374[1], 96375[1], 96376[1], 96377[1], 96523[0], 97597[1], 97598[1], 97602[1], 97605[1], 97606[1], 97607[1], 97608[1], 99155[0], 99156[0], 99157[0], 99211[1], 99212[1], 99213[1], 99214[1], 99215[1], 99217[1], 99218[1], 99219[1], 99220[1], 99221[1], 99222[1], 99223[1], 99231[1], 99232[1], 99233[1], 99234[1], 99235[1], 99236[1], 99238[1], 99239[1], 99241[1], 99242[1], 99243[1], 99244[1], 99245[1], 99251[1], 99252[1], 99253[1], 99254[1], 99255[1], 99291[1], 99292[1], 99304[1], 99305[1], 99306[1], 99307[1], 99308[1], 99309[1], 99310[1], 99315[1], 99316[1], 99334[1], 99335[1], 99336[1], 99337[1], 99347[1], 99348[1], 99349[1], 99350[1], 99374[1], 99375[1], 99377[1], 99378[1], 99446[0], 99447[0], 99448[0], 99449[0], 99451[0], 99452[0], 99495[0], 99496[0], G0168[1], G0463[1], G0471[1], J0670[1], J2001[1]
12042	0213T[0], 0216T[0], 0567T[1], 0568T[1], 0569T[1], 0570T[1], 0571T[1], 0572T[1], 0573T[1], 0574T[1], 0580T[1], 0581T[1], 0582T[1], 0655T[1], 11042[1], 11740[1], 11900[1], 11901[1], 12041[0], 15772[1], 15774[1], 20560[1], 20561[1], 20700[1], 20701[1], 36000[1], 36400[1], 36405[1], 36406[1], 36410[1], 36420[1], 36425[1], 36430[1], 36440[1], 36591[0], 36592[0], 36600[1], 36640[1], 43752[1], 51701[1], 51702[1], 51703[1], 64400[0], 64405[0], 64408[0], 64415[0], 64416[0], 64417[0], 64418[0], 64420[0], 64421[0], 64425[0], 64430[0], 64435[0], 64445[0], 64446[0], 64447[0], 64448[0], 64449[0], 64450[1], 64451[1], 64479[0], 64480[0], 64483[0], 64484[0], 64490[0], 64491[0], 64492[0], 64493[0], 64494[0], 64495[0], 64505[0], 64510[0], 64517[0], 64520[0], 64530[0], 66987[1], 66988[1], 69990[0], 92012[1], 92014[1], 93000[1], 93005[1], 93010[1], 93040[1], 93041[1], 93042[1], 93318[1], 93355[1], 94002[1], 94200[1], 94680[1], 94681[1], 94690[1], 95812[1], 95813[1], 95816[1], 95819[1], 95822[1], 95829[1], 95955[1], 96360[1], 96361[1], 96365[1], 96366[1], 96367[1], 96368[1], 96372[1], 96374[1], 96375[1], 96376[1], 96377[1], 96523[0], 97597[1], 97598[1], 97602[1], 97605[1], 97606[1], 97607[1], 97608[1], 99155[0], 99156[0], 99157[0], 99211[1], 99212[1], 99213[1], 99214[1], 99215[1], 99217[1], 99218[1], 99219[1], 99220[1], 99221[1], 99222[1], 99223[1], 99231[1], 99232[1], 99233[1], 99234[1], 99235[1], 99236[1], 99238[1], 99239[1], 99241[1], 99242[1], 99243[1], 99244[1], 99245[1], 99251[1], 99252[1], 99253[1], 99254[1], 99255[1], 99291[1], 99292[1], 99304[1], 99305[1], 99306[1], 99307[1], 99308[1],

0 = Modifier usage not allowed or inappropriate 1 = Modifier usage allowed

Code 1	Code 2
	99309[1], 99310[1], 99315[1], 99316[1], 99334[1], 99335[1], 99336[1], 99337[1], 99347[1], 99348[1], 99349[1], 99350[1], 99374[1], 99375[1], 99377[1], 99378[1], 99446[0], 99447[0], 99448[0], 99449[0], 99451[0], 99452[0], 99495[0], 99496[0], G0168[1], G0463[1], G0471[1], J0670[1], J2001[1]
12044	0213T[0], 0216T[0], 0567T[1], 0568T[1], 0569T[1], 0570T[1], 0571T[1], 0572T[1], 0573T[1], 0574T[1], 0580T[1], 0581T[1], 0582T[1], 0655T[1], 11043[1], 11044[1], 11900[1], 11901[1], 12041[0], 12042[0], 12054[1], 15772[1], 15774[1], 20560[1], 20561[1], 20700[1], 20701[1], 36000[1], 36400[1], 36405[1], 36406[1], 36410[1], 36420[1], 36425[1], 36430[1], 36440[1], 36591[0], 36592[0], 36600[1], 36640[1], 43752[1], 51701[1], 51702[1], 51703[1], 64400[0], 64405[0], 64408[0], 64415[0], 64416[0], 64417[0], 64418[0], 64420[0], 64421[0], 64425[0], 64430[0], 64435[0], 64445[0], 64446[0], 64447[0], 64448[0], 64449[0], 64450[1], 64451[1], 64479[0], 64480[0], 64483[0], 64484[0], 64490[0], 64491[0], 64492[0], 64493[0], 64494[0], 64495[0], 64505[0], 64510[0], 64517[0], 64520[0], 64530[0], 66987[1], 66988[1], 69990[0], 92012[1], 92014[1], 93000[1], 93005[1], 93010[1], 93040[1], 93041[1], 93042[1], 93318[1], 93355[1], 94002[1], 94200[1], 94680[1], 94681[1], 94690[1], 95812[1], 95813[1], 95816[1], 95819[1], 95822[1], 95829[1], 95955[1], 96360[1], 96361[1], 96365[1], 96366[1], 96367[1], 96368[1], 96372[1], 96374[1], 96375[1], 96376[1], 96377[1], 96523[0], 97597[1], 97598[1], 97602[1], 97605[1], 97606[1], 97607[1], 97608[1], 99155[0], 99156[0], 99157[0], 99211[1], 99212[1], 99213[1], 99214[1], 99215[1], 99217[1], 99218[1], 99219[1], 99220[1], 99221[1], 99222[1], 99223[1], 99231[1], 99232[1], 99233[1], 99234[1], 99235[1], 99236[1], 99238[1], 99239[1], 99241[1], 99242[1], 99243[1], 99244[1], 99245[1], 99251[1], 99252[1], 99253[1], 99254[1], 99255[1], 99291[1], 99292[1], 99304[1], 99305[1], 99306[1], 99307[1], 99308[1], 99309[1], 99310[1], 99315[1], 99316[1], 99334[1], 99335[1], 99336[1], 99337[1], 99347[1], 99348[1], 99349[1], 99350[1], 99374[1], 99375[1], 99377[1], 99378[1], 99446[0], 99447[0], 99448[0], 99449[0], 99451[0], 99452[0], 99495[0], 99496[0], G0168[1], G0463[1], G0471[1], J0670[1], J2001[1]
12045	0213T[0], 0216T[0], 0567T[1], 0568T[1], 0569T[1], 0570T[1], 0571T[1], 0572T[1], 0573T[1], 0574T[1], 0580T[1], 0581T[1], 0582T[1], 0655T[1], 11042[1], 11900[1], 11901[1], 12041[0], 12042[0], 12044[0], 12055[1], 15772[1], 15774[1], 20560[1], 20561[1], 20700[1], 20701[1], 36000[1], 36400[1], 36405[1], 36406[1], 36410[1], 36420[1], 36425[1], 36430[1], 36440[1], 36591[0], 36592[0], 36600[1], 36640[1], 43752[1], 51701[1], 51702[1], 51703[1], 64400[0], 64405[0], 64408[0], 64415[0], 64416[0], 64417[0], 64418[0], 64420[0], 64421[0], 64425[0], 64430[0], 64435[0], 64445[0], 64446[0], 64447[0], 64448[0], 64449[0], 64450[1], 64451[1], 64479[0], 64480[0], 64483[0], 64484[0], 64490[0], 64491[0], 64492[0], 64493[0], 64494[0], 64495[0], 64505[0], 64510[0], 64517[0], 64520[0], 64530[0], 64625[1], 66987[1], 66988[1], 69990[0], 92012[1], 92014[1], 93000[1], 93005[1], 93010[1], 93040[1], 93041[1], 93042[1], 93318[1], 93355[1], 94002[1], 94200[1], 94680[1], 94681[1], 94690[1], 95812[1], 95813[1], 95816[1], 95819[1], 95822[1], 95829[1], 95955[1], 96360[1], 96361[1], 96365[1], 96366[1], 96367[1], 96368[1], 96372[1], 96374[1], 96375[1], 96376[1], 96377[1], 96523[0], 97597[1], 97598[1], 97602[1], 97605[1], 97606[1], 97607[1], 97608[1], 99155[0], 99156[0], 99157[0], 99211[1], 99212[1], 99213[1], 99214[1], 99215[1], 99217[1], 99218[1], 99219[1], 99220[1], 99221[1], 99222[1], 99223[1], 99231[1], 99232[1], 99233[1], 99234[1], 99235[1], 99236[1], 99238[1], 99239[1], 99241[1], 99242[1], 99243[1], 99244[1], 99245[1], 99251[1], 99252[1], 99253[1], 99254[1], 99255[1], 99291[1], 99292[1], 99304[1], 99305[1], 99306[1], 99307[1], 99308[1], 99309[1], 99310[1], 99315[1], 99316[1], 99334[1], 99335[1], 99336[1], 99337[1], 99347[1], 99348[1], 99349[1], 99350[1], 99374[1], 99375[1], 99377[1], 99378[1], 99446[0], 99447[0], 99448[0], 99449[0], 99451[0], 99452[0], 99495[0], 99496[0], G0168[1], G0463[1], G0471[1], J0670[1], J2001[1]
12046	0213T[0], 0216T[0], 0567T[1], 0568T[1], 0569T[1], 0570T[1], 0571T[1], 0572T[1], 0573T[1], 0574T[1], 0580T[1], 0581T[1], 0582T[1], 0655T[1], 11043[1], 11044[1], 11900[1], 11901[1], 12041[0], 12042[0], 12044[0], 12045[0], 12056[1], 15772[1], 15774[1], 20560[1], 20561[1], 20700[1], 20701[1], 36000[1], 36400[1], 36405[1], 36406[1], 36410[1], 36420[1], 36425[1], 36430[1], 36440[1], 36591[0], 36592[0], 36600[1], 36640[1], 43752[1], 51701[1], 51702[1], 51703[1], 64400[0], 64405[0], 64408[0], 64415[0], 64416[0], 64417[0], 64418[0], 64420[0], 64421[0], 64425[0], 64430[0], 64435[0], 64445[0], 64446[0], 64447[0], 64448[0], 64449[0], 64450[1], 64451[1], 64479[0], 64480[0], 64483[0], 64484[0], 64490[0], 64491[0], 64492[0], 64493[0], 64494[0], 64495[0], 64505[0], 64510[0], 64517[0], 64520[0], 64530[0], 64625[1], 66987[1], 66988[1], 69990[0], 92012[1], 92014[1], 93000[1], 93005[1], 93010[1], 93040[1], 93041[1], 93042[1], 93318[1], 93355[1], 94002[1], 94200[1], 94680[1], 94681[1], 94690[1], 95812[1], 95813[1], 95816[1], 95819[1], 95822[1], 95829[1], 95955[1], 96360[1], 96361[1], 96365[1], 96366[1], 96367[1], 96368[1], 96372[1], 96374[1], 96375[1], 96376[1], 96377[1], 96523[0], 97597[1], 97598[1], 97602[1], 97605[1], 97606[1], 97607[1], 97608[1], 99155[0], 99156[0], 99157[0], 99211[1], 99212[1], 99213[1], 99214[1], 99215[1], 99217[1], 99218[1], 99219[1], 99220[1], 99221[1], 99222[1], 99223[1], 99231[1], 99232[1], 99233[1], 99234[1], 99235[1], 99236[1], 99238[1], 99239[1], 99241[1], 99242[1], 99243[1], 99244[1], 99245[1], 99251[1], 99252[1], 99253[1], 99254[1], 99255[1], 99291[1], 99292[1], 99304[1], 99305[1], 99306[1], 99307[1], 99308[1], 99309[1], 99310[1], 99315[1], 99316[1], 99334[1], 99335[1], 99336[1], 99337[1], 99347[1], 99348[1], 99349[1], 99350[1], 99374[1], 99375[1], 99377[1], 99378[1], 99446[0], 99447[0], 99448[0], 99449[0], 99451[0], 99452[0], 99495[0], 99496[0], G0168[1], G0463[1], G0471[1], J0670[1], J2001[1]
12047	0213T[0], 0216T[0], 0567T[1], 0568T[1], 0569T[1], 0570T[1], 0571T[1], 0572T[1], 0573T[1], 0574T[1], 0580T[1], 0581T[1], 0582T[1], 0655T[1], 11900[1], 11901[1], 12037[1], 12041[0], 12042[0], 12044[0], 12045[0], 12046[0], 12057[1], 15772[1], 15774[1], 20560[1], 20561[1], 20700[1], 20701[1], 36000[1], 36400[1], 36405[1], 36406[1], 36410[1], 36420[1], 36425[1], 36430[1], 36440[1], 36591[0], 36592[0], 36600[1], 36640[1], 43752[1], 51701[1], 51702[1], 51703[1], 64400[0], 64405[0], 64408[0], 64415[0], 64416[0], 64417[0], 64418[0], 64420[0], 64421[0], 64425[0], 64430[0], 64435[0], 64445[0], 64446[0], 64447[0], 64448[0], 64449[0], 64450[1], 64451[1], 64479[0], 64480[0], 64483[0], 64484[0], 64490[0], 64491[0], 64492[0], 64493[0], 64494[0], 64495[0], 64505[0], 64510[0], 64517[0], 64520[0], 64530[0], 64625[1], 66987[1], 66988[1], 69990[0], 92012[1], 92014[1], 93000[1], 93005[1], 93010[1], 93040[1], 93041[1], 93042[1], 93318[1], 93355[1], 94002[1], 94200[1], 94680[1], 94681[1], 94690[1], 95812[1], 95813[1], 95816[1], 95819[1], 95822[1], 95829[1], 95955[1], 96360[1], 96361[1], 96365[1], 96366[1], 96367[1], 96368[1], 96372[1], 96374[1], 96375[1], 96376[1], 96377[1], 96523[0], 97597[1], 97598[1], 97602[1], 97605[1], 97606[1], 97607[1], 97608[1], 99155[0], 99156[0], 99157[0], 99211[1], 99212[1], 99213[1], 99214[1], 99215[1], 99217[1], 99218[1], 99219[1], 99220[1], 99221[1], 99222[1], 99223[1], 99231[1], 99232[1], 99233[1], 99234[1], 99235[1], 99236[1], 99238[1], 99239[1], 99241[1], 99242[1], 99243[1], 99244[1], 99245[1], 99251[1], 99252[1], 99253[1], 99254[1], 99255[1], 99291[1], 99292[1], 99304[1], 99305[1], 99306[1], 99307[1], 99308[1], 99309[1], 99310[1], 99315[1], 99316[1], 99334[1], 99335[1], 99336[1], 99337[1], 99347[1], 99348[1], 99349[1], 99350[1], 99374[1], 99375[1], 99377[1], 99378[1], 99446[0], 99447[0], 99448[0], 99449[0], 99451[0], 99452[0], 99495[0], 99496[0], G0168[1], G0463[1], G0471[1], J0670[1], J2001[1]
13131	0213T[0], 0216T[0], 0567T[1], 0568T[1], 0569T[1], 0570T[1], 0571T[1], 0572T[1], 0573T[1], 0574T[1], 0580T[1], 0581T[1], 0582T[1], 0655T[1], 11000[1], 11010[1], 11011[1], 11012[1], 11042[1], 11043[1], 11044[1], 11900[1], 11901[1], 13133[0], 13160[1], 15772[1], 15774[1], 20560[1], 20561[1], 20700[1], 20701[1], 36000[1], 36400[1], 36405[1], 36406[1], 36410[1], 36420[1], 36425[1], 36430[1], 36440[1], 36591[0], 36592[0], 36600[1], 36640[1], 43752[1], 51701[1], 51702[1], 51703[1], 64400[0], 64405[0], 64408[0], 64415[0], 64416[0], 64417[0], 64418[0], 64420[0], 64421[0], 64425[0], 64430[0], 64435[0], 64445[0], 64446[0], 64447[0], 64448[0], 64449[0], 64450[1], 64451[1], 64479[0], 64480[0], 64483[0], 64484[0], 64490[0], 64491[0], 64492[0], 64493[0], 64494[0], 64495[0], 64505[0], 64510[0], 64517[0], 64520[0], 64530[0], 64625[1], 66987[1], 66988[1], 69990[1], 92012[1], 92014[1], 93000[1], 93005[1], 93010[1], 93040[1], 93041[1], 93042[1], 93318[1], 93355[1], 94002[1], 94200[1], 94680[1], 94681[1], 94690[1], 95812[1], 95813[1], 95816[1], 95819[1], 95822[1], 95829[1], 95955[1], 96360[1], 96361[1], 96365[1], 96366[1], 96367[1], 96368[1], 96372[1], 96374[1], 96375[1], 96376[1], 96377[1], 96523[0], 97597[1], 97598[1], 97602[1], 97605[1], 97606[1], 97607[1], 97608[1], 99155[0], 99156[0], 99157[0], 99211[1], 99212[1], 99213[1], 99214[1], 99215[1], 99217[1], 99218[1], 99219[1], 99220[1], 99221[1], 99222[1], 99223[1], 99231[1], 99232[1], 99233[1], 99234[1], 99235[1], 99236[1], 99238[1], 99239[1], 99241[1], 99242[1], 99243[1], 99244[1], 99245[1], 99251[1], 99252[1], 99253[1], 99254[1], 99255[1], 99291[1], 99292[1], 99304[1], 99305[1], 99306[1], 99307[1], 99308[1], 99309[1], 99310[1], 99315[1], 99316[1], 99334[1], 99335[1], 99336[1], 99337[1], 99347[1], 99348[1], 99349[1], 99350[1], 99374[1], 99375[1], 99377[1], 99378[1], 99446[0], 99447[0], 99448[0], 99449[0], 99451[0], 99452[0], 99495[0], 99496[0], G0168[1], G0463[1], G0471[1], J0670[1], J2001[1]
13132	0213T[0], 0216T[0], 0567T[1], 0568T[1], 0569T[1], 0570T[1], 0571T[1], 0572T[1], 0573T[1], 0574T[1], 0580T[1], 0581T[1], 0582T[1], 0655T[1], 11000[1], 11010[1], 11011[1], 11012[1], 11042[1], 11043[1], 11044[1], 11056[1], 11900[1], 11901[1], 13131[0], 13160[1], 15772[1], 15774[1], 20560[1], 20561[1], 20700[1], 20701[1], 36000[1], 36400[1], 36405[1], 36406[1], 36410[1], 36420[1], 36425[1], 36430[1], 36440[1], 36591[0], 36592[0], 36600[1], 36640[1], 43752[1], 51701[1], 51702[1], 51703[1], 64400[0], 64405[0], 64408[0], 64415[0], 64416[0], 64417[0], 64418[0], 64420[0], 64421[0], 64425[0], 64430[0], 64435[0], 64445[0], 64446[0], 64447[0], 64448[0], 64449[0], 64450[1], 64451[1], 64479[0], 64480[0], 64483[0], 64484[0], 64490[0], 64491[0], 64492[0], 64493[0], 64494[0], 64495[0], 64505[0], 64510[0], 64517[0], 64520[0], 64530[0], 64625[1], 66987[1], 66988[1], 69990[1], 92012[1], 92014[1], 93000[1], 93005[1], 93010[1], 93040[1], 93041[1], 93042[1], 93318[1], 93355[1], 94002[1], 94200[1], 94680[1], 94681[1], 94690[1], 95812[1], 95813[1], 95816[1], 95819[1], 95822[1], 95829[1], 95955[1], 96360[1], 96361[1], 96365[1], 96366[1], 96367[1], 96368[1], 96372[1], 96374[1], 96375[1], 96376[1], 96377[1], 96523[0], 97597[1], 97598[1], 97602[1], 97605[1], 97606[1], 97607[1], 97608[1], 99155[0], 99156[0], 99157[0], 99211[1], 99212[1], 99213[1], 99214[1], 99215[1], 99217[1], 99218[1], 99219[1], 99220[1], 99221[1], 99222[1], 99223[1], 99231[1], 99232[1], 99233[1], 99234[1], 99235[1], 99236[1], 99238[1], 99239[1], 99241[1], 99242[1], 99243[1], 99244[1], 99245[1], 99251[1], 99252[1], 99253[1], 99254[1], 99255[1], 99291[1], 99292[1], 99304[1], 99305[1], 99306[1], 99307[1], 99308[1], 99309[1], 99310[1], 99315[1], 99316[1], 99334[1], 99335[1], 99336[1], 99337[1], 99347[1], 99348[1], 99349[1], 99350[1], 99374[1], 99375[1], 99377[1], 99378[1], 99446[0], 99447[0], 99448[0], 99449[0], 99451[0], 99452[0], 99495[0], 99496[0], G0168[1], G0463[1], G0471[1], J0670[1], J2001[1]
13133	0567T[1], 0568T[1], 0569T[1], 0570T[1], 0571T[1], 0572T[1], 0573T[1], 0574T[1], 0580T[1], 0581T[1], 0582T[1], 0655T[1], 11900[1], 11901[1], 13160[1], 20560[1], 20561[1], 20700[1], 20701[1], 36591[0], 36592[0], 64451[1], 66987[1], 66988[1], 69990[1], 96523[0], J0670[1], J2001[1]
13160	0213T[0], 0216T[0], 0596T[1], 0597T[1], 10180[1], 11000[1], 11001[1], 11004[1], 11005[1], 11006[1], 11010[1], 11011[1], 11012[1], 11042[1], 11043[1], 11044[1], 11045[1], 11046[1], 11047[1], 11102[1], 11104[1], 11106[1], 11900[1], 11901[1], 12001[1], 12002[1], 12004[1], 12005[1], 12006[1], 12007[1], 12011[1], 12013[1], 12014[1], 12015[1], 12016[1], 12017[1], 12018[1], 12020[1], 12021[1], 12031[1],

Appendix A: NCCI - CPT Codes

0 = Modifier usage not allowed or inappropriate   1 = Modifier usage allowed

Code 1	Code 2
	12032[1], 12034[1], 12035[1], 12036[1], 12037[1], 12041[1], 12042[1], 12044[1], 12045[1], 12046[1], 12047[1], 12051[1], 12052[1], 12053[1], 12054[1], 12055[1], 12056[1], 12057[1], 36000[1], 36400[1], 36405[1], 36406[1], 36410[1], 36420[1], 36425[1], 36430[1], 36440[1], 36591[0], 36592[0], 36600[1], 36640[1], 43752[1], 51701[1], 51702[1], 51703[1], 62320[0], 62321[0], 62322[0], 62323[0], 62324[0], 62325[0], 62326[0], 62327[0], 64400[0], 64405[0], 64408[0], 64415[0], 64416[0], 64417[0], 64418[0], 64420[0], 64421[0], 64425[0], 64430[0], 64435[0], 64445[0], 64446[0], 64447[0], 64448[0], 64449[0], 64450[1], 64451[0], 64454[1], 64461[0], 64462[0], 64463[0], 64479[0], 64480[0], 64483[0], 64484[0], 64486[0], 64487[0], 64488[0], 64489[0], 64490[0], 64491[0], 64492[0], 64493[0], 64494[0], 64495[0], 64505[0], 64510[0], 64517[0], 64520[0], 64530[0], 69990[0], 92012[1], 92014[1], 93000[1], 93005[1], 93010[1], 93040[1], 93041[1], 93042[1], 93318[1], 93355[1], 94002[1], 94200[1], 94680[1], 94681[1], 94690[1], 95812[1], 95813[1], 95816[1], 95819[1], 95822[1], 95829[1], 95955[1], 96360[1], 96361[1], 96365[1], 96366[1], 96367[1], 96368[1], 96372[1], 96374[1], 96375[1], 96376[1], 96377[1], 96523[0], 97597[1], 97598[1], 97602[1], 97605[1], 97606[1], 97607[1], 97608[1], 99155[0], 99156[0], 99157[0], 99211[1], 99212[1], 99213[1], 99214[1], 99215[1], 99217[1], 99218[1], 99219[1], 99220[1], 99221[1], 99222[1], 99223[1], 99231[1], 99232[1], 99233[1], 99234[1], 99235[1], 99236[1], 99238[1], 99239[1], 99241[1], 99242[1], 99243[1], 99244[1], 99245[1], 99251[1], 99252[1], 99253[1], 99254[1], 99255[1], 99291[1], 99292[1], 99304[1], 99305[1], 99306[1], 99307[1], 99308[1], 99309[1], 99310[1], 99315[1], 99316[1], 99334[1], 99335[1], 99336[1], 99337[1], 99347[1], 99348[1], 99349[1], 99350[1], 99374[1], 99375[1], 99377[1], 99378[1], 99446[0], 99447[0], 99448[0], 99449[0], 99451[0], 99452[0], 99495[0], 99496[0], G0168[1], G0463[1], G0471[1]
17270	0213T[0], 0216T[0], 0419T[1], 0420T[1], 0596T[1], 0597T[1], 11102[1], 11104[1], 11106[1], 11600[1], 11601[1], 11602[1], 11603[1], 11604[1], 11606[1], 11620[1], 11621[1], 11622[1], 11623[1], 11624[1], 11626[1], 11640[1], 11641[1], 11642[1], 11643[1], 11644[1], 11646[1], 11900[1], 11901[1], 12001[1], 12002[1], 12004[1], 12005[1], 12006[1], 12007[1], 12011[1], 12013[1], 12014[1], 12015[1], 12016[1], 12017[1], 12018[1], 12020[1], 12021[1], 12031[1], 12032[1], 12034[1], 12035[1], 12036[1], 12037[1], 12041[1], 12042[1], 12044[1], 12045[1], 12046[1], 12047[1], 12051[1], 12052[1], 12053[1], 12054[1], 12055[1], 12056[1], 12057[1], 13100[1], 13101[1], 13102[1], 13120[1], 13121[1], 13122[1], 13131[1], 13132[1], 13133[1], 13151[1], 13152[1], 13153[1], 17000[1], 17004[1], 17110[1], 17111[1], 17340[1], 36000[1], 36400[1], 36405[1], 36406[1], 36410[1], 36420[1], 36425[1], 36430[1], 36440[1], 36591[0], 36592[0], 36600[1], 36640[1], 43752[1], 51701[1], 51702[1], 51703[1], 62320[0], 62321[0], 62322[0], 62323[0], 62324[0], 62325[0], 62326[0], 62327[0], 64400[0], 64405[0], 64408[0], 64415[0], 64416[0], 64417[0], 64418[0], 64420[0], 64421[0], 64425[0], 64430[0], 64435[0], 64445[0], 64446[0], 64447[0], 64448[0], 64449[0], 64450[1], 64451[0], 64454[1], 64461[0], 64462[0], 64463[0], 64479[0], 64480[0], 64483[0], 64484[0], 64486[0], 64487[0], 64488[0], 64489[0], 64490[0], 64491[0], 64492[0], 64493[0], 64494[0], 64495[0], 64505[0], 64510[0], 64517[0], 64520[0], 64530[0], 69990[0], 92012[1], 92014[1], 93000[1], 93005[1], 93010[1], 93040[1], 93041[1], 93042[1], 93318[1], 93355[1], 94002[1], 94200[1], 94680[1], 94681[1], 94690[1], 95812[1], 95813[1], 95816[1], 95819[1], 95822[1], 95829[1], 95955[1], 96360[1], 96361[1], 96365[1], 96366[1], 96367[1], 96368[1], 96372[1], 96374[1], 96375[1], 96376[1], 96377[1], 96523[0], 99155[0], 99156[0], 99157[0], 99211[1], 99212[1], 99213[1], 99214[1], 99215[1], 99217[1], 99218[1], 99219[1], 99220[1], 99221[1], 99222[1], 99223[1], 99231[1], 99232[1], 99233[1], 99234[1], 99235[1], 99236[1], 99238[1], 99239[1], 99241[1], 99242[1], 99243[1], 99244[1], 99245[1], 99251[1], 99252[1], 99253[1], 99254[1], 99255[1], 99291[1], 99292[1], 99304[1], 99305[1], 99306[1], 99307[1], 99308[1], 99309[1], 99310[1], 99315[1], 99316[1], 99334[1], 99335[1], 99336[1], 99337[1], 99347[1], 99348[1], 99349[1], 99350[1], 99374[1], 99375[1], 99377[1], 99378[1], 99446[0], 99447[0], 99448[0], 99449[0], 99451[0], 99452[0], 99495[0], 99496[0], G0463[1], G0471[1], J0670[1], J2001[1]
17271	0213T[0], 0216T[0], 0596T[1], 0597T[1], 11102[1], 11104[1], 11106[1], 11601[1], 11602[1], 11603[1], 11604[1], 11606[1], 11621[1], 11622[1], 11623[1], 11624[1], 11626[1], 11640[1], 11641[1], 11642[1], 11643[1], 11644[1], 11646[1], 11900[1], 11901[1], 12001[1], 12002[1], 12004[1], 12005[1], 12006[1], 12007[1], 12011[1], 12013[1], 12014[1], 12015[1], 12016[1], 12017[1], 12018[1], 12020[1], 12021[1], 12031[1], 12032[1], 12034[1], 12035[1], 12036[1], 12037[1], 12041[1], 12042[1], 12044[1], 12045[1], 12046[1], 12047[1], 12051[1], 12052[1], 12053[1], 12054[1], 12055[1], 12056[1], 12057[1], 13100[1], 13101[1], 13102[1], 13120[1], 13121[1], 13122[1], 13131[1], 13132[1], 13133[1], 13151[1], 13152[1], 13153[1], 17000[1], 17004[1], 17110[1], 17111[1], 17340[1], 36000[1], 36400[1], 36405[1], 36406[1], 36410[1], 36420[1], 36425[1], 36430[1], 36440[1], 36591[0], 36592[0], 36600[1], 36640[1], 43752[1], 51701[1], 51702[1], 51703[1], 62320[0], 62321[0], 62322[0], 62323[0], 62324[0], 62325[0], 62326[0], 62327[0], 64400[0], 64405[0], 64408[0], 64415[0], 64416[0], 64417[0], 64418[0], 64420[0], 64421[0], 64425[0], 64430[0], 64435[0], 64445[0], 64446[0], 64447[0], 64448[0], 64449[0], 64450[1], 64451[0], 64454[1], 64461[0], 64462[0], 64463[0], 64479[0], 64480[0], 64483[0], 64484[0], 64486[0], 64487[0], 64488[0], 64489[0], 64490[0], 64491[0], 64492[0], 64493[0], 64494[0], 64495[0], 64505[0], 64510[0], 64517[0], 64520[0], 64530[0], 69990[0], 92012[1], 92014[1], 93000[1], 93005[1], 93010[1], 93040[1], 93041[1], 93042[1], 93318[1], 93355[1], 94002[1], 94200[1], 94680[1], 94681[1], 94690[1], 95812[1], 95813[1], 95816[1], 95819[1], 95822[1], 95829[1], 95955[1], 96360[1], 96361[1], 96365[1], 96366[1], 96367[1], 96368[1], 96372[1], 96374[1], 96375[1], 96376[1], 96377[1], 96523[0], 99155[0], 99156[0], 99157[0], 99211[1], 99212[1], 99213[1], 99214[1], 99215[1], 99217[1], 99218[1], 99219[1], 99220[1], 99221[1], 99222[1], 99223[1], 99231[1], 99232[1], 99233[1], 99234[1], 99235[1], 99236[1], 99238[1], 99239[1], 99241[1], 99242[1], 99243[1], 99244[1], 99245[1], 99251[1], 99252[1], 99253[1], 99254[1], 99255[1], 99291[1], 99292[1], 99304[1], 99305[1], 99306[1], 99307[1], 99308[1], 99309[1], 99310[1], 99315[1], 99316[1], 99334[1], 99335[1], 99336[1], 99337[1], 99347[1], 99348[1], 99349[1], 99350[1], 99374[1], 99375[1], 99377[1], 99378[1], 99446[0], 99447[0], 99448[0], 99449[0], 99451[0], 99452[0], 99495[0], 99496[0], G0463[1], G0471[1], J0670[1], J2001[1]
17272	0213T[0], 0216T[0], 0596T[1], 0597T[1], 11102[1], 11104[1], 11106[1], 11601[1], 11602[1], 11603[1], 11604[1], 11606[1], 11621[1], 11622[1], 11623[1], 11624[1], 11626[1], 11641[1], 11642[1], 11643[1], 11644[1], 11646[1], 11900[1], 11901[1], 12001[1], 12002[1], 12004[1], 12005[1], 12006[1], 12007[1], 12011[1], 12013[1], 12014[1], 12015[1], 12016[1], 12017[1], 12018[1], 12020[1], 12021[1], 12031[1], 12032[1], 12034[1], 12035[1], 12036[1], 12037[1], 12041[1], 12042[1], 12044[1], 12045[1], 12046[1], 12047[1], 12051[1], 12052[1], 12053[1], 12054[1], 12055[1], 12056[1], 12057[1], 13100[1], 13101[1], 13102[1], 13120[1], 13121[1], 13122[1], 13131[1], 13132[1], 13133[1], 13151[1], 13152[1], 13153[1], 17000[1], 17004[1], 17110[1], 17111[1], 17340[1], 36000[1], 36400[1], 36405[1], 36406[1], 36410[1], 36420[1], 36425[1], 36430[1], 36440[1], 36591[0], 36592[0], 36600[1], 36640[1], 43752[1], 51701[1], 51702[1], 51703[1], 62320[0], 62321[0], 62322[0], 62323[0], 62324[0], 62325[0], 62326[0], 62327[0], 64400[0], 64405[0], 64408[0], 64415[0], 64416[0], 64417[0], 64418[0], 64420[0], 64421[0], 64425[0], 64430[0], 64435[0], 64445[0], 64446[0], 64447[0], 64448[0], 64449[0], 64450[1], 64451[0], 64454[1], 64461[0], 64462[0], 64463[0], 64479[0], 64480[0], 64483[0], 64484[0], 64486[0], 64487[0], 64488[0], 64489[0], 64490[0], 64491[0], 64492[0], 64493[0], 64494[0], 64495[0], 64505[0], 64510[0], 64517[0], 64520[0], 64530[0], 69990[0], 92012[1], 92014[1], 93000[1], 93005[1], 93010[1], 93040[1], 93041[1], 93042[1], 93318[1], 93355[1], 94002[1], 94200[1], 94680[1], 94681[1], 94690[1], 95812[1], 95813[1], 95816[1], 95819[1], 95822[1], 95829[1], 95955[1], 96360[1], 96361[1], 96365[1], 96366[1], 96367[1], 96368[1], 96372[1], 96374[1], 96375[1], 96376[1], 96377[1], 96523[0], 99155[0], 99156[0], 99157[0], 99211[1], 99212[1], 99213[1], 99214[1], 99215[1], 99217[1], 99218[1], 99219[1], 99220[1], 99221[1], 99222[1], 99223[1], 99231[1], 99232[1], 99233[1], 99234[1], 99235[1], 99236[1], 99238[1], 99239[1], 99241[1], 99242[1], 99243[1], 99244[1], 99245[1], 99251[1], 99252[1], 99253[1], 99254[1], 99255[1], 99291[1], 99292[1], 99304[1], 99305[1], 99306[1], 99307[1], 99308[1], 99309[1], 99310[1], 99315[1], 99316[1], 99334[1], 99335[1], 99336[1], 99337[1], 99347[1], 99348[1], 99349[1], 99350[1], 99374[1], 99375[1], 99377[1], 99378[1], 99446[0], 99447[0], 99448[0], 99449[0], 99451[0], 99452[0], 99495[0], 99496[0], G0463[1], G0471[1], J0670[1], J2001[1]
17273	0213T[0], 0216T[0], 0596T[1], 0597T[1], 11102[1], 11104[1], 11106[1], 11602[1], 11603[1], 11604[1], 11606[1], 11622[1], 11623[1], 11624[1], 11626[1], 11641[1], 11642[1], 11643[1], 11644[1], 11646[1], 11900[1], 11901[1], 12001[1], 12002[1], 12004[1], 12005[1], 12006[1], 12007[1], 12011[1], 12013[1], 12014[1], 12015[1], 12016[1], 12017[1], 12018[1], 12020[1], 12021[1], 12031[1], 12032[1], 12034[1], 12035[1], 12036[1], 12037[1], 12041[1], 12042[1], 12044[1], 12045[1], 12046[1], 12047[1], 12051[1], 12052[1], 12053[1], 12054[1], 12055[1], 12056[1], 12057[1], 13100[1], 13101[1], 13102[1], 13120[1], 13121[1], 13122[1], 13131[1], 13132[1], 13133[1], 13151[1], 13152[1], 13153[1], 17000[1], 17004[1], 17110[1], 17111[1], 17340[1], 36000[1], 36400[1], 36405[1], 36406[1], 36410[1], 36420[1], 36425[1], 36430[1], 36440[1], 36591[0], 36592[0], 36600[1], 36640[1], 43752[1], 51701[1], 51702[1], 51703[1], 62320[0], 62321[0], 62322[0], 62323[0], 62324[0], 62325[0], 62326[0], 62327[0], 64400[0], 64405[0], 64408[0], 64415[0], 64416[0], 64417[0], 64418[0], 64420[0], 64421[0], 64425[0], 64430[0], 64435[0], 64445[0], 64446[0], 64447[0], 64448[0], 64449[0], 64450[1], 64451[0], 64454[1], 64461[0], 64462[0], 64463[0], 64479[0], 64480[0], 64483[0], 64484[0], 64486[0], 64487[0], 64488[0], 64489[0], 64490[0], 64491[0], 64492[0], 64493[0], 64494[0], 64495[0], 64505[0], 64510[0], 64517[0], 64520[0], 64530[0], 69990[0], 92012[1], 92014[1], 93000[1], 93005[1], 93010[1], 93040[1], 93041[1], 93042[1], 93318[1], 93355[1], 94002[1], 94200[1], 94680[1], 94681[1], 94690[1], 95812[1], 95813[1], 95816[1], 95819[1], 95822[1], 95829[1], 95955[1], 96360[1], 96361[1], 96365[1], 96366[1], 96367[1], 96368[1], 96372[1], 96374[1], 96375[1], 96376[1], 96377[1], 96523[0], 99155[0], 99156[0], 99157[0], 99211[1], 99212[1], 99213[1], 99214[1], 99215[1], 99217[1], 99218[1], 99219[1], 99220[1], 99221[1], 99222[1], 99223[1], 99231[1], 99232[1], 99233[1], 99234[1], 99235[1], 99236[1], 99238[1], 99239[1], 99241[1], 99242[1], 99243[1], 99244[1], 99245[1], 99251[1], 99252[1], 99253[1], 99254[1], 99255[1], 99291[1], 99292[1], 99304[1], 99305[1], 99306[1], 99307[1], 99308[1], 99309[1], 99310[1], 99315[1], 99316[1], 99334[1], 99335[1], 99336[1], 99337[1], 99347[1], 99348[1], 99349[1], 99350[1], 99374[1], 99375[1], 99377[1], 99378[1], 99446[0], 99447[0], 99448[0], 99449[0], 99451[0], 99452[0], 99495[0], 99496[0], G0463[1], G0471[1], J0670[1], J2001[1]
17274	0213T[0], 0216T[0], 0596T[1], 0597T[1], 11102[1], 11104[1], 11106[1], 11606[1], 11623[1], 11624[1], 11626[1], 11642[1], 11643[1], 11644[1], 11646[1], 11900[1], 11901[1], 12001[1], 12002[1], 12004[1], 12005[1], 12006[1], 12007[1], 12011[1], 12013[1], 12014[1], 12015[1], 12016[1], 12017[1], 12018[1], 12020[1], 12021[1], 12031[1], 12032[1], 12034[1], 12035[1], 12036[1], 12037[1], 12041[1], 12042[1], 12044[1], 12045[1], 12046[1], 12047[1], 12051[1], 12052[1], 12053[1], 12054[1], 12055[1], 12056[1], 12057[1], 13100[1], 13101[1], 13102[1], 13120[1], 13121[1], 13122[1], 13131[1], 13132[1], 13133[1], 13151[1], 13152[1], 13153[1], 17000[1], 17004[1], 17110[1], 17111[1], 17340[1], 36000[1], 36400[1], 36405[1], 36406[1], 36410[1], 36420[1], 36425[1], 36430[1], 36440[1], 36591[0], 36592[0], 36600[1], 36640[1], 43752[1], 51701[1], 51702[1], 51703[1], 62320[0], 62321[0], 62322[0], 62323[0], 62324[0], 62325[0], 62326[0], 62327[0], 64400[0], 64405[0], 64408[0], 64415[0], 64416[0], 64417[0], 64418[0], 64420[0], 64421[0], 64425[0], 64430[0], 64435[0], 64445[0], 64446[0], 64447[0], 64448[0], 64449[0],

0 = Modifier usage not allowed or inappropriate 1 = Modifier usage allowed

Code 1	Code 2
	64450[1], 64451[0], 64454[1], 64461[0], 64462[0], 64463[0], 64479[0], 64480[0], 64483[0], 64484[0], 64486[0], 64487[0], 64488[0], 64489[0], 64490[0], 64491[0], 64492[0], 64493[0], 64494[0], 64495[0], 64505[0], 64510[0], 64517[0], 64520[0], 64530[0], 69990[0], 92012[1], 92014[1], 93000[1], 93005[1], 93010[1], 93040[1], 93041[1], 93042[1], 93318[1], 93355[1], 94002[1], 94200[1], 94680[1], 94681[1], 94690[1], 95812[1], 95813[1], 95816[1], 95819[1], 95822[1], 95829[1], 95955[1], 96360[1], 96361[1], 96365[1], 96366[1], 96367[1], 96368[1], 96372[1], 96374[1], 96375[1], 96376[1], 96377[1], 96523[0], 99155[0], 99156[0], 99157[0], 99211[1], 99212[1], 99213[1], 99214[1], 99215[1], 99217[1], 99218[1], 99219[1], 99220[1], 99221[1], 99222[1], 99223[1], 99231[1], 99232[1], 99233[1], 99234[1], 99235[1], 99236[1], 99238[1], 99239[1], 99241[1], 99242[1], 99243[1], 99244[1], 99245[1], 99251[1], 99252[1], 99253[1], 99254[1], 99255[1], 99291[1], 99292[1], 99304[1], 99305[1], 99306[1], 99307[1], 99308[1], 99309[1], 99310[1], 99315[1], 99316[1], 99334[1], 99335[1], 99336[1], 99337[1], 99347[1], 99348[1], 99349[1], 99350[1], 99374[1], 99375[1], 99377[1], 99378[1], 99446[0], 99447[0], 99448[0], 99449[0], 99451[0], 99452[0], 99495[0], 99496[0], G0463[1], G0471[1], J0670[1], J2001[1]
17276	0213T[0], 0216T[0], 0596T[1], 0597T[1], 11102[1], 11104[1], 11106[1], 11606[1], 11624[1], 11626[1], 11643[1], 11644[1], 11646[1], 11900[1], 11901[1], 12001[1], 12002[1], 12004[1], 12005[1], 12006[1], 12007[1], 12011[1], 12013[1], 12014[1], 12015[1], 12016[1], 12017[1], 12018[1], 12020[1], 12021[1], 12031[1], 12032[1], 12034[1], 12035[1], 12036[1], 12037[1], 12041[1], 12042[1], 12044[1], 12045[1], 12046[1], 12047[1], 12051[1], 12052[1], 12053[1], 12054[1], 12055[1], 12056[1], 12057[1], 13100[1], 13101[1], 13102[1], 13120[1], 13121[1], 13122[1], 13131[1], 13132[1], 13133[1], 13151[1], 13152[1], 13153[1], 17000[1], 17004[1], 17110[1], 17111[1], 17340[1], 36000[1], 36400[1], 36405[1], 36406[1], 36410[1], 36420[1], 36425[1], 36430[1], 36440[1], 36591[0], 36592[0], 36600[1], 36640[1], 43752[1], 51701[1], 51702[1], 51703[1], 62320[0], 62321[0], 62322[0], 62323[0], 62324[0], 62325[0], 62326[0], 62327[0], 64400[0], 64405[0], 64408[0], 64415[0], 64416[0], 64417[0], 64418[0], 64420[0], 64421[0], 64425[0], 64430[0], 64435[0], 64445[0], 64446[0], 64447[0], 64448[0], 64449[0], 64450[1], 64451[0], 64454[1], 64461[0], 64462[0], 64463[0], 64479[0], 64480[0], 64483[0], 64484[0], 64486[0], 64487[0], 64488[0], 64489[0], 64490[0], 64491[0], 64492[0], 64493[0], 64494[0], 64495[0], 64505[0], 64510[0], 64517[0], 64520[0], 64530[0], 69990[0], 92012[1], 92014[1], 93000[1], 93005[1], 93010[1], 93040[1], 93041[1], 93042[1], 93318[1], 93355[1], 94002[1], 94200[1], 94680[1], 94681[1], 94690[1], 95812[1], 95813[1], 95816[1], 95819[1], 95822[1], 95829[1], 95955[1], 96360[1], 96361[1], 96365[1], 96366[1], 96367[1], 96368[1], 96372[1], 96374[1], 96375[1], 96376[1], 96377[1], 96523[0], 99155[0], 99156[0], 99157[0], 99211[1], 99212[1], 99213[1], 99214[1], 99215[1], 99217[1], 99218[1], 99219[1], 99220[1], 99221[1], 99222[1], 99223[1], 99231[1], 99232[1], 99233[1], 99234[1], 99235[1], 99236[1], 99238[1], 99239[1], 99241[1], 99242[1], 99243[1], 99244[1], 99245[1], 99251[1], 99252[1], 99253[1], 99254[1], 99255[1], 99291[1], 99292[1], 99304[1], 99305[1], 99306[1], 99307[1], 99308[1], 99309[1], 99310[1], 99315[1], 99316[1], 99334[1], 99335[1], 99336[1], 99337[1], 99347[1], 99348[1], 99349[1], 99350[1], 99374[1], 99375[1], 99377[1], 99378[1], 99446[0], 99447[0], 99448[0], 99449[0], 99451[0], 99452[0], 99495[0], 99496[0], G0463[1], G0471[1], J0670[1], J2001[1]
35800	0213T[0], 0216T[0], 0596T[1], 0597T[1], 0708T[1], 0709T[1], 12001[1], 12002[1], 12004[1], 12005[1], 12006[1], 12007[1], 12011[1], 12013[1], 12014[1], 12015[1], 12016[1], 12017[1], 12018[1], 12020[1], 12021[1], 12031[1], 12032[1], 12034[1], 12035[1], 12036[1], 12037[1], 12041[1], 12042[1], 12044[1], 12045[1], 12046[1], 12047[1], 12051[1], 12052[1], 12053[1], 12054[1], 12055[1], 12056[1], 12057[1], 13100[1], 13101[1], 13102[1], 13120[1], 13121[1], 13122[1], 13131[1], 13132[1], 13133[1], 13151[1], 13152[1], 13153[1], 36000[1], 36002[1], 36400[1], 36405[1], 36406[1], 36410[1], 36420[1], 36425[1], 36430[1], 36440[1], 36591[0], 36592[0], 36595[1], 36596[1], 36600[1], 36640[1], 43752[1], 51701[1], 51702[1], 51703[1], 62320[0], 62321[0], 62322[0], 62323[0], 62324[0], 62325[0], 62326[0], 62327[0], 64400[0], 64405[0], 64408[0], 64415[0], 64416[0], 64417[0], 64418[0], 64420[0], 64421[0], 64425[0], 64430[0], 64435[0], 64445[0], 64446[0], 64447[0], 64448[0], 64449[0], 64450[0], 64451[0], 64454[0], 64461[0], 64462[0], 64463[0], 64479[0], 64480[0], 64483[0], 64484[0], 64486[0], 64487[0], 64488[0], 64489[0], 64490[0], 64491[0], 64492[0], 64493[0], 64494[0], 64495[0], 64505[0], 64510[0], 64517[0], 64520[0], 64530[0], 69990[0], 92012[1], 92014[1], 93000[1], 93005[1], 93010[1], 93040[1], 93041[1], 93042[1], 93318[1], 93355[1], 94002[1], 94200[1], 94680[1], 94681[1], 94690[1], 95812[1], 95813[1], 95816[1], 95819[1], 95822[1], 95829[1], 95955[1], 96360[1], 96361[1], 96365[1], 96366[1], 96367[1], 96368[1], 96372[1], 96374[1], 96375[1], 96376[1], 96377[1], 96523[0], 99155[0], 99156[0], 99157[0], 99211[1], 99212[1], 99213[1], 99214[1], 99215[1], 99217[1], 99218[1], 99219[1], 99220[1], 99221[1], 99222[1], 99223[1], 99231[1], 99232[1], 99233[1], 99234[1], 99235[1], 99236[1], 99238[1], 99239[1], 99241[1], 99242[1], 99243[1], 99244[1], 99245[1], 99251[1], 99252[1], 99253[1], 99254[1], 99255[1], 99291[1], 99292[1], 99304[1], 99305[1], 99306[1], 99307[1], 99308[1], 99309[1], 99310[1], 99315[1], 99316[1], 99334[1], 99335[1], 99336[1], 99337[1], 99347[1], 99348[1], 99349[1], 99350[1], 99374[1], 99375[1], 99377[1], 99378[1], 99446[0], 99447[0], 99448[0], 99449[0], 99451[0], 99452[0], 99495[0], 99496[0], G0463[1], G0471[1]
35820	0213T[0], 0216T[0], 0596T[1], 0597T[1], 0708T[1], 0709T[1], 12001[1], 12002[1], 12004[1], 12005[1], 12006[1], 12007[1], 12011[1], 12013[1], 12014[1], 12015[1], 12016[1], 12017[1], 12018[1], 12020[1], 12021[1], 12031[1], 12032[1], 12034[1], 12035[1], 12036[1], 12037[1], 12041[1], 12042[1], 12044[1], 12045[1], 12046[1], 12047[1], 12051[1], 12052[1], 12053[1], 12054[1], 12055[1], 12056[1], 12057[1], 13100[1], 13101[1], 13102[1], 13120[1], 13121[1], 13122[1], 13131[1], 13132[1], 13133[1], 13151[1], 13152[1], 13153[1], 32100[1], 32551[1], 36000[1], 36002[1], 36400[1], 36405[1], 36406[1], 36410[1], 36420[1], 36425[1], 36430[1], 36440[1], 36591[0], 36592[0], 36595[1], 36596[1], 36600[1], 36640[1], 39000[1], 39010[1], 43752[1], 51701[1], 51702[1], 51703[1], 62320[0], 62321[0], 62322[0], 62323[0], 62324[0], 62325[0], 62326[0], 62327[0], 64400[0], 64405[0], 64408[0], 64415[0], 64416[0], 64417[0], 64418[0], 64420[0], 64421[0], 64425[0], 64430[0], 64435[0], 64445[0], 64446[0], 64447[0], 64448[0], 64449[0], 64450[0], 64451[0], 64454[0], 64461[0], 64462[0], 64463[0], 64479[0], 64480[0], 64483[0], 64484[0], 64486[0], 64487[0], 64488[0], 64489[0], 64490[0], 64491[0], 64492[0], 64493[0], 64494[0], 64495[0], 64505[0], 64510[0], 64517[0], 64520[0], 64530[0], 69990[0], 75600[1], 75605[1], 75741[1], 75743[1], 75746[1], 75756[1], 75825[1], 75827[1], 92012[1], 92014[1], 93000[1], 93005[1], 93010[1], 93040[1], 93041[1], 93042[1], 93318[1], 93355[1], 94002[1], 94200[1], 94680[1], 94681[1], 94690[1], 95812[1], 95813[1], 95816[1], 95819[1], 95822[1], 95829[1], 95955[1], 96360[1], 96361[1], 96365[1], 96366[1], 96367[1], 96368[1], 96372[1], 96374[1], 96375[1], 96376[1], 96377[1], 96523[0], 99155[0], 99156[0], 99157[0], 99211[1], 99212[1], 99213[1], 99214[1], 99215[1], 99217[1], 99218[1], 99219[1], 99220[1], 99221[1], 99222[1], 99223[1], 99231[1], 99232[1], 99233[1], 99234[1], 99235[1], 99236[1], 99238[1], 99239[1], 99241[1], 99242[1], 99243[1], 99244[1], 99245[1], 99251[1], 99252[1], 99253[1], 99254[1], 99255[1], 99291[1], 99292[1], 99304[1], 99305[1], 99306[1], 99307[1], 99308[1], 99309[1], 99310[1], 99315[1], 99316[1], 99334[1], 99335[1], 99336[1], 99337[1], 99347[1], 99348[1], 99349[1], 99350[1], 99374[1], 99375[1], 99377[1], 99378[1], 99446[0], 99447[0], 99448[0], 99449[0], 99451[0], 99452[0], 99495[0], 99496[0], G0463[1], G0471[1]
35840	0213T[0], 0216T[0], 0596T[1], 0597T[1], 0645T[1], 0708T[1], 0709T[1], 12001[1], 12002[1], 12004[1], 12005[1], 12006[1], 12007[1], 12011[1], 12013[1], 12014[1], 12015[1], 12016[1], 12017[1], 12018[1], 12020[1], 12021[1], 12031[1], 12032[1], 12034[1], 12035[1], 12036[1], 12037[1], 12041[1], 12042[1], 12044[1], 12045[1], 12046[1], 12047[1], 12051[1], 12052[1], 12053[1], 12054[1], 12055[1], 12056[1], 12057[1], 13100[1], 13101[1], 13102[1], 13120[1], 13121[1], 13122[1], 13131[1], 13132[1], 13133[1], 13151[1], 13152[1], 13153[1], 36000[1], 36002[1], 36400[1], 36405[1], 36406[1], 36410[1], 36420[1], 36425[1], 36430[1], 36440[1], 36591[0], 36592[0], 36595[1], 36596[1], 36600[1], 36640[1], 43752[1], 49000[0], 49002[1], 51701[1], 51702[1], 51703[1], 62320[0], 62321[0], 62322[0], 62323[0], 62324[0], 62325[0], 62326[0], 62327[0], 64400[0], 64405[0], 64408[0], 64415[0], 64416[0], 64417[0], 64418[0], 64420[0], 64421[0], 64425[0], 64430[0], 64435[0], 64445[0], 64446[0], 64447[0], 64448[0], 64449[0], 64450[0], 64451[0], 64454[0], 64461[0], 64462[0], 64463[0], 64479[0], 64480[0], 64483[0], 64484[0], 64486[0], 64487[0], 64488[0], 64489[0], 64490[0], 64491[0], 64492[0], 64493[0], 64494[0], 64495[0], 64505[0], 64510[0], 64517[0], 64520[0], 64530[0], 69990[0], 75625[1], 75630[1], 75635[1], 75726[1], 75731[1], 75733[1], 75810[1], 75825[1], 75831[1], 75833[1], 75840[1], 75842[1], 75885[1], 75887[1], 75889[1], 75891[1], 92012[1], 92014[1], 93000[1], 93005[1], 93010[1], 93040[1], 93041[1], 93042[1], 93318[1], 93355[1], 94002[1], 94200[1], 94680[1], 94681[1], 94690[1], 95812[1], 95813[1], 95816[1], 95819[1], 95822[1], 95829[1], 95955[1], 96360[1], 96361[1], 96365[1], 96366[1], 96367[1], 96368[1], 96372[1], 96374[1], 96375[1], 96376[1], 96377[1], 96523[0], 99155[0], 99156[0], 99157[0], 99211[1], 99212[1], 99213[1], 99214[1], 99215[1], 99217[1], 99218[1], 99219[1], 99220[1], 99221[1], 99222[1], 99223[1], 99231[1], 99232[1], 99233[1], 99234[1], 99235[1], 99236[1], 99238[1], 99239[1], 99241[1], 99242[1], 99243[1], 99244[1], 99245[1], 99251[1], 99252[1], 99253[1], 99254[1], 99255[1], 99291[1], 99292[1], 99304[1], 99305[1], 99306[1], 99307[1], 99308[1], 99309[1], 99310[1], 99315[1], 99316[1], 99334[1], 99335[1], 99336[1], 99337[1], 99347[1], 99348[1], 99349[1], 99350[1], 99374[1], 99375[1], 99377[1], 99378[1], 99446[0], 99447[0], 99448[0], 99449[0], 99451[0], 99452[0], 99495[0], 99496[0], G0463[1], G0471[1]
35860	0213T[0], 0216T[0], 0596T[1], 0597T[1], 0708T[1], 0709T[1], 12001[1], 12002[1], 12004[1], 12005[1], 12006[1], 12007[1], 12011[1], 12013[1], 12014[1], 12015[1], 12016[1], 12017[1], 12018[1], 12020[1], 12021[1], 12031[1], 12032[1], 12034[1], 12035[1], 12036[1], 12037[1], 12041[1], 12042[1], 12044[1], 12045[1], 12046[1], 12047[1], 12051[1], 12052[1], 12053[1], 12054[1], 12055[1], 12056[1], 12057[1], 13100[1], 13101[1], 13102[1], 13120[1], 13121[1], 13122[1], 13131[1], 13132[1], 13133[1], 13151[1], 13152[1], 13153[1], 36000[1], 36002[1], 36400[1], 36405[1], 36406[1], 36410[1], 36420[1], 36425[1], 36430[1], 36440[1], 36591[0], 36592[0], 36595[1], 36596[1], 36600[1], 36640[1], 43752[1], 51701[1], 51702[1], 51703[1], 62320[0], 62321[0], 62322[0], 62323[0], 62324[0], 62325[0], 62326[0], 62327[0], 64400[0], 64405[0], 64408[0], 64415[0], 64416[0], 64417[0], 64418[0], 64420[0], 64421[0], 64425[0], 64430[0], 64435[0], 64445[0], 64446[0], 64447[0], 64448[0], 64449[0], 64450[0], 64451[0], 64454[0], 64461[0], 64462[0], 64463[0], 64479[0], 64480[0], 64483[0], 64484[0], 64486[0], 64487[0], 64488[0], 64489[0], 64490[0], 64491[0], 64492[0], 64493[0], 64494[0], 64495[0], 64505[0], 64510[0], 64517[0], 64520[0], 64530[0], 69990[0], 75710[1], 75716[1], 75820[1], 75822[1], 92012[1], 92014[1], 93000[1], 93005[1], 93010[1], 93040[1], 93041[1], 93042[1], 93318[1], 93355[1], 94002[1], 94200[1], 94680[1], 94681[1], 94690[1], 95812[1], 95813[1], 95816[1], 95819[1], 95822[1], 95829[1], 95955[1], 96360[1], 96361[1], 96365[1], 96366[1], 96367[1], 96368[1], 96372[1], 96374[1], 96375[1], 96376[1], 96377[1], 96523[0], 99155[0], 99156[0], 99157[0], 99211[1], 99212[1], 99213[1], 99214[1], 99215[1], 99217[1], 99218[1], 99219[1], 99220[1], 99221[1], 99222[1], 99223[1], 99231[1], 99232[1], 99233[1], 99234[1], 99235[1], 99236[1], 99238[1], 99239[1], 99241[1], 99242[1], 99243[1], 99244[1], 99245[1], 99251[1], 99252[1], 99253[1], 99254[1], 99255[1], 99291[1], 99292[1], 99304[1], 99305[1], 99306[1], 99307[1], 99308[1], 99309[1], 99310[1], 99315[1], 99316[1], 99334[1], 99335[1], 99336[1], 99337[1], 99347[1],

0 = Modifier usage not allowed or inappropriate 1 = Modifier usage allowed

Code 1	Code 2
	99348[1], 99349[1], 99350[1], 99374[1], 99375[1], 99377[1], 99378[1], 99446[0], 99447[0], 99448[0], 99449[0], 99451[0], 99452[0], 99495[0], 99496[0], G0463[1], G0471[1]
36000	0543T[1], 0544T[1], 0567T[1], 0568T[1], 0569T[1], 0570T[1], 0571T[1], 0572T[1], 0573T[1], 0574T[1], 0580T[1], 0581T[1], 0655T[1], 36591[0], 36592[0], 66987[1], 66988[1], 69990[0], 77001[1], 77002[1], 96523[0]
36011	35201[1], 35206[1], 35226[1], 35231[1], 35236[1], 35256[1], 35261[1], 35266[1], 35286[1], 36000[1], 36005[1], 36010[1], 36400[1], 36405[1], 36406[1], 36410[1], 36420[1], 36425[1], 36555[1], 36556[1], 36568[1], 36569[1], 36572[1], 36573[1], 36591[0], 36592[0], 69990[0], 75893[1], 77001[1], 77002[1], 96523[0], J0670[1], J1642[1], J1644[1], J2001[1]
36012	35201[1], 35206[1], 35226[1], 35231[1], 35236[1], 35256[1], 35261[1], 35266[1], 35286[1], 36000[1], 36002[1], 36005[1], 36010[1], 36011[1], 36400[1], 36405[1], 36406[1], 36410[1], 36420[1], 36425[1], 36555[1], 36556[1], 36568[1], 36569[1], 36572[1], 36573[1], 36591[0], 36592[0], 69990[0], 75893[1], 76000[1], 77001[1], 77002[1], 96523[0], J0670[1], J1642[1], J1644[1], J2001[1]
36245	01916[0], 01924[0], 01925[0], 01926[0], 34713[1], 34714[1], 34812[1], 34813[1], 35201[1], 35206[1], 35226[1], 35231[1], 35236[1], 35256[1], 35261[1], 35266[1], 35286[1], 36002[1], 36140[1], 36160[1], 36200[1], 36500[1], 36591[0], 36592[0], 69990[0], 75893[1], 76000[1], 77001[1], 77002[1], 93050[0], 96523[0], J0670[1], J1642[1], J1644[1], J2001[1]
36246	01916[0], 01924[0], 01925[0], 01926[0], 12001[1], 12002[1], 12004[1], 12005[1], 12006[1], 12007[1], 12011[1], 12013[1], 12014[1], 12015[1], 12016[1], 12017[1], 12018[1], 12020[1], 12021[1], 12031[1], 12032[1], 12034[1], 12035[1], 12036[1], 12037[1], 12041[1], 12042[1], 12044[1], 12045[1], 12046[1], 12047[1], 12051[1], 12052[1], 12053[1], 12054[1], 12055[1], 12056[1], 12057[1], 13100[1], 13101[1], 13102[1], 13120[1], 13121[1], 13122[1], 13131[1], 13132[1], 13133[1], 13151[1], 13152[1], 13153[1], 34713[1], 34714[1], 34812[1], 34813[1], 35201[1], 35206[1], 35226[1], 35231[1], 35236[1], 35256[1], 35261[1], 35266[1], 35286[1], 36002[1], 36140[1], 36160[1], 36200[1], 36245[1], 36500[1], 36591[0], 36592[0], 64461[0], 64462[0], 64463[0], 64486[0], 64487[0], 64488[0], 64489[0], 69990[0], 75893[1], 92012[1], 92014[1], 93050[0], 96361[1], 96366[1], 96367[1], 96368[1], 96523[0], 99211[1], 99212[1], 99213[1], 99214[1], 99215[1], 99217[1], 99218[1], 99219[1], 99220[1], 99221[1], 99222[1], 99223[1], 99231[1], 99232[1], 99233[1], 99234[1], 99235[1], 99236[1], 99238[1], 99239[1], 99241[1], 99242[1], 99243[1], 99244[1], 99245[1], 99251[1], 99252[1], 99253[1], 99254[1], 99255[1], 99291[1], 99292[1], 99304[1], 99305[1], 99306[1], 99307[1], 99308[1], 99309[1], 99310[1], 99315[1], 99316[1], 99334[1], 99335[1], 99336[1], 99337[1], 99347[1], 99348[1], 99349[1], 99350[1], 99374[1], 99375[1], 99377[1], 99378[1], 99446[0], 99447[0], 99448[0], 99449[0], 99451[0], 99452[0], 99495[1], 99496[1], G0463[1], J0670[1], J1642[1], J1644[1], J2001[1]
36247	01916[0], 01924[0], 01925[0], 01926[0], 12001[1], 12002[1], 12004[1], 12005[1], 12006[1], 12007[1], 12011[1], 12013[1], 12014[1], 12015[1], 12016[1], 12017[1], 12018[1], 12020[1], 12021[1], 12031[1], 12032[1], 12034[1], 12035[1], 12036[1], 12037[1], 12041[1], 12042[1], 12044[1], 12045[1], 12046[1], 12047[1], 12051[1], 12052[1], 12053[1], 12054[1], 12055[1], 12056[1], 12057[1], 13100[1], 13101[1], 13102[1], 13120[1], 13121[1], 13122[1], 13131[1], 13132[1], 13133[1], 13151[1], 13152[1], 13153[1], 34713[1], 34714[1], 34812[1], 34813[1], 35201[1], 35206[1], 35226[1], 35231[1], 35236[1], 35256[1], 35261[1], 35266[1], 35286[1], 35840[1], 36002[1], 36140[1], 36160[1], 36200[1], 36245[1], 36246[1], 36500[1], 36591[0], 36592[0], 64461[0], 64462[0], 64463[0], 64486[0], 64487[0], 64488[0], 64489[0], 69990[0], 75893[1], 92012[1], 92014[1], 93050[0], 96361[1], 96366[1], 96367[1], 96368[1], 96523[0], 99211[1], 99212[1], 99213[1], 99214[1], 99215[1], 99217[1], 99218[1], 99219[1], 99220[1], 99221[1], 99222[1], 99223[1], 99231[1], 99232[1], 99233[1], 99234[1], 99235[1], 99236[1], 99238[1], 99239[1], 99241[1], 99242[1], 99243[1], 99244[1], 99245[1], 99251[1], 99252[1], 99253[1], 99254[1], 99255[1], 99291[1], 99292[1], 99304[1], 99305[1], 99306[1], 99307[1], 99308[1], 99309[1], 99310[1], 99315[1], 99316[1], 99334[1], 99335[1], 99336[1], 99337[1], 99347[1], 99348[1], 99349[1], 99350[1], 99374[1], 99375[1], 99377[1], 99378[1], 99446[0], 99447[0], 99448[0], 99449[0], 99451[0], 99452[0], 99495[1], 99496[1], G0463[1], J0670[1], J1642[1], J1644[1], J2001[1]
36248	36002[1], 36200[1], 36591[0], 36592[0], 93050[0], 96523[0]
36251	01916[0], 01924[0], 01925[0], 01926[0], 0213T[0], 0216T[0], 0596T[1], 0597T[1], 0708T[1], 0709T[1], 12001[1], 12002[1], 12004[1], 12005[1], 12006[1], 12007[1], 12011[1], 12013[1], 12014[1], 12015[1], 12016[1], 12017[1], 12018[1], 12020[1], 12021[1], 12031[1], 12032[1], 12034[1], 12035[1], 12036[1], 12037[1], 12041[1], 12042[1], 12044[1], 12045[1], 12046[1], 12047[1], 12051[1], 12052[1], 12053[1], 12054[1], 12055[1], 12056[1], 12057[1], 13100[1], 13101[1], 13102[1], 13120[1], 13121[1], 13122[1], 13131[1], 13132[1], 13133[1], 13151[1], 13152[1], 13153[1], 35201[1], 35206[1], 35226[1], 35231[1], 35236[1], 35256[1], 35261[1], 35266[1], 35286[1], 36000[1], 36005[1], 36140[1], 36160[1], 36200[1], 36245[1], 36246[1], 36247[1], 36400[1], 36405[1], 36406[1], 36410[1], 36420[1], 36425[1], 36430[1], 36440[1], 36500[1], 36591[0], 36592[0], 36600[1], 36640[1], 43752[1], 51701[1], 51702[1], 51703[1], 62320[0], 62321[0], 62322[0], 62323[0], 62324[0], 62325[0], 62326[0], 62327[0], 64400[0], 64405[0], 64408[0], 64415[0], 64416[0], 64417[0], 64418[0], 64420[0], 64421[0], 64425[0], 64430[0], 64435[0], 64445[0], 64446[0], 64447[0], 64448[0], 64449[0], 64450[0], 64451[0], 64454[0], 64461[0], 64462[0], 64463[0], 64479[0], 64480[0], 64483[0], 64484[0], 64486[0], 64487[0], 64488[0], 64489[0], 64490[0], 64491[0], 64492[0], 64493[0], 64494[0], 64495[0], 64505[0], 64510[0], 64517[0], 64520[0], 64530[0], 69990[0], 75625[1], 75831[1], 75833[1], 75893[1], 76000[1], 76942[1], 76998[1], 77001[1], 77002[1], 92012[1], 92014[1], 93000[1], 93005[1], 93010[1], 93040[1], 93041[1], 93042[1], 93050[0], 93318[1], 93355[1], 94002[1], 94200[1], 94680[1], 94681[1], 94690[1], 95812[1], 95813[1], 95816[1], 95819[1], 95822[1], 95829[1], 95955[1], 96360[1], 96361[1], 96365[1], 96366[1], 96367[1], 96368[1], 96372[1], 96374[1], 96375[1], 96376[1], 96377[1], 96523[0], 99155[0], 99156[0], 99157[0], 99211[1], 99212[1], 99213[1], 99214[1], 99215[1], 99217[1], 99218[1], 99219[1], 99220[1], 99221[1], 99222[1], 99223[1], 99231[1], 99232[1], 99233[1], 99234[1], 99235[1], 99236[1], 99238[1], 99239[1], 99241[1], 99242[1], 99243[1], 99244[1], 99245[1], 99251[1], 99252[1], 99253[1], 99254[1], 99255[1], 99291[1], 99292[1], 99304[1], 99305[1], 99306[1], 99307[1], 99308[1], 99309[1], 99310[1], 99315[1], 99316[1], 99334[1], 99335[1], 99336[1], 99337[1], 99347[1], 99348[1], 99349[1], 99350[1], 99374[1], 99375[1], 99377[1], 99378[1], 99446[0], 99447[0], 99448[0], 99449[0], 99451[0], 99452[0], 99495[1], 99496[1], G0269[1], G0463[1], G0471[1], J0670[1], J1642[1], J1644[1], J2001[1]
36252	01916[0], 01924[0], 01925[0], 01926[0], 0213T[0], 0216T[0], 0596T[1], 0597T[1], 0708T[1], 0709T[1], 12001[1], 12002[1], 12004[1], 12005[1], 12006[1], 12007[1], 12011[1], 12013[1], 12014[1], 12015[1], 12016[1], 12017[1], 12018[1], 12020[1], 12021[1], 12031[1], 12032[1], 12034[1], 12035[1], 12036[1], 12037[1], 12041[1], 12042[1], 12044[1], 12045[1], 12046[1], 12047[1], 12051[1], 12052[1], 12053[1], 12054[1], 12055[1], 12056[1], 12057[1], 13100[1], 13101[1], 13102[1], 13120[1], 13121[1], 13122[1], 13131[1], 13132[1], 13133[1], 13151[1], 13152[1], 13153[1], 35201[1], 35206[1], 35226[1], 35231[1], 35236[1], 35256[1], 35261[1], 35266[1], 35286[1], 36000[1], 36005[1], 36140[1], 36160[1], 36200[1], 36245[1], 36246[1], 36247[1], 36251[1], 36400[1], 36405[1], 36406[1], 36410[1], 36420[1], 36425[1], 36430[1], 36440[1], 36500[1], 36591[0], 36592[0], 36600[1], 36640[1], 43752[1], 51701[1], 51702[1], 51703[1], 62320[0], 62321[0], 62322[0], 62323[0], 62324[0], 62325[0], 62326[0], 62327[0], 64400[0], 64405[0], 64408[0], 64415[0], 64416[0], 64417[0], 64418[0], 64420[0], 64421[0], 64425[0], 64430[0], 64435[0], 64445[0], 64446[0], 64447[0], 64448[0], 64449[0], 64450[0], 64451[0], 64454[0], 64461[0], 64462[0], 64463[0], 64479[0], 64480[0], 64483[0], 64484[0], 64486[0], 64487[0], 64488[0], 64489[0], 64490[0], 64491[0], 64492[0], 64493[0], 64494[0], 64495[0], 64505[0], 64510[0], 64517[0], 64520[0], 64530[0], 69990[0], 75625[1], 75831[1], 75833[1], 75893[1], 76000[1], 76942[1], 76998[1], 77001[1], 77002[1], 92012[1], 92014[1], 93000[1], 93005[1], 93010[1], 93040[1], 93041[1], 93042[1], 93050[0], 93318[1], 93355[1], 94002[1], 94200[1], 94680[1], 94681[1], 94690[1], 95812[1], 95813[1], 95816[1], 95819[1], 95822[1], 95829[1], 95955[1], 96360[1], 96361[1], 96365[1], 96366[1], 96367[1], 96368[1], 96372[1], 96374[1], 96375[1], 96376[1], 96377[1], 96523[0], 99155[0], 99156[0], 99157[0], 99211[1], 99212[1], 99213[1], 99214[1], 99215[1], 99217[1], 99218[1], 99219[1], 99220[1], 99221[1], 99222[1], 99223[1], 99231[1], 99232[1], 99233[1], 99234[1], 99235[1], 99236[1], 99238[1], 99239[1], 99241[1], 99242[1], 99243[1], 99244[1], 99245[1], 99251[1], 99252[1], 99253[1], 99254[1], 99255[1], 99291[1], 99292[1], 99304[1], 99305[1], 99306[1], 99307[1], 99308[1], 99309[1], 99310[1], 99315[1], 99316[1], 99334[1], 99335[1], 99336[1], 99337[1], 99347[1], 99348[1], 99349[1], 99350[1], 99374[1], 99375[1], 99377[1], 99378[1], 99446[0], 99447[0], 99448[0], 99449[0], 99451[0], 99452[0], 99495[1], 99496[1], G0269[1], G0463[1], G0471[1], J0670[1], J1642[1], J1644[1], J2001[1]
36253	01916[0], 01924[0], 01925[0], 01926[0], 0213T[0], 0216T[0], 0596T[1], 0597T[1], 0708T[1], 0709T[1], 12001[1], 12002[1], 12004[1], 12005[1], 12006[1], 12007[1], 12011[1], 12013[1], 12014[1], 12015[1], 12016[1], 12017[1], 12018[1], 12020[1], 12021[1], 12031[1], 12032[1], 12034[1], 12035[1], 12036[1], 12037[1], 12041[1], 12042[1], 12044[1], 12045[1], 12046[1], 12047[1], 12051[1], 12052[1], 12053[1], 12054[1], 12055[1], 12056[1], 12057[1], 13100[1], 13101[1], 13102[1], 13120[1], 13121[1], 13122[1], 13131[1], 13132[1], 13133[1], 13151[1], 13152[1], 13153[1], 35201[1], 35206[1], 35226[1], 35231[1], 35236[1], 35256[1], 35261[1], 35266[1], 35286[1], 36000[1], 36005[1], 36140[1], 36160[1], 36200[1], 36245[1], 36246[1], 36247[1], 36251[1], 36252[1], 36400[1], 36405[1], 36406[1], 36410[1], 36420[1], 36425[1], 36430[1], 36440[1], 36500[1], 36591[0], 36592[0], 36600[1], 36640[1], 43752[1], 51701[1], 51702[1], 51703[1], 62320[0], 62321[0], 62322[0], 62323[0], 62324[0], 62325[0], 62326[0], 62327[0], 64400[0], 64405[0], 64408[0], 64415[0], 64416[0], 64417[0], 64418[0], 64420[0], 64421[0], 64425[0], 64430[0], 64435[0], 64445[0], 64446[0], 64447[0], 64448[0], 64449[0], 64450[0], 64451[0], 64454[0], 64461[0], 64462[0], 64463[0], 64479[0], 64480[0], 64483[0], 64484[0], 64486[0], 64487[0], 64488[0], 64489[0], 64490[0], 64491[0], 64492[0], 64493[0], 64494[0], 64495[0], 64505[0], 64510[0], 64517[0], 64520[0], 64530[0], 69990[0], 75625[1], 75831[1], 75833[1], 75893[1], 76000[1], 76942[1], 76998[1], 77001[1], 77002[1], 92012[1], 92014[1], 93000[1], 93005[1], 93010[1], 93040[1], 93041[1], 93042[1], 93050[0], 93318[1], 93355[1], 94002[1], 94200[1], 94680[1], 94681[1], 94690[1], 95812[1], 95813[1], 95816[1], 95819[1], 95822[1], 95829[1], 95955[1], 96360[1], 96361[1], 96365[1], 96366[1], 96367[1], 96368[1], 96372[1], 96374[1], 96375[1], 96376[1], 96377[1], 96523[0], 99155[0], 99156[0], 99157[0], 99211[1], 99212[1], 99213[1], 99214[1], 99215[1], 99217[1], 99218[1], 99219[1], 99220[1], 99221[1], 99222[1], 99223[1], 99231[1], 99232[1], 99233[1], 99234[1], 99235[1], 99236[1], 99238[1], 99239[1], 99241[1], 99242[1], 99243[1], 99244[1], 99245[1], 99251[1], 99252[1], 99253[1], 99254[1], 99255[1], 99291[1], 99292[1], 99304[1], 99305[1], 99306[1], 99307[1], 99308[1], 99309[1], 99310[1], 99315[1], 99316[1], 99334[1], 99335[1], 99336[1], 99337[1], 99347[1], 99348[1], 99349[1], 99350[1], 99374[1], 99375[1], 99377[1], 99378[1], 99446[0], 99447[0], 99448[0], 99449[0], 99451[0], 99452[0], 99495[1], 99496[1], G0269[1], G0463[1], G0471[1], J0670[1], J1642[1], J1644[1], J2001[1]

0 = Modifier usage not allowed or inappropriate 1 = Modifier usage allowed

Appendix A: NCCI - CPT Codes

Code 1	Code 2
36254	01916[0], 01924[0], 01925[0], 01926[0], 0213T[0], 0216T[0], 0596T[1], 0597T[1], 0708T[1], 0709T[1], 12001[1], 12002[1], 12004[1], 12005[1], 12006[1], 12007[1], 12011[1], 12013[1], 12014[1], 12015[1], 12016[1], 12017[1], 12018[1], 12020[1], 12021[1], 12031[1], 12032[1], 12034[1], 12035[1], 12036[1], 12037[1], 12041[1], 12042[1], 12044[1], 12045[1], 12046[1], 12047[1], 12051[1], 12052[1], 12053[1], 12054[1], 12055[1], 12056[1], 12057[1], 13100[1], 13101[1], 13102[1], 13120[1], 13121[1], 13122[1], 13131[1], 13132[1], 13133[1], 13151[1], 13152[1], 13153[1], 35201[1], 35206[1], 35226[1], 35231[1], 35236[1], 35256[1], 35261[1], 35266[1], 35286[1], 36000[1], 36005[1], 36140[1], 36160[1], 36200[1], 36245[1], 36246[1], 36247[1], 36251[1], 36252[1], 36253[1], 36400[1], 36405[1], 36406[1], 36410[1], 36420[1], 36425[1], 36430[1], 36440[1], 36500[1], 36591[0], 36592[0], 36600[1], 36640[1], 43752[1], 51701[1], 51702[1], 51703[1], 62320[0], 62321[0], 62322[0], 62323[0], 62324[0], 62325[0], 62326[0], 62327[0], 64400[0], 64405[0], 64408[0], 64415[0], 64416[0], 64417[0], 64418[0], 64420[0], 64421[0], 64425[0], 64430[0], 64435[0], 64445[0], 64446[0], 64447[0], 64448[0], 64449[0], 64450[0], 64451[0], 64454[0], 64461[0], 64462[0], 64463[0], 64479[0], 64480[0], 64483[0], 64484[0], 64486[0], 64487[0], 64488[0], 64489[0], 64490[0], 64491[0], 64492[0], 64493[0], 64494[0], 64495[0], 64505[0], 64510[0], 64517[0], 64520[0], 64530[0], 69990[0], 75625[1], 75831[1], 75833[1], 75893[1], 76000[1], 76942[1], 76998[1], 77001[1], 77002[1], 92012[1], 92014[1], 93000[1], 93005[1], 93010[1], 93040[1], 93041[1], 93042[1], 93050[0], 93318[1], 93355[1], 94002[1], 94200[1], 94680[1], 94681[1], 94690[1], 95812[1], 95813[1], 95816[1], 95819[1], 95822[1], 95829[1], 95955[1], 96360[1], 96361[1], 96365[1], 96366[1], 96367[1], 96368[1], 96372[1], 96374[1], 96375[1], 96376[1], 96377[1], 96523[0], 99155[0], 99156[0], 99157[0], 99211[1], 99212[1], 99213[1], 99214[1], 99215[1], 99217[1], 99218[1], 99219[1], 99220[1], 99221[1], 99222[1], 99223[1], 99231[1], 99232[1], 99233[1], 99234[1], 99235[1], 99236[1], 99238[1], 99239[1], 99241[1], 99242[1], 99243[1], 99244[1], 99245[1], 99251[1], 99252[1], 99253[1], 99254[1], 99255[1], 99291[1], 99292[1], 99304[1], 99305[1], 99306[1], 99307[1], 99308[1], 99309[1], 99310[1], 99315[1], 99316[1], 99334[1], 99335[1], 99336[1], 99337[1], 99347[1], 99348[1], 99349[1], 99350[1], 99374[1], 99375[1], 99377[1], 99378[1], 99446[0], 99447[0], 99448[0], 99449[0], 99451[0], 99452[0], 99495[1], 99496[1], G0269[1], G0463[1], G0471[1], J0670[1], J1642[1], J1644[1], J2001[1]
36415	36591[0], 36592[0], 96523[0], 99211[1]
36416	36591[0], 36592[0], 96523[0]
36593	35201[1], 35206[1], 35226[1], 35231[1], 35236[1], 35256[1], 35261[1], 35266[1], 35286[1], 36005[1], 36591[0], 36592[0], 69990[0], 96523[0], J1642[1], J1644[1]
36600	0543T[1], 0544T[1], 0567T[1], 0568T[1], 0569T[1], 0570T[1], 0571T[1], 0572T[1], 0573T[1], 0574T[1], 0580T[1], 0581T[1], 0655T[1], 20560[1], 36002[1], 36005[1], 36140[1], 36591[0], 36592[0], 36625[1], 66987[1], 66988[1], 69990[0], 76000[1], 77001[1], 77002[1], 93050[0], 96523[0], J0670[1], J2001[1]
36800	01844[0], 01924[0], 01925[0], 01926[0], 0213T[0], 0216T[0], 0596T[1], 0597T[1], 0708T[1], 0709T[1], 11000[1], 11001[1], 11004[1], 11005[1], 11006[1], 11042[1], 11043[1], 11044[1], 11045[1], 11046[1], 11047[1], 12001[1], 12002[1], 12004[1], 12005[1], 12006[1], 12007[1], 12011[1], 12013[1], 12014[1], 12015[1], 12016[1], 12017[1], 12018[1], 12020[1], 12021[1], 12031[1], 12032[1], 12034[1], 12035[1], 12036[1], 12037[1], 12041[1], 12042[1], 12044[1], 12045[1], 12046[1], 12047[1], 12051[1], 12052[1], 12053[1], 12054[1], 12055[1], 12056[1], 12057[1], 13100[1], 13101[1], 13102[1], 13120[1], 13121[1], 13122[1], 13131[1], 13132[1], 13133[1], 13151[1], 13152[1], 13153[1], 35201[1], 35206[1], 35226[1], 35231[1], 35236[1], 35256[1], 35261[1], 35266[1], 35286[1], 35800[1], 35860[1], 36000[1], 36002[1], 36005[1], 36400[1], 36405[1], 36406[1], 36410[1], 36420[1], 36425[1], 36430[1], 36440[1], 36591[0], 36592[0], 36600[1], 36640[1], 36810[1], 36815[1], 36819[1], 36820[1], 36821[1], 36831[1], 36832[1], 36833[1], 36835[1], 36861[1], 43752[1], 49421[1], 51701[1], 51702[1], 51703[1], 62320[0], 62321[0], 62322[0], 62323[0], 62324[0], 62325[0], 62326[0], 62327[0], 64400[0], 64405[0], 64408[0], 64415[0], 64416[0], 64417[0], 64418[0], 64420[0], 64421[0], 64425[0], 64430[0], 64435[0], 64445[0], 64446[0], 64447[0], 64448[0], 64449[0], 64450[0], 64451[0], 64454[0], 64461[0], 64462[0], 64463[0], 64479[0], 64480[0], 64483[0], 64484[0], 64486[0], 64487[0], 64488[0], 64489[0], 64490[0], 64491[0], 64492[0], 64493[0], 64494[0], 64495[0], 64505[0], 64510[0], 64517[0], 64520[0], 64530[0], 69990[0], 92012[1], 92014[1], 93000[1], 93005[1], 93010[1], 93040[1], 93041[1], 93042[1], 93318[1], 93355[1], 94002[1], 94200[1], 94680[1], 94681[1], 94690[1], 95812[1], 95813[1], 95816[1], 95819[1], 95822[1], 95829[1], 95955[1], 96360[1], 96361[1], 96365[1], 96366[1], 96367[1], 96368[1], 96372[1], 96374[1], 96375[1], 96376[1], 96377[1], 96523[0], 97597[1], 97598[1], 97602[1], 99155[0], 99156[0], 99157[0], 99211[1], 99212[1], 99213[1], 99214[1], 99215[1], 99217[1], 99218[1], 99219[1], 99220[1], 99221[1], 99222[1], 99223[1], 99231[1], 99232[1], 99233[1], 99234[1], 99235[1], 99236[1], 99238[1], 99239[1], 99241[1], 99242[1], 99243[1], 99244[1], 99245[1], 99251[1], 99252[1], 99253[1], 99254[1], 99255[1], 99291[1], 99292[1], 99304[1], 99305[1], 99306[1], 99307[1], 99308[1], 99309[1], 99310[1], 99315[1], 99316[1], 99334[1], 99335[1], 99336[1], 99337[1], 99347[1], 99348[1], 99349[1], 99350[1], 99374[1], 99375[1], 99377[1], 99378[1], 99446[0], 99447[0], 99448[0], 99449[0], 99451[0], 99452[0], 99495[1], 99496[1], G0463[1], G0471[1]
36810	01844[0], 01924[0], 01925[0], 01926[0], 0213T[0], 0216T[0], 0596T[1], 0597T[1], 0708T[1], 0709T[1], 11000[1], 11001[1], 11004[1], 11005[1], 11006[1], 11042[1], 11043[1], 11044[1], 11045[1], 11046[1], 11047[1], 12001[1], 12002[1], 12004[1], 12005[1], 12006[1], 12007[1], 12011[1], 12013[1], 12014[1], 12015[1], 12016[1], 12017[1], 12018[1], 12020[1], 12021[1], 12031[1], 12032[1], 12034[1], 12035[1], 12036[1], 12037[1], 12041[1], 12042[1], 12044[1], 12045[1], 12046[1], 12047[1], 12051[1], 12052[1], 12053[1], 12054[1], 12055[1], 12056[1], 12057[1], 13100[1], 13101[1], 13102[1], 13120[1], 13121[1], 13122[1], 13131[1], 13132[1], 13133[1], 13151[1], 13152[1], 13153[1], 35201[1], 35206[1], 35226[1], 35231[1], 35236[1], 35256[1], 35261[1], 35266[1], 35286[1], 36000[1], 36002[1], 36005[1], 36400[1], 36405[1], 36406[1], 36410[1], 36420[1], 36425[1], 36430[1], 36440[1], 36591[0], 36592[0], 36600[1], 36640[1], 36819[1], 36820[1], 36821[1], 36823[1], 36825[1], 36830[1], 36831[1], 36832[1], 36833[1], 36835[1], 43752[1], 51701[1], 51702[1], 51703[1], 62320[0], 62321[0], 62322[0], 62323[0], 62324[0], 62325[0], 62326[0], 62327[0], 64400[0], 64405[0], 64408[0], 64415[0], 64416[0], 64417[0], 64418[0], 64420[0], 64421[0], 64425[0], 64430[0], 64435[0], 64445[0], 64446[0], 64447[0], 64448[0], 64449[0], 64450[0], 64451[0], 64454[0], 64461[0], 64462[0], 64463[0], 64479[0], 64480[0], 64483[0], 64484[0], 64486[0], 64487[0], 64488[0], 64489[0], 64490[0], 64491[0], 64492[0], 64493[0], 64494[0], 64495[0], 64505[0], 64510[0], 64517[0], 64520[0], 64530[0], 69990[0], 92012[1], 92014[1], 93000[1], 93005[1], 93010[1], 93040[1], 93041[1], 93042[1], 93050[0], 93318[1], 93355[1], 94002[1], 94200[1], 94680[1], 94681[1], 94690[1], 95812[1], 95813[1], 95816[1], 95819[1], 95822[1], 95829[1], 95955[1], 96360[1], 96361[1], 96365[1], 96366[1], 96367[1], 96368[1], 96372[1], 96374[1], 96375[1], 96376[1], 96377[1], 96523[0], 97597[1], 97598[1], 97602[1], 99155[0], 99156[0], 99157[0], 99211[1], 99212[1], 99213[1], 99214[1], 99215[1], 99217[1], 99218[1], 99219[1], 99220[1], 99221[1], 99222[1], 99223[1], 99231[1], 99232[1], 99233[1], 99234[1], 99235[1], 99236[1], 99238[1], 99239[1], 99241[1], 99242[1], 99243[1], 99244[1], 99245[1], 99251[1], 99252[1], 99253[1], 99254[1], 99255[1], 99291[1], 99292[1], 99304[1], 99305[1], 99306[1], 99307[1], 99308[1], 99309[1], 99310[1], 99315[1], 99316[1], 99334[1], 99335[1], 99336[1], 99337[1], 99347[1], 99348[1], 99349[1], 99350[1], 99374[1], 99375[1], 99377[1], 99378[1], 99446[0], 99447[0], 99448[0], 99449[0], 99451[0], 99452[0], 99495[1], 99496[1], G0463[1], G0471[1]
36815	01844[0], 01924[0], 01925[0], 01926[0], 0213T[0], 0216T[0], 0596T[1], 0597T[1], 0708T[1], 0709T[1], 11000[1], 11001[1], 11004[1], 11005[1], 11006[1], 11042[1], 11043[1], 11044[1], 11045[1], 11046[1], 11047[1], 12001[1], 12002[1], 12004[1], 12005[1], 12006[1], 12007[1], 12011[1], 12013[1], 12014[1], 12015[1], 12016[1], 12017[1], 12018[1], 12020[1], 12021[1], 12031[1], 12032[1], 12034[1], 12035[1], 12036[1], 12037[1], 12041[1], 12042[1], 12044[1], 12045[1], 12046[1], 12047[1], 12051[1], 12052[1], 12053[1], 12054[1], 12055[1], 12056[1], 12057[1], 13100[1], 13101[1], 13102[1], 13120[1], 13121[1], 13122[1], 13131[1], 13132[1], 13133[1], 13151[1], 13152[1], 13153[1], 35201[1], 35206[1], 35226[1], 35231[1], 35236[1], 35256[1], 35261[1], 35266[1], 35286[1], 36000[1], 36002[1], 36005[1], 36400[1], 36405[1], 36406[1], 36410[1], 36420[1], 36425[1], 36430[1], 36440[1], 36591[0], 36592[0], 36600[1], 36640[1], 36810[1], 36819[1], 36820[1], 36821[1], 36823[1], 36825[1], 36830[1], 36831[1], 36832[1], 36833[1], 36835[1], 43752[1], 51701[1], 51702[1], 51703[1], 62320[0], 62321[0], 62322[0], 62323[0], 62324[0], 62325[0], 62326[0], 62327[0], 64400[0], 64405[0], 64408[0], 64415[0], 64416[0], 64417[0], 64418[0], 64420[0], 64421[0], 64425[0], 64430[0], 64435[0], 64445[0], 64446[0], 64447[0], 64448[0], 64449[0], 64450[0], 64451[0], 64454[0], 64461[0], 64462[0], 64463[0], 64479[0], 64480[0], 64483[0], 64484[0], 64486[0], 64487[0], 64488[0], 64489[0], 64490[0], 64491[0], 64492[0], 64493[0], 64494[0], 64495[0], 64505[0], 64510[0], 64517[0], 64520[0], 64530[0], 69990[0], 92012[1], 92014[1], 93000[1], 93005[1], 93010[1], 93040[1], 93041[1], 93042[1], 93050[0], 93318[1], 93355[1], 94002[1], 94200[1], 94680[1], 94681[1], 94690[1], 95812[1], 95813[1], 95816[1], 95819[1], 95822[1], 95829[1], 95955[1], 96360[1], 96361[1], 96365[1], 96366[1], 96367[1], 96368[1], 96372[1], 96374[1], 96375[1], 96376[1], 96377[1], 96523[0], 97597[1], 97598[1], 97602[1], 99155[0], 99156[0], 99157[0], 99211[1], 99212[1], 99213[1], 99214[1], 99215[1], 99217[1], 99218[1], 99219[1], 99220[1], 99221[1], 99222[1], 99223[1], 99231[1], 99232[1], 99233[1], 99234[1], 99235[1], 99236[1], 99238[1], 99239[1], 99241[1], 99242[1], 99243[1], 99244[1], 99245[1], 99251[1], 99252[1], 99253[1], 99254[1], 99255[1], 99291[1], 99292[1], 99304[1], 99305[1], 99306[1], 99307[1], 99308[1], 99309[1], 99310[1], 99315[1], 99316[1], 99334[1], 99335[1], 99336[1], 99337[1], 99347[1], 99348[1], 99349[1], 99350[1], 99374[1], 99375[1], 99377[1], 99378[1], 99446[0], 99447[0], 99448[0], 99449[0], 99451[0], 99452[0], 99495[1], 99496[1], G0463[1], G0471[1]
36818	01844[0], 01924[0], 01925[0], 01926[0], 0213T[0], 0216T[0], 0596T[1], 0597T[1], 0708T[1], 0709T[1], 12001[1], 12002[1], 12004[1], 12005[1], 12006[1], 12007[1], 12011[1], 12013[1], 12014[1], 12015[1], 12016[1], 12017[1], 12018[1], 12020[1], 12021[1], 12031[1], 12032[1], 12034[1], 12035[1], 12036[1], 12037[1], 12041[1], 12042[1], 12044[1], 12045[1], 12046[1], 12047[1], 12051[1], 12052[1], 12053[1], 12054[1], 12055[1], 12056[1], 12057[1], 13100[1], 13101[1], 13102[1], 13120[1], 13121[1], 13122[1], 13131[1], 13132[1], 13133[1], 13151[1], 13152[1], 13153[1], 33951[1], 33952[1], 33953[1], 33954[1], 35206[1], 35226[1], 35236[1], 35256[1], 35266[1], 35286[1], 35702[1], 35703[1], 35860[1], 36000[1], 36002[1], 36005[1], 36400[1], 36405[1], 36406[1], 36410[1], 36420[1], 36425[1], 36430[1], 36440[1], 36591[0], 36592[0], 36600[1], 36640[1], 36800[1], 36810[1], 36815[1], 36821[1], 36825[1], 36830[1], 36831[1], 36832[1], 36833[1], 36835[1], 36860[1], 36861[1], 36901[1], 36902[1], 36903[1], 36904[1], 36905[1], 36906[1], 43752[1], 51701[1], 51702[1], 51703[1], 62320[0], 62321[0], 62322[0], 62323[0], 62324[0], 62325[0], 62326[0], 62327[0], 64400[0], 64405[0], 64408[0], 64415[0], 64416[0], 64417[0], 64418[0], 64420[0], 64421[0], 64425[0], 64430[0], 64435[0], 64445[0], 64446[0], 64447[0], 64448[0], 64449[0], 64450[0], 64451[0], 64454[0], 64461[0], 64462[0], 64463[0], 64479[0], 64480[0], 64483[0], 64484[0], 64486[0], 64487[0], 64488[0], 64489[0], 64490[0], 64491[0], 64492[0], 64493[0], 64494[0], 64495[0], 64505[0], 64510[0], 64517[0], 64520[0], 64530[0], 69990[0], 92012[1], 92014[1], 93000[1], 93005[1], 93010[1], 93040[1], 93041[1], 93042[1], 93318[1], 93355[1], 94002[1], 94200[1], 94680[1], 94681[1], 94690[1], 95812[1], 95813[1], 95816[1], 95819[1], 95822[1], 95829[1], 95955[1], 96360[1],

0 = Modifier usage not allowed or inappropriate   1 = Modifier usage allowed

Appendix A: NCCI - CPT Codes

Code 1	Code 2
	96361[1], 96365[1], 96366[1], 96367[1], 96368[1], 96372[1], 96374[1], 96375[1], 96376[1], 96377[1], 96523[0], 99155[0], 99156[0], 99157[0], 99211[1], 99212[1], 99213[1], 99214[1], 99215[1], 99217[1], 99218[1], 99219[1], 99220[1], 99221[1], 99222[1], 99223[1], 99231[1], 99232[1], 99233[1], 99234[1], 99235[1], 99236[1], 99238[1], 99239[1], 99241[1], 99242[1], 99243[1], 99244[1], 99245[1], 99251[1], 99252[1], 99253[1], 99254[1], 99255[1], 99291[1], 99292[1], 99304[1], 99305[1], 99306[1], 99307[1], 99308[1], 99309[1], 99310[1], 99315[1], 99316[1], 99334[1], 99335[1], 99336[1], 99337[1], 99347[1], 99348[1], 99349[1], 99350[1], 99374[1], 99375[1], 99377[1], 99378[1], 99446[0], 99447[0], 99448[0], 99449[0], 99451[0], 99452[0], 99495[0], 99496[0], G0463[1], G0471[1]
36819	01844[0], 01924[0], 01925[0], 01926[0], 0213T[0], 0216T[0], 0596T[1], 0597T[1], 0708T[1], 0709T[1], 12001[1], 12002[1], 12004[1], 12005[1], 12006[1], 12007[1], 12011[1], 12013[1], 12014[1], 12015[1], 12016[1], 12017[1], 12018[1], 12020[1], 12021[1], 12031[1], 12032[1], 12034[1], 12035[1], 12036[1], 12037[1], 12041[1], 12042[1], 12044[1], 12045[1], 12046[1], 12047[1], 12051[1], 12052[1], 12053[1], 12054[1], 12055[1], 12056[1], 12057[1], 13100[1], 13101[1], 13102[1], 13120[1], 13121[1], 13122[1], 13131[1], 13132[1], 13133[1], 13151[1], 13152[1], 13153[1], 33951[1], 33952[1], 33953[1], 33954[1], 35206[1], 35226[1], 35236[1], 35256[1], 35266[1], 35286[1], 35702[1], 35703[1], 35860[1], 36000[1], 36002[1], 36005[1], 36400[1], 36405[1], 36406[1], 36410[1], 36420[1], 36425[1], 36430[1], 36440[1], 36591[0], 36592[0], 36600[1], 36640[1], 36818[1], 36821[1], 36823[1], 36830[1], 36901[1], 36902[1], 36903[1], 36904[1], 36905[1], 36906[1], 43752[1], 51701[1], 51702[1], 51703[1], 62320[0], 62321[0], 62322[0], 62323[0], 62324[0], 62325[0], 62326[0], 62327[0], 64400[0], 64405[0], 64408[0], 64415[0], 64416[0], 64417[0], 64418[0], 64420[0], 64421[0], 64425[0], 64430[0], 64435[0], 64445[0], 64446[0], 64447[0], 64448[0], 64449[0], 64450[0], 64451[0], 64454[0], 64461[0], 64462[0], 64463[0], 64479[0], 64480[0], 64483[0], 64484[0], 64486[0], 64487[0], 64488[0], 64489[0], 64490[0], 64491[0], 64492[0], 64493[0], 64494[0], 64495[0], 64505[0], 64510[0], 64517[0], 64520[0], 64530[0], 69990[0], 92012[1], 92014[1], 93000[1], 93005[1], 93010[1], 93040[1], 93041[1], 93042[1], 93318[1], 93355[1], 94002[1], 94200[1], 94680[1], 94681[1], 94690[1], 95812[1], 95813[1], 95816[1], 95819[1], 95822[1], 95829[1], 95955[1], 96360[1], 96361[1], 96365[1], 96366[1], 96367[1], 96368[1], 96372[1], 96374[1], 96375[1], 96376[1], 96377[1], 96523[0], 99155[0], 99156[0], 99157[0], 99211[1], 99212[1], 99213[1], 99214[1], 99215[1], 99217[1], 99218[1], 99219[1], 99220[1], 99221[1], 99222[1], 99223[1], 99231[1], 99232[1], 99233[1], 99234[1], 99235[1], 99236[1], 99238[1], 99239[1], 99241[1], 99242[1], 99243[1], 99244[1], 99245[1], 99251[1], 99252[1], 99253[1], 99254[1], 99255[1], 99291[1], 99292[1], 99304[1], 99305[1], 99306[1], 99307[1], 99308[1], 99309[1], 99310[1], 99315[1], 99316[1], 99334[1], 99335[1], 99336[1], 99337[1], 99347[1], 99348[1], 99349[1], 99350[1], 99374[1], 99375[1], 99377[1], 99378[1], 99446[0], 99447[0], 99448[0], 99449[0], 99451[0], 99452[0], 99495[0], 99496[0], G0463[1], G0471[1]
36820	01844[0], 01924[0], 01925[0], 01926[0], 0213T[0], 0216T[0], 0596T[1], 0597T[1], 0708T[1], 0709T[1], 12001[1], 12002[1], 12004[1], 12005[1], 12006[1], 12007[1], 12011[1], 12013[1], 12014[1], 12015[1], 12016[1], 12017[1], 12018[1], 12020[1], 12021[1], 12031[1], 12032[1], 12034[1], 12035[1], 12036[1], 12037[1], 12041[1], 12042[1], 12044[1], 12045[1], 12046[1], 12047[1], 12051[1], 12052[1], 12053[1], 12054[1], 12055[1], 12056[1], 12057[1], 13100[1], 13101[1], 13102[1], 13120[1], 13121[1], 13122[1], 13131[1], 13132[1], 13133[1], 13151[1], 13152[1], 13153[1], 33951[1], 33952[1], 33953[1], 33954[1], 35206[1], 35226[1], 35236[1], 35256[1], 35266[1], 35286[1], 35702[1], 35703[1], 35860[1], 36000[1], 36005[1], 36400[1], 36405[1], 36406[1], 36410[1], 36420[1], 36425[1], 36430[1], 36440[1], 36591[0], 36592[0], 36600[1], 36640[1], 36818[1], 36819[1], 36823[1], 36901[1], 36902[1], 36903[1], 43752[1], 51701[1], 51702[1], 51703[1], 62320[0], 62321[0], 62322[0], 62323[0], 62324[0], 62325[0], 62326[0], 62327[0], 64400[0], 64405[0], 64408[0], 64415[0], 64416[0], 64417[0], 64418[0], 64420[0], 64421[0], 64425[0], 64430[0], 64435[0], 64445[0], 64446[0], 64447[0], 64448[0], 64449[0], 64450[0], 64451[0], 64454[0], 64461[0], 64462[0], 64463[0], 64479[0], 64480[0], 64483[0], 64484[0], 64486[0], 64487[0], 64488[0], 64489[0], 64490[0], 64491[0], 64492[0], 64493[0], 64494[0], 64495[0], 64505[0], 64510[0], 64517[0], 64520[0], 64530[0], 69990[0], 92012[1], 92014[1], 93000[1], 93005[1], 93010[1], 93040[1], 93041[1], 93042[1], 93318[1], 93355[1], 94002[1], 94200[1], 94680[1], 94681[1], 94690[1], 95812[1], 95813[1], 95816[1], 95819[1], 95822[1], 95829[1], 95955[1], 96360[1], 96361[1], 96365[1], 96366[1], 96367[1], 96368[1], 96372[1], 96374[1], 96375[1], 96376[1], 96377[1], 96523[0], 99155[0], 99156[0], 99157[0], 99211[1], 99212[1], 99213[1], 99214[1], 99215[1], 99217[1], 99218[1], 99219[1], 99220[1], 99221[1], 99222[1], 99223[1], 99231[1], 99232[1], 99233[1], 99234[1], 99235[1], 99236[1], 99238[1], 99239[1], 99241[1], 99242[1], 99243[1], 99244[1], 99245[1], 99251[1], 99252[1], 99253[1], 99254[1], 99255[1], 99291[1], 99292[1], 99304[1], 99305[1], 99306[1], 99307[1], 99308[1], 99309[1], 99310[1], 99315[1], 99316[1], 99334[1], 99335[1], 99336[1], 99337[1], 99347[1], 99348[1], 99349[1], 99350[1], 99374[1], 99375[1], 99377[1], 99378[1], 99446[0], 99447[0], 99448[0], 99449[0], 99451[0], 99452[0], 99495[0], 99496[0], G0463[1], G0471[1]
36821	01844[0], 01924[0], 01925[0], 01926[0], 0213T[0], 0216T[0], 0596T[1], 0597T[1], 0708T[1], 0709T[1], 12001[1], 12002[1], 12004[1], 12005[1], 12006[1], 12007[1], 12011[1], 12013[1], 12014[1], 12015[1], 12016[1], 12017[1], 12018[1], 12020[1], 12021[1], 12031[1], 12032[1], 12034[1], 12035[1], 12036[1], 12037[1], 12041[1], 12042[1], 12044[1], 12045[1], 12046[1], 12047[1], 12051[1], 12052[1], 12053[1], 12054[1], 12055[1], 12056[1], 12057[1], 13100[1], 13101[1], 13102[1], 13120[1], 13121[1], 13122[1], 13131[1], 13132[1], 13133[1], 13151[1], 13152[1], 13153[1], 35206[1], 35226[1], 35236[1], 35256[1], 35266[1], 35286[1], 35702[1], 35703[1], 35860[1], 36000[1], 36002[1], 36005[1], 36400[1], 36405[1], 36406[1], 36410[1], 36420[1], 36425[1], 36430[1], 36440[1], 36591[0], 36592[0], 36600[1], 36640[1], 36820[0], 36823[1], 36825[1], 36833[1], 36901[1], 36902[1], 36903[1], 43752[1], 51701[1], 51702[1], 51703[1], 62320[0], 62321[0], 62322[0], 62323[0], 62324[0], 62325[0], 62326[0], 62327[0], 64400[0], 64405[0], 64408[0], 64415[0], 64416[0], 64417[0], 64418[0], 64420[0], 64421[0], 64425[0], 64430[0], 64435[0], 64445[0], 64446[0], 64447[0], 64448[0], 64449[0], 64450[0], 64451[0], 64454[0], 64461[0], 64462[0], 64463[0], 64479[0], 64480[0], 64483[0], 64484[0], 64486[0], 64487[0], 64488[0], 64489[0], 64490[0], 64491[0], 64492[0], 64493[0], 64494[0], 64495[0], 64505[0], 64510[0], 64517[0], 64520[0], 64530[0], 69990[0], 92012[1], 92014[1], 93000[1], 93005[1], 93010[1], 93040[1], 93041[1], 93042[1], 93318[1], 93355[1], 94002[1], 94200[1], 94680[1], 94681[1], 94690[1], 95812[1], 95813[1], 95816[1], 95819[1], 95822[1], 95829[1], 95955[1], 96360[1], 96361[1], 96365[1], 96366[1], 96367[1], 96368[1], 96372[1], 96374[1], 96375[1], 96376[1], 96377[1], 96523[0], 99155[0], 99156[0], 99157[0], 99211[1], 99212[1], 99213[1], 99214[1], 99215[1], 99217[1], 99218[1], 99219[1], 99220[1], 99221[1], 99222[1], 99223[1], 99231[1], 99232[1], 99233[1], 99234[1], 99235[1], 99236[1], 99238[1], 99239[1], 99241[1], 99242[1], 99243[1], 99244[1], 99245[1], 99251[1], 99252[1], 99253[1], 99254[1], 99255[1], 99291[1], 99292[1], 99304[1], 99305[1], 99306[1], 99307[1], 99308[1], 99309[1], 99310[1], 99315[1], 99316[1], 99334[1], 99335[1], 99336[1], 99337[1], 99347[1], 99348[1], 99349[1], 99350[1], 99374[1], 99375[1], 99377[1], 99378[1], 99446[0], 99447[0], 99448[0], 99449[0], 99451[0], 99452[0], 99495[0], 99496[0], G0463[1], G0471[1]
36825	01844[0], 01924[0], 01925[0], 01926[0], 0213T[0], 0216T[0], 0596T[1], 0597T[1], 0708T[1], 0709T[1], 12001[1], 12002[1], 12004[1], 12005[1], 12006[1], 12007[1], 12011[1], 12013[1], 12014[1], 12015[1], 12016[1], 12017[1], 12018[1], 12020[1], 12021[1], 12031[1], 12032[1], 12034[1], 12035[1], 12036[1], 12037[1], 12041[1], 12042[1], 12044[1], 12045[1], 12046[1], 12047[1], 12051[1], 12052[1], 12053[1], 12054[1], 12055[1], 12056[1], 12057[1], 13100[1], 13101[1], 13102[1], 13120[1], 13121[1], 13122[1], 13131[1], 13132[1], 13133[1], 13151[1], 13152[1], 13153[1], 35206[1], 35226[1], 35236[1], 35256[1], 35266[1], 35286[1], 35702[1], 35703[1], 35860[1], 36000[1], 36002[1], 36005[1], 36400[1], 36405[1], 36406[1], 36410[1], 36420[1], 36425[1], 36430[1], 36440[1], 36591[0], 36592[0], 36600[1], 36640[1], 36819[1], 36820[1], 36833[1], 36901[1], 36902[1], 36903[1], 43752[1], 51701[1], 51702[1], 51703[1], 62320[0], 62321[0], 62322[0], 62323[0], 62324[0], 62325[0], 62326[0], 62327[0], 64400[0], 64405[0], 64408[0], 64415[0], 64416[0], 64417[0], 64418[0], 64420[0], 64421[0], 64425[0], 64430[0], 64435[0], 64445[0], 64446[0], 64447[0], 64448[0], 64449[0], 64450[0], 64451[0], 64454[0], 64461[0], 64462[0], 64463[0], 64479[0], 64480[0], 64483[0], 64484[0], 64486[0], 64487[0], 64488[0], 64489[0], 64490[0], 64491[0], 64492[0], 64493[0], 64494[0], 64495[0], 64505[0], 64510[0], 64517[0], 64520[0], 64530[0], 69990[0], 92012[1], 92014[1], 93000[1], 93005[1], 93010[1], 93040[1], 93041[1], 93042[1], 93318[1], 93355[1], 94002[1], 94200[1], 94680[1], 94681[1], 94690[1], 95812[1], 95813[1], 95816[1], 95819[1], 95822[1], 95829[1], 95955[1], 96360[1], 96361[1], 96365[1], 96366[1], 96367[1], 96368[1], 96372[1], 96374[1], 96375[1], 96376[1], 96377[1], 96523[0], 99155[0], 99156[0], 99157[0], 99211[1], 99212[1], 99213[1], 99214[1], 99215[1], 99217[1], 99218[1], 99219[1], 99220[1], 99221[1], 99222[1], 99223[1], 99231[1], 99232[1], 99233[1], 99234[1], 99235[1], 99236[1], 99238[1], 99239[1], 99241[1], 99242[1], 99243[1], 99244[1], 99245[1], 99251[1], 99252[1], 99253[1], 99254[1], 99255[1], 99291[1], 99292[1], 99304[1], 99305[1], 99306[1], 99307[1], 99308[1], 99309[1], 99310[1], 99315[1], 99316[1], 99334[1], 99335[1], 99336[1], 99337[1], 99347[1], 99348[1], 99349[1], 99350[1], 99374[1], 99375[1], 99377[1], 99378[1], 99446[0], 99447[0], 99448[0], 99449[0], 99451[0], 99452[0], 99495[0], 99496[0], G0463[1], G0471[1]
36830	01844[0], 01924[0], 01925[0], 01926[0], 0213T[0], 0216T[0], 0596T[1], 0597T[1], 0708T[1], 0709T[1], 12001[1], 12002[1], 12004[1], 12005[1], 12006[1], 12007[1], 12011[1], 12013[1], 12014[1], 12015[1], 12016[1], 12017[1], 12018[1], 12020[1], 12021[1], 12031[1], 12032[1], 12034[1], 12035[1], 12036[1], 12037[1], 12041[1], 12042[1], 12044[1], 12045[1], 12046[1], 12047[1], 12051[1], 12052[1], 12053[1], 12054[1], 12055[1], 12056[1], 12057[1], 13100[1], 13101[1], 13102[1], 13120[1], 13121[1], 13122[1], 13131[1], 13132[1], 13133[1], 13151[1], 13152[1], 13153[1], 35206[1], 35226[1], 35236[1], 35256[1], 35266[1], 35286[1], 35702[1], 35703[1], 35800[1], 35860[1], 36000[1], 36002[1], 36005[1], 36400[1], 36405[1], 36406[1], 36410[1], 36420[1], 36425[1], 36430[1], 36440[1], 36591[0], 36592[0], 36600[1], 36640[1], 36820[1], 36821[1], 36825[1], 36901[1], 36902[1], 36903[1], 43752[1], 51701[1], 51702[1], 51703[1], 62320[0], 62321[0], 62322[0], 62323[0], 62324[0], 62325[0], 62326[0], 62327[0], 64400[0], 64405[0], 64408[0], 64415[0], 64416[0], 64417[0], 64418[0], 64420[0], 64421[0], 64425[0], 64430[0], 64435[0], 64445[0], 64446[0], 64447[0], 64448[0], 64449[0], 64450[0], 64451[0], 64454[0], 64461[0], 64462[0], 64463[0], 64479[0], 64480[0], 64483[0], 64484[0], 64486[0], 64487[0], 64488[0], 64489[0], 64490[0], 64491[0], 64492[0], 64493[0], 64494[0], 64495[0], 64505[0], 64510[0], 64517[0], 64520[0], 64530[0], 69990[0], 92012[1], 92014[1], 93000[1], 93005[1], 93010[1], 93040[1], 93041[1], 93042[1], 93318[1], 93355[1], 94002[1], 94200[1], 94680[1], 94681[1], 94690[1], 95812[1], 95813[1], 95816[1], 95819[1], 95822[1], 95829[1], 95955[1], 96360[1], 96361[1], 96365[1], 96366[1], 96367[1], 96368[1], 96372[1], 96374[1], 96375[1], 96376[1], 96377[1], 96523[0], 99155[0], 99156[0], 99157[0], 99211[1], 99212[1], 99213[1], 99214[1], 99215[1], 99217[1], 99218[1], 99219[1], 99220[1], 99221[1], 99222[1], 99223[1], 99231[1], 99232[1], 99233[1], 99234[1], 99235[1], 99236[1], 99238[1], 99239[1], 99241[1], 99242[1], 99243[1], 99244[1], 99245[1], 99251[1], 99252[1], 99253[1], 99254[1], 99255[1], 99291[1], 99292[1], 99304[1], 99305[1], 99306[1], 99307[1], 99308[1], 99309[1], 99310[1], 99315[1], 99316[1], 99334[1], 99335[1], 99336[1], 99337[1], 99347[1], 99348[1], 99349[1], 99350[1], 99374[1], 99375[1],

0 = Modifier usage not allowed or inappropriate   1 = Modifier usage allowed

Code 1	Code 2
	99377[1], 99378[1], 99446[0], 99447[0], 99448[0], 99449[0], 99451[0], 99452[0], 99495[0], 99496[0], G0463[1], G0471[1]
36831	01844[0], 01924[0], 01925[0], 01926[0], 0213T[0], 0216T[0], 0596T[1], 0597T[1], 0708T[1], 0709T[1], 11000[1], 11001[1], 11004[1], 11005[1], 11006[1], 11042[1], 11043[1], 11044[1], 11045[1], 11046[1], 11047[1], 12001[1], 12002[1], 12004[1], 12005[1], 12006[1], 12007[1], 12011[1], 12013[1], 12014[1], 12015[1], 12016[1], 12017[1], 12018[1], 12020[1], 12021[1], 12031[1], 12032[1], 12034[1], 12035[1], 12036[1], 12037[1], 12041[1], 12042[1], 12044[1], 12045[1], 12046[1], 12047[1], 12051[1], 12052[1], 12053[1], 12054[1], 12055[1], 12056[1], 12057[1], 13100[1], 13101[1], 13102[1], 13120[1], 13121[1], 13122[1], 13131[1], 13132[1], 13133[1], 13151[1], 13152[1], 13153[1], 34001[1], 34101[1], 34111[1], 34201[1], 34203[1], 34421[1], 34451[1], 35206[1], 35226[1], 35236[1], 35256[1], 35266[1], 35286[1], 35702[1], 35703[1], 35800[1], 35860[1], 35875[1], 35876[1], 36000[1], 36002[1], 36005[1], 36400[1], 36405[1], 36406[1], 36410[1], 36420[1], 36425[1], 36430[1], 36440[1], 36591[0], 36592[0], 36593[1], 36600[1], 36640[1], 36819[1], 36820[1], 36821[1], 36825[1], 36830[1], 36832[0], 36833[1], 36901[1], 36902[1], 36903[1], 36904[0], 36905[0], 36906[0], 36909[1], 37211[1], 37212[1], 37213[1], 37214[1], 43752[1], 51701[1], 51702[1], 51703[1], 61645[1], 62320[0], 62321[0], 62322[0], 62323[0], 62324[0], 62325[0], 62326[0], 62327[0], 64400[0], 64405[0], 64408[0], 64415[0], 64416[0], 64417[0], 64418[0], 64420[0], 64421[0], 64425[0], 64430[0], 64435[0], 64445[0], 64446[0], 64447[0], 64448[0], 64449[0], 64450[0], 64451[0], 64454[0], 64461[0], 64462[0], 64463[0], 64479[0], 64480[0], 64483[0], 64484[0], 64486[0], 64487[0], 64488[0], 64489[0], 64490[0], 64491[0], 64492[0], 64493[0], 64494[0], 64495[0], 64505[0], 64510[0], 64517[0], 64520[0], 64530[0], 69990[0], 92012[1], 92014[1], 93000[1], 93005[1], 93010[1], 93040[1], 93041[1], 93042[1], 93318[1], 93355[1], 94002[1], 94200[1], 94680[1], 94681[1], 94690[1], 95812[1], 95813[1], 95816[1], 95819[1], 95822[1], 95829[1], 95955[1], 96360[1], 96361[1], 96365[1], 96366[1], 96367[1], 96368[1], 96372[1], 96374[1], 96375[1], 96376[1], 96377[1], 96523[0], 97597[1], 97598[1], 97602[1], 99155[0], 99156[0], 99157[0], 99211[1], 99212[1], 99213[1], 99214[1], 99215[1], 99217[1], 99218[1], 99219[1], 99220[1], 99221[1], 99222[1], 99223[1], 99231[1], 99232[1], 99233[1], 99234[1], 99235[1], 99236[1], 99238[1], 99239[1], 99241[1], 99242[1], 99243[1], 99244[1], 99245[1], 99251[1], 99252[1], 99253[1], 99254[1], 99255[1], 99291[1], 99292[1], 99304[1], 99305[1], 99306[1], 99307[1], 99308[1], 99309[1], 99310[1], 99315[1], 99316[1], 99334[1], 99335[1], 99336[1], 99337[1], 99347[1], 99348[1], 99349[1], 99350[1], 99374[1], 99375[1], 99377[1], 99378[1], 99446[0], 99447[0], 99448[0], 99449[0], 99451[0], 99452[0], 99495[0], 99496[0], G0463[1], G0471[1]
36832	01844[0], 01924[0], 01925[0], 01926[0], 0213T[0], 0216T[0], 0596T[1], 0597T[1], 0708T[1], 0709T[1], 11000[1], 11001[1], 11004[1], 11005[1], 11006[1], 11042[1], 11043[1], 11044[1], 11045[1], 11046[1], 11047[1], 12001[1], 12002[1], 12004[1], 12005[1], 12006[1], 12007[1], 12011[1], 12013[1], 12014[1], 12015[1], 12016[1], 12017[1], 12018[1], 12020[1], 12021[1], 12031[1], 12032[1], 12034[1], 12035[1], 12036[1], 12037[1], 12041[1], 12042[1], 12044[1], 12045[1], 12046[1], 12047[1], 12051[1], 12052[1], 12053[1], 12054[1], 12055[1], 12056[1], 12057[1], 13100[1], 13101[1], 13102[1], 13120[1], 13121[1], 13122[1], 13131[1], 13132[1], 13133[1], 13151[1], 13152[1], 13153[1], 35206[1], 35226[1], 35236[1], 35256[1], 35266[1], 35286[1], 35702[1], 35703[1], 35860[1], 36000[1], 36002[1], 36005[1], 36400[1], 36405[1], 36406[1], 36410[1], 36420[1], 36425[1], 36430[1], 36440[1], 36591[0], 36592[0], 36600[1], 36640[1], 36819[1], 36820[1], 36821[1], 36825[1], 36830[1], 36833[1], 36835[1], 43752[1], 51701[1], 51702[1], 51703[1], 62320[0], 62321[0], 62322[0], 62323[0], 62324[0], 62325[0], 62326[0], 62327[0], 64400[0], 64405[0], 64408[0], 64415[0], 64416[0], 64417[0], 64418[0], 64420[0], 64421[0], 64425[0], 64430[0], 64435[0], 64445[0], 64446[0], 64447[0], 64448[0], 64449[0], 64450[0], 64451[0], 64454[0], 64461[0], 64462[0], 64463[0], 64479[0], 64480[0], 64483[0], 64484[0], 64486[0], 64487[0], 64488[0], 64489[0], 64490[0], 64491[0], 64492[0], 64493[0], 64494[0], 64495[0], 64505[0], 64510[0], 64517[0], 64520[0], 64530[0], 69990[0], 92012[1], 92014[1], 93000[1], 93005[1], 93010[1], 93040[1], 93041[1], 93042[1], 93318[1], 93355[1], 94002[1], 94200[1], 94680[1], 94681[1], 94690[1], 95812[1], 95813[1], 95816[1], 95819[1], 95822[1], 95829[1], 95955[1], 96360[1], 96361[1], 96365[1], 96366[1], 96367[1], 96368[1], 96372[1], 96374[1], 96375[1], 96376[1], 96377[1], 96523[0], 97597[1], 97598[1], 97602[1], 99155[0], 99156[0], 99157[0], 99211[1], 99212[1], 99213[1], 99214[1], 99215[1], 99217[1], 99218[1], 99219[1], 99220[1], 99221[1], 99222[1], 99223[1], 99231[1], 99232[1], 99233[1], 99234[1], 99235[1], 99236[1], 99238[1], 99239[1], 99241[1], 99242[1], 99243[1], 99244[1], 99245[1], 99251[1], 99252[1], 99253[1], 99254[1], 99255[1], 99291[1], 99292[1], 99304[1], 99305[1], 99306[1], 99307[1], 99308[1], 99309[1], 99310[1], 99315[1], 99316[1], 99334[1], 99335[1], 99336[1], 99337[1], 99347[1], 99348[1], 99349[1], 99350[1], 99374[1], 99375[1], 99377[1], 99378[1], 99446[0], 99447[0], 99448[0], 99449[0], 99451[0], 99452[0], 99495[0], 99496[0], G0463[1], G0471[1]
36833	01844[0], 01924[0], 01925[0], 01926[0], 0213T[0], 0216T[0], 0596T[1], 0597T[1], 0708T[1], 0709T[1], 11000[1], 11001[1], 11004[1], 11005[1], 11006[1], 11042[1], 11043[1], 11044[1], 11045[1], 11046[1], 11047[1], 12001[1], 12002[1], 12004[1], 12005[1], 12006[1], 12007[1], 12011[1], 12013[1], 12014[1], 12015[1], 12016[1], 12017[1], 12018[1], 12020[1], 12021[1], 12031[1], 12032[1], 12034[1], 12035[1], 12036[1], 12037[1], 12041[1], 12042[1], 12044[1], 12045[1], 12046[1], 12047[1], 12051[1], 12052[1], 12053[1], 12054[1], 12055[1], 12056[1], 12057[1], 13100[1], 13101[1], 13102[1], 13120[1], 13121[1], 13122[1], 13131[1], 13132[1], 13133[1], 13151[1], 13152[1], 13153[1], 34001[1], 34101[1], 34111[1], 34201[1], 34203[1], 34421[1], 34451[1], 34490[1], 35206[1], 35226[1], 35236[1], 35256[1], 35266[1], 35286[1], 35800[1], 35860[1], 35876[1], 36000[1], 36002[1], 36005[1], 36400[1], 36405[1], 36406[1], 36410[1], 36420[1], 36425[1], 36430[1], 36440[1], 36591[0], 36592[0], 36593[1], 36600[1], 36640[1], 36819[1], 36820[1], 36830[1], 37211[1], 37212[1], 37213[1], 37214[1], 43752[1], 51701[1], 51702[1], 51703[1], 61645[1], 62320[0], 62321[0], 62322[0], 62323[0], 62324[0], 62325[0], 62326[0], 62327[0], 64400[0], 64405[0], 64408[0], 64415[0], 64416[0], 64417[0], 64418[0], 64420[0], 64421[0], 64425[0], 64430[0], 64435[0], 64445[0], 64446[0], 64447[0], 64448[0], 64449[0], 64450[0], 64451[0], 64454[0], 64461[0], 64462[0], 64463[0], 64479[0], 64480[0], 64483[0], 64484[0], 64486[0], 64487[0], 64488[0], 64489[0], 64490[0], 64491[0], 64492[0], 64493[0], 64494[0], 64495[0], 64505[0], 64510[0], 64517[0], 64520[0], 64530[0], 69990[0], 92012[1], 92014[1], 93000[1], 93005[1], 93010[1], 93040[1], 93041[1], 93042[1], 93318[1], 93355[1], 94002[1], 94200[1], 94680[1], 94681[1], 94690[1], 95812[1], 95813[1], 95816[1], 95819[1], 95822[1], 95829[1], 95955[1], 96360[1], 96361[1], 96365[1], 96366[1], 96367[1], 96368[1], 96372[1], 96374[1], 96375[1], 96376[1], 96377[1], 96523[0], 97597[1], 97598[1], 97602[1], 99155[0], 99156[0], 99157[0], 99211[1], 99212[1], 99213[1], 99214[1], 99215[1], 99217[1], 99218[1], 99219[1], 99220[1], 99221[1], 99222[1], 99223[1], 99231[1], 99232[1], 99233[1], 99234[1], 99235[1], 99236[1], 99238[1], 99239[1], 99241[1], 99242[1], 99243[1], 99244[1], 99245[1], 99251[1], 99252[1], 99253[1], 99254[1], 99255[1], 99291[1], 99292[1], 99304[1], 99305[1], 99306[1], 99307[1], 99308[1], 99309[1], 99310[1], 99315[1], 99316[1], 99334[1], 99335[1], 99336[1], 99337[1], 99347[1], 99348[1], 99349[1], 99350[1], 99374[1], 99375[1], 99377[1], 99378[1], 99446[0], 99447[0], 99448[0], 99449[0], 99451[0], 99452[0], 99495[0], 99496[0], G0463[1], G0471[1]
36835	01844[0], 01924[0], 01925[0], 01926[0], 0213T[0], 0216T[0], 0596T[1], 0597T[1], 0708T[1], 0709T[1], 11000[1], 11001[1], 11004[1], 11005[1], 11006[1], 11042[1], 11043[1], 11044[1], 11045[1], 11046[1], 11047[1], 12001[1], 12002[1], 12004[1], 12005[1], 12006[1], 12007[1], 12011[1], 12013[1], 12014[1], 12015[1], 12016[1], 12017[1], 12018[1], 12020[1], 12021[1], 12031[1], 12032[1], 12034[1], 12035[1], 12036[1], 12037[1], 12041[1], 12042[1], 12044[1], 12045[1], 12046[1], 12047[1], 12051[1], 12052[1], 12053[1], 12054[1], 12055[1], 12056[1], 12057[1], 13100[1], 13101[1], 13102[1], 13120[1], 13121[1], 13122[1], 13131[1], 13132[1], 13133[1], 13151[1], 13152[1], 13153[1], 35206[1], 35226[1], 35236[1], 35256[1], 35266[1], 35286[1], 36000[1], 36002[1], 36005[1], 36400[1], 36405[1], 36406[1], 36410[1], 36420[1], 36425[1], 36430[1], 36440[1], 36591[0], 36592[0], 36600[1], 36640[1], 36819[1], 36820[1], 36825[1], 36830[1], 36831[1], 36833[1], 43752[1], 51701[1], 51702[1], 51703[1], 62320[0], 62321[0], 62322[0], 62323[0], 62324[0], 62325[0], 62326[0], 62327[0], 64400[0], 64405[0], 64408[0], 64415[0], 64416[0], 64417[0], 64418[0], 64420[0], 64421[0], 64425[0], 64430[0], 64435[0], 64445[0], 64446[0], 64447[0], 64448[0], 64449[0], 64450[0], 64451[0], 64454[0], 64461[0], 64462[0], 64463[0], 64479[0], 64480[0], 64483[0], 64484[0], 64486[0], 64487[0], 64488[0], 64489[0], 64490[0], 64491[0], 64492[0], 64493[0], 64494[0], 64495[0], 64505[0], 64510[0], 64517[0], 64520[0], 64530[0], 69990[0], 92012[1], 92014[1], 93000[1], 93005[1], 93010[1], 93040[1], 93041[1], 93042[1], 93318[1], 93355[1], 94002[1], 94200[1], 94680[1], 94681[1], 94690[1], 95812[1], 95813[1], 95816[1], 95819[1], 95822[1], 95829[1], 95955[1], 96360[1], 96361[1], 96365[1], 96366[1], 96367[1], 96368[1], 96372[1], 96374[1], 96375[1], 96376[1], 96377[1], 96523[0], 97597[1], 97598[1], 97602[1], 99155[0], 99156[0], 99157[0], 99211[1], 99212[1], 99213[1], 99214[1], 99215[1], 99217[1], 99218[1], 99219[1], 99220[1], 99221[1], 99222[1], 99223[1], 99231[1], 99232[1], 99233[1], 99234[1], 99235[1], 99236[1], 99238[1], 99239[1], 99241[1], 99242[1], 99243[1], 99244[1], 99245[1], 99251[1], 99252[1], 99253[1], 99254[1], 99255[1], 99291[1], 99292[1], 99304[1], 99305[1], 99306[1], 99307[1], 99308[1], 99309[1], 99310[1], 99315[1], 99316[1], 99334[1], 99335[1], 99336[1], 99337[1], 99347[1], 99348[1], 99349[1], 99350[1], 99374[1], 99375[1], 99377[1], 99378[1], 99446[0], 99447[0], 99448[0], 99449[0], 99451[0], 99452[0], 99495[0], 99496[0], G0463[1], G0471[1]
36838	01844[0], 0213T[0], 0216T[0], 0596T[1], 0597T[1], 0708T[1], 0709T[1], 12001[1], 12002[1], 12004[1], 12005[1], 12006[1], 12007[1], 12011[1], 12013[1], 12014[1], 12015[1], 12016[1], 12017[1], 12018[1], 12020[1], 12021[1], 12031[1], 12032[1], 12034[1], 12035[1], 12036[1], 12037[1], 12041[1], 12042[1], 12044[1], 12045[1], 12046[1], 12047[1], 12051[1], 12052[1], 12053[1], 12054[1], 12055[1], 12056[1], 12057[1], 13100[1], 13101[1], 13102[1], 13120[1], 13121[1], 13122[1], 13131[1], 13132[1], 13133[1], 13151[1], 13152[1], 13153[1], 35206[1], 35226[1], 35512[1], 35522[1], 36000[1], 36002[1], 36005[1], 36400[1], 36405[1], 36406[1], 36410[1], 36420[1], 36425[1], 36430[1], 36440[1], 36591[0], 36592[0], 36600[1], 36640[1], 36831[1], 36832[1], 36833[1], 36860[1], 36861[1], 36904[1], 36905[1], 36906[1], 37607[1], 37618[1], 43752[1], 51701[1], 51702[1], 51703[1], 62320[0], 62321[0], 62322[0], 62323[0], 62324[0], 62325[0], 62326[0], 62327[0], 64400[0], 64405[0], 64408[0], 64415[0], 64416[0], 64417[0], 64418[0], 64420[0], 64421[0], 64425[0], 64430[0], 64435[0], 64445[0], 64446[0], 64447[0], 64448[0], 64449[0], 64450[0], 64451[0], 64454[0], 64461[0], 64462[0], 64463[0], 64479[0], 64480[0], 64483[0], 64484[0], 64486[0], 64487[0], 64488[0], 64489[0], 64490[0], 64491[0], 64492[0], 64493[0], 64494[0], 64495[0], 64505[0], 64510[0], 64517[0], 64520[0], 64530[0], 69990[0], 92012[1], 92014[1], 93000[1], 93005[1], 93010[1], 93040[1], 93041[1], 93042[1], 93318[1], 93355[1], 94002[1], 94200[1], 94680[1], 94681[1], 94690[1], 95812[1], 95813[1], 95816[1], 95819[1], 95822[1], 95829[1], 95955[1], 96360[1], 96361[1], 96365[1], 96366[1], 96367[1], 96368[1], 96372[1], 96374[1], 96375[1], 96376[1], 96377[1], 96523[0], 99155[0], 99156[0], 99157[0], 99211[1], 99212[1], 99213[1], 99214[1], 99215[1], 99217[1], 99218[1], 99219[1], 99220[1], 99221[1], 99222[1], 99223[1], 99231[1], 99232[1], 99233[1], 99234[1], 99235[1], 99236[1], 99238[1], 99239[1], 99241[1], 99242[1], 99243[1], 99244[1], 99245[1], 99251[1], 99252[1], 99253[1], 99254[1], 99255[1], 99291[1], 99292[1], 99304[1], 99305[1], 99306[1], 99307[1], 99308[1], 99309[1], 99310[1], 99315[1], 99316[1], 99334[1], 99335[1], 99336[1], 99337[1], 99347[1],

0 = Modifier usage not allowed or inappropriate 1 = Modifier usage allowed

Appendix A: NCCI - CPT Codes

Code 1	Code 2
	99348[1], 99349[1], 99350[1], 99374[1], 99375[1], 99377[1], 99378[1], 99446[0], 99447[0], 99448[0], 99449[0], 99451[0], 99452[0], 99495[0], 99496[0], G0463[1], G0471[1]
36860	01844[0], 01924[0], 01925[0], 01926[0], 0213T[0], 0216T[0], 0596T[1], 0597T[1], 0708T[1], 0709T[1], 12001[1], 12002[1], 12004[1], 12005[1], 12006[1], 12007[1], 12011[1], 12013[1], 12014[1], 12015[1], 12016[1], 12017[1], 12018[1], 12020[1], 12021[1], 12031[1], 12032[1], 12034[1], 12035[1], 12036[1], 12037[1], 12041[1], 12042[1], 12044[1], 12045[1], 12046[1], 12047[1], 12051[1], 12052[1], 12053[1], 12054[1], 12055[1], 12056[1], 12057[1], 13100[1], 13101[1], 13102[1], 13120[1], 13121[1], 13122[1], 13131[1], 13132[1], 13133[1], 13151[1], 13152[1], 13153[1], 35201[1], 35206[1], 35226[1], 35231[1], 35236[1], 35256[1], 35261[1], 35266[1], 35286[1], 35860[1], 36000[1], 36002[1], 36005[1], 36400[1], 36405[1], 36406[1], 36410[1], 36420[1], 36425[1], 36430[1], 36440[1], 36591[0], 36592[0], 36593[1], 36600[1], 36640[1], 36800[1], 36810[1], 36815[1], 36819[1], 36820[1], 36821[1], 36825[1], 36830[1], 36831[1], 36832[1], 36833[1], 36835[1], 36861[1], 36901[1], 36902[1], 36903[1], 36907[1], 36908[1], 36909[1], 37211[1], 37212[1], 37213[1], 37214[1], 43752[1], 51701[1], 51702[1], 51703[1], 62320[0], 62321[0], 62322[0], 62323[0], 62324[0], 62325[0], 62326[0], 62327[0], 64400[0], 64405[0], 64408[0], 64415[0], 64416[0], 64417[0], 64418[0], 64420[0], 64421[0], 64425[0], 64430[0], 64435[0], 64445[0], 64446[0], 64447[0], 64448[0], 64449[0], 64450[0], 64451[0], 64454[0], 64461[0], 64462[0], 64463[0], 64479[0], 64480[0], 64483[0], 64484[0], 64486[0], 64487[0], 64488[0], 64489[0], 64490[0], 64491[0], 64492[0], 64493[0], 64494[0], 64495[0], 64505[0], 64510[0], 64517[0], 64520[0], 64530[0], 69990[0], 76942[1], 76998[1], 77001[1], 77002[1], 92012[1], 92014[1], 93000[1], 93005[1], 93010[1], 93040[1], 93041[1], 93042[1], 93318[1], 93355[1], 94002[1], 94200[1], 94680[1], 94681[1], 94690[1], 95812[1], 95813[1], 95816[1], 95819[1], 95822[1], 95829[1], 95955[1], 96360[1], 96361[1], 96365[1], 96366[1], 96367[1], 96368[1], 96372[1], 96374[1], 96375[1], 96376[1], 96377[1], 96523[0], 99155[0], 99156[0], 99157[0], 99211[1], 99212[1], 99213[1], 99214[1], 99215[1], 99217[1], 99218[1], 99219[1], 99220[1], 99221[1], 99222[1], 99223[1], 99231[1], 99232[1], 99233[1], 99234[1], 99235[1], 99236[1], 99238[1], 99239[1], 99241[1], 99242[1], 99243[1], 99244[1], 99245[1], 99251[1], 99252[1], 99253[1], 99254[1], 99255[1], 99291[1], 99292[1], 99304[1], 99305[1], 99306[1], 99307[1], 99308[1], 99309[1], 99310[1], 99315[1], 99316[1], 99334[1], 99335[1], 99336[1], 99337[1], 99347[1], 99348[1], 99349[1], 99350[1], 99374[1], 99375[1], 99377[1], 99378[1], 99446[0], 99447[0], 99448[0], 99449[0], 99451[0], 99452[0], 99495[1], 99496[1], G0463[1], G0471[1], J0670[1], J1642[1], J1644[1], J2001[1]
36861	01844[0], 01924[0], 01925[0], 01926[0], 0213T[0], 0216T[0], 0596T[1], 0597T[1], 0708T[1], 0709T[1], 12001[1], 12002[1], 12004[1], 12005[1], 12006[1], 12007[1], 12011[1], 12013[1], 12014[1], 12015[1], 12016[1], 12017[1], 12018[1], 12020[1], 12021[1], 12031[1], 12032[1], 12034[1], 12035[1], 12036[1], 12037[1], 12041[1], 12042[1], 12044[1], 12045[1], 12046[1], 12047[1], 12051[1], 12052[1], 12053[1], 12054[1], 12055[1], 12056[1], 12057[1], 13100[1], 13101[1], 13102[1], 13120[1], 13121[1], 13122[1], 13131[1], 13132[1], 13133[1], 13151[1], 13152[1], 13153[1], 35201[1], 35206[1], 35226[1], 35231[1], 35236[1], 35256[1], 35261[1], 35266[1], 35286[1], 36000[1], 36002[1], 36005[1], 36400[1], 36405[1], 36406[1], 36410[1], 36420[1], 36425[1], 36430[1], 36440[1], 36591[0], 36592[0], 36593[1], 36600[1], 36640[1], 36810[1], 36815[1], 36819[1], 36820[1], 36821[1], 36825[1], 36830[1], 36831[1], 36832[1], 36833[1], 36901[1], 36902[1], 36903[1], 36907[1], 36908[1], 36909[1], 37211[1], 37212[1], 37213[1], 37214[1], 43752[1], 51701[1], 51702[1], 51703[1], 62320[0], 62321[0], 62322[0], 62323[0], 62324[0], 62325[0], 62326[0], 62327[0], 64400[0], 64405[0], 64408[0], 64415[0], 64416[0], 64417[0], 64418[0], 64420[0], 64421[0], 64425[0], 64430[0], 64435[0], 64445[0], 64446[0], 64447[0], 64448[0], 64449[0], 64450[0], 64451[0], 64454[0], 64461[0], 64462[0], 64463[0], 64479[0], 64480[0], 64483[0], 64484[0], 64486[0], 64487[0], 64488[0], 64489[0], 64490[0], 64491[0], 64492[0], 64493[0], 64494[0], 64495[0], 64505[0], 64510[0], 64517[0], 64520[0], 64530[0], 69990[0], 76942[1], 76998[1], 77001[1], 77002[1], 92012[1], 92014[1], 93000[1], 93005[1], 93010[1], 93040[1], 93041[1], 93042[1], 93318[1], 93355[1], 94002[1], 94200[1], 94680[1], 94681[1], 94690[1], 95812[1], 95813[1], 95816[1], 95819[1], 95822[1], 95829[1], 95955[1], 96360[1], 96361[1], 96365[1], 96366[1], 96367[1], 96368[1], 96372[1], 96374[1], 96375[1], 96376[1], 96377[1], 96523[0], 99155[0], 99156[0], 99157[0], 99211[1], 99212[1], 99213[1], 99214[1], 99215[1], 99217[1], 99218[1], 99219[1], 99220[1], 99221[1], 99222[1], 99223[1], 99231[1], 99232[1], 99233[1], 99234[1], 99235[1], 99236[1], 99238[1], 99239[1], 99241[1], 99242[1], 99243[1], 99244[1], 99245[1], 99251[1], 99252[1], 99253[1], 99254[1], 99255[1], 99291[1], 99292[1], 99304[1], 99305[1], 99306[1], 99307[1], 99308[1], 99309[1], 99310[1], 99315[1], 99316[1], 99334[1], 99335[1], 99336[1], 99337[1], 99347[1], 99348[1], 99349[1], 99350[1], 99374[1], 99375[1], 99377[1], 99378[1], 99446[0], 99447[0], 99448[0], 99449[0], 99451[0], 99452[0], 99495[1], 99496[1], G0463[1], G0471[1]
36901	01916[0], 01924[0], 01925[0], 01926[0], 01930[1], 0213T[0], 0216T[0], 0596T[1], 0597T[1], 0645T[1], 0708T[1], 0709T[1], 12001[1], 12002[1], 12004[1], 12005[1], 12006[1], 12007[1], 12011[1], 12013[1], 12014[1], 12015[1], 12016[1], 12017[1], 12018[1], 12020[1], 12021[1], 12031[1], 12032[1], 12034[1], 12035[1], 12036[1], 12037[1], 12041[1], 12042[1], 12044[1], 12045[1], 12046[1], 12047[1], 12051[1], 12052[1], 12053[1], 12054[1], 12055[1], 12056[1], 12057[1], 13100[1], 13101[1], 13102[1], 13120[1], 13121[1], 13122[1], 13131[1], 13132[1], 13133[1], 13151[1], 13152[1], 13153[1], 35201[1], 35206[1], 35207[1], 35211[1], 35216[1], 35221[1], 35226[1], 35231[1], 35236[1], 35241[1], 35246[1], 35251[1], 35256[1], 35261[1], 35266[1], 35271[1], 35276[1], 35281[1], 35286[1], 36000[1], 36002[1], 36005[1], 36010[1], 36011[1], 36012[1], 36140[1], 36200[1], 36261[1], 36400[1], 36405[1], 36406[1], 36410[1], 36420[1], 36425[1], 36430[1], 36440[1], 36500[1], 36591[0], 36592[0], 36600[1], 36640[1], 36832[1], 36833[1], 43752[1], 51701[1], 51702[1], 51703[1], 62320[0], 62321[0], 62322[0], 62323[0], 62324[0], 62325[0], 62326[0], 62327[0], 64400[0], 64405[0], 64408[0], 64415[0], 64416[0], 64417[0], 64418[0], 64420[0], 64421[0], 64425[0], 64430[0], 64435[0], 64445[0], 64446[0], 64447[0], 64448[0], 64449[0], 64450[0], 64451[0], 64454[0], 64461[0], 64462[0], 64463[0], 64479[0], 64480[0], 64483[0], 64484[0], 64486[0], 64487[0], 64488[0], 64489[0], 64490[0], 64491[0], 64492[0], 64493[0], 64494[0], 64495[0], 64505[0], 64510[0], 64517[0], 64520[0], 64530[0], 69990[0], 75820[1], 75822[1], 75825[1], 75827[1], 75893[1], 76000[1], 76942[1], 76998[1], 77001[1], 77002[1], 77012[1], 77021[1], 92012[1], 92014[1], 93000[1], 93005[1], 93010[1], 93040[1], 93041[1], 93042[1], 93318[1], 94002[1], 94200[1], 94680[1], 94681[1], 94690[1], 95812[1], 95813[1], 95816[1], 95819[1], 95822[1], 95829[1], 95955[1], 96360[1], 96361[1], 96365[1], 96366[1], 96367[1], 96368[1], 96372[1], 96374[1], 96375[1], 96376[1], 96377[1], 96523[0], 99155[0], 99156[0], 99157[0], 99211[1], 99212[1], 99213[1], 99214[1], 99215[1], 99217[1], 99218[1], 99219[1], 99220[1], 99221[1], 99222[1], 99223[1], 99231[1], 99232[1], 99233[1], 99234[1], 99235[1], 99236[1], 99238[1], 99239[1], 99241[1], 99242[1], 99243[1], 99244[1], 99245[1], 99251[1], 99252[1], 99253[1], 99254[1], 99255[1], 99291[1], 99292[1], 99304[1], 99305[1], 99306[1], 99307[1], 99308[1], 99309[1], 99310[1], 99315[1], 99316[1], 99334[1], 99335[1], 99336[1], 99337[1], 99347[1], 99348[1], 99349[1], 99350[1], 99374[1], 99375[1], 99377[1], 99378[1], J0670[1], J1644[1], J2001[1]
36902	01916[0], 01924[0], 01925[0], 01926[0], 01930[1], 0213T[0], 0216T[0], 0596T[1], 0597T[1], 0645T[1], 0708T[1], 0709T[1], 12001[1], 12002[1], 12004[1], 12005[1], 12006[1], 12007[1], 12011[1], 12013[1], 12014[1], 12015[1], 12016[1], 12017[1], 12018[1], 12020[1], 12021[1], 12031[1], 12032[1], 12034[1], 12035[1], 12036[1], 12037[1], 12041[1], 12042[1], 12044[1], 12045[1], 12046[1], 12047[1], 12051[1], 12052[1], 12053[1], 12054[1], 12055[1], 12056[1], 12057[1], 13100[1], 13101[1], 13102[1], 13120[1], 13121[1], 13122[1], 13131[1], 13132[1], 13133[1], 13151[1], 13152[1], 13153[1], 35201[1], 35206[1], 35207[1], 35211[1], 35216[1], 35221[1], 35226[1], 35231[1], 35236[1], 35241[1], 35246[1], 35251[1], 35256[1], 35261[1], 35266[1], 35271[1], 35276[1], 35281[1], 35286[1], 36000[1], 36002[1], 36005[1], 36010[1], 36011[1], 36012[1], 36140[1], 36200[1], 36261[1], 36400[1], 36405[1], 36406[1], 36410[1], 36420[1], 36425[1], 36430[1], 36440[1], 36500[1], 36591[0], 36592[0], 36600[1], 36640[1], 36832[1], 36833[1], 36901[1], 43752[1], 51701[1], 51702[1], 51703[1], 62320[0], 62321[0], 62322[0], 62323[0], 62324[0], 62325[0], 62326[0], 62327[0], 64400[0], 64405[0], 64408[0], 64415[0], 64416[0], 64417[0], 64418[0], 64420[0], 64421[0], 64425[0], 64430[0], 64435[0], 64445[0], 64446[0], 64447[0], 64448[0], 64449[0], 64450[0], 64451[0], 64454[0], 64461[0], 64462[0], 64463[0], 64479[0], 64480[0], 64483[0], 64484[0], 64486[0], 64487[0], 64488[0], 64489[0], 64490[0], 64491[0], 64492[0], 64493[0], 64494[0], 64495[0], 64505[0], 64510[0], 64517[0], 64520[0], 64530[0], 69990[0], 75820[1], 75822[1], 75825[1], 75827[1], 75893[1], 76000[1], 76942[1], 76998[1], 77001[1], 77002[1], 77012[1], 77021[1], 92012[1], 92014[1], 93000[1], 93005[1], 93010[1], 93040[1], 93041[1], 93042[1], 93318[1], 94002[1], 94200[1], 94680[1], 94681[1], 94690[1], 95812[1], 95813[1], 95816[1], 95819[1], 95822[1], 95829[1], 95955[1], 96360[1], 96361[1], 96365[1], 96366[1], 96367[1], 96368[1], 96372[1], 96374[1], 96375[1], 96376[1], 96377[1], 96523[0], 99155[0], 99156[0], 99157[0], 99211[1], 99212[1], 99213[1], 99214[1], 99215[1], 99217[1], 99218[1], 99219[1], 99220[1], 99221[1], 99222[1], 99223[1], 99231[1], 99232[1], 99233[1], 99234[1], 99235[1], 99236[1], 99238[1], 99239[1], 99241[1], 99242[1], 99243[1], 99244[1], 99245[1], 99251[1], 99252[1], 99253[1], 99254[1], 99255[1], 99291[1], 99292[1], 99304[1], 99305[1], 99306[1], 99307[1], 99308[1], 99309[1], 99310[1], 99315[1], 99316[1], 99334[1], 99335[1], 99336[1], 99337[1], 99347[1], 99348[1], 99349[1], 99350[1], 99374[1], 99375[1], 99377[1], 99378[1], J0670[1], J1642[1], J1644[1], J2001[1]
36903	01916[0], 01924[0], 01925[0], 01926[0], 01930[1], 0213T[0], 0216T[0], 0596T[1], 0597T[1], 0645T[1], 0708T[1], 0709T[1], 12001[1], 12002[1], 12004[1], 12005[1], 12006[1], 12007[1], 12011[1], 12013[1], 12014[1], 12015[1], 12016[1], 12017[1], 12018[1], 12020[1], 12021[1], 12031[1], 12032[1], 12034[1], 12035[1], 12036[1], 12037[1], 12041[1], 12042[1], 12044[1], 12045[1], 12046[1], 12047[1], 12051[1], 12052[1], 12053[1], 12054[1], 12055[1], 12056[1], 12057[1], 13100[1], 13101[1], 13102[1], 13120[1], 13121[1], 13122[1], 13131[1], 13132[1], 13133[1], 13151[1], 13152[1], 13153[1], 35201[1], 35206[1], 35207[1], 35211[1], 35216[1], 35221[1], 35226[1], 35231[1], 35236[1], 35241[1], 35246[1], 35251[1], 35256[1], 35261[1], 35266[1], 35271[1], 35276[1], 35281[1], 35286[1], 36000[1], 36002[1], 36005[1], 36010[1], 36011[1], 36012[1], 36140[1], 36200[1], 36261[1], 36400[1], 36405[1], 36406[1], 36410[1], 36420[1], 36425[1], 36430[1], 36440[1], 36500[1], 36591[0], 36592[0], 36600[1], 36640[1], 36832[1], 36833[1], 36901[1], 36902[1], 37237[1], 37239[1], 43752[1], 51701[1], 51702[1], 51703[1], 62320[0], 62321[0], 62322[0], 62323[0], 62324[0], 62325[0], 62326[0], 62327[0], 64400[0], 64405[0], 64408[0], 64415[0], 64416[0], 64417[0], 64418[0], 64420[0], 64421[0], 64425[0], 64430[0], 64435[0], 64445[0], 64446[0], 64447[0], 64448[0], 64449[0], 64450[0], 64451[0], 64454[0], 64461[0], 64462[0], 64463[0], 64479[0], 64480[0], 64483[0], 64484[0], 64486[0], 64487[0], 64488[0], 64489[0], 64490[0], 64491[0], 64492[0], 64493[0], 64494[0], 64495[0], 64505[0], 64510[0], 64517[0], 64520[0], 64530[0], 69990[0], 75820[1], 75822[1], 75825[1], 75827[1], 75893[1], 76000[1], 76942[1], 76998[1], 77001[1], 77002[1], 77012[1], 77021[1], 92012[1], 92014[1], 93000[1], 93005[1], 93010[1], 93040[1], 93041[1], 93042[1], 93318[1], 94002[1], 94200[1], 94680[1], 94681[1], 94690[1], 95812[1], 95813[1], 95816[1], 95819[1], 95822[1], 95829[1], 95955[1], 96360[1], 96361[1], 96365[1], 96366[1], 96367[1], 96368[1], 96372[1], 96374[1], 96375[1], 96376[1], 96377[1], 96523[0], 99155[0], 99156[0], 99157[0], 99211[1], 99212[1], 99213[1], 99214[1], 99215[1], 99217[1], 99218[1], 99219[1], 99220[1], 99221[1], 99222[1], 99223[1], 99231[1], 99232[1], 99233[1], 99234[1], 99235[1], 99236[1], 99238[1], 99239[1], 99241[1], 99242[1],

0 = Modifier usage not allowed or inappropriate   1 = Modifier usage allowed

Code 1	Code 2
	99243[1], 99244[1], 99245[1], 99251[1], 99252[1], 99253[1], 99254[1], 99255[1], 99291[1], 99292[1], 99304[1], 99305[1], 99306[1], 99307[1], 99308[1], 99309[1], 99310[1], 99315[1], 99316[1], 99334[1], 99335[1], 99336[1], 99337[1], 99347[1], 99348[1], 99349[1], 99350[1], 99374[1], 99375[1], 99377[1], 99378[1], J0670[1], J1642[1], J1644[1], J2001[1]
36904	01844[0], 01916[0], 01924[0], 01925[0], 01926[0], 01930[1], 0213T[0], 0216T[0], 0596T[1], 0597T[1], 0645T[1], 0708T[1], 0709T[1], 11000[1], 11001[1], 11004[1], 11005[1], 11006[1], 11042[1], 11043[1], 11044[1], 11045[1], 11046[1], 11047[1], 12001[1], 12002[1], 12004[1], 12005[1], 12006[1], 12007[1], 12011[1], 12013[1], 12014[1], 12015[1], 12016[1], 12017[1], 12018[1], 12020[1], 12021[1], 12031[1], 12032[1], 12034[1], 12035[1], 12036[1], 12037[1], 12041[1], 12042[1], 12044[1], 12045[1], 12046[1], 12047[1], 12051[1], 12052[1], 12053[1], 12054[1], 12055[1], 12056[1], 12057[1], 13100[1], 13101[1], 13102[1], 13120[1], 13121[1], 13122[1], 13131[1], 13132[1], 13133[1], 13151[1], 13152[1], 13153[1], 35201[1], 35206[1], 35207[1], 35211[1], 35216[1], 35221[1], 35226[1], 35231[1], 35236[1], 35241[1], 35246[1], 35251[1], 35256[1], 35261[1], 35266[1], 35271[1], 35276[1], 35281[1], 35286[1], 35800[1], 35860[1], 36000[1], 36002[1], 36005[1], 36010[1], 36011[1], 36012[1], 36140[1], 36200[1], 36261[1], 36400[1], 36405[1], 36406[1], 36410[1], 36420[1], 36425[1], 36430[1], 36440[1], 36500[1], 36591[0], 36592[0], 36593[1], 36600[1], 36640[1], 36800[1], 36810[1], 36815[1], 36821[1], 36825[1], 36830[1], 36832[0], 36833[0], 36835[1], 36860[1], 36861[1], 36901[1], 36902[1], 36903[1], 37186[1], 37188[1], 37211[1], 37212[1], 37213[1], 37214[1], 43752[1], 51701[1], 51702[1], 51703[1], 62320[0], 62321[0], 62322[0], 62323[0], 62324[0], 62325[0], 62326[0], 62327[0], 64400[0], 64405[0], 64408[0], 64415[0], 64416[0], 64417[0], 64418[0], 64420[0], 64421[0], 64425[0], 64430[0], 64435[0], 64445[0], 64446[0], 64447[0], 64448[0], 64449[0], 64450[0], 64451[0], 64454[0], 64461[0], 64462[0], 64463[0], 64479[0], 64480[0], 64483[0], 64484[0], 64486[0], 64487[0], 64488[0], 64489[0], 64490[0], 64491[0], 64492[0], 64493[0], 64494[0], 64495[0], 64505[0], 64510[0], 64517[0], 64520[0], 64530[0], 69990[0], 75820[1], 75822[1], 75825[1], 75827[1], 75893[1], 76000[1], 76942[1], 76998[1], 77001[1], 77002[1], 77012[1], 77021[1], 92012[1], 92014[1], 93000[1], 93005[1], 93010[1], 93040[1], 93041[1], 93042[1], 93050[0], 93318[1], 93355[1], 94002[1], 94200[1], 94680[1], 94681[1], 94690[1], 95812[1], 95813[1], 95816[1], 95819[1], 95822[1], 95829[1], 95955[1], 96360[1], 96361[1], 96365[1], 96366[1], 96367[1], 96368[1], 96372[1], 96374[1], 96375[1], 96376[1], 96377[1], 96523[0], 97597[1], 97598[1], 97602[1], 99155[0], 99156[0], 99157[0], 99211[1], 99212[1], 99213[1], 99214[1], 99215[1], 99217[1], 99218[1], 99219[1], 99220[1], 99221[1], 99222[1], 99223[1], 99231[1], 99232[1], 99233[1], 99234[1], 99235[1], 99236[1], 99238[1], 99239[1], 99241[1], 99242[1], 99243[1], 99244[1], 99245[1], 99251[1], 99252[1], 99253[1], 99254[1], 99255[1], 99291[1], 99292[1], 99304[1], 99305[1], 99306[1], 99307[1], 99308[1], 99309[1], 99310[1], 99315[1], 99316[1], 99334[1], 99335[1], 99336[1], 99337[1], 99347[1], 99348[1], 99349[1], 99350[1], 99374[1], 99375[1], 99377[1], 99378[1], 99446[0], 99447[0], 99448[0], 99449[0], 99451[0], 99452[0], 99495[0], 99496[0], G0463[1], G0471[1], J0670[1], J1642[1], J1644[1], J2001[1]
36905	01844[0], 01916[0], 01924[0], 01925[0], 01926[0], 01930[1], 0213T[0], 0216T[0], 0596T[1], 0597T[1], 0645T[1], 0708T[1], 0709T[1], 11000[1], 11001[1], 11004[1], 11005[1], 11006[1], 11042[1], 11043[1], 11044[1], 11045[1], 11046[1], 11047[1], 12001[1], 12002[1], 12004[1], 12005[1], 12006[1], 12007[1], 12011[1], 12013[1], 12014[1], 12015[1], 12016[1], 12017[1], 12018[1], 12020[1], 12021[1], 12031[1], 12032[1], 12034[1], 12035[1], 12036[1], 12037[1], 12041[1], 12042[1], 12044[1], 12045[1], 12046[1], 12047[1], 12051[1], 12052[1], 12053[1], 12054[1], 12055[1], 12056[1], 12057[1], 13100[1], 13101[1], 13102[1], 13120[1], 13121[1], 13122[1], 13131[1], 13132[1], 13133[1], 13151[1], 13152[1], 13153[1], 35201[1], 35206[1], 35207[1], 35211[1], 35216[1], 35221[1], 35226[1], 35231[1], 35236[1], 35241[1], 35246[1], 35251[1], 35256[1], 35261[1], 35266[1], 35271[1], 35276[1], 35281[1], 35286[1], 35800[1], 35860[1], 36000[1], 36002[1], 36005[1], 36010[1], 36011[1], 36012[1], 36140[1], 36200[1], 36261[1], 36400[1], 36405[1], 36406[1], 36410[1], 36420[1], 36425[1], 36430[1], 36440[1], 36500[1], 36591[0], 36592[0], 36593[1], 36600[1], 36640[1], 36800[1], 36810[1], 36815[1], 36821[1], 36825[1], 36830[1], 36832[0], 36833[0], 36835[1], 36860[1], 36861[1], 36901[1], 36902[1], 36903[1], 36904[1], 37186[1], 37187[1], 37188[1], 37211[1], 37212[1], 37213[1], 37214[1], 37246[1], 37247[1], 37248[1], 37249[1], 43752[1], 51701[1], 51702[1], 51703[1], 62320[0], 62321[0], 62322[0], 62323[0], 62324[0], 62325[0], 62326[0], 62327[0], 64400[0], 64405[0], 64408[0], 64415[0], 64416[0], 64417[0], 64418[0], 64420[0], 64421[0], 64425[0], 64430[0], 64435[0], 64445[0], 64446[0], 64447[0], 64448[0], 64449[0], 64450[0], 64451[0], 64454[0], 64461[0], 64462[0], 64463[0], 64479[0], 64480[0], 64483[0], 64484[0], 64486[0], 64487[0], 64488[0], 64489[0], 64490[0], 64491[0], 64492[0], 64493[0], 64494[0], 64495[0], 64505[0], 64510[0], 64517[0], 64520[0], 64530[0], 69990[0], 75820[1], 75822[1], 75825[1], 75827[1], 75893[1], 76000[1], 76942[1], 76998[1], 77001[1], 77002[1], 77012[1], 77021[1], 92012[1], 92014[1], 93000[1], 93005[1], 93010[1], 93040[1], 93041[1], 93042[1], 93050[0], 93318[1], 93355[1], 94002[1], 94200[1], 94680[1], 94681[1], 94690[1], 95812[1], 95813[1], 95816[1], 95819[1], 95822[1], 95829[1], 95955[1], 96360[1], 96361[1], 96365[1], 96366[1], 96367[1], 96368[1], 96372[1], 96374[1], 96375[1], 96376[1], 96377[1], 96523[0], 97597[1], 97598[1], 97602[1], 99155[0], 99156[0], 99157[0], 99211[1], 99212[1], 99213[1], 99214[1], 99215[1], 99217[1], 99218[1], 99219[1], 99220[1], 99221[1], 99222[1], 99223[1], 99231[1], 99232[1], 99233[1], 99234[1], 99235[1], 99236[1], 99238[1], 99239[1], 99241[1], 99242[1], 99243[1], 99244[1], 99245[1], 99251[1], 99252[1], 99253[1], 99254[1], 99255[1], 99291[1], 99292[1], 99304[1], 99305[1], 99306[1], 99307[1], 99308[1], 99309[1], 99310[1], 99315[1], 99316[1], 99334[1], 99335[1], 99336[1], 99337[1], 99347[1], 99348[1], 99349[1], 99350[1], 99374[1], 99375[1], 99377[1], 99378[1], 99446[0], 99447[0], 99448[0], 99449[0], 99451[0], 99452[0], 99495[0], 99496[0], G0463[1], G0471[1], J0670[1], J1642[1], J1644[1], J2001[1]
36906	01844[0], 01916[0], 01924[0], 01925[0], 01926[0], 01930[1], 0213T[0], 0216T[0], 0596T[1], 0597T[1], 0645T[1], 0708T[1], 0709T[1], 11000[1], 11001[1], 11004[1], 11005[1], 11006[1], 11042[1], 11043[1], 11044[1], 11045[1], 11046[1], 11047[1], 12001[1], 12002[1], 12004[1], 12005[1], 12006[1], 12007[1], 12011[1], 12013[1], 12014[1], 12015[1], 12016[1], 12017[1], 12018[1], 12020[1], 12021[1], 12031[1], 12032[1], 12034[1], 12035[1], 12036[1], 12037[1], 12041[1], 12042[1], 12044[1], 12045[1], 12046[1], 12047[1], 12051[1], 12052[1], 12053[1], 12054[1], 12055[1], 12056[1], 12057[1], 13100[1], 13101[1], 13102[1], 13120[1], 13121[1], 13122[1], 13131[1], 13132[1], 13133[1], 13151[1], 13152[1], 13153[1], 33951[1], 33952[1], 33953[1], 33954[1], 35201[1], 35206[1], 35207[1], 35211[1], 35216[1], 35221[1], 35226[1], 35231[1], 35236[1], 35241[1], 35246[1], 35251[1], 35256[1], 35261[1], 35266[1], 35271[1], 35276[1], 35281[1], 35286[1], 35800[1], 35860[1], 36000[1], 36002[1], 36005[1], 36010[1], 36011[1], 36012[1], 36140[1], 36200[1], 36261[1], 36400[1], 36405[1], 36406[1], 36410[1], 36420[1], 36425[1], 36430[1], 36440[1], 36500[1], 36591[0], 36592[0], 36593[1], 36600[1], 36640[1], 36800[1], 36810[1], 36815[1], 36821[1], 36825[1], 36830[1], 36832[0], 36833[0], 36835[1], 36860[1], 36861[1], 36901[1], 36902[1], 36903[1], 36904[1], 36905[1], 37184[1], 37186[1], 37187[1], 37188[1], 37211[1], 37212[1], 37213[1], 37214[1], 37236[1], 37237[1], 37238[1], 37239[1], 37246[1], 37247[1], 37248[1], 37249[1], 43752[1], 51701[1], 51702[1], 51703[1], 62320[0], 62321[0], 62322[0], 62323[0], 62324[0], 62325[0], 62326[0], 62327[0], 64400[0], 64405[0], 64408[0], 64415[0], 64416[0], 64417[0], 64418[0], 64420[0], 64421[0], 64425[0], 64430[0], 64435[0], 64445[0], 64446[0], 64447[0], 64448[0], 64449[0], 64450[0], 64451[0], 64454[0], 64461[0], 64462[0], 64463[0], 64479[0], 64480[0], 64483[0], 64484[0], 64486[0], 64487[0], 64488[0], 64489[0], 64490[0], 64491[0], 64492[0], 64493[0], 64494[0], 64495[0], 64505[0], 64510[0], 64517[0], 64520[0], 64530[0], 69990[0], 75820[1], 75822[1], 75825[1], 75827[1], 75893[1], 76000[1], 76942[1], 76998[1], 77001[1], 77002[1], 77012[1], 77021[1], 92012[1], 92014[1], 93000[1], 93005[1], 93010[1], 93040[1], 93041[1], 93042[1], 93050[0], 93318[1], 93355[1], 94002[1], 94200[1], 94680[1], 94681[1], 94690[1], 95812[1], 95813[1], 95816[1], 95819[1], 95822[1], 95829[1], 95955[1], 96360[1], 96361[1], 96365[1], 96366[1], 96367[1], 96368[1], 96372[1], 96374[1], 96375[1], 96376[1], 96377[1], 96523[0], 97597[1], 97598[1], 97602[1], 99155[0], 99156[0], 99157[0], 99211[1], 99212[1], 99213[1], 99214[1], 99215[1], 99217[1], 99218[1], 99219[1], 99220[1], 99221[1], 99222[1], 99223[1], 99231[1], 99232[1], 99233[1], 99234[1], 99235[1], 99236[1], 99238[1], 99239[1], 99241[1], 99242[1], 99243[1], 99244[1], 99245[1], 99251[1], 99252[1], 99253[1], 99254[1], 99255[1], 99291[1], 99292[1], 99304[1], 99305[1], 99306[1], 99307[1], 99308[1], 99309[1], 99310[1], 99315[1], 99316[1], 99334[1], 99335[1], 99336[1], 99337[1], 99347[1], 99348[1], 99349[1], 99350[1], 99374[1], 99375[1], 99377[1], 99378[1], 99446[0], 99447[0], 99448[0], 99449[0], 99451[0], 99452[0], 99495[0], 99496[0], G0463[1], G0471[1], J0670[1], J1642[1], J1644[1], J2001[1]
36907	01916[0], 01924[0], 01925[0], 01926[0], 01930[1], 0213T[0], 0216T[0], 0596T[1], 0597T[1], 0645T[1], 0708T[1], 0709T[1], 12001[1], 12002[1], 12004[1], 12005[1], 12006[1], 12007[1], 12011[1], 12013[1], 12014[1], 12015[1], 12016[1], 12017[1], 12018[1], 12020[1], 12021[1], 12031[1], 12032[1], 12034[1], 12035[1], 12036[1], 12037[1], 12041[1], 12042[1], 12044[1], 12045[1], 12046[1], 12047[1], 12051[1], 12052[1], 12053[1], 12054[1], 12055[1], 12056[1], 12057[1], 13100[1], 13101[1], 13102[1], 13120[1], 13121[1], 13122[1], 13131[1], 13132[1], 13133[1], 13151[1], 13152[1], 13153[1], 35201[1], 35206[1], 35207[1], 35211[1], 35216[1], 35221[1], 35226[1], 35231[1], 35236[1], 35241[1], 35246[1], 35251[1], 35256[1], 35261[1], 35266[1], 35271[1], 35276[1], 35281[1], 35286[1], 36000[1], 36002[1], 36005[1], 36010[1], 36011[1], 36012[1], 36140[1], 36200[1], 36261[1], 36400[1], 36405[1], 36406[1], 36410[1], 36420[1], 36425[1], 36430[1], 36440[1], 36500[1], 36591[0], 36592[0], 36600[1], 36640[1], 43752[1], 51701[1], 51702[1], 51703[1], 62320[0], 62321[0], 62322[0], 62323[0], 62324[0], 62325[0], 62326[0], 62327[0], 64400[0], 64405[0], 64408[0], 64415[0], 64416[0], 64417[0], 64418[0], 64420[0], 64421[0], 64425[0], 64430[0], 64435[0], 64445[0], 64446[0], 64447[0], 64448[0], 64449[0], 64450[0], 64451[0], 64454[0], 64461[0], 64462[0], 64463[0], 64479[0], 64480[0], 64483[0], 64484[0], 64486[0], 64487[0], 64488[0], 64489[0], 64490[0], 64491[0], 64492[0], 64493[0], 64494[0], 64495[0], 64505[0], 64510[0], 64517[0], 64520[0], 64530[0], 69990[0], 75820[1], 75822[1], 75825[1], 75827[1], 75893[1], 76000[1], 76942[1], 76998[1], 77001[1], 77002[1], 77012[1], 77021[1], 92012[1], 92014[1], 93000[1], 93005[1], 93010[1], 93040[1], 93041[1], 93042[1], 93318[1], 94002[1], 94200[1], 94680[1], 94681[1], 94690[1], 95812[1], 95813[1], 95816[1], 95819[1], 95822[1], 95829[1], 95955[1], 96360[1], 96361[1], 96365[1], 96366[1], 96367[1], 96368[1], 96372[1], 96374[1], 96375[1], 96376[1], 96377[1], 96523[0], 99155[0], 99156[0], 99157[0], 99211[1], 99212[1], 99213[1], 99214[1], 99215[1], 99217[1], 99218[1], 99219[1], 99220[1], 99221[1], 99222[1], 99223[1], 99231[1], 99232[1], 99233[1], 99234[1], 99235[1], 99236[1], 99238[1], 99239[1], 99241[1], 99242[1], 99243[1], 99244[1], 99245[1], 99251[1], 99252[1], 99253[1], 99254[1], 99255[1], 99291[1], 99292[1], 99304[1], 99305[1], 99306[1], 99307[1], 99308[1], 99309[1], 99310[1], 99315[1], 99316[1], 99334[1], 99335[1], 99336[1], 99337[1], 99347[1], 99348[1], 99349[1], 99350[1], 99374[1], 99375[1], 99377[1], 99378[1], J0670[1], J1642[1], J1644[1], J2001[1]
36908	01916[0], 01924[0], 01925[0], 01926[0], 01930[1], 0213T[0], 0216T[0], 0596T[1], 0597T[1], 0645T[1], 0708T[1], 0709T[1], 12001[1], 12002[1], 12004[1], 12005[1], 12006[1], 12007[1], 12011[1], 12013[1], 12014[1], 12015[1], 12016[1], 12017[1], 12018[1], 12020[1], 12021[1], 12031[1], 12032[1], 12034[1], 12035[1], 12036[1], 12037[1], 12041[1], 12042[1], 12044[1], 12045[1], 12046[1], 12047[1], 12051[1],

0 = Modifier usage not allowed or inappropriate 1 = Modifier usage allowed

Code 1	Code 2
	12052[1], 12053[1], 12054[1], 12055[1], 12056[1], 12057[1], 13100[1], 13101[1], 13102[1], 13120[1], 13121[1], 13122[1], 13131[1], 13132[1], 13133[1], 13151[1], 13152[1], 13153[1], 35201[1], 35206[1], 35207[1], 35211[1], 35216[1], 35221[1], 35226[1], 35231[1], 35236[1], 35241[1], 35246[1], 35251[1], 35256[1], 35261[1], 35266[1], 35271[1], 35276[1], 35281[1], 35286[1], 36000[1], 36002[1], 36005[1], 36010[1], 36011[1], 36012[1], 36140[1], 36200[1], 36261[1], 36400[1], 36405[1], 36406[1], 36410[1], 36420[1], 36425[1], 36430[1], 36440[1], 36500[1], 36591[0], 36592[0], 36600[1], 36640[1], 36907[1], 37239[1], 43752[1], 51701[1], 51702[1], 51703[1], 62320[0], 62321[0], 62322[0], 62323[0], 62324[0], 62325[0], 62326[0], 62327[0], 64400[0], 64405[0], 64408[0], 64415[0], 64416[0], 64417[0], 64418[0], 64420[0], 64421[0], 64425[0], 64430[0], 64435[0], 64445[0], 64446[0], 64447[0], 64448[0], 64449[0], 64450[0], 64451[0], 64454[0], 64461[0], 64462[0], 64463[0], 64479[0], 64480[0], 64483[0], 64484[0], 64486[0], 64487[0], 64488[0], 64489[0], 64490[0], 64491[0], 64492[0], 64493[0], 64494[0], 64495[0], 64505[0], 64510[0], 64517[0], 64520[0], 64530[0], 69990[0], 75820[1], 75822[1], 75825[1], 75827[1], 75893[1], 76000[1], 76942[1], 76998[1], 77001[1], 77002[1], 77012[1], 77021[1], 92012[1], 92014[1], 93000[1], 93005[1], 93010[1], 93040[1], 93041[1], 93042[1], 93318[1], 94002[1], 94200[1], 94680[1], 94681[1], 94690[1], 95812[1], 95813[1], 95816[1], 95819[1], 95822[1], 95829[1], 95955[1], 96360[1], 96361[1], 96365[1], 96366[1], 96367[1], 96368[1], 96372[1], 96374[1], 96375[1], 96376[1], 96377[1], 96523[0], 99155[0], 99156[0], 99157[0], 99211[1], 99212[1], 99213[1], 99214[1], 99215[1], 99217[1], 99218[1], 99219[1], 99220[1], 99221[1], 99222[1], 99223[1], 99231[1], 99232[1], 99233[1], 99234[1], 99235[1], 99236[1], 99238[1], 99239[1], 99241[1], 99242[1], 99243[1], 99244[1], 99245[1], 99251[1], 99252[1], 99253[1], 99254[1], 99255[1], 99291[1], 99292[1], 99304[1], 99305[1], 99306[1], 99307[1], 99308[1], 99309[1], 99310[1], 99315[1], 99316[1], 99334[1], 99335[1], 99336[1], 99337[1], 99347[1], 99348[1], 99349[1], 99350[1], 99374[1], 99375[1], 99377[1], 99378[1], J0670[1], J1642[1], J1644[1], J2001[1]
36909	01916[0], 01924[0], 01925[0], 01926[0], 01930[1], 0213T[0], 0216T[0], 0596T[1], 0597T[1], 0645T[1], 0708T[1], 0709T[1], 12001[1], 12002[1], 12004[1], 12005[1], 12006[1], 12007[1], 12011[1], 12013[1], 12014[1], 12015[1], 12016[1], 12017[1], 12018[1], 12020[1], 12021[1], 12031[1], 12032[1], 12034[1], 12035[1], 12036[1], 12037[1], 12041[1], 12042[1], 12044[1], 12045[1], 12046[1], 12047[1], 12051[1], 12052[1], 12053[1], 12054[1], 12055[1], 12056[1], 12057[1], 13100[1], 13101[1], 13102[1], 13120[1], 13121[1], 13122[1], 13131[1], 13132[1], 13133[1], 13151[1], 13152[1], 13153[1], 35201[1], 35206[1], 35207[1], 35211[1], 35216[1], 35221[1], 35226[1], 35231[1], 35236[1], 35241[1], 35246[1], 35251[1], 35256[1], 35261[1], 35266[1], 35271[1], 35276[1], 35281[1], 35286[1], 36000[1], 36002[1], 36005[1], 36010[1], 36011[1], 36012[1], 36140[1], 36200[1], 36261[1], 36400[1], 36405[1], 36406[1], 36410[1], 36420[1], 36425[1], 36430[1], 36440[1], 36465[1], 36466[1], 36470[1], 36471[1], 36500[1], 36591[0], 36592[0], 36600[1], 36640[1], 43752[1], 51701[1], 51702[1], 51703[1], 62320[0], 62321[0], 62322[0], 62323[0], 62324[0], 62325[0], 62326[0], 62327[0], 64400[0], 64405[0], 64408[0], 64415[0], 64416[0], 64417[0], 64418[0], 64420[0], 64421[0], 64425[0], 64430[0], 64435[0], 64445[0], 64446[0], 64447[0], 64448[0], 64449[0], 64450[0], 64451[0], 64454[0], 64461[0], 64462[0], 64463[0], 64479[0], 64480[0], 64483[0], 64484[0], 64486[0], 64487[0], 64488[0], 64489[0], 64490[0], 64491[0], 64492[0], 64493[0], 64494[0], 64495[0], 64505[0], 64510[0], 64517[0], 64520[0], 64530[0], 69990[0], 75820[1], 75822[1], 75825[1], 75827[1], 75893[1], 76000[1], 76942[1], 76998[1], 77001[1], 77002[1], 77012[1], 77021[1], 92012[1], 92014[1], 93000[1], 93005[1], 93010[1], 93040[1], 93041[1], 93042[1], 93318[1], 94002[1], 94200[1], 94680[1], 94681[1], 94690[1], 95812[1], 95813[1], 95816[1], 95819[1], 95822[1], 95829[1], 95955[1], 96360[1], 96361[1], 96365[1], 96366[1], 96367[1], 96368[1], 96372[1], 96374[1], 96375[1], 96376[1], 96377[1], 96523[0], 99155[0], 99156[0], 99157[0], 99211[1], 99212[1], 99213[1], 99214[1], 99215[1], 99217[1], 99218[1], 99219[1], 99220[1], 99221[1], 99222[1], 99223[1], 99231[1], 99232[1], 99233[1], 99234[1], 99235[1], 99236[1], 99238[1], 99239[1], 99241[1], 99242[1], 99243[1], 99244[1], 99245[1], 99251[1], 99252[1], 99253[1], 99254[1], 99255[1], 99291[1], 99292[1], 99304[1], 99305[1], 99306[1], 99307[1], 99308[1], 99309[1], 99310[1], 99315[1], 99316[1], 99334[1], 99335[1], 99336[1], 99337[1], 99347[1], 99348[1], 99349[1], 99350[1], 99374[1], 99375[1], 99377[1], 99378[1], J0670[1], J1644[1], J2001[1]
37788	0213T[0], 0216T[0], 0596T[1], 0597T[1], 0708T[1], 0709T[1], 12001[1], 12002[1], 12004[1], 12005[1], 12006[1], 12007[1], 12011[1], 12013[1], 12014[1], 12015[1], 12016[1], 12017[1], 12018[1], 12020[1], 12021[1], 12031[1], 12032[1], 12034[1], 12035[1], 12036[1], 12037[1], 12041[1], 12042[1], 12044[1], 12045[1], 12046[1], 12047[1], 12051[1], 12052[1], 12053[1], 12054[1], 12055[1], 12056[1], 12057[1], 13100[1], 13101[1], 13102[1], 13120[1], 13121[1], 13122[1], 13131[1], 13132[1], 13133[1], 13151[1], 13152[1], 13153[1], 36000[1], 36400[1], 36405[1], 36406[1], 36410[1], 36420[1], 36425[1], 36430[1], 36440[1], 36591[0], 36592[0], 36600[1], 36640[1], 43752[1], 51701[1], 51702[1], 51703[1], 62320[0], 62321[0], 62322[0], 62323[0], 62324[0], 62325[0], 62326[0], 62327[0], 64400[0], 64405[0], 64408[0], 64415[0], 64416[0], 64417[0], 64418[0], 64420[0], 64421[0], 64425[0], 64430[0], 64435[0], 64445[0], 64446[0], 64447[0], 64448[0], 64449[0], 64450[0], 64451[0], 64454[0], 64461[0], 64462[0], 64463[0], 64479[0], 64480[0], 64483[0], 64484[0], 64486[0], 64487[0], 64488[0], 64489[0], 64490[0], 64491[0], 64492[0], 64493[0], 64494[0], 64495[0], 64505[0], 64510[0], 64517[0], 64520[0], 64530[0], 69990[0], 92012[1], 92014[1], 93000[1], 93005[1], 93010[1], 93040[1], 93041[1], 93042[1], 93318[1], 93355[1], 94002[1], 94200[1], 94680[1], 94681[1], 94690[1], 95812[1], 95813[1], 95816[1], 95819[1], 95822[1], 95829[1], 95955[1], 96360[1], 96361[1], 96365[1], 96366[1], 96367[1], 96368[1], 96372[1], 96374[1], 96375[1], 96376[1], 96377[1], 96523[0], 99155[0], 99156[0], 99157[0], 99211[1], 99212[1], 99213[1], 99214[1], 99215[1], 99217[1], 99218[1], 99219[1], 99220[1], 99221[1], 99222[1], 99223[1], 99231[1], 99232[1], 99233[1], 99234[1], 99235[1], 99236[1], 99238[1], 99239[1], 99241[1], 99242[1], 99243[1], 99244[1], 99245[1], 99251[1], 99252[1], 99253[1], 99254[1], 99255[1], 99291[1], 99292[1], 99304[1], 99305[1], 99306[1], 99307[1], 99308[1], 99309[1], 99310[1], 99315[1], 99316[1], 99334[1], 99335[1], 99336[1], 99337[1], 99347[1], 99348[1], 99349[1], 99350[1], 99374[1], 99375[1], 99377[1], 99378[1], 99446[0], 99447[0], 99448[0], 99449[0], 99451[0], 99452[0], 99495[0], 99496[0], G0463[1], G0471[1]
37790	0213T[0], 0216T[0], 0596T[1], 0597T[1], 0708T[1], 0709T[1], 12001[1], 12002[1], 12004[1], 12005[1], 12006[1], 12007[1], 12011[1], 12013[1], 12014[1], 12015[1], 12016[1], 12017[1], 12018[1], 12020[1], 12021[1], 12031[1], 12032[1], 12034[1], 12035[1], 12036[1], 12037[1], 12041[1], 12042[1], 12044[1], 12045[1], 12046[1], 12047[1], 12051[1], 12052[1], 12053[1], 12054[1], 12055[1], 12056[1], 12057[1], 13100[1], 13101[1], 13102[1], 13120[1], 13121[1], 13122[1], 13131[1], 13132[1], 13133[1], 13151[1], 13152[1], 13153[1], 36000[1], 36400[1], 36405[1], 36406[1], 36410[1], 36420[1], 36425[1], 36430[1], 36440[1], 36591[0], 36592[0], 36600[1], 36640[1], 43752[1], 51701[1], 51702[1], 51703[1], 62320[0], 62321[0], 62322[0], 62323[0], 62324[0], 62325[0], 62326[0], 62327[0], 64400[0], 64405[0], 64408[0], 64415[0], 64416[0], 64417[0], 64418[0], 64420[0], 64421[0], 64425[0], 64430[0], 64435[0], 64445[0], 64446[0], 64447[0], 64448[0], 64449[0], 64450[0], 64451[0], 64454[0], 64461[0], 64462[0], 64463[0], 64479[0], 64480[0], 64483[0], 64484[0], 64486[0], 64487[0], 64488[0], 64489[0], 64490[0], 64491[0], 64492[0], 64493[0], 64494[0], 64495[0], 64505[0], 64510[0], 64517[0], 64520[0], 64530[0], 69990[0], 92012[1], 92014[1], 93000[1], 93005[1], 93010[1], 93040[1], 93041[1], 93042[1], 93318[1], 93355[1], 94002[1], 94200[1], 94680[1], 94681[1], 94690[1], 95812[1], 95813[1], 95816[1], 95819[1], 95822[1], 95829[1], 95955[1], 96360[1], 96361[1], 96365[1], 96366[1], 96367[1], 96368[1], 96372[1], 96374[1], 96375[1], 96376[1], 96377[1], 96523[0], 99155[0], 99156[0], 99157[0], 99211[1], 99212[1], 99213[1], 99214[1], 99215[1], 99217[1], 99218[1], 99219[1], 99220[1], 99221[1], 99222[1], 99223[1], 99231[1], 99232[1], 99233[1], 99234[1], 99235[1], 99236[1], 99238[1], 99239[1], 99241[1], 99242[1], 99243[1], 99244[1], 99245[1], 99251[1], 99252[1], 99253[1], 99254[1], 99255[1], 99291[1], 99292[1], 99304[1], 99305[1], 99306[1], 99307[1], 99308[1], 99309[1], 99310[1], 99315[1], 99316[1], 99334[1], 99335[1], 99336[1], 99337[1], 99347[1], 99348[1], 99349[1], 99350[1], 99374[1], 99375[1], 99377[1], 99378[1], 99446[0], 99447[0], 99448[0], 99449[0], 99451[0], 99452[0], 99495[0], 99496[0], G0463[1], G0471[1]
38500	0213T[0], 0216T[0], 0596T[1], 0597T[1], 0708T[1], 0709T[1], 10005[1], 10007[1], 10009[1], 10011[1], 10021[1], 11000[1], 11001[1], 11004[1], 11005[1], 11006[1], 11042[1], 11043[1], 11044[1], 11045[1], 11046[1], 11047[1], 12001[1], 12002[1], 12004[1], 12005[1], 12006[1], 12007[1], 12011[1], 12013[1], 12014[1], 12015[1], 12016[1], 12017[1], 12018[1], 12020[1], 12021[1], 12031[1], 12032[1], 12034[1], 12035[1], 12036[1], 12037[1], 12041[1], 12042[1], 12044[1], 12045[1], 12046[1], 12047[1], 12051[1], 12052[1], 12053[1], 12054[1], 12055[1], 12056[1], 12057[1], 13100[1], 13101[1], 13102[1], 13120[1], 13121[1], 13122[1], 13131[1], 13132[1], 13133[1], 13151[1], 13152[1], 13153[1], 36000[1], 36400[1], 36405[1], 36406[1], 36410[1], 36420[1], 36425[1], 36430[1], 36440[1], 36591[0], 36592[0], 36600[1], 36640[1], 38505[1], 43752[1], 51701[1], 51702[1], 51703[1], 62320[0], 62321[0], 62322[0], 62323[0], 62324[0], 62325[0], 62326[0], 62327[0], 64400[0], 64405[0], 64408[0], 64415[0], 64416[0], 64417[0], 64418[0], 64420[0], 64421[0], 64425[0], 64430[0], 64435[0], 64445[0], 64446[0], 64447[0], 64448[0], 64449[0], 64450[0], 64451[0], 64454[0], 64461[0], 64462[0], 64463[0], 64479[0], 64480[0], 64483[0], 64484[0], 64486[0], 64487[0], 64488[0], 64489[0], 64490[0], 64491[0], 64492[0], 64493[0], 64494[0], 64495[0], 64505[0], 64510[0], 64517[0], 64520[0], 64530[0], 69990[0], 92012[1], 92014[1], 93000[1], 93005[1], 93010[1], 93040[1], 93041[1], 93042[1], 93318[1], 93355[1], 94002[1], 94200[1], 94680[1], 94681[1], 94690[1], 95812[1], 95813[1], 95816[1], 95819[1], 95822[1], 95829[1], 95955[1], 96360[1], 96361[1], 96365[1], 96366[1], 96367[1], 96368[1], 96372[1], 96374[1], 96375[1], 96376[1], 96377[1], 96523[0], 97597[1], 97598[1], 97602[1], 99155[0], 99156[0], 99157[0], 99211[1], 99212[1], 99213[1], 99214[1], 99215[1], 99217[1], 99218[1], 99219[1], 99220[1], 99221[1], 99222[1], 99223[1], 99231[1], 99232[1], 99233[1], 99234[1], 99235[1], 99236[1], 99238[1], 99239[1], 99241[1], 99242[1], 99243[1], 99244[1], 99245[1], 99251[1], 99252[1], 99253[1], 99254[1], 99255[1], 99291[1], 99292[1], 99304[1], 99305[1], 99306[1], 99307[1], 99308[1], 99309[1], 99310[1], 99315[1], 99316[1], 99334[1], 99335[1], 99336[1], 99337[1], 99347[1], 99348[1], 99349[1], 99350[1], 99374[1], 99375[1], 99377[1], 99378[1], 99446[0], 99447[0], 99448[0], 99449[0], 99451[0], 99452[0], 99495[0], 99496[0], G0463[1], G0471[1], J0670[1], J2001[1]
38505	0213T[0], 0216T[0], 0596T[1], 0597T[1], 0708T[1], 0709T[1], 10005[1], 10007[1], 10009[1], 10011[1], 10021[1], 11000[1], 11001[1], 11004[1], 11005[1], 11006[1], 11042[1], 11043[1], 11044[1], 11045[1], 11046[1], 11047[1], 12001[1], 12002[1], 12004[1], 12005[1], 12006[1], 12007[1], 12011[1], 12013[1], 12014[1], 12015[1], 12016[1], 12017[1], 12018[1], 12020[1], 12021[1], 12031[1], 12032[1], 12034[1], 12035[1], 12036[1], 12037[1], 12041[1], 12042[1], 12044[1], 12045[1], 12046[1], 12047[1], 12051[1], 12052[1], 12053[1], 12054[1], 12055[1], 12056[1], 12057[1], 13100[1], 13101[1], 13102[1], 13120[1], 13121[1], 13122[1], 13131[1], 13132[1], 13133[1], 13151[1], 13152[1], 13153[1], 36000[1], 36400[1], 36405[1], 36406[1], 36410[1], 36420[1], 36425[1], 36430[1], 36440[1], 36591[0], 36592[0], 36600[1], 36640[1], 43752[1], 51701[1], 51702[1], 51703[1], 62320[0], 62321[0], 62322[0], 62323[0], 62324[0], 62325[0], 62326[0], 62327[0], 64400[0], 64405[0], 64408[0], 64415[0], 64416[0], 64417[0], 64418[0], 64420[0], 64421[0], 64425[0], 64430[0], 64435[0], 64445[0], 64446[0], 64447[0], 64448[0], 64449[0], 64450[0], 64451[0], 64454[0], 64461[0], 64462[0], 64463[0], 64479[0], 64480[0], 64483[0], 64484[0],

0 = Modifier usage not allowed or inappropriate 1 = Modifier usage allowed

Code 1	Code 2
	64486[0], 64487[0], 64488[0], 64489[0], 64490[0], 64491[0], 64492[0], 64493[0], 64494[0], 64495[0], 64505[0], 64510[0], 64517[0], 64520[0], 64530[0], 69990[0], 76000[1], 77001[1], 92012[1], 92014[1], 93000[1], 93005[1], 93010[1], 93040[1], 93041[1], 93042[1], 93318[1], 93355[1], 94002[1], 94200[1], 94680[1], 94681[1], 94690[1], 95812[1], 95813[1], 95816[1], 95819[1], 95822[1], 95829[1], 95955[1], 96360[1], 96361[1], 96365[1], 96366[1], 96367[1], 96368[1], 96372[1], 96374[1], 96375[1], 96376[1], 96377[1], 96523[0], 97597[1], 97598[1], 97602[1], 99155[0], 99156[0], 99157[0], 99211[1], 99212[1], 99213[1], 99214[1], 99215[1], 99217[1], 99218[1], 99219[1], 99220[1], 99221[1], 99222[1], 99223[1], 99231[1], 99232[1], 99233[1], 99234[1], 99235[1], 99236[1], 99238[1], 99239[1], 99241[1], 99242[1], 99243[1], 99244[1], 99245[1], 99251[1], 99252[1], 99253[1], 99254[1], 99255[1], 99291[1], 99292[1], 99304[1], 99305[1], 99306[1], 99307[1], 99308[1], 99309[1], 99310[1], 99315[1], 99316[1], 99334[1], 99335[1], 99336[1], 99337[1], 99347[1], 99348[1], 99349[1], 99350[1], 99374[1], 99375[1], 99377[1], 99378[1], 99446[0], 99447[0], 99448[0], 99449[0], 99451[0], 99452[0], 99495[1], 99496[1], G0463[1], G0471[1], J2001[1]
38531	0213T[0], 0216T[0], 0596T[1], 0597T[1], 0708T[1], 0709T[1], 10021[1], 11000[1], 11001[1], 11004[1], 11005[1], 11006[1], 11042[1], 11043[1], 11044[1], 11045[1], 11046[1], 11047[1], 12001[1], 12002[1], 12004[1], 12005[1], 12006[1], 12007[1], 12011[1], 12013[1], 12014[1], 12015[1], 12016[1], 12017[1], 12018[1], 12020[1], 12021[1], 12031[1], 12032[1], 12034[1], 12035[1], 12036[1], 12037[1], 12041[1], 12042[1], 12044[1], 12045[1], 12046[1], 12047[1], 12051[1], 12052[1], 12053[1], 12054[1], 12055[1], 12056[1], 12057[1], 13100[1], 13101[1], 13102[1], 13120[1], 13121[1], 13122[1], 13131[1], 13132[1], 13133[1], 13151[1], 13152[1], 13153[1], 22902[1], 36000[1], 36400[1], 36405[1], 36406[1], 36410[1], 36420[1], 36425[1], 36430[1], 36440[1], 36591[0], 36592[0], 36600[1], 36640[1], 38500[1], 38505[1], 43752[1], 51701[1], 51702[1], 51703[1], 62320[0], 62321[0], 62322[0], 62323[0], 62324[0], 62325[0], 62326[0], 62327[0], 64400[0], 64405[0], 64408[0], 64415[0], 64416[0], 64417[0], 64418[0], 64420[0], 64421[0], 64425[0], 64430[0], 64435[0], 64445[0], 64446[0], 64447[0], 64448[0], 64449[0], 64450[0], 64451[0], 64454[0], 64461[0], 64462[0], 64463[0], 64479[0], 64480[0], 64483[0], 64484[0], 64486[0], 64487[0], 64488[0], 64489[0], 64490[0], 64491[0], 64492[0], 64493[0], 64494[0], 64495[0], 64505[0], 64510[0], 64517[0], 64520[0], 64530[0], 69990[0], 92012[1], 92014[1], 93000[1], 93005[1], 93010[1], 93040[1], 93041[1], 93042[1], 93318[1], 93355[1], 94002[1], 94200[1], 94680[1], 94681[1], 94690[1], 95812[1], 95813[1], 95816[1], 95819[1], 95822[1], 95829[1], 95955[1], 96360[1], 96361[1], 96365[1], 96366[1], 96367[1], 96368[1], 96372[1], 96374[1], 96375[1], 96376[1], 96377[1], 96523[0], 97597[1], 97598[1], 97602[1], 99155[0], 99156[0], 99157[0], 99211[1], 99212[1], 99213[1], 99214[1], 99215[1], 99217[1], 99218[1], 99219[1], 99220[1], 99221[1], 99222[1], 99223[1], 99231[1], 99232[1], 99233[1], 99234[1], 99235[1], 99236[1], 99238[1], 99239[1], 99241[1], 99242[1], 99243[1], 99244[1], 99245[1], 99251[1], 99252[1], 99253[1], 99254[1], 99255[1], 99291[1], 99292[1], 99304[1], 99305[1], 99306[1], 99307[1], 99308[1], 99309[1], 99310[1], 99315[1], 99316[1], 99334[1], 99335[1], 99336[1], 99337[1], 99347[1], 99348[1], 99349[1], 99350[1], 99374[1], 99375[1], 99377[1], 99378[1], 99446[0], 99447[0], 99448[0], 99449[0], 99495[0], 99496[0], G0463[1], G0471[1], J0670[1], J2001[1]
38562	0213T[0], 0216T[0], 0596T[1], 0597T[1], 0708T[1], 0709T[1], 11000[1], 11001[1], 11004[1], 11005[1], 11006[1], 11042[1], 11043[1], 11044[1], 11045[1], 11046[1], 11047[1], 12001[1], 12002[1], 12004[1], 12005[1], 12006[1], 12007[1], 12011[1], 12013[1], 12014[1], 12015[1], 12016[1], 12017[1], 12018[1], 12020[1], 12021[1], 12031[1], 12032[1], 12034[1], 12035[1], 12036[1], 12037[1], 12041[1], 12042[1], 12044[1], 12045[1], 12046[1], 12047[1], 12051[1], 12052[1], 12053[1], 12054[1], 12055[1], 12056[1], 12057[1], 13100[1], 13101[1], 13102[1], 13120[1], 13121[1], 13122[1], 13131[1], 13132[1], 13133[1], 13151[1], 13152[1], 13153[1], 36000[1], 36400[1], 36405[1], 36406[1], 36410[1], 36420[1], 36425[1], 36430[1], 36440[1], 36591[0], 36592[0], 36600[1], 36640[1], 43752[1], 44005[0], 44180[0], 44602[1], 44603[1], 44604[1], 44605[1], 44820[0], 44850[0], 44950[0], 44970[0], 49000[0], 49002[1], 49010[0], 49255[0], 49320[1], 49321[1], 49570[0], 51701[1], 51702[1], 51703[1], 52000[1], 62320[0], 62321[0], 62322[0], 62323[0], 62324[0], 62325[0], 62326[0], 62327[0], 64400[0], 64405[0], 64408[0], 64415[0], 64416[0], 64417[0], 64418[0], 64420[0], 64421[0], 64425[0], 64430[0], 64435[0], 64445[0], 64446[0], 64447[0], 64448[0], 64449[0], 64450[0], 64451[0], 64454[0], 64461[0], 64462[0], 64463[0], 64479[0], 64480[0], 64483[0], 64484[0], 64486[0], 64487[0], 64488[0], 64489[0], 64490[0], 64491[0], 64492[0], 64493[0], 64494[0], 64495[0], 64505[0], 64510[0], 64517[0], 64520[0], 64530[0], 69990[0], 92012[1], 92014[1], 93000[1], 93005[1], 93010[1], 93040[1], 93041[1], 93042[1], 93318[1], 93355[1], 94002[1], 94200[1], 94680[1], 94681[1], 94690[1], 95812[1], 95813[1], 95816[1], 95819[1], 95822[1], 95829[1], 95955[1], 96360[1], 96361[1], 96365[1], 96366[1], 96367[1], 96368[1], 96372[1], 96374[1], 96375[1], 96376[1], 96377[1], 96523[0], 97597[1], 97598[1], 97602[1], 99155[0], 99156[0], 99157[0], 99211[1], 99212[1], 99213[1], 99214[1], 99215[1], 99217[1], 99218[1], 99219[1], 99220[1], 99221[1], 99222[1], 99223[1], 99231[1], 99232[1], 99233[1], 99234[1], 99235[1], 99236[1], 99238[1], 99239[1], 99241[1], 99242[1], 99243[1], 99244[1], 99245[1], 99251[1], 99252[1], 99253[1], 99254[1], 99255[1], 99291[1], 99292[1], 99304[1], 99305[1], 99306[1], 99307[1], 99308[1], 99309[1], 99310[1], 99315[1], 99316[1], 99334[1], 99335[1], 99336[1], 99337[1], 99347[1], 99348[1], 99349[1], 99350[1], 99374[1], 99375[1], 99377[1], 99378[1], 99446[0], 99447[0], 99448[0], 99449[0], 99451[0], 99452[0], 99495[0], 99496[0], G0463[1], G0471[1]
38564	0213T[0], 0216T[0], 0596T[1], 0597T[1], 0708T[1], 0709T[1], 11000[1], 11001[1], 11004[1], 11005[1], 11006[1], 11042[1], 11043[1], 11044[1], 11045[1], 11046[1], 11047[1], 12001[1], 12002[1], 12004[1], 12005[1], 12006[1], 12007[1], 12011[1], 12013[1], 12014[1], 12015[1], 12016[1], 12017[1], 12018[1], 12020[1], 12021[1], 12031[1], 12032[1], 12034[1], 12035[1], 12036[1], 12037[1], 12041[1], 12042[1], 12044[1], 12045[1], 12046[1], 12047[1], 12051[1], 12052[1], 12053[1], 12054[1], 12055[1], 12056[1], 12057[1], 13100[1], 13101[1], 13102[1], 13120[1], 13121[1], 13122[1], 13131[1], 13132[1], 13133[1], 13151[1], 13152[1], 13153[1], 36000[1], 36400[1], 36405[1], 36406[1], 36410[1], 36420[1], 36425[1], 36430[1], 36440[1], 36591[0], 36592[0], 36600[1], 36640[1], 38570[0], 43752[1], 44602[1], 44603[1], 44604[1], 44605[1], 44950[0], 44970[0], 49000[0], 49002[1], 49320[1], 49321[1], 51701[1], 51702[1], 51703[1], 52000[1], 62320[0], 62321[0], 62322[0], 62323[0], 62324[0], 62325[0], 62326[0], 62327[0], 64400[0], 64405[0], 64408[0], 64415[0], 64416[0], 64417[0], 64418[0], 64420[0], 64421[0], 64425[0], 64430[0], 64435[0], 64445[0], 64446[0], 64447[0], 64448[0], 64449[0], 64450[0], 64451[0], 64454[0], 64461[0], 64462[0], 64463[0], 64479[0], 64480[0], 64483[0], 64484[0], 64486[0], 64487[0], 64488[0], 64489[0], 64490[0], 64491[0], 64492[0], 64493[0], 64494[0], 64495[0], 64505[0], 64510[0], 64517[0], 64520[0], 64530[0], 69990[0], 92012[1], 92014[1], 93000[1], 93005[1], 93010[1], 93040[1], 93041[1], 93042[1], 93318[1], 93355[1], 94002[1], 94200[1], 94680[1], 94681[1], 94690[1], 95812[1], 95813[1], 95816[1], 95819[1], 95822[1], 95829[1], 95955[1], 96360[1], 96361[1], 96365[1], 96366[1], 96367[1], 96368[1], 96372[1], 96374[1], 96375[1], 96376[1], 96377[1], 96523[0], 97597[1], 97598[1], 97602[1], 99155[0], 99156[0], 99157[0], 99211[1], 99212[1], 99213[1], 99214[1], 99215[1], 99217[1], 99218[1], 99219[1], 99220[1], 99221[1], 99222[1], 99223[1], 99231[1], 99232[1], 99233[1], 99234[1], 99235[1], 99236[1], 99238[1], 99239[1], 99241[1], 99242[1], 99243[1], 99244[1], 99245[1], 99251[1], 99252[1], 99253[1], 99254[1], 99255[1], 99291[1], 99292[1], 99304[1], 99305[1], 99306[1], 99307[1], 99308[1], 99309[1], 99310[1], 99315[1], 99316[1], 99334[1], 99335[1], 99336[1], 99337[1], 99347[1], 99348[1], 99349[1], 99350[1], 99374[1], 99375[1], 99377[1], 99378[1], 99446[0], 99447[0], 99448[0], 99449[0], 99451[0], 99452[0], 99495[0], 99496[0], G0463[1], G0471[1]
38570	0213T[0], 0216T[0], 0596T[1], 0597T[1], 0708T[1], 0709T[1], 10005[1], 10007[1], 10009[1], 10011[1], 10021[1], 12001[1], 12002[1], 12004[1], 12005[1], 12006[1], 12007[1], 12011[1], 12013[1], 12014[1], 12015[1], 12016[1], 12017[1], 12018[1], 12020[1], 12021[1], 12031[1], 12032[1], 12034[1], 12035[1], 12036[1], 12037[1], 12041[1], 12042[1], 12044[1], 12045[1], 12046[1], 12047[1], 12051[1], 12052[1], 12053[1], 12054[1], 12055[1], 12056[1], 12057[1], 13100[1], 13101[1], 13102[1], 13120[1], 13121[1], 13122[1], 13131[1], 13132[1], 13133[1], 13151[1], 13152[1], 13153[1], 36000[1], 36400[1], 36405[1], 36406[1], 36410[1], 36420[1], 36425[1], 36430[1], 36440[1], 36591[0], 36592[0], 36600[1], 36640[1], 38562[0], 43752[1], 44602[1], 44603[1], 44604[1], 44605[1], 44950[0], 44970[1], 49010[1], 49082[1], 49083[1], 49084[1], 49320[0], 49321[1], 49400[0], 51701[1], 51702[1], 51703[1], 57410[1], 62320[0], 62321[0], 62322[0], 62323[0], 62324[0], 62325[0], 62326[0], 62327[0], 64400[0], 64405[0], 64408[0], 64415[0], 64416[0], 64417[0], 64418[0], 64420[0], 64421[0], 64425[0], 64430[0], 64435[0], 64445[0], 64446[0], 64447[0], 64448[0], 64449[0], 64450[0], 64451[0], 64454[0], 64461[0], 64462[0], 64463[0], 64479[0], 64480[0], 64483[0], 64484[0], 64486[0], 64487[0], 64488[0], 64489[0], 64490[0], 64491[0], 64492[0], 64493[0], 64494[0], 64495[0], 64505[0], 64510[0], 64517[0], 64520[0], 64530[0], 69990[0], 76000[1], 77001[1], 77002[1], 92012[1], 92014[1], 93000[1], 93005[1], 93010[1], 93040[1], 93041[1], 93042[1], 93318[1], 93355[1], 94002[1], 94200[1], 94680[1], 94681[1], 94690[1], 95812[1], 95813[1], 95816[1], 95819[1], 95822[1], 95829[1], 95955[1], 96360[1], 96361[1], 96365[1], 96366[1], 96367[1], 96368[1], 96372[1], 96374[1], 96375[1], 96376[1], 96377[1], 96523[0], 99155[0], 99156[0], 99157[0], 99211[1], 99212[1], 99213[1], 99214[1], 99215[1], 99217[1], 99218[1], 99219[1], 99220[1], 99221[1], 99222[1], 99223[1], 99231[1], 99232[1], 99233[1], 99234[1], 99235[1], 99236[1], 99238[1], 99239[1], 99241[1], 99242[1], 99243[1], 99244[1], 99245[1], 99251[1], 99252[1], 99253[1], 99254[1], 99255[1], 99291[1], 99292[1], 99304[1], 99305[1], 99306[1], 99307[1], 99308[1], 99309[1], 99310[1], 99315[1], 99316[1], 99334[1], 99335[1], 99336[1], 99337[1], 99347[1], 99348[1], 99349[1], 99350[1], 99374[1], 99375[1], 99377[1], 99378[1], 99446[0], 99447[0], 99448[0], 99449[0], 99451[0], 99452[0], 99495[0], 99496[0], G0463[1], G0471[1]
38760	0213T[0], 0216T[0], 0596T[1], 0597T[1], 0708T[1], 0709T[1], 11000[1], 11001[1], 11004[1], 11005[1], 11006[1], 11042[1], 11043[1], 11044[1], 11045[1], 11046[1], 11047[1], 12001[1], 12002[1], 12004[1], 12005[1], 12006[1], 12007[1], 12011[1], 12013[1], 12014[1], 12015[1], 12016[1], 12017[1], 12018[1], 12020[1], 12021[1], 12031[1], 12032[1], 12034[1], 12035[1], 12036[1], 12037[1], 12041[1], 12042[1], 12044[1], 12045[1], 12046[1], 12047[1], 12051[1], 12052[1], 12053[1], 12054[1], 12055[1], 12056[1], 12057[1], 13100[1], 13101[1], 13102[1], 13120[1], 13121[1], 13122[1], 13131[1], 13132[1], 13133[1], 13151[1], 13152[1], 13153[1], 36000[1], 36400[1], 36405[1], 36406[1], 36410[1], 36420[1], 36425[1], 36430[1], 36440[1], 36591[0], 36592[0], 36600[1], 36640[1], 38500[1], 38531[0], 43752[1], 51701[1], 51702[1], 51703[1], 62320[0], 62321[0], 62322[0], 62323[0], 62324[0], 62325[0], 62326[0], 62327[0], 64400[0], 64405[0], 64408[0], 64415[0], 64416[0], 64417[0], 64418[0], 64420[0], 64421[0], 64425[0], 64430[0], 64435[0], 64445[0], 64446[0], 64447[0], 64448[0], 64449[0], 64450[0], 64451[0], 64454[0], 64461[0], 64462[0], 64463[0], 64479[0], 64480[0], 64483[0], 64484[0], 64486[0], 64487[0], 64488[0], 64489[0], 64490[0], 64491[0], 64492[0], 64493[0], 64494[0], 64495[0], 64505[0], 64510[0], 64517[0], 64520[0], 64530[0], 69990[0], 92012[1], 92014[1], 93000[1], 93005[1], 93010[1], 93040[1], 93041[1], 93042[1], 93318[1], 93355[1], 94002[1], 94200[1], 94680[1], 94681[1], 94690[1], 95812[1], 95813[1], 95816[1], 95819[1], 95822[1], 95829[1], 95955[1], 96360[1], 96361[1], 96365[1], 96366[1], 96367[1], 96368[1], 96372[1], 96374[1], 96375[1], 96376[1], 96377[1], 96523[0], 97597[1], 97598[1], 97602[1], 99155[0], 99156[0], 99157[0], 99211[1], 99212[1], 99213[1], 99214[1], 99215[1], 99217[1], 99218[1],

0 = Modifier usage not allowed or inappropriate 1 = Modifier usage allowed

Code 1	Code 2
	99219[1], 99220[1], 99221[1], 99222[1], 99223[1], 99231[1], 99232[1], 99233[1], 99234[1], 99235[1], 99236[1], 99238[1], 99239[1], 99241[1], 99242[1], 99243[1], 99244[1], 99245[1], 99251[1], 99252[1], 99253[1], 99254[1], 99255[1], 99291[1], 99292[1], 99304[1], 99305[1], 99306[1], 99307[1], 99308[1], 99309[1], 99310[1], 99315[1], 99316[1], 99334[1], 99335[1], 99336[1], 99337[1], 99347[1], 99348[1], 99349[1], 99350[1], 99374[1], 99375[1], 99377[1], 99378[1], 99446[0], 99447[0], 99448[0], 99449[0], 99451[0], 99452[0], 99495[0], 99496[0], G0463[1], G0471[1]
38765	0213T[0], 0216T[0], 0596T[1], 0597T[1], 0708T[1], 0709T[1], 11000[1], 11001[1], 11004[1], 11005[1], 11006[1], 11042[1], 11043[1], 11044[1], 11045[1], 11046[1], 11047[1], 12001[1], 12002[1], 12004[1], 12005[1], 12006[1], 12007[1], 12011[1], 12013[1], 12014[1], 12015[1], 12016[1], 12017[1], 12018[1], 12020[1], 12021[1], 12031[1], 12032[1], 12034[1], 12035[1], 12036[1], 12037[1], 12041[1], 12042[1], 12044[1], 12045[1], 12046[1], 12047[1], 12051[1], 12052[1], 12053[1], 12054[1], 12055[1], 12056[1], 12057[1], 13100[1], 13101[1], 13102[1], 13120[1], 13121[1], 13122[1], 13131[1], 13132[1], 13133[1], 13151[1], 13152[1], 13153[1], 36000[1], 36400[1], 36405[1], 36406[1], 36410[1], 36420[1], 36425[1], 36430[1], 36440[1], 36591[0], 36592[0], 36600[1], 36640[1], 38500[1], 38531[0], 38562[1], 38571[1], 38760[1], 38770[1], 43752[1], 51701[1], 51702[1], 51703[1], 52000[1], 62320[0], 62321[0], 62322[0], 62323[0], 62324[0], 62325[0], 62326[0], 62327[0], 64400[0], 64405[0], 64408[0], 64415[0], 64416[0], 64417[0], 64418[0], 64420[0], 64421[0], 64425[0], 64430[0], 64435[0], 64445[0], 64446[0], 64447[0], 64448[0], 64449[0], 64450[0], 64451[0], 64454[0], 64461[0], 64462[0], 64463[0], 64479[0], 64480[0], 64483[0], 64484[0], 64486[0], 64487[0], 64488[0], 64489[0], 64490[0], 64491[0], 64492[0], 64493[0], 64494[0], 64495[0], 64505[0], 64510[0], 64517[0], 64520[0], 64530[0], 69990[0], 92012[1], 92014[1], 93000[1], 93005[1], 93010[1], 93040[1], 93041[1], 93042[1], 93318[1], 93355[1], 94002[1], 94200[1], 94680[1], 94681[1], 94690[1], 95812[1], 95813[1], 95816[1], 95819[1], 95822[1], 95829[1], 95955[1], 96360[1], 96361[1], 96365[1], 96366[1], 96367[1], 96368[1], 96372[1], 96374[1], 96375[1], 96376[1], 96377[1], 96523[0], 97597[1], 97598[1], 97602[1], 99155[0], 99156[0], 99157[0], 99211[1], 99212[1], 99213[1], 99214[1], 99215[1], 99217[1], 99218[1], 99219[1], 99220[1], 99221[1], 99222[1], 99223[1], 99231[1], 99232[1], 99233[1], 99234[1], 99235[1], 99236[1], 99238[1], 99239[1], 99241[1], 99242[1], 99243[1], 99244[1], 99245[1], 99251[1], 99252[1], 99253[1], 99254[1], 99255[1], 99291[1], 99292[1], 99304[1], 99305[1], 99306[1], 99307[1], 99308[1], 99309[1], 99310[1], 99315[1], 99316[1], 99334[1], 99335[1], 99336[1], 99337[1], 99347[1], 99348[1], 99349[1], 99350[1], 99374[1], 99375[1], 99377[1], 99378[1], 99446[0], 99447[0], 99448[0], 99449[0], 99451[0], 99452[0], 99495[0], 99496[0], G0463[1], G0471[1], J0670[1], J2001[1]
38770	0213T[0], 0216T[0], 0596T[1], 0597T[1], 0708T[1], 0709T[1], 11000[1], 11001[1], 11004[1], 11005[1], 11006[1], 11042[1], 11043[1], 11044[1], 11045[1], 11046[1], 11047[1], 12001[1], 12002[1], 12004[1], 12005[1], 12006[1], 12007[1], 12011[1], 12013[1], 12014[1], 12015[1], 12016[1], 12017[1], 12018[1], 12020[1], 12021[1], 12031[1], 12032[1], 12034[1], 12035[1], 12036[1], 12037[1], 12041[1], 12042[1], 12044[1], 12045[1], 12046[1], 12047[1], 12051[1], 12052[1], 12053[1], 12054[1], 12055[1], 12056[1], 12057[1], 13100[1], 13101[1], 13102[1], 13120[1], 13121[1], 13122[1], 13131[1], 13132[1], 13133[1], 13151[1], 13152[1], 13153[1], 36000[1], 36400[1], 36405[1], 36406[1], 36410[1], 36420[1], 36425[1], 36430[1], 36440[1], 36591[0], 36592[0], 36600[1], 36640[1], 38500[1], 38531[1], 38562[1], 38564[0], 38571[0], 38760[1], 43752[1], 44005[0], 44180[0], 44602[1], 44603[1], 44604[1], 44605[1], 44820[0], 44850[0], 44950[0], 44970[0], 49000[0], 49002[1], 49010[0], 49320[1], 49321[1], 49570[0], 51701[1], 51702[1], 51703[1], 52000[1], 62320[0], 62321[0], 62322[0], 62323[0], 62324[0], 62325[0], 62326[0], 62327[0], 64400[0], 64405[0], 64408[0], 64415[0], 64416[0], 64417[0], 64418[0], 64420[0], 64421[0], 64425[0], 64430[0], 64435[0], 64445[0], 64446[0], 64447[0], 64448[0], 64449[0], 64450[0], 64451[0], 64454[0], 64461[0], 64462[0], 64463[0], 64479[0], 64480[0], 64483[0], 64484[0], 64486[0], 64487[0], 64488[0], 64489[0], 64490[0], 64491[0], 64492[0], 64493[0], 64494[0], 64495[0], 64505[0], 64510[0], 64517[0], 64520[0], 64530[0], 69990[0], 92012[1], 92014[1], 93000[1], 93005[1], 93010[1], 93040[1], 93041[1], 93042[1], 93318[1], 93355[1], 94002[1], 94200[1], 94680[1], 94681[1], 94690[1], 95812[1], 95813[1], 95816[1], 95819[1], 95822[1], 95829[1], 95955[1], 96360[1], 96361[1], 96365[1], 96366[1], 96367[1], 96368[1], 96372[1], 96374[1], 96375[1], 96376[1], 96377[1], 96523[0], 97597[1], 97598[1], 97602[1], 99155[0], 99156[0], 99157[0], 99211[1], 99212[1], 99213[1], 99214[1], 99215[1], 99217[1], 99218[1], 99219[1], 99220[1], 99221[1], 99222[1], 99223[1], 99231[1], 99232[1], 99233[1], 99234[1], 99235[1], 99236[1], 99238[1], 99239[1], 99241[1], 99242[1], 99243[1], 99244[1], 99245[1], 99251[1], 99252[1], 99253[1], 99254[1], 99255[1], 99291[1], 99292[1], 99304[1], 99305[1], 99306[1], 99307[1], 99308[1], 99309[1], 99310[1], 99315[1], 99316[1], 99334[1], 99335[1], 99336[1], 99337[1], 99347[1], 99348[1], 99349[1], 99350[1], 99374[1], 99375[1], 99377[1], 99378[1], 99446[0], 99447[0], 99448[0], 99449[0], 99451[0], 99452[0], 99495[0], 99496[0], G0463[1], G0471[1]
38780	0213T[0], 0216T[0], 0596T[1], 0597T[1], 0708T[1], 0709T[1], 11000[1], 11001[1], 11004[1], 11005[1], 11006[1], 11042[1], 11043[1], 11044[1], 11045[1], 11046[1], 11047[1], 12001[1], 12002[1], 12004[1], 12005[1], 12006[1], 12007[1], 12011[1], 12013[1], 12014[1], 12015[1], 12016[1], 12017[1], 12018[1], 12020[1], 12021[1], 12031[1], 12032[1], 12034[1], 12035[1], 12036[1], 12037[1], 12041[1], 12042[1], 12044[1], 12045[1], 12046[1], 12047[1], 12051[1], 12052[1], 12053[1], 12054[1], 12055[1], 12056[1], 12057[1], 13100[1], 13101[1], 13102[1], 13120[1], 13121[1], 13122[1], 13131[1], 13132[1], 13133[1], 13151[1], 13152[1], 13153[1], 36000[1], 36400[1], 36405[1], 36406[1], 36410[1], 36420[1], 36425[1], 36430[1], 36440[1], 36591[0], 36592[0], 36600[1], 36640[1], 38500[1], 38531[1], 38562[1], 38564[0], 38570[1], 38571[0], 38572[0], 38765[1], 38770[0], 43752[1], 44005[0], 44180[0], 44602[1], 44603[1], 44604[1], 44605[1], 44820[0], 44850[0], 44950[0], 44970[0], 49000[0], 49002[1], 49010[0], 49320[1], 49321[1], 49570[0], 51701[1], 51702[1], 51703[1], 52000[1], 62320[0], 62321[0], 62322[0], 62323[0], 62324[0], 62325[0], 62326[0], 62327[0], 64400[0], 64405[0], 64408[0], 64415[0], 64416[0], 64417[0], 64418[0], 64420[0], 64421[0], 64425[0], 64430[0], 64435[0], 64445[0], 64446[0], 64447[0], 64448[0], 64449[0], 64450[0], 64451[0], 64454[0], 64461[0], 64462[0], 64463[0], 64479[0], 64480[0], 64483[0], 64484[0], 64486[0], 64487[0], 64488[0], 64489[0], 64490[0], 64491[0], 64492[0], 64493[0], 64494[0], 64495[0], 64505[0], 64510[0], 64517[0], 64520[0], 64530[0], 69990[0], 92012[1], 92014[1], 93000[1], 93005[1], 93010[1], 93040[1], 93041[1], 93042[1], 93318[1], 93355[1], 94002[1], 94200[1], 94680[1], 94681[1], 94690[1], 95812[1], 95813[1], 95816[1], 95819[1], 95822[1], 95829[1], 95955[1], 96360[1], 96361[1], 96365[1], 96366[1], 96367[1], 96368[1], 96372[1], 96374[1], 96375[1], 96376[1], 96377[1], 96523[0], 97597[1], 97598[1], 97602[1], 99155[0], 99156[0], 99157[0], 99211[1], 99212[1], 99213[1], 99214[1], 99215[1], 99217[1], 99218[1], 99219[1], 99220[1], 99221[1], 99222[1], 99223[1], 99231[1], 99232[1], 99233[1], 99234[1], 99235[1], 99236[1], 99238[1], 99239[1], 99241[1], 99242[1], 99243[1], 99244[1], 99245[1], 99251[1], 99252[1], 99253[1], 99254[1], 99255[1], 99291[1], 99292[1], 99304[1], 99305[1], 99306[1], 99307[1], 99308[1], 99309[1], 99310[1], 99315[1], 99316[1], 99334[1], 99335[1], 99336[1], 99337[1], 99347[1], 99348[1], 99349[1], 99350[1], 99374[1], 99375[1], 99377[1], 99378[1], 99446[0], 99447[0], 99448[0], 99449[0], 99451[0], 99452[0], 99495[0], 99496[0], G0463[1], G0471[1]
44660	0213T[0], 0216T[0], 0596T[1], 0597T[1], 0708T[1], 0709T[1], 11000[1], 11001[1], 11004[1], 11005[1], 11006[1], 11042[1], 11043[1], 11044[1], 11045[1], 11046[1], 11047[1], 12001[1], 12002[1], 12004[1], 12005[1], 12006[1], 12007[1], 12011[1], 12013[1], 12014[1], 12015[1], 12016[1], 12017[1], 12018[1], 12020[1], 12021[1], 12031[1], 12032[1], 12034[1], 12035[1], 12036[1], 12037[1], 12041[1], 12042[1], 12044[1], 12045[1], 12046[1], 12047[1], 12051[1], 12052[1], 12053[1], 12054[1], 12055[1], 12056[1], 12057[1], 13100[1], 13101[1], 13102[1], 13120[1], 13121[1], 13122[1], 13131[1], 13132[1], 13133[1], 13151[1], 13152[1], 13153[1], 36000[1], 36400[1], 36405[1], 36406[1], 36410[1], 36420[1], 36425[1], 36430[1], 36440[1], 36591[0], 36592[0], 36600[1], 36640[1], 43752[1], 44005[0], 44120[1], 44140[1], 44141[1], 44143[1], 44144[1], 44145[1], 44146[1], 44147[1], 44150[0], 44151[0], 44155[0], 44156[0], 44157[0], 44158[0], 44160[1], 44180[0], 44500[1], 44602[1], 44603[1], 44604[1], 44605[1], 44661[1], 44701[1], 44820[0], 44850[0], 44950[0], 44970[0], 49000[0], 49002[1], 49010[0], 49255[0], 49320[1], 49560[1], 49561[1], 49565[1], 49566[1], 49570[0], 50715[1], 51550[1], 51555[1], 51565[1], 51701[1], 51702[1], 51703[1], 62320[0], 62321[0], 62322[0], 62323[0], 62324[0], 62325[0], 62326[0], 62327[0], 64400[0], 64405[0], 64408[0], 64415[0], 64416[0], 64417[0], 64418[0], 64420[0], 64421[0], 64425[0], 64430[0], 64435[0], 64445[0], 64446[0], 64447[0], 64448[0], 64449[0], 64450[0], 64451[0], 64454[0], 64461[0], 64462[0], 64463[0], 64479[0], 64480[0], 64483[0], 64484[0], 64486[0], 64487[0], 64488[0], 64489[0], 64490[0], 64491[0], 64492[0], 64493[0], 64494[0], 64495[0], 64505[0], 64510[0], 64517[0], 64520[0], 64530[0], 69990[0], 92012[1], 92014[1], 93000[1], 93005[1], 93010[1], 93040[1], 93041[1], 93042[1], 93318[1], 93355[1], 94002[1], 94200[1], 94680[1], 94681[1], 94690[1], 95812[1], 95813[1], 95816[1], 95819[1], 95822[1], 95829[1], 95955[1], 96360[1], 96361[1], 96365[1], 96366[1], 96367[1], 96368[1], 96372[1], 96374[1], 96375[1], 96376[1], 96377[1], 96523[0], 97597[1], 97598[1], 97602[1], 99155[0], 99156[0], 99157[0], 99211[1], 99212[1], 99213[1], 99214[1], 99215[1], 99217[1], 99218[1], 99219[1], 99220[1], 99221[1], 99222[1], 99223[1], 99231[1], 99232[1], 99233[1], 99234[1], 99235[1], 99236[1], 99238[1], 99239[1], 99241[1], 99242[1], 99243[1], 99244[1], 99245[1], 99251[1], 99252[1], 99253[1], 99254[1], 99255[1], 99291[1], 99292[1], 99304[1], 99305[1], 99306[1], 99307[1], 99308[1], 99309[1], 99310[1], 99315[1], 99316[1], 99334[1], 99335[1], 99336[1], 99337[1], 99347[1], 99348[1], 99349[1], 99350[1], 99374[1], 99375[1], 99377[1], 99378[1], 99446[0], 99447[0], 99448[0], 99449[0], 99451[0], 99452[0], 99495[0], 99496[0], G0463[1], G0471[1]
44661	0213T[0], 0216T[0], 0596T[1], 0597T[1], 0708T[1], 0709T[1], 11000[1], 11001[1], 11004[1], 11005[1], 11006[1], 11042[1], 11043[1], 11044[1], 11045[1], 11046[1], 11047[1], 12001[1], 12002[1], 12004[1], 12005[1], 12006[1], 12007[1], 12011[1], 12013[1], 12014[1], 12015[1], 12016[1], 12017[1], 12018[1], 12020[1], 12021[1], 12031[1], 12032[1], 12034[1], 12035[1], 12036[1], 12037[1], 12041[1], 12042[1], 12044[1], 12045[1], 12046[1], 12047[1], 12051[1], 12052[1], 12053[1], 12054[1], 12055[1], 12056[1], 12057[1], 13100[1], 13101[1], 13102[1], 13120[1], 13121[1], 13122[1], 13131[1], 13132[1], 13133[1], 13151[1], 13152[1], 13153[1], 36000[1], 36400[1], 36405[1], 36406[1], 36410[1], 36420[1], 36425[1], 36430[1], 36440[1], 36591[0], 36592[0], 36600[1], 36640[1], 43752[1], 44005[0], 44021[1], 44120[1], 44140[1], 44141[1], 44143[1], 44144[1], 44145[1], 44146[1], 44147[1], 44150[0], 44151[0], 44155[0], 44156[0], 44157[0], 44158[0], 44160[1], 44180[0], 44500[1], 44602[1], 44603[1], 44604[1], 44605[1], 44620[1], 44701[1], 44820[0], 44850[0], 44950[0], 44970[0], 45380[1], 49000[0], 49002[1], 49010[0], 49020[1], 49040[1], 49060[1], 49255[0], 49320[1], 49560[1], 49561[1], 49565[1], 49566[1], 49570[0], 49572[1], 49585[1], 49587[1], 51550[1], 51555[1], 51565[1], 51701[1], 51702[1], 51703[1], 62320[0], 62321[0], 62322[0], 62323[0], 62324[0], 62325[0], 62326[0], 62327[0], 64400[0], 64405[0], 64408[0], 64415[0], 64416[0], 64417[0], 64418[0], 64420[0], 64421[0], 64425[0], 64430[0], 64435[0], 64445[0], 64446[0], 64447[0], 64448[0], 64449[0], 64450[0], 64451[0], 64454[0], 64461[0], 64462[0], 64463[0], 64479[0], 64480[0], 64483[0], 64484[0], 64486[0], 64487[0], 64488[0], 64489[0], 64490[0], 64491[0], 64492[0], 64493[0], 64494[0], 64495[0], 64505[0], 64510[0], 64517[0], 64520[0], 64530[0], 69990[0], 92012[1], 92014[1], 93000[1], 93005[1], 93010[1], 93040[1], 93041[1], 93042[1], 93318[1], 93355[1], 94002[1], 94200[1], 94680[1], 94681[1], 94690[1], 95812[1], 95813[1], 95816[1], 95819[1], 95822[1],

0 = Modifier usage not allowed or inappropriate 1 = Modifier usage allowed

Code 1	Code 2
	95829[1], 95955[1], 96360[1], 96361[1], 96365[1], 96366[1], 96367[1], 96368[1], 96372[1], 96374[1], 96375[1], 96376[1], 96377[1], 96523[0], 97597[1], 97598[1], 97602[1], 99155[0], 99156[0], 99157[0], 99211[1], 99212[1], 99213[1], 99214[1], 99215[1], 99217[1], 99218[1], 99219[1], 99220[1], 99221[1], 99222[1], 99223[1], 99231[1], 99232[1], 99233[1], 99234[1], 99235[1], 99236[1], 99238[1], 99239[1], 99241[1], 99242[1], 99243[1], 99244[1], 99245[1], 99251[1], 99252[1], 99253[1], 99254[1], 99255[1], 99291[1], 99292[1], 99304[1], 99305[1], 99306[1], 99307[1], 99308[1], 99309[1], 99310[1], 99315[1], 99316[1], 99334[1], 99335[1], 99336[1], 99337[1], 99347[1], 99348[1], 99349[1], 99350[1], 99374[1], 99375[1], 99377[1], 99378[1], 99446[0], 99447[0], 99448[0], 99449[0], 99451[0], 99452[0], 99495[0], 99496[0], G0463[1], G0471[1]
49000	0213T[0], 0216T[0], 0596T[1], 0597T[1], 0708T[1], 0709T[1], 10005[1], 10007[1], 10009[1], 10011[1], 10021[1], 11000[1], 11001[1], 11004[1], 11005[1], 11006[1], 11042[1], 11043[1], 11044[1], 11045[1], 11046[1], 11047[1], 12001[1], 12002[1], 12004[1], 12005[1], 12006[1], 12007[1], 12011[1], 12013[1], 12014[1], 12015[1], 12016[1], 12017[1], 12018[1], 12020[1], 12021[1], 12031[1], 12032[1], 12034[1], 12035[1], 12036[1], 12037[1], 12041[1], 12042[1], 12044[1], 12045[1], 12046[1], 12047[1], 12051[1], 12052[1], 12053[1], 12054[1], 12055[1], 12056[1], 12057[1], 13100[1], 13101[1], 13102[1], 13120[1], 13121[1], 13122[1], 13131[1], 13132[1], 13133[1], 13151[1], 13152[1], 13153[1], 20102[1], 36000[1], 36400[1], 36405[1], 36406[1], 36410[1], 36420[1], 36425[1], 36430[1], 36440[1], 36591[0], 36592[0], 36600[1], 36640[1], 43752[1], 44015[0], 44180[0], 44950[0], 44970[0], 49013[1], 49014[1], 49255[0], 51701[1], 51702[1], 51703[1], 57410[0], 62320[0], 62321[0], 62322[0], 62323[0], 62324[0], 62325[0], 62326[0], 62327[0], 64400[0], 64405[0], 64408[0], 64415[0], 64416[0], 64417[0], 64418[0], 64420[0], 64421[0], 64425[0], 64430[0], 64435[0], 64445[0], 64446[0], 64447[0], 64448[0], 64449[0], 64450[0], 64451[0], 64454[0], 64461[0], 64462[0], 64463[0], 64479[0], 64480[0], 64483[0], 64484[0], 64486[0], 64487[0], 64488[0], 64489[0], 64490[0], 64491[0], 64492[0], 64493[0], 64494[0], 64495[0], 64505[0], 64510[0], 64517[0], 64520[0], 64530[0], 69990[0], 92012[1], 92014[1], 93000[1], 93005[1], 93010[1], 93040[1], 93041[1], 93042[1], 93318[1], 93355[1], 94002[1], 94200[1], 94680[1], 94681[1], 94690[1], 95812[1], 95813[1], 95816[1], 95819[1], 95822[1], 95829[1], 95955[1], 96360[1], 96361[1], 96365[1], 96366[1], 96367[1], 96368[1], 96372[1], 96374[1], 96375[1], 96376[1], 96377[1], 96523[0], 97597[1], 97598[1], 97602[1], 99155[0], 99156[0], 99157[0], 99211[1], 99212[1], 99213[1], 99214[1], 99215[1], 99217[1], 99218[1], 99219[1], 99220[1], 99221[1], 99222[1], 99223[1], 99231[1], 99232[1], 99233[1], 99234[1], 99235[1], 99236[1], 99238[1], 99239[1], 99241[1], 99242[1], 99243[1], 99244[1], 99245[1], 99251[1], 99252[1], 99253[1], 99254[1], 99255[1], 99291[1], 99292[1], 99304[1], 99305[1], 99306[1], 99307[1], 99308[1], 99309[1], 99310[1], 99315[1], 99316[1], 99334[1], 99335[1], 99336[1], 99337[1], 99347[1], 99348[1], 99349[1], 99350[1], 99374[1], 99375[1], 99377[1], 99378[1], 99446[0], 99447[0], 99448[0], 99449[0], 99451[0], 99452[0], 99495[0], 99496[0], G0463[1], G0471[1]
49002	0213T[0], 0216T[0], 0596T[1], 0597T[1], 0708T[1], 0709T[1], 11000[1], 11001[1], 11004[1], 11005[1], 11006[1], 11042[1], 11043[1], 11044[1], 11045[1], 11046[1], 11047[1], 12001[1], 12002[1], 12004[1], 12005[1], 12006[1], 12007[1], 12011[1], 12013[1], 12014[1], 12015[1], 12016[1], 12017[1], 12018[1], 12020[1], 12021[1], 12031[1], 12032[1], 12034[1], 12035[1], 12036[1], 12037[1], 12041[1], 12042[1], 12044[1], 12045[1], 12046[1], 12047[1], 12051[1], 12052[1], 12053[1], 12054[1], 12055[1], 12056[1], 12057[1], 13100[1], 13101[1], 13102[1], 13120[1], 13121[1], 13122[1], 13131[1], 13132[1], 13133[1], 13151[1], 13152[1], 13153[1], 20102[1], 36000[1], 36400[1], 36405[1], 36406[1], 36410[1], 36420[1], 36425[1], 36430[1], 36440[1], 36591[0], 36592[0], 36600[1], 36640[1], 43752[1], 44005[0], 44180[0], 44820[0], 44850[0], 44950[0], 44970[0], 49000[0], 49010[0], 49013[1], 49014[1], 49255[0], 49570[1], 51701[1], 51702[1], 51703[1], 62320[0], 62321[0], 62322[0], 62323[0], 62324[0], 62325[0], 62326[0], 62327[0], 64400[0], 64405[0], 64408[0], 64415[0], 64416[0], 64417[0], 64418[0], 64420[0], 64421[0], 64425[0], 64430[0], 64435[0], 64445[0], 64446[0], 64447[0], 64448[0], 64449[0], 64450[0], 64451[0], 64454[0], 64461[0], 64462[0], 64463[0], 64479[0], 64480[0], 64483[0], 64484[0], 64486[0], 64487[0], 64488[0], 64489[0], 64490[0], 64491[0], 64492[0], 64493[0], 64494[0], 64495[0], 64505[0], 64510[0], 64517[0], 64520[0], 64530[0], 69990[0], 92012[1], 92014[1], 93000[1], 93005[1], 93010[1], 93040[1], 93041[1], 93042[1], 93318[1], 93355[1], 94002[1], 94200[1], 94680[1], 94681[1], 94690[1], 95812[1], 95813[1], 95816[1], 95819[1], 95822[1], 95829[1], 95955[1], 96360[1], 96361[1], 96365[1], 96366[1], 96367[1], 96368[1], 96372[1], 96374[1], 96375[1], 96376[1], 96377[1], 96523[0], 97597[1], 97598[1], 97602[1], 99155[0], 99156[0], 99157[0], 99211[1], 99212[1], 99213[1], 99214[1], 99215[1], 99217[1], 99218[1], 99219[1], 99220[1], 99221[1], 99222[1], 99223[1], 99231[1], 99232[1], 99233[1], 99234[1], 99235[1], 99236[1], 99238[1], 99239[1], 99241[1], 99242[1], 99243[1], 99244[1], 99245[1], 99251[1], 99252[1], 99253[1], 99254[1], 99255[1], 99291[1], 99292[1], 99304[1], 99305[1], 99306[1], 99307[1], 99308[1], 99309[1], 99310[1], 99315[1], 99316[1], 99334[1], 99335[1], 99336[1], 99337[1], 99347[1], 99348[1], 99349[1], 99350[1], 99374[1], 99375[1], 99377[1], 99378[1], 99446[0], 99447[0], 99448[0], 99449[0], 99451[0], 99452[0], 99495[0], 99496[0], G0463[1], G0471[1]
49010	0213T[0], 0216T[0], 0596T[1], 0597T[1], 0708T[1], 0709T[1], 10005[1], 10007[1], 10009[1], 10011[1], 10021[1], 12001[1], 12002[1], 12004[1], 12005[1], 12006[1], 12007[1], 12011[1], 12013[1], 12014[1], 12015[1], 12016[1], 12017[1], 12018[1], 12020[1], 12021[1], 12031[1], 12032[1], 12034[1], 12035[1], 12036[1], 12037[1], 12041[1], 12042[1], 12044[1], 12045[1], 12046[1], 12047[1], 12051[1], 12052[1], 12053[1], 12054[1], 12055[1], 12056[1], 12057[1], 13100[1], 13101[1], 13102[1], 13120[1], 13121[1], 13122[1], 13131[1], 13132[1], 13133[1], 13151[1], 13152[1], 13153[1], 20102[1], 36000[1], 36400[1], 36405[1], 36406[1], 36410[1], 36420[1], 36425[1], 36430[1], 36440[1], 36591[0], 36592[0], 36600[1], 36640[1], 43752[1], 44180[0], 44950[0], 44970[0], 49000[0], 49013[1], 49014[1], 49255[0], 49320[1], 51701[1], 51702[1], 51703[1], 62320[0], 62321[0], 62322[0], 62323[0], 62324[0], 62325[0], 62326[0], 62327[0], 64400[0], 64405[0], 64408[0], 64415[0], 64416[0], 64417[0], 64418[0], 64420[0], 64421[0], 64425[0], 64430[0], 64435[0], 64445[0], 64446[0], 64447[0], 64448[0], 64449[0], 64450[0], 64451[0], 64454[0], 64461[0], 64462[0], 64463[0], 64479[0], 64480[0], 64483[0], 64484[0], 64486[0], 64487[0], 64488[0], 64489[0], 64490[0], 64491[0], 64492[0], 64493[0], 64494[0], 64495[0], 64505[0], 64510[0], 64517[0], 64520[0], 64530[0], 69990[0], 92012[1], 92014[1], 93000[1], 93005[1], 93010[1], 93040[1], 93041[1], 93042[1], 93318[1], 93355[1], 94002[1], 94200[1], 94680[1], 94681[1], 94690[1], 95812[1], 95813[1], 95816[1], 95819[1], 95822[1], 95829[1], 95955[1], 96360[1], 96361[1], 96365[1], 96366[1], 96367[1], 96368[1], 96372[1], 96374[1], 96375[1], 96376[1], 96377[1], 96523[0], 99155[0], 99156[0], 99157[0], 99211[1], 99212[1], 99213[1], 99214[1], 99215[1], 99217[1], 99218[1], 99219[1], 99220[1], 99221[1], 99222[1], 99223[1], 99231[1], 99232[1], 99233[1], 99234[1], 99235[1], 99236[1], 99238[1], 99239[1], 99241[1], 99242[1], 99243[1], 99244[1], 99245[1], 99251[1], 99252[1], 99253[1], 99254[1], 99255[1], 99291[1], 99292[1], 99304[1], 99305[1], 99306[1], 99307[1], 99308[1], 99309[1], 99310[1], 99315[1], 99316[1], 99334[1], 99335[1], 99336[1], 99337[1], 99347[1], 99348[1], 99349[1], 99350[1], 99374[1], 99375[1], 99377[1], 99378[1], 99446[0], 99447[0], 99448[0], 99449[0], 99451[0], 99452[0], 99495[0], 99496[0], G0463[1], G0471[1]
49020	0213T[0], 0216T[0], 0596T[1], 0597T[1], 0708T[1], 0709T[1], 12001[1], 12002[1], 12004[1], 12005[1], 12006[1], 12007[1], 12011[1], 12013[1], 12014[1], 12015[1], 12016[1], 12017[1], 12018[1], 12020[1], 12021[1], 12031[1], 12032[1], 12034[1], 12035[1], 12036[1], 12037[1], 12041[1], 12042[1], 12044[1], 12045[1], 12046[1], 12047[1], 12051[1], 12052[1], 12053[1], 12054[1], 12055[1], 12056[1], 12057[1], 13100[1], 13101[1], 13102[1], 13120[1], 13121[1], 13122[1], 13131[1], 13132[1], 13133[1], 13151[1], 13152[1], 13153[1], 20102[1], 36000[1], 36400[1], 36405[1], 36406[1], 36410[1], 36420[1], 36425[1], 36430[1], 36440[1], 36591[0], 36592[0], 36600[1], 36640[1], 43752[1], 44005[0], 44180[0], 44602[1], 44603[1], 44604[1], 44605[1], 44820[0], 44850[0], 44950[0], 44970[0], 49000[0], 49002[1], 49010[0], 49013[1], 49014[1], 49185[1], 49203[1], 49204[1], 49255[0], 49320[1], 49402[1], 49406[1], 49407[1], 49424[1], 49570[1], 51701[1], 51702[1], 51703[1], 62320[0], 62321[0], 62322[0], 62323[0], 62324[0], 62325[0], 62326[0], 62327[0], 64400[0], 64405[0], 64408[0], 64415[0], 64416[0], 64417[0], 64418[0], 64420[0], 64421[0], 64425[0], 64430[0], 64435[0], 64445[0], 64446[0], 64447[0], 64448[0], 64449[0], 64450[0], 64451[0], 64454[0], 64461[0], 64462[0], 64463[0], 64479[0], 64480[0], 64483[0], 64484[0], 64486[0], 64487[0], 64488[0], 64489[0], 64490[0], 64491[0], 64492[0], 64493[0], 64494[0], 64495[0], 64505[0], 64510[0], 64517[0], 64520[0], 64530[0], 69990[0], 76000[1], 77001[1], 77002[1], 92012[1], 92014[1], 93000[1], 93005[1], 93010[1], 93040[1], 93041[1], 93042[1], 93318[1], 93355[1], 94002[1], 94200[1], 94680[1], 94681[1], 94690[1], 95812[1], 95813[1], 95816[1], 95819[1], 95822[1], 95829[1], 95955[1], 96360[1], 96361[1], 96365[1], 96366[1], 96367[1], 96368[1], 96372[1], 96374[1], 96375[1], 96376[1], 96377[1], 96523[0], 99155[0], 99156[0], 99157[0], 99211[1], 99212[1], 99213[1], 99214[1], 99215[1], 99217[1], 99218[1], 99219[1], 99220[1], 99221[1], 99222[1], 99223[1], 99231[1], 99232[1], 99233[1], 99234[1], 99235[1], 99236[1], 99238[1], 99239[1], 99241[1], 99242[1], 99243[1], 99244[1], 99245[1], 99251[1], 99252[1], 99253[1], 99254[1], 99255[1], 99291[1], 99292[1], 99304[1], 99305[1], 99306[1], 99307[1], 99308[1], 99309[1], 99310[1], 99315[1], 99316[1], 99334[1], 99335[1], 99336[1], 99337[1], 99347[1], 99348[1], 99349[1], 99350[1], 99374[1], 99375[1], 99377[1], 99378[1], 99446[0], 99447[0], 99448[0], 99449[0], 99451[0], 99452[0], 99495[0], 99496[0], G0463[1], G0471[1]
49060	0213T[0], 0216T[0], 0596T[1], 0597T[1], 0708T[1], 0709T[1], 12001[1], 12002[1], 12004[1], 12005[1], 12006[1], 12007[1], 12011[1], 12013[1], 12014[1], 12015[1], 12016[1], 12017[1], 12018[1], 12020[1], 12021[1], 12031[1], 12032[1], 12034[1], 12035[1], 12036[1], 12037[1], 12041[1], 12042[1], 12044[1], 12045[1], 12046[1], 12047[1], 12051[1], 12052[1], 12053[1], 12054[1], 12055[1], 12056[1], 12057[1], 13100[1], 13101[1], 13102[1], 13120[1], 13121[1], 13122[1], 13131[1], 13132[1], 13133[1], 13151[1], 13152[1], 13153[1], 20102[1], 36000[1], 36400[1], 36405[1], 36406[1], 36410[1], 36420[1], 36425[1], 36430[1], 36440[1], 36591[0], 36592[0], 36600[1], 36640[1], 43752[1], 44005[0], 44180[0], 44602[1], 44603[1], 44604[1], 44605[1], 44820[0], 44850[0], 44950[0], 44970[0], 49000[0], 49002[1], 49010[0], 49013[1], 49014[1], 49020[1], 49185[1], 49255[0], 49320[1], 49406[1], 49407[1], 49423[1], 49424[1], 49570[0], 51701[1], 51702[1], 51703[1], 60540[1], 60545[1], 62320[0], 62321[0], 62322[0], 62323[0], 62324[0], 62325[0], 62326[0], 62327[0], 64400[0], 64405[0], 64408[0], 64415[0], 64416[0], 64417[0], 64418[0], 64420[0], 64421[0], 64425[0], 64430[0], 64435[0], 64445[0], 64446[0], 64447[0], 64448[0], 64449[0], 64450[0], 64451[0], 64454[0], 64461[0], 64462[0], 64463[0], 64479[0], 64480[0], 64483[0], 64484[0], 64486[0], 64487[0], 64488[0], 64489[0], 64490[0], 64491[0], 64492[0], 64493[0], 64494[0], 64495[0], 64505[0], 64510[0], 64517[0], 64520[0], 64530[0], 69990[0], 92012[1], 92014[1], 93000[1], 93005[1], 93010[1], 93040[1], 93041[1], 93042[1], 93318[1], 93355[1], 94002[1], 94200[1], 94680[1], 94681[1], 94690[1], 95812[1], 95813[1], 95816[1], 95819[1], 95822[1], 95829[1], 95955[1], 96360[1], 96361[1], 96365[1], 96366[1], 96367[1], 96368[1], 96372[1], 96374[1], 96375[1], 96376[1], 96377[1], 96523[0], 99155[0], 99156[0], 99157[0], 99211[1], 99212[1], 99213[1], 99214[1], 99215[1], 99217[1], 99218[1], 99219[1], 99220[1], 99221[1], 99222[1], 99223[1], 99231[1], 99232[1], 99233[1], 99234[1], 99235[1], 99236[1], 99238[1], 99239[1], 99241[1], 99242[1], 99243[1], 99244[1], 99245[1], 99251[1], 99252[1], 99253[1], 99254[1], 99255[1], 99291[1], 99292[1], 99304[1], 99305[1], 99306[1], 99307[1], 99308[1], 99309[1], 99310[1], 99315[1], 99316[1], 99334[1], 99335[1], 99336[1], 99337[1], 99347[1],

0 = Modifier usage not allowed or inappropriate 1 = Modifier usage allowed

Code 1	Code 2
	99348[1], 99349[1], 99350[1], 99374[1], 99375[1], 99377[1], 99378[1], 99446[0], 99447[0], 99448[0], 99449[0], 99451[0], 99452[0], 99495[0], 99496[0], G0463[1], G0471[1]
49082	0213T[0], 0216T[0], 0596T[1], 0597T[1], 0708T[1], 0709T[1], 12001[1], 12002[1], 12004[1], 12005[1], 12006[1], 12007[1], 12011[1], 12013[1], 12014[1], 12015[1], 12016[1], 12017[1], 12018[1], 12020[1], 12021[1], 12031[1], 12032[1], 12034[1], 12035[1], 12036[1], 12037[1], 12041[1], 12042[1], 12044[1], 12045[1], 12046[1], 12047[1], 12051[1], 12052[1], 12053[1], 12054[1], 12055[1], 12056[1], 12057[1], 13100[1], 13101[1], 13102[1], 13120[1], 13121[1], 13122[1], 13131[1], 13132[1], 13133[1], 13151[1], 13152[1], 13153[1], 20102[1], 36000[1], 36400[1], 36405[1], 36406[1], 36410[1], 36420[1], 36425[1], 36430[1], 36440[1], 36591[0], 36592[0], 36600[1], 36640[1], 43752[1], 49013[1], 49014[1], 51701[1], 51702[1], 51703[1], 62320[0], 62321[0], 62322[0], 62323[0], 62324[0], 62325[0], 62326[0], 62327[0], 64400[0], 64405[0], 64408[0], 64415[0], 64416[0], 64417[0], 64418[0], 64420[0], 64421[0], 64425[0], 64430[0], 64435[0], 64445[0], 64446[0], 64447[0], 64448[0], 64449[0], 64450[0], 64451[0], 64454[0], 64461[0], 64462[0], 64463[0], 64479[0], 64480[0], 64483[0], 64484[0], 64486[0], 64487[0], 64488[0], 64489[0], 64490[0], 64491[0], 64492[0], 64493[0], 64494[0], 64495[0], 64505[0], 64510[0], 64517[0], 64520[0], 64530[0], 69990[0], 76000[1], 76380[1], 76942[1], 76998[1], 77001[1], 77002[1], 77012[1], 77021[1], 92012[1], 92014[1], 93000[1], 93005[1], 93010[1], 93040[1], 93041[1], 93042[1], 93318[1], 93355[1], 94002[1], 94200[1], 94680[1], 94681[1], 94690[1], 95812[1], 95813[1], 95816[1], 95819[1], 95822[1], 95829[1], 95955[1], 96360[1], 96361[1], 96365[1], 96366[1], 96367[1], 96368[1], 96372[1], 96374[1], 96375[1], 96376[1], 96377[1], 96523[0], 99155[0], 99156[0], 99157[0], 99211[1], 99212[1], 99213[1], 99214[1], 99215[1], 99217[1], 99218[1], 99219[1], 99220[1], 99221[1], 99222[1], 99223[1], 99231[1], 99232[1], 99233[1], 99234[1], 99235[1], 99236[1], 99238[1], 99239[1], 99241[1], 99242[1], 99243[1], 99244[1], 99245[1], 99251[1], 99252[1], 99253[1], 99254[1], 99255[1], 99291[1], 99292[1], 99304[1], 99305[1], 99306[1], 99307[1], 99308[1], 99309[1], 99310[1], 99315[1], 99316[1], 99334[1], 99335[1], 99336[1], 99337[1], 99347[1], 99348[1], 99349[1], 99350[1], 99374[1], 99375[1], 99377[1], 99378[1], 99446[0], 99447[0], 99448[0], 99449[0], 99451[0], 99452[0], 99495[1], 99496[1], G0463[1], G0471[1]
49083	0213T[0], 0216T[0], 0596T[1], 0597T[1], 0708T[1], 0709T[1], 12001[1], 12002[1], 12004[1], 12005[1], 12006[1], 12007[1], 12011[1], 12013[1], 12014[1], 12015[1], 12016[1], 12017[1], 12018[1], 12020[1], 12021[1], 12031[1], 12032[1], 12034[1], 12035[1], 12036[1], 12037[1], 12041[1], 12042[1], 12044[1], 12045[1], 12046[1], 12047[1], 12051[1], 12052[1], 12053[1], 12054[1], 12055[1], 12056[1], 12057[1], 13100[1], 13101[1], 13102[1], 13120[1], 13121[1], 13122[1], 13131[1], 13132[1], 13133[1], 13151[1], 13152[1], 13153[1], 20102[1], 36000[1], 36400[1], 36405[1], 36406[1], 36410[1], 36420[1], 36425[1], 36430[1], 36440[1], 36591[0], 36592[0], 36600[1], 36640[1], 43752[1], 49013[1], 49014[1], 49082[0], 51701[1], 51702[1], 51703[1], 62320[0], 62321[0], 62322[0], 62323[0], 62324[0], 62325[0], 62326[0], 62327[0], 64400[0], 64405[0], 64408[0], 64415[0], 64416[0], 64417[0], 64418[0], 64420[0], 64421[0], 64425[0], 64430[0], 64435[0], 64445[0], 64446[0], 64447[0], 64448[0], 64449[0], 64450[0], 64451[0], 64454[0], 64461[0], 64462[0], 64463[0], 64479[0], 64480[0], 64483[0], 64484[0], 64486[0], 64487[0], 64488[0], 64489[0], 64490[0], 64491[0], 64492[0], 64493[0], 64494[0], 64495[0], 64505[0], 64510[0], 64517[0], 64520[0], 64530[0], 69990[0], 76000[1], 76380[1], 76942[1], 76998[1], 77001[1], 77002[1], 77012[1], 77021[1], 92012[1], 92014[1], 93000[1], 93005[1], 93010[1], 93040[1], 93041[1], 93042[1], 93318[1], 93355[1], 94002[1], 94200[1], 94680[1], 94681[1], 94690[1], 95812[1], 95813[1], 95816[1], 95819[1], 95822[1], 95829[1], 95955[1], 96360[1], 96361[1], 96365[1], 96366[1], 96367[1], 96368[1], 96372[1], 96374[1], 96375[1], 96376[1], 96377[1], 96523[0], 99155[0], 99156[0], 99157[0], 99211[1], 99212[1], 99213[1], 99214[1], 99215[1], 99217[1], 99218[1], 99219[1], 99220[1], 99221[1], 99222[1], 99223[1], 99231[1], 99232[1], 99233[1], 99234[1], 99235[1], 99236[1], 99238[1], 99239[1], 99241[1], 99242[1], 99243[1], 99244[1], 99245[1], 99251[1], 99252[1], 99253[1], 99254[1], 99255[1], 99291[1], 99292[1], 99304[1], 99305[1], 99306[1], 99307[1], 99308[1], 99309[1], 99310[1], 99315[1], 99316[1], 99334[1], 99335[1], 99336[1], 99337[1], 99347[1], 99348[1], 99349[1], 99350[1], 99374[1], 99375[1], 99377[1], 99378[1], 99446[0], 99447[0], 99448[0], 99449[0], 99451[0], 99452[0], 99495[1], 99496[1], G0463[1], G0471[1]
49084	0213T[0], 0216T[0], 0596T[1], 0597T[1], 0708T[1], 0709T[1], 12001[1], 12002[1], 12004[1], 12005[1], 12006[1], 12007[1], 12011[1], 12013[1], 12014[1], 12015[1], 12016[1], 12017[1], 12018[1], 12020[1], 12021[1], 12031[1], 12032[1], 12034[1], 12035[1], 12036[1], 12037[1], 12041[1], 12042[1], 12044[1], 12045[1], 12046[1], 12047[1], 12051[1], 12052[1], 12053[1], 12054[1], 12055[1], 12056[1], 12057[1], 13100[1], 13101[1], 13102[1], 13120[1], 13121[1], 13122[1], 13131[1], 13132[1], 13133[1], 13151[1], 13152[1], 13153[1], 20102[1], 36000[1], 36400[1], 36405[1], 36406[1], 36410[1], 36420[1], 36425[1], 36430[1], 36440[1], 36591[0], 36592[0], 36600[1], 36640[1], 43752[1], 49013[1], 49014[1], 49082[0], 49083[0], 51701[1], 51702[1], 51703[1], 62320[0], 62321[0], 62322[0], 62323[0], 62324[0], 62325[0], 62326[0], 62327[0], 64400[0], 64405[0], 64408[0], 64415[0], 64416[0], 64417[0], 64418[0], 64420[0], 64421[0], 64425[0], 64430[0], 64435[0], 64445[0], 64446[0], 64447[0], 64448[0], 64449[0], 64450[0], 64451[0], 64454[0], 64461[0], 64462[0], 64463[0], 64479[0], 64480[0], 64483[0], 64484[0], 64486[0], 64487[0], 64488[0], 64489[0], 64490[0], 64491[0], 64492[0], 64493[0], 64494[0], 64495[0], 64505[0], 64510[0], 64517[0], 64520[0], 64530[0], 69990[0], 76000[1], 76380[1], 76942[1], 76998[1], 77001[1], 77002[1], 77012[1], 77021[1], 92012[1], 92014[1], 93000[1], 93005[1], 93010[1], 93040[1], 93041[1], 93042[1], 93318[1], 93355[1], 94002[1], 94200[1], 94680[1], 94681[1], 94690[1], 95812[1], 95813[1], 95816[1], 95819[1], 95822[1], 95829[1], 95955[1], 96360[1], 96361[1], 96365[1], 96366[1], 96367[1], 96368[1], 96372[1], 96374[1], 96375[1], 96376[1], 96377[1], 96523[0], 99155[0], 99156[0], 99157[0], 99211[1], 99212[1], 99213[1], 99214[1], 99215[1], 99217[1], 99218[1], 99219[1], 99220[1], 99221[1], 99222[1], 99223[1], 99231[1], 99232[1], 99233[1], 99234[1], 99235[1], 99236[1], 99238[1], 99239[1], 99241[1], 99242[1], 99243[1], 99244[1], 99245[1], 99251[1], 99252[1], 99253[1], 99254[1], 99255[1], 99291[1], 99292[1], 99304[1], 99305[1], 99306[1], 99307[1], 99308[1], 99309[1], 99310[1], 99315[1], 99316[1], 99334[1], 99335[1], 99336[1], 99337[1], 99347[1], 99348[1], 99349[1], 99350[1], 99374[1], 99375[1], 99377[1], 99378[1], 99446[0], 99447[0], 99448[0], 99449[0], 99451[0], 99452[0], 99495[1], 99496[1], G0463[1], G0471[1]
49180	0213T[0], 0216T[0], 0596T[1], 0597T[1], 0708T[1], 0709T[1], 10005[1], 10007[1], 10009[1], 10011[1], 10021[1], 12001[1], 12002[1], 12004[1], 12005[1], 12006[1], 12007[1], 12011[1], 12013[1], 12014[1], 12015[1], 12016[1], 12017[1], 12018[1], 12020[1], 12021[1], 12031[1], 12032[1], 12034[1], 12035[1], 12036[1], 12037[1], 12041[1], 12042[1], 12044[1], 12045[1], 12046[1], 12047[1], 12051[1], 12052[1], 12053[1], 12054[1], 12055[1], 12056[1], 12057[1], 13100[1], 13101[1], 13102[1], 13120[1], 13121[1], 13122[1], 13131[1], 13132[1], 13133[1], 13151[1], 13152[1], 13153[1], 36000[1], 36400[1], 36405[1], 36406[1], 36410[1], 36420[1], 36425[1], 36430[1], 36440[1], 36591[0], 36592[0], 36600[1], 36640[1], 43752[1], 44950[0], 44970[0], 51701[1], 51702[1], 51703[1], 62320[0], 62321[0], 62322[0], 62323[0], 62324[0], 62325[0], 62326[0], 62327[0], 64400[0], 64405[0], 64408[0], 64415[0], 64416[0], 64417[0], 64418[0], 64420[0], 64421[0], 64425[0], 64430[0], 64435[0], 64445[0], 64446[0], 64447[0], 64448[0], 64449[0], 64450[0], 64451[0], 64454[0], 64461[0], 64462[0], 64463[0], 64479[0], 64480[0], 64483[0], 64484[0], 64486[0], 64487[0], 64488[0], 64489[0], 64490[0], 64491[0], 64492[0], 64493[0], 64494[0], 64495[0], 64505[0], 64510[0], 64517[0], 64520[0], 64530[0], 69990[0], 92012[1], 92014[1], 93000[1], 93005[1], 93010[1], 93040[1], 93041[1], 93042[1], 93318[1], 93355[1], 94002[1], 94200[1], 94680[1], 94681[1], 94690[1], 95812[1], 95813[1], 95816[1], 95819[1], 95822[1], 95829[1], 95955[1], 96360[1], 96361[1], 96365[1], 96366[1], 96367[1], 96368[1], 96372[1], 96374[1], 96375[1], 96376[1], 96377[1], 96523[0], 99155[0], 99156[0], 99157[0], 99211[1], 99212[1], 99213[1], 99214[1], 99215[1], 99217[1], 99218[1], 99219[1], 99220[1], 99221[1], 99222[1], 99223[1], 99231[1], 99232[1], 99233[1], 99234[1], 99235[1], 99236[1], 99238[1], 99239[1], 99241[1], 99242[1], 99243[1], 99244[1], 99245[1], 99251[1], 99252[1], 99253[1], 99254[1], 99255[1], 99291[1], 99292[1], 99304[1], 99305[1], 99306[1], 99307[1], 99308[1], 99309[1], 99310[1], 99315[1], 99316[1], 99334[1], 99335[1], 99336[1], 99337[1], 99347[1], 99348[1], 99349[1], 99350[1], 99374[1], 99375[1], 99377[1], 99378[1], 99446[0], 99447[0], 99448[0], 99449[0], 99451[0], 99452[0], 99495[1], 99496[1], G0463[1], G0471[1], J0670[1], J1642[1], J1644[1], J2001[1]
49185	0213T[0], 0216T[0], 0524T[1], 0596T[1], 0597T[1], 0708T[1], 0709T[1], 12001[1], 12002[1], 12004[1], 12005[1], 12006[1], 12007[1], 12011[1], 12013[1], 12014[1], 12015[1], 12016[1], 12017[1], 12018[1], 12020[1], 12021[1], 12031[1], 12032[1], 12034[1], 12035[1], 12036[1], 12037[1], 12041[1], 12042[1], 12044[1], 12045[1], 12046[1], 12047[1], 12051[1], 12052[1], 12053[1], 12054[1], 12055[1], 12056[1], 12057[1], 13100[1], 13101[1], 13102[1], 13120[1], 13121[1], 13122[1], 13131[1], 13132[1], 13133[1], 13151[1], 13152[1], 13153[1], 32560[1], 36000[1], 36400[1], 36405[1], 36406[1], 36410[1], 36420[1], 36425[1], 36430[1], 36440[1], 36465[1], 36468[1], 36470[1], 36471[1], 36591[0], 36592[0], 36600[1], 36640[1], 43752[1], 44602[1], 44603[1], 44604[1], 44605[1], 49320[1], 49424[1], 51701[1], 51702[1], 51703[1], 62320[0], 62321[0], 62322[0], 62323[0], 62324[0], 62325[0], 62326[0], 62327[0], 64400[0], 64405[0], 64408[0], 64415[0], 64416[0], 64417[0], 64418[0], 64420[0], 64421[0], 64425[0], 64430[0], 64435[0], 64445[0], 64446[0], 64447[0], 64448[0], 64449[0], 64450[0], 64451[0], 64454[0], 64461[0], 64462[0], 64463[0], 64479[0], 64480[0], 64483[0], 64484[0], 64486[0], 64487[0], 64488[0], 64489[0], 64490[0], 64491[0], 64492[0], 64493[0], 64494[0], 64495[0], 64505[0], 64510[0], 64517[0], 64520[0], 64530[0], 69990[0], 76000[1], 76080[1], 76380[1], 76942[1], 76998[1], 77001[1], 77002[1], 77012[1], 77021[1], 92012[1], 92014[1], 93000[1], 93005[1], 93010[1], 93040[1], 93041[1], 93042[1], 93318[1], 93355[1], 94002[1], 94200[1], 94680[1], 94681[1], 94690[1], 95812[1], 95813[1], 95816[1], 95819[1], 95822[1], 95829[1], 95955[1], 96360[1], 96361[1], 96365[1], 96366[1], 96367[1], 96368[1], 96372[1], 96374[1], 96375[1], 96376[1], 96377[1], 96523[0], 99155[0], 99156[0], 99157[0], 99211[1], 99212[1], 99213[1], 99214[1], 99215[1], 99217[1], 99218[1], 99219[1], 99220[1], 99221[1], 99222[1], 99223[1], 99231[1], 99232[1], 99233[1], 99234[1], 99235[1], 99236[1], 99238[1], 99239[1], 99241[1], 99242[1], 99243[1], 99244[1], 99245[1], 99251[1], 99252[1], 99253[1], 99254[1], 99255[1], 99291[1], 99292[1], 99304[1], 99305[1], 99306[1], 99307[1], 99308[1], 99309[1], 99310[1], 99315[1], 99316[1], 99334[1], 99335[1], 99336[1], 99337[1], 99347[1], 99348[1], 99349[1], 99350[1], 99374[1], 99375[1], 99377[1], 99378[1], 99446[0], 99447[0], 99448[0], 99449[0], 99451[0], 99452[0], 99495[1], 99496[1], G0463[1], G0471[1], J0670[1], J2001[1]
49320	0213T[0], 0216T[0], 0596T[1], 0597T[1], 0708T[1], 0709T[1], 12001[1], 12002[1], 12004[1], 12005[1], 12006[1], 12007[1], 12011[1], 12013[1], 12014[1], 12015[1], 12016[1], 12017[1], 12018[1], 12020[1], 12021[1], 12031[1], 12032[1], 12034[1], 12035[1], 12036[1], 12037[1], 12041[1], 12042[1], 12044[1], 12045[1], 12046[1], 12047[1], 12051[1], 12052[1], 12053[1], 12054[1], 12055[1], 12056[1], 12057[1], 13100[1], 13101[1], 13102[1], 13120[1], 13121[1], 13122[1], 13131[1], 13132[1], 13133[1], 13151[1], 13152[1], 13153[1], 36000[1], 36400[1], 36405[1], 36406[1], 36410[1], 36420[1], 36425[1], 36430[1], 36440[1], 36591[0], 36592[0], 36600[1], 36640[1], 43752[1], 44005[0], 47001[1], 49082[1], 49083[1],

0 = Modifier usage not allowed or inappropriate 1 = Modifier usage allowed

Appendix A: NCCI - CPT Codes

Code 1	Code 2
	49084[1], 49400[0], 50715[1], 51701[1], 51702[1], 51703[1], 57410[1], 62320[0], 62321[0], 62322[0], 62323[0], 62324[0], 62325[0], 62326[0], 62327[0], 64400[0], 64405[0], 64408[0], 64415[0], 64416[0], 64417[0], 64418[0], 64420[0], 64421[0], 64425[0], 64430[0], 64435[0], 64445[0], 64446[0], 64447[0], 64448[0], 64449[0], 64450[0], 64451[0], 64454[0], 64461[0], 64462[0], 64463[0], 64479[0], 64480[0], 64483[0], 64484[0], 64486[0], 64487[0], 64488[0], 64489[0], 64490[0], 64491[0], 64492[0], 64493[0], 64494[0], 64495[0], 64505[0], 64510[0], 64517[0], 64520[0], 64530[0], 69990[0], 76000[1], 77001[1], 77002[1], 92012[1], 92014[1], 93000[1], 93005[1], 93010[1], 93040[1], 93041[1], 93042[1], 93318[1], 93355[1], 94002[1], 94200[1], 94680[1], 94681[1], 94690[1], 95812[1], 95813[1], 95816[1], 95819[1], 95822[1], 95829[1], 95955[1], 96360[1], 96361[1], 96365[1], 96366[1], 96367[1], 96368[1], 96372[1], 96374[1], 96375[1], 96376[1], 96377[1], 96523[0], 99155[0], 99156[0], 99157[0], 99211[1], 99212[1], 99213[1], 99214[1], 99215[1], 99217[1], 99218[1], 99219[1], 99220[1], 99221[1], 99222[1], 99223[1], 99231[1], 99232[1], 99233[1], 99234[1], 99235[1], 99236[1], 99238[1], 99239[1], 99241[1], 99242[1], 99243[1], 99244[1], 99245[1], 99251[1], 99252[1], 99253[1], 99254[1], 99255[1], 99291[1], 99292[1], 99304[1], 99305[1], 99306[1], 99307[1], 99308[1], 99309[1], 99310[1], 99315[1], 99316[1], 99334[1], 99335[1], 99336[1], 99337[1], 99347[1], 99348[1], 99349[1], 99350[1], 99374[1], 99375[1], 99377[1], 99378[1], 99446[0], 99447[0], 99448[0], 99449[0], 99451[0], 99452[0], 99495[0], 99496[0], G0463[1], G0471[1]
49321	0213T[0], 0216T[0], 0596T[1], 0597T[1], 0708T[1], 0709T[1], 10005[1], 10007[1], 10009[1], 10011[1], 10021[1], 12001[1], 12002[1], 12004[1], 12005[1], 12006[1], 12007[1], 12011[1], 12013[1], 12014[1], 12015[1], 12016[1], 12017[1], 12018[1], 12020[1], 12021[1], 12031[1], 12032[1], 12034[1], 12035[1], 12036[1], 12037[1], 12041[1], 12042[1], 12044[1], 12045[1], 12046[1], 12047[1], 12051[1], 12052[1], 12053[1], 12054[1], 12055[1], 12056[1], 12057[1], 13100[1], 13101[1], 13102[1], 13120[1], 13121[1], 13122[1], 13131[1], 13132[1], 13133[1], 13151[1], 13152[1], 13153[1], 36000[1], 36400[1], 36405[1], 36406[1], 36410[1], 36420[1], 36425[1], 36430[1], 36440[1], 36591[0], 36592[0], 36600[1], 36640[1], 43653[0], 43752[1], 44005[0], 44180[0], 44602[1], 44603[1], 44604[1], 44605[1], 44950[0], 47001[1], 49082[1], 49083[1], 49084[1], 49320[0], 49400[0], 50715[1], 51701[1], 51702[1], 51703[1], 57410[1], 62320[0], 62321[0], 62322[0], 62323[0], 62324[0], 62325[0], 62326[0], 62327[0], 64400[0], 64405[0], 64408[0], 64415[0], 64416[0], 64417[0], 64418[0], 64420[0], 64421[0], 64425[0], 64430[0], 64435[0], 64445[0], 64446[0], 64447[0], 64448[0], 64449[0], 64450[0], 64451[0], 64454[0], 64461[0], 64462[0], 64463[0], 64479[0], 64480[0], 64483[0], 64484[0], 64486[0], 64487[0], 64488[0], 64489[0], 64490[0], 64491[0], 64492[0], 64493[0], 64494[0], 64495[0], 64505[0], 64510[0], 64517[0], 64520[0], 64530[0], 69990[0], 76000[1], 77001[1], 77002[1], 92012[1], 92014[1], 93000[1], 93005[1], 93010[1], 93040[1], 93041[1], 93042[1], 93318[1], 93355[1], 94002[1], 94200[1], 94680[1], 94681[1], 94690[1], 95812[1], 95813[1], 95816[1], 95819[1], 95822[1], 95829[1], 95955[1], 96360[1], 96361[1], 96365[1], 96366[1], 96367[1], 96368[1], 96372[1], 96374[1], 96375[1], 96376[1], 96377[1], 96523[0], 99155[0], 99156[0], 99157[0], 99211[1], 99212[1], 99213[1], 99214[1], 99215[1], 99217[1], 99218[1], 99219[1], 99220[1], 99221[1], 99222[1], 99223[1], 99231[1], 99232[1], 99233[1], 99234[1], 99235[1], 99236[1], 99238[1], 99239[1], 99241[1], 99242[1], 99243[1], 99244[1], 99245[1], 99251[1], 99252[1], 99253[1], 99254[1], 99255[1], 99291[1], 99292[1], 99304[1], 99305[1], 99306[1], 99307[1], 99308[1], 99309[1], 99310[1], 99315[1], 99316[1], 99334[1], 99335[1], 99336[1], 99337[1], 99347[1], 99348[1], 99349[1], 99350[1], 99374[1], 99375[1], 99377[1], 99378[1], 99446[0], 99447[0], 99448[0], 99449[0], 99451[0], 99452[0], 99495[0], 99496[0], G0463[1], G0471[1]
49324	0213T[0], 0216T[0], 0596T[1], 0597T[1], 0708T[1], 0709T[1], 11000[1], 11001[1], 11004[1], 11005[1], 11006[1], 11042[1], 11043[1], 11044[1], 11045[1], 11046[1], 11047[1], 12001[1], 12002[1], 12004[1], 12005[1], 12006[1], 12007[1], 12011[1], 12013[1], 12014[1], 12015[1], 12016[1], 12017[1], 12018[1], 12020[1], 12021[1], 12031[1], 12032[1], 12034[1], 12035[1], 12036[1], 12037[1], 12041[1], 12042[1], 12044[1], 12045[1], 12046[1], 12047[1], 12051[1], 12052[1], 12053[1], 12054[1], 12055[1], 12056[1], 12057[1], 13100[1], 13101[1], 13102[1], 13120[1], 13121[1], 13122[1], 13131[1], 13132[1], 13133[1], 13151[1], 13152[1], 13153[1], 36000[1], 36400[1], 36405[1], 36406[1], 36410[1], 36420[1], 36425[1], 36430[1], 36440[1], 36591[0], 36592[0], 36600[1], 36640[1], 43653[0], 43752[1], 44005[0], 44180[0], 44602[1], 44603[1], 44604[1], 44605[1], 44950[0], 44970[1], 49000[0], 49082[1], 49083[1], 49084[1], 49320[0], 49400[0], 49421[1], 49422[1], 49436[1], 50715[1], 51701[1], 51702[1], 51703[1], 58660[0], 62320[0], 62321[0], 62322[0], 62323[0], 62324[0], 62325[0], 62326[0], 62327[0], 64400[0], 64405[0], 64408[0], 64415[0], 64416[0], 64417[0], 64418[0], 64420[0], 64421[0], 64425[0], 64430[0], 64435[0], 64445[0], 64446[0], 64447[0], 64448[0], 64449[0], 64450[0], 64451[0], 64454[0], 64461[0], 64462[0], 64463[0], 64479[0], 64480[0], 64483[0], 64484[0], 64486[0], 64487[0], 64488[0], 64489[0], 64490[0], 64491[0], 64492[0], 64493[0], 64494[0], 64495[0], 64505[0], 64510[0], 64517[0], 64520[0], 64530[0], 69990[0], 76000[1], 77001[1], 77002[1], 92012[1], 92014[1], 93000[1], 93005[1], 93010[1], 93040[1], 93041[1], 93042[1], 93318[1], 93355[1], 94002[1], 94200[1], 94680[1], 94681[1], 94690[1], 95812[1], 95813[1], 95816[1], 95819[1], 95822[1], 95829[1], 95955[1], 96360[1], 96361[1], 96365[1], 96366[1], 96367[1], 96368[1], 96372[1], 96374[1], 96375[1], 96376[1], 96377[1], 96523[0], 97597[1], 97598[1], 97602[1], 99155[0], 99156[0], 99157[0], 99211[1], 99212[1], 99213[1], 99214[1], 99215[1], 99217[1], 99218[1], 99219[1], 99220[1], 99221[1], 99222[1], 99223[1], 99231[1], 99232[1], 99233[1], 99234[1], 99235[1], 99236[1], 99238[1], 99239[1], 99241[1], 99242[1], 99243[1], 99244[1], 99245[1], 99251[1], 99252[1], 99253[1], 99254[1], 99255[1], 99291[1], 99292[1], 99304[1], 99305[1], 99306[1], 99307[1], 99308[1], 99309[1], 99310[1], 99315[1], 99316[1], 99334[1], 99335[1], 99336[1], 99337[1], 99347[1], 99348[1], 99349[1], 99350[1], 99374[1], 99375[1], 99377[1], 99378[1], 99446[0], 99447[0], 99448[0], 99449[0], 99451[0], 99452[0], 99495[0], 99496[0], G0463[1], G0471[1]
49325	0213T[0], 0216T[0], 0596T[1], 0597T[1], 0708T[1], 0709T[1], 11000[1], 11001[1], 11004[1], 11005[1], 11006[1], 11042[1], 11043[1], 11044[1], 11045[1], 11046[1], 11047[1], 12001[1], 12002[1], 12004[1], 12005[1], 12006[1], 12007[1], 12011[1], 12013[1], 12014[1], 12015[1], 12016[1], 12017[1], 12018[1], 12020[1], 12021[1], 12031[1], 12032[1], 12034[1], 12035[1], 12036[1], 12037[1], 12041[1], 12042[1], 12044[1], 12045[1], 12046[1], 12047[1], 12051[1], 12052[1], 12053[1], 12054[1], 12055[1], 12056[1], 12057[1], 13100[1], 13101[1], 13102[1], 13120[1], 13121[1], 13122[1], 13131[1], 13132[1], 13133[1], 13151[1], 13152[1], 13153[1], 36000[1], 36400[1], 36405[1], 36406[1], 36410[1], 36420[1], 36425[1], 36430[1], 36440[1], 36591[0], 36592[0], 36600[1], 36640[1], 43653[0], 43752[1], 44005[0], 44180[0], 44602[1], 44603[1], 44604[1], 44605[1], 44950[0], 44970[1], 49000[0], 49082[1], 49083[1], 49084[1], 49320[0], 49324[1], 49400[0], 49421[1], 49422[1], 50715[1], 51701[1], 51702[1], 51703[1], 58660[0], 62320[0], 62321[0], 62322[0], 62323[0], 62324[0], 62325[0], 62326[0], 62327[0], 64400[0], 64405[0], 64408[0], 64415[0], 64416[0], 64417[0], 64418[0], 64420[0], 64421[0], 64425[0], 64430[0], 64435[0], 64445[0], 64446[0], 64447[0], 64448[0], 64449[0], 64450[0], 64451[0], 64454[0], 64461[0], 64462[0], 64463[0], 64479[0], 64480[0], 64483[0], 64484[0], 64486[0], 64487[0], 64488[0], 64489[0], 64490[0], 64491[0], 64492[0], 64493[0], 64494[0], 64495[0], 64505[0], 64510[0], 64517[0], 64520[0], 64530[0], 69990[0], 76000[1], 77001[1], 77002[1], 92012[1], 92014[1], 93000[1], 93005[1], 93010[1], 93040[1], 93041[1], 93042[1], 93318[1], 93355[1], 94002[1], 94200[1], 94680[1], 94681[1], 94690[1], 95812[1], 95813[1], 95816[1], 95819[1], 95822[1], 95829[1], 95955[1], 96360[1], 96361[1], 96365[1], 96366[1], 96367[1], 96368[1], 96372[1], 96374[1], 96375[1], 96376[1], 96377[1], 96523[0], 97597[1], 97598[1], 97602[1], 99155[0], 99156[0], 99157[0], 99211[1], 99212[1], 99213[1], 99214[1], 99215[1], 99217[1], 99218[1], 99219[1], 99220[1], 99221[1], 99222[1], 99223[1], 99231[1], 99232[1], 99233[1], 99234[1], 99235[1], 99236[1], 99238[1], 99239[1], 99241[1], 99242[1], 99243[1], 99244[1], 99245[1], 99251[1], 99252[1], 99253[1], 99254[1], 99255[1], 99291[1], 99292[1], 99304[1], 99305[1], 99306[1], 99307[1], 99308[1], 99309[1], 99310[1], 99315[1], 99316[1], 99334[1], 99335[1], 99336[1], 99337[1], 99347[1], 99348[1], 99349[1], 99350[1], 99374[1], 99375[1], 99377[1], 99378[1], 99446[0], 99447[0], 99448[0], 99449[0], 99451[0], 99452[0], 99495[0], 99496[0], G0463[1], G0471[1]
49327	36591[0], 36592[0], 43653[0], 44005[0], 44180[0], 44970[1], 49082[1], 49083[1], 49084[1], 49320[1], 49400[0], 50715[1], 57410[0], 58660[0], 76000[1], 76380[1], 76942[1], 76998[1], 77002[1], 77012[1], 77021[1], 96523[0]
49400	0213T[1], 0216T[1], 0596T[1], 0597T[1], 0708T[1], 0709T[1], 12001[1], 12002[1], 12004[1], 12005[1], 12006[1], 12007[1], 12011[1], 12013[1], 12014[1], 12015[1], 12016[1], 12017[1], 12018[1], 12020[1], 12021[1], 12031[1], 12032[1], 12034[1], 12035[1], 12036[1], 12037[1], 12041[1], 12042[1], 12044[1], 12045[1], 12046[1], 12047[1], 12051[1], 12052[1], 12053[1], 12054[1], 12055[1], 12056[1], 12057[1], 13100[1], 13101[1], 13102[1], 13120[1], 13121[1], 13122[1], 13131[1], 13132[1], 13133[1], 13151[1], 13152[1], 13153[1], 36000[1], 36400[1], 36405[1], 36406[1], 36410[1], 36420[1], 36425[1], 36430[1], 36440[1], 36591[0], 36592[0], 36600[1], 36640[1], 43752[1], 51701[1], 51702[1], 51703[1], 62320[0], 62321[0], 62322[0], 62323[0], 62324[0], 62325[0], 62326[0], 62327[0], 64400[0], 64405[0], 64408[0], 64415[1], 64416[1], 64417[1], 64418[0], 64420[0], 64421[0], 64425[0], 64430[0], 64435[0], 64445[0], 64446[0], 64447[0], 64448[0], 64449[0], 64450[1], 64451[0], 64454[1], 64461[0], 64462[0], 64463[0], 64479[0], 64480[0], 64483[0], 64484[0], 64486[0], 64487[0], 64488[0], 64489[0], 64490[1], 64491[0], 64492[0], 64493[1], 64494[0], 64495[0], 64505[0], 64510[0], 64517[0], 64520[0], 64530[0], 69990[0], 76000[1], 76942[1], 76998[1], 77001[1], 77002[1], 92012[1], 92014[1], 93000[1], 93005[1], 93010[1], 93040[1], 93041[1], 93042[1], 93318[1], 93355[1], 94002[1], 94200[1], 94680[1], 94681[1], 94690[1], 95812[1], 95813[1], 95816[1], 95819[1], 95822[1], 95829[1], 95955[1], 96360[1], 96361[1], 96365[1], 96366[1], 96367[1], 96368[1], 96372[1], 96374[1], 96375[1], 96376[1], 96377[1], 96523[0], 99155[0], 99156[0], 99157[0], 99211[1], 99212[1], 99213[1], 99214[1], 99215[1], 99217[1], 99218[1], 99219[1], 99220[1], 99221[1], 99222[1], 99223[1], 99231[1], 99232[1], 99233[1], 99234[1], 99235[1], 99236[1], 99238[1], 99239[1], 99241[1], 99242[1], 99243[1], 99244[1], 99245[1], 99251[1], 99252[1], 99253[1], 99254[1], 99255[1], 99291[1], 99292[1], 99304[1], 99305[1], 99306[1], 99307[1], 99308[1], 99309[1], 99310[1], 99315[1], 99316[1], 99334[1], 99335[1], 99336[1], 99337[1], 99347[1], 99348[1], 99349[1], 99350[1], 99374[1], 99375[1], 99377[1], 99378[1], 99446[0], 99447[0], 99448[0], 99449[0], 99451[0], 99452[0], 99495[1], 99496[1], G0463[1], G0471[1]
49402	0213T[1], 0216T[1], 0596T[1], 0597T[1], 0708T[1], 0709T[1], 11000[1], 11001[1], 11004[1], 11005[1], 11006[1], 11042[1], 11043[1], 11044[1], 11045[1], 11046[1], 11047[1], 12001[1], 12002[1], 12004[1], 12005[1], 12006[1], 12007[1], 12011[1], 12013[1], 12014[1], 12015[1], 12016[1], 12017[1], 12018[1], 12020[1], 12021[1], 12031[1], 12032[1], 12034[1], 12035[1], 12036[1], 12037[1], 12041[1], 12042[1], 12044[1], 12045[1], 12046[1], 12047[1], 12051[1], 12052[1], 12053[1], 12054[1], 12055[1], 12056[1], 12057[1], 13100[1], 13101[1], 13102[1], 13120[1], 13121[1], 13122[1], 13131[1], 13132[1], 13133[1], 13151[1], 13152[1], 13153[1], 20102[1], 36000[1], 36400[1], 36405[1], 36406[1], 36410[1], 36420[1], 36425[1], 36430[1], 36440[1], 36591[0], 36592[0], 36600[1], 36640[1], 43752[1], 44005[0], 44180[0], 44602[1], 44603[1], 44604[1], 44605[1], 44820[0], 44850[0], 44950[0], 44970[0], 49000[0], 49002[1], 49010[0], 49013[1], 49014[1], 49255[0], 49320[1], 49429[1], 49560[1], 49561[1], 49565[1], 49566[1], 49570[0], 49572[1], 49580[1], 49582[1], 49585[1], 49587[1], 51701[1], 51702[1], 51703[1], 62320[0],

0 = Modifier usage not allowed or inappropriate 1 = Modifier usage allowed

Code 1	Code 2
	62321[0], 62322[0], 62323[0], 62324[0], 62325[0], 62326[0], 62327[0], 64400[0], 64405[0], 64408[0], 64415[1], 64416[1], 64417[1], 64418[0], 64420[0], 64421[0], 64425[0], 64430[0], 64435[0], 64445[0], 64446[0], 64447[0], 64448[0], 64449[0], 64450[1], 64451[0], 64454[1], 64461[0], 64462[0], 64463[0], 64479[0], 64480[0], 64483[0], 64484[0], 64486[0], 64487[0], 64488[0], 64489[0], 64490[1], 64491[0], 64492[0], 64493[1], 64494[0], 64495[0], 64505[0], 64510[0], 64517[0], 64520[0], 64530[0], 69990[0], 92012[1], 92014[1], 93000[1], 93005[1], 93010[1], 93040[1], 93041[1], 93042[1], 93318[1], 93355[1], 94002[1], 94200[1], 94680[1], 94681[1], 94690[1], 95812[1], 95813[1], 95816[1], 95819[1], 95822[1], 95829[1], 95955[1], 96360[1], 96361[1], 96365[1], 96366[1], 96367[1], 96368[1], 96372[1], 96374[1], 96375[1], 96376[1], 96377[1], 96523[0], 97597[1], 97598[1], 97602[1], 99155[0], 99156[0], 99157[0], 99211[1], 99212[1], 99213[1], 99214[1], 99215[1], 99217[1], 99218[1], 99219[1], 99220[1], 99221[1], 99222[1], 99223[1], 99231[1], 99232[1], 99233[1], 99234[1], 99235[1], 99236[1], 99238[1], 99239[1], 99241[1], 99242[1], 99243[1], 99244[1], 99245[1], 99251[1], 99252[1], 99253[1], 99254[1], 99255[1], 99291[1], 99292[1], 99304[1], 99305[1], 99306[1], 99307[1], 99308[1], 99309[1], 99310[1], 99315[1], 99316[1], 99334[1], 99335[1], 99336[1], 99337[1], 99347[1], 99348[1], 99349[1], 99350[1], 99374[1], 99375[1], 99377[1], 99378[1], 99446[0], 99447[0], 99448[0], 99449[0], 99451[0], 99452[0], 99495[0], 99496[0], G0463[1], G0471[1]
49405	0213T[0], 0216T[0], 0596T[1], 0597T[1], 0708T[1], 0709T[1], 12001[1], 12002[1], 12004[1], 12005[1], 12006[1], 12007[1], 12011[1], 12013[1], 12014[1], 12015[1], 12016[1], 12017[1], 12018[1], 12020[1], 12021[1], 12031[1], 12032[1], 12034[1], 12035[1], 12036[1], 12037[1], 12041[1], 12042[1], 12044[1], 12045[1], 12046[1], 12047[1], 12051[1], 12052[1], 12053[1], 12054[1], 12055[1], 12056[1], 12057[1], 13100[1], 13101[1], 13102[1], 13120[1], 13121[1], 13122[1], 13131[1], 13132[1], 13133[1], 13151[1], 13152[1], 13153[1], 32551[1], 32554[1], 32555[1], 32556[1], 32557[1], 32601[1], 32607[1], 32608[1], 32609[1], 36000[1], 36400[1], 36405[1], 36406[1], 36410[1], 36420[1], 36425[1], 36430[1], 36440[1], 36591[0], 36592[0], 36600[1], 36640[1], 43752[1], 44602[1], 44603[1], 44604[1], 44605[1], 44950[0], 44970[0], 47000[1], 47001[0], 48102[1], 49000[0], 49002[1], 49185[1], 49320[1], 49406[1], 49423[1], 49424[1], 51701[1], 51702[1], 51703[1], 62320[0], 62321[0], 62322[0], 62323[0], 62324[0], 62325[0], 62326[0], 62327[0], 64400[0], 64405[0], 64408[0], 64415[0], 64416[0], 64417[0], 64418[0], 64420[0], 64421[0], 64425[0], 64430[0], 64435[0], 64445[0], 64446[0], 64447[0], 64448[0], 64449[0], 64450[0], 64451[0], 64454[0], 64461[0], 64462[0], 64463[0], 64479[0], 64480[0], 64483[0], 64484[0], 64486[0], 64487[0], 64488[0], 64489[0], 64490[0], 64491[0], 64492[0], 64493[0], 64494[0], 64495[0], 64505[0], 64510[0], 64517[0], 64520[0], 64530[0], 69990[0], 75989[1], 76000[1], 76380[1], 76942[1], 76998[1], 77001[1], 77002[1], 77003[1], 77012[1], 77021[1], 92012[1], 92014[1], 93000[1], 93005[1], 93010[1], 93040[1], 93041[1], 93042[1], 93318[1], 93355[1], 94002[1], 94200[1], 94680[1], 94681[1], 94690[1], 95812[1], 95813[1], 95816[1], 95819[1], 95822[1], 95829[1], 95955[1], 96360[1], 96361[1], 96365[1], 96366[1], 96367[1], 96368[1], 96372[1], 96374[1], 96375[1], 96376[1], 96377[1], 96523[0], 99155[0], 99156[0], 99157[0], 99211[1], 99212[1], 99213[1], 99214[1], 99215[1], 99217[1], 99218[1], 99219[1], 99220[1], 99221[1], 99222[1], 99223[1], 99231[1], 99232[1], 99233[1], 99234[1], 99235[1], 99236[1], 99238[1], 99239[1], 99241[1], 99242[1], 99243[1], 99244[1], 99245[1], 99251[1], 99252[1], 99253[1], 99254[1], 99255[1], 99291[1], 99292[1], 99304[1], 99305[1], 99306[1], 99307[1], 99308[1], 99309[1], 99310[1], 99315[1], 99316[1], 99334[1], 99335[1], 99336[1], 99337[1], 99347[1], 99348[1], 99349[1], 99350[1], 99374[1], 99375[1], 99377[1], 99378[1], 99446[0], 99447[0], 99448[0], 99449[0], 99451[0], 99452[0], G0463[1], G0471[1], J0670[1], J2001[1]
49406	00910[0], 0213T[0], 0216T[0], 0596T[1], 0597T[1], 0708T[1], 0709T[1], 12001[1], 12002[1], 12004[1], 12005[1], 12006[1], 12007[1], 12011[1], 12013[1], 12014[1], 12015[1], 12016[1], 12017[1], 12018[1], 12020[1], 12021[1], 12031[1], 12032[1], 12034[1], 12035[1], 12036[1], 12037[1], 12041[1], 12042[1], 12044[1], 12045[1], 12046[1], 12047[1], 12051[1], 12052[1], 12053[1], 12054[1], 12055[1], 12056[1], 12057[1], 13100[1], 13101[1], 13102[1], 13120[1], 13121[1], 13122[1], 13131[1], 13132[1], 13133[1], 13151[1], 13152[1], 13153[1], 36000[1], 36400[1], 36405[1], 36406[1], 36410[1], 36420[1], 36425[1], 36430[1], 36440[1], 36591[0], 36592[0], 36600[1], 36640[1], 43752[1], 44005[0], 44180[0], 44602[1], 44603[1], 44604[1], 44605[1], 44701[1], 44820[0], 44850[0], 44950[0], 44970[0], 49000[0], 49002[1], 49010[0], 49082[1], 49083[1], 49084[1], 49180[1], 49185[1], 49255[0], 49320[1], 49322[1], 49400[1], 49402[1], 49423[1], 49424[1], 49570[0], 50010[1], 50205[1], 50715[1], 51045[1], 51570[1], 51701[1], 51702[1], 51703[1], 57410[0], 58660[1], 58700[0], 58800[0], 58900[0], 62320[0], 62321[0], 62322[0], 62323[0], 62324[0], 62325[0], 62326[0], 62327[0], 64400[0], 64405[0], 64408[0], 64415[0], 64416[0], 64417[0], 64418[0], 64420[0], 64421[0], 64425[0], 64430[0], 64435[0], 64445[0], 64446[0], 64447[0], 64448[0], 64449[0], 64450[0], 64451[0], 64454[0], 64461[0], 64462[0], 64463[0], 64479[0], 64480[0], 64483[0], 64484[0], 64486[0], 64487[0], 64488[0], 64489[0], 64490[0], 64491[0], 64492[0], 64493[0], 64494[0], 64495[0], 64505[0], 64510[0], 64517[0], 64520[0], 64530[0], 69990[0], 75989[1], 76000[1], 76380[1], 76942[1], 76998[1], 77001[1], 77002[1], 77003[1], 77012[1], 77021[1], 92012[1], 92014[1], 93000[1], 93005[1], 93010[1], 93040[1], 93041[1], 93042[1], 93318[1], 93355[1], 94002[1], 94200[1], 94680[1], 94681[1], 94690[1], 95812[1], 95813[1], 95816[1], 95819[1], 95822[1], 95829[1], 95955[1], 96360[1], 96361[1], 96365[1], 96366[1], 96367[1], 96368[1], 96372[1], 96374[1], 96375[1], 96376[1], 96377[1], 96523[0], 99155[0], 99156[0], 99157[0], 99211[1], 99212[1], 99213[1], 99214[1], 99215[1], 99217[1], 99218[1], 99219[1], 99220[1], 99221[1], 99222[1], 99223[1], 99231[1], 99232[1], 99233[1], 99234[1], 99235[1], 99236[1], 99238[1], 99239[1], 99241[1], 99242[1], 99243[1], 99244[1], 99245[1], 99251[1], 99252[1], 99253[1], 99254[1], 99255[1], 99291[1], 99292[1], 99304[1], 99305[1], 99306[1], 99307[1], 99308[1], 99309[1], 99310[1], 99315[1], 99316[1], 99334[1], 99335[1], 99336[1], 99337[1], 99347[1], 99348[1], 99349[1], 99350[1], 99374[1], 99375[1], 99377[1], 99378[1], 99446[0], 99447[0], 99448[0], 99449[0], 99451[0], 99452[0], G0463[1], G0471[1], J0670[1], J2001[1]
49407	0213T[0], 0216T[0], 0596T[1], 0597T[1], 0708T[1], 0709T[1], 12001[1], 12002[1], 12004[1], 12005[1], 12006[1], 12007[1], 12011[1], 12013[1], 12014[1], 12015[1], 12016[1], 12017[1], 12018[1], 12020[1], 12021[1], 12031[1], 12032[1], 12034[1], 12035[1], 12036[1], 12037[1], 12041[1], 12042[1], 12044[1], 12045[1], 12046[1], 12047[1], 12051[1], 12052[1], 12053[1], 12054[1], 12055[1], 12056[1], 12057[1], 13100[1], 13101[1], 13102[1], 13120[1], 13121[1], 13122[1], 13131[1], 13132[1], 13133[1], 13151[1], 13152[1], 13153[1], 36000[1], 36400[1], 36405[1], 36406[1], 36410[1], 36420[1], 36425[1], 36430[1], 36440[1], 36591[0], 36592[0], 36600[1], 36640[1], 43752[1], 44701[1], 45005[1], 45900[0], 45905[0], 45910[0], 45915[0], 45990[1], 46040[0], 46080[0], 46220[0], 46600[1], 46601[1], 46940[0], 46942[0], 49082[1], 49083[1], 49084[1], 49185[1], 49322[1], 49406[1], 49423[1], 49424[1], 50715[1], 51701[1], 51702[1], 51703[1], 57410[0], 58660[1], 58805[0], 58900[0], 62320[0], 62321[0], 62322[0], 62323[0], 62324[0], 62325[0], 62326[0], 62327[0], 64400[0], 64405[0], 64408[0], 64415[0], 64416[0], 64417[0], 64418[0], 64420[0], 64421[0], 64425[0], 64430[0], 64435[0], 64445[0], 64446[0], 64447[0], 64448[0], 64449[0], 64450[0], 64451[0], 64454[0], 64461[0], 64462[0], 64463[0], 64479[0], 64480[0], 64483[0], 64484[0], 64486[0], 64487[0], 64488[0], 64489[0], 64490[0], 64491[0], 64492[0], 64493[0], 64494[0], 64495[0], 64505[0], 64510[0], 64517[0], 64520[0], 64530[0], 69990[0], 75989[1], 76000[1], 76380[1], 76942[1], 76998[1], 77001[1], 77002[1], 77003[1], 77012[1], 77021[1], 92012[1], 92014[1], 93000[1], 93005[1], 93010[1], 93040[1], 93041[1], 93042[1], 93318[1], 93355[1], 94002[1], 94200[1], 94680[1], 94681[1], 94690[1], 95812[1], 95813[1], 95816[1], 95819[1], 95822[1], 95829[1], 95955[1], 96360[1], 96361[1], 96365[1], 96366[1], 96367[1], 96368[1], 96372[1], 96374[1], 96375[1], 96376[1], 96377[1], 96523[0], 99155[0], 99156[0], 99157[0], 99211[1], 99212[1], 99213[1], 99214[1], 99215[1], 99217[1], 99218[1], 99219[1], 99220[1], 99221[1], 99222[1], 99223[1], 99231[1], 99232[1], 99233[1], 99234[1], 99235[1], 99236[1], 99238[1], 99239[1], 99241[1], 99242[1], 99243[1], 99244[1], 99245[1], 99251[1], 99252[1], 99253[1], 99254[1], 99255[1], 99291[1], 99292[1], 99304[1], 99305[1], 99306[1], 99307[1], 99308[1], 99309[1], 99310[1], 99315[1], 99316[1], 99334[1], 99335[1], 99336[1], 99337[1], 99347[1], 99348[1], 99349[1], 99350[1], 99374[1], 99375[1], 99377[1], 99378[1], 99446[0], 99447[0], 99448[0], 99449[0], 99451[0], 99452[0], G0463[1], G0471[1], J0670[1], J2001[1]
49411	0213T[0], 0216T[0], 0596T[1], 0597T[1], 0708T[1], 0709T[1], 10035[1], 10036[1], 12001[1], 12002[1], 12004[1], 12005[1], 12006[1], 12007[1], 12011[1], 12013[1], 12014[1], 12015[1], 12016[1], 12017[1], 12018[1], 12020[1], 12021[1], 12031[1], 12032[1], 12034[1], 12035[1], 12036[1], 12037[1], 12041[1], 12042[1], 12044[1], 12045[1], 12046[1], 12047[1], 12051[1], 12052[1], 12053[1], 12054[1], 12055[1], 12056[1], 12057[1], 13100[1], 13101[1], 13102[1], 13120[1], 13121[1], 13122[1], 13131[1], 13132[1], 13133[1], 13151[1], 13152[1], 13153[1], 36000[1], 36400[1], 36405[1], 36406[1], 36410[1], 36420[1], 36425[1], 36430[1], 36440[1], 36591[0], 36592[0], 36600[1], 36640[1], 43752[1], 44602[1], 44603[1], 44604[1], 44605[1], 49320[0], 49327[0], 49412[1], 51701[1], 51702[1], 51703[1], 62320[0], 62321[0], 62322[0], 62323[0], 62324[0], 62325[0], 62326[0], 62327[0], 64400[0], 64405[0], 64408[0], 64415[0], 64416[0], 64417[0], 64418[0], 64420[0], 64421[0], 64425[0], 64430[0], 64435[0], 64445[0], 64446[0], 64447[0], 64448[0], 64449[0], 64450[0], 64451[0], 64454[0], 64461[0], 64462[0], 64463[0], 64479[0], 64480[0], 64483[0], 64484[0], 64486[0], 64487[0], 64488[0], 64489[0], 64490[0], 64491[0], 64492[0], 64493[0], 64494[0], 64495[0], 64505[0], 64510[0], 64517[0], 64520[0], 64530[0], 69990[0], 76000[1], 76998[1], 77001[1], 92012[1], 92014[1], 93000[1], 93005[1], 93010[1], 93040[1], 93041[1], 93042[1], 93318[1], 93355[1], 94002[1], 94200[1], 94680[1], 94681[1], 94690[1], 95812[1], 95813[1], 95816[1], 95819[1], 95822[1], 95829[1], 95955[1], 96360[1], 96361[1], 96365[1], 96366[1], 96367[1], 96368[1], 96372[1], 96374[1], 96375[1], 96376[1], 96377[1], 96523[0], 99155[0], 99156[0], 99157[0], 99211[1], 99212[1], 99213[1], 99214[1], 99215[1], 99217[1], 99218[1], 99219[1], 99220[1], 99221[1], 99222[1], 99223[1], 99231[1], 99232[1], 99233[1], 99234[1], 99235[1], 99236[1], 99238[1], 99239[1], 99241[1], 99242[1], 99243[1], 99244[1], 99245[1], 99251[1], 99252[1], 99253[1], 99254[1], 99255[1], 99291[1], 99292[1], 99304[1], 99305[1], 99306[1], 99307[1], 99308[1], 99309[1], 99310[1], 99315[1], 99316[1], 99334[1], 99335[1], 99336[1], 99337[1], 99347[1], 99348[1], 99349[1], 99350[1], 99374[1], 99375[1], 99377[1], 99378[1], 99446[0], 99447[0], 99448[0], 99449[0], 99451[0], 99452[0], 99495[1], 99496[1], G0463[1], G0471[1], J0670[1], J2001[1]
49412	10036[1], 36591[0], 36592[0], 49327[1], 76000[1], 76380[1], 76942[1], 76998[1], 77002[1], 77012[1], 77021[1], 96523[0]
49418	0596T[1], 0597T[1], 0708T[1], 0709T[1], 11000[1], 11001[1], 11004[1], 11005[1], 11006[1], 11042[1], 11043[1], 11044[1], 11045[1], 11046[1], 11047[1], 12001[1], 12002[1], 12004[1], 12005[1], 12006[1], 12007[1], 12011[1], 12013[1], 12014[1], 12015[1], 12016[1], 12017[1], 12018[1], 12020[1], 12021[1], 12031[1], 12032[1], 12034[1], 12035[1], 12036[1], 12037[1], 12041[1], 12042[1], 12044[1], 12045[1], 12046[1], 12047[1], 12051[1], 12052[1], 12053[1], 12054[1], 12055[1], 12056[1], 12057[1], 13100[1], 13101[1], 13102[1], 13120[1], 13121[1], 13122[1], 13131[1], 13132[1], 13133[1], 13151[1], 13152[1], 13153[1], 36000[1], 36400[1], 36405[1], 36406[1], 36410[1], 36420[1], 36425[1], 36430[1], 36440[1], 36591[0], 36592[0], 36600[1], 36640[1], 43752[1], 49324[1], 49325[1], 49400[1], 49421[0], 51701[1], 51702[1], 51703[1], 62320[0], 62321[0], 62322[0], 62323[0], 62324[0], 62325[0], 62326[0], 62327[0], 64400[0], 64405[0], 64408[0], 64415[0], 64416[0], 64417[0], 64418[0], 64420[0], 64421[0], 64425[0],

Code 1	Code 2
	64430[0], 64435[0], 64445[0], 64446[0], 64447[0], 64448[0], 64449[0], 64450[0], 64451[0], 64454[0], 64461[0], 64462[0], 64463[0], 64479[0], 64480[0], 64483[0], 64484[0], 64486[0], 64487[0], 64488[0], 64489[0], 64490[0], 64491[0], 64492[0], 64493[0], 64494[0], 64495[0], 64505[0], 64510[0], 64517[0], 64520[0], 64530[0], 69990[0], 76000[1], 76380[1], 76942[1], 76998[1], 77001[1], 77002[1], 77012[1], 77021[1], 92012[1], 92014[1], 93000[1], 93005[1], 93010[1], 93040[1], 93041[1], 93042[1], 93318[1], 93355[1], 94002[1], 94200[1], 94680[1], 94681[1], 94690[1], 95812[1], 95813[1], 95816[1], 95819[1], 95822[1], 95829[1], 95955[1], 96360[1], 96361[1], 96365[1], 96366[1], 96367[1], 96368[1], 96372[1], 96374[1], 96375[1], 96376[1], 96377[1], 96523[0], 97597[1], 97598[1], 97602[1], 99155[0], 99156[0], 99157[0], 99211[1], 99212[1], 99213[1], 99214[1], 99215[1], 99217[1], 99218[1], 99219[1], 99220[1], 99221[1], 99222[1], 99223[1], 99231[1], 99232[1], 99233[1], 99234[1], 99235[1], 99236[1], 99238[1], 99239[1], 99241[1], 99242[1], 99243[1], 99244[1], 99245[1], 99251[1], 99252[1], 99253[1], 99254[1], 99255[1], 99291[1], 99292[1], 99304[1], 99305[1], 99306[1], 99307[1], 99308[1], 99309[1], 99310[1], 99315[1], 99316[1], 99334[1], 99335[1], 99336[1], 99337[1], 99347[1], 99348[1], 99349[1], 99350[1], 99374[1], 99375[1], 99377[1], 99378[1], 99446[0], 99447[0], 99448[0], 99449[0], 99451[0], 99452[0], 99495[1], 99496[1], G0463[1], G0471[1], J0670[1], J2001[1]
49419	0213T[1], 0216T[1], 0596T[1], 0597T[1], 0708T[1], 0709T[1], 11000[1], 11001[1], 11004[1], 11005[1], 11006[1], 11042[1], 11043[1], 11044[1], 11045[1], 11046[1], 11047[1], 12001[1], 12002[1], 12004[1], 12005[1], 12006[1], 12007[1], 12011[1], 12013[1], 12014[1], 12015[1], 12016[1], 12017[1], 12018[1], 12020[1], 12021[1], 12031[1], 12032[1], 12034[1], 12035[1], 12036[1], 12037[1], 12041[1], 12042[1], 12044[1], 12045[1], 12046[1], 12047[1], 12051[1], 12052[1], 12053[1], 12054[1], 12055[1], 12056[1], 12057[1], 13100[1], 13101[1], 13102[1], 13120[1], 13121[1], 13122[1], 13131[1], 13132[1], 13133[1], 13151[1], 13152[1], 13153[1], 36000[1], 36400[1], 36405[1], 36406[1], 36410[1], 36420[1], 36425[1], 36430[1], 36440[1], 36591[0], 36592[0], 36600[1], 36640[1], 43752[1], 44005[0], 44180[0], 44602[1], 44603[1], 44604[1], 44605[1], 44820[1], 44850[1], 49000[0], 49002[1], 49010[1], 49255[1], 49320[1], 49324[1], 49325[1], 49400[1], 49402[1], 49418[0], 49421[0], 49422[1], 49436[1], 49570[1], 51701[1], 51702[1], 51703[1], 62320[0], 62321[0], 62322[0], 62323[0], 62324[0], 62325[0], 62326[0], 62327[0], 64400[0], 64405[0], 64408[0], 64415[1], 64416[0], 64417[1], 64418[0], 64420[0], 64421[0], 64425[0], 64430[0], 64435[0], 64445[0], 64446[0], 64447[0], 64448[0], 64449[0], 64450[1], 64451[0], 64454[1], 64461[0], 64462[0], 64463[0], 64479[0], 64480[0], 64483[0], 64484[0], 64486[0], 64487[0], 64488[0], 64489[0], 64490[1], 64491[0], 64492[0], 64493[1], 64494[0], 64495[0], 64505[0], 64510[0], 64517[0], 64520[0], 64530[0], 69990[0], 92012[1], 92014[1], 93000[1], 93005[1], 93010[1], 93040[1], 93041[1], 93042[1], 93318[1], 93355[1], 94002[1], 94200[1], 94680[1], 94681[1], 94690[1], 95812[1], 95813[1], 95816[1], 95819[1], 95822[1], 95829[1], 95955[1], 96360[1], 96361[1], 96365[1], 96366[1], 96367[1], 96368[1], 96372[1], 96374[1], 96375[1], 96376[1], 96377[1], 96523[0], 97597[1], 97598[1], 97602[1], 99155[0], 99156[0], 99157[0], 99211[1], 99212[1], 99213[1], 99214[1], 99215[1], 99217[1], 99218[1], 99219[1], 99220[1], 99221[1], 99222[1], 99223[1], 99231[1], 99232[1], 99233[1], 99234[1], 99235[1], 99236[1], 99238[1], 99239[1], 99241[1], 99242[1], 99243[1], 99244[1], 99245[1], 99251[1], 99252[1], 99253[1], 99254[1], 99255[1], 99291[1], 99292[1], 99304[1], 99305[1], 99306[1], 99307[1], 99308[1], 99309[1], 99310[1], 99315[1], 99316[1], 99334[1], 99335[1], 99336[1], 99337[1], 99347[1], 99348[1], 99349[1], 99350[1], 99374[1], 99375[1], 99377[1], 99378[1], 99446[0], 99447[0], 99448[0], 99449[0], 99451[0], 99452[0], 99495[0], 99496[0], G0463[1], G0471[1], J1642[1], J1644[1]
49421	0213T[1], 0216T[1], 0596T[1], 0597T[1], 0708T[1], 0709T[1], 11000[1], 11001[1], 11004[1], 11005[1], 11006[1], 11042[1], 11043[1], 11044[1], 11045[1], 11046[1], 11047[1], 12001[1], 12002[1], 12004[1], 12005[1], 12006[1], 12007[1], 12011[1], 12013[1], 12014[1], 12015[1], 12016[1], 12017[1], 12018[1], 12020[1], 12021[1], 12031[1], 12032[1], 12034[1], 12035[1], 12036[1], 12037[1], 12041[1], 12042[1], 12044[1], 12045[1], 12046[1], 12047[1], 12051[1], 12052[1], 12053[1], 12054[1], 12055[1], 12056[1], 12057[1], 13100[1], 13101[1], 13102[1], 13120[1], 13121[1], 13122[1], 13131[1], 13132[1], 13133[1], 13151[1], 13152[1], 13153[1], 36000[1], 36400[1], 36405[1], 36406[1], 36410[1], 36420[1], 36425[1], 36430[1], 36440[1], 36591[0], 36592[0], 36600[1], 36640[1], 43752[1], 44005[0], 44180[0], 44602[1], 44603[1], 44604[1], 44605[1], 44820[0], 44850[0], 49000[1], 49002[1], 49010[1], 49255[0], 49320[0], 49400[1], 49402[1], 49422[1], 49436[1], 49570[1], 51701[1], 51702[1], 51703[1], 62320[0], 62321[0], 62322[0], 62323[0], 62324[0], 62325[0], 62326[0], 62327[0], 64400[0], 64405[0], 64408[0], 64415[1], 64416[1], 64417[1], 64418[0], 64420[0], 64421[0], 64425[0], 64430[0], 64435[0], 64445[0], 64446[0], 64447[0], 64448[0], 64449[0], 64450[1], 64451[0], 64454[1], 64461[0], 64462[0], 64463[0], 64479[0], 64480[0], 64483[0], 64484[0], 64486[0], 64487[0], 64488[0], 64489[0], 64490[1], 64491[0], 64492[0], 64493[1], 64494[0], 64495[0], 64505[0], 64510[0], 64517[0], 64520[0], 64530[0], 69990[0], 92012[1], 92014[1], 93000[1], 93005[1], 93010[1], 93040[1], 93041[1], 93042[1], 93318[1], 93355[1], 94002[1], 94200[1], 94680[1], 94681[1], 94690[1], 95812[1], 95813[1], 95816[1], 95819[1], 95822[1], 95829[1], 95955[1], 96360[1], 96361[1], 96365[1], 96366[1], 96367[1], 96368[1], 96372[1], 96374[1], 96375[1], 96376[1], 96377[1], 96523[0], 97597[1], 97598[1], 97602[1], 99155[0], 99156[0], 99157[0], 99211[1], 99212[1], 99213[1], 99214[1], 99215[1], 99217[1], 99218[1], 99219[1], 99220[1], 99221[1], 99222[1], 99223[1], 99231[1], 99232[1], 99233[1], 99234[1], 99235[1], 99236[1], 99238[1], 99239[1], 99241[1], 99242[1], 99243[1], 99244[1], 99245[1], 99251[1], 99252[1], 99253[1], 99254[1], 99255[1], 99291[1], 99292[1], 99304[1], 99305[1], 99306[1], 99307[1], 99308[1], 99309[1], 99310[1], 99315[1], 99316[1], 99334[1], 99335[1], 99336[1], 99337[1], 99347[1], 99348[1], 99349[1], 99350[1], 99374[1], 99375[1], 99377[1], 99378[1], 99446[0], 99447[0], 99448[0], 99449[0], 99451[0], 99452[0], 99495[1], 99496[1], G0463[1], G0471[1]
49422	0213T[1], 0216T[1], 0596T[1], 0597T[1], 0708T[1], 0709T[1], 11000[1], 11001[1], 11004[1], 11005[1], 11006[1], 11042[1], 11043[1], 11044[1], 11045[1], 11046[1], 11047[1], 12001[1], 12002[1], 12004[1], 12005[1], 12006[1], 12007[1], 12011[1], 12013[1], 12014[1], 12015[1], 12016[1], 12017[1], 12018[1], 12020[1], 12021[1], 12031[1], 12032[1], 12034[1], 12035[1], 12036[1], 12037[1], 12041[1], 12042[1], 12044[1], 12045[1], 12046[1], 12047[1], 12051[1], 12052[1], 12053[1], 12054[1], 12055[1], 12056[1], 12057[1], 13100[1], 13101[1], 13102[1], 13120[1], 13121[1], 13122[1], 13131[1], 13132[1], 13133[1], 13151[1], 13152[1], 13153[1], 36000[1], 36400[1], 36405[1], 36406[1], 36410[1], 36420[1], 36425[1], 36430[1], 36440[1], 36591[0], 36592[0], 36600[1], 36640[1], 43752[1], 44005[0], 44180[0], 44602[1], 44603[1], 44604[1], 44605[1], 44820[0], 44850[0], 49000[1], 49002[1], 49010[1], 49255[1], 49320[1], 49400[1], 49436[1], 49570[1], 51701[1], 51702[1], 51703[1], 62320[0], 62321[0], 62322[0], 62323[0], 62324[0], 62325[0], 62326[0], 62327[0], 64400[0], 64405[0], 64408[0], 64415[1], 64416[1], 64417[1], 64418[0], 64420[0], 64421[0], 64425[0], 64430[0], 64435[0], 64445[0], 64446[0], 64447[0], 64448[0], 64449[0], 64450[1], 64451[0], 64454[1], 64461[0], 64462[0], 64463[0], 64479[0], 64480[0], 64483[0], 64484[0], 64486[0], 64487[0], 64488[0], 64489[0], 64490[1], 64491[0], 64492[0], 64493[1], 64494[0], 64495[0], 64505[0], 64510[0], 64517[0], 64520[0], 64530[0], 69990[0], 92012[1], 92014[1], 93000[1], 93005[1], 93010[1], 93040[1], 93041[1], 93042[1], 93318[1], 93355[1], 94002[1], 94200[1], 94680[1], 94681[1], 94690[1], 95812[1], 95813[1], 95816[1], 95819[1], 95822[1], 95829[1], 95955[1], 96360[1], 96361[1], 96365[1], 96366[1], 96367[1], 96368[1], 96372[1], 96374[1], 96375[1], 96376[1], 96377[1], 96523[0], 97597[1], 97598[1], 97602[1], 99155[0], 99156[0], 99157[0], 99211[1], 99212[1], 99213[1], 99214[1], 99215[1], 99217[1], 99218[1], 99219[1], 99220[1], 99221[1], 99222[1], 99223[1], 99231[1], 99232[1], 99233[1], 99234[1], 99235[1], 99236[1], 99238[1], 99239[1], 99241[1], 99242[1], 99243[1], 99244[1], 99245[1], 99251[1], 99252[1], 99253[1], 99254[1], 99255[1], 99291[1], 99292[1], 99304[1], 99305[1], 99306[1], 99307[1], 99308[1], 99309[1], 99310[1], 99315[1], 99316[1], 99334[1], 99335[1], 99336[1], 99337[1], 99347[1], 99348[1], 99349[1], 99350[1], 99374[1], 99375[1], 99377[1], 99378[1], 99446[0], 99447[0], 99448[0], 99449[0], 99451[0], 99452[0], 99495[0], 99496[0], G0463[1], G0471[1]
49423	0213T[1], 0216T[1], 0596T[1], 0597T[1], 0708T[1], 0709T[1], 12001[1], 12002[1], 12004[1], 12005[1], 12006[1], 12007[1], 12011[1], 12013[1], 12014[1], 12015[1], 12016[1], 12017[1], 12018[1], 12020[1], 12021[1], 12031[1], 12032[1], 12034[1], 12035[1], 12036[1], 12037[1], 12041[1], 12042[1], 12044[1], 12045[1], 12046[1], 12047[1], 12051[1], 12052[1], 12053[1], 12054[1], 12055[1], 12056[1], 12057[1], 13100[1], 13101[1], 13102[1], 13120[1], 13121[1], 13122[1], 13131[1], 13132[1], 13133[1], 13151[1], 13152[1], 13153[1], 36000[1], 36400[1], 36405[1], 36406[1], 36410[1], 36420[1], 36425[1], 36430[1], 36440[1], 36591[0], 36592[0], 36600[1], 36640[1], 43752[1], 44602[1], 44603[1], 44604[1], 44605[1], 49320[1], 51701[1], 51702[1], 51703[1], 62320[0], 62321[0], 62322[0], 62323[0], 62324[0], 62325[0], 62326[0], 62327[0], 64400[0], 64405[0], 64408[0], 64415[1], 64416[1], 64417[1], 64418[0], 64420[0], 64421[0], 64425[0], 64430[0], 64435[0], 64445[0], 64446[0], 64447[0], 64448[0], 64449[0], 64450[1], 64451[0], 64454[1], 64461[0], 64462[0], 64463[0], 64479[0], 64480[0], 64483[0], 64484[0], 64486[0], 64487[0], 64488[0], 64489[0], 64490[1], 64491[0], 64492[0], 64493[1], 64494[0], 64495[0], 64505[0], 64510[0], 64517[0], 64520[0], 64530[0], 69990[0], 76000[1], 76942[1], 76998[1], 77001[1], 77002[1], 92012[1], 92014[1], 93000[1], 93005[1], 93010[1], 93040[1], 93041[1], 93042[1], 93318[1], 93355[1], 94002[1], 94200[1], 94680[1], 94681[1], 94690[1], 95812[1], 95813[1], 95816[1], 95819[1], 95822[1], 95829[1], 95955[1], 96360[1], 96361[1], 96365[1], 96366[1], 96367[1], 96368[1], 96372[1], 96374[1], 96375[1], 96376[1], 96377[1], 96523[0], 99155[0], 99156[0], 99157[0], 99211[1], 99212[1], 99213[1], 99214[1], 99215[1], 99217[1], 99218[1], 99219[1], 99220[1], 99221[1], 99222[1], 99223[1], 99231[1], 99232[1], 99233[1], 99234[1], 99235[1], 99236[1], 99238[1], 99239[1], 99241[1], 99242[1], 99243[1], 99244[1], 99245[1], 99251[1], 99252[1], 99253[1], 99254[1], 99255[1], 99291[1], 99292[1], 99304[1], 99305[1], 99306[1], 99307[1], 99308[1], 99309[1], 99310[1], 99315[1], 99316[1], 99334[1], 99335[1], 99336[1], 99337[1], 99347[1], 99348[1], 99349[1], 99350[1], 99374[1], 99375[1], 99377[1], 99378[1], 99446[0], 99447[0], 99448[0], 99449[0], 99451[0], 99452[0], 99495[1], 99496[1], G0463[1], G0471[1], J0670[1], J2001[1]
49424	0213T[1], 0216T[1], 0596T[1], 0597T[1], 0708T[1], 0709T[1], 12001[1], 12002[1], 12004[1], 12005[1], 12006[1], 12007[1], 12011[1], 12013[1], 12014[1], 12015[1], 12016[1], 12017[1], 12018[1], 12020[1], 12021[1], 12031[1], 12032[1], 12034[1], 12035[1], 12036[1], 12037[1], 12041[1], 12042[1], 12044[1], 12045[1], 12046[1], 12047[1], 12051[1], 12052[1], 12053[1], 12054[1], 12055[1], 12056[1], 12057[1], 13100[1], 13101[1], 13102[1], 13120[1], 13121[1], 13122[1], 13131[1], 13132[1], 13133[1], 13151[1], 13152[1], 13153[1], 36000[1], 36400[1], 36405[1], 36406[1], 36410[1], 36420[1], 36425[1], 36430[1], 36440[1], 36591[0], 36592[0], 36600[1], 36640[1], 43752[1], 44602[1], 44603[1], 44604[1], 44605[1], 49320[1], 51701[1], 51702[1], 51703[1], 62320[0], 62321[0], 62322[0], 62323[0], 62324[0], 62325[0], 62326[0], 62327[0], 64400[0], 64405[0], 64408[0], 64415[1], 64416[1], 64417[1], 64418[0], 64420[0], 64421[0], 64425[0], 64430[0], 64435[0], 64445[0], 64446[0], 64447[0], 64448[0], 64449[0], 64450[1], 64451[0], 64454[1], 64461[0], 64462[0], 64463[0], 64479[0], 64480[0], 64483[0], 64484[0], 64486[0], 64487[0], 64488[0], 64489[0], 64490[1], 64491[0], 64492[0], 64493[1], 64494[0], 64495[0], 64505[0], 64510[0], 64517[0], 64520[0], 64530[0], 69990[0], 76000[1], 77001[1], 77002[1], 92012[1], 92014[1], 93000[1], 93005[1], 93010[1], 93040[1], 93041[1], 93042[1], 93318[1], 93355[1], 94002[1], 94200[1],

0 = Modifier usage not allowed or inappropriate 1 = Modifier usage allowed

Code 1	Code 2
	94680[1], 94681[1], 94690[1], 95812[1], 95813[1], 95816[1], 95819[1], 95822[1], 95829[1], 95955[1], 96360[1], 96361[1], 96365[1], 96366[1], 96367[1], 96368[1], 96372[1], 96374[1], 96375[1], 96376[1], 96377[1], 96523[0], 99155[0], 99156[0], 99157[0], 99211[1], 99212[1], 99213[1], 99214[1], 99215[1], 99217[1], 99218[1], 99219[1], 99220[1], 99221[1], 99222[1], 99223[1], 99231[1], 99232[1], 99233[1], 99234[1], 99235[1], 99236[1], 99238[1], 99239[1], 99241[1], 99242[1], 99243[1], 99244[1], 99245[1], 99251[1], 99252[1], 99253[1], 99254[1], 99255[1], 99291[1], 99292[1], 99304[1], 99305[1], 99306[1], 99307[1], 99308[1], 99309[1], 99310[1], 99315[1], 99316[1], 99334[1], 99335[1], 99336[1], 99337[1], 99347[1], 99348[1], 99349[1], 99350[1], 99374[1], 99375[1], 99377[1], 99378[1], 99446[0], 99447[0], 99448[0], 99449[0], 99451[0], 99452[0], 99495[1], 99496[1], G0463[1], G0471[1], J0670[1], J2001[1]
49435	11000[1], 11001[1], 11004[1], 11005[1], 11006[1], 11042[1], 11043[1], 11044[1], 11045[1], 11046[1], 11047[1], 36591[0], 36592[0], 96523[0], 97597[1], 97598[1], 97602[1]
49436	0213T[1], 0216T[1], 0596T[1], 0597T[1], 0708T[1], 0709T[1], 12001[1], 12002[1], 12004[1], 12005[1], 12006[1], 12007[1], 12011[1], 12013[1], 12014[1], 12015[1], 12016[1], 12017[1], 12018[1], 12020[1], 12021[1], 12031[1], 12032[1], 12034[1], 12035[1], 12036[1], 12037[1], 12041[1], 12042[1], 12044[1], 12045[1], 12046[1], 12047[1], 12051[1], 12052[1], 12053[1], 12054[1], 12055[1], 12056[1], 12057[1], 13100[1], 13101[1], 13102[1], 13120[1], 13121[1], 13122[1], 13131[1], 13132[1], 13133[1], 13151[1], 13152[1], 13153[1], 36000[1], 36400[1], 36405[1], 36406[1], 36410[1], 36420[1], 36425[1], 36430[1], 36440[1], 36591[0], 36592[0], 36600[1], 36640[1], 43752[1], 51701[1], 51702[1], 51703[1], 62320[0], 62321[0], 62322[0], 62323[0], 62324[0], 62325[0], 62326[0], 62327[0], 64400[0], 64405[0], 64408[0], 64415[1], 64416[1], 64417[1], 64418[0], 64420[0], 64421[0], 64425[0], 64430[0], 64435[0], 64445[0], 64446[0], 64447[0], 64448[0], 64449[0], 64450[1], 64451[0], 64454[1], 64461[0], 64462[0], 64463[0], 64479[0], 64480[0], 64483[0], 64484[0], 64486[0], 64487[0], 64488[0], 64489[0], 64490[1], 64491[0], 64492[0], 64493[1], 64494[0], 64495[0], 64505[0], 64510[0], 64517[0], 64520[0], 64530[0], 69990[0], 92012[1], 92014[1], 93000[1], 93005[1], 93010[1], 93040[1], 93041[1], 93042[1], 93318[1], 93355[1], 94002[1], 94200[1], 94680[1], 94681[1], 94690[1], 95812[1], 95813[1], 95816[1], 95819[1], 95822[1], 95829[1], 95955[1], 96360[1], 96361[1], 96365[1], 96366[1], 96367[1], 96368[1], 96372[1], 96374[1], 96375[1], 96376[1], 96377[1], 96523[0], 99155[0], 99156[0], 99157[0], 99211[1], 99212[1], 99213[1], 99214[1], 99215[1], 99217[1], 99218[1], 99219[1], 99220[1], 99221[1], 99222[1], 99223[1], 99231[1], 99232[1], 99233[1], 99234[1], 99235[1], 99236[1], 99238[1], 99239[1], 99241[1], 99242[1], 99243[1], 99244[1], 99245[1], 99251[1], 99252[1], 99253[1], 99254[1], 99255[1], 99291[1], 99292[1], 99304[1], 99305[1], 99306[1], 99307[1], 99308[1], 99309[1], 99310[1], 99315[1], 99316[1], 99334[1], 99335[1], 99336[1], 99337[1], 99347[1], 99348[1], 99349[1], 99350[1], 99374[1], 99375[1], 99377[1], 99378[1], 99446[0], 99447[0], 99448[0], 99449[0], 99451[0], 99452[0], 99495[0], 99496[0], G0463[1], G0471[1]
50010	0213T[0], 0216T[0], 0596T[1], 0597T[1], 0708T[1], 0709T[1], 12001[1], 12002[1], 12004[1], 12005[1], 12006[1], 12007[1], 12011[1], 12013[1], 12014[1], 12015[1], 12016[1], 12017[1], 12018[1], 12020[1], 12021[1], 12031[1], 12032[1], 12034[1], 12035[1], 12036[1], 12037[1], 12041[1], 12042[1], 12044[1], 12045[1], 12046[1], 12047[1], 12051[1], 12052[1], 12053[1], 12054[1], 12055[1], 12056[1], 12057[1], 13100[1], 13101[1], 13102[1], 13120[1], 13121[1], 13122[1], 13131[1], 13132[1], 13133[1], 13151[1], 13152[1], 13153[1], 36000[1], 36400[1], 36405[1], 36406[1], 36410[1], 36420[1], 36425[1], 36430[1], 36440[1], 36591[0], 36592[0], 36600[1], 36640[1], 43752[1], 44602[1], 44603[1], 44604[1], 44605[1], 44950[0], 44970[0], 49000[0], 49002[1], 49010[0], 50100[1], 51701[1], 51702[1], 51703[1], 60540[1], 60545[1], 62320[0], 62321[0], 62322[0], 62323[0], 62324[0], 62325[0], 62326[0], 62327[0], 64400[0], 64405[0], 64408[0], 64415[0], 64416[0], 64417[0], 64418[0], 64420[0], 64421[0], 64425[0], 64430[0], 64435[0], 64445[0], 64446[0], 64447[0], 64448[0], 64449[0], 64450[0], 64451[0], 64454[0], 64461[0], 64462[0], 64463[0], 64479[0], 64480[0], 64483[0], 64484[0], 64486[0], 64487[0], 64488[0], 64489[0], 64490[0], 64491[0], 64492[0], 64493[0], 64494[0], 64495[0], 64505[0], 64510[0], 64517[0], 64520[0], 64530[0], 69990[0], 92012[1], 92014[1], 93000[1], 93005[1], 93010[1], 93040[1], 93041[1], 93042[1], 93318[1], 93355[1], 94002[1], 94200[1], 94680[1], 94681[1], 94690[1], 95812[1], 95813[1], 95816[1], 95819[1], 95822[1], 95829[1], 95955[1], 96360[1], 96361[1], 96365[1], 96366[1], 96367[1], 96368[1], 96372[1], 96374[1], 96375[1], 96376[1], 96377[1], 96523[0], 99155[0], 99156[0], 99157[0], 99211[1], 99212[1], 99213[1], 99214[1], 99215[1], 99217[1], 99218[1], 99219[1], 99220[1], 99221[1], 99222[1], 99223[1], 99231[1], 99232[1], 99233[1], 99234[1], 99235[1], 99236[1], 99238[1], 99239[1], 99241[1], 99242[1], 99243[1], 99244[1], 99245[1], 99251[1], 99252[1], 99253[1], 99254[1], 99255[1], 99291[1], 99292[1], 99304[1], 99305[1], 99306[1], 99307[1], 99308[1], 99309[1], 99310[1], 99315[1], 99316[1], 99334[1], 99335[1], 99336[1], 99337[1], 99347[1], 99348[1], 99349[1], 99350[1], 99374[1], 99375[1], 99377[1], 99378[1], 99446[0], 99447[0], 99448[0], 99449[0], 99451[0], 99452[0], 99495[0], 99496[0], G0463[1], G0471[1]
50020	0213T[0], 0216T[0], 0596T[1], 0597T[1], 0708T[1], 0709T[1], 12001[1], 12002[1], 12004[1], 12005[1], 12006[1], 12007[1], 12011[1], 12013[1], 12014[1], 12015[1], 12016[1], 12017[1], 12018[1], 12020[1], 12021[1], 12031[1], 12032[1], 12034[1], 12035[1], 12036[1], 12037[1], 12041[1], 12042[1], 12044[1], 12045[1], 12046[1], 12047[1], 12051[1], 12052[1], 12053[1], 12054[1], 12055[1], 12056[1], 12057[1], 13100[1], 13101[1], 13102[1], 13120[1], 13121[1], 13122[1], 13131[1], 13132[1], 13133[1], 13151[1], 13152[1], 13153[1], 36000[1], 36400[1], 36405[1], 36406[1], 36410[1], 36420[1], 36425[1], 36430[1], 36440[1], 36591[0], 36592[0], 36600[1], 36640[1], 43752[1], 44602[1], 44603[1], 44604[1], 44605[1], 44950[0], 44970[0], 49000[0], 49002[1], 49010[0], 49020[1], 49405[1], 49406[1], 50010[1], 50205[1], 51701[1], 51702[1], 51703[1], 62320[0], 62321[0], 62322[0], 62323[0], 62324[0], 62325[0], 62326[0], 62327[0], 64400[0], 64405[0], 64408[0], 64415[0], 64416[0], 64417[0], 64418[0], 64420[0], 64421[0], 64425[0], 64430[0], 64435[0], 64445[0], 64446[0], 64447[0], 64448[0], 64449[0], 64450[0], 64451[0], 64454[0], 64461[0], 64462[0], 64463[0], 64479[0], 64480[0], 64483[0], 64484[0], 64486[0], 64487[0], 64488[0], 64489[0], 64490[0], 64491[0], 64492[0], 64493[0], 64494[0], 64495[0], 64505[0], 64510[0], 64517[0], 64520[0], 64530[0], 69990[0], 92012[1], 92014[1], 93000[1], 93005[1], 93010[1], 93040[1], 93041[1], 93042[1], 93318[1], 93355[1], 94002[1], 94200[1], 94680[1], 94681[1], 94690[1], 95812[1], 95813[1], 95816[1], 95819[1], 95822[1], 95829[1], 95955[1], 96360[1], 96361[1], 96365[1], 96366[1], 96367[1], 96368[1], 96372[1], 96374[1], 96375[1], 96376[1], 96377[1], 96523[0], 99155[0], 99156[0], 99157[0], 99211[1], 99212[1], 99213[1], 99214[1], 99215[1], 99217[1], 99218[1], 99219[1], 99220[1], 99221[1], 99222[1], 99223[1], 99231[1], 99232[1], 99233[1], 99234[1], 99235[1], 99236[1], 99238[1], 99239[1], 99241[1], 99242[1], 99243[1], 99244[1], 99245[1], 99251[1], 99252[1], 99253[1], 99254[1], 99255[1], 99291[1], 99292[1], 99304[1], 99305[1], 99306[1], 99307[1], 99308[1], 99309[1], 99310[1], 99315[1], 99316[1], 99334[1], 99335[1], 99336[1], 99337[1], 99347[1], 99348[1], 99349[1], 99350[1], 99374[1], 99375[1], 99377[1], 99378[1], 99446[0], 99447[0], 99448[0], 99449[0], 99451[0], 99452[0], 99495[0], 99496[0], G0463[1], G0471[1]
50040	0213T[0], 0216T[0], 0596T[1], 0597T[1], 0708T[1], 0709T[1], 11000[1], 11001[1], 11004[1], 11005[1], 11006[1], 11042[1], 11043[1], 11044[1], 11045[1], 11046[1], 11047[1], 12001[1], 12002[1], 12004[1], 12005[1], 12006[1], 12007[1], 12011[1], 12013[1], 12014[1], 12015[1], 12016[1], 12017[1], 12018[1], 12020[1], 12021[1], 12031[1], 12032[1], 12034[1], 12035[1], 12036[1], 12037[1], 12041[1], 12042[1], 12044[1], 12045[1], 12046[1], 12047[1], 12051[1], 12052[1], 12053[1], 12054[1], 12055[1], 12056[1], 12057[1], 13100[1], 13101[1], 13102[1], 13120[1], 13121[1], 13122[1], 13131[1], 13132[1], 13133[1], 13151[1], 13152[1], 13153[1], 36000[1], 36400[1], 36405[1], 36406[1], 36410[1], 36420[1], 36425[1], 36430[1], 36440[1], 36591[0], 36592[0], 36600[1], 36640[1], 43752[1], 44602[1], 44603[1], 44604[1], 44605[1], 44950[0], 44970[0], 49000[0], 49002[1], 49010[0], 49406[1], 50010[1], 50020[1], 50045[1], 50500[1], 50541[1], 51701[1], 51702[1], 51703[1], 62320[0], 62321[0], 62322[0], 62323[0], 62324[0], 62325[0], 62326[0], 62327[0], 64400[0], 64405[0], 64408[0], 64415[0], 64416[0], 64417[0], 64418[0], 64420[0], 64421[0], 64425[0], 64430[0], 64435[0], 64445[0], 64446[0], 64447[0], 64448[0], 64449[0], 64450[0], 64451[0], 64454[0], 64461[0], 64462[0], 64463[0], 64479[0], 64480[0], 64483[0], 64484[0], 64486[0], 64487[0], 64488[0], 64489[0], 64490[0], 64491[0], 64492[0], 64493[0], 64494[0], 64495[0], 64505[0], 64510[0], 64517[0], 64520[0], 64530[0], 69990[0], 92012[1], 92014[1], 93000[1], 93005[1], 93010[1], 93040[1], 93041[1], 93042[1], 93318[1], 93355[1], 94002[1], 94200[1], 94680[1], 94681[1], 94690[1], 95812[1], 95813[1], 95816[1], 95819[1], 95822[1], 95829[1], 95955[1], 96360[1], 96361[1], 96365[1], 96366[1], 96367[1], 96368[1], 96372[1], 96374[1], 96375[1], 96376[1], 96377[1], 96523[0], 97597[1], 97598[1], 97602[1], 99155[0], 99156[0], 99157[0], 99211[1], 99212[1], 99213[1], 99214[1], 99215[1], 99217[1], 99218[1], 99219[1], 99220[1], 99221[1], 99222[1], 99223[1], 99231[1], 99232[1], 99233[1], 99234[1], 99235[1], 99236[1], 99238[1], 99239[1], 99241[1], 99242[1], 99243[1], 99244[1], 99245[1], 99251[1], 99252[1], 99253[1], 99254[1], 99255[1], 99291[1], 99292[1], 99304[1], 99305[1], 99306[1], 99307[1], 99308[1], 99309[1], 99310[1], 99315[1], 99316[1], 99334[1], 99335[1], 99336[1], 99337[1], 99347[1], 99348[1], 99349[1], 99350[1], 99374[1], 99375[1], 99377[1], 99378[1], 99446[0], 99447[0], 99448[0], 99449[0], 99451[0], 99452[0], 99495[0], 99496[0], G0463[1], G0471[1]
50045	0213T[0], 0216T[0], 0596T[1], 0597T[1], 0708T[1], 0709T[1], 11000[1], 11001[1], 11004[1], 11005[1], 11006[1], 11042[1], 11043[1], 11044[1], 11045[1], 11046[1], 11047[1], 12001[1], 12002[1], 12004[1], 12005[1], 12006[1], 12007[1], 12011[1], 12013[1], 12014[1], 12015[1], 12016[1], 12017[1], 12018[1], 12020[1], 12021[1], 12031[1], 12032[1], 12034[1], 12035[1], 12036[1], 12037[1], 12041[1], 12042[1], 12044[1], 12045[1], 12046[1], 12047[1], 12051[1], 12052[1], 12053[1], 12054[1], 12055[1], 12056[1], 12057[1], 13100[1], 13101[1], 13102[1], 13120[1], 13121[1], 13122[1], 13131[1], 13132[1], 13133[1], 13151[1], 13152[1], 13153[1], 36000[1], 36400[1], 36405[1], 36406[1], 36410[1], 36420[1], 36425[1], 36430[1], 36440[1], 36591[0], 36592[0], 36600[1], 36640[1], 43752[1], 44602[1], 44603[1], 44604[1], 44605[1], 44950[0], 44970[0], 49000[0], 49002[1], 49010[0], 49406[1], 50010[1], 50020[1], 50541[1], 51701[1], 51702[1], 51703[1], 62320[0], 62321[0], 62322[0], 62323[0], 62324[0], 62325[0], 62326[0], 62327[0], 64400[0], 64405[0], 64408[0], 64415[0], 64416[0], 64417[0], 64418[0], 64420[0], 64421[0], 64425[0], 64430[0], 64435[0], 64445[0], 64446[0], 64447[0], 64448[0], 64449[0], 64450[0], 64451[0], 64454[0], 64461[0], 64462[0], 64463[0], 64479[0], 64480[0], 64483[0], 64484[0], 64486[0], 64487[0], 64488[0], 64489[0], 64490[0], 64491[0], 64492[0], 64493[0], 64494[0], 64495[0], 64505[0], 64510[0], 64517[0], 64520[0], 64530[0], 69990[0], 92012[1], 92014[1], 93000[1], 93005[1], 93010[1], 93040[1], 93041[1], 93042[1], 93318[1], 93355[1], 94002[1], 94200[1], 94680[1], 94681[1], 94690[1], 95812[1], 95813[1], 95816[1], 95819[1], 95822[1], 95829[1], 95955[1], 96360[1], 96361[1], 96365[1], 96366[1], 96367[1], 96368[1], 96372[1], 96374[1], 96375[1], 96376[1], 96377[1], 96523[0], 97597[1], 97598[1], 97602[1], 99155[0], 99156[0], 99157[0], 99211[1], 99212[1], 99213[1], 99214[1], 99215[1], 99217[1], 99218[1], 99219[1], 99220[1], 99221[1], 99222[1], 99223[1], 99231[1], 99232[1], 99233[1], 99234[1], 99235[1], 99236[1], 99238[1], 99239[1], 99241[1], 99242[1], 99243[1], 99244[1], 99245[1], 99251[1], 99252[1], 99253[1], 99254[1], 99255[1], 99291[1], 99292[1], 99304[1], 99305[1], 99306[1], 99307[1], 99308[1], 99309[1], 99310[1], 99315[1], 99316[1], 99334[1], 99335[1], 99336[1], 99337[1], 99347[1], 99348[1], 99349[1], 99350[1], 99374[1], 99375[1], 99377[1], 99378[1], 99446[0], 99447[0], 99448[0], 99449[0], 99451[0], 99452[0], 99495[0], 99496[0], G0463[1], G0471[1]

0 = Modifier usage not allowed or inappropriate   1 = Modifier usage allowed

Code 1	Code 2
50060	0213T[0], 0216T[0], 0596T[1], 0597T[1], 0708T[1], 0709T[1], 11000[1], 11001[1], 11004[1], 11005[1], 11006[1], 11042[1], 11043[1], 11044[1], 11045[1], 11046[1], 11047[1], 12001[1], 12002[1], 12004[1], 12005[1], 12006[1], 12007[1], 12011[1], 12013[1], 12014[1], 12015[1], 12016[1], 12017[1], 12018[1], 12020[1], 12021[1], 12031[1], 12032[1], 12034[1], 12035[1], 12036[1], 12037[1], 12041[1], 12042[1], 12044[1], 12045[1], 12046[1], 12047[1], 12051[1], 12052[1], 12053[1], 12054[1], 12055[1], 12056[1], 12057[1], 13100[1], 13101[1], 13102[1], 13120[1], 13121[1], 13122[1], 13131[1], 13132[1], 13133[1], 13151[1], 13152[1], 13153[1], 36000[1], 36400[1], 36405[1], 36406[1], 36410[1], 36420[1], 36425[1], 36430[1], 36440[1], 36591[0], 36592[0], 36600[1], 36640[1], 43752[1], 44602[1], 44603[1], 44604[1], 44605[1], 44950[0], 44970[0], 49000[0], 49002[1], 49010[0], 49406[1], 50020[1], 50040[1], 50045[1], 50065[1], 50070[1], 50075[1], 50500[1], 51701[1], 51702[1], 51703[1], 62320[0], 62321[0], 62322[0], 62323[0], 62324[0], 62325[0], 62326[0], 62327[0], 64400[0], 64405[0], 64408[0], 64415[0], 64416[0], 64417[0], 64418[0], 64420[0], 64421[0], 64425[0], 64430[0], 64435[0], 64445[0], 64446[0], 64447[0], 64448[0], 64449[0], 64450[0], 64451[0], 64454[0], 64461[0], 64462[0], 64463[0], 64479[0], 64480[0], 64483[0], 64484[0], 64486[0], 64487[0], 64488[0], 64489[0], 64490[0], 64491[0], 64492[0], 64493[0], 64494[0], 64495[0], 64505[0], 64510[0], 64517[0], 64520[0], 64530[0], 69990[0], 92012[1], 92014[1], 93000[1], 93005[1], 93010[1], 93040[1], 93041[1], 93042[1], 93318[1], 93355[1], 94002[1], 94200[1], 94680[1], 94681[1], 94690[1], 95812[1], 95813[1], 95816[1], 95819[1], 95822[1], 95829[1], 95955[1], 96360[1], 96361[1], 96365[1], 96366[1], 96367[1], 96368[1], 96372[1], 96374[1], 96375[1], 96376[1], 96377[1], 96523[0], 97597[1], 97598[1], 97602[1], 99155[0], 99156[0], 99157[0], 99211[1], 99212[1], 99213[1], 99214[1], 99215[1], 99217[1], 99218[1], 99219[1], 99220[1], 99221[1], 99222[1], 99223[1], 99231[1], 99232[1], 99233[1], 99234[1], 99235[1], 99236[1], 99238[1], 99239[1], 99241[1], 99242[1], 99243[1], 99244[1], 99245[1], 99251[1], 99252[1], 99253[1], 99254[1], 99255[1], 99291[1], 99292[1], 99304[1], 99305[1], 99306[1], 99307[1], 99308[1], 99309[1], 99310[1], 99315[1], 99316[1], 99334[1], 99335[1], 99336[1], 99337[1], 99347[1], 99348[1], 99349[1], 99350[1], 99374[1], 99375[1], 99377[1], 99378[1], 99446[0], 99447[0], 99448[0], 99449[0], 99451[0], 99452[0], 99495[0], 99496[0], G0463[1], G0471[1]
50065	0213T[0], 0216T[0], 0596T[1], 0597T[1], 0708T[1], 0709T[1], 11000[1], 11001[1], 11004[1], 11005[1], 11006[1], 11042[1], 11043[1], 11044[1], 11045[1], 11046[1], 11047[1], 12001[1], 12002[1], 12004[1], 12005[1], 12006[1], 12007[1], 12011[1], 12013[1], 12014[1], 12015[1], 12016[1], 12017[1], 12018[1], 12020[1], 12021[1], 12031[1], 12032[1], 12034[1], 12035[1], 12036[1], 12037[1], 12041[1], 12042[1], 12044[1], 12045[1], 12046[1], 12047[1], 12051[1], 12052[1], 12053[1], 12054[1], 12055[1], 12056[1], 12057[1], 13100[1], 13101[1], 13102[1], 13120[1], 13121[1], 13122[1], 13131[1], 13132[1], 13133[1], 13151[1], 13152[1], 13153[1], 36000[1], 36400[1], 36405[1], 36406[1], 36410[1], 36420[1], 36425[1], 36430[1], 36440[1], 36591[0], 36592[0], 36600[1], 36640[1], 43752[1], 44602[1], 44603[1], 44604[1], 44605[1], 44950[0], 44970[0], 49000[0], 49002[1], 49010[0], 49406[1], 50020[1], 50040[1], 50045[1], 50075[1], 50500[1], 51701[1], 51702[1], 51703[1], 62320[0], 62321[0], 62322[0], 62323[0], 62324[0], 62325[0], 62326[0], 62327[0], 64400[0], 64405[0], 64408[0], 64415[0], 64416[0], 64417[0], 64418[0], 64420[0], 64421[0], 64425[0], 64430[0], 64435[0], 64445[0], 64446[0], 64447[0], 64448[0], 64449[0], 64450[0], 64451[0], 64454[0], 64461[0], 64462[0], 64463[0], 64479[0], 64480[0], 64483[0], 64484[0], 64486[0], 64487[0], 64488[0], 64489[0], 64490[0], 64491[0], 64492[0], 64493[0], 64494[0], 64495[0], 64505[0], 64510[0], 64517[0], 64520[0], 64530[0], 69990[0], 92012[1], 92014[1], 93000[1], 93005[1], 93010[1], 93040[1], 93041[1], 93042[1], 93318[1], 93355[1], 94002[1], 94200[1], 94680[1], 94681[1], 94690[1], 95812[1], 95813[1], 95816[1], 95819[1], 95822[1], 95829[1], 95955[1], 96360[1], 96361[1], 96365[1], 96366[1], 96367[1], 96368[1], 96372[1], 96374[1], 96375[1], 96376[1], 96377[1], 96523[0], 97597[1], 97598[1], 97602[1], 99155[0], 99156[0], 99157[0], 99211[1], 99212[1], 99213[1], 99214[1], 99215[1], 99217[1], 99218[1], 99219[1], 99220[1], 99221[1], 99222[1], 99223[1], 99231[1], 99232[1], 99233[1], 99234[1], 99235[1], 99236[1], 99238[1], 99239[1], 99241[1], 99242[1], 99243[1], 99244[1], 99245[1], 99251[1], 99252[1], 99253[1], 99254[1], 99255[1], 99291[1], 99292[1], 99304[1], 99305[1], 99306[1], 99307[1], 99308[1], 99309[1], 99310[1], 99315[1], 99316[1], 99334[1], 99335[1], 99336[1], 99337[1], 99347[1], 99348[1], 99349[1], 99350[1], 99374[1], 99375[1], 99377[1], 99378[1], 99446[0], 99447[0], 99448[0], 99449[0], 99451[0], 99452[0], 99495[0], 99496[0], G0463[1], G0471[1]
50070	0213T[0], 0216T[0], 0596T[1], 0597T[1], 0708T[1], 0709T[1], 11000[1], 11001[1], 11004[1], 11005[1], 11006[1], 11042[1], 11043[1], 11044[1], 11045[1], 11046[1], 11047[1], 12001[1], 12002[1], 12004[1], 12005[1], 12006[1], 12007[1], 12011[1], 12013[1], 12014[1], 12015[1], 12016[1], 12017[1], 12018[1], 12020[1], 12021[1], 12031[1], 12032[1], 12034[1], 12035[1], 12036[1], 12037[1], 12041[1], 12042[1], 12044[1], 12045[1], 12046[1], 12047[1], 12051[1], 12052[1], 12053[1], 12054[1], 12055[1], 12056[1], 12057[1], 13100[1], 13101[1], 13102[1], 13120[1], 13121[1], 13122[1], 13131[1], 13132[1], 13133[1], 13151[1], 13152[1], 13153[1], 36000[1], 36400[1], 36405[1], 36406[1], 36410[1], 36420[1], 36425[1], 36430[1], 36440[1], 36591[0], 36592[0], 36600[1], 36640[1], 43752[1], 44602[1], 44603[1], 44604[1], 44605[1], 44950[0], 44970[0], 49000[0], 49002[1], 49010[0], 49406[1], 50020[1], 50040[1], 50045[1], 50065[1], 50075[1], 50500[1], 51701[1], 51702[1], 51703[1], 62320[0], 62321[0], 62322[0], 62323[0], 62324[0], 62325[0], 62326[0], 62327[0], 64400[0], 64405[0], 64408[0], 64415[0], 64416[0], 64417[0], 64418[0], 64420[0], 64421[0], 64425[0], 64430[0], 64435[0], 64445[0], 64446[0], 64447[0], 64448[0], 64449[0], 64450[0], 64451[0], 64454[0], 64461[0], 64462[0], 64463[0], 64479[0], 64480[0], 64483[0], 64484[0], 64486[0], 64487[0], 64488[0], 64489[0], 64490[0], 64491[0], 64492[0], 64493[0], 64494[0], 64495[0], 64505[0], 64510[0], 64517[0], 64520[0], 64530[0], 69990[0], 92012[1], 92014[1], 93000[1], 93005[1], 93010[1], 93040[1], 93041[1], 93042[1], 93318[1], 93355[1], 94002[1], 94200[1], 94680[1], 94681[1], 94690[1], 95812[1], 95813[1], 95816[1], 95819[1], 95822[1], 95829[1], 95955[1], 96360[1], 96361[1], 96365[1], 96366[1], 96367[1], 96368[1], 96372[1], 96374[1], 96375[1], 96376[1], 96377[1], 96523[0], 97597[1], 97598[1], 97602[1], 99155[0], 99156[0], 99157[0], 99211[1], 99212[1], 99213[1], 99214[1], 99215[1], 99217[1], 99218[1], 99219[1], 99220[1], 99221[1], 99222[1], 99223[1], 99231[1], 99232[1], 99233[1], 99234[1], 99235[1], 99236[1], 99238[1], 99239[1], 99241[1], 99242[1], 99243[1], 99244[1], 99245[1], 99251[1], 99252[1], 99253[1], 99254[1], 99255[1], 99291[1], 99292[1], 99304[1], 99305[1], 99306[1], 99307[1], 99308[1], 99309[1], 99310[1], 99315[1], 99316[1], 99334[1], 99335[1], 99336[1], 99337[1], 99347[1], 99348[1], 99349[1], 99350[1], 99374[1], 99375[1], 99377[1], 99378[1], 99446[0], 99447[0], 99448[0], 99449[0], 99451[0], 99452[0], 99495[0], 99496[0], G0463[1], G0471[1]
50075	0213T[0], 0216T[0], 0596T[1], 0597T[1], 0708T[1], 0709T[1], 11000[1], 11001[1], 11004[1], 11005[1], 11006[1], 11042[1], 11043[1], 11044[1], 11045[1], 11046[1], 11047[1], 12001[1], 12002[1], 12004[1], 12005[1], 12006[1], 12007[1], 12011[1], 12013[1], 12014[1], 12015[1], 12016[1], 12017[1], 12018[1], 12020[1], 12021[1], 12031[1], 12032[1], 12034[1], 12035[1], 12036[1], 12037[1], 12041[1], 12042[1], 12044[1], 12045[1], 12046[1], 12047[1], 12051[1], 12052[1], 12053[1], 12054[1], 12055[1], 12056[1], 12057[1], 13100[1], 13101[1], 13102[1], 13120[1], 13121[1], 13122[1], 13131[1], 13132[1], 13133[1], 13151[1], 13152[1], 13153[1], 36000[1], 36400[1], 36405[1], 36406[1], 36410[1], 36420[1], 36425[1], 36430[1], 36440[1], 36591[0], 36592[0], 36600[1], 36640[1], 43752[1], 44602[1], 44603[1], 44604[1], 44605[1], 44950[0], 44970[0], 49000[0], 49002[1], 49010[0], 49406[1], 50020[1], 50040[1], 50045[1], 50500[1], 51701[1], 51702[1], 51703[1], 62320[0], 62321[0], 62322[0], 62323[0], 62324[0], 62325[0], 62326[0], 62327[0], 64400[0], 64405[0], 64408[0], 64415[0], 64416[0], 64417[0], 64418[0], 64420[0], 64421[0], 64425[0], 64430[0], 64435[0], 64445[0], 64446[0], 64447[0], 64448[0], 64449[0], 64450[0], 64451[0], 64454[0], 64461[0], 64462[0], 64463[0], 64479[0], 64480[0], 64483[0], 64484[0], 64486[0], 64487[0], 64488[0], 64489[0], 64490[0], 64491[0], 64492[0], 64493[0], 64494[0], 64495[0], 64505[0], 64510[0], 64517[0], 64520[0], 64530[0], 69990[0], 92012[1], 92014[1], 93000[1], 93005[1], 93010[1], 93040[1], 93041[1], 93042[1], 93318[1], 93355[1], 94002[1], 94200[1], 94680[1], 94681[1], 94690[1], 95812[1], 95813[1], 95816[1], 95819[1], 95822[1], 95829[1], 95955[1], 96360[1], 96361[1], 96365[1], 96366[1], 96367[1], 96368[1], 96372[1], 96374[1], 96375[1], 96376[1], 96377[1], 96523[0], 97597[1], 97598[1], 97602[1], 99155[0], 99156[0], 99157[0], 99211[1], 99212[1], 99213[1], 99214[1], 99215[1], 99217[1], 99218[1], 99219[1], 99220[1], 99221[1], 99222[1], 99223[1], 99231[1], 99232[1], 99233[1], 99234[1], 99235[1], 99236[1], 99238[1], 99239[1], 99241[1], 99242[1], 99243[1], 99244[1], 99245[1], 99251[1], 99252[1], 99253[1], 99254[1], 99255[1], 99291[1], 99292[1], 99304[1], 99305[1], 99306[1], 99307[1], 99308[1], 99309[1], 99310[1], 99315[1], 99316[1], 99334[1], 99335[1], 99336[1], 99337[1], 99347[1], 99348[1], 99349[1], 99350[1], 99374[1], 99375[1], 99377[1], 99378[1], 99446[0], 99447[0], 99448[0], 99449[0], 99451[0], 99452[0], 99495[0], 99496[0], G0463[1], G0471[1]
50080	0213T[0], 0216T[0], 0596T[1], 0597T[1], 0708T[1], 0709T[1], 11000[1], 11001[1], 11004[1], 11005[1], 11006[1], 11042[1], 11043[1], 11044[1], 11045[1], 11046[1], 11047[1], 12001[1], 12002[1], 12004[1], 12005[1], 12006[1], 12007[1], 12011[1], 12013[1], 12014[1], 12015[1], 12016[1], 12017[1], 12018[1], 12020[1], 12021[1], 12031[1], 12032[1], 12034[1], 12035[1], 12036[1], 12037[1], 12041[1], 12042[1], 12044[1], 12045[1], 12046[1], 12047[1], 12051[1], 12052[1], 12053[1], 12054[1], 12055[1], 12056[1], 12057[1], 13100[1], 13101[1], 13102[1], 13120[1], 13121[1], 13122[1], 13131[1], 13132[1], 13133[1], 13151[1], 13152[1], 13153[1], 36000[1], 36400[1], 36405[1], 36406[1], 36410[1], 36420[1], 36425[1], 36430[1], 36440[1], 36591[0], 36592[0], 36600[1], 36640[1], 43752[1], 50081[1], 50382[1], 50436[1], 50437[1], 50561[1], 50693[1], 50694[1], 50695[1], 50961[1], 50980[1], 51701[1], 51702[1], 51703[1], 52320[1], 52325[1], 52330[1], 52352[1], 52353[1], 52356[1], 62320[0], 62321[0], 62322[0], 62323[0], 62324[0], 62325[0], 62326[0], 62327[0], 64400[0], 64405[0], 64408[0], 64415[0], 64416[0], 64417[0], 64418[0], 64420[0], 64421[0], 64425[0], 64430[0], 64435[0], 64445[0], 64446[0], 64447[0], 64448[0], 64449[0], 64450[0], 64451[0], 64454[0], 64461[0], 64462[0], 64463[0], 64479[0], 64480[0], 64483[0], 64484[0], 64486[0], 64487[0], 64488[0], 64489[0], 64490[0], 64491[0], 64492[0], 64493[0], 64494[0], 64495[0], 64505[0], 64510[0], 64517[0], 64520[0], 64530[0], 69990[0], 76380[1], 76942[1], 76998[1], 77001[1], 77002[1], 77012[1], 77021[1], 92012[1], 92014[1], 93000[1], 93005[1], 93010[1], 93040[1], 93041[1], 93042[1], 93318[1], 93355[1], 94002[1], 94200[1], 94680[1], 94681[1], 94690[1], 95812[1], 95813[1], 95816[1], 95819[1], 95822[1], 95829[1], 95955[1], 96360[1], 96361[1], 96365[1], 96366[1], 96367[1], 96368[1], 96372[1], 96374[1], 96375[1], 96376[1], 96377[1], 96523[0], 97597[1], 97598[1], 97602[1], 99155[0], 99156[0], 99157[0], 99211[1], 99212[1], 99213[1], 99214[1], 99215[1], 99217[1], 99218[1], 99219[1], 99220[1], 99221[1], 99222[1], 99223[1], 99231[1], 99232[1], 99233[1], 99234[1], 99235[1], 99236[1], 99238[1], 99239[1], 99241[1], 99242[1], 99243[1], 99244[1], 99245[1], 99251[1], 99252[1], 99253[1], 99254[1], 99255[1], 99291[1], 99292[1], 99304[1], 99305[1], 99306[1], 99307[1], 99308[1], 99309[1], 99310[1], 99315[1], 99316[1], 99334[1], 99335[1], 99336[1], 99337[1], 99347[1], 99348[1], 99349[1], 99350[1], 99374[1], 99375[1], 99377[1], 99378[1], 99446[0], 99447[0], 99448[0], 99449[0], 99451[0], 99452[0], 99495[0], 99496[0], G0463[1], G0471[1]
50081	0213T[0], 0216T[0], 0596T[1], 0597T[1], 0708T[1], 0709T[1], 11000[1], 11001[1], 11004[1], 11005[1], 11006[1], 11042[1], 11043[1], 11044[1], 11045[1], 11046[1], 11047[1], 12001[1], 12002[1], 12004[1], 12005[1], 12006[1], 12007[1], 12011[1], 12013[1], 12014[1], 12015[1], 12016[1], 12017[1], 12018[1], 12020[1], 12021[1], 12031[1], 12032[1], 12034[1], 12035[1], 12036[1], 12037[1], 12041[1], 12042[1],

0 = Modifier usage not allowed or inappropriate   1 = Modifier usage allowed

Code 1	Code 2
	12044[1], 12045[1], 12046[1], 12047[1], 12051[1], 12052[1], 12053[1], 12054[1], 12055[1], 12056[1], 12057[1], 13100[1], 13101[1], 13102[1], 13120[1], 13121[1], 13122[1], 13131[1], 13132[1], 13133[1], 13151[1], 13152[1], 13153[1], 36000[1], 36400[1], 36405[1], 36406[1], 36410[1], 36420[1], 36425[1], 36430[1], 36440[1], 36591[0], 36592[0], 36600[1], 36640[1], 43752[1], 50382[1], 50436[1], 50437[1], 50561[1], 50693[1], 50694[1], 50695[1], 50961[1], 50980[1], 51701[1], 51702[1], 51703[1], 52320[1], 52325[1], 52330[1], 52352[1], 52353[1], 52356[1], 62320[0], 62321[0], 62322[0], 62323[0], 62324[0], 62325[0], 62326[0], 62327[0], 64400[0], 64405[0], 64408[0], 64415[0], 64416[0], 64417[0], 64418[0], 64420[0], 64421[0], 64425[0], 64430[0], 64435[0], 64445[0], 64446[0], 64447[0], 64448[0], 64449[0], 64450[0], 64451[0], 64454[0], 64461[0], 64462[0], 64463[0], 64479[0], 64480[0], 64483[0], 64484[0], 64486[0], 64487[0], 64488[0], 64489[0], 64490[0], 64491[0], 64492[0], 64493[0], 64494[0], 64495[0], 64505[0], 64510[0], 64517[0], 64520[0], 64530[0], 69990[0], 76380[1], 76942[1], 76998[1], 77001[1], 77002[1], 77012[1], 77021[1], 92012[1], 92014[1], 93000[1], 93005[1], 93010[1], 93040[1], 93041[1], 93042[1], 93318[1], 93355[1], 94002[1], 94200[1], 94680[1], 94681[1], 94690[1], 95812[1], 95813[1], 95816[1], 95819[1], 95822[1], 95829[1], 95955[1], 96360[1], 96361[1], 96365[1], 96366[1], 96367[1], 96368[1], 96372[1], 96374[1], 96375[1], 96376[1], 96377[1], 96523[0], 97597[1], 97598[1], 97602[1], 99155[0], 99156[0], 99157[0], 99211[1], 99212[1], 99213[1], 99214[1], 99215[1], 99217[1], 99218[1], 99219[1], 99220[1], 99221[1], 99222[1], 99223[1], 99231[1], 99232[1], 99233[1], 99234[1], 99235[1], 99236[1], 99238[1], 99239[1], 99241[1], 99242[1], 99243[1], 99244[1], 99245[1], 99251[1], 99252[1], 99253[1], 99254[1], 99255[1], 99291[1], 99292[1], 99304[1], 99305[1], 99306[1], 99307[1], 99308[1], 99309[1], 99310[1], 99315[1], 99316[1], 99334[1], 99335[1], 99336[1], 99337[1], 99347[1], 99348[1], 99349[1], 99350[1], 99374[1], 99375[1], 99377[1], 99378[1], 99446[0], 99447[0], 99448[0], 99449[0], 99451[0], 99452[0], 99495[0], 99496[0], G0463[1], G0471[1]
50100	0213T[0], 0216T[0], 0596T[1], 0597T[1], 0708T[1], 0709T[1], 12001[1], 12002[1], 12004[1], 12005[1], 12006[1], 12007[1], 12011[1], 12013[1], 12014[1], 12015[1], 12016[1], 12017[1], 12018[1], 12020[1], 12021[1], 12031[1], 12032[1], 12034[1], 12035[1], 12036[1], 12037[1], 12041[1], 12042[1], 12044[1], 12045[1], 12046[1], 12047[1], 12051[1], 12052[1], 12053[1], 12054[1], 12055[1], 12056[1], 12057[1], 13100[1], 13101[1], 13102[1], 13120[1], 13121[1], 13122[1], 13131[1], 13132[1], 13133[1], 13151[1], 13152[1], 13153[1], 36000[1], 36400[1], 36405[1], 36406[1], 36410[1], 36420[1], 36425[1], 36430[1], 36440[1], 36591[0], 36592[0], 36600[1], 36640[1], 43752[1], 44602[1], 44603[1], 44604[1], 44605[1], 44950[0], 44970[0], 49000[0], 49002[1], 49010[0], 49406[1], 50020[1], 51701[1], 51702[1], 51703[1], 62320[0], 62321[0], 62322[0], 62323[0], 62324[0], 62325[0], 62326[0], 62327[0], 64400[0], 64405[0], 64408[0], 64415[0], 64416[0], 64417[0], 64418[0], 64420[0], 64421[0], 64425[0], 64430[0], 64435[0], 64445[0], 64446[0], 64447[0], 64448[0], 64449[0], 64450[0], 64451[0], 64454[0], 64461[0], 64462[0], 64463[0], 64479[0], 64480[0], 64483[0], 64484[0], 64486[0], 64487[0], 64488[0], 64489[0], 64490[0], 64491[0], 64492[0], 64493[0], 64494[0], 64495[0], 64505[0], 64510[0], 64517[0], 64520[0], 64530[0], 69990[0], 92012[1], 92014[1], 93000[1], 93005[1], 93010[1], 93040[1], 93041[1], 93042[1], 93318[1], 93355[1], 94002[1], 94200[1], 94680[1], 94681[1], 94690[1], 95812[1], 95813[1], 95816[1], 95819[1], 95822[1], 95829[1], 95955[1], 96360[1], 96361[1], 96365[1], 96366[1], 96367[1], 96368[1], 96372[1], 96374[1], 96375[1], 96376[1], 96377[1], 96523[0], 99155[0], 99156[0], 99157[0], 99211[1], 99212[1], 99213[1], 99214[1], 99215[1], 99217[1], 99218[1], 99219[1], 99220[1], 99221[1], 99222[1], 99223[1], 99231[1], 99232[1], 99233[1], 99234[1], 99235[1], 99236[1], 99238[1], 99239[1], 99241[1], 99242[1], 99243[1], 99244[1], 99245[1], 99251[1], 99252[1], 99253[1], 99254[1], 99255[1], 99291[1], 99292[1], 99304[1], 99305[1], 99306[1], 99307[1], 99308[1], 99309[1], 99310[1], 99315[1], 99316[1], 99334[1], 99335[1], 99336[1], 99337[1], 99347[1], 99348[1], 99349[1], 99350[1], 99374[1], 99375[1], 99377[1], 99378[1], 99446[0], 99447[0], 99448[0], 99449[0], 99451[0], 99452[0], 99495[0], 99496[0], G0463[1], G0471[1]
50120	0213T[0], 0216T[0], 0596T[1], 0597T[1], 0708T[1], 0709T[1], 11000[1], 11001[1], 11004[1], 11005[1], 11006[1], 11042[1], 11043[1], 11044[1], 11045[1], 11046[1], 11047[1], 12001[1], 12002[1], 12004[1], 12005[1], 12006[1], 12007[1], 12011[1], 12013[1], 12014[1], 12015[1], 12016[1], 12017[1], 12018[1], 12020[1], 12021[1], 12031[1], 12032[1], 12034[1], 12035[1], 12036[1], 12037[1], 12041[1], 12042[1], 12044[1], 12045[1], 12046[1], 12047[1], 12051[1], 12052[1], 12053[1], 12054[1], 12055[1], 12056[1], 12057[1], 13100[1], 13101[1], 13102[1], 13120[1], 13121[1], 13122[1], 13131[1], 13132[1], 13133[1], 13151[1], 13152[1], 13153[1], 36000[1], 36400[1], 36405[1], 36406[1], 36410[1], 36420[1], 36425[1], 36430[1], 36440[1], 36591[0], 36592[0], 36600[1], 36640[1], 43752[1], 44602[1], 44603[1], 44604[1], 44605[1], 44950[0], 44970[0], 49000[0], 49002[1], 49010[0], 49406[1], 50020[1], 50544[1], 51701[1], 51702[1], 51703[1], 62320[0], 62321[0], 62322[0], 62323[0], 62324[0], 62325[0], 62326[0], 62327[0], 64400[0], 64405[0], 64408[0], 64415[0], 64416[0], 64417[0], 64418[0], 64420[0], 64421[0], 64425[0], 64430[0], 64435[0], 64445[0], 64446[0], 64447[0], 64448[0], 64449[0], 64450[0], 64451[0], 64454[0], 64461[0], 64462[0], 64463[0], 64479[0], 64480[0], 64483[0], 64484[0], 64486[0], 64487[0], 64488[0], 64489[0], 64490[0], 64491[0], 64492[0], 64493[0], 64494[0], 64495[0], 64505[0], 64510[0], 64517[0], 64520[0], 64530[0], 69990[0], 92012[1], 92014[1], 93000[1], 93005[1], 93010[1], 93040[1], 93041[1], 93042[1], 93318[1], 93355[1], 94002[1], 94200[1], 94680[1], 94681[1], 94690[1], 95812[1], 95813[1], 95816[1], 95819[1], 95822[1], 95829[1], 95955[1], 96360[1], 96361[1], 96365[1], 96366[1], 96367[1], 96368[1], 96372[1], 96374[1], 96375[1], 96376[1], 96377[1], 96523[0], 97597[1], 97598[1], 97602[1], 99155[0], 99156[0], 99157[0], 99211[1], 99212[1], 99213[1], 99214[1], 99215[1], 99217[1], 99218[1], 99219[1], 99220[1], 99221[1], 99222[1], 99223[1], 99231[1], 99232[1], 99233[1], 99234[1], 99235[1], 99236[1], 99238[1], 99239[1], 99241[1], 99242[1], 99243[1], 99244[1], 99245[1], 99251[1], 99252[1], 99253[1], 99254[1], 99255[1], 99291[1], 99292[1], 99304[1], 99305[1], 99306[1], 99307[1], 99308[1], 99309[1], 99310[1], 99315[1], 99316[1], 99334[1], 99335[1], 99336[1], 99337[1], 99347[1], 99348[1], 99349[1], 99350[1], 99374[1], 99375[1], 99377[1], 99378[1], 99446[0], 99447[0], 99448[0], 99449[0], 99451[0], 99452[0], 99495[0], 99496[0], G0463[1], G0471[1]
50125	0213T[0], 0216T[0], 0596T[1], 0597T[1], 0708T[1], 0709T[1], 11000[1], 11001[1], 11004[1], 11005[1], 11006[1], 11042[1], 11043[1], 11044[1], 11045[1], 11046[1], 11047[1], 12001[1], 12002[1], 12004[1], 12005[1], 12006[1], 12007[1], 12011[1], 12013[1], 12014[1], 12015[1], 12016[1], 12017[1], 12018[1], 12020[1], 12021[1], 12031[1], 12032[1], 12034[1], 12035[1], 12036[1], 12037[1], 12041[1], 12042[1], 12044[1], 12045[1], 12046[1], 12047[1], 12051[1], 12052[1], 12053[1], 12054[1], 12055[1], 12056[1], 12057[1], 13100[1], 13101[1], 13102[1], 13120[1], 13121[1], 13122[1], 13131[1], 13132[1], 13133[1], 13151[1], 13152[1], 13153[1], 36000[1], 36400[1], 36405[1], 36406[1], 36410[1], 36420[1], 36425[1], 36430[1], 36440[1], 36591[0], 36592[0], 36600[1], 36640[1], 43752[1], 44602[1], 44603[1], 44604[1], 44605[1], 44950[0], 44970[0], 49000[0], 49002[1], 49010[0], 49406[1], 50020[1], 50120[1], 50544[1], 51701[1], 51702[1], 51703[1], 62320[0], 62321[0], 62322[0], 62323[0], 62324[0], 62325[0], 62326[0], 62327[0], 64400[0], 64405[0], 64408[0], 64415[0], 64416[0], 64417[0], 64418[0], 64420[0], 64421[0], 64425[0], 64430[0], 64435[0], 64445[0], 64446[0], 64447[0], 64448[0], 64449[0], 64450[0], 64451[0], 64454[0], 64461[0], 64462[0], 64463[0], 64479[0], 64480[0], 64483[0], 64484[0], 64486[0], 64487[0], 64488[0], 64489[0], 64490[0], 64491[0], 64492[0], 64493[0], 64494[0], 64495[0], 64505[0], 64510[0], 64517[0], 64520[0], 64530[0], 69990[0], 92012[1], 92014[1], 93000[1], 93005[1], 93010[1], 93040[1], 93041[1], 93042[1], 93318[1], 93355[1], 94002[1], 94200[1], 94680[1], 94681[1], 94690[1], 95812[1], 95813[1], 95816[1], 95819[1], 95822[1], 95829[1], 95955[1], 96360[1], 96361[1], 96365[1], 96366[1], 96367[1], 96368[1], 96372[1], 96374[1], 96375[1], 96376[1], 96377[1], 96523[0], 97597[1], 97598[1], 97602[1], 99155[0], 99156[0], 99157[0], 99211[1], 99212[1], 99213[1], 99214[1], 99215[1], 99217[1], 99218[1], 99219[1], 99220[1], 99221[1], 99222[1], 99223[1], 99231[1], 99232[1], 99233[1], 99234[1], 99235[1], 99236[1], 99238[1], 99239[1], 99241[1], 99242[1], 99243[1], 99244[1], 99245[1], 99251[1], 99252[1], 99253[1], 99254[1], 99255[1], 99291[1], 99292[1], 99304[1], 99305[1], 99306[1], 99307[1], 99308[1], 99309[1], 99310[1], 99315[1], 99316[1], 99334[1], 99335[1], 99336[1], 99337[1], 99347[1], 99348[1], 99349[1], 99350[1], 99374[1], 99375[1], 99377[1], 99378[1], 99446[0], 99447[0], 99448[0], 99449[0], 99451[0], 99452[0], 99495[0], 99496[0], G0463[1], G0471[1]
50130	0213T[0], 0216T[0], 0596T[1], 0597T[1], 0708T[1], 0709T[1], 11000[1], 11001[1], 11004[1], 11005[1], 11006[1], 11042[1], 11043[1], 11044[1], 11045[1], 11046[1], 11047[1], 12001[1], 12002[1], 12004[1], 12005[1], 12006[1], 12007[1], 12011[1], 12013[1], 12014[1], 12015[1], 12016[1], 12017[1], 12018[1], 12020[1], 12021[1], 12031[1], 12032[1], 12034[1], 12035[1], 12036[1], 12037[1], 12041[1], 12042[1], 12044[1], 12045[1], 12046[1], 12047[1], 12051[1], 12052[1], 12053[1], 12054[1], 12055[1], 12056[1], 12057[1], 13100[1], 13101[1], 13102[1], 13120[1], 13121[1], 13122[1], 13131[1], 13132[1], 13133[1], 13151[1], 13152[1], 13153[1], 36000[1], 36400[1], 36405[1], 36406[1], 36410[1], 36420[1], 36425[1], 36430[1], 36440[1], 36591[0], 36592[0], 36600[1], 36640[1], 43752[1], 44602[1], 44603[1], 44604[1], 44605[1], 44950[0], 44970[0], 49000[0], 49002[1], 49010[0], 49406[1], 50020[1], 50120[1], 50125[1], 50544[1], 51701[1], 51702[1], 51703[1], 62320[0], 62321[0], 62322[0], 62323[0], 62324[0], 62325[0], 62326[0], 62327[0], 64400[0], 64405[0], 64408[0], 64415[0], 64416[0], 64417[0], 64418[0], 64420[0], 64421[0], 64425[0], 64430[0], 64435[0], 64445[0], 64446[0], 64447[0], 64448[0], 64449[0], 64450[0], 64451[0], 64454[0], 64461[0], 64462[0], 64463[0], 64479[0], 64480[0], 64483[0], 64484[0], 64486[0], 64487[0], 64488[0], 64489[0], 64490[0], 64491[0], 64492[0], 64493[0], 64494[0], 64495[0], 64505[0], 64510[0], 64517[0], 64520[0], 64530[0], 69990[0], 92012[1], 92014[1], 93000[1], 93005[1], 93010[1], 93040[1], 93041[1], 93042[1], 93318[1], 93355[1], 94002[1], 94200[1], 94680[1], 94681[1], 94690[1], 95812[1], 95813[1], 95816[1], 95819[1], 95822[1], 95829[1], 95955[1], 96360[1], 96361[1], 96365[1], 96366[1], 96367[1], 96368[1], 96372[1], 96374[1], 96375[1], 96376[1], 96377[1], 96523[0], 97597[1], 97598[1], 97602[1], 99155[0], 99156[0], 99157[0], 99211[1], 99212[1], 99213[1], 99214[1], 99215[1], 99217[1], 99218[1], 99219[1], 99220[1], 99221[1], 99222[1], 99223[1], 99231[1], 99232[1], 99233[1], 99234[1], 99235[1], 99236[1], 99238[1], 99239[1], 99241[1], 99242[1], 99243[1], 99244[1], 99245[1], 99251[1], 99252[1], 99253[1], 99254[1], 99255[1], 99291[1], 99292[1], 99304[1], 99305[1], 99306[1], 99307[1], 99308[1], 99309[1], 99310[1], 99315[1], 99316[1], 99334[1], 99335[1], 99336[1], 99337[1], 99347[1], 99348[1], 99349[1], 99350[1], 99374[1], 99375[1], 99377[1], 99378[1], 99446[0], 99447[0], 99448[0], 99449[0], 99451[0], 99452[0], 99495[0], 99496[0], G0463[1], G0471[1]
50135	0213T[0], 0216T[0], 0596T[1], 0597T[1], 0708T[1], 0709T[1], 11000[1], 11001[1], 11004[1], 11005[1], 11006[1], 11042[1], 11043[1], 11044[1], 11045[1], 11046[1], 11047[1], 12001[1], 12002[1], 12004[1], 12005[1], 12006[1], 12007[1], 12011[1], 12013[1], 12014[1], 12015[1], 12016[1], 12017[1], 12018[1], 12020[1], 12021[1], 12031[1], 12032[1], 12034[1], 12035[1], 12036[1], 12037[1], 12041[1], 12042[1], 12044[1], 12045[1], 12046[1], 12047[1], 12051[1], 12052[1], 12053[1], 12054[1], 12055[1], 12056[1], 12057[1], 13100[1], 13101[1], 13102[1], 13120[1], 13121[1], 13122[1], 13131[1], 13132[1], 13133[1], 13151[1], 13152[1], 13153[1], 36000[1], 36400[1], 36405[1], 36406[1], 36410[1], 36420[1], 36425[1], 36430[1], 36440[1], 36591[0], 36592[0], 36600[1], 36640[1], 43752[1], 44602[1], 44603[1], 44604[1], 44605[1], 44950[0], 44970[0], 49000[0], 49002[1], 49010[0], 49406[1], 50020[1], 50120[1], 50125[1], 50130[1], 50544[1], 51701[1], 51702[1], 51703[1], 62320[0], 62321[0], 62322[0], 62323[0], 62324[0],

0 = Modifier usage not allowed or inappropriate 1 = Modifier usage allowed

Code 1	Code 2
	62325[0], 62326[0], 62327[0], 64400[0], 64405[0], 64408[0], 64415[0], 64416[0], 64417[0], 64418[0], 64420[0], 64421[0], 64425[0], 64430[0], 64435[0], 64445[0], 64446[0], 64447[0], 64448[0], 64449[0], 64450[0], 64451[0], 64454[0], 64461[0], 64462[0], 64463[0], 64479[0], 64480[0], 64483[0], 64484[0], 64486[0], 64487[0], 64488[0], 64489[0], 64490[0], 64491[0], 64492[0], 64493[0], 64494[0], 64495[0], 64505[0], 64510[0], 64517[0], 64520[0], 64530[0], 69990[0], 92012[1], 92014[1], 93000[1], 93005[1], 93010[1], 93040[1], 93041[1], 93042[1], 93318[1], 93355[1], 94002[1], 94200[1], 94680[1], 94681[1], 94690[1], 95812[1], 95813[1], 95816[1], 95819[1], 95822[1], 95829[1], 95955[1], 96360[1], 96361[1], 96365[1], 96366[1], 96367[1], 96368[1], 96372[1], 96374[1], 96375[1], 96376[1], 96377[1], 96523[0], 97597[1], 97598[1], 97602[1], 99155[0], 99156[0], 99157[0], 99211[1], 99212[1], 99213[1], 99214[1], 99215[1], 99217[1], 99218[1], 99219[1], 99220[1], 99221[1], 99222[1], 99223[1], 99231[1], 99232[1], 99233[1], 99234[1], 99235[1], 99236[1], 99238[1], 99239[1], 99241[1], 99242[1], 99243[1], 99244[1], 99245[1], 99251[1], 99252[1], 99253[1], 99254[1], 99255[1], 99291[1], 99292[1], 99304[1], 99305[1], 99306[1], 99307[1], 99308[1], 99309[1], 99310[1], 99315[1], 99316[1], 99334[1], 99335[1], 99336[1], 99337[1], 99347[1], 99348[1], 99349[1], 99350[1], 99374[1], 99375[1], 99377[1], 99378[1], 99446[0], 99447[0], 99448[0], 99449[0], 99451[0], 99452[0], 99495[0], 99496[0], G0463[1], G0471[1]
50200	0213T[0], 0216T[0], 0596T[1], 0597T[1], 0708T[1], 0709T[1], 10005[1], 10007[1], 10009[1], 10011[1], 10021[1], 12001[1], 12002[1], 12004[1], 12005[1], 12006[1], 12007[1], 12011[1], 12013[1], 12014[1], 12015[1], 12016[1], 12017[1], 12018[1], 12020[1], 12021[1], 12031[1], 12032[1], 12034[1], 12035[1], 12036[1], 12037[1], 12041[1], 12042[1], 12044[1], 12045[1], 12046[1], 12047[1], 12051[1], 12052[1], 12053[1], 12054[1], 12055[1], 12056[1], 12057[1], 13100[1], 13101[1], 13102[1], 13120[1], 13121[1], 13122[1], 13131[1], 13132[1], 13133[1], 13151[1], 13152[1], 13153[1], 36000[1], 36400[1], 36405[1], 36406[1], 36410[1], 36420[1], 36425[1], 36430[1], 36440[1], 36591[0], 36592[0], 36600[1], 36640[1], 43752[1], 44950[0], 44970[0], 50205[1], 51701[1], 51702[1], 51703[1], 62320[0], 62321[0], 62322[0], 62323[0], 62324[0], 62325[0], 62326[0], 62327[0], 64400[0], 64405[0], 64408[0], 64415[0], 64416[0], 64417[0], 64418[0], 64420[0], 64421[0], 64425[0], 64430[0], 64435[0], 64445[0], 64446[0], 64447[0], 64448[0], 64449[0], 64450[0], 64451[0], 64454[0], 64461[0], 64462[0], 64463[0], 64479[0], 64480[0], 64483[0], 64484[0], 64486[0], 64487[0], 64488[0], 64489[0], 64490[0], 64491[0], 64492[0], 64493[0], 64494[0], 64495[0], 64505[0], 64510[0], 64517[0], 64520[0], 64530[0], 69990[0], 76000[1], 76998[1], 92012[1], 92014[1], 93000[1], 93005[1], 93010[1], 93040[1], 93041[1], 93042[1], 93318[1], 93355[1], 94002[1], 94200[1], 94680[1], 94681[1], 94690[1], 95812[1], 95813[1], 95816[1], 95819[1], 95822[1], 95829[1], 95955[1], 96360[1], 96361[1], 96365[1], 96366[1], 96367[1], 96368[1], 96372[1], 96374[1], 96375[1], 96376[1], 96377[1], 96523[0], 99155[0], 99156[0], 99157[0], 99211[1], 99212[1], 99213[1], 99214[1], 99215[1], 99217[1], 99218[1], 99219[1], 99220[1], 99221[1], 99222[1], 99223[1], 99231[1], 99232[1], 99233[1], 99234[1], 99235[1], 99236[1], 99238[1], 99239[1], 99241[1], 99242[1], 99243[1], 99244[1], 99245[1], 99251[1], 99252[1], 99253[1], 99254[1], 99255[1], 99291[1], 99292[1], 99304[1], 99305[1], 99306[1], 99307[1], 99308[1], 99309[1], 99310[1], 99315[1], 99316[1], 99334[1], 99335[1], 99336[1], 99337[1], 99347[1], 99348[1], 99349[1], 99350[1], 99374[1], 99375[1], 99377[1], 99378[1], 99446[0], 99447[0], 99448[0], 99449[0], 99451[0], 99452[0], 99495[1], 99496[1], G0463[1], G0471[1], J0670[1], J1642[1], J1644[1], J2001[1]
50205	0213T[0], 0216T[0], 0596T[1], 0597T[1], 0708T[1], 0709T[1], 10005[1], 10007[1], 10009[1], 10011[1], 10021[1], 12001[1], 12002[1], 12004[1], 12005[1], 12006[1], 12007[1], 12011[1], 12013[1], 12014[1], 12015[1], 12016[1], 12017[1], 12018[1], 12020[1], 12021[1], 12031[1], 12032[1], 12034[1], 12035[1], 12036[1], 12037[1], 12041[1], 12042[1], 12044[1], 12045[1], 12046[1], 12047[1], 12051[1], 12052[1], 12053[1], 12054[1], 12055[1], 12056[1], 12057[1], 13100[1], 13101[1], 13102[1], 13120[1], 13121[1], 13122[1], 13131[1], 13132[1], 13133[1], 13151[1], 13152[1], 13153[1], 36000[1], 36400[1], 36405[1], 36406[1], 36410[1], 36420[1], 36425[1], 36430[1], 36440[1], 36591[0], 36592[0], 36600[1], 36640[1], 43752[1], 44950[0], 44970[0], 49010[0], 50500[1], 51701[1], 51702[1], 51703[1], 62320[0], 62321[0], 62322[0], 62323[0], 62324[0], 62325[0], 62326[0], 62327[0], 64400[0], 64405[0], 64408[0], 64415[0], 64416[0], 64417[0], 64418[0], 64420[0], 64421[0], 64425[0], 64430[0], 64435[0], 64445[0], 64446[0], 64447[0], 64448[0], 64449[0], 64450[0], 64451[0], 64454[0], 64461[0], 64462[0], 64463[0], 64479[0], 64480[0], 64483[0], 64484[0], 64486[0], 64487[0], 64488[0], 64489[0], 64490[0], 64491[0], 64492[0], 64493[0], 64494[0], 64495[0], 64505[0], 64510[0], 64517[0], 64520[0], 64530[0], 69990[0], 92012[1], 92014[1], 93000[1], 93005[1], 93010[1], 93040[1], 93041[1], 93042[1], 93318[1], 93355[1], 94002[1], 94200[1], 94680[1], 94681[1], 94690[1], 95812[1], 95813[1], 95816[1], 95819[1], 95822[1], 95829[1], 95955[1], 96360[1], 96361[1], 96365[1], 96366[1], 96367[1], 96368[1], 96372[1], 96374[1], 96375[1], 96376[1], 96377[1], 96523[0], 99155[0], 99156[0], 99157[0], 99211[1], 99212[1], 99213[1], 99214[1], 99215[1], 99217[1], 99218[1], 99219[1], 99220[1], 99221[1], 99222[1], 99223[1], 99231[1], 99232[1], 99233[1], 99234[1], 99235[1], 99236[1], 99238[1], 99239[1], 99241[1], 99242[1], 99243[1], 99244[1], 99245[1], 99251[1], 99252[1], 99253[1], 99254[1], 99255[1], 99291[1], 99292[1], 99304[1], 99305[1], 99306[1], 99307[1], 99308[1], 99309[1], 99310[1], 99315[1], 99316[1], 99334[1], 99335[1], 99336[1], 99337[1], 99347[1], 99348[1], 99349[1], 99350[1], 99374[1], 99375[1], 99377[1], 99378[1], 99446[0], 99447[0], 99448[0], 99449[0], 99451[0], 99452[0], 99495[0], 99496[0], G0463[1], G0471[1]
50220	0213T[0], 0216T[0], 0596T[1], 0597T[1], 0600T[1], 0601T[1], 0708T[1], 0709T[1], 11000[1], 11001[1], 11004[1], 11005[1], 11006[1], 11042[1], 11043[1], 11044[1], 11045[1], 11046[1], 11047[1], 12001[1], 12002[1], 12004[1], 12005[1], 12006[1], 12007[1], 12011[1], 12013[1], 12014[1], 12015[1], 12016[1], 12017[1], 12018[1], 12020[1], 12021[1], 12031[1], 12032[1], 12034[1], 12035[1], 12036[1], 12037[1], 12041[1], 12042[1], 12044[1], 12045[1], 12046[1], 12047[1], 12051[1], 12052[1], 12053[1], 12054[1], 12055[1], 12056[1], 12057[1], 13100[1], 13101[1], 13102[1], 13120[1], 13121[1], 13122[1], 13131[1], 13132[1], 13133[1], 13151[1], 13152[1], 13153[1], 32551[1], 32556[1], 32557[1], 36000[1], 36400[1], 36405[1], 36406[1], 36410[1], 36420[1], 36425[1], 36430[1], 36440[1], 36591[0], 36592[0], 36600[1], 36640[1], 38747[1], 43752[1], 44602[1], 44603[1], 44604[1], 44605[1], 44950[0], 44970[0], 49000[0], 49002[1], 49010[0], 50100[1], 50205[1], 50250[1], 50280[1], 50290[1], 50541[1], 50542[1], 50543[1], 50544[1], 50545[0], 50546[1], 50548[1], 50605[1], 50650[1], 51701[1], 51702[1], 51703[1], 52005[1], 60540[1], 60545[1], 60650[1], 62320[0], 62321[0], 62322[0], 62323[0], 62324[0], 62325[0], 62326[0], 62327[0], 64400[0], 64405[0], 64408[0], 64415[0], 64416[0], 64417[0], 64418[0], 64420[0], 64421[0], 64425[0], 64430[0], 64435[0], 64445[0], 64446[0], 64447[0], 64448[0], 64449[0], 64450[0], 64451[0], 64454[0], 64461[0], 64462[0], 64463[0], 64479[0], 64480[0], 64483[0], 64484[0], 64486[0], 64487[0], 64488[0], 64489[0], 64490[0], 64491[0], 64492[0], 64493[0], 64494[0], 64495[0], 64505[0], 64510[0], 64517[0], 64520[0], 64530[0], 69990[0], 92012[1], 92014[1], 93000[1], 93005[1], 93010[1], 93040[1], 93041[1], 93042[1], 93318[1], 93355[1], 94002[1], 94200[1], 94680[1], 94681[1], 94690[1], 95812[1], 95813[1], 95816[1], 95819[1], 95822[1], 95829[1], 95955[1], 96360[1], 96361[1], 96365[1], 96366[1], 96367[1], 96368[1], 96372[1], 96374[1], 96375[1], 96376[1], 96377[1], 96523[0], 97597[1], 97598[1], 97602[1], 99155[0], 99156[0], 99157[0], 99211[1], 99212[1], 99213[1], 99214[1], 99215[1], 99217[1], 99218[1], 99219[1], 99220[1], 99221[1], 99222[1], 99223[1], 99231[1], 99232[1], 99233[1], 99234[1], 99235[1], 99236[1], 99238[1], 99239[1], 99241[1], 99242[1], 99243[1], 99244[1], 99245[1], 99251[1], 99252[1], 99253[1], 99254[1], 99255[1], 99291[1], 99292[1], 99304[1], 99305[1], 99306[1], 99307[1], 99308[1], 99309[1], 99310[1], 99315[1], 99316[1], 99334[1], 99335[1], 99336[1], 99337[1], 99347[1], 99348[1], 99349[1], 99350[1], 99374[1], 99375[1], 99377[1], 99378[1], 99446[0], 99447[0], 99448[0], 99449[0], 99451[0], 99452[0], 99495[0], 99496[0], G0463[1], G0471[1]
50225	0213T[0], 0216T[0], 0596T[1], 0597T[1], 0600T[1], 0601T[1], 0708T[1], 0709T[1], 11000[1], 11001[1], 11004[1], 11005[1], 11006[1], 11042[1], 11043[1], 11044[1], 11045[1], 11046[1], 11047[1], 12001[1], 12002[1], 12004[1], 12005[1], 12006[1], 12007[1], 12011[1], 12013[1], 12014[1], 12015[1], 12016[1], 12017[1], 12018[1], 12020[1], 12021[1], 12031[1], 12032[1], 12034[1], 12035[1], 12036[1], 12037[1], 12041[1], 12042[1], 12044[1], 12045[1], 12046[1], 12047[1], 12051[1], 12052[1], 12053[1], 12054[1], 12055[1], 12056[1], 12057[1], 13100[1], 13101[1], 13102[1], 13120[1], 13121[1], 13122[1], 13131[1], 13132[1], 13133[1], 13151[1], 13152[1], 13153[1], 20650[1], 32556[1], 32557[1], 36000[1], 36400[1], 36405[1], 36406[1], 36410[1], 36420[1], 36425[1], 36430[1], 36440[1], 36591[0], 36592[0], 36600[1], 36640[1], 38747[1], 43752[1], 44602[1], 44603[1], 44604[1], 44605[1], 44950[0], 44970[0], 49000[0], 49002[1], 49010[0], 49203[1], 50100[1], 50205[1], 50220[1], 50250[1], 50280[1], 50290[1], 50541[1], 50542[1], 50543[1], 50544[1], 50545[1], 50546[1], 50548[1], 50605[1], 50650[0], 51701[1], 51702[1], 51703[1], 60540[1], 60545[1], 60650[1], 62320[0], 62321[0], 62322[0], 62323[0], 62324[0], 62325[0], 62326[0], 62327[0], 64400[0], 64405[0], 64408[0], 64415[0], 64416[0], 64417[0], 64418[0], 64420[0], 64421[0], 64425[0], 64430[0], 64435[0], 64445[0], 64446[0], 64447[0], 64448[0], 64449[0], 64450[0], 64451[0], 64454[0], 64461[0], 64462[0], 64463[0], 64479[0], 64480[0], 64483[0], 64484[0], 64486[0], 64487[0], 64488[0], 64489[0], 64490[0], 64491[0], 64492[0], 64493[0], 64494[0], 64495[0], 64505[0], 64510[0], 64517[0], 64520[0], 64530[0], 69990[0], 92012[1], 92014[1], 93000[1], 93005[1], 93010[1], 93040[1], 93041[1], 93042[1], 93318[1], 93355[1], 94002[1], 94200[1], 94680[1], 94681[1], 94690[1], 95812[1], 95813[1], 95816[1], 95819[1], 95822[1], 95829[1], 95955[1], 96360[1], 96361[1], 96365[1], 96366[1], 96367[1], 96368[1], 96372[1], 96374[1], 96375[1], 96376[1], 96377[1], 96523[0], 97597[1], 97598[1], 97602[1], 99155[0], 99156[0], 99157[0], 99211[1], 99212[1], 99213[1], 99214[1], 99215[1], 99217[1], 99218[1], 99219[1], 99220[1], 99221[1], 99222[1], 99223[1], 99231[1], 99232[1], 99233[1], 99234[1], 99235[1], 99236[1], 99238[1], 99239[1], 99241[1], 99242[1], 99243[1], 99244[1], 99245[1], 99251[1], 99252[1], 99253[1], 99254[1], 99255[1], 99291[1], 99292[1], 99304[1], 99305[1], 99306[1], 99307[1], 99308[1], 99309[1], 99310[1], 99315[1], 99316[1], 99334[1], 99335[1], 99336[1], 99337[1], 99347[1], 99348[1], 99349[1], 99350[1], 99374[1], 99375[1], 99377[1], 99378[1], 99446[0], 99447[0], 99448[0], 99449[0], 99451[0], 99452[0], 99495[0], 99496[0], G0463[1], G0471[1]
50230	0213T[0], 0216T[0], 0596T[1], 0597T[1], 0600T[1], 0601T[1], 0708T[1], 0709T[1], 11000[1], 11001[1], 11004[1], 11005[1], 11006[1], 11042[1], 11043[1], 11044[1], 11045[1], 11046[1], 11047[1], 12001[1], 12002[1], 12004[1], 12005[1], 12006[1], 12007[1], 12011[1], 12013[1], 12014[1], 12015[1], 12016[1], 12017[1], 12018[1], 12020[1], 12021[1], 12031[1], 12032[1], 12034[1], 12035[1], 12036[1], 12037[1], 12041[1], 12042[1], 12044[1], 12045[1], 12046[1], 12047[1], 12051[1], 12052[1], 12053[1], 12054[1], 12055[1], 12056[1], 12057[1], 13100[1], 13101[1], 13102[1], 13120[1], 13121[1], 13122[1], 13131[1], 13132[1], 13133[1], 13151[1], 13152[1], 13153[1], 32551[1], 32556[1], 32557[1], 35702[1], 35703[1], 36000[1], 36400[1], 36405[1], 36406[1], 36410[1], 36420[1], 36425[1], 36430[1], 36440[1], 36591[0], 36592[0], 36600[1], 36640[1], 38100[1], 38101[1], 38120[1], 38562[0], 38564[0], 38570[1], 38780[1], 43752[1], 44950[0], 44970[0], 49010[0], 49203[1], 49255[0], 50080[1], 50081[1], 50100[1], 50205[1], 50220[1], 50250[1], 50280[1], 50290[1], 50526[1], 50541[1], 50542[1], 50543[1], 50544[1], 50545[0], 50546[1], 50548[1], 50605[1], 50650[1], 51701[1], 51702[1], 51703[1], 52281[1], 52332[1], 52356[1], 60540[1], 60545[1], 60650[1], 62320[0], 62321[0], 62322[0], 62323[0], 62324[0], 62325[0], 62326[0], 62327[0], 64400[0], 64405[0], 64408[0], 64415[0], 64416[0], 64417[0], 64418[0], 64420[0], 64421[0], 64425[0], 64430[0], 64435[0], 64445[0], 64446[0], 64447[0], 64448[0], 64449[0], 64450[0], 64451[0],

0 = Modifier usage not allowed or inappropriate 1 = Modifier usage allowed

Appendix A: NCCI - CPT Codes

Code 1	Code 2
	64454[0], 64461[0], 64462[0], 64463[0], 64479[0], 64480[0], 64483[0], 64484[0], 64486[0], 64487[0], 64488[0], 64489[0], 64490[0], 64491[0], 64492[0], 64493[0], 64494[0], 64495[0], 64505[0], 64510[0], 64517[0], 64520[0], 64530[0], 69990[0], 92012[1], 92014[1], 93000[1], 93005[1], 93010[1], 93040[1], 93041[1], 93042[1], 93318[1], 93355[1], 94002[1], 94200[1], 94680[1], 94681[1], 94690[1], 95812[1], 95813[1], 95816[1], 95819[1], 95822[1], 95829[1], 95955[1], 96360[1], 96361[1], 96365[1], 96366[1], 96367[1], 96368[1], 96372[1], 96374[1], 96375[1], 96376[1], 96377[1], 96523[0], 97597[1], 97598[1], 97602[1], 99155[0], 99156[0], 99157[0], 99211[1], 99212[1], 99213[1], 99214[1], 99215[1], 99217[1], 99218[1], 99219[1], 99220[1], 99221[1], 99222[1], 99223[1], 99231[1], 99232[1], 99233[1], 99234[1], 99235[1], 99236[1], 99238[1], 99239[1], 99241[1], 99242[1], 99243[1], 99244[1], 99245[1], 99251[1], 99252[1], 99253[1], 99254[1], 99255[1], 99291[1], 99292[1], 99304[1], 99305[1], 99306[1], 99307[1], 99308[1], 99309[1], 99310[1], 99315[1], 99316[1], 99334[1], 99335[1], 99336[1], 99337[1], 99347[1], 99348[1], 99349[1], 99350[1], 99374[1], 99375[1], 99377[1], 99378[1], 99446[0], 99447[0], 99448[0], 99449[0], 99451[0], 99452[0], 99495[0], 99496[0], G0463[1], G0471[1]
50234	0213T[0], 0216T[0], 0596T[1], 0597T[1], 0600T[1], 0601T[1], 0708T[1], 0709T[1], 11000[1], 11001[1], 11004[1], 11005[1], 11006[1], 11042[1], 11043[1], 11044[1], 11045[1], 11046[1], 11047[1], 12001[1], 12002[1], 12004[1], 12005[1], 12006[1], 12007[1], 12011[1], 12013[1], 12014[1], 12015[1], 12016[1], 12017[1], 12018[1], 12020[1], 12021[1], 12031[1], 12032[1], 12034[1], 12035[1], 12036[1], 12037[1], 12041[1], 12042[1], 12044[1], 12045[1], 12046[1], 12047[1], 12051[1], 12052[1], 12053[1], 12054[1], 12055[1], 12056[1], 12057[1], 13100[1], 13101[1], 13102[1], 13120[1], 13121[1], 13122[1], 13131[1], 13132[1], 13133[1], 13151[1], 13152[1], 13153[1], 32551[1], 32556[1], 32557[1], 36000[1], 36400[1], 36405[1], 36406[1], 36410[1], 36420[1], 36425[1], 36430[1], 36440[1], 36591[0], 36592[0], 36600[1], 36640[1], 38747[1], 43752[1], 44602[1], 44603[1], 44604[1], 44605[1], 44950[0], 44970[0], 49000[0], 49002[1], 49010[0], 49203[1], 50100[1], 50236[1], 50250[1], 50280[1], 50290[1], 50500[1], 50541[1], 50542[1], 50543[1], 50544[1], 50545[1], 50546[1], 50548[1], 50650[1], 50660[1], 51701[1], 51702[1], 51703[1], 52000[0], 52240[1], 60540[1], 60545[1], 60650[1], 62320[0], 62321[0], 62322[0], 62323[0], 62324[0], 62325[0], 62326[0], 62327[0], 64400[0], 64405[0], 64408[0], 64415[0], 64416[0], 64417[0], 64418[0], 64420[0], 64421[0], 64425[0], 64430[0], 64435[0], 64445[0], 64446[0], 64447[0], 64448[0], 64449[0], 64450[0], 64451[0], 64454[0], 64461[0], 64462[0], 64463[0], 64479[0], 64480[0], 64483[0], 64484[0], 64486[0], 64487[0], 64488[0], 64489[0], 64490[0], 64491[0], 64492[0], 64493[0], 64494[0], 64495[0], 64505[0], 64510[0], 64517[0], 64520[0], 64530[0], 69990[0], 92012[1], 92014[1], 93000[1], 93005[1], 93010[1], 93040[1], 93041[1], 93042[1], 93318[1], 93355[1], 94002[1], 94200[1], 94680[1], 94681[1], 94690[1], 95812[1], 95813[1], 95816[1], 95819[1], 95822[1], 95829[1], 95955[1], 96360[1], 96361[1], 96365[1], 96366[1], 96367[1], 96368[1], 96372[1], 96374[1], 96375[1], 96376[1], 96377[1], 96523[0], 97597[1], 97598[1], 97602[1], 99155[0], 99156[0], 99157[0], 99211[1], 99212[1], 99213[1], 99214[1], 99215[1], 99217[1], 99218[1], 99219[1], 99220[1], 99221[1], 99222[1], 99223[1], 99231[1], 99232[1], 99233[1], 99234[1], 99235[1], 99236[1], 99238[1], 99239[1], 99241[1], 99242[1], 99243[1], 99244[1], 99245[1], 99251[1], 99252[1], 99253[1], 99254[1], 99255[1], 99291[1], 99292[1], 99304[1], 99305[1], 99306[1], 99307[1], 99308[1], 99309[1], 99310[1], 99315[1], 99316[1], 99334[1], 99335[1], 99336[1], 99337[1], 99347[1], 99348[1], 99349[1], 99350[1], 99374[1], 99375[1], 99377[1], 99378[1], 99446[0], 99447[0], 99448[0], 99449[0], 99451[0], 99452[0], 99495[0], 99496[0], G0463[1], G0471[1]
50236	0213T[0], 0216T[0], 0596T[1], 0597T[1], 0600T[1], 0601T[1], 0708T[1], 0709T[1], 11000[1], 11001[1], 11004[1], 11005[1], 11006[1], 11042[1], 11043[1], 11044[1], 11045[1], 11046[1], 11047[1], 12001[1], 12002[1], 12004[1], 12005[1], 12006[1], 12007[1], 12011[1], 12013[1], 12014[1], 12015[1], 12016[1], 12017[1], 12018[1], 12020[1], 12021[1], 12031[1], 12032[1], 12034[1], 12035[1], 12036[1], 12037[1], 12041[1], 12042[1], 12044[1], 12045[1], 12046[1], 12047[1], 12051[1], 12052[1], 12053[1], 12054[1], 12055[1], 12056[1], 12057[1], 13100[1], 13101[1], 13102[1], 13120[1], 13121[1], 13122[1], 13131[1], 13132[1], 13133[1], 13151[1], 13152[1], 13153[1], 32551[1], 32556[1], 32557[1], 36000[1], 36400[1], 36405[1], 36406[1], 36410[1], 36420[1], 36425[1], 36430[1], 36440[1], 36591[0], 36592[0], 36600[1], 36640[1], 38747[1], 43752[1], 44602[1], 44603[1], 44604[1], 44605[1], 44950[0], 44970[0], 49000[0], 49002[1], 49010[0], 49203[1], 49204[1], 50100[1], 50250[1], 50280[1], 50290[1], 50500[1], 50541[1], 50542[1], 50543[1], 50544[1], 50545[1], 50546[1], 50548[1], 50650[1], 50660[1], 51701[1], 51702[1], 51703[1], 52000[0], 52240[1], 60540[1], 60545[1], 60650[1], 62320[0], 62321[0], 62322[0], 62323[0], 62324[0], 62325[0], 62326[0], 62327[0], 64400[0], 64405[0], 64408[0], 64415[0], 64416[0], 64417[0], 64418[0], 64420[0], 64421[0], 64425[0], 64430[0], 64435[0], 64445[0], 64446[0], 64447[0], 64448[0], 64449[0], 64450[0], 64451[0], 64454[0], 64461[0], 64462[0], 64463[0], 64479[0], 64480[0], 64483[0], 64484[0], 64486[0], 64487[0], 64488[0], 64489[0], 64490[0], 64491[0], 64492[0], 64493[0], 64494[0], 64495[0], 64505[0], 64510[0], 64517[0], 64520[0], 64530[0], 69990[0], 92012[1], 92014[1], 93000[1], 93005[1], 93010[1], 93040[1], 93041[1], 93042[1], 93318[1], 93355[1], 94002[1], 94200[1], 94680[1], 94681[1], 94690[1], 95812[1], 95813[1], 95816[1], 95819[1], 95822[1], 95829[1], 95955[1], 96360[1], 96361[1], 96365[1], 96366[1], 96367[1], 96368[1], 96372[1], 96374[1], 96375[1], 96376[1], 96377[1], 96523[0], 97597[1], 97598[1], 97602[1], 99155[0], 99156[0], 99157[0], 99211[1], 99212[1], 99213[1], 99214[1], 99215[1], 99217[1], 99218[1], 99219[1], 99220[1], 99221[1], 99222[1], 99223[1], 99231[1], 99232[1], 99233[1], 99234[1], 99235[1], 99236[1], 99238[1], 99239[1], 99241[1], 99242[1], 99243[1], 99244[1], 99245[1], 99251[1], 99252[1], 99253[1], 99254[1], 99255[1], 99291[1], 99292[1], 99304[1], 99305[1], 99306[1], 99307[1], 99308[1], 99309[1], 99310[1], 99315[1], 99316[1], 99334[1], 99335[1], 99336[1], 99337[1], 99347[1], 99348[1], 99349[1], 99350[1], 99374[1], 99375[1], 99377[1], 99378[1], 99446[0], 99447[0], 99448[0], 99449[0], 99451[0], 99452[0], 99495[0], 99496[0], G0463[1], G0471[1]
50240	0213T[0], 0216T[0], 0596T[1], 0597T[1], 0600T[1], 0601T[1], 0708T[1], 0709T[1], 11000[1], 11001[1], 11004[1], 11005[1], 11006[1], 11042[1], 11043[1], 11044[1], 11045[1], 11046[1], 11047[1], 12001[1], 12002[1], 12004[1], 12005[1], 12006[1], 12007[1], 12011[1], 12013[1], 12014[1], 12015[1], 12016[1], 12017[1], 12018[1], 12020[1], 12021[1], 12031[1], 12032[1], 12034[1], 12035[1], 12036[1], 12037[1], 12041[1], 12042[1], 12044[1], 12045[1], 12046[1], 12047[1], 12051[1], 12052[1], 12053[1], 12054[1], 12055[1], 12056[1], 12057[1], 13100[1], 13101[1], 13102[1], 13120[1], 13121[1], 13122[1], 13131[1], 13132[1], 13133[1], 13151[1], 13152[1], 13153[1], 32551[1], 32556[1], 32557[1], 35840[1], 36000[1], 36400[1], 36405[1], 36406[1], 36410[1], 36420[1], 36425[1], 36430[1], 36440[1], 36591[0], 36592[0], 36600[1], 36640[1], 38100[1], 38101[1], 38120[1], 43752[1], 44602[1], 44603[1], 44604[1], 44605[1], 44950[0], 44970[0], 49000[0], 49002[1], 49010[0], 50100[1], 50250[1], 50280[1], 50290[1], 50500[1], 50541[1], 50542[1], 50543[1], 50544[1], 51701[1], 51702[1], 51703[1], 60540[1], 60545[1], 60650[1], 62320[0], 62321[0], 62322[0], 62323[0], 62324[0], 62325[0], 62326[0], 62327[0], 64400[0], 64405[0], 64408[0], 64415[0], 64416[0], 64417[0], 64418[0], 64420[0], 64421[0], 64425[0], 64430[0], 64435[0], 64445[0], 64446[0], 64447[0], 64448[0], 64449[0], 64450[0], 64451[0], 64454[0], 64461[0], 64462[0], 64463[0], 64479[0], 64480[0], 64483[0], 64484[0], 64486[0], 64487[0], 64488[0], 64489[0], 64490[0], 64491[0], 64492[0], 64493[0], 64494[0], 64495[0], 64505[0], 64510[0], 64517[0], 64520[0], 64530[0], 69990[0], 92012[1], 92014[1], 93000[1], 93005[1], 93010[1], 93040[1], 93041[1], 93042[1], 93318[1], 93355[1], 94002[1], 94200[1], 94680[1], 94681[1], 94690[1], 95812[1], 95813[1], 95816[1], 95819[1], 95822[1], 95829[1], 95955[1], 96360[1], 96361[1], 96365[1], 96366[1], 96367[1], 96368[1], 96372[1], 96374[1], 96375[1], 96376[1], 96377[1], 96523[0], 97597[1], 97598[1], 97602[1], 99155[0], 99156[0], 99157[0], 99211[1], 99212[1], 99213[1], 99214[1], 99215[1], 99217[1], 99218[1], 99219[1], 99220[1], 99221[1], 99222[1], 99223[1], 99231[1], 99232[1], 99233[1], 99234[1], 99235[1], 99236[1], 99238[1], 99239[1], 99241[1], 99242[1], 99243[1], 99244[1], 99245[1], 99251[1], 99252[1], 99253[1], 99254[1], 99255[1], 99291[1], 99292[1], 99304[1], 99305[1], 99306[1], 99307[1], 99308[1], 99309[1], 99310[1], 99315[1], 99316[1], 99334[1], 99335[1], 99336[1], 99337[1], 99347[1], 99348[1], 99349[1], 99350[1], 99374[1], 99375[1], 99377[1], 99378[1], 99446[0], 99447[0], 99448[0], 99449[0], 99451[0], 99452[0], 99495[0], 99496[0], G0463[1], G0471[1]
50250	0213T[0], 0216T[0], 0596T[1], 0597T[1], 0708T[1], 0709T[1], 12001[1], 12002[1], 12004[1], 12005[1], 12006[1], 12007[1], 12011[1], 12013[1], 12014[1], 12015[1], 12016[1], 12017[1], 12018[1], 12020[1], 12021[1], 12031[1], 12032[1], 12034[1], 12035[1], 12036[1], 12037[1], 12041[1], 12042[1], 12044[1], 12045[1], 12046[1], 12047[1], 12051[1], 12052[1], 12053[1], 12054[1], 12055[1], 12056[1], 12057[1], 13100[1], 13101[1], 13102[1], 13120[1], 13121[1], 13122[1], 13131[1], 13132[1], 13133[1], 13151[1], 13152[1], 13153[1], 36000[1], 36400[1], 36405[1], 36406[1], 36410[1], 36420[1], 36425[1], 36430[1], 36440[1], 36591[0], 36592[0], 36600[1], 36640[1], 43653[0], 43752[1], 44820[1], 44850[1], 44950[1], 44970[0], 49000[0], 49002[1], 49010[0], 49203[1], 50040[1], 50045[1], 50100[1], 50500[1], 50541[1], 50542[1], 50544[1], 50592[1], 50593[1], 50715[1], 51701[1], 51702[1], 51703[1], 62320[0], 62321[0], 62322[0], 62323[0], 62324[0], 62325[0], 62326[0], 62327[0], 64400[0], 64405[0], 64408[0], 64415[0], 64416[0], 64417[0], 64418[0], 64420[0], 64421[0], 64425[0], 64430[0], 64435[0], 64445[0], 64446[0], 64447[0], 64448[0], 64449[0], 64450[0], 64451[0], 64454[0], 64461[0], 64462[0], 64463[0], 64479[0], 64480[0], 64483[0], 64484[0], 64486[0], 64487[0], 64488[0], 64489[0], 64490[0], 64491[0], 64492[0], 64493[0], 64494[0], 64495[0], 64505[0], 64510[0], 64517[0], 64520[0], 64530[0], 69990[0], 76940[1], 76942[1], 76998[1], 92012[1], 92014[1], 93000[1], 93005[1], 93010[1], 93040[1], 93041[1], 93042[1], 93318[1], 93355[1], 94002[1], 94200[1], 94680[1], 94681[1], 94690[1], 95812[1], 95813[1], 95816[1], 95819[1], 95822[1], 95829[1], 95955[1], 96360[1], 96361[1], 96365[1], 96366[1], 96367[1], 96368[1], 96372[1], 96374[1], 96375[1], 96376[1], 96377[1], 96523[0], 99155[0], 99156[0], 99157[0], 99211[1], 99212[1], 99213[1], 99214[1], 99215[1], 99217[1], 99218[1], 99219[1], 99220[1], 99221[1], 99222[1], 99223[1], 99231[1], 99232[1], 99233[1], 99234[1], 99235[1], 99236[1], 99238[1], 99239[1], 99241[1], 99242[1], 99243[1], 99244[1], 99245[1], 99251[1], 99252[1], 99253[1], 99254[1], 99255[1], 99291[1], 99292[1], 99304[1], 99305[1], 99306[1], 99307[1], 99308[1], 99309[1], 99310[1], 99315[1], 99316[1], 99334[1], 99335[1], 99336[1], 99337[1], 99347[1], 99348[1], 99349[1], 99350[1], 99374[1], 99375[1], 99377[1], 99378[1], 99446[0], 99447[0], 99448[0], 99449[0], 99451[0], 99452[0], 99495[0], 99496[0], G0463[1], G0471[1]
50280	0213T[0], 0216T[0], 0596T[1], 0597T[1], 0708T[1], 0709T[1], 11000[1], 11001[1], 11004[1], 11005[1], 11006[1], 11042[1], 11043[1], 11044[1], 11045[1], 11046[1], 11047[1], 12001[1], 12002[1], 12004[1], 12005[1], 12006[1], 12007[1], 12011[1], 12013[1], 12014[1], 12015[1], 12016[1], 12017[1], 12018[1], 12020[1], 12021[1], 12031[1], 12032[1], 12034[1], 12035[1], 12036[1], 12037[1], 12041[1], 12042[1], 12044[1], 12045[1], 12046[1], 12047[1], 12051[1], 12052[1], 12053[1], 12054[1], 12055[1], 12056[1], 12057[1], 13100[1], 13101[1], 13102[1], 13120[1], 13121[1], 13122[1], 13131[1], 13132[1], 13133[1], 13151[1], 13152[1], 13153[1], 36000[1], 36400[1], 36405[1], 36406[1], 36410[1], 36420[1], 36425[1], 36430[1], 36440[1], 36591[0], 36592[0], 36600[1], 36640[1], 43752[1], 44602[1], 44603[1], 44604[1], 44605[1], 44950[0], 44970[0], 49000[0], 49002[1], 49010[0], 50040[1], 50045[1], 50100[1], 50500[1], 50541[1], 50544[1], 51701[1], 51702[1], 51703[1], 62320[0], 62321[0], 62322[0], 62323[0], 62324[0], 62325[0], 62326[0], 62327[0], 64400[0], 64405[0], 64408[0], 64415[0], 64416[0], 64417[0], 64418[0],

0 = Modifier usage not allowed or inappropriate   1 = Modifier usage allowed

Code 1	Code 2
	64420[0], 64421[0], 64425[0], 64430[0], 64435[0], 64445[0], 64446[0], 64447[0], 64448[0], 64449[0], 64450[0], 64451[0], 64454[0], 64461[0], 64462[0], 64463[0], 64479[0], 64480[0], 64483[0], 64484[0], 64486[0], 64487[0], 64488[0], 64489[0], 64490[0], 64491[0], 64492[0], 64493[0], 64494[0], 64495[0], 64505[0], 64510[0], 64517[0], 64520[0], 64530[0], 69990[0], 92012[1], 92014[1], 93000[1], 93005[1], 93010[1], 93040[1], 93041[1], 93042[1], 93318[1], 93355[1], 94002[1], 94200[1], 94680[1], 94681[1], 94690[1], 95812[1], 95813[1], 95816[1], 95819[1], 95822[1], 95829[1], 95955[1], 96360[1], 96361[1], 96365[1], 96366[1], 96367[1], 96368[1], 96372[1], 96374[1], 96375[1], 96376[1], 96377[1], 96523[0], 97597[1], 97598[1], 97602[1], 99155[0], 99156[0], 99157[0], 99211[1], 99212[1], 99213[1], 99214[1], 99215[1], 99217[1], 99218[1], 99219[1], 99220[1], 99221[1], 99222[1], 99223[1], 99231[1], 99232[1], 99233[1], 99234[1], 99235[1], 99236[1], 99238[1], 99239[1], 99241[1], 99242[1], 99243[1], 99244[1], 99245[1], 99251[1], 99252[1], 99253[1], 99254[1], 99255[1], 99291[1], 99292[1], 99304[1], 99305[1], 99306[1], 99307[1], 99308[1], 99309[1], 99310[1], 99315[1], 99316[1], 99334[1], 99335[1], 99336[1], 99337[1], 99347[1], 99348[1], 99349[1], 99350[1], 99374[1], 99375[1], 99377[1], 99378[1], 99446[0], 99447[0], 99448[0], 99449[0], 99451[0], 99452[0], 99495[0], 99496[0], G0463[1], G0471[1]
50290	0213T[0], 0216T[0], 0596T[1], 0597T[1], 0708T[1], 0709T[1], 11000[1], 11001[1], 11004[1], 11005[1], 11006[1], 11042[1], 11043[1], 11044[1], 11045[1], 11046[1], 11047[1], 12001[1], 12002[1], 12004[1], 12005[1], 12006[1], 12007[1], 12011[1], 12013[1], 12014[1], 12015[1], 12016[1], 12017[1], 12018[1], 12020[1], 12021[1], 12031[1], 12032[1], 12034[1], 12035[1], 12036[1], 12037[1], 12041[1], 12042[1], 12044[1], 12045[1], 12046[1], 12047[1], 12051[1], 12052[1], 12053[1], 12054[1], 12055[1], 12056[1], 12057[1], 13100[1], 13101[1], 13102[1], 13120[1], 13121[1], 13122[1], 13131[1], 13132[1], 13133[1], 13151[1], 13152[1], 13153[1], 36000[1], 36400[1], 36405[1], 36406[1], 36410[1], 36420[1], 36425[1], 36430[1], 36440[1], 36591[0], 36592[0], 36600[1], 36640[1], 43752[1], 44602[1], 44603[1], 44604[1], 44605[1], 44950[0], 44970[0], 49000[0], 49002[1], 49010[0], 50100[1], 50500[1], 50544[1], 51701[1], 51702[1], 51703[1], 62320[0], 62321[0], 62322[0], 62323[0], 62324[0], 62325[0], 62326[0], 62327[0], 64400[0], 64405[0], 64408[0], 64415[0], 64416[0], 64417[0], 64418[0], 64420[0], 64421[0], 64425[0], 64430[0], 64435[0], 64445[0], 64446[0], 64447[0], 64448[0], 64449[0], 64450[0], 64451[0], 64454[0], 64461[0], 64462[0], 64463[0], 64479[0], 64480[0], 64483[0], 64484[0], 64486[0], 64487[0], 64488[0], 64489[0], 64490[0], 64491[0], 64492[0], 64493[0], 64494[0], 64495[0], 64505[0], 64510[0], 64517[0], 64520[0], 64530[0], 69990[0], 92012[1], 92014[1], 93000[1], 93005[1], 93010[1], 93040[1], 93041[1], 93042[1], 93318[1], 93355[1], 94002[1], 94200[1], 94680[1], 94681[1], 94690[1], 95812[1], 95813[1], 95816[1], 95819[1], 95822[1], 95829[1], 95955[1], 96360[1], 96361[1], 96365[1], 96366[1], 96367[1], 96368[1], 96372[1], 96374[1], 96375[1], 96376[1], 96377[1], 96523[0], 97597[1], 97598[1], 97602[1], 99155[0], 99156[0], 99157[0], 99211[1], 99212[1], 99213[1], 99214[1], 99215[1], 99217[1], 99218[1], 99219[1], 99220[1], 99221[1], 99222[1], 99223[1], 99231[1], 99232[1], 99233[1], 99234[1], 99235[1], 99236[1], 99238[1], 99239[1], 99241[1], 99242[1], 99243[1], 99244[1], 99245[1], 99251[1], 99252[1], 99253[1], 99254[1], 99255[1], 99291[1], 99292[1], 99304[1], 99305[1], 99306[1], 99307[1], 99308[1], 99309[1], 99310[1], 99315[1], 99316[1], 99334[1], 99335[1], 99336[1], 99337[1], 99347[1], 99348[1], 99349[1], 99350[1], 99374[1], 99375[1], 99377[1], 99378[1], 99446[0], 99447[0], 99448[0], 99449[0], 99451[0], 99452[0], 99495[0], 99496[0], G0463[1], G0471[1]
50300	0213T[1], 0216T[1], 11000[1], 11001[1], 11004[1], 11005[1], 11006[1], 11042[1], 11043[1], 11044[1], 11045[1], 11046[1], 11047[1], 36000[1], 36410[1], 36591[0], 36592[0], 44602[1], 44603[1], 44604[1], 44605[1], 44950[0], 44970[0], 49000[0], 49002[1], 49010[0], 50220[0], 50225[0], 50230[0], 50234[0], 50236[0], 50240[0], 50541[1], 50542[0], 50543[0], 50544[1], 50545[1], 50546[1], 50548[1], 50605[1], 61650[1], 62324[1], 62325[1], 62326[1], 62327[1], 64415[1], 64416[1], 64417[1], 64450[1], 64454[1], 64486[1], 64487[1], 64488[1], 64489[1], 64490[1], 64493[1], 69990[0], 96523[0], 97597[1], 97598[1], 97602[1]
50320	0213T[0], 0216T[0], 0596T[1], 0597T[1], 0708T[1], 0709T[1], 11000[1], 11001[1], 11004[1], 11005[1], 11006[1], 11042[1], 11043[1], 11044[1], 11045[1], 11046[1], 11047[1], 12001[1], 12002[1], 12004[1], 12005[1], 12006[1], 12007[1], 12011[1], 12013[1], 12014[1], 12015[1], 12016[1], 12017[1], 12018[1], 12020[1], 12021[1], 12031[1], 12032[1], 12034[1], 12035[1], 12036[1], 12037[1], 12041[1], 12042[1], 12044[1], 12045[1], 12046[1], 12047[1], 12051[1], 12052[1], 12053[1], 12054[1], 12055[1], 12056[1], 12057[1], 13100[1], 13101[1], 13102[1], 13120[1], 13121[1], 13122[1], 13131[1], 13132[1], 13133[1], 13151[1], 13152[1], 13153[1], 36000[1], 36400[1], 36405[1], 36406[1], 36410[1], 36420[1], 36425[1], 36430[1], 36440[1], 36591[0], 36592[0], 36600[1], 36640[1], 43752[1], 44602[1], 44603[1], 44604[1], 44605[1], 44950[0], 44970[0], 49000[0], 49002[1], 49010[0], 50220[0], 50225[0], 50230[0], 50234[0], 50236[0], 50240[0], 50541[1], 50542[0], 50543[0], 50544[1], 50545[1], 50546[1], 50547[1], 50548[1], 50605[1], 50650[1], 51701[1], 51702[1], 51703[1], 62320[0], 62321[0], 62322[0], 62323[0], 62324[0], 62325[0], 62326[0], 62327[0], 64400[0], 64405[0], 64408[0], 64415[0], 64416[0], 64417[0], 64418[0], 64420[0], 64421[0], 64425[0], 64430[0], 64435[0], 64445[0], 64446[0], 64447[0], 64448[0], 64449[0], 64450[0], 64451[0], 64454[0], 64461[0], 64462[0], 64463[0], 64479[0], 64480[0], 64483[0], 64484[0], 64486[0], 64487[0], 64488[0], 64489[0], 64490[0], 64491[0], 64492[0], 64493[0], 64494[0], 64495[0], 64505[0], 64510[0], 64517[0], 64520[0], 64530[0], 69990[0], 92012[1], 92014[1], 93000[1], 93005[1], 93010[1], 93040[1], 93041[1], 93042[1], 93318[1], 93355[1], 94002[1], 94200[1], 94680[1], 94681[1], 94690[1], 95812[1], 95813[1], 95816[1], 95819[1], 95822[1], 95829[1], 95955[1], 96360[1], 96361[1], 96365[1], 96366[1], 96367[1], 96368[1], 96372[1], 96374[1], 96375[1], 96376[1], 96377[1], 96523[0], 97597[1], 97598[1], 97602[1], 99155[0], 99156[0], 99157[0], 99211[1], 99212[1], 99213[1], 99214[1], 99215[1], 99217[1], 99218[1], 99219[1], 99220[1], 99221[1], 99222[1], 99223[1], 99231[1], 99232[1], 99233[1], 99234[1], 99235[1], 99236[1], 99238[1], 99239[1], 99241[1], 99242[1], 99243[1], 99244[1], 99245[1], 99251[1], 99252[1], 99253[1], 99254[1], 99255[1], 99291[1], 99292[1], 99304[1], 99305[1], 99306[1], 99307[1], 99308[1], 99309[1], 99310[1], 99315[1], 99316[1], 99334[1], 99335[1], 99336[1], 99337[1], 99347[1], 99348[1], 99349[1], 99350[1], 99374[1], 99375[1], 99377[1], 99378[1], 99446[0], 99447[0], 99448[0], 99449[0], 99451[0], 99452[0], 99495[0], 99496[0], G0463[1], G0471[1]
50323	11000[1], 11001[1], 11004[1], 11005[1], 11006[1], 11042[1], 11043[1], 11044[1], 11045[1], 11046[1], 11047[1], 36591[0], 36592[0], 60540[1], 60545[1], 69990[0], 96523[0], 97597[1], 97598[1], 97602[1]
50325	11000[1], 11001[1], 11004[1], 11005[1], 11006[1], 11042[1], 11043[1], 11044[1], 11045[1], 11046[1], 11047[1], 36591[0], 36592[0], 49400[0], 50323[0], 69990[0], 96523[0], 97597[1], 97598[1], 97602[1]
50327	36591[0], 36592[0], 69990[0], 96523[0]
50328	36591[0], 36592[0], 69990[0], 96523[0]
50329	36591[0], 36592[0], 69990[0], 96523[0]
50340	0213T[0], 0216T[0], 0596T[1], 0597T[1], 0708T[1], 0709T[1], 11000[1], 11001[1], 11004[1], 11005[1], 11006[1], 11042[1], 11043[1], 11044[1], 11045[1], 11046[1], 11047[1], 12001[1], 12002[1], 12004[1], 12005[1], 12006[1], 12007[1], 12011[1], 12013[1], 12014[1], 12015[1], 12016[1], 12017[1], 12018[1], 12020[1], 12021[1], 12031[1], 12032[1], 12034[1], 12035[1], 12036[1], 12037[1], 12041[1], 12042[1], 12044[1], 12045[1], 12046[1], 12047[1], 12051[1], 12052[1], 12053[1], 12054[1], 12055[1], 12056[1], 12057[1], 13100[1], 13101[1], 13102[1], 13120[1], 13121[1], 13122[1], 13131[1], 13132[1], 13133[1], 13151[1], 13152[1], 13153[1], 36000[1], 36400[1], 36405[1], 36406[1], 36410[1], 36420[1], 36425[1], 36430[1], 36440[1], 36591[0], 36592[0], 36600[1], 36640[1], 38100[1], 38101[1], 38120[1], 43752[1], 44602[1], 44603[1], 44604[1], 44605[1], 44950[0], 44970[0], 49000[0], 49002[1], 49010[0], 50220[0], 50225[0], 50230[0], 50234[0], 50236[0], 50240[0], 50541[1], 50542[1], 50543[1], 50544[1], 50545[1], 50546[1], 50548[1], 50605[1], 50650[1], 51701[1], 51702[1], 51703[1], 62320[0], 62321[0], 62322[0], 62323[0], 62324[0], 62325[0], 62326[0], 62327[0], 64400[0], 64405[0], 64408[0], 64415[0], 64416[0], 64417[0], 64418[0], 64420[0], 64421[0], 64425[0], 64430[0], 64435[0], 64445[0], 64446[0], 64447[0], 64448[0], 64449[0], 64450[0], 64451[0], 64454[0], 64461[0], 64462[0], 64463[0], 64479[0], 64480[0], 64483[0], 64484[0], 64486[0], 64487[0], 64488[0], 64489[0], 64490[0], 64491[0], 64492[0], 64493[0], 64494[0], 64495[0], 64505[0], 64510[0], 64517[0], 64520[0], 64530[0], 69990[0], 92012[1], 92014[1], 93000[1], 93005[1], 93010[1], 93040[1], 93041[1], 93042[1], 93318[1], 93355[1], 94002[1], 94200[1], 94680[1], 94681[1], 94690[1], 95812[1], 95813[1], 95816[1], 95819[1], 95822[1], 95829[1], 95955[1], 96360[1], 96361[1], 96365[1], 96366[1], 96367[1], 96368[1], 96372[1], 96374[1], 96375[1], 96376[1], 96377[1], 96523[0], 97597[1], 97598[1], 97602[1], 99155[0], 99156[0], 99157[0], 99211[1], 99212[1], 99213[1], 99214[1], 99215[1], 99217[1], 99218[1], 99219[1], 99220[1], 99221[1], 99222[1], 99223[1], 99231[1], 99232[1], 99233[1], 99234[1], 99235[1], 99236[1], 99238[1], 99239[1], 99241[1], 99242[1], 99243[1], 99244[1], 99245[1], 99251[1], 99252[1], 99253[1], 99254[1], 99255[1], 99291[1], 99292[1], 99304[1], 99305[1], 99306[1], 99307[1], 99308[1], 99309[1], 99310[1], 99315[1], 99316[1], 99334[1], 99335[1], 99336[1], 99337[1], 99347[1], 99348[1], 99349[1], 99350[1], 99374[1], 99375[1], 99377[1], 99378[1], 99446[0], 99447[0], 99448[0], 99449[0], 99451[0], 99452[0], 99495[0], 99496[0], G0463[1], G0471[1]
50360	0213T[0], 0216T[0], 0596T[1], 0597T[1], 0708T[1], 0709T[1], 11000[1], 11001[1], 11004[1], 11005[1], 11006[1], 11042[1], 11043[1], 11044[1], 11045[1], 11046[1], 11047[1], 12001[1], 12002[1], 12004[1], 12005[1], 12006[1], 12007[1], 12011[1], 12013[1], 12014[1], 12015[1], 12016[1], 12017[1], 12018[1], 12020[1], 12021[1], 12031[1], 12032[1], 12034[1], 12035[1], 12036[1], 12037[1], 12041[1], 12042[1], 12044[1], 12045[1], 12046[1], 12047[1], 12051[1], 12052[1], 12053[1], 12054[1], 12055[1], 12056[1], 12057[1], 13100[1], 13101[1], 13102[1], 13120[1], 13121[1], 13122[1], 13131[1], 13132[1], 13133[1], 13151[1], 13152[1], 13153[1], 35221[1], 35840[1], 36000[1], 36400[1], 36405[1], 36406[1], 36410[1], 36420[1], 36425[1], 36430[1], 36440[1], 36591[0], 36592[0], 36600[1], 36640[1], 43752[1], 44602[1], 44603[1], 44604[1], 44605[1], 44950[0], 44970[0], 49000[0], 49002[1], 49010[0], 49421[1], 50200[1], 50220[0], 50225[0], 50230[0], 50234[0], 50236[0], 50240[0], 50400[1], 50780[1], 51701[1], 51702[1], 51703[1], 62320[0], 62321[0], 62322[0], 62323[0], 62324[0], 62325[0], 62326[0], 62327[0], 64400[0], 64405[0], 64408[0], 64415[0], 64416[0], 64417[0], 64418[0], 64420[0], 64421[0], 64425[0], 64430[0], 64435[0], 64445[0], 64446[0], 64447[0], 64448[0], 64449[0], 64450[0], 64451[0], 64454[0], 64461[0], 64462[0], 64463[0], 64479[0], 64480[0], 64483[0], 64484[0], 64486[0], 64487[0], 64488[0], 64489[0], 64490[0], 64491[0], 64492[0], 64493[0], 64494[0], 64495[0], 64505[0], 64510[0], 64517[0], 64520[0], 64530[0], 69990[0], 92012[1], 92014[1], 93000[1], 93005[1], 93010[1], 93040[1], 93041[1], 93042[1], 93318[1], 93355[1], 94002[1], 94200[1], 94680[1], 94681[1], 94690[1], 95812[1], 95813[1], 95816[1], 95819[1], 95822[1], 95829[1], 95955[1], 96360[1], 96361[1], 96365[1], 96366[1], 96367[1], 96368[1], 96372[1], 96374[1], 96375[1], 96376[1], 96377[1], 96523[0], 97597[1], 97598[1], 97602[1], 99155[0], 99156[0], 99157[0], 99211[1], 99212[1], 99213[1], 99214[1], 99215[1], 99217[1], 99218[1], 99219[1], 99220[1], 99221[1], 99222[1], 99223[1], 99231[1], 99232[1], 99233[1], 99234[1], 99235[1], 99236[1], 99238[1], 99239[1], 99241[1], 99242[1], 99243[1], 99244[1], 99245[1], 99251[1], 99252[1], 99253[1], 99254[1], 99255[1], 99291[1], 99292[1], 99304[1], 99305[1], 99306[1], 99307[1], 99308[1], 99309[1],

0 = Modifier usage not allowed or inappropriate 1 = Modifier usage allowed

Code 1	Code 2
	99310[1], 99315[1], 99316[1], 99334[1], 99335[1], 99336[1], 99337[1], 99347[1], 99348[1], 99349[1], 99350[1], 99374[1], 99375[1], 99377[1], 99378[1], 99446[0], 99447[0], 99448[0], 99449[0], 99451[0], 99452[0], 99495[0], 99496[0], G0463[1], G0471[1]
50365	0213T[0], 0216T[0], 0596T[1], 0597T[1], 0708T[1], 0709T[1], 11000[1], 11001[1], 11004[1], 11005[1], 11006[1], 11042[1], 11043[1], 11044[1], 11045[1], 11046[1], 11047[1], 12001[1], 12002[1], 12004[1], 12005[1], 12006[1], 12007[1], 12011[1], 12013[1], 12014[1], 12015[1], 12016[1], 12017[1], 12018[1], 12020[1], 12021[1], 12031[1], 12032[1], 12034[1], 12035[1], 12036[1], 12037[1], 12041[1], 12042[1], 12044[1], 12045[1], 12046[1], 12047[1], 12051[1], 12052[1], 12053[1], 12054[1], 12055[1], 12056[1], 12057[1], 13100[1], 13101[1], 13102[1], 13120[1], 13121[1], 13122[1], 13131[1], 13132[1], 13133[1], 13151[1], 13152[1], 13153[1], 36000[1], 36400[1], 36405[1], 36406[1], 36410[1], 36420[1], 36425[1], 36430[1], 36440[1], 36591[0], 36592[0], 36600[1], 36640[1], 38100[1], 38101[1], 38120[1], 43752[1], 44602[1], 44603[1], 44604[1], 44605[1], 44950[0], 44970[0], 49000[0], 49002[1], 49010[0], 50220[0], 50225[0], 50230[0], 50234[0], 50236[0], 50240[0], 50340[0], 50541[1], 50542[1], 50543[1], 50544[1], 50545[1], 50546[1], 50548[1], 50605[1], 50650[1], 50780[0], 51701[1], 51702[1], 51703[1], 62320[0], 62321[0], 62322[0], 62323[0], 62324[0], 62325[0], 62326[0], 62327[0], 64400[0], 64405[0], 64408[0], 64415[0], 64416[0], 64417[0], 64418[0], 64420[0], 64421[0], 64425[0], 64430[0], 64435[0], 64445[0], 64446[0], 64447[0], 64448[0], 64449[0], 64450[0], 64451[0], 64454[0], 64461[0], 64462[0], 64463[0], 64479[0], 64480[0], 64483[0], 64484[0], 64486[0], 64487[0], 64488[0], 64489[0], 64490[0], 64491[0], 64492[0], 64493[0], 64494[0], 64495[0], 64505[0], 64510[0], 64517[0], 64520[0], 64530[0], 69990[0], 92012[1], 92014[1], 93000[1], 93005[1], 93010[1], 93040[1], 93041[1], 93042[1], 93318[1], 93355[1], 94002[1], 94200[1], 94680[1], 94681[1], 94690[1], 95812[1], 95813[1], 95816[1], 95819[1], 95822[1], 95829[1], 95955[1], 96360[1], 96361[1], 96365[1], 96366[1], 96367[1], 96368[1], 96372[1], 96374[1], 96375[1], 96376[1], 96377[1], 96523[0], 97597[1], 97598[1], 97602[1], 99155[0], 99156[0], 99157[0], 99211[1], 99212[1], 99213[1], 99214[1], 99215[1], 99217[1], 99218[1], 99219[1], 99220[1], 99221[1], 99222[1], 99223[1], 99231[1], 99232[1], 99233[1], 99234[1], 99235[1], 99236[1], 99238[1], 99239[1], 99241[1], 99242[1], 99243[1], 99244[1], 99245[1], 99251[1], 99252[1], 99253[1], 99254[1], 99255[1], 99291[1], 99292[1], 99304[1], 99305[1], 99306[1], 99307[1], 99308[1], 99309[1], 99310[1], 99315[1], 99316[1], 99334[1], 99335[1], 99336[1], 99337[1], 99347[1], 99348[1], 99349[1], 99350[1], 99374[1], 99375[1], 99377[1], 99378[1], 99446[0], 99447[0], 99448[0], 99449[0], 99451[0], 99452[0], 99495[0], 99496[0], G0463[1], G0471[1]
50370	0213T[0], 0216T[0], 0596T[1], 0597T[1], 0708T[1], 0709T[1], 11000[1], 11001[1], 11004[1], 11005[1], 11006[1], 11042[1], 11043[1], 11044[1], 11045[1], 11046[1], 11047[1], 12001[1], 12002[1], 12004[1], 12005[1], 12006[1], 12007[1], 12011[1], 12013[1], 12014[1], 12015[1], 12016[1], 12017[1], 12018[1], 12020[1], 12021[1], 12031[1], 12032[1], 12034[1], 12035[1], 12036[1], 12037[1], 12041[1], 12042[1], 12044[1], 12045[1], 12046[1], 12047[1], 12051[1], 12052[1], 12053[1], 12054[1], 12055[1], 12056[1], 12057[1], 13100[1], 13101[1], 13102[1], 13120[1], 13121[1], 13122[1], 13131[1], 13132[1], 13133[1], 13151[1], 13152[1], 13153[1], 36000[1], 36400[1], 36405[1], 36406[1], 36410[1], 36420[1], 36425[1], 36430[1], 36440[1], 36591[0], 36592[0], 36600[1], 36640[1], 38100[1], 38101[1], 38120[1], 43752[1], 44602[1], 44603[1], 44604[1], 44605[1], 44950[0], 44970[0], 49000[0], 49002[1], 49010[0], 50220[0], 50225[0], 50230[0], 50234[0], 50236[0], 50240[0], 50340[1], 50541[1], 50542[1], 50543[1], 50544[1], 50545[1], 50546[1], 50548[1], 50605[1], 51701[1], 51702[1], 51703[1], 62320[0], 62321[0], 62322[0], 62323[0], 62324[0], 62325[0], 62326[0], 62327[0], 64400[0], 64405[0], 64408[0], 64415[0], 64416[0], 64417[0], 64418[0], 64420[0], 64421[0], 64425[0], 64430[0], 64435[0], 64445[0], 64446[0], 64447[0], 64448[0], 64449[0], 64450[0], 64451[0], 64454[0], 64461[0], 64462[0], 64463[0], 64479[0], 64480[0], 64483[0], 64484[0], 64486[0], 64487[0], 64488[0], 64489[0], 64490[0], 64491[0], 64492[0], 64493[0], 64494[0], 64495[0], 64505[0], 64510[0], 64517[0], 64520[0], 64530[0], 69990[0], 92012[1], 92014[1], 93000[1], 93005[1], 93010[1], 93040[1], 93041[1], 93042[1], 93318[1], 93355[1], 94002[1], 94200[1], 94680[1], 94681[1], 94690[1], 95812[1], 95813[1], 95816[1], 95819[1], 95822[1], 95829[1], 95955[1], 96360[1], 96361[1], 96365[1], 96366[1], 96367[1], 96368[1], 96372[1], 96374[1], 96375[1], 96376[1], 96377[1], 96523[0], 97597[1], 97598[1], 97602[1], 99155[0], 99156[0], 99157[0], 99211[1], 99212[1], 99213[1], 99214[1], 99215[1], 99217[1], 99218[1], 99219[1], 99220[1], 99221[1], 99222[1], 99223[1], 99231[1], 99232[1], 99233[1], 99234[1], 99235[1], 99236[1], 99238[1], 99239[1], 99241[1], 99242[1], 99243[1], 99244[1], 99245[1], 99251[1], 99252[1], 99253[1], 99254[1], 99255[1], 99291[1], 99292[1], 99304[1], 99305[1], 99306[1], 99307[1], 99308[1], 99309[1], 99310[1], 99315[1], 99316[1], 99334[1], 99335[1], 99336[1], 99337[1], 99347[1], 99348[1], 99349[1], 99350[1], 99374[1], 99375[1], 99377[1], 99378[1], 99446[0], 99447[0], 99448[0], 99449[0], 99451[0], 99452[0], 99495[0], 99496[0], G0463[1], G0471[1]
50380	0213T[0], 0216T[0], 0596T[1], 0597T[1], 0708T[1], 0709T[1], 12001[1], 12002[1], 12004[1], 12005[1], 12006[1], 12007[1], 12011[1], 12013[1], 12014[1], 12015[1], 12016[1], 12017[1], 12018[1], 12020[1], 12021[1], 12031[1], 12032[1], 12034[1], 12035[1], 12036[1], 12037[1], 12041[1], 12042[1], 12044[1], 12045[1], 12046[1], 12047[1], 12051[1], 12052[1], 12053[1], 12054[1], 12055[1], 12056[1], 12057[1], 13100[1], 13101[1], 13102[1], 13120[1], 13121[1], 13122[1], 13131[1], 13132[1], 13133[1], 13151[1], 13152[1], 13153[1], 35840[1], 36000[1], 36400[1], 36405[1], 36406[1], 36410[1], 36420[1], 36425[1], 36430[1], 36440[1], 36591[0], 36592[0], 36600[1], 36640[1], 38100[1], 38101[1], 38120[1], 43752[1], 44602[1], 44603[1], 44604[1], 44605[1], 44950[0], 44970[0], 49000[0], 49002[1], 49010[0], 50340[1], 50544[1], 50605[1], 50780[0], 51701[1], 51702[1], 51703[1], 62320[0], 62321[0], 62322[0], 62323[0], 62324[0], 62325[0], 62326[0], 62327[0], 64400[0], 64405[0], 64408[0], 64415[0], 64416[0], 64417[0], 64418[0], 64420[0], 64421[0], 64425[0], 64430[0], 64435[0], 64445[0], 64446[0], 64447[0], 64448[0], 64449[0], 64450[0], 64451[0], 64454[0], 64461[0], 64462[0], 64463[0], 64479[0], 64480[0], 64483[0], 64484[0], 64486[0], 64487[0], 64488[0], 64489[0], 64490[0], 64491[0], 64492[0], 64493[0], 64494[0], 64495[0], 64505[0], 64510[0], 64517[0], 64520[0], 64530[0], 69990[0], 92012[1], 92014[1], 93000[1], 93005[1], 93010[1], 93040[1], 93041[1], 93042[1], 93318[1], 93355[1], 94002[1], 94200[1], 94680[1], 94681[1], 94690[1], 95812[1], 95813[1], 95816[1], 95819[1], 95822[1], 95829[1], 95955[1], 96360[1], 96361[1], 96365[1], 96366[1], 96367[1], 96368[1], 96372[1], 96374[1], 96375[1], 96376[1], 96377[1], 96523[0], 99155[0], 99156[0], 99157[0], 99211[1], 99212[1], 99213[1], 99214[1], 99215[1], 99217[1], 99218[1], 99219[1], 99220[1], 99221[1], 99222[1], 99223[1], 99231[1], 99232[1], 99233[1], 99234[1], 99235[1], 99236[1], 99238[1], 99239[1], 99241[1], 99242[1], 99243[1], 99244[1], 99245[1], 99251[1], 99252[1], 99253[1], 99254[1], 99255[1], 99291[1], 99292[1], 99304[1], 99305[1], 99306[1], 99307[1], 99308[1], 99309[1], 99310[1], 99315[1], 99316[1], 99334[1], 99335[1], 99336[1], 99337[1], 99347[1], 99348[1], 99349[1], 99350[1], 99374[1], 99375[1], 99377[1], 99378[1], 99446[0], 99447[0], 99448[0], 99449[0], 99451[0], 99452[0], 99495[0], 99496[0], G0463[1], G0471[1]
50382	0213T[0], 0216T[0], 0596T[1], 0597T[1], 0708T[1], 0709T[1], 11000[1], 11001[1], 11004[1], 11005[1], 11006[1], 11042[1], 11043[1], 11044[1], 11045[1], 11046[1], 11047[1], 12001[1], 12002[1], 12004[1], 12005[1], 12006[1], 12007[1], 12011[1], 12013[1], 12014[1], 12015[1], 12016[1], 12017[1], 12018[1], 12020[1], 12021[1], 12031[1], 12032[1], 12034[1], 12035[1], 12036[1], 12037[1], 12041[1], 12042[1], 12044[1], 12045[1], 12046[1], 12047[1], 12051[1], 12052[1], 12053[1], 12054[1], 12055[1], 12056[1], 12057[1], 13100[1], 13101[1], 13102[1], 13120[1], 13121[1], 13122[1], 13131[1], 13132[1], 13133[1], 13151[1], 13152[1], 13153[1], 36000[1], 36400[1], 36405[1], 36406[1], 36410[1], 36420[1], 36425[1], 36430[1], 36440[1], 36591[0], 36592[0], 36600[1], 36640[1], 43752[1], 50384[1], 50385[1], 50386[1], 50387[1], 50390[1], 50430[1], 50431[1], 50432[1], 50436[1], 50437[1], 50688[1], 50693[1], 50694[1], 50695[1], 51701[1], 51702[1], 51703[1], 52332[1], 52356[1], 62320[0], 62321[0], 62322[0], 62323[0], 62324[0], 62325[0], 62326[0], 62327[0], 64400[0], 64405[0], 64408[0], 64415[0], 64416[0], 64417[0], 64418[0], 64420[0], 64421[0], 64425[0], 64430[0], 64435[0], 64445[0], 64446[0], 64447[0], 64448[0], 64449[0], 64450[0], 64451[0], 64454[0], 64461[0], 64462[0], 64463[0], 64479[0], 64480[0], 64483[0], 64484[0], 64486[0], 64487[0], 64488[0], 64489[0], 64490[0], 64491[0], 64492[0], 64493[0], 64494[0], 64495[0], 64505[0], 64510[0], 64517[0], 64520[0], 64530[0], 69990[0], 76000[1], 76380[1], 76942[1], 76998[1], 77001[1], 77002[1], 77012[1], 77021[1], 92012[1], 92014[1], 93000[1], 93005[1], 93010[1], 93040[1], 93041[1], 93042[1], 93318[1], 93355[1], 94002[1], 94200[1], 94680[1], 94681[1], 94690[1], 95812[1], 95813[1], 95816[1], 95819[1], 95822[1], 95829[1], 95955[1], 96360[1], 96361[1], 96365[1], 96366[1], 96367[1], 96368[1], 96372[1], 96374[1], 96375[1], 96376[1], 96377[1], 96523[0], 97597[1], 97598[1], 97602[1], 99155[0], 99156[0], 99157[0], 99211[1], 99212[1], 99213[1], 99214[1], 99215[1], 99217[1], 99218[1], 99219[1], 99220[1], 99221[1], 99222[1], 99223[1], 99231[1], 99232[1], 99233[1], 99234[1], 99235[1], 99236[1], 99238[1], 99239[1], 99241[1], 99242[1], 99243[1], 99244[1], 99245[1], 99251[1], 99252[1], 99253[1], 99254[1], 99255[1], 99291[1], 99292[1], 99304[1], 99305[1], 99306[1], 99307[1], 99308[1], 99309[1], 99310[1], 99315[1], 99316[1], 99334[1], 99335[1], 99336[1], 99337[1], 99347[1], 99348[1], 99349[1], 99350[1], 99374[1], 99375[1], 99377[1], 99378[1], 99446[0], 99447[0], 99448[0], 99449[0], 99451[0], 99452[0], 99495[1], 99496[1], G0463[1], G0471[1], J0670[1], J2001[1]
50384	0213T[0], 0216T[0], 0596T[1], 0597T[1], 0708T[1], 0709T[1], 11000[1], 11001[1], 11004[1], 11005[1], 11006[1], 11042[1], 11043[1], 11044[1], 11045[1], 11046[1], 11047[1], 12001[1], 12002[1], 12004[1], 12005[1], 12006[1], 12007[1], 12011[1], 12013[1], 12014[1], 12015[1], 12016[1], 12017[1], 12018[1], 12020[1], 12021[1], 12031[1], 12032[1], 12034[1], 12035[1], 12036[1], 12037[1], 12041[1], 12042[1], 12044[1], 12045[1], 12046[1], 12047[1], 12051[1], 12052[1], 12053[1], 12054[1], 12055[1], 12056[1], 12057[1], 13100[1], 13101[1], 13102[1], 13120[1], 13121[1], 13122[1], 13131[1], 13132[1], 13133[1], 13151[1], 13152[1], 13153[1], 36000[1], 36400[1], 36405[1], 36406[1], 36410[1], 36420[1], 36425[1], 36430[1], 36440[1], 36591[0], 36592[0], 36600[1], 36640[1], 43752[1], 50385[1], 50386[1], 50387[1], 50390[1], 50430[1], 50431[1], 50432[1], 50436[1], 50688[1], 50693[1], 50694[1], 50695[1], 51701[1], 51702[1], 51703[1], 52332[1], 52356[1], 62320[0], 62321[0], 62322[0], 62323[0], 62324[0], 62325[0], 62326[0], 62327[0], 64400[0], 64405[0], 64408[0], 64415[0], 64416[0], 64417[0], 64418[0], 64420[0], 64421[0], 64425[0], 64430[0], 64435[0], 64445[0], 64446[0], 64447[0], 64448[0], 64449[0], 64450[0], 64451[0], 64454[0], 64461[0], 64462[0], 64463[0], 64479[0], 64480[0], 64483[0], 64484[0], 64486[0], 64487[0], 64488[0], 64489[0], 64490[0], 64491[0], 64492[0], 64493[0], 64494[0], 64495[0], 64505[0], 64510[0], 64517[0], 64520[0], 64530[0], 69990[0], 76000[1], 76380[1], 76942[1], 76998[1], 77001[1], 77002[1], 77012[1], 77021[1], 92012[1], 92014[1], 93000[1], 93005[1], 93010[1], 93040[1], 93041[1], 93042[1], 93318[1], 93355[1], 94002[1], 94200[1], 94680[1], 94681[1], 94690[1], 95812[1], 95813[1], 95816[1], 95819[1], 95822[1], 95829[1], 95955[1], 96360[1], 96361[1], 96365[1], 96366[1], 96367[1], 96368[1], 96372[1], 96374[1], 96375[1], 96376[1], 96377[1], 96523[0], 97597[1], 97598[1], 97602[1], 99155[0], 99156[0], 99157[0], 99211[1], 99212[1], 99213[1], 99214[1], 99215[1], 99217[1], 99218[1], 99219[1], 99220[1], 99221[1], 99222[1], 99223[1], 99231[1], 99232[1], 99233[1], 99234[1], 99235[1], 99236[1], 99238[1], 99239[1], 99241[1], 99242[1], 99243[1], 99244[1], 99245[1], 99251[1], 99252[1], 99253[1], 99254[1], 99255[1], 99291[1], 99292[1], 99304[1], 99305[1], 99306[1], 99307[1], 99308[1], 99309[1], 99310[1], 99315[1], 99316[1], 99334[1], 99335[1], 99336[1], 99337[1], 99347[1], 99348[1],

0 = Modifier usage not allowed or inappropriate 1 = Modifier usage allowed

Code 1	Code 2
	99349[1], 99350[1], 99374[1], 99375[1], 99377[1], 99378[1], 99446[0], 99447[0], 99448[0], 99449[0], 99451[0], 99452[0], 99495[1], 99496[1], G0463[1], G0471[1], J0670[1], J2001[1]
50385	0213T[0], 0216T[0], 0708T[1], 0709T[1], 11000[1], 11001[1], 11004[1], 11005[1], 11006[1], 11042[1], 11043[1], 11044[1], 11045[1], 11046[1], 11047[1], 12001[1], 12002[1], 12004[1], 12005[1], 12006[1], 12007[1], 12011[1], 12013[1], 12014[1], 12015[1], 12016[1], 12017[1], 12018[1], 12020[1], 12021[1], 12031[1], 12032[1], 12034[1], 12035[1], 12036[1], 12037[1], 12041[1], 12042[1], 12044[1], 12045[1], 12046[1], 12047[1], 12051[1], 12052[1], 12053[1], 12054[1], 12055[1], 12056[1], 12057[1], 13100[1], 13101[1], 13102[1], 13120[1], 13121[1], 13122[1], 13131[1], 13132[1], 13133[1], 13151[1], 13152[1], 13153[1], 36000[1], 36400[1], 36405[1], 36406[1], 36410[1], 36420[1], 36425[1], 36430[1], 36440[1], 36591[0], 36592[0], 36600[1], 36640[1], 43752[1], 50386[1], 50693[1], 50694[1], 50695[1], 52310[1], 52332[1], 52356[1], 62320[0], 62321[0], 62322[0], 62323[0], 62324[0], 62325[0], 62326[0], 62327[0], 64400[0], 64405[0], 64408[0], 64415[0], 64416[0], 64417[0], 64418[0], 64420[0], 64421[0], 64425[0], 64430[0], 64435[0], 64445[0], 64446[0], 64447[0], 64448[0], 64449[0], 64450[0], 64451[0], 64454[0], 64461[0], 64462[0], 64463[0], 64479[0], 64480[0], 64483[0], 64484[0], 64486[0], 64487[0], 64488[0], 64489[0], 64490[0], 64491[0], 64492[0], 64493[0], 64494[0], 64495[0], 64505[0], 64510[0], 64517[0], 64520[0], 64530[0], 69990[0], 75984[1], 76000[1], 76942[1], 76998[1], 77001[1], 77002[1], 92012[1], 92014[1], 93000[1], 93005[1], 93010[1], 93040[1], 93041[1], 93042[1], 93318[1], 93355[1], 94002[1], 94200[1], 94680[1], 94681[1], 94690[1], 95812[1], 95813[1], 95816[1], 95819[1], 95822[1], 95829[1], 95955[1], 96360[1], 96361[1], 96365[1], 96366[1], 96367[1], 96368[1], 96372[1], 96374[1], 96375[1], 96376[1], 96377[1], 96523[0], 97597[1], 97598[1], 97602[1], 99155[0], 99156[0], 99157[0], 99211[1], 99212[1], 99213[1], 99214[1], 99215[1], 99217[1], 99218[1], 99219[1], 99220[1], 99221[1], 99222[1], 99223[1], 99231[1], 99232[1], 99233[1], 99234[1], 99235[1], 99236[1], 99238[1], 99239[1], 99241[1], 99242[1], 99243[1], 99244[1], 99245[1], 99251[1], 99252[1], 99253[1], 99254[1], 99255[1], 99291[1], 99292[1], 99304[1], 99305[1], 99306[1], 99307[1], 99308[1], 99309[1], 99310[1], 99315[1], 99316[1], 99334[1], 99335[1], 99336[1], 99337[1], 99347[1], 99348[1], 99349[1], 99350[1], 99374[1], 99375[1], 99377[1], 99378[1], 99446[0], 99447[0], 99448[0], 99449[0], 99451[0], 99452[0], 99495[1], 99496[1], G0463[1]
50386	0213T[0], 0216T[0], 0708T[1], 0709T[1], 11000[1], 11001[1], 11004[1], 11005[1], 11006[1], 11042[1], 11043[1], 11044[1], 11045[1], 11046[1], 11047[1], 12001[1], 12002[1], 12004[1], 12005[1], 12006[1], 12007[1], 12011[1], 12013[1], 12014[1], 12015[1], 12016[1], 12017[1], 12018[1], 12020[1], 12021[1], 12031[1], 12032[1], 12034[1], 12035[1], 12036[1], 12037[1], 12041[1], 12042[1], 12044[1], 12045[1], 12046[1], 12047[1], 12051[1], 12052[1], 12053[1], 12054[1], 12055[1], 12056[1], 12057[1], 13100[1], 13101[1], 13102[1], 13120[1], 13121[1], 13122[1], 13131[1], 13132[1], 13133[1], 13151[1], 13152[1], 13153[1], 36000[1], 36400[1], 36405[1], 36406[1], 36410[1], 36420[1], 36425[1], 36430[1], 36440[1], 36591[0], 36592[0], 36600[1], 36640[1], 43752[1], 52310[1], 52332[1], 52356[1], 62320[0], 62321[0], 62322[0], 62323[0], 62324[0], 62325[0], 62326[0], 62327[0], 64400[0], 64405[0], 64408[0], 64415[0], 64416[0], 64417[0], 64418[0], 64420[0], 64421[0], 64425[0], 64430[0], 64435[0], 64445[0], 64446[0], 64447[0], 64448[0], 64449[0], 64450[0], 64451[0], 64454[0], 64461[0], 64462[0], 64463[0], 64479[0], 64480[0], 64483[0], 64484[0], 64486[0], 64487[0], 64488[0], 64489[0], 64490[0], 64491[0], 64492[0], 64493[0], 64494[0], 64495[0], 64505[0], 64510[0], 64517[0], 64520[0], 64530[0], 69990[0], 75984[1], 76000[1], 76942[1], 76998[1], 77001[1], 77002[1], 92012[1], 92014[1], 93000[1], 93005[1], 93010[1], 93040[1], 93041[1], 93042[1], 93318[1], 93355[1], 94002[1], 94200[1], 94680[1], 94681[1], 94690[1], 95812[1], 95813[1], 95816[1], 95819[1], 95822[1], 95829[1], 95955[1], 96360[1], 96361[1], 96365[1], 96366[1], 96367[1], 96368[1], 96372[1], 96374[1], 96375[1], 96376[1], 96377[1], 96523[0], 97597[1], 97598[1], 97602[1], 99155[0], 99156[0], 99157[0], 99211[1], 99212[1], 99213[1], 99214[1], 99215[1], 99217[1], 99218[1], 99219[1], 99220[1], 99221[1], 99222[1], 99223[1], 99231[1], 99232[1], 99233[1], 99234[1], 99235[1], 99236[1], 99238[1], 99239[1], 99241[1], 99242[1], 99243[1], 99244[1], 99245[1], 99251[1], 99252[1], 99253[1], 99254[1], 99255[1], 99291[1], 99292[1], 99304[1], 99305[1], 99306[1], 99307[1], 99308[1], 99309[1], 99310[1], 99315[1], 99316[1], 99334[1], 99335[1], 99336[1], 99337[1], 99347[1], 99348[1], 99349[1], 99350[1], 99374[1], 99375[1], 99377[1], 99378[1], 99446[0], 99447[0], 99448[0], 99449[0], 99451[0], 99452[0], 99495[1], 99496[1], G0463[1]
50387	0213T[0], 0216T[0], 0596T[1], 0597T[1], 0708T[1], 0709T[1], 11000[1], 11001[1], 11004[1], 11005[1], 11006[1], 11042[1], 11043[1], 11044[1], 11045[1], 11046[1], 11047[1], 12001[1], 12002[1], 12004[1], 12005[1], 12006[1], 12007[1], 12011[1], 12013[1], 12014[1], 12015[1], 12016[1], 12017[1], 12018[1], 12020[1], 12021[1], 12031[1], 12032[1], 12034[1], 12035[1], 12036[1], 12037[1], 12041[1], 12042[1], 12044[1], 12045[1], 12046[1], 12047[1], 12051[1], 12052[1], 12053[1], 12054[1], 12055[1], 12056[1], 12057[1], 13100[1], 13101[1], 13102[1], 13120[1], 13121[1], 13122[1], 13131[1], 13132[1], 13133[1], 13151[1], 13152[1], 13153[1], 36000[1], 36400[1], 36405[1], 36406[1], 36410[1], 36420[1], 36425[1], 36430[1], 36440[1], 36591[0], 36592[0], 36600[1], 36640[1], 43752[1], 50430[1], 50431[1], 50432[1], 50433[1], 50435[1], 50436[1], 50437[1], 50688[1], 50693[1], 50694[1], 50695[1], 51701[1], 51702[1], 51703[1], 62320[0], 62321[0], 62322[0], 62323[0], 62324[0], 62325[0], 62326[0], 62327[0], 64400[0], 64405[0], 64408[0], 64415[0], 64416[0], 64417[0], 64418[0], 64420[0], 64421[0], 64425[0], 64430[0], 64435[0], 64445[0], 64446[0], 64447[0], 64448[0], 64449[0], 64450[0], 64451[0], 64454[0], 64461[0], 64462[0], 64463[0], 64479[0], 64480[0], 64483[0], 64484[0], 64486[0], 64487[0], 64488[0], 64489[0], 64490[0], 64491[0], 64492[0], 64493[0], 64494[0], 64495[0], 64505[0], 64510[0], 64517[0], 64520[0], 64530[0], 69990[0], 74485[1], 76000[1], 77001[1], 77002[1], 92012[1], 92014[1], 93000[1], 93005[1], 93010[1], 93040[1], 93041[1], 93042[1], 93318[1], 93355[1], 94002[1], 94200[1], 94680[1], 94681[1], 94690[1], 95812[1], 95813[1], 95816[1], 95819[1], 95822[1], 95829[1], 95955[1], 96360[1], 96361[1], 96365[1], 96366[1], 96367[1], 96368[1], 96372[1], 96374[1], 96375[1], 96376[1], 96377[1], 96523[0], 97597[1], 97598[1], 97602[1], 99155[0], 99156[0], 99157[0], 99211[1], 99212[1], 99213[1], 99214[1], 99215[1], 99217[1], 99218[1], 99219[1], 99220[1], 99221[1], 99222[1], 99223[1], 99231[1], 99232[1], 99233[1], 99234[1], 99235[1], 99236[1], 99238[1], 99239[1], 99241[1], 99242[1], 99243[1], 99244[1], 99245[1], 99251[1], 99252[1], 99253[1], 99254[1], 99255[1], 99291[1], 99292[1], 99304[1], 99305[1], 99306[1], 99307[1], 99308[1], 99309[1], 99310[1], 99315[1], 99316[1], 99334[1], 99335[1], 99336[1], 99337[1], 99347[1], 99348[1], 99349[1], 99350[1], 99374[1], 99375[1], 99377[1], 99378[1], 99446[0], 99447[0], 99448[0], 99449[0], 99451[0], 99452[0], 99495[1], 99496[1], G0463[1], G0471[1], J0670[1], J2001[1]
50389	0213T[0], 0216T[0], 0596T[1], 0597T[1], 0708T[1], 0709T[1], 11000[1], 11001[1], 11004[1], 11005[1], 11006[1], 11042[1], 11043[1], 11044[1], 11045[1], 11046[1], 11047[1], 12001[1], 12002[1], 12004[1], 12005[1], 12006[1], 12007[1], 12011[1], 12013[1], 12014[1], 12015[1], 12016[1], 12017[1], 12018[1], 12020[1], 12021[1], 12031[1], 12032[1], 12034[1], 12035[1], 12036[1], 12037[1], 12041[1], 12042[1], 12044[1], 12045[1], 12046[1], 12047[1], 12051[1], 12052[1], 12053[1], 12054[1], 12055[1], 12056[1], 12057[1], 13100[1], 13101[1], 13102[1], 13120[1], 13121[1], 13122[1], 13131[1], 13132[1], 13133[1], 13151[1], 13152[1], 13153[1], 36000[1], 36400[1], 36405[1], 36406[1], 36410[1], 36420[1], 36425[1], 36430[1], 36440[1], 36591[0], 36592[0], 36600[1], 36640[1], 43752[1], 50430[1], 50431[1], 50436[1], 50437[1], 50693[1], 50694[1], 50695[1], 51701[1], 51702[1], 51703[1], 62320[0], 62321[0], 62322[0], 62323[0], 62324[0], 62325[0], 62326[0], 62327[0], 64400[0], 64405[0], 64408[0], 64415[0], 64416[0], 64417[0], 64418[0], 64420[0], 64421[0], 64425[0], 64430[0], 64435[0], 64445[0], 64446[0], 64447[0], 64448[0], 64449[0], 64450[0], 64451[0], 64454[0], 64461[0], 64462[0], 64463[0], 64479[0], 64480[0], 64483[0], 64484[0], 64486[0], 64487[0], 64488[0], 64489[0], 64490[0], 64491[0], 64492[0], 64493[0], 64494[0], 64495[0], 64505[0], 64510[0], 64517[0], 64520[0], 64530[0], 69990[0], 76000[1], 77001[1], 77002[1], 92012[1], 92014[1], 93000[1], 93005[1], 93010[1], 93040[1], 93041[1], 93042[1], 93318[1], 93355[1], 94002[1], 94200[1], 94680[1], 94681[1], 94690[1], 95812[1], 95813[1], 95816[1], 95819[1], 95822[1], 95829[1], 95955[1], 96360[1], 96361[1], 96365[1], 96366[1], 96367[1], 96368[1], 96372[1], 96374[1], 96375[1], 96376[1], 96377[1], 96523[0], 97597[1], 97598[1], 97602[1], 99155[0], 99156[0], 99157[0], 99211[1], 99212[1], 99213[1], 99214[1], 99215[1], 99217[1], 99218[1], 99219[1], 99220[1], 99221[1], 99222[1], 99223[1], 99231[1], 99232[1], 99233[1], 99234[1], 99235[1], 99236[1], 99238[1], 99239[1], 99241[1], 99242[1], 99243[1], 99244[1], 99245[1], 99251[1], 99252[1], 99253[1], 99254[1], 99255[1], 99291[1], 99292[1], 99304[1], 99305[1], 99306[1], 99307[1], 99308[1], 99309[1], 99310[1], 99315[1], 99316[1], 99334[1], 99335[1], 99336[1], 99337[1], 99347[1], 99348[1], 99349[1], 99350[1], 99374[1], 99375[1], 99377[1], 99378[1], 99446[0], 99447[0], 99448[0], 99449[0], 99451[0], 99452[0], 99495[1], 99496[1], G0463[1], G0471[1], J0670[1], J2001[1]
50390	0213T[0], 0216T[0], 0596T[1], 0597T[1], 0708T[1], 0709T[1], 12001[1], 12002[1], 12004[1], 12005[1], 12006[1], 12007[1], 12011[1], 12013[1], 12014[1], 12015[1], 12016[1], 12017[1], 12018[1], 12020[1], 12021[1], 12031[1], 12032[1], 12034[1], 12035[1], 12036[1], 12037[1], 12041[1], 12042[1], 12044[1], 12045[1], 12046[1], 12047[1], 12051[1], 12052[1], 12053[1], 12054[1], 12055[1], 12056[1], 12057[1], 13100[1], 13101[1], 13102[1], 13120[1], 13121[1], 13122[1], 13131[1], 13132[1], 13133[1], 13151[1], 13152[1], 13153[1], 36000[1], 36400[1], 36405[1], 36406[1], 36410[1], 36420[1], 36425[1], 36430[1], 36440[1], 36591[0], 36592[0], 36600[1], 36640[1], 43752[1], 51701[1], 51702[1], 51703[1], 62320[0], 62321[0], 62322[0], 62323[0], 62324[0], 62325[0], 62326[0], 62327[0], 64400[0], 64405[0], 64408[0], 64415[0], 64416[0], 64417[0], 64418[0], 64420[0], 64421[0], 64425[0], 64430[0], 64435[0], 64445[0], 64446[0], 64447[0], 64448[0], 64449[0], 64450[0], 64451[0], 64454[0], 64461[0], 64462[0], 64463[0], 64479[0], 64480[0], 64483[0], 64484[0], 64486[0], 64487[0], 64488[0], 64489[0], 64490[0], 64491[0], 64492[0], 64493[0], 64494[0], 64495[0], 64505[0], 64510[0], 64517[0], 64520[0], 64530[0], 69990[0], 76000[1], 76998[1], 77001[1], 92012[1], 92014[1], 93000[1], 93005[1], 93010[1], 93040[1], 93041[1], 93042[1], 93318[1], 93355[1], 94002[1], 94200[1], 94680[1], 94681[1], 94690[1], 95812[1], 95813[1], 95816[1], 95819[1], 95822[1], 95829[1], 95955[1], 96360[1], 96361[1], 96365[1], 96366[1], 96367[1], 96368[1], 96372[1], 96374[1], 96375[1], 96376[1], 96377[1], 96523[0], 99155[0], 99156[0], 99157[0], 99211[1], 99212[1], 99213[1], 99214[1], 99215[1], 99217[1], 99218[1], 99219[1], 99220[1], 99221[1], 99222[1], 99223[1], 99231[1], 99232[1], 99233[1], 99234[1], 99235[1], 99236[1], 99238[1], 99239[1], 99241[1], 99242[1], 99243[1], 99244[1], 99245[1], 99251[1], 99252[1], 99253[1], 99254[1], 99255[1], 99291[1], 99292[1], 99304[1], 99305[1], 99306[1], 99307[1], 99308[1], 99309[1], 99310[1], 99315[1], 99316[1], 99334[1], 99335[1], 99336[1], 99337[1], 99347[1], 99348[1], 99349[1], 99350[1], 99374[1], 99375[1], 99377[1], 99378[1], 99446[0], 99447[0], 99448[0], 99449[0], 99451[0], 99452[0], 99495[1], 99496[1], G0463[1], G0471[1]
50391	00860[0], 00862[0], 0213T[0], 0216T[0], 0596T[1], 0597T[1], 0708T[1], 0709T[1], 12001[1], 12002[1], 12004[1], 12005[1], 12006[1], 12007[1], 12011[1], 12013[1], 12014[1], 12015[1], 12016[1], 12017[1], 12018[1], 12020[1], 12021[1], 12031[1], 12032[1], 12034[1], 12035[1], 12036[1], 12037[1], 12041[1], 12042[1], 12044[1], 12045[1], 12046[1], 12047[1], 12051[1], 12052[1], 12053[1], 12054[1], 12055[1], 12056[1], 12057[1], 13100[1], 13101[1], 13102[1], 13120[1], 13121[1], 13122[1], 13131[1], 13132[1],

Appendix A: NCCI - CPT Codes

0 = Modifier usage not allowed or inappropriate 1 = Modifier usage allowed

Code 1	Code 2
	13133[1], 13151[1], 13152[1], 13153[1], 36000[1], 36400[1], 36405[1], 36406[1], 36410[1], 36420[1], 36425[1], 36430[1], 36440[1], 36591[0], 36592[0], 36600[1], 36640[1], 43752[1], 50390[1], 50432[1], 50436[1], 50437[1], 50693[1], 50694[1], 50695[1], 51701[0], 51702[0], 51703[1], 62320[0], 62321[0], 62322[0], 62323[0], 62324[0], 62325[0], 62326[0], 62327[0], 64400[0], 64405[0], 64408[0], 64415[0], 64416[0], 64417[0], 64418[0], 64420[0], 64421[0], 64425[0], 64430[0], 64435[0], 64445[0], 64446[0], 64447[0], 64448[0], 64449[0], 64450[0], 64451[0], 64454[0], 64461[0], 64462[0], 64463[0], 64479[0], 64480[0], 64483[0], 64484[0], 64486[0], 64487[0], 64488[0], 64489[0], 64490[0], 64491[0], 64492[0], 64493[0], 64494[0], 64495[0], 64505[0], 64510[0], 64517[0], 64520[0], 64530[0], 69990[0], 76000[1], 92012[1], 92014[1], 93000[1], 93005[1], 93010[1], 93040[1], 93041[1], 93042[1], 93318[1], 93355[1], 94002[1], 94200[1], 94680[1], 94681[1], 94690[1], 95812[1], 95813[1], 95816[1], 95819[1], 95822[1], 95829[1], 95955[1], 96360[1], 96361[1], 96365[1], 96366[1], 96367[1], 96368[1], 96372[1], 96374[1], 96375[1], 96376[1], 96377[1], 96523[0], 99155[0], 99156[0], 99157[0], 99211[1], 99212[1], 99213[1], 99214[1], 99215[1], 99217[1], 99218[1], 99219[1], 99220[1], 99221[1], 99222[1], 99223[1], 99231[1], 99232[1], 99233[1], 99234[1], 99235[1], 99236[1], 99238[1], 99239[1], 99241[1], 99242[1], 99243[1], 99244[1], 99245[1], 99251[1], 99252[1], 99253[1], 99254[1], 99255[1], 99291[1], 99292[1], 99304[1], 99305[1], 99306[1], 99307[1], 99308[1], 99309[1], 99310[1], 99315[1], 99316[1], 99334[1], 99335[1], 99336[1], 99337[1], 99347[1], 99348[1], 99349[1], 99350[1], 99374[1], 99375[1], 99377[1], 99378[1], 99446[0], 99447[0], 99448[0], 99449[0], 99451[0], 99452[0], 99495[1], 99496[1], G0463[1], G0471[0]
50396	0213T[0], 0216T[0], 0596T[1], 0597T[1], 0708T[1], 0709T[1], 12001[1], 12002[1], 12004[1], 12005[1], 12006[1], 12007[1], 12011[1], 12013[1], 12014[1], 12015[1], 12016[1], 12017[1], 12018[1], 12020[1], 12021[1], 12031[1], 12032[1], 12034[1], 12035[1], 12036[1], 12037[1], 12041[1], 12042[1], 12044[1], 12045[1], 12046[1], 12047[1], 12051[1], 12052[1], 12053[1], 12054[1], 12055[1], 12056[1], 12057[1], 13100[1], 13101[1], 13102[1], 13120[1], 13121[1], 13122[1], 13131[1], 13132[1], 13133[1], 13151[1], 13152[1], 13153[1], 36000[1], 36400[1], 36405[1], 36406[1], 36410[1], 36420[1], 36425[1], 36430[1], 36440[1], 36591[0], 36592[0], 36600[1], 36640[1], 43752[1], 50436[1], 50437[1], 51701[1], 51702[1], 51703[1], 62320[0], 62321[0], 62322[0], 62323[0], 62324[0], 62325[0], 62326[0], 62327[0], 64400[0], 64405[0], 64408[0], 64415[0], 64416[0], 64417[0], 64418[0], 64420[0], 64421[0], 64425[0], 64430[0], 64435[0], 64445[0], 64446[0], 64447[0], 64448[0], 64449[0], 64450[0], 64451[0], 64454[0], 64461[0], 64462[0], 64463[0], 64479[0], 64480[0], 64483[0], 64484[0], 64486[0], 64487[0], 64488[0], 64489[0], 64490[0], 64491[0], 64492[0], 64493[0], 64494[0], 64495[0], 64505[0], 64510[0], 64517[0], 64520[0], 64530[0], 69990[0], 76000[1], 76942[1], 76998[1], 77001[1], 77002[1], 92012[1], 92014[1], 93000[1], 93005[1], 93010[1], 93040[1], 93041[1], 93042[1], 93318[1], 93355[1], 94002[1], 94200[1], 94680[1], 94681[1], 94690[1], 95812[1], 95813[1], 95816[1], 95819[1], 95822[1], 95829[1], 95955[1], 96360[1], 96361[1], 96365[1], 96366[1], 96367[1], 96368[1], 96372[1], 96374[1], 96375[1], 96376[1], 96377[1], 96523[0], 99155[0], 99156[0], 99157[0], 99211[1], 99212[1], 99213[1], 99214[1], 99215[1], 99217[1], 99218[1], 99219[1], 99220[1], 99221[1], 99222[1], 99223[1], 99231[1], 99232[1], 99233[1], 99234[1], 99235[1], 99236[1], 99238[1], 99239[1], 99241[1], 99242[1], 99243[1], 99244[1], 99245[1], 99251[1], 99252[1], 99253[1], 99254[1], 99255[1], 99291[1], 99292[1], 99304[1], 99305[1], 99306[1], 99307[1], 99308[1], 99309[1], 99310[1], 99315[1], 99316[1], 99334[1], 99335[1], 99336[1], 99337[1], 99347[1], 99348[1], 99349[1], 99350[1], 99374[1], 99375[1], 99377[1], 99378[1], 99446[0], 99447[0], 99448[0], 99449[0], 99451[0], 99452[0], 99495[1], 99496[1], G0463[1], G0471[1]
50400	0213T[0], 0216T[0], 0596T[1], 0597T[1], 0708T[1], 0709T[1], 11000[1], 11001[1], 11004[1], 11005[1], 11006[1], 11042[1], 11043[1], 11044[1], 11045[1], 11046[1], 11047[1], 12001[1], 12002[1], 12004[1], 12005[1], 12006[1], 12007[1], 12011[1], 12013[1], 12014[1], 12015[1], 12016[1], 12017[1], 12018[1], 12020[1], 12021[1], 12031[1], 12032[1], 12034[1], 12035[1], 12036[1], 12037[1], 12041[1], 12042[1], 12044[1], 12045[1], 12046[1], 12047[1], 12051[1], 12052[1], 12053[1], 12054[1], 12055[1], 12056[1], 12057[1], 13100[1], 13101[1], 13102[1], 13120[1], 13121[1], 13122[1], 13131[1], 13132[1], 13133[1], 13151[1], 13152[1], 13153[1], 36000[1], 36400[1], 36405[1], 36406[1], 36410[1], 36420[1], 36425[1], 36430[1], 36440[1], 36591[0], 36592[0], 36600[1], 36640[1], 43752[1], 44602[1], 44603[1], 44604[1], 44605[1], 44950[0], 44970[0], 49000[0], 49002[1], 49010[0], 50544[1], 50605[1], 50715[1], 51701[1], 51702[1], 51703[1], 52005[1], 62320[0], 62321[0], 62322[0], 62323[0], 62324[0], 62325[0], 62326[0], 62327[0], 64400[0], 64405[0], 64408[0], 64415[0], 64416[0], 64417[0], 64418[0], 64420[0], 64421[0], 64425[0], 64430[0], 64435[0], 64445[0], 64446[0], 64447[0], 64448[0], 64449[0], 64450[0], 64451[0], 64454[0], 64461[0], 64462[0], 64463[0], 64479[0], 64480[0], 64483[0], 64484[0], 64486[0], 64487[0], 64488[0], 64489[0], 64490[0], 64491[0], 64492[0], 64493[0], 64494[0], 64495[0], 64505[0], 64510[0], 64517[0], 64520[0], 64530[0], 69990[0], 92012[1], 92014[1], 93000[1], 93005[1], 93010[1], 93040[1], 93041[1], 93042[1], 93318[1], 93355[1], 94002[1], 94200[1], 94680[1], 94681[1], 94690[1], 95812[1], 95813[1], 95816[1], 95819[1], 95822[1], 95829[1], 95955[1], 96360[1], 96361[1], 96365[1], 96366[1], 96367[1], 96368[1], 96372[1], 96374[1], 96375[1], 96376[1], 96377[1], 96523[0], 97597[1], 97598[1], 97602[1], 99155[0], 99156[0], 99157[0], 99211[1], 99212[1], 99213[1], 99214[1], 99215[1], 99217[1], 99218[1], 99219[1], 99220[1], 99221[1], 99222[1], 99223[1], 99231[1], 99232[1], 99233[1], 99234[1], 99235[1], 99236[1], 99238[1], 99239[1], 99241[1], 99242[1], 99243[1], 99244[1], 99245[1], 99251[1], 99252[1], 99253[1], 99254[1], 99255[1], 99291[1], 99292[1], 99304[1], 99305[1], 99306[1], 99307[1], 99308[1], 99309[1], 99310[1], 99315[1], 99316[1], 99334[1], 99335[1], 99336[1], 99337[1], 99347[1], 99348[1], 99349[1], 99350[1], 99374[1], 99375[1], 99377[1], 99378[1], 99446[0], 99447[0], 99448[0], 99449[0], 99451[0], 99452[0], 99495[0], 99496[0], G0463[1], G0471[1]
50405	0213T[0], 0216T[0], 0596T[1], 0597T[1], 0708T[1], 0709T[1], 11000[1], 11001[1], 11004[1], 11005[1], 11006[1], 11042[1], 11043[1], 11044[1], 11045[1], 11046[1], 11047[1], 12001[1], 12002[1], 12004[1], 12005[1], 12006[1], 12007[1], 12011[1], 12013[1], 12014[1], 12015[1], 12016[1], 12017[1], 12018[1], 12020[1], 12021[1], 12031[1], 12032[1], 12034[1], 12035[1], 12036[1], 12037[1], 12041[1], 12042[1], 12044[1], 12045[1], 12046[1], 12047[1], 12051[1], 12052[1], 12053[1], 12054[1], 12055[1], 12056[1], 12057[1], 13100[1], 13101[1], 13102[1], 13120[1], 13121[1], 13122[1], 13131[1], 13132[1], 13133[1], 13151[1], 13152[1], 13153[1], 36000[1], 36400[1], 36405[1], 36406[1], 36410[1], 36420[1], 36425[1], 36430[1], 36440[1], 36591[0], 36592[0], 36600[1], 36640[1], 43752[1], 44602[1], 44603[1], 44604[1], 44605[1], 44950[0], 44970[0], 49000[0], 49002[1], 49010[0], 50100[1], 50400[1], 50544[1], 50605[1], 50715[1], 51701[1], 51702[1], 51703[1], 52005[1], 62320[0], 62321[0], 62322[0], 62323[0], 62324[0], 62325[0], 62326[0], 62327[0], 64400[0], 64405[0], 64408[0], 64415[0], 64416[0], 64417[0], 64418[0], 64420[0], 64421[0], 64425[0], 64430[0], 64435[0], 64445[0], 64446[0], 64447[0], 64448[0], 64449[0], 64450[0], 64451[0], 64454[0], 64461[0], 64462[0], 64463[0], 64479[0], 64480[0], 64483[0], 64484[0], 64486[0], 64487[0], 64488[0], 64489[0], 64490[0], 64491[0], 64492[0], 64493[0], 64494[0], 64495[0], 64505[0], 64510[0], 64517[0], 64520[0], 64530[0], 69990[0], 92012[1], 92014[1], 93000[1], 93005[1], 93010[1], 93040[1], 93041[1], 93042[1], 93318[1], 93355[1], 94002[1], 94200[1], 94680[1], 94681[1], 94690[1], 95812[1], 95813[1], 95816[1], 95819[1], 95822[1], 95829[1], 95955[1], 96360[1], 96361[1], 96365[1], 96366[1], 96367[1], 96368[1], 96372[1], 96374[1], 96375[1], 96376[1], 96377[1], 96523[0], 97597[1], 97598[1], 97602[1], 99155[0], 99156[0], 99157[0], 99211[1], 99212[1], 99213[1], 99214[1], 99215[1], 99217[1], 99218[1], 99219[1], 99220[1], 99221[1], 99222[1], 99223[1], 99231[1], 99232[1], 99233[1], 99234[1], 99235[1], 99236[1], 99238[1], 99239[1], 99241[1], 99242[1], 99243[1], 99244[1], 99245[1], 99251[1], 99252[1], 99253[1], 99254[1], 99255[1], 99291[1], 99292[1], 99304[1], 99305[1], 99306[1], 99307[1], 99308[1], 99309[1], 99310[1], 99315[1], 99316[1], 99334[1], 99335[1], 99336[1], 99337[1], 99347[1], 99348[1], 99349[1], 99350[1], 99374[1], 99375[1], 99377[1], 99378[1], 99446[0], 99447[0], 99448[0], 99449[0], 99451[0], 99452[0], 99495[0], 99496[0], G0463[1], G0471[1]
50430	0213T[0], 0216T[0], 0596T[1], 0597T[1], 0708T[1], 0709T[1], 12001[1], 12002[1], 12004[1], 12005[1], 12006[1], 12007[1], 12011[1], 12013[1], 12014[1], 12015[1], 12016[1], 12017[1], 12018[1], 12020[1], 12021[1], 12031[1], 12032[1], 12034[1], 12035[1], 12036[1], 12037[1], 12041[1], 12042[1], 12044[1], 12045[1], 12046[1], 12047[1], 12051[1], 12052[1], 12053[1], 12054[1], 12055[1], 12056[1], 12057[1], 13100[1], 13101[1], 13102[1], 13120[1], 13121[1], 13122[1], 13131[1], 13132[1], 13133[1], 13151[1], 13152[1], 13153[1], 36000[1], 36011[1], 36400[1], 36405[1], 36406[1], 36410[1], 36420[1], 36425[1], 36430[1], 36440[1], 36591[0], 36592[0], 36600[1], 36640[1], 43752[1], 50431[1], 50436[1], 51701[1], 51702[1], 51703[1], 62320[0], 62321[0], 62322[0], 62323[0], 62324[0], 62325[0], 62326[0], 62327[0], 64400[0], 64405[0], 64408[0], 64415[0], 64416[0], 64417[0], 64418[0], 64420[0], 64421[0], 64425[0], 64430[0], 64435[0], 64445[0], 64446[0], 64447[0], 64448[0], 64449[0], 64450[0], 64451[0], 64454[0], 64461[0], 64462[0], 64463[0], 64479[0], 64480[0], 64483[0], 64484[0], 64486[0], 64487[0], 64488[0], 64489[0], 64490[0], 64491[0], 64492[0], 64493[0], 64494[0], 64495[0], 64505[0], 64510[0], 64517[0], 64520[0], 64530[0], 69990[0], 74425[1], 76000[1], 76942[1], 76998[1], 77001[1], 77002[1], 92012[1], 92014[1], 93000[1], 93005[1], 93010[1], 93040[1], 93041[1], 93042[1], 93318[1], 93355[1], 94002[1], 94200[1], 94680[1], 94681[1], 94690[1], 95812[1], 95813[1], 95816[1], 95819[1], 95822[1], 95829[1], 95955[1], 96360[1], 96361[1], 96365[1], 96366[1], 96367[1], 96368[1], 96372[1], 96374[1], 96375[1], 96376[1], 96377[1], 96523[0], 99155[0], 99156[0], 99157[0], 99211[1], 99212[1], 99213[1], 99214[1], 99215[1], 99217[1], 99218[1], 99219[1], 99220[1], 99221[1], 99222[1], 99223[1], 99231[1], 99232[1], 99233[1], 99234[1], 99235[1], 99236[1], 99238[1], 99239[1], 99241[1], 99242[1], 99243[1], 99244[1], 99245[1], 99251[1], 99252[1], 99253[1], 99254[1], 99255[1], 99291[1], 99292[1], 99304[1], 99305[1], 99306[1], 99307[1], 99308[1], 99309[1], 99310[1], 99315[1], 99316[1], 99334[1], 99335[1], 99336[1], 99337[1], 99347[1], 99348[1], 99349[1], 99350[1], 99374[1], 99375[1], 99377[1], 99378[1], 99446[0], 99447[0], 99448[0], 99449[0], 99451[0], 99452[0], 99495[1], 99496[1], G0463[1], G0471[1], J0670[1], J2001[1]
50431	0213T[0], 0216T[0], 0596T[1], 0597T[1], 0708T[1], 0709T[1], 12001[1], 12002[1], 12004[1], 12005[1], 12006[1], 12007[1], 12011[1], 12013[1], 12014[1], 12015[1], 12016[1], 12017[1], 12018[1], 12020[1], 12021[1], 12031[1], 12032[1], 12034[1], 12035[1], 12036[1], 12037[1], 12041[1], 12042[1], 12044[1], 12045[1], 12046[1], 12047[1], 12051[1], 12052[1], 12053[1], 12054[1], 12055[1], 12056[1], 12057[1], 13100[1], 13101[1], 13102[1], 13120[1], 13121[1], 13122[1], 13131[1], 13132[1], 13133[1], 13151[1], 13152[1], 13153[1], 36000[1], 36011[1], 36400[1], 36405[1], 36406[1], 36410[1], 36420[1], 36425[1], 36430[1], 36440[1], 36591[0], 36592[0], 36600[1], 36640[1], 43752[1], 51701[1], 51702[1], 51703[1], 62320[0], 62321[0], 62322[0], 62323[0], 62324[0], 62325[0], 62326[0], 62327[0], 64400[0], 64405[0], 64408[0], 64415[0], 64416[0], 64417[0], 64418[0], 64420[0], 64421[0], 64425[0], 64430[0], 64435[0], 64445[0], 64446[0], 64447[0], 64448[0], 64449[0], 64450[0], 64451[0], 64454[0], 64461[0], 64462[0], 64463[0], 64479[0], 64480[0], 64483[0], 64484[0], 64486[0], 64487[0], 64488[0], 64489[0], 64490[0], 64491[0], 64492[0], 64493[0], 64494[0], 64495[0], 64505[0], 64510[0], 64517[0], 64520[0], 64530[0], 69990[0], 74425[1], 76000[1], 76942[1], 76998[1], 77001[1], 77002[1], 92012[1], 92014[1], 93000[1], 93005[1], 93010[1], 93040[1], 93041[1], 93042[1], 93318[1], 93355[1], 94002[1], 94200[1], 94680[1], 94681[1], 94690[1], 95812[1], 95813[1], 95816[1], 95819[1], 95822[1], 95829[1], 95955[1], 96360[1], 96361[1], 96365[1], 96366[1], 96367[1], 96368[1], 96372[1], 96374[1], 96375[1], 96376[1], 96377[1], 96523[0], 99155[0], 99156[0], 99157[0], 99211[1], 99212[1], 99213[1], 99214[1], 99215[1], 99217[1],

0 = Modifier usage not allowed or inappropriate   1 = Modifier usage allowed

Code 1	Code 2
	99218[1], 99219[1], 99220[1], 99221[1], 99222[1], 99223[1], 99231[1], 99232[1], 99233[1], 99234[1], 99235[1], 99236[1], 99238[1], 99239[1], 99241[1], 99242[1], 99243[1], 99244[1], 99245[1], 99251[1], 99252[1], 99253[1], 99254[1], 99255[1], 99291[1], 99292[1], 99304[1], 99305[1], 99306[1], 99307[1], 99308[1], 99309[1], 99310[1], 99315[1], 99316[1], 99334[1], 99335[1], 99336[1], 99337[1], 99347[1], 99348[1], 99349[1], 99350[1], 99374[1], 99375[1], 99377[1], 99378[1], 99446[0], 99447[0], 99448[0], 99449[0], 99451[0], 99452[0], 99495[1], 99496[1], G0463[1], G0471[1]
50432	0213T[0], 0216T[0], 0596T[1], 0597T[1], 0708T[1], 0709T[1], 12001[1], 12002[1], 12004[1], 12005[1], 12006[1], 12007[1], 12011[1], 12013[1], 12014[1], 12015[1], 12016[1], 12017[1], 12018[1], 12020[1], 12021[1], 12031[1], 12032[1], 12034[1], 12035[1], 12036[1], 12037[1], 12041[1], 12042[1], 12044[1], 12045[1], 12046[1], 12047[1], 12051[1], 12052[1], 12053[1], 12054[1], 12055[1], 12056[1], 12057[1], 13100[1], 13101[1], 13102[1], 13120[1], 13121[1], 13122[1], 13131[1], 13132[1], 13133[1], 13151[1], 13152[1], 13153[1], 36000[1], 36011[1], 36400[1], 36405[1], 36406[1], 36410[1], 36420[1], 36425[1], 36430[1], 36440[1], 36591[0], 36592[0], 36600[1], 36640[1], 43752[1], 50390[1], 50430[1], 50431[1], 50434[1], 50435[1], 50436[1], 50437[1], 51701[1], 51702[1], 51703[1], 62320[0], 62321[0], 62322[0], 62323[0], 62324[0], 62325[0], 62326[0], 62327[0], 64400[0], 64405[0], 64408[0], 64415[0], 64416[0], 64417[0], 64418[0], 64420[0], 64421[0], 64425[0], 64430[0], 64435[0], 64445[0], 64446[0], 64447[0], 64448[0], 64449[0], 64450[0], 64451[0], 64454[0], 64461[0], 64462[0], 64463[0], 64479[0], 64480[0], 64483[0], 64484[0], 64486[0], 64487[0], 64488[0], 64489[0], 64490[0], 64491[0], 64492[0], 64493[0], 64494[0], 64495[0], 64505[0], 64510[0], 64517[0], 64520[0], 64530[0], 69990[0], 74425[1], 76000[1], 76380[1], 76942[1], 76998[1], 77001[1], 77002[1], 77012[1], 77021[1], 92012[1], 92014[1], 93000[1], 93005[1], 93010[1], 93040[1], 93041[1], 93042[1], 93318[1], 93355[1], 94002[1], 94200[1], 94680[1], 94681[1], 94690[1], 95812[1], 95813[1], 95816[1], 95819[1], 95822[1], 95829[1], 95955[1], 96360[1], 96361[1], 96365[1], 96366[1], 96367[1], 96368[1], 96372[1], 96374[1], 96375[1], 96376[1], 96377[1], 96523[0], 99155[0], 99156[0], 99157[0], 99211[1], 99212[1], 99213[1], 99214[1], 99215[1], 99217[1], 99218[1], 99219[1], 99220[1], 99221[1], 99222[1], 99223[1], 99231[1], 99232[1], 99233[1], 99234[1], 99235[1], 99236[1], 99238[1], 99239[1], 99241[1], 99242[1], 99243[1], 99244[1], 99245[1], 99251[1], 99252[1], 99253[1], 99254[1], 99255[1], 99291[1], 99292[1], 99304[1], 99305[1], 99306[1], 99307[1], 99308[1], 99309[1], 99310[1], 99315[1], 99316[1], 99334[1], 99335[1], 99336[1], 99337[1], 99347[1], 99348[1], 99349[1], 99350[1], 99374[1], 99375[1], 99377[1], 99378[1], 99446[0], 99447[0], 99448[0], 99449[0], 99451[0], 99452[0], 99495[1], 99496[1], G0463[1], G0471[1], J0670[1], J2001[1]
50433	0213T[0], 0216T[0], 0596T[1], 0597T[1], 0708T[1], 0709T[1], 12001[0], 12002[1], 12004[1], 12005[1], 12006[1], 12007[1], 12011[1], 12013[1], 12014[1], 12015[1], 12016[1], 12017[1], 12018[1], 12020[1], 12021[1], 12031[1], 12032[1], 12034[1], 12035[1], 12036[1], 12037[1], 12041[1], 12042[1], 12044[1], 12045[1], 12046[1], 12047[1], 12051[1], 12052[1], 12053[1], 12054[1], 12055[1], 12056[1], 12057[1], 13100[1], 13101[1], 13102[1], 13120[1], 13121[1], 13122[1], 13131[1], 13132[1], 13133[1], 13151[1], 13152[1], 13153[1], 36000[1], 36011[1], 36400[1], 36405[1], 36406[1], 36410[1], 36420[1], 36425[1], 36430[1], 36440[1], 36591[0], 36592[0], 36600[1], 36640[1], 43752[1], 50430[1], 50431[1], 50432[1], 50436[1], 50437[1], 50684[1], 51701[1], 51702[1], 51703[1], 62320[0], 62321[0], 62322[0], 62323[0], 62324[0], 62325[0], 62326[0], 62327[0], 64400[0], 64405[0], 64408[0], 64415[0], 64416[0], 64417[0], 64418[0], 64420[0], 64421[0], 64425[0], 64430[0], 64435[0], 64445[0], 64446[0], 64447[0], 64448[0], 64449[0], 64450[0], 64451[0], 64454[0], 64461[0], 64462[0], 64463[0], 64479[0], 64480[0], 64483[0], 64484[0], 64486[0], 64487[0], 64488[0], 64489[0], 64490[0], 64491[0], 64492[0], 64493[0], 64494[0], 64495[0], 64505[0], 64510[0], 64517[0], 64520[0], 64530[0], 69990[0], 74425[1], 76000[1], 76380[1], 76942[1], 76998[1], 77001[1], 77002[1], 77012[1], 77021[1], 92012[1], 92014[1], 93000[1], 93005[1], 93010[1], 93040[1], 93041[1], 93042[1], 93318[1], 94002[1], 94200[1], 94680[1], 94681[1], 94690[1], 95812[1], 95813[1], 95816[1], 95819[1], 95822[1], 95829[1], 95955[1], 96360[1], 96361[1], 96365[1], 96366[1], 96367[1], 96368[1], 96372[1], 96374[1], 96375[1], 96376[1], 96377[1], 96523[0], 99155[0], 99156[0], 99157[0], 99211[1], 99212[1], 99213[1], 99214[1], 99215[1], 99217[1], 99218[1], 99219[1], 99220[1], 99221[1], 99222[1], 99223[1], 99231[1], 99232[1], 99233[1], 99234[1], 99235[1], 99236[1], 99238[1], 99239[1], 99241[1], 99242[1], 99243[1], 99244[1], 99245[1], 99251[1], 99252[1], 99253[1], 99254[1], 99255[1], 99291[1], 99292[1], 99304[1], 99305[1], 99306[1], 99307[1], 99308[1], 99309[1], 99310[1], 99315[1], 99316[1], 99334[1], 99335[1], 99336[1], 99337[1], 99347[1], 99348[1], 99349[1], 99350[1], 99374[1], 99375[1], 99377[1], 99378[1], 99446[1], 99447[1], 99448[1], 99449[1], 99451[1], 99452[1], J0670[1], J2001[1]
50434	0213T[0], 0216T[0], 0596T[1], 0597T[1], 0708T[1], 0709T[1], 12001[1], 12002[1], 12004[1], 12005[1], 12006[1], 12007[1], 12011[1], 12013[1], 12014[1], 12015[1], 12016[1], 12017[1], 12018[1], 12020[1], 12021[1], 12031[1], 12032[1], 12034[1], 12035[1], 12036[1], 12037[1], 12041[1], 12042[1], 12044[1], 12045[1], 12046[1], 12047[1], 12051[1], 12052[1], 12053[1], 12054[1], 12055[1], 12056[1], 12057[1], 13100[1], 13101[1], 13102[1], 13120[1], 13121[1], 13122[1], 13131[1], 13132[1], 13133[1], 13151[1], 13152[1], 13153[1], 36000[1], 36011[1], 36400[1], 36405[1], 36406[1], 36410[1], 36420[1], 36425[1], 36430[1], 36440[1], 36591[0], 36592[0], 36600[1], 36640[1], 43752[1], 49185[1], 49424[1], 50387[1], 50430[1], 50431[1], 50435[1], 50436[1], 50684[1], 51701[1], 51702[1], 51703[1], 62320[0], 62321[0], 62322[0], 62323[0], 62324[0], 62325[0], 62326[0], 62327[0], 64400[0], 64405[0], 64408[0], 64415[0], 64416[0], 64417[0], 64418[0], 64420[0], 64421[0], 64425[0], 64430[0], 64435[0], 64445[0], 64446[0], 64447[0], 64448[0], 64449[0], 64450[0], 64451[0], 64454[0], 64461[0], 64462[0], 64463[0], 64479[0], 64480[0], 64483[0], 64484[0], 64486[0], 64487[0], 64488[0], 64489[0], 64490[0], 64491[0], 64492[0], 64493[0], 64494[0], 64495[0], 64505[0], 64510[0], 64517[0], 64520[0], 64530[0], 69990[0], 74425[1], 76000[1], 76380[1], 76942[1], 76998[1], 77001[1], 77002[1], 77012[1], 77021[1], 92012[1], 92014[1], 93000[1], 93005[1], 93010[1], 93040[1], 93041[1], 93042[1], 93318[1], 93355[1], 94002[1], 94200[1], 94680[1], 94681[1], 94690[1], 95812[1], 95813[1], 95816[1], 95819[1], 95822[1], 95829[1], 95955[1], 96360[1], 96361[1], 96365[1], 96366[1], 96367[1], 96368[1], 96372[1], 96374[1], 96375[1], 96376[1], 96377[1], 96523[0], 99155[0], 99156[0], 99157[0], 99211[1], 99212[1], 99213[1], 99214[1], 99215[1], 99217[1], 99218[1], 99219[1], 99220[1], 99221[1], 99222[1], 99223[1], 99231[1], 99232[1], 99233[1], 99234[1], 99235[1], 99236[1], 99238[1], 99239[1], 99241[1], 99242[1], 99243[1], 99244[1], 99245[1], 99251[1], 99252[1], 99253[1], 99254[1], 99255[1], 99291[1], 99292[1], 99304[1], 99305[1], 99306[1], 99307[1], 99308[1], 99309[1], 99310[1], 99315[1], 99316[1], 99334[1], 99335[1], 99336[1], 99337[1], 99347[1], 99348[1], 99349[1], 99350[1], 99374[1], 99375[1], 99377[1], 99378[1], 99446[0], 99447[0], 99448[0], 99449[0], 99451[0], 99452[0], 99495[1], 99496[1], G0463[1], G0471[1], J0670[1], J2001[1]
50435	0213T[0], 0216T[0], 0596T[1], 0597T[1], 0708T[1], 0709T[1], 12001[1], 12002[1], 12004[1], 12005[1], 12006[1], 12007[1], 12011[1], 12013[1], 12014[1], 12015[1], 12016[1], 12017[1], 12018[1], 12020[1], 12021[1], 12031[1], 12032[1], 12034[1], 12035[1], 12036[1], 12037[1], 12041[1], 12042[1], 12044[1], 12045[1], 12046[1], 12047[1], 12051[1], 12052[1], 12053[1], 12054[1], 12055[1], 12056[1], 12057[1], 13100[1], 13101[1], 13102[1], 13120[1], 13121[1], 13122[1], 13131[1], 13132[1], 13133[1], 13151[1], 13152[1], 13153[1], 36000[1], 36011[1], 36400[1], 36405[1], 36406[1], 36410[1], 36420[1], 36425[1], 36430[1], 36440[1], 36591[0], 36592[0], 36600[1], 36640[1], 43752[1], 49185[1], 49424[1], 50389[1], 50430[1], 50431[1], 51701[1], 51702[1], 51703[1], 62320[0], 62321[0], 62322[0], 62323[0], 62324[0], 62325[0], 62326[0], 62327[0], 64400[0], 64405[0], 64408[0], 64415[0], 64416[0], 64417[0], 64418[0], 64420[0], 64421[0], 64425[0], 64430[0], 64435[0], 64445[0], 64446[0], 64447[0], 64448[0], 64449[0], 64450[0], 64451[0], 64454[0], 64461[0], 64462[0], 64463[0], 64479[0], 64480[0], 64483[0], 64484[0], 64486[0], 64487[0], 64488[0], 64489[0], 64490[0], 64491[0], 64492[0], 64493[0], 64494[0], 64495[0], 64505[0], 64510[0], 64517[0], 64520[0], 64530[0], 69990[0], 74425[1], 76000[1], 76380[1], 76942[1], 76998[1], 77001[1], 77002[1], 77012[1], 77021[1], 92012[1], 92014[1], 93000[1], 93005[1], 93010[1], 93040[1], 93041[1], 93042[1], 93318[1], 93355[1], 94002[1], 94200[1], 94680[1], 94681[1], 94690[1], 95812[1], 95813[1], 95816[1], 95819[1], 95822[1], 95829[1], 95955[1], 96360[1], 96361[1], 96365[1], 96366[1], 96367[1], 96368[1], 96372[1], 96374[1], 96375[1], 96376[1], 96377[1], 96523[0], 99155[0], 99156[0], 99157[0], 99211[1], 99212[1], 99213[1], 99214[1], 99215[1], 99217[1], 99218[1], 99219[1], 99220[1], 99221[1], 99222[1], 99223[1], 99231[1], 99232[1], 99233[1], 99234[1], 99235[1], 99236[1], 99238[1], 99239[1], 99241[1], 99242[1], 99243[1], 99244[1], 99245[1], 99251[1], 99252[1], 99253[1], 99254[1], 99255[1], 99291[1], 99292[1], 99304[1], 99305[1], 99306[1], 99307[1], 99308[1], 99309[1], 99310[1], 99315[1], 99316[1], 99334[1], 99335[1], 99336[1], 99337[1], 99347[1], 99348[1], 99349[1], 99350[1], 99374[1], 99375[1], 99377[1], 99378[1], 99446[0], 99447[0], 99448[0], 99449[0], 99451[0], 99452[0], 99495[1], 99496[1], G0463[1], G0471[1], J0670[1], J2001[1]
50436	0213T[0], 0216T[0], 0596T[1], 0597T[1], 0708T[1], 0709T[1], 12001[1], 12002[1], 12004[1], 12005[1], 12006[1], 12007[1], 12011[1], 12013[1], 12014[1], 12015[1], 12016[1], 12017[1], 12018[1], 12020[1], 12021[1], 12031[1], 12032[1], 12034[1], 12035[1], 12036[1], 12037[1], 12041[1], 12042[1], 12044[1], 12045[1], 12046[1], 12047[1], 12051[1], 12052[1], 12053[1], 12054[1], 12055[1], 12056[1], 12057[1], 13100[1], 13101[1], 13102[1], 13120[1], 13121[1], 13122[1], 13131[1], 13132[1], 13133[1], 13151[1], 13152[1], 13153[1], 36000[1], 36400[1], 36405[1], 36406[1], 36410[1], 36420[1], 36425[1], 36430[1], 36440[1], 36591[0], 36592[0], 36600[1], 36640[1], 43752[1], 50390[1], 50431[1], 50435[1], 51701[1], 51702[1], 51703[1], 62320[0], 62321[0], 62322[0], 62323[0], 62324[0], 62325[0], 62326[0], 62327[0], 64400[0], 64405[0], 64408[0], 64415[0], 64416[0], 64417[0], 64418[0], 64420[0], 64421[0], 64425[0], 64430[0], 64435[0], 64445[0], 64446[0], 64447[0], 64448[0], 64449[0], 64450[0], 64451[0], 64454[0], 64461[0], 64462[0], 64463[0], 64479[0], 64480[0], 64483[0], 64484[0], 64486[0], 64487[0], 64488[0], 64489[0], 64490[0], 64491[0], 64492[0], 64493[0], 64494[0], 64495[0], 64505[0], 64510[0], 64517[0], 64520[0], 64530[0], 69990[0], 74485[1], 76000[1], 76380[1], 76942[1], 76998[1], 77001[1], 77002[1], 77012[1], 77021[1], 92012[1], 92014[1], 93000[1], 93005[1], 93010[1], 93040[1], 93041[1], 93042[1], 93318[1], 93355[1], 94002[1], 94200[1], 94680[1], 94681[1], 94690[1], 95812[1], 95813[1], 95816[1], 95819[1], 95822[1], 95829[1], 95955[1], 96360[1], 96361[1], 96365[1], 96366[1], 96367[1], 96368[1], 96372[1], 96374[1], 96375[1], 96376[1], 96377[1], 96523[0], 99155[0], 99156[0], 99157[0], 99211[1], 99212[1], 99213[1], 99214[1], 99215[1], 99217[1], 99218[1], 99219[1], 99220[1], 99221[1], 99222[1], 99223[1], 99231[1], 99232[1], 99233[1], 99234[1], 99235[1], 99236[1], 99238[1], 99239[1], 99241[1], 99242[1], 99243[1], 99244[1], 99245[1], 99251[1], 99252[1], 99253[1], 99254[1], 99255[1], 99291[1], 99292[1], 99304[1], 99305[1], 99306[1], 99307[1], 99308[1], 99309[1], 99310[1], 99315[1], 99316[1], 99334[1], 99335[1], 99336[1], 99337[1], 99347[1], 99348[1], 99349[1], 99350[1], 99374[1], 99375[1], 99377[1], 99378[1], 99446[0], 99447[0], 99448[0], 99449[0], 99495[1], 99496[1], G0463[1], G0471[1]
50437	0213T[0], 0216T[0], 0596T[1], 0597T[1], 0708T[1], 0709T[1], 12001[1], 12002[1], 12004[1], 12005[1], 12006[1], 12007[1], 12011[1], 12013[1], 12014[1], 12015[1], 12016[1], 12017[1], 12018[1], 12020[1], 12021[1], 12031[1], 12032[1], 12034[1], 12035[1], 12036[1], 12037[1], 12041[1], 12042[1], 12044[1], 12045[1], 12046[1], 12047[1], 12051[1], 12052[1], 12053[1], 12054[1], 12055[1], 12056[1], 12057[1], 13100[1], 13101[1], 13102[1], 13120[1], 13121[1], 13122[1], 13131[1], 13132[1], 13133[1], 13151[1],

Appendix A: NCCI - CPT Codes

0 = Modifier usage not allowed or inappropriate 1 = Modifier usage allowed

Code 1	Code 2
	13152^1, 13153^1, 36000^1, 36400^1, 36405^1, 36406^1, 36410^1, 36420^1, 36425^1, 36430^1, 36440^1, 36591^0, 36592^0, 36600^1, 36640^1, 43752^1, 50384^1, 50390^1, 50430^1, 50431^1, 50434^1, 50435^1, 51701^1, 51702^1, 51703^1, 52334^1, 62320^0, 62321^0, 62322^0, 62323^0, 62324^0, 62325^0, 62326^0, 62327^0, 64400^0, 64405^0, 64408^0, 64415^0, 64416^0, 64417^0, 64418^0, 64420^0, 64421^0, 64425^0, 64430^0, 64435^0, 64445^0, 64446^0, 64447^0, 64448^0, 64449^0, 64450^0, 64451^0, 64454^0, 64461^0, 64462^0, 64463^0, 64479^0, 64480^0, 64483^0, 64484^0, 64486^0, 64487^0, 64488^0, 64489^0, 64490^0, 64491^0, 64492^0, 64493^0, 64494^0, 64495^0, 64505^0, 64510^0, 64517^0, 64520^0, 64530^0, 69990^0, 74485^1, 76000^1, 76380^1, 76942^1, 76998^1, 77001^1, 77002^1, 77012^1, 77021^1, 92012^1, 92014^1, 93000^1, 93005^1, 93010^1, 93040^1, 93041^1, 93042^1, 93318^1, 93355^1, 94002^1, 94200^1, 94680^1, 94681^1, 94690^1, 95812^1, 95813^1, 95816^1, 95819^1, 95822^1, 95829^1, 95955^1, 96360^1, 96361^1, 96365^1, 96366^1, 96367^1, 96368^1, 96372^1, 96374^1, 96375^1, 96376^1, 96377^1, 96523^0, 99155^0, 99156^0, 99157^0, 99211^1, 99212^1, 99213^1, 99214^1, 99215^1, 99217^1, 99218^1, 99219^1, 99220^1, 99221^1, 99222^1, 99223^1, 99231^1, 99232^1, 99233^1, 99234^1, 99235^1, 99236^1, 99238^1, 99239^1, 99241^1, 99242^1, 99243^1, 99244^1, 99245^1, 99251^1, 99252^1, 99253^1, 99254^1, 99255^1, 99291^1, 99292^1, 99304^1, 99305^1, 99306^1, 99307^1, 99308^1, 99309^1, 99310^1, 99315^1, 99316^1, 99334^1, 99335^1, 99336^1, 99337^1, 99347^1, 99348^1, 99349^1, 99350^1, 99374^1, 99375^1, 99377^1, 99378^1, 99446^0, 99447^0, 99448^0, 99449^0, 99495^1, 99496^1, G0463^1, G0471^1
50500	0213T^0, 0216T^0, 0596T^1, 0597T^1, 0708T^1, 0709T^1, 12001^1, 12002^1, 12004^1, 12005^1, 12006^1, 12007^1, 12011^1, 12013^1, 12014^1, 12015^1, 12016^1, 12017^1, 12018^1, 12020^1, 12021^1, 12031^1, 12032^1, 12034^1, 12035^1, 12036^1, 12037^1, 12041^1, 12042^1, 12044^1, 12045^1, 12046^1, 12047^1, 12051^1, 12052^1, 12053^1, 12054^1, 12055^1, 12056^1, 12057^1, 13100^1, 13101^1, 13102^1, 13120^1, 13121^1, 13122^1, 13131^1, 13132^1, 13133^1, 13151^1, 13152^1, 13153^1, 36000^1, 36400^1, 36405^1, 36406^1, 36410^1, 36420^1, 36425^1, 36430^1, 36440^1, 36591^0, 36592^0, 36600^1, 36640^1, 43752^1, 44602^1, 44603^1, 44604^1, 44605^1, 44950^0, 44970^0, 49000^0, 49002^1, 49010^0, 51701^1, 51702^1, 51703^1, 62320^0, 62321^0, 62322^0, 62323^0, 62324^0, 62325^0, 62326^0, 62327^0, 64400^0, 64405^0, 64408^0, 64415^0, 64416^0, 64417^0, 64418^0, 64420^0, 64421^0, 64425^0, 64430^0, 64435^0, 64445^0, 64446^0, 64447^0, 64448^0, 64449^0, 64450^0, 64451^0, 64454^0, 64461^0, 64462^0, 64463^0, 64479^0, 64480^0, 64483^0, 64484^0, 64486^0, 64487^0, 64488^0, 64489^0, 64490^0, 64491^0, 64492^0, 64493^0, 64494^0, 64495^0, 64505^0, 64510^0, 64517^0, 64520^0, 64530^0, 69990^0, 92012^1, 92014^1, 93000^1, 93005^1, 93010^1, 93040^1, 93041^1, 93042^1, 93318^1, 93355^1, 94002^1, 94200^1, 94680^1, 94681^1, 94690^1, 95812^1, 95813^1, 95816^1, 95819^1, 95822^1, 95829^1, 95955^1, 96360^1, 96361^1, 96365^1, 96366^1, 96367^1, 96368^1, 96372^1, 96374^1, 96375^1, 96376^1, 96377^1, 96523^0, 99155^0, 99156^0, 99157^0, 99211^1, 99212^1, 99213^1, 99214^1, 99215^1, 99217^1, 99218^1, 99219^1, 99220^1, 99221^1, 99222^1, 99223^1, 99231^1, 99232^1, 99233^1, 99234^1, 99235^1, 99236^1, 99238^1, 99239^1, 99241^1, 99242^1, 99243^1, 99244^1, 99245^1, 99251^1, 99252^1, 99253^1, 99254^1, 99255^1, 99291^1, 99292^1, 99304^1, 99305^1, 99306^1, 99307^1, 99308^1, 99309^1, 99310^1, 99315^1, 99316^1, 99334^1, 99335^1, 99336^1, 99337^1, 99347^1, 99348^1, 99349^1, 99350^1, 99374^1, 99375^1, 99377^1, 99378^1, 99446^0, 99447^0, 99448^0, 99449^0, 99451^0, 99452^0, 99495^0, 99496^0, G0463^1, G0471^1
50520	0213T^0, 0216T^0, 0596T^1, 0597T^1, 0708T^1, 0709T^1, 11000^1, 11001^1, 11004^1, 11005^1, 11006^1, 11042^1, 11043^1, 11044^1, 11045^1, 11046^1, 11047^1, 12001^1, 12002^1, 12004^1, 12005^1, 12006^1, 12007^1, 12011^1, 12013^1, 12014^1, 12015^1, 12016^1, 12017^1, 12018^1, 12020^1, 12021^1, 12031^1, 12032^1, 12034^1, 12035^1, 12036^1, 12037^1, 12041^1, 12042^1, 12044^1, 12045^1, 12046^1, 12047^1, 12051^1, 12052^1, 12053^1, 12054^1, 12055^1, 12056^1, 12057^1, 13100^1, 13101^1, 13102^1, 13120^1, 13121^1, 13122^1, 13131^1, 13132^1, 13133^1, 13151^1, 13152^1, 13153^1, 36000^1, 36400^1, 36405^1, 36406^1, 36410^1, 36420^1, 36425^1, 36430^1, 36440^1, 36591^0, 36592^0, 36600^1, 36640^1, 43752^1, 44602^1, 44603^1, 44604^1, 44605^1, 44950^0, 44970^0, 49000^0, 49002^1, 49010^0, 50544^1, 51701^1, 51702^1, 51703^1, 62320^0, 62321^0, 62322^0, 62323^0, 62324^0, 62325^0, 62326^0, 62327^0, 64400^0, 64405^0, 64408^0, 64415^0, 64416^0, 64417^0, 64418^0, 64420^0, 64421^0, 64425^0, 64430^0, 64435^0, 64445^0, 64446^0, 64447^0, 64448^0, 64449^0, 64450^0, 64451^0, 64454^0, 64461^0, 64462^0, 64463^0, 64479^0, 64480^0, 64483^0, 64484^0, 64486^0, 64487^0, 64488^0, 64489^0, 64490^0, 64491^0, 64492^0, 64493^0, 64494^0, 64495^0, 64505^0, 64510^0, 64517^0, 64520^0, 64530^0, 69990^0, 92012^1, 92014^1, 93000^1, 93005^1, 93010^1, 93040^1, 93041^1, 93042^1, 93318^1, 93355^1, 94002^1, 94200^1, 94680^1, 94681^1, 94690^1, 95812^1, 95813^1, 95816^1, 95819^1, 95822^1, 95829^1, 95955^1, 96360^1, 96361^1, 96365^1, 96366^1, 96367^1, 96368^1, 96372^1, 96374^1, 96375^1, 96376^1, 96377^1, 96523^0, 97597^1, 97598^1, 97602^1, 99155^0, 99156^0, 99157^0, 99211^1, 99212^1, 99213^1, 99214^1, 99215^1, 99217^1, 99218^1, 99219^1, 99220^1, 99221^1, 99222^1, 99223^1, 99231^1, 99232^1, 99233^1, 99234^1, 99235^1, 99236^1, 99238^1, 99239^1, 99241^1, 99242^1, 99243^1, 99244^1, 99245^1, 99251^1, 99252^1, 99253^1, 99254^1, 99255^1, 99291^1, 99292^1, 99304^1, 99305^1, 99306^1, 99307^1, 99308^1, 99309^1, 99310^1, 99315^1, 99316^1, 99334^1, 99335^1, 99336^1, 99337^1, 99347^1, 99348^1, 99349^1, 99350^1, 99374^1, 99375^1, 99377^1, 99378^1, 99446^0, 99447^0, 99448^0, 99449^0, 99451^0, 99452^0, 99495^0, 99496^0, G0463^1, G0471^1
50525	0213T^0, 0216T^0, 0596T^1, 0597T^1, 0708T^1, 0709T^1, 11000^1, 11001^1, 11004^1, 11005^1, 11006^1, 11042^1, 11043^1, 11044^1, 11045^1, 11046^1, 11047^1, 12001^1, 12002^1, 12004^1, 12005^1, 12006^1, 12007^1, 12011^1, 12013^1, 12014^1, 12015^1, 12016^1, 12017^1, 12018^1, 12020^1, 12021^1, 12031^1, 12032^1, 12034^1, 12035^1, 12036^1, 12037^1, 12041^1, 12042^1, 12044^1, 12045^1, 12046^1, 12047^1, 12051^1, 12052^1, 12053^1, 12054^1, 12055^1, 12056^1, 12057^1, 13100^1, 13101^1, 13102^1, 13120^1, 13121^1, 13122^1, 13131^1, 13132^1, 13133^1, 13151^1, 13152^1, 13153^1, 36000^1, 36400^1, 36405^1, 36406^1, 36410^1, 36420^1, 36425^1, 36430^1, 36440^1, 36591^0, 36592^0, 36600^1, 36640^1, 43752^1, 44602^1, 44603^1, 44604^1, 44605^1, 44950^0, 44970^0, 49000^0, 49002^1, 49010^0, 49320^1, 50520^1, 50526^1, 51701^1, 51702^1, 51703^1, 62320^0, 62321^0, 62322^0, 62323^0, 62324^0, 62325^0, 62326^0, 62327^0, 64400^0, 64405^0, 64408^0, 64415^0, 64416^0, 64417^0, 64418^0, 64420^0, 64421^0, 64425^0, 64430^0, 64435^0, 64445^0, 64446^0, 64447^0, 64448^0, 64449^0, 64450^0, 64451^0, 64454^0, 64461^0, 64462^0, 64463^0, 64479^0, 64480^0, 64483^0, 64484^0, 64486^0, 64487^0, 64488^0, 64489^0, 64490^0, 64491^0, 64492^0, 64493^0, 64494^0, 64495^0, 64505^0, 64510^0, 64517^0, 64520^0, 64530^0, 69990^0, 92012^1, 92014^1, 93000^1, 93005^1, 93010^1, 93040^1, 93041^1, 93042^1, 93318^1, 93355^1, 94002^1, 94200^1, 94680^1, 94681^1, 94690^1, 95812^1, 95813^1, 95816^1, 95819^1, 95822^1, 95829^1, 95955^1, 96360^1, 96361^1, 96365^1, 96366^1, 96367^1, 96368^1, 96372^1, 96374^1, 96375^1, 96376^1, 96377^1, 96523^0, 97597^1, 97598^1, 97602^1, 99155^0, 99156^0, 99157^0, 99211^1, 99212^1, 99213^1, 99214^1, 99215^1, 99217^1, 99218^1, 99219^1, 99220^1, 99221^1, 99222^1, 99223^1, 99231^1, 99232^1, 99233^1, 99234^1, 99235^1, 99236^1, 99238^1, 99239^1, 99241^1, 99242^1, 99243^1, 99244^1, 99245^1, 99251^1, 99252^1, 99253^1, 99254^1, 99255^1, 99291^1, 99292^1, 99304^1, 99305^1, 99306^1, 99307^1, 99308^1, 99309^1, 99310^1, 99315^1, 99316^1, 99334^1, 99335^1, 99336^1, 99337^1, 99347^1, 99348^1, 99349^1, 99350^1, 99374^1, 99375^1, 99377^1, 99378^1, 99446^0, 99447^0, 99448^0, 99449^0, 99451^0, 99452^0, 99495^0, 99496^0, G0463^1, G0471^1
50526	0213T^0, 0216T^0, 0596T^1, 0597T^1, 0708T^1, 0709T^1, 11000^1, 11001^1, 11004^1, 11005^1, 11006^1, 11042^1, 11043^1, 11044^1, 11045^1, 11046^1, 11047^1, 12001^1, 12002^1, 12004^1, 12005^1, 12006^1, 12007^1, 12011^1, 12013^1, 12014^1, 12015^1, 12016^1, 12017^1, 12018^1, 12020^1, 12021^1, 12031^1, 12032^1, 12034^1, 12035^1, 12036^1, 12037^1, 12041^1, 12042^1, 12044^1, 12045^1, 12046^1, 12047^1, 12051^1, 12052^1, 12053^1, 12054^1, 12055^1, 12056^1, 12057^1, 13100^1, 13101^1, 13102^1, 13120^1, 13121^1, 13122^1, 13131^1, 13132^1, 13133^1, 13151^1, 13152^1, 13153^1, 36000^1, 36400^1, 36405^1, 36406^1, 36410^1, 36420^1, 36425^1, 36430^1, 36440^1, 36591^0, 36592^0, 36600^1, 36640^1, 43752^1, 49000^0, 49002^1, 49010^0, 51701^1, 51702^1, 51703^1, 62320^0, 62321^0, 62322^0, 62323^0, 62324^0, 62325^0, 62326^0, 62327^0, 64400^0, 64405^0, 64408^0, 64415^0, 64416^0, 64417^0, 64418^0, 64420^0, 64421^0, 64425^0, 64430^0, 64435^0, 64445^0, 64446^0, 64447^0, 64448^0, 64449^0, 64450^0, 64451^0, 64454^0, 64461^0, 64462^0, 64463^0, 64479^0, 64480^0, 64483^0, 64484^0, 64486^0, 64487^0, 64488^0, 64489^0, 64490^0, 64491^0, 64492^0, 64493^0, 64494^0, 64495^0, 64505^0, 64510^0, 64517^0, 64520^0, 64530^0, 69990^0, 92012^1, 92014^1, 93000^1, 93005^1, 93010^1, 93040^1, 93041^1, 93042^1, 93318^1, 93355^1, 94002^1, 94200^1, 94680^1, 94681^1, 94690^1, 95812^1, 95813^1, 95816^1, 95819^1, 95822^1, 95829^1, 95955^1, 96360^1, 96361^1, 96365^1, 96366^1, 96367^1, 96368^1, 96372^1, 96374^1, 96375^1, 96376^1, 96377^1, 96523^0, 97597^1, 97598^1, 97602^1, 99155^0, 99156^0, 99157^0, 99211^1, 99212^1, 99213^1, 99214^1, 99215^1, 99217^1, 99218^1, 99219^1, 99220^1, 99221^1, 99222^1, 99223^1, 99231^1, 99232^1, 99233^1, 99234^1, 99235^1, 99236^1, 99238^1, 99239^1, 99241^1, 99242^1, 99243^1, 99244^1, 99245^1, 99251^1, 99252^1, 99253^1, 99254^1, 99255^1, 99291^1, 99292^1, 99304^1, 99305^1, 99306^1, 99307^1, 99308^1, 99309^1, 99310^1, 99315^1, 99316^1, 99334^1, 99335^1, 99336^1, 99337^1, 99347^1, 99348^1, 99349^1, 99350^1, 99374^1, 99375^1, 99377^1, 99378^1, 99446^0, 99447^0, 99448^0, 99449^0, 99451^0, 99452^0, 99495^0, 99496^0, G0463^1, G0471^1
50540	0213T^0, 0216T^0, 0596T^1, 0597T^1, 0708T^1, 0709T^1, 11000^1, 11001^1, 11004^1, 11005^1, 11006^1, 11042^1, 11043^1, 11044^1, 11045^1, 11046^1, 11047^1, 12001^1, 12002^1, 12004^1, 12005^1, 12006^1, 12007^1, 12011^1, 12013^1, 12014^1, 12015^1, 12016^1, 12017^1, 12018^1, 12020^1, 12021^1, 12031^1, 12032^1, 12034^1, 12035^1, 12036^1, 12037^1, 12041^1, 12042^1, 12044^1, 12045^1, 12046^1, 12047^1, 12051^1, 12052^1, 12053^1, 12054^1, 12055^1, 12056^1, 12057^1, 13100^1, 13101^1, 13102^1, 13120^1, 13121^1, 13122^1, 13131^1, 13132^1, 13133^1, 13151^1, 13152^1, 13153^1, 36000^1, 36400^1, 36405^1, 36406^1, 36410^1, 36420^1, 36425^1, 36430^1, 36440^1, 36591^0, 36592^0, 36600^1, 36640^1, 43752^1, 44602^1, 44603^1, 44604^1, 44605^1, 44950^0, 44970^0, 49000^0, 49002^1, 49010^0, 50100^1, 50400^1, 50405^1, 50544^1, 51701^1, 51702^1, 51703^1, 62320^0, 62321^0, 62322^0, 62323^0, 62324^0, 62325^0, 62326^0, 62327^0, 64400^0, 64405^0, 64408^0, 64415^0, 64416^0, 64417^0, 64418^0, 64420^0, 64421^0, 64425^0, 64430^0, 64435^0, 64445^0, 64446^0, 64447^0, 64448^0, 64449^0, 64450^0, 64451^0, 64454^0, 64461^0, 64462^0, 64463^0, 64479^0, 64480^0, 64483^0, 64484^0, 64486^0, 64487^0, 64488^0, 64489^0, 64490^0, 64491^0, 64492^0, 64493^0, 64494^0, 64495^0, 64505^0, 64510^0,

0 = Modifier usage not allowed or inappropriate 1 = Modifier usage allowed

Code 1	Code 2
	64517[0], 64520[0], 64530[0], 69990[0], 92012[1], 92014[1], 93000[1], 93005[1], 93010[1], 93040[1], 93041[1], 93042[1], 93318[1], 93355[1], 94002[1], 94200[1], 94680[1], 94681[1], 94690[1], 95812[1], 95813[1], 95816[1], 95819[1], 95822[1], 95829[1], 95955[1], 96360[1], 96361[1], 96365[1], 96366[1], 96367[1], 96368[1], 96372[1], 96374[1], 96375[1], 96376[1], 96377[1], 96523[0], 97597[1], 97598[1], 97602[1], 99155[0], 99156[0], 99157[0], 99211[1], 99212[1], 99213[1], 99214[1], 99215[1], 99217[1], 99218[1], 99219[1], 99220[1], 99221[1], 99222[1], 99223[1], 99231[1], 99232[1], 99233[1], 99234[1], 99235[1], 99236[1], 99238[1], 99239[1], 99241[1], 99242[1], 99243[1], 99244[1], 99245[1], 99251[1], 99252[1], 99253[1], 99254[1], 99255[1], 99291[1], 99292[1], 99304[1], 99305[1], 99306[1], 99307[1], 99308[1], 99309[1], 99310[1], 99315[1], 99316[1], 99334[1], 99335[1], 99336[1], 99337[1], 99347[1], 99348[1], 99349[1], 99350[1], 99374[1], 99375[1], 99377[1], 99378[1], 99446[0], 99447[0], 99448[0], 99449[0], 99451[0], 99452[0], 99495[0], 99496[0], G0463[1], G0471[1]
50541	0213T[0], 0216T[0], 0596T[1], 0597T[1], 0708T[1], 0709T[1], 12001[1], 12002[1], 12004[1], 12005[1], 12006[1], 12007[1], 12011[1], 12013[1], 12014[1], 12015[1], 12016[1], 12017[1], 12018[1], 12020[1], 12021[1], 12031[1], 12032[1], 12034[1], 12035[1], 12036[1], 12037[1], 12041[1], 12042[1], 12044[1], 12045[1], 12046[1], 12047[1], 12051[1], 12052[1], 12053[1], 12054[1], 12055[1], 12056[1], 12057[1], 13100[1], 13101[1], 13102[1], 13120[1], 13121[1], 13122[1], 13131[1], 13132[1], 13133[1], 13151[1], 13152[1], 13153[1], 36000[1], 36400[1], 36405[1], 36406[1], 36410[1], 36420[1], 36425[1], 36430[1], 36440[1], 36591[0], 36592[0], 36600[1], 36640[1], 43653[0], 43752[1], 44005[0], 44180[0], 44602[1], 44603[1], 44604[1], 44605[1], 44950[0], 44970[1], 49082[1], 49083[1], 49084[1], 49320[0], 49400[0], 50390[1], 50592[1], 50593[1], 50715[1], 51701[1], 51702[1], 51703[1], 58660[0], 62320[0], 62321[0], 62322[0], 62323[0], 62324[0], 62325[0], 62326[0], 62327[0], 64400[0], 64405[0], 64408[0], 64415[0], 64416[0], 64417[0], 64418[0], 64420[0], 64421[0], 64425[0], 64430[0], 64435[0], 64445[0], 64446[0], 64447[0], 64448[0], 64449[0], 64450[0], 64451[0], 64454[0], 64461[0], 64462[0], 64463[0], 64479[0], 64480[0], 64483[0], 64484[0], 64486[0], 64487[0], 64488[0], 64489[0], 64490[0], 64491[0], 64492[0], 64493[0], 64494[0], 64495[0], 64505[0], 64510[0], 64517[0], 64520[0], 64530[0], 69990[0], 76000[1], 77001[1], 77002[1], 92012[1], 92014[1], 93000[1], 93005[1], 93010[1], 93040[1], 93041[1], 93042[1], 93318[1], 93355[1], 94002[1], 94200[1], 94680[1], 94681[1], 94690[1], 95812[1], 95813[1], 95816[1], 95819[1], 95822[1], 95829[1], 95955[1], 96360[1], 96361[1], 96365[1], 96366[1], 96367[1], 96368[1], 96372[1], 96374[1], 96375[1], 96376[1], 96377[1], 96523[0], 99155[0], 99156[0], 99157[0], 99211[1], 99212[1], 99213[1], 99214[1], 99215[1], 99217[1], 99218[1], 99219[1], 99220[1], 99221[1], 99222[1], 99223[1], 99231[1], 99232[1], 99233[1], 99234[1], 99235[1], 99236[1], 99238[1], 99239[1], 99241[1], 99242[1], 99243[1], 99244[1], 99245[1], 99251[1], 99252[1], 99253[1], 99254[1], 99255[1], 99291[1], 99292[1], 99304[1], 99305[1], 99306[1], 99307[1], 99308[1], 99309[1], 99310[1], 99315[1], 99316[1], 99334[1], 99335[1], 99336[1], 99337[1], 99347[1], 99348[1], 99349[1], 99350[1], 99374[1], 99375[1], 99377[1], 99378[1], 99446[0], 99447[0], 99448[0], 99449[0], 99451[0], 99452[0], 99495[0], 99496[0], G0463[1], G0471[1]
50542	0213T[0], 0216T[0], 0596T[1], 0597T[1], 0708T[1], 0709T[1], 12001[1], 12002[1], 12004[1], 12005[1], 12006[1], 12007[1], 12011[1], 12013[1], 12014[1], 12015[1], 12016[1], 12017[1], 12018[1], 12020[1], 12021[1], 12031[1], 12032[1], 12034[1], 12035[1], 12036[1], 12037[1], 12041[1], 12042[1], 12044[1], 12045[1], 12046[1], 12047[1], 12051[1], 12052[1], 12053[1], 12054[1], 12055[1], 12056[1], 12057[1], 13100[1], 13101[1], 13102[1], 13120[1], 13121[1], 13122[1], 13131[1], 13132[1], 13133[1], 13151[1], 13152[1], 13153[1], 35840[1], 36000[1], 36400[1], 36405[1], 36406[1], 36410[1], 36420[1], 36425[1], 36430[1], 36440[1], 36591[0], 36592[0], 36600[1], 36640[1], 43653[0], 43752[1], 44005[0], 44180[0], 44602[1], 44603[1], 44604[1], 44605[1], 44950[0], 44970[1], 49082[1], 49083[1], 49084[1], 49203[1], 49320[0], 49400[0], 50205[0], 50541[0], 50592[1], 50593[1], 50715[1], 51701[1], 51702[1], 51703[1], 58660[0], 60540[1], 60545[1], 62320[0], 62321[0], 62322[0], 62323[0], 62324[0], 62325[0], 62326[0], 62327[0], 64400[0], 64405[0], 64408[0], 64415[0], 64416[0], 64417[0], 64418[0], 64420[0], 64421[0], 64425[0], 64430[0], 64435[0], 64445[0], 64446[0], 64447[0], 64448[0], 64449[0], 64450[0], 64451[0], 64454[0], 64461[0], 64462[0], 64463[0], 64479[0], 64480[0], 64483[0], 64484[0], 64486[0], 64487[0], 64488[0], 64489[0], 64490[0], 64491[0], 64492[0], 64493[0], 64494[0], 64495[0], 64505[0], 64510[0], 64517[0], 64520[0], 64530[0], 69990[0], 76000[1], 76940[1], 76942[1], 76998[1], 77001[1], 77002[1], 92012[1], 92014[1], 93000[1], 93005[1], 93010[1], 93040[1], 93041[1], 93042[1], 93318[1], 93355[1], 94002[1], 94200[1], 94680[1], 94681[1], 94690[1], 95812[1], 95813[1], 95816[1], 95819[1], 95822[1], 95829[1], 95955[1], 96360[1], 96361[1], 96365[1], 96366[1], 96367[1], 96368[1], 96372[1], 96374[1], 96375[1], 96376[1], 96377[1], 96523[0], 99155[0], 99156[0], 99157[0], 99211[1], 99212[1], 99213[1], 99214[1], 99215[1], 99217[1], 99218[1], 99219[1], 99220[1], 99221[1], 99222[1], 99223[1], 99231[1], 99232[1], 99233[1], 99234[1], 99235[1], 99236[1], 99238[1], 99239[1], 99241[1], 99242[1], 99243[1], 99244[1], 99245[1], 99251[1], 99252[1], 99253[1], 99254[1], 99255[1], 99291[1], 99292[1], 99304[1], 99305[1], 99306[1], 99307[1], 99308[1], 99309[1], 99310[1], 99315[1], 99316[1], 99334[1], 99335[1], 99336[1], 99337[1], 99347[1], 99348[1], 99349[1], 99350[1], 99374[1], 99375[1], 99377[1], 99378[1], 99446[0], 99447[0], 99448[0], 99449[0], 99451[0], 99452[0], 99495[0], 99496[0], G0463[1], G0471[1]
50543	0213T[0], 0216T[0], 0596T[1], 0597T[1], 0708T[1], 0709T[1], 11000[1], 11001[1], 11004[1], 11005[1], 11006[1], 11042[1], 11043[1], 11044[1], 11045[1], 11046[1], 11047[1], 12001[1], 12002[1], 12004[1], 12005[1], 12006[1], 12007[1], 12011[1], 12013[1], 12014[1], 12015[1], 12016[1], 12017[1], 12018[1], 12020[1], 12021[1], 12031[1], 12032[1], 12034[1], 12035[1], 12036[1], 12037[1], 12041[1], 12042[1], 12044[1], 12045[1], 12046[1], 12047[1], 12051[1], 12052[1], 12053[1], 12054[1], 12055[1], 12056[1], 12057[1], 13100[1], 13101[1], 13102[1], 13120[1], 13121[1], 13122[1], 13131[1], 13132[1], 13133[1], 13151[1], 13152[1], 13153[1], 35840[1], 36000[1], 36400[1], 36405[1], 36406[1], 36410[1], 36420[1], 36425[1], 36430[1], 36440[1], 36591[0], 36592[0], 36600[1], 36640[1], 38100[1], 38101[1], 38120[1], 43653[0], 43752[1], 44005[0], 44180[0], 44602[1], 44603[1], 44604[1], 44605[1], 44950[0], 44970[1], 49082[1], 49083[1], 49084[1], 49320[0], 49321[1], 49400[0], 50205[1], 50541[1], 50542[1], 50715[1], 51701[1], 51702[1], 51703[1], 58660[0], 60540[1], 60545[1], 60650[1], 62320[0], 62321[0], 62322[0], 62323[0], 62324[0], 62325[0], 62326[0], 62327[0], 64400[0], 64405[0], 64408[0], 64415[0], 64416[0], 64417[0], 64418[0], 64420[0], 64421[0], 64425[0], 64430[0], 64435[0], 64445[0], 64446[0], 64447[0], 64448[0], 64449[0], 64450[0], 64451[0], 64454[0], 64461[0], 64462[0], 64463[0], 64479[0], 64480[0], 64483[0], 64484[0], 64486[0], 64487[0], 64488[0], 64489[0], 64490[0], 64491[0], 64492[0], 64493[0], 64494[0], 64495[0], 64505[0], 64510[0], 64517[0], 64520[0], 64530[0], 69990[0], 76000[1], 77001[1], 77002[1], 92012[1], 92014[1], 93000[1], 93005[1], 93010[1], 93040[1], 93041[1], 93042[1], 93318[1], 93355[1], 94002[1], 94200[1], 94680[1], 94681[1], 94690[1], 95812[1], 95813[1], 95816[1], 95819[1], 95822[1], 95829[1], 95955[1], 96360[1], 96361[1], 96365[1], 96366[1], 96367[1], 96368[1], 96372[1], 96374[1], 96375[1], 96376[1], 96377[1], 96523[0], 97597[1], 97598[1], 97602[1], 99155[0], 99156[0], 99157[0], 99211[1], 99212[1], 99213[1], 99214[1], 99215[1], 99217[1], 99218[1], 99219[1], 99220[1], 99221[1], 99222[1], 99223[1], 99231[1], 99232[1], 99233[1], 99234[1], 99235[1], 99236[1], 99238[1], 99239[1], 99241[1], 99242[1], 99243[1], 99244[1], 99245[1], 99251[1], 99252[1], 99253[1], 99254[1], 99255[1], 99291[1], 99292[1], 99304[1], 99305[1], 99306[1], 99307[1], 99308[1], 99309[1], 99310[1], 99315[1], 99316[1], 99334[1], 99335[1], 99336[1], 99337[1], 99347[1], 99348[1], 99349[1], 99350[1], 99374[1], 99375[1], 99377[1], 99378[1], 99446[0], 99447[0], 99448[0], 99449[0], 99451[0], 99452[0], 99495[0], 99496[0], G0463[1], G0471[1]
50544	0213T[0], 0216T[0], 0596T[1], 0597T[1], 0708T[1], 0709T[1], 11000[1], 11001[1], 11004[1], 11005[1], 11006[1], 11042[1], 11043[1], 11044[1], 11045[1], 11046[1], 11047[1], 12001[1], 12002[1], 12004[1], 12005[1], 12006[1], 12007[1], 12011[1], 12013[1], 12014[1], 12015[1], 12016[1], 12017[1], 12018[1], 12020[1], 12021[1], 12031[1], 12032[1], 12034[1], 12035[1], 12036[1], 12037[1], 12041[1], 12042[1], 12044[1], 12045[1], 12046[1], 12047[1], 12051[1], 12052[1], 12053[1], 12054[1], 12055[1], 12056[1], 12057[1], 13100[1], 13101[1], 13102[1], 13120[1], 13121[1], 13122[1], 13131[1], 13132[1], 13133[1], 13151[1], 13152[1], 13153[1], 36000[1], 36400[1], 36405[1], 36406[1], 36410[1], 36420[1], 36425[1], 36430[1], 36440[1], 36591[0], 36592[0], 36600[1], 36640[1], 43653[0], 43752[1], 44005[0], 44180[0], 44602[1], 44603[1], 44604[1], 44605[1], 44950[0], 44970[1], 49082[1], 49083[1], 49084[1], 49320[0], 49400[0], 50390[1], 50715[1], 51701[1], 51702[1], 51703[1], 58660[0], 62320[0], 62321[0], 62322[0], 62323[0], 62324[0], 62325[0], 62326[0], 62327[0], 64400[0], 64405[0], 64408[0], 64415[0], 64416[0], 64417[0], 64418[0], 64420[0], 64421[0], 64425[0], 64430[0], 64435[0], 64445[0], 64446[0], 64447[0], 64448[0], 64449[0], 64450[0], 64451[0], 64454[0], 64461[0], 64462[0], 64463[0], 64479[0], 64480[0], 64483[0], 64484[0], 64486[0], 64487[0], 64488[0], 64489[0], 64490[0], 64491[0], 64492[0], 64493[0], 64494[0], 64495[0], 64505[0], 64510[0], 64517[0], 64520[0], 64530[0], 69990[0], 76000[1], 77001[1], 77002[1], 92012[1], 92014[1], 93000[1], 93005[1], 93010[1], 93040[1], 93041[1], 93042[1], 93318[1], 93355[1], 94002[1], 94200[1], 94680[1], 94681[1], 94690[1], 95812[1], 95813[1], 95816[1], 95819[1], 95822[1], 95829[1], 95955[1], 96360[1], 96361[1], 96365[1], 96366[1], 96367[1], 96368[1], 96372[1], 96374[1], 96375[1], 96376[1], 96377[1], 96523[0], 97597[1], 97598[1], 97602[1], 99155[0], 99156[0], 99157[0], 99211[1], 99212[1], 99213[1], 99214[1], 99215[1], 99217[1], 99218[1], 99219[1], 99220[1], 99221[1], 99222[1], 99223[1], 99231[1], 99232[1], 99233[1], 99234[1], 99235[1], 99236[1], 99238[1], 99239[1], 99241[1], 99242[1], 99243[1], 99244[1], 99245[1], 99251[1], 99252[1], 99253[1], 99254[1], 99255[1], 99291[1], 99292[1], 99304[1], 99305[1], 99306[1], 99307[1], 99308[1], 99309[1], 99310[1], 99315[1], 99316[1], 99334[1], 99335[1], 99336[1], 99337[1], 99347[1], 99348[1], 99349[1], 99350[1], 99374[1], 99375[1], 99377[1], 99378[1], 99446[0], 99447[0], 99448[0], 99449[0], 99451[0], 99452[0], 99495[0], 99496[0], G0463[1], G0471[1]
50545	0213T[0], 0216T[0], 0596T[1], 0597T[1], 0708T[1], 0709T[1], 11000[1], 11001[1], 11004[1], 11005[1], 11006[1], 11042[1], 11043[1], 11044[1], 11045[1], 11046[1], 11047[1], 12001[1], 12002[1], 12004[1], 12005[1], 12006[1], 12007[1], 12011[1], 12013[1], 12014[1], 12015[1], 12016[1], 12017[1], 12018[1], 12020[1], 12021[1], 12031[1], 12032[1], 12034[1], 12035[1], 12036[1], 12037[1], 12041[1], 12042[1], 12044[1], 12045[1], 12046[1], 12047[1], 12051[1], 12052[1], 12053[1], 12054[1], 12055[1], 12056[1], 12057[1], 13100[1], 13101[1], 13102[1], 13120[1], 13121[1], 13122[1], 13131[1], 13132[1], 13133[1], 13151[1], 13152[1], 13153[1], 35840[1], 36000[1], 36400[1], 36405[1], 36406[1], 36410[1], 36420[1], 36425[1], 36430[1], 36440[1], 36591[0], 36592[0], 36600[1], 36640[1], 38100[1], 38101[1], 38120[1], 38562[1], 38564[1], 38570[1], 43653[0], 43752[1], 44005[0], 44180[0], 44602[1], 44603[1], 44604[1], 44605[1], 44950[0], 44970[1], 49082[1], 49083[1], 49084[1], 49320[0], 49321[1], 49400[0], 49405[1], 49406[1], 50020[1], 50040[1], 50045[1], 50060[1], 50065[1], 50070[1], 50075[1], 50080[1], 50081[1], 50100[1], 50205[1], 50240[1], 50390[1], 50541[1], 50542[1], 50543[1], 50544[1], 50546[1], 50547[1], 50548[1], 50605[1], 50650[0], 50715[1], 51701[1], 51702[1], 51703[1], 58660[0], 60540[1], 60545[1], 60650[1], 62320[0], 62321[0], 62322[0], 62323[0], 62324[0], 62325[0], 62326[0], 62327[0], 64400[0], 64405[0], 64408[0], 64415[0], 64416[0], 64417[0], 64418[0], 64420[0], 64421[0], 64425[0], 64430[0], 64435[0], 64445[0], 64446[0], 64447[0], 64448[0], 64449[0], 64450[0], 64451[0], 64454[0], 64461[0], 64462[0], 64463[0], 64479[0], 64480[0], 64483[0], 64484[0], 64486[0], 64487[0], 64488[0], 64489[0],

Appendix A: NCCI - CPT Codes

0 = Modifier usage not allowed or inappropriate 1 = Modifier usage allowed

Code 1	Code 2
	64490[0], 64491[0], 64492[0], 64493[0], 64494[0], 64495[0], 64505[0], 64510[0], 64517[0], 64520[0], 64530[0], 69990[0], 76000[1], 77001[1], 77002[1], 92012[1], 92014[1], 93000[1], 93005[1], 93010[1], 93040[1], 93041[1], 93042[1], 93318[1], 93355[1], 94002[1], 94200[1], 94680[1], 94681[1], 94690[1], 95812[1], 95813[1], 95816[1], 95819[1], 95822[1], 95829[1], 95955[1], 96360[1], 96361[1], 96365[1], 96366[1], 96367[1], 96368[1], 96372[1], 96374[1], 96375[1], 96376[1], 96377[1], 96523[0], 97597[1], 97598[1], 97602[1], 99155[0], 99156[0], 99157[0], 99211[1], 99212[1], 99213[1], 99214[1], 99215[1], 99217[1], 99218[1], 99219[1], 99220[1], 99221[1], 99222[1], 99223[1], 99231[1], 99232[1], 99233[1], 99234[1], 99235[1], 99236[1], 99238[1], 99239[1], 99241[1], 99242[1], 99243[1], 99244[1], 99245[1], 99251[1], 99252[1], 99253[1], 99254[1], 99255[1], 99291[1], 99292[1], 99304[1], 99305[1], 99306[1], 99307[1], 99308[1], 99309[1], 99310[1], 99315[1], 99316[1], 99334[1], 99335[1], 99336[1], 99337[1], 99347[1], 99348[1], 99349[1], 99350[1], 99374[1], 99375[1], 99377[1], 99378[1], 99446[0], 99447[0], 99448[0], 99449[0], 99451[0], 99452[0], 99495[0], 99496[0], G0463[1], G0471[1]
50546	0213T[0], 0216T[0], 0596T[1], 0597T[1], 0708T[1], 0709T[1], 11000[1], 11001[1], 11004[1], 11005[1], 11006[1], 11042[1], 11043[1], 11044[1], 11045[1], 11046[1], 11047[1], 12001[1], 12002[1], 12004[1], 12005[1], 12006[1], 12007[1], 12011[1], 12013[1], 12014[1], 12015[1], 12016[1], 12017[1], 12018[1], 12020[1], 12021[1], 12031[1], 12032[1], 12034[1], 12035[1], 12036[1], 12037[1], 12041[1], 12042[1], 12044[1], 12045[1], 12046[1], 12047[1], 12051[1], 12052[1], 12053[1], 12054[1], 12055[1], 12056[1], 12057[1], 13100[1], 13101[1], 13102[1], 13120[1], 13121[1], 13122[1], 13131[1], 13132[1], 13133[1], 13151[1], 13152[1], 13153[1], 36000[1], 36400[1], 36405[1], 36406[1], 36410[1], 36420[1], 36425[1], 36430[1], 36440[1], 36591[0], 36592[0], 36600[1], 36640[1], 38100[1], 38101[1], 38120[1], 43653[0], 43752[1], 44005[0], 44180[0], 44602[1], 44603[1], 44604[1], 44605[1], 44950[0], 44970[1], 49082[1], 49083[1], 49084[1], 49320[0], 49321[1], 49400[0], 49405[1], 49406[1], 50020[1], 50040[1], 50045[1], 50060[1], 50065[1], 50070[1], 50075[1], 50080[1], 50081[1], 50100[1], 50205[1], 50240[1], 50390[1], 50542[1], 50543[1], 50605[1], 50650[1], 50715[1], 51701[1], 51702[1], 51703[1], 58660[0], 60540[1], 60545[1], 60650[1], 62320[0], 62321[0], 62322[0], 62323[0], 62324[0], 62325[0], 62326[0], 62327[0], 64400[0], 64405[0], 64408[0], 64415[0], 64416[0], 64417[0], 64418[0], 64420[0], 64421[0], 64425[0], 64430[0], 64435[0], 64445[0], 64446[0], 64447[0], 64448[0], 64449[0], 64450[0], 64451[0], 64454[0], 64461[0], 64462[0], 64463[0], 64479[0], 64480[0], 64483[0], 64484[0], 64486[0], 64487[0], 64488[0], 64489[0], 64490[0], 64491[0], 64492[0], 64493[0], 64494[0], 64495[0], 64505[0], 64510[0], 64517[0], 64520[0], 64530[0], 69990[0], 76000[1], 77001[1], 77002[1], 92012[1], 92014[1], 93000[1], 93005[1], 93010[1], 93040[1], 93041[1], 93042[1], 93318[1], 93355[1], 94002[1], 94200[1], 94680[1], 94681[1], 94690[1], 95812[1], 95813[1], 95816[1], 95819[1], 95822[1], 95829[1], 95955[1], 96360[1], 96361[1], 96365[1], 96366[1], 96367[1], 96368[1], 96372[1], 96374[1], 96375[1], 96376[1], 96377[1], 96523[0], 97597[1], 97598[1], 97602[1], 99155[0], 99156[0], 99157[0], 99211[1], 99212[1], 99213[1], 99214[1], 99215[1], 99217[1], 99218[1], 99219[1], 99220[1], 99221[1], 99222[1], 99223[1], 99231[1], 99232[1], 99233[1], 99234[1], 99235[1], 99236[1], 99238[1], 99239[1], 99241[1], 99242[1], 99243[1], 99244[1], 99245[1], 99251[1], 99252[1], 99253[1], 99254[1], 99255[1], 99291[1], 99292[1], 99304[1], 99305[1], 99306[1], 99307[1], 99308[1], 99309[1], 99310[1], 99315[1], 99316[1], 99334[1], 99335[1], 99336[1], 99337[1], 99347[1], 99348[1], 99349[1], 99350[1], 99374[1], 99375[1], 99377[1], 99378[1], 99446[0], 99447[0], 99448[0], 99449[0], 99451[0], 99452[0], 99495[0], 99496[0], G0463[1], G0471[1]
50547	0213T[0], 0216T[0], 0596T[1], 0597T[1], 0708T[1], 0709T[1], 11000[1], 11001[1], 11004[1], 11005[1], 11006[1], 11042[1], 11043[1], 11044[1], 11045[1], 11046[1], 11047[1], 12001[1], 12002[1], 12004[1], 12005[1], 12006[1], 12007[1], 12011[1], 12013[1], 12014[1], 12015[1], 12016[1], 12017[1], 12018[1], 12020[1], 12021[1], 12031[1], 12032[1], 12034[1], 12035[1], 12036[1], 12037[1], 12041[1], 12042[1], 12044[1], 12045[1], 12046[1], 12047[1], 12051[1], 12052[1], 12053[1], 12054[1], 12055[1], 12056[1], 12057[1], 13100[1], 13101[1], 13102[1], 13120[1], 13121[1], 13122[1], 13131[1], 13132[1], 13133[1], 13151[1], 13152[1], 13153[1], 36000[1], 36400[1], 36405[1], 36406[1], 36410[1], 36420[1], 36425[1], 36430[1], 36440[1], 36591[0], 36592[0], 36600[1], 36640[1], 38100[1], 38101[1], 38120[1], 43653[0], 43752[1], 44005[0], 44180[0], 44602[1], 44603[1], 44604[1], 44605[1], 44950[0], 44970[1], 49082[1], 49083[1], 49084[1], 49320[0], 49321[1], 49400[0], 50542[1], 50543[1], 50546[1], 50605[1], 50650[0], 50715[1], 51701[1], 51702[1], 51703[1], 58660[0], 62320[0], 62321[0], 62322[0], 62323[0], 62324[0], 62325[0], 62326[0], 62327[0], 64400[0], 64405[0], 64408[0], 64415[0], 64416[0], 64417[0], 64418[0], 64420[0], 64421[0], 64425[0], 64430[0], 64435[0], 64445[0], 64446[0], 64447[0], 64448[0], 64449[0], 64450[0], 64451[0], 64454[0], 64461[0], 64462[0], 64463[0], 64479[0], 64480[0], 64483[0], 64484[0], 64486[0], 64487[0], 64488[0], 64489[0], 64490[0], 64491[0], 64492[0], 64493[0], 64494[0], 64495[0], 64505[0], 64510[0], 64517[0], 64520[0], 64530[0], 69990[0], 76000[1], 77001[1], 77002[1], 92012[1], 92014[1], 93000[1], 93005[1], 93010[1], 93040[1], 93041[1], 93042[1], 93318[1], 93355[1], 94002[1], 94200[1], 94680[1], 94681[1], 94690[1], 95812[1], 95813[1], 95816[1], 95819[1], 95822[1], 95829[1], 95955[1], 96360[1], 96361[1], 96365[1], 96366[1], 96367[1], 96368[1], 96372[1], 96374[1], 96375[1], 96376[1], 96377[1], 96523[0], 97597[1], 97598[1], 97602[1], 99155[0], 99156[0], 99157[0], 99211[1], 99212[1], 99213[1], 99214[1], 99215[1], 99217[1], 99218[1], 99219[1], 99220[1], 99221[1], 99222[1], 99223[1], 99231[1], 99232[1], 99233[1], 99234[1], 99235[1], 99236[1], 99238[1], 99239[1], 99241[1], 99242[1], 99243[1], 99244[1], 99245[1], 99251[1], 99252[1], 99253[1], 99254[1], 99255[1], 99291[1], 99292[1], 99304[1], 99305[1], 99306[1], 99307[1], 99308[1], 99309[1], 99310[1], 99315[1], 99316[1], 99334[1], 99335[1], 99336[1], 99337[1], 99347[1], 99348[1], 99349[1], 99350[1], 99374[1], 99375[1], 99377[1], 99378[1], 99446[0], 99447[0], 99448[0], 99449[0], 99451[0], 99452[0], 99495[0], 99496[0], G0463[1], G0471[1]
50548	0213T[0], 0216T[0], 0596T[1], 0597T[1], 0708T[1], 0709T[1], 11000[1], 11001[1], 11004[1], 11005[1], 11006[1], 11042[1], 11043[1], 11044[1], 11045[1], 11046[1], 11047[1], 12001[1], 12002[1], 12004[1], 12005[1], 12006[1], 12007[1], 12011[1], 12013[1], 12014[1], 12015[1], 12016[1], 12017[1], 12018[1], 12020[1], 12021[1], 12031[1], 12032[1], 12034[1], 12035[1], 12036[1], 12037[1], 12041[1], 12042[1], 12044[1], 12045[1], 12046[1], 12047[1], 12051[1], 12052[1], 12053[1], 12054[1], 12055[1], 12056[1], 12057[1], 13100[1], 13101[1], 13102[1], 13120[1], 13121[1], 13122[1], 13131[1], 13132[1], 13133[1], 13151[1], 13152[1], 13153[1], 36000[1], 36400[1], 36405[1], 36406[1], 36410[1], 36420[1], 36425[1], 36430[1], 36440[1], 36591[0], 36592[0], 36600[1], 36640[1], 38100[1], 38101[1], 38120[1], 43653[0], 43752[1], 44005[0], 44180[0], 44602[1], 44603[1], 44604[1], 44605[1], 44950[0], 44970[1], 49082[1], 49083[1], 49084[1], 49320[0], 49321[1], 49400[0], 49405[1], 49406[1], 50020[1], 50040[1], 50045[1], 50060[1], 50065[1], 50070[1], 50075[1], 50080[1], 50081[1], 50100[1], 50205[1], 50240[1], 50390[1], 50542[1], 50543[1], 50546[1], 50605[1], 50650[1], 50660[1], 50715[1], 51701[1], 51702[1], 51703[1], 58660[0], 60540[1], 60545[1], 60650[1], 62320[0], 62321[0], 62322[0], 62323[0], 62324[0], 62325[0], 62326[0], 62327[0], 64400[0], 64405[0], 64408[0], 64415[0], 64416[0], 64417[0], 64418[0], 64420[0], 64421[0], 64425[0], 64430[0], 64435[0], 64445[0], 64446[0], 64447[0], 64448[0], 64449[0], 64450[0], 64451[0], 64454[0], 64461[0], 64462[0], 64463[0], 64479[0], 64480[0], 64483[0], 64484[0], 64486[0], 64487[0], 64488[0], 64489[0], 64490[0], 64491[0], 64492[0], 64493[0], 64494[0], 64495[0], 64505[0], 64510[0], 64517[0], 64520[0], 64530[0], 69990[0], 76000[1], 77001[1], 77002[1], 92012[1], 92014[1], 93000[1], 93005[1], 93010[1], 93040[1], 93041[1], 93042[1], 93318[1], 93355[1], 94002[1], 94200[1], 94680[1], 94681[1], 94690[1], 95812[1], 95813[1], 95816[1], 95819[1], 95822[1], 95829[1], 95955[1], 96360[1], 96361[1], 96365[1], 96366[1], 96367[1], 96368[1], 96372[1], 96374[1], 96375[1], 96376[1], 96377[1], 96523[0], 97597[1], 97598[1], 97602[1], 99155[0], 99156[0], 99157[0], 99211[1], 99212[1], 99213[1], 99214[1], 99215[1], 99217[1], 99218[1], 99219[1], 99220[1], 99221[1], 99222[1], 99223[1], 99231[1], 99232[1], 99233[1], 99234[1], 99235[1], 99236[1], 99238[1], 99239[1], 99241[1], 99242[1], 99243[1], 99244[1], 99245[1], 99251[1], 99252[1], 99253[1], 99254[1], 99255[1], 99291[1], 99292[1], 99304[1], 99305[1], 99306[1], 99307[1], 99308[1], 99309[1], 99310[1], 99315[1], 99316[1], 99334[1], 99335[1], 99336[1], 99337[1], 99347[1], 99348[1], 99349[1], 99350[1], 99374[1], 99375[1], 99377[1], 99378[1], 99446[0], 99447[0], 99448[0], 99449[0], 99451[0], 99452[0], 99495[0], 99496[0], G0463[1], G0471[1]
50551	0213T[0], 0216T[0], 0596T[1], 0597T[1], 0708T[1], 0709T[1], 12001[1], 12002[1], 12004[1], 12005[1], 12006[1], 12007[1], 12011[1], 12013[1], 12014[1], 12015[1], 12016[1], 12017[1], 12018[1], 12020[1], 12021[1], 12031[1], 12032[1], 12034[1], 12035[1], 12036[1], 12037[1], 12041[1], 12042[1], 12044[1], 12045[1], 12046[1], 12047[1], 12051[1], 12052[1], 12053[1], 12054[1], 12055[1], 12056[1], 12057[1], 13100[1], 13101[1], 13102[1], 13120[1], 13121[1], 13122[1], 13131[1], 13132[1], 13133[1], 13151[1], 13152[1], 13153[1], 36000[1], 36400[1], 36405[1], 36406[1], 36410[1], 36420[1], 36425[1], 36430[1], 36440[1], 36591[0], 36592[0], 36600[1], 36640[1], 43752[1], 50391[1], 50430[1], 50431[1], 50436[1], 50437[1], 50570[1], 50572[1], 50574[1], 50575[1], 50576[1], 50580[1], 50684[1], 51701[1], 51702[1], 51703[1], 62320[0], 62321[0], 62322[0], 62323[0], 62324[0], 62325[0], 62326[0], 62327[0], 64400[0], 64405[0], 64408[0], 64415[0], 64416[0], 64417[0], 64418[0], 64420[0], 64421[0], 64425[0], 64430[0], 64435[0], 64445[0], 64446[0], 64447[0], 64448[0], 64449[0], 64450[0], 64451[0], 64454[0], 64461[0], 64462[0], 64463[0], 64479[0], 64480[0], 64483[0], 64484[0], 64486[0], 64487[0], 64488[0], 64489[0], 64490[0], 64491[0], 64492[0], 64493[0], 64494[0], 64495[0], 64505[0], 64510[0], 64517[0], 64520[0], 64530[0], 69990[0], 76000[1], 77001[1], 77002[1], 92012[1], 92014[1], 93000[1], 93005[1], 93010[1], 93040[1], 93041[1], 93042[1], 93318[1], 93355[1], 94002[1], 94200[1], 94680[1], 94681[1], 94690[1], 95812[1], 95813[1], 95816[1], 95819[1], 95822[1], 95829[1], 95955[1], 96360[1], 96361[1], 96365[1], 96366[1], 96367[1], 96368[1], 96372[1], 96374[1], 96375[1], 96376[1], 96377[1], 96523[0], 99155[0], 99156[0], 99157[0], 99211[1], 99212[1], 99213[1], 99214[1], 99215[1], 99217[1], 99218[1], 99219[1], 99220[1], 99221[1], 99222[1], 99223[1], 99231[1], 99232[1], 99233[1], 99234[1], 99235[1], 99236[1], 99238[1], 99239[1], 99241[1], 99242[1], 99243[1], 99244[1], 99245[1], 99251[1], 99252[1], 99253[1], 99254[1], 99255[1], 99291[1], 99292[1], 99304[1], 99305[1], 99306[1], 99307[1], 99308[1], 99309[1], 99310[1], 99315[1], 99316[1], 99334[1], 99335[1], 99336[1], 99337[1], 99347[1], 99348[1], 99349[1], 99350[1], 99374[1], 99375[1], 99377[1], 99378[1], 99446[0], 99447[0], 99448[0], 99449[0], 99451[0], 99452[0], 99495[1], 99496[1], G0463[1], G0471[1], J2001[1]
50553	0213T[0], 0216T[0], 0596T[1], 0597T[1], 0708T[1], 0709T[1], 12001[1], 12002[1], 12004[1], 12005[1], 12006[1], 12007[1], 12011[1], 12013[1], 12014[1], 12015[1], 12016[1], 12017[1], 12018[1], 12020[1], 12021[1], 12031[1], 12032[1], 12034[1], 12035[1], 12036[1], 12037[1], 12041[1], 12042[1], 12044[1], 12045[1], 12046[1], 12047[1], 12051[1], 12052[1], 12053[1], 12054[1], 12055[1], 12056[1], 12057[1], 13100[1], 13101[1], 13102[1], 13120[1], 13121[1], 13122[1], 13131[1], 13132[1], 13133[1], 13151[1], 13152[1], 13153[1], 36000[1], 36400[1], 36405[1], 36406[1], 36410[1], 36420[1], 36425[1], 36430[1], 36440[1], 36591[0], 36592[0], 36600[1], 36640[1], 43752[1], 50432[1], 50436[1], 50437[1], 50551[1], 50570[1], 50572[1], 50574[0], 50575[1], 50576[0], 50580[1], 50684[1], 50706[1], 51701[1], 51702[1], 51703[1], 62320[0], 62321[0], 62322[0], 62323[0], 62324[0], 62325[0], 62326[0], 62327[0], 64400[0], 64405[0], 64408[0], 64415[0], 64416[0], 64417[0], 64418[0], 64420[0], 64421[0], 64425[0], 64430[0],

0 = Modifier usage not allowed or inappropriate   1 = Modifier usage allowed

Code 1	Code 2
	64435[0], 64445[0], 64446[0], 64447[0], 64448[0], 64449[0], 64450[0], 64451[0], 64454[0], 64461[0], 64462[0], 64463[0], 64479[0], 64480[0], 64483[0], 64484[0], 64486[0], 64487[0], 64488[0], 64489[0], 64490[0], 64491[0], 64492[0], 64493[0], 64494[0], 64495[0], 64505[0], 64510[0], 64517[0], 64520[0], 64530[0], 69990[0], 76000[1], 77001[1], 77002[1], 92012[1], 92014[1], 93000[1], 93005[1], 93010[1], 93040[1], 93041[1], 93042[1], 93318[1], 93355[1], 94002[1], 94200[1], 94680[1], 94681[1], 94690[1], 95812[1], 95813[1], 95816[1], 95819[1], 95822[1], 95829[1], 95955[1], 96360[1], 96361[1], 96365[1], 96366[1], 96367[1], 96368[1], 96372[1], 96374[1], 96375[1], 96376[1], 96377[1], 96523[0], 99155[0], 99156[0], 99157[0], 99211[1], 99212[1], 99213[1], 99214[1], 99215[1], 99217[1], 99218[1], 99219[1], 99220[1], 99221[1], 99222[1], 99223[1], 99231[1], 99232[1], 99233[1], 99234[1], 99235[1], 99236[1], 99238[1], 99239[1], 99241[1], 99242[1], 99243[1], 99244[1], 99245[1], 99251[1], 99252[1], 99253[1], 99254[1], 99255[1], 99291[1], 99292[1], 99304[1], 99305[1], 99306[1], 99307[1], 99308[1], 99309[1], 99310[1], 99315[1], 99316[1], 99334[1], 99335[1], 99336[1], 99337[1], 99347[1], 99348[1], 99349[1], 99350[1], 99374[1], 99375[1], 99377[1], 99378[1], 99446[0], 99447[0], 99448[0], 99449[0], 99451[0], 99452[0], 99495[1], 99496[1], G0463[1], G0471[1], J2001[1]
50555	0213T[0], 0216T[0], 0596T[1], 0597T[1], 0708T[1], 0709T[1], 10005[1], 10007[1], 10009[1], 10011[1], 10021[1], 12001[1], 12002[1], 12004[1], 12005[1], 12006[1], 12007[1], 12011[1], 12013[1], 12014[1], 12015[1], 12016[1], 12017[1], 12018[1], 12020[1], 12021[1], 12031[1], 12032[1], 12034[1], 12035[1], 12036[1], 12037[1], 12041[1], 12042[1], 12044[1], 12045[1], 12046[1], 12047[1], 12051[1], 12052[1], 12053[1], 12054[1], 12055[1], 12056[1], 12057[1], 13100[1], 13101[1], 13102[1], 13120[1], 13121[1], 13122[1], 13131[1], 13132[1], 13133[1], 13151[1], 13152[1], 13153[1], 36000[1], 36400[1], 36405[1], 36406[1], 36410[1], 36420[1], 36425[1], 36430[1], 36440[1], 36591[0], 36592[0], 36600[1], 36640[1], 43752[1], 50430[1], 50431[1], 50432[1], 50436[1], 50437[1], 50551[1], 50570[1], 50572[1], 50574[1], 50575[0], 50580[0], 50606[1], 50684[1], 51701[1], 51702[1], 51703[1], 62320[0], 62321[0], 62322[0], 62323[0], 62324[0], 62325[0], 62326[0], 62327[0], 64400[0], 64405[0], 64408[0], 64415[0], 64416[0], 64417[0], 64418[0], 64420[0], 64421[0], 64425[0], 64430[0], 64435[0], 64445[0], 64446[0], 64447[0], 64448[0], 64449[0], 64450[0], 64451[0], 64454[0], 64461[0], 64462[0], 64463[0], 64479[0], 64480[0], 64483[0], 64484[0], 64486[0], 64487[0], 64488[0], 64489[0], 64490[0], 64491[0], 64492[0], 64493[0], 64494[0], 64495[0], 64505[0], 64510[0], 64517[0], 64520[0], 64530[0], 69990[0], 76000[1], 77001[1], 77002[1], 92012[1], 92014[1], 93000[1], 93005[1], 93010[1], 93040[1], 93041[1], 93042[1], 93318[1], 93355[1], 94002[1], 94200[1], 94680[1], 94681[1], 94690[1], 95812[1], 95813[1], 95816[1], 95819[1], 95822[1], 95829[1], 95955[1], 96360[1], 96361[1], 96365[1], 96366[1], 96367[1], 96368[1], 96372[1], 96374[1], 96375[1], 96376[1], 96377[1], 96523[0], 99155[0], 99156[0], 99157[0], 99211[1], 99212[1], 99213[1], 99214[1], 99215[1], 99217[1], 99218[1], 99219[1], 99220[1], 99221[1], 99222[1], 99223[1], 99231[1], 99232[1], 99233[1], 99234[1], 99235[1], 99236[1], 99238[1], 99239[1], 99241[1], 99242[1], 99243[1], 99244[1], 99245[1], 99251[1], 99252[1], 99253[1], 99254[1], 99255[1], 99291[1], 99292[1], 99304[1], 99305[1], 99306[1], 99307[1], 99308[1], 99309[1], 99310[1], 99315[1], 99316[1], 99334[1], 99335[1], 99336[1], 99337[1], 99347[1], 99348[1], 99349[1], 99350[1], 99374[1], 99375[1], 99377[1], 99378[1], 99446[0], 99447[0], 99448[0], 99449[0], 99451[0], 99452[0], 99495[1], 99496[1], G0463[1], G0471[1], J2001[1]
50557	0213T[0], 0216T[0], 0596T[1], 0597T[1], 0708T[1], 0709T[1], 10005[1], 10007[1], 10009[1], 10011[1], 10021[1], 12001[1], 12002[1], 12004[1], 12005[1], 12006[1], 12007[1], 12011[1], 12013[1], 12014[1], 12015[1], 12016[1], 12017[1], 12018[1], 12020[1], 12021[1], 12031[1], 12032[1], 12034[1], 12035[1], 12036[1], 12037[1], 12041[1], 12042[1], 12044[1], 12045[1], 12046[1], 12047[1], 12051[1], 12052[1], 12053[1], 12054[1], 12055[1], 12056[1], 12057[1], 13100[1], 13101[1], 13102[1], 13120[1], 13121[1], 13122[1], 13131[1], 13132[1], 13133[1], 13151[1], 13152[1], 13153[1], 36000[1], 36400[1], 36405[1], 36406[1], 36410[1], 36420[1], 36425[1], 36430[1], 36440[1], 36591[0], 36592[0], 36600[1], 36640[1], 43752[1], 50430[1], 50431[1], 50432[1], 50436[1], 50437[1], 50551[1], 50555[0], 50570[1], 50572[1], 50574[1], 50575[0], 50576[1], 50580[0], 50684[1], 50955[1], 50974[1], 51701[1], 51702[1], 51703[1], 62320[0], 62321[0], 62322[0], 62323[0], 62324[0], 62325[0], 62326[0], 62327[0], 64400[0], 64405[0], 64408[0], 64415[0], 64416[0], 64417[0], 64418[0], 64420[0], 64421[0], 64425[0], 64430[0], 64435[0], 64445[0], 64446[0], 64447[0], 64448[0], 64449[0], 64450[0], 64451[0], 64454[0], 64461[0], 64462[0], 64463[0], 64479[0], 64480[0], 64483[0], 64484[0], 64486[0], 64487[0], 64488[0], 64489[0], 64490[0], 64491[0], 64492[0], 64493[0], 64494[0], 64495[0], 64505[0], 64510[0], 64517[0], 64520[0], 64530[0], 69990[0], 76000[1], 77001[1], 77002[1], 92012[1], 92014[1], 93000[1], 93005[1], 93010[1], 93040[1], 93041[1], 93042[1], 93318[1], 93355[1], 94002[1], 94200[1], 94680[1], 94681[1], 94690[1], 95812[1], 95813[1], 95816[1], 95819[1], 95822[1], 95829[1], 95955[1], 96360[1], 96361[1], 96365[1], 96366[1], 96367[1], 96368[1], 96372[1], 96374[1], 96375[1], 96376[1], 96377[1], 96523[0], 99155[0], 99156[0], 99157[0], 99211[1], 99212[1], 99213[1], 99214[1], 99215[1], 99217[1], 99218[1], 99219[1], 99220[1], 99221[1], 99222[1], 99223[1], 99231[1], 99232[1], 99233[1], 99234[1], 99235[1], 99236[1], 99238[1], 99239[1], 99241[1], 99242[1], 99243[1], 99244[1], 99245[1], 99251[1], 99252[1], 99253[1], 99254[1], 99255[1], 99291[1], 99292[1], 99304[1], 99305[1], 99306[1], 99307[1], 99308[1], 99309[1], 99310[1], 99315[1], 99316[1], 99334[1], 99335[1], 99336[1], 99337[1], 99347[1], 99348[1], 99349[1], 99350[1], 99374[1], 99375[1], 99377[1], 99378[1], 99446[0], 99447[0], 99448[0], 99449[0], 99451[0], 99452[0], 99495[1], 99496[1], G0463[1], G0471[1], J2001[1]
50561	0213T[0], 0216T[0], 0596T[1], 0597T[1], 0708T[1], 0709T[1], 11000[1], 11001[1], 11004[1], 11005[1], 11006[1], 11042[1], 11043[1], 11044[1], 11045[1], 11046[1], 11047[1], 12001[1], 12002[1], 12004[1], 12005[1], 12006[1], 12007[1], 12011[1], 12013[1], 12014[1], 12015[1], 12016[1], 12017[1], 12018[1], 12020[1], 12021[1], 12031[1], 12032[1], 12034[1], 12035[1], 12036[1], 12037[1], 12041[1], 12042[1], 12044[1], 12045[1], 12046[1], 12047[1], 12051[1], 12052[1], 12053[1], 12054[1], 12055[1], 12056[1], 12057[1], 13100[1], 13101[1], 13102[1], 13120[1], 13121[1], 13122[1], 13131[1], 13132[1], 13133[1], 13151[1], 13152[1], 13153[1], 36000[1], 36400[1], 36405[1], 36406[1], 36410[1], 36420[1], 36425[1], 36430[1], 36440[1], 36591[0], 36592[0], 36600[1], 36640[1], 43752[1], 50430[1], 50431[1], 50432[1], 50436[1], 50437[1], 50551[1], 50570[1], 50572[1], 50574[0], 50575[0], 50576[0], 50580[1], 50684[1], 50961[1], 50980[1], 51701[1], 51702[1], 51703[1], 52320[1], 52325[1], 52330[1], 52352[1], 52353[1], 62320[0], 62321[0], 62322[0], 62323[0], 62324[0], 62325[0], 62326[0], 62327[0], 64400[0], 64405[0], 64408[0], 64415[0], 64416[0], 64417[0], 64418[0], 64420[0], 64421[0], 64425[0], 64430[0], 64435[0], 64445[0], 64446[0], 64447[0], 64448[0], 64449[0], 64450[0], 64451[0], 64454[0], 64461[0], 64462[0], 64463[0], 64479[0], 64480[0], 64483[0], 64484[0], 64486[0], 64487[0], 64488[0], 64489[0], 64490[0], 64491[0], 64492[0], 64493[0], 64494[0], 64495[0], 64505[0], 64510[0], 64517[0], 64520[0], 64530[0], 69990[0], 76000[1], 77001[1], 77002[1], 92012[1], 92014[1], 93000[1], 93005[1], 93010[1], 93040[1], 93041[1], 93042[1], 93318[1], 93355[1], 94002[1], 94200[1], 94680[1], 94681[1], 94690[1], 95812[1], 95813[1], 95816[1], 95819[1], 95822[1], 95829[1], 95955[1], 96360[1], 96361[1], 96365[1], 96366[1], 96367[1], 96368[1], 96372[1], 96374[1], 96375[1], 96376[1], 96377[1], 96523[0], 97597[1], 97598[1], 97602[1], 99155[0], 99156[0], 99157[0], 99211[1], 99212[1], 99213[1], 99214[1], 99215[1], 99217[1], 99218[1], 99219[1], 99220[1], 99221[1], 99222[1], 99223[1], 99231[1], 99232[1], 99233[1], 99234[1], 99235[1], 99236[1], 99238[1], 99239[1], 99241[1], 99242[1], 99243[1], 99244[1], 99245[1], 99251[1], 99252[1], 99253[1], 99254[1], 99255[1], 99291[1], 99292[1], 99304[1], 99305[1], 99306[1], 99307[1], 99308[1], 99309[1], 99310[1], 99315[1], 99316[1], 99334[1], 99335[1], 99336[1], 99337[1], 99347[1], 99348[1], 99349[1], 99350[1], 99374[1], 99375[1], 99377[1], 99378[1], 99446[0], 99447[0], 99448[0], 99449[0], 99451[0], 99452[0], 99495[1], 99496[1], G0463[1], G0471[1], J2001[1]
50562	0213T[0], 0216T[0], 0596T[1], 0597T[1], 0708T[1], 0709T[1], 11000[1], 11001[1], 11004[1], 11005[1], 11006[1], 11042[1], 11043[1], 11044[1], 11045[1], 11046[1], 11047[1], 12001[1], 12002[1], 12004[1], 12005[1], 12006[1], 12007[1], 12011[1], 12013[1], 12014[1], 12015[1], 12016[1], 12017[1], 12018[1], 12020[1], 12021[1], 12031[1], 12032[1], 12034[1], 12035[1], 12036[1], 12037[1], 12041[1], 12042[1], 12044[1], 12045[1], 12046[1], 12047[1], 12051[1], 12052[1], 12053[1], 12054[1], 12055[1], 12056[1], 12057[1], 13100[1], 13101[1], 13102[1], 13120[1], 13121[1], 13122[1], 13131[1], 13132[1], 13133[1], 13151[1], 13152[1], 13153[1], 36000[1], 36400[1], 36405[1], 36406[1], 36410[1], 36420[1], 36425[1], 36430[1], 36440[1], 36591[0], 36592[0], 36600[1], 36640[1], 43752[1], 50430[1], 50431[1], 50432[1], 50436[1], 50437[1], 50551[1], 50555[1], 50557[1], 50570[1], 50572[1], 50684[1], 50955[1], 50974[1], 51701[1], 51702[1], 51703[1], 62320[0], 62321[0], 62322[0], 62323[0], 62324[0], 62325[0], 62326[0], 62327[0], 64400[0], 64405[0], 64408[0], 64415[0], 64416[0], 64417[0], 64418[0], 64420[0], 64421[0], 64425[0], 64430[0], 64435[0], 64445[0], 64446[0], 64447[0], 64448[0], 64449[0], 64450[0], 64451[0], 64454[0], 64461[0], 64462[0], 64463[0], 64479[0], 64480[0], 64483[0], 64484[0], 64486[0], 64487[0], 64488[0], 64489[0], 64490[0], 64491[0], 64492[0], 64493[0], 64494[0], 64495[0], 64505[0], 64510[0], 64517[0], 64520[0], 64530[0], 69990[0], 76000[1], 77001[1], 77002[1], 92012[1], 92014[1], 93000[1], 93005[1], 93010[1], 93040[1], 93041[1], 93042[1], 93318[1], 93355[1], 94002[1], 94200[1], 94680[1], 94681[1], 94690[1], 95812[1], 95813[1], 95816[1], 95819[1], 95822[1], 95829[1], 95955[1], 96360[1], 96361[1], 96365[1], 96366[1], 96367[1], 96368[1], 96372[1], 96374[1], 96375[1], 96376[1], 96377[1], 96523[0], 97597[1], 97598[1], 97602[1], 99155[0], 99156[0], 99157[0], 99211[1], 99212[1], 99213[1], 99214[1], 99215[1], 99217[1], 99218[1], 99219[1], 99220[1], 99221[1], 99222[1], 99223[1], 99231[1], 99232[1], 99233[1], 99234[1], 99235[1], 99236[1], 99238[1], 99239[1], 99241[1], 99242[1], 99243[1], 99244[1], 99245[1], 99251[1], 99252[1], 99253[1], 99254[1], 99255[1], 99291[1], 99292[1], 99304[1], 99305[1], 99306[1], 99307[1], 99308[1], 99309[1], 99310[1], 99315[1], 99316[1], 99334[1], 99335[1], 99336[1], 99337[1], 99347[1], 99348[1], 99349[1], 99350[1], 99374[1], 99375[1], 99377[1], 99378[1], 99446[0], 99447[0], 99448[0], 99449[0], 99451[0], 99452[0], 99495[0], 99496[0], G0463[1], G0471[1]
50570	0213T[0], 0216T[0], 0596T[1], 0597T[1], 0708T[1], 0709T[1], 11000[1], 11001[1], 11004[1], 11005[1], 11006[1], 11042[1], 11043[1], 11044[1], 11045[1], 11046[1], 11047[1], 12001[1], 12002[1], 12004[1], 12005[1], 12006[1], 12007[1], 12011[1], 12013[1], 12014[1], 12015[1], 12016[1], 12017[1], 12018[1], 12020[1], 12021[1], 12031[1], 12032[1], 12034[1], 12035[1], 12036[1], 12037[1], 12041[1], 12042[1], 12044[1], 12045[1], 12046[1], 12047[1], 12051[1], 12052[1], 12053[1], 12054[1], 12055[1], 12056[1], 12057[1], 13100[1], 13101[1], 13102[1], 13120[1], 13121[1], 13122[1], 13131[1], 13132[1], 13133[1], 13151[1], 13152[1], 13153[1], 36000[1], 36400[1], 36405[1], 36406[1], 36410[1], 36420[1], 36425[1], 36430[1], 36440[1], 36591[0], 36592[0], 36600[1], 36640[1], 43752[1], 50391[1], 50430[1], 50431[1], 50432[1], 50436[1], 50437[1], 50684[1], 51701[1], 51702[1], 51703[1], 62320[0], 62321[0], 62322[0], 62323[0], 62324[0], 62325[0], 62326[0], 62327[0], 64400[0], 64405[0], 64408[0], 64415[0], 64416[0], 64417[0], 64418[0], 64420[0], 64421[0], 64425[0], 64430[0], 64435[0], 64445[0], 64446[0], 64447[0], 64448[0], 64449[0], 64450[0], 64451[0], 64454[0], 64461[0], 64462[0], 64463[0], 64479[0], 64480[0], 64483[0], 64484[0], 64486[0], 64487[0], 64488[0], 64489[0], 64490[0], 64491[0], 64492[0], 64493[0], 64494[0], 64495[0], 64505[0], 64510[0], 64517[0], 64520[0], 64530[0], 69990[0], 76000[1], 77001[1], 77002[1], 92012[1], 92014[1], 93000[1], 93005[1], 93010[1], 93040[1], 93041[1], 93042[1], 93318[1],

0 = Modifier usage not allowed or inappropriate 1 = Modifier usage allowed

Appendix A: NCCI - CPT Codes

Code 1	Code 2
	93355[1], 94002[1], 94200[1], 94680[1], 94681[1], 94690[1], 95812[1], 95813[1], 95816[1], 95819[1], 95822[1], 95829[1], 95955[1], 96360[1], 96361[1], 96365[1], 96366[1], 96367[1], 96368[1], 96372[1], 96374[1], 96375[1], 96376[1], 96377[1], 96523[0], 97597[1], 97598[1], 97602[1], 99155[0], 99156[0], 99157[0], 99211[1], 99212[1], 99213[1], 99214[1], 99215[1], 99217[1], 99218[1], 99219[1], 99220[1], 99221[1], 99222[1], 99223[1], 99231[1], 99232[1], 99233[1], 99234[1], 99235[1], 99236[1], 99238[1], 99239[1], 99241[1], 99242[1], 99243[1], 99244[1], 99245[1], 99251[1], 99252[1], 99253[1], 99254[1], 99255[1], 99291[1], 99292[1], 99304[1], 99305[1], 99306[1], 99307[1], 99308[1], 99309[1], 99310[1], 99315[1], 99316[1], 99334[1], 99335[1], 99336[1], 99337[1], 99347[1], 99348[1], 99349[1], 99350[1], 99374[1], 99375[1], 99377[1], 99378[1], 99446[0], 99447[0], 99448[0], 99449[0], 99451[0], 99452[0], 99495[1], 99496[1], G0463[1], G0471[1]
50572	0213T[0], 0216T[0], 0596T[1], 0597T[1], 0708T[1], 0709T[1], 11000[1], 11001[1], 11004[1], 11005[1], 11006[1], 11042[1], 11043[1], 11044[1], 11045[1], 11046[1], 11047[1], 12001[1], 12002[1], 12004[1], 12005[1], 12006[1], 12007[1], 12011[1], 12013[1], 12014[1], 12015[1], 12016[1], 12017[1], 12018[1], 12020[1], 12021[1], 12031[1], 12032[1], 12034[1], 12035[1], 12036[1], 12037[1], 12041[1], 12042[1], 12044[1], 12045[1], 12046[1], 12047[1], 12051[1], 12052[1], 12053[1], 12054[1], 12055[1], 12056[1], 12057[1], 13100[1], 13101[1], 13102[1], 13120[1], 13121[1], 13122[1], 13131[1], 13132[1], 13133[1], 13151[1], 13152[1], 13153[1], 36000[1], 36400[1], 36405[1], 36406[1], 36410[1], 36420[1], 36425[1], 36430[1], 36440[1], 36591[0], 36592[0], 36600[1], 36640[1], 43752[1], 50432[1], 50436[1], 50437[1], 50570[1], 50684[1], 50706[1], 51701[1], 51702[1], 51703[1], 62320[0], 62321[0], 62322[0], 62323[0], 62324[0], 62325[0], 62326[0], 62327[0], 64400[0], 64405[0], 64408[0], 64415[0], 64416[0], 64417[0], 64418[0], 64420[0], 64421[0], 64425[0], 64430[0], 64435[0], 64445[0], 64446[0], 64447[0], 64448[0], 64449[0], 64450[0], 64451[0], 64454[0], 64461[0], 64462[0], 64463[0], 64479[0], 64480[0], 64483[0], 64484[0], 64486[0], 64487[0], 64488[0], 64489[0], 64490[0], 64491[0], 64492[0], 64493[0], 64494[0], 64495[0], 64505[0], 64510[0], 64517[0], 64520[0], 64530[0], 69990[0], 76000[1], 77001[1], 77002[1], 92012[1], 92014[1], 93000[1], 93005[1], 93010[1], 93040[1], 93041[1], 93042[1], 93318[1], 93355[1], 94002[1], 94200[1], 94680[1], 94681[1], 94690[1], 95812[1], 95813[1], 95816[1], 95819[1], 95822[1], 95829[1], 95955[1], 96360[1], 96361[1], 96365[1], 96366[1], 96367[1], 96368[1], 96372[1], 96374[1], 96375[1], 96376[1], 96377[1], 96523[0], 97597[1], 97598[1], 97602[1], 99155[0], 99156[0], 99157[0], 99211[1], 99212[1], 99213[1], 99214[1], 99215[1], 99217[1], 99218[1], 99219[1], 99220[1], 99221[1], 99222[1], 99223[1], 99231[1], 99232[1], 99233[1], 99234[1], 99235[1], 99236[1], 99238[1], 99239[1], 99241[1], 99242[1], 99243[1], 99244[1], 99245[1], 99251[1], 99252[1], 99253[1], 99254[1], 99255[1], 99291[1], 99292[1], 99304[1], 99305[1], 99306[1], 99307[1], 99308[1], 99309[1], 99310[1], 99315[1], 99316[1], 99334[1], 99335[1], 99336[1], 99337[1], 99347[1], 99348[1], 99349[1], 99350[1], 99374[1], 99375[1], 99377[1], 99378[1], 99446[0], 99447[0], 99448[0], 99449[0], 99451[0], 99452[0], 99495[1], 99496[1], G0463[1], G0471[1]
50574	0213T[0], 0216T[0], 0596T[1], 0597T[1], 0708T[1], 0709T[1], 10005[1], 10007[1], 10009[1], 10011[1], 10021[1], 11000[1], 11001[1], 11004[1], 11005[1], 11006[1], 11042[1], 11043[1], 11044[1], 11045[1], 11046[1], 11047[1], 12001[1], 12002[1], 12004[1], 12005[1], 12006[1], 12007[1], 12011[1], 12013[1], 12014[1], 12015[1], 12016[1], 12017[1], 12018[1], 12020[1], 12021[1], 12031[1], 12032[1], 12034[1], 12035[1], 12036[1], 12037[1], 12041[1], 12042[1], 12044[1], 12045[1], 12046[1], 12047[1], 12051[1], 12052[1], 12053[1], 12054[1], 12055[1], 12056[1], 12057[1], 13100[1], 13101[1], 13102[1], 13120[1], 13121[1], 13122[1], 13131[1], 13132[1], 13133[1], 13151[1], 13152[1], 13153[1], 36000[1], 36400[1], 36405[1], 36406[1], 36410[1], 36420[1], 36425[1], 36430[1], 36440[1], 36591[0], 36592[0], 36600[1], 36640[1], 43752[1], 50430[1], 50431[1], 50432[1], 50436[1], 50437[1], 50562[1], 50570[1], 50606[1], 50684[1], 51701[1], 51702[1], 51703[1], 62320[0], 62321[0], 62322[0], 62323[0], 62324[0], 62325[0], 62326[0], 62327[0], 64400[0], 64405[0], 64408[0], 64415[0], 64416[0], 64417[0], 64418[0], 64420[0], 64421[0], 64425[0], 64430[0], 64435[0], 64445[0], 64446[0], 64447[0], 64448[0], 64449[0], 64450[0], 64451[0], 64454[0], 64461[0], 64462[0], 64463[0], 64479[0], 64480[0], 64483[0], 64484[0], 64486[0], 64487[0], 64488[0], 64489[0], 64490[0], 64491[0], 64492[0], 64493[0], 64494[0], 64495[0], 64505[0], 64510[0], 64517[0], 64520[0], 64530[0], 69990[0], 76000[1], 77001[1], 77002[1], 92012[1], 92014[1], 93000[1], 93005[1], 93010[1], 93040[1], 93041[1], 93042[1], 93318[1], 93355[1], 94002[1], 94200[1], 94680[1], 94681[1], 94690[1], 95812[1], 95813[1], 95816[1], 95819[1], 95822[1], 95829[1], 95955[1], 96360[1], 96361[1], 96365[1], 96366[1], 96367[1], 96368[1], 96372[1], 96374[1], 96375[1], 96376[1], 96377[1], 96523[0], 97597[1], 97598[1], 97602[1], 99155[0], 99156[0], 99157[0], 99211[1], 99212[1], 99213[1], 99214[1], 99215[1], 99217[1], 99218[1], 99219[1], 99220[1], 99221[1], 99222[1], 99223[1], 99231[1], 99232[1], 99233[1], 99234[1], 99235[1], 99236[1], 99238[1], 99239[1], 99241[1], 99242[1], 99243[1], 99244[1], 99245[1], 99251[1], 99252[1], 99253[1], 99254[1], 99255[1], 99291[1], 99292[1], 99304[1], 99305[1], 99306[1], 99307[1], 99308[1], 99309[1], 99310[1], 99315[1], 99316[1], 99334[1], 99335[1], 99336[1], 99337[1], 99347[1], 99348[1], 99349[1], 99350[1], 99374[1], 99375[1], 99377[1], 99378[1], 99446[0], 99447[0], 99448[0], 99449[0], 99451[0], 99452[0], 99495[1], 99496[1], G0463[1], G0471[1]
50575	0213T[0], 0216T[0], 0596T[1], 0597T[1], 0708T[1], 0709T[1], 11000[1], 11001[1], 11004[1], 11005[1], 11006[1], 11042[1], 11043[1], 11044[1], 11045[1], 11046[1], 11047[1], 12001[1], 12002[1], 12004[1], 12005[1], 12006[1], 12007[1], 12011[1], 12013[1], 12014[1], 12015[1], 12016[1], 12017[1], 12018[1], 12020[1], 12021[1], 12031[1], 12032[1], 12034[1], 12035[1], 12036[1], 12037[1], 12041[1], 12042[1], 12044[1], 12045[1], 12046[1], 12047[1], 12051[1], 12052[1], 12053[1], 12054[1], 12055[1], 12056[1], 12057[1], 13100[1], 13101[1], 13102[1], 13120[1], 13121[1], 13122[1], 13131[1], 13132[1], 13133[1], 13151[1], 13152[1], 13153[1], 36000[1], 36400[1], 36405[1], 36406[1], 36410[1], 36420[1], 36425[1], 36430[1], 36440[1], 36591[0], 36592[0], 36600[1], 36640[1], 43752[1], 50382[1], 50384[1], 50387[1], 50436[1], 50437[1], 50562[1], 50570[1], 50605[1], 50684[1], 50693[1], 50694[1], 50695[1], 51701[1], 51702[1], 51703[1], 62320[0], 62321[0], 62322[0], 62323[0], 62324[0], 62325[0], 62326[0], 62327[0], 64400[0], 64405[0], 64408[0], 64415[0], 64416[0], 64417[0], 64418[0], 64420[0], 64421[0], 64425[0], 64430[0], 64435[0], 64445[0], 64446[0], 64447[0], 64448[0], 64449[0], 64450[0], 64451[0], 64454[0], 64461[0], 64462[0], 64463[0], 64479[0], 64480[0], 64483[0], 64484[0], 64486[0], 64487[0], 64488[0], 64489[0], 64490[0], 64491[0], 64492[0], 64493[0], 64494[0], 64495[0], 64505[0], 64510[0], 64517[0], 64520[0], 64530[0], 69990[0], 76000[1], 77001[1], 77002[1], 92012[1], 92014[1], 93000[1], 93005[1], 93010[1], 93040[1], 93041[1], 93042[1], 93318[1], 93355[1], 94002[1], 94200[1], 94680[1], 94681[1], 94690[1], 95812[1], 95813[1], 95816[1], 95819[1], 95822[1], 95829[1], 95955[1], 96360[1], 96361[1], 96365[1], 96366[1], 96367[1], 96368[1], 96372[1], 96374[1], 96375[1], 96376[1], 96377[1], 96523[0], 97597[1], 97598[1], 97602[1], 99155[0], 99156[0], 99157[0], 99211[1], 99212[1], 99213[1], 99214[1], 99215[1], 99217[1], 99218[1], 99219[1], 99220[1], 99221[1], 99222[1], 99223[1], 99231[1], 99232[1], 99233[1], 99234[1], 99235[1], 99236[1], 99238[1], 99239[1], 99241[1], 99242[1], 99243[1], 99244[1], 99245[1], 99251[1], 99252[1], 99253[1], 99254[1], 99255[1], 99291[1], 99292[1], 99304[1], 99305[1], 99306[1], 99307[1], 99308[1], 99309[1], 99310[1], 99315[1], 99316[1], 99334[1], 99335[1], 99336[1], 99337[1], 99347[1], 99348[1], 99349[1], 99350[1], 99374[1], 99375[1], 99377[1], 99378[1], 99446[0], 99447[0], 99448[0], 99449[0], 99451[0], 99452[0], 99495[1], 99496[1], G0463[1], G0471[1]
50576	0213T[0], 0216T[0], 0596T[1], 0597T[1], 0708T[1], 0709T[1], 10005[1], 10007[1], 10009[1], 10011[1], 10021[1], 11000[1], 11001[1], 11004[1], 11005[1], 11006[1], 11042[1], 11043[1], 11044[1], 11045[1], 11046[1], 11047[1], 12001[1], 12002[1], 12004[1], 12005[1], 12006[1], 12007[1], 12011[1], 12013[1], 12014[1], 12015[1], 12016[1], 12017[1], 12018[1], 12020[1], 12021[1], 12031[1], 12032[1], 12034[1], 12035[1], 12036[1], 12037[1], 12041[1], 12042[1], 12044[1], 12045[1], 12046[1], 12047[1], 12051[1], 12052[1], 12053[1], 12054[1], 12055[1], 12056[1], 12057[1], 13100[1], 13101[1], 13102[1], 13120[1], 13121[1], 13122[1], 13131[1], 13132[1], 13133[1], 13151[1], 13152[1], 13153[1], 36000[1], 36400[1], 36405[1], 36406[1], 36410[1], 36420[1], 36425[1], 36430[1], 36440[1], 36591[0], 36592[0], 36600[1], 36640[1], 43752[1], 50432[1], 50436[1], 50437[1], 50555[0], 50562[1], 50570[1], 50574[1], 50684[1], 50955[1], 50974[1], 51701[1], 51702[1], 51703[1], 62320[0], 62321[0], 62322[0], 62323[0], 62324[0], 62325[0], 62326[0], 62327[0], 64400[0], 64405[0], 64408[0], 64415[0], 64416[0], 64417[0], 64418[0], 64420[0], 64421[0], 64425[0], 64430[0], 64435[0], 64445[0], 64446[0], 64447[0], 64448[0], 64449[0], 64450[0], 64451[0], 64454[0], 64461[0], 64462[0], 64463[0], 64479[0], 64480[0], 64483[0], 64484[0], 64486[0], 64487[0], 64488[0], 64489[0], 64490[0], 64491[0], 64492[0], 64493[0], 64494[0], 64495[0], 64505[0], 64510[0], 64517[0], 64520[0], 64530[0], 69990[0], 76000[1], 77001[1], 77002[1], 92012[1], 92014[1], 93000[1], 93005[1], 93010[1], 93040[1], 93041[1], 93042[1], 93318[1], 93355[1], 94002[1], 94200[1], 94680[1], 94681[1], 94690[1], 95812[1], 95813[1], 95816[1], 95819[1], 95822[1], 95829[1], 95955[1], 96360[1], 96361[1], 96365[1], 96366[1], 96367[1], 96368[1], 96372[1], 96374[1], 96375[1], 96376[1], 96377[1], 96523[0], 97597[1], 97598[1], 97602[1], 99155[0], 99156[0], 99157[0], 99211[1], 99212[1], 99213[1], 99214[1], 99215[1], 99217[1], 99218[1], 99219[1], 99220[1], 99221[1], 99222[1], 99223[1], 99231[1], 99232[1], 99233[1], 99234[1], 99235[1], 99236[1], 99238[1], 99239[1], 99241[1], 99242[1], 99243[1], 99244[1], 99245[1], 99251[1], 99252[1], 99253[1], 99254[1], 99255[1], 99291[1], 99292[1], 99304[1], 99305[1], 99306[1], 99307[1], 99308[1], 99309[1], 99310[1], 99315[1], 99316[1], 99334[1], 99335[1], 99336[1], 99337[1], 99347[1], 99348[1], 99349[1], 99350[1], 99374[1], 99375[1], 99377[1], 99378[1], 99446[0], 99447[0], 99448[0], 99449[0], 99451[0], 99452[0], 99495[1], 99496[1], G0463[1], G0471[1]
50580	0213T[0], 0216T[0], 0596T[1], 0597T[1], 0708T[1], 0709T[1], 11000[1], 11001[1], 11004[1], 11005[1], 11006[1], 11042[1], 11043[1], 11044[1], 11045[1], 11046[1], 11047[1], 12001[1], 12002[1], 12004[1], 12005[1], 12006[1], 12007[1], 12011[1], 12013[1], 12014[1], 12015[1], 12016[1], 12017[1], 12018[1], 12020[1], 12021[1], 12031[1], 12032[1], 12034[1], 12035[1], 12036[1], 12037[1], 12041[1], 12042[1], 12044[1], 12045[1], 12046[1], 12047[1], 12051[1], 12052[1], 12053[1], 12054[1], 12055[1], 12056[1], 12057[1], 13100[1], 13101[1], 13102[1], 13120[1], 13121[1], 13122[1], 13131[1], 13132[1], 13133[1], 13151[1], 13152[1], 13153[1], 36000[1], 36400[1], 36405[1], 36406[1], 36410[1], 36420[1], 36425[1], 36430[1], 36440[1], 36591[0], 36592[0], 36600[1], 36640[1], 43752[1], 50432[1], 50436[1], 50437[1], 50562[1], 50570[1], 50684[1], 51701[1], 51702[1], 51703[1], 62320[0], 62321[0], 62322[0], 62323[0], 62324[0], 62325[0], 62326[0], 62327[0], 64400[0], 64405[0], 64408[0], 64415[0], 64416[0], 64417[0], 64418[0], 64420[0], 64421[0], 64425[0], 64430[0], 64435[0], 64445[0], 64446[0], 64447[0], 64448[0], 64449[0], 64450[0], 64451[0], 64454[0], 64461[0], 64462[0], 64463[0], 64479[0], 64480[0], 64483[0], 64484[0], 64486[0], 64487[0], 64488[0], 64489[0], 64490[0], 64491[0], 64492[0], 64493[0], 64494[0], 64495[0], 64505[0], 64510[0], 64517[0], 64520[0], 64530[0], 69990[0], 76000[1], 77001[1], 77002[1], 92012[1], 92014[1], 93000[1], 93005[1], 93010[1], 93040[1], 93041[1], 93042[1], 93318[1], 93355[1], 94002[1], 94200[1], 94680[1], 94681[1], 94690[1], 95812[1], 95813[1], 95816[1], 95819[1], 95822[1], 95829[1], 95955[1], 96360[1], 96361[1], 96365[1], 96366[1], 96367[1], 96368[1], 96372[1], 96374[1], 96375[1], 96376[1], 96377[1], 96523[0], 97597[1], 97598[1], 97602[1], 99155[0], 99156[0], 99157[0], 99211[1], 99212[1], 99213[1], 99214[1], 99215[1], 99217[1], 99218[1], 99219[1], 99220[1], 99221[1],

0 = Modifier usage not allowed or inappropriate 1 = Modifier usage allowed

Code 1	Code 2
	99222[1], 99223[1], 99231[1], 99232[1], 99233[1], 99234[1], 99235[1], 99236[1], 99238[1], 99239[1], 99241[1], 99242[1], 99243[1], 99244[1], 99245[1], 99251[1], 99252[1], 99253[1], 99254[1], 99255[1], 99291[1], 99292[1], 99304[1], 99305[1], 99306[1], 99307[1], 99308[1], 99309[1], 99310[1], 99315[1], 99316[1], 99334[1], 99335[1], 99336[1], 99337[1], 99347[1], 99348[1], 99349[1], 99350[1], 99374[1], 99375[1], 99377[1], 99378[1], 99446[0], 99447[0], 99448[0], 99449[0], 99451[0], 99452[0], 99495[1], 99496[1], G0463[1], G0471[1]
50590	0213T[0], 0216T[0], 0596T[1], 0597T[1], 0708T[1], 0709T[1], 12001[1], 12002[1], 12004[1], 12005[1], 12006[1], 12007[1], 12011[1], 12013[1], 12014[1], 12015[1], 12016[1], 12017[1], 12018[1], 12020[1], 12021[1], 12031[1], 12032[1], 12034[1], 12035[1], 12036[1], 12037[1], 12041[1], 12042[1], 12044[1], 12045[1], 12046[1], 12047[1], 12051[1], 12052[1], 12053[1], 12054[1], 12055[1], 12056[1], 12057[1], 13100[1], 13101[1], 13102[1], 13120[1], 13121[1], 13122[1], 13131[1], 13132[1], 13133[1], 13151[1], 13152[1], 13153[1], 36000[1], 36400[1], 36405[1], 36406[1], 36410[1], 36420[1], 36425[1], 36430[1], 36440[1], 36591[0], 36592[0], 36600[1], 36640[1], 43752[1], 51701[1], 51702[1], 51703[1], 52005[1], 52320[1], 52325[1], 52330[1], 52351[1], 52352[1], 52353[1], 52356[1], 62320[0], 62321[0], 62322[0], 62323[0], 62324[0], 62325[0], 62326[0], 62327[0], 64400[0], 64405[0], 64408[0], 64415[0], 64416[0], 64417[0], 64418[0], 64420[0], 64421[0], 64425[0], 64430[0], 64435[0], 64445[0], 64446[0], 64447[0], 64448[0], 64449[0], 64450[0], 64451[0], 64454[0], 64461[0], 64462[0], 64463[0], 64479[0], 64480[0], 64483[0], 64484[0], 64486[0], 64487[0], 64488[0], 64489[0], 64490[0], 64491[0], 64492[0], 64493[0], 64494[0], 64495[0], 64505[0], 64510[0], 64517[0], 64520[0], 64530[0], 69990[0], 76000[1], 77001[1], 92012[1], 92014[1], 93000[1], 93005[1], 93010[1], 93040[1], 93041[1], 93042[1], 93318[1], 93355[1], 94002[1], 94200[1], 94680[1], 94681[1], 94690[1], 95812[1], 95813[1], 95816[1], 95819[1], 95822[1], 95829[1], 95955[1], 96360[1], 96361[1], 96365[1], 96366[1], 96367[1], 96368[1], 96372[1], 96374[1], 96375[1], 96376[1], 96377[1], 96523[0], 99155[0], 99156[0], 99157[0], 99211[1], 99212[1], 99213[1], 99214[1], 99215[1], 99217[1], 99218[1], 99219[1], 99220[1], 99221[1], 99222[1], 99223[1], 99231[1], 99232[1], 99233[1], 99234[1], 99235[1], 99236[1], 99238[1], 99239[1], 99241[1], 99242[1], 99243[1], 99244[1], 99245[1], 99251[1], 99252[1], 99253[1], 99254[1], 99255[1], 99291[1], 99292[1], 99304[1], 99305[1], 99306[1], 99307[1], 99308[1], 99309[1], 99310[1], 99315[1], 99316[1], 99334[1], 99335[1], 99336[1], 99337[1], 99347[1], 99348[1], 99349[1], 99350[1], 99374[1], 99375[1], 99377[1], 99378[1], 99446[0], 99447[0], 99448[0], 99449[0], 99451[0], 99452[0], 99495[0], 99496[0], G0463[1], G0471[1]
50592	0213T[0], 0216T[0], 0596T[1], 0597T[1], 0708T[1], 0709T[1], 12001[1], 12002[1], 12004[1], 12005[1], 12006[1], 12007[1], 12011[1], 12013[1], 12014[1], 12015[1], 12016[1], 12017[1], 12018[1], 12020[1], 12021[1], 12031[1], 12032[1], 12034[1], 12035[1], 12036[1], 12037[1], 12041[1], 12042[1], 12044[1], 12045[1], 12046[1], 12047[1], 12051[1], 12052[1], 12053[1], 12054[1], 12055[1], 12056[1], 12057[1], 13100[1], 13101[1], 13102[1], 13120[1], 13121[1], 13122[1], 13131[1], 13132[1], 13133[1], 13151[1], 13152[1], 13153[1], 36000[1], 36400[1], 36405[1], 36406[1], 36410[1], 36420[1], 36425[1], 36430[1], 36440[1], 36591[0], 36592[0], 36600[1], 36640[1], 43752[1], 51701[1], 51702[1], 51703[1], 62320[0], 62321[0], 62322[0], 62323[0], 62324[0], 62325[0], 62326[0], 62327[0], 64400[0], 64405[0], 64408[0], 64415[0], 64416[0], 64417[0], 64418[0], 64420[0], 64421[0], 64425[0], 64430[0], 64435[0], 64445[0], 64446[0], 64447[0], 64448[0], 64449[0], 64450[0], 64451[0], 64454[0], 64461[0], 64462[0], 64463[0], 64479[0], 64480[0], 64483[0], 64484[0], 64486[0], 64487[0], 64488[0], 64489[0], 64490[0], 64491[0], 64492[0], 64493[0], 64494[0], 64495[0], 64505[0], 64510[0], 64517[0], 64520[0], 64530[0], 69990[0], 76000[1], 76380[1], 76942[1], 76998[1], 77001[1], 77002[1], 77012[1], 77021[1], 92012[1], 92014[1], 93000[1], 93005[1], 93010[1], 93040[1], 93041[1], 93042[1], 93318[1], 93355[1], 94002[1], 94200[1], 94680[1], 94681[1], 94690[1], 95812[1], 95813[1], 95816[1], 95819[1], 95822[1], 95829[1], 95955[1], 96360[1], 96361[1], 96365[1], 96366[1], 96367[1], 96368[1], 96372[1], 96374[1], 96375[1], 96376[1], 96377[1], 96523[0], 99155[0], 99156[0], 99157[0], 99211[1], 99212[1], 99213[1], 99214[1], 99215[1], 99217[1], 99218[1], 99219[1], 99220[1], 99221[1], 99222[1], 99223[1], 99231[1], 99232[1], 99233[1], 99234[1], 99235[1], 99236[1], 99238[1], 99239[1], 99241[1], 99242[1], 99243[1], 99244[1], 99245[1], 99251[1], 99252[1], 99253[1], 99254[1], 99255[1], 99291[1], 99292[1], 99304[1], 99305[1], 99306[1], 99307[1], 99308[1], 99309[1], 99310[1], 99315[1], 99316[1], 99334[1], 99335[1], 99336[1], 99337[1], 99347[1], 99348[1], 99349[1], 99350[1], 99374[1], 99375[1], 99377[1], 99378[1], 99446[0], 99447[0], 99448[0], 99449[0], 99451[0], 99452[0], 99495[0], 99496[0], G0463[1], G0471[1], J0670[1], J2001[1]
50593	0213T[0], 0216T[0], 0708T[1], 0709T[1], 12001[1], 12002[1], 12004[1], 12005[1], 12006[1], 12007[1], 12011[1], 12013[1], 12014[1], 12015[1], 12016[1], 12017[1], 12018[1], 12020[1], 12021[1], 12031[1], 12032[1], 12034[1], 12035[1], 12036[1], 12037[1], 12041[1], 12042[1], 12044[1], 12045[1], 12046[1], 12047[1], 12051[1], 12052[1], 12053[1], 12054[1], 12055[1], 12056[1], 12057[1], 13100[1], 13101[1], 13102[1], 13120[1], 13121[1], 13122[1], 13131[1], 13132[1], 13133[1], 13151[1], 13152[1], 13153[1], 36000[1], 36400[1], 36405[1], 36406[1], 36410[1], 36420[1], 36425[1], 36430[1], 36440[1], 36591[0], 36592[0], 36600[1], 36640[1], 43752[1], 50592[0], 62320[0], 62321[0], 62322[0], 62323[0], 62324[0], 62325[0], 62326[0], 62327[0], 64400[0], 64405[0], 64408[0], 64415[0], 64416[0], 64417[0], 64418[0], 64420[0], 64421[0], 64425[0], 64430[0], 64435[0], 64445[0], 64446[0], 64447[0], 64448[0], 64449[0], 64450[0], 64451[0], 64454[0], 64461[0], 64462[0], 64463[0], 64479[0], 64480[0], 64483[0], 64484[0], 64486[0], 64487[0], 64488[0], 64489[0], 64490[0], 64491[0], 64492[0], 64493[0], 64494[0], 64495[0], 64505[0], 64510[0], 64517[0], 64520[0], 64530[0], 69990[0], 76000[1], 76380[1], 76942[1], 76998[1], 77001[1], 77002[1], 77012[1], 77021[1], 92012[1], 92014[1], 93000[1], 93005[1], 93010[1], 93040[1], 93041[1], 93042[1], 93318[1], 93355[1], 94002[1], 94200[1], 94680[1], 94681[1], 94690[1], 95812[1], 95813[1], 95816[1], 95819[1], 95822[1], 95829[1], 95955[1], 96360[1], 96361[1], 96365[1], 96366[1], 96367[1], 96368[1], 96372[1], 96374[1], 96375[1], 96376[1], 96377[1], 96523[0], 99155[0], 99156[0], 99157[0], 99211[1], 99212[1], 99213[1], 99214[1], 99215[1], 99217[1], 99218[1], 99219[1], 99220[1], 99221[1], 99222[1], 99223[1], 99231[1], 99232[1], 99233[1], 99234[1], 99235[1], 99236[1], 99238[1], 99239[1], 99241[1], 99242[1], 99243[1], 99244[1], 99245[1], 99251[1], 99252[1], 99253[1], 99254[1], 99255[1], 99291[1], 99292[1], 99304[1], 99305[1], 99306[1], 99307[1], 99308[1], 99309[1], 99310[1], 99315[1], 99316[1], 99334[1], 99335[1], 99336[1], 99337[1], 99347[1], 99348[1], 99349[1], 99350[1], 99374[1], 99375[1], 99377[1], 99378[1], 99446[0], 99447[0], 99448[0], 99449[0], 99451[0], 99452[0], 99495[0], 99496[0], G0463[1], J0670[1], J2001[1]
50600	00910[0], 0213T[0], 0216T[0], 0596T[1], 0597T[1], 0708T[1], 0709T[1], 11000[1], 11001[1], 11004[1], 11005[1], 11006[1], 11042[1], 11043[1], 11044[1], 11045[1], 11046[1], 11047[1], 12001[1], 12002[1], 12004[1], 12005[1], 12006[1], 12007[1], 12011[1], 12013[1], 12014[1], 12015[1], 12016[1], 12017[1], 12018[1], 12020[1], 12021[1], 12031[1], 12032[1], 12034[1], 12035[1], 12036[1], 12037[1], 12041[1], 12042[1], 12044[1], 12045[1], 12046[1], 12047[1], 12051[1], 12052[1], 12053[1], 12054[1], 12055[1], 12056[1], 12057[1], 13100[1], 13101[1], 13102[1], 13120[1], 13121[1], 13122[1], 13131[1], 13132[1], 13133[1], 13151[1], 13152[1], 13153[1], 36000[1], 36400[1], 36405[1], 36406[1], 36410[1], 36420[1], 36425[1], 36430[1], 36440[1], 36591[0], 36592[0], 36600[1], 36640[1], 43752[1], 44602[1], 44603[1], 44604[1], 44605[1], 44950[0], 44970[0], 49000[0], 49002[1], 49010[0], 50100[1], 50650[1], 51701[1], 51702[1], 51703[1], 62320[0], 62321[0], 62322[0], 62323[0], 62324[0], 62325[0], 62326[0], 62327[0], 64400[0], 64405[0], 64408[0], 64415[0], 64416[0], 64417[0], 64418[0], 64420[0], 64421[0], 64425[0], 64430[0], 64435[0], 64445[0], 64446[0], 64447[0], 64448[0], 64449[0], 64450[0], 64451[0], 64454[0], 64461[0], 64462[0], 64463[0], 64479[0], 64480[0], 64483[0], 64484[0], 64486[0], 64487[0], 64488[0], 64489[0], 64490[0], 64491[0], 64492[0], 64493[0], 64494[0], 64495[0], 64505[0], 64510[0], 64517[0], 64520[0], 64530[0], 69990[0], 92012[1], 92014[1], 93000[1], 93005[1], 93010[1], 93040[1], 93041[1], 93042[1], 93318[1], 93355[1], 94002[1], 94200[1], 94680[1], 94681[1], 94690[1], 95812[1], 95813[1], 95816[1], 95819[1], 95822[1], 95829[1], 95955[1], 96360[1], 96361[1], 96365[1], 96366[1], 96367[1], 96368[1], 96372[1], 96374[1], 96375[1], 96376[1], 96377[1], 96523[0], 97597[1], 97598[1], 97602[1], 99155[0], 99156[0], 99157[0], 99211[1], 99212[1], 99213[1], 99214[1], 99215[1], 99217[1], 99218[1], 99219[1], 99220[1], 99221[1], 99222[1], 99223[1], 99231[1], 99232[1], 99233[1], 99234[1], 99235[1], 99236[1], 99238[1], 99239[1], 99241[1], 99242[1], 99243[1], 99244[1], 99245[1], 99251[1], 99252[1], 99253[1], 99254[1], 99255[1], 99291[1], 99292[1], 99304[1], 99305[1], 99306[1], 99307[1], 99308[1], 99309[1], 99310[1], 99315[1], 99316[1], 99334[1], 99335[1], 99336[1], 99337[1], 99347[1], 99348[1], 99349[1], 99350[1], 99374[1], 99375[1], 99377[1], 99378[1], 99446[0], 99447[0], 99448[0], 99449[0], 99451[0], 99452[0], 99495[0], 99496[0], G0463[1], G0471[1]
50605	00910[0], 0213T[0], 0216T[0], 0596T[1], 0597T[1], 0708T[1], 0709T[1], 11000[1], 11001[1], 11004[1], 11005[1], 11006[1], 11042[1], 11043[1], 11044[1], 11045[1], 11046[1], 11047[1], 12001[1], 12002[1], 12004[1], 12005[1], 12006[1], 12007[1], 12011[1], 12013[1], 12014[1], 12015[1], 12016[1], 12017[1], 12018[1], 12020[1], 12021[1], 12031[1], 12032[1], 12034[1], 12035[1], 12036[1], 12037[1], 12041[1], 12042[1], 12044[1], 12045[1], 12046[1], 12047[1], 12051[1], 12052[1], 12053[1], 12054[1], 12055[1], 12056[1], 12057[1], 13100[1], 13101[1], 13102[1], 13120[1], 13121[1], 13122[1], 13131[1], 13132[1], 13133[1], 13151[1], 13152[1], 13153[1], 36000[1], 36400[1], 36405[1], 36406[1], 36410[1], 36420[1], 36425[1], 36430[1], 36440[1], 36591[0], 36592[0], 36600[1], 36640[1], 43752[1], 44602[1], 44603[1], 44604[1], 44605[1], 44950[0], 44970[0], 49000[0], 49002[1], 49010[0], 50100[1], 50382[1], 50384[1], 50387[1], 50600[1], 50715[1], 51701[1], 51702[1], 51703[1], 62320[0], 62321[0], 62322[0], 62323[0], 62324[0], 62325[0], 62326[0], 62327[0], 64400[0], 64405[0], 64408[0], 64415[0], 64416[0], 64417[0], 64418[0], 64420[0], 64421[0], 64425[0], 64430[0], 64435[0], 64445[0], 64446[0], 64447[0], 64448[0], 64449[0], 64450[0], 64451[0], 64454[0], 64461[0], 64462[0], 64463[0], 64479[0], 64480[0], 64483[0], 64484[0], 64486[0], 64487[0], 64488[0], 64489[0], 64490[0], 64491[0], 64492[0], 64493[0], 64494[0], 64495[0], 64505[0], 64510[0], 64517[0], 64520[0], 64530[0], 69990[0], 92012[1], 92014[1], 93000[1], 93005[1], 93010[1], 93040[1], 93041[1], 93042[1], 93318[1], 93355[1], 94002[1], 94200[1], 94680[1], 94681[1], 94690[1], 95812[1], 95813[1], 95816[1], 95819[1], 95822[1], 95829[1], 95955[1], 96360[1], 96361[1], 96365[1], 96366[1], 96367[1], 96368[1], 96372[1], 96374[1], 96375[1], 96376[1], 96377[1], 96523[0], 97597[1], 97598[1], 97602[1], 99155[0], 99156[0], 99157[0], 99211[1], 99212[1], 99213[1], 99214[1], 99215[1], 99217[1], 99218[1], 99219[1], 99220[1], 99221[1], 99222[1], 99223[1], 99231[1], 99232[1], 99233[1], 99234[1], 99235[1], 99236[1], 99238[1], 99239[1], 99241[1], 99242[1], 99243[1], 99244[1], 99245[1], 99251[1], 99252[1], 99253[1], 99254[1], 99255[1], 99291[1], 99292[1], 99304[1], 99305[1], 99306[1], 99307[1], 99308[1], 99309[1], 99310[1], 99315[1], 99316[1], 99334[1], 99335[1], 99336[1], 99337[1], 99347[1], 99348[1], 99349[1], 99350[1], 99374[1], 99375[1], 99377[1], 99378[1], 99446[0], 99447[0], 99448[0], 99449[0], 99451[0], 99452[0], 99495[0], 99496[0], G0463[1], G0471[1]
50606	0213T[0], 0216T[0], 0596T[1], 0597T[1], 0708T[1], 0709T[1], 10005[1], 10007[1], 10009[1], 10011[1], 10021[1], 12001[0], 12002[1], 12004[1], 12005[1], 12006[1], 12007[1], 12011[1], 12013[1], 12014[1], 12015[1], 12016[1], 12017[1], 12018[1], 12020[1], 12021[1], 12031[1], 12032[1], 12034[1], 12035[1], 12036[1], 12037[1], 12041[1], 12042[1], 12044[1], 12045[1], 12046[1], 12047[1], 12051[1], 12052[1], 12053[1], 12054[1], 12055[1], 12056[1], 12057[1], 13100[1], 13101[1], 13102[1], 13120[1], 13121[1],

Appendix A: NCCI - CPT Codes

0 = Modifier usage not allowed or inappropriate 1 = Modifier usage allowed

Code 1	Code 2
	13122[1], 13131[1], 13132[1], 13133[1], 13151[1], 13152[1], 13153[1], 36000[1], 36400[1], 36405[1], 36406[1], 36410[1], 36420[1], 36425[1], 36430[1], 36440[1], 36600[1], 36640[1], 43752[1], 51701[1], 51702[1], 51703[1], 62320[0], 62321[0], 62322[0], 62323[0], 62324[0], 62325[0], 62326[0], 62327[0], 64400[0], 64405[0], 64408[0], 64415[0], 64416[0], 64417[0], 64418[0], 64420[0], 64421[0], 64425[0], 64430[0], 64435[0], 64445[0], 64446[0], 64447[0], 64448[0], 64449[0], 64450[0], 64451[0], 64454[0], 64461[0], 64463[0], 64479[0], 64483[0], 64486[0], 64487[0], 64488[0], 64489[0], 64490[0], 64493[0], 64505[0], 64510[0], 64517[0], 64520[0], 64530[0], 69990[0], 74425[1], 76000[1], 76380[1], 76942[1], 76998[1], 77002[1], 77012[1], 77021[1], 92012[1], 92014[1], 93000[1], 93005[1], 93010[1], 93040[1], 93041[1], 93042[1], 93318[1], 94002[1], 94200[1], 94680[1], 94681[1], 94690[1], 95812[1], 95813[1], 95816[1], 95819[1], 95822[1], 95829[1], 95955[1], 96360[1], 96365[1], 96372[1], 96374[1], 96375[1], 96376[1], 96377[1], 96523[0], 99155[0], 99156[0], 99157[0], 99211[1], 99212[1], 99213[1], 99214[1], 99215[1], 99217[1], 99218[1], 99219[1], 99220[1], 99221[1], 99222[1], 99223[1], 99231[1], 99232[1], 99233[1], 99234[1], 99235[1], 99236[1], 99238[1], 99239[1], 99241[1], 99242[1], 99243[1], 99244[1], 99245[1], 99251[1], 99252[1], 99253[1], 99254[1], 99255[1], 99291[1], 99292[1], 99304[1], 99305[1], 99306[1], 99307[1], 99308[1], 99309[1], 99310[1], 99315[1], 99316[1], 99334[1], 99335[1], 99336[1], 99337[1], 99347[1], 99348[1], 99349[1], 99350[1], 99374[1], 99375[1], 99377[1], 99378[1]
50610	00910[0], 0213T[0], 0216T[0], 0596T[1], 0597T[1], 0708T[1], 0709T[1], 11000[1], 11001[1], 11004[1], 11005[1], 11006[1], 11042[1], 11043[1], 11044[1], 11045[1], 11046[1], 11047[1], 12001[1], 12002[1], 12004[1], 12005[1], 12006[1], 12007[1], 12011[1], 12013[1], 12014[1], 12015[1], 12016[1], 12017[1], 12018[1], 12020[1], 12021[1], 12031[1], 12032[1], 12034[1], 12035[1], 12036[1], 12037[1], 12041[1], 12042[1], 12044[1], 12045[1], 12046[1], 12047[1], 12051[1], 12052[1], 12053[1], 12054[1], 12055[1], 12056[1], 12057[1], 13100[1], 13101[1], 13102[1], 13120[1], 13121[1], 13122[1], 13131[1], 13132[1], 13133[1], 13151[1], 13152[1], 13153[1], 36000[1], 36400[1], 36405[1], 36406[1], 36410[1], 36420[1], 36425[1], 36430[1], 36440[1], 36591[0], 36592[0], 36600[1], 36640[1], 43752[1], 44602[1], 44603[1], 44604[1], 44605[1], 44950[0], 44970[0], 49000[0], 49002[1], 49010[0], 50600[1], 50605[1], 50715[1], 50945[1], 51701[1], 51702[1], 51703[1], 62320[0], 62321[0], 62322[0], 62323[0], 62324[0], 62325[0], 62326[0], 62327[0], 64400[0], 64405[0], 64408[0], 64415[0], 64416[0], 64417[0], 64418[0], 64420[0], 64421[0], 64425[0], 64430[0], 64435[0], 64445[0], 64446[0], 64447[0], 64448[0], 64449[0], 64450[0], 64451[0], 64454[0], 64461[0], 64462[0], 64463[0], 64479[0], 64480[0], 64483[0], 64484[0], 64486[0], 64487[0], 64488[0], 64489[0], 64490[0], 64491[0], 64492[0], 64493[0], 64494[0], 64495[0], 64505[0], 64510[0], 64517[0], 64520[0], 64530[0], 69990[0], 92012[1], 92014[1], 93000[1], 93005[1], 93010[1], 93040[1], 93041[1], 93042[1], 93318[1], 93355[1], 94002[1], 94200[1], 94680[1], 94681[1], 94690[1], 95812[1], 95813[1], 95816[1], 95819[1], 95822[1], 95829[1], 95955[1], 96360[1], 96361[1], 96365[1], 96366[1], 96367[1], 96368[1], 96372[1], 96374[1], 96375[1], 96376[1], 96377[1], 96523[0], 97597[1], 97598[1], 97602[1], 99155[0], 99156[0], 99157[0], 99211[1], 99212[1], 99213[1], 99214[1], 99215[1], 99217[1], 99218[1], 99219[1], 99220[1], 99221[1], 99222[1], 99223[1], 99231[1], 99232[1], 99233[1], 99234[1], 99235[1], 99236[1], 99238[1], 99239[1], 99241[1], 99242[1], 99243[1], 99244[1], 99245[1], 99251[1], 99252[1], 99253[1], 99254[1], 99255[1], 99291[1], 99292[1], 99304[1], 99305[1], 99306[1], 99307[1], 99308[1], 99309[1], 99310[1], 99315[1], 99316[1], 99334[1], 99335[1], 99336[1], 99337[1], 99347[1], 99348[1], 99349[1], 99350[1], 99374[1], 99375[1], 99377[1], 99378[1], 99446[0], 99447[0], 99448[0], 99449[0], 99451[0], 99452[0], 99495[0], 99496[0], G0463[1], G0471[1]
50620	00910[0], 0213T[0], 0216T[0], 0596T[1], 0597T[1], 0708T[1], 0709T[1], 11000[1], 11001[1], 11004[1], 11005[1], 11006[1], 11042[1], 11043[1], 11044[1], 11045[1], 11046[1], 11047[1], 12001[1], 12002[1], 12004[1], 12005[1], 12006[1], 12007[1], 12011[1], 12013[1], 12014[1], 12015[1], 12016[1], 12017[1], 12018[1], 12020[1], 12021[1], 12031[1], 12032[1], 12034[1], 12035[1], 12036[1], 12037[1], 12041[1], 12042[1], 12044[1], 12045[1], 12046[1], 12047[1], 12051[1], 12052[1], 12053[1], 12054[1], 12055[1], 12056[1], 12057[1], 13100[1], 13101[1], 13102[1], 13120[1], 13121[1], 13122[1], 13131[1], 13132[1], 13133[1], 13151[1], 13152[1], 13153[1], 36000[1], 36400[1], 36405[1], 36406[1], 36410[1], 36420[1], 36425[1], 36430[1], 36440[1], 36591[0], 36592[0], 36600[1], 36640[1], 43752[1], 44602[1], 44603[1], 44604[1], 44605[1], 44950[0], 44970[0], 49000[0], 49002[1], 49010[0], 50600[1], 50605[1], 50715[1], 50945[1], 51701[1], 51702[1], 51703[1], 62320[0], 62321[0], 62322[0], 62323[0], 62324[0], 62325[0], 62326[0], 62327[0], 64400[0], 64405[0], 64408[0], 64415[0], 64416[0], 64417[0], 64418[0], 64420[0], 64421[0], 64425[0], 64430[0], 64435[0], 64445[0], 64446[0], 64447[0], 64448[0], 64449[0], 64450[0], 64451[0], 64454[0], 64461[0], 64462[0], 64463[0], 64479[0], 64480[0], 64483[0], 64484[0], 64486[0], 64487[0], 64488[0], 64489[0], 64490[0], 64491[0], 64492[0], 64493[0], 64494[0], 64495[0], 64505[0], 64510[0], 64517[0], 64520[0], 64530[0], 69990[0], 92012[1], 92014[1], 93000[1], 93005[1], 93010[1], 93040[1], 93041[1], 93042[1], 93318[1], 93355[1], 94002[1], 94200[1], 94680[1], 94681[1], 94690[1], 95812[1], 95813[1], 95816[1], 95819[1], 95822[1], 95829[1], 95955[1], 96360[1], 96361[1], 96365[1], 96366[1], 96367[1], 96368[1], 96372[1], 96374[1], 96375[1], 96376[1], 96377[1], 96523[0], 97597[1], 97598[1], 97602[1], 99155[0], 99156[0], 99157[0], 99211[1], 99212[1], 99213[1], 99214[1], 99215[1], 99217[1], 99218[1], 99219[1], 99220[1], 99221[1], 99222[1], 99223[1], 99231[1], 99232[1], 99233[1], 99234[1], 99235[1], 99236[1], 99238[1], 99239[1], 99241[1], 99242[1], 99243[1], 99244[1], 99245[1], 99251[1], 99252[1], 99253[1], 99254[1], 99255[1], 99291[1], 99292[1], 99304[1], 99305[1], 99306[1], 99307[1], 99308[1], 99309[1], 99310[1], 99315[1], 99316[1], 99334[1], 99335[1], 99336[1], 99337[1], 99347[1], 99348[1], 99349[1], 99350[1], 99374[1], 99375[1], 99377[1], 99378[1], 99446[0], 99447[0], 99448[0], 99449[0], 99451[0], 99452[0], 99495[0], 99496[0], G0463[1], G0471[1]
50630	00910[0], 0213T[0], 0216T[0], 0596T[1], 0597T[1], 0708T[1], 0709T[1], 11000[1], 11001[1], 11004[1], 11005[1], 11006[1], 11042[1], 11043[1], 11044[1], 11045[1], 11046[1], 11047[1], 12001[1], 12002[1], 12004[1], 12005[1], 12006[1], 12007[1], 12011[1], 12013[1], 12014[1], 12015[1], 12016[1], 12017[1], 12018[1], 12020[1], 12021[1], 12031[1], 12032[1], 12034[1], 12035[1], 12036[1], 12037[1], 12041[1], 12042[1], 12044[1], 12045[1], 12046[1], 12047[1], 12051[1], 12052[1], 12053[1], 12054[1], 12055[1], 12056[1], 12057[1], 13100[1], 13101[1], 13102[1], 13120[1], 13121[1], 13122[1], 13131[1], 13132[1], 13133[1], 13151[1], 13152[1], 13153[1], 36000[1], 36400[1], 36405[1], 36406[1], 36410[1], 36420[1], 36425[1], 36430[1], 36440[1], 36591[0], 36592[0], 36600[1], 36640[1], 43752[1], 44602[1], 44603[1], 44604[1], 44605[1], 44950[0], 44970[0], 49000[0], 49002[1], 49010[0], 50600[1], 50605[1], 50715[1], 50945[1], 51701[1], 51702[1], 51703[1], 52000[0], 62320[0], 62321[0], 62322[0], 62323[0], 62324[0], 62325[0], 62326[0], 62327[0], 64400[0], 64405[0], 64408[0], 64415[0], 64416[0], 64417[0], 64418[0], 64420[0], 64421[0], 64425[0], 64430[0], 64435[0], 64445[0], 64446[0], 64447[0], 64448[0], 64449[0], 64450[0], 64451[0], 64454[0], 64461[0], 64462[0], 64463[0], 64479[0], 64480[0], 64483[0], 64484[0], 64486[0], 64487[0], 64488[0], 64489[0], 64490[0], 64491[0], 64492[0], 64493[0], 64494[0], 64495[0], 64505[0], 64510[0], 64517[0], 64520[0], 64530[0], 69990[0], 92012[1], 92014[1], 93000[1], 93005[1], 93010[1], 93040[1], 93041[1], 93042[1], 93318[1], 93355[1], 94002[1], 94200[1], 94680[1], 94681[1], 94690[1], 95812[1], 95813[1], 95816[1], 95819[1], 95822[1], 95829[1], 95955[1], 96360[1], 96361[1], 96365[1], 96366[1], 96367[1], 96368[1], 96372[1], 96374[1], 96375[1], 96376[1], 96377[1], 96523[0], 97597[1], 97598[1], 97602[1], 99155[0], 99156[0], 99157[0], 99211[1], 99212[1], 99213[1], 99214[1], 99215[1], 99217[1], 99218[1], 99219[1], 99220[1], 99221[1], 99222[1], 99223[1], 99231[1], 99232[1], 99233[1], 99234[1], 99235[1], 99236[1], 99238[1], 99239[1], 99241[1], 99242[1], 99243[1], 99244[1], 99245[1], 99251[1], 99252[1], 99253[1], 99254[1], 99255[1], 99291[1], 99292[1], 99304[1], 99305[1], 99306[1], 99307[1], 99308[1], 99309[1], 99310[1], 99315[1], 99316[1], 99334[1], 99335[1], 99336[1], 99337[1], 99347[1], 99348[1], 99349[1], 99350[1], 99374[1], 99375[1], 99377[1], 99378[1], 99446[0], 99447[0], 99448[0], 99449[0], 99451[0], 99452[0], 99495[0], 99496[0], G0463[1], G0471[1]
50650	00910[0], 0213T[0], 0216T[0], 0596T[1], 0597T[1], 0708T[1], 0709T[1], 11000[1], 11001[1], 11004[1], 11005[1], 11006[1], 11042[1], 11043[1], 11044[1], 11045[1], 11046[1], 11047[1], 12001[1], 12002[1], 12004[1], 12005[1], 12006[1], 12007[1], 12011[1], 12013[1], 12014[1], 12015[1], 12016[1], 12017[1], 12018[1], 12020[1], 12021[1], 12031[1], 12032[1], 12034[1], 12035[1], 12036[1], 12037[1], 12041[1], 12042[1], 12044[1], 12045[1], 12046[1], 12047[1], 12051[1], 12052[1], 12053[1], 12054[1], 12055[1], 12056[1], 12057[1], 13100[1], 13101[1], 13102[1], 13120[1], 13121[1], 13122[1], 13131[1], 13132[1], 13133[1], 13151[1], 13152[1], 13153[1], 36000[1], 36400[1], 36405[1], 36406[1], 36410[1], 36420[1], 36425[1], 36430[1], 36440[1], 36591[0], 36592[0], 36600[1], 36640[1], 43752[1], 44950[0], 44970[0], 49010[0], 49320[1], 49321[1], 50715[1], 51701[0], 51702[0], 51703[1], 52000[0], 62320[0], 62321[0], 62322[0], 62323[0], 62324[0], 62325[0], 62326[0], 62327[0], 64400[0], 64405[0], 64408[0], 64415[0], 64416[0], 64417[0], 64418[0], 64420[0], 64421[0], 64425[0], 64430[0], 64435[0], 64445[0], 64446[0], 64447[0], 64448[0], 64449[0], 64450[0], 64451[0], 64454[0], 64461[0], 64462[0], 64463[0], 64479[0], 64480[0], 64483[0], 64484[0], 64486[0], 64487[0], 64488[0], 64489[0], 64490[0], 64491[0], 64492[0], 64493[0], 64494[0], 64495[0], 64505[0], 64510[0], 64517[0], 64520[0], 64530[0], 69990[0], 92012[1], 92014[1], 93000[1], 93005[1], 93010[1], 93040[1], 93041[1], 93042[1], 93318[1], 93355[1], 94002[1], 94200[1], 94680[1], 94681[1], 94690[1], 95812[1], 95813[1], 95816[1], 95819[1], 95822[1], 95829[1], 95955[1], 96360[1], 96361[1], 96365[1], 96366[1], 96367[1], 96368[1], 96372[1], 96374[1], 96375[1], 96376[1], 96377[1], 96523[0], 97597[1], 97598[1], 97602[1], 99155[0], 99156[0], 99157[0], 99211[1], 99212[1], 99213[1], 99214[1], 99215[1], 99217[1], 99218[1], 99219[1], 99220[1], 99221[1], 99222[1], 99223[1], 99231[1], 99232[1], 99233[1], 99234[1], 99235[1], 99236[1], 99238[1], 99239[1], 99241[1], 99242[1], 99243[1], 99244[1], 99245[1], 99251[1], 99252[1], 99253[1], 99254[1], 99255[1], 99291[1], 99292[1], 99304[1], 99305[1], 99306[1], 99307[1], 99308[1], 99309[1], 99310[1], 99315[1], 99316[1], 99334[1], 99335[1], 99336[1], 99337[1], 99347[1], 99348[1], 99349[1], 99350[1], 99374[1], 99375[1], 99377[1], 99378[1], 99446[0], 99447[0], 99448[0], 99449[0], 99451[0], 99452[0], 99495[0], 99496[0], G0463[1], G0471[0]
50660	00910[0], 0213T[0], 0216T[0], 0596T[1], 0597T[1], 0708T[1], 0709T[1], 11000[1], 11001[1], 11004[1], 11005[1], 11006[1], 11042[1], 11043[1], 11044[1], 11045[1], 11046[1], 11047[1], 12001[1], 12002[1], 12004[1], 12005[1], 12006[1], 12007[1], 12011[1], 12013[1], 12014[1], 12015[1], 12016[1], 12017[1], 12018[1], 12020[1], 12021[1], 12031[1], 12032[1], 12034[1], 12035[1], 12036[1], 12037[1], 12041[1], 12042[1], 12044[1], 12045[1], 12046[1], 12047[1], 12051[1], 12052[1], 12053[1], 12054[1], 12055[1], 12056[1], 12057[1], 13100[1], 13101[1], 13102[1], 13120[1], 13121[1], 13122[1], 13131[1], 13132[1], 13133[1], 13151[1], 13152[1], 13153[1], 36000[1], 36400[1], 36405[1], 36406[1], 36410[1], 36420[1], 36425[1], 36430[1], 36440[1], 36591[0], 36592[0], 36600[1], 36640[1], 43752[1], 44602[1], 44603[1], 44604[1], 44605[1], 44950[0], 44970[0], 49000[0], 49002[1], 49010[0], 49320[1], 49321[1], 50605[1], 50650[1], 50715[1], 51701[0], 51702[0], 51703[1], 52000[0], 62320[0], 62321[0], 62322[0], 62323[0], 62324[0], 62325[0], 62326[0], 62327[0], 64400[0], 64405[0], 64408[0], 64415[0], 64416[0], 64417[0], 64418[0], 64420[0], 64421[0], 64425[0], 64430[0], 64435[0], 64445[0], 64446[0], 64447[0], 64448[0], 64449[0], 64450[0], 64451[0], 64454[0], 64461[0], 64462[0], 64463[0], 64479[0], 64480[0], 64483[0], 64484[0], 64486[0], 64487[0], 64488[0], 64489[0], 64490[0], 64491[0], 64492[0], 64493[0], 64494[0], 64495[0], 64505[0], 64510[0], 64517[0], 64520[0], 64530[0], 69990[0], 92012[1], 92014[1], 93000[1], 93005[1], 93010[1], 93040[1], 93041[1], 93042[1], 93318[1], 93355[1], 94002[1], 94200[1], 94680[1],

0 = Modifier usage not allowed or inappropriate 1 = Modifier usage allowed

Code 1	Code 2
	94681[1], 94690[1], 95812[1], 95813[1], 95816[1], 95819[1], 95822[1], 95829[1], 95955[1], 96360[1], 96361[1], 96365[1], 96366[1], 96367[1], 96368[1], 96372[1], 96374[1], 96375[1], 96376[1], 96377[1], 96523[0], 97597[1], 97598[1], 97602[1], 99155[0], 99156[0], 99157[0], 99211[1], 99212[1], 99213[1], 99214[1], 99215[1], 99217[1], 99218[1], 99219[1], 99220[1], 99221[1], 99222[1], 99223[1], 99231[1], 99232[1], 99233[1], 99234[1], 99235[1], 99236[1], 99238[1], 99239[1], 99241[1], 99242[1], 99243[1], 99244[1], 99245[1], 99251[1], 99252[1], 99253[1], 99254[1], 99255[1], 99291[1], 99292[1], 99304[1], 99305[1], 99306[1], 99307[1], 99308[1], 99309[1], 99310[1], 99315[1], 99316[1], 99334[1], 99335[1], 99336[1], 99337[1], 99347[1], 99348[1], 99349[1], 99350[1], 99374[1], 99375[1], 99377[1], 99378[1], 99446[0], 99447[0], 99448[0], 99449[0], 99451[0], 99452[0], 99495[0], 99496[0], G0463[1], G0471[0]
50684	00910[0], 0213T[0], 0216T[0], 0708T[1], 0709T[1], 12001[1], 12002[1], 12004[1], 12005[1], 12006[1], 12007[1], 12011[1], 12013[1], 12014[1], 12015[1], 12016[1], 12017[1], 12018[1], 12020[1], 12021[1], 12031[1], 12032[1], 12034[1], 12035[1], 12036[1], 12037[1], 12041[1], 12042[1], 12044[1], 12045[1], 12046[1], 12047[1], 12051[1], 12052[1], 12053[1], 12054[1], 12055[1], 12056[1], 12057[1], 13100[1], 13101[1], 13102[1], 13120[1], 13121[1], 13122[1], 13131[1], 13132[1], 13133[1], 13151[1], 13152[1], 13153[1], 36000[1], 36400[1], 36405[1], 36406[1], 36410[1], 36420[1], 36425[1], 36430[1], 36440[1], 36591[0], 36592[0], 36600[1], 36640[1], 43752[1], 50436[1], 50437[1], 50715[1], 51701[1], 51702[1], 51703[1], 62320[0], 62321[0], 62322[0], 62323[0], 62324[0], 62325[0], 62326[0], 62327[0], 64400[0], 64405[0], 64408[0], 64415[0], 64416[0], 64417[0], 64418[0], 64420[0], 64421[0], 64425[0], 64430[0], 64435[0], 64445[0], 64446[0], 64447[0], 64448[0], 64449[0], 64450[0], 64451[0], 64454[0], 64461[0], 64462[0], 64463[0], 64479[0], 64480[0], 64483[0], 64484[0], 64486[0], 64487[0], 64488[0], 64489[0], 64490[0], 64491[0], 64492[0], 64493[0], 64494[0], 64495[0], 64505[0], 64510[0], 64517[0], 64520[0], 64530[0], 69990[0], 76000[1], 77001[1], 92012[1], 92014[1], 93000[1], 93005[1], 93010[1], 93040[1], 93041[1], 93042[1], 93318[1], 93355[1], 94002[1], 94200[1], 94680[1], 94681[1], 94690[1], 95812[1], 95813[1], 95816[1], 95819[1], 95822[1], 95829[1], 95955[1], 96360[1], 96361[1], 96365[1], 96366[1], 96367[1], 96368[1], 96372[1], 96374[1], 96375[1], 96376[1], 96377[1], 96523[0], 99155[0], 99156[0], 99157[0], 99211[1], 99212[1], 99213[1], 99214[1], 99215[1], 99217[1], 99218[1], 99219[1], 99220[1], 99221[1], 99222[1], 99223[1], 99231[1], 99232[1], 99233[1], 99234[1], 99235[1], 99236[1], 99238[1], 99239[1], 99241[1], 99242[1], 99243[1], 99244[1], 99245[1], 99251[1], 99252[1], 99253[1], 99254[1], 99255[1], 99291[1], 99292[1], 99304[1], 99305[1], 99306[1], 99307[1], 99308[1], 99309[1], 99310[1], 99315[1], 99316[1], 99334[1], 99335[1], 99336[1], 99337[1], 99347[1], 99348[1], 99349[1], 99350[1], 99374[1], 99375[1], 99377[1], 99378[1], 99446[0], 99447[0], 99448[0], 99449[0], 99451[0], 99452[0], 99495[1], 99496[1], G0463[1], G0471[1], J1644[1], J2001[1]
50686	00910[0], 0213T[0], 0216T[0], 0596T[1], 0597T[1], 0708T[1], 0709T[1], 12001[1], 12002[1], 12004[1], 12005[1], 12006[1], 12007[1], 12011[1], 12013[1], 12014[1], 12015[1], 12016[1], 12017[1], 12018[1], 12020[1], 12021[1], 12031[1], 12032[1], 12034[1], 12035[1], 12036[1], 12037[1], 12041[1], 12042[1], 12044[1], 12045[1], 12046[1], 12047[1], 12051[1], 12052[1], 12053[1], 12054[1], 12055[1], 12056[1], 12057[1], 13100[1], 13101[1], 13102[1], 13120[1], 13121[1], 13122[1], 13131[1], 13132[1], 13133[1], 13151[1], 13152[1], 13153[1], 36000[1], 36400[1], 36405[1], 36406[1], 36410[1], 36420[1], 36425[1], 36430[1], 36440[1], 36591[0], 36592[0], 36600[1], 36640[1], 43752[1], 50436[1], 50437[1], 50715[1], 51701[1], 51702[1], 51703[1], 62320[0], 62321[0], 62322[0], 62323[0], 62324[0], 62325[0], 62326[0], 62327[0], 64400[0], 64405[0], 64408[0], 64415[0], 64416[0], 64417[0], 64418[0], 64420[0], 64421[0], 64425[0], 64430[0], 64435[0], 64445[0], 64446[0], 64447[0], 64448[0], 64449[0], 64450[0], 64451[0], 64454[0], 64461[0], 64462[0], 64463[0], 64479[0], 64480[0], 64483[0], 64484[0], 64486[0], 64487[0], 64488[0], 64489[0], 64490[0], 64491[0], 64492[0], 64493[0], 64494[0], 64495[0], 64505[0], 64510[0], 64517[0], 64520[0], 64530[0], 69990[0], 92012[1], 92014[1], 93000[1], 93005[1], 93010[1], 93040[1], 93041[1], 93042[1], 93318[1], 93355[1], 94002[1], 94200[1], 94680[1], 94681[1], 94690[1], 95812[1], 95813[1], 95816[1], 95819[1], 95822[1], 95829[1], 95955[1], 96360[1], 96361[1], 96365[1], 96366[1], 96367[1], 96368[1], 96372[1], 96374[1], 96375[1], 96376[1], 96377[1], 96523[0], 99155[0], 99156[0], 99157[0], 99211[1], 99212[1], 99213[1], 99214[1], 99215[1], 99217[1], 99218[1], 99219[1], 99220[1], 99221[1], 99222[1], 99223[1], 99231[1], 99232[1], 99233[1], 99234[1], 99235[1], 99236[1], 99238[1], 99239[1], 99241[1], 99242[1], 99243[1], 99244[1], 99245[1], 99251[1], 99252[1], 99253[1], 99254[1], 99255[1], 99291[1], 99292[1], 99304[1], 99305[1], 99306[1], 99307[1], 99308[1], 99309[1], 99310[1], 99315[1], 99316[1], 99334[1], 99335[1], 99336[1], 99337[1], 99347[1], 99348[1], 99349[1], 99350[1], 99374[1], 99375[1], 99377[1], 99378[1], 99446[0], 99447[0], 99448[0], 99449[0], 99451[0], 99452[0], 99495[1], 99496[1], G0463[1], G0471[1]
50688	00910[0], 0213T[0], 0216T[0], 0596T[1], 0597T[1], 0708T[1], 0709T[1], 12001[1], 12002[1], 12004[1], 12005[1], 12006[1], 12007[1], 12011[1], 12013[1], 12014[1], 12015[1], 12016[1], 12017[1], 12018[1], 12020[1], 12021[1], 12031[1], 12032[1], 12034[1], 12035[1], 12036[1], 12037[1], 12041[1], 12042[1], 12044[1], 12045[1], 12046[1], 12047[1], 12051[1], 12052[1], 12053[1], 12054[1], 12055[1], 12056[1], 12057[1], 13100[1], 13101[1], 13102[1], 13120[1], 13121[1], 13122[1], 13131[1], 13132[1], 13133[1], 13151[1], 13152[1], 13153[1], 36000[1], 36400[1], 36405[1], 36406[1], 36410[1], 36420[1], 36425[1], 36430[1], 36440[1], 36591[0], 36592[0], 36600[1], 36640[1], 43752[1], 50693[1], 50694[1], 50695[1], 50715[1], 51701[1], 51702[1], 51703[1], 62320[0], 62321[0], 62322[0], 62323[0], 62324[0], 62325[0], 62326[0], 62327[0], 64400[0], 64405[0], 64408[0], 64415[0], 64416[0], 64417[0], 64418[0], 64420[0], 64421[0], 64425[0], 64430[0], 64435[0], 64445[0], 64446[0], 64447[0], 64448[0], 64449[0], 64450[0], 64451[0], 64454[0], 64461[0], 64462[0], 64463[0], 64479[0], 64480[0], 64483[0], 64484[0], 64486[0], 64487[0], 64488[0], 64489[0], 64490[0], 64491[0], 64492[0], 64493[0], 64494[0], 64495[0], 64505[0], 64510[0], 64517[0], 64520[0], 64530[0], 69990[0], 74425[1], 76000[1], 77001[1], 77002[1], 92012[1], 92014[1], 93000[1], 93005[1], 93010[1], 93040[1], 93041[1], 93042[1], 93318[1], 93355[1], 94002[1], 94200[1], 94680[1], 94681[1], 94690[1], 95812[1], 95813[1], 95816[1], 95819[1], 95822[1], 95829[1], 95955[1], 96360[1], 96361[1], 96365[1], 96366[1], 96367[1], 96368[1], 96372[1], 96374[1], 96375[1], 96376[1], 96377[1], 96523[0], 99155[0], 99156[0], 99157[0], 99211[1], 99212[1], 99213[1], 99214[1], 99215[1], 99217[1], 99218[1], 99219[1], 99220[1], 99221[1], 99222[1], 99223[1], 99231[1], 99232[1], 99233[1], 99234[1], 99235[1], 99236[1], 99238[1], 99239[1], 99241[1], 99242[1], 99243[1], 99244[1], 99245[1], 99251[1], 99252[1], 99253[1], 99254[1], 99255[1], 99291[1], 99292[1], 99304[1], 99305[1], 99306[1], 99307[1], 99308[1], 99309[1], 99310[1], 99315[1], 99316[1], 99334[1], 99335[1], 99336[1], 99337[1], 99347[1], 99348[1], 99349[1], 99350[1], 99374[1], 99375[1], 99377[1], 99378[1], 99446[0], 99447[0], 99448[0], 99449[0], 99451[0], 99452[0], 99495[0], 99496[0], G0463[1], G0471[1]
50690	00910[0], 0213T[0], 0216T[0], 0596T[1], 0597T[1], 0708T[1], 0709T[1], 12001[1], 12002[1], 12004[1], 12005[1], 12006[1], 12007[1], 12011[1], 12013[1], 12014[1], 12015[1], 12016[1], 12017[1], 12018[1], 12020[1], 12021[1], 12031[1], 12032[1], 12034[1], 12035[1], 12036[1], 12037[1], 12041[1], 12042[1], 12044[1], 12045[1], 12046[1], 12047[1], 12051[1], 12052[1], 12053[1], 12054[1], 12055[1], 12056[1], 12057[1], 13100[1], 13101[1], 13102[1], 13120[1], 13121[1], 13122[1], 13131[1], 13132[1], 13133[1], 13151[1], 13152[1], 13153[1], 36000[1], 36400[1], 36405[1], 36406[1], 36410[1], 36420[1], 36425[1], 36430[1], 36440[1], 36591[0], 36592[0], 36600[1], 36640[1], 43752[1], 50715[1], 51701[1], 51702[1], 51703[1], 62320[0], 62321[0], 62322[0], 62323[0], 62324[0], 62325[0], 62326[0], 62327[0], 64400[0], 64405[0], 64408[0], 64415[0], 64416[0], 64417[0], 64418[0], 64420[0], 64421[0], 64425[0], 64430[0], 64435[0], 64445[0], 64446[0], 64447[0], 64448[0], 64449[0], 64450[0], 64451[0], 64454[0], 64461[0], 64462[0], 64463[0], 64479[0], 64480[0], 64483[0], 64484[0], 64486[0], 64487[0], 64488[0], 64489[0], 64490[0], 64491[0], 64492[0], 64493[0], 64494[0], 64495[0], 64505[0], 64510[0], 64517[0], 64520[0], 64530[0], 69990[0], 92012[1], 92014[1], 93000[1], 93005[1], 93010[1], 93040[1], 93041[1], 93042[1], 93318[1], 93355[1], 94002[1], 94200[1], 94680[1], 94681[1], 94690[1], 95812[1], 95813[1], 95816[1], 95819[1], 95822[1], 95829[1], 95955[1], 96360[1], 96361[1], 96365[1], 96366[1], 96367[1], 96368[1], 96372[1], 96374[1], 96375[1], 96376[1], 96377[1], 96523[0], 99155[0], 99156[0], 99157[0], 99211[1], 99212[1], 99213[1], 99214[1], 99215[1], 99217[1], 99218[1], 99219[1], 99220[1], 99221[1], 99222[1], 99223[1], 99231[1], 99232[1], 99233[1], 99234[1], 99235[1], 99236[1], 99238[1], 99239[1], 99241[1], 99242[1], 99243[1], 99244[1], 99245[1], 99251[1], 99252[1], 99253[1], 99254[1], 99255[1], 99291[1], 99292[1], 99304[1], 99305[1], 99306[1], 99307[1], 99308[1], 99309[1], 99310[1], 99315[1], 99316[1], 99334[1], 99335[1], 99336[1], 99337[1], 99347[1], 99348[1], 99349[1], 99350[1], 99374[1], 99375[1], 99377[1], 99378[1], 99446[0], 99447[0], 99448[0], 99449[0], 99451[0], 99452[0], 99495[1], 99496[1], G0463[1], G0471[1], J1644[1], J2001[1]
50693	0213T[0], 0216T[0], 0596T[1], 0597T[1], 0708T[1], 0709T[1], 12001[1], 12002[1], 12004[1], 12005[1], 12006[1], 12007[1], 12011[1], 12013[1], 12014[1], 12015[1], 12016[1], 12017[1], 12018[1], 12020[1], 12021[1], 12031[1], 12032[1], 12034[1], 12035[1], 12036[1], 12037[1], 12041[1], 12042[1], 12044[1], 12045[1], 12046[1], 12047[1], 12051[1], 12052[1], 12053[1], 12054[1], 12055[1], 12056[1], 12057[1], 13100[1], 13101[1], 13102[1], 13120[1], 13121[1], 13122[1], 13131[1], 13132[1], 13133[1], 13151[1], 13152[1], 13153[1], 36000[1], 36011[1], 36400[1], 36405[1], 36406[1], 36410[1], 36420[1], 36425[1], 36430[1], 36440[1], 36591[0], 36592[0], 36600[1], 36640[1], 43752[1], 49185[1], 49424[1], 50390[1], 50430[1], 50431[1], 50432[1], 50433[1], 50434[1], 50435[1], 50436[1], 50437[1], 50684[1], 51701[1], 51702[1], 51703[1], 62320[0], 62321[0], 62322[0], 62323[0], 62324[0], 62325[0], 62326[0], 62327[0], 64400[0], 64405[0], 64408[0], 64415[0], 64416[0], 64417[0], 64418[0], 64420[0], 64421[0], 64425[0], 64430[0], 64435[0], 64445[0], 64446[0], 64447[0], 64448[0], 64449[0], 64450[0], 64451[0], 64454[0], 64461[0], 64462[0], 64463[0], 64479[0], 64480[0], 64483[0], 64484[0], 64486[0], 64487[0], 64488[0], 64489[0], 64490[0], 64491[0], 64492[0], 64493[0], 64494[0], 64495[0], 64505[0], 64510[0], 64517[0], 64520[0], 64530[0], 69990[0], 74425[1], 76000[1], 76380[1], 76942[1], 76998[1], 77001[1], 77002[1], 77012[1], 77021[1], 92012[1], 92014[1], 93000[1], 93005[1], 93010[1], 93040[1], 93041[1], 93042[1], 93318[1], 93355[1], 94002[1], 94200[1], 94680[1], 94681[1], 94690[1], 95812[1], 95813[1], 95816[1], 95819[1], 95822[1], 95829[1], 95955[1], 96360[1], 96361[1], 96365[1], 96366[1], 96367[1], 96368[1], 96372[1], 96374[1], 96375[1], 96376[1], 96377[1], 96523[0], 99155[0], 99156[0], 99157[0], 99211[1], 99212[1], 99213[1], 99214[1], 99215[1], 99217[1], 99218[1], 99219[1], 99220[1], 99221[1], 99222[1], 99223[1], 99231[1], 99232[1], 99233[1], 99234[1], 99235[1], 99236[1], 99238[1], 99239[1], 99241[1], 99242[1], 99243[1], 99244[1], 99245[1], 99251[1], 99252[1], 99253[1], 99254[1], 99255[1], 99291[1], 99292[1], 99304[1], 99305[1], 99306[1], 99307[1], 99308[1], 99309[1], 99310[1], 99315[1], 99316[1], 99334[1], 99335[1], 99336[1], 99337[1], 99347[1], 99348[1], 99349[1], 99350[1], 99374[1], 99375[1], 99377[1], 99378[1], 99446[0], 99447[0], 99448[0], 99449[0], 99451[0], 99452[0], 99495[1], 99496[1], G0463[1], G0471[1], J0670[1], J2001[1]
50694	0213T[0], 0216T[0], 0596T[1], 0597T[1], 0708T[1], 0709T[1], 12001[1], 12002[1], 12004[1], 12005[1], 12006[1], 12007[1], 12011[1], 12013[1], 12014[1], 12015[1], 12016[1], 12017[1], 12018[1], 12020[1], 12021[1], 12031[1], 12032[1], 12034[1], 12035[1], 12036[1], 12037[1], 12041[1], 12042[1], 12044[1], 12045[1], 12046[1], 12047[1], 12051[1], 12052[1], 12053[1], 12054[1], 12055[1], 12056[1], 12057[1],

0 = Modifier usage not allowed or inappropriate 1 = Modifier usage allowed

Code 1	Code 2
	13100[1], 13101[1], 13102[1], 13120[1], 13121[1], 13122[1], 13131[1], 13132[1], 13133[1], 13151[1], 13152[1], 13153[1], 36000[1], 36011[1], 36400[1], 36405[1], 36406[1], 36410[1], 36420[1], 36425[1], 36430[1], 36440[1], 36591[0], 36592[0], 36600[1], 36640[1], 43752[1], 49185[1], 49424[1], 50390[1], 50430[1], 50431[1], 50432[1], 50433[1], 50434[1], 50435[1], 50436[1], 50437[1], 50684[1], 50693[1], 51701[1], 51702[1], 51703[1], 62320[0], 62321[0], 62322[0], 62323[0], 62324[0], 62325[0], 62326[0], 62327[0], 64400[0], 64405[0], 64408[0], 64415[0], 64416[0], 64417[0], 64418[0], 64420[0], 64421[0], 64425[0], 64430[0], 64435[0], 64445[0], 64446[0], 64447[0], 64448[0], 64449[0], 64450[0], 64451[0], 64454[0], 64461[0], 64462[0], 64463[0], 64479[0], 64480[0], 64483[0], 64484[0], 64486[0], 64487[0], 64488[0], 64489[0], 64490[0], 64491[0], 64492[0], 64493[0], 64494[0], 64495[0], 64505[0], 64510[0], 64517[0], 64520[0], 64530[0], 69990[0], 74425[1], 76000[1], 76380[1], 76942[1], 76998[1], 77001[1], 77002[1], 77012[1], 77021[1], 92012[1], 92014[1], 93000[1], 93005[1], 93010[1], 93040[1], 93041[1], 93042[1], 93318[1], 93355[1], 94002[1], 94200[1], 94680[1], 94681[1], 94690[1], 95812[1], 95813[1], 95816[1], 95819[1], 95822[1], 95829[1], 95955[1], 96360[1], 96361[1], 96365[1], 96366[1], 96367[1], 96368[1], 96372[1], 96374[1], 96375[1], 96376[1], 96377[1], 96523[0], 99155[0], 99156[0], 99157[0], 99211[1], 99212[1], 99213[1], 99214[1], 99215[1], 99217[1], 99218[1], 99219[1], 99220[1], 99221[1], 99222[1], 99223[1], 99231[1], 99232[1], 99233[1], 99234[1], 99235[1], 99236[1], 99238[1], 99239[1], 99241[1], 99242[1], 99243[1], 99244[1], 99245[1], 99251[1], 99252[1], 99253[1], 99254[1], 99255[1], 99291[1], 99292[1], 99304[1], 99305[1], 99306[1], 99307[1], 99308[1], 99309[1], 99310[1], 99315[1], 99316[1], 99334[1], 99335[1], 99336[1], 99337[1], 99347[1], 99348[1], 99349[1], 99350[1], 99374[1], 99375[1], 99377[1], 99378[1], 99446[0], 99447[0], 99448[0], 99449[0], 99451[0], 99452[0], 99495[1], 99496[1], G0463[1], G0471[1], J0670[1], J2001[1]
50695	0213T[0], 0216T[0], 0596T[1], 0597T[1], 0708T[1], 0709T[1], 12001[1], 12002[1], 12004[1], 12005[1], 12006[1], 12007[1], 12011[1], 12013[1], 12014[1], 12015[1], 12016[1], 12017[1], 12018[1], 12020[1], 12021[1], 12031[1], 12032[1], 12034[1], 12035[1], 12036[1], 12037[1], 12041[1], 12042[1], 12044[1], 12045[1], 12046[1], 12047[1], 12051[1], 12052[1], 12053[1], 12054[1], 12055[1], 12056[1], 12057[1], 13100[1], 13101[1], 13102[1], 13120[1], 13121[1], 13122[1], 13131[1], 13132[1], 13133[1], 13151[1], 13152[1], 13153[1], 36000[1], 36011[1], 36400[1], 36405[1], 36406[1], 36410[1], 36420[1], 36425[1], 36430[1], 36440[1], 36591[0], 36592[0], 36600[1], 36640[1], 43752[1], 49185[1], 49424[1], 50390[1], 50430[1], 50431[1], 50432[1], 50433[1], 50434[1], 50435[1], 50436[1], 50437[1], 50684[1], 50693[1], 50694[1], 51701[1], 51702[1], 51703[1], 62320[0], 62321[0], 62322[0], 62323[0], 62324[0], 62325[0], 62326[0], 62327[0], 64400[0], 64405[0], 64408[0], 64415[0], 64416[0], 64417[0], 64418[0], 64420[0], 64421[0], 64425[0], 64430[0], 64435[0], 64445[0], 64446[0], 64447[0], 64448[0], 64449[0], 64450[0], 64451[0], 64454[0], 64461[0], 64462[0], 64463[0], 64479[0], 64480[0], 64483[0], 64484[0], 64486[0], 64487[0], 64488[0], 64489[0], 64490[0], 64491[0], 64492[0], 64493[0], 64494[0], 64495[0], 64505[0], 64510[0], 64517[0], 64520[0], 64530[0], 69990[0], 74425[1], 76000[1], 76380[1], 76942[1], 76998[1], 77001[1], 77002[1], 77012[1], 77021[1], 92012[1], 92014[1], 93000[1], 93005[1], 93010[1], 93040[1], 93041[1], 93042[1], 93318[1], 93355[1], 94002[1], 94200[1], 94680[1], 94681[1], 94690[1], 95812[1], 95813[1], 95816[1], 95819[1], 95822[1], 95829[1], 95955[1], 96360[1], 96361[1], 96365[1], 96366[1], 96367[1], 96368[1], 96372[1], 96374[1], 96375[1], 96376[1], 96377[1], 96523[0], 99155[0], 99156[0], 99157[0], 99211[1], 99212[1], 99213[1], 99214[1], 99215[1], 99217[1], 99218[1], 99219[1], 99220[1], 99221[1], 99222[1], 99223[1], 99231[1], 99232[1], 99233[1], 99234[1], 99235[1], 99236[1], 99238[1], 99239[1], 99241[1], 99242[1], 99243[1], 99244[1], 99245[1], 99251[1], 99252[1], 99253[1], 99254[1], 99255[1], 99291[1], 99292[1], 99304[1], 99305[1], 99306[1], 99307[1], 99308[1], 99309[1], 99310[1], 99315[1], 99316[1], 99334[1], 99335[1], 99336[1], 99337[1], 99347[1], 99348[1], 99349[1], 99350[1], 99374[1], 99375[1], 99377[1], 99378[1], 99446[0], 99447[0], 99448[0], 99449[0], 99451[0], 99452[0], 99495[1], 99496[1], G0463[1], G0471[1], J0670[1], J2001[1]
50700	00910[0], 0213T[0], 0216T[0], 0596T[1], 0597T[1], 0708T[1], 0709T[1], 11000[1], 11001[1], 11004[1], 11005[1], 11006[1], 11042[1], 11043[1], 11044[1], 11045[1], 11046[1], 11047[1], 12001[1], 12002[1], 12004[1], 12005[1], 12006[1], 12007[1], 12011[1], 12013[1], 12014[1], 12015[1], 12016[1], 12017[1], 12018[1], 12020[1], 12021[1], 12031[1], 12032[1], 12034[1], 12035[1], 12036[1], 12037[1], 12041[1], 12042[1], 12044[1], 12045[1], 12046[1], 12047[1], 12051[1], 12052[1], 12053[1], 12054[1], 12055[1], 12056[1], 12057[1], 13100[1], 13101[1], 13102[1], 13120[1], 13121[1], 13122[1], 13131[1], 13132[1], 13133[1], 13151[1], 13152[1], 13153[1], 36000[1], 36400[1], 36405[1], 36406[1], 36410[1], 36420[1], 36425[1], 36430[1], 36440[1], 36591[0], 36592[0], 36600[1], 36640[1], 43752[1], 44602[1], 44603[1], 44604[1], 44605[1], 44850[0], 44950[0], 44970[0], 49000[0], 49002[1], 49010[0], 50100[1], 50600[1], 50605[1], 50715[1], 50722[1], 50900[1], 51701[1], 51702[1], 51703[1], 62320[0], 62321[0], 62322[0], 62323[0], 62324[0], 62325[0], 62326[0], 62327[0], 64400[0], 64405[0], 64408[0], 64415[0], 64416[0], 64417[0], 64418[0], 64420[0], 64421[0], 64425[0], 64430[0], 64435[0], 64445[0], 64446[0], 64447[0], 64448[0], 64449[0], 64450[0], 64451[0], 64454[0], 64461[0], 64462[0], 64463[0], 64479[0], 64480[0], 64483[0], 64484[0], 64486[0], 64487[0], 64488[0], 64489[0], 64490[0], 64491[0], 64492[0], 64493[0], 64494[0], 64495[0], 64505[0], 64510[0], 64517[0], 64520[0], 64530[0], 69990[0], 92012[1], 92014[1], 93000[1], 93005[1], 93010[1], 93040[1], 93041[1], 93042[1], 93318[1], 93355[1], 94002[1], 94200[1], 94680[1], 94681[1], 94690[1], 95812[1], 95813[1], 95816[1], 95819[1], 95822[1], 95829[1], 95955[1], 96360[1], 96361[1], 96365[1], 96366[1], 96367[1], 96368[1], 96372[1], 96374[1], 96375[1], 96376[1], 96377[1], 96523[0], 97597[1], 97598[1], 97602[1], 99155[0], 99156[0], 99157[0], 99211[1], 99212[1], 99213[1], 99214[1], 99215[1], 99217[1], 99218[1], 99219[1], 99220[1], 99221[1], 99222[1], 99223[1], 99231[1], 99232[1], 99233[1], 99234[1], 99235[1], 99236[1], 99238[1], 99239[1], 99241[1], 99242[1], 99243[1], 99244[1], 99245[1], 99251[1], 99252[1], 99253[1], 99254[1], 99255[1], 99291[1], 99292[1], 99304[1], 99305[1], 99306[1], 99307[1], 99308[1], 99309[1], 99310[1], 99315[1], 99316[1], 99334[1], 99335[1], 99336[1], 99337[1], 99347[1], 99348[1], 99349[1], 99350[1], 99374[1], 99375[1], 99377[1], 99378[1], 99446[0], 99447[0], 99448[0], 99449[0], 99451[0], 99452[0], 99495[0], 99496[0], G0463[1], G0471[1]
50705	0213T[0], 0216T[0], 0596T[1], 0597T[1], 0708T[1], 0709T[1], 12001[0], 12002[1], 12004[1], 12005[1], 12006[1], 12007[1], 12011[1], 12013[1], 12014[1], 12015[1], 12016[1], 12017[1], 12018[1], 12020[1], 12021[1], 12031[1], 12032[1], 12034[1], 12035[1], 12036[1], 12037[1], 12041[1], 12042[1], 12044[1], 12045[1], 12046[1], 12047[1], 12051[1], 12052[1], 12053[1], 12054[1], 12055[1], 12056[1], 12057[1], 13100[1], 13101[1], 13102[1], 13120[1], 13121[1], 13122[1], 13131[1], 13132[1], 13133[1], 13151[1], 13152[1], 13153[1], 36000[1], 36400[1], 36405[1], 36406[1], 36410[1], 36420[1], 36425[1], 36430[1], 36440[1], 36600[1], 36640[1], 43752[1], 50436[1], 50437[1], 51701[1], 51702[1], 51703[1], 62320[0], 62321[0], 62322[0], 62323[0], 62324[0], 62325[0], 62326[0], 62327[0], 64400[0], 64405[0], 64408[0], 64415[0], 64416[0], 64417[0], 64418[0], 64420[0], 64421[0], 64425[0], 64430[0], 64435[0], 64445[0], 64446[0], 64447[0], 64448[0], 64449[0], 64450[0], 64451[0], 64454[0], 64461[0], 64463[0], 64479[0], 64483[0], 64486[0], 64487[0], 64488[0], 64489[0], 64490[0], 64493[0], 64505[0], 64510[0], 64517[0], 64520[0], 64530[0], 69990[0], 74425[1], 76000[1], 76380[1], 76942[1], 76998[1], 77002[1], 77012[1], 77021[1], 92012[1], 92014[1], 93000[1], 93005[1], 93010[1], 93040[1], 93041[1], 93042[1], 93318[1], 94002[1], 94200[1], 94680[1], 94681[1], 94690[1], 95812[1], 95813[1], 95816[1], 95819[1], 95822[1], 95829[1], 95955[1], 96360[1], 96365[1], 96372[1], 96374[1], 96375[1], 96376[1], 96377[1], 96523[0], 99155[0], 99156[0], 99157[0], 99211[1], 99212[1], 99213[1], 99214[1], 99215[1], 99217[1], 99218[1], 99219[1], 99220[1], 99221[1], 99222[1], 99223[1], 99231[1], 99232[1], 99233[1], 99234[1], 99235[1], 99236[1], 99238[1], 99239[1], 99241[1], 99242[1], 99243[1], 99244[1], 99245[1], 99251[1], 99252[1], 99253[1], 99254[1], 99255[1], 99291[1], 99292[1], 99304[1], 99305[1], 99306[1], 99307[1], 99308[1], 99309[1], 99310[1], 99315[1], 99316[1], 99334[1], 99335[1], 99336[1], 99337[1], 99347[1], 99348[1], 99349[1], 99350[1], 99374[1], 99375[1], 99377[1], 99378[1]
50706	0213T[0], 0216T[0], 0596T[1], 0597T[1], 0708T[1], 0709T[1], 12001[0], 12002[1], 12004[1], 12005[1], 12006[1], 12007[1], 12011[1], 12013[1], 12014[1], 12015[1], 12016[1], 12017[1], 12018[1], 12020[1], 12021[1], 12031[1], 12032[1], 12034[1], 12035[1], 12036[1], 12037[1], 12041[1], 12042[1], 12044[1], 12045[1], 12046[1], 12047[1], 12051[1], 12052[1], 12053[1], 12054[1], 12055[1], 12056[1], 12057[1], 13100[1], 13101[1], 13102[1], 13120[1], 13121[1], 13122[1], 13131[1], 13132[1], 13133[1], 13151[1], 13152[1], 13153[1], 36000[1], 36400[1], 36405[1], 36406[1], 36410[1], 36420[1], 36425[1], 36430[1], 36440[1], 36600[1], 36640[1], 43752[1], 50436[1], 50437[1], 51701[1], 51702[1], 51703[1], 62320[0], 62321[0], 62322[0], 62323[0], 62324[0], 62325[0], 62326[0], 62327[0], 64400[0], 64405[0], 64408[0], 64415[0], 64416[0], 64417[0], 64418[0], 64420[0], 64421[0], 64425[0], 64430[0], 64435[0], 64445[0], 64446[0], 64447[0], 64448[0], 64449[0], 64450[0], 64451[0], 64454[0], 64461[0], 64463[0], 64479[0], 64483[0], 64486[0], 64487[0], 64488[0], 64489[0], 64490[0], 64493[0], 64505[0], 64510[0], 64517[0], 64520[0], 64530[0], 69990[0], 74425[1], 74485[1], 76000[1], 76380[1], 76942[1], 76998[1], 77002[1], 77012[1], 77021[1], 92012[1], 92014[1], 93000[1], 93005[1], 93010[1], 93040[1], 93041[1], 93042[1], 93318[1], 94002[1], 94200[1], 94680[1], 94681[1], 94690[1], 95812[1], 95813[1], 95816[1], 95819[1], 95822[1], 95829[1], 95955[1], 96360[1], 96365[1], 96372[1], 96374[1], 96375[1], 96376[1], 96377[1], 96523[0], 99155[0], 99156[0], 99157[0], 99211[1], 99212[1], 99213[1], 99214[1], 99215[1], 99217[1], 99218[1], 99219[1], 99220[1], 99221[1], 99222[1], 99223[1], 99231[1], 99232[1], 99233[1], 99234[1], 99235[1], 99236[1], 99238[1], 99239[1], 99241[1], 99242[1], 99243[1], 99244[1], 99245[1], 99251[1], 99252[1], 99253[1], 99254[1], 99255[1], 99291[1], 99292[1], 99304[1], 99305[1], 99306[1], 99307[1], 99308[1], 99309[1], 99310[1], 99315[1], 99316[1], 99334[1], 99335[1], 99336[1], 99337[1], 99347[1], 99348[1], 99349[1], 99350[1], 99374[1], 99375[1], 99377[1], 99378[1]
50715	00910[0], 0213T[0], 0216T[0], 0666T[1], 0708T[1], 0709T[1], 12001[1], 12002[1], 12004[1], 12005[1], 12006[1], 12007[1], 12011[1], 12013[1], 12014[1], 12015[1], 12016[1], 12017[1], 12018[1], 12020[1], 12021[1], 12031[1], 12032[1], 12034[1], 12035[1], 12036[1], 12037[1], 12041[1], 12042[1], 12044[1], 12045[1], 12046[1], 12047[1], 12051[1], 12052[1], 12053[1], 12054[1], 12055[1], 12056[1], 12057[1], 13100[1], 13101[1], 13102[1], 13120[1], 13121[1], 13122[1], 13131[1], 13132[1], 13133[1], 13151[1], 13152[1], 13153[1], 36000[1], 36400[1], 36405[1], 36406[1], 36410[1], 36420[1], 36425[1], 36430[1], 36440[1], 36591[0], 36592[0], 36600[1], 36640[1], 43752[1], 44005[0], 44180[0], 44850[0], 44950[0], 44970[0], 49000[0], 49002[1], 49010[0], 49203[1], 50100[1], 50600[1], 50900[1], 51100[1], 51101[1], 51102[1], 51701[1], 51702[1], 51703[1], 52005[1], 57423[1], 58570[1], 58571[1], 62320[0], 62321[0], 62322[0], 62323[0], 62324[0], 62325[0], 62326[0], 62327[0], 64400[0], 64405[0], 64408[0], 64415[0], 64416[0], 64417[0], 64418[0], 64420[0], 64421[0], 64425[0], 64430[0], 64435[0], 64445[0], 64446[0], 64447[0], 64448[0], 64449[0], 64450[0], 64451[0], 64454[0], 64461[0], 64462[0], 64463[0], 64479[0], 64480[0], 64483[0], 64484[0], 64486[0], 64487[0], 64488[0], 64489[0], 64490[0], 64491[0], 64492[0], 64493[0], 64494[0], 64495[0], 64505[0], 64510[0], 64517[0], 64520[0], 64530[0], 69990[0], 92012[1], 92014[1], 93000[1], 93005[1], 93010[1], 93040[1], 93041[1], 93042[1], 93318[1], 93355[1], 94002[1], 94200[1], 94680[1], 94681[1], 94690[1], 95812[1], 95813[1], 95816[1], 95819[1], 95822[1], 95829[1], 95955[1], 96360[1], 96361[1], 96365[1], 96366[1], 96367[1], 96368[1], 96372[1], 96374[1], 96375[1],

0 = Modifier usage not allowed or inappropriate 1 = Modifier usage allowed

Code 1	Code 2
	96376[1], 96377[1], 96523[0], 99155[0], 99156[0], 99157[0], 99211[1], 99212[1], 99213[1], 99214[1], 99215[1], 99217[1], 99218[1], 99219[1], 99220[1], 99221[1], 99222[1], 99223[1], 99231[1], 99232[1], 99233[1], 99234[1], 99235[1], 99236[1], 99238[1], 99239[1], 99241[1], 99242[1], 99243[1], 99244[1], 99245[1], 99251[1], 99252[1], 99253[1], 99254[1], 99255[1], 99291[1], 99292[1], 99304[1], 99305[1], 99306[1], 99307[1], 99308[1], 99309[1], 99310[1], 99315[1], 99316[1], 99334[1], 99335[1], 99336[1], 99337[1], 99347[1], 99348[1], 99349[1], 99350[1], 99374[1], 99375[1], 99377[1], 99378[1], 99446[0], 99447[0], 99448[0], 99449[0], 99451[0], 99452[0], 99495[0], 99496[0], G0463[1], G0471[1]
50722	00910[0], 0213T[0], 0216T[0], 0596T[1], 0597T[1], 0708T[1], 0709T[1], 12001[1], 12002[1], 12004[1], 12005[1], 12006[1], 12007[1], 12011[1], 12013[1], 12014[1], 12015[1], 12016[1], 12017[1], 12018[1], 12020[1], 12021[1], 12031[1], 12032[1], 12034[1], 12035[1], 12036[1], 12037[1], 12041[1], 12042[1], 12044[1], 12045[1], 12046[1], 12047[1], 12051[1], 12052[1], 12053[1], 12054[1], 12055[1], 12056[1], 12057[1], 13100[1], 13101[1], 13102[1], 13120[1], 13121[1], 13122[1], 13131[1], 13132[1], 13133[1], 13151[1], 13152[1], 13153[1], 36000[1], 36400[1], 36405[1], 36406[1], 36410[1], 36420[1], 36425[1], 36430[1], 36440[1], 36591[0], 36592[0], 36600[1], 36640[1], 43752[1], 44602[1], 44603[1], 44604[1], 44605[1], 44850[0], 44950[0], 44970[0], 49000[0], 49002[1], 49010[0], 50600[1], 50605[1], 50715[1], 50900[1], 51701[1], 51702[1], 51703[1], 62320[0], 62321[0], 62322[0], 62323[0], 62324[0], 62325[0], 62326[0], 62327[0], 64400[0], 64405[0], 64408[0], 64415[0], 64416[0], 64417[0], 64418[0], 64420[0], 64421[0], 64425[0], 64430[0], 64435[0], 64445[0], 64446[0], 64447[0], 64448[0], 64449[0], 64450[0], 64451[0], 64454[0], 64461[0], 64462[0], 64463[0], 64479[0], 64480[0], 64483[0], 64484[0], 64486[0], 64487[0], 64488[0], 64489[0], 64490[0], 64491[0], 64492[0], 64493[0], 64494[0], 64495[0], 64505[0], 64510[0], 64517[0], 64520[0], 64530[0], 69990[0], 92012[1], 92014[1], 93000[1], 93005[1], 93010[1], 93040[1], 93041[1], 93042[1], 93318[1], 93355[1], 94002[1], 94200[1], 94680[1], 94681[1], 94690[1], 95812[1], 95813[1], 95816[1], 95819[1], 95822[1], 95829[1], 95955[1], 96360[1], 96361[1], 96365[1], 96366[1], 96367[1], 96368[1], 96372[1], 96374[1], 96375[1], 96376[1], 96377[1], 96523[0], 99155[0], 99156[0], 99157[0], 99211[1], 99212[1], 99213[1], 99214[1], 99215[1], 99217[1], 99218[1], 99219[1], 99220[1], 99221[1], 99222[1], 99223[1], 99231[1], 99232[1], 99233[1], 99234[1], 99235[1], 99236[1], 99238[1], 99239[1], 99241[1], 99242[1], 99243[1], 99244[1], 99245[1], 99251[1], 99252[1], 99253[1], 99254[1], 99255[1], 99291[1], 99292[1], 99304[1], 99305[1], 99306[1], 99307[1], 99308[1], 99309[1], 99310[1], 99315[1], 99316[1], 99334[1], 99335[1], 99336[1], 99337[1], 99347[1], 99348[1], 99349[1], 99350[1], 99374[1], 99375[1], 99377[1], 99378[1], 99446[0], 99447[0], 99448[0], 99449[0], 99451[0], 99452[0], 99495[0], 99496[0], G0463[1], G0471[1]
50725	00910[0], 0213T[0], 0216T[0], 0596T[1], 0597T[1], 0708T[1], 0709T[1], 12001[1], 12002[1], 12004[1], 12005[1], 12006[1], 12007[1], 12011[1], 12013[1], 12014[1], 12015[1], 12016[1], 12017[1], 12018[1], 12020[1], 12021[1], 12031[1], 12032[1], 12034[1], 12035[1], 12036[1], 12037[1], 12041[1], 12042[1], 12044[1], 12045[1], 12046[1], 12047[1], 12051[1], 12052[1], 12053[1], 12054[1], 12055[1], 12056[1], 12057[1], 13100[1], 13101[1], 13102[1], 13120[1], 13121[1], 13122[1], 13131[1], 13132[1], 13133[1], 13151[1], 13152[1], 13153[1], 36000[1], 36400[1], 36405[1], 36406[1], 36410[1], 36420[1], 36425[1], 36430[1], 36440[1], 36591[0], 36592[0], 36600[1], 36640[1], 43752[1], 44602[1], 44603[1], 44604[1], 44605[1], 44850[0], 44950[0], 44970[0], 49000[0], 49002[1], 49010[0], 50100[1], 50600[1], 50605[1], 50715[1], 50900[1], 51701[1], 51702[1], 51703[1], 62320[0], 62321[0], 62322[0], 62323[0], 62324[0], 62325[0], 62326[0], 62327[0], 64400[0], 64405[0], 64408[0], 64415[0], 64416[0], 64417[0], 64418[0], 64420[0], 64421[0], 64425[0], 64430[0], 64435[0], 64445[0], 64446[0], 64447[0], 64448[0], 64449[0], 64450[0], 64451[0], 64454[0], 64461[0], 64462[0], 64463[0], 64479[0], 64480[0], 64483[0], 64484[0], 64486[0], 64487[0], 64488[0], 64489[0], 64490[0], 64491[0], 64492[0], 64493[0], 64494[0], 64495[0], 64505[0], 64510[0], 64517[0], 64520[0], 64530[0], 69990[0], 92012[1], 92014[1], 93000[1], 93005[1], 93010[1], 93040[1], 93041[1], 93042[1], 93318[1], 93355[1], 94002[1], 94200[1], 94680[1], 94681[1], 94690[1], 95812[1], 95813[1], 95816[1], 95819[1], 95822[1], 95829[1], 95955[1], 96360[1], 96361[1], 96365[1], 96366[1], 96367[1], 96368[1], 96372[1], 96374[1], 96375[1], 96376[1], 96377[1], 96523[0], 99155[0], 99156[0], 99157[0], 99211[1], 99212[1], 99213[1], 99214[1], 99215[1], 99217[1], 99218[1], 99219[1], 99220[1], 99221[1], 99222[1], 99223[1], 99231[1], 99232[1], 99233[1], 99234[1], 99235[1], 99236[1], 99238[1], 99239[1], 99241[1], 99242[1], 99243[1], 99244[1], 99245[1], 99251[1], 99252[1], 99253[1], 99254[1], 99255[1], 99291[1], 99292[1], 99304[1], 99305[1], 99306[1], 99307[1], 99308[1], 99309[1], 99310[1], 99315[1], 99316[1], 99334[1], 99335[1], 99336[1], 99337[1], 99347[1], 99348[1], 99349[1], 99350[1], 99374[1], 99375[1], 99377[1], 99378[1], 99446[0], 99447[0], 99448[0], 99449[0], 99451[0], 99452[0], 99495[0], 99496[0], G0463[1], G0471[1]
50727	00910[0], 0213T[0], 0216T[0], 0596T[1], 0597T[1], 0708T[1], 0709T[1], 11000[1], 11001[1], 11004[1], 11005[1], 11006[1], 11042[1], 11043[1], 11044[1], 11045[1], 11046[1], 11047[1], 12001[1], 12002[1], 12004[1], 12005[1], 12006[1], 12007[1], 12011[1], 12013[1], 12014[1], 12015[1], 12016[1], 12017[1], 12018[1], 12020[1], 12021[1], 12031[1], 12032[1], 12034[1], 12035[1], 12036[1], 12037[1], 12041[1], 12042[1], 12044[1], 12045[1], 12046[1], 12047[1], 12051[1], 12052[1], 12053[1], 12054[1], 12055[1], 12056[1], 12057[1], 13100[1], 13101[1], 13102[1], 13120[1], 13121[1], 13122[1], 13131[1], 13132[1], 13133[1], 13151[1], 13152[1], 13153[1], 36000[1], 36400[1], 36405[1], 36406[1], 36410[1], 36420[1], 36425[1], 36430[1], 36440[1], 36591[0], 36592[0], 36600[1], 36640[1], 43752[1], 44602[1], 44603[1], 44604[1], 44605[1], 44850[0], 44950[0], 44970[0], 49000[0], 49002[1], 49010[0], 50605[1], 50715[1], 51701[1], 51702[1], 51703[1], 53520[0], 62320[0], 62321[0], 62322[0], 62323[0], 62324[0], 62325[0], 62326[0], 62327[0], 64400[0], 64405[0], 64408[0], 64415[0], 64416[0], 64417[0], 64418[0], 64420[0], 64421[0], 64425[0], 64430[0], 64435[0], 64445[0], 64446[0], 64447[0], 64448[0], 64449[0], 64450[0], 64451[0], 64454[0], 64461[0], 64462[0], 64463[0], 64479[0], 64480[0], 64483[0], 64484[0], 64486[0], 64487[0], 64488[0], 64489[0], 64490[0], 64491[0], 64492[0], 64493[0], 64494[0], 64495[0], 64505[0], 64510[0], 64517[0], 64520[0], 64530[0], 69990[0], 92012[1], 92014[1], 93000[1], 93005[1], 93010[1], 93040[1], 93041[1], 93042[1], 93318[1], 93355[1], 94002[1], 94200[1], 94680[1], 94681[1], 94690[1], 95812[1], 95813[1], 95816[1], 95819[1], 95822[1], 95829[1], 95955[1], 96360[1], 96361[1], 96365[1], 96366[1], 96367[1], 96368[1], 96372[1], 96374[1], 96375[1], 96376[1], 96377[1], 96523[0], 97597[1], 97598[1], 97602[1], 99155[0], 99156[0], 99157[0], 99211[1], 99212[1], 99213[1], 99214[1], 99215[1], 99217[1], 99218[1], 99219[1], 99220[1], 99221[1], 99222[1], 99223[1], 99231[1], 99232[1], 99233[1], 99234[1], 99235[1], 99236[1], 99238[1], 99239[1], 99241[1], 99242[1], 99243[1], 99244[1], 99245[1], 99251[1], 99252[1], 99253[1], 99254[1], 99255[1], 99291[1], 99292[1], 99304[1], 99305[1], 99306[1], 99307[1], 99308[1], 99309[1], 99310[1], 99315[1], 99316[1], 99334[1], 99335[1], 99336[1], 99337[1], 99347[1], 99348[1], 99349[1], 99350[1], 99374[1], 99375[1], 99377[1], 99378[1], 99446[0], 99447[0], 99448[0], 99449[0], 99451[0], 99452[0], 99495[0], 99496[0], G0463[1], G0471[1]
50728	00910[0], 0213T[0], 0216T[0], 0437T[1], 0596T[1], 0597T[1], 0708T[1], 0709T[1], 11000[1], 11001[1], 11004[1], 11005[1], 11006[1], 11042[1], 11043[1], 11044[1], 11045[1], 11046[1], 11047[1], 12001[1], 12002[1], 12004[1], 12005[1], 12006[1], 12007[1], 12011[1], 12013[1], 12014[1], 12015[1], 12016[1], 12017[1], 12018[1], 12020[1], 12021[1], 12031[1], 12032[1], 12034[1], 12035[1], 12036[1], 12037[1], 12041[1], 12042[1], 12044[1], 12045[1], 12046[1], 12047[1], 12051[1], 12052[1], 12053[1], 12054[1], 12055[1], 12056[1], 12057[1], 13100[1], 13101[1], 13102[1], 13120[1], 13121[1], 13122[1], 13131[1], 13132[1], 13133[1], 13151[1], 13152[1], 13153[1], 15777[1], 36000[1], 36400[1], 36405[1], 36406[1], 36410[1], 36420[1], 36425[1], 36430[1], 36440[1], 36591[0], 36592[0], 36600[1], 36640[1], 43752[1], 44602[1], 44603[1], 44604[1], 44605[1], 44820[0], 44850[0], 44950[0], 44970[0], 49000[0], 49002[1], 49010[0], 49568[1], 50605[1], 50715[1], 50727[1], 51701[1], 51702[1], 51703[1], 53520[0], 57267[1], 62320[0], 62321[0], 62322[0], 62323[0], 62324[0], 62325[0], 62326[0], 62327[0], 64400[0], 64405[0], 64408[0], 64415[0], 64416[0], 64417[0], 64418[0], 64420[0], 64421[0], 64425[0], 64430[0], 64435[0], 64445[0], 64446[0], 64447[0], 64448[0], 64449[0], 64450[0], 64451[0], 64454[0], 64461[0], 64462[0], 64463[0], 64479[0], 64480[0], 64483[0], 64484[0], 64486[0], 64487[0], 64488[0], 64489[0], 64490[0], 64491[0], 64492[0], 64493[0], 64494[0], 64495[0], 64505[0], 64510[0], 64517[0], 64520[0], 64530[0], 69990[0], 92012[1], 92014[1], 93000[1], 93005[1], 93010[1], 93040[1], 93041[1], 93042[1], 93318[1], 93355[1], 94002[1], 94200[1], 94680[1], 94681[1], 94690[1], 95812[1], 95813[1], 95816[1], 95819[1], 95822[1], 95829[1], 95955[1], 96360[1], 96361[1], 96365[1], 96366[1], 96367[1], 96368[1], 96372[1], 96374[1], 96375[1], 96376[1], 96377[1], 96523[0], 97597[1], 97598[1], 97602[1], 99155[0], 99156[0], 99157[0], 99211[1], 99212[1], 99213[1], 99214[1], 99215[1], 99217[1], 99218[1], 99219[1], 99220[1], 99221[1], 99222[1], 99223[1], 99231[1], 99232[1], 99233[1], 99234[1], 99235[1], 99236[1], 99238[1], 99239[1], 99241[1], 99242[1], 99243[1], 99244[1], 99245[1], 99251[1], 99252[1], 99253[1], 99254[1], 99255[1], 99291[1], 99292[1], 99304[1], 99305[1], 99306[1], 99307[1], 99308[1], 99309[1], 99310[1], 99315[1], 99316[1], 99334[1], 99335[1], 99336[1], 99337[1], 99347[1], 99348[1], 99349[1], 99350[1], 99374[1], 99375[1], 99377[1], 99378[1], 99446[0], 99447[0], 99448[0], 99449[0], 99451[0], 99452[0], 99495[0], 99496[0], G0463[1], G0471[1]
50740	00910[0], 0213T[0], 0216T[0], 0596T[1], 0597T[1], 0708T[1], 0709T[1], 12001[1], 12002[1], 12004[1], 12005[1], 12006[1], 12007[1], 12011[1], 12013[1], 12014[1], 12015[1], 12016[1], 12017[1], 12018[1], 12020[1], 12021[1], 12031[1], 12032[1], 12034[1], 12035[1], 12036[1], 12037[1], 12041[1], 12042[1], 12044[1], 12045[1], 12046[1], 12047[1], 12051[1], 12052[1], 12053[1], 12054[1], 12055[1], 12056[1], 12057[1], 13100[1], 13101[1], 13102[1], 13120[1], 13121[1], 13122[1], 13131[1], 13132[1], 13133[1], 13151[1], 13152[1], 13153[1], 36000[1], 36400[1], 36405[1], 36406[1], 36410[1], 36420[1], 36425[1], 36430[1], 36440[1], 36591[0], 36592[0], 36600[1], 36640[1], 43752[1], 44602[1], 44603[1], 44604[1], 44605[1], 44850[0], 44950[0], 44970[0], 49000[0], 49002[1], 49010[0], 50100[1], 50605[1], 50650[0], 50782[1], 50800[1], 50860[1], 51701[1], 51702[1], 51703[1], 62320[0], 62321[0], 62322[0], 62323[0], 62324[0], 62325[0], 62326[0], 62327[0], 64400[0], 64405[0], 64408[0], 64415[0], 64416[0], 64417[0], 64418[0], 64420[0], 64421[0], 64425[0], 64430[0], 64435[0], 64445[0], 64446[0], 64447[0], 64448[0], 64449[0], 64450[0], 64451[0], 64454[0], 64461[0], 64462[0], 64463[0], 64479[0], 64480[0], 64483[0], 64484[0], 64486[0], 64487[0], 64488[0], 64489[0], 64490[0], 64491[0], 64492[0], 64493[0], 64494[0], 64495[0], 64505[0], 64510[0], 64517[0], 64520[0], 64530[0], 69990[0], 92012[1], 92014[1], 93000[1], 93005[1], 93010[1], 93040[1], 93041[1], 93042[1], 93318[1], 93355[1], 94002[1], 94200[1], 94680[1], 94681[1], 94690[1], 95812[1], 95813[1], 95816[1], 95819[1], 95822[1], 95829[1], 95955[1], 96360[1], 96361[1], 96365[1], 96366[1], 96367[1], 96368[1], 96372[1], 96374[1], 96375[1], 96376[1], 96377[1], 96523[0], 99155[0], 99156[0], 99157[0], 99211[1], 99212[1], 99213[1], 99214[1], 99215[1], 99217[1], 99218[1], 99219[1], 99220[1], 99221[1], 99222[1], 99223[1], 99231[1], 99232[1], 99233[1], 99234[1], 99235[1], 99236[1], 99238[1], 99239[1], 99241[1], 99242[1], 99243[1], 99244[1], 99245[1], 99251[1], 99252[1], 99253[1], 99254[1], 99255[1], 99291[1], 99292[1], 99304[1], 99305[1], 99306[1], 99307[1], 99308[1], 99309[1], 99310[1], 99315[1], 99316[1], 99334[1], 99335[1], 99336[1], 99337[1], 99347[1], 99348[1], 99349[1], 99350[1], 99374[1], 99375[1], 99377[1], 99378[1], 99446[0], 99447[0], 99448[0], 99449[0], 99451[0], 99452[0], 99495[0], 99496[0], G0463[1], G0471[1]

0 = Modifier usage not allowed or inappropriate 1 = Modifier usage allowed

Code 1	Code 2
50750	00910[0], 0213T[0], 0216T[0], 0596T[1], 0597T[1], 0708T[1], 0709T[1], 12001[1], 12002[1], 12004[1], 12005[1], 12006[1], 12007[1], 12011[1], 12013[1], 12014[1], 12015[1], 12016[1], 12017[1], 12018[1], 12020[1], 12021[1], 12031[1], 12032[1], 12034[1], 12035[1], 12036[1], 12037[1], 12041[1], 12042[1], 12044[1], 12045[1], 12046[1], 12047[1], 12051[1], 12052[1], 12053[1], 12054[1], 12055[1], 12056[1], 12057[1], 13100[1], 13101[1], 13102[1], 13120[1], 13121[1], 13122[1], 13131[1], 13132[1], 13133[1], 13151[1], 13152[1], 13153[1], 36000[1], 36400[1], 36405[1], 36406[1], 36410[1], 36420[1], 36425[1], 36430[1], 36440[1], 36591[0], 36592[0], 36600[1], 36640[1], 43752[1], 44602[1], 44603[1], 44604[1], 44605[1], 44850[0], 44950[0], 44970[0], 49000[0], 49002[1], 49010[0], 50605[1], 50650[0], 50740[1], 50760[1], 50780[1], 50782[1], 50800[1], 50860[1], 51701[1], 51702[1], 51703[1], 62320[0], 62321[0], 62322[0], 62323[0], 62324[0], 62325[0], 62326[0], 62327[0], 64400[0], 64405[0], 64408[0], 64415[0], 64416[0], 64417[0], 64418[0], 64420[0], 64421[0], 64425[0], 64430[0], 64435[0], 64445[0], 64446[0], 64447[0], 64448[0], 64449[0], 64450[0], 64451[0], 64454[0], 64461[0], 64462[0], 64463[0], 64479[0], 64480[0], 64483[0], 64484[0], 64486[0], 64487[0], 64488[0], 64489[0], 64490[0], 64491[0], 64492[0], 64493[0], 64494[0], 64495[0], 64505[0], 64510[0], 64517[0], 64520[0], 64530[0], 69990[0], 92012[1], 92014[1], 93000[1], 93005[1], 93010[1], 93040[1], 93041[1], 93042[1], 93318[1], 93355[1], 94002[1], 94200[1], 94680[1], 94681[1], 94690[1], 95812[1], 95813[1], 95816[1], 95819[1], 95822[1], 95829[1], 95955[1], 96360[1], 96361[1], 96365[1], 96366[1], 96367[1], 96368[1], 96372[1], 96374[1], 96375[1], 96376[1], 96377[1], 96523[0], 99155[0], 99156[0], 99157[0], 99211[1], 99212[1], 99213[1], 99214[1], 99215[1], 99217[1], 99218[1], 99219[1], 99220[1], 99221[1], 99222[1], 99223[1], 99231[1], 99232[1], 99233[1], 99234[1], 99235[1], 99236[1], 99238[1], 99239[1], 99241[1], 99242[1], 99243[1], 99244[1], 99245[1], 99251[1], 99252[1], 99253[1], 99254[1], 99255[1], 99291[1], 99292[1], 99304[1], 99305[1], 99306[1], 99307[1], 99308[1], 99309[1], 99310[1], 99315[1], 99316[1], 99334[1], 99335[1], 99336[1], 99337[1], 99347[1], 99348[1], 99349[1], 99350[1], 99374[1], 99375[1], 99377[1], 99378[1], 99446[0], 99447[0], 99448[0], 99449[0], 99451[0], 99452[0], 99495[0], 99496[0], G0463[1], G0471[1]
50760	00910[0], 0213T[0], 0216T[0], 0596T[1], 0597T[1], 0708T[1], 0709T[1], 12001[1], 12002[1], 12004[1], 12005[1], 12006[1], 12007[1], 12011[1], 12013[1], 12014[1], 12015[1], 12016[1], 12017[1], 12018[1], 12020[1], 12021[1], 12031[1], 12032[1], 12034[1], 12035[1], 12036[1], 12037[1], 12041[1], 12042[1], 12044[1], 12045[1], 12046[1], 12047[1], 12051[1], 12052[1], 12053[1], 12054[1], 12055[1], 12056[1], 12057[1], 13100[1], 13101[1], 13102[1], 13120[1], 13121[1], 13122[1], 13131[1], 13132[1], 13133[1], 13151[1], 13152[1], 13153[1], 36000[1], 36400[1], 36405[1], 36406[1], 36410[1], 36420[1], 36425[1], 36430[1], 36440[1], 36591[0], 36592[0], 36600[1], 36640[1], 43752[1], 44602[1], 44603[1], 44604[1], 44605[1], 44850[0], 44950[0], 44970[0], 49000[0], 49002[1], 49010[0], 50605[1], 50650[0], 50740[1], 50782[1], 50800[1], 50860[1], 51701[1], 51702[1], 51703[1], 62320[0], 62321[0], 62322[0], 62323[0], 62324[0], 62325[0], 62326[0], 62327[0], 64400[0], 64405[0], 64408[0], 64415[0], 64416[0], 64417[0], 64418[0], 64420[0], 64421[0], 64425[0], 64430[0], 64435[0], 64445[0], 64446[0], 64447[0], 64448[0], 64449[0], 64450[0], 64451[0], 64454[0], 64461[0], 64462[0], 64463[0], 64479[0], 64480[0], 64483[0], 64484[0], 64486[0], 64487[0], 64488[0], 64489[0], 64490[0], 64491[0], 64492[0], 64493[0], 64494[0], 64495[0], 64505[0], 64510[0], 64517[0], 64520[0], 64530[0], 69990[0], 92012[1], 92014[1], 93000[1], 93005[1], 93010[1], 93040[1], 93041[1], 93042[1], 93318[1], 93355[1], 94002[1], 94200[1], 94680[1], 94681[1], 94690[1], 95812[1], 95813[1], 95816[1], 95819[1], 95822[1], 95829[1], 95955[1], 96360[1], 96361[1], 96365[1], 96366[1], 96367[1], 96368[1], 96372[1], 96374[1], 96375[1], 96376[1], 96377[1], 96523[0], 99155[0], 99156[0], 99157[0], 99211[1], 99212[1], 99213[1], 99214[1], 99215[1], 99217[1], 99218[1], 99219[1], 99220[1], 99221[1], 99222[1], 99223[1], 99231[1], 99232[1], 99233[1], 99234[1], 99235[1], 99236[1], 99238[1], 99239[1], 99241[1], 99242[1], 99243[1], 99244[1], 99245[1], 99251[1], 99252[1], 99253[1], 99254[1], 99255[1], 99291[1], 99292[1], 99304[1], 99305[1], 99306[1], 99307[1], 99308[1], 99309[1], 99310[1], 99315[1], 99316[1], 99334[1], 99335[1], 99336[1], 99337[1], 99347[1], 99348[1], 99349[1], 99350[1], 99374[1], 99375[1], 99377[1], 99378[1], 99446[0], 99447[0], 99448[0], 99449[0], 99451[0], 99452[0], 99495[0], 99496[0], G0463[1], G0471[1]
50770	00910[0], 0213T[0], 0216T[0], 0596T[1], 0597T[1], 0708T[1], 0709T[1], 12001[1], 12002[1], 12004[1], 12005[1], 12006[1], 12007[1], 12011[1], 12013[1], 12014[1], 12015[1], 12016[1], 12017[1], 12018[1], 12020[1], 12021[1], 12031[1], 12032[1], 12034[1], 12035[1], 12036[1], 12037[1], 12041[1], 12042[1], 12044[1], 12045[1], 12046[1], 12047[1], 12051[1], 12052[1], 12053[1], 12054[1], 12055[1], 12056[1], 12057[1], 13100[1], 13101[1], 13102[1], 13120[1], 13121[1], 13122[1], 13131[1], 13132[1], 13133[1], 13151[1], 13152[1], 13153[1], 36000[1], 36400[1], 36405[1], 36406[1], 36410[1], 36420[1], 36425[1], 36430[1], 36440[1], 36591[0], 36592[0], 36600[1], 36640[1], 43752[1], 44602[1], 44603[1], 44604[1], 44605[1], 44850[0], 44950[0], 44970[0], 49000[0], 49002[1], 49010[0], 50605[1], 50650[0], 50740[1], 50750[1], 50760[1], 50780[1], 50782[1], 50783[1], 50800[1], 50860[1], 51701[1], 51702[1], 51703[1], 62320[0], 62321[0], 62322[0], 62323[0], 62324[0], 62325[0], 62326[0], 62327[0], 64400[0], 64405[0], 64408[0], 64415[0], 64416[0], 64417[0], 64418[0], 64420[0], 64421[0], 64425[0], 64430[0], 64435[0], 64445[0], 64446[0], 64447[0], 64448[0], 64449[0], 64450[0], 64451[0], 64454[0], 64461[0], 64462[0], 64463[0], 64479[0], 64480[0], 64483[0], 64484[0], 64486[0], 64487[0], 64488[0], 64489[0], 64490[0], 64491[0], 64492[0], 64493[0], 64494[0], 64495[0], 64505[0], 64510[0], 64517[0], 64520[0], 64530[0], 69990[0], 92012[1], 92014[1], 93000[1], 93005[1], 93010[1], 93040[1], 93041[1], 93042[1], 93318[1], 93355[1], 94002[1], 94200[1], 94680[1], 94681[1], 94690[1], 95812[1], 95813[1], 95816[1], 95819[1], 95822[1], 95829[1], 95955[1], 96360[1], 96361[1], 96365[1], 96366[1], 96367[1], 96368[1], 96372[1], 96374[1], 96375[1], 96376[1], 96377[1], 96523[0], 99155[0], 99156[0], 99157[0], 99211[1], 99212[1], 99213[1], 99214[1], 99215[1], 99217[1], 99218[1], 99219[1], 99220[1], 99221[1], 99222[1], 99223[1], 99231[1], 99232[1], 99233[1], 99234[1], 99235[1], 99236[1], 99238[1], 99239[1], 99241[1], 99242[1], 99243[1], 99244[1], 99245[1], 99251[1], 99252[1], 99253[1], 99254[1], 99255[1], 99291[1], 99292[1], 99304[1], 99305[1], 99306[1], 99307[1], 99308[1], 99309[1], 99310[1], 99315[1], 99316[1], 99334[1], 99335[1], 99336[1], 99337[1], 99347[1], 99348[1], 99349[1], 99350[1], 99374[1], 99375[1], 99377[1], 99378[1], 99446[0], 99447[0], 99448[0], 99449[0], 99451[0], 99452[0], 99495[0], 99496[0], G0463[1], G0471[1]
50780	00910[0], 0213T[0], 0216T[0], 0596T[1], 0597T[1], 0708T[1], 0709T[1], 12001[1], 12002[1], 12004[1], 12005[1], 12006[1], 12007[1], 12011[1], 12013[1], 12014[1], 12015[1], 12016[1], 12017[1], 12018[1], 12020[1], 12021[1], 12031[1], 12032[1], 12034[1], 12035[1], 12036[1], 12037[1], 12041[1], 12042[1], 12044[1], 12045[1], 12046[1], 12047[1], 12051[1], 12052[1], 12053[1], 12054[1], 12055[1], 12056[1], 12057[1], 13100[1], 13101[1], 13102[1], 13120[1], 13121[1], 13122[1], 13131[1], 13132[1], 13133[1], 13151[1], 13152[1], 13153[1], 36000[1], 36400[1], 36405[1], 36406[1], 36410[1], 36420[1], 36425[1], 36430[1], 36440[1], 36591[0], 36592[0], 36600[1], 36640[1], 43752[1], 44602[1], 44603[1], 44604[1], 44605[1], 44850[0], 44950[0], 44970[0], 49000[0], 49002[1], 49010[0], 50605[1], 50650[0], 50715[1], 50740[1], 50760[1], 50947[1], 50948[1], 51701[0], 51702[0], 51703[1], 52000[0], 62320[0], 62321[0], 62322[0], 62323[0], 62324[0], 62325[0], 62326[0], 62327[0], 64400[0], 64405[0], 64408[0], 64415[0], 64416[0], 64417[0], 64418[0], 64420[0], 64421[0], 64425[0], 64430[0], 64435[0], 64445[0], 64446[0], 64447[0], 64448[0], 64449[0], 64450[0], 64451[0], 64454[0], 64461[0], 64462[0], 64463[0], 64479[0], 64480[0], 64483[0], 64484[0], 64486[0], 64487[0], 64488[0], 64489[0], 64490[0], 64491[0], 64492[0], 64493[0], 64494[0], 64495[0], 64505[0], 64510[0], 64517[0], 64520[0], 64530[0], 69990[0], 92012[1], 92014[1], 93000[1], 93005[1], 93010[1], 93040[1], 93041[1], 93042[1], 93318[1], 93355[1], 94002[1], 94200[1], 94680[1], 94681[1], 94690[1], 95812[1], 95813[1], 95816[1], 95819[1], 95822[1], 95829[1], 95955[1], 96360[1], 96361[1], 96365[1], 96366[1], 96367[1], 96368[1], 96372[1], 96374[1], 96375[1], 96376[1], 96377[1], 96523[0], 99155[0], 99156[0], 99157[0], 99211[1], 99212[1], 99213[1], 99214[1], 99215[1], 99217[1], 99218[1], 99219[1], 99220[1], 99221[1], 99222[1], 99223[1], 99231[1], 99232[1], 99233[1], 99234[1], 99235[1], 99236[1], 99238[1], 99239[1], 99241[1], 99242[1], 99243[1], 99244[1], 99245[1], 99251[1], 99252[1], 99253[1], 99254[1], 99255[1], 99291[1], 99292[1], 99304[1], 99305[1], 99306[1], 99307[1], 99308[1], 99309[1], 99310[1], 99315[1], 99316[1], 99334[1], 99335[1], 99336[1], 99337[1], 99347[1], 99348[1], 99349[1], 99350[1], 99374[1], 99375[1], 99377[1], 99378[1], 99446[0], 99447[0], 99448[0], 99449[0], 99451[0], 99452[0], 99495[0], 99496[0], G0463[1], G0471[0]
50782	00910[0], 0213T[0], 0216T[0], 0596T[1], 0597T[1], 0708T[1], 0709T[1], 12001[1], 12002[1], 12004[1], 12005[1], 12006[1], 12007[1], 12011[1], 12013[1], 12014[1], 12015[1], 12016[1], 12017[1], 12018[1], 12020[1], 12021[1], 12031[1], 12032[1], 12034[1], 12035[1], 12036[1], 12037[1], 12041[1], 12042[1], 12044[1], 12045[1], 12046[1], 12047[1], 12051[1], 12052[1], 12053[1], 12054[1], 12055[1], 12056[1], 12057[1], 13100[1], 13101[1], 13102[1], 13120[1], 13121[1], 13122[1], 13131[1], 13132[1], 13133[1], 13151[1], 13152[1], 13153[1], 36000[1], 36400[1], 36405[1], 36406[1], 36410[1], 36420[1], 36425[1], 36430[1], 36440[1], 36591[0], 36592[0], 36600[1], 36640[1], 43752[1], 44602[1], 44603[1], 44604[1], 44605[1], 44850[0], 44950[0], 44970[0], 49000[0], 49002[1], 49010[0], 50605[1], 50650[0], 50715[1], 50780[1], 50785[1], 51701[0], 51702[0], 51703[1], 51820[0], 52000[0], 62320[0], 62321[0], 62322[0], 62323[0], 62324[0], 62325[0], 62326[0], 62327[0], 64400[0], 64405[0], 64408[0], 64415[0], 64416[0], 64417[0], 64418[0], 64420[0], 64421[0], 64425[0], 64430[0], 64435[0], 64445[0], 64446[0], 64447[0], 64448[0], 64449[0], 64450[0], 64451[0], 64454[0], 64461[0], 64462[0], 64463[0], 64479[0], 64480[0], 64483[0], 64484[0], 64486[0], 64487[0], 64488[0], 64489[0], 64490[0], 64491[0], 64492[0], 64493[0], 64494[0], 64495[0], 64505[0], 64510[0], 64517[0], 64520[0], 64530[0], 69990[0], 92012[1], 92014[1], 93000[1], 93005[1], 93010[1], 93040[1], 93041[1], 93042[1], 93318[1], 93355[1], 94002[1], 94200[1], 94680[1], 94681[1], 94690[1], 95812[1], 95813[1], 95816[1], 95819[1], 95822[1], 95829[1], 95955[1], 96360[1], 96361[1], 96365[1], 96366[1], 96367[1], 96368[1], 96372[1], 96374[1], 96375[1], 96376[1], 96377[1], 96523[0], 99155[0], 99156[0], 99157[0], 99211[1], 99212[1], 99213[1], 99214[1], 99215[1], 99217[1], 99218[1], 99219[1], 99220[1], 99221[1], 99222[1], 99223[1], 99231[1], 99232[1], 99233[1], 99234[1], 99235[1], 99236[1], 99238[1], 99239[1], 99241[1], 99242[1], 99243[1], 99244[1], 99245[1], 99251[1], 99252[1], 99253[1], 99254[1], 99255[1], 99291[1], 99292[1], 99304[1], 99305[1], 99306[1], 99307[1], 99308[1], 99309[1], 99310[1], 99315[1], 99316[1], 99334[1], 99335[1], 99336[1], 99337[1], 99347[1], 99348[1], 99349[1], 99350[1], 99374[1], 99375[1], 99377[1], 99378[1], 99446[0], 99447[0], 99448[0], 99449[0], 99451[0], 99452[0], 99495[0], 99496[0], G0463[1], G0471[0]
50783	00910[0], 0213T[0], 0216T[0], 0596T[1], 0597T[1], 0708T[1], 0709T[1], 12001[1], 12002[1], 12004[1], 12005[1], 12006[1], 12007[1], 12011[1], 12013[1], 12014[1], 12015[1], 12016[1], 12017[1], 12018[1], 12020[1], 12021[1], 12031[1], 12032[1], 12034[1], 12035[1], 12036[1], 12037[1], 12041[1], 12042[1], 12044[1], 12045[1], 12046[1], 12047[1], 12051[1], 12052[1], 12053[1], 12054[1], 12055[1], 12056[1], 12057[1], 13100[1], 13101[1], 13102[1], 13120[1], 13121[1], 13122[1], 13131[1], 13132[1], 13133[1], 13151[1], 13152[1], 13153[1], 36000[1], 36400[1], 36405[1], 36406[1], 36410[1], 36420[1], 36425[1], 36430[1], 36440[1], 36591[0], 36592[0], 36600[1], 36640[1], 43752[1], 44602[1], 44603[1], 44604[1], 44605[1], 44850[0], 44950[0], 44970[0], 49000[0], 49002[1], 49010[0], 50605[1], 50650[0], 50715[1], 50740[1], 50750[1], 50760[1], 50780[1], 50782[1], 50785[1], 51701[0], 51702[0], 51703[1], 51820[0], 52000[0], 62320[0], 62321[0], 62322[0], 62323[0], 62324[0], 62325[0], 62326[0], 62327[0], 64400[0],

0 = Modifier usage not allowed or inappropriate 1 = Modifier usage allowed

Code 1	Code 2
	64405[0], 64408[0], 64415[0], 64416[0], 64417[0], 64418[0], 64420[0], 64421[0], 64425[0], 64430[0], 64435[0], 64445[0], 64446[0], 64447[0], 64448[0], 64449[0], 64450[0], 64451[0], 64454[0], 64461[0], 64462[0], 64463[0], 64479[0], 64480[0], 64483[0], 64484[0], 64486[0], 64487[0], 64488[0], 64489[0], 64490[0], 64491[0], 64492[0], 64493[0], 64494[0], 64495[0], 64505[0], 64510[0], 64517[0], 64520[0], 64530[0], 69990[0], 92012[1], 92014[1], 93000[1], 93005[1], 93010[1], 93040[1], 93041[1], 93042[1], 93318[1], 93355[1], 94002[1], 94200[1], 94680[1], 94681[1], 94690[1], 95812[1], 95813[1], 95816[1], 95819[1], 95822[1], 95829[1], 95955[1], 96360[1], 96361[1], 96365[1], 96366[1], 96367[1], 96368[1], 96372[1], 96374[1], 96375[1], 96376[1], 96377[1], 96523[0], 99155[0], 99156[0], 99157[0], 99211[1], 99212[1], 99213[1], 99214[1], 99215[1], 99217[1], 99218[1], 99219[1], 99220[1], 99221[1], 99222[1], 99223[1], 99231[1], 99232[1], 99233[1], 99234[1], 99235[1], 99236[1], 99238[1], 99239[1], 99241[1], 99242[1], 99243[1], 99244[1], 99245[1], 99251[1], 99252[1], 99253[1], 99254[1], 99255[1], 99291[1], 99292[1], 99304[1], 99305[1], 99306[1], 99307[1], 99308[1], 99309[1], 99310[1], 99315[1], 99316[1], 99334[1], 99335[1], 99336[1], 99337[1], 99347[1], 99348[1], 99349[1], 99350[1], 99374[1], 99375[1], 99377[1], 99378[1], 99446[0], 99447[0], 99448[0], 99449[0], 99451[0], 99452[0], 99495[0], 99496[0], G0463[1], G0471[0]
50785	00910[0], 0213T[0], 0216T[0], 0596T[1], 0597T[1], 0708T[1], 0709T[1], 12001[1], 12002[1], 12004[1], 12005[1], 12006[1], 12007[1], 12011[1], 12013[1], 12014[1], 12015[1], 12016[1], 12017[1], 12018[1], 12020[1], 12021[1], 12031[1], 12032[1], 12034[1], 12035[1], 12036[1], 12037[1], 12041[1], 12042[1], 12044[1], 12045[1], 12046[1], 12047[1], 12051[1], 12052[1], 12053[1], 12054[1], 12055[1], 12056[1], 12057[1], 13100[1], 13101[1], 13102[1], 13120[1], 13121[1], 13122[1], 13131[1], 13132[1], 13133[1], 13151[1], 13152[1], 13153[1], 36000[1], 36400[1], 36405[1], 36406[1], 36410[1], 36420[1], 36425[1], 36430[1], 36440[1], 36591[0], 36592[0], 36600[1], 36640[1], 43752[1], 44602[1], 44603[1], 44604[1], 44605[1], 44850[0], 44950[0], 44970[0], 49000[0], 49002[1], 49010[0], 49320[1], 50605[1], 50650[0], 50715[1], 50740[1], 50750[1], 50760[1], 50770[1], 50780[1], 51701[0], 51702[0], 51703[1], 51820[0], 52000[0], 62320[0], 62321[0], 62322[0], 62323[0], 62324[0], 62325[0], 62326[0], 62327[0], 64400[0], 64405[0], 64408[0], 64415[0], 64416[0], 64417[0], 64418[0], 64420[0], 64421[0], 64425[0], 64430[0], 64435[0], 64445[0], 64446[0], 64447[0], 64448[0], 64449[0], 64450[0], 64451[0], 64454[0], 64461[0], 64462[0], 64463[0], 64479[0], 64480[0], 64483[0], 64484[0], 64486[0], 64487[0], 64488[0], 64489[0], 64490[0], 64491[0], 64492[0], 64493[0], 64494[0], 64495[0], 64505[0], 64510[0], 64517[0], 64520[0], 64530[0], 69990[0], 92012[1], 92014[1], 93000[1], 93005[1], 93010[1], 93040[1], 93041[1], 93042[1], 93318[1], 93355[1], 94002[1], 94200[1], 94680[1], 94681[1], 94690[1], 95812[1], 95813[1], 95816[1], 95819[1], 95822[1], 95829[1], 95955[1], 96360[1], 96361[1], 96365[1], 96366[1], 96367[1], 96368[1], 96372[1], 96374[1], 96375[1], 96376[1], 96377[1], 96523[0], 99155[0], 99156[0], 99157[0], 99211[1], 99212[1], 99213[1], 99214[1], 99215[1], 99217[1], 99218[1], 99219[1], 99220[1], 99221[1], 99222[1], 99223[1], 99231[1], 99232[1], 99233[1], 99234[1], 99235[1], 99236[1], 99238[1], 99239[1], 99241[1], 99242[1], 99243[1], 99244[1], 99245[1], 99251[1], 99252[1], 99253[1], 99254[1], 99255[1], 99291[1], 99292[1], 99304[1], 99305[1], 99306[1], 99307[1], 99308[1], 99309[1], 99310[1], 99315[1], 99316[1], 99334[1], 99335[1], 99336[1], 99337[1], 99347[1], 99348[1], 99349[1], 99350[1], 99374[1], 99375[1], 99377[1], 99378[1], 99446[0], 99447[0], 99448[0], 99449[0], 99451[0], 99452[0], 99495[0], 99496[0], G0463[1], G0471[0]
50800	00910[0], 0213T[0], 0216T[0], 0596T[1], 0597T[1], 0708T[1], 0709T[1], 12001[1], 12002[1], 12004[1], 12005[1], 12006[1], 12007[1], 12011[1], 12013[1], 12014[1], 12015[1], 12016[1], 12017[1], 12018[1], 12020[1], 12021[1], 12031[1], 12032[1], 12034[1], 12035[1], 12036[1], 12037[1], 12041[1], 12042[1], 12044[1], 12045[1], 12046[1], 12047[1], 12051[1], 12052[1], 12053[1], 12054[1], 12055[1], 12056[1], 12057[1], 13100[1], 13101[1], 13102[1], 13120[1], 13121[1], 13122[1], 13131[1], 13132[1], 13133[1], 13151[1], 13152[1], 13153[1], 36000[1], 36400[1], 36405[1], 36406[1], 36410[1], 36420[1], 36425[1], 36430[1], 36440[1], 36591[0], 36592[0], 36600[1], 36640[1], 43752[1], 44005[0], 44180[0], 44602[1], 44603[1], 44604[1], 44605[1], 44820[0], 44850[0], 44950[0], 44970[0], 49000[0], 49002[1], 49010[0], 49255[0], 49320[1], 50605[0], 50650[0], 50715[1], 50820[0], 50825[1], 50860[1], 51701[0], 51702[0], 51703[1], 62320[0], 62321[0], 62322[0], 62323[0], 62324[0], 62325[0], 62326[0], 62327[0], 64400[0], 64405[0], 64408[0], 64415[0], 64416[0], 64417[0], 64418[0], 64420[0], 64421[0], 64425[0], 64430[0], 64435[0], 64445[0], 64446[0], 64447[0], 64448[0], 64449[0], 64450[0], 64451[0], 64454[0], 64461[0], 64462[0], 64463[0], 64479[0], 64480[0], 64483[0], 64484[0], 64486[0], 64487[0], 64488[0], 64489[0], 64490[0], 64491[0], 64492[0], 64493[0], 64494[0], 64495[0], 64505[0], 64510[0], 64517[0], 64520[0], 64530[0], 69990[0], 92012[1], 92014[1], 93000[1], 93005[1], 93010[1], 93040[1], 93041[1], 93042[1], 93318[1], 93355[1], 94002[1], 94200[1], 94680[1], 94681[1], 94690[1], 95812[1], 95813[1], 95816[1], 95819[1], 95822[1], 95829[1], 95955[1], 96360[1], 96361[1], 96365[1], 96366[1], 96367[1], 96368[1], 96372[1], 96374[1], 96375[1], 96376[1], 96377[1], 96523[0], 99155[0], 99156[0], 99157[0], 99211[1], 99212[1], 99213[1], 99214[1], 99215[1], 99217[1], 99218[1], 99219[1], 99220[1], 99221[1], 99222[1], 99223[1], 99231[1], 99232[1], 99233[1], 99234[1], 99235[1], 99236[1], 99238[1], 99239[1], 99241[1], 99242[1], 99243[1], 99244[1], 99245[1], 99251[1], 99252[1], 99253[1], 99254[1], 99255[1], 99291[1], 99292[1], 99304[1], 99305[1], 99306[1], 99307[1], 99308[1], 99309[1], 99310[1], 99315[1], 99316[1], 99334[1], 99335[1], 99336[1], 99337[1], 99347[1], 99348[1], 99349[1], 99350[1], 99374[1], 99375[1], 99377[1], 99378[1], 99446[0], 99447[0], 99448[0], 99449[0], 99451[0], 99452[0], 99495[0], 99496[0], G0463[1], G0471[0]
50810	00910[0], 0213T[0], 0216T[0], 0596T[1], 0597T[1], 0708T[1], 0709T[1], 12001[1], 12002[1], 12004[1], 12005[1], 12006[1], 12007[1], 12011[1], 12013[1], 12014[1], 12015[1], 12016[1], 12017[1], 12018[1], 12020[1], 12021[1], 12031[1], 12032[1], 12034[1], 12035[1], 12036[1], 12037[1], 12041[1], 12042[1], 12044[1], 12045[1], 12046[1], 12047[1], 12051[1], 12052[1], 12053[1], 12054[1], 12055[1], 12056[1], 12057[1], 13100[1], 13101[1], 13102[1], 13120[1], 13121[1], 13122[1], 13131[1], 13132[1], 13133[1], 13151[1], 13152[1], 13153[1], 36000[1], 36400[1], 36405[1], 36406[1], 36410[1], 36420[1], 36425[1], 36430[1], 36440[1], 36591[0], 36592[0], 36600[1], 36640[1], 43752[1], 44005[0], 44180[0], 44188[1], 44320[1], 44602[1], 44603[1], 44604[1], 44605[1], 44820[0], 44850[0], 44950[0], 44970[0], 49000[0], 49002[1], 49010[0], 49255[0], 49320[1], 50605[0], 50650[0], 50715[1], 50740[1], 50750[1], 50760[1], 50770[1], 50800[1], 50820[1], 50825[1], 51701[0], 51702[0], 51703[1], 62320[0], 62321[0], 62322[0], 62323[0], 62324[0], 62325[0], 62326[0], 62327[0], 64400[0], 64405[0], 64408[0], 64415[0], 64416[0], 64417[0], 64418[0], 64420[0], 64421[0], 64425[0], 64430[0], 64435[0], 64445[0], 64446[0], 64447[0], 64448[0], 64449[0], 64450[0], 64451[0], 64454[0], 64461[0], 64462[0], 64463[0], 64479[0], 64480[0], 64483[0], 64484[0], 64486[0], 64487[0], 64488[0], 64489[0], 64490[0], 64491[0], 64492[0], 64493[0], 64494[0], 64495[0], 64505[0], 64510[0], 64517[0], 64520[0], 64530[0], 69990[0], 92012[1], 92014[1], 93000[1], 93005[1], 93010[1], 93040[1], 93041[1], 93042[1], 93318[1], 93355[1], 94002[1], 94200[1], 94680[1], 94681[1], 94690[1], 95812[1], 95813[1], 95816[1], 95819[1], 95822[1], 95829[1], 95955[1], 96360[1], 96361[1], 96365[1], 96366[1], 96367[1], 96368[1], 96372[1], 96374[1], 96375[1], 96376[1], 96377[1], 96523[0], 99155[0], 99156[0], 99157[0], 99211[1], 99212[1], 99213[1], 99214[1], 99215[1], 99217[1], 99218[1], 99219[1], 99220[1], 99221[1], 99222[1], 99223[1], 99231[1], 99232[1], 99233[1], 99234[1], 99235[1], 99236[1], 99238[1], 99239[1], 99241[1], 99242[1], 99243[1], 99244[1], 99245[1], 99251[1], 99252[1], 99253[1], 99254[1], 99255[1], 99291[1], 99292[1], 99304[1], 99305[1], 99306[1], 99307[1], 99308[1], 99309[1], 99310[1], 99315[1], 99316[1], 99334[1], 99335[1], 99336[1], 99337[1], 99347[1], 99348[1], 99349[1], 99350[1], 99374[1], 99375[1], 99377[1], 99378[1], 99446[0], 99447[0], 99448[0], 99449[0], 99451[0], 99452[0], 99495[0], 99496[0], G0463[1], G0471[0]
50815	00910[0], 0213T[0], 0216T[0], 0596T[1], 0597T[1], 0708T[1], 0709T[1], 12001[1], 12002[1], 12004[1], 12005[1], 12006[1], 12007[1], 12011[1], 12013[1], 12014[1], 12015[1], 12016[1], 12017[1], 12018[1], 12020[1], 12021[1], 12031[1], 12032[1], 12034[1], 12035[1], 12036[1], 12037[1], 12041[1], 12042[1], 12044[1], 12045[1], 12046[1], 12047[1], 12051[1], 12052[1], 12053[1], 12054[1], 12055[1], 12056[1], 12057[1], 13100[1], 13101[1], 13102[1], 13120[1], 13121[1], 13122[1], 13131[1], 13132[1], 13133[1], 13151[1], 13152[1], 13153[1], 36000[1], 36400[1], 36405[1], 36406[1], 36410[1], 36420[1], 36425[1], 36430[1], 36440[1], 36591[0], 36592[0], 36600[1], 36640[1], 43752[1], 44005[0], 44180[0], 44602[1], 44603[1], 44604[1], 44605[1], 44820[0], 44850[0], 44950[0], 44970[0], 49000[0], 49002[1], 49010[0], 49255[0], 49320[1], 50605[0], 50650[0], 50715[1], 50740[1], 50750[1], 50760[1], 50770[1], 50820[1], 50825[1], 51701[0], 51702[0], 51703[1], 62320[0], 62321[0], 62322[0], 62323[0], 62324[0], 62325[0], 62326[0], 62327[0], 64400[0], 64405[0], 64408[0], 64415[0], 64416[0], 64417[0], 64418[0], 64420[0], 64421[0], 64425[0], 64430[0], 64435[0], 64445[0], 64446[0], 64447[0], 64448[0], 64449[0], 64450[0], 64451[0], 64454[0], 64461[0], 64462[0], 64463[0], 64479[0], 64480[0], 64483[0], 64484[0], 64486[0], 64487[0], 64488[0], 64489[0], 64490[0], 64491[0], 64492[0], 64493[0], 64494[0], 64495[0], 64505[0], 64510[0], 64517[0], 64520[0], 64530[0], 69990[0], 92012[1], 92014[1], 93000[1], 93005[1], 93010[1], 93040[1], 93041[1], 93042[1], 93318[1], 93355[1], 94002[1], 94200[1], 94680[1], 94681[1], 94690[1], 95812[1], 95813[1], 95816[1], 95819[1], 95822[1], 95829[1], 95955[1], 96360[1], 96361[1], 96365[1], 96366[1], 96367[1], 96368[1], 96372[1], 96374[1], 96375[1], 96376[1], 96377[1], 96523[0], 99155[0], 99156[0], 99157[0], 99211[1], 99212[1], 99213[1], 99214[1], 99215[1], 99217[1], 99218[1], 99219[1], 99220[1], 99221[1], 99222[1], 99223[1], 99231[1], 99232[1], 99233[1], 99234[1], 99235[1], 99236[1], 99238[1], 99239[1], 99241[1], 99242[1], 99243[1], 99244[1], 99245[1], 99251[1], 99252[1], 99253[1], 99254[1], 99255[1], 99291[1], 99292[1], 99304[1], 99305[1], 99306[1], 99307[1], 99308[1], 99309[1], 99310[1], 99315[1], 99316[1], 99334[1], 99335[1], 99336[1], 99337[1], 99347[1], 99348[1], 99349[1], 99350[1], 99374[1], 99375[1], 99377[1], 99378[1], 99446[0], 99447[0], 99448[0], 99449[0], 99451[0], 99452[0], 99495[0], 99496[0], G0463[1], G0471[0]
50820	00910[0], 0213T[0], 0216T[0], 0596T[1], 0597T[1], 0708T[1], 0709T[1], 12001[1], 12002[1], 12004[1], 12005[1], 12006[1], 12007[1], 12011[1], 12013[1], 12014[1], 12015[1], 12016[1], 12017[1], 12018[1], 12020[1], 12021[1], 12031[1], 12032[1], 12034[1], 12035[1], 12036[1], 12037[1], 12041[1], 12042[1], 12044[1], 12045[1], 12046[1], 12047[1], 12051[1], 12052[1], 12053[1], 12054[1], 12055[1], 12056[1], 12057[1], 13100[1], 13101[1], 13102[1], 13120[1], 13121[1], 13122[1], 13131[1], 13132[1], 13133[1], 13151[1], 13152[1], 13153[1], 36000[1], 36400[1], 36405[1], 36406[1], 36410[1], 36420[1], 36425[1], 36430[1], 36440[1], 36591[0], 36592[0], 36600[1], 36640[1], 43752[1], 44005[0], 44180[0], 44602[1], 44603[1], 44604[1], 44605[1], 44820[0], 44850[0], 44950[0], 44970[0], 49000[0], 49002[1], 49010[0], 49255[0], 49320[1], 50605[0], 50650[0], 50715[1], 50740[1], 50750[1], 50760[1], 50770[1], 50825[1], 51580[0], 51585[0], 51701[0], 51702[0], 51703[1], 62320[0], 62321[0], 62322[0], 62323[0], 62324[0], 62325[0], 62326[0], 62327[0], 64400[0], 64405[0], 64408[0], 64415[0], 64416[0], 64417[0], 64418[0], 64420[0], 64421[0], 64425[0], 64430[0], 64435[0], 64445[0], 64446[0], 64447[0], 64448[0], 64449[0], 64450[0], 64451[0], 64454[0], 64461[0], 64462[0], 64463[0], 64479[0], 64480[0], 64483[0], 64484[0], 64486[0], 64487[0], 64488[0], 64489[0], 64490[0], 64491[0], 64492[0], 64493[0], 64494[0], 64495[0], 64505[0], 64510[0], 64517[0], 64520[0], 64530[0], 69990[0], 92012[1], 92014[1], 93000[1], 93005[1], 93010[1], 93040[1], 93041[1], 93042[1], 93318[1], 93355[1], 94002[1], 94200[1], 94680[1], 94681[1],

0 = Modifier usage not allowed or inappropriate 1 = Modifier usage allowed

Code 1	Code 2
	94690[1], 95812[1], 95813[1], 95816[1], 95819[1], 95822[1], 95829[1], 95955[1], 96360[1], 96361[1], 96365[1], 96366[1], 96367[1], 96368[1], 96372[1], 96374[1], 96375[1], 96376[1], 96377[1], 96523[0], 99155[0], 99156[0], 99157[0], 99211[1], 99212[1], 99213[1], 99214[1], 99215[1], 99217[1], 99218[1], 99219[1], 99220[1], 99221[1], 99222[1], 99223[1], 99231[1], 99232[1], 99233[1], 99234[1], 99235[1], 99236[1], 99238[1], 99239[1], 99241[1], 99242[1], 99243[1], 99244[1], 99245[1], 99251[1], 99252[1], 99253[1], 99254[1], 99255[1], 99291[1], 99292[1], 99304[1], 99305[1], 99306[1], 99307[1], 99308[1], 99309[1], 99310[1], 99315[1], 99316[1], 99334[1], 99335[1], 99336[1], 99337[1], 99347[1], 99348[1], 99349[1], 99350[1], 99374[1], 99375[1], 99377[1], 99378[1], 99446[0], 99447[0], 99448[0], 99449[0], 99451[0], 99452[0], 99495[0], 99496[0], G0463[1], G0471[0]
50825	00910[0], 0213T[0], 0216T[0], 0596T[1], 0597T[1], 0708T[1], 0709T[1], 11000[1], 11001[1], 11004[1], 11005[1], 11006[1], 11042[1], 11043[1], 11044[1], 11045[1], 11046[1], 11047[1], 12001[1], 12002[1], 12004[1], 12005[1], 12006[1], 12007[1], 12011[1], 12013[1], 12014[1], 12015[1], 12016[1], 12017[1], 12018[1], 12020[1], 12021[1], 12031[1], 12032[1], 12034[1], 12035[1], 12036[1], 12037[1], 12041[1], 12042[1], 12044[1], 12045[1], 12046[1], 12047[1], 12051[1], 12052[1], 12053[1], 12054[1], 12055[1], 12056[1], 12057[1], 13100[1], 13101[1], 13102[1], 13120[1], 13121[1], 13122[1], 13131[1], 13132[1], 13133[1], 13151[1], 13152[1], 13153[1], 36000[1], 36400[1], 36405[1], 36406[1], 36410[1], 36420[1], 36425[1], 36430[1], 36440[1], 36591[0], 36592[0], 36600[1], 36640[1], 43752[1], 44005[0], 44180[0], 44602[1], 44603[1], 44604[1], 44605[1], 44820[0], 44850[0], 44950[0], 44970[0], 49000[0], 49002[1], 49010[0], 49255[0], 49320[1], 50605[0], 50650[0], 50715[1], 50740[1], 50750[1], 50760[1], 50770[1], 51701[0], 51702[0], 51703[1], 62320[0], 62321[0], 62322[0], 62323[0], 62324[0], 62325[0], 62326[0], 62327[0], 64400[0], 64405[0], 64408[0], 64415[0], 64416[0], 64417[0], 64418[0], 64420[0], 64421[0], 64425[0], 64430[0], 64435[0], 64445[0], 64446[0], 64447[0], 64448[0], 64449[0], 64450[0], 64451[0], 64454[0], 64461[0], 64462[0], 64463[0], 64479[0], 64480[0], 64483[0], 64484[0], 64486[0], 64487[0], 64488[0], 64489[0], 64490[0], 64491[0], 64492[0], 64493[0], 64494[0], 64495[0], 64505[0], 64510[0], 64517[0], 64520[0], 64530[0], 69990[0], 92012[1], 92014[1], 93000[1], 93005[1], 93010[1], 93040[1], 93041[1], 93042[1], 93318[1], 93355[1], 94002[1], 94200[1], 94680[1], 94681[1], 94690[1], 95812[1], 95813[1], 95816[1], 95819[1], 95822[1], 95829[1], 95955[1], 96360[1], 96361[1], 96365[1], 96366[1], 96367[1], 96368[1], 96372[1], 96374[1], 96375[1], 96376[1], 96377[1], 96523[0], 97597[1], 97598[1], 97602[1], 99155[0], 99156[0], 99157[0], 99211[1], 99212[1], 99213[1], 99214[1], 99215[1], 99217[1], 99218[1], 99219[1], 99220[1], 99221[1], 99222[1], 99223[1], 99231[1], 99232[1], 99233[1], 99234[1], 99235[1], 99236[1], 99238[1], 99239[1], 99241[1], 99242[1], 99243[1], 99244[1], 99245[1], 99251[1], 99252[1], 99253[1], 99254[1], 99255[1], 99291[1], 99292[1], 99304[1], 99305[1], 99306[1], 99307[1], 99308[1], 99309[1], 99310[1], 99315[1], 99316[1], 99334[1], 99335[1], 99336[1], 99337[1], 99347[1], 99348[1], 99349[1], 99350[1], 99374[1], 99375[1], 99377[1], 99378[1], 99446[0], 99447[0], 99448[0], 99449[0], 99451[0], 99452[0], 99495[0], 99496[0], G0463[1], G0471[0]
50830	00910[0], 0213T[0], 0216T[0], 0596T[1], 0597T[1], 0708T[1], 0709T[1], 12001[1], 12002[1], 12004[1], 12005[1], 12006[1], 12007[1], 12011[1], 12013[1], 12014[1], 12015[1], 12016[1], 12017[1], 12018[1], 12020[1], 12021[1], 12031[1], 12032[1], 12034[1], 12035[1], 12036[1], 12037[1], 12041[1], 12042[1], 12044[1], 12045[1], 12046[1], 12047[1], 12051[1], 12052[1], 12053[1], 12054[1], 12055[1], 12056[1], 12057[1], 13100[1], 13101[1], 13102[1], 13120[1], 13121[1], 13122[1], 13131[1], 13132[1], 13133[1], 13151[1], 13152[1], 13153[1], 36000[1], 36400[1], 36405[1], 36406[1], 36410[1], 36420[1], 36425[1], 36430[1], 36440[1], 36591[0], 36592[0], 36600[1], 36640[1], 43752[1], 44005[0], 44180[0], 44602[1], 44603[1], 44604[1], 44605[1], 44820[0], 44850[0], 44950[0], 44970[0], 49000[0], 49002[1], 49010[0], 49255[0], 50605[0], 50650[0], 50715[1], 50780[0], 50782[0], 50783[0], 50785[0], 50800[1], 50810[1], 50815[1], 50860[0], 50947[0], 50948[0], 51565[0], 51701[0], 51702[0], 51703[1], 52000[1], 62320[0], 62321[0], 62322[0], 62323[0], 62324[0], 62325[0], 62326[0], 62327[0], 64400[0], 64405[0], 64408[0], 64415[0], 64416[0], 64417[0], 64418[0], 64420[0], 64421[0], 64425[0], 64430[0], 64435[0], 64445[0], 64446[0], 64447[0], 64448[0], 64449[0], 64450[0], 64451[0], 64454[0], 64461[0], 64462[0], 64463[0], 64479[0], 64480[0], 64483[0], 64484[0], 64486[0], 64487[0], 64488[0], 64489[0], 64490[0], 64491[0], 64492[0], 64493[0], 64494[0], 64495[0], 64505[0], 64510[0], 64517[0], 64520[0], 64530[0], 69990[0], 92012[1], 92014[1], 93000[1], 93005[1], 93010[1], 93040[1], 93041[1], 93042[1], 93318[1], 93355[1], 94002[1], 94200[1], 94680[1], 94681[1], 94690[1], 95812[1], 95813[1], 95816[1], 95819[1], 95822[1], 95829[1], 95955[1], 96360[1], 96361[1], 96365[1], 96366[1], 96367[1], 96368[1], 96372[1], 96374[1], 96375[1], 96376[1], 96377[1], 96523[0], 99155[0], 99156[0], 99157[0], 99211[1], 99212[1], 99213[1], 99214[1], 99215[1], 99217[1], 99218[1], 99219[1], 99220[1], 99221[1], 99222[1], 99223[1], 99231[1], 99232[1], 99233[1], 99234[1], 99235[1], 99236[1], 99238[1], 99239[1], 99241[1], 99242[1], 99243[1], 99244[1], 99245[1], 99251[1], 99252[1], 99253[1], 99254[1], 99255[1], 99291[1], 99292[1], 99304[1], 99305[1], 99306[1], 99307[1], 99308[1], 99309[1], 99310[1], 99315[1], 99316[1], 99334[1], 99335[1], 99336[1], 99337[1], 99347[1], 99348[1], 99349[1], 99350[1], 99374[1], 99375[1], 99377[1], 99378[1], 99446[0], 99447[0], 99448[0], 99449[0], 99451[0], 99452[0], 99495[0], 99496[0], G0463[1], G0471[0]
50840	00910[0], 0213T[0], 0216T[0], 0596T[1], 0597T[1], 0708T[1], 0709T[1], 11000[1], 11001[1], 11004[1], 11005[1], 11006[1], 11042[1], 11043[1], 11044[1], 11045[1], 11046[1], 11047[1], 12001[1], 12002[1], 12004[1], 12005[1], 12006[1], 12007[1], 12011[1], 12013[1], 12014[1], 12015[1], 12016[1], 12017[1], 12018[1], 12020[1], 12021[1], 12031[1], 12032[1], 12034[1], 12035[1], 12036[1], 12037[1], 12041[1], 12042[1], 12044[1], 12045[1], 12046[1], 12047[1], 12051[1], 12052[1], 12053[1], 12054[1], 12055[1], 12056[1], 12057[1], 13100[1], 13101[1], 13102[1], 13120[1], 13121[1], 13122[1], 13131[1], 13132[1], 13133[1], 13151[1], 13152[1], 13153[1], 36000[1], 36400[1], 36405[1], 36406[1], 36410[1], 36420[1], 36425[1], 36430[1], 36440[1], 36591[0], 36592[0], 36600[1], 36640[1], 43752[1], 44005[0], 44180[0], 44602[1], 44603[1], 44604[1], 44605[1], 44820[0], 44850[0], 44950[0], 44970[0], 49000[0], 49002[1], 49010[0], 49255[0], 49320[1], 50605[1], 50650[0], 50715[1], 51701[0], 51702[0], 51703[1], 62320[0], 62321[0], 62322[0], 62323[0], 62324[0], 62325[0], 62326[0], 62327[0], 64400[0], 64405[0], 64408[0], 64415[0], 64416[0], 64417[0], 64418[0], 64420[0], 64421[0], 64425[0], 64430[0], 64435[0], 64445[0], 64446[0], 64447[0], 64448[0], 64449[0], 64450[0], 64451[0], 64454[0], 64461[0], 64462[0], 64463[0], 64479[0], 64480[0], 64483[0], 64484[0], 64486[0], 64487[0], 64488[0], 64489[0], 64490[0], 64491[0], 64492[0], 64493[0], 64494[0], 64495[0], 64505[0], 64510[0], 64517[0], 64520[0], 64530[0], 69990[0], 92012[1], 92014[1], 93000[1], 93005[1], 93010[1], 93040[1], 93041[1], 93042[1], 93318[1], 93355[1], 94002[1], 94200[1], 94680[1], 94681[1], 94690[1], 95812[1], 95813[1], 95816[1], 95819[1], 95822[1], 95829[1], 95955[1], 96360[1], 96361[1], 96365[1], 96366[1], 96367[1], 96368[1], 96372[1], 96374[1], 96375[1], 96376[1], 96377[1], 96523[0], 97597[1], 97598[1], 97602[1], 99155[0], 99156[0], 99157[0], 99211[1], 99212[1], 99213[1], 99214[1], 99215[1], 99217[1], 99218[1], 99219[1], 99220[1], 99221[1], 99222[1], 99223[1], 99231[1], 99232[1], 99233[1], 99234[1], 99235[1], 99236[1], 99238[1], 99239[1], 99241[1], 99242[1], 99243[1], 99244[1], 99245[1], 99251[1], 99252[1], 99253[1], 99254[1], 99255[1], 99291[1], 99292[1], 99304[1], 99305[1], 99306[1], 99307[1], 99308[1], 99309[1], 99310[1], 99315[1], 99316[1], 99334[1], 99335[1], 99336[1], 99337[1], 99347[1], 99348[1], 99349[1], 99350[1], 99374[1], 99375[1], 99377[1], 99378[1], 99446[0], 99447[0], 99448[0], 99449[0], 99451[0], 99452[0], 99495[0], 99496[0], G0463[1], G0471[0]
50845	00910[0], 0213T[0], 0216T[0], 0596T[1], 0597T[1], 0708T[1], 0709T[1], 12001[1], 12002[1], 12004[1], 12005[1], 12006[1], 12007[1], 12011[1], 12013[1], 12014[1], 12015[1], 12016[1], 12017[1], 12018[1], 12020[1], 12021[1], 12031[1], 12032[1], 12034[1], 12035[1], 12036[1], 12037[1], 12041[1], 12042[1], 12044[1], 12045[1], 12046[1], 12047[1], 12051[1], 12052[1], 12053[1], 12054[1], 12055[1], 12056[1], 12057[1], 13100[1], 13101[1], 13102[1], 13120[1], 13121[1], 13122[1], 13131[1], 13132[1], 13133[1], 13151[1], 13152[1], 13153[1], 36000[1], 36400[1], 36405[1], 36406[1], 36410[1], 36420[1], 36425[1], 36430[1], 36440[1], 36591[0], 36592[0], 36600[1], 36640[1], 43752[1], 44005[0], 44180[0], 44602[1], 44603[1], 44604[1], 44605[1], 44820[0], 44850[0], 44950[0], 44970[0], 49000[0], 49002[1], 49010[0], 49255[0], 50650[0], 50715[1], 51701[0], 51702[0], 51703[1], 62320[0], 62321[0], 62322[0], 62323[0], 62324[0], 62325[0], 62326[0], 62327[0], 64400[0], 64405[0], 64408[0], 64415[0], 64416[0], 64417[0], 64418[0], 64420[0], 64421[0], 64425[0], 64430[0], 64435[0], 64445[0], 64446[0], 64447[0], 64448[0], 64449[0], 64450[0], 64451[0], 64454[0], 64461[0], 64462[0], 64463[0], 64479[0], 64480[0], 64483[0], 64484[0], 64486[0], 64487[0], 64488[0], 64489[0], 64490[0], 64491[0], 64492[0], 64493[0], 64494[0], 64495[0], 64505[0], 64510[0], 64517[0], 64520[0], 64530[0], 69990[0], 92012[1], 92014[1], 93000[1], 93005[1], 93010[1], 93040[1], 93041[1], 93042[1], 93318[1], 93355[1], 94002[1], 94200[1], 94680[1], 94681[1], 94690[1], 95812[1], 95813[1], 95816[1], 95819[1], 95822[1], 95829[1], 95955[1], 96360[1], 96361[1], 96365[1], 96366[1], 96367[1], 96368[1], 96372[1], 96374[1], 96375[1], 96376[1], 96377[1], 96523[0], 99155[0], 99156[0], 99157[0], 99211[1], 99212[1], 99213[1], 99214[1], 99215[1], 99217[1], 99218[1], 99219[1], 99220[1], 99221[1], 99222[1], 99223[1], 99231[1], 99232[1], 99233[1], 99234[1], 99235[1], 99236[1], 99238[1], 99239[1], 99241[1], 99242[1], 99243[1], 99244[1], 99245[1], 99251[1], 99252[1], 99253[1], 99254[1], 99255[1], 99291[1], 99292[1], 99304[1], 99305[1], 99306[1], 99307[1], 99308[1], 99309[1], 99310[1], 99315[1], 99316[1], 99334[1], 99335[1], 99336[1], 99337[1], 99347[1], 99348[1], 99349[1], 99350[1], 99374[1], 99375[1], 99377[1], 99378[1], 99446[0], 99447[0], 99448[0], 99449[0], 99451[0], 99452[0], 99495[0], 99496[0], G0463[1], G0471[0]
50860	00910[0], 0213T[0], 0216T[0], 0596T[1], 0597T[1], 0708T[1], 0709T[1], 12001[1], 12002[1], 12004[1], 12005[1], 12006[1], 12007[1], 12011[1], 12013[1], 12014[1], 12015[1], 12016[1], 12017[1], 12018[1], 12020[1], 12021[1], 12031[1], 12032[1], 12034[1], 12035[1], 12036[1], 12037[1], 12041[1], 12042[1], 12044[1], 12045[1], 12046[1], 12047[1], 12051[1], 12052[1], 12053[1], 12054[1], 12055[1], 12056[1], 12057[1], 13100[1], 13101[1], 13102[1], 13120[1], 13121[1], 13122[1], 13131[1], 13132[1], 13133[1], 13151[1], 13152[1], 13153[1], 36000[1], 36400[1], 36405[1], 36406[1], 36410[1], 36420[1], 36425[1], 36430[1], 36440[1], 36591[0], 36592[0], 36600[1], 36640[1], 43752[1], 44602[1], 44603[1], 44604[1], 44605[1], 44850[0], 44950[0], 44970[0], 49000[0], 49002[1], 49010[0], 50605[1], 50650[0], 50715[1], 50810[1], 50815[1], 50820[1], 50825[1], 51701[0], 51702[0], 51703[1], 62320[0], 62321[0], 62322[0], 62323[0], 62324[0], 62325[0], 62326[0], 62327[0], 64400[0], 64405[0], 64408[0], 64415[0], 64416[0], 64417[0], 64418[0], 64420[0], 64421[0], 64425[0], 64430[0], 64435[0], 64445[0], 64446[0], 64447[0], 64448[0], 64449[0], 64450[0], 64451[0], 64454[0], 64461[0], 64462[0], 64463[0], 64479[0], 64480[0], 64483[0], 64484[0], 64486[0], 64487[0], 64488[0], 64489[0], 64490[0], 64491[0], 64492[0], 64493[0], 64494[0], 64495[0], 64505[0], 64510[0], 64517[0], 64520[0], 64530[0], 69990[0], 92012[1], 92014[1], 93000[1], 93005[1], 93010[1], 93040[1], 93041[1], 93042[1], 93318[1], 93355[1], 94002[1], 94200[1], 94680[1], 94681[1], 94690[1], 95812[1], 95813[1], 95816[1], 95819[1], 95822[1], 95829[1], 95955[1], 96360[1], 96361[1], 96365[1], 96366[1], 96367[1], 96368[1], 96372[1], 96374[1], 96375[1], 96376[1], 96377[1], 96523[0], 99155[0], 99156[0], 99157[0], 99211[1], 99212[1], 99213[1], 99214[1], 99215[1], 99217[1], 99218[1], 99219[1], 99220[1], 99221[1], 99222[1], 99223[1], 99231[1], 99232[1], 99233[1], 99234[1], 99235[1], 99236[1], 99238[1], 99239[1], 99241[1], 99242[1], 99243[1], 99244[1], 99245[1], 99251[1], 99252[1], 99253[1], 99254[1], 99255[1], 99291[1], 99292[1], 99304[1], 99305[1], 99306[1],

0 = Modifier usage not allowed or inappropriate 1 = Modifier usage allowed

Code 1	Code 2
	99307[1], 99308[1], 99309[1], 99310[1], 99315[1], 99316[1], 99334[1], 99335[1], 99336[1], 99337[1], 99347[1], 99348[1], 99349[1], 99350[1], 99374[1], 99375[1], 99377[1], 99378[1], 99446[0], 99447[0], 99448[0], 99449[0], 99451[0], 99452[0], 99495[0], 99496[0], G0463[1], G0471[0]
50900	00910[0], 0213T[0], 0216T[0], 0596T[1], 0597T[1], 0708T[1], 0709T[1], 12001[1], 12002[1], 12004[1], 12005[1], 12006[1], 12007[1], 12011[1], 12013[1], 12014[1], 12015[1], 12016[1], 12017[1], 12018[1], 12020[1], 12021[1], 12031[1], 12032[1], 12034[1], 12035[1], 12036[1], 12037[1], 12041[1], 12042[1], 12044[1], 12045[1], 12046[1], 12047[1], 12051[1], 12052[1], 12053[1], 12054[1], 12055[1], 12056[1], 12057[1], 13100[1], 13101[1], 13102[1], 13120[1], 13121[1], 13122[1], 13131[1], 13132[1], 13133[1], 13151[1], 13152[1], 13153[1], 36000[1], 36400[1], 36405[1], 36406[1], 36410[1], 36420[1], 36425[1], 36430[1], 36440[1], 36591[0], 36592[0], 36600[1], 36640[1], 43752[1], 44602[1], 44603[1], 44604[1], 44605[1], 44850[0], 44950[0], 44970[0], 49000[0], 49002[1], 49010[0], 50650[0], 51701[0], 51702[0], 51703[1], 62320[0], 62321[0], 62322[0], 62323[0], 62324[0], 62325[0], 62326[0], 62327[0], 64400[0], 64405[0], 64408[0], 64415[0], 64416[0], 64417[0], 64418[0], 64420[0], 64421[0], 64425[0], 64430[0], 64435[0], 64445[0], 64446[0], 64447[0], 64448[0], 64449[0], 64450[0], 64451[0], 64454[0], 64461[0], 64462[0], 64463[0], 64479[0], 64480[0], 64483[0], 64484[0], 64486[0], 64487[0], 64488[0], 64489[0], 64490[0], 64491[0], 64492[0], 64493[0], 64494[0], 64495[0], 64505[0], 64510[0], 64517[0], 64520[0], 64530[0], 69990[0], 92012[1], 92014[1], 93000[1], 93005[1], 93010[1], 93040[1], 93041[1], 93042[1], 93318[1], 93355[1], 94002[1], 94200[1], 94680[1], 94681[1], 94690[1], 95812[1], 95813[1], 95816[1], 95819[1], 95822[1], 95829[1], 95955[1], 96360[1], 96361[1], 96365[1], 96366[1], 96367[1], 96368[1], 96372[1], 96374[1], 96375[1], 96376[1], 96377[1], 96523[0], 99155[0], 99156[0], 99157[0], 99211[1], 99212[1], 99213[1], 99214[1], 99215[1], 99217[1], 99218[1], 99219[1], 99220[1], 99221[1], 99222[1], 99223[1], 99231[1], 99232[1], 99233[1], 99234[1], 99235[1], 99236[1], 99238[1], 99239[1], 99241[1], 99242[1], 99243[1], 99244[1], 99245[1], 99251[1], 99252[1], 99253[1], 99254[1], 99255[1], 99291[1], 99292[1], 99304[1], 99305[1], 99306[1], 99307[1], 99308[1], 99309[1], 99310[1], 99315[1], 99316[1], 99334[1], 99335[1], 99336[1], 99337[1], 99347[1], 99348[1], 99349[1], 99350[1], 99374[1], 99375[1], 99377[1], 99378[1], 99446[0], 99447[0], 99448[0], 99449[0], 99451[0], 99452[0], 99495[0], 99496[0], G0463[1], G0471[0]
50920	00910[0], 0213T[0], 0216T[0], 0596T[1], 0597T[1], 0708T[1], 0709T[1], 11000[1], 11001[1], 11004[1], 11005[1], 11006[1], 11042[1], 11043[1], 11044[1], 11045[1], 11046[1], 11047[1], 12001[1], 12002[1], 12004[1], 12005[1], 12006[1], 12007[1], 12011[1], 12013[1], 12014[1], 12015[1], 12016[1], 12017[1], 12018[1], 12020[1], 12021[1], 12031[1], 12032[1], 12034[1], 12035[1], 12036[1], 12037[1], 12041[1], 12042[1], 12044[1], 12045[1], 12046[1], 12047[1], 12051[1], 12052[1], 12053[1], 12054[1], 12055[1], 12056[1], 12057[1], 13100[1], 13101[1], 13102[1], 13120[1], 13121[1], 13122[1], 13131[1], 13132[1], 13133[1], 13151[1], 13152[1], 13153[1], 36000[1], 36400[1], 36405[1], 36406[1], 36410[1], 36420[1], 36425[1], 36430[1], 36440[1], 36591[0], 36592[0], 36600[1], 36640[1], 43752[1], 44602[1], 44603[1], 44604[1], 44605[1], 44850[0], 44950[0], 44970[0], 49000[0], 49002[1], 49010[0], 50605[1], 50650[0], 50715[1], 50900[1], 51701[0], 51702[0], 51703[1], 62320[0], 62321[0], 62322[0], 62323[0], 62324[0], 62325[0], 62326[0], 62327[0], 64400[0], 64405[0], 64408[0], 64415[0], 64416[0], 64417[0], 64418[0], 64420[0], 64421[0], 64425[0], 64430[0], 64435[0], 64445[0], 64446[0], 64447[0], 64448[0], 64449[0], 64450[0], 64451[0], 64454[0], 64461[0], 64462[0], 64463[0], 64479[0], 64480[0], 64483[0], 64484[0], 64486[0], 64487[0], 64488[0], 64489[0], 64490[0], 64491[0], 64492[0], 64493[0], 64494[0], 64495[0], 64505[0], 64510[0], 64517[0], 64520[0], 64530[0], 69990[0], 92012[1], 92014[1], 93000[1], 93005[1], 93010[1], 93040[1], 93041[1], 93042[1], 93318[1], 93355[1], 94002[1], 94200[1], 94680[1], 94681[1], 94690[1], 95812[1], 95813[1], 95816[1], 95819[1], 95822[1], 95829[1], 95955[1], 96360[1], 96361[1], 96365[1], 96366[1], 96367[1], 96368[1], 96372[1], 96374[1], 96375[1], 96376[1], 96377[1], 96523[0], 97597[1], 97598[1], 97602[1], 99155[0], 99156[0], 99157[0], 99211[1], 99212[1], 99213[1], 99214[1], 99215[1], 99217[1], 99218[1], 99219[1], 99220[1], 99221[1], 99222[1], 99223[1], 99231[1], 99232[1], 99233[1], 99234[1], 99235[1], 99236[1], 99238[1], 99239[1], 99241[1], 99242[1], 99243[1], 99244[1], 99245[1], 99251[1], 99252[1], 99253[1], 99254[1], 99255[1], 99291[1], 99292[1], 99304[1], 99305[1], 99306[1], 99307[1], 99308[1], 99309[1], 99310[1], 99315[1], 99316[1], 99334[1], 99335[1], 99336[1], 99337[1], 99347[1], 99348[1], 99349[1], 99350[1], 99374[1], 99375[1], 99377[1], 99378[1], 99446[0], 99447[0], 99448[0], 99449[0], 99451[0], 99452[0], 99495[0], 99496[0], G0463[1], G0471[0]
50930	00910[0], 0213T[0], 0216T[0], 0596T[1], 0597T[1], 0708T[1], 0709T[1], 11000[1], 11001[1], 11004[1], 11005[1], 11006[1], 11042[1], 11043[1], 11044[1], 11045[1], 11046[1], 11047[1], 12001[1], 12002[1], 12004[1], 12005[1], 12006[1], 12007[1], 12011[1], 12013[1], 12014[1], 12015[1], 12016[1], 12017[1], 12018[1], 12020[1], 12021[1], 12031[1], 12032[1], 12034[1], 12035[1], 12036[1], 12037[1], 12041[1], 12042[1], 12044[1], 12045[1], 12046[1], 12047[1], 12051[1], 12052[1], 12053[1], 12054[1], 12055[1], 12056[1], 12057[1], 13100[1], 13101[1], 13102[1], 13120[1], 13121[1], 13122[1], 13131[1], 13132[1], 13133[1], 13151[1], 13152[1], 13153[1], 36000[1], 36400[1], 36405[1], 36406[1], 36410[1], 36420[1], 36425[1], 36430[1], 36440[1], 36591[0], 36592[0], 36600[1], 36640[1], 43752[1], 44005[0], 44180[0], 44602[1], 44603[1], 44604[1], 44605[1], 44850[0], 44950[0], 44970[0], 49000[0], 49002[1], 49010[0], 49255[0], 50605[1], 50650[0], 50715[1], 50900[1], 51701[0], 51702[0], 51703[1], 62320[0], 62321[0], 62322[0], 62323[0], 62324[0], 62325[0], 62326[0], 62327[0], 64400[0], 64405[0], 64408[0], 64415[0], 64416[0], 64417[0], 64418[0], 64420[0], 64421[0], 64425[0], 64430[0], 64435[0], 64445[0], 64446[0], 64447[0], 64448[0], 64449[0], 64450[0], 64451[0], 64454[0], 64461[0], 64462[0], 64463[0], 64479[0], 64480[0], 64483[0], 64484[0], 64486[0], 64487[0], 64488[0], 64489[0], 64490[0], 64491[0], 64492[0], 64493[0], 64494[0], 64495[0], 64505[0], 64510[0], 64517[0], 64520[0], 64530[0], 69990[0], 92012[1], 92014[1], 93000[1], 93005[1], 93010[1], 93040[1], 93041[1], 93042[1], 93318[1], 93355[1], 94002[1], 94200[1], 94680[1], 94681[1], 94690[1], 95812[1], 95813[1], 95816[1], 95819[1], 95822[1], 95829[1], 95955[1], 96360[1], 96361[1], 96365[1], 96366[1], 96367[1], 96368[1], 96372[1], 96374[1], 96375[1], 96376[1], 96377[1], 96523[0], 97597[1], 97598[1], 97602[1], 99155[0], 99156[0], 99157[0], 99211[1], 99212[1], 99213[1], 99214[1], 99215[1], 99217[1], 99218[1], 99219[1], 99220[1], 99221[1], 99222[1], 99223[1], 99231[1], 99232[1], 99233[1], 99234[1], 99235[1], 99236[1], 99238[1], 99239[1], 99241[1], 99242[1], 99243[1], 99244[1], 99245[1], 99251[1], 99252[1], 99253[1], 99254[1], 99255[1], 99291[1], 99292[1], 99304[1], 99305[1], 99306[1], 99307[1], 99308[1], 99309[1], 99310[1], 99315[1], 99316[1], 99334[1], 99335[1], 99336[1], 99337[1], 99347[1], 99348[1], 99349[1], 99350[1], 99374[1], 99375[1], 99377[1], 99378[1], 99446[0], 99447[0], 99448[0], 99449[0], 99451[0], 99452[0], 99495[0], 99496[0], G0463[1], G0471[0]
50940	00910[0], 0213T[0], 0216T[0], 0596T[1], 0597T[1], 0708T[1], 0709T[1], 12001[1], 12002[1], 12004[1], 12005[1], 12006[1], 12007[1], 12011[1], 12013[1], 12014[1], 12015[1], 12016[1], 12017[1], 12018[1], 12020[1], 12021[1], 12031[1], 12032[1], 12034[1], 12035[1], 12036[1], 12037[1], 12041[1], 12042[1], 12044[1], 12045[1], 12046[1], 12047[1], 12051[1], 12052[1], 12053[1], 12054[1], 12055[1], 12056[1], 12057[1], 13100[1], 13101[1], 13102[1], 13120[1], 13121[1], 13122[1], 13131[1], 13132[1], 13133[1], 13151[1], 13152[1], 13153[1], 36000[1], 36400[1], 36405[1], 36406[1], 36410[1], 36420[1], 36425[1], 36430[1], 36440[1], 36591[0], 36592[0], 36600[1], 36640[1], 43752[1], 44602[1], 44603[1], 44604[1], 44605[1], 44850[0], 44950[0], 44970[0], 49000[0], 49002[1], 49010[0], 50605[1], 50650[0], 50715[1], 50900[1], 51701[0], 51702[0], 51703[1], 62320[0], 62321[0], 62322[0], 62323[0], 62324[0], 62325[0], 62326[0], 62327[0], 64400[0], 64405[0], 64408[0], 64415[0], 64416[0], 64417[0], 64418[0], 64420[0], 64421[0], 64425[0], 64430[0], 64435[0], 64445[0], 64446[0], 64447[0], 64448[0], 64449[0], 64450[0], 64451[0], 64454[0], 64461[0], 64462[0], 64463[0], 64479[0], 64480[0], 64483[0], 64484[0], 64486[0], 64487[0], 64488[0], 64489[0], 64490[0], 64491[0], 64492[0], 64493[0], 64494[0], 64495[0], 64505[0], 64510[0], 64517[0], 64520[0], 64530[0], 69990[0], 92012[1], 92014[1], 93000[1], 93005[1], 93010[1], 93040[1], 93041[1], 93042[1], 93318[1], 93355[1], 94002[1], 94200[1], 94680[1], 94681[1], 94690[1], 95812[1], 95813[1], 95816[1], 95819[1], 95822[1], 95829[1], 95955[1], 96360[1], 96361[1], 96365[1], 96366[1], 96367[1], 96368[1], 96372[1], 96374[1], 96375[1], 96376[1], 96377[1], 96523[0], 99155[0], 99156[0], 99157[0], 99211[1], 99212[1], 99213[1], 99214[1], 99215[1], 99217[1], 99218[1], 99219[1], 99220[1], 99221[1], 99222[1], 99223[1], 99231[1], 99232[1], 99233[1], 99234[1], 99235[1], 99236[1], 99238[1], 99239[1], 99241[1], 99242[1], 99243[1], 99244[1], 99245[1], 99251[1], 99252[1], 99253[1], 99254[1], 99255[1], 99291[1], 99292[1], 99304[1], 99305[1], 99306[1], 99307[1], 99308[1], 99309[1], 99310[1], 99315[1], 99316[1], 99334[1], 99335[1], 99336[1], 99337[1], 99347[1], 99348[1], 99349[1], 99350[1], 99374[1], 99375[1], 99377[1], 99378[1], 99446[0], 99447[0], 99448[0], 99449[0], 99451[0], 99452[0], 99495[0], 99496[0], G0463[1], G0471[0]
50945	00910[0], 0213T[0], 0216T[0], 0596T[1], 0597T[1], 0708T[1], 0709T[1], 11000[1], 11001[1], 11004[1], 11005[1], 11006[1], 11042[1], 11043[1], 11044[1], 11045[1], 11046[1], 11047[1], 12001[1], 12002[1], 12004[1], 12005[1], 12006[1], 12007[1], 12011[1], 12013[1], 12014[1], 12015[1], 12016[1], 12017[1], 12018[1], 12020[1], 12021[1], 12031[1], 12032[1], 12034[1], 12035[1], 12036[1], 12037[1], 12041[1], 12042[1], 12044[1], 12045[1], 12046[1], 12047[1], 12051[1], 12052[1], 12053[1], 12054[1], 12055[1], 12056[1], 12057[1], 13100[1], 13101[1], 13102[1], 13120[1], 13121[1], 13122[1], 13131[1], 13132[1], 13133[1], 13151[1], 13152[1], 13153[1], 36000[1], 36400[1], 36405[1], 36406[1], 36410[1], 36420[1], 36425[1], 36430[1], 36440[1], 36591[0], 36592[0], 36600[1], 36640[1], 43653[0], 43752[1], 44005[0], 44180[0], 44602[1], 44603[1], 44604[1], 44605[1], 44950[0], 44970[1], 49082[1], 49083[1], 49084[1], 49320[0], 49400[0], 50715[1], 51701[1], 51702[1], 51703[1], 58660[0], 62320[0], 62321[0], 62322[0], 62323[0], 62324[0], 62325[0], 62326[0], 62327[0], 64400[0], 64405[0], 64408[0], 64415[0], 64416[0], 64417[0], 64418[0], 64420[0], 64421[0], 64425[0], 64430[0], 64435[0], 64445[0], 64446[0], 64447[0], 64448[0], 64449[0], 64450[0], 64451[0], 64454[0], 64461[0], 64462[0], 64463[0], 64479[0], 64480[0], 64483[0], 64484[0], 64486[0], 64487[0], 64488[0], 64489[0], 64490[0], 64491[0], 64492[0], 64493[0], 64494[0], 64495[0], 64505[0], 64510[0], 64517[0], 64520[0], 64530[0], 69990[0], 76000[1], 77001[1], 77002[1], 92012[1], 92014[1], 93000[1], 93005[1], 93010[1], 93040[1], 93041[1], 93042[1], 93318[1], 93355[1], 94002[1], 94200[1], 94680[1], 94681[1], 94690[1], 95812[1], 95813[1], 95816[1], 95819[1], 95822[1], 95829[1], 95955[1], 96360[1], 96361[1], 96365[1], 96366[1], 96367[1], 96368[1], 96372[1], 96374[1], 96375[1], 96376[1], 96377[1], 96523[0], 97597[1], 97598[1], 97602[1], 99155[0], 99156[0], 99157[0], 99211[1], 99212[1], 99213[1], 99214[1], 99215[1], 99217[1], 99218[1], 99219[1], 99220[1], 99221[1], 99222[1], 99223[1], 99231[1], 99232[1], 99233[1], 99234[1], 99235[1], 99236[1], 99238[1], 99239[1], 99241[1], 99242[1], 99243[1], 99244[1], 99245[1], 99251[1], 99252[1], 99253[1], 99254[1], 99255[1], 99291[1], 99292[1], 99304[1], 99305[1], 99306[1], 99307[1], 99308[1], 99309[1], 99310[1], 99315[1], 99316[1], 99334[1], 99335[1], 99336[1], 99337[1], 99347[1], 99348[1], 99349[1], 99350[1], 99374[1], 99375[1], 99377[1], 99378[1], 99446[0], 99447[0], 99448[0], 99449[0], 99451[0], 99452[0], 99495[0], 99496[0], G0463[1], G0471[1]
50947	00910[0], 0213T[0], 0216T[0], 0596T[1], 0597T[1], 0708T[1], 0709T[1], 12001[1], 12002[1], 12004[1], 12005[1], 12006[1], 12007[1], 12011[1], 12013[1], 12014[1], 12015[1], 12016[1], 12017[1], 12018[1],

Appendix A: NCCI - CPT Codes

0 = Modifier usage not allowed or inappropriate 1 = Modifier usage allowed

Code 1	Code 2
	12020[1], 12021[1], 12031[1], 12032[1], 12034[1], 12035[1], 12036[1], 12037[1], 12041[1], 12042[1], 12044[1], 12045[1], 12046[1], 12047[1], 12051[1], 12052[1], 12053[1], 12054[1], 12055[1], 12056[1], 12057[1], 13100[1], 13101[1], 13102[1], 13120[1], 13121[1], 13122[1], 13131[1], 13132[1], 13133[1], 13151[1], 13152[1], 13153[1], 35840[1], 36000[1], 36400[1], 36405[1], 36406[1], 36410[1], 36420[1], 36425[1], 36430[1], 36440[1], 36591[0], 36592[0], 36600[1], 36640[1], 43653[0], 43752[1], 44005[0], 44180[0], 44602[1], 44603[1], 44604[1], 44605[1], 44950[0], 44970[1], 49082[1], 49083[1], 49084[1], 49320[0], 49400[0], 50382[1], 50384[1], 50387[1], 50430[1], 50431[1], 50605[1], 50650[0], 50684[1], 50715[1], 50782[0], 50783[0], 50785[0], 51565[0], 51700[1], 51701[1], 51702[1], 51703[1], 51820[0], 52000[0], 52310[0], 52315[0], 52332[1], 52356[1], 53000[0], 53010[0], 53020[0], 53025[0], 53660[1], 53661[1], 53665[1], 58660[0], 62320[0], 62321[0], 62322[0], 62323[0], 62324[0], 62325[0], 62326[0], 62327[0], 64400[0], 64405[0], 64408[0], 64415[0], 64416[0], 64417[0], 64418[0], 64420[0], 64421[0], 64425[0], 64430[0], 64435[0], 64445[0], 64446[0], 64447[0], 64448[0], 64449[0], 64450[0], 64451[0], 64454[0], 64461[0], 64462[0], 64463[0], 64479[0], 64480[0], 64483[0], 64484[0], 64486[0], 64487[0], 64488[0], 64489[0], 64490[0], 64491[0], 64492[0], 64493[0], 64494[0], 64495[0], 64505[0], 64510[0], 64517[0], 64520[0], 64530[0], 69990[0], 76000[1], 77001[1], 77002[1], 92012[1], 92014[1], 93000[1], 93005[1], 93010[1], 93040[1], 93041[1], 93042[1], 93318[1], 93355[1], 94002[1], 94200[1], 94680[1], 94681[1], 94690[1], 95812[1], 95813[1], 95816[1], 95819[1], 95822[1], 95829[1], 95955[1], 96360[1], 96361[1], 96365[1], 96366[1], 96367[1], 96368[1], 96372[1], 96374[1], 96375[1], 96376[1], 96377[1], 96523[0], 99155[0], 99156[0], 99157[0], 99211[1], 99212[1], 99213[1], 99214[1], 99215[1], 99217[1], 99218[1], 99219[1], 99220[1], 99221[1], 99222[1], 99223[1], 99231[1], 99232[1], 99233[1], 99234[1], 99235[1], 99236[1], 99238[1], 99239[1], 99241[1], 99242[1], 99243[1], 99244[1], 99245[1], 99251[1], 99252[1], 99253[1], 99254[1], 99255[1], 99291[1], 99292[1], 99304[1], 99305[1], 99306[1], 99307[1], 99308[1], 99309[1], 99310[1], 99315[1], 99316[1], 99334[1], 99335[1], 99336[1], 99337[1], 99347[1], 99348[1], 99349[1], 99350[1], 99374[1], 99375[1], 99377[1], 99378[1], 99446[0], 99447[0], 99448[0], 99449[0], 99451[0], 99452[0], 99495[0], 99496[0], G0463[1], G0471[1], P9612[1]
50948	00910[0], 0213T[0], 0216T[0], 0596T[1], 0597T[1], 0708T[1], 0709T[1], 12001[1], 12002[1], 12004[1], 12005[1], 12006[1], 12007[1], 12011[1], 12013[1], 12014[1], 12015[1], 12016[1], 12017[1], 12018[1], 12020[1], 12021[1], 12031[1], 12032[1], 12034[1], 12035[1], 12036[1], 12037[1], 12041[1], 12042[1], 12044[1], 12045[1], 12046[1], 12047[1], 12051[1], 12052[1], 12053[1], 12054[1], 12055[1], 12056[1], 12057[1], 13100[1], 13101[1], 13102[1], 13120[1], 13121[1], 13122[1], 13131[1], 13132[1], 13133[1], 13151[1], 13152[1], 13153[1], 35840[1], 36000[1], 36400[1], 36405[1], 36406[1], 36410[1], 36420[1], 36425[1], 36430[1], 36440[1], 36591[0], 36592[0], 36600[1], 36640[1], 43653[0], 43752[1], 44005[0], 44180[0], 44602[1], 44603[1], 44604[1], 44605[1], 44950[0], 44970[1], 49082[1], 49083[1], 49084[1], 49320[0], 49400[0], 50430[1], 50431[1], 50605[1], 50650[0], 50684[1], 50715[1], 50782[0], 50783[0], 50785[0], 51565[0], 51700[1], 51701[1], 51702[1], 51703[1], 51820[0], 52000[0], 52332[1], 52356[1], 53660[1], 53661[1], 53665[1], 58660[0], 62320[0], 62321[0], 62322[0], 62323[0], 62324[0], 62325[0], 62326[0], 62327[0], 64400[0], 64405[0], 64408[0], 64415[0], 64416[0], 64417[0], 64418[0], 64420[0], 64421[0], 64425[0], 64430[0], 64435[0], 64445[0], 64446[0], 64447[0], 64448[0], 64449[0], 64450[0], 64451[0], 64454[0], 64461[0], 64462[0], 64463[0], 64479[0], 64480[0], 64483[0], 64484[0], 64486[0], 64487[0], 64488[0], 64489[0], 64490[0], 64491[0], 64492[0], 64493[0], 64494[0], 64495[0], 64505[0], 64510[0], 64517[0], 64520[0], 64530[0], 69990[0], 76000[1], 77001[1], 77002[1], 92012[1], 92014[1], 93000[1], 93005[1], 93010[1], 93040[1], 93041[1], 93042[1], 93318[1], 93355[1], 94002[1], 94200[1], 94680[1], 94681[1], 94690[1], 95812[1], 95813[1], 95816[1], 95819[1], 95822[1], 95829[1], 95955[1], 96360[1], 96361[1], 96365[1], 96366[1], 96367[1], 96368[1], 96372[1], 96374[1], 96375[1], 96376[1], 96377[1], 96523[0], 99155[0], 99156[0], 99157[0], 99211[1], 99212[1], 99213[1], 99214[1], 99215[1], 99217[1], 99218[1], 99219[1], 99220[1], 99221[1], 99222[1], 99223[1], 99231[1], 99232[1], 99233[1], 99234[1], 99235[1], 99236[1], 99238[1], 99239[1], 99241[1], 99242[1], 99243[1], 99244[1], 99245[1], 99251[1], 99252[1], 99253[1], 99254[1], 99255[1], 99291[1], 99292[1], 99304[1], 99305[1], 99306[1], 99307[1], 99308[1], 99309[1], 99310[1], 99315[1], 99316[1], 99334[1], 99335[1], 99336[1], 99337[1], 99347[1], 99348[1], 99349[1], 99350[1], 99374[1], 99375[1], 99377[1], 99378[1], 99446[0], 99447[0], 99448[0], 99449[0], 99451[0], 99452[0], 99495[0], 99496[0], G0463[1], G0471[1], P9612[1]
50951	00910[0], 0213T[0], 0216T[0], 0596T[1], 0597T[1], 0708T[1], 0709T[1], 12001[1], 12002[1], 12004[1], 12005[1], 12006[1], 12007[1], 12011[1], 12013[1], 12014[1], 12015[1], 12016[1], 12017[1], 12018[1], 12020[1], 12021[1], 12031[1], 12032[1], 12034[1], 12035[1], 12036[1], 12037[1], 12041[1], 12042[1], 12044[1], 12045[1], 12046[1], 12047[1], 12051[1], 12052[1], 12053[1], 12054[1], 12055[1], 12056[1], 12057[1], 13100[1], 13101[1], 13102[1], 13120[1], 13121[1], 13122[1], 13131[1], 13132[1], 13133[1], 13151[1], 13152[1], 13153[1], 36000[1], 36400[1], 36405[1], 36406[1], 36410[1], 36420[1], 36425[1], 36430[1], 36440[1], 36591[0], 36592[0], 36600[1], 36640[1], 43752[1], 50391[1], 50436[1], 50437[1], 50684[1], 51701[1], 51702[1], 51703[1], 62320[0], 62321[0], 62322[0], 62323[0], 62324[0], 62325[0], 62326[0], 62327[0], 64400[0], 64405[0], 64408[0], 64415[0], 64416[0], 64417[0], 64418[0], 64420[0], 64421[0], 64425[0], 64430[0], 64435[0], 64445[0], 64446[0], 64447[0], 64448[0], 64449[0], 64450[0], 64451[0], 64454[0], 64461[0], 64462[0], 64463[0], 64479[0], 64480[0], 64483[0], 64484[0], 64486[0], 64487[0], 64488[0], 64489[0], 64490[0], 64491[0], 64492[0], 64493[0], 64494[0], 64495[0], 64505[0], 64510[0], 64517[0], 64520[0], 64530[0], 69990[0], 76000[1], 77001[1], 77002[1], 92012[1], 92014[1], 93000[1], 93005[1], 93010[1], 93040[1], 93041[1], 93042[1], 93318[1], 93355[1], 94002[1], 94200[1], 94680[1], 94681[1], 94690[1], 95812[1], 95813[1], 95816[1], 95819[1], 95822[1], 95829[1], 95955[1], 96360[1], 96361[1], 96365[1], 96366[1], 96367[1], 96368[1], 96372[1], 96374[1], 96375[1], 96376[1], 96377[1], 96523[0], 99155[0], 99156[0], 99157[0], 99211[1], 99212[1], 99213[1], 99214[1], 99215[1], 99217[1], 99218[1], 99219[1], 99220[1], 99221[1], 99222[1], 99223[1], 99231[1], 99232[1], 99233[1], 99234[1], 99235[1], 99236[1], 99238[1], 99239[1], 99241[1], 99242[1], 99243[1], 99244[1], 99245[1], 99251[1], 99252[1], 99253[1], 99254[1], 99255[1], 99291[1], 99292[1], 99304[1], 99305[1], 99306[1], 99307[1], 99308[1], 99309[1], 99310[1], 99315[1], 99316[1], 99334[1], 99335[1], 99336[1], 99337[1], 99347[1], 99348[1], 99349[1], 99350[1], 99374[1], 99375[1], 99377[1], 99378[1], 99446[0], 99447[0], 99448[0], 99449[0], 99451[0], 99452[0], 99495[1], 99496[1], G0463[1], G0471[1], J2001[1]
50953	00910[0], 0213T[0], 0216T[0], 0596T[1], 0597T[1], 0708T[1], 0709T[1], 12001[1], 12002[1], 12004[1], 12005[1], 12006[1], 12007[1], 12011[1], 12013[1], 12014[1], 12015[1], 12016[1], 12017[1], 12018[1], 12020[1], 12021[1], 12031[1], 12032[1], 12034[1], 12035[1], 12036[1], 12037[1], 12041[1], 12042[1], 12044[1], 12045[1], 12046[1], 12047[1], 12051[1], 12052[1], 12053[1], 12054[1], 12055[1], 12056[1], 12057[1], 13100[1], 13101[1], 13102[1], 13120[1], 13121[1], 13122[1], 13131[1], 13132[1], 13133[1], 13151[1], 13152[1], 13153[1], 36000[1], 36400[1], 36405[1], 36406[1], 36410[1], 36420[1], 36425[1], 36430[1], 36440[1], 36591[0], 36592[0], 36600[1], 36640[1], 43752[1], 50436[1], 50437[1], 50684[1], 50706[1], 50951[1], 51701[1], 51702[1], 51703[1], 62320[0], 62321[0], 62322[0], 62323[0], 62324[0], 62325[0], 62326[0], 62327[0], 64400[0], 64405[0], 64408[0], 64415[0], 64416[0], 64417[0], 64418[0], 64420[0], 64421[0], 64425[0], 64430[0], 64435[0], 64445[0], 64446[0], 64447[0], 64448[0], 64449[0], 64450[0], 64451[0], 64454[0], 64461[0], 64462[0], 64463[0], 64479[0], 64480[0], 64483[0], 64484[0], 64486[0], 64487[0], 64488[0], 64489[0], 64490[0], 64491[0], 64492[0], 64493[0], 64494[0], 64495[0], 64505[0], 64510[0], 64517[0], 64520[0], 64530[0], 69990[0], 76000[1], 77001[1], 77002[1], 92012[1], 92014[1], 93000[1], 93005[1], 93010[1], 93040[1], 93041[1], 93042[1], 93318[1], 93355[1], 94002[1], 94200[1], 94680[1], 94681[1], 94690[1], 95812[1], 95813[1], 95816[1], 95819[1], 95822[1], 95829[1], 95955[1], 96360[1], 96361[1], 96365[1], 96366[1], 96367[1], 96368[1], 96372[1], 96374[1], 96375[1], 96376[1], 96377[1], 96523[0], 99155[0], 99156[0], 99157[0], 99211[1], 99212[1], 99213[1], 99214[1], 99215[1], 99217[1], 99218[1], 99219[1], 99220[1], 99221[1], 99222[1], 99223[1], 99231[1], 99232[1], 99233[1], 99234[1], 99235[1], 99236[1], 99238[1], 99239[1], 99241[1], 99242[1], 99243[1], 99244[1], 99245[1], 99251[1], 99252[1], 99253[1], 99254[1], 99255[1], 99291[1], 99292[1], 99304[1], 99305[1], 99306[1], 99307[1], 99308[1], 99309[1], 99310[1], 99315[1], 99316[1], 99334[1], 99335[1], 99336[1], 99337[1], 99347[1], 99348[1], 99349[1], 99350[1], 99374[1], 99375[1], 99377[1], 99378[1], 99446[0], 99447[0], 99448[0], 99449[0], 99451[0], 99452[0], 99495[1], 99496[1], G0463[1], G0471[1], J2001[1]
50955	00910[0], 0213T[0], 0216T[0], 0596T[1], 0597T[1], 0708T[1], 0709T[1], 10005[1], 10007[1], 10009[1], 10011[1], 10021[1], 12001[1], 12002[1], 12004[1], 12005[1], 12006[1], 12007[1], 12011[1], 12013[1], 12014[1], 12015[1], 12016[1], 12017[1], 12018[1], 12020[1], 12021[1], 12031[1], 12032[1], 12034[1], 12035[1], 12036[1], 12037[1], 12041[1], 12042[1], 12044[1], 12045[1], 12046[1], 12047[1], 12051[1], 12052[1], 12053[1], 12054[1], 12055[1], 12056[1], 12057[1], 13100[1], 13101[1], 13102[1], 13120[1], 13121[1], 13122[1], 13131[1], 13132[1], 13133[1], 13151[1], 13152[1], 13153[1], 36000[1], 36400[1], 36405[1], 36406[1], 36410[1], 36420[1], 36425[1], 36430[1], 36440[1], 36591[0], 36592[0], 36600[1], 36640[1], 43752[1], 50436[1], 50437[1], 50606[1], 50684[1], 50715[1], 50951[1], 51701[1], 51702[1], 51703[1], 62320[0], 62321[0], 62322[0], 62323[0], 62324[0], 62325[0], 62326[0], 62327[0], 64400[0], 64405[0], 64408[0], 64415[0], 64416[0], 64417[0], 64418[0], 64420[0], 64421[0], 64425[0], 64430[0], 64435[0], 64445[0], 64446[0], 64447[0], 64448[0], 64449[0], 64450[0], 64451[0], 64454[0], 64461[0], 64462[0], 64463[0], 64479[0], 64480[0], 64483[0], 64484[0], 64486[0], 64487[0], 64488[0], 64489[0], 64490[0], 64491[0], 64492[0], 64493[0], 64494[0], 64495[0], 64505[0], 64510[0], 64517[0], 64520[0], 64530[0], 69990[0], 76000[1], 77001[1], 77002[1], 92012[1], 92014[1], 93000[1], 93005[1], 93010[1], 93040[1], 93041[1], 93042[1], 93318[1], 93355[1], 94002[1], 94200[1], 94680[1], 94681[1], 94690[1], 95812[1], 95813[1], 95816[1], 95819[1], 95822[1], 95829[1], 95955[1], 96360[1], 96361[1], 96365[1], 96366[1], 96367[1], 96368[1], 96372[1], 96374[1], 96375[1], 96376[1], 96377[1], 96523[0], 99155[0], 99156[0], 99157[0], 99211[1], 99212[1], 99213[1], 99214[1], 99215[1], 99217[1], 99218[1], 99219[1], 99220[1], 99221[1], 99222[1], 99223[1], 99231[1], 99232[1], 99233[1], 99234[1], 99235[1], 99236[1], 99238[1], 99239[1], 99241[1], 99242[1], 99243[1], 99244[1], 99245[1], 99251[1], 99252[1], 99253[1], 99254[1], 99255[1], 99291[1], 99292[1], 99304[1], 99305[1], 99306[1], 99307[1], 99308[1], 99309[1], 99310[1], 99315[1], 99316[1], 99334[1], 99335[1], 99336[1], 99337[1], 99347[1], 99348[1], 99349[1], 99350[1], 99374[1], 99375[1], 99377[1], 99378[1], 99446[0], 99447[0], 99448[0], 99449[0], 99451[0], 99452[0], 99495[1], 99496[1], G0463[1], G0471[1], J2001[1]
50957	00910[0], 0213T[0], 0216T[0], 0596T[1], 0597T[1], 0708T[1], 0709T[1], 10005[1], 10007[1], 10009[1], 10011[1], 10021[1], 12001[1], 12002[1], 12004[1], 12005[1], 12006[1], 12007[1], 12011[1], 12013[1], 12014[1], 12015[1], 12016[1], 12017[1], 12018[1], 12020[1], 12021[1], 12031[1], 12032[1], 12034[1], 12035[1], 12036[1], 12037[1], 12041[1], 12042[1], 12044[1], 12045[1], 12046[1], 12047[1], 12051[1], 12052[1], 12053[1], 12054[1], 12055[1], 12056[1], 12057[1], 13100[1], 13101[1], 13102[1], 13120[1], 13121[1], 13122[1], 13131[1], 13132[1], 13133[1], 13151[1], 13152[1], 13153[1], 36000[1], 36400[1], 36405[1], 36406[1], 36410[1], 36420[1], 36425[1], 36430[1], 36440[1], 36591[0], 36592[0], 36600[1], 36640[1], 43752[1], 50436[1], 50437[1], 50684[1], 50715[1], 50951[1], 50955[0], 50974[0], 51701[1], 51702[1], 51703[1], 62320[0], 62321[0], 62322[0], 62323[0], 62324[0], 62325[0], 62326[0], 62327[0], 64400[0], 64405[0], 64408[0], 64415[0], 64416[0], 64417[0], 64418[0], 64420[0], 64421[0], 64425[0],

0 = Modifier usage not allowed or inappropriate 1 = Modifier usage allowed

Code 1	Code 2
	64430^0, 64435^0, 64445^0, 64446^0, 64447^0, 64448^0, 64449^0, 64450^0, 64451^0, 64454^0, 64461^0, 64462^0, 64463^0, 64479^0, 64480^0, 64483^0, 64484^0, 64486^0, 64487^0, 64488^0, 64489^0, 64490^0, 64491^0, 64492^0, 64493^0, 64494^0, 64495^0, 64505^0, 64510^0, 64517^0, 64520^0, 64530^0, 69990^0, 76000^1, 77001^1, 77002^1, 92012^1, 92014^1, 93000^1, 93005^1, 93010^1, 93040^1, 93041^1, 93042^1, 93318^1, 93355^1, 94002^1, 94200^1, 94680^1, 94681^1, 94690^1, 95812^1, 95813^1, 95816^1, 95819^1, 95822^1, 95829^1, 95955^1, 96360^1, 96361^1, 96365^1, 96366^1, 96367^1, 96368^1, 96372^1, 96374^1, 96375^1, 96376^1, 96377^1, 96523^0, 99155^0, 99156^0, 99157^0, 99211^1, 99212^1, 99213^1, 99214^1, 99215^1, 99217^1, 99218^1, 99219^1, 99220^1, 99221^1, 99222^1, 99223^1, 99231^1, 99232^1, 99233^1, 99234^1, 99235^1, 99236^1, 99238^1, 99239^1, 99241^1, 99242^1, 99243^1, 99244^1, 99245^1, 99251^1, 99252^1, 99253^1, 99254^1, 99255^1, 99291^1, 99292^1, 99304^1, 99305^1, 99306^1, 99307^1, 99308^1, 99309^1, 99310^1, 99315^1, 99316^1, 99334^1, 99335^1, 99336^1, 99337^1, 99347^1, 99348^1, 99349^1, 99350^1, 99374^1, 99375^1, 99377^1, 99378^1, 99446^0, 99447^0, 99448^0, 99449^0, 99451^0, 99452^0, 99495^1, 99496^1, G0463^1, G0471^1, J2001^1
50961	00910^0, 0213T^0, 0216T^0, 0596T^1, 0597T^1, 0708T^1, 0709T^1, 11000^1, 11001^1, 11004^1, 11005^1, 11006^1, 11042^1, 11043^1, 11044^1, 11045^1, 11046^1, 11047^1, 12001^1, 12002^1, 12004^1, 12005^1, 12006^1, 12007^1, 12011^1, 12013^1, 12014^1, 12015^1, 12016^1, 12017^1, 12018^1, 12020^1, 12021^1, 12031^1, 12032^1, 12034^1, 12035^1, 12036^1, 12037^1, 12041^1, 12042^1, 12044^1, 12045^1, 12046^1, 12047^1, 12051^1, 12052^1, 12053^1, 12054^1, 12055^1, 12056^1, 12057^1, 13100^1, 13101^1, 13102^1, 13120^1, 13121^1, 13122^1, 13131^1, 13132^1, 13133^1, 13151^1, 13152^1, 13153^1, 36000^1, 36400^1, 36405^1, 36406^1, 36410^1, 36420^1, 36425^1, 36430^1, 36440^1, 36591^0, 36592^0, 36600^1, 36640^1, 43752^1, 50436^1, 50437^1, 50684^1, 50715^1, 50951^1, 51701^1, 51702^1, 51703^1, 52320^1, 52330^1, 62320^0, 62321^0, 62322^0, 62323^0, 62324^0, 62325^0, 62326^0, 62327^0, 64400^0, 64405^0, 64408^0, 64415^0, 64416^0, 64417^0, 64418^0, 64420^0, 64421^0, 64425^0, 64430^0, 64435^0, 64445^0, 64446^0, 64447^0, 64448^0, 64449^0, 64450^0, 64451^0, 64454^0, 64461^0, 64462^0, 64463^0, 64479^0, 64480^0, 64483^0, 64484^0, 64486^0, 64487^0, 64488^0, 64489^0, 64490^0, 64491^0, 64492^0, 64493^0, 64494^0, 64495^0, 64505^0, 64510^0, 64517^0, 64520^0, 64530^0, 69990^0, 76000^1, 77001^1, 77002^1, 92012^1, 92014^1, 93000^1, 93005^1, 93010^1, 93040^1, 93041^1, 93042^1, 93318^1, 93355^1, 94002^1, 94200^1, 94680^1, 94681^1, 94690^1, 95812^1, 95813^1, 95816^1, 95819^1, 95822^1, 95829^1, 95955^1, 96360^1, 96361^1, 96365^1, 96366^1, 96367^1, 96368^1, 96372^1, 96374^1, 96375^1, 96376^1, 96377^1, 96523^0, 97597^1, 97598^1, 97602^1, 99155^0, 99156^0, 99157^0, 99211^1, 99212^1, 99213^1, 99214^1, 99215^1, 99217^1, 99218^1, 99219^1, 99220^1, 99221^1, 99222^1, 99223^1, 99231^1, 99232^1, 99233^1, 99234^1, 99235^1, 99236^1, 99238^1, 99239^1, 99241^1, 99242^1, 99243^1, 99244^1, 99245^1, 99251^1, 99252^1, 99253^1, 99254^1, 99255^1, 99291^1, 99292^1, 99304^1, 99305^1, 99306^1, 99307^1, 99308^1, 99309^1, 99310^1, 99315^1, 99316^1, 99334^1, 99335^1, 99336^1, 99337^1, 99347^1, 99348^1, 99349^1, 99350^1, 99374^1, 99375^1, 99377^1, 99378^1, 99446^0, 99447^0, 99448^0, 99449^0, 99451^0, 99452^0, 99495^1, 99496^1, G0463^1, G0471^1, J2001^1
50970	00910^0, 0213T^0, 0216T^0, 0596T^1, 0597T^1, 0708T^1, 0709T^1, 11000^1, 11001^1, 11004^1, 11005^1, 11006^1, 11042^1, 11043^1, 11044^1, 11045^1, 11046^1, 11047^1, 12001^1, 12002^1, 12004^1, 12005^1, 12006^1, 12007^1, 12011^1, 12013^1, 12014^1, 12015^1, 12016^1, 12017^1, 12018^1, 12020^1, 12021^1, 12031^1, 12032^1, 12034^1, 12035^1, 12036^1, 12037^1, 12041^1, 12042^1, 12044^1, 12045^1, 12046^1, 12047^1, 12051^1, 12052^1, 12053^1, 12054^1, 12055^1, 12056^1, 12057^1, 13100^1, 13101^1, 13102^1, 13120^1, 13121^1, 13122^1, 13131^1, 13132^1, 13133^1, 13151^1, 13152^1, 13153^1, 36000^1, 36400^1, 36405^1, 36406^1, 36410^1, 36420^1, 36425^1, 36430^1, 36440^1, 36591^0, 36592^0, 36600^1, 36640^1, 43752^1, 50391^1, 50684^1, 51701^1, 51702^1, 51703^1, 62320^0, 62321^0, 62322^0, 62323^0, 62324^0, 62325^0, 62326^0, 62327^0, 64400^0, 64405^0, 64408^0, 64415^0, 64416^0, 64417^0, 64418^0, 64420^0, 64421^0, 64425^0, 64430^0, 64435^0, 64445^0, 64446^0, 64447^0, 64448^0, 64449^0, 64450^0, 64451^0, 64454^0, 64461^0, 64462^0, 64463^0, 64479^0, 64480^0, 64483^0, 64484^0, 64486^0, 64487^0, 64488^0, 64489^0, 64490^0, 64491^0, 64492^0, 64493^0, 64494^0, 64495^0, 64505^0, 64510^0, 64517^0, 64520^0, 64530^0, 69990^0, 76000^1, 77001^1, 77002^1, 92012^1, 92014^1, 93000^1, 93005^1, 93010^1, 93040^1, 93041^1, 93042^1, 93318^1, 93355^1, 94002^1, 94200^1, 94680^1, 94681^1, 94690^1, 95812^1, 95813^1, 95816^1, 95819^1, 95822^1, 95829^1, 95955^1, 96360^1, 96361^1, 96365^1, 96366^1, 96367^1, 96368^1, 96372^1, 96374^1, 96375^1, 96376^1, 96377^1, 96523^0, 97597^1, 97598^1, 97602^1, 99155^0, 99156^0, 99157^0, 99211^1, 99212^1, 99213^1, 99214^1, 99215^1, 99217^1, 99218^1, 99219^1, 99220^1, 99221^1, 99222^1, 99223^1, 99231^1, 99232^1, 99233^1, 99234^1, 99235^1, 99236^1, 99238^1, 99239^1, 99241^1, 99242^1, 99243^1, 99244^1, 99245^1, 99251^1, 99252^1, 99253^1, 99254^1, 99255^1, 99291^1, 99292^1, 99304^1, 99305^1, 99306^1, 99307^1, 99308^1, 99309^1, 99310^1, 99315^1, 99316^1, 99334^1, 99335^1, 99336^1, 99337^1, 99347^1, 99348^1, 99349^1, 99350^1, 99374^1, 99375^1, 99377^1, 99378^1, 99446^0, 99447^0, 99448^0, 99449^0, 99451^0, 99452^0, 99495^1, 99496^1, G0463^1, G0471^1
50972	00910^0, 0213T^0, 0216T^0, 0596T^1, 0597T^1, 0708T^1, 0709T^1, 11000^1, 11001^1, 11004^1, 11005^1, 11006^1, 11042^1, 11043^1, 11044^1, 11045^1, 11046^1, 11047^1, 12001^1, 12002^1, 12004^1, 12005^1, 12006^1, 12007^1, 12011^1, 12013^1, 12014^1, 12015^1, 12016^1, 12017^1, 12018^1, 12020^1, 12021^1, 12031^1, 12032^1, 12034^1, 12035^1, 12036^1, 12037^1, 12041^1, 12042^1, 12044^1, 12045^1, 12046^1, 12047^1, 12051^1, 12052^1, 12053^1, 12054^1, 12055^1, 12056^1, 12057^1, 13100^1, 13101^1, 13102^1, 13120^1, 13121^1, 13122^1, 13131^1, 13132^1, 13133^1, 13151^1, 13152^1, 13153^1, 36000^1, 36400^1, 36405^1, 36406^1, 36410^1, 36420^1, 36425^1, 36430^1, 36440^1, 36591^0, 36592^0, 36600^1, 36640^1, 43752^1, 50684^1, 50706^1, 50970^1, 51701^1, 51702^1, 51703^1, 62320^0, 62321^0, 62322^0, 62323^0, 62324^0, 62325^0, 62326^0, 62327^0, 64400^0, 64405^0, 64408^0, 64415^0, 64416^0, 64417^0, 64418^0, 64420^0, 64421^0, 64425^0, 64430^0, 64435^0, 64445^0, 64446^0, 64447^0, 64448^0, 64449^0, 64450^0, 64451^0, 64454^0, 64461^0, 64462^0, 64463^0, 64479^0, 64480^0, 64483^0, 64484^0, 64486^0, 64487^0, 64488^0, 64489^0, 64490^0, 64491^0, 64492^0, 64493^0, 64494^0, 64495^0, 64505^0, 64510^0, 64517^0, 64520^0, 64530^0, 69990^0, 76000^1, 77001^1, 77002^1, 92012^1, 92014^1, 93000^1, 93005^1, 93010^1, 93040^1, 93041^1, 93042^1, 93318^1, 93355^1, 94002^1, 94200^1, 94680^1, 94681^1, 94690^1, 95812^1, 95813^1, 95816^1, 95819^1, 95822^1, 95829^1, 95955^1, 96360^1, 96361^1, 96365^1, 96366^1, 96367^1, 96368^1, 96372^1, 96374^1, 96375^1, 96376^1, 96377^1, 96523^0, 97597^1, 97598^1, 97602^1, 99155^0, 99156^0, 99157^0, 99211^1, 99212^1, 99213^1, 99214^1, 99215^1, 99217^1, 99218^1, 99219^1, 99220^1, 99221^1, 99222^1, 99223^1, 99231^1, 99232^1, 99233^1, 99234^1, 99235^1, 99236^1, 99238^1, 99239^1, 99241^1, 99242^1, 99243^1, 99244^1, 99245^1, 99251^1, 99252^1, 99253^1, 99254^1, 99255^1, 99291^1, 99292^1, 99304^1, 99305^1, 99306^1, 99307^1, 99308^1, 99309^1, 99310^1, 99315^1, 99316^1, 99334^1, 99335^1, 99336^1, 99337^1, 99347^1, 99348^1, 99349^1, 99350^1, 99374^1, 99375^1, 99377^1, 99378^1, 99446^0, 99447^0, 99448^0, 99449^0, 99451^0, 99452^0, 99495^1, 99496^1, G0463^1, G0471^1
50974	00910^0, 0213T^0, 0216T^0, 0596T^1, 0597T^1, 0708T^1, 0709T^1, 10005^1, 10007^1, 10009^1, 10011^1, 10021^1, 11000^1, 11001^1, 11004^1, 11005^1, 11006^1, 11042^1, 11043^1, 11044^1, 11045^1, 11046^1, 11047^1, 12001^1, 12002^1, 12004^1, 12005^1, 12006^1, 12007^1, 12011^1, 12013^1, 12014^1, 12015^1, 12016^1, 12017^1, 12018^1, 12020^1, 12021^1, 12031^1, 12032^1, 12034^1, 12035^1, 12036^1, 12037^1, 12041^1, 12042^1, 12044^1, 12045^1, 12046^1, 12047^1, 12051^1, 12052^1, 12053^1, 12054^1, 12055^1, 12056^1, 12057^1, 13100^1, 13101^1, 13102^1, 13120^1, 13121^1, 13122^1, 13131^1, 13132^1, 13133^1, 13151^1, 13152^1, 13153^1, 36000^1, 36400^1, 36405^1, 36406^1, 36410^1, 36420^1, 36425^1, 36430^1, 36440^1, 36591^0, 36592^0, 36600^1, 36640^1, 43752^1, 50606^1, 50684^1, 50715^1, 50970^1, 51701^1, 51702^1, 51703^1, 62320^0, 62321^0, 62322^0, 62323^0, 62324^0, 62325^0, 62326^0, 62327^0, 64400^0, 64405^0, 64408^0, 64415^0, 64416^0, 64417^0, 64418^0, 64420^0, 64421^0, 64425^0, 64430^0, 64435^0, 64445^0, 64446^0, 64447^0, 64448^0, 64449^0, 64450^0, 64451^0, 64454^0, 64461^0, 64462^0, 64463^0, 64479^0, 64480^0, 64483^0, 64484^0, 64486^0, 64487^0, 64488^0, 64489^0, 64490^0, 64491^0, 64492^0, 64493^0, 64494^0, 64495^0, 64505^0, 64510^0, 64517^0, 64520^0, 64530^0, 69990^0, 76000^1, 77001^1, 77002^1, 92012^1, 92014^1, 93000^1, 93005^1, 93010^1, 93040^1, 93041^1, 93042^1, 93318^1, 93355^1, 94002^1, 94200^1, 94680^1, 94681^1, 94690^1, 95812^1, 95813^1, 95816^1, 95819^1, 95822^1, 95829^1, 95955^1, 96360^1, 96361^1, 96365^1, 96366^1, 96367^1, 96368^1, 96372^1, 96374^1, 96375^1, 96376^1, 96377^1, 96523^0, 97597^1, 97598^1, 97602^1, 99155^0, 99156^0, 99157^0, 99211^1, 99212^1, 99213^1, 99214^1, 99215^1, 99217^1, 99218^1, 99219^1, 99220^1, 99221^1, 99222^1, 99223^1, 99231^1, 99232^1, 99233^1, 99234^1, 99235^1, 99236^1, 99238^1, 99239^1, 99241^1, 99242^1, 99243^1, 99244^1, 99245^1, 99251^1, 99252^1, 99253^1, 99254^1, 99255^1, 99291^1, 99292^1, 99304^1, 99305^1, 99306^1, 99307^1, 99308^1, 99309^1, 99310^1, 99315^1, 99316^1, 99334^1, 99335^1, 99336^1, 99337^1, 99347^1, 99348^1, 99349^1, 99350^1, 99374^1, 99375^1, 99377^1, 99378^1, 99446^0, 99447^0, 99448^0, 99449^0, 99451^0, 99452^0, 99495^1, 99496^1, G0463^1, G0471^1
50976	00910^0, 0213T^0, 0216T^0, 0596T^1, 0597T^1, 0708T^1, 0709T^1, 10005^1, 10007^1, 10009^1, 10011^1, 10021^1, 11000^1, 11001^1, 11004^1, 11005^1, 11006^1, 11042^1, 11043^1, 11044^1, 11045^1, 11046^1, 11047^1, 12001^1, 12002^1, 12004^1, 12005^1, 12006^1, 12007^1, 12011^1, 12013^1, 12014^1, 12015^1, 12016^1, 12017^1, 12018^1, 12020^1, 12021^1, 12031^1, 12032^1, 12034^1, 12035^1, 12036^1, 12037^1, 12041^1, 12042^1, 12044^1, 12045^1, 12046^1, 12047^1, 12051^1, 12052^1, 12053^1, 12054^1, 12055^1, 12056^1, 12057^1, 13100^1, 13101^1, 13102^1, 13120^1, 13121^1, 13122^1, 13131^1, 13132^1, 13133^1, 13151^1, 13152^1, 13153^1, 36000^1, 36400^1, 36405^1, 36406^1, 36410^1, 36420^1, 36425^1, 36430^1, 36440^1, 36591^0, 36592^0, 36600^1, 36640^1, 43752^1, 50684^1, 50715^1, 50955^0, 50970^1, 50974^1, 51701^1, 51702^1, 51703^1, 62320^0, 62321^0, 62322^0, 62323^0, 62324^0, 62325^0, 62326^0, 62327^0, 64400^0, 64405^0, 64408^0, 64415^0, 64416^0, 64417^0, 64418^0, 64420^0, 64421^0, 64425^0, 64430^0, 64435^0, 64445^0, 64446^0, 64447^0, 64448^0, 64449^0, 64450^0, 64451^0, 64454^0, 64461^0, 64462^0, 64463^0, 64479^0, 64480^0, 64483^0, 64484^0, 64486^0, 64487^0, 64488^0, 64489^0, 64490^0, 64491^0, 64492^0, 64493^0, 64494^0, 64495^0, 64505^0, 64510^0, 64517^0, 64520^0, 64530^0, 69990^0, 76000^1, 77001^1, 77002^1, 92012^1, 92014^1, 93000^1, 93005^1, 93010^1, 93040^1, 93041^1, 93042^1, 93318^1, 93355^1, 94002^1, 94200^1, 94680^1, 94681^1, 94690^1, 95812^1, 95813^1, 95816^1, 95819^1, 95822^1, 95829^1, 95955^1, 96360^1, 96361^1, 96365^1, 96366^1, 96367^1, 96368^1, 96372^1, 96374^1, 96375^1, 96376^1, 96377^1, 96523^0, 97597^1,

Appendix A: NCCI - CPT Codes

0 = Modifier usage not allowed or inappropriate 1 = Modifier usage allowed

Code 1	Code 2
	97598[1], 97602[1], 99155[0], 99156[0], 99157[0], 99211[1], 99212[1], 99213[1], 99214[1], 99215[1], 99217[1], 99218[1], 99219[1], 99220[1], 99221[1], 99222[1], 99223[1], 99231[1], 99232[1], 99233[1], 99234[1], 99235[1], 99236[1], 99238[1], 99239[1], 99241[1], 99242[1], 99243[1], 99244[1], 99245[1], 99251[1], 99252[1], 99253[1], 99254[1], 99255[1], 99291[1], 99292[1], 99304[1], 99305[1], 99306[1], 99307[1], 99308[1], 99309[1], 99310[1], 99315[1], 99316[1], 99334[1], 99335[1], 99336[1], 99337[1], 99347[1], 99348[1], 99349[1], 99350[1], 99374[1], 99375[1], 99377[1], 99378[1], 99446[0], 99447[0], 99448[0], 99449[0], 99451[0], 99452[0], 99495[1], 99496[1], G0463[1], G0471[1]
50980	00910[0], 0213T[0], 0216T[0], 0596T[1], 0597T[1], 0708T[1], 0709T[1], 11000[1], 11001[1], 11004[1], 11005[1], 11006[1], 11042[1], 11043[1], 11044[1], 11045[1], 11046[1], 11047[1], 12001[1], 12002[1], 12004[1], 12005[1], 12006[1], 12007[1], 12011[1], 12013[1], 12014[1], 12015[1], 12016[1], 12017[1], 12018[1], 12020[1], 12021[1], 12031[1], 12032[1], 12034[1], 12035[1], 12036[1], 12037[1], 12041[1], 12042[1], 12044[1], 12045[1], 12046[1], 12047[1], 12051[1], 12052[1], 12053[1], 12054[1], 12055[1], 12056[1], 12057[1], 13100[1], 13101[1], 13102[1], 13120[1], 13121[1], 13122[1], 13131[1], 13132[1], 13133[1], 13151[1], 13152[1], 13153[1], 36000[1], 36400[1], 36405[1], 36406[1], 36410[1], 36420[1], 36425[1], 36430[1], 36440[1], 36591[0], 36592[0], 36600[1], 36640[1], 43752[1], 50684[1], 50715[1], 50961[1], 50970[1], 51701[1], 51702[1], 51703[1], 52320[1], 52325[1], 52330[1], 52352[1], 62320[0], 62321[0], 62322[0], 62323[0], 62324[0], 62325[0], 62326[0], 62327[0], 64400[0], 64405[0], 64408[0], 64415[0], 64416[0], 64417[0], 64418[0], 64420[0], 64421[0], 64425[0], 64430[0], 64435[0], 64445[0], 64446[0], 64447[0], 64448[0], 64449[0], 64450[0], 64451[0], 64454[0], 64461[0], 64462[0], 64463[0], 64479[0], 64480[0], 64483[0], 64484[0], 64486[0], 64487[0], 64488[0], 64489[0], 64490[0], 64491[0], 64492[0], 64493[0], 64494[0], 64495[0], 64505[0], 64510[0], 64517[0], 64520[0], 64530[0], 69990[0], 76000[1], 77001[1], 77002[1], 92012[1], 92014[1], 93000[1], 93005[1], 93010[1], 93040[1], 93041[1], 93042[1], 93318[1], 93355[1], 94002[1], 94200[1], 94680[1], 94681[1], 94690[1], 95812[1], 95813[1], 95816[1], 95819[1], 95822[1], 95829[1], 95955[1], 96360[1], 96361[1], 96365[1], 96366[1], 96367[1], 96368[1], 96372[1], 96374[1], 96375[1], 96376[1], 96377[1], 96523[0], 97597[1], 97598[1], 97602[1], 99155[0], 99156[0], 99157[0], 99211[1], 99212[1], 99213[1], 99214[1], 99215[1], 99217[1], 99218[1], 99219[1], 99220[1], 99221[1], 99222[1], 99223[1], 99231[1], 99232[1], 99233[1], 99234[1], 99235[1], 99236[1], 99238[1], 99239[1], 99241[1], 99242[1], 99243[1], 99244[1], 99245[1], 99251[1], 99252[1], 99253[1], 99254[1], 99255[1], 99291[1], 99292[1], 99304[1], 99305[1], 99306[1], 99307[1], 99308[1], 99309[1], 99310[1], 99315[1], 99316[1], 99334[1], 99335[1], 99336[1], 99337[1], 99347[1], 99348[1], 99349[1], 99350[1], 99374[1], 99375[1], 99377[1], 99378[1], 99446[0], 99447[0], 99448[0], 99449[0], 99451[0], 99452[0], 99495[1], 99496[1], G0463[1], G0471[1]
51020	00910[0], 0213T[0], 0216T[0], 0596T[1], 0597T[1], 0708T[1], 0709T[1], 11000[1], 11001[1], 11004[1], 11005[1], 11006[1], 11042[1], 11043[1], 11044[1], 11045[1], 11046[1], 11047[1], 12001[1], 12002[1], 12004[1], 12005[1], 12006[1], 12007[1], 12011[1], 12013[1], 12014[1], 12015[1], 12016[1], 12017[1], 12018[1], 12020[1], 12021[1], 12031[1], 12032[1], 12034[1], 12035[1], 12036[1], 12037[1], 12041[1], 12042[1], 12044[1], 12045[1], 12046[1], 12047[1], 12051[1], 12052[1], 12053[1], 12054[1], 12055[1], 12056[1], 12057[1], 13100[1], 13101[1], 13102[1], 13120[1], 13121[1], 13122[1], 13131[1], 13132[1], 13133[1], 13151[1], 13152[1], 13153[1], 36000[1], 36400[1], 36405[1], 36406[1], 36410[1], 36420[1], 36425[1], 36430[1], 36440[1], 36591[0], 36592[0], 36600[1], 36640[1], 43752[1], 44602[1], 44603[1], 44604[1], 44605[1], 44950[0], 44970[0], 49000[0], 49002[1], 49320[1], 50715[1], 51045[0], 51100[1], 51101[1], 51102[1], 51520[0], 51525[0], 51701[0], 51702[0], 51703[1], 52000[0], 62320[0], 62321[0], 62322[0], 62323[0], 62324[0], 62325[0], 62326[0], 62327[0], 64400[0], 64405[0], 64408[0], 64415[0], 64416[0], 64417[0], 64418[0], 64420[0], 64421[0], 64425[0], 64430[0], 64435[0], 64445[0], 64446[0], 64447[0], 64448[0], 64449[0], 64450[0], 64451[0], 64454[0], 64461[0], 64462[0], 64463[0], 64479[0], 64480[0], 64483[0], 64484[0], 64486[0], 64487[0], 64488[0], 64489[0], 64490[0], 64491[0], 64492[0], 64493[0], 64494[0], 64495[0], 64505[0], 64510[0], 64517[0], 64520[0], 64530[0], 69990[0], 92012[1], 92014[1], 93000[1], 93005[1], 93010[1], 93040[1], 93041[1], 93042[1], 93318[1], 93355[1], 94002[1], 94200[1], 94680[1], 94681[1], 94690[1], 95812[1], 95813[1], 95816[1], 95819[1], 95822[1], 95829[1], 95955[1], 96360[1], 96361[1], 96365[1], 96366[1], 96367[1], 96368[1], 96372[1], 96374[1], 96375[1], 96376[1], 96377[1], 96523[0], 97597[1], 97598[1], 97602[1], 99155[0], 99156[0], 99157[0], 99211[1], 99212[1], 99213[1], 99214[1], 99215[1], 99217[1], 99218[1], 99219[1], 99220[1], 99221[1], 99222[1], 99223[1], 99231[1], 99232[1], 99233[1], 99234[1], 99235[1], 99236[1], 99238[1], 99239[1], 99241[1], 99242[1], 99243[1], 99244[1], 99245[1], 99251[1], 99252[1], 99253[1], 99254[1], 99255[1], 99291[1], 99292[1], 99304[1], 99305[1], 99306[1], 99307[1], 99308[1], 99309[1], 99310[1], 99315[1], 99316[1], 99334[1], 99335[1], 99336[1], 99337[1], 99347[1], 99348[1], 99349[1], 99350[1], 99374[1], 99375[1], 99377[1], 99378[1], 99446[0], 99447[0], 99448[0], 99449[0], 99451[0], 99452[0], 99495[0], 99496[0], G0463[1], G0471[0]
51030	00910[0], 0213T[0], 0216T[0], 0596T[1], 0597T[1], 0708T[1], 0709T[1], 11000[1], 11001[1], 11004[1], 11005[1], 11006[1], 11042[1], 11043[1], 11044[1], 11045[1], 11046[1], 11047[1], 12001[1], 12002[1], 12004[1], 12005[1], 12006[1], 12007[1], 12011[1], 12013[1], 12014[1], 12015[1], 12016[1], 12017[1], 12018[1], 12020[1], 12021[1], 12031[1], 12032[1], 12034[1], 12035[1], 12036[1], 12037[1], 12041[1], 12042[1], 12044[1], 12045[1], 12046[1], 12047[1], 12051[1], 12052[1], 12053[1], 12054[1], 12055[1], 12056[1], 12057[1], 13100[1], 13101[1], 13102[1], 13120[1], 13121[1], 13122[1], 13131[1], 13132[1], 13133[1], 13151[1], 13152[1], 13153[1], 36000[1], 36400[1], 36405[1], 36406[1], 36410[1], 36420[1], 36425[1], 36430[1], 36440[1], 36591[0], 36592[0], 36600[1], 36640[1], 43752[1], 44602[1], 44603[1], 44604[1], 44605[1], 44950[0], 44970[0], 49000[0], 49002[1], 49320[1], 50715[1], 51045[0], 51100[1], 51101[1], 51102[1], 51520[0], 51525[0], 51701[0], 51702[0], 51703[1], 52000[0], 62320[0], 62321[0], 62322[0], 62323[0], 62324[0], 62325[0], 62326[0], 62327[0], 64400[0], 64405[0], 64408[0], 64415[0], 64416[0], 64417[0], 64418[0], 64420[0], 64421[0], 64425[0], 64430[0], 64435[0], 64445[0], 64446[0], 64447[0], 64448[0], 64449[0], 64450[0], 64451[0], 64454[0], 64461[0], 64462[0], 64463[0], 64479[0], 64480[0], 64483[0], 64484[0], 64486[0], 64487[0], 64488[0], 64489[0], 64490[0], 64491[0], 64492[0], 64493[0], 64494[0], 64495[0], 64505[0], 64510[0], 64517[0], 64520[0], 64530[0], 69990[0], 92012[1], 92014[1], 93000[1], 93005[1], 93010[1], 93040[1], 93041[1], 93042[1], 93318[1], 93355[1], 94002[1], 94200[1], 94680[1], 94681[1], 94690[1], 95812[1], 95813[1], 95816[1], 95819[1], 95822[1], 95829[1], 95955[1], 96360[1], 96361[1], 96365[1], 96366[1], 96367[1], 96368[1], 96372[1], 96374[1], 96375[1], 96376[1], 96377[1], 96523[0], 97597[1], 97598[1], 97602[1], 99155[0], 99156[0], 99157[0], 99211[1], 99212[1], 99213[1], 99214[1], 99215[1], 99217[1], 99218[1], 99219[1], 99220[1], 99221[1], 99222[1], 99223[1], 99231[1], 99232[1], 99233[1], 99234[1], 99235[1], 99236[1], 99238[1], 99239[1], 99241[1], 99242[1], 99243[1], 99244[1], 99245[1], 99251[1], 99252[1], 99253[1], 99254[1], 99255[1], 99291[1], 99292[1], 99304[1], 99305[1], 99306[1], 99307[1], 99308[1], 99309[1], 99310[1], 99315[1], 99316[1], 99334[1], 99335[1], 99336[1], 99337[1], 99347[1], 99348[1], 99349[1], 99350[1], 99374[1], 99375[1], 99377[1], 99378[1], 99446[0], 99447[0], 99448[0], 99449[0], 99451[0], 99452[0], 99495[0], 99496[0], G0463[1], G0471[0]
51040	00910[0], 0213T[0], 0216T[0], 0596T[1], 0597T[1], 0708T[1], 0709T[1], 11000[1], 11001[1], 11004[1], 11005[1], 11006[1], 11042[1], 11043[1], 11044[1], 11045[1], 11046[1], 11047[1], 12001[1], 12002[1], 12004[1], 12005[1], 12006[1], 12007[1], 12011[1], 12013[1], 12014[1], 12015[1], 12016[1], 12017[1], 12018[1], 12020[1], 12021[1], 12031[1], 12032[1], 12034[1], 12035[1], 12036[1], 12037[1], 12041[1], 12042[1], 12044[1], 12045[1], 12046[1], 12047[1], 12051[1], 12052[1], 12053[1], 12054[1], 12055[1], 12056[1], 12057[1], 13100[1], 13101[1], 13102[1], 13120[1], 13121[1], 13122[1], 13131[1], 13132[1], 13133[1], 13151[1], 13152[1], 13153[1], 36000[1], 36400[1], 36405[1], 36406[1], 36410[1], 36420[1], 36425[1], 36430[1], 36440[1], 36591[0], 36592[0], 36600[1], 36640[1], 43752[1], 44602[1], 44603[1], 44604[1], 44605[1], 44950[0], 44970[0], 49000[0], 49002[1], 49320[1], 50715[1], 51045[0], 51100[1], 51101[1], 51102[1], 51520[0], 51525[0], 51570[0], 51701[0], 51702[0], 51703[1], 52000[0], 52005[1], 52276[1], 52281[1], 62320[0], 62321[0], 62322[0], 62323[0], 62324[0], 62325[0], 62326[0], 62327[0], 64400[0], 64405[0], 64408[0], 64415[0], 64416[0], 64417[0], 64418[0], 64420[0], 64421[0], 64425[0], 64430[0], 64435[0], 64445[0], 64446[0], 64447[0], 64448[0], 64449[0], 64450[0], 64451[0], 64454[0], 64461[0], 64462[0], 64463[0], 64479[0], 64480[0], 64483[0], 64484[0], 64486[0], 64487[0], 64488[0], 64489[0], 64490[0], 64491[0], 64492[0], 64493[0], 64494[0], 64495[0], 64505[0], 64510[0], 64517[0], 64520[0], 64530[0], 69990[0], 92012[1], 92014[1], 93000[1], 93005[1], 93010[1], 93040[1], 93041[1], 93042[1], 93318[1], 93355[1], 94002[1], 94200[1], 94680[1], 94681[1], 94690[1], 95812[1], 95813[1], 95816[1], 95819[1], 95822[1], 95829[1], 95955[1], 96360[1], 96361[1], 96365[1], 96366[1], 96367[1], 96368[1], 96372[1], 96374[1], 96375[1], 96376[1], 96377[1], 96523[0], 97597[1], 97598[1], 97602[1], 99155[0], 99156[0], 99157[0], 99211[1], 99212[1], 99213[1], 99214[1], 99215[1], 99217[1], 99218[1], 99219[1], 99220[1], 99221[1], 99222[1], 99223[1], 99231[1], 99232[1], 99233[1], 99234[1], 99235[1], 99236[1], 99238[1], 99239[1], 99241[1], 99242[1], 99243[1], 99244[1], 99245[1], 99251[1], 99252[1], 99253[1], 99254[1], 99255[1], 99291[1], 99292[1], 99304[1], 99305[1], 99306[1], 99307[1], 99308[1], 99309[1], 99310[1], 99315[1], 99316[1], 99334[1], 99335[1], 99336[1], 99337[1], 99347[1], 99348[1], 99349[1], 99350[1], 99374[1], 99375[1], 99377[1], 99378[1], 99446[0], 99447[0], 99448[0], 99449[0], 99451[0], 99452[0], 99495[0], 99496[0], G0463[1], G0471[0]
51045	00910[0], 0213T[0], 0216T[0], 0596T[1], 0597T[1], 0708T[1], 0709T[1], 11000[1], 11001[1], 11004[1], 11005[1], 11006[1], 11042[1], 11043[1], 11044[1], 11045[1], 11046[1], 11047[1], 12001[1], 12002[1], 12004[1], 12005[1], 12006[1], 12007[1], 12011[1], 12013[1], 12014[1], 12015[1], 12016[1], 12017[1], 12018[1], 12020[1], 12021[1], 12031[1], 12032[1], 12034[1], 12035[1], 12036[1], 12037[1], 12041[1], 12042[1], 12044[1], 12045[1], 12046[1], 12047[1], 12051[1], 12052[1], 12053[1], 12054[1], 12055[1], 12056[1], 12057[1], 13100[1], 13101[1], 13102[1], 13120[1], 13121[1], 13122[1], 13131[1], 13132[1], 13133[1], 13151[1], 13152[1], 13153[1], 36000[1], 36400[1], 36405[1], 36406[1], 36410[1], 36420[1], 36425[1], 36430[1], 36440[1], 36591[0], 36592[0], 36600[1], 36640[1], 43752[1], 44602[1], 44603[1], 44604[1], 44605[1], 44950[0], 44970[0], 49000[0], 49002[1], 49320[1], 50715[1], 51701[0], 51702[0], 51703[1], 52000[0], 62320[0], 62321[0], 62322[0], 62323[0], 62324[0], 62325[0], 62326[0], 62327[0], 64400[0], 64405[0], 64408[0], 64415[0], 64416[0], 64417[0], 64418[0], 64420[0], 64421[0], 64425[0], 64430[0], 64435[0], 64445[0], 64446[0], 64447[0], 64448[0], 64449[0], 64450[0], 64451[0], 64454[0], 64461[0], 64462[0], 64463[0], 64479[0], 64480[0], 64483[0], 64484[0], 64486[0], 64487[0], 64488[0], 64489[0], 64490[0], 64491[0], 64492[0], 64493[0], 64494[0], 64495[0], 64505[0], 64510[0], 64517[0], 64520[0], 64530[0], 69990[0], 92012[1], 92014[1], 93000[1], 93005[1], 93010[1], 93040[1], 93041[1], 93042[1], 93318[1], 93355[1], 94002[1], 94200[1], 94680[1], 94681[1], 94690[1], 95812[1], 95813[1], 95816[1], 95819[1], 95822[1], 95829[1], 95955[1], 96360[1], 96361[1], 96365[1], 96366[1], 96367[1], 96368[1], 96372[1], 96374[1], 96375[1], 96376[1], 96377[1], 96523[0], 97597[1], 97598[1], 97602[1], 99155[0], 99156[0], 99157[0], 99211[1], 99212[1], 99213[1], 99214[1], 99215[1], 99217[1], 99218[1], 99219[1], 99220[1], 99221[1], 99222[1], 99223[1], 99231[1], 99232[1], 99233[1], 99234[1], 99235[1], 99236[1], 99238[1], 99239[1], 99241[1], 99242[1], 99243[1], 99244[1], 99245[1], 99251[1], 99252[1],

0 = Modifier usage not allowed or inappropriate 1 = Modifier usage allowed

Code 1	Code 2
	99253[1], 99254[1], 99255[1], 99291[1], 99292[1], 99304[1], 99305[1], 99306[1], 99307[1], 99308[1], 99309[1], 99310[1], 99315[1], 99316[1], 99334[1], 99335[1], 99336[1], 99337[1], 99347[1], 99348[1], 99349[1], 99350[1], 99374[1], 99375[1], 99377[1], 99378[1], 99446[0], 99447[0], 99448[0], 99449[0], 99451[0], 99452[0], 99495[0], 99496[0], G0463[1], G0471[0]
51050	00910[0], 0213T[0], 0216T[0], 0596T[1], 0597T[1], 0708T[1], 0709T[1], 11000[1], 11001[1], 11004[1], 11005[1], 11006[1], 11042[1], 11043[1], 11044[1], 11045[1], 11046[1], 11047[1], 12001[1], 12002[1], 12004[1], 12005[1], 12006[1], 12007[1], 12011[1], 12013[1], 12014[1], 12015[1], 12016[1], 12017[1], 12018[1], 12020[1], 12021[1], 12031[1], 12032[1], 12034[1], 12035[1], 12036[1], 12037[1], 12041[1], 12042[1], 12044[1], 12045[1], 12046[1], 12047[1], 12051[1], 12052[1], 12053[1], 12054[1], 12055[1], 12056[1], 12057[1], 13100[1], 13101[1], 13102[1], 13120[1], 13121[1], 13122[1], 13131[1], 13132[1], 13133[1], 13151[1], 13152[1], 13153[1], 36000[1], 36400[1], 36405[1], 36406[1], 36410[1], 36420[1], 36425[1], 36430[1], 36440[1], 36591[0], 36592[0], 36600[1], 36640[1], 43752[1], 44602[1], 44603[1], 44604[1], 44605[1], 44950[0], 44970[0], 49000[0], 49002[1], 49320[1], 50715[1], 51045[0], 51520[0], 51525[0], 51570[0], 51701[0], 51702[0], 51703[1], 52000[0], 62320[0], 62321[0], 62322[0], 62323[0], 62324[0], 62325[0], 62326[0], 62327[0], 64400[0], 64405[0], 64408[0], 64415[0], 64416[0], 64417[0], 64418[0], 64420[0], 64421[0], 64425[0], 64430[0], 64435[0], 64445[0], 64446[0], 64447[0], 64448[0], 64449[0], 64450[0], 64451[0], 64454[0], 64461[0], 64462[0], 64463[0], 64479[0], 64480[0], 64483[0], 64484[0], 64486[0], 64487[0], 64488[0], 64489[0], 64490[0], 64491[0], 64492[0], 64493[0], 64494[0], 64495[0], 64505[0], 64510[0], 64517[0], 64520[0], 64530[0], 69990[0], 92012[1], 92014[1], 93000[1], 93005[1], 93010[1], 93040[1], 93041[1], 93042[1], 93318[1], 93355[1], 94002[1], 94200[1], 94680[1], 94681[1], 94690[1], 95812[1], 95813[1], 95816[1], 95819[1], 95822[1], 95829[1], 95955[1], 96360[1], 96361[1], 96365[1], 96366[1], 96367[1], 96368[1], 96372[1], 96374[1], 96375[1], 96376[1], 96377[1], 96523[0], 97597[1], 97598[1], 97602[1], 99155[0], 99156[0], 99157[0], 99211[1], 99212[1], 99213[1], 99214[1], 99215[1], 99217[1], 99218[1], 99219[1], 99220[1], 99221[1], 99222[1], 99223[1], 99231[1], 99232[1], 99233[1], 99234[1], 99235[1], 99236[1], 99238[1], 99239[1], 99241[1], 99242[1], 99243[1], 99244[1], 99245[1], 99251[1], 99252[1], 99253[1], 99254[1], 99255[1], 99291[1], 99292[1], 99304[1], 99305[1], 99306[1], 99307[1], 99308[1], 99309[1], 99310[1], 99315[1], 99316[1], 99334[1], 99335[1], 99336[1], 99337[1], 99347[1], 99348[1], 99349[1], 99350[1], 99374[1], 99375[1], 99377[1], 99378[1], 99446[0], 99447[0], 99448[0], 99449[0], 99451[0], 99452[0], 99495[0], 99496[0], G0463[1], G0471[0]
51060	00910[0], 0213T[0], 0216T[0], 0596T[1], 0597T[1], 0708T[1], 0709T[1], 11000[1], 11001[1], 11004[1], 11005[1], 11006[1], 11042[1], 11043[1], 11044[1], 11045[1], 11046[1], 11047[1], 12001[1], 12002[1], 12004[1], 12005[1], 12006[1], 12007[1], 12011[1], 12013[1], 12014[1], 12015[1], 12016[1], 12017[1], 12018[1], 12020[1], 12021[1], 12031[1], 12032[1], 12034[1], 12035[1], 12036[1], 12037[1], 12041[1], 12042[1], 12044[1], 12045[1], 12046[1], 12047[1], 12051[1], 12052[1], 12053[1], 12054[1], 12055[1], 12056[1], 12057[1], 13100[1], 13101[1], 13102[1], 13120[1], 13121[1], 13122[1], 13131[1], 13132[1], 13133[1], 13151[1], 13152[1], 13153[1], 36000[1], 36400[1], 36405[1], 36406[1], 36410[1], 36420[1], 36425[1], 36430[1], 36440[1], 36591[0], 36592[0], 36600[1], 36640[1], 43752[1], 44602[1], 44603[1], 44604[1], 44605[1], 44950[0], 44970[0], 49000[0], 49002[1], 49320[1], 50715[1], 51045[0], 51520[0], 51525[0], 51570[0], 51701[0], 51702[0], 51703[1], 52000[0], 62320[0], 62321[0], 62322[0], 62323[0], 62324[0], 62325[0], 62326[0], 62327[0], 64400[0], 64405[0], 64408[0], 64415[0], 64416[0], 64417[0], 64418[0], 64420[0], 64421[0], 64425[0], 64430[0], 64435[0], 64445[0], 64446[0], 64447[0], 64448[0], 64449[0], 64450[0], 64451[0], 64454[0], 64461[0], 64462[0], 64463[0], 64479[0], 64480[0], 64483[0], 64484[0], 64486[0], 64487[0], 64488[0], 64489[0], 64490[0], 64491[0], 64492[0], 64493[0], 64494[0], 64495[0], 64505[0], 64510[0], 64517[0], 64520[0], 64530[0], 69990[0], 92012[1], 92014[1], 93000[1], 93005[1], 93010[1], 93040[1], 93041[1], 93042[1], 93318[1], 93355[1], 94002[1], 94200[1], 94680[1], 94681[1], 94690[1], 95812[1], 95813[1], 95816[1], 95819[1], 95822[1], 95829[1], 95955[1], 96360[1], 96361[1], 96365[1], 96366[1], 96367[1], 96368[1], 96372[1], 96374[1], 96375[1], 96376[1], 96377[1], 96523[0], 97597[1], 97598[1], 97602[1], 99155[0], 99156[0], 99157[0], 99211[1], 99212[1], 99213[1], 99214[1], 99215[1], 99217[1], 99218[1], 99219[1], 99220[1], 99221[1], 99222[1], 99223[1], 99231[1], 99232[1], 99233[1], 99234[1], 99235[1], 99236[1], 99238[1], 99239[1], 99241[1], 99242[1], 99243[1], 99244[1], 99245[1], 99251[1], 99252[1], 99253[1], 99254[1], 99255[1], 99291[1], 99292[1], 99304[1], 99305[1], 99306[1], 99307[1], 99308[1], 99309[1], 99310[1], 99315[1], 99316[1], 99334[1], 99335[1], 99336[1], 99337[1], 99347[1], 99348[1], 99349[1], 99350[1], 99374[1], 99375[1], 99377[1], 99378[1], 99446[0], 99447[0], 99448[0], 99449[0], 99451[0], 99452[0], 99495[0], 99496[0], G0463[1], G0471[0]
51065	00910[0], 0213T[0], 0216T[0], 0596T[1], 0597T[1], 0708T[1], 0709T[1], 11000[1], 11001[1], 11004[1], 11005[1], 11006[1], 11042[1], 11043[1], 11044[1], 11045[1], 11046[1], 11047[1], 12001[1], 12002[1], 12004[1], 12005[1], 12006[1], 12007[1], 12011[1], 12013[1], 12014[1], 12015[1], 12016[1], 12017[1], 12018[1], 12020[1], 12021[1], 12031[1], 12032[1], 12034[1], 12035[1], 12036[1], 12037[1], 12041[1], 12042[1], 12044[1], 12045[1], 12046[1], 12047[1], 12051[1], 12052[1], 12053[1], 12054[1], 12055[1], 12056[1], 12057[1], 13100[1], 13101[1], 13102[1], 13120[1], 13121[1], 13122[1], 13131[1], 13132[1], 13133[1], 13151[1], 13152[1], 13153[1], 36000[1], 36400[1], 36405[1], 36406[1], 36410[1], 36420[1], 36425[1], 36430[1], 36440[1], 36591[0], 36592[0], 36600[1], 36640[1], 43752[1], 44602[1], 44603[1], 44604[1], 44605[1], 44950[0], 44970[0], 49000[0], 49002[1], 49320[1], 50715[1], 51045[0], 51520[0], 51525[0], 51570[0], 51701[0], 51702[0], 51703[1], 52000[0], 62320[0], 62321[0], 62322[0], 62323[0], 62324[0], 62325[0], 62326[0], 62327[0], 64400[0], 64405[0], 64408[0], 64415[0], 64416[0], 64417[0], 64418[0], 64420[0], 64421[0], 64425[0], 64430[0], 64435[0], 64445[0], 64446[0], 64447[0], 64448[0], 64449[0], 64450[0], 64451[0], 64454[0], 64461[0], 64462[0], 64463[0], 64479[0], 64480[0], 64483[0], 64484[0], 64486[0], 64487[0], 64488[0], 64489[0], 64490[0], 64491[0], 64492[0], 64493[0], 64494[0], 64495[0], 64505[0], 64510[0], 64517[0], 64520[0], 64530[0], 69990[0], 92012[1], 92014[1], 93000[1], 93005[1], 93010[1], 93040[1], 93041[1], 93042[1], 93318[1], 93355[1], 94002[1], 94200[1], 94680[1], 94681[1], 94690[1], 95812[1], 95813[1], 95816[1], 95819[1], 95822[1], 95829[1], 95955[1], 96360[1], 96361[1], 96365[1], 96366[1], 96367[1], 96368[1], 96372[1], 96374[1], 96375[1], 96376[1], 96377[1], 96523[0], 97597[1], 97598[1], 97602[1], 99155[0], 99156[0], 99157[0], 99211[1], 99212[1], 99213[1], 99214[1], 99215[1], 99217[1], 99218[1], 99219[1], 99220[1], 99221[1], 99222[1], 99223[1], 99231[1], 99232[1], 99233[1], 99234[1], 99235[1], 99236[1], 99238[1], 99239[1], 99241[1], 99242[1], 99243[1], 99244[1], 99245[1], 99251[1], 99252[1], 99253[1], 99254[1], 99255[1], 99291[1], 99292[1], 99304[1], 99305[1], 99306[1], 99307[1], 99308[1], 99309[1], 99310[1], 99315[1], 99316[1], 99334[1], 99335[1], 99336[1], 99337[1], 99347[1], 99348[1], 99349[1], 99350[1], 99374[1], 99375[1], 99377[1], 99378[1], 99446[0], 99447[0], 99448[0], 99449[0], 99451[0], 99452[0], 99495[0], 99496[0], G0463[1], G0471[0]
51080	00910[0], 0213T[0], 0216T[0], 0596T[1], 0597T[1], 0708T[1], 0709T[1], 12001[1], 12002[1], 12004[1], 12005[1], 12006[1], 12007[1], 12011[1], 12013[1], 12014[1], 12015[1], 12016[1], 12017[1], 12018[1], 12020[1], 12021[1], 12031[1], 12032[1], 12034[1], 12035[1], 12036[1], 12037[1], 12041[1], 12042[1], 12044[1], 12045[1], 12046[1], 12047[1], 12051[1], 12052[1], 12053[1], 12054[1], 12055[1], 12056[1], 12057[1], 13100[1], 13101[1], 13102[1], 13120[1], 13121[1], 13122[1], 13131[1], 13132[1], 13133[1], 13151[1], 13152[1], 13153[1], 36000[1], 36400[1], 36405[1], 36406[1], 36410[1], 36420[1], 36425[1], 36430[1], 36440[1], 36591[0], 36592[0], 36600[1], 36640[1], 43752[1], 44602[1], 44603[1], 44604[1], 44605[1], 44950[0], 44970[0], 49000[0], 49002[1], 49320[1], 49406[1], 50715[1], 51045[1], 51570[1], 51701[0], 51702[0], 51703[1], 52000[0], 62320[0], 62321[0], 62322[0], 62323[0], 62324[0], 62325[0], 62326[0], 62327[0], 64400[0], 64405[0], 64408[0], 64415[0], 64416[0], 64417[0], 64418[0], 64420[0], 64421[0], 64425[0], 64430[0], 64435[0], 64445[0], 64446[0], 64447[0], 64448[0], 64449[0], 64450[0], 64451[0], 64454[0], 64461[0], 64462[0], 64463[0], 64479[0], 64480[0], 64483[0], 64484[0], 64486[0], 64487[0], 64488[0], 64489[0], 64490[0], 64491[0], 64492[0], 64493[0], 64494[0], 64495[0], 64505[0], 64510[0], 64517[0], 64520[0], 64530[0], 69990[0], 92012[1], 92014[1], 93000[1], 93005[1], 93010[1], 93040[1], 93041[1], 93042[1], 93318[1], 93355[1], 94002[1], 94200[1], 94680[1], 94681[1], 94690[1], 95812[1], 95813[1], 95816[1], 95819[1], 95822[1], 95829[1], 95955[1], 96360[1], 96361[1], 96365[1], 96366[1], 96367[1], 96368[1], 96372[1], 96374[1], 96375[1], 96376[1], 96377[1], 96523[0], 99155[0], 99156[0], 99157[0], 99211[1], 99212[1], 99213[1], 99214[1], 99215[1], 99217[1], 99218[1], 99219[1], 99220[1], 99221[1], 99222[1], 99223[1], 99231[1], 99232[1], 99233[1], 99234[1], 99235[1], 99236[1], 99238[1], 99239[1], 99241[1], 99242[1], 99243[1], 99244[1], 99245[1], 99251[1], 99252[1], 99253[1], 99254[1], 99255[1], 99291[1], 99292[1], 99304[1], 99305[1], 99306[1], 99307[1], 99308[1], 99309[1], 99310[1], 99315[1], 99316[1], 99334[1], 99335[1], 99336[1], 99337[1], 99347[1], 99348[1], 99349[1], 99350[1], 99374[1], 99375[1], 99377[1], 99378[1], 99446[0], 99447[0], 99448[0], 99449[0], 99451[0], 99452[0], 99495[0], 99496[0], G0463[1], G0471[0]
51100	00910[0], 0213T[0], 0216T[0], 0708T[1], 0709T[1], 12001[1], 12002[1], 12004[1], 12005[1], 12006[1], 12007[1], 12011[1], 12013[1], 12014[1], 12015[1], 12016[1], 12017[1], 12018[1], 12020[1], 12021[1], 12031[1], 12032[1], 12034[1], 12035[1], 12036[1], 12037[1], 12041[1], 12042[1], 12044[1], 12045[1], 12046[1], 12047[1], 12051[1], 12052[1], 12053[1], 12054[1], 12055[1], 12056[1], 12057[1], 13100[1], 13101[1], 13102[1], 13120[1], 13121[1], 13122[1], 13131[1], 13132[1], 13133[1], 13151[1], 13152[1], 13153[1], 36000[1], 36400[1], 36405[1], 36406[1], 36410[1], 36420[1], 36425[1], 36430[1], 36440[1], 36591[0], 36592[0], 36600[1], 36640[1], 43752[1], 44970[0], 51701[0], 52000[1], 62320[0], 62321[0], 62322[0], 62323[0], 62324[0], 62325[0], 62326[0], 62327[0], 64400[0], 64405[0], 64408[0], 64415[0], 64416[0], 64417[0], 64418[0], 64420[0], 64421[0], 64425[0], 64430[0], 64435[0], 64445[0], 64446[0], 64447[0], 64448[0], 64449[0], 64450[0], 64451[0], 64454[0], 64461[0], 64462[0], 64463[0], 64479[0], 64480[0], 64483[0], 64484[0], 64486[0], 64487[0], 64488[0], 64489[0], 64490[0], 64491[0], 64492[0], 64493[0], 64494[0], 64495[0], 64505[0], 64510[0], 64517[0], 64520[0], 64530[0], 69990[0], 92012[1], 92014[1], 93000[1], 93005[1], 93010[1], 93040[1], 93041[1], 93042[1], 93318[1], 93355[1], 94002[1], 94200[1], 94680[1], 94681[1], 94690[1], 95812[1], 95813[1], 95816[1], 95819[1], 95822[1], 95829[1], 95955[1], 96360[1], 96361[1], 96365[1], 96366[1], 96367[1], 96368[1], 96372[1], 96374[1], 96375[1], 96376[1], 96377[1], 96523[0], 99155[0], 99156[0], 99157[0], 99211[1], 99212[1], 99213[1], 99214[1], 99215[1], 99217[1], 99218[1], 99219[1], 99220[1], 99221[1], 99222[1], 99223[1], 99231[1], 99232[1], 99233[1], 99234[1], 99235[1], 99236[1], 99238[1], 99239[1], 99241[1], 99242[1], 99243[1], 99244[1], 99245[1], 99251[1], 99252[1], 99253[1], 99254[1], 99255[1], 99291[1], 99292[1], 99304[1], 99305[1], 99306[1], 99307[1], 99308[1], 99309[1], 99310[1], 99315[1], 99316[1], 99334[1], 99335[1], 99336[1], 99337[1], 99347[1], 99348[1], 99349[1], 99350[1], 99374[1], 99375[1], 99377[1], 99378[1], 99446[0], 99447[0], 99448[0], 99449[0], 99451[0], 99452[0], 99495[1], 99496[1], G0463[1], J0670[1], J2001[1]
51101	00910[0], 0213T[0], 0216T[0], 0708T[1], 0709T[1], 12001[1], 12002[1], 12004[1], 12005[1], 12006[1], 12007[1], 12011[1], 12013[1], 12014[1], 12015[1], 12016[1], 12017[1], 12018[1], 12020[1], 12021[1], 12031[1], 12032[1], 12034[1], 12035[1], 12036[1], 12037[1], 12041[1], 12042[1], 12044[1], 12045[1], 12046[1], 12047[1], 12051[1], 12052[1], 12053[1], 12054[1], 12055[1], 12056[1], 12057[1], 13100[1], 13101[1], 13102[1], 13120[1], 13121[1], 13122[1], 13131[1], 13132[1], 13133[1], 13151[1], 13152[1],

0 = Modifier usage not allowed or inappropriate 1 = Modifier usage allowed

Code 1	Code 2
	13153[1], 36000[1], 36400[1], 36405[1], 36406[1], 36410[1], 36420[1], 36425[1], 36430[1], 36440[1], 36591[0], 36592[0], 36600[1], 36640[1], 43752[1], 44970[0], 51100[1], 51701[0], 52000[0], 62320[0], 62321[0], 62322[0], 62323[0], 62324[0], 62325[0], 62326[0], 62327[0], 64400[0], 64405[0], 64408[0], 64415[0], 64416[0], 64417[0], 64418[0], 64420[0], 64421[0], 64425[0], 64430[0], 64435[0], 64445[0], 64446[0], 64447[0], 64448[0], 64449[0], 64450[0], 64451[0], 64454[0], 64461[0], 64462[0], 64463[0], 64479[0], 64480[0], 64483[0], 64484[0], 64486[0], 64487[0], 64488[0], 64489[0], 64490[0], 64491[0], 64492[0], 64493[0], 64494[0], 64495[0], 64505[0], 64510[0], 64517[0], 64520[0], 64530[0], 69990[0], 76000[1], 77001[1], 92012[1], 92014[1], 93000[1], 93005[1], 93010[1], 93040[1], 93041[1], 93042[1], 93318[1], 93355[1], 94002[1], 94200[1], 94680[1], 94681[1], 94690[1], 95812[1], 95813[1], 95816[1], 95819[1], 95822[1], 95829[1], 95955[1], 96360[1], 96361[1], 96365[1], 96366[1], 96367[1], 96368[1], 96372[1], 96374[1], 96375[1], 96376[1], 96377[1], 96523[0], 99155[0], 99156[0], 99157[0], 99211[1], 99212[1], 99213[1], 99214[1], 99215[1], 99217[1], 99218[1], 99219[1], 99220[1], 99221[1], 99222[1], 99223[1], 99231[1], 99232[1], 99233[1], 99234[1], 99235[1], 99236[1], 99238[1], 99239[1], 99241[1], 99242[1], 99243[1], 99244[1], 99245[1], 99251[1], 99252[1], 99253[1], 99254[1], 99255[1], 99291[1], 99292[1], 99304[1], 99305[1], 99306[1], 99307[1], 99308[1], 99309[1], 99310[1], 99315[1], 99316[1], 99334[1], 99335[1], 99336[1], 99337[1], 99347[1], 99348[1], 99349[1], 99350[1], 99374[1], 99375[1], 99377[1], 99378[1], 99446[0], 99447[0], 99448[0], 99449[0], 99451[0], 99452[0], 99495[1], 99496[1], G0463[1], J0670[1], J2001[1]
51102	00910[0], 0213T[0], 0216T[0], 0708T[1], 0709T[1], 11000[1], 11001[1], 11004[1], 11005[1], 11006[1], 11042[1], 11043[1], 11044[1], 11045[1], 11046[1], 11047[1], 12001[1], 12002[1], 12004[1], 12005[1], 12006[1], 12007[1], 12011[1], 12013[1], 12014[1], 12015[1], 12016[1], 12017[1], 12018[1], 12020[1], 12021[1], 12031[1], 12032[1], 12034[1], 12035[1], 12036[1], 12037[1], 12041[1], 12042[1], 12044[1], 12045[1], 12046[1], 12047[1], 12051[1], 12052[1], 12053[1], 12054[1], 12055[1], 12056[1], 12057[1], 13100[1], 13101[1], 13102[1], 13120[1], 13121[1], 13122[1], 13131[1], 13132[1], 13133[1], 13151[1], 13152[1], 13153[1], 36000[1], 36400[1], 36405[1], 36406[1], 36410[1], 36420[1], 36425[1], 36430[1], 36440[1], 36591[0], 36592[0], 36600[1], 36640[1], 43752[1], 44970[0], 51100[1], 51101[1], 51701[0], 51702[0], 52000[0], 52281[1], 62320[0], 62321[0], 62322[0], 62323[0], 62324[0], 62325[0], 62326[0], 62327[0], 64400[0], 64405[0], 64408[0], 64415[0], 64416[0], 64417[0], 64418[0], 64420[0], 64421[0], 64425[0], 64430[0], 64435[0], 64445[0], 64446[0], 64447[0], 64448[0], 64449[0], 64450[0], 64451[0], 64454[0], 64461[0], 64462[0], 64463[0], 64479[0], 64480[0], 64483[0], 64484[0], 64486[0], 64487[0], 64488[0], 64489[0], 64490[0], 64491[0], 64492[0], 64493[0], 64494[0], 64495[0], 64505[0], 64510[0], 64517[0], 64520[0], 64530[0], 69990[0], 76000[1], 77001[1], 92012[1], 92014[1], 93000[1], 93005[1], 93010[1], 93040[1], 93041[1], 93042[1], 93318[1], 93355[1], 94002[1], 94200[1], 94680[1], 94681[1], 94690[1], 95812[1], 95813[1], 95816[1], 95819[1], 95822[1], 95829[1], 95955[1], 96360[1], 96361[1], 96365[1], 96366[1], 96367[1], 96368[1], 96372[1], 96374[1], 96375[1], 96376[1], 96377[1], 96523[0], 97597[1], 97598[1], 97602[1], 99155[0], 99156[0], 99157[0], 99211[1], 99212[1], 99213[1], 99214[1], 99215[1], 99217[1], 99218[1], 99219[1], 99220[1], 99221[1], 99222[1], 99223[1], 99231[1], 99232[1], 99233[1], 99234[1], 99235[1], 99236[1], 99238[1], 99239[1], 99241[1], 99242[1], 99243[1], 99244[1], 99245[1], 99251[1], 99252[1], 99253[1], 99254[1], 99255[1], 99291[1], 99292[1], 99304[1], 99305[1], 99306[1], 99307[1], 99308[1], 99309[1], 99310[1], 99315[1], 99316[1], 99334[1], 99335[1], 99336[1], 99337[1], 99347[1], 99348[1], 99349[1], 99350[1], 99374[1], 99375[1], 99377[1], 99378[1], 99446[0], 99447[0], 99448[0], 99449[0], 99451[0], 99452[0], 99495[1], 99496[1], G0463[1], G0471[0], J0670[1], J2001[1]
51500	00910[0], 0213T[0], 0216T[0], 0437T[1], 0596T[1], 0597T[1], 0708T[1], 0709T[1], 11000[1], 11001[1], 11004[1], 11005[1], 11006[1], 11042[1], 11043[1], 11044[1], 11045[1], 11046[1], 11047[1], 12001[1], 12002[1], 12004[1], 12005[1], 12006[1], 12007[1], 12011[1], 12013[1], 12014[1], 12015[1], 12016[1], 12017[1], 12018[1], 12020[1], 12021[1], 12031[1], 12032[1], 12034[1], 12035[1], 12036[1], 12037[1], 12041[1], 12042[1], 12044[1], 12045[1], 12046[1], 12047[1], 12051[1], 12052[1], 12053[1], 12054[1], 12055[1], 12056[1], 12057[1], 13100[1], 13101[1], 13102[1], 13120[1], 13121[1], 13122[1], 13131[1], 13132[1], 13133[1], 13151[1], 13152[1], 13153[1], 15777[1], 36000[1], 36400[1], 36405[1], 36406[1], 36410[1], 36420[1], 36425[1], 36430[1], 36440[1], 36591[0], 36592[0], 36600[1], 36640[1], 43752[1], 44602[1], 44603[1], 44604[1], 44605[1], 44950[0], 44970[0], 49000[0], 49002[1], 49320[1], 49568[1], 49580[1], 49582[1], 49585[1], 49587[1], 50715[1], 51045[0], 51570[0], 51701[0], 51702[0], 51703[1], 52000[1], 57267[1], 62320[0], 62321[0], 62322[0], 62323[0], 62324[0], 62325[0], 62326[0], 62327[0], 64400[0], 64405[0], 64408[0], 64415[0], 64416[0], 64417[0], 64418[0], 64420[0], 64421[0], 64425[0], 64430[0], 64435[0], 64445[0], 64446[0], 64447[0], 64448[0], 64449[0], 64450[0], 64451[0], 64454[0], 64461[0], 64462[0], 64463[0], 64479[0], 64480[0], 64483[0], 64484[0], 64486[0], 64487[0], 64488[0], 64489[0], 64490[0], 64491[0], 64492[0], 64493[0], 64494[0], 64495[0], 64505[0], 64510[0], 64517[0], 64520[0], 64530[0], 69990[0], 92012[1], 92014[1], 93000[1], 93005[1], 93010[1], 93040[1], 93041[1], 93042[1], 93318[1], 93355[1], 94002[1], 94200[1], 94680[1], 94681[1], 94690[1], 95812[1], 95813[1], 95816[1], 95819[1], 95822[1], 95829[1], 95955[1], 96360[1], 96361[1], 96365[1], 96366[1], 96367[1], 96368[1], 96372[1], 96374[1], 96375[1], 96376[1], 96377[1], 96523[0], 97597[1], 97598[1], 97602[1], 99155[0], 99156[0], 99157[0], 99211[1], 99212[1], 99213[1], 99214[1], 99215[1], 99217[1], 99218[1], 99219[1], 99220[1], 99221[1], 99222[1], 99223[1], 99231[1], 99232[1], 99233[1], 99234[1], 99235[1], 99236[1], 99238[1], 99239[1], 99241[1], 99242[1], 99243[1], 99244[1], 99245[1], 99251[1], 99252[1], 99253[1], 99254[1], 99255[1], 99291[1], 99292[1], 99304[1], 99305[1], 99306[1], 99307[1], 99308[1], 99309[1], 99310[1], 99315[1], 99316[1], 99334[1], 99335[1], 99336[1], 99337[1], 99347[1], 99348[1], 99349[1], 99350[1], 99374[1], 99375[1], 99377[1], 99378[1], 99446[0], 99447[0], 99448[0], 99449[0], 99451[0], 99452[0], 99495[0], 99496[0], G0463[1], G0471[0]
51520	00910[0], 0213T[0], 0216T[0], 0596T[1], 0597T[1], 0708T[1], 0709T[1], 11000[1], 11001[1], 11004[1], 11005[1], 11006[1], 11042[1], 11043[1], 11044[1], 11045[1], 11046[1], 11047[1], 12001[1], 12002[1], 12004[1], 12005[1], 12006[1], 12007[1], 12011[1], 12013[1], 12014[1], 12015[1], 12016[1], 12017[1], 12018[1], 12020[1], 12021[1], 12031[1], 12032[1], 12034[1], 12035[1], 12036[1], 12037[1], 12041[1], 12042[1], 12044[1], 12045[1], 12046[1], 12047[1], 12051[1], 12052[1], 12053[1], 12054[1], 12055[1], 12056[1], 12057[1], 13100[1], 13101[1], 13102[1], 13120[1], 13121[1], 13122[1], 13131[1], 13132[1], 13133[1], 13151[1], 13152[1], 13153[1], 36000[1], 36400[1], 36405[1], 36406[1], 36410[1], 36420[1], 36425[1], 36430[1], 36440[1], 36591[0], 36592[0], 36600[1], 36640[1], 43752[1], 44602[1], 44603[1], 44604[1], 44605[1], 44950[0], 44970[0], 49000[0], 49002[1], 49320[1], 50715[1], 51045[0], 51701[0], 51702[0], 51703[1], 52000[0], 62320[0], 62321[0], 62322[0], 62323[0], 62324[0], 62325[0], 62326[0], 62327[0], 64400[0], 64405[0], 64408[0], 64415[0], 64416[0], 64417[0], 64418[0], 64420[0], 64421[0], 64425[0], 64430[0], 64435[0], 64445[0], 64446[0], 64447[0], 64448[0], 64449[0], 64450[0], 64451[0], 64454[0], 64461[0], 64462[0], 64463[0], 64479[0], 64480[0], 64483[0], 64484[0], 64486[0], 64487[0], 64488[0], 64489[0], 64490[0], 64491[0], 64492[0], 64493[0], 64494[0], 64495[0], 64505[0], 64510[0], 64517[0], 64520[0], 64530[0], 69990[0], 92012[1], 92014[1], 93000[1], 93005[1], 93010[1], 93040[1], 93041[1], 93042[1], 93318[1], 93355[1], 94002[1], 94200[1], 94680[1], 94681[1], 94690[1], 95812[1], 95813[1], 95816[1], 95819[1], 95822[1], 95829[1], 95955[1], 96360[1], 96361[1], 96365[1], 96366[1], 96367[1], 96368[1], 96372[1], 96374[1], 96375[1], 96376[1], 96377[1], 96523[0], 97597[1], 97598[1], 97602[1], 99155[0], 99156[0], 99157[0], 99211[1], 99212[1], 99213[1], 99214[1], 99215[1], 99217[1], 99218[1], 99219[1], 99220[1], 99221[1], 99222[1], 99223[1], 99231[1], 99232[1], 99233[1], 99234[1], 99235[1], 99236[1], 99238[1], 99239[1], 99241[1], 99242[1], 99243[1], 99244[1], 99245[1], 99251[1], 99252[1], 99253[1], 99254[1], 99255[1], 99291[1], 99292[1], 99304[1], 99305[1], 99306[1], 99307[1], 99308[1], 99309[1], 99310[1], 99315[1], 99316[1], 99334[1], 99335[1], 99336[1], 99337[1], 99347[1], 99348[1], 99349[1], 99350[1], 99374[1], 99375[1], 99377[1], 99378[1], 99446[0], 99447[0], 99448[0], 99449[0], 99451[0], 99452[0], 99495[0], 99496[0], G0463[1], G0471[0]
51525	00910[0], 0213T[0], 0216T[0], 0596T[1], 0597T[1], 0708T[1], 0709T[1], 11000[1], 11001[1], 11004[1], 11005[1], 11006[1], 11042[1], 11043[1], 11044[1], 11045[1], 11046[1], 11047[1], 12001[1], 12002[1], 12004[1], 12005[1], 12006[1], 12007[1], 12011[1], 12013[1], 12014[1], 12015[1], 12016[1], 12017[1], 12018[1], 12020[1], 12021[1], 12031[1], 12032[1], 12034[1], 12035[1], 12036[1], 12037[1], 12041[1], 12042[1], 12044[1], 12045[1], 12046[1], 12047[1], 12051[1], 12052[1], 12053[1], 12054[1], 12055[1], 12056[1], 12057[1], 13100[1], 13101[1], 13102[1], 13120[1], 13121[1], 13122[1], 13131[1], 13132[1], 13133[1], 13151[1], 13152[1], 13153[1], 36000[1], 36400[1], 36405[1], 36406[1], 36410[1], 36420[1], 36425[1], 36430[1], 36440[1], 36591[0], 36592[0], 36600[1], 36640[1], 43752[1], 44602[1], 44603[1], 44604[1], 44605[1], 44950[0], 44970[0], 49000[0], 49002[1], 49320[1], 50715[1], 51045[0], 51520[0], 51701[0], 51702[0], 51703[1], 52000[0], 62320[0], 62321[0], 62322[0], 62323[0], 62324[0], 62325[0], 62326[0], 62327[0], 64400[0], 64405[0], 64408[0], 64415[0], 64416[0], 64417[0], 64418[0], 64420[0], 64421[0], 64425[0], 64430[0], 64435[0], 64445[0], 64446[0], 64447[0], 64448[0], 64449[0], 64450[0], 64451[0], 64454[0], 64461[0], 64462[0], 64463[0], 64479[0], 64480[0], 64483[0], 64484[0], 64486[0], 64487[0], 64488[0], 64489[0], 64490[0], 64491[0], 64492[0], 64493[0], 64494[0], 64495[0], 64505[0], 64510[0], 64517[0], 64520[0], 64530[0], 69990[0], 92012[1], 92014[1], 93000[1], 93005[1], 93010[1], 93040[1], 93041[1], 93042[1], 93318[1], 93355[1], 94002[1], 94200[1], 94680[1], 94681[1], 94690[1], 95812[1], 95813[1], 95816[1], 95819[1], 95822[1], 95829[1], 95955[1], 96360[1], 96361[1], 96365[1], 96366[1], 96367[1], 96368[1], 96372[1], 96374[1], 96375[1], 96376[1], 96377[1], 96523[0], 97597[1], 97598[1], 97602[1], 99155[0], 99156[0], 99157[0], 99211[1], 99212[1], 99213[1], 99214[1], 99215[1], 99217[1], 99218[1], 99219[1], 99220[1], 99221[1], 99222[1], 99223[1], 99231[1], 99232[1], 99233[1], 99234[1], 99235[1], 99236[1], 99238[1], 99239[1], 99241[1], 99242[1], 99243[1], 99244[1], 99245[1], 99251[1], 99252[1], 99253[1], 99254[1], 99255[1], 99291[1], 99292[1], 99304[1], 99305[1], 99306[1], 99307[1], 99308[1], 99309[1], 99310[1], 99315[1], 99316[1], 99334[1], 99335[1], 99336[1], 99337[1], 99347[1], 99348[1], 99349[1], 99350[1], 99374[1], 99375[1], 99377[1], 99378[1], 99446[0], 99447[0], 99448[0], 99449[0], 99451[0], 99452[0], 99495[0], 99496[0], G0463[1], G0471[0]
51530	00910[0], 0213T[0], 0216T[0], 0596T[1], 0597T[1], 0708T[1], 0709T[1], 11000[1], 11001[1], 11004[1], 11005[1], 11006[1], 11042[1], 11043[1], 11044[1], 11045[1], 11046[1], 11047[1], 12001[1], 12002[1], 12004[1], 12005[1], 12006[1], 12007[1], 12011[1], 12013[1], 12014[1], 12015[1], 12016[1], 12017[1], 12018[1], 12020[1], 12021[1], 12031[1], 12032[1], 12034[1], 12035[1], 12036[1], 12037[1], 12041[1], 12042[1], 12044[1], 12045[1], 12046[1], 12047[1], 12051[1], 12052[1], 12053[1], 12054[1], 12055[1], 12056[1], 12057[1], 13100[1], 13101[1], 13102[1], 13120[1], 13121[1], 13122[1], 13131[1], 13132[1], 13133[1], 13151[1], 13152[1], 13153[1], 36000[1], 36400[1], 36405[1], 36406[1], 36410[1], 36420[1], 36425[1], 36430[1], 36440[1], 36591[0], 36592[0], 36600[1], 36640[1], 43752[1], 44602[1], 44603[1], 44604[1], 44605[1], 44950[0], 44970[0], 49000[0], 49002[1], 49320[1], 50715[1], 51045[0], 51520[0], 51525[0], 51570[0], 51701[0], 51702[0], 51703[1], 52000[0], 62320[0], 62321[0], 62322[0], 62323[0], 62324[0], 62325[0], 62326[0], 62327[0], 64400[0], 64405[0], 64408[0], 64415[0], 64416[0], 64417[0], 64418[0], 64420[0], 64421[0], 64425[0], 64430[0], 64435[0], 64445[0], 64446[0], 64447[0], 64448[0],

0 = Modifier usage not allowed or inappropriate 1 = Modifier usage allowed

Appendix A: NCCI - CPT Codes

Code 1	Code 2
	64449[0], 64450[0], 64451[0], 64454[0], 64461[0], 64462[0], 64463[0], 64479[0], 64480[0], 64483[0], 64484[0], 64486[0], 64487[0], 64488[0], 64489[0], 64490[0], 64491[0], 64492[0], 64493[0], 64494[0], 64495[0], 64505[0], 64510[0], 64517[0], 64520[0], 64530[0], 69990[0], 92012[1], 92014[1], 93000[1], 93005[1], 93010[1], 93040[1], 93041[1], 93042[1], 93318[1], 93355[1], 94002[1], 94200[1], 94680[1], 94681[1], 94690[1], 95812[1], 95813[1], 95816[1], 95819[1], 95822[1], 95829[1], 95955[1], 96360[1], 96361[1], 96365[1], 96366[1], 96367[1], 96368[1], 96372[1], 96374[1], 96375[1], 96376[1], 96377[1], 96523[0], 97597[1], 97598[1], 97602[1], 99155[0], 99156[0], 99157[0], 99211[1], 99212[1], 99213[1], 99214[1], 99215[1], 99217[1], 99218[1], 99219[1], 99220[1], 99221[1], 99222[1], 99223[1], 99231[1], 99232[1], 99233[1], 99234[1], 99235[1], 99236[1], 99238[1], 99239[1], 99241[1], 99242[1], 99243[1], 99244[1], 99245[1], 99251[1], 99252[1], 99253[1], 99254[1], 99255[1], 99291[1], 99292[1], 99304[1], 99305[1], 99306[1], 99307[1], 99308[1], 99309[1], 99310[1], 99315[1], 99316[1], 99334[1], 99335[1], 99336[1], 99337[1], 99347[1], 99348[1], 99349[1], 99350[1], 99374[1], 99375[1], 99377[1], 99378[1], 99446[0], 99447[0], 99448[0], 99449[0], 99451[0], 99452[0], 99495[0], 99496[0], G0463[1], G0471[0]
51535	00910[0], 0213T[0], 0216T[0], 0596T[1], 0597T[1], 0708T[1], 0709T[1], 11000[1], 11001[1], 11004[1], 11005[1], 11006[1], 11042[1], 11043[1], 11044[1], 11045[1], 11046[1], 11047[1], 12001[1], 12002[1], 12004[1], 12005[1], 12006[1], 12007[1], 12011[1], 12013[1], 12014[1], 12015[1], 12016[1], 12017[1], 12018[1], 12020[1], 12021[1], 12031[1], 12032[1], 12034[1], 12035[1], 12036[1], 12037[1], 12041[1], 12042[1], 12044[1], 12045[1], 12046[1], 12047[1], 12051[1], 12052[1], 12053[1], 12054[1], 12055[1], 12056[1], 12057[1], 13100[1], 13101[1], 13102[1], 13120[1], 13121[1], 13122[1], 13131[1], 13132[1], 13133[1], 13151[1], 13152[1], 13153[1], 36000[1], 36400[1], 36405[1], 36406[1], 36410[1], 36420[1], 36425[1], 36430[1], 36440[1], 36591[0], 36592[0], 36600[1], 36640[1], 43752[1], 44602[1], 44603[1], 44604[1], 44605[1], 44950[0], 44970[0], 49000[0], 49002[1], 49320[1], 50715[1], 51045[0], 51520[0], 51525[0], 51570[0], 51701[0], 51702[0], 51703[1], 52000[0], 62320[0], 62321[0], 62322[0], 62323[0], 62324[0], 62325[0], 62326[0], 62327[0], 64400[0], 64405[0], 64408[0], 64415[0], 64416[0], 64417[0], 64418[0], 64420[0], 64421[0], 64425[0], 64430[0], 64435[0], 64445[0], 64446[0], 64447[0], 64448[0], 64449[0], 64450[0], 64451[0], 64454[0], 64461[0], 64462[0], 64463[0], 64479[0], 64480[0], 64483[0], 64484[0], 64486[0], 64487[0], 64488[0], 64489[0], 64490[0], 64491[0], 64492[0], 64493[0], 64494[0], 64495[0], 64505[0], 64510[0], 64517[0], 64520[0], 64530[0], 69990[0], 92012[1], 92014[1], 93000[1], 93005[1], 93010[1], 93040[1], 93041[1], 93042[1], 93318[1], 93355[1], 94002[1], 94200[1], 94680[1], 94681[1], 94690[1], 95812[1], 95813[1], 95816[1], 95819[1], 95822[1], 95829[1], 95955[1], 96360[1], 96361[1], 96365[1], 96366[1], 96367[1], 96368[1], 96372[1], 96374[1], 96375[1], 96376[1], 96377[1], 96523[0], 97597[1], 97598[1], 97602[1], 99155[0], 99156[0], 99157[0], 99211[1], 99212[1], 99213[1], 99214[1], 99215[1], 99217[1], 99218[1], 99219[1], 99220[1], 99221[1], 99222[1], 99223[1], 99231[1], 99232[1], 99233[1], 99234[1], 99235[1], 99236[1], 99238[1], 99239[1], 99241[1], 99242[1], 99243[1], 99244[1], 99245[1], 99251[1], 99252[1], 99253[1], 99254[1], 99255[1], 99291[1], 99292[1], 99304[1], 99305[1], 99306[1], 99307[1], 99308[1], 99309[1], 99310[1], 99315[1], 99316[1], 99334[1], 99335[1], 99336[1], 99337[1], 99347[1], 99348[1], 99349[1], 99350[1], 99374[1], 99375[1], 99377[1], 99378[1], 99446[0], 99447[0], 99448[0], 99449[0], 99451[0], 99452[0], 99495[0], 99496[0], G0463[1], G0471[0]
51550	00910[0], 0213T[0], 0216T[0], 0596T[1], 0597T[1], 0708T[1], 0709T[1], 11000[1], 11001[1], 11004[1], 11005[1], 11006[1], 11042[1], 11043[1], 11044[1], 11045[1], 11046[1], 11047[1], 12001[1], 12002[1], 12004[1], 12005[1], 12006[1], 12007[1], 12011[1], 12013[1], 12014[1], 12015[1], 12016[1], 12017[1], 12018[1], 12020[1], 12021[1], 12031[1], 12032[1], 12034[1], 12035[1], 12036[1], 12037[1], 12041[1], 12042[1], 12044[1], 12045[1], 12046[1], 12047[1], 12051[1], 12052[1], 12053[1], 12054[1], 12055[1], 12056[1], 12057[1], 13100[1], 13101[1], 13102[1], 13120[1], 13121[1], 13122[1], 13131[1], 13132[1], 13133[1], 13151[1], 13152[1], 13153[1], 36000[1], 36400[1], 36405[1], 36406[1], 36410[1], 36420[1], 36425[1], 36430[1], 36440[1], 36591[0], 36592[0], 36600[1], 36640[1], 43752[1], 44005[0], 44180[0], 44602[1], 44603[1], 44604[1], 44605[1], 44850[0], 44950[0], 44970[0], 49000[0], 49002[1], 49010[0], 49255[0], 49320[1], 49321[1], 50650[0], 50715[1], 51045[0], 51520[0], 51525[0], 51570[0], 51701[0], 51702[0], 51703[1], 52000[0], 58662[1], 62320[0], 62321[0], 62322[0], 62323[0], 62324[0], 62325[0], 62326[0], 62327[0], 64400[0], 64405[0], 64408[0], 64415[0], 64416[0], 64417[0], 64418[0], 64420[0], 64421[0], 64425[0], 64430[0], 64435[0], 64445[0], 64446[0], 64447[0], 64448[0], 64449[0], 64450[0], 64451[0], 64454[0], 64461[0], 64462[0], 64463[0], 64479[0], 64480[0], 64483[0], 64484[0], 64486[0], 64487[0], 64488[0], 64489[0], 64490[0], 64491[0], 64492[0], 64493[0], 64494[0], 64495[0], 64505[0], 64510[0], 64517[0], 64520[0], 64530[0], 69990[0], 92012[1], 92014[1], 93000[1], 93005[1], 93010[1], 93040[1], 93041[1], 93042[1], 93318[1], 93355[1], 94002[1], 94200[1], 94680[1], 94681[1], 94690[1], 95812[1], 95813[1], 95816[1], 95819[1], 95822[1], 95829[1], 95955[1], 96360[1], 96361[1], 96365[1], 96366[1], 96367[1], 96368[1], 96372[1], 96374[1], 96375[1], 96376[1], 96377[1], 96523[0], 97597[1], 97598[1], 97602[1], 99155[0], 99156[0], 99157[0], 99211[1], 99212[1], 99213[1], 99214[1], 99215[1], 99217[1], 99218[1], 99219[1], 99220[1], 99221[1], 99222[1], 99223[1], 99231[1], 99232[1], 99233[1], 99234[1], 99235[1], 99236[1], 99238[1], 99239[1], 99241[1], 99242[1], 99243[1], 99244[1], 99245[1], 99251[1], 99252[1], 99253[1], 99254[1], 99255[1], 99291[1], 99292[1], 99304[1], 99305[1], 99306[1], 99307[1], 99308[1], 99309[1], 99310[1], 99315[1], 99316[1], 99334[1], 99335[1], 99336[1], 99337[1], 99347[1], 99348[1], 99349[1], 99350[1], 99374[1], 99375[1], 99377[1], 99378[1], 99446[0], 99447[0], 99448[0], 99449[0], 99451[0], 99452[0], 99495[0], 99496[0], G0463[1], G0471[0]
51555	00910[0], 0213T[0], 0216T[0], 0596T[1], 0597T[1], 0708T[1], 0709T[1], 11000[1], 11001[1], 11004[1], 11005[1], 11006[1], 11042[1], 11043[1], 11044[1], 11045[1], 11046[1], 11047[1], 12001[1], 12002[1], 12004[1], 12005[1], 12006[1], 12007[1], 12011[1], 12013[1], 12014[1], 12015[1], 12016[1], 12017[1], 12018[1], 12020[1], 12021[1], 12031[1], 12032[1], 12034[1], 12035[1], 12036[1], 12037[1], 12041[1], 12042[1], 12044[1], 12045[1], 12046[1], 12047[1], 12051[1], 12052[1], 12053[1], 12054[1], 12055[1], 12056[1], 12057[1], 13100[1], 13101[1], 13102[1], 13120[1], 13121[1], 13122[1], 13131[1], 13132[1], 13133[1], 13151[1], 13152[1], 13153[1], 36000[1], 36400[1], 36405[1], 36406[1], 36410[1], 36420[1], 36425[1], 36430[1], 36440[1], 36591[0], 36592[0], 36600[1], 36640[1], 43752[1], 44005[0], 44180[0], 44602[1], 44603[1], 44604[1], 44605[1], 44850[0], 44950[0], 44970[0], 49000[0], 49002[1], 49010[0], 49255[0], 49320[1], 49321[1], 50650[0], 50715[1], 51045[0], 51520[0], 51525[0], 51550[0], 51570[0], 51700[0], 51701[0], 51702[0], 51703[1], 52000[0], 58662[1], 62320[0], 62321[0], 62322[0], 62323[0], 62324[0], 62325[0], 62326[0], 62327[0], 64400[0], 64405[0], 64408[0], 64415[0], 64416[0], 64417[0], 64418[0], 64420[0], 64421[0], 64425[0], 64430[0], 64435[0], 64445[0], 64446[0], 64447[0], 64448[0], 64449[0], 64450[0], 64451[0], 64454[0], 64461[0], 64462[0], 64463[0], 64479[0], 64480[0], 64483[0], 64484[0], 64486[0], 64487[0], 64488[0], 64489[0], 64490[0], 64491[0], 64492[0], 64493[0], 64494[0], 64495[0], 64505[0], 64510[0], 64517[0], 64520[0], 64530[0], 69990[0], 92012[1], 92014[1], 93000[1], 93005[1], 93010[1], 93040[1], 93041[1], 93042[1], 93318[1], 93355[1], 94002[1], 94200[1], 94680[1], 94681[1], 94690[1], 95812[1], 95813[1], 95816[1], 95819[1], 95822[1], 95829[1], 95955[1], 96360[1], 96361[1], 96365[1], 96366[1], 96367[1], 96368[1], 96372[1], 96374[1], 96375[1], 96376[1], 96377[1], 96523[0], 97597[1], 97598[1], 97602[1], 99155[0], 99156[0], 99157[0], 99211[1], 99212[1], 99213[1], 99214[1], 99215[1], 99217[1], 99218[1], 99219[1], 99220[1], 99221[1], 99222[1], 99223[1], 99231[1], 99232[1], 99233[1], 99234[1], 99235[1], 99236[1], 99238[1], 99239[1], 99241[1], 99242[1], 99243[1], 99244[1], 99245[1], 99251[1], 99252[1], 99253[1], 99254[1], 99255[1], 99291[1], 99292[1], 99304[1], 99305[1], 99306[1], 99307[1], 99308[1], 99309[1], 99310[1], 99315[1], 99316[1], 99334[1], 99335[1], 99336[1], 99337[1], 99347[1], 99348[1], 99349[1], 99350[1], 99374[1], 99375[1], 99377[1], 99378[1], 99446[0], 99447[0], 99448[0], 99449[0], 99451[0], 99452[0], 99495[0], 99496[0], G0463[1], G0471[0]
51565	00910[0], 0213T[0], 0216T[0], 0596T[1], 0597T[1], 0708T[1], 0709T[1], 11000[1], 11001[1], 11004[1], 11005[1], 11006[1], 11042[1], 11043[1], 11044[1], 11045[1], 11046[1], 11047[1], 12001[1], 12002[1], 12004[1], 12005[1], 12006[1], 12007[1], 12011[1], 12013[1], 12014[1], 12015[1], 12016[1], 12017[1], 12018[1], 12020[1], 12021[1], 12031[1], 12032[1], 12034[1], 12035[1], 12036[1], 12037[1], 12041[1], 12042[1], 12044[1], 12045[1], 12046[1], 12047[1], 12051[1], 12052[1], 12053[1], 12054[1], 12055[1], 12056[1], 12057[1], 13100[1], 13101[1], 13102[1], 13120[1], 13121[1], 13122[1], 13131[1], 13132[1], 13133[1], 13151[1], 13152[1], 13153[1], 36000[1], 36400[1], 36405[1], 36406[1], 36410[1], 36420[1], 36425[1], 36430[1], 36440[1], 36591[0], 36592[0], 36600[1], 36640[1], 43752[1], 44602[1], 44603[1], 44604[1], 44605[1], 44850[0], 44950[0], 44970[0], 49000[0], 49002[1], 49010[0], 49255[0], 49320[1], 49321[1], 50605[1], 50650[0], 50715[1], 50780[0], 50782[0], 50783[0], 50785[0], 51045[0], 51520[0], 51525[0], 51550[0], 51555[0], 51570[0], 51701[0], 51702[0], 51703[1], 52000[0], 58662[1], 62320[0], 62321[0], 62322[0], 62323[0], 62324[0], 62325[0], 62326[0], 62327[0], 64400[0], 64405[0], 64408[0], 64415[0], 64416[0], 64417[0], 64418[0], 64420[0], 64421[0], 64425[0], 64430[0], 64435[0], 64445[0], 64446[0], 64447[0], 64448[0], 64449[0], 64450[0], 64451[0], 64454[0], 64461[0], 64462[0], 64463[0], 64479[0], 64480[0], 64483[0], 64484[0], 64486[0], 64487[0], 64488[0], 64489[0], 64490[0], 64491[0], 64492[0], 64493[0], 64494[0], 64495[0], 64505[0], 64510[0], 64517[0], 64520[0], 64530[0], 69990[0], 92012[1], 92014[1], 93000[1], 93005[1], 93010[1], 93040[1], 93041[1], 93042[1], 93318[1], 93355[1], 94002[1], 94200[1], 94680[1], 94681[1], 94690[1], 95812[1], 95813[1], 95816[1], 95819[1], 95822[1], 95829[1], 95955[1], 96360[1], 96361[1], 96365[1], 96366[1], 96367[1], 96368[1], 96372[1], 96374[1], 96375[1], 96376[1], 96377[1], 96523[0], 97597[1], 97598[1], 97602[1], 99155[0], 99156[0], 99157[0], 99211[1], 99212[1], 99213[1], 99214[1], 99215[1], 99217[1], 99218[1], 99219[1], 99220[1], 99221[1], 99222[1], 99223[1], 99231[1], 99232[1], 99233[1], 99234[1], 99235[1], 99236[1], 99238[1], 99239[1], 99241[1], 99242[1], 99243[1], 99244[1], 99245[1], 99251[1], 99252[1], 99253[1], 99254[1], 99255[1], 99291[1], 99292[1], 99304[1], 99305[1], 99306[1], 99307[1], 99308[1], 99309[1], 99310[1], 99315[1], 99316[1], 99334[1], 99335[1], 99336[1], 99337[1], 99347[1], 99348[1], 99349[1], 99350[1], 99374[1], 99375[1], 99377[1], 99378[1], 99446[0], 99447[0], 99448[0], 99449[0], 99451[0], 99452[0], 99495[0], 99496[0], G0463[1], G0471[0]
51570	00910[0], 0213T[0], 0216T[0], 0596T[1], 0597T[1], 0708T[1], 0709T[1], 11000[1], 11001[1], 11004[1], 11005[1], 11006[1], 11042[1], 11043[1], 11044[1], 11045[1], 11046[1], 11047[1], 12001[1], 12002[1], 12004[1], 12005[1], 12006[1], 12007[1], 12011[1], 12013[1], 12014[1], 12015[1], 12016[1], 12017[1], 12018[1], 12020[1], 12021[1], 12031[1], 12032[1], 12034[1], 12035[1], 12036[1], 12037[1], 12041[1], 12042[1], 12044[1], 12045[1], 12046[1], 12047[1], 12051[1], 12052[1], 12053[1], 12054[1], 12055[1], 12056[1], 12057[1], 13100[1], 13101[1], 13102[1], 13120[1], 13121[1], 13122[1], 13131[1], 13132[1], 13133[1], 13151[1], 13152[1], 13153[1], 36000[1], 36400[1], 36405[1], 36406[1], 36410[1], 36420[1], 36425[1], 36430[1], 36440[1], 36591[0], 36592[0], 36600[1], 36640[1], 38573[0], 43752[1], 44602[1], 44603[1], 44604[1], 44605[1], 44850[0], 44950[0], 44970[0], 49000[0], 49002[1], 49010[0], 49255[0], 49320[1], 49321[1], 50605[1], 50650[0], 50715[1], 50800[1], 50810[1], 50825[1], 51045[0], 51520[0], 51525[0], 51701[0], 51702[0], 51703[1], 52000[0], 52204[0], 58662[1], 62320[0], 62321[0], 62322[0], 62323[0], 62324[0], 62325[0], 62326[0], 62327[0], 64400[0], 64405[0], 64408[0], 64415[0], 64416[0], 64417[0], 64418[0], 64420[0], 64421[0], 64425[0], 64430[0], 64435[0], 64445[0], 64446[0], 64447[0],

Appendix A: NCCI - CPT Codes

0 = Modifier usage not allowed or inappropriate 1 = Modifier usage allowed

Code 1	Code 2
	64448[0], 64449[0], 64450[0], 64451[0], 64454[0], 64461[0], 64462[0], 64463[0], 64479[0], 64480[0], 64483[0], 64484[0], 64486[0], 64487[0], 64488[0], 64489[0], 64490[0], 64491[0], 64492[0], 64493[0], 64494[0], 64495[0], 64505[0], 64510[0], 64517[0], 64520[0], 64530[0], 69990[0], 92012[1], 92014[1], 93000[1], 93005[1], 93010[1], 93040[1], 93041[1], 93042[1], 93318[1], 93355[1], 94002[1], 94200[1], 94680[1], 94681[1], 94690[1], 95812[1], 95813[1], 95816[1], 95819[1], 95822[1], 95829[1], 95955[1], 96360[1], 96361[1], 96365[1], 96366[1], 96367[1], 96368[1], 96372[1], 96374[1], 96375[1], 96376[1], 96377[1], 96523[0], 97597[1], 97598[1], 97602[1], 99155[0], 99156[0], 99157[0], 99211[1], 99212[1], 99213[1], 99214[1], 99215[1], 99217[1], 99218[1], 99219[1], 99220[1], 99221[1], 99222[1], 99223[1], 99231[1], 99232[1], 99233[1], 99234[1], 99235[1], 99236[1], 99238[1], 99239[1], 99241[1], 99242[1], 99243[1], 99244[1], 99245[1], 99251[1], 99252[1], 99253[1], 99254[1], 99255[1], 99291[1], 99292[1], 99304[1], 99305[1], 99306[1], 99307[1], 99308[1], 99309[1], 99310[1], 99315[1], 99316[1], 99334[1], 99335[1], 99336[1], 99337[1], 99347[1], 99348[1], 99349[1], 99350[1], 99374[1], 99375[1], 99377[1], 99378[1], 99446[0], 99447[0], 99448[0], 99449[0], 99451[0], 99452[0], 99495[0], 99496[0], G0463[1], G0471[0]
51575	00910[0], 0213T[0], 0216T[0], 0596T[1], 0597T[1], 0708T[1], 0709T[1], 11000[1], 11001[1], 11004[1], 11005[1], 11006[1], 11042[1], 11043[1], 11044[1], 11045[1], 11046[1], 11047[1], 12001[1], 12002[1], 12004[1], 12005[1], 12006[1], 12007[1], 12011[1], 12013[1], 12014[1], 12015[1], 12016[1], 12017[1], 12018[1], 12020[1], 12021[1], 12031[1], 12032[1], 12034[1], 12035[1], 12036[1], 12037[1], 12041[1], 12042[1], 12044[1], 12045[1], 12046[1], 12047[1], 12051[1], 12052[1], 12053[1], 12054[1], 12055[1], 12056[1], 12057[1], 13100[1], 13101[1], 13102[1], 13120[1], 13121[1], 13122[1], 13131[1], 13132[1], 13133[1], 13151[1], 13152[1], 13153[1], 36000[1], 36400[1], 36405[1], 36406[1], 36410[1], 36420[1], 36425[1], 36430[1], 36440[1], 36591[0], 36592[0], 36600[1], 36640[1], 38571[1], 38572[1], 38573[0], 38770[1], 38780[1], 43752[1], 44005[0], 44180[0], 44602[1], 44603[1], 44604[1], 44605[1], 44820[0], 44850[0], 44950[0], 44970[0], 49000[0], 49002[1], 49010[0], 49255[0], 49320[1], 49321[1], 50605[1], 50650[0], 50715[1], 50800[1], 50810[1], 50825[1], 51045[0], 51520[0], 51550[0], 51555[0], 51565[0], 51570[0], 51701[0], 51702[0], 51703[1], 52000[1], 52204[0], 58662[1], 62320[0], 62321[0], 62322[0], 62323[0], 62324[0], 62325[0], 62326[0], 62327[0], 64400[0], 64405[0], 64408[0], 64415[0], 64416[0], 64417[0], 64418[0], 64420[0], 64421[0], 64425[0], 64430[0], 64435[0], 64445[0], 64446[0], 64447[0], 64448[0], 64449[0], 64450[0], 64451[0], 64454[0], 64461[0], 64462[0], 64463[0], 64479[0], 64480[0], 64483[0], 64484[0], 64486[0], 64487[0], 64488[0], 64489[0], 64490[0], 64491[0], 64492[0], 64493[0], 64494[0], 64495[0], 64505[0], 64510[0], 64517[0], 64520[0], 64530[0], 69990[0], 92012[1], 92014[1], 93000[1], 93005[1], 93010[1], 93040[1], 93041[1], 93042[1], 93318[1], 93355[1], 94002[1], 94200[1], 94680[1], 94681[1], 94690[1], 95812[1], 95813[1], 95816[1], 95819[1], 95822[1], 95829[1], 95955[1], 96360[1], 96361[1], 96365[1], 96366[1], 96367[1], 96368[1], 96372[1], 96374[1], 96375[1], 96376[1], 96377[1], 96523[0], 97597[1], 97598[1], 97602[1], 99155[0], 99156[0], 99157[0], 99211[1], 99212[1], 99213[1], 99214[1], 99215[1], 99217[1], 99218[1], 99219[1], 99220[1], 99221[1], 99222[1], 99223[1], 99231[1], 99232[1], 99233[1], 99234[1], 99235[1], 99236[1], 99238[1], 99239[1], 99241[1], 99242[1], 99243[1], 99244[1], 99245[1], 99251[1], 99252[1], 99253[1], 99254[1], 99255[1], 99291[1], 99292[1], 99304[1], 99305[1], 99306[1], 99307[1], 99308[1], 99309[1], 99310[1], 99315[1], 99316[1], 99334[1], 99335[1], 99336[1], 99337[1], 99347[1], 99348[1], 99349[1], 99350[1], 99374[1], 99375[1], 99377[1], 99378[1], 99446[0], 99447[0], 99448[0], 99449[0], 99451[0], 99452[0], 99495[0], 99496[0], G0463[1], G0471[0]
51580	00910[0], 0213T[0], 0216T[0], 0596T[1], 0597T[1], 0708T[1], 0709T[1], 11000[1], 11001[1], 11004[1], 11005[1], 11006[1], 11042[1], 11043[1], 11044[1], 11045[1], 11046[1], 11047[1], 12001[1], 12002[1], 12004[1], 12005[1], 12006[1], 12007[1], 12011[1], 12013[1], 12014[1], 12015[1], 12016[1], 12017[1], 12018[1], 12020[1], 12021[1], 12031[1], 12032[1], 12034[1], 12035[1], 12036[1], 12037[1], 12041[1], 12042[1], 12044[1], 12045[1], 12046[1], 12047[1], 12051[1], 12052[1], 12053[1], 12054[1], 12055[1], 12056[1], 12057[1], 13100[1], 13101[1], 13102[1], 13120[1], 13121[1], 13122[1], 13131[1], 13132[1], 13133[1], 13151[1], 13152[1], 13153[1], 36000[1], 36400[1], 36405[1], 36406[1], 36410[1], 36420[1], 36425[1], 36430[1], 36440[1], 36591[0], 36592[0], 36600[1], 36640[1], 38573[0], 43752[1], 44005[0], 44180[0], 44602[1], 44603[1], 44604[1], 44605[1], 44820[0], 44850[0], 44950[0], 44970[0], 49000[0], 49002[1], 49010[0], 49255[0], 49320[1], 49321[1], 50605[1], 50650[0], 50715[1], 50800[1], 50810[1], 50825[1], 51045[0], 51520[0], 51525[0], 51550[0], 51555[0], 51565[0], 51570[0], 51575[0], 51701[0], 51702[0], 51703[1], 52000[0], 52204[0], 58662[1], 62320[0], 62321[0], 62322[0], 62323[0], 62324[0], 62325[0], 62326[0], 62327[0], 64400[0], 64405[0], 64408[0], 64415[0], 64416[0], 64417[0], 64418[0], 64420[0], 64421[0], 64425[0], 64430[0], 64435[0], 64445[0], 64446[0], 64447[0], 64448[0], 64449[0], 64450[0], 64451[0], 64454[0], 64461[0], 64462[0], 64463[0], 64479[0], 64480[0], 64483[0], 64484[0], 64486[0], 64487[0], 64488[0], 64489[0], 64490[0], 64491[0], 64492[0], 64493[0], 64494[0], 64495[0], 64505[0], 64510[0], 64517[0], 64520[0], 64530[0], 69990[0], 92012[1], 92014[1], 93000[1], 93005[1], 93010[1], 93040[1], 93041[1], 93042[1], 93318[1], 93355[1], 94002[1], 94200[1], 94680[1], 94681[1], 94690[1], 95812[1], 95813[1], 95816[1], 95819[1], 95822[1], 95829[1], 95955[1], 96360[1], 96361[1], 96365[1], 96366[1], 96367[1], 96368[1], 96372[1], 96374[1], 96375[1], 96376[1], 96377[1], 96523[0], 97597[1], 97598[1], 97602[1], 99155[0], 99156[0], 99157[0], 99211[1], 99212[1], 99213[1], 99214[1], 99215[1], 99217[1], 99218[1], 99219[1], 99220[1], 99221[1], 99222[1], 99223[1], 99231[1], 99232[1], 99233[1], 99234[1], 99235[1], 99236[1], 99238[1], 99239[1], 99241[1], 99242[1], 99243[1], 99244[1], 99245[1], 99251[1], 99252[1], 99253[1], 99254[1], 99255[1], 99291[1], 99292[1], 99304[1], 99305[1], 99306[1], 99307[1], 99308[1], 99309[1], 99310[1], 99315[1], 99316[1], 99334[1], 99335[1], 99336[1], 99337[1], 99347[1], 99348[1], 99349[1], 99350[1], 99374[1], 99375[1], 99377[1], 99378[1], 99446[0], 99447[0], 99448[0], 99449[0], 99451[0], 99452[0], 99495[0], 99496[0], G0463[1], G0471[0]
51585	00910[0], 0213T[0], 0216T[0], 0596T[1], 0597T[1], 0708T[1], 0709T[1], 11000[1], 11001[1], 11004[1], 11005[1], 11006[1], 11042[1], 11043[1], 11044[1], 11045[1], 11046[1], 11047[1], 12001[1], 12002[1], 12004[1], 12005[1], 12006[1], 12007[1], 12011[1], 12013[1], 12014[1], 12015[1], 12016[1], 12017[1], 12018[1], 12020[1], 12021[1], 12031[1], 12032[1], 12034[1], 12035[1], 12036[1], 12037[1], 12041[1], 12042[1], 12044[1], 12045[1], 12046[1], 12047[1], 12051[1], 12052[1], 12053[1], 12054[1], 12055[1], 12056[1], 12057[1], 13100[1], 13101[1], 13102[1], 13120[1], 13121[1], 13122[1], 13131[1], 13132[1], 13133[1], 13151[1], 13152[1], 13153[1], 36000[1], 36400[1], 36405[1], 36406[1], 36410[1], 36420[1], 36425[1], 36430[1], 36440[1], 36591[0], 36592[0], 36600[1], 36640[1], 38571[1], 38572[1], 38573[0], 38770[1], 38780[1], 43752[1], 44005[0], 44180[0], 44602[1], 44603[1], 44604[1], 44605[1], 44820[0], 44850[0], 44950[0], 44970[0], 49000[0], 49002[1], 49255[0], 49320[1], 49321[1], 50605[1], 50650[0], 50715[1], 50800[1], 50810[1], 50825[1], 51045[0], 51525[0], 51550[0], 51555[0], 51565[0], 51570[0], 51575[0], 51580[0], 51701[0], 51702[0], 51703[1], 52000[1], 52204[0], 58662[1], 62320[0], 62321[0], 62322[0], 62323[0], 62324[0], 62325[0], 62326[0], 62327[0], 64400[0], 64405[0], 64408[0], 64415[0], 64416[0], 64417[0], 64418[0], 64420[0], 64421[0], 64425[0], 64430[0], 64435[0], 64445[0], 64446[0], 64447[0], 64448[0], 64449[0], 64450[0], 64451[0], 64454[0], 64461[0], 64462[0], 64463[0], 64479[0], 64480[0], 64483[0], 64484[0], 64486[0], 64487[0], 64488[0], 64489[0], 64490[0], 64491[0], 64492[0], 64493[0], 64494[0], 64495[0], 64505[0], 64510[0], 64517[0], 64520[0], 64530[0], 69990[0], 92012[1], 92014[1], 93000[1], 93005[1], 93010[1], 93040[1], 93041[1], 93042[1], 93318[1], 93355[1], 94002[1], 94200[1], 94680[1], 94681[1], 94690[1], 95812[1], 95813[1], 95816[1], 95819[1], 95822[1], 95829[1], 95955[1], 96360[1], 96361[1], 96365[1], 96366[1], 96367[1], 96368[1], 96372[1], 96374[1], 96375[1], 96376[1], 96377[1], 96523[0], 97597[1], 97598[1], 97602[1], 99155[0], 99156[0], 99157[0], 99211[1], 99212[1], 99213[1], 99214[1], 99215[1], 99217[1], 99218[1], 99219[1], 99220[1], 99221[1], 99222[1], 99223[1], 99231[1], 99232[1], 99233[1], 99234[1], 99235[1], 99236[1], 99238[1], 99239[1], 99241[1], 99242[1], 99243[1], 99244[1], 99245[1], 99251[1], 99252[1], 99253[1], 99254[1], 99255[1], 99291[1], 99292[1], 99304[1], 99305[1], 99306[1], 99307[1], 99308[1], 99309[1], 99310[1], 99315[1], 99316[1], 99334[1], 99335[1], 99336[1], 99337[1], 99347[1], 99348[1], 99349[1], 99350[1], 99374[1], 99375[1], 99377[1], 99378[1], 99446[0], 99447[0], 99448[0], 99449[0], 99451[0], 99452[0], 99495[0], 99496[0], G0463[1], G0471[0]
51590	00910[0], 0213T[0], 0216T[0], 0596T[1], 0597T[1], 0708T[1], 0709T[1], 11000[1], 11001[1], 11004[1], 11005[1], 11006[1], 11042[1], 11043[1], 11044[1], 11045[1], 11046[1], 11047[1], 12001[1], 12002[1], 12004[1], 12005[1], 12006[1], 12007[1], 12011[1], 12013[1], 12014[1], 12015[1], 12016[1], 12017[1], 12018[1], 12020[1], 12021[1], 12031[1], 12032[1], 12034[1], 12035[1], 12036[1], 12037[1], 12041[1], 12042[1], 12044[1], 12045[1], 12046[1], 12047[1], 12051[1], 12052[1], 12053[1], 12054[1], 12055[1], 12056[1], 12057[1], 13100[1], 13101[1], 13102[1], 13120[1], 13121[1], 13122[1], 13131[1], 13132[1], 13133[1], 13151[1], 13152[1], 13153[1], 36000[1], 36400[1], 36405[1], 36406[1], 36410[1], 36420[1], 36425[1], 36430[1], 36440[1], 36591[0], 36592[0], 36600[1], 36640[1], 38573[0], 43752[1], 44005[0], 44180[0], 44602[1], 44603[1], 44604[1], 44605[1], 44820[0], 44850[0], 44950[0], 44970[0], 49000[0], 49002[1], 49010[0], 49255[0], 49320[1], 49321[1], 50605[1], 50650[0], 50715[1], 50800[1], 50810[1], 50820[0], 50825[1], 51045[0], 51520[0], 51525[0], 51550[0], 51555[0], 51565[0], 51570[0], 51575[0], 51580[0], 51585[0], 51701[0], 51702[0], 51703[1], 52000[0], 52204[0], 58662[1], 62320[0], 62321[0], 62322[0], 62323[0], 62324[0], 62325[0], 62326[0], 62327[0], 64400[0], 64405[0], 64408[0], 64415[0], 64416[0], 64417[0], 64418[0], 64420[0], 64421[0], 64425[0], 64430[0], 64435[0], 64445[0], 64446[0], 64447[0], 64448[0], 64449[0], 64450[0], 64451[0], 64454[0], 64461[0], 64462[0], 64463[0], 64479[0], 64480[0], 64483[0], 64484[0], 64486[0], 64487[0], 64488[0], 64489[0], 64490[0], 64491[0], 64492[0], 64493[0], 64494[0], 64495[0], 64505[0], 64510[0], 64517[0], 64520[0], 64530[0], 69990[0], 92012[1], 92014[1], 93000[1], 93005[1], 93010[1], 93040[1], 93041[1], 93042[1], 93318[1], 93355[1], 94002[1], 94200[1], 94680[1], 94681[1], 94690[1], 95812[1], 95813[1], 95816[1], 95819[1], 95822[1], 95829[1], 95955[1], 96360[1], 96361[1], 96365[1], 96366[1], 96367[1], 96368[1], 96372[1], 96374[1], 96375[1], 96376[1], 96377[1], 96523[0], 97597[1], 97598[1], 97602[1], 99155[0], 99156[0], 99157[0], 99211[1], 99212[1], 99213[1], 99214[1], 99215[1], 99217[1], 99218[1], 99219[1], 99220[1], 99221[1], 99222[1], 99223[1], 99231[1], 99232[1], 99233[1], 99234[1], 99235[1], 99236[1], 99238[1], 99239[1], 99241[1], 99242[1], 99243[1], 99244[1], 99245[1], 99251[1], 99252[1], 99253[1], 99254[1], 99255[1], 99291[1], 99292[1], 99304[1], 99305[1], 99306[1], 99307[1], 99308[1], 99309[1], 99310[1], 99315[1], 99316[1], 99334[1], 99335[1], 99336[1], 99337[1], 99347[1], 99348[1], 99349[1], 99350[1], 99374[1], 99375[1], 99377[1], 99378[1], 99446[0], 99447[0], 99448[0], 99449[0], 99451[0], 99452[0], 99495[0], 99496[0], G0463[1], G0471[0]
51595	00910[0], 0213T[0], 0216T[0], 0596T[1], 0597T[1], 0708T[1], 0709T[1], 11000[1], 11001[1], 11004[1], 11005[1], 11006[1], 11042[1], 11043[1], 11044[1], 11045[1], 11046[1], 11047[1], 12001[1], 12002[1], 12004[1], 12005[1], 12006[1], 12007[1], 12011[1], 12013[1], 12014[1], 12015[1], 12016[1], 12017[1], 12018[1], 12020[1], 12021[1], 12031[1], 12032[1], 12034[1], 12035[1], 12036[1], 12037[1], 12041[1], 12042[1], 12044[1], 12045[1], 12046[1], 12047[1], 12051[1], 12052[1], 12053[1], 12054[1], 12055[1], 12056[1], 12057[1], 13100[1], 13101[1], 13102[1], 13120[1], 13121[1], 13122[1], 13131[1], 13132[1],

0 = Modifier usage not allowed or inappropriate 1 = Modifier usage allowed

Code 1	Code 2
	13133[1], 13151[1], 13152[1], 13153[1], 36000[1], 36400[1], 36405[1], 36406[1], 36410[1], 36420[1], 36425[1], 36430[1], 36440[1], 36591[0], 36592[0], 36600[1], 36640[1], 38571[1], 38572[1], 38573[0], 38770[1], 38780[1], 43752[1], 44005[0], 44130[1], 44180[0], 44602[1], 44603[1], 44604[1], 44605[1], 44820[0], 44850[0], 44950[0], 44970[0], 49000[0], 49002[1], 49010[0], 49255[0], 49320[1], 49321[1], 50605[0], 50650[0], 50715[1], 50800[1], 50810[1], 50820[0], 50825[1], 51045[0], 51525[0], 51550[0], 51555[0], 51565[0], 51570[0], 51575[0], 51580[0], 51585[0], 51590[0], 51701[0], 51702[0], 51703[1], 52000[1], 52204[0], 53210[1], 55842[0], 55845[0], 58200[0], 58210[0], 58662[1], 62320[0], 62321[0], 62322[0], 62323[0], 62324[0], 62325[0], 62326[0], 62327[0], 64400[0], 64405[0], 64408[0], 64415[0], 64416[0], 64417[0], 64418[0], 64420[0], 64421[0], 64425[0], 64430[0], 64435[0], 64445[0], 64446[0], 64447[0], 64448[0], 64449[0], 64450[0], 64451[0], 64454[0], 64461[0], 64462[0], 64463[0], 64479[0], 64480[0], 64483[0], 64484[0], 64486[0], 64487[0], 64488[0], 64489[0], 64490[0], 64491[0], 64492[0], 64493[0], 64494[0], 64495[0], 64505[0], 64510[0], 64517[0], 64520[0], 64530[0], 69990[0], 92012[1], 92014[1], 93000[1], 93005[1], 93010[1], 93040[1], 93041[1], 93042[1], 93318[1], 93355[1], 94002[1], 94200[1], 94680[1], 94681[1], 94690[1], 95812[1], 95813[1], 95816[1], 95819[1], 95822[1], 95829[1], 95955[1], 96360[1], 96361[1], 96365[1], 96366[1], 96367[1], 96368[1], 96372[1], 96374[1], 96375[1], 96376[1], 96377[1], 96523[0], 97597[1], 97598[1], 97602[1], 99155[0], 99156[0], 99157[0], 99211[1], 99212[1], 99213[1], 99214[1], 99215[1], 99217[1], 99218[1], 99219[1], 99220[1], 99221[1], 99222[1], 99223[1], 99231[1], 99232[1], 99233[1], 99234[1], 99235[1], 99236[1], 99238[1], 99239[1], 99241[1], 99242[1], 99243[1], 99244[1], 99245[1], 99251[1], 99252[1], 99253[1], 99254[1], 99255[1], 99291[1], 99292[1], 99304[1], 99305[1], 99306[1], 99307[1], 99308[1], 99309[1], 99310[1], 99315[1], 99316[1], 99334[1], 99335[1], 99336[1], 99337[1], 99347[1], 99348[1], 99349[1], 99350[1], 99374[1], 99375[1], 99377[1], 99378[1], 99446[0], 99447[0], 99448[0], 99449[0], 99451[0], 99452[0], 99495[0], 99496[0], G0463[1], G0471[0]
51596	00910[0], 0213T[0], 0216T[0], 0596T[1], 0597T[1], 0708T[1], 0709T[1], 11000[1], 11001[1], 11004[1], 11005[1], 11006[1], 11042[1], 11043[1], 11044[1], 11045[1], 11046[1], 11047[1], 12001[1], 12002[1], 12004[1], 12005[1], 12006[1], 12007[1], 12011[1], 12013[1], 12014[1], 12015[1], 12016[1], 12017[1], 12018[1], 12020[1], 12021[1], 12031[1], 12032[1], 12034[1], 12035[1], 12036[1], 12037[1], 12041[1], 12042[1], 12044[1], 12045[1], 12046[1], 12047[1], 12051[1], 12052[1], 12053[1], 12054[1], 12055[1], 12056[1], 12057[1], 13100[1], 13101[1], 13102[1], 13120[1], 13121[1], 13122[1], 13131[1], 13132[1], 13133[1], 13151[1], 13152[1], 13153[1], 36000[1], 36400[1], 36405[1], 36406[1], 36410[1], 36420[1], 36425[1], 36430[1], 36440[1], 36591[0], 36592[0], 36600[1], 36640[1], 43752[1], 44005[0], 44180[0], 44602[1], 44603[1], 44604[1], 44605[1], 44820[0], 44850[0], 44950[0], 44970[0], 49000[0], 49002[1], 49010[0], 49255[0], 49320[1], 49321[1], 50605[0], 50650[0], 50715[1], 50800[1], 50810[1], 50820[0], 50825[1], 51045[0], 51520[0], 51525[0], 51550[0], 51555[0], 51565[0], 51570[0], 51575[0], 51580[0], 51585[0], 51590[0], 51595[0], 51701[0], 51702[0], 51703[1], 52000[0], 52204[0], 58662[1], 62320[0], 62321[0], 62322[0], 62323[0], 62324[0], 62325[0], 62326[0], 62327[0], 64400[0], 64405[0], 64408[0], 64415[0], 64416[0], 64417[0], 64418[0], 64420[0], 64421[0], 64425[0], 64430[0], 64435[0], 64445[0], 64446[0], 64447[0], 64448[0], 64449[0], 64450[0], 64451[0], 64454[0], 64461[0], 64462[0], 64463[0], 64479[0], 64480[0], 64483[0], 64484[0], 64486[0], 64487[0], 64488[0], 64489[0], 64490[0], 64491[0], 64492[0], 64493[0], 64494[0], 64495[0], 64505[0], 64510[0], 64517[0], 64520[0], 64530[0], 69990[0], 92012[1], 92014[1], 93000[1], 93005[1], 93010[1], 93040[1], 93041[1], 93042[1], 93318[1], 93355[1], 94002[1], 94200[1], 94680[1], 94681[1], 94690[1], 95812[1], 95813[1], 95816[1], 95819[1], 95822[1], 95829[1], 95955[1], 96360[1], 96361[1], 96365[1], 96366[1], 96367[1], 96368[1], 96372[1], 96374[1], 96375[1], 96376[1], 96377[1], 96523[0], 97597[1], 97598[1], 97602[1], 99155[0], 99156[0], 99157[0], 99211[1], 99212[1], 99213[1], 99214[1], 99215[1], 99217[1], 99218[1], 99219[1], 99220[1], 99221[1], 99222[1], 99223[1], 99231[1], 99232[1], 99233[1], 99234[1], 99235[1], 99236[1], 99238[1], 99239[1], 99241[1], 99242[1], 99243[1], 99244[1], 99245[1], 99251[1], 99252[1], 99253[1], 99254[1], 99255[1], 99291[1], 99292[1], 99304[1], 99305[1], 99306[1], 99307[1], 99308[1], 99309[1], 99310[1], 99315[1], 99316[1], 99334[1], 99335[1], 99336[1], 99337[1], 99347[1], 99348[1], 99349[1], 99350[1], 99374[1], 99375[1], 99377[1], 99378[1], 99446[0], 99447[0], 99448[0], 99449[0], 99451[0], 99452[0], 99495[0], 99496[0], G0463[1], G0471[0]
51597	00910[0], 0213T[0], 0216T[0], 0596T[0], 0597T[0], 0664T[1], 0665T[1], 0666T[1], 0667T[1], 0708T[1], 0709T[1], 11000[1], 11001[1], 11004[1], 11005[1], 11006[1], 11042[1], 11043[1], 11044[1], 11045[1], 11046[1], 11047[1], 12001[1], 12002[1], 12004[1], 12005[1], 12006[1], 12007[1], 12011[1], 12013[1], 12014[1], 12015[1], 12016[1], 12017[1], 12018[1], 12020[1], 12021[1], 12031[1], 12032[1], 12034[1], 12035[1], 12036[1], 12037[1], 12041[1], 12042[1], 12044[1], 12045[1], 12046[1], 12047[1], 12051[1], 12052[1], 12053[1], 12054[1], 12055[1], 12056[1], 12057[1], 13100[1], 13101[1], 13102[1], 13120[1], 13121[1], 13122[1], 13131[1], 13132[1], 13133[1], 13151[1], 13152[1], 13153[1], 36000[1], 36400[1], 36405[1], 36406[1], 36410[1], 36420[1], 36425[1], 36430[1], 36440[1], 36591[0], 36592[0], 36600[1], 36640[1], 38562[0], 38564[0], 38571[0], 38572[0], 38573[0], 38770[0], 38780[0], 43752[1], 44005[0], 44140[1], 44141[1], 44143[1], 44144[1], 44145[1], 44146[1], 44147[1], 44150[1], 44151[1], 44155[1], 44156[1], 44157[1], 44158[1], 44180[0], 44188[1], 44320[0], 44322[1], 44340[0], 44345[1], 44346[1], 44602[1], 44603[1], 44604[1], 44605[1], 44620[1], 44625[1], 44820[0], 44850[0], 44950[0], 44955[0], 44960[0], 44970[0], 45110[1], 45111[1], 45112[1], 45113[1], 45114[1], 45116[1], 45119[1], 45120[1], 45121[1], 45123[1], 45126[1], 45130[1], 45135[1], 45160[1], 45171[1], 45172[1], 45190[1], 45395[1], 45397[1], 45505[1], 45540[1], 46080[1], 46083[1], 46200[1], 46220[1], 46221[1], 46230[1], 46250[1], 46255[1], 46257[1], 46258[1], 46260[1], 46261[1], 46262[1], 46270[1], 46275[1], 46280[1], 46285[1], 46600[1], 46601[1], 46940[1], 46942[1], 46947[1], 46948[1], 49000[0], 49002[1], 49010[0], 49020[1], 49040[1], 49082[1], 49083[1], 49084[1], 49203[1], 49204[1], 49205[1], 49255[0], 49320[1], 49321[1], 49560[1], 49561[1], 49565[1], 49566[1], 49570[1], 49580[1], 49582[1], 49585[1], 49587[1], 50650[0], 50715[1], 50800[0], 50810[0], 50860[0], 51040[1], 51045[0], 51520[0], 51525[0], 51550[0], 51555[0], 51565[0], 51570[0], 51575[0], 51580[0], 51585[0], 51590[0], 51595[0], 51596[0], 51701[0], 51702[0], 51703[0], 52000[1], 52204[0], 55821[0], 55831[0], 55840[0], 55842[0], 55845[0], 55866[0], 57106[0], 57410[0], 57530[1], 57531[1], 57540[1], 57545[1], 57550[1], 57555[1], 57556[1], 58100[0], 58120[0], 58140[1], 58145[1], 58146[1], 58150[1], 58152[1], 58180[1], 58200[1], 58210[1], 58240[1], 58260[1], 58262[1], 58263[1], 58267[1], 58270[1], 58275[1], 58280[1], 58290[1], 58291[1], 58292[1], 58294[1], 58541[1], 58542[1], 58543[1], 58544[1], 58548[1], 58558[0], 58570[1], 58571[1], 58572[1], 58573[1], 58575[1], 58660[0], 58662[1], 58950[1], 58951[1], 58952[1], 58953[0], 58954[0], 58956[1], 58957[1], 58958[1], 62320[0], 62321[0], 62322[0], 62323[0], 62324[0], 62325[0], 62326[0], 62327[0], 64400[0], 64405[0], 64408[0], 64415[0], 64416[0], 64417[0], 64418[0], 64420[0], 64421[0], 64425[0], 64430[0], 64435[0], 64445[0], 64446[0], 64447[0], 64448[0], 64449[0], 64450[0], 64451[0], 64454[0], 64461[0], 64462[0], 64463[0], 64479[0], 64480[0], 64483[0], 64484[0], 64486[0], 64487[0], 64488[0], 64489[0], 64490[0], 64491[0], 64492[0], 64493[0], 64494[0], 64495[0], 64505[0], 64510[0], 64517[0], 64520[0], 64530[0], 69990[0], 92012[1], 92014[1], 93000[1], 93005[1], 93010[1], 93040[1], 93041[1], 93042[1], 93318[1], 93355[1], 94002[1], 94200[1], 94680[1], 94681[1], 94690[1], 95812[1], 95813[1], 95816[1], 95819[1], 95822[1], 95829[1], 95955[1], 96360[1], 96361[1], 96365[1], 96366[1], 96367[1], 96368[1], 96372[1], 96374[1], 96375[1], 96376[1], 96377[1], 96523[0], 97597[1], 97598[1], 97602[1], 99155[0], 99156[0], 99157[0], 99211[1], 99212[1], 99213[1], 99214[1], 99215[1], 99217[1], 99218[1], 99219[1], 99220[1], 99221[1], 99222[1], 99223[1], 99231[1], 99232[1], 99233[1], 99234[1], 99235[1], 99236[1], 99238[1], 99239[1], 99241[1], 99242[1], 99243[1], 99244[1], 99245[1], 99251[1], 99252[1], 99253[1], 99254[1], 99255[1], 99291[1], 99292[1], 99304[1], 99305[1], 99306[1], 99307[1], 99308[1], 99309[1], 99310[1], 99315[1], 99316[1], 99334[1], 99335[1], 99336[1], 99337[1], 99347[1], 99348[1], 99349[1], 99350[1], 99374[1], 99375[1], 99377[1], 99378[1], 99446[0], 99447[0], 99448[0], 99449[0], 99451[0], 99452[0], 99495[0], 99496[0], G0463[1], G0471[0], P9612[0]
51600	00910[0], 0213T[0], 0216T[0], 0708T[1], 0709T[1], 12001[1], 12002[1], 12004[1], 12005[1], 12006[1], 12007[1], 12011[1], 12013[1], 12014[1], 12015[1], 12016[1], 12017[1], 12018[1], 12020[1], 12021[1], 12031[1], 12032[1], 12034[1], 12035[1], 12036[1], 12037[1], 12041[1], 12042[1], 12044[1], 12045[1], 12046[1], 12047[1], 12051[1], 12052[1], 12053[1], 12054[1], 12055[1], 12056[1], 12057[1], 13100[1], 13101[1], 13102[1], 13120[1], 13121[1], 13122[1], 13131[1], 13132[1], 13133[1], 13151[1], 13152[1], 13153[1], 36000[1], 36400[1], 36405[1], 36406[1], 36410[1], 36420[1], 36425[1], 36430[1], 36440[1], 36591[0], 36592[0], 36600[1], 36640[1], 43752[1], 50715[1], 51700[0], 51701[0], 51702[0], 51703[0], 62320[0], 62321[0], 62322[0], 62323[0], 62324[0], 62325[0], 62326[0], 62327[0], 64400[0], 64405[0], 64408[0], 64415[0], 64416[0], 64417[0], 64418[0], 64420[0], 64421[0], 64425[0], 64430[0], 64435[0], 64445[0], 64446[0], 64447[0], 64448[0], 64449[0], 64450[0], 64451[0], 64454[0], 64461[0], 64462[0], 64463[0], 64479[0], 64480[0], 64483[0], 64484[0], 64486[0], 64487[0], 64488[0], 64489[0], 64490[0], 64491[0], 64492[0], 64493[0], 64494[0], 64495[0], 64505[0], 64510[0], 64517[0], 64520[0], 64530[0], 69990[0], 76000[1], 77001[1], 77002[1], 92012[1], 92014[1], 93000[1], 93005[1], 93010[1], 93040[1], 93041[1], 93042[1], 93318[1], 93355[1], 94002[1], 94200[1], 94680[1], 94681[1], 94690[1], 95812[1], 95813[1], 95816[1], 95819[1], 95822[1], 95829[1], 95955[1], 96360[1], 96361[1], 96365[1], 96366[1], 96367[1], 96368[1], 96372[1], 96374[1], 96375[1], 96376[1], 96377[1], 96523[0], 99155[0], 99156[0], 99157[0], 99211[1], 99212[1], 99213[1], 99214[1], 99215[1], 99217[1], 99218[1], 99219[1], 99220[1], 99221[1], 99222[1], 99223[1], 99231[1], 99232[1], 99233[1], 99234[1], 99235[1], 99236[1], 99238[1], 99239[1], 99241[1], 99242[1], 99243[1], 99244[1], 99245[1], 99251[1], 99252[1], 99253[1], 99254[1], 99255[1], 99291[1], 99292[1], 99304[1], 99305[1], 99306[1], 99307[1], 99308[1], 99309[1], 99310[1], 99315[1], 99316[1], 99334[1], 99335[1], 99336[1], 99337[1], 99347[1], 99348[1], 99349[1], 99350[1], 99374[1], 99375[1], 99377[1], 99378[1], 99446[0], 99447[0], 99448[0], 99449[0], 99451[0], 99452[0], 99495[1], 99496[1], G0463[1], G0471[0], J0670[1], J2001[1], P9612[0]
51605	00910[0], 0213T[0], 0216T[0], 0596T[0], 0597T[0], 0708T[1], 0709T[1], 12001[1], 12002[1], 12004[1], 12005[1], 12006[1], 12007[1], 12011[1], 12013[1], 12014[1], 12015[1], 12016[1], 12017[1], 12018[1], 12020[1], 12021[1], 12031[1], 12032[1], 12034[1], 12035[1], 12036[1], 12037[1], 12041[1], 12042[1], 12044[1], 12045[1], 12046[1], 12047[1], 12051[1], 12052[1], 12053[1], 12054[1], 12055[1], 12056[1], 12057[1], 13100[1], 13101[1], 13102[1], 13120[1], 13121[1], 13122[1], 13131[1], 13132[1], 13133[1], 13151[1], 13152[1], 13153[1], 36000[1], 36400[1], 36405[1], 36406[1], 36410[1], 36420[1], 36425[1], 36430[1], 36440[1], 36591[0], 36592[0], 36600[1], 36640[1], 43752[1], 50715[1], 51700[0], 51701[0], 51702[0], 51703[0], 62320[0], 62321[0], 62322[0], 62323[0], 62324[0], 62325[0], 62326[0], 62327[0], 64400[0], 64405[0], 64408[0], 64415[0], 64416[0], 64417[0], 64418[0], 64420[0], 64421[0], 64425[0], 64430[0], 64435[0], 64445[0], 64446[0], 64447[0], 64448[0], 64449[0], 64450[0], 64451[0], 64454[0], 64461[0], 64462[0], 64463[0], 64479[0], 64480[0], 64483[0], 64484[0], 64486[0], 64487[0], 64488[0], 64489[0], 64490[0], 64491[0], 64492[0], 64493[0], 64494[0], 64495[0], 64505[0], 64510[0], 64517[0], 64520[0], 64530[0], 69990[0], 76000[1], 77001[1], 77002[1], 92012[1], 92014[1], 93000[1], 93005[1], 93010[1], 93040[1], 93041[1], 93042[1], 93318[1], 93355[1], 94002[1], 94200[1], 94680[1], 94681[1], 94690[1], 95812[1], 95813[1], 95816[1], 95819[1], 95822[1], 95829[1], 95955[1], 96360[1], 96361[1],

0 = Modifier usage not allowed or inappropriate 1 = Modifier usage allowed

Appendix A: NCCI - CPT Codes

Code 1	Code 2
	96365[1], 96366[1], 96367[1], 96368[1], 96372[1], 96374[1], 96375[1], 96376[1], 96377[1], 96523[0], 99155[0], 99156[0], 99157[0], 99211[1], 99212[1], 99213[1], 99214[1], 99215[1], 99217[1], 99218[1], 99219[1], 99220[1], 99221[1], 99222[1], 99223[1], 99231[1], 99232[1], 99233[1], 99234[1], 99235[1], 99236[1], 99238[1], 99239[1], 99241[1], 99242[1], 99243[1], 99244[1], 99245[1], 99251[1], 99252[1], 99253[1], 99254[1], 99255[1], 99291[1], 99292[1], 99304[1], 99305[1], 99306[1], 99307[1], 99308[1], 99309[1], 99310[1], 99315[1], 99316[1], 99334[1], 99335[1], 99336[1], 99337[1], 99347[1], 99348[1], 99349[1], 99350[1], 99374[1], 99375[1], 99377[1], 99378[1], 99446[0], 99447[0], 99448[0], 99449[0], 99451[0], 99452[0], 99495[1], 99496[1], G0463[1], G0471[0], J0670[1], J1644[1], J2001[1], P9612[0]
51610	00910[0], 0213T[0], 0216T[0], 0708T[1], 0709T[1], 12001[1], 12002[1], 12004[1], 12005[1], 12006[1], 12007[1], 12011[1], 12013[1], 12014[1], 12015[1], 12016[1], 12017[1], 12018[1], 12020[1], 12021[1], 12031[1], 12032[1], 12034[1], 12035[1], 12036[1], 12037[1], 12041[1], 12042[1], 12044[1], 12045[1], 12046[1], 12047[1], 12051[1], 12052[1], 12053[1], 12054[1], 12055[1], 12056[1], 12057[1], 13100[1], 13101[1], 13102[1], 13120[1], 13121[1], 13122[1], 13131[1], 13132[1], 13133[1], 13151[1], 13152[1], 13153[1], 36000[1], 36400[1], 36405[1], 36406[1], 36410[1], 36420[1], 36425[1], 36430[1], 36440[1], 36591[0], 36592[0], 36600[1], 36640[1], 43752[1], 50715[1], 51600[1], 51700[0], 51701[0], 51702[0], 51703[0], 62320[0], 62321[0], 62322[0], 62323[0], 62324[0], 62325[0], 62326[0], 62327[0], 64400[0], 64405[0], 64408[0], 64415[0], 64416[0], 64417[0], 64418[0], 64420[0], 64421[0], 64425[0], 64430[0], 64435[0], 64445[0], 64446[0], 64447[0], 64448[0], 64449[0], 64450[0], 64451[0], 64454[0], 64461[0], 64462[0], 64463[0], 64479[0], 64480[0], 64483[0], 64484[0], 64486[0], 64487[0], 64488[0], 64489[0], 64490[0], 64491[0], 64492[0], 64493[0], 64494[0], 64495[0], 64505[0], 64510[0], 64517[0], 64520[0], 64530[0], 69990[0], 76000[1], 77001[1], 77002[1], 92012[1], 92014[1], 93000[1], 93005[1], 93010[1], 93040[1], 93041[1], 93042[1], 93318[1], 93355[1], 94002[1], 94200[1], 94680[1], 94681[1], 94690[1], 95812[1], 95813[1], 95816[1], 95819[1], 95822[1], 95829[1], 95955[1], 96360[1], 96361[1], 96365[1], 96366[1], 96367[1], 96368[1], 96372[1], 96374[1], 96375[1], 96376[1], 96377[1], 96523[0], 99155[0], 99156[0], 99157[0], 99211[1], 99212[1], 99213[1], 99214[1], 99215[1], 99217[1], 99218[1], 99219[1], 99220[1], 99221[1], 99222[1], 99223[1], 99231[1], 99232[1], 99233[1], 99234[1], 99235[1], 99236[1], 99238[1], 99239[1], 99241[1], 99242[1], 99243[1], 99244[1], 99245[1], 99251[1], 99252[1], 99253[1], 99254[1], 99255[1], 99291[1], 99292[1], 99304[1], 99305[1], 99306[1], 99307[1], 99308[1], 99309[1], 99310[1], 99315[1], 99316[1], 99334[1], 99335[1], 99336[1], 99337[1], 99347[1], 99348[1], 99349[1], 99350[1], 99374[1], 99375[1], 99377[1], 99378[1], 99446[0], 99447[0], 99448[0], 99449[0], 99451[0], 99452[0], 99495[1], 99496[1], G0463[1], G0471[0], J2001[1], P9612[0]
51700	00910[0], 0213T[0], 0216T[0], 0708T[1], 0709T[1], 12001[1], 12002[1], 12004[1], 12005[1], 12006[1], 12007[1], 12011[1], 12013[1], 12014[1], 12015[1], 12016[1], 12017[1], 12018[1], 12020[1], 12021[1], 12031[1], 12032[1], 12034[1], 12035[1], 12036[1], 12037[1], 12041[1], 12042[1], 12044[1], 12045[1], 12046[1], 12047[1], 12051[1], 12052[1], 12053[1], 12054[1], 12055[1], 12056[1], 12057[1], 13100[1], 13101[1], 13102[1], 13120[1], 13121[1], 13122[1], 13131[1], 13132[1], 13133[1], 13151[1], 13152[1], 13153[1], 36000[1], 36400[1], 36405[1], 36406[1], 36410[1], 36420[1], 36425[1], 36430[1], 36440[1], 36591[0], 36592[0], 36600[1], 36640[1], 43752[1], 50715[1], 51701[0], 51702[0], 62320[0], 62321[0], 62322[0], 62323[0], 62324[0], 62325[0], 62326[0], 62327[0], 64400[0], 64405[0], 64408[0], 64415[0], 64416[0], 64417[0], 64418[0], 64420[0], 64421[0], 64425[0], 64430[0], 64435[0], 64445[0], 64446[0], 64447[0], 64448[0], 64449[0], 64450[0], 64451[0], 64454[0], 64461[0], 64462[0], 64463[0], 64479[0], 64480[0], 64483[0], 64484[0], 64486[0], 64487[0], 64488[0], 64489[0], 64490[0], 64491[0], 64492[0], 64493[0], 64494[0], 64495[0], 64505[0], 64510[0], 64517[0], 64520[0], 64530[0], 69990[0], 92012[1], 92014[1], 93000[1], 93005[1], 93010[1], 93040[1], 93041[1], 93042[1], 93318[1], 93355[1], 94002[1], 94200[1], 94680[1], 94681[1], 94690[1], 95812[1], 95813[1], 95816[1], 95819[1], 95822[1], 95829[1], 95955[1], 96360[1], 96361[1], 96365[1], 96366[1], 96367[1], 96368[1], 96372[1], 96374[1], 96375[1], 96376[1], 96377[1], 96523[0], 99155[0], 99156[0], 99157[0], 99211[1], 99212[1], 99213[1], 99214[1], 99215[1], 99217[1], 99218[1], 99219[1], 99220[1], 99221[1], 99222[1], 99223[1], 99231[1], 99232[1], 99233[1], 99234[1], 99235[1], 99236[1], 99238[1], 99239[1], 99241[1], 99242[1], 99243[1], 99244[1], 99245[1], 99251[1], 99252[1], 99253[1], 99254[1], 99255[1], 99291[1], 99292[1], 99304[1], 99305[1], 99306[1], 99307[1], 99308[1], 99309[1], 99310[1], 99315[1], 99316[1], 99334[1], 99335[1], 99336[1], 99337[1], 99347[1], 99348[1], 99349[1], 99350[1], 99374[1], 99375[1], 99377[1], 99378[1], 99446[0], 99447[0], 99448[0], 99449[0], 99451[0], 99452[0], 99495[1], 99496[1], G0463[1], G0471[0], J0670[1], J2001[1], P9612[0]
51701	0543T[1], 0544T[1], 0567T[1], 0568T[1], 0569T[1], 0570T[1], 0571T[1], 0572T[1], 0573T[1], 0574T[1], 0580T[1], 0581T[1], 0655T[1], 11000[1], 11001[1], 11004[1], 11005[1], 11006[1], 11042[1], 11043[1], 11044[1], 11045[1], 11046[1], 11047[1], 13102[1], 13122[1], 13133[1], 13153[1], 20560[1], 20561[1], 36400[1], 36405[1], 36406[1], 36420[1], 36425[1], 36430[1], 36440[1], 36591[0], 36592[0], 36600[1], 64480[0], 64484[0], 66987[1], 66988[1], 69990[0], 92012[1], 92014[1], 93000[1], 93005[1], 93010[1], 93040[1], 93041[1], 93042[1], 93318[1], 93355[1], 94002[1], 94200[1], 94680[1], 94681[1], 94690[1], 95812[1], 95813[1], 95816[1], 95819[1], 95822[1], 95829[1], 95955[1], 96360[1], 96361[1], 96365[1], 96366[1], 96367[1], 96368[1], 96372[1], 96374[1], 96375[1], 96376[1], 96377[1], 96523[0], 97597[1], 97598[1], 97602[1], 99155[0], 99156[0], 99157[0], 99211[1], 99212[1], 99213[1], 99214[1], 99215[1], 99217[1], 99218[1], 99219[1], 99220[1], 99221[1], 99222[1], 99223[1], 99231[1], 99232[1], 99233[1], 99234[1], 99235[1], 99236[1], 99238[1], 99239[1], 99241[1], 99242[1], 99243[1], 99244[1], 99245[1], 99251[1], 99252[1], 99253[1], 99254[1], 99255[1], 99291[1], 99292[1], 99304[1], 99305[1], 99306[1], 99307[1], 99308[1], 99309[1], 99310[1], 99315[1], 99316[1], 99334[1], 99335[1], 99336[1], 99337[1], 99347[1], 99348[1], 99349[1], 99350[1], 99374[1], 99375[1], 99377[1], 99378[1], 99446[0], 99447[0], 99448[0], 99449[0], 99451[0], 99452[0], 99495[1], 99496[1], G0463[1], J0670[1], J2001[1], P9612[0], P9615[0]
51702	0543T[1], 0544T[1], 0567T[1], 0568T[1], 0569T[1], 0570T[1], 0571T[1], 0572T[1], 0573T[1], 0574T[1], 0580T[1], 0581T[1], 0655T[1], 11000[1], 11001[1], 11004[1], 11005[1], 11006[1], 11042[1], 11043[1], 11044[1], 11045[1], 11046[1], 11047[1], 13102[1], 13122[1], 13133[1], 13153[1], 20560[1], 20561[1], 36400[1], 36405[1], 36406[1], 36420[1], 36425[1], 36430[1], 36440[1], 36591[0], 36592[0], 36600[1], 51701[0], 64480[0], 64484[0], 66987[1], 66988[1], 69990[0], 92012[1], 92014[1], 93000[1], 93005[1], 93010[1], 93040[1], 93041[1], 93042[1], 93318[1], 93355[1], 94002[1], 94200[1], 94680[1], 94681[1], 94690[1], 95812[1], 95813[1], 95816[1], 95819[1], 95822[1], 95829[1], 95955[1], 96360[1], 96361[1], 96365[1], 96366[1], 96367[1], 96368[1], 96372[1], 96374[1], 96375[1], 96376[1], 96377[1], 96523[0], 97597[1], 97598[1], 97602[1], 99155[0], 99156[0], 99157[0], 99211[1], 99212[1], 99213[1], 99214[1], 99215[1], 99217[1], 99218[1], 99219[1], 99220[1], 99221[1], 99222[1], 99223[1], 99231[1], 99232[1], 99233[1], 99234[1], 99235[1], 99236[1], 99238[1], 99239[1], 99241[1], 99242[1], 99243[1], 99244[1], 99245[1], 99251[1], 99252[1], 99253[1], 99254[1], 99255[1], 99291[1], 99292[1], 99304[1], 99305[1], 99306[1], 99307[1], 99308[1], 99309[1], 99310[1], 99315[1], 99316[1], 99334[1], 99335[1], 99336[1], 99337[1], 99347[1], 99348[1], 99349[1], 99350[1], 99374[1], 99375[1], 99377[1], 99378[1], 99446[0], 99447[0], 99448[0], 99449[0], 99451[0], 99452[0], 99495[1], 99496[1], G0463[1], J0670[1], J2001[1], P9612[0]
51703	0543T[1], 0544T[1], 0567T[1], 0568T[1], 0569T[1], 0570T[1], 0571T[1], 0572T[1], 0573T[1], 0574T[1], 0580T[1], 0581T[1], 0655T[1], 11000[1], 11001[1], 11004[1], 11005[1], 11006[1], 11042[1], 11043[1], 11044[1], 11045[1], 11046[1], 11047[1], 13102[1], 13122[1], 13133[1], 13153[1], 20560[1], 20561[1], 20701[1], 36400[1], 36405[1], 36406[1], 36420[1], 36425[1], 36430[1], 36440[1], 36591[0], 36592[0], 36600[1], 51700[0], 51701[0], 51702[0], 53080[1], 64415[0], 64417[0], 64450[0], 64480[0], 64484[0], 64486[0], 64487[0], 64488[0], 64489[0], 66987[1], 66988[1], 69990[0], 92012[1], 92014[1], 93000[1], 93005[1], 93010[1], 93040[1], 93041[1], 93042[1], 93318[1], 93355[1], 94002[1], 94200[1], 94680[1], 94681[1], 94690[1], 95812[1], 95813[1], 95816[1], 95819[1], 95822[1], 95829[1], 95955[1], 96360[1], 96361[1], 96365[1], 96366[1], 96367[1], 96368[1], 96372[1], 96374[1], 96375[1], 96376[1], 96377[1], 96523[0], 97597[1], 97598[1], 97602[1], 99155[0], 99156[0], 99157[0], 99211[1], 99212[1], 99213[1], 99214[1], 99215[1], 99217[1], 99218[1], 99219[1], 99220[1], 99221[1], 99222[1], 99223[1], 99231[1], 99232[1], 99233[1], 99234[1], 99235[1], 99236[1], 99238[1], 99239[1], 99241[1], 99242[1], 99243[1], 99244[1], 99245[1], 99251[1], 99252[1], 99253[1], 99254[1], 99255[1], 99291[1], 99292[1], 99304[1], 99305[1], 99306[1], 99307[1], 99308[1], 99309[1], 99310[1], 99315[1], 99316[1], 99334[1], 99335[1], 99336[1], 99337[1], 99347[1], 99348[1], 99349[1], 99350[1], 99374[1], 99375[1], 99377[1], 99378[1], 99446[0], 99447[0], 99448[0], 99449[0], 99451[0], 99452[0], 99495[1], 99496[1], G0463[1], G0471[0], J0670[1], J2001[1], P9612[0]
51705	00910[0], 0213T[0], 0216T[0], 0708T[1], 0709T[1], 12001[1], 12002[1], 12004[1], 12005[1], 12006[1], 12007[1], 12011[1], 12013[1], 12014[1], 12015[1], 12016[1], 12017[1], 12018[1], 12020[1], 12021[1], 12031[1], 12032[1], 12034[1], 12035[1], 12036[1], 12037[1], 12041[1], 12042[1], 12044[1], 12045[1], 12046[1], 12047[1], 12051[1], 12052[1], 12053[1], 12054[1], 12055[1], 12056[1], 12057[1], 13100[1], 13101[1], 13102[1], 13120[1], 13121[1], 13122[1], 13131[1], 13132[1], 13133[1], 13151[1], 13152[1], 13153[1], 36000[1], 36400[1], 36405[1], 36406[1], 36410[1], 36420[1], 36425[1], 36430[1], 36440[1], 36591[0], 36592[0], 36600[1], 36640[1], 43752[1], 50715[1], 51700[0], 51701[0], 51702[0], 51703[1], 52000[0], 62320[0], 62321[0], 62322[0], 62323[0], 62324[0], 62325[0], 62326[0], 62327[0], 64400[0], 64405[0], 64408[0], 64415[0], 64416[0], 64417[0], 64418[0], 64420[0], 64421[0], 64425[0], 64430[0], 64435[0], 64445[0], 64446[0], 64447[0], 64448[0], 64449[0], 64450[0], 64451[0], 64454[0], 64461[0], 64462[0], 64463[0], 64479[0], 64480[0], 64483[0], 64484[0], 64486[0], 64487[0], 64488[0], 64489[0], 64490[0], 64491[0], 64492[0], 64493[0], 64494[0], 64495[0], 64505[0], 64510[0], 64517[0], 64520[0], 64530[0], 69990[0], 76000[1], 76942[1], 76998[1], 77001[1], 77002[1], 92012[1], 92014[1], 93000[1], 93005[1], 93010[1], 93040[1], 93041[1], 93042[1], 93318[1], 93355[1], 94002[1], 94200[1], 94680[1], 94681[1], 94690[1], 95812[1], 95813[1], 95816[1], 95819[1], 95822[1], 95829[1], 95955[1], 96360[1], 96361[1], 96365[1], 96366[1], 96367[1], 96368[1], 96372[1], 96374[1], 96375[1], 96376[1], 96377[1], 96523[0], 99155[0], 99156[0], 99157[0], 99211[1], 99212[1], 99213[1], 99214[1], 99215[1], 99217[1], 99218[1], 99219[1], 99220[1], 99221[1], 99222[1], 99223[1], 99231[1], 99232[1], 99233[1], 99234[1], 99235[1], 99236[1], 99238[1], 99239[1], 99241[1], 99242[1], 99243[1], 99244[1], 99245[1], 99251[1], 99252[1], 99253[1], 99254[1], 99255[1], 99291[1], 99292[1], 99304[1], 99305[1], 99306[1], 99307[1], 99308[1], 99309[1], 99310[1], 99315[1], 99316[1], 99334[1], 99335[1], 99336[1], 99337[1], 99347[1], 99348[1], 99349[1], 99350[1], 99374[1], 99375[1], 99377[1], 99378[1], 99446[0], 99447[0], 99448[0], 99449[0], 99451[0], 99452[0], 99495[1], 99496[1], G0463[1], G0471[0]
51710	00910[0], 0213T[0], 0216T[0], 0596T[1], 0708T[1], 0709T[1], 12001[1], 12002[1], 12004[1], 12005[1], 12006[1], 12007[1], 12011[1], 12013[1], 12014[1], 12015[1], 12016[1], 12017[1], 12018[1], 12020[1], 12021[1], 12031[1], 12032[1], 12034[1], 12035[1], 12036[1], 12037[1], 12041[1], 12042[1], 12044[1], 12045[1], 12046[1], 12047[1], 12051[1], 12052[1], 12053[1], 12054[1], 12055[1], 12056[1], 12057[1],

Appendix A: NCCI - CPT Codes

0 = Modifier usage not allowed or inappropriate 1 = Modifier usage allowed

Code 1	Code 2
	13100[1], 13101[1], 13102[1], 13120[1], 13121[1], 13122[1], 13131[1], 13132[1], 13133[1], 13151[1], 13152[1], 13153[1], 36000[1], 36400[1], 36405[1], 36406[1], 36410[1], 36420[1], 36425[1], 36430[1], 36440[1], 36591[0], 36592[0], 36600[1], 36640[1], 43752[1], 50715[1], 51701[0], 51702[0], 51703[1], 51705[1], 52000[0], 62320[0], 62321[0], 62322[0], 62323[0], 62324[0], 62325[0], 62326[0], 62327[0], 64400[0], 64405[0], 64408[0], 64415[0], 64416[0], 64417[0], 64418[0], 64420[0], 64421[0], 64425[0], 64430[0], 64435[0], 64445[0], 64446[0], 64447[0], 64448[0], 64449[0], 64450[0], 64451[0], 64454[0], 64461[0], 64462[0], 64463[0], 64479[0], 64480[0], 64483[0], 64484[0], 64486[0], 64487[0], 64488[0], 64489[0], 64490[0], 64491[0], 64492[0], 64493[0], 64494[0], 64495[0], 64505[0], 64510[0], 64517[0], 64520[0], 64530[0], 69990[0], 76000[1], 76942[1], 76998[1], 77001[1], 77002[1], 92012[1], 92014[1], 93000[1], 93005[1], 93010[1], 93040[1], 93041[1], 93042[1], 93318[1], 93355[1], 94002[1], 94200[1], 94680[1], 94681[1], 94690[1], 95812[1], 95813[1], 95816[1], 95819[1], 95822[1], 95829[1], 95955[1], 96360[1], 96361[1], 96365[1], 96366[1], 96367[1], 96368[1], 96372[1], 96374[1], 96375[1], 96376[1], 96377[1], 96523[0], 99155[0], 99156[0], 99157[0], 99211[1], 99212[1], 99213[1], 99214[1], 99215[1], 99217[1], 99218[1], 99219[1], 99220[1], 99221[1], 99222[1], 99223[1], 99231[1], 99232[1], 99233[1], 99234[1], 99235[1], 99236[1], 99238[1], 99239[1], 99241[1], 99242[1], 99243[1], 99244[1], 99245[1], 99251[1], 99252[1], 99253[1], 99254[1], 99255[1], 99291[1], 99292[1], 99304[1], 99305[1], 99306[1], 99307[1], 99308[1], 99309[1], 99310[1], 99315[1], 99316[1], 99334[1], 99335[1], 99336[1], 99337[1], 99347[1], 99348[1], 99349[1], 99350[1], 99374[1], 99375[1], 99377[1], 99378[1], 99446[0], 99447[0], 99448[0], 99449[0], 99451[0], 99452[0], 99495[1], 99496[1], G0463[1], G0471[0]
51715	00910[0], 0213T[0], 0216T[0], 0499T[1], 0596T[0], 0597T[0], 0708T[1], 0709T[1], 12001[1], 12002[1], 12004[1], 12005[1], 12006[1], 12007[1], 12011[1], 12013[1], 12014[1], 12015[1], 12016[1], 12017[1], 12018[1], 12020[1], 12021[1], 12031[1], 12032[1], 12034[1], 12035[1], 12036[1], 12037[1], 12041[1], 12042[1], 12044[1], 12045[1], 12046[1], 12047[1], 12051[1], 12052[1], 12053[1], 12054[1], 12055[1], 12056[1], 12057[1], 13100[1], 13101[1], 13102[1], 13120[1], 13121[1], 13122[1], 13131[1], 13132[1], 13133[1], 13151[1], 13152[1], 13153[1], 36000[1], 36400[1], 36405[1], 36406[1], 36410[1], 36420[1], 36425[1], 36430[1], 36440[1], 36591[0], 36592[0], 36600[1], 36640[1], 43752[1], 50715[1], 51701[0], 51702[0], 51703[0], 52000[0], 52001[1], 52005[1], 52007[1], 52010[1], 52204[1], 52214[1], 52224[1], 52281[1], 52283[1], 52285[1], 52287[1], 52332[1], 52356[1], 53000[0], 53010[0], 53020[0], 53025[0], 62320[0], 62321[0], 62322[0], 62323[0], 62324[0], 62325[0], 62326[0], 62327[0], 64400[0], 64405[0], 64408[0], 64415[0], 64416[0], 64417[0], 64418[0], 64420[0], 64421[0], 64425[0], 64430[0], 64435[0], 64445[0], 64446[0], 64447[0], 64448[0], 64449[0], 64450[0], 64451[0], 64454[0], 64461[0], 64462[0], 64463[0], 64479[0], 64480[0], 64483[0], 64484[0], 64486[0], 64487[0], 64488[0], 64489[0], 64490[0], 64491[0], 64492[0], 64493[0], 64494[0], 64495[0], 64505[0], 64510[0], 64517[0], 64520[0], 64530[0], 69990[0], 92012[1], 92014[1], 93000[1], 93005[1], 93010[1], 93040[1], 93041[1], 93042[1], 93318[1], 93355[1], 94002[1], 94200[1], 94680[1], 94681[1], 94690[1], 95812[1], 95813[1], 95816[1], 95819[1], 95822[1], 95829[1], 95955[1], 96360[1], 96361[1], 96365[1], 96366[1], 96367[1], 96368[1], 96372[1], 96374[1], 96375[1], 96376[1], 96377[1], 96523[0], 99155[0], 99156[0], 99157[0], 99211[1], 99212[1], 99213[1], 99214[1], 99215[1], 99217[1], 99218[1], 99219[1], 99220[1], 99221[1], 99222[1], 99223[1], 99231[1], 99232[1], 99233[1], 99234[1], 99235[1], 99236[1], 99238[1], 99239[1], 99241[1], 99242[1], 99243[1], 99244[1], 99245[1], 99251[1], 99252[1], 99253[1], 99254[1], 99255[1], 99291[1], 99292[1], 99304[1], 99305[1], 99306[1], 99307[1], 99308[1], 99309[1], 99310[1], 99315[1], 99316[1], 99334[1], 99335[1], 99336[1], 99337[1], 99347[1], 99348[1], 99349[1], 99350[1], 99374[1], 99375[1], 99377[1], 99378[1], 99446[0], 99447[0], 99448[0], 99449[0], 99451[0], 99452[0], 99495[1], 99496[1], G0463[1], G0471[0], J2001[1], P9612[0]
51720	00910[0], 0213T[0], 0216T[0], 0596T[0], 0597T[0], 0708T[1], 0709T[1], 12001[1], 12002[1], 12004[1], 12005[1], 12006[1], 12007[1], 12011[1], 12013[1], 12014[1], 12015[1], 12016[1], 12017[1], 12018[1], 12020[1], 12021[1], 12031[1], 12032[1], 12034[1], 12035[1], 12036[1], 12037[1], 12041[1], 12042[1], 12044[1], 12045[1], 12046[1], 12047[1], 12051[1], 12052[1], 12053[1], 12054[1], 12055[1], 12056[1], 12057[1], 13100[1], 13101[1], 13102[1], 13120[1], 13121[1], 13122[1], 13131[1], 13132[1], 13133[1], 13151[1], 13152[1], 13153[1], 36000[1], 36400[1], 36405[1], 36406[1], 36410[1], 36420[1], 36425[1], 36430[1], 36440[1], 36591[0], 36592[0], 36600[1], 36640[1], 43752[1], 50715[1], 51700[0], 51701[0], 51702[0], 51703[0], 52000[0], 62320[0], 62321[0], 62322[0], 62323[0], 62324[0], 62325[0], 62326[0], 62327[0], 64400[0], 64405[0], 64408[0], 64415[0], 64416[0], 64417[0], 64418[0], 64420[0], 64421[0], 64425[0], 64430[0], 64435[0], 64445[0], 64446[0], 64447[0], 64448[0], 64449[0], 64450[0], 64451[0], 64454[0], 64461[0], 64462[0], 64463[0], 64479[0], 64480[0], 64483[0], 64484[0], 64486[0], 64487[0], 64488[0], 64489[0], 64490[0], 64491[0], 64492[0], 64493[0], 64494[0], 64495[0], 64505[0], 64510[0], 64517[0], 64520[0], 64530[0], 69990[0], 92012[1], 92014[1], 93000[1], 93005[1], 93010[1], 93040[1], 93041[1], 93042[1], 93318[1], 93355[1], 94002[1], 94200[1], 94680[1], 94681[1], 94690[1], 95812[1], 95813[1], 95816[1], 95819[1], 95822[1], 95829[1], 95955[1], 96360[1], 96361[1], 96365[1], 96366[1], 96367[1], 96368[1], 96372[1], 96374[1], 96375[1], 96376[1], 96377[1], 96523[0], 99155[0], 99156[0], 99157[0], 99211[1], 99212[1], 99213[1], 99214[1], 99215[1], 99217[1], 99218[1], 99219[1], 99220[1], 99221[1], 99222[1], 99223[1], 99231[1], 99232[1], 99233[1], 99234[1], 99235[1], 99236[1], 99238[1], 99239[1], 99241[1], 99242[1], 99243[1], 99244[1], 99245[1], 99251[1], 99252[1], 99253[1], 99254[1], 99255[1], 99291[1], 99292[1], 99304[1], 99305[1], 99306[1], 99307[1], 99308[1], 99309[1], 99310[1], 99315[1], 99316[1], 99334[1], 99335[1], 99336[1], 99337[1], 99347[1], 99348[1], 99349[1], 99350[1], 99374[1], 99375[1], 99377[1], 99378[1], 99446[0], 99447[0], 99448[0], 99449[0], 99451[0], 99452[0], 99495[1], 99496[1], G0463[1], G0471[0], J0670[1], J2001[1], P9612[0]
51725	00910[0], 0213T[0], 0216T[0], 0708T[1], 0709T[1], 12001[1], 12002[1], 12004[1], 12005[1], 12006[1], 12007[1], 12011[1], 12013[1], 12014[1], 12015[1], 12016[1], 12017[1], 12018[1], 12020[1], 12021[1], 12031[1], 12032[1], 12034[1], 12035[1], 12036[1], 12037[1], 12041[1], 12042[1], 12044[1], 12045[1], 12046[1], 12047[1], 12051[1], 12052[1], 12053[1], 12054[1], 12055[1], 12056[1], 12057[1], 13100[1], 13101[1], 13102[1], 13120[1], 13121[1], 13122[1], 13131[1], 13132[1], 13133[1], 13151[1], 13152[1], 13153[1], 36000[1], 36400[1], 36405[1], 36406[1], 36410[1], 36420[1], 36425[1], 36430[1], 36440[1], 36591[0], 36592[0], 36600[1], 36640[1], 43752[1], 50715[1], 51701[0], 51702[0], 51703[0], 62320[0], 62321[0], 62322[0], 62323[0], 62324[0], 62325[0], 62326[0], 62327[0], 64400[0], 64405[0], 64408[0], 64415[0], 64416[0], 64417[0], 64418[0], 64420[0], 64421[0], 64425[0], 64430[0], 64435[0], 64445[0], 64446[0], 64447[0], 64448[0], 64449[0], 64450[0], 64451[0], 64454[0], 64461[0], 64462[0], 64463[0], 64479[0], 64480[0], 64483[0], 64484[0], 64486[0], 64487[0], 64488[0], 64489[0], 64490[0], 64491[0], 64492[0], 64493[0], 64494[0], 64495[0], 64505[0], 64510[0], 64517[0], 64520[0], 64530[0], 69990[0], 92012[1], 92014[1], 93000[1], 93005[1], 93010[1], 93040[1], 93041[1], 93042[1], 93318[1], 93355[1], 94002[1], 94200[1], 94680[1], 94681[1], 94690[1], 95812[1], 95813[1], 95816[1], 95819[1], 95822[1], 95829[1], 95955[1], 96360[1], 96361[1], 96365[1], 96366[1], 96367[1], 96368[1], 96372[1], 96374[1], 96375[1], 96376[1], 96377[1], 96523[0], 99155[0], 99156[0], 99157[0], 99211[1], 99212[1], 99213[1], 99214[1], 99215[1], 99217[1], 99218[1], 99219[1], 99220[1], 99221[1], 99222[1], 99223[1], 99231[1], 99232[1], 99233[1], 99234[1], 99235[1], 99236[1], 99238[1], 99239[1], 99241[1], 99242[1], 99243[1], 99244[1], 99245[1], 99251[1], 99252[1], 99253[1], 99254[1], 99255[1], 99291[1], 99292[1], 99304[1], 99305[1], 99306[1], 99307[1], 99308[1], 99309[1], 99310[1], 99315[1], 99316[1], 99334[1], 99335[1], 99336[1], 99337[1], 99347[1], 99348[1], 99349[1], 99350[1], 99374[1], 99375[1], 99377[1], 99378[1], 99446[0], 99447[0], 99448[0], 99449[0], 99451[0], 99452[0], 99495[1], 99496[1], G0463[1], G0471[0], P9612[0]
51726	00910[0], 0708T[1], 0709T[1], 12001[1], 12002[1], 12004[1], 12005[1], 12006[1], 12007[1], 12011[1], 12013[1], 12014[1], 12015[1], 12016[1], 12017[1], 12018[1], 12020[1], 12021[1], 12031[1], 12032[1], 12034[1], 12035[1], 12036[1], 12037[1], 12041[1], 12042[1], 12044[1], 12045[1], 12046[1], 12047[1], 12051[1], 12052[1], 12053[1], 12054[1], 12055[1], 12056[1], 12057[1], 13100[1], 13101[1], 13102[1], 13120[1], 13121[1], 13122[1], 13131[1], 13132[1], 13133[1], 13151[1], 13152[1], 13153[1], 36000[1], 36400[1], 36405[1], 36406[1], 36410[1], 36420[1], 36425[1], 36430[1], 36440[1], 36591[0], 36592[0], 36600[1], 36640[1], 43752[1], 50715[1], 51701[0], 51702[0], 51703[0], 51725[0], 62320[0], 62321[0], 62322[0], 62323[0], 62324[0], 62325[0], 62326[0], 62327[0], 64400[0], 64405[0], 64408[0], 64415[0], 64416[0], 64417[0], 64418[0], 64420[0], 64421[0], 64425[0], 64430[0], 64435[0], 64445[0], 64446[0], 64447[0], 64448[0], 64449[0], 64450[0], 64451[0], 64454[0], 64461[0], 64462[0], 64463[0], 64479[0], 64480[0], 64483[0], 64484[0], 64486[0], 64487[0], 64488[0], 64489[0], 64490[0], 64491[0], 64492[0], 64493[0], 64494[0], 64495[0], 64505[0], 64510[0], 64517[0], 64520[0], 64530[0], 69990[0], 92012[1], 92014[1], 93000[1], 93005[1], 93010[1], 93040[1], 93041[1], 93042[1], 93318[1], 93355[1], 94002[1], 94200[1], 94680[1], 94681[1], 94690[1], 95812[1], 95813[1], 95816[1], 95819[1], 95822[1], 95829[1], 95955[1], 96360[1], 96361[1], 96365[1], 96366[1], 96367[1], 96368[1], 96372[1], 96374[1], 96375[1], 96376[1], 96377[1], 96523[0], 99155[0], 99156[0], 99157[0], 99211[1], 99212[1], 99213[1], 99214[1], 99215[1], 99217[1], 99218[1], 99219[1], 99220[1], 99221[1], 99222[1], 99223[1], 99231[1], 99232[1], 99233[1], 99234[1], 99235[1], 99236[1], 99238[1], 99239[1], 99241[1], 99242[1], 99243[1], 99244[1], 99245[1], 99251[1], 99252[1], 99253[1], 99254[1], 99255[1], 99291[1], 99292[1], 99304[1], 99305[1], 99306[1], 99307[1], 99308[1], 99309[1], 99310[1], 99315[1], 99316[1], 99334[1], 99335[1], 99336[1], 99337[1], 99347[1], 99348[1], 99349[1], 99350[1], 99374[1], 99375[1], 99377[1], 99378[1], 99446[0], 99447[0], 99448[0], 99449[0], 99451[0], 99452[0], 99495[1], 99496[1], G0463[1], G0471[0], P9612[0]
51727	00910[0], 0213T[0], 0216T[0], 0708T[1], 0709T[1], 11000[1], 11001[1], 11004[1], 11005[1], 11006[1], 11042[1], 11043[1], 11044[1], 11045[1], 11046[1], 11047[1], 12001[1], 12002[1], 12004[1], 12005[1], 12006[1], 12007[1], 12011[1], 12013[1], 12014[1], 12015[1], 12016[1], 12017[1], 12018[1], 12020[1], 12021[1], 12031[1], 12032[1], 12034[1], 12035[1], 12036[1], 12037[1], 12041[1], 12042[1], 12044[1], 12045[1], 12046[1], 12047[1], 12051[1], 12052[1], 12053[1], 12054[1], 12055[1], 12056[1], 12057[1], 13100[1], 13101[1], 13102[1], 13120[1], 13121[1], 13122[1], 13131[1], 13132[1], 13133[1], 13151[1], 13152[1], 13153[1], 36000[1], 36400[1], 36405[1], 36406[1], 36410[1], 36420[1], 36425[1], 36430[1], 36440[1], 36591[0], 36592[0], 36600[1], 36640[1], 43752[1], 50715[1], 51701[0], 51702[0], 51703[1], 51725[0], 51726[0], 62320[0], 62321[0], 62322[0], 62323[0], 62324[0], 62325[0], 62326[0], 62327[0], 64400[0], 64405[0], 64408[0], 64415[0], 64416[0], 64417[0], 64418[0], 64420[0], 64421[0], 64425[0], 64430[0], 64435[0], 64445[0], 64446[0], 64447[0], 64448[0], 64449[0], 64450[0], 64451[0], 64454[0], 64461[0], 64462[0], 64463[0], 64479[0], 64480[0], 64483[0], 64484[0], 64486[0], 64487[0], 64488[0], 64489[0], 64490[0], 64491[0], 64492[0], 64493[0], 64494[0], 64495[0], 64505[0], 64510[0], 64517[0], 64520[0], 64530[0], 69990[0], 92012[1], 92014[1], 93000[1], 93005[1], 93010[1], 93040[1], 93041[1], 93042[1], 93318[1], 93355[1], 94002[1], 94200[1], 94680[1], 94681[1], 94690[1], 95812[1], 95813[1], 95816[1], 95819[1], 95822[1], 95829[1], 95955[1], 96360[1], 96361[1], 96365[1], 96366[1], 96367[1], 96368[1], 96372[1], 96374[1], 96375[1], 96376[1], 96377[1], 96523[0], 97597[1], 97598[1], 97602[1], 99155[0], 99156[0], 99157[0], 99211[1], 99212[1], 99213[1], 99214[1], 99215[1], 99217[1], 99218[1],

0 = Modifier usage not allowed or inappropriate 1 = Modifier usage allowed

Code 1	Code 2
	99219[1], 99220[1], 99221[1], 99222[1], 99223[1], 99231[1], 99232[1], 99233[1], 99234[1], 99235[1], 99236[1], 99238[1], 99239[1], 99241[1], 99242[1], 99243[1], 99244[1], 99245[1], 99251[1], 99252[1], 99253[1], 99254[1], 99255[1], 99291[1], 99292[1], 99304[1], 99305[1], 99306[1], 99307[1], 99308[1], 99309[1], 99310[1], 99315[1], 99316[1], 99334[1], 99335[1], 99336[1], 99337[1], 99347[1], 99348[1], 99349[1], 99350[1], 99374[1], 99375[1], 99377[1], 99378[1], 99446[0], 99447[0], 99448[0], 99449[0], 99451[0], 99452[0], 99495[1], 99496[1], G0463[1], G0471[0], J0670[1], J2001[1], P9612[0]
51728	00910[0], 0213T[0], 0216T[0], 0708T[1], 0709T[1], 12001[1], 12002[1], 12004[1], 12005[1], 12006[1], 12007[1], 12011[1], 12013[1], 12014[1], 12015[1], 12016[1], 12017[1], 12018[1], 12020[1], 12021[1], 12031[1], 12032[1], 12034[1], 12035[1], 12036[1], 12037[1], 12041[1], 12042[1], 12044[1], 12045[1], 12046[1], 12047[1], 12051[1], 12052[1], 12053[1], 12054[1], 12055[1], 12056[1], 12057[1], 13100[1], 13101[1], 13102[1], 13120[1], 13121[1], 13122[1], 13131[1], 13132[1], 13133[1], 13151[1], 13152[1], 13153[1], 36000[1], 36400[1], 36405[1], 36406[1], 36410[1], 36420[1], 36425[1], 36430[1], 36440[1], 36591[0], 36592[0], 36600[1], 36640[1], 43752[1], 50715[1], 51701[0], 51702[0], 51703[1], 51725[0], 51726[0], 51727[0], 62320[0], 62321[0], 62322[0], 62323[0], 62324[0], 62325[0], 62326[0], 62327[0], 64400[0], 64405[0], 64408[0], 64415[0], 64416[0], 64417[0], 64418[0], 64420[0], 64421[0], 64425[0], 64430[0], 64435[0], 64445[0], 64446[0], 64447[0], 64448[0], 64449[0], 64450[0], 64451[0], 64454[0], 64461[0], 64462[0], 64463[0], 64479[0], 64480[0], 64483[0], 64484[0], 64486[0], 64487[0], 64488[0], 64489[0], 64490[0], 64491[0], 64492[0], 64493[0], 64494[0], 64495[0], 64505[0], 64510[0], 64517[0], 64520[0], 64530[0], 69990[0], 90901[1], 92012[1], 92014[1], 93000[1], 93005[1], 93010[1], 93040[1], 93041[1], 93042[1], 93318[1], 93355[1], 94002[1], 94200[1], 94680[1], 94681[1], 94690[1], 95812[1], 95813[1], 95816[1], 95819[1], 95822[1], 95829[1], 95955[1], 96360[1], 96361[1], 96365[1], 96366[1], 96367[1], 96368[1], 96372[1], 96374[1], 96375[1], 96376[1], 96377[1], 96523[0], 99155[0], 99156[0], 99157[0], 99211[1], 99212[1], 99213[1], 99214[1], 99215[1], 99217[1], 99218[1], 99219[1], 99220[1], 99221[1], 99222[1], 99223[1], 99231[1], 99232[1], 99233[1], 99234[1], 99235[1], 99236[1], 99238[1], 99239[1], 99241[1], 99242[1], 99243[1], 99244[1], 99245[1], 99251[1], 99252[1], 99253[1], 99254[1], 99255[1], 99291[1], 99292[1], 99304[1], 99305[1], 99306[1], 99307[1], 99308[1], 99309[1], 99310[1], 99315[1], 99316[1], 99334[1], 99335[1], 99336[1], 99337[1], 99347[1], 99348[1], 99349[1], 99350[1], 99374[1], 99375[1], 99377[1], 99378[1], 99446[0], 99447[0], 99448[0], 99449[0], 99451[0], 99452[0], 99495[1], 99496[1], G0463[1], G0471[0], J0670[1], J2001[1], P9612[0]
51729	00910[0], 0213T[0], 0216T[0], 0596T[0], 0597T[0], 0708T[1], 0709T[1], 11000[1], 11001[1], 11004[1], 11005[1], 11006[1], 11042[1], 11043[1], 11044[1], 11045[1], 11046[1], 11047[1], 12001[1], 12002[1], 12004[1], 12005[1], 12006[1], 12007[1], 12011[1], 12013[1], 12014[1], 12015[1], 12016[1], 12017[1], 12018[1], 12020[1], 12021[1], 12031[1], 12032[1], 12034[1], 12035[1], 12036[1], 12037[1], 12041[1], 12042[1], 12044[1], 12045[1], 12046[1], 12047[1], 12051[1], 12052[1], 12053[1], 12054[1], 12055[1], 12056[1], 12057[1], 13100[1], 13101[1], 13102[1], 13120[1], 13121[1], 13122[1], 13131[1], 13132[1], 13133[1], 13151[1], 13152[1], 13153[1], 36000[1], 36400[1], 36405[1], 36406[1], 36410[1], 36420[1], 36425[1], 36430[1], 36440[1], 36591[0], 36592[0], 36600[1], 36640[1], 43752[1], 50715[1], 51701[0], 51702[0], 51703[1], 51725[0], 51726[0], 51727[0], 51728[0], 62320[0], 62321[0], 62322[0], 62323[0], 62324[0], 62325[0], 62326[0], 62327[0], 64400[0], 64405[0], 64408[0], 64415[0], 64416[0], 64417[0], 64418[0], 64420[0], 64421[0], 64425[0], 64430[0], 64435[0], 64445[0], 64446[0], 64447[0], 64448[0], 64449[0], 64450[0], 64451[0], 64454[0], 64461[0], 64462[0], 64463[0], 64479[0], 64480[0], 64483[0], 64484[0], 64486[0], 64487[0], 64488[0], 64489[0], 64490[0], 64491[0], 64492[0], 64493[0], 64494[0], 64495[0], 64505[0], 64510[0], 64517[0], 64520[0], 64530[0], 69990[0], 90901[1], 92012[1], 92014[1], 93000[1], 93005[1], 93010[1], 93040[1], 93041[1], 93042[1], 93318[1], 93355[1], 94002[1], 94200[1], 94680[1], 94681[1], 94690[1], 95812[1], 95813[1], 95816[1], 95819[1], 95822[1], 95829[1], 95955[1], 96360[1], 96361[1], 96365[1], 96366[1], 96367[1], 96368[1], 96372[1], 96374[1], 96375[1], 96376[1], 96377[1], 96523[0], 97597[1], 97598[1], 97602[1], 99155[0], 99156[0], 99157[0], 99211[1], 99212[1], 99213[1], 99214[1], 99215[1], 99217[1], 99218[1], 99219[1], 99220[1], 99221[1], 99222[1], 99223[1], 99231[1], 99232[1], 99233[1], 99234[1], 99235[1], 99236[1], 99238[1], 99239[1], 99241[1], 99242[1], 99243[1], 99244[1], 99245[1], 99251[1], 99252[1], 99253[1], 99254[1], 99255[1], 99291[1], 99292[1], 99304[1], 99305[1], 99306[1], 99307[1], 99308[1], 99309[1], 99310[1], 99315[1], 99316[1], 99334[1], 99335[1], 99336[1], 99337[1], 99347[1], 99348[1], 99349[1], 99350[1], 99374[1], 99375[1], 99377[1], 99378[1], 99446[0], 99447[0], 99448[0], 99449[0], 99451[0], 99452[0], 99495[1], 99496[1], G0463[1], G0471[0], J0670[1], J2001[1], P9612[0]
51736	00910[0], 0213T[0], 0216T[0], 0596T[0], 0597T[0], 0708T[1], 0709T[1], 36000[1], 36400[1], 36405[1], 36406[1], 36410[1], 36420[1], 36425[1], 36430[1], 36440[1], 36591[0], 36592[0], 36600[1], 36640[1], 43752[1], 50715[1], 51701[0], 51702[0], 51703[0], 61650[1], 62320[0], 62321[0], 62322[0], 62323[0], 62324[0], 62325[0], 62326[0], 62327[0], 64400[0], 64405[0], 64408[0], 64415[0], 64416[0], 64417[0], 64418[0], 64420[0], 64421[0], 64425[0], 64430[0], 64435[0], 64445[0], 64446[0], 64447[0], 64448[0], 64449[0], 64450[0], 64451[0], 64454[0], 64461[0], 64463[0], 64479[0], 64483[0], 64486[0], 64487[0], 64488[0], 64489[0], 64490[0], 64493[0], 64505[0], 64510[0], 64517[0], 64520[0], 64530[0], 69990[0], 93000[1], 93005[1], 93010[1], 93040[1], 93041[1], 93042[1], 93318[1], 93355[1], 94002[1], 94200[1], 94680[1], 94681[1], 94690[1], 95812[1], 95813[1], 95816[1], 95819[1], 95822[1], 95829[1], 95955[1], 96360[1], 96365[1], 96372[1], 96374[1], 96375[1], 96376[1], 96377[1], 96523[0], 99155[0], 99156[0], 99157[0], G0471[0], P9612[0]
51741	00910[0], 0213T[0], 0216T[0], 0596T[1], 0597T[1], 0708T[1], 0709T[1], 36000[1], 36400[1], 36405[1], 36406[1], 36410[1], 36420[1], 36425[1], 36430[1], 36440[1], 36591[0], 36592[0], 36600[1], 36640[1], 43752[1], 50715[1], 51701[0], 51702[1], 51703[1], 51736[0], 61650[1], 62320[0], 62321[0], 62322[0], 62323[0], 62324[0], 62325[0], 62326[0], 62327[0], 64400[0], 64405[0], 64408[0], 64415[0], 64416[0], 64417[0], 64418[0], 64420[0], 64421[0], 64425[0], 64430[0], 64435[0], 64445[0], 64446[0], 64447[0], 64448[0], 64449[0], 64450[0], 64451[0], 64454[0], 64461[0], 64463[0], 64479[0], 64483[0], 64486[0], 64487[0], 64488[0], 64489[0], 64490[0], 64493[0], 64505[0], 64510[0], 64517[0], 64520[0], 64530[0], 69990[0], 93000[1], 93005[1], 93010[1], 93040[1], 93041[1], 93042[1], 93318[1], 93355[1], 94002[1], 94200[1], 94680[1], 94681[1], 94690[1], 95812[1], 95813[1], 95816[1], 95819[1], 95822[1], 95829[1], 95955[1], 96360[1], 96365[1], 96372[1], 96374[1], 96375[1], 96376[1], 96377[1], 96523[0], 99155[0], 99156[0], 99157[0], G0471[1], P9612[0]
51784	00910[0], 0213T[0], 0216T[0], 0333T[1], 0464T[1], 0596T[1], 0597T[1], 0708T[1], 0709T[1], 12001[1], 12002[1], 12004[1], 12005[1], 12006[1], 12007[1], 12011[1], 12013[1], 12014[1], 12015[1], 12016[1], 12017[1], 12018[1], 12020[1], 12021[1], 12031[1], 12032[1], 12034[1], 12035[1], 12036[1], 12037[1], 12041[1], 12042[1], 12044[1], 12045[1], 12046[1], 12047[1], 12051[1], 12052[1], 12053[1], 12054[1], 12055[1], 12056[1], 12057[1], 13100[1], 13101[1], 13102[1], 13120[1], 13121[1], 13122[1], 13131[1], 13132[1], 13133[1], 13151[1], 13152[1], 13153[1], 36000[1], 36400[1], 36405[1], 36406[1], 36410[1], 36420[1], 36425[1], 36430[1], 36440[1], 36591[0], 36592[0], 36600[1], 36640[1], 43752[1], 50715[1], 51701[0], 51703[1], 51785[1], 62320[0], 62321[0], 62322[0], 62323[0], 62324[0], 62325[0], 62326[0], 62327[0], 64400[0], 64405[0], 64408[0], 64415[0], 64416[0], 64417[0], 64418[0], 64420[0], 64421[0], 64425[0], 64430[0], 64435[0], 64445[0], 64446[0], 64447[0], 64448[0], 64449[0], 64450[0], 64451[0], 64454[0], 64461[0], 64463[0], 64479[0], 64483[0], 64486[0], 64487[0], 64488[0], 64489[0], 64490[0], 64493[0], 64505[0], 64510[0], 64517[0], 64520[0], 64530[0], 69990[0], 92012[1], 92014[1], 92652[1], 92653[1], 93000[1], 93005[1], 93010[1], 93040[1], 93041[1], 93042[1], 93318[1], 93355[1], 94002[1], 94200[1], 94680[1], 94681[1], 94690[1], 95812[1], 95813[1], 95816[1], 95819[1], 95822[1], 95829[1], 95860[1], 95861[1], 95867[1], 95868[1], 95870[1], 95907[1], 95908[1], 95909[1], 95910[1], 95911[1], 95912[1], 95913[1], 95925[1], 95926[1], 95927[1], 95930[1], 95933[1], 95937[1], 95940[1], 95955[1], 96360[1], 96361[1], 96365[1], 96366[1], 96367[1], 96368[1], 96372[1], 96374[1], 96375[1], 96376[1], 96377[1], 96523[0], 99155[0], 99156[0], 99157[0], 99211[1], 99212[1], 99213[1], 99214[1], 99215[1], 99217[1], 99218[1], 99219[1], 99220[1], 99221[1], 99222[1], 99223[1], 99231[1], 99232[1], 99233[1], 99234[1], 99235[1], 99236[1], 99238[1], 99239[1], 99241[1], 99242[1], 99243[1], 99244[1], 99245[1], 99251[1], 99252[1], 99253[1], 99254[1], 99255[1], 99291[1], 99292[1], 99304[1], 99305[1], 99306[1], 99307[1], 99308[1], 99309[1], 99310[1], 99315[1], 99316[1], 99334[1], 99335[1], 99336[1], 99337[1], 99347[1], 99348[1], 99349[1], 99350[1], 99374[1], 99375[1], 99377[1], 99378[1], 99446[0], 99447[0], 99448[0], 99449[0], 99451[0], 99452[0], 99495[1], 99496[1], G0453[1], G0463[1]
51785	00910[0], 0213T[0], 0216T[0], 0333T[1], 0464T[1], 0596T[0], 0597T[0], 0708T[1], 0709T[1], 12001[1], 12002[1], 12004[1], 12005[1], 12006[1], 12007[1], 12011[1], 12013[1], 12014[1], 12015[1], 12016[1], 12017[1], 12018[1], 12020[1], 12021[1], 12031[1], 12032[1], 12034[1], 12035[1], 12036[1], 12037[1], 12041[1], 12042[1], 12044[1], 12045[1], 12046[1], 12047[1], 12051[1], 12052[1], 12053[1], 12054[1], 12055[1], 12056[1], 12057[1], 13100[1], 13101[1], 13102[1], 13120[1], 13121[1], 13122[1], 13131[1], 13132[1], 13133[1], 13151[1], 13152[1], 13153[1], 36000[1], 36400[1], 36405[1], 36406[1], 36410[1], 36420[1], 36425[1], 36430[1], 36440[1], 36591[0], 36592[0], 36600[1], 36640[1], 43752[1], 50715[1], 51701[0], 51702[0], 51703[0], 62320[0], 62321[0], 62322[0], 62323[0], 62324[0], 62325[0], 62326[0], 62327[0], 64400[0], 64405[0], 64408[0], 64415[0], 64416[0], 64417[0], 64418[0], 64420[0], 64421[0], 64425[0], 64430[0], 64435[0], 64445[0], 64446[0], 64447[0], 64448[0], 64449[0], 64450[0], 64451[0], 64454[0], 64461[0], 64463[0], 64479[0], 64483[0], 64486[0], 64487[0], 64488[0], 64489[0], 64490[0], 64493[0], 64505[0], 64510[0], 64517[0], 64520[0], 64530[0], 69990[0], 92012[1], 92014[1], 92652[1], 92653[1], 93000[1], 93005[1], 93010[1], 93040[1], 93041[1], 93042[1], 93318[1], 93355[1], 94002[1], 94200[1], 94680[1], 94681[1], 94690[1], 95812[1], 95813[1], 95816[1], 95819[1], 95822[1], 95829[1], 95860[1], 95861[1], 95867[1], 95868[1], 95870[1], 95907[1], 95908[1], 95909[1], 95910[1], 95911[1], 95912[1], 95913[1], 95925[1], 95926[1], 95927[1], 95930[1], 95933[1], 95937[1], 95940[1], 95955[1], 96360[1], 96361[1], 96365[1], 96366[1], 96367[1], 96368[1], 96372[1], 96374[1], 96375[1], 96376[1], 96377[1], 96523[0], 99155[0], 99156[0], 99157[0], 99211[1], 99212[1], 99213[1], 99214[1], 99215[1], 99217[1], 99218[1], 99219[1], 99220[1], 99221[1], 99222[1], 99223[1], 99231[1], 99232[1], 99233[1], 99234[1], 99235[1], 99236[1], 99238[1], 99239[1], 99241[1], 99242[1], 99243[1], 99244[1], 99245[1], 99251[1], 99252[1], 99253[1], 99254[1], 99255[1], 99291[1], 99292[1], 99304[1], 99305[1], 99306[1], 99307[1], 99308[1], 99309[1], 99310[1], 99315[1], 99316[1], 99334[1], 99335[1], 99336[1], 99337[1], 99347[1], 99348[1], 99349[1], 99350[1], 99374[1], 99375[1], 99377[1], 99378[1], 99446[0], 99447[0], 99448[0], 99449[0], 99451[0], 99452[0], 99495[1], 99496[1], G0453[1], G0463[1], G0471[0], P9612[0]
51792	00910[0], 0213T[0], 0216T[0], 0596T[0], 0597T[0], 0708T[1], 0709T[1], 12001[1], 12002[1], 12004[1], 12005[1], 12006[1], 12007[1], 12011[1], 12013[1], 12014[1], 12015[1], 12016[1], 12017[1], 12018[1], 12020[1], 12021[1], 12031[1], 12032[1], 12034[1], 12035[1], 12036[1], 12037[1], 12041[1], 12042[1], 12044[1], 12045[1], 12046[1], 12047[1], 12051[1], 12052[1], 12053[1], 12054[1], 12055[1], 12056[1], 12057[1], 13100[1], 13101[1], 13102[1], 13120[1], 13121[1], 13122[1], 13131[1], 13132[1], 13133[1], 13151[1], 13152[1], 13153[1], 36000[1], 36400[1], 36405[1], 36406[1], 36410[1], 36420[1], 36425[1],

0 = Modifier usage not allowed or inappropriate 1 = Modifier usage allowed

Code 1	Code 2
	36430[1], 36440[1], 36591[0], 36592[0], 36600[1], 36640[1], 43752[1], 50715[1], 51701[0], 51702[0], 51703[0], 51784[0], 62320[0], 62321[0], 62322[0], 62323[0], 62324[0], 62325[0], 62326[0], 62327[0], 64400[0], 64405[0], 64408[0], 64415[0], 64416[0], 64417[0], 64418[0], 64420[0], 64421[0], 64425[0], 64430[0], 64435[0], 64445[0], 64446[0], 64447[0], 64448[0], 64449[0], 64450[0], 64451[0], 64454[0], 64461[0], 64462[0], 64463[0], 64479[0], 64480[0], 64483[0], 64484[0], 64486[0], 64487[0], 64488[0], 64489[0], 64490[0], 64491[0], 64492[0], 64493[0], 64494[0], 64495[0], 64505[0], 64510[0], 64517[0], 64520[0], 64530[0], 69990[0], 92012[1], 92014[1], 93000[1], 93005[1], 93010[1], 93040[1], 93041[1], 93042[1], 93318[1], 93355[1], 94002[1], 94200[1], 94680[1], 94681[1], 94690[1], 95812[1], 95813[1], 95816[1], 95819[1], 95822[1], 95829[1], 95870[1], 95955[1], 96360[1], 96361[1], 96365[1], 96366[1], 96367[1], 96368[1], 96372[1], 96374[1], 96375[1], 96376[1], 96377[1], 96523[0], 99155[0], 99156[0], 99157[0], 99211[1], 99212[1], 99213[1], 99214[1], 99215[1], 99217[1], 99218[1], 99219[1], 99220[1], 99221[1], 99222[1], 99223[1], 99231[1], 99232[1], 99233[1], 99234[1], 99235[1], 99236[1], 99238[1], 99239[1], 99241[1], 99242[1], 99243[1], 99244[1], 99245[1], 99251[1], 99252[1], 99253[1], 99254[1], 99255[1], 99291[1], 99292[1], 99304[1], 99305[1], 99306[1], 99307[1], 99308[1], 99309[1], 99310[1], 99315[1], 99316[1], 99334[1], 99335[1], 99336[1], 99337[1], 99347[1], 99348[1], 99349[1], 99350[1], 99374[1], 99375[1], 99377[1], 99378[1], 99446[0], 99447[0], 99448[0], 99449[0], 99451[0], 99452[0], 99495[1], 99496[1], G0463[1], G0471[0], P9612[0]
51797	36591[0], 36592[0], 96523[0]
51798	0213T[1], 0216T[1], 36591[0], 36592[0], 61650[1], 62324[1], 62325[1], 62326[1], 62327[1], 64415[1], 64417[1], 64450[1], 64454[1], 64486[1], 64487[1], 64488[1], 64489[1], 64490[1], 64493[1], 69990[0], 96523[0], 99211[1]
51800	00910[0], 0213T[0], 0216T[0], 0596T[1], 0597T[1], 0708T[1], 0709T[1], 11000[1], 11001[1], 11004[1], 11005[1], 11006[1], 11042[1], 11043[1], 11044[1], 11045[1], 11046[1], 11047[1], 12001[1], 12002[1], 12004[1], 12005[1], 12006[1], 12007[1], 12011[1], 12013[1], 12014[1], 12015[1], 12016[1], 12017[1], 12018[1], 12020[1], 12021[1], 12031[1], 12032[1], 12034[1], 12035[1], 12036[1], 12037[1], 12041[1], 12042[1], 12044[1], 12045[1], 12046[1], 12047[1], 12051[1], 12052[1], 12053[1], 12054[1], 12055[1], 12056[1], 12057[1], 13100[1], 13101[1], 13102[1], 13120[1], 13121[1], 13122[1], 13131[1], 13132[1], 13133[1], 13151[1], 13152[1], 13153[1], 36000[1], 36400[1], 36405[1], 36406[1], 36410[1], 36420[1], 36425[1], 36430[1], 36440[1], 36591[0], 36592[0], 36600[1], 36640[1], 43752[1], 44602[1], 44603[1], 44604[1], 44605[1], 44950[0], 44970[0], 49000[0], 49002[1], 49320[1], 50605[1], 50715[1], 51550[1], 51701[0], 51702[0], 51703[1], 51860[1], 51865[1], 52000[0], 53000[0], 53010[0], 53020[0], 53025[0], 62320[0], 62321[0], 62322[0], 62323[0], 62324[0], 62325[0], 62326[0], 62327[0], 64400[0], 64405[0], 64408[0], 64415[0], 64416[0], 64417[0], 64418[0], 64420[0], 64421[0], 64425[0], 64430[0], 64435[0], 64445[0], 64446[0], 64447[0], 64448[0], 64449[0], 64450[0], 64451[0], 64454[0], 64461[0], 64462[0], 64463[0], 64479[0], 64480[0], 64483[0], 64484[0], 64486[0], 64487[0], 64488[0], 64489[0], 64490[0], 64491[0], 64492[0], 64493[0], 64494[0], 64495[0], 64505[0], 64510[0], 64517[0], 64520[0], 64530[0], 69990[0], 92012[1], 92014[1], 93000[1], 93005[1], 93010[1], 93040[1], 93041[1], 93042[1], 93318[1], 93355[1], 94002[1], 94200[1], 94680[1], 94681[1], 94690[1], 95812[1], 95813[1], 95816[1], 95819[1], 95822[1], 95829[1], 95955[1], 96360[1], 96361[1], 96365[1], 96366[1], 96367[1], 96368[1], 96372[1], 96374[1], 96375[1], 96376[1], 96377[1], 96523[0], 97597[1], 97598[1], 97602[1], 99155[0], 99156[0], 99157[0], 99211[1], 99212[1], 99213[1], 99214[1], 99215[1], 99217[1], 99218[1], 99219[1], 99220[1], 99221[1], 99222[1], 99223[1], 99231[1], 99232[1], 99233[1], 99234[1], 99235[1], 99236[1], 99238[1], 99239[1], 99241[1], 99242[1], 99243[1], 99244[1], 99245[1], 99251[1], 99252[1], 99253[1], 99254[1], 99255[1], 99291[1], 99292[1], 99304[1], 99305[1], 99306[1], 99307[1], 99308[1], 99309[1], 99310[1], 99315[1], 99316[1], 99334[1], 99335[1], 99336[1], 99337[1], 99347[1], 99348[1], 99349[1], 99350[1], 99374[1], 99375[1], 99377[1], 99378[1], 99446[0], 99447[0], 99448[0], 99449[0], 99451[0], 99452[0], 99495[0], 99496[0], G0463[1], G0471[0]
51820	00910[0], 0213T[0], 0216T[0], 0596T[1], 0597T[1], 0708T[1], 0709T[1], 11000[1], 11001[1], 11004[1], 11005[1], 11006[1], 11042[1], 11043[1], 11044[1], 11045[1], 11046[1], 11047[1], 12001[1], 12002[1], 12004[1], 12005[1], 12006[1], 12007[1], 12011[1], 12013[1], 12014[1], 12015[1], 12016[1], 12017[1], 12018[1], 12020[1], 12021[1], 12031[1], 12032[1], 12034[1], 12035[1], 12036[1], 12037[1], 12041[1], 12042[1], 12044[1], 12045[1], 12046[1], 12047[1], 12051[1], 12052[1], 12053[1], 12054[1], 12055[1], 12056[1], 12057[1], 13100[1], 13101[1], 13102[1], 13120[1], 13121[1], 13122[1], 13131[1], 13132[1], 13133[1], 13151[1], 13152[1], 13153[1], 36000[1], 36400[1], 36405[1], 36406[1], 36410[1], 36420[1], 36425[1], 36430[1], 36440[1], 36591[0], 36592[0], 36600[1], 36640[1], 43752[1], 44602[1], 44603[1], 44604[1], 44605[1], 44850[0], 44950[0], 44970[0], 49000[0], 49002[1], 49010[0], 49320[1], 50605[1], 50715[1], 50780[0], 51701[0], 51702[0], 51703[1], 51800[1], 51860[1], 51865[1], 52000[0], 53000[0], 53010[0], 53020[0], 53025[0], 62320[0], 62321[0], 62322[0], 62323[0], 62324[0], 62325[0], 62326[0], 62327[0], 64400[0], 64405[0], 64408[0], 64415[0], 64416[0], 64417[0], 64418[0], 64420[0], 64421[0], 64425[0], 64430[0], 64435[0], 64445[0], 64446[0], 64447[0], 64448[0], 64449[0], 64450[0], 64451[0], 64454[0], 64461[0], 64462[0], 64463[0], 64479[0], 64480[0], 64483[0], 64484[0], 64486[0], 64487[0], 64488[0], 64489[0], 64490[0], 64491[0], 64492[0], 64493[0], 64494[0], 64495[0], 64505[0], 64510[0], 64517[0], 64520[0], 64530[0], 69990[0], 92012[1], 92014[1], 93000[1], 93005[1], 93010[1], 93040[1], 93041[1], 93042[1], 93318[1], 93355[1], 94002[1], 94200[1], 94680[1], 94681[1], 94690[1], 95812[1], 95813[1], 95816[1], 95819[1], 95822[1], 95829[1], 95955[1], 96360[1], 96361[1], 96365[1], 96366[1], 96367[1], 96368[1], 96372[1], 96374[1], 96375[1], 96376[1], 96377[1], 96523[0], 97597[1], 97598[1], 97602[1], 99155[0], 99156[0], 99157[0], 99211[1], 99212[1], 99213[1], 99214[1], 99215[1], 99217[1], 99218[1], 99219[1], 99220[1], 99221[1], 99222[1], 99223[1], 99231[1], 99232[1], 99233[1], 99234[1], 99235[1], 99236[1], 99238[1], 99239[1], 99241[1], 99242[1], 99243[1], 99244[1], 99245[1], 99251[1], 99252[1], 99253[1], 99254[1], 99255[1], 99291[1], 99292[1], 99304[1], 99305[1], 99306[1], 99307[1], 99308[1], 99309[1], 99310[1], 99315[1], 99316[1], 99334[1], 99335[1], 99336[1], 99337[1], 99347[1], 99348[1], 99349[1], 99350[1], 99374[1], 99375[1], 99377[1], 99378[1], 99446[0], 99447[0], 99448[0], 99449[0], 99451[0], 99452[0], 99495[0], 99496[0], G0463[1], G0471[0]
51840	00910[0], 0213T[0], 0216T[0], 0596T[1], 0597T[1], 0708T[1], 0709T[1], 12001[1], 12002[1], 12004[1], 12005[1], 12006[1], 12007[1], 12011[1], 12013[1], 12014[1], 12015[1], 12016[1], 12017[1], 12018[1], 12020[1], 12021[1], 12031[1], 12032[1], 12034[1], 12035[1], 12036[1], 12037[1], 12041[1], 12042[1], 12044[1], 12045[1], 12046[1], 12047[1], 12051[1], 12052[1], 12053[1], 12054[1], 12055[1], 12056[1], 12057[1], 13100[1], 13101[1], 13102[1], 13120[1], 13121[1], 13122[1], 13131[1], 13132[1], 13133[1], 13151[1], 13152[1], 13153[1], 36000[1], 36400[1], 36405[1], 36406[1], 36410[1], 36420[1], 36425[1], 36430[1], 36440[1], 36591[0], 36592[0], 36600[1], 36640[1], 43752[1], 44602[1], 44603[1], 44604[1], 44605[1], 44950[0], 44970[0], 49000[0], 49002[1], 49320[1], 50715[1], 51040[1], 51595[1], 51701[0], 51702[0], 51703[1], 52000[0], 52001[1], 52005[1], 53000[0], 53010[0], 53020[0], 53025[0], 53660[1], 53661[1], 62320[0], 62321[0], 62322[0], 62323[0], 62324[0], 62325[0], 62326[0], 62327[0], 64400[0], 64405[0], 64408[0], 64415[0], 64416[0], 64417[0], 64418[0], 64420[0], 64421[0], 64425[0], 64430[0], 64435[0], 64445[0], 64446[0], 64447[0], 64448[0], 64449[0], 64450[0], 64451[0], 64454[0], 64461[0], 64462[0], 64463[0], 64479[0], 64480[0], 64483[0], 64484[0], 64486[0], 64487[0], 64488[0], 64489[0], 64490[0], 64491[0], 64492[0], 64493[0], 64494[0], 64495[0], 64505[0], 64510[0], 64517[0], 64520[0], 64530[0], 69990[0], 92012[1], 92014[1], 93000[1], 93005[1], 93010[1], 93040[1], 93041[1], 93042[1], 93318[1], 93355[1], 94002[1], 94200[1], 94680[1], 94681[1], 94690[1], 95812[1], 95813[1], 95816[1], 95819[1], 95822[1], 95829[1], 95955[1], 96360[1], 96361[1], 96365[1], 96366[1], 96367[1], 96368[1], 96372[1], 96374[1], 96375[1], 96376[1], 96377[1], 96523[0], 99155[0], 99156[0], 99157[0], 99211[1], 99212[1], 99213[1], 99214[1], 99215[1], 99217[1], 99218[1], 99219[1], 99220[1], 99221[1], 99222[1], 99223[1], 99231[1], 99232[1], 99233[1], 99234[1], 99235[1], 99236[1], 99238[1], 99239[1], 99241[1], 99242[1], 99243[1], 99244[1], 99245[1], 99251[1], 99252[1], 99253[1], 99254[1], 99255[1], 99291[1], 99292[1], 99304[1], 99305[1], 99306[1], 99307[1], 99308[1], 99309[1], 99310[1], 99315[1], 99316[1], 99334[1], 99335[1], 99336[1], 99337[1], 99347[1], 99348[1], 99349[1], 99350[1], 99374[1], 99375[1], 99377[1], 99378[1], 99446[0], 99447[0], 99448[0], 99449[0], 99451[0], 99452[0], 99495[0], 99496[0], G0463[1], G0471[0]
51841	00910[0], 0213T[0], 0216T[0], 0596T[1], 0597T[1], 0708T[1], 0709T[1], 12001[1], 12002[1], 12004[1], 12005[1], 12006[1], 12007[1], 12011[1], 12013[1], 12014[1], 12015[1], 12016[1], 12017[1], 12018[1], 12020[1], 12021[1], 12031[1], 12032[1], 12034[1], 12035[1], 12036[1], 12037[1], 12041[1], 12042[1], 12044[1], 12045[1], 12046[1], 12047[1], 12051[1], 12052[1], 12053[1], 12054[1], 12055[1], 12056[1], 12057[1], 13100[1], 13101[1], 13102[1], 13120[1], 13121[1], 13122[1], 13131[1], 13132[1], 13133[1], 13151[1], 13152[1], 13153[1], 36000[1], 36400[1], 36405[1], 36406[1], 36410[1], 36420[1], 36425[1], 36430[1], 36440[1], 36591[0], 36592[0], 36600[1], 36640[1], 43752[1], 44602[1], 44603[1], 44604[1], 44605[1], 44950[0], 44970[0], 49000[0], 49002[1], 49320[1], 50715[1], 51595[1], 51701[0], 51702[0], 51703[1], 51840[1], 52000[0], 52001[1], 53000[0], 53010[0], 53020[0], 53025[0], 57285[1], 62320[0], 62321[0], 62322[0], 62323[0], 62324[0], 62325[0], 62326[0], 62327[0], 64400[0], 64405[0], 64408[0], 64415[0], 64416[0], 64417[0], 64418[0], 64420[0], 64421[0], 64425[0], 64430[0], 64435[0], 64445[0], 64446[0], 64447[0], 64448[0], 64449[0], 64450[0], 64451[0], 64454[0], 64461[0], 64462[0], 64463[0], 64479[0], 64480[0], 64483[0], 64484[0], 64486[0], 64487[0], 64488[0], 64489[0], 64490[0], 64491[0], 64492[0], 64493[0], 64494[0], 64495[0], 64505[0], 64510[0], 64517[0], 64520[0], 64530[0], 69990[0], 92012[1], 92014[1], 93000[1], 93005[1], 93010[1], 93040[1], 93041[1], 93042[1], 93318[1], 93355[1], 94002[1], 94200[1], 94680[1], 94681[1], 94690[1], 95812[1], 95813[1], 95816[1], 95819[1], 95822[1], 95829[1], 95955[1], 96360[1], 96361[1], 96365[1], 96366[1], 96367[1], 96368[1], 96372[1], 96374[1], 96375[1], 96376[1], 96377[1], 96523[0], 99155[0], 99156[0], 99157[0], 99211[1], 99212[1], 99213[1], 99214[1], 99215[1], 99217[1], 99218[1], 99219[1], 99220[1], 99221[1], 99222[1], 99223[1], 99231[1], 99232[1], 99233[1], 99234[1], 99235[1], 99236[1], 99238[1], 99239[1], 99241[1], 99242[1], 99243[1], 99244[1], 99245[1], 99251[1], 99252[1], 99253[1], 99254[1], 99255[1], 99291[1], 99292[1], 99304[1], 99305[1], 99306[1], 99307[1], 99308[1], 99309[1], 99310[1], 99315[1], 99316[1], 99334[1], 99335[1], 99336[1], 99337[1], 99347[1], 99348[1], 99349[1], 99350[1], 99374[1], 99375[1], 99377[1], 99378[1], 99446[0], 99447[0], 99448[0], 99449[0], 99451[0], 99452[0], 99495[0], 99496[0], G0463[1], G0471[0]
51860	00910[0], 0213T[0], 0216T[0], 0596T[1], 0597T[1], 0708T[1], 0709T[1], 12001[1], 12002[1], 12004[1], 12005[1], 12006[1], 12007[1], 12011[1], 12013[1], 12014[1], 12015[1], 12016[1], 12017[1], 12018[1], 12020[1], 12021[1], 12031[1], 12032[1], 12034[1], 12035[1], 12036[1], 12037[1], 12041[1], 12042[1], 12044[1], 12045[1], 12046[1], 12047[1], 12051[1], 12052[1], 12053[1], 12054[1], 12055[1], 12056[1], 12057[1], 13100[1], 13101[1], 13102[1], 13120[1], 13121[1], 13122[1], 13131[1], 13132[1], 13133[1], 13151[1], 13152[1], 13153[1], 36000[1], 36400[1], 36405[1], 36406[1], 36410[1], 36420[1], 36425[1], 36430[1], 36440[1], 36591[0], 36592[0], 36600[1], 36640[1], 43752[1], 44602[1], 44603[1], 44604[1], 44605[1], 44850[0], 44950[0], 44970[0], 49000[0], 49002[1], 49010[0], 49255[0], 49320[1], 50715[1],

Code 1	Code 2
	51701[0], 51702[0], 51703[1], 52000[1], 62320[0], 62321[0], 62322[0], 62323[0], 62324[0], 62325[0], 62326[0], 62327[0], 64400[0], 64405[0], 64408[0], 64415[0], 64416[0], 64417[0], 64418[0], 64420[0], 64421[0], 64425[0], 64430[0], 64435[0], 64445[0], 64446[0], 64447[0], 64448[0], 64449[0], 64450[0], 64451[0], 64454[0], 64461[0], 64462[0], 64463[0], 64479[0], 64480[0], 64483[0], 64484[0], 64486[0], 64487[0], 64488[0], 64489[0], 64490[0], 64491[0], 64492[0], 64493[0], 64494[0], 64495[0], 64505[0], 64510[0], 64517[0], 64520[0], 64530[0], 69990[0], 92012[1], 92014[1], 93000[1], 93005[1], 93010[1], 93040[1], 93041[1], 93042[1], 93318[1], 93355[1], 94002[1], 94200[1], 94680[1], 94681[1], 94690[1], 95812[1], 95813[1], 95816[1], 95819[1], 95822[1], 95829[1], 95955[1], 96360[1], 96361[1], 96365[1], 96366[1], 96367[1], 96368[1], 96372[1], 96374[1], 96375[1], 96376[1], 96377[1], 96523[0], 99155[0], 99156[0], 99157[0], 99211[1], 99212[1], 99213[1], 99214[1], 99215[1], 99217[1], 99218[1], 99219[1], 99220[1], 99221[1], 99222[1], 99223[1], 99231[1], 99232[1], 99233[1], 99234[1], 99235[1], 99236[1], 99238[1], 99239[1], 99241[1], 99242[1], 99243[1], 99244[1], 99245[1], 99251[1], 99252[1], 99253[1], 99254[1], 99255[1], 99291[1], 99292[1], 99304[1], 99305[1], 99306[1], 99307[1], 99308[1], 99309[1], 99310[1], 99315[1], 99316[1], 99334[1], 99335[1], 99336[1], 99337[1], 99347[1], 99348[1], 99349[1], 99350[1], 99374[1], 99375[1], 99377[1], 99378[1], 99446[0], 99447[0], 99448[0], 99449[0], 99451[0], 99452[0], 99495[0], 99496[0], G0463[1], G0471[0]
51865	00910[0], 0213T[0], 0216T[0], 0596T[1], 0597T[1], 0708T[1], 0709T[1], 12001[1], 12002[1], 12004[1], 12005[1], 12006[1], 12007[1], 12011[1], 12013[1], 12014[1], 12015[1], 12016[1], 12017[1], 12018[1], 12020[1], 12021[1], 12031[1], 12032[1], 12034[1], 12035[1], 12036[1], 12037[1], 12041[1], 12042[1], 12044[1], 12045[1], 12046[1], 12047[1], 12051[1], 12052[1], 12053[1], 12054[1], 12055[1], 12056[1], 12057[1], 13100[1], 13101[1], 13102[1], 13120[1], 13121[1], 13122[1], 13131[1], 13132[1], 13133[1], 13151[1], 13152[1], 13153[1], 36000[1], 36400[1], 36405[1], 36406[1], 36410[1], 36420[1], 36425[1], 36430[1], 36440[1], 36591[0], 36592[0], 36600[1], 36640[1], 43752[1], 44005[0], 44180[0], 44602[1], 44603[1], 44604[1], 44605[1], 44850[0], 44950[0], 44970[0], 49000[0], 49002[1], 49010[0], 49255[0], 49320[1], 50715[1], 51040[1], 51701[0], 51702[0], 51703[1], 51860[1], 52000[1], 62320[0], 62321[0], 62322[0], 62323[0], 62324[0], 62325[0], 62326[0], 62327[0], 64400[0], 64405[0], 64408[0], 64415[0], 64416[0], 64417[0], 64418[0], 64420[0], 64421[0], 64425[0], 64430[0], 64435[0], 64445[0], 64446[0], 64447[0], 64448[0], 64449[0], 64450[0], 64451[0], 64454[0], 64461[0], 64462[0], 64463[0], 64479[0], 64480[0], 64483[0], 64484[0], 64486[0], 64487[0], 64488[0], 64489[0], 64490[0], 64491[0], 64492[0], 64493[0], 64494[0], 64495[0], 64505[0], 64510[0], 64517[0], 64520[0], 64530[0], 69990[0], 92012[1], 92014[1], 93000[1], 93005[1], 93010[1], 93040[1], 93041[1], 93042[1], 93318[1], 93355[1], 94002[1], 94200[1], 94680[1], 94681[1], 94690[1], 95812[1], 95813[1], 95816[1], 95819[1], 95822[1], 95829[1], 95955[1], 96360[1], 96361[1], 96365[1], 96366[1], 96367[1], 96368[1], 96372[1], 96374[1], 96375[1], 96376[1], 96377[1], 96523[0], 99155[0], 99156[0], 99157[0], 99211[1], 99212[1], 99213[1], 99214[1], 99215[1], 99217[1], 99218[1], 99219[1], 99220[1], 99221[1], 99222[1], 99223[1], 99231[1], 99232[1], 99233[1], 99234[1], 99235[1], 99236[1], 99238[1], 99239[1], 99241[1], 99242[1], 99243[1], 99244[1], 99245[1], 99251[1], 99252[1], 99253[1], 99254[1], 99255[1], 99291[1], 99292[1], 99304[1], 99305[1], 99306[1], 99307[1], 99308[1], 99309[1], 99310[1], 99315[1], 99316[1], 99334[1], 99335[1], 99336[1], 99337[1], 99347[1], 99348[1], 99349[1], 99350[1], 99374[1], 99375[1], 99377[1], 99378[1], 99446[0], 99447[0], 99448[0], 99449[0], 99451[0], 99452[0], 99495[0], 99496[0], G0463[1], G0471[0]
51880	00910[0], 0213T[0], 0216T[0], 0596T[1], 0597T[1], 0708T[1], 0709T[1], 11000[1], 11001[1], 11004[1], 11005[1], 11006[1], 11042[1], 11043[1], 11044[1], 11045[1], 11046[1], 11047[1], 12001[1], 12002[1], 12004[1], 12005[1], 12006[1], 12007[1], 12011[1], 12013[1], 12014[1], 12015[1], 12016[1], 12017[1], 12018[1], 12020[1], 12021[1], 12031[1], 12032[1], 12034[1], 12035[1], 12036[1], 12037[1], 12041[1], 12042[1], 12044[1], 12045[1], 12046[1], 12047[1], 12051[1], 12052[1], 12053[1], 12054[1], 12055[1], 12056[1], 12057[1], 13100[1], 13101[1], 13102[1], 13120[1], 13121[1], 13122[1], 13131[1], 13132[1], 13133[1], 13151[1], 13152[1], 13153[1], 36000[1], 36400[1], 36405[1], 36406[1], 36410[1], 36420[1], 36425[1], 36430[1], 36440[1], 36591[0], 36592[0], 36600[1], 36640[1], 43752[1], 44950[0], 44970[0], 50715[1], 51701[0], 51702[0], 51703[1], 52000[1], 62320[0], 62321[0], 62322[0], 62323[0], 62324[0], 62325[0], 62326[0], 62327[0], 64400[0], 64405[0], 64408[0], 64415[0], 64416[0], 64417[0], 64418[0], 64420[0], 64421[0], 64425[0], 64430[0], 64435[0], 64445[0], 64446[0], 64447[0], 64448[0], 64449[0], 64450[0], 64451[0], 64454[0], 64461[0], 64462[0], 64463[0], 64479[0], 64480[0], 64483[0], 64484[0], 64486[0], 64487[0], 64488[0], 64489[0], 64490[0], 64491[0], 64492[0], 64493[0], 64494[0], 64495[0], 64505[0], 64510[0], 64517[0], 64520[0], 64530[0], 69990[0], 92012[1], 92014[1], 93000[1], 93005[1], 93010[1], 93040[1], 93041[1], 93042[1], 93318[1], 93355[1], 94002[1], 94200[1], 94680[1], 94681[1], 94690[1], 95812[1], 95813[1], 95816[1], 95819[1], 95822[1], 95829[1], 95955[1], 96360[1], 96361[1], 96365[1], 96366[1], 96367[1], 96368[1], 96372[1], 96374[1], 96375[1], 96376[1], 96377[1], 96523[0], 97597[1], 97598[1], 97602[1], 99155[0], 99156[0], 99157[0], 99211[1], 99212[1], 99213[1], 99214[1], 99215[1], 99217[1], 99218[1], 99219[1], 99220[1], 99221[1], 99222[1], 99223[1], 99231[1], 99232[1], 99233[1], 99234[1], 99235[1], 99236[1], 99238[1], 99239[1], 99241[1], 99242[1], 99243[1], 99244[1], 99245[1], 99251[1], 99252[1], 99253[1], 99254[1], 99255[1], 99291[1], 99292[1], 99304[1], 99305[1], 99306[1], 99307[1], 99308[1], 99309[1], 99310[1], 99315[1], 99316[1], 99334[1], 99335[1], 99336[1], 99337[1], 99347[1], 99348[1], 99349[1], 99350[1], 99374[1], 99375[1], 99377[1], 99378[1], 99446[0], 99447[0], 99448[0], 99449[0], 99451[0], 99452[0], 99495[0], 99496[0], G0463[1], G0471[0]
51900	00910[0], 0213T[0], 0216T[0], 0596T[1], 0597T[1], 0708T[1], 0709T[1], 11000[1], 11001[1], 11004[1], 11005[1], 11006[1], 11042[1], 11043[1], 11044[1], 11045[1], 11046[1], 11047[1], 12001[1], 12002[1], 12004[1], 12005[1], 12006[1], 12007[1], 12011[1], 12013[1], 12014[1], 12015[1], 12016[1], 12017[1], 12018[1], 12020[1], 12021[1], 12031[1], 12032[1], 12034[1], 12035[1], 12036[1], 12037[1], 12041[1], 12042[1], 12044[1], 12045[1], 12046[1], 12047[1], 12051[1], 12052[1], 12053[1], 12054[1], 12055[1], 12056[1], 12057[1], 13100[1], 13101[1], 13102[1], 13120[1], 13121[1], 13122[1], 13131[1], 13132[1], 13133[1], 13151[1], 13152[1], 13153[1], 36000[1], 36400[1], 36405[1], 36406[1], 36410[1], 36420[1], 36425[1], 36430[1], 36440[1], 36591[0], 36592[0], 36600[1], 36640[1], 43752[1], 44602[1], 44603[1], 44604[1], 44605[1], 44850[0], 44950[0], 44970[0], 49000[0], 49002[1], 49010[0], 49255[0], 49320[1], 50715[1], 51701[0], 51702[0], 51703[1], 51860[1], 51865[1], 51880[0], 52000[0], 62320[0], 62321[0], 62322[0], 62323[0], 62324[0], 62325[0], 62326[0], 62327[0], 64400[0], 64405[0], 64408[0], 64415[0], 64416[0], 64417[0], 64418[0], 64420[0], 64421[0], 64425[0], 64430[0], 64435[0], 64445[0], 64446[0], 64447[0], 64448[0], 64449[0], 64450[0], 64451[0], 64454[0], 64461[0], 64462[0], 64463[0], 64479[0], 64480[0], 64483[0], 64484[0], 64486[0], 64487[0], 64488[0], 64489[0], 64490[0], 64491[0], 64492[0], 64493[0], 64494[0], 64495[0], 64505[0], 64510[0], 64517[0], 64520[0], 64530[0], 69990[0], 92012[1], 92014[1], 93000[1], 93005[1], 93010[1], 93040[1], 93041[1], 93042[1], 93318[1], 93355[1], 94002[1], 94200[1], 94680[1], 94681[1], 94690[1], 95812[1], 95813[1], 95816[1], 95819[1], 95822[1], 95829[1], 95955[1], 96360[1], 96361[1], 96365[1], 96366[1], 96367[1], 96368[1], 96372[1], 96374[1], 96375[1], 96376[1], 96377[1], 96523[0], 97597[1], 97598[1], 97602[1], 99155[0], 99156[0], 99157[0], 99211[1], 99212[1], 99213[1], 99214[1], 99215[1], 99217[1], 99218[1], 99219[1], 99220[1], 99221[1], 99222[1], 99223[1], 99231[1], 99232[1], 99233[1], 99234[1], 99235[1], 99236[1], 99238[1], 99239[1], 99241[1], 99242[1], 99243[1], 99244[1], 99245[1], 99251[1], 99252[1], 99253[1], 99254[1], 99255[1], 99291[1], 99292[1], 99304[1], 99305[1], 99306[1], 99307[1], 99308[1], 99309[1], 99310[1], 99315[1], 99316[1], 99334[1], 99335[1], 99336[1], 99337[1], 99347[1], 99348[1], 99349[1], 99350[1], 99374[1], 99375[1], 99377[1], 99378[1], 99446[0], 99447[0], 99448[0], 99449[0], 99451[0], 99452[0], 99495[0], 99496[0], G0463[1], G0471[0]
51920	00910[0], 0213T[0], 0216T[0], 0596T[1], 0597T[1], 0708T[1], 0709T[1], 11000[1], 11001[1], 11004[1], 11005[1], 11006[1], 11042[1], 11043[1], 11044[1], 11045[1], 11046[1], 11047[1], 12001[1], 12002[1], 12004[1], 12005[1], 12006[1], 12007[1], 12011[1], 12013[1], 12014[1], 12015[1], 12016[1], 12017[1], 12018[1], 12020[1], 12021[1], 12031[1], 12032[1], 12034[1], 12035[1], 12036[1], 12037[1], 12041[1], 12042[1], 12044[1], 12045[1], 12046[1], 12047[1], 12051[1], 12052[1], 12053[1], 12054[1], 12055[1], 12056[1], 12057[1], 13100[1], 13101[1], 13102[1], 13120[1], 13121[1], 13122[1], 13131[1], 13132[1], 13133[1], 13151[1], 13152[1], 13153[1], 36000[1], 36400[1], 36405[1], 36406[1], 36410[1], 36420[1], 36425[1], 36430[1], 36440[1], 36591[0], 36592[0], 36600[1], 36640[1], 43752[1], 44602[1], 44603[1], 44604[1], 44605[1], 44850[0], 44950[0], 44970[0], 49000[0], 49002[1], 49010[0], 49255[0], 49320[1], 50715[1], 51701[0], 51702[0], 51703[1], 51860[1], 51865[1], 51880[0], 52000[0], 62320[0], 62321[0], 62322[0], 62323[0], 62324[0], 62325[0], 62326[0], 62327[0], 64400[0], 64405[0], 64408[0], 64415[0], 64416[0], 64417[0], 64418[0], 64420[0], 64421[0], 64425[0], 64430[0], 64435[0], 64445[0], 64446[0], 64447[0], 64448[0], 64449[0], 64450[0], 64451[0], 64454[0], 64461[0], 64462[0], 64463[0], 64479[0], 64480[0], 64483[0], 64484[0], 64486[0], 64487[0], 64488[0], 64489[0], 64490[0], 64491[0], 64492[0], 64493[0], 64494[0], 64495[0], 64505[0], 64510[0], 64517[0], 64520[0], 64530[0], 69990[0], 92012[1], 92014[1], 93000[1], 93005[1], 93010[1], 93040[1], 93041[1], 93042[1], 93318[1], 93355[1], 94002[1], 94200[1], 94680[1], 94681[1], 94690[1], 95812[1], 95813[1], 95816[1], 95819[1], 95822[1], 95829[1], 95955[1], 96360[1], 96361[1], 96365[1], 96366[1], 96367[1], 96368[1], 96372[1], 96374[1], 96375[1], 96376[1], 96377[1], 96523[0], 97597[1], 97598[1], 97602[1], 99155[0], 99156[0], 99157[0], 99211[1], 99212[1], 99213[1], 99214[1], 99215[1], 99217[1], 99218[1], 99219[1], 99220[1], 99221[1], 99222[1], 99223[1], 99231[1], 99232[1], 99233[1], 99234[1], 99235[1], 99236[1], 99238[1], 99239[1], 99241[1], 99242[1], 99243[1], 99244[1], 99245[1], 99251[1], 99252[1], 99253[1], 99254[1], 99255[1], 99291[1], 99292[1], 99304[1], 99305[1], 99306[1], 99307[1], 99308[1], 99309[1], 99310[1], 99315[1], 99316[1], 99334[1], 99335[1], 99336[1], 99337[1], 99347[1], 99348[1], 99349[1], 99350[1], 99374[1], 99375[1], 99377[1], 99378[1], 99446[0], 99447[0], 99448[0], 99449[0], 99451[0], 99452[0], 99495[0], 99496[0], G0463[1], G0471[0]
51925	00910[0], 0213T[0], 0216T[0], 0596T[1], 0597T[1], 0664T[1], 0665T[1], 0667T[1], 0708T[1], 0709T[1], 11000[1], 11001[1], 11004[1], 11005[1], 11006[1], 11042[1], 11043[1], 11044[1], 11045[1], 11046[1], 11047[1], 12001[1], 12002[1], 12004[1], 12005[1], 12006[1], 12007[1], 12011[1], 12013[1], 12014[1], 12015[1], 12016[1], 12017[1], 12018[1], 12020[1], 12021[1], 12031[1], 12032[1], 12034[1], 12035[1], 12036[1], 12037[1], 12041[1], 12042[1], 12044[1], 12045[1], 12046[1], 12047[1], 12051[1], 12052[1], 12053[1], 12054[1], 12055[1], 12056[1], 12057[1], 13100[1], 13101[1], 13102[1], 13120[1], 13121[1], 13122[1], 13131[1], 13132[1], 13133[1], 13151[1], 13152[1], 13153[1], 36000[1], 36400[1], 36405[1], 36406[1], 36410[1], 36420[1], 36425[1], 36430[1], 36440[1], 36591[0], 36592[0], 36600[1], 36640[1], 43752[1], 44005[0], 44180[0], 44602[1], 44603[1], 44604[1], 44605[1], 44850[0], 44950[0], 44970[0], 49000[0], 49002[1], 49010[0], 49255[0], 49320[1], 49321[1], 50715[1], 51701[0], 51702[0], 51703[1], 51860[1], 51865[1], 51880[0], 51920[1], 52000[0], 57505[0], 57530[0], 57550[0], 57555[0], 57558[0], 58120[0], 58140[0], 58146[0], 58150[1], 58152[1], 58180[1], 58260[1], 58262[1], 58263[1], 58267[1], 58270[1], 58275[1], 58280[1], 58290[1], 58291[1], 58292[1], 58294[1], 58545[0], 58546[0], 58561[0], 62320[0], 62321[0], 62322[0], 62323[0], 62324[0], 62325[0], 62326[0], 62327[0], 64400[0], 64405[0],

0 = Modifier usage not allowed or inappropriate 1 = Modifier usage allowed

Code 1	Code 2
	64408[0], 64415[0], 64416[0], 64417[0], 64418[0], 64420[0], 64421[0], 64425[0], 64430[0], 64435[0], 64445[0], 64446[0], 64447[0], 64448[0], 64449[0], 64450[0], 64451[0], 64454[0], 64461[0], 64462[0], 64463[0], 64479[0], 64480[0], 64483[0], 64484[0], 64486[0], 64487[0], 64488[0], 64489[0], 64490[0], 64491[0], 64492[0], 64493[0], 64494[0], 64495[0], 64505[0], 64510[0], 64517[0], 64520[0], 64530[0], 69990[0], 92012[1], 92014[1], 93000[1], 93005[1], 93010[1], 93040[1], 93041[1], 93042[1], 93318[1], 93355[1], 94002[1], 94200[1], 94680[1], 94681[1], 94690[1], 95812[1], 95813[1], 95816[1], 95819[1], 95822[1], 95829[1], 95955[1], 96360[1], 96361[1], 96365[1], 96366[1], 96367[1], 96368[1], 96372[1], 96374[1], 96375[1], 96376[1], 96377[1], 96523[0], 97597[1], 97598[1], 97602[1], 99155[0], 99156[0], 99157[0], 99211[1], 99212[1], 99213[1], 99214[1], 99215[1], 99217[1], 99218[1], 99219[1], 99220[1], 99221[1], 99222[1], 99223[1], 99231[1], 99232[1], 99233[1], 99234[1], 99235[1], 99236[1], 99238[1], 99239[1], 99241[1], 99242[1], 99243[1], 99244[1], 99245[1], 99251[1], 99252[1], 99253[1], 99254[1], 99255[1], 99291[1], 99292[1], 99304[1], 99305[1], 99306[1], 99307[1], 99308[1], 99309[1], 99310[1], 99315[1], 99316[1], 99334[1], 99335[1], 99336[1], 99337[1], 99347[1], 99348[1], 99349[1], 99350[1], 99374[1], 99375[1], 99377[1], 99378[1], 99446[0], 99447[0], 99448[0], 99449[0], 99451[0], 99452[0], 99495[0], 99496[0], G0463[1], G0471[0]
51940	00910[0], 0213T[0], 0216T[0], 0596T[1], 0597T[1], 0708T[1], 0709T[1], 11000[1], 11001[1], 11004[1], 11005[1], 11006[1], 11042[1], 11043[1], 11044[1], 11045[1], 11046[1], 11047[1], 12001[1], 12002[1], 12004[1], 12005[1], 12006[1], 12007[1], 12011[1], 12013[1], 12014[1], 12015[1], 12016[1], 12017[1], 12018[1], 12020[1], 12021[1], 12031[1], 12032[1], 12034[1], 12035[1], 12036[1], 12037[1], 12041[1], 12042[1], 12044[1], 12045[1], 12046[1], 12047[1], 12051[1], 12052[1], 12053[1], 12054[1], 12055[1], 12056[1], 12057[1], 13100[1], 13101[1], 13102[1], 13120[1], 13121[1], 13122[1], 13131[1], 13132[1], 13133[1], 13151[1], 13152[1], 13153[1], 36000[1], 36400[1], 36405[1], 36406[1], 36410[1], 36420[1], 36425[1], 36430[1], 36440[1], 36591[0], 36592[0], 36600[1], 36640[1], 43752[1], 44602[1], 44603[1], 44604[1], 44605[1], 44850[0], 44950[0], 44970[0], 49000[0], 49002[1], 49010[0], 49255[0], 50715[1], 51701[0], 51702[0], 51703[1], 51880[0], 52000[0], 62320[0], 62321[0], 62322[0], 62323[0], 62324[0], 62325[0], 62326[0], 62327[0], 64400[0], 64405[0], 64408[0], 64415[0], 64416[0], 64417[0], 64418[0], 64420[0], 64421[0], 64425[0], 64430[0], 64435[0], 64445[0], 64446[0], 64447[0], 64448[0], 64449[0], 64450[0], 64451[0], 64454[0], 64461[0], 64462[0], 64463[0], 64479[0], 64480[0], 64483[0], 64484[0], 64486[0], 64487[0], 64488[0], 64489[0], 64490[0], 64491[0], 64492[0], 64493[0], 64494[0], 64495[0], 64505[0], 64510[0], 64517[0], 64520[0], 64530[0], 69990[0], 92012[1], 92014[1], 93000[1], 93005[1], 93010[1], 93040[1], 93041[1], 93042[1], 93318[1], 93355[1], 94002[1], 94200[1], 94680[1], 94681[1], 94690[1], 95812[1], 95813[1], 95816[1], 95819[1], 95822[1], 95829[1], 95955[1], 96360[1], 96361[1], 96365[1], 96366[1], 96367[1], 96368[1], 96372[1], 96374[1], 96375[1], 96376[1], 96377[1], 96523[0], 97597[1], 97598[1], 97602[1], 99155[0], 99156[0], 99157[0], 99211[1], 99212[1], 99213[1], 99214[1], 99215[1], 99217[1], 99218[1], 99219[1], 99220[1], 99221[1], 99222[1], 99223[1], 99231[1], 99232[1], 99233[1], 99234[1], 99235[1], 99236[1], 99238[1], 99239[1], 99241[1], 99242[1], 99243[1], 99244[1], 99245[1], 99251[1], 99252[1], 99253[1], 99254[1], 99255[1], 99291[1], 99292[1], 99304[1], 99305[1], 99306[1], 99307[1], 99308[1], 99309[1], 99310[1], 99315[1], 99316[1], 99334[1], 99335[1], 99336[1], 99337[1], 99347[1], 99348[1], 99349[1], 99350[1], 99374[1], 99375[1], 99377[1], 99378[1], 99446[0], 99447[0], 99448[0], 99449[0], 99451[0], 99452[0], 99495[0], 99496[0], G0463[1], G0471[0]
51960	00910[0], 0213T[0], 0216T[0], 0596T[1], 0597T[1], 0708T[1], 0709T[1], 11000[1], 11001[1], 11004[1], 11005[1], 11006[1], 11042[1], 11043[1], 11044[1], 11045[1], 11046[1], 11047[1], 12001[1], 12002[1], 12004[1], 12005[1], 12006[1], 12007[1], 12011[1], 12013[1], 12014[1], 12015[1], 12016[1], 12017[1], 12018[1], 12020[1], 12021[1], 12031[1], 12032[1], 12034[1], 12035[1], 12036[1], 12037[1], 12041[1], 12042[1], 12044[1], 12045[1], 12046[1], 12047[1], 12051[1], 12052[1], 12053[1], 12054[1], 12055[1], 12056[1], 12057[1], 13100[1], 13101[1], 13102[1], 13120[1], 13121[1], 13122[1], 13131[1], 13132[1], 13133[1], 13151[1], 13152[1], 13153[1], 36000[1], 36400[1], 36405[1], 36406[1], 36410[1], 36420[1], 36425[1], 36430[1], 36440[1], 36591[0], 36592[0], 36600[1], 36640[1], 43752[1], 44005[0], 44180[0], 44602[1], 44603[1], 44604[1], 44605[1], 44661[1], 44820[0], 44850[0], 44950[0], 44970[0], 45800[1], 49000[0], 49002[1], 49010[0], 49255[0], 49320[1], 50715[1], 51701[0], 51702[0], 51703[1], 52000[0], 62320[0], 62321[0], 62322[0], 62323[0], 62324[0], 62325[0], 62326[0], 62327[0], 64400[0], 64405[0], 64408[0], 64415[0], 64416[0], 64417[0], 64418[0], 64420[0], 64421[0], 64425[0], 64430[0], 64435[0], 64445[0], 64446[0], 64447[0], 64448[0], 64449[0], 64450[0], 64451[0], 64454[0], 64461[0], 64462[0], 64463[0], 64479[0], 64480[0], 64483[0], 64484[0], 64486[0], 64487[0], 64488[0], 64489[0], 64490[0], 64491[0], 64492[0], 64493[0], 64494[0], 64495[0], 64505[0], 64510[0], 64517[0], 64520[0], 64530[0], 69990[0], 92012[1], 92014[1], 93000[1], 93005[1], 93010[1], 93040[1], 93041[1], 93042[1], 93318[1], 93355[1], 94002[1], 94200[1], 94680[1], 94681[1], 94690[1], 95812[1], 95813[1], 95816[1], 95819[1], 95822[1], 95829[1], 95955[1], 96360[1], 96361[1], 96365[1], 96366[1], 96367[1], 96368[1], 96372[1], 96374[1], 96375[1], 96376[1], 96377[1], 96523[0], 97597[1], 97598[1], 97602[1], 99155[0], 99156[0], 99157[0], 99211[1], 99212[1], 99213[1], 99214[1], 99215[1], 99217[1], 99218[1], 99219[1], 99220[1], 99221[1], 99222[1], 99223[1], 99231[1], 99232[1], 99233[1], 99234[1], 99235[1], 99236[1], 99238[1], 99239[1], 99241[1], 99242[1], 99243[1], 99244[1], 99245[1], 99251[1], 99252[1], 99253[1], 99254[1], 99255[1], 99291[1], 99292[1], 99304[1], 99305[1], 99306[1], 99307[1], 99308[1], 99309[1], 99310[1], 99315[1], 99316[1], 99334[1], 99335[1], 99336[1], 99337[1], 99347[1], 99348[1], 99349[1], 99350[1], 99374[1], 99375[1], 99377[1], 99378[1], 99446[0], 99447[0], 99448[0], 99449[0], 99451[0], 99452[0], 99495[0], 99496[0], G0463[1], G0471[0]
51980	00910[0], 0213T[0], 0216T[0], 0596T[1], 0597T[1], 0708T[1], 0709T[1], 12001[1], 12002[1], 12004[1], 12005[1], 12006[1], 12007[1], 12011[1], 12013[1], 12014[1], 12015[1], 12016[1], 12017[1], 12018[1], 12020[1], 12021[1], 12031[1], 12032[1], 12034[1], 12035[1], 12036[1], 12037[1], 12041[1], 12042[1], 12044[1], 12045[1], 12046[1], 12047[1], 12051[1], 12052[1], 12053[1], 12054[1], 12055[1], 12056[1], 12057[1], 13100[1], 13101[1], 13102[1], 13120[1], 13121[1], 13122[1], 13131[1], 13132[1], 13133[1], 13151[1], 13152[1], 13153[1], 36000[1], 36400[1], 36405[1], 36406[1], 36410[1], 36420[1], 36425[1], 36430[1], 36440[1], 36591[0], 36592[0], 36600[1], 36640[1], 43752[1], 44602[1], 44603[1], 44604[1], 44605[1], 44850[0], 44950[0], 44970[0], 49000[0], 49002[1], 49320[1], 50715[1], 51701[0], 51702[0], 51703[1], 51880[0], 52000[0], 62320[0], 62321[0], 62322[0], 62323[0], 62324[0], 62325[0], 62326[0], 62327[0], 64400[0], 64405[0], 64408[0], 64415[0], 64416[0], 64417[0], 64418[0], 64420[0], 64421[0], 64425[0], 64430[0], 64435[0], 64445[0], 64446[0], 64447[0], 64448[0], 64449[0], 64450[0], 64451[0], 64454[0], 64461[0], 64462[0], 64463[0], 64479[0], 64480[0], 64483[0], 64484[0], 64486[0], 64487[0], 64488[0], 64489[0], 64490[0], 64491[0], 64492[0], 64493[0], 64494[0], 64495[0], 64505[0], 64510[0], 64517[0], 64520[0], 64530[0], 69990[0], 92012[1], 92014[1], 93000[1], 93005[1], 93010[1], 93040[1], 93041[1], 93042[1], 93318[1], 93355[1], 94002[1], 94200[1], 94680[1], 94681[1], 94690[1], 95812[1], 95813[1], 95816[1], 95819[1], 95822[1], 95829[1], 95955[1], 96360[1], 96361[1], 96365[1], 96366[1], 96367[1], 96368[1], 96372[1], 96374[1], 96375[1], 96376[1], 96377[1], 96523[0], 99155[0], 99156[0], 99157[0], 99211[1], 99212[1], 99213[1], 99214[1], 99215[1], 99217[1], 99218[1], 99219[1], 99220[1], 99221[1], 99222[1], 99223[1], 99231[1], 99232[1], 99233[1], 99234[1], 99235[1], 99236[1], 99238[1], 99239[1], 99241[1], 99242[1], 99243[1], 99244[1], 99245[1], 99251[1], 99252[1], 99253[1], 99254[1], 99255[1], 99291[1], 99292[1], 99304[1], 99305[1], 99306[1], 99307[1], 99308[1], 99309[1], 99310[1], 99315[1], 99316[1], 99334[1], 99335[1], 99336[1], 99337[1], 99347[1], 99348[1], 99349[1], 99350[1], 99374[1], 99375[1], 99377[1], 99378[1], 99446[0], 99447[0], 99448[0], 99449[0], 99451[0], 99452[0], 99495[0], 99496[0], G0463[1], G0471[0]
51990	00910[0], 0213T[0], 0216T[0], 0596T[1], 0597T[1], 0708T[1], 0709T[1], 12001[1], 12002[1], 12004[1], 12005[1], 12006[1], 12007[1], 12011[1], 12013[1], 12014[1], 12015[1], 12016[1], 12017[1], 12018[1], 12020[1], 12021[1], 12031[1], 12032[1], 12034[1], 12035[1], 12036[1], 12037[1], 12041[1], 12042[1], 12044[1], 12045[1], 12046[1], 12047[1], 12051[1], 12052[1], 12053[1], 12054[1], 12055[1], 12056[1], 12057[1], 13100[1], 13101[1], 13102[1], 13120[1], 13121[1], 13122[1], 13131[1], 13132[1], 13133[1], 13151[1], 13152[1], 13153[1], 36000[1], 36400[1], 36405[1], 36406[1], 36410[1], 36420[1], 36425[1], 36430[1], 36440[1], 36591[0], 36592[0], 36600[1], 36640[1], 43653[0], 43752[1], 44005[0], 44180[0], 44602[1], 44603[1], 44604[1], 44605[1], 44950[0], 44970[1], 49082[1], 49083[1], 49084[1], 49320[0], 49400[0], 50715[1], 51701[0], 51702[0], 51703[1], 51992[0], 52000[1], 57285[1], 58660[0], 62320[0], 62321[0], 62322[0], 62323[0], 62324[0], 62325[0], 62326[0], 62327[0], 64400[0], 64405[0], 64408[0], 64415[0], 64416[0], 64417[0], 64418[0], 64420[0], 64421[0], 64425[0], 64430[0], 64435[0], 64445[0], 64446[0], 64447[0], 64448[0], 64449[0], 64450[0], 64451[0], 64454[0], 64461[0], 64462[0], 64463[0], 64479[0], 64480[0], 64483[0], 64484[0], 64486[0], 64487[0], 64488[0], 64489[0], 64490[0], 64491[0], 64492[0], 64493[0], 64494[0], 64495[0], 64505[0], 64510[0], 64517[0], 64520[0], 64530[0], 69990[0], 76000[1], 77001[1], 77002[1], 92012[1], 92014[1], 93000[1], 93005[1], 93010[1], 93040[1], 93041[1], 93042[1], 93318[1], 93355[1], 94002[1], 94200[1], 94680[1], 94681[1], 94690[1], 95812[1], 95813[1], 95816[1], 95819[1], 95822[1], 95829[1], 95955[1], 96360[1], 96361[1], 96365[1], 96366[1], 96367[1], 96368[1], 96372[1], 96374[1], 96375[1], 96376[1], 96377[1], 96523[0], 99155[0], 99156[0], 99157[0], 99211[1], 99212[1], 99213[1], 99214[1], 99215[1], 99217[1], 99218[1], 99219[1], 99220[1], 99221[1], 99222[1], 99223[1], 99231[1], 99232[1], 99233[1], 99234[1], 99235[1], 99236[1], 99238[1], 99239[1], 99241[1], 99242[1], 99243[1], 99244[1], 99245[1], 99251[1], 99252[1], 99253[1], 99254[1], 99255[1], 99291[1], 99292[1], 99304[1], 99305[1], 99306[1], 99307[1], 99308[1], 99309[1], 99310[1], 99315[1], 99316[1], 99334[1], 99335[1], 99336[1], 99337[1], 99347[1], 99348[1], 99349[1], 99350[1], 99374[1], 99375[1], 99377[1], 99378[1], 99446[0], 99447[0], 99448[0], 99449[0], 99451[0], 99452[0], 99495[0], 99496[0], G0463[1], G0471[0]
52000	00910[0], 00916[0], 0213T[0], 0216T[0], 0596T[0], 0597T[0], 0708T[1], 0709T[1], 12001[1], 12002[1], 12004[1], 12005[1], 12006[1], 12007[1], 12011[1], 12013[1], 12014[1], 12015[1], 12016[1], 12017[1], 12018[1], 12020[1], 12021[1], 12031[1], 12032[1], 12034[1], 12035[1], 12036[1], 12037[1], 12041[1], 12042[1], 12044[1], 12045[1], 12046[1], 12047[1], 12051[1], 12052[1], 12053[1], 12054[1], 12055[1], 12056[1], 12057[1], 13100[1], 13101[1], 13102[1], 13120[1], 13121[1], 13122[1], 13131[1], 13132[1], 13133[1], 13151[1], 13152[1], 13153[1], 36000[1], 36400[1], 36405[1], 36406[1], 36410[1], 36420[1], 36425[1], 36430[1], 36440[1], 36591[0], 36592[0], 36600[1], 36640[1], 43752[1], 51700[1], 51701[0], 51702[0], 51703[0], 53000[0], 53010[0], 53020[0], 53025[0], 53600[0], 53601[0], 53605[0], 53620[0], 53621[0], 53660[0], 53661[0], 53665[0], 57410[0], 62320[0], 62321[0], 62322[0], 62323[0], 62324[0], 62325[0], 62326[0], 62327[0], 64400[0], 64405[0], 64408[0], 64415[0], 64416[0], 64417[0], 64418[0], 64420[0], 64421[0], 64425[0], 64430[0], 64435[0], 64445[0], 64446[0], 64447[0], 64448[0], 64449[0], 64450[0], 64451[0], 64454[0], 64461[0], 64462[0], 64463[0], 64479[0], 64480[0], 64483[0], 64484[0], 64486[0], 64487[0], 64488[0], 64489[0], 64490[0], 64491[0], 64492[0], 64493[0], 64494[0], 64495[0], 64505[0], 64510[0], 64517[0], 64520[0], 64530[0], 69990[0], 76000[1], 77001[1], 77002[1], 92012[1], 92014[1], 93000[1], 93005[1], 93010[1], 93040[1], 93041[1], 93042[1], 93318[1], 93355[1], 94002[1], 94200[1], 94680[1], 94681[1], 94690[1], 95812[1], 95813[1], 95816[1], 95819[1], 95822[1], 95829[1], 95955[1], 96360[1], 96361[1], 96365[1], 96366[1], 96367[1], 96368[1], 96372[1], 96374[1], 96375[1],

0 = Modifier usage not allowed or inappropriate 1 = Modifier usage allowed

Code 1	Code 2
	96376[1], 96377[1], 96523[0], 99155[0], 99156[0], 99157[0], 99211[1], 99212[1], 99213[1], 99214[1], 99215[1], 99217[1], 99218[1], 99219[1], 99220[1], 99221[1], 99222[1], 99223[1], 99231[1], 99232[1], 99233[1], 99234[1], 99235[1], 99236[1], 99238[1], 99239[1], 99241[1], 99242[1], 99243[1], 99244[1], 99245[1], 99251[1], 99252[1], 99253[1], 99254[1], 99255[1], 99291[1], 99292[1], 99304[1], 99305[1], 99306[1], 99307[1], 99308[1], 99309[1], 99310[1], 99315[1], 99316[1], 99334[1], 99335[1], 99336[1], 99337[1], 99347[1], 99348[1], 99349[1], 99350[1], 99374[1], 99375[1], 99377[1], 99378[1], 99446[0], 99447[0], 99448[0], 99449[0], 99451[0], 99452[0], 99495[1], 99496[1], C9738[1], G0463[1], G0471[0], J2001[1], P9612[0]
52001	00910[0], 00916[0], 0213T[0], 0216T[0], 0596T[0], 0597T[0], 0708T[1], 0709T[1], 12001[1], 12002[1], 12004[1], 12005[1], 12006[1], 12007[1], 12011[1], 12013[1], 12014[1], 12015[1], 12016[1], 12017[1], 12018[1], 12020[1], 12021[1], 12031[1], 12032[1], 12034[1], 12035[1], 12036[1], 12037[1], 12041[1], 12042[1], 12044[1], 12045[1], 12046[1], 12047[1], 12051[1], 12052[1], 12053[1], 12054[1], 12055[1], 12056[1], 12057[1], 13100[1], 13101[1], 13102[1], 13120[1], 13121[1], 13122[1], 13131[1], 13132[1], 13133[1], 13151[1], 13152[1], 13153[1], 36000[1], 36400[1], 36405[1], 36406[1], 36410[1], 36420[1], 36425[1], 36430[1], 36440[1], 36591[0], 36592[0], 36600[1], 36640[1], 43752[1], 51700[0], 51701[0], 51702[0], 51703[0], 52000[0], 52281[0], 53000[0], 53010[0], 53020[0], 53025[0], 53600[0], 53601[0], 53605[0], 53620[0], 53621[0], 53660[0], 53661[0], 57410[0], 62320[0], 62321[0], 62322[0], 62323[0], 62324[0], 62325[0], 62326[0], 62327[0], 64400[0], 64405[0], 64408[0], 64415[0], 64416[0], 64417[0], 64418[0], 64420[0], 64421[0], 64425[0], 64430[0], 64435[0], 64445[0], 64446[0], 64447[0], 64448[0], 64449[0], 64450[0], 64451[0], 64454[0], 64461[0], 64462[0], 64463[0], 64479[0], 64480[0], 64483[0], 64484[0], 64486[0], 64487[0], 64488[0], 64489[0], 64490[0], 64491[0], 64492[0], 64493[0], 64494[0], 64495[0], 64505[0], 64510[0], 64517[0], 64520[0], 64530[0], 76000[1], 77001[1], 77002[1], 92012[1], 92014[1], 93000[1], 93005[1], 93010[1], 93040[1], 93041[1], 93042[1], 93318[1], 93355[1], 94002[1], 94200[1], 94680[1], 94681[1], 94690[1], 95812[1], 95813[1], 95816[1], 95819[1], 95822[1], 95829[1], 95955[1], 96360[1], 96361[1], 96365[1], 96366[1], 96367[1], 96368[1], 96372[1], 96374[1], 96375[1], 96376[1], 96377[1], 96523[0], 99155[0], 99156[0], 99157[0], 99211[1], 99212[1], 99213[1], 99214[1], 99215[1], 99217[1], 99218[1], 99219[1], 99220[1], 99221[1], 99222[1], 99223[1], 99231[1], 99232[1], 99233[1], 99234[1], 99235[1], 99236[1], 99238[1], 99239[1], 99241[1], 99242[1], 99243[1], 99244[1], 99245[1], 99251[1], 99252[1], 99253[1], 99254[1], 99255[1], 99291[1], 99292[1], 99304[1], 99305[1], 99306[1], 99307[1], 99308[1], 99309[1], 99310[1], 99315[1], 99316[1], 99334[1], 99335[1], 99336[1], 99337[1], 99347[1], 99348[1], 99349[1], 99350[1], 99374[1], 99375[1], 99377[1], 99378[1], 99446[0], 99447[0], 99448[0], 99449[0], 99451[0], 99452[0], 99495[1], 99496[1], G0463[1], G0471[0], P9612[0]
52005	00910[0], 00916[0], 0213T[0], 0216T[0], 0708T[1], 0709T[1], 12001[1], 12002[1], 12004[1], 12005[1], 12006[1], 12007[1], 12011[1], 12013[1], 12014[1], 12015[1], 12016[1], 12017[1], 12018[1], 12020[1], 12021[1], 12031[1], 12032[1], 12034[1], 12035[1], 12036[1], 12037[1], 12041[1], 12042[1], 12044[1], 12045[1], 12046[1], 12047[1], 12051[1], 12052[1], 12053[1], 12054[1], 12055[1], 12056[1], 12057[1], 13100[1], 13101[1], 13102[1], 13120[1], 13121[1], 13122[1], 13131[1], 13132[1], 13133[1], 13151[1], 13152[1], 13153[1], 36000[1], 36400[1], 36405[1], 36406[1], 36410[1], 36420[1], 36425[1], 36430[1], 36440[1], 36591[0], 36592[0], 36600[1], 36640[1], 43752[1], 50684[1], 51600[0], 51610[0], 51700[0], 51701[0], 51702[0], 51703[0], 52000[0], 52001[1], 52265[1], 52310[0], 52315[0], 53000[0], 53010[0], 53020[0], 53025[0], 53600[0], 53601[0], 53605[0], 53620[0], 53621[0], 53660[0], 53661[0], 53665[0], 57410[0], 62320[0], 62321[0], 62322[0], 62323[0], 62324[0], 62325[0], 62326[0], 62327[0], 64400[0], 64405[0], 64408[0], 64415[0], 64416[0], 64417[0], 64418[0], 64420[0], 64421[0], 64425[0], 64430[0], 64435[0], 64445[0], 64446[0], 64447[0], 64448[0], 64449[0], 64450[0], 64451[0], 64454[0], 64461[0], 64462[0], 64463[0], 64479[0], 64480[0], 64483[0], 64484[0], 64486[0], 64487[0], 64488[0], 64489[0], 64490[0], 64491[0], 64492[0], 64493[0], 64494[0], 64495[0], 64505[0], 64510[0], 64517[0], 64520[0], 64530[0], 69990[0], 76000[1], 77001[1], 77002[1], 92012[1], 92014[1], 93000[1], 93005[1], 93010[1], 93040[1], 93041[1], 93042[1], 93318[1], 93355[1], 94002[1], 94200[1], 94680[1], 94681[1], 94690[1], 95812[1], 95813[1], 95816[1], 95819[1], 95822[1], 95829[1], 95955[1], 96360[1], 96361[1], 96365[1], 96366[1], 96367[1], 96368[1], 96372[1], 96374[1], 96375[1], 96376[1], 96377[1], 96523[0], 99155[0], 99156[0], 99157[0], 99211[1], 99212[1], 99213[1], 99214[1], 99215[1], 99217[1], 99218[1], 99219[1], 99220[1], 99221[1], 99222[1], 99223[1], 99231[1], 99232[1], 99233[1], 99234[1], 99235[1], 99236[1], 99238[1], 99239[1], 99241[1], 99242[1], 99243[1], 99244[1], 99245[1], 99251[1], 99252[1], 99253[1], 99254[1], 99255[1], 99291[1], 99292[1], 99304[1], 99305[1], 99306[1], 99307[1], 99308[1], 99309[1], 99310[1], 99315[1], 99316[1], 99334[1], 99335[1], 99336[1], 99337[1], 99347[1], 99348[1], 99349[1], 99350[1], 99374[1], 99375[1], 99377[1], 99378[1], 99446[0], 99447[0], 99448[0], 99449[0], 99451[0], 99452[0], 99495[1], 99496[1], G0463[1], G0471[0], P9612[0]
52007	00910[0], 00916[0], 0213T[0], 0216T[0], 0596T[0], 0597T[0], 0708T[1], 0709T[1], 10005[1], 10007[1], 10009[1], 10011[1], 10021[1], 12001[1], 12002[1], 12004[1], 12005[1], 12006[1], 12007[1], 12011[1], 12013[1], 12014[1], 12015[1], 12016[1], 12017[1], 12018[1], 12020[1], 12021[1], 12031[1], 12032[1], 12034[1], 12035[1], 12036[1], 12037[1], 12041[1], 12042[1], 12044[1], 12045[1], 12046[1], 12047[1], 12051[1], 12052[1], 12053[1], 12054[1], 12055[1], 12056[1], 12057[1], 13100[1], 13101[1], 13102[1], 13120[1], 13121[1], 13122[1], 13131[1], 13132[1], 13133[1], 13151[1], 13152[1], 13153[1], 36000[1], 36400[1], 36405[1], 36406[1], 36410[1], 36420[1], 36425[1], 36430[1], 36440[1], 36591[0], 36592[0], 36600[1], 36640[1], 43752[1], 50606[1], 50684[1], 51700[0], 51701[0], 51702[0], 51703[0], 52000[0], 52001[1], 52005[1], 52204[1], 52281[0], 52310[0], 52315[0], 53000[0], 53010[0], 53020[0], 53025[0], 53600[0], 53601[0], 53605[0], 53620[0], 53621[0], 53660[0], 53661[0], 53665[0], 57410[0], 62320[0], 62321[0], 62322[0], 62323[0], 62324[0], 62325[0], 62326[0], 62327[0], 64400[0], 64405[0], 64408[0], 64415[0], 64416[0], 64417[0], 64418[0], 64420[0], 64421[0], 64425[0], 64430[0], 64435[0], 64445[0], 64446[0], 64447[0], 64448[0], 64449[0], 64450[0], 64451[0], 64454[0], 64461[0], 64462[0], 64463[0], 64479[0], 64480[0], 64483[0], 64484[0], 64486[0], 64487[0], 64488[0], 64489[0], 64490[0], 64491[0], 64492[0], 64493[0], 64494[0], 64495[0], 64505[0], 64510[0], 64517[0], 64520[0], 64530[0], 69990[0], 76000[1], 77001[1], 77002[1], 92012[1], 92014[1], 93000[1], 93005[1], 93010[1], 93040[1], 93041[1], 93042[1], 93318[1], 93355[1], 94002[1], 94200[1], 94680[1], 94681[1], 94690[1], 95812[1], 95813[1], 95816[1], 95819[1], 95822[1], 95829[1], 95955[1], 96360[1], 96361[1], 96365[1], 96366[1], 96367[1], 96368[1], 96372[1], 96374[1], 96375[1], 96376[1], 96377[1], 96523[0], 99155[0], 99156[0], 99157[0], 99211[1], 99212[1], 99213[1], 99214[1], 99215[1], 99217[1], 99218[1], 99219[1], 99220[1], 99221[1], 99222[1], 99223[1], 99231[1], 99232[1], 99233[1], 99234[1], 99235[1], 99236[1], 99238[1], 99239[1], 99241[1], 99242[1], 99243[1], 99244[1], 99245[1], 99251[1], 99252[1], 99253[1], 99254[1], 99255[1], 99291[1], 99292[1], 99304[1], 99305[1], 99306[1], 99307[1], 99308[1], 99309[1], 99310[1], 99315[1], 99316[1], 99334[1], 99335[1], 99336[1], 99337[1], 99347[1], 99348[1], 99349[1], 99350[1], 99374[1], 99375[1], 99377[1], 99378[1], 99446[0], 99447[0], 99448[0], 99449[0], 99451[0], 99452[0], 99495[1], 99496[1], G0463[1], G0471[0], P9612[0]
52010	00910[0], 00916[0], 0213T[0], 0216T[0], 0596T[0], 0597T[0], 0708T[1], 0709T[1], 12001[1], 12002[1], 12004[1], 12005[1], 12006[1], 12007[1], 12011[1], 12013[1], 12014[1], 12015[1], 12016[1], 12017[1], 12018[1], 12020[1], 12021[1], 12031[1], 12032[1], 12034[1], 12035[1], 12036[1], 12037[1], 12041[1], 12042[1], 12044[1], 12045[1], 12046[1], 12047[1], 12051[1], 12052[1], 12053[1], 12054[1], 12055[1], 12056[1], 12057[1], 13100[1], 13101[1], 13102[1], 13120[1], 13121[1], 13122[1], 13131[1], 13132[1], 13133[1], 13151[1], 13152[1], 13153[1], 36000[1], 36400[1], 36405[1], 36406[1], 36410[1], 36420[1], 36425[1], 36430[1], 36440[1], 36591[0], 36592[0], 36600[1], 36640[1], 43752[1], 51701[0], 51702[0], 51703[0], 52000[0], 52001[1], 52250[1], 52281[0], 52310[0], 52315[0], 53000[0], 53010[0], 53020[0], 53025[0], 53600[0], 53601[0], 53605[0], 53620[0], 53621[0], 53660[0], 53661[0], 53665[0], 57410[0], 62320[0], 62321[0], 62322[0], 62323[0], 62324[0], 62325[0], 62326[0], 62327[0], 64400[0], 64405[0], 64408[0], 64415[0], 64416[0], 64417[0], 64418[0], 64420[0], 64421[0], 64425[0], 64430[0], 64435[0], 64445[0], 64446[0], 64447[0], 64448[0], 64449[0], 64450[0], 64451[0], 64454[0], 64461[0], 64462[0], 64463[0], 64479[0], 64480[0], 64483[0], 64484[0], 64486[0], 64487[0], 64488[0], 64489[0], 64490[0], 64491[0], 64492[0], 64493[0], 64494[0], 64495[0], 64505[0], 64510[0], 64517[0], 64520[0], 64530[0], 69990[0], 76000[1], 77001[1], 77002[1], 92012[1], 92014[1], 93000[1], 93005[1], 93010[1], 93040[1], 93041[1], 93042[1], 93318[1], 93355[1], 94002[1], 94200[1], 94680[1], 94681[1], 94690[1], 95812[1], 95813[1], 95816[1], 95819[1], 95822[1], 95829[1], 95955[1], 96360[1], 96361[1], 96365[1], 96366[1], 96367[1], 96368[1], 96372[1], 96374[1], 96375[1], 96376[1], 96377[1], 96523[0], 99155[0], 99156[0], 99157[0], 99211[1], 99212[1], 99213[1], 99214[1], 99215[1], 99217[1], 99218[1], 99219[1], 99220[1], 99221[1], 99222[1], 99223[1], 99231[1], 99232[1], 99233[1], 99234[1], 99235[1], 99236[1], 99238[1], 99239[1], 99241[1], 99242[1], 99243[1], 99244[1], 99245[1], 99251[1], 99252[1], 99253[1], 99254[1], 99255[1], 99291[1], 99292[1], 99304[1], 99305[1], 99306[1], 99307[1], 99308[1], 99309[1], 99310[1], 99315[1], 99316[1], 99334[1], 99335[1], 99336[1], 99337[1], 99347[1], 99348[1], 99349[1], 99350[1], 99374[1], 99375[1], 99377[1], 99378[1], 99446[0], 99447[0], 99448[0], 99449[0], 99451[0], 99452[0], 99495[1], 99496[1], G0463[1], G0471[0], J2001[1], P9612[0]
52204	00910[0], 00916[0], 0213T[0], 0216T[0], 0596T[0], 0597T[0], 0708T[1], 0709T[1], 10005[1], 10007[1], 10009[1], 10011[1], 10021[1], 12001[1], 12002[1], 12004[1], 12005[1], 12006[1], 12007[1], 12011[1], 12013[1], 12014[1], 12015[1], 12016[1], 12017[1], 12018[1], 12020[1], 12021[1], 12031[1], 12032[1], 12034[1], 12035[1], 12036[1], 12037[1], 12041[1], 12042[1], 12044[1], 12045[1], 12046[1], 12047[1], 12051[1], 12052[1], 12053[1], 12054[1], 12055[1], 12056[1], 12057[1], 13100[1], 13101[1], 13102[1], 13120[1], 13121[1], 13122[1], 13131[1], 13132[1], 13133[1], 13151[1], 13152[1], 13153[1], 36000[1], 36400[1], 36405[1], 36406[1], 36410[1], 36420[1], 36425[1], 36430[1], 36440[1], 36591[0], 36592[0], 36600[1], 36640[1], 43752[1], 51700[0], 51701[0], 51702[0], 51703[0], 52000[0], 52001[1], 52005[1], 52310[0], 52315[0], 53000[0], 53010[0], 53020[0], 53025[0], 53600[0], 53601[0], 53605[0], 53620[0], 53621[0], 53660[0], 53661[0], 53665[0], 57410[0], 62320[0], 62321[0], 62322[0], 62323[0], 62324[0], 62325[0], 62326[0], 62327[0], 64400[0], 64405[0], 64408[0], 64415[0], 64416[0], 64417[0], 64418[0], 64420[0], 64421[0], 64425[0], 64430[0], 64435[0], 64445[0], 64446[0], 64447[0], 64448[0], 64449[0], 64450[0], 64451[0], 64454[0], 64461[0], 64462[0], 64463[0], 64479[0], 64480[0], 64483[0], 64484[0], 64486[0], 64487[0], 64488[0], 64489[0], 64490[0], 64491[0], 64492[0], 64493[0], 64494[0], 64495[0], 64505[0], 64510[0], 64517[0], 64520[0], 64530[0], 69990[0], 76000[1], 77001[1], 77002[1], 92012[1], 92014[1], 93000[1], 93005[1], 93010[1], 93040[1], 93041[1], 93042[1], 93318[1], 93355[1], 94002[1], 94200[1], 94680[1], 94681[1], 94690[1], 95812[1], 95813[1], 95816[1], 95819[1], 95822[1], 95829[1], 95955[1], 96360[1], 96361[1], 96365[1], 96366[1], 96367[1], 96368[1], 96372[1], 96374[1], 96375[1], 96376[1], 96377[1], 96523[0], 99155[0], 99156[0], 99157[0], 99211[1], 99212[1], 99213[1], 99214[1], 99215[1], 99217[1], 99218[1], 99219[1], 99220[1], 99221[1], 99222[1], 99223[1], 99231[1], 99232[1], 99233[1], 99234[1], 99235[1], 99236[1], 99238[1], 99239[1], 99241[1], 99242[1], 99243[1], 99244[1], 99245[1], 99251[1], 99252[1], 99253[1], 99254[1], 99255[1], 99291[1], 99292[1], 99304[1], 99305[1], 99306[1], 99307[1], 99308[1], 99309[1], 99310[1], 99315[1], 99316[1], 99334[1], 99335[1], 99336[1],

0 = Modifier usage not allowed or inappropriate 1 = Modifier usage allowed

Code 1	Code 2
	99337[1], 99347[1], 99348[1], 99349[1], 99350[1], 99374[1], 99375[1], 99377[1], 99378[1], 99446[0], 99447[0], 99448[0], 99449[0], 99451[0], 99452[0], 99495[1], 99496[1], G0463[1], G0471[0], P9612[0]
52214	00910[0], 00912[0], 00916[0], 0213T[0], 0216T[0], 0596T[0], 0597T[0], 0708T[1], 0709T[1], 12001[1], 12002[1], 12004[1], 12005[1], 12006[1], 12007[1], 12011[1], 12013[1], 12014[1], 12015[1], 12016[1], 12017[1], 12018[1], 12020[1], 12021[1], 12031[1], 12032[1], 12034[1], 12035[1], 12036[1], 12037[1], 12041[1], 12042[1], 12044[1], 12045[1], 12046[1], 12047[1], 12051[1], 12052[1], 12053[1], 12054[1], 12055[1], 12056[1], 12057[1], 13100[1], 13101[1], 13102[1], 13120[1], 13121[1], 13122[1], 13131[1], 13132[1], 13133[1], 13151[1], 13152[1], 13153[1], 36000[1], 36400[1], 36405[1], 36406[1], 36410[1], 36420[1], 36425[1], 36430[1], 36440[1], 36591[0], 36592[0], 36600[1], 36640[1], 43752[1], 51701[0], 51702[0], 51703[0], 52000[0], 52001[1], 52005[1], 52204[1], 52224[1], 52250[0], 52260[1], 52265[1], 52281[0], 52310[0], 52315[0], 52500[1], 53000[0], 53010[0], 53020[0], 53025[0], 53600[0], 53601[0], 53605[0], 53620[0], 53621[0], 53660[0], 53661[0], 53665[0], 57410[0], 62320[0], 62321[0], 62322[0], 62323[0], 62324[0], 62325[0], 62326[0], 62327[0], 64400[0], 64405[0], 64408[0], 64415[0], 64416[0], 64417[0], 64418[0], 64420[0], 64421[0], 64425[0], 64430[0], 64435[0], 64445[0], 64446[0], 64447[0], 64448[0], 64449[0], 64450[0], 64451[0], 64454[0], 64461[0], 64462[0], 64463[0], 64479[0], 64480[0], 64483[0], 64484[0], 64486[0], 64487[0], 64488[0], 64489[0], 64490[0], 64491[0], 64492[0], 64493[0], 64494[0], 64495[0], 64505[0], 64510[0], 64517[0], 64520[0], 64530[0], 69990[0], 76000[1], 77001[1], 77002[1], 92012[1], 92014[1], 93000[1], 93005[1], 93010[1], 93040[1], 93041[1], 93042[1], 93318[1], 93355[1], 94002[1], 94200[1], 94680[1], 94681[1], 94690[1], 95812[1], 95813[1], 95816[1], 95819[1], 95822[1], 95829[1], 95955[1], 96360[1], 96361[1], 96365[1], 96366[1], 96367[1], 96368[1], 96372[1], 96374[1], 96375[1], 96376[1], 96377[1], 96523[0], 99155[0], 99156[0], 99157[0], 99211[1], 99212[1], 99213[1], 99214[1], 99215[1], 99217[1], 99218[1], 99219[1], 99220[1], 99221[1], 99222[1], 99223[1], 99231[1], 99232[1], 99233[1], 99234[1], 99235[1], 99236[1], 99238[1], 99239[1], 99241[1], 99242[1], 99243[1], 99244[1], 99245[1], 99251[1], 99252[1], 99253[1], 99254[1], 99255[1], 99291[1], 99292[1], 99304[1], 99305[1], 99306[1], 99307[1], 99308[1], 99309[1], 99310[1], 99315[1], 99316[1], 99334[1], 99335[1], 99336[1], 99337[1], 99347[1], 99348[1], 99349[1], 99350[1], 99374[1], 99375[1], 99377[1], 99378[1], 99446[0], 99447[0], 99448[0], 99449[0], 99451[0], 99452[0], 99495[1], 99496[1], G0463[1], G0471[0], J0670[1], J2001[1], P9612[0]
52224	00910[0], 00912[0], 00916[0], 0213T[0], 0216T[0], 0596T[0], 0597T[0], 0708T[1], 0709T[1], 10005[1], 10007[1], 10009[1], 10011[1], 10021[1], 12001[1], 12002[1], 12004[1], 12005[1], 12006[1], 12007[1], 12011[1], 12013[1], 12014[1], 12015[1], 12016[1], 12017[1], 12018[1], 12020[1], 12021[1], 12031[1], 12032[1], 12034[1], 12035[1], 12036[1], 12037[1], 12041[1], 12042[1], 12044[1], 12045[1], 12046[1], 12047[1], 12051[1], 12052[1], 12053[1], 12054[1], 12055[1], 12056[1], 12057[1], 13100[1], 13101[1], 13102[1], 13120[1], 13121[1], 13122[1], 13131[1], 13132[1], 13133[1], 13151[1], 13152[1], 13153[1], 36000[1], 36400[1], 36405[1], 36406[1], 36410[1], 36420[1], 36425[1], 36430[1], 36440[1], 36591[0], 36592[0], 36600[1], 36640[1], 43752[1], 51701[0], 51702[0], 51703[0], 51720[1], 52000[0], 52001[1], 52005[1], 52204[0], 52260[0], 52281[0], 52310[0], 52315[0], 53000[0], 53010[0], 53020[0], 53025[0], 53600[0], 53601[0], 53605[0], 53620[0], 53621[0], 53660[0], 53661[0], 53665[0], 57410[0], 62320[0], 62321[0], 62322[0], 62323[0], 62324[0], 62325[0], 62326[0], 62327[0], 64400[0], 64405[0], 64408[0], 64415[0], 64416[0], 64417[0], 64418[0], 64420[0], 64421[0], 64425[0], 64430[0], 64435[0], 64445[0], 64446[0], 64447[0], 64448[0], 64449[0], 64450[0], 64451[0], 64454[0], 64461[0], 64462[0], 64463[0], 64479[0], 64480[0], 64483[0], 64484[0], 64486[0], 64487[0], 64488[0], 64489[0], 64490[0], 64491[0], 64492[0], 64493[0], 64494[0], 64495[0], 64505[0], 64510[0], 64517[0], 64520[0], 64530[0], 69990[0], 76000[1], 77001[1], 77002[1], 92012[1], 92014[1], 93000[1], 93005[1], 93010[1], 93040[1], 93041[1], 93042[1], 93318[1], 93355[1], 94002[1], 94200[1], 94680[1], 94681[1], 94690[1], 95812[1], 95813[1], 95816[1], 95819[1], 95822[1], 95829[1], 95955[1], 96360[1], 96361[1], 96365[1], 96366[1], 96367[1], 96368[1], 96372[1], 96374[1], 96375[1], 96376[1], 96377[1], 96523[0], 99155[0], 99156[0], 99157[0], 99211[1], 99212[1], 99213[1], 99214[1], 99215[1], 99217[1], 99218[1], 99219[1], 99220[1], 99221[1], 99222[1], 99223[1], 99231[1], 99232[1], 99233[1], 99234[1], 99235[1], 99236[1], 99238[1], 99239[1], 99241[1], 99242[1], 99243[1], 99244[1], 99245[1], 99251[1], 99252[1], 99253[1], 99254[1], 99255[1], 99291[1], 99292[1], 99304[1], 99305[1], 99306[1], 99307[1], 99308[1], 99309[1], 99310[1], 99315[1], 99316[1], 99334[1], 99335[1], 99336[1], 99337[1], 99347[1], 99348[1], 99349[1], 99350[1], 99374[1], 99375[1], 99377[1], 99378[1], 99446[0], 99447[0], 99448[0], 99449[0], 99451[0], 99452[0], 99495[1], 99496[1], G0463[1], G0471[0], J0670[1], J2001[1], P9612[0]
52234	00910[0], 00912[0], 00916[0], 0213T[0], 0216T[0], 0596T[0], 0597T[0], 0708T[1], 0709T[1], 11000[1], 11001[1], 11004[1], 11005[1], 11006[1], 11042[1], 11043[1], 11044[1], 11045[1], 11046[1], 11047[1], 12001[1], 12002[1], 12004[1], 12005[1], 12006[1], 12007[1], 12011[1], 12013[1], 12014[1], 12015[1], 12016[1], 12017[1], 12018[1], 12020[1], 12021[1], 12031[1], 12032[1], 12034[1], 12035[1], 12036[1], 12037[1], 12041[1], 12042[1], 12044[1], 12045[1], 12046[1], 12047[1], 12051[1], 12052[1], 12053[1], 12054[1], 12055[1], 12056[1], 12057[1], 13100[1], 13101[1], 13102[1], 13120[1], 13121[1], 13122[1], 13131[1], 13132[1], 13133[1], 13151[1], 13152[1], 13153[1], 36000[1], 36400[1], 36405[1], 36406[1], 36410[1], 36420[1], 36425[1], 36430[1], 36440[1], 36591[0], 36592[0], 36600[1], 36640[1], 43752[1], 51700[0], 51701[0], 51702[0], 51703[0], 51720[1], 52000[0], 52001[1], 52005[1], 52204[1], 52214[1], 52224[1], 52276[1], 52281[0], 52310[0], 52315[0], 52332[1], 52356[1], 53000[0], 53010[0], 53020[0], 53025[0], 53600[0], 53601[0], 53605[0], 53620[0], 53621[0], 53660[0], 53661[0], 53665[0], 57410[0], 62320[0], 62321[0], 62322[0], 62323[0], 62324[0], 62325[0], 62326[0], 62327[0], 64400[0], 64405[0], 64408[0], 64415[0], 64416[0], 64417[0], 64418[0], 64420[0], 64421[0], 64425[0], 64430[0], 64435[0], 64445[0], 64446[0], 64447[0], 64448[0], 64449[0], 64450[0], 64451[0], 64454[0], 64461[0], 64462[0], 64463[0], 64479[0], 64480[0], 64483[0], 64484[0], 64486[0], 64487[0], 64488[0], 64489[0], 64490[0], 64491[0], 64492[0], 64493[0], 64494[0], 64495[0], 64505[0], 64510[0], 64517[0], 64520[0], 64530[0], 69990[0], 76000[1], 77001[1], 77002[1], 92012[1], 92014[1], 93000[1], 93005[1], 93010[1], 93040[1], 93041[1], 93042[1], 93318[1], 93355[1], 94002[1], 94200[1], 94680[1], 94681[1], 94690[1], 95812[1], 95813[1], 95816[1], 95819[1], 95822[1], 95829[1], 95955[1], 96360[1], 96361[1], 96365[1], 96366[1], 96367[1], 96368[1], 96372[1], 96374[1], 96375[1], 96376[1], 96377[1], 96523[0], 97597[1], 97598[1], 97602[1], 99155[0], 99156[0], 99157[0], 99211[1], 99212[1], 99213[1], 99214[1], 99215[1], 99217[1], 99218[1], 99219[1], 99220[1], 99221[1], 99222[1], 99223[1], 99231[1], 99232[1], 99233[1], 99234[1], 99235[1], 99236[1], 99238[1], 99239[1], 99241[1], 99242[1], 99243[1], 99244[1], 99245[1], 99251[1], 99252[1], 99253[1], 99254[1], 99255[1], 99291[1], 99292[1], 99304[1], 99305[1], 99306[1], 99307[1], 99308[1], 99309[1], 99310[1], 99315[1], 99316[1], 99334[1], 99335[1], 99336[1], 99337[1], 99347[1], 99348[1], 99349[1], 99350[1], 99374[1], 99375[1], 99377[1], 99378[1], 99446[0], 99447[0], 99448[0], 99449[0], 99451[0], 99452[0], 99495[1], 99496[1], G0463[1], G0471[0], P9612[0]
52235	00910[0], 00912[0], 00916[0], 0213T[0], 0216T[0], 0596T[0], 0597T[0], 0708T[1], 0709T[1], 11000[1], 11001[1], 11004[1], 11005[1], 11006[1], 11042[1], 11043[1], 11044[1], 11045[1], 11046[1], 11047[1], 12001[1], 12002[1], 12004[1], 12005[1], 12006[1], 12007[1], 12011[1], 12013[1], 12014[1], 12015[1], 12016[1], 12017[1], 12018[1], 12020[1], 12021[1], 12031[1], 12032[1], 12034[1], 12035[1], 12036[1], 12037[1], 12041[1], 12042[1], 12044[1], 12045[1], 12046[1], 12047[1], 12051[1], 12052[1], 12053[1], 12054[1], 12055[1], 12056[1], 12057[1], 13100[1], 13101[1], 13102[1], 13120[1], 13121[1], 13122[1], 13131[1], 13132[1], 13133[1], 13151[1], 13152[1], 13153[1], 36000[1], 36400[1], 36405[1], 36406[1], 36410[1], 36420[1], 36425[1], 36430[1], 36440[1], 36591[0], 36592[0], 36600[1], 36640[1], 43752[1], 51700[0], 51701[0], 51702[0], 51703[0], 51720[1], 52000[0], 52001[1], 52005[1], 52204[1], 52214[1], 52224[1], 52234[0], 52276[1], 52281[0], 52310[0], 52315[0], 52332[1], 53000[0], 53010[0], 53020[0], 53025[0], 53600[0], 53601[0], 53605[0], 53620[0], 53621[0], 53660[0], 53661[0], 53665[0], 57410[0], 62320[0], 62321[0], 62322[0], 62323[0], 62324[0], 62325[0], 62326[0], 62327[0], 64400[0], 64405[0], 64408[0], 64415[0], 64416[0], 64417[0], 64418[0], 64420[0], 64421[0], 64425[0], 64430[0], 64435[0], 64445[0], 64446[0], 64447[0], 64448[0], 64449[0], 64450[0], 64451[0], 64454[0], 64461[0], 64462[0], 64463[0], 64479[0], 64480[0], 64483[0], 64484[0], 64486[0], 64487[0], 64488[0], 64489[0], 64490[0], 64491[0], 64492[0], 64493[0], 64494[0], 64495[0], 64505[0], 64510[0], 64517[0], 64520[0], 64530[0], 69990[0], 76000[1], 77001[1], 77002[1], 92012[1], 92014[1], 93000[1], 93005[1], 93010[1], 93040[1], 93041[1], 93042[1], 93318[1], 93355[1], 94002[1], 94200[1], 94680[1], 94681[1], 94690[1], 95812[1], 95813[1], 95816[1], 95819[1], 95822[1], 95829[1], 95955[1], 96360[1], 96361[1], 96365[1], 96366[1], 96367[1], 96368[1], 96372[1], 96374[1], 96375[1], 96376[1], 96377[1], 96523[0], 97597[1], 97598[1], 97602[1], 99155[0], 99156[0], 99157[0], 99211[1], 99212[1], 99213[1], 99214[1], 99215[1], 99217[1], 99218[1], 99219[1], 99220[1], 99221[1], 99222[1], 99223[1], 99231[1], 99232[1], 99233[1], 99234[1], 99235[1], 99236[1], 99238[1], 99239[1], 99241[1], 99242[1], 99243[1], 99244[1], 99245[1], 99251[1], 99252[1], 99253[1], 99254[1], 99255[1], 99291[1], 99292[1], 99304[1], 99305[1], 99306[1], 99307[1], 99308[1], 99309[1], 99310[1], 99315[1], 99316[1], 99334[1], 99335[1], 99336[1], 99337[1], 99347[1], 99348[1], 99349[1], 99350[1], 99374[1], 99375[1], 99377[1], 99378[1], 99446[0], 99447[0], 99448[0], 99449[0], 99451[0], 99452[0], 99495[1], 99496[1], G0463[1], G0471[0], P9612[0]
52240	00910[0], 00912[0], 00916[0], 0213T[0], 0216T[0], 0596T[0], 0597T[0], 0708T[1], 0709T[1], 11000[1], 11001[1], 11004[1], 11005[1], 11006[1], 11042[1], 11043[1], 11044[1], 11045[1], 11046[1], 11047[1], 12001[1], 12002[1], 12004[1], 12005[1], 12006[1], 12007[1], 12011[1], 12013[1], 12014[1], 12015[1], 12016[1], 12017[1], 12018[1], 12020[1], 12021[1], 12031[1], 12032[1], 12034[1], 12035[1], 12036[1], 12037[1], 12041[1], 12042[1], 12044[1], 12045[1], 12046[1], 12047[1], 12051[1], 12052[1], 12053[1], 12054[1], 12055[1], 12056[1], 12057[1], 13100[1], 13101[1], 13102[1], 13120[1], 13121[1], 13122[1], 13131[1], 13132[1], 13133[1], 13151[1], 13152[1], 13153[1], 36000[1], 36400[1], 36405[1], 36406[1], 36410[1], 36420[1], 36425[1], 36430[1], 36440[1], 36591[0], 36592[0], 36600[1], 36640[1], 43752[1], 51700[0], 51701[0], 51702[0], 51703[0], 51720[1], 52000[0], 52001[1], 52005[1], 52204[1], 52214[1], 52224[1], 52234[0], 52235[0], 52276[1], 52281[0], 52310[0], 52315[0], 52317[1], 52332[1], 52356[1], 52400[0], 53000[0], 53010[0], 53020[0], 53025[0], 53600[0], 53601[0], 53605[0], 53620[0], 53621[0], 53660[0], 53661[0], 53665[0], 57410[0], 62320[0], 62321[0], 62322[0], 62323[0], 62324[0], 62325[0], 62326[0], 62327[0], 64400[0], 64405[0], 64408[0], 64415[0], 64416[0], 64417[0], 64418[0], 64420[0], 64421[0], 64425[0], 64430[0], 64435[0], 64445[0], 64446[0], 64447[0], 64448[0], 64449[0], 64450[0], 64451[0], 64454[0], 64461[0], 64462[0], 64463[0], 64479[0], 64480[0], 64483[0], 64484[0], 64486[0], 64487[0], 64488[0], 64489[0], 64490[0], 64491[0], 64492[0], 64493[0], 64494[0], 64495[0], 64505[0], 64510[0], 64517[0], 64520[0], 64530[0], 69990[0], 76000[1], 77001[1], 77002[1], 92012[1], 92014[1], 93000[1], 93005[1], 93010[1], 93040[1], 93041[1], 93042[1], 93318[1], 93355[1], 94002[1], 94200[1], 94680[1], 94681[1], 94690[1], 95812[1], 95813[1], 95816[1], 95819[1], 95822[1], 95829[1], 95955[1], 96360[1], 96361[1], 96365[1], 96366[1], 96367[1], 96368[1], 96372[1], 96374[1], 96375[1], 96376[1], 96377[1], 96523[0], 97597[1], 97598[1], 97602[1], 99155[0], 99156[0], 99157[0], 99211[1], 99212[1], 99213[1], 99214[1], 99215[1], 99217[1], 99218[1], 99219[1], 99220[1], 99221[1], 99222[1], 99223[1], 99231[1], 99232[1], 99233[1], 99234[1], 99235[1], 99236[1], 99238[1], 99239[1], 99241[1], 99242[1],

0 = Modifier usage not allowed or inappropriate   1 = Modifier usage allowed

Code 1	Code 2
	99243[1], 99244[1], 99245[1], 99251[1], 99252[1], 99253[1], 99254[1], 99255[1], 99291[1], 99292[1], 99304[1], 99305[1], 99306[1], 99307[1], 99308[1], 99309[1], 99310[1], 99315[1], 99316[1], 99334[1], 99335[1], 99336[1], 99337[1], 99347[1], 99348[1], 99349[1], 99350[1], 99374[1], 99375[1], 99377[1], 99378[1], 99446[0], 99447[0], 99448[0], 99449[0], 99451[0], 99452[0], 99495[1], 99496[1], G0463[1], G0471[0], P9612[0]
52250	00910[0], 00916[0], 0213T[0], 0216T[0], 0596T[0], 0597T[0], 0708T[1], 0709T[1], 10005[1], 10007[1], 10009[1], 10011[1], 10021[1], 11000[1], 11001[1], 11004[1], 11005[1], 11006[1], 11042[1], 11043[1], 11044[1], 11045[1], 11046[1], 11047[1], 12001[1], 12002[1], 12004[1], 12005[1], 12006[1], 12007[1], 12011[1], 12013[1], 12014[1], 12015[1], 12016[1], 12017[1], 12018[1], 12020[1], 12021[1], 12031[1], 12032[1], 12034[1], 12035[1], 12036[1], 12037[1], 12041[1], 12042[1], 12044[1], 12045[1], 12046[1], 12047[1], 12051[1], 12052[1], 12053[1], 12054[1], 12055[1], 12056[1], 12057[1], 13100[1], 13101[1], 13102[1], 13120[1], 13121[1], 13122[1], 13131[1], 13132[1], 13133[1], 13151[1], 13152[1], 13153[1], 36000[1], 36400[1], 36405[1], 36406[1], 36410[1], 36420[1], 36425[1], 36430[1], 36440[1], 36591[0], 36592[0], 36600[1], 36640[1], 43752[1], 51701[0], 51702[0], 51703[0], 52000[0], 52001[1], 52204[0], 52224[0], 52234[1], 52235[1], 52240[1], 52281[0], 52310[0], 52315[0], 53000[0], 53010[0], 53020[0], 53025[0], 53600[0], 53601[0], 53605[0], 53620[0], 53621[0], 53660[0], 53661[0], 53665[0], 57410[0], 62320[0], 62321[0], 62322[0], 62323[0], 62324[0], 62325[0], 62326[0], 62327[0], 64400[0], 64405[0], 64408[0], 64415[0], 64416[0], 64417[0], 64418[0], 64420[0], 64421[0], 64425[0], 64430[0], 64435[0], 64445[0], 64446[0], 64447[0], 64448[0], 64449[0], 64450[0], 64451[0], 64454[0], 64461[0], 64462[0], 64463[0], 64479[0], 64480[0], 64483[0], 64484[0], 64486[0], 64487[0], 64488[0], 64489[0], 64490[0], 64491[0], 64492[0], 64493[0], 64494[0], 64495[0], 64505[0], 64510[0], 64517[0], 64520[0], 64530[0], 69990[0], 76000[1], 77001[1], 77002[1], 92012[1], 92014[1], 93000[1], 93005[1], 93010[1], 93040[1], 93041[1], 93042[1], 93318[1], 93355[1], 94002[1], 94200[1], 94680[1], 94681[1], 94690[1], 95812[1], 95813[1], 95816[1], 95819[1], 95822[1], 95829[1], 95955[1], 96360[1], 96361[1], 96365[1], 96366[1], 96367[1], 96368[1], 96372[1], 96374[1], 96375[1], 96376[1], 96377[1], 96523[0], 97597[1], 97598[1], 97602[1], 99155[0], 99156[0], 99157[0], 99211[1], 99212[1], 99213[1], 99214[1], 99215[1], 99217[1], 99218[1], 99219[1], 99220[1], 99221[1], 99222[1], 99223[1], 99231[1], 99232[1], 99233[1], 99234[1], 99235[1], 99236[1], 99238[1], 99239[1], 99241[1], 99242[1], 99243[1], 99244[1], 99245[1], 99251[1], 99252[1], 99253[1], 99254[1], 99255[1], 99291[1], 99292[1], 99304[1], 99305[1], 99306[1], 99307[1], 99308[1], 99309[1], 99310[1], 99315[1], 99316[1], 99334[1], 99335[1], 99336[1], 99337[1], 99347[1], 99348[1], 99349[1], 99350[1], 99374[1], 99375[1], 99377[1], 99378[1], 99446[0], 99447[0], 99448[0], 99449[0], 99451[0], 99452[0], 99495[1], 99496[1], G0463[1], G0471[0], P9612[0]
52260	00910[0], 00916[0], 0213T[0], 0216T[0], 0596T[0], 0597T[0], 0708T[1], 0709T[1], 12001[1], 12002[1], 12004[1], 12005[1], 12006[1], 12007[1], 12011[1], 12013[1], 12014[1], 12015[1], 12016[1], 12017[1], 12018[1], 12020[1], 12021[1], 12031[1], 12032[1], 12034[1], 12035[1], 12036[1], 12037[1], 12041[1], 12042[1], 12044[1], 12045[1], 12046[1], 12047[1], 12051[1], 12052[1], 12053[1], 12054[1], 12055[1], 12056[1], 12057[1], 13100[1], 13101[1], 13102[1], 13120[1], 13121[1], 13122[1], 13131[1], 13132[1], 13133[1], 13151[1], 13152[1], 13153[1], 36000[1], 36400[1], 36405[1], 36406[1], 36410[1], 36420[1], 36425[1], 36430[1], 36440[1], 36591[0], 36592[0], 36600[1], 36640[1], 43752[1], 50715[1], 51701[0], 51702[0], 51703[0], 52000[0], 52001[1], 52005[0], 52204[1], 52281[0], 52310[0], 52315[0], 53000[0], 53010[0], 53020[0], 53025[0], 53600[0], 53601[0], 53605[0], 53620[0], 53621[0], 53660[0], 53661[0], 53665[0], 57410[0], 62320[0], 62321[0], 62322[0], 62323[0], 62324[0], 62325[0], 62326[0], 62327[0], 64400[0], 64405[0], 64408[0], 64415[0], 64416[0], 64417[0], 64418[0], 64420[0], 64421[0], 64425[0], 64430[0], 64435[0], 64445[0], 64446[0], 64447[0], 64448[0], 64449[0], 64450[0], 64451[0], 64454[0], 64461[0], 64462[0], 64463[0], 64479[0], 64480[0], 64483[0], 64484[0], 64486[0], 64487[0], 64488[0], 64489[0], 64490[0], 64491[0], 64492[0], 64493[0], 64494[0], 64495[0], 64505[0], 64510[0], 64517[0], 64520[0], 64530[0], 69990[0], 76000[1], 77001[1], 77002[1], 92012[1], 92014[1], 93000[1], 93005[1], 93010[1], 93040[1], 93041[1], 93042[1], 93318[1], 93355[1], 94002[1], 94200[1], 94680[1], 94681[1], 94690[1], 95812[1], 95813[1], 95816[1], 95819[1], 95822[1], 95829[1], 95955[1], 96360[1], 96361[1], 96365[1], 96366[1], 96367[1], 96368[1], 96372[1], 96374[1], 96375[1], 96376[1], 96377[1], 96523[0], 99151[0], 99152[0], 99153[0], 99155[0], 99156[0], 99157[0], 99211[1], 99212[1], 99213[1], 99214[1], 99215[1], 99217[1], 99218[1], 99219[1], 99220[1], 99221[1], 99222[1], 99223[1], 99231[1], 99232[1], 99233[1], 99234[1], 99235[1], 99236[1], 99238[1], 99239[1], 99241[1], 99242[1], 99243[1], 99244[1], 99245[1], 99251[1], 99252[1], 99253[1], 99254[1], 99255[1], 99291[1], 99292[1], 99304[1], 99305[1], 99306[1], 99307[1], 99308[1], 99309[1], 99310[1], 99315[1], 99316[1], 99334[1], 99335[1], 99336[1], 99337[1], 99347[1], 99348[1], 99349[1], 99350[1], 99374[1], 99375[1], 99377[1], 99378[1], 99446[0], 99447[0], 99448[0], 99449[0], 99451[0], 99452[0], 99495[1], 99496[1], G0463[1], G0471[0], P9612[0]
52265	00910[0], 00916[0], 0213T[0], 0216T[0], 0596T[0], 0597T[0], 0708T[1], 0709T[1], 12001[1], 12002[1], 12004[1], 12005[1], 12006[1], 12007[1], 12011[1], 12013[1], 12014[1], 12015[1], 12016[1], 12017[1], 12018[1], 12020[1], 12021[1], 12031[1], 12032[1], 12034[1], 12035[1], 12036[1], 12037[1], 12041[1], 12042[1], 12044[1], 12045[1], 12046[1], 12047[1], 12051[1], 12052[1], 12053[1], 12054[1], 12055[1], 12056[1], 12057[1], 13100[1], 13101[1], 13102[1], 13120[1], 13121[1], 13122[1], 13131[1], 13132[1], 13133[1], 13151[1], 13152[1], 13153[1], 36000[1], 36400[1], 36405[1], 36406[1], 36410[1], 36420[1], 36425[1], 36430[1], 36440[1], 36591[0], 36592[0], 36600[1], 36640[1], 43752[1], 51701[0], 51702[0], 51703[0], 52000[0], 52001[1], 52204[1], 52260[1], 52281[0], 52310[0], 52315[0], 53000[0], 53010[0], 53020[0], 53025[0], 53600[0], 53601[0], 53605[0], 53620[0], 53621[0], 53660[0], 53661[0], 53665[0], 57410[0], 62320[0], 62321[0], 62322[0], 62323[0], 62324[0], 62325[0], 62326[0], 62327[0], 64400[0], 64405[0], 64408[0], 64415[0], 64416[0], 64417[0], 64418[0], 64420[0], 64421[0], 64425[0], 64430[0], 64435[0], 64445[0], 64446[0], 64447[0], 64448[0], 64449[0], 64450[0], 64451[0], 64454[0], 64461[0], 64462[0], 64463[0], 64479[0], 64480[0], 64483[0], 64484[0], 64486[0], 64487[0], 64488[0], 64489[0], 64490[0], 64491[0], 64492[0], 64493[0], 64494[0], 64495[0], 64505[0], 64510[0], 64517[0], 64520[0], 64530[0], 69990[0], 76000[1], 77001[1], 77002[1], 92012[1], 92014[1], 93000[1], 93005[1], 93010[1], 93040[1], 93041[1], 93042[1], 93318[1], 93355[1], 94002[1], 94200[1], 94680[1], 94681[1], 94690[1], 95812[1], 95813[1], 95816[1], 95819[1], 95822[1], 95829[1], 95955[1], 96360[1], 96361[1], 96365[1], 96366[1], 96367[1], 96368[1], 96372[1], 96374[1], 96375[1], 96376[1], 96377[1], 96523[0], 99155[0], 99156[0], 99157[0], 99211[1], 99212[1], 99213[1], 99214[1], 99215[1], 99217[1], 99218[1], 99219[1], 99220[1], 99221[1], 99222[1], 99223[1], 99231[1], 99232[1], 99233[1], 99234[1], 99235[1], 99236[1], 99238[1], 99239[1], 99241[1], 99242[1], 99243[1], 99244[1], 99245[1], 99251[1], 99252[1], 99253[1], 99254[1], 99255[1], 99291[1], 99292[1], 99304[1], 99305[1], 99306[1], 99307[1], 99308[1], 99309[1], 99310[1], 99315[1], 99316[1], 99334[1], 99335[1], 99336[1], 99337[1], 99347[1], 99348[1], 99349[1], 99350[1], 99374[1], 99375[1], 99377[1], 99378[1], 99446[0], 99447[0], 99448[0], 99449[0], 99451[0], 99452[0], 99495[1], 99496[1], G0463[1], G0471[0], J2001[1], P9612[0]
52270	00910[0], 00916[0], 0213T[0], 0216T[0], 0596T[0], 0597T[0], 0708T[1], 0709T[1], 11000[1], 11001[1], 11004[1], 11005[1], 11006[1], 11042[1], 11043[1], 11044[1], 11045[1], 11046[1], 11047[1], 12001[1], 12002[1], 12004[1], 12005[1], 12006[1], 12007[1], 12011[1], 12013[1], 12014[1], 12015[1], 12016[1], 12017[1], 12018[1], 12020[1], 12021[1], 12031[1], 12032[1], 12034[1], 12035[1], 12036[1], 12037[1], 12041[1], 12042[1], 12044[1], 12045[1], 12046[1], 12047[1], 12051[1], 12052[1], 12053[1], 12054[1], 12055[1], 12056[1], 12057[1], 13100[1], 13101[1], 13102[1], 13120[1], 13121[1], 13122[1], 13131[1], 13132[1], 13133[1], 13151[1], 13152[1], 13153[1], 36000[1], 36400[1], 36405[1], 36406[1], 36410[1], 36420[1], 36425[1], 36430[1], 36440[1], 36591[0], 36592[0], 36600[1], 36640[1], 43752[1], 51701[0], 51702[0], 51703[0], 52000[0], 52001[1], 52281[0], 52310[0], 52315[0], 53000[0], 53010[0], 53020[0], 53025[0], 53600[0], 53601[0], 53605[0], 53620[0], 53621[0], 53660[0], 53661[0], 53665[0], 57410[0], 62320[0], 62321[0], 62322[0], 62323[0], 62324[0], 62325[0], 62326[0], 62327[0], 64400[0], 64405[0], 64408[0], 64415[0], 64416[0], 64417[0], 64418[0], 64420[0], 64421[0], 64425[0], 64430[0], 64435[0], 64445[0], 64446[0], 64447[0], 64448[0], 64449[0], 64450[0], 64451[0], 64454[0], 64461[0], 64462[0], 64463[0], 64479[0], 64480[0], 64483[0], 64484[0], 64486[0], 64487[0], 64488[0], 64489[0], 64490[0], 64491[0], 64492[0], 64493[0], 64494[0], 64495[0], 64505[0], 64510[0], 64517[0], 64520[0], 64530[0], 69990[0], 76000[1], 77001[1], 77002[1], 92012[1], 92014[1], 93000[1], 93005[1], 93010[1], 93040[1], 93041[1], 93042[1], 93318[1], 93355[1], 94002[1], 94200[1], 94680[1], 94681[1], 94690[1], 95812[1], 95813[1], 95816[1], 95819[1], 95822[1], 95829[1], 95955[1], 96360[1], 96361[1], 96365[1], 96366[1], 96367[1], 96368[1], 96372[1], 96374[1], 96375[1], 96376[1], 96377[1], 96523[0], 97597[1], 97598[1], 97602[1], 99155[0], 99156[0], 99157[0], 99211[1], 99212[1], 99213[1], 99214[1], 99215[1], 99217[1], 99218[1], 99219[1], 99220[1], 99221[1], 99222[1], 99223[1], 99231[1], 99232[1], 99233[1], 99234[1], 99235[1], 99236[1], 99238[1], 99239[1], 99241[1], 99242[1], 99243[1], 99244[1], 99245[1], 99251[1], 99252[1], 99253[1], 99254[1], 99255[1], 99291[1], 99292[1], 99304[1], 99305[1], 99306[1], 99307[1], 99308[1], 99309[1], 99310[1], 99315[1], 99316[1], 99334[1], 99335[1], 99336[1], 99337[1], 99347[1], 99348[1], 99349[1], 99350[1], 99374[1], 99375[1], 99377[1], 99378[1], 99446[0], 99447[0], 99448[0], 99449[0], 99451[0], 99452[0], 99495[1], 99496[1], G0463[1], G0471[0], J2001[1], P9612[0]
52275	00910[0], 00916[0], 0213T[0], 0216T[0], 0596T[0], 0597T[0], 0708T[1], 0709T[1], 11000[1], 11001[1], 11004[1], 11005[1], 11006[1], 11042[1], 11043[1], 11044[1], 11045[1], 11046[1], 11047[1], 12001[1], 12002[1], 12004[1], 12005[1], 12006[1], 12007[1], 12011[1], 12013[1], 12014[1], 12015[1], 12016[1], 12017[1], 12018[1], 12020[1], 12021[1], 12031[1], 12032[1], 12034[1], 12035[1], 12036[1], 12037[1], 12041[1], 12042[1], 12044[1], 12045[1], 12046[1], 12047[1], 12051[1], 12052[1], 12053[1], 12054[1], 12055[1], 12056[1], 12057[1], 13100[1], 13101[1], 13102[1], 13120[1], 13121[1], 13122[1], 13131[1], 13132[1], 13133[1], 13151[1], 13152[1], 13153[1], 36000[1], 36400[1], 36405[1], 36406[1], 36410[1], 36420[1], 36425[1], 36430[1], 36440[1], 36591[0], 36592[0], 36600[1], 36640[1], 43752[1], 51701[0], 51702[0], 51703[0], 52000[0], 52001[1], 52270[1], 52276[1], 52281[0], 52310[0], 52315[0], 53000[0], 53010[0], 53020[0], 53025[0], 53600[0], 53601[0], 53605[0], 53620[0], 53621[0], 53660[0], 53661[0], 53665[0], 57410[0], 62320[0], 62321[0], 62322[0], 62323[0], 62324[0], 62325[0], 62326[0], 62327[0], 64400[0], 64405[0], 64408[0], 64415[0], 64416[0], 64417[0], 64418[0], 64420[0], 64421[0], 64425[0], 64430[0], 64435[0], 64445[0], 64446[0], 64447[0], 64448[0], 64449[0], 64450[0], 64451[0], 64454[0], 64461[0], 64462[0], 64463[0], 64479[0], 64480[0], 64483[0], 64484[0], 64486[0], 64487[0], 64488[0], 64489[0], 64490[0], 64491[0], 64492[0], 64493[0], 64494[0], 64495[0], 64505[0], 64510[0], 64517[0], 64520[0], 64530[0], 69990[0], 76000[1], 77001[1], 77002[1], 92012[1], 92014[1], 93000[1], 93005[1], 93010[1], 93040[1], 93041[1], 93042[1], 93318[1], 93355[1], 94002[1], 94200[1], 94680[1], 94681[1], 94690[1], 95812[1], 95813[1], 95816[1], 95819[1], 95822[1], 95829[1], 95955[1], 96360[1], 96361[1], 96365[1], 96366[1], 96367[1], 96368[1], 96372[1], 96374[1], 96375[1], 96376[1], 96377[1], 96523[0], 97597[1], 97598[1], 97602[1], 99155[0], 99156[0], 99157[0], 99211[1], 99212[1], 99213[1], 99214[1], 99215[1], 99217[1], 99218[1], 99219[1], 99220[1], 99221[1], 99222[1], 99223[1], 99231[1], 99232[1], 99233[1], 99234[1], 99235[1], 99236[1], 99238[1], 99239[1], 99241[1], 99242[1], 99243[1], 99244[1], 99245[1], 99251[1], 99252[1], 99253[1], 99254[1], 99255[1], 99291[1], 99292[1], 99304[1], 99305[1],

0 = Modifier usage not allowed or inappropriate 1 = Modifier usage allowed

Code 1	Code 2
	99306[1], 99307[1], 99308[1], 99309[1], 99310[1], 99315[1], 99316[1], 99334[1], 99335[1], 99336[1], 99337[1], 99347[1], 99348[1], 99349[1], 99350[1], 99374[1], 99375[1], 99377[1], 99378[1], 99446[0], 99447[0], 99448[0], 99449[0], 99451[0], 99452[0], 99495[1], 99496[1], G0463[1], G0471[0], J2001[1], P9612[0]
52276	00910[0], 00916[0], 0213T[0], 0216T[0], 0596T[0], 0597T[0], 0708T[1], 0709T[1], 11000[1], 11001[1], 11004[1], 11005[1], 11006[1], 11042[1], 11043[1], 11044[1], 11045[1], 11046[1], 11047[1], 12001[1], 12002[1], 12004[1], 12005[1], 12006[1], 12007[1], 12011[1], 12013[1], 12014[1], 12015[1], 12016[1], 12017[1], 12018[1], 12020[1], 12021[1], 12031[1], 12032[1], 12034[1], 12035[1], 12036[1], 12037[1], 12041[1], 12042[1], 12044[1], 12045[1], 12046[1], 12047[1], 12051[1], 12052[1], 12053[1], 12054[1], 12055[1], 12056[1], 12057[1], 13100[1], 13101[1], 13102[1], 13120[1], 13121[1], 13122[1], 13131[1], 13132[1], 13133[1], 13151[1], 13152[1], 13153[1], 36000[1], 36400[1], 36405[1], 36406[1], 36410[1], 36420[1], 36425[1], 36430[1], 36440[1], 36591[0], 36592[0], 36600[1], 36640[1], 43752[1], 51102[1], 51700[0], 51701[0], 51702[0], 51703[0], 52000[0], 52001[1], 52204[1], 52270[1], 52281[0], 52310[0], 52315[0], 53000[0], 53010[0], 53020[0], 53025[0], 53600[0], 53601[0], 53605[0], 53620[0], 53621[0], 53660[0], 53661[0], 53665[0], 57410[0], 62320[0], 62321[0], 62322[0], 62323[0], 62324[0], 62325[0], 62326[0], 62327[0], 64400[0], 64405[0], 64408[0], 64415[0], 64416[0], 64417[0], 64418[0], 64420[0], 64421[0], 64425[0], 64430[0], 64435[0], 64445[0], 64446[0], 64447[0], 64448[0], 64449[0], 64450[0], 64451[0], 64454[0], 64461[0], 64462[0], 64463[0], 64479[0], 64480[0], 64483[0], 64484[0], 64486[0], 64487[0], 64488[0], 64489[0], 64490[0], 64491[0], 64492[0], 64493[0], 64494[0], 64495[0], 64505[0], 64510[0], 64517[0], 64520[0], 64530[0], 69990[0], 76000[1], 77001[1], 77002[1], 92012[1], 92014[1], 93000[1], 93005[1], 93010[1], 93040[1], 93041[1], 93042[1], 93318[1], 93355[1], 94002[1], 94200[1], 94680[1], 94681[1], 94690[1], 95812[1], 95813[1], 95816[1], 95819[1], 95822[1], 95829[1], 95955[1], 96360[1], 96361[1], 96365[1], 96366[1], 96367[1], 96368[1], 96372[1], 96374[1], 96375[1], 96376[1], 96377[1], 96523[0], 97597[1], 97598[1], 97602[1], 99155[0], 99156[0], 99157[0], 99211[1], 99212[1], 99213[1], 99214[1], 99215[1], 99217[1], 99218[1], 99219[1], 99220[1], 99221[1], 99222[1], 99223[1], 99231[1], 99232[1], 99233[1], 99234[1], 99235[1], 99236[1], 99238[1], 99239[1], 99241[1], 99242[1], 99243[1], 99244[1], 99245[1], 99251[1], 99252[1], 99253[1], 99254[1], 99255[1], 99291[1], 99292[1], 99304[1], 99305[1], 99306[1], 99307[1], 99308[1], 99309[1], 99310[1], 99315[1], 99316[1], 99334[1], 99335[1], 99336[1], 99337[1], 99347[1], 99348[1], 99349[1], 99350[1], 99374[1], 99375[1], 99377[1], 99378[1], 99446[0], 99447[0], 99448[0], 99449[0], 99451[0], 99452[0], 99495[1], 99496[1], G0463[1], G0471[0], J2001[1], P9612[0]
52277	00910[0], 00916[0], 0213T[0], 0216T[0], 0596T[0], 0597T[0], 0708T[1], 0709T[1], 11000[1], 11001[1], 11004[1], 11005[1], 11006[1], 11042[1], 11043[1], 11044[1], 11045[1], 11046[1], 11047[1], 12001[1], 12002[1], 12004[1], 12005[1], 12006[1], 12007[1], 12011[1], 12013[1], 12014[1], 12015[1], 12016[1], 12017[1], 12018[1], 12020[1], 12021[1], 12031[1], 12032[1], 12034[1], 12035[1], 12036[1], 12037[1], 12041[1], 12042[1], 12044[1], 12045[1], 12046[1], 12047[1], 12051[1], 12052[1], 12053[1], 12054[1], 12055[1], 12056[1], 12057[1], 13100[1], 13101[1], 13102[1], 13120[1], 13121[1], 13122[1], 13131[1], 13132[1], 13133[1], 13151[1], 13152[1], 13153[1], 36000[1], 36400[1], 36405[1], 36406[1], 36410[1], 36420[1], 36425[1], 36430[1], 36440[1], 36591[0], 36592[0], 36600[1], 36640[1], 43752[1], 51701[0], 51702[0], 51703[0], 52000[0], 52001[1], 52281[0], 52301[1], 52310[0], 52315[0], 53000[0], 53010[0], 53020[0], 53025[0], 53600[0], 53601[0], 53605[0], 53620[0], 53621[0], 53660[0], 53661[0], 53665[0], 57410[0], 62320[0], 62321[0], 62322[0], 62323[0], 62324[0], 62325[0], 62326[0], 62327[0], 64400[0], 64405[0], 64408[0], 64415[0], 64416[0], 64417[0], 64418[0], 64420[0], 64421[0], 64425[0], 64430[0], 64435[0], 64445[0], 64446[0], 64447[0], 64448[0], 64449[0], 64450[0], 64451[0], 64454[0], 64461[0], 64462[0], 64463[0], 64479[0], 64480[0], 64483[0], 64484[0], 64486[0], 64487[0], 64488[0], 64489[0], 64490[0], 64491[0], 64492[0], 64493[0], 64494[0], 64495[0], 64505[0], 64510[0], 64517[0], 64520[0], 64530[0], 69990[0], 76000[1], 77001[1], 77002[1], 92012[1], 92014[1], 93000[1], 93005[1], 93010[1], 93040[1], 93041[1], 93042[1], 93318[1], 93355[1], 94002[1], 94200[1], 94680[1], 94681[1], 94690[1], 95812[1], 95813[1], 95816[1], 95819[1], 95822[1], 95829[1], 95955[1], 96360[1], 96361[1], 96365[1], 96366[1], 96367[1], 96368[1], 96372[1], 96374[1], 96375[1], 96376[1], 96377[1], 96523[0], 97597[1], 97598[1], 97602[1], 99155[0], 99156[0], 99157[0], 99211[1], 99212[1], 99213[1], 99214[1], 99215[1], 99217[1], 99218[1], 99219[1], 99220[1], 99221[1], 99222[1], 99223[1], 99231[1], 99232[1], 99233[1], 99234[1], 99235[1], 99236[1], 99238[1], 99239[1], 99241[1], 99242[1], 99243[1], 99244[1], 99245[1], 99251[1], 99252[1], 99253[1], 99254[1], 99255[1], 99291[1], 99292[1], 99304[1], 99305[1], 99306[1], 99307[1], 99308[1], 99309[1], 99310[1], 99315[1], 99316[1], 99334[1], 99335[1], 99336[1], 99337[1], 99347[1], 99348[1], 99349[1], 99350[1], 99374[1], 99375[1], 99377[1], 99378[1], 99446[0], 99447[0], 99448[0], 99449[0], 99451[0], 99452[0], 99495[1], 99496[1], G0463[1], G0471[0], P9612[0]
52281	00910[0], 00916[0], 0213T[0], 0216T[0], 0596T[0], 0597T[0], 0708T[1], 0709T[1], 11000[1], 11001[1], 11004[1], 11005[1], 11006[1], 11042[1], 11043[1], 11044[1], 11045[1], 11046[1], 11047[1], 12001[1], 12002[1], 12004[1], 12005[1], 12006[1], 12007[1], 12011[1], 12013[1], 12014[1], 12015[1], 12016[1], 12017[1], 12018[1], 12020[1], 12021[1], 12031[1], 12032[1], 12034[1], 12035[1], 12036[1], 12037[1], 12041[1], 12042[1], 12044[1], 12045[1], 12046[1], 12047[1], 12051[1], 12052[1], 12053[1], 12054[1], 12055[1], 12056[1], 12057[1], 13100[1], 13101[1], 13102[1], 13120[1], 13121[1], 13122[1], 13131[1], 13132[1], 13133[1], 13151[1], 13152[1], 13153[1], 36000[1], 36400[1], 36405[1], 36406[1], 36410[1], 36420[1], 36425[1], 36430[1], 36440[1], 36591[0], 36592[0], 36600[1], 36640[1], 43752[1], 51600[1], 51605[1], 51610[1], 51700[0], 51701[0], 51702[0], 51703[0], 51720[1], 52000[0], 52005[0], 52204[0], 52283[0], 52287[0], 52310[0], 53000[0], 53010[0], 53020[0], 53025[0], 53600[0], 53601[0], 53605[0], 53620[0], 53621[0], 53660[0], 53661[0], 53665[0], 57410[0], 62320[0], 62321[0], 62322[0], 62323[0], 62324[0], 62325[0], 62326[0], 62327[0], 64400[0], 64405[0], 64408[0], 64415[0], 64416[0], 64417[0], 64418[0], 64420[0], 64421[0], 64425[0], 64430[0], 64435[0], 64445[0], 64446[0], 64447[0], 64448[0], 64449[0], 64450[0], 64451[0], 64454[0], 64461[0], 64462[0], 64463[0], 64479[0], 64480[0], 64483[0], 64484[0], 64486[0], 64487[0], 64488[0], 64489[0], 64490[0], 64491[0], 64492[0], 64493[0], 64494[0], 64495[0], 64505[0], 64510[0], 64517[0], 64520[0], 64530[0], 69990[0], 76000[1], 77001[1], 77002[1], 92012[1], 92014[1], 93000[1], 93005[1], 93010[1], 93040[1], 93041[1], 93042[1], 93318[1], 93355[1], 94002[1], 94200[1], 94680[1], 94681[1], 94690[1], 95812[1], 95813[1], 95816[1], 95819[1], 95822[1], 95829[1], 95955[1], 96360[1], 96361[1], 96365[1], 96366[1], 96367[1], 96368[1], 96372[1], 96374[1], 96375[1], 96376[1], 96377[1], 96523[0], 97597[1], 97598[1], 97602[1], 99155[0], 99156[0], 99157[0], 99211[1], 99212[1], 99213[1], 99214[1], 99215[1], 99217[1], 99218[1], 99219[1], 99220[1], 99221[1], 99222[1], 99223[1], 99231[1], 99232[1], 99233[1], 99234[1], 99235[1], 99236[1], 99238[1], 99239[1], 99241[1], 99242[1], 99243[1], 99244[1], 99245[1], 99251[1], 99252[1], 99253[1], 99254[1], 99255[1], 99291[1], 99292[1], 99304[1], 99305[1], 99306[1], 99307[1], 99308[1], 99309[1], 99310[1], 99315[1], 99316[1], 99334[1], 99335[1], 99336[1], 99337[1], 99347[1], 99348[1], 99349[1], 99350[1], 99374[1], 99375[1], 99377[1], 99378[1], 99446[0], 99447[0], 99448[0], 99449[0], 99451[0], 99452[0], 99495[1], 99496[1], G0463[1], G0471[0], P9612[0]
52282	00910[0], 00916[0], 0213T[0], 0216T[0], 0596T[0], 0597T[0], 0619T[0], 0708T[1], 0709T[1], 11000[1], 11001[1], 11004[1], 11005[1], 11006[1], 11042[1], 11043[1], 11044[1], 11045[1], 11046[1], 11047[1], 12001[1], 12002[1], 12004[1], 12005[1], 12006[1], 12007[1], 12011[1], 12013[1], 12014[1], 12015[1], 12016[1], 12017[1], 12018[1], 12020[1], 12021[1], 12031[1], 12032[1], 12034[1], 12035[1], 12036[1], 12037[1], 12041[1], 12042[1], 12044[1], 12045[1], 12046[1], 12047[1], 12051[1], 12052[1], 12053[1], 12054[1], 12055[1], 12056[1], 12057[1], 13100[1], 13101[1], 13102[1], 13120[1], 13121[1], 13122[1], 13131[1], 13132[1], 13133[1], 13151[1], 13152[1], 13153[1], 36000[1], 36400[1], 36405[1], 36406[1], 36410[1], 36420[1], 36425[1], 36430[1], 36440[1], 36591[0], 36592[0], 36600[1], 36640[1], 43752[1], 51701[0], 51702[0], 51703[0], 52000[0], 52001[1], 52281[0], 52310[0], 52315[0], 52441[0], 53000[0], 53010[0], 53020[0], 53025[0], 53600[0], 53601[0], 53605[0], 53620[0], 53621[0], 53660[0], 53661[0], 53665[0], 53855[1], 57410[0], 62320[0], 62321[0], 62322[0], 62323[0], 62324[0], 62325[0], 62326[0], 62327[0], 64400[0], 64405[0], 64408[0], 64415[0], 64416[0], 64417[0], 64418[0], 64420[0], 64421[0], 64425[0], 64430[0], 64435[0], 64445[0], 64446[0], 64447[0], 64448[0], 64449[0], 64450[0], 64451[0], 64454[0], 64461[0], 64462[0], 64463[0], 64479[0], 64480[0], 64483[0], 64484[0], 64486[0], 64487[0], 64488[0], 64489[0], 64490[0], 64491[0], 64492[0], 64493[0], 64494[0], 64495[0], 64505[0], 64510[0], 64517[0], 64520[0], 64530[0], 69990[0], 76000[1], 77001[1], 77002[1], 92012[1], 92014[1], 93000[1], 93005[1], 93010[1], 93040[1], 93041[1], 93042[1], 93318[1], 93355[1], 94002[1], 94200[1], 94680[1], 94681[1], 94690[1], 95812[1], 95813[1], 95816[1], 95819[1], 95822[1], 95829[1], 95955[1], 96360[1], 96361[1], 96365[1], 96366[1], 96367[1], 96368[1], 96372[1], 96374[1], 96375[1], 96376[1], 96377[1], 96523[0], 97597[1], 97598[1], 97602[1], 99155[0], 99156[0], 99157[0], 99211[1], 99212[1], 99213[1], 99214[1], 99215[1], 99217[1], 99218[1], 99219[1], 99220[1], 99221[1], 99222[1], 99223[1], 99231[1], 99232[1], 99233[1], 99234[1], 99235[1], 99236[1], 99238[1], 99239[1], 99241[1], 99242[1], 99243[1], 99244[1], 99245[1], 99251[1], 99252[1], 99253[1], 99254[1], 99255[1], 99291[1], 99292[1], 99304[1], 99305[1], 99306[1], 99307[1], 99308[1], 99309[1], 99310[1], 99315[1], 99316[1], 99334[1], 99335[1], 99336[1], 99337[1], 99347[1], 99348[1], 99349[1], 99350[1], 99374[1], 99375[1], 99377[1], 99378[1], 99446[0], 99447[0], 99448[0], 99449[0], 99451[0], 99452[0], 99495[1], 99496[1], G0463[1], G0471[0], J2001[1], P9612[0]
52283	00910[0], 00916[0], 0213T[0], 0216T[0], 0596T[0], 0597T[0], 0708T[1], 0709T[1], 12001[1], 12002[1], 12004[1], 12005[1], 12006[1], 12007[1], 12011[1], 12013[1], 12014[1], 12015[1], 12016[1], 12017[1], 12018[1], 12020[1], 12021[1], 12031[1], 12032[1], 12034[1], 12035[1], 12036[1], 12037[1], 12041[1], 12042[1], 12044[1], 12045[1], 12046[1], 12047[1], 12051[1], 12052[1], 12053[1], 12054[1], 12055[1], 12056[1], 12057[1], 13100[1], 13101[1], 13102[1], 13120[1], 13121[1], 13122[1], 13131[1], 13132[1], 13133[1], 13151[1], 13152[1], 13153[1], 36000[1], 36400[1], 36405[1], 36406[1], 36410[1], 36420[1], 36425[1], 36430[1], 36440[1], 36591[0], 36592[0], 36600[1], 36640[1], 43752[1], 51701[0], 51702[0], 51703[0], 52000[0], 52001[1], 52310[0], 52315[0], 53000[0], 53010[0], 53020[0], 53025[0], 53600[0], 53601[0], 53605[0], 53620[0], 53621[0], 53660[0], 53661[0], 53665[0], 57410[0], 62320[0], 62321[0], 62322[0], 62323[0], 62324[0], 62325[0], 62326[0], 62327[0], 64400[0], 64405[0], 64408[0], 64415[0], 64416[0], 64417[0], 64418[0], 64420[0], 64421[0], 64425[0], 64430[0], 64435[0], 64445[0], 64446[0], 64447[0], 64448[0], 64449[0], 64450[0], 64451[0], 64454[0], 64461[0], 64462[0], 64463[0], 64479[0], 64480[0], 64483[0], 64484[0], 64486[0], 64487[0], 64488[0], 64489[0], 64490[0], 64491[0], 64492[0], 64493[0], 64494[0], 64495[0], 64505[0], 64510[0], 64517[0], 64520[0], 64530[0], 69990[0], 76000[1], 77001[1], 77002[1], 92012[1], 92014[1], 93000[1], 93005[1], 93010[1], 93040[1], 93041[1], 93042[1], 93318[1], 93355[1], 94002[1], 94200[1], 94680[1], 94681[1], 94690[1], 95812[1], 95813[1], 95816[1], 95819[1], 95822[1], 95829[1], 95955[1], 96360[1], 96361[1], 96365[1], 96366[1], 96367[1], 96368[1], 96372[1], 96374[1], 96375[1], 96376[1], 96377[1], 96523[0], 99155[0], 99156[0], 99157[0], 99211[1], 99212[1], 99213[1], 99214[1], 99215[1], 99217[1], 99218[1], 99219[1], 99220[1], 99221[1], 99222[1], 99223[1], 99231[1], 99232[1], 99233[1], 99234[1], 99235[1], 99236[1], 99238[1], 99239[1], 99241[1],

0 = Modifier usage not allowed or inappropriate   1 = Modifier usage allowed

Code 1	Code 2
	99242[1], 99243[1], 99244[1], 99245[1], 99251[1], 99252[1], 99253[1], 99254[1], 99255[1], 99291[1], 99292[1], 99304[1], 99305[1], 99306[1], 99307[1], 99308[1], 99309[1], 99310[1], 99315[1], 99316[1], 99334[1], 99335[1], 99336[1], 99337[1], 99347[1], 99348[1], 99349[1], 99350[1], 99374[1], 99375[1], 99377[1], 99378[1], 99446[0], 99447[0], 99448[0], 99449[0], 99451[0], 99452[0], 99495[1], 99496[1], G0463[1], G0471[0], J2001[1], P9612[0]
52285	00910[0], 00916[0], 0213T[0], 0216T[0], 0596T[0], 0597T[0], 0708T[1], 0709T[1], 11000[1], 11001[1], 11004[1], 11005[1], 11006[1], 11042[1], 11043[1], 11044[1], 11045[1], 11046[1], 11047[1], 12001[1], 12002[1], 12004[1], 12005[1], 12006[1], 12007[1], 12011[1], 12013[1], 12014[1], 12015[1], 12016[1], 12017[1], 12018[1], 12020[1], 12021[1], 12031[1], 12032[1], 12034[1], 12035[1], 12036[1], 12037[1], 12041[1], 12042[1], 12044[1], 12045[1], 12046[1], 12047[1], 12051[1], 12052[1], 12053[1], 12054[1], 12055[1], 12056[1], 12057[1], 13100[1], 13101[1], 13102[1], 13120[1], 13121[1], 13122[1], 13131[1], 13132[1], 13133[1], 13151[1], 13152[1], 13153[1], 36000[1], 36400[1], 36405[1], 36406[1], 36410[1], 36420[1], 36425[1], 36430[1], 36440[1], 36591[0], 36592[0], 36600[1], 36640[1], 43752[1], 51701[0], 51702[0], 51703[0], 52000[0], 52001[1], 52005[1], 52214[1], 52270[1], 52276[1], 52281[0], 52310[0], 52315[0], 53000[0], 53010[0], 53020[0], 53025[0], 53600[0], 53601[0], 53605[0], 53620[0], 53621[0], 53660[0], 53661[0], 53665[0], 57410[0], 62320[0], 62321[0], 62322[0], 62323[0], 62324[0], 62325[0], 62326[0], 62327[0], 64400[0], 64405[0], 64408[0], 64415[0], 64416[0], 64417[0], 64418[0], 64420[0], 64421[0], 64425[0], 64430[0], 64435[0], 64445[0], 64446[0], 64447[0], 64448[0], 64449[0], 64450[0], 64451[0], 64454[0], 64461[0], 64462[0], 64463[0], 64479[0], 64480[0], 64483[0], 64484[0], 64486[0], 64487[0], 64488[0], 64489[0], 64490[0], 64491[0], 64492[0], 64493[0], 64494[0], 64495[0], 64505[0], 64510[0], 64517[0], 64520[0], 64530[0], 69990[0], 76000[1], 77001[1], 77002[1], 92012[1], 92014[1], 93000[1], 93005[1], 93010[1], 93040[1], 93041[1], 93042[1], 93318[1], 93355[1], 94002[1], 94200[1], 94680[1], 94681[1], 94690[1], 95812[1], 95813[1], 95816[1], 95819[1], 95822[1], 95829[1], 95955[1], 96360[1], 96361[1], 96365[1], 96366[1], 96367[1], 96368[1], 96372[1], 96374[1], 96375[1], 96376[1], 96377[1], 96523[0], 97597[1], 97598[1], 97602[1], 99155[0], 99156[0], 99157[0], 99211[1], 99212[1], 99213[1], 99214[1], 99215[1], 99217[1], 99218[1], 99219[1], 99220[1], 99221[1], 99222[1], 99223[1], 99231[1], 99232[1], 99233[1], 99234[1], 99235[1], 99236[1], 99238[1], 99239[1], 99241[1], 99242[1], 99243[1], 99244[1], 99245[1], 99251[1], 99252[1], 99253[1], 99254[1], 99255[1], 99291[1], 99292[1], 99304[1], 99305[1], 99306[1], 99307[1], 99308[1], 99309[1], 99310[1], 99315[1], 99316[1], 99334[1], 99335[1], 99336[1], 99337[1], 99347[1], 99348[1], 99349[1], 99350[1], 99374[1], 99375[1], 99377[1], 99378[1], 99446[0], 99447[0], 99448[0], 99449[0], 99451[0], 99452[0], 99495[1], 99496[1], G0463[1], G0471[0], J2001[1], P9612[0]
52287	00910[0], 00916[0], 0213T[0], 0216T[0], 0596T[0], 0597T[0], 0708T[1], 0709T[1], 12001[1], 12002[1], 12004[1], 12005[1], 12006[1], 12007[1], 12011[1], 12013[1], 12014[1], 12015[1], 12016[1], 12017[1], 12018[1], 12020[1], 12021[1], 12031[1], 12032[1], 12034[1], 12035[1], 12036[1], 12037[1], 12041[1], 12042[1], 12044[1], 12045[1], 12046[1], 12047[1], 12051[1], 12052[1], 12053[1], 12054[1], 12055[1], 12056[1], 12057[1], 13100[1], 13101[1], 13102[1], 13120[1], 13121[1], 13122[1], 13131[1], 13132[1], 13133[1], 13151[1], 13152[1], 13153[1], 36000[1], 36400[1], 36405[1], 36406[1], 36410[1], 36420[1], 36425[1], 36430[1], 36440[1], 36591[0], 36592[0], 36600[1], 36640[1], 43752[1], 51701[0], 51702[0], 51703[0], 52000[0], 52001[1], 52310[0], 52315[0], 53000[0], 53010[0], 53020[0], 53025[0], 53600[0], 53601[0], 53605[0], 53620[0], 53621[0], 53660[0], 53661[0], 53665[0], 57410[0], 62320[0], 62321[0], 62322[0], 62323[0], 62324[0], 62325[0], 62326[0], 62327[0], 64400[0], 64405[0], 64408[0], 64415[0], 64416[0], 64417[0], 64418[0], 64420[0], 64421[0], 64425[0], 64430[0], 64435[0], 64445[0], 64446[0], 64447[0], 64448[0], 64449[0], 64450[0], 64451[0], 64454[0], 64461[0], 64462[0], 64463[0], 64479[0], 64480[0], 64483[0], 64484[0], 64486[0], 64487[0], 64488[0], 64489[0], 64490[0], 64491[0], 64492[0], 64493[0], 64494[0], 64495[0], 64505[0], 64510[0], 64517[0], 64520[0], 64530[0], 69990[0], 76000[1], 77001[1], 77002[1], 92012[1], 92014[1], 93000[1], 93005[1], 93010[1], 93040[1], 93041[1], 93042[1], 93318[1], 93355[1], 94002[1], 94200[1], 94680[1], 94681[1], 94690[1], 95812[1], 95813[1], 95816[1], 95819[1], 95822[1], 95829[1], 95955[1], 96360[1], 96361[1], 96365[1], 96366[1], 96367[1], 96368[1], 96372[1], 96374[1], 96375[1], 96376[1], 96377[1], 96523[0], 99155[0], 99156[0], 99157[0], 99211[1], 99212[1], 99213[1], 99214[1], 99215[1], 99217[1], 99218[1], 99219[1], 99220[1], 99221[1], 99222[1], 99223[1], 99231[1], 99232[1], 99233[1], 99234[1], 99235[1], 99236[1], 99238[1], 99239[1], 99241[1], 99242[1], 99243[1], 99244[1], 99245[1], 99251[1], 99252[1], 99253[1], 99254[1], 99255[1], 99291[1], 99292[1], 99304[1], 99305[1], 99306[1], 99307[1], 99308[1], 99309[1], 99310[1], 99315[1], 99316[1], 99334[1], 99335[1], 99336[1], 99337[1], 99347[1], 99348[1], 99349[1], 99350[1], 99374[1], 99375[1], 99377[1], 99378[1], 99446[0], 99447[0], 99448[0], 99449[0], 99451[0], 99452[0], 99495[1], 99496[1], G0463[1], G0471[0], J0670[1], J2001[1], P9612[0]
52290	00910[0], 00916[0], 0213T[0], 0216T[0], 0596T[0], 0597T[0], 0708T[1], 0709T[1], 11000[1], 11001[1], 11004[1], 11005[1], 11006[1], 11042[1], 11043[1], 11044[1], 11045[1], 11046[1], 11047[1], 12001[1], 12002[1], 12004[1], 12005[1], 12006[1], 12007[1], 12011[1], 12013[1], 12014[1], 12015[1], 12016[1], 12017[1], 12018[1], 12020[1], 12021[1], 12031[1], 12032[1], 12034[1], 12035[1], 12036[1], 12037[1], 12041[1], 12042[1], 12044[1], 12045[1], 12046[1], 12047[1], 12051[1], 12052[1], 12053[1], 12054[1], 12055[1], 12056[1], 12057[1], 13100[1], 13101[1], 13102[1], 13120[1], 13121[1], 13122[1], 13131[1], 13132[1], 13133[1], 13151[1], 13152[1], 13153[1], 36000[1], 36400[1], 36405[1], 36406[1], 36410[1], 36420[1], 36425[1], 36430[1], 36440[1], 36591[0], 36592[0], 36600[1], 36640[1], 43752[1], 51701[0], 51702[0], 51703[0], 52000[0], 52001[1], 52281[0], 52310[0], 52315[0], 53000[0], 53010[0], 53020[0], 53025[0], 53600[0], 53601[0], 53605[0], 53620[0], 53621[0], 53660[0], 53661[0], 53665[0], 57410[0], 62320[0], 62321[0], 62322[0], 62323[0], 62324[0], 62325[0], 62326[0], 62327[0], 64400[0], 64405[0], 64408[0], 64415[0], 64416[0], 64417[0], 64418[0], 64420[0], 64421[0], 64425[0], 64430[0], 64435[0], 64445[0], 64446[0], 64447[0], 64448[0], 64449[0], 64450[0], 64451[0], 64454[0], 64461[0], 64462[0], 64463[0], 64479[0], 64480[0], 64483[0], 64484[0], 64486[0], 64487[0], 64488[0], 64489[0], 64490[0], 64491[0], 64492[0], 64493[0], 64494[0], 64495[0], 64505[0], 64510[0], 64517[0], 64520[0], 64530[0], 69990[0], 76000[1], 77001[1], 77002[1], 92012[1], 92014[1], 93000[1], 93005[1], 93010[1], 93040[1], 93041[1], 93042[1], 93318[1], 93355[1], 94002[1], 94200[1], 94680[1], 94681[1], 94690[1], 95812[1], 95813[1], 95816[1], 95819[1], 95822[1], 95829[1], 95955[1], 96360[1], 96361[1], 96365[1], 96366[1], 96367[1], 96368[1], 96372[1], 96374[1], 96375[1], 96376[1], 96377[1], 96523[0], 97597[1], 97598[1], 97602[1], 99155[0], 99156[0], 99157[0], 99211[1], 99212[1], 99213[1], 99214[1], 99215[1], 99217[1], 99218[1], 99219[1], 99220[1], 99221[1], 99222[1], 99223[1], 99231[1], 99232[1], 99233[1], 99234[1], 99235[1], 99236[1], 99238[1], 99239[1], 99241[1], 99242[1], 99243[1], 99244[1], 99245[1], 99251[1], 99252[1], 99253[1], 99254[1], 99255[1], 99291[1], 99292[1], 99304[1], 99305[1], 99306[1], 99307[1], 99308[1], 99309[1], 99310[1], 99315[1], 99316[1], 99334[1], 99335[1], 99336[1], 99337[1], 99347[1], 99348[1], 99349[1], 99350[1], 99374[1], 99375[1], 99377[1], 99378[1], 99446[0], 99447[0], 99448[0], 99449[0], 99451[0], 99452[0], 99495[1], 99496[1], G0463[1], G0471[0], P9612[0]
52300	00910[0], 00916[0], 0213T[0], 0216T[0], 0596T[0], 0597T[0], 0708T[1], 0709T[1], 11000[1], 11001[1], 11004[1], 11005[1], 11006[1], 11042[1], 11043[1], 11044[1], 11045[1], 11046[1], 11047[1], 12001[1], 12002[1], 12004[1], 12005[1], 12006[1], 12007[1], 12011[1], 12013[1], 12014[1], 12015[1], 12016[1], 12017[1], 12018[1], 12020[1], 12021[1], 12031[1], 12032[1], 12034[1], 12035[1], 12036[1], 12037[1], 12041[1], 12042[1], 12044[1], 12045[1], 12046[1], 12047[1], 12051[1], 12052[1], 12053[1], 12054[1], 12055[1], 12056[1], 12057[1], 13100[1], 13101[1], 13102[1], 13120[1], 13121[1], 13122[1], 13131[1], 13132[1], 13133[1], 13151[1], 13152[1], 13153[1], 36000[1], 36400[1], 36405[1], 36406[1], 36410[1], 36420[1], 36425[1], 36430[1], 36440[1], 36591[0], 36592[0], 36600[1], 36640[1], 43752[1], 51701[0], 51702[0], 51703[0], 52000[0], 52001[1], 52281[0], 52290[1], 52310[0], 52315[0], 53000[0], 53010[0], 53020[0], 53025[0], 53600[0], 53601[0], 53605[0], 53620[0], 53621[0], 53660[0], 53661[0], 53665[0], 57410[0], 62320[0], 62321[0], 62322[0], 62323[0], 62324[0], 62325[0], 62326[0], 62327[0], 64400[0], 64405[0], 64408[0], 64415[0], 64416[0], 64417[0], 64418[0], 64420[0], 64421[0], 64425[0], 64430[0], 64435[0], 64445[0], 64446[0], 64447[0], 64448[0], 64449[0], 64450[0], 64451[0], 64454[0], 64461[0], 64462[0], 64463[0], 64479[0], 64480[0], 64483[0], 64484[0], 64486[0], 64487[0], 64488[0], 64489[0], 64490[0], 64491[0], 64492[0], 64493[0], 64494[0], 64495[0], 64505[0], 64510[0], 64517[0], 64520[0], 64530[0], 69990[0], 76000[1], 77001[1], 77002[1], 92012[1], 92014[1], 93000[1], 93005[1], 93010[1], 93040[1], 93041[1], 93042[1], 93318[1], 93355[1], 94002[1], 94200[1], 94680[1], 94681[1], 94690[1], 95812[1], 95813[1], 95816[1], 95819[1], 95822[1], 95829[1], 95955[1], 96360[1], 96361[1], 96365[1], 96366[1], 96367[1], 96368[1], 96372[1], 96374[1], 96375[1], 96376[1], 96377[1], 96523[0], 97597[1], 97598[1], 97602[1], 99155[0], 99156[0], 99157[0], 99211[1], 99212[1], 99213[1], 99214[1], 99215[1], 99217[1], 99218[1], 99219[1], 99220[1], 99221[1], 99222[1], 99223[1], 99231[1], 99232[1], 99233[1], 99234[1], 99235[1], 99236[1], 99238[1], 99239[1], 99241[1], 99242[1], 99243[1], 99244[1], 99245[1], 99251[1], 99252[1], 99253[1], 99254[1], 99255[1], 99291[1], 99292[1], 99304[1], 99305[1], 99306[1], 99307[1], 99308[1], 99309[1], 99310[1], 99315[1], 99316[1], 99334[1], 99335[1], 99336[1], 99337[1], 99347[1], 99348[1], 99349[1], 99350[1], 99374[1], 99375[1], 99377[1], 99378[1], 99446[0], 99447[0], 99448[0], 99449[0], 99451[0], 99452[0], 99495[1], 99496[1], G0463[1], G0471[0], P9612[0]
52301	00910[0], 00916[0], 0213T[0], 0216T[0], 0596T[0], 0597T[0], 0708T[1], 0709T[1], 11000[1], 11001[1], 11004[1], 11005[1], 11006[1], 11042[1], 11043[1], 11044[1], 11045[1], 11046[1], 11047[1], 12001[1], 12002[1], 12004[1], 12005[1], 12006[1], 12007[1], 12011[1], 12013[1], 12014[1], 12015[1], 12016[1], 12017[1], 12018[1], 12020[1], 12021[1], 12031[1], 12032[1], 12034[1], 12035[1], 12036[1], 12037[1], 12041[1], 12042[1], 12044[1], 12045[1], 12046[1], 12047[1], 12051[1], 12052[1], 12053[1], 12054[1], 12055[1], 12056[1], 12057[1], 13100[1], 13101[1], 13102[1], 13120[1], 13121[1], 13122[1], 13131[1], 13132[1], 13133[1], 13151[1], 13152[1], 13153[1], 36000[1], 36400[1], 36405[1], 36406[1], 36410[1], 36420[1], 36425[1], 36430[1], 36440[1], 36591[0], 36592[0], 36600[1], 36640[1], 43752[1], 51701[0], 51702[0], 51703[0], 52000[0], 52001[1], 52204[1], 52270[1], 52275[1], 52276[1], 52281[0], 52290[1], 52300[1], 52305[1], 52310[0], 52315[0], 52332[1], 52356[1], 53000[0], 53010[0], 53020[0], 53025[0], 53200[1], 53600[0], 53601[0], 53605[0], 53620[0], 53621[0], 53660[0], 53661[0], 53665[0], 57410[0], 62320[0], 62321[0], 62322[0], 62323[0], 62324[0], 62325[0], 62326[0], 62327[0], 64400[0], 64405[0], 64408[0], 64415[0], 64416[0], 64417[0], 64418[0], 64420[0], 64421[0], 64425[0], 64430[0], 64435[0], 64445[0], 64446[0], 64447[0], 64448[0], 64449[0], 64450[0], 64451[0], 64454[0], 64461[0], 64462[0], 64463[0], 64479[0], 64480[0], 64483[0], 64484[0], 64486[0], 64487[0], 64488[0], 64489[0], 64490[0], 64491[0], 64492[0], 64493[0], 64494[0], 64495[0], 64505[0], 64510[0], 64517[0], 64520[0], 64530[0], 69990[0], 76000[1], 77001[1], 77002[1], 92012[1], 92014[1], 93000[1], 93005[1], 93010[1], 93040[1], 93041[1], 93042[1], 93318[1], 93355[1], 94002[1], 94200[1], 94680[1], 94681[1], 94690[1], 95812[1], 95813[1], 95816[1], 95819[1], 95822[1], 95829[1], 95955[1], 96360[1], 96361[1], 96365[1], 96366[1], 96367[1], 96368[1], 96372[1], 96374[1], 96375[1], 96376[1], 96377[1], 96523[0], 97597[1], 97598[1], 97602[1], 99155[0], 99156[0], 99157[0], 99211[1], 99212[1], 99213[1], 99214[1], 99215[1], 99217[1], 99218[1], 99219[1], 99220[1], 99221[1], 99222[1], 99223[1], 99231[1], 99232[1], 99233[1], 99234[1],

0 = Modifier usage not allowed or inappropriate 1 = Modifier usage allowed

Code 1	Code 2
	99235[1], 99236[1], 99238[1], 99239[1], 99241[1], 99242[1], 99243[1], 99244[1], 99245[1], 99251[1], 99252[1], 99253[1], 99254[1], 99255[1], 99291[1], 99292[1], 99304[1], 99305[1], 99306[1], 99307[1], 99308[1], 99309[1], 99310[1], 99315[1], 99316[1], 99334[1], 99335[1], 99336[1], 99337[1], 99347[1], 99348[1], 99349[1], 99350[1], 99374[1], 99375[1], 99377[1], 99378[1], 99446[0], 99447[0], 99448[0], 99449[0], 99451[0], 99452[0], 99495[1], 99496[1], G0463[1], G0471[0], P9612[0]
52305	00910[0], 00916[0], 0213T[0], 0216T[0], 0596T[0], 0597T[0], 0708T[1], 0709T[1], 11000[1], 11001[1], 11004[1], 11005[1], 11006[1], 11042[1], 11043[1], 11044[1], 11045[1], 11046[1], 11047[1], 12001[1], 12002[1], 12004[1], 12005[1], 12006[1], 12007[1], 12011[1], 12013[1], 12014[1], 12015[1], 12016[1], 12017[1], 12018[1], 12020[1], 12021[1], 12031[1], 12032[1], 12034[1], 12035[1], 12036[1], 12037[1], 12041[1], 12042[1], 12044[1], 12045[1], 12046[1], 12047[1], 12051[1], 12052[1], 12053[1], 12054[1], 12055[1], 12056[1], 12057[1], 13100[1], 13101[1], 13102[1], 13120[1], 13121[1], 13122[1], 13131[1], 13132[1], 13133[1], 13151[1], 13152[1], 13153[1], 36000[1], 36400[1], 36405[1], 36406[1], 36410[1], 36420[1], 36425[1], 36430[1], 36440[1], 36591[0], 36592[0], 36600[1], 36640[1], 43752[1], 51701[0], 51702[0], 51703[0], 52000[0], 52001[1], 52281[0], 52310[0], 52315[0], 53000[0], 53010[0], 53020[0], 53025[0], 53600[0], 53601[0], 53605[0], 53620[0], 53621[0], 53660[0], 53661[0], 53665[0], 57410[0], 62320[0], 62321[0], 62322[0], 62323[0], 62324[0], 62325[0], 62326[0], 62327[0], 64400[0], 64405[0], 64408[0], 64415[0], 64416[0], 64417[0], 64418[0], 64420[0], 64421[0], 64425[0], 64430[0], 64435[0], 64445[0], 64446[0], 64447[0], 64448[0], 64449[0], 64450[0], 64451[0], 64454[0], 64461[0], 64462[0], 64463[0], 64479[0], 64480[0], 64483[0], 64484[0], 64486[0], 64487[0], 64488[0], 64489[0], 64490[0], 64491[0], 64492[0], 64493[0], 64494[0], 64495[0], 64505[0], 64510[0], 64517[0], 64520[0], 64530[0], 69990[0], 76000[1], 77001[1], 77002[1], 92012[1], 92014[1], 93000[1], 93005[1], 93010[1], 93040[1], 93041[1], 93042[1], 93318[1], 93355[1], 94002[1], 94200[1], 94680[1], 94681[1], 94690[1], 95812[1], 95813[1], 95816[1], 95819[1], 95822[1], 95829[1], 95955[1], 96360[1], 96361[1], 96365[1], 96366[1], 96367[1], 96368[1], 96372[1], 96374[1], 96375[1], 96376[1], 96377[1], 96523[0], 97597[1], 97598[1], 97602[1], 99155[0], 99156[0], 99157[0], 99211[1], 99212[1], 99213[1], 99214[1], 99215[1], 99217[1], 99218[1], 99219[1], 99220[1], 99221[1], 99222[1], 99223[1], 99231[1], 99232[1], 99233[1], 99234[1], 99235[1], 99236[1], 99238[1], 99239[1], 99241[1], 99242[1], 99243[1], 99244[1], 99245[1], 99251[1], 99252[1], 99253[1], 99254[1], 99255[1], 99291[1], 99292[1], 99304[1], 99305[1], 99306[1], 99307[1], 99308[1], 99309[1], 99310[1], 99315[1], 99316[1], 99334[1], 99335[1], 99336[1], 99337[1], 99347[1], 99348[1], 99349[1], 99350[1], 99374[1], 99375[1], 99377[1], 99378[1], 99446[0], 99447[0], 99448[0], 99449[0], 99451[0], 99452[0], 99495[1], 99496[1], G0463[1], G0471[0], P9612[0]
52310	00910[0], 00916[0], 00918[0], 0213T[0], 0216T[0], 0596T[0], 0597T[0], 0708T[1], 0709T[1], 11000[1], 11001[1], 11004[1], 11005[1], 11006[1], 11042[1], 11043[1], 11044[1], 11045[1], 11046[1], 11047[1], 12001[1], 12002[1], 12004[1], 12005[1], 12006[1], 12007[1], 12011[1], 12013[1], 12014[1], 12015[1], 12016[1], 12017[1], 12018[1], 12020[1], 12021[1], 12031[1], 12032[1], 12034[1], 12035[1], 12036[1], 12037[1], 12041[1], 12042[1], 12044[1], 12045[1], 12046[1], 12047[1], 12051[1], 12052[1], 12053[1], 12054[1], 12055[1], 12056[1], 12057[1], 13100[1], 13101[1], 13102[1], 13120[1], 13121[1], 13122[1], 13131[1], 13132[1], 13133[1], 13151[1], 13152[1], 13153[1], 20102[1], 36000[1], 36400[1], 36405[1], 36406[1], 36410[1], 36420[1], 36425[1], 36430[1], 36440[1], 36591[0], 36592[0], 36600[1], 36640[1], 43752[1], 49013[1], 49014[1], 50715[1], 51700[0], 51701[0], 51702[0], 51703[0], 52000[0], 52001[1], 53000[0], 53010[0], 53020[0], 53025[0], 53600[0], 53601[0], 53605[0], 53620[0], 53621[0], 53660[0], 53661[0], 53665[0], 57410[0], 62320[0], 62321[0], 62322[0], 62323[0], 62324[0], 62325[0], 62326[0], 62327[0], 64400[0], 64405[0], 64408[0], 64415[0], 64416[0], 64417[0], 64418[0], 64420[0], 64421[0], 64425[0], 64430[0], 64435[0], 64445[0], 64446[0], 64447[0], 64448[0], 64449[0], 64450[0], 64451[0], 64454[0], 64461[0], 64462[0], 64463[0], 64479[0], 64480[0], 64483[0], 64484[0], 64486[0], 64487[0], 64488[0], 64489[0], 64490[0], 64491[0], 64492[0], 64493[0], 64494[0], 64495[0], 64505[0], 64510[0], 64517[0], 64520[0], 64530[0], 69990[0], 76000[1], 77001[1], 77002[1], 92012[1], 92014[1], 93000[1], 93005[1], 93010[1], 93040[1], 93041[1], 93042[1], 93318[1], 93355[1], 94002[1], 94200[1], 94680[1], 94681[1], 94690[1], 95812[1], 95813[1], 95816[1], 95819[1], 95822[1], 95829[1], 95955[1], 96360[1], 96361[1], 96365[1], 96366[1], 96367[1], 96368[1], 96372[1], 96374[1], 96375[1], 96376[1], 96377[1], 96523[0], 97597[1], 97598[1], 97602[1], 99155[0], 99156[0], 99157[0], 99211[1], 99212[1], 99213[1], 99214[1], 99215[1], 99217[1], 99218[1], 99219[1], 99220[1], 99221[1], 99222[1], 99223[1], 99231[1], 99232[1], 99233[1], 99234[1], 99235[1], 99236[1], 99238[1], 99239[1], 99241[1], 99242[1], 99243[1], 99244[1], 99245[1], 99251[1], 99252[1], 99253[1], 99254[1], 99255[1], 99291[1], 99292[1], 99304[1], 99305[1], 99306[1], 99307[1], 99308[1], 99309[1], 99310[1], 99315[1], 99316[1], 99334[1], 99335[1], 99336[1], 99337[1], 99347[1], 99348[1], 99349[1], 99350[1], 99374[1], 99375[1], 99377[1], 99378[1], 99446[0], 99447[0], 99448[0], 99449[0], 99451[0], 99452[0], 99495[1], 99496[1], G0463[1], G0471[0], J2001[1], P9612[0]
52315	00910[0], 00916[0], 00918[0], 0213T[0], 0216T[0], 0596T[0], 0597T[0], 0708T[1], 0709T[1], 11000[1], 11001[1], 11004[1], 11005[1], 11006[1], 11042[1], 11043[1], 11044[1], 11045[1], 11046[1], 11047[1], 12001[1], 12002[1], 12004[1], 12005[1], 12006[1], 12007[1], 12011[1], 12013[1], 12014[1], 12015[1], 12016[1], 12017[1], 12018[1], 12020[1], 12021[1], 12031[1], 12032[1], 12034[1], 12035[1], 12036[1], 12037[1], 12041[1], 12042[1], 12044[1], 12045[1], 12046[1], 12047[1], 12051[1], 12052[1], 12053[1], 12054[1], 12055[1], 12056[1], 12057[1], 13100[1], 13101[1], 13102[1], 13120[1], 13121[1], 13122[1], 13131[1], 13132[1], 13133[1], 13151[1], 13152[1], 13153[1], 20102[1], 36000[1], 36400[1], 36405[1], 36406[1], 36410[1], 36420[1], 36425[1], 36430[1], 36440[1], 36591[0], 36592[0], 36600[1], 36640[1], 43752[1], 49013[1], 49014[1], 50385[1], 50386[1], 50715[1], 51701[0], 51702[0], 51703[0], 52000[0], 52001[1], 52281[0], 52310[0], 53000[0], 53010[0], 53020[0], 53025[0], 53600[0], 53601[0], 53605[0], 53620[0], 53621[0], 53660[0], 53661[0], 53665[0], 57410[0], 62320[0], 62321[0], 62322[0], 62323[0], 62324[0], 62325[0], 62326[0], 62327[0], 64400[0], 64405[0], 64408[0], 64415[0], 64416[0], 64417[0], 64418[0], 64420[0], 64421[0], 64425[0], 64430[0], 64435[0], 64445[0], 64446[0], 64447[0], 64448[0], 64449[0], 64450[0], 64451[0], 64454[0], 64461[0], 64462[0], 64463[0], 64479[0], 64480[0], 64483[0], 64484[0], 64486[0], 64487[0], 64488[0], 64489[0], 64490[0], 64491[0], 64492[0], 64493[0], 64494[0], 64495[0], 64505[0], 64510[0], 64517[0], 64520[0], 64530[0], 69990[0], 76000[1], 77001[1], 77002[1], 92012[1], 92014[1], 93000[1], 93005[1], 93010[1], 93040[1], 93041[1], 93042[1], 93318[1], 93355[1], 94002[1], 94200[1], 94680[1], 94681[1], 94690[1], 95812[1], 95813[1], 95816[1], 95819[1], 95822[1], 95829[1], 95955[1], 96360[1], 96361[1], 96365[1], 96366[1], 96367[1], 96368[1], 96372[1], 96374[1], 96375[1], 96376[1], 96377[1], 96523[0], 97597[1], 97598[1], 97602[1], 99155[0], 99156[0], 99157[0], 99211[1], 99212[1], 99213[1], 99214[1], 99215[1], 99217[1], 99218[1], 99219[1], 99220[1], 99221[1], 99222[1], 99223[1], 99231[1], 99232[1], 99233[1], 99234[1], 99235[1], 99236[1], 99238[1], 99239[1], 99241[1], 99242[1], 99243[1], 99244[1], 99245[1], 99251[1], 99252[1], 99253[1], 99254[1], 99255[1], 99291[1], 99292[1], 99304[1], 99305[1], 99306[1], 99307[1], 99308[1], 99309[1], 99310[1], 99315[1], 99316[1], 99334[1], 99335[1], 99336[1], 99337[1], 99347[1], 99348[1], 99349[1], 99350[1], 99374[1], 99375[1], 99377[1], 99378[1], 99446[0], 99447[0], 99448[0], 99449[0], 99451[0], 99452[0], 99495[1], 99496[1], G0463[1], G0471[0], J2001[1], P9612[0]
52317	00910[0], 00916[0], 00918[0], 0213T[0], 0216T[0], 0596T[0], 0597T[0], 0708T[1], 0709T[1], 11000[1], 11001[1], 11004[1], 11005[1], 11006[1], 11042[1], 11043[1], 11044[1], 11045[1], 11046[1], 11047[1], 12001[1], 12002[1], 12004[1], 12005[1], 12006[1], 12007[1], 12011[1], 12013[1], 12014[1], 12015[1], 12016[1], 12017[1], 12018[1], 12020[1], 12021[1], 12031[1], 12032[1], 12034[1], 12035[1], 12036[1], 12037[1], 12041[1], 12042[1], 12044[1], 12045[1], 12046[1], 12047[1], 12051[1], 12052[1], 12053[1], 12054[1], 12055[1], 12056[1], 12057[1], 13100[1], 13101[1], 13102[1], 13120[1], 13121[1], 13122[1], 13131[1], 13132[1], 13133[1], 13151[1], 13152[1], 13153[1], 36000[1], 36400[1], 36405[1], 36406[1], 36410[1], 36420[1], 36425[1], 36430[1], 36440[1], 36591[0], 36592[0], 36600[1], 36640[1], 43752[1], 51701[0], 51702[0], 51703[0], 52000[0], 52204[1], 52276[1], 52281[0], 52310[1], 52315[1], 53000[0], 53010[0], 53020[0], 53025[0], 53600[0], 53601[0], 53605[0], 53620[0], 53621[0], 53660[0], 53661[0], 53665[0], 57410[0], 62320[0], 62321[0], 62322[0], 62323[0], 62324[0], 62325[0], 62326[0], 62327[0], 64400[0], 64405[0], 64408[0], 64415[0], 64416[0], 64417[0], 64418[0], 64420[0], 64421[0], 64425[0], 64430[0], 64435[0], 64445[0], 64446[0], 64447[0], 64448[0], 64449[0], 64450[0], 64451[0], 64454[0], 64461[0], 64462[0], 64463[0], 64479[0], 64480[0], 64483[0], 64484[0], 64486[0], 64487[0], 64488[0], 64489[0], 64490[0], 64491[0], 64492[0], 64493[0], 64494[0], 64495[0], 64505[0], 64510[0], 64517[0], 64520[0], 64530[0], 69990[0], 76000[1], 77001[1], 77002[1], 92012[1], 92014[1], 93000[1], 93005[1], 93010[1], 93040[1], 93041[1], 93042[1], 93318[1], 93355[1], 94002[1], 94200[1], 94680[1], 94681[1], 94690[1], 95812[1], 95813[1], 95816[1], 95819[1], 95822[1], 95829[1], 95955[1], 96360[1], 96361[1], 96365[1], 96366[1], 96367[1], 96368[1], 96372[1], 96374[1], 96375[1], 96376[1], 96377[1], 96523[0], 97597[1], 97598[1], 97602[1], 99155[0], 99156[0], 99157[0], 99211[1], 99212[1], 99213[1], 99214[1], 99215[1], 99217[1], 99218[1], 99219[1], 99220[1], 99221[1], 99222[1], 99223[1], 99231[1], 99232[1], 99233[1], 99234[1], 99235[1], 99236[1], 99238[1], 99239[1], 99241[1], 99242[1], 99243[1], 99244[1], 99245[1], 99251[1], 99252[1], 99253[1], 99254[1], 99255[1], 99291[1], 99292[1], 99304[1], 99305[1], 99306[1], 99307[1], 99308[1], 99309[1], 99310[1], 99315[1], 99316[1], 99334[1], 99335[1], 99336[1], 99337[1], 99347[1], 99348[1], 99349[1], 99350[1], 99374[1], 99375[1], 99377[1], 99378[1], 99446[0], 99447[0], 99448[0], 99449[0], 99451[0], 99452[0], 99495[1], 99496[1], G0463[1], G0471[0], J2001[1], P9612[0]
52318	00910[0], 00916[0], 00918[0], 0213T[0], 0216T[0], 0596T[0], 0597T[0], 0708T[1], 0709T[1], 11000[1], 11001[1], 11004[1], 11005[1], 11006[1], 11042[1], 11043[1], 11044[1], 11045[1], 11046[1], 11047[1], 12001[1], 12002[1], 12004[1], 12005[1], 12006[1], 12007[1], 12011[1], 12013[1], 12014[1], 12015[1], 12016[1], 12017[1], 12018[1], 12020[1], 12021[1], 12031[1], 12032[1], 12034[1], 12035[1], 12036[1], 12037[1], 12041[1], 12042[1], 12044[1], 12045[1], 12046[1], 12047[1], 12051[1], 12052[1], 12053[1], 12054[1], 12055[1], 12056[1], 12057[1], 13100[1], 13101[1], 13102[1], 13120[1], 13121[1], 13122[1], 13131[1], 13132[1], 13133[1], 13151[1], 13152[1], 13153[1], 36000[1], 36400[1], 36405[1], 36406[1], 36410[1], 36420[1], 36425[1], 36430[1], 36440[1], 36591[0], 36592[0], 36600[1], 36640[1], 43752[1], 51701[0], 51702[0], 51703[0], 52000[0], 52005[1], 52204[1], 52281[0], 52310[1], 52315[1], 52317[1], 53000[0], 53010[0], 53020[0], 53025[0], 53600[0], 53601[0], 53605[0], 53620[0], 53621[0], 53660[0], 53661[0], 53665[0], 57410[0], 62320[0], 62321[0], 62322[0], 62323[0], 62324[0], 62325[0], 62326[0], 62327[0], 64400[0], 64405[0], 64408[0], 64415[0], 64416[0], 64417[0], 64418[0], 64420[0], 64421[0], 64425[0], 64430[0], 64435[0], 64445[0], 64446[0], 64447[0], 64448[0], 64449[0], 64450[0], 64451[0], 64454[0], 64461[0], 64462[0], 64463[0], 64479[0], 64480[0], 64483[0], 64484[0], 64486[0], 64487[0], 64488[0], 64489[0], 64490[0], 64491[0], 64492[0], 64493[0], 64494[0], 64495[0], 64505[0], 64510[0], 64517[0], 64520[0], 64530[0], 69990[0], 76000[1], 77001[1], 77002[1], 92012[1], 92014[1], 93000[1], 93005[1], 93010[1], 93040[1], 93041[1], 93042[1], 93318[1], 93355[1], 94002[1], 94200[1], 94680[1], 94681[1], 94690[1], 95812[1], 95813[1], 95816[1], 95819[1], 95822[1], 95829[1], 95955[1], 96360[1], 96361[1], 96365[1], 96366[1], 96367[1], 96368[1], 96372[1], 96374[1], 96375[1], 96376[1], 96377[1],

0 = Modifier usage not allowed or inappropriate 1 = Modifier usage allowed

Code 1	Code 2
	96523[0], 97597[1], 97598[1], 97602[1], 99155[0], 99156[0], 99157[0], 99211[1], 99212[1], 99213[1], 99214[1], 99215[1], 99217[1], 99218[1], 99219[1], 99220[1], 99221[1], 99222[1], 99223[1], 99231[1], 99232[1], 99233[1], 99234[1], 99235[1], 99236[1], 99238[1], 99239[1], 99241[1], 99242[1], 99243[1], 99244[1], 99245[1], 99251[1], 99252[1], 99253[1], 99254[1], 99255[1], 99291[1], 99292[1], 99304[1], 99305[1], 99306[1], 99307[1], 99308[1], 99309[1], 99310[1], 99315[1], 99316[1], 99334[1], 99335[1], 99336[1], 99337[1], 99347[1], 99348[1], 99349[1], 99350[1], 99374[1], 99375[1], 99377[1], 99378[1], 99446[0], 99447[0], 99448[0], 99449[0], 99451[0], 99452[0], 99495[1], 99496[1], G0463[1], G0471[0], P9612[0]
52320	00910[0], 00916[0], 00918[0], 0213T[0], 0216T[0], 0596T[0], 0597T[0], 0708T[1], 0709T[1], 11000[1], 11001[1], 11004[1], 11005[1], 11006[1], 11042[1], 11043[1], 11044[1], 11045[1], 11046[1], 11047[1], 12001[1], 12002[1], 12004[1], 12005[1], 12006[1], 12007[1], 12011[1], 12013[1], 12014[1], 12015[1], 12016[1], 12017[1], 12018[1], 12020[1], 12021[1], 12031[1], 12032[1], 12034[1], 12035[1], 12036[1], 12037[1], 12041[1], 12042[1], 12044[1], 12045[1], 12046[1], 12047[1], 12051[1], 12052[1], 12053[1], 12054[1], 12055[1], 12056[1], 12057[1], 13100[1], 13101[1], 13102[1], 13120[1], 13121[1], 13122[1], 13131[1], 13132[1], 13133[1], 13151[1], 13152[1], 13153[1], 36000[1], 36400[1], 36405[1], 36406[1], 36410[1], 36420[1], 36425[1], 36430[1], 36440[1], 36591[0], 36592[0], 36600[1], 36640[1], 43752[1], 50715[1], 50945[1], 51701[0], 51702[0], 51703[0], 52000[0], 52001[1], 52005[0], 52007[0], 52204[1], 52281[0], 52310[0], 52315[0], 52317[1], 52318[1], 53000[0], 53010[0], 53020[0], 53025[0], 53600[0], 53601[0], 53605[0], 53620[0], 53621[0], 53660[0], 53661[0], 53665[0], 57410[0], 62320[0], 62321[0], 62322[0], 62323[0], 62324[0], 62325[0], 62326[0], 62327[0], 64400[0], 64405[0], 64408[0], 64415[0], 64416[0], 64417[0], 64418[0], 64420[0], 64421[0], 64425[0], 64430[0], 64435[0], 64445[0], 64446[0], 64447[0], 64448[0], 64449[0], 64450[0], 64451[0], 64454[0], 64461[0], 64462[0], 64463[0], 64479[0], 64480[0], 64483[0], 64484[0], 64486[0], 64487[0], 64488[0], 64489[0], 64490[0], 64491[0], 64492[0], 64493[0], 64494[0], 64495[0], 64505[0], 64510[0], 64517[0], 64520[0], 64530[0], 69990[0], 76000[1], 77001[1], 77002[1], 92012[1], 92014[1], 93000[1], 93005[1], 93010[1], 93040[1], 93041[1], 93042[1], 93318[1], 93355[1], 94002[1], 94200[1], 94680[1], 94681[1], 94690[1], 95812[1], 95813[1], 95816[1], 95819[1], 95822[1], 95829[1], 95955[1], 96360[1], 96361[1], 96365[1], 96366[1], 96367[1], 96368[1], 96372[1], 96374[1], 96375[1], 96376[1], 96377[1], 96523[0], 97597[1], 97598[1], 97602[1], 99155[0], 99156[0], 99157[0], 99211[1], 99212[1], 99213[1], 99214[1], 99215[1], 99217[1], 99218[1], 99219[1], 99220[1], 99221[1], 99222[1], 99223[1], 99231[1], 99232[1], 99233[1], 99234[1], 99235[1], 99236[1], 99238[1], 99239[1], 99241[1], 99242[1], 99243[1], 99244[1], 99245[1], 99251[1], 99252[1], 99253[1], 99254[1], 99255[1], 99291[1], 99292[1], 99304[1], 99305[1], 99306[1], 99307[1], 99308[1], 99309[1], 99310[1], 99315[1], 99316[1], 99334[1], 99335[1], 99336[1], 99337[1], 99347[1], 99348[1], 99349[1], 99350[1], 99374[1], 99375[1], 99377[1], 99378[1], 99446[0], 99447[0], 99448[0], 99449[0], 99451[0], 99452[0], 99495[1], 99496[1], G0463[1], G0471[0], P9612[0]
52325	00910[0], 00916[0], 00918[0], 0213T[0], 0216T[0], 0596T[0], 0597T[0], 0708T[1], 0709T[1], 12001[1], 12002[1], 12004[1], 12005[1], 12006[1], 12007[1], 12011[1], 12013[1], 12014[1], 12015[1], 12016[1], 12017[1], 12018[1], 12020[1], 12021[1], 12031[1], 12032[1], 12034[1], 12035[1], 12036[1], 12037[1], 12041[1], 12042[1], 12044[1], 12045[1], 12046[1], 12047[1], 12051[1], 12052[1], 12053[1], 12054[1], 12055[1], 12056[1], 12057[1], 13100[1], 13101[1], 13102[1], 13120[1], 13121[1], 13122[1], 13131[1], 13132[1], 13133[1], 13151[1], 13152[1], 13153[1], 36000[1], 36400[1], 36405[1], 36406[1], 36410[1], 36420[1], 36425[1], 36430[1], 36440[1], 36591[0], 36592[0], 36600[1], 36640[1], 43752[1], 50715[1], 50945[1], 50961[1], 51701[0], 51702[0], 51703[0], 52000[0], 52001[1], 52005[0], 52007[0], 52281[0], 52310[0], 52315[0], 52317[1], 52318[1], 52320[1], 53000[0], 53010[0], 53020[0], 53025[0], 53600[0], 53601[0], 53605[0], 53620[0], 53621[0], 53660[0], 53661[0], 53665[0], 57410[0], 62320[0], 62321[0], 62322[0], 62323[0], 62324[0], 62325[0], 62326[0], 62327[0], 64400[0], 64405[0], 64408[0], 64415[0], 64416[0], 64417[0], 64418[0], 64420[0], 64421[0], 64425[0], 64430[0], 64435[0], 64445[0], 64446[0], 64447[0], 64448[0], 64449[0], 64450[0], 64451[0], 64454[0], 64461[0], 64462[0], 64463[0], 64479[0], 64480[0], 64483[0], 64484[0], 64486[0], 64487[0], 64488[0], 64489[0], 64490[0], 64491[0], 64492[0], 64493[0], 64494[0], 64495[0], 64505[0], 64510[0], 64517[0], 64520[0], 64530[0], 69990[0], 76000[1], 77001[1], 77002[1], 92012[1], 92014[1], 93000[1], 93005[1], 93010[1], 93040[1], 93041[1], 93042[1], 93318[1], 93355[1], 94002[1], 94200[1], 94680[1], 94681[1], 94690[1], 95812[1], 95813[1], 95816[1], 95819[1], 95822[1], 95829[1], 95955[1], 96360[1], 96361[1], 96365[1], 96366[1], 96367[1], 96368[1], 96372[1], 96374[1], 96375[1], 96376[1], 96377[1], 96523[0], 99155[0], 99156[0], 99157[0], 99211[1], 99212[1], 99213[1], 99214[1], 99215[1], 99217[1], 99218[1], 99219[1], 99220[1], 99221[1], 99222[1], 99223[1], 99231[1], 99232[1], 99233[1], 99234[1], 99235[1], 99236[1], 99238[1], 99239[1], 99241[1], 99242[1], 99243[1], 99244[1], 99245[1], 99251[1], 99252[1], 99253[1], 99254[1], 99255[1], 99291[1], 99292[1], 99304[1], 99305[1], 99306[1], 99307[1], 99308[1], 99309[1], 99310[1], 99315[1], 99316[1], 99334[1], 99335[1], 99336[1], 99337[1], 99347[1], 99348[1], 99349[1], 99350[1], 99374[1], 99375[1], 99377[1], 99378[1], 99446[0], 99447[0], 99448[0], 99449[0], 99451[0], 99452[0], 99495[1], 99496[1], G0463[1], G0471[0], P9612[0]
52327	00910[0], 00916[0], 00918[0], 0213T[0], 0216T[0], 0596T[0], 0597T[0], 0708T[1], 0709T[1], 12001[1], 12002[1], 12004[1], 12005[1], 12006[1], 12007[1], 12011[1], 12013[1], 12014[1], 12015[1], 12016[1], 12017[1], 12018[1], 12020[1], 12021[1], 12031[1], 12032[1], 12034[1], 12035[1], 12036[1], 12037[1], 12041[1], 12042[1], 12044[1], 12045[1], 12046[1], 12047[1], 12051[1], 12052[1], 12053[1], 12054[1], 12055[1], 12056[1], 12057[1], 13100[1], 13101[1], 13102[1], 13120[1], 13121[1], 13122[1], 13131[1], 13132[1], 13133[1], 13151[1], 13152[1], 13153[1], 36000[1], 36400[1], 36405[1], 36406[1], 36410[1], 36420[1], 36425[1], 36430[1], 36440[1], 36591[0], 36592[0], 36600[1], 36640[1], 43752[1], 50715[1], 51701[0], 51702[0], 51703[0], 52000[0], 52001[1], 52005[0], 52007[0], 52281[0], 52310[0], 52315[0], 53000[0], 53010[0], 53020[0], 53025[0], 53600[0], 53601[0], 53605[0], 53620[0], 53621[0], 53660[0], 53661[0], 53665[0], 57410[0], 62320[0], 62321[0], 62322[0], 62323[0], 62324[0], 62325[0], 62326[0], 62327[0], 64400[0], 64405[0], 64408[0], 64415[0], 64416[0], 64417[0], 64418[0], 64420[0], 64421[0], 64425[0], 64430[0], 64435[0], 64445[0], 64446[0], 64447[0], 64448[0], 64449[0], 64450[0], 64451[0], 64454[0], 64461[0], 64462[0], 64463[0], 64479[0], 64480[0], 64483[0], 64484[0], 64486[0], 64487[0], 64488[0], 64489[0], 64490[0], 64491[0], 64492[0], 64493[0], 64494[0], 64495[0], 64505[0], 64510[0], 64517[0], 64520[0], 64530[0], 69990[0], 76000[1], 77001[1], 77002[1], 92012[1], 92014[1], 93000[1], 93005[1], 93010[1], 93040[1], 93041[1], 93042[1], 93318[1], 93355[1], 94002[1], 94200[1], 94680[1], 94681[1], 94690[1], 95812[1], 95813[1], 95816[1], 95819[1], 95822[1], 95829[1], 95955[1], 96360[1], 96361[1], 96365[1], 96366[1], 96367[1], 96368[1], 96372[1], 96374[1], 96375[1], 96376[1], 96377[1], 96523[0], 99155[0], 99156[0], 99157[0], 99211[1], 99212[1], 99213[1], 99214[1], 99215[1], 99217[1], 99218[1], 99219[1], 99220[1], 99221[1], 99222[1], 99223[1], 99231[1], 99232[1], 99233[1], 99234[1], 99235[1], 99236[1], 99238[1], 99239[1], 99241[1], 99242[1], 99243[1], 99244[1], 99245[1], 99251[1], 99252[1], 99253[1], 99254[1], 99255[1], 99291[1], 99292[1], 99304[1], 99305[1], 99306[1], 99307[1], 99308[1], 99309[1], 99310[1], 99315[1], 99316[1], 99334[1], 99335[1], 99336[1], 99337[1], 99347[1], 99348[1], 99349[1], 99350[1], 99374[1], 99375[1], 99377[1], 99378[1], 99446[0], 99447[0], 99448[0], 99449[0], 99451[0], 99452[0], 99495[1], 99496[1], G0463[1], G0471[0], P9612[0]
52330	00910[0], 00916[0], 00918[0], 0213T[0], 0216T[0], 0596T[0], 0597T[0], 0708T[1], 0709T[1], 11000[1], 11001[1], 11004[1], 11005[1], 11006[1], 11042[1], 11043[1], 11044[1], 11045[1], 11046[1], 11047[1], 12001[1], 12002[1], 12004[1], 12005[1], 12006[1], 12007[1], 12011[1], 12013[1], 12014[1], 12015[1], 12016[1], 12017[1], 12018[1], 12020[1], 12021[1], 12031[1], 12032[1], 12034[1], 12035[1], 12036[1], 12037[1], 12041[1], 12042[1], 12044[1], 12045[1], 12046[1], 12047[1], 12051[1], 12052[1], 12053[1], 12054[1], 12055[1], 12056[1], 12057[1], 13100[1], 13101[1], 13102[1], 13120[1], 13121[1], 13122[1], 13131[1], 13132[1], 13133[1], 13151[1], 13152[1], 13153[1], 36000[1], 36400[1], 36405[1], 36406[1], 36410[1], 36420[1], 36425[1], 36430[1], 36440[1], 36591[0], 36592[0], 36600[1], 36640[1], 43752[1], 50715[1], 51701[0], 51702[0], 51703[0], 52000[0], 52001[1], 52005[0], 52007[0], 52281[0], 52310[0], 52315[0], 52320[1], 52325[1], 53000[0], 53010[0], 53020[0], 53025[0], 53600[0], 53601[0], 53605[0], 53620[0], 53621[0], 53660[0], 53661[0], 53665[0], 57410[0], 62320[0], 62321[0], 62322[0], 62323[0], 62324[0], 62325[0], 62326[0], 62327[0], 64400[0], 64405[0], 64408[0], 64415[0], 64416[0], 64417[0], 64418[0], 64420[0], 64421[0], 64425[0], 64430[0], 64435[0], 64445[0], 64446[0], 64447[0], 64448[0], 64449[0], 64450[0], 64451[0], 64454[0], 64461[0], 64462[0], 64463[0], 64479[0], 64480[0], 64483[0], 64484[0], 64486[0], 64487[0], 64488[0], 64489[0], 64490[0], 64491[0], 64492[0], 64493[0], 64494[0], 64495[0], 64505[0], 64510[0], 64517[0], 64520[0], 64530[0], 69990[0], 76000[1], 77001[1], 77002[1], 92012[1], 92014[1], 93000[1], 93005[1], 93010[1], 93040[1], 93041[1], 93042[1], 93318[1], 93355[1], 94002[1], 94200[1], 94680[1], 94681[1], 94690[1], 95812[1], 95813[1], 95816[1], 95819[1], 95822[1], 95829[1], 95955[1], 96360[1], 96361[1], 96365[1], 96366[1], 96367[1], 96368[1], 96372[1], 96374[1], 96375[1], 96376[1], 96377[1], 96523[0], 97597[1], 97598[1], 97602[1], 99155[0], 99156[0], 99157[0], 99211[1], 99212[1], 99213[1], 99214[1], 99215[1], 99217[1], 99218[1], 99219[1], 99220[1], 99221[1], 99222[1], 99223[1], 99231[1], 99232[1], 99233[1], 99234[1], 99235[1], 99236[1], 99238[1], 99239[1], 99241[1], 99242[1], 99243[1], 99244[1], 99245[1], 99251[1], 99252[1], 99253[1], 99254[1], 99255[1], 99291[1], 99292[1], 99304[1], 99305[1], 99306[1], 99307[1], 99308[1], 99309[1], 99310[1], 99315[1], 99316[1], 99334[1], 99335[1], 99336[1], 99337[1], 99347[1], 99348[1], 99349[1], 99350[1], 99374[1], 99375[1], 99377[1], 99378[1], 99446[0], 99447[0], 99448[0], 99449[0], 99451[0], 99452[0], 99495[1], 99496[1], G0463[1], G0471[0], J2001[1], P9612[0]
52332	00910[0], 00916[0], 0213T[0], 0216T[0], 0596T[0], 0597T[0], 0708T[1], 0709T[1], 11000[1], 11001[1], 11004[1], 11005[1], 11006[1], 11042[1], 11043[1], 11044[1], 11045[1], 11046[1], 11047[1], 12001[1], 12002[1], 12004[1], 12005[1], 12006[1], 12007[1], 12011[1], 12013[1], 12014[1], 12015[1], 12016[1], 12017[1], 12018[1], 12020[1], 12021[1], 12031[1], 12032[1], 12034[1], 12035[1], 12036[1], 12037[1], 12041[1], 12042[1], 12044[1], 12045[1], 12046[1], 12047[1], 12051[1], 12052[1], 12053[1], 12054[1], 12055[1], 12056[1], 12057[1], 13100[1], 13101[1], 13102[1], 13120[1], 13121[1], 13122[1], 13131[1], 13132[1], 13133[1], 13151[1], 13152[1], 13153[1], 36000[1], 36400[1], 36405[1], 36406[1], 36410[1], 36420[1], 36425[1], 36430[1], 36440[1], 36591[0], 36592[0], 36600[1], 36640[1], 43752[1], 50387[1], 50430[1], 50431[1], 50684[1], 50693[1], 50694[1], 50695[1], 50715[1], 51700[0], 51701[0], 51702[0], 51703[0], 52000[0], 52001[1], 52005[1], 52007[1], 52204[1], 52281[0], 52310[0], 52315[0], 53000[0], 53010[0], 53020[0], 53025[0], 53600[0], 53601[0], 53605[0], 53620[0], 53621[0], 53660[0], 53661[0], 53665[0], 57410[0], 62320[0], 62321[0], 62322[0], 62323[0], 62324[0], 62325[0], 62326[0], 62327[0], 64400[0], 64405[0], 64408[0], 64415[0], 64416[0], 64417[0], 64418[0], 64420[0], 64421[0], 64425[0], 64430[0], 64435[0], 64445[0], 64446[0], 64447[0], 64448[0], 64449[0], 64450[0], 64451[0], 64454[0], 64461[0], 64462[0], 64463[0], 64479[0], 64480[0], 64483[0], 64484[0], 64486[0], 64487[0], 64488[0], 64489[0], 64490[0], 64491[0], 64492[0], 64493[0], 64494[0], 64495[0], 64505[0], 64510[0], 64517[0], 64520[0], 64530[0], 69990[0], 76000[1], 77001[1], 77002[1], 92012[1], 92014[1], 93000[1], 93005[1], 93010[1], 93040[1], 93041[1], 93042[1], 93318[1], 93355[1], 94002[1], 94200[1], 94680[1], 94681[1],

0 = Modifier usage not allowed or inappropriate   1 = Modifier usage allowed

Code 1	Code 2
	94690[1], 95812[1], 95813[1], 95816[1], 95819[1], 95822[1], 95829[1], 95955[1], 96360[1], 96361[1], 96365[1], 96366[1], 96367[1], 96368[1], 96372[1], 96374[1], 96375[1], 96376[1], 96377[1], 96523[0], 97597[1], 97598[1], 97602[1], 99155[0], 99156[0], 99157[0], 99211[1], 99212[1], 99213[1], 99214[1], 99215[1], 99217[1], 99218[1], 99219[1], 99220[1], 99221[1], 99222[1], 99223[1], 99231[1], 99232[1], 99233[1], 99234[1], 99235[1], 99236[1], 99238[1], 99239[1], 99241[1], 99242[1], 99243[1], 99244[1], 99245[1], 99251[1], 99252[1], 99253[1], 99254[1], 99255[1], 99291[1], 99292[1], 99304[1], 99305[1], 99306[1], 99307[1], 99308[1], 99309[1], 99310[1], 99315[1], 99316[1], 99334[1], 99335[1], 99336[1], 99337[1], 99347[1], 99348[1], 99349[1], 99350[1], 99374[1], 99375[1], 99377[1], 99378[1], 99446[0], 99447[0], 99448[0], 99449[0], 99451[0], 99452[0], 99495[1], 99496[1], G0463[1], G0471[0], J2001[1], P9612[0]
52334	00910[0], 00916[0], 0213T[0], 0216T[0], 0596T[0], 0597T[0], 0708T[1], 0709T[1], 11000[1], 11001[1], 11004[1], 11005[1], 11006[1], 11042[1], 11043[1], 11044[1], 11045[1], 11046[1], 11047[1], 12001[1], 12002[1], 12004[1], 12005[1], 12006[1], 12007[1], 12011[1], 12013[1], 12014[1], 12015[1], 12016[1], 12017[1], 12018[1], 12020[1], 12021[1], 12031[1], 12032[1], 12034[1], 12035[1], 12036[1], 12037[1], 12041[1], 12042[1], 12044[1], 12045[1], 12046[1], 12047[1], 12051[1], 12052[1], 12053[1], 12054[1], 12055[1], 12056[1], 12057[1], 13100[1], 13101[1], 13102[1], 13120[1], 13121[1], 13122[1], 13131[1], 13132[1], 13133[1], 13151[1], 13152[1], 13153[1], 36000[1], 36400[1], 36405[1], 36406[1], 36410[1], 36420[1], 36425[1], 36430[1], 36440[1], 36591[0], 36592[0], 36600[1], 36640[1], 43752[1], 50436[1], 50715[1], 51701[0], 51702[0], 51703[0], 52000[0], 52001[1], 52005[0], 52007[0], 52281[0], 52310[0], 52315[0], 52351[0], 53000[0], 53010[0], 53020[0], 53025[0], 53600[0], 53601[0], 53605[0], 53620[0], 53621[0], 53660[0], 53661[0], 53665[0], 57410[0], 62320[0], 62321[0], 62322[0], 62323[0], 62324[0], 62325[0], 62326[0], 62327[0], 64400[0], 64405[0], 64408[0], 64415[0], 64416[0], 64417[0], 64418[0], 64420[0], 64421[0], 64425[0], 64430[0], 64435[0], 64445[0], 64446[0], 64447[0], 64448[0], 64449[0], 64450[0], 64451[0], 64454[0], 64461[0], 64462[0], 64463[0], 64479[0], 64480[0], 64483[0], 64484[0], 64486[0], 64487[0], 64488[0], 64489[0], 64490[0], 64491[0], 64492[0], 64493[0], 64494[0], 64495[0], 64505[0], 64510[0], 64517[0], 64520[0], 64530[0], 69990[0], 76000[1], 77001[1], 77002[1], 92012[1], 92014[1], 93000[1], 93005[1], 93010[1], 93040[1], 93041[1], 93042[1], 93318[1], 93355[1], 94002[1], 94200[1], 94680[1], 94681[1], 94690[1], 95812[1], 95813[1], 95816[1], 95819[1], 95822[1], 95829[1], 95955[1], 96360[1], 96361[1], 96365[1], 96366[1], 96367[1], 96368[1], 96372[1], 96374[1], 96375[1], 96376[1], 96377[1], 96523[0], 97597[1], 97598[1], 97602[1], 99155[0], 99156[0], 99157[0], 99211[1], 99212[1], 99213[1], 99214[1], 99215[1], 99217[1], 99218[1], 99219[1], 99220[1], 99221[1], 99222[1], 99223[1], 99231[1], 99232[1], 99233[1], 99234[1], 99235[1], 99236[1], 99238[1], 99239[1], 99241[1], 99242[1], 99243[1], 99244[1], 99245[1], 99251[1], 99252[1], 99253[1], 99254[1], 99255[1], 99291[1], 99292[1], 99304[1], 99305[1], 99306[1], 99307[1], 99308[1], 99309[1], 99310[1], 99315[1], 99316[1], 99334[1], 99335[1], 99336[1], 99337[1], 99347[1], 99348[1], 99349[1], 99350[1], 99374[1], 99375[1], 99377[1], 99378[1], 99446[0], 99447[0], 99448[0], 99449[0], 99451[0], 99452[0], 99495[1], 99496[1], G0463[1], G0471[0], P9612[0]
52341	00910[0], 00916[0], 0213T[0], 0216T[0], 0596T[0], 0597T[0], 0708T[1], 0709T[1], 12001[1], 12002[1], 12004[1], 12005[1], 12006[1], 12007[1], 12011[1], 12013[1], 12014[1], 12015[1], 12016[1], 12017[1], 12018[1], 12020[1], 12021[1], 12031[1], 12032[1], 12034[1], 12035[1], 12036[1], 12037[1], 12041[1], 12042[1], 12044[1], 12045[1], 12046[1], 12047[1], 12051[1], 12052[1], 12053[1], 12054[1], 12055[1], 12056[1], 12057[1], 13100[1], 13101[1], 13102[1], 13120[1], 13121[1], 13122[1], 13131[1], 13132[1], 13133[1], 13151[1], 13152[1], 13153[1], 36000[1], 36400[1], 36405[1], 36406[1], 36410[1], 36420[1], 36425[1], 36430[1], 36440[1], 36591[0], 36592[0], 36600[1], 36640[1], 43752[1], 50706[1], 50715[1], 50953[1], 50972[1], 51701[0], 51702[0], 51703[0], 52000[0], 52001[1], 52005[0], 52007[0], 52204[1], 52281[0], 52310[0], 52315[0], 52351[0], 53000[0], 53010[0], 53020[0], 53025[0], 53600[0], 53601[0], 53605[0], 53620[0], 53621[0], 53660[0], 53661[0], 53665[0], 57410[0], 62320[0], 62321[0], 62322[0], 62323[0], 62324[0], 62325[0], 62326[0], 62327[0], 64400[0], 64405[0], 64408[0], 64415[0], 64416[0], 64417[0], 64418[0], 64420[0], 64421[0], 64425[0], 64430[0], 64435[0], 64445[0], 64446[0], 64447[0], 64448[0], 64449[0], 64450[0], 64451[0], 64454[0], 64461[0], 64462[0], 64463[0], 64479[0], 64480[0], 64483[0], 64484[0], 64486[0], 64487[0], 64488[0], 64489[0], 64490[0], 64491[0], 64492[0], 64493[0], 64494[0], 64495[0], 64505[0], 64510[0], 64517[0], 64520[0], 64530[0], 69990[0], 76000[1], 77001[1], 77002[1], 92012[1], 92014[1], 93000[1], 93005[1], 93010[1], 93040[1], 93041[1], 93042[1], 93318[1], 93355[1], 94002[1], 94200[1], 94680[1], 94681[1], 94690[1], 95812[1], 95813[1], 95816[1], 95819[1], 95822[1], 95829[1], 95955[1], 96360[1], 96361[1], 96365[1], 96366[1], 96367[1], 96368[1], 96372[1], 96374[1], 96375[1], 96376[1], 96377[1], 96523[0], 99155[0], 99156[0], 99157[0], 99211[1], 99212[1], 99213[1], 99214[1], 99215[1], 99217[1], 99218[1], 99219[1], 99220[1], 99221[1], 99222[1], 99223[1], 99231[1], 99232[1], 99233[1], 99234[1], 99235[1], 99236[1], 99238[1], 99239[1], 99241[1], 99242[1], 99243[1], 99244[1], 99245[1], 99251[1], 99252[1], 99253[1], 99254[1], 99255[1], 99291[1], 99292[1], 99304[1], 99305[1], 99306[1], 99307[1], 99308[1], 99309[1], 99310[1], 99315[1], 99316[1], 99334[1], 99335[1], 99336[1], 99337[1], 99347[1], 99348[1], 99349[1], 99350[1], 99374[1], 99375[1], 99377[1], 99378[1], 99446[0], 99447[0], 99448[0], 99449[0], 99451[0], 99452[0], 99495[1], 99496[1], G0463[1], G0471[0], P9612[1]
52342	00910[0], 00916[0], 0213T[0], 0216T[0], 0596T[0], 0597T[0], 0708T[1], 0709T[1], 12001[1], 12002[1], 12004[1], 12005[1], 12006[1], 12007[1], 12011[1], 12013[1], 12014[1], 12015[1], 12016[1], 12017[1], 12018[1], 12020[1], 12021[1], 12031[1], 12032[1], 12034[1], 12035[1], 12036[1], 12037[1], 12041[1], 12042[1], 12044[1], 12045[1], 12046[1], 12047[1], 12051[1], 12052[1], 12053[1], 12054[1], 12055[1], 12056[1], 12057[1], 13100[1], 13101[1], 13102[1], 13120[1], 13121[1], 13122[1], 13131[1], 13132[1], 13133[1], 13151[1], 13152[1], 13153[1], 36000[1], 36400[1], 36405[1], 36406[1], 36410[1], 36420[1], 36425[1], 36430[1], 36440[1], 36591[0], 36592[0], 36600[1], 36640[1], 43752[1], 50706[1], 50715[1], 50953[1], 50972[1], 51701[0], 51702[0], 51703[0], 52000[0], 52001[1], 52005[0], 52007[0], 52204[1], 52281[0], 52310[0], 52315[0], 52351[0], 53000[0], 53010[0], 53020[0], 53025[0], 53600[0], 53601[0], 53605[0], 53620[0], 53621[0], 53660[0], 53661[0], 53665[0], 57410[0], 62320[0], 62321[0], 62322[0], 62323[0], 62324[0], 62325[0], 62326[0], 62327[0], 64400[0], 64405[0], 64408[0], 64415[0], 64416[0], 64417[0], 64418[0], 64420[0], 64421[0], 64425[0], 64430[0], 64435[0], 64445[0], 64446[0], 64447[0], 64448[0], 64449[0], 64450[0], 64451[0], 64454[0], 64461[0], 64462[0], 64463[0], 64479[0], 64480[0], 64483[0], 64484[0], 64486[0], 64487[0], 64488[0], 64489[0], 64490[0], 64491[0], 64492[0], 64493[0], 64494[0], 64495[0], 64505[0], 64510[0], 64517[0], 64520[0], 64530[0], 69990[0], 76000[1], 77001[1], 77002[1], 92012[1], 92014[1], 93000[1], 93005[1], 93010[1], 93040[1], 93041[1], 93042[1], 93318[1], 93355[1], 94002[1], 94200[1], 94680[1], 94681[1], 94690[1], 95812[1], 95813[1], 95816[1], 95819[1], 95822[1], 95829[1], 95955[1], 96360[1], 96361[1], 96365[1], 96366[1], 96367[1], 96368[1], 96372[1], 96374[1], 96375[1], 96376[1], 96377[1], 96523[0], 99155[0], 99156[0], 99157[0], 99211[1], 99212[1], 99213[1], 99214[1], 99215[1], 99217[1], 99218[1], 99219[1], 99220[1], 99221[1], 99222[1], 99223[1], 99231[1], 99232[1], 99233[1], 99234[1], 99235[1], 99236[1], 99238[1], 99239[1], 99241[1], 99242[1], 99243[1], 99244[1], 99245[1], 99251[1], 99252[1], 99253[1], 99254[1], 99255[1], 99291[1], 99292[1], 99304[1], 99305[1], 99306[1], 99307[1], 99308[1], 99309[1], 99310[1], 99315[1], 99316[1], 99334[1], 99335[1], 99336[1], 99337[1], 99347[1], 99348[1], 99349[1], 99350[1], 99374[1], 99375[1], 99377[1], 99378[1], 99446[0], 99447[0], 99448[0], 99449[0], 99451[0], 99452[0], 99495[1], 99496[1], G0463[1], G0471[0], P9612[1]
52343	00910[0], 00916[0], 0213T[0], 0216T[0], 0596T[0], 0597T[0], 0708T[1], 0709T[1], 12001[1], 12002[1], 12004[1], 12005[1], 12006[1], 12007[1], 12011[1], 12013[1], 12014[1], 12015[1], 12016[1], 12017[1], 12018[1], 12020[1], 12021[1], 12031[1], 12032[1], 12034[1], 12035[1], 12036[1], 12037[1], 12041[1], 12042[1], 12044[1], 12045[1], 12046[1], 12047[1], 12051[1], 12052[1], 12053[1], 12054[1], 12055[1], 12056[1], 12057[1], 13100[1], 13101[1], 13102[1], 13120[1], 13121[1], 13122[1], 13131[1], 13132[1], 13133[1], 13151[1], 13152[1], 13153[1], 36000[1], 36400[1], 36405[1], 36406[1], 36410[1], 36420[1], 36425[1], 36430[1], 36440[1], 36591[0], 36592[0], 36600[1], 36640[1], 43752[1], 50706[1], 50715[1], 50953[1], 50972[1], 51701[0], 51702[0], 51703[0], 52000[0], 52001[1], 52005[0], 52007[0], 52204[1], 52281[0], 52310[0], 52315[0], 52351[0], 53000[0], 53010[0], 53020[0], 53025[0], 53600[0], 53601[0], 53605[0], 53620[0], 53621[0], 53660[0], 53661[0], 53665[0], 57410[0], 62320[0], 62321[0], 62322[0], 62323[0], 62324[0], 62325[0], 62326[0], 62327[0], 64400[0], 64405[0], 64408[0], 64415[0], 64416[0], 64417[0], 64418[0], 64420[0], 64421[0], 64425[0], 64430[0], 64435[0], 64445[0], 64446[0], 64447[0], 64448[0], 64449[0], 64450[0], 64451[0], 64454[0], 64461[0], 64462[0], 64463[0], 64479[0], 64480[0], 64483[0], 64484[0], 64486[0], 64487[0], 64488[0], 64489[0], 64490[0], 64491[0], 64492[0], 64493[0], 64494[0], 64495[0], 64505[0], 64510[0], 64517[0], 64520[0], 64530[0], 69990[0], 76000[1], 77001[1], 77002[1], 92012[1], 92014[1], 93000[1], 93005[1], 93010[1], 93040[1], 93041[1], 93042[1], 93318[1], 93355[1], 94002[1], 94200[1], 94680[1], 94681[1], 94690[1], 95812[1], 95813[1], 95816[1], 95819[1], 95822[1], 95829[1], 95955[1], 96360[1], 96361[1], 96365[1], 96366[1], 96367[1], 96368[1], 96372[1], 96374[1], 96375[1], 96376[1], 96377[1], 96523[0], 99155[0], 99156[0], 99157[0], 99211[1], 99212[1], 99213[1], 99214[1], 99215[1], 99217[1], 99218[1], 99219[1], 99220[1], 99221[1], 99222[1], 99223[1], 99231[1], 99232[1], 99233[1], 99234[1], 99235[1], 99236[1], 99238[1], 99239[1], 99241[1], 99242[1], 99243[1], 99244[1], 99245[1], 99251[1], 99252[1], 99253[1], 99254[1], 99255[1], 99291[1], 99292[1], 99304[1], 99305[1], 99306[1], 99307[1], 99308[1], 99309[1], 99310[1], 99315[1], 99316[1], 99334[1], 99335[1], 99336[1], 99337[1], 99347[1], 99348[1], 99349[1], 99350[1], 99374[1], 99375[1], 99377[1], 99378[1], 99446[0], 99447[0], 99448[0], 99449[0], 99451[0], 99452[0], 99495[1], 99496[1], G0463[1], G0471[0], P9612[1]
52344	00910[0], 00916[0], 0213T[0], 0216T[0], 0596T[0], 0597T[0], 0708T[1], 0709T[1], 12001[1], 12002[1], 12004[1], 12005[1], 12006[1], 12007[1], 12011[1], 12013[1], 12014[1], 12015[1], 12016[1], 12017[1], 12018[1], 12020[1], 12021[1], 12031[1], 12032[1], 12034[1], 12035[1], 12036[1], 12037[1], 12041[1], 12042[1], 12044[1], 12045[1], 12046[1], 12047[1], 12051[1], 12052[1], 12053[1], 12054[1], 12055[1], 12056[1], 12057[1], 13100[1], 13101[1], 13102[1], 13120[1], 13121[1], 13122[1], 13131[1], 13132[1], 13133[1], 13151[1], 13152[1], 13153[1], 36000[1], 36400[1], 36405[1], 36406[1], 36410[1], 36420[1], 36425[1], 36430[1], 36440[1], 36591[0], 36592[0], 36600[1], 36640[1], 43752[1], 50706[1], 50715[1], 50953[1], 50972[1], 51701[0], 51702[0], 51703[0], 52000[0], 52001[1], 52005[0], 52007[0], 52204[1], 52281[0], 52310[0], 52315[0], 52341[1], 52351[0], 53000[0], 53010[0], 53020[0], 53025[0], 53600[0], 53601[0], 53605[0], 53620[0], 53621[0], 53660[0], 53661[0], 53665[0], 57410[0], 62320[0], 62321[0], 62322[0], 62323[0], 62324[0], 62325[0], 62326[0], 62327[0], 64400[0], 64405[0], 64408[0], 64415[0], 64416[0], 64417[0], 64418[0], 64420[0], 64421[0], 64425[0], 64430[0], 64435[0], 64445[0], 64446[0], 64447[0], 64448[0], 64449[0], 64450[0], 64451[0], 64454[0], 64461[0], 64462[0], 64463[0], 64479[0], 64480[0], 64483[0], 64484[0], 64486[0], 64487[0], 64488[0], 64489[0], 64490[0], 64491[0], 64492[0], 64493[0], 64494[0], 64495[0], 64505[0], 64510[0], 64517[0], 64520[0], 64530[0], 69990[0], 76000[1], 77001[1], 77002[1], 92012[1], 92014[1], 93000[1], 93005[1], 93010[1], 93040[1], 93041[1], 93042[1],

Code 1	Code 2
	93318[1], 93355[1], 94002[1], 94200[1], 94680[1], 94681[1], 94690[1], 95812[1], 95813[1], 95816[1], 95819[1], 95822[1], 95829[1], 95955[1], 96360[1], 96361[1], 96365[1], 96366[1], 96367[1], 96368[1], 96372[1], 96374[1], 96375[1], 96376[1], 96377[1], 96523[0], 99155[0], 99156[0], 99157[0], 99211[1], 99212[1], 99213[1], 99214[1], 99215[1], 99217[1], 99218[1], 99219[1], 99220[1], 99221[1], 99222[1], 99223[1], 99231[1], 99232[1], 99233[1], 99234[1], 99235[1], 99236[1], 99238[1], 99239[1], 99241[1], 99242[1], 99243[1], 99244[1], 99245[1], 99251[1], 99252[1], 99253[1], 99254[1], 99255[1], 99291[1], 99292[1], 99304[1], 99305[1], 99306[1], 99307[1], 99308[1], 99309[1], 99310[1], 99315[1], 99316[1], 99334[1], 99335[1], 99336[1], 99337[1], 99347[1], 99348[1], 99349[1], 99350[1], 99374[1], 99375[1], 99377[1], 99378[1], 99446[0], 99447[0], 99448[0], 99449[0], 99451[0], 99452[0], 99495[1], 99496[1], G0463[1], G0471[0], P9612[1]
52345	00910[0], 00916[0], 0213T[0], 0216T[0], 0596T[0], 0597T[0], 0708T[1], 0709T[1], 12001[1], 12002[1], 12004[1], 12005[1], 12006[1], 12007[1], 12011[1], 12013[1], 12014[1], 12015[1], 12016[1], 12017[1], 12018[1], 12020[1], 12021[1], 12031[1], 12032[1], 12034[1], 12035[1], 12036[1], 12037[1], 12041[1], 12042[1], 12044[1], 12045[1], 12046[1], 12047[1], 12051[1], 12052[1], 12053[1], 12054[1], 12055[1], 12056[1], 12057[1], 13100[1], 13101[1], 13102[1], 13120[1], 13121[1], 13122[1], 13131[1], 13132[1], 13133[1], 13151[1], 13152[1], 13153[1], 36000[1], 36400[1], 36405[1], 36406[1], 36410[1], 36420[1], 36425[1], 36430[1], 36440[1], 36591[0], 36592[0], 36600[1], 36640[1], 43752[1], 50706[1], 50715[1], 50953[1], 50972[1], 51701[0], 51702[0], 51703[0], 52000[0], 52001[1], 52005[0], 52007[0], 52204[1], 52281[0], 52310[0], 52315[0], 52342[1], 52351[0], 53000[0], 53010[0], 53020[0], 53025[0], 53600[0], 53601[0], 53605[0], 53620[0], 53621[0], 53660[0], 53661[0], 53665[0], 57410[0], 62320[0], 62321[0], 62322[0], 62323[0], 62324[0], 62325[0], 62326[0], 62327[0], 64400[0], 64405[0], 64408[0], 64415[0], 64416[0], 64417[0], 64418[0], 64420[0], 64421[0], 64425[0], 64430[0], 64435[0], 64445[0], 64446[0], 64447[0], 64448[0], 64449[0], 64450[0], 64451[0], 64454[0], 64461[0], 64462[0], 64463[0], 64479[0], 64480[0], 64483[0], 64484[0], 64486[0], 64487[0], 64488[0], 64489[0], 64490[0], 64491[0], 64492[0], 64493[0], 64494[0], 64495[0], 64505[0], 64510[0], 64517[0], 64520[0], 64530[0], 69990[0], 76000[1], 77001[1], 77002[1], 92012[1], 92014[1], 93000[1], 93005[1], 93010[1], 93040[1], 93041[1], 93042[1], 93318[1], 93355[1], 94002[1], 94200[1], 94680[1], 94681[1], 94690[1], 95812[1], 95813[1], 95816[1], 95819[1], 95822[1], 95829[1], 95955[1], 96360[1], 96361[1], 96365[1], 96366[1], 96367[1], 96368[1], 96372[1], 96374[1], 96375[1], 96376[1], 96377[1], 96523[0], 99155[0], 99156[0], 99157[0], 99211[1], 99212[1], 99213[1], 99214[1], 99215[1], 99217[1], 99218[1], 99219[1], 99220[1], 99221[1], 99222[1], 99223[1], 99231[1], 99232[1], 99233[1], 99234[1], 99235[1], 99236[1], 99238[1], 99239[1], 99241[1], 99242[1], 99243[1], 99244[1], 99245[1], 99251[1], 99252[1], 99253[1], 99254[1], 99255[1], 99291[1], 99292[1], 99304[1], 99305[1], 99306[1], 99307[1], 99308[1], 99309[1], 99310[1], 99315[1], 99316[1], 99334[1], 99335[1], 99336[1], 99337[1], 99347[1], 99348[1], 99349[1], 99350[1], 99374[1], 99375[1], 99377[1], 99378[1], 99446[0], 99447[0], 99448[0], 99449[0], 99451[0], 99452[0], 99495[1], 99496[1], G0463[1], G0471[0], P9612[1]
52346	00910[0], 00916[0], 0213T[0], 0216T[0], 0596T[0], 0597T[0], 0708T[1], 0709T[1], 12001[1], 12002[1], 12004[1], 12005[1], 12006[1], 12007[1], 12011[1], 12013[1], 12014[1], 12015[1], 12016[1], 12017[1], 12018[1], 12020[1], 12021[1], 12031[1], 12032[1], 12034[1], 12035[1], 12036[1], 12037[1], 12041[1], 12042[1], 12044[1], 12045[1], 12046[1], 12047[1], 12051[1], 12052[1], 12053[1], 12054[1], 12055[1], 12056[1], 12057[1], 13100[1], 13101[1], 13102[1], 13120[1], 13121[1], 13122[1], 13131[1], 13132[1], 13133[1], 13151[1], 13152[1], 13153[1], 36000[1], 36400[1], 36405[1], 36406[1], 36410[1], 36420[1], 36425[1], 36430[1], 36440[1], 36591[0], 36592[0], 36600[1], 36640[1], 43752[1], 50706[1], 50715[1], 50953[1], 50972[1], 51701[0], 51702[0], 51703[0], 52000[0], 52001[1], 52005[0], 52007[0], 52204[1], 52281[0], 52310[0], 52315[0], 52343[1], 52351[0], 53000[0], 53010[0], 53020[0], 53025[0], 53600[0], 53601[0], 53605[0], 53620[0], 53621[0], 53660[0], 53661[0], 53665[0], 57410[0], 62320[0], 62321[0], 62322[0], 62323[0], 62324[0], 62325[0], 62326[0], 62327[0], 64400[0], 64405[0], 64408[0], 64415[0], 64416[0], 64417[0], 64418[0], 64420[0], 64421[0], 64425[0], 64430[0], 64435[0], 64445[0], 64446[0], 64447[0], 64448[0], 64449[0], 64450[0], 64451[0], 64454[0], 64461[0], 64462[0], 64463[0], 64479[0], 64480[0], 64483[0], 64484[0], 64486[0], 64487[0], 64488[0], 64489[0], 64490[0], 64491[0], 64492[0], 64493[0], 64494[0], 64495[0], 64505[0], 64510[0], 64517[0], 64520[0], 64530[0], 69990[0], 76000[1], 77001[1], 77002[1], 92012[1], 92014[1], 93000[1], 93005[1], 93010[1], 93040[1], 93041[1], 93042[1], 93318[1], 93355[1], 94002[1], 94200[1], 94680[1], 94681[1], 94690[1], 95812[1], 95813[1], 95816[1], 95819[1], 95822[1], 95829[1], 95955[1], 96360[1], 96361[1], 96365[1], 96366[1], 96367[1], 96368[1], 96372[1], 96374[1], 96375[1], 96376[1], 96377[1], 96523[0], 99155[0], 99156[0], 99157[0], 99211[1], 99212[1], 99213[1], 99214[1], 99215[1], 99217[1], 99218[1], 99219[1], 99220[1], 99221[1], 99222[1], 99223[1], 99231[1], 99232[1], 99233[1], 99234[1], 99235[1], 99236[1], 99238[1], 99239[1], 99241[1], 99242[1], 99243[1], 99244[1], 99245[1], 99251[1], 99252[1], 99253[1], 99254[1], 99255[1], 99291[1], 99292[1], 99304[1], 99305[1], 99306[1], 99307[1], 99308[1], 99309[1], 99310[1], 99315[1], 99316[1], 99334[1], 99335[1], 99336[1], 99337[1], 99347[1], 99348[1], 99349[1], 99350[1], 99374[1], 99375[1], 99377[1], 99378[1], 99446[0], 99447[0], 99448[0], 99449[0], 99451[0], 99452[0], 99495[1], 99496[1], G0463[1], G0471[0], P9612[1]
52351	00910[0], 00916[0], 0213T[0], 0216T[0], 0596T[0], 0597T[0], 0708T[1], 0709T[1], 12001[1], 12002[1], 12004[1], 12005[1], 12006[1], 12007[1], 12011[1], 12013[1], 12014[1], 12015[1], 12016[1], 12017[1], 12018[1], 12020[1], 12021[1], 12031[1], 12032[1], 12034[1], 12035[1], 12036[1], 12037[1], 12041[1], 12042[1], 12044[1], 12045[1], 12046[1], 12047[1], 12051[1], 12052[1], 12053[1], 12054[1], 12055[1], 12056[1], 12057[1], 13100[1], 13101[1], 13102[1], 13120[1], 13121[1], 13122[1], 13131[1], 13132[1], 13133[1], 13151[1], 13152[1], 13153[1], 36000[1], 36400[1], 36405[1], 36406[1], 36410[1], 36420[1], 36425[1], 36430[1], 36440[1], 36591[0], 36592[0], 36600[1], 36640[1], 43752[1], 51701[0], 51702[0], 51703[0], 52000[0], 52001[1], 52005[0], 52007[0], 52204[1], 52281[0], 52310[0], 52315[0], 53000[0], 53010[0], 53020[0], 53025[0], 53600[0], 53601[0], 53605[0], 53620[0], 53621[0], 53660[0], 53661[0], 53665[0], 57410[0], 62320[0], 62321[0], 62322[0], 62323[0], 62324[0], 62325[0], 62326[0], 62327[0], 64400[0], 64405[0], 64408[0], 64415[0], 64416[0], 64417[0], 64418[0], 64420[0], 64421[0], 64425[0], 64430[0], 64435[0], 64445[0], 64446[0], 64447[0], 64448[0], 64449[0], 64450[0], 64451[0], 64454[0], 64461[0], 64462[0], 64463[0], 64479[0], 64480[0], 64483[0], 64484[0], 64486[0], 64487[0], 64488[0], 64489[0], 64490[0], 64491[0], 64492[0], 64493[0], 64494[0], 64495[0], 64505[0], 64510[0], 64517[0], 64520[0], 64530[0], 69990[0], 76000[1], 77001[1], 77002[1], 92012[1], 92014[1], 93000[1], 93005[1], 93010[1], 93040[1], 93041[1], 93042[1], 93318[1], 93355[1], 94002[1], 94200[1], 94680[1], 94681[1], 94690[1], 95812[1], 95813[1], 95816[1], 95819[1], 95822[1], 95829[1], 95955[1], 96360[1], 96361[1], 96365[1], 96366[1], 96367[1], 96368[1], 96372[1], 96374[1], 96375[1], 96376[1], 96377[1], 96523[0], 99155[0], 99156[0], 99157[0], 99211[1], 99212[1], 99213[1], 99214[1], 99215[1], 99217[1], 99218[1], 99219[1], 99220[1], 99221[1], 99222[1], 99223[1], 99231[1], 99232[1], 99233[1], 99234[1], 99235[1], 99236[1], 99238[1], 99239[1], 99241[1], 99242[1], 99243[1], 99244[1], 99245[1], 99251[1], 99252[1], 99253[1], 99254[1], 99255[1], 99291[1], 99292[1], 99304[1], 99305[1], 99306[1], 99307[1], 99308[1], 99309[1], 99310[1], 99315[1], 99316[1], 99334[1], 99335[1], 99336[1], 99337[1], 99347[1], 99348[1], 99349[1], 99350[1], 99374[1], 99375[1], 99377[1], 99378[1], 99446[0], 99447[0], 99448[0], 99449[0], 99451[0], 99452[0], 99495[1], 99496[1], G0463[1], G0471[0], P9612[1]
52352	00910[0], 00916[0], 00918[0], 0213T[0], 0216T[0], 0596T[0], 0597T[0], 0708T[1], 0709T[1], 11000[1], 11001[1], 11004[1], 11005[1], 11006[1], 11042[1], 11043[1], 11044[1], 11045[1], 11046[1], 11047[1], 12001[1], 12002[1], 12004[1], 12005[1], 12006[1], 12007[1], 12011[1], 12013[1], 12014[1], 12015[1], 12016[1], 12017[1], 12018[1], 12020[1], 12021[1], 12031[1], 12032[1], 12034[1], 12035[1], 12036[1], 12037[1], 12041[1], 12042[1], 12044[1], 12045[1], 12046[1], 12047[1], 12051[1], 12052[1], 12053[1], 12054[1], 12055[1], 12056[1], 12057[1], 13100[1], 13101[1], 13102[1], 13120[1], 13121[1], 13122[1], 13131[1], 13132[1], 13133[1], 13151[1], 13152[1], 13153[1], 36000[1], 36400[1], 36405[1], 36406[1], 36410[1], 36420[1], 36425[1], 36430[1], 36440[1], 36591[0], 36592[0], 36600[1], 36640[1], 43752[1], 50945[1], 50961[1], 51700[0], 51701[0], 51702[0], 51703[0], 52000[0], 52001[1], 52005[0], 52007[0], 52235[1], 52281[0], 52310[0], 52315[0], 52317[1], 52318[1], 52320[1], 52325[1], 52330[1], 52341[1], 52342[1], 52343[1], 52344[1], 52345[1], 52346[1], 52351[0], 53000[0], 53010[0], 53020[0], 53025[0], 53600[0], 53601[0], 53605[0], 53620[0], 53621[0], 53660[0], 53661[0], 53665[0], 57410[0], 62320[0], 62321[0], 62322[0], 62323[0], 62324[0], 62325[0], 62326[0], 62327[0], 64400[0], 64405[0], 64408[0], 64415[0], 64416[0], 64417[0], 64418[0], 64420[0], 64421[0], 64425[0], 64430[0], 64435[0], 64445[0], 64446[0], 64447[0], 64448[0], 64449[0], 64450[0], 64451[0], 64454[0], 64461[0], 64462[0], 64463[0], 64479[0], 64480[0], 64483[0], 64484[0], 64486[0], 64487[0], 64488[0], 64489[0], 64490[0], 64491[0], 64492[0], 64493[0], 64494[0], 64495[0], 64505[0], 64510[0], 64517[0], 64520[0], 64530[0], 69990[0], 76000[1], 77001[1], 77002[1], 92012[1], 92014[1], 93000[1], 93005[1], 93010[1], 93040[1], 93041[1], 93042[1], 93318[1], 93355[1], 94002[1], 94200[1], 94680[1], 94681[1], 94690[1], 95812[1], 95813[1], 95816[1], 95819[1], 95822[1], 95829[1], 95955[1], 96360[1], 96361[1], 96365[1], 96366[1], 96367[1], 96368[1], 96372[1], 96374[1], 96375[1], 96376[1], 96377[1], 96523[0], 97597[1], 97598[1], 97602[1], 99155[0], 99156[0], 99157[0], 99211[1], 99212[1], 99213[1], 99214[1], 99215[1], 99217[1], 99218[1], 99219[1], 99220[1], 99221[1], 99222[1], 99223[1], 99231[1], 99232[1], 99233[1], 99234[1], 99235[1], 99236[1], 99238[1], 99239[1], 99241[1], 99242[1], 99243[1], 99244[1], 99245[1], 99251[1], 99252[1], 99253[1], 99254[1], 99255[1], 99291[1], 99292[1], 99304[1], 99305[1], 99306[1], 99307[1], 99308[1], 99309[1], 99310[1], 99315[1], 99316[1], 99334[1], 99335[1], 99336[1], 99337[1], 99347[1], 99348[1], 99349[1], 99350[1], 99374[1], 99375[1], 99377[1], 99378[1], 99446[0], 99447[0], 99448[0], 99449[0], 99451[0], 99452[0], 99495[1], 99496[1], G0463[1], G0471[0], P9612[1]
52353	00910[0], 00916[0], 00918[0], 0213T[0], 0216T[0], 0596T[0], 0597T[0], 0708T[1], 0709T[1], 12001[1], 12002[1], 12004[1], 12005[1], 12006[1], 12007[1], 12011[1], 12013[1], 12014[1], 12015[1], 12016[1], 12017[1], 12018[1], 12020[1], 12021[1], 12031[1], 12032[1], 12034[1], 12035[1], 12036[1], 12037[1], 12041[1], 12042[1], 12044[1], 12045[1], 12046[1], 12047[1], 12051[1], 12052[1], 12053[1], 12054[1], 12055[1], 12056[1], 12057[1], 13100[1], 13101[1], 13102[1], 13120[1], 13121[1], 13122[1], 13131[1], 13132[1], 13133[1], 13151[1], 13152[1], 13153[1], 36000[1], 36400[1], 36405[1], 36406[1], 36410[1], 36420[1], 36425[1], 36430[1], 36440[1], 36591[0], 36592[0], 36600[1], 36640[1], 43752[1], 50945[1], 50961[1], 50980[1], 51700[1], 51701[0], 51702[0], 51703[0], 52000[0], 52001[1], 52005[0], 52007[0], 52235[1], 52281[0], 52310[0], 52315[0], 52317[1], 52318[1], 52320[1], 52325[1], 52330[1], 52332[1], 52341[1], 52342[1], 52343[1], 52344[1], 52345[1], 52346[1], 52351[0], 52352[0], 53000[0], 53010[0], 53020[0], 53025[0], 53600[0], 53601[0], 53605[0], 53620[0], 53621[0], 53660[0], 53661[0], 53665[0], 57410[0], 62320[0], 62321[0], 62322[0], 62323[0], 62324[0], 62325[0], 62326[0], 62327[0], 64400[0], 64405[0], 64408[0], 64415[0], 64416[0], 64417[0], 64418[0], 64420[0], 64421[0], 64425[0], 64430[0], 64435[0], 64445[0], 64446[0], 64447[0], 64448[0], 64449[0], 64450[0], 64451[0], 64454[0], 64461[0], 64462[0], 64463[0], 64479[0], 64480[0], 64483[0], 64484[0], 64486[0], 64487[0], 64488[0], 64489[0], 64490[0], 64491[0], 64492[0], 64493[0], 64494[0], 64495[0], 64505[0], 64510[0], 64517[0], 64520[0],

0 = Modifier usage not allowed or inappropriate 1 = Modifier usage allowed

Code 1	Code 2
	64530[0], 69990[0], 76000[1], 77001[1], 77002[1], 92012[1], 92014[1], 93000[1], 93005[1], 93010[1], 93040[1], 93041[1], 93042[1], 93318[1], 93355[1], 94002[1], 94200[1], 94680[1], 94681[1], 94690[1], 95812[1], 95813[1], 95816[1], 95819[1], 95822[1], 95829[1], 95955[1], 96360[1], 96361[1], 96365[1], 96366[1], 96367[1], 96368[1], 96372[1], 96374[1], 96375[1], 96376[1], 96377[1], 96523[0], 99155[0], 99156[0], 99157[0], 99211[1], 99212[1], 99213[1], 99214[1], 99215[1], 99217[1], 99218[1], 99219[1], 99220[1], 99221[1], 99222[1], 99223[1], 99231[1], 99232[1], 99233[1], 99234[1], 99235[1], 99236[1], 99238[1], 99239[1], 99241[1], 99242[1], 99243[1], 99244[1], 99245[1], 99251[1], 99252[1], 99253[1], 99254[1], 99255[1], 99291[1], 99292[1], 99304[1], 99305[1], 99306[1], 99307[1], 99308[1], 99309[1], 99310[1], 99315[1], 99316[1], 99334[1], 99335[1], 99336[1], 99337[1], 99347[1], 99348[1], 99349[1], 99350[1], 99374[1], 99375[1], 99377[1], 99378[1], 99446[0], 99447[0], 99448[0], 99449[0], 99451[0], 99452[0], 99495[1], 99496[1], G0463[1], G0471[0], P9612[1]
52354	00910[0], 00912[0], 00916[0], 0213T[0], 0216T[0], 0596T[0], 0597T[0], 0708T[1], 0709T[1], 10005[1], 10007[1], 10009[1], 10011[1], 10021[1], 12001[1], 12002[1], 12004[1], 12005[1], 12006[1], 12007[1], 12011[1], 12013[1], 12014[1], 12015[1], 12016[1], 12017[1], 12018[1], 12020[1], 12021[1], 12031[1], 12032[1], 12034[1], 12035[1], 12036[1], 12037[1], 12041[1], 12042[1], 12044[1], 12045[1], 12046[1], 12047[1], 12051[1], 12052[1], 12053[1], 12054[1], 12055[1], 12056[1], 12057[1], 13100[1], 13101[1], 13102[1], 13120[1], 13121[1], 13122[1], 13131[1], 13132[1], 13133[1], 13151[1], 13152[1], 13153[1], 36000[1], 36400[1], 36405[1], 36406[1], 36410[1], 36420[1], 36425[1], 36430[1], 36440[1], 36591[0], 36592[0], 36600[1], 36640[1], 43752[1], 50606[1], 51701[0], 51702[0], 51703[0], 52000[0], 52001[1], 52005[0], 52007[0], 52204[1], 52234[1], 52235[1], 52240[1], 52281[0], 52301[1], 52310[0], 52315[0], 52341[1], 52342[1], 52343[1], 52344[1], 52345[1], 52346[1], 52351[0], 53000[0], 53010[0], 53020[0], 53025[0], 53600[0], 53601[0], 53605[0], 53620[0], 53621[0], 53660[0], 53661[0], 53665[0], 57410[0], 62320[0], 62321[0], 62322[0], 62323[0], 62324[0], 62325[0], 62326[0], 62327[0], 64400[0], 64405[0], 64408[0], 64415[0], 64416[0], 64417[0], 64418[0], 64420[0], 64421[0], 64425[0], 64430[0], 64435[0], 64445[0], 64446[0], 64447[0], 64448[0], 64449[0], 64450[0], 64451[0], 64454[0], 64461[0], 64462[0], 64463[0], 64479[0], 64480[0], 64483[0], 64484[0], 64486[0], 64487[0], 64488[0], 64489[0], 64490[0], 64491[0], 64492[0], 64493[0], 64494[0], 64495[0], 64505[0], 64510[0], 64517[0], 64520[0], 64530[0], 69990[0], 76000[1], 77001[1], 77002[1], 92012[1], 92014[1], 93000[1], 93005[1], 93010[1], 93040[1], 93041[1], 93042[1], 93318[1], 93355[1], 94002[1], 94200[1], 94680[1], 94681[1], 94690[1], 95812[1], 95813[1], 95816[1], 95819[1], 95822[1], 95829[1], 95955[1], 96360[1], 96361[1], 96365[1], 96366[1], 96367[1], 96368[1], 96372[1], 96374[1], 96375[1], 96376[1], 96377[1], 96523[0], 99155[0], 99156[0], 99157[0], 99211[1], 99212[1], 99213[1], 99214[1], 99215[1], 99217[1], 99218[1], 99219[1], 99220[1], 99221[1], 99222[1], 99223[1], 99231[1], 99232[1], 99233[1], 99234[1], 99235[1], 99236[1], 99238[1], 99239[1], 99241[1], 99242[1], 99243[1], 99244[1], 99245[1], 99251[1], 99252[1], 99253[1], 99254[1], 99255[1], 99291[1], 99292[1], 99304[1], 99305[1], 99306[1], 99307[1], 99308[1], 99309[1], 99310[1], 99315[1], 99316[1], 99334[1], 99335[1], 99336[1], 99337[1], 99347[1], 99348[1], 99349[1], 99350[1], 99374[1], 99375[1], 99377[1], 99378[1], 99446[0], 99447[0], 99448[0], 99449[0], 99451[0], 99452[0], 99495[1], 99496[1], G0463[1], G0471[0], P9612[1]
52355	00910[0], 00912[0], 00916[0], 0213T[0], 0216T[0], 0596T[0], 0597T[0], 0708T[1], 0709T[1], 11000[1], 11001[1], 11004[1], 11005[1], 11006[1], 11042[1], 11043[1], 11044[1], 11045[1], 11046[1], 11047[1], 12001[1], 12002[1], 12004[1], 12005[1], 12006[1], 12007[1], 12011[1], 12013[1], 12014[1], 12015[1], 12016[1], 12017[1], 12018[1], 12020[1], 12021[1], 12031[1], 12032[1], 12034[1], 12035[1], 12036[1], 12037[1], 12041[1], 12042[1], 12044[1], 12045[1], 12046[1], 12047[1], 12051[1], 12052[1], 12053[1], 12054[1], 12055[1], 12056[1], 12057[1], 13100[1], 13101[1], 13102[1], 13120[1], 13121[1], 13122[1], 13131[1], 13132[1], 13133[1], 13151[1], 13152[1], 13153[1], 36000[1], 36400[1], 36405[1], 36406[1], 36410[1], 36420[1], 36425[1], 36430[1], 36440[1], 36591[0], 36592[0], 36600[1], 36640[1], 43752[1], 51701[0], 51702[0], 51703[0], 52000[0], 52001[1], 52005[0], 52007[0], 52204[1], 52224[1], 52281[0], 52310[0], 52315[0], 52341[1], 52342[1], 52343[1], 52344[1], 52345[1], 52346[1], 52351[0], 52354[1], 53000[0], 53010[0], 53020[0], 53025[0], 53600[0], 53601[0], 53605[0], 53620[0], 53621[0], 53660[0], 53661[0], 53665[0], 57410[0], 62320[0], 62321[0], 62322[0], 62323[0], 62324[0], 62325[0], 62326[0], 62327[0], 64400[0], 64405[0], 64408[0], 64415[0], 64416[0], 64417[0], 64418[0], 64420[0], 64421[0], 64425[0], 64430[0], 64435[0], 64445[0], 64446[0], 64447[0], 64448[0], 64449[0], 64450[0], 64451[0], 64454[0], 64461[0], 64462[0], 64463[0], 64479[0], 64480[0], 64483[0], 64484[0], 64486[0], 64487[0], 64488[0], 64489[0], 64490[0], 64491[0], 64492[0], 64493[0], 64494[0], 64495[0], 64505[0], 64510[0], 64517[0], 64520[0], 64530[0], 69990[0], 76000[1], 77001[1], 77002[1], 92012[1], 92014[1], 93000[1], 93005[1], 93010[1], 93040[1], 93041[1], 93042[1], 93318[1], 93355[1], 94002[1], 94200[1], 94680[1], 94681[1], 94690[1], 95812[1], 95813[1], 95816[1], 95819[1], 95822[1], 95829[1], 95955[1], 96360[1], 96361[1], 96365[1], 96366[1], 96367[1], 96368[1], 96372[1], 96374[1], 96375[1], 96376[1], 96377[1], 96523[0], 97597[1], 97598[1], 97602[1], 99155[0], 99156[0], 99157[0], 99211[1], 99212[1], 99213[1], 99214[1], 99215[1], 99217[1], 99218[1], 99219[1], 99220[1], 99221[1], 99222[1], 99223[1], 99231[1], 99232[1], 99233[1], 99234[1], 99235[1], 99236[1], 99238[1], 99239[1], 99241[1], 99242[1], 99243[1], 99244[1], 99245[1], 99251[1], 99252[1], 99253[1], 99254[1], 99255[1], 99291[1], 99292[1], 99304[1], 99305[1], 99306[1], 99307[1], 99308[1], 99309[1], 99310[1], 99315[1], 99316[1], 99334[1], 99335[1], 99336[1], 99337[1], 99347[1], 99348[1], 99349[1], 99350[1], 99374[1], 99375[1], 99377[1], 99378[1], 99446[0], 99447[0], 99448[0], 99449[0], 99451[0], 99452[0], 99495[1], 99496[1], G0463[1], G0471[0], P9612[1]
52356	00910[0], 00916[0], 00918[0], 0213T[0], 0216T[0], 0596T[0], 0597T[0], 0708T[1], 0709T[1], 11000[1], 11001[1], 11004[1], 11005[1], 11006[1], 11042[1], 11043[1], 11044[1], 11045[1], 11046[1], 11047[1], 12001[1], 12002[1], 12004[1], 12005[1], 12006[1], 12007[1], 12011[1], 12013[1], 12014[1], 12015[1], 12016[1], 12017[1], 12018[1], 12020[1], 12021[1], 12031[1], 12032[1], 12034[1], 12035[1], 12036[1], 12037[1], 12041[1], 12042[1], 12044[1], 12045[1], 12046[1], 12047[1], 12051[1], 12052[1], 12053[1], 12054[1], 12055[1], 12056[1], 12057[1], 13100[1], 13101[1], 13102[1], 13120[1], 13121[1], 13122[1], 13131[1], 13132[1], 13133[1], 13151[1], 13152[1], 13153[1], 36000[1], 36400[1], 36405[1], 36406[1], 36410[1], 36420[1], 36425[1], 36430[1], 36440[1], 36591[0], 36592[0], 36600[1], 36640[1], 43752[1], 50387[1], 50430[1], 50431[1], 50561[1], 50684[1], 50715[1], 50945[1], 50961[1], 50980[1], 51700[1], 51701[0], 51702[0], 51703[0], 52000[0], 52001[1], 52005[0], 52007[1], 52204[1], 52235[1], 52281[0], 52310[0], 52315[0], 52317[1], 52318[1], 52320[1], 52325[1], 52330[1], 52332[1], 52341[1], 52342[1], 52343[1], 52344[1], 52345[1], 52346[1], 52351[1], 52352[1], 52353[1], 53000[0], 53010[0], 53020[0], 53025[0], 53600[0], 53601[0], 53605[0], 53620[0], 53621[0], 53660[0], 53661[0], 53665[0], 57410[0], 62320[0], 62321[0], 62322[0], 62323[0], 62324[0], 62325[0], 62326[0], 62327[0], 64400[0], 64405[0], 64408[0], 64415[0], 64416[0], 64417[0], 64418[0], 64420[0], 64421[0], 64425[0], 64430[0], 64435[0], 64445[0], 64446[0], 64447[0], 64448[0], 64449[0], 64450[0], 64451[0], 64454[0], 64461[0], 64462[0], 64463[0], 64479[0], 64480[0], 64483[0], 64484[0], 64486[0], 64487[0], 64488[0], 64489[0], 64490[0], 64491[0], 64492[0], 64493[0], 64494[0], 64495[0], 64505[0], 64510[0], 64517[0], 64520[0], 64530[0], 69990[0], 76000[1], 77001[1], 77002[1], 92012[1], 92014[1], 93000[1], 93005[1], 93010[1], 93040[1], 93041[1], 93042[1], 93318[1], 93355[1], 94002[1], 94200[1], 94680[1], 94681[1], 94690[1], 95812[1], 95813[1], 95816[1], 95819[1], 95822[1], 95829[1], 95955[1], 96360[1], 96361[1], 96365[1], 96366[1], 96367[1], 96368[1], 96372[1], 96374[1], 96375[1], 96376[1], 96377[1], 96523[0], 97597[1], 97598[1], 97602[1], 99155[0], 99156[0], 99157[0], 99211[1], 99212[1], 99213[1], 99214[1], 99215[1], 99217[1], 99218[1], 99219[1], 99220[1], 99221[1], 99222[1], 99223[1], 99231[1], 99232[1], 99233[1], 99234[1], 99235[1], 99236[1], 99238[1], 99239[1], 99241[1], 99242[1], 99243[1], 99244[1], 99245[1], 99251[1], 99252[1], 99253[1], 99254[1], 99255[1], 99291[1], 99292[1], 99304[1], 99305[1], 99306[1], 99307[1], 99308[1], 99309[1], 99310[1], 99315[1], 99316[1], 99334[1], 99335[1], 99336[1], 99337[1], 99347[1], 99348[1], 99349[1], 99350[1], 99374[1], 99375[1], 99377[1], 99378[1], 99446[0], 99447[0], 99448[0], 99449[0], 99451[0], 99452[0], G0463[1], G0471[0], J2001[1], P9612[1]
52400	00910[0], 00916[0], 0213T[0], 0216T[0], 0499T[0], 0596T[0], 0597T[0], 0619T[1], 0708T[1], 0709T[1], 11000[1], 11001[1], 11004[1], 11005[1], 11006[1], 11042[1], 11043[1], 11044[1], 11045[1], 11046[1], 11047[1], 12001[1], 12002[1], 12004[1], 12005[1], 12006[1], 12007[1], 12011[1], 12013[1], 12014[1], 12015[1], 12016[1], 12017[1], 12018[1], 12020[1], 12021[1], 12031[1], 12032[1], 12034[1], 12035[1], 12036[1], 12037[1], 12041[1], 12042[1], 12044[1], 12045[1], 12046[1], 12047[1], 12051[1], 12052[1], 12053[1], 12054[1], 12055[1], 12056[1], 12057[1], 13100[1], 13101[1], 13102[1], 13120[1], 13121[1], 13122[1], 13131[1], 13132[1], 13133[1], 13151[1], 13152[1], 13153[1], 36000[1], 36400[1], 36405[1], 36406[1], 36410[1], 36420[1], 36425[1], 36430[1], 36440[1], 36591[0], 36592[0], 36600[1], 36640[1], 43752[1], 51701[0], 51702[0], 51703[0], 52000[0], 52001[1], 52270[1], 52275[0], 52276[0], 52281[0], 52283[0], 52287[0], 52310[0], 52315[0], 52441[1], 52500[0], 52630[0], 53000[0], 53010[0], 53020[0], 53025[0], 53600[0], 53601[0], 53605[0], 53620[0], 53621[0], 53660[0], 53661[0], 53855[1], 57410[0], 62320[0], 62321[0], 62322[0], 62323[0], 62324[0], 62325[0], 62326[0], 62327[0], 64400[0], 64405[0], 64408[0], 64415[0], 64416[0], 64417[0], 64418[0], 64420[0], 64421[0], 64425[0], 64430[0], 64435[0], 64445[0], 64446[0], 64447[0], 64448[0], 64449[0], 64450[0], 64451[0], 64454[0], 64461[0], 64462[0], 64463[0], 64479[0], 64480[0], 64483[0], 64484[0], 64486[0], 64487[0], 64488[0], 64489[0], 64490[0], 64491[0], 64492[0], 64493[0], 64494[0], 64495[0], 64505[0], 64510[0], 64517[0], 64520[0], 64530[0], 69990[0], 76000[1], 77001[1], 77002[1], 92012[1], 92014[1], 93000[1], 93005[1], 93010[1], 93040[1], 93041[1], 93042[1], 93318[1], 93355[1], 94002[1], 94200[1], 94680[1], 94681[1], 94690[1], 95812[1], 95813[1], 95816[1], 95819[1], 95822[1], 95829[1], 95955[1], 96360[1], 96361[1], 96365[1], 96366[1], 96367[1], 96368[1], 96372[1], 96374[1], 96375[1], 96376[1], 96377[1], 96523[0], 97597[1], 97598[1], 97602[1], 99155[0], 99156[0], 99157[0], 99211[1], 99212[1], 99213[1], 99214[1], 99215[1], 99217[1], 99218[1], 99219[1], 99220[1], 99221[1], 99222[1], 99223[1], 99231[1], 99232[1], 99233[1], 99234[1], 99235[1], 99236[1], 99238[1], 99239[1], 99241[1], 99242[1], 99243[1], 99244[1], 99245[1], 99251[1], 99252[1], 99253[1], 99254[1], 99255[1], 99291[1], 99292[1], 99304[1], 99305[1], 99306[1], 99307[1], 99308[1], 99309[1], 99310[1], 99315[1], 99316[1], 99334[1], 99335[1], 99336[1], 99337[1], 99347[1], 99348[1], 99349[1], 99350[1], 99374[1], 99375[1], 99377[1], 99378[1], 99446[0], 99447[0], 99448[0], 99449[0], 99451[0], 99452[0], 99495[0], 99496[0], G0463[1], G0471[0], P9612[1]
52402	00910[0], 00916[0], 0213T[0], 0216T[0], 0596T[0], 0597T[0], 0619T[1], 0708T[1], 0709T[1], 11000[1], 11001[1], 11004[1], 11005[1], 11006[1], 11042[1], 11043[1], 11044[1], 11045[1], 11046[1], 11047[1], 12001[1], 12002[1], 12004[1], 12005[1], 12006[1], 12007[1], 12011[1], 12013[1], 12014[1], 12015[1], 12016[1], 12017[1], 12018[1], 12020[1], 12021[1], 12031[1], 12032[1], 12034[1], 12035[1], 12036[1], 12037[1], 12041[1], 12042[1], 12044[1], 12045[1], 12046[1], 12047[1], 12051[1], 12052[1], 12053[1], 12054[1], 12055[1], 12056[1], 12057[1], 13100[1], 13101[1], 13102[1], 13120[1], 13121[1], 13122[1], 13131[1], 13132[1], 13133[1], 13151[1], 13152[1], 13153[1], 36000[1], 36400[1], 36405[1], 36406[1], 36410[1], 36420[1], 36425[1], 36430[1], 36440[1], 36591[0], 36592[0], 36600[1], 36640[1], 43752[1], 51701[0], 51702[0], 51703[0], 52000[0], 52001[1], 52010[0], 52281[0], 52310[0], 52315[0], 52441[1], 53000[0], 53010[0], 53020[0], 53025[0], 53080[1], 53600[1], 53601[1], 53605[1], 53620[1], 53621[1],

0 = Modifier usage not allowed or inappropriate 1 = Modifier usage allowed

Appendix A: NCCI - CPT Codes

Code 1	Code 2
	53660[1], 53661[1], 53665[1], 53855[1], 62320[0], 62321[0], 62322[0], 62323[0], 62324[0], 62325[0], 62326[0], 62327[0], 64400[0], 64405[0], 64408[0], 64415[0], 64416[0], 64417[0], 64418[0], 64420[0], 64421[0], 64425[0], 64430[0], 64435[0], 64445[0], 64446[0], 64447[0], 64448[0], 64449[0], 64450[0], 64451[0], 64454[0], 64461[0], 64462[0], 64463[0], 64479[0], 64480[0], 64483[0], 64484[0], 64486[0], 64487[0], 64488[0], 64489[0], 64490[0], 64491[0], 64492[0], 64493[0], 64494[0], 64495[0], 64505[0], 64510[0], 64517[0], 64520[0], 64530[0], 69990[0], 76000[1], 77001[1], 77002[1], 92012[1], 92014[1], 93000[1], 93005[1], 93010[1], 93040[1], 93041[1], 93042[1], 93318[1], 93355[1], 94002[1], 94200[1], 94680[1], 94681[1], 94690[1], 95812[1], 95813[1], 95816[1], 95819[1], 95822[1], 95829[1], 95955[1], 96360[1], 96361[1], 96365[1], 96366[1], 96367[1], 96368[1], 96372[1], 96374[1], 96375[1], 96376[1], 96377[1], 96523[0], 97597[1], 97598[1], 97602[1], 99155[0], 99156[0], 99157[0], 99211[1], 99212[1], 99213[1], 99214[1], 99215[1], 99217[1], 99218[1], 99219[1], 99220[1], 99221[1], 99222[1], 99223[1], 99231[1], 99232[1], 99233[1], 99234[1], 99235[1], 99236[1], 99238[1], 99239[1], 99241[1], 99242[1], 99243[1], 99244[1], 99245[1], 99251[1], 99252[1], 99253[1], 99254[1], 99255[1], 99291[1], 99292[1], 99304[1], 99305[1], 99306[1], 99307[1], 99308[1], 99309[1], 99310[1], 99315[1], 99316[1], 99334[1], 99335[1], 99336[1], 99337[1], 99347[1], 99348[1], 99349[1], 99350[1], 99374[1], 99375[1], 99377[1], 99378[1], 99446[0], 99447[0], 99448[0], 99449[0], 99451[0], 99452[0], 99495[1], 99496[1], G0463[1], G0471[0], P9612[0]
52441	00910[0], 00916[0], 0213T[0], 0216T[0], 0596T[0], 0597T[0], 0708T[1], 0709T[1], 11000[1], 11001[1], 11004[1], 11005[1], 11006[1], 11042[1], 11043[1], 11044[1], 11045[1], 11046[1], 11047[1], 12001[1], 12002[1], 12004[1], 12005[1], 12006[1], 12007[1], 12011[1], 12013[1], 12014[1], 12015[1], 12016[1], 12017[1], 12018[1], 12020[1], 12021[1], 12031[1], 12032[1], 12034[1], 12035[1], 12036[1], 12037[1], 12041[1], 12042[1], 12044[1], 12045[1], 12046[1], 12047[1], 12051[1], 12052[1], 12053[1], 12054[1], 12055[1], 12056[1], 12057[1], 13100[1], 13101[1], 13102[1], 13120[1], 13121[1], 13122[1], 13131[1], 13132[1], 13133[1], 13151[1], 13152[1], 13153[1], 36000[1], 36400[1], 36405[1], 36406[1], 36410[1], 36420[1], 36425[1], 36430[1], 36440[1], 36591[0], 36592[0], 36600[1], 36640[1], 43752[1], 51701[0], 51702[0], 51703[0], 52000[0], 52001[1], 52281[0], 52310[0], 52315[0], 53000[0], 53010[0], 53020[0], 53025[0], 53080[1], 53520[1], 53600[0], 53601[0], 53605[0], 53620[0], 53621[0], 53660[0], 53661[0], 53665[0], 53855[0], 57410[0], 62320[0], 62321[0], 62322[0], 62323[0], 62324[0], 62325[0], 62326[0], 62327[0], 64400[0], 64405[0], 64408[0], 64415[0], 64416[0], 64417[0], 64418[0], 64420[0], 64421[0], 64425[0], 64430[0], 64435[0], 64445[0], 64446[0], 64447[0], 64448[0], 64449[0], 64450[0], 64451[0], 64454[0], 64461[0], 64462[0], 64463[0], 64479[0], 64480[0], 64483[0], 64484[0], 64486[0], 64487[0], 64488[0], 64489[0], 64490[0], 64491[0], 64492[0], 64493[0], 64494[0], 64495[0], 64505[0], 64510[0], 64517[0], 64520[0], 64530[0], 69990[0], 76000[1], 77001[1], 77002[1], 92012[1], 92014[1], 93000[1], 93005[1], 93010[1], 93040[1], 93041[1], 93042[1], 93318[1], 93355[1], 94002[1], 94200[1], 94680[1], 94681[1], 94690[1], 95812[1], 95813[1], 95816[1], 95819[1], 95822[1], 95829[1], 95955[1], 96360[1], 96361[1], 96365[1], 96366[1], 96367[1], 96368[1], 96372[1], 96374[1], 96375[1], 96376[1], 96377[1], 96523[0], 97597[1], 97598[1], 97602[1], 99155[0], 99156[0], 99157[0], 99211[1], 99212[1], 99213[1], 99214[1], 99215[1], 99217[1], 99218[1], 99219[1], 99220[1], 99221[1], 99222[1], 99223[1], 99231[1], 99232[1], 99233[1], 99234[1], 99235[1], 99236[1], 99238[1], 99239[1], 99241[1], 99242[1], 99243[1], 99244[1], 99245[1], 99251[1], 99252[1], 99253[1], 99254[1], 99255[1], 99291[1], 99292[1], 99304[1], 99305[1], 99306[1], 99307[1], 99308[1], 99309[1], 99310[1], 99315[1], 99316[1], 99334[1], 99335[1], 99336[1], 99337[1], 99347[1], 99348[1], 99349[1], 99350[1], 99374[1], 99375[1], 99377[1], 99378[1], 99446[0], 99447[0], 99448[0], 99449[0], 99451[0], 99452[0], 99495[1], 99496[1], C9739[1], C9740[1], G0463[1], G0471[0], J0670[1], J2001[1], P9612[0]
52442	00910[0], 00916[0], 0213T[0], 0216T[0], 0708T[1], 0709T[1], 11000[1], 11001[1], 11004[1], 11005[1], 11006[1], 11042[1], 11043[1], 11044[1], 11045[1], 11046[1], 11047[1], 12001[1], 12002[1], 12004[1], 12005[1], 12006[1], 12007[1], 12011[1], 12013[1], 12014[1], 12015[1], 12016[1], 12017[1], 12018[1], 12020[1], 12021[1], 12031[1], 12032[1], 12034[1], 12035[1], 12036[1], 12037[1], 12041[1], 12042[1], 12044[1], 12045[1], 12046[1], 12047[1], 12051[1], 12052[1], 12053[1], 12054[1], 12055[1], 12056[1], 12057[1], 13100[1], 13101[1], 13102[1], 13120[1], 13121[1], 13122[1], 13131[1], 13132[1], 13133[1], 13151[1], 13152[1], 13153[1], 36000[1], 36400[1], 36405[1], 36406[1], 36410[1], 36420[1], 36425[1], 36430[1], 36440[1], 36591[0], 36592[0], 36600[1], 36640[1], 43752[1], 51701[1], 51702[1], 51703[1], 52000[0], 52001[1], 52281[0], 52310[0], 52315[0], 53000[0], 53010[0], 53020[0], 53025[0], 53080[1], 53520[1], 53600[1], 53601[1], 53605[1], 53620[1], 53621[1], 53660[1], 53661[1], 53665[1], 57410[0], 61650[1], 62320[0], 62321[0], 62322[0], 62323[0], 62324[0], 62325[0], 62326[0], 62327[0], 64400[0], 64405[0], 64408[0], 64415[0], 64416[0], 64417[0], 64418[0], 64420[0], 64421[0], 64425[0], 64430[0], 64435[0], 64445[0], 64446[0], 64447[0], 64448[0], 64449[0], 64450[0], 64451[0], 64454[0], 64461[0], 64463[0], 64479[0], 64483[0], 64486[0], 64487[0], 64488[0], 64489[0], 64490[0], 64493[0], 64505[0], 64510[0], 64517[0], 64520[0], 64530[0], 69990[0], 76000[1], 77001[1], 77002[1], 92012[1], 92014[1], 93000[1], 93005[1], 93010[1], 93040[1], 93041[1], 93042[1], 93318[1], 93355[1], 94002[1], 94200[1], 94680[1], 94681[1], 94690[1], 95812[1], 95813[1], 95816[1], 95819[1], 95822[1], 95829[1], 95955[1], 96360[1], 96365[1], 96372[1], 96374[1], 96375[1], 96376[1], 96377[1], 96523[0], 97597[1], 97598[1], 97602[1], 99155[0], 99156[0], 99157[0], 99211[1], 99212[1], 99213[1], 99214[1], 99215[1], 99217[1], 99218[1], 99219[1], 99220[1], 99221[1], 99222[1], 99223[1], 99231[1], 99232[1], 99233[1], 99234[1], 99235[1], 99236[1], 99238[1], 99239[1], 99241[1], 99242[1], 99243[1], 99244[1], 99245[1], 99251[1], 99252[1], 99253[1], 99254[1], 99255[1], 99291[1], 99292[1], 99304[1], 99305[1], 99306[1], 99307[1], 99308[1], 99309[1], 99310[1], 99315[1], 99316[1], 99334[1], 99335[1], 99336[1], 99337[1], 99347[1], 99348[1], 99349[1], 99350[1], 99374[1], 99375[1], 99377[1], 99378[1], 99446[0], 99447[0], 99448[0], 99449[0], 99451[0], 99452[0], 99495[1], 99496[1], G0463[1], G0471[1], J0670[1], J2001[1], P9612[0]
52450	00910[0], 00914[0], 00916[0], 0213T[0], 0216T[0], 0421T[1], 0596T[0], 0597T[0], 0708T[1], 0709T[1], 12001[1], 12002[1], 12004[1], 12005[1], 12006[1], 12007[1], 12011[1], 12013[1], 12014[1], 12015[1], 12016[1], 12017[1], 12018[1], 12020[1], 12021[1], 12031[1], 12032[1], 12034[1], 12035[1], 12036[1], 12037[1], 12041[1], 12042[1], 12044[1], 12045[1], 12046[1], 12047[1], 12051[1], 12052[1], 12053[1], 12054[1], 12055[1], 12056[1], 12057[1], 13100[1], 13101[1], 13102[1], 13120[1], 13121[1], 13122[1], 13131[1], 13132[1], 13133[1], 13151[1], 13152[1], 13153[1], 36000[1], 36400[1], 36405[1], 36406[1], 36410[1], 36420[1], 36425[1], 36430[1], 36440[1], 36591[0], 36592[0], 36600[1], 36640[1], 43752[1], 51701[0], 51702[0], 51703[0], 52000[0], 52001[1], 52281[0], 52441[1], 52500[0], 52647[1], 52648[1], 53000[0], 53010[0], 53020[0], 53025[0], 53600[0], 53601[0], 53605[0], 53620[0], 53621[0], 53855[1], 62320[0], 62321[0], 62322[0], 62323[0], 62324[0], 62325[0], 62326[0], 62327[0], 64400[0], 64405[0], 64408[0], 64415[0], 64416[0], 64417[0], 64418[0], 64420[0], 64421[0], 64425[0], 64430[0], 64435[0], 64445[0], 64446[0], 64447[0], 64448[0], 64449[0], 64450[0], 64451[0], 64454[0], 64461[0], 64462[0], 64463[0], 64479[0], 64480[0], 64483[0], 64484[0], 64486[0], 64487[0], 64488[0], 64489[0], 64490[0], 64491[0], 64492[0], 64493[0], 64494[0], 64495[0], 64505[0], 64510[0], 64517[0], 64520[0], 64530[0], 69990[0], 76000[1], 77001[1], 77002[1], 92012[1], 92014[1], 93000[1], 93005[1], 93010[1], 93040[1], 93041[1], 93042[1], 93318[1], 93355[1], 94002[1], 94200[1], 94680[1], 94681[1], 94690[1], 95812[1], 95813[1], 95816[1], 95819[1], 95822[1], 95829[1], 95955[1], 96360[1], 96361[1], 96365[1], 96366[1], 96367[1], 96368[1], 96372[1], 96374[1], 96375[1], 96376[1], 96377[1], 96523[0], 99155[0], 99156[0], 99157[0], 99211[1], 99212[1], 99213[1], 99214[1], 99215[1], 99217[1], 99218[1], 99219[1], 99220[1], 99221[1], 99222[1], 99223[1], 99231[1], 99232[1], 99233[1], 99234[1], 99235[1], 99236[1], 99238[1], 99239[1], 99241[1], 99242[1], 99243[1], 99244[1], 99245[1], 99251[1], 99252[1], 99253[1], 99254[1], 99255[1], 99291[1], 99292[1], 99304[1], 99305[1], 99306[1], 99307[1], 99308[1], 99309[1], 99310[1], 99315[1], 99316[1], 99334[1], 99335[1], 99336[1], 99337[1], 99347[1], 99348[1], 99349[1], 99350[1], 99374[1], 99375[1], 99377[1], 99378[1], 99446[0], 99447[0], 99448[0], 99449[0], 99451[0], 99452[0], 99495[0], 99496[0], G0463[1], G0471[0], P9612[0]
52500	00910[0], 00912[0], 00914[0], 00916[0], 0213T[0], 0216T[0], 0596T[0], 0597T[0], 0708T[1], 0709T[1], 11000[1], 11001[1], 11004[1], 11005[1], 11006[1], 11042[1], 11043[1], 11044[1], 11045[1], 11046[1], 11047[1], 12001[1], 12002[1], 12004[1], 12005[1], 12006[1], 12007[1], 12011[1], 12013[1], 12014[1], 12015[1], 12016[1], 12017[1], 12018[1], 12020[1], 12021[1], 12031[1], 12032[1], 12034[1], 12035[1], 12036[1], 12037[1], 12041[1], 12042[1], 12044[1], 12045[1], 12046[1], 12047[1], 12051[1], 12052[1], 12053[1], 12054[1], 12055[1], 12056[1], 12057[1], 13100[1], 13101[1], 13102[1], 13120[1], 13121[1], 13122[1], 13131[1], 13132[1], 13133[1], 13151[1], 13152[1], 13153[1], 36000[1], 36400[1], 36405[1], 36406[1], 36410[1], 36420[1], 36425[1], 36430[1], 36440[1], 36591[0], 36592[0], 36600[1], 36640[1], 43752[1], 51701[0], 51702[0], 51703[0], 52000[0], 52001[1], 52281[0], 52441[1], 53000[0], 53010[0], 53020[0], 53025[0], 53600[0], 53601[0], 53605[0], 53620[0], 53621[0], 53855[1], 62320[0], 62321[0], 62322[0], 62323[0], 62324[0], 62325[0], 62326[0], 62327[0], 64400[0], 64405[0], 64408[0], 64415[0], 64416[0], 64417[0], 64418[0], 64420[0], 64421[0], 64425[0], 64430[0], 64435[0], 64445[0], 64446[0], 64447[0], 64448[0], 64449[0], 64450[0], 64451[0], 64454[0], 64461[0], 64462[0], 64463[0], 64479[0], 64480[0], 64483[0], 64484[0], 64486[0], 64487[0], 64488[0], 64489[0], 64490[0], 64491[0], 64492[0], 64493[0], 64494[0], 64495[0], 64505[0], 64510[0], 64517[0], 64520[0], 64530[0], 69990[0], 76000[1], 77001[1], 77002[1], 92012[1], 92014[1], 93000[1], 93005[1], 93010[1], 93040[1], 93041[1], 93042[1], 93318[1], 93355[1], 94002[1], 94200[1], 94680[1], 94681[1], 94690[1], 95812[1], 95813[1], 95816[1], 95819[1], 95822[1], 95829[1], 95955[1], 96360[1], 96361[1], 96365[1], 96366[1], 96367[1], 96368[1], 96372[1], 96374[1], 96375[1], 96376[1], 96377[1], 96523[0], 97597[1], 97598[1], 97602[1], 99155[0], 99156[0], 99157[0], 99211[1], 99212[1], 99213[1], 99214[1], 99215[1], 99217[1], 99218[1], 99219[1], 99220[1], 99221[1], 99222[1], 99223[1], 99231[1], 99232[1], 99233[1], 99234[1], 99235[1], 99236[1], 99238[1], 99239[1], 99241[1], 99242[1], 99243[1], 99244[1], 99245[1], 99251[1], 99252[1], 99253[1], 99254[1], 99255[1], 99291[1], 99292[1], 99304[1], 99305[1], 99306[1], 99307[1], 99308[1], 99309[1], 99310[1], 99315[1], 99316[1], 99334[1], 99335[1], 99336[1], 99337[1], 99347[1], 99348[1], 99349[1], 99350[1], 99374[1], 99375[1], 99377[1], 99378[1], 99446[0], 99447[0], 99448[0], 99449[0], 99451[0], 99452[0], 99495[0], 99496[0], G0463[1], G0471[0], P9612[0]
52601	00910[0], 00914[0], 00916[0], 0213T[0], 0216T[0], 0421T[0], 0499T[1], 0582T[0], 0596T[0], 0597T[0], 0600T[1], 0601T[1], 0655T[0], 0708T[1], 0709T[1], 11000[1], 11001[1], 11004[1], 11005[1], 11006[1], 11042[1], 11043[1], 11044[1], 11045[1], 11046[1], 11047[1], 12001[1], 12002[1], 12004[1], 12005[1], 12006[1], 12007[1], 12011[1], 12013[1], 12014[1], 12015[1], 12016[1], 12017[1], 12018[1], 12020[1], 12021[1], 12031[1], 12032[1], 12034[1], 12035[1], 12036[1], 12037[1], 12041[1], 12042[1], 12044[1], 12045[1], 12046[1], 12047[1], 12051[1], 12052[1], 12053[1], 12054[1], 12055[1], 12056[1], 12057[1], 13100[1], 13101[1], 13102[1], 13120[1], 13121[1], 13122[1], 13131[1], 13132[1], 13133[1], 13151[1], 13152[1], 13153[1], 36000[1], 36400[1], 36405[1], 36406[1], 36410[1], 36420[1], 36425[1], 36430[1], 36440[1], 36591[0], 36592[0], 36600[1], 36640[1], 43752[1], 51040[1], 51102[1], 51700[0], 51701[0], 51702[0], 51703[0], 52000[0], 52001[1], 52005[1], 52204[1], 52214[1], 52224[1], 52270[1], 52275[1], 52276[1], 52281[0], 52283[1], 52287[1], 52310[0], 52315[0], 52400[0], 52441[1], 52450[1], 52500[1],

0 = Modifier usage not allowed or inappropriate 1 = Modifier usage allowed

Code 1	Code 2
	52630[0], 52640[0], 52647[0], 52648[0], 53000[0], 53010[0], 53020[0], 53025[0], 53600[0], 53601[0], 53605[0], 53620[0], 53621[0], 53850[0], 53852[0], 53854[0], 53855[1], 55000[1], 55250[1], 55700[1], 55705[1], 55706[0], 55873[1], 55880[1], 62320[0], 62321[0], 62322[0], 62323[0], 62324[0], 62325[0], 62326[0], 62327[0], 64400[0], 64405[0], 64408[0], 64415[0], 64416[0], 64417[0], 64418[0], 64420[0], 64421[0], 64425[0], 64430[0], 64435[0], 64445[0], 64446[0], 64447[0], 64448[0], 64449[0], 64450[0], 64451[0], 64454[0], 64461[0], 64462[0], 64463[0], 64479[0], 64480[0], 64483[0], 64484[0], 64486[0], 64487[0], 64488[0], 64489[0], 64490[0], 64491[0], 64492[0], 64493[0], 64494[0], 64495[0], 64505[0], 64510[0], 64517[0], 64520[0], 64530[0], 69990[0], 76000[1], 77001[1], 77002[1], 92012[1], 92014[1], 93000[1], 93005[1], 93010[1], 93040[1], 93041[1], 93042[1], 93318[1], 93355[1], 94002[1], 94200[1], 94680[1], 94681[1], 94690[1], 95812[1], 95813[1], 95816[1], 95819[1], 95822[1], 95829[1], 95955[1], 96360[1], 96361[1], 96365[1], 96366[1], 96367[1], 96368[1], 96372[1], 96374[1], 96375[1], 96376[1], 96377[1], 96523[0], 97597[1], 97598[1], 97602[1], 99155[0], 99156[0], 99157[0], 99211[1], 99212[1], 99213[1], 99214[1], 99215[1], 99217[1], 99218[1], 99219[1], 99220[1], 99221[1], 99222[1], 99223[1], 99231[1], 99232[1], 99233[1], 99234[1], 99235[1], 99236[1], 99238[1], 99239[1], 99241[1], 99242[1], 99243[1], 99244[1], 99245[1], 99251[1], 99252[1], 99253[1], 99254[1], 99255[1], 99291[1], 99292[1], 99304[1], 99305[1], 99306[1], 99307[1], 99308[1], 99309[1], 99310[1], 99315[1], 99316[1], 99334[1], 99335[1], 99336[1], 99337[1], 99347[1], 99348[1], 99349[1], 99350[1], 99374[1], 99375[1], 99377[1], 99378[1], 99446[0], 99447[0], 99448[0], 99449[0], 99451[0], 99452[0], 99495[0], 99496[0], G0463[1], G0471[0], P9612[0]
52630	00910[0], 00914[0], 00916[0], 0213T[0], 0216T[0], 0582T[0], 0596T[0], 0597T[0], 0600T[1], 0601T[1], 0655T[0], 0708T[1], 0709T[1], 11000[1], 11001[1], 11004[1], 11005[1], 11006[1], 11042[1], 11043[1], 11044[1], 11045[1], 11046[1], 11047[1], 12001[1], 12002[1], 12004[1], 12005[1], 12006[1], 12007[1], 12011[1], 12013[1], 12014[1], 12015[1], 12016[1], 12017[1], 12018[1], 12020[1], 12021[1], 12031[1], 12032[1], 12034[1], 12035[1], 12036[1], 12037[1], 12041[1], 12042[1], 12044[1], 12045[1], 12046[1], 12047[1], 12051[1], 12052[1], 12053[1], 12054[1], 12055[1], 12056[1], 12057[1], 13100[1], 13101[1], 13102[1], 13120[1], 13121[1], 13122[1], 13131[1], 13132[1], 13133[1], 13151[1], 13152[1], 13153[1], 36000[1], 36400[1], 36405[1], 36406[1], 36410[1], 36420[1], 36425[1], 36430[1], 36440[1], 36591[0], 36592[0], 36600[1], 36640[1], 43752[1], 51102[1], 51700[1], 51701[0], 51702[0], 51703[0], 52000[0], 52001[1], 52005[1], 52204[1], 52214[1], 52224[1], 52270[1], 52275[0], 52276[1], 52281[0], 52310[0], 52315[0], 52441[1], 52450[1], 52500[0], 52640[0], 53000[0], 53010[0], 53020[0], 53025[0], 53600[0], 53601[0], 53605[0], 53620[0], 53621[0], 53854[0], 53855[1], 55250[1], 55700[0], 55705[1], 55706[0], 55873[1], 55880[1], 62320[0], 62321[0], 62322[0], 62323[0], 62324[0], 62325[0], 62326[0], 62327[0], 64400[0], 64405[0], 64408[0], 64415[0], 64416[0], 64417[0], 64418[0], 64420[0], 64421[0], 64425[0], 64430[0], 64435[0], 64445[0], 64446[0], 64447[0], 64448[0], 64449[0], 64450[0], 64451[0], 64454[0], 64461[0], 64462[0], 64463[0], 64479[0], 64480[0], 64483[0], 64484[0], 64486[0], 64487[0], 64488[0], 64489[0], 64490[0], 64491[0], 64492[0], 64493[0], 64494[0], 64495[0], 64505[0], 64510[0], 64517[0], 64520[0], 64530[0], 76000[1], 77001[1], 77002[1], 92012[1], 92014[1], 93000[1], 93005[1], 93010[1], 93040[1], 93041[1], 93042[1], 93318[1], 93355[1], 94002[1], 94200[1], 94680[1], 94681[1], 94690[1], 95812[1], 95813[1], 95816[1], 95819[1], 95822[1], 95829[1], 95955[1], 96360[1], 96361[1], 96365[1], 96366[1], 96367[1], 96368[1], 96372[1], 96374[1], 96375[1], 96376[1], 96377[1], 96523[0], 97597[1], 97598[1], 97602[1], 99155[0], 99156[0], 99157[0], 99211[1], 99212[1], 99213[1], 99214[1], 99215[1], 99217[1], 99218[1], 99219[1], 99220[1], 99221[1], 99222[1], 99223[1], 99231[1], 99232[1], 99233[1], 99234[1], 99235[1], 99236[1], 99238[1], 99239[1], 99241[1], 99242[1], 99243[1], 99244[1], 99245[1], 99251[1], 99252[1], 99253[1], 99254[1], 99255[1], 99291[1], 99292[1], 99304[1], 99305[1], 99306[1], 99307[1], 99308[1], 99309[1], 99310[1], 99315[1], 99316[1], 99334[1], 99335[1], 99336[1], 99337[1], 99347[1], 99348[1], 99349[1], 99350[1], 99374[1], 99375[1], 99377[1], 99378[1], 99446[0], 99447[0], 99448[0], 99449[0], 99451[0], 99452[0], 99495[0], 99496[0], G0463[1], G0471[0], P9612[0]
52640	00910[0], 00914[0], 00916[0], 0213T[0], 0216T[0], 0421T[0], 0499T[1], 0596T[0], 0597T[0], 0600T[1], 0601T[1], 0708T[1], 0709T[1], 11000[1], 11001[1], 11004[1], 11005[1], 11006[1], 11042[1], 11043[1], 11044[1], 11045[1], 11046[1], 11047[1], 12001[1], 12002[1], 12004[1], 12005[1], 12006[1], 12007[1], 12011[1], 12013[1], 12014[1], 12015[1], 12016[1], 12017[1], 12018[1], 12020[1], 12021[1], 12031[1], 12032[1], 12034[1], 12035[1], 12036[1], 12037[1], 12041[1], 12042[1], 12044[1], 12045[1], 12046[1], 12047[1], 12051[1], 12052[1], 12053[1], 12054[1], 12055[1], 12056[1], 12057[1], 13100[1], 13101[1], 13102[1], 13120[1], 13121[1], 13122[1], 13131[1], 13132[1], 13133[1], 13151[1], 13152[1], 13153[1], 36000[1], 36400[1], 36405[1], 36406[1], 36410[1], 36420[1], 36425[1], 36430[1], 36440[1], 36591[0], 36592[0], 36600[1], 36640[1], 43752[1], 51701[0], 51702[0], 51703[0], 52000[0], 52001[1], 52276[1], 52281[0], 52283[1], 52287[1], 52441[1], 52450[1], 52500[1], 53000[0], 53010[0], 53020[0], 53025[0], 53600[0], 53601[0], 53605[0], 53620[0], 53621[0], 53855[1], 55873[1], 55880[1], 62320[0], 62321[0], 62322[0], 62323[0], 62324[0], 62325[0], 62326[0], 62327[0], 64400[0], 64405[0], 64408[0], 64415[0], 64416[0], 64417[0], 64418[0], 64420[0], 64421[0], 64425[0], 64430[0], 64435[0], 64445[0], 64446[0], 64447[0], 64448[0], 64449[0], 64450[0], 64451[0], 64454[0], 64461[0], 64462[0], 64463[0], 64479[0], 64480[0], 64483[0], 64484[0], 64486[0], 64487[0], 64488[0], 64489[0], 64490[0], 64491[0], 64492[0], 64493[0], 64494[0], 64495[0], 64505[0], 64510[0], 64517[0], 64520[0], 64530[0], 69990[0], 76000[1], 77001[1], 77002[1], 92012[1], 92014[1], 93000[1], 93005[1], 93010[1], 93040[1], 93041[1], 93042[1], 93318[1], 93355[1], 94002[1], 94200[1], 94680[1], 94681[1], 94690[1], 95812[1], 95813[1], 95816[1], 95819[1], 95822[1], 95829[1], 95955[1], 96360[1], 96361[1], 96365[1], 96366[1], 96367[1], 96368[1], 96372[1], 96374[1], 96375[1], 96376[1], 96377[1], 96523[0], 97597[1], 97598[1], 97602[1], 99155[0], 99156[0], 99157[0], 99211[1], 99212[1], 99213[1], 99214[1], 99215[1], 99217[1], 99218[1], 99219[1], 99220[1], 99221[1], 99222[1], 99223[1], 99231[1], 99232[1], 99233[1], 99234[1], 99235[1], 99236[1], 99238[1], 99239[1], 99241[1], 99242[1], 99243[1], 99244[1], 99245[1], 99251[1], 99252[1], 99253[1], 99254[1], 99255[1], 99291[1], 99292[1], 99304[1], 99305[1], 99306[1], 99307[1], 99308[1], 99309[1], 99310[1], 99315[1], 99316[1], 99334[1], 99335[1], 99336[1], 99337[1], 99347[1], 99348[1], 99349[1], 99350[1], 99374[1], 99375[1], 99377[1], 99378[1], 99446[0], 99447[0], 99448[0], 99449[0], 99451[0], 99452[0], 99495[0], 99496[0], G0463[1], G0471[0], P9612[0]
52647	00910[0], 00914[0], 00916[0], 0213T[0], 0216T[0], 0421T[0], 0499T[1], 0582T[0], 0596T[0], 0597T[0], 0600T[1], 0601T[1], 0655T[0], 0708T[1], 0709T[1], 11000[1], 11001[1], 11004[1], 11005[1], 11006[1], 11042[1], 11043[1], 11044[1], 11045[1], 11046[1], 11047[1], 12001[1], 12002[1], 12004[1], 12005[1], 12006[1], 12007[1], 12011[1], 12013[1], 12014[1], 12015[1], 12016[1], 12017[1], 12018[1], 12020[1], 12021[1], 12031[1], 12032[1], 12034[1], 12035[1], 12036[1], 12037[1], 12041[1], 12042[1], 12044[1], 12045[1], 12046[1], 12047[1], 12051[1], 12052[1], 12053[1], 12054[1], 12055[1], 12056[1], 12057[1], 13100[1], 13101[1], 13102[1], 13120[1], 13121[1], 13122[1], 13131[1], 13132[1], 13133[1], 13151[1], 13152[1], 13153[1], 36000[1], 36400[1], 36405[1], 36406[1], 36410[1], 36420[1], 36425[1], 36430[1], 36440[1], 36591[0], 36592[0], 36600[1], 36640[1], 43752[1], 51040[1], 51102[1], 51700[0], 51701[0], 51702[0], 51703[0], 52000[0], 52001[1], 52005[1], 52204[1], 52214[1], 52224[1], 52234[1], 52235[1], 52240[1], 52270[0], 52275[1], 52276[0], 52281[0], 52283[1], 52287[1], 52305[1], 52310[0], 52315[0], 52400[0], 52441[1], 52500[0], 52630[0], 52640[0], 52700[1], 53000[0], 53010[0], 53020[0], 53025[0], 53600[0], 53601[0], 53605[0], 53620[0], 53621[0], 53660[0], 53661[0], 53665[0], 53850[0], 53852[0], 53854[0], 53855[1], 55000[1], 55200[1], 55250[0], 55700[1], 55705[1], 55706[1], 55873[1], 55880[1], 62320[0], 62321[0], 62322[0], 62323[0], 62324[0], 62325[0], 62326[0], 62327[0], 64400[0], 64405[0], 64408[0], 64415[0], 64416[0], 64417[0], 64418[0], 64420[0], 64421[0], 64425[0], 64430[0], 64435[0], 64445[0], 64446[0], 64447[0], 64448[0], 64449[0], 64450[0], 64451[0], 64454[0], 64461[0], 64462[0], 64463[0], 64479[0], 64480[0], 64483[0], 64484[0], 64486[0], 64487[0], 64488[0], 64489[0], 64490[0], 64491[0], 64492[0], 64493[0], 64494[0], 64495[0], 64505[0], 64510[0], 64517[0], 64520[0], 64530[0], 69990[0], 76000[1], 77001[1], 77002[1], 92012[1], 92014[1], 93000[1], 93005[1], 93010[1], 93040[1], 93041[1], 93042[1], 93318[1], 93355[1], 94002[1], 94200[1], 94680[1], 94681[1], 94690[1], 95812[1], 95813[1], 95816[1], 95819[1], 95822[1], 95829[1], 95955[1], 96360[1], 96361[1], 96365[1], 96366[1], 96367[1], 96368[1], 96372[1], 96374[1], 96375[1], 96376[1], 96377[1], 96523[0], 97597[1], 97598[1], 97602[1], 99155[0], 99156[0], 99157[0], 99211[1], 99212[1], 99213[1], 99214[1], 99215[1], 99217[1], 99218[1], 99219[1], 99220[1], 99221[1], 99222[1], 99223[1], 99231[1], 99232[1], 99233[1], 99234[1], 99235[1], 99236[1], 99238[1], 99239[1], 99241[1], 99242[1], 99243[1], 99244[1], 99245[1], 99251[1], 99252[1], 99253[1], 99254[1], 99255[1], 99291[1], 99292[1], 99304[1], 99305[1], 99306[1], 99307[1], 99308[1], 99309[1], 99310[1], 99315[1], 99316[1], 99334[1], 99335[1], 99336[1], 99337[1], 99347[1], 99348[1], 99349[1], 99350[1], 99374[1], 99375[1], 99377[1], 99378[1], 99446[0], 99447[0], 99448[0], 99449[0], 99451[0], 99452[0], 99495[0], 99496[0], G0463[1], G0471[0], J2001[1], P9612[0]
52648	00910[0], 00914[0], 00916[0], 0213T[0], 0216T[0], 0421T[0], 0499T[1], 0582T[0], 0596T[0], 0597T[0], 0600T[1], 0601T[1], 0655T[0], 0708T[1], 0709T[1], 11000[1], 11001[1], 11004[1], 11005[1], 11006[1], 11042[1], 11043[1], 11044[1], 11045[1], 11046[1], 11047[1], 12001[1], 12002[1], 12004[1], 12005[1], 12006[1], 12007[1], 12011[1], 12013[1], 12014[1], 12015[1], 12016[1], 12017[1], 12018[1], 12020[1], 12021[1], 12031[1], 12032[1], 12034[1], 12035[1], 12036[1], 12037[1], 12041[1], 12042[1], 12044[1], 12045[1], 12046[1], 12047[1], 12051[1], 12052[1], 12053[1], 12054[1], 12055[1], 12056[1], 12057[1], 13100[1], 13101[1], 13102[1], 13120[1], 13121[1], 13122[1], 13131[1], 13132[1], 13133[1], 13151[1], 13152[1], 13153[1], 36000[1], 36400[1], 36405[1], 36406[1], 36410[1], 36420[1], 36425[1], 36430[1], 36440[1], 36591[0], 36592[0], 36600[1], 36640[1], 43752[1], 51040[1], 51700[0], 51701[0], 51702[0], 51703[0], 52000[0], 52001[1], 52005[1], 52204[1], 52214[1], 52224[1], 52234[1], 52235[1], 52240[1], 52270[0], 52275[1], 52276[0], 52281[0], 52283[1], 52287[1], 52305[1], 52310[0], 52315[0], 52400[0], 52441[1], 52500[0], 52630[0], 52640[0], 52647[0], 52700[1], 53000[0], 53010[0], 53020[0], 53025[0], 53600[0], 53601[0], 53605[0], 53620[0], 53621[0], 53660[0], 53661[0], 53665[0], 53850[0], 53852[0], 53854[0], 53855[1], 55000[1], 55200[1], 55250[0], 55700[0], 55705[1], 55706[0], 55873[1], 55880[1], 62320[0], 62321[0], 62322[0], 62323[0], 62324[0], 62325[0], 62326[0], 62327[0], 64400[0], 64405[0], 64408[0], 64415[0], 64416[0], 64417[0], 64418[0], 64420[0], 64421[0], 64425[0], 64430[0], 64435[0], 64445[0], 64446[0], 64447[0], 64448[0], 64449[0], 64450[0], 64451[0], 64454[0], 64461[0], 64462[0], 64463[0], 64479[0], 64480[0], 64483[0], 64484[0], 64486[0], 64487[0], 64488[0], 64489[0], 64490[0], 64491[0], 64492[0], 64493[0], 64494[0], 64495[0], 64505[0], 64510[0], 64517[0], 64520[0], 64530[0], 69990[0], 76000[1], 77001[1], 77002[1], 92012[1], 92014[1], 93000[1], 93005[1], 93010[1], 93040[1], 93041[1], 93042[1], 93318[1], 93355[1], 94002[1], 94200[1], 94680[1], 94681[1], 94690[1], 95812[1], 95813[1], 95816[1], 95819[1], 95822[1], 95829[1], 95955[1], 96360[1], 96361[1], 96365[1], 96366[1], 96367[1], 96368[1], 96372[1], 96374[1], 96375[1], 96376[1], 96377[1], 96523[0], 97597[1], 97598[1], 97602[1], 99155[0], 99156[0], 99157[0], 99211[1], 99212[1], 99213[1], 99214[1], 99215[1], 99217[1], 99218[1], 99219[1], 99220[1], 99221[1], 99222[1], 99223[1], 99231[1], 99232[1], 99233[1], 99234[1], 99235[1], 99236[1], 99238[1], 99239[1], 99241[1], 99242[1], 99243[1], 99244[1], 99245[1], 99251[1], 99252[1], 99253[1], 99254[1], 99255[1], 99291[1], 99292[1], 99304[1], 99305[1], 99306[1], 99307[1], 99308[1], 99309[1], 99310[1], 99315[1], 99316[1], 99334[1], 99335[1], 99336[1], 99337[1], 99347[1],

0 = Modifier usage not allowed or inappropriate 1 = Modifier usage allowed

Code 1	Code 2
	99348[1], 99349[1], 99350[1], 99374[1], 99375[1], 99377[1], 99378[1], 99446[0], 99447[0], 99448[0], 99449[0], 99451[0], 99452[0], 99495[0], 99496[0], G0463[1], G0471[0], P9612[0]
52649	00910[0], 00914[0], 00916[0], 0213T[0], 0216T[0], 0421T[0], 0499T[1], 0596T[0], 0597T[0], 0708T[1], 0709T[1], 11000[1], 11001[1], 11004[1], 11005[1], 11006[1], 11042[1], 11043[1], 11044[1], 11045[1], 11046[1], 11047[1], 12001[1], 12002[1], 12004[1], 12005[1], 12006[1], 12007[1], 12011[1], 12013[1], 12014[1], 12015[1], 12016[1], 12017[1], 12018[1], 12020[1], 12021[1], 12031[1], 12032[1], 12034[1], 12035[1], 12036[1], 12037[1], 12041[1], 12042[1], 12044[1], 12045[1], 12046[1], 12047[1], 12051[1], 12052[1], 12053[1], 12054[1], 12055[1], 12056[1], 12057[1], 13100[1], 13101[1], 13102[1], 13120[1], 13121[1], 13122[1], 13131[1], 13132[1], 13133[1], 13151[1], 13152[1], 13153[1], 36000[1], 36400[1], 36405[1], 36406[1], 36410[1], 36420[1], 36425[1], 36430[1], 36440[1], 36591[0], 36592[0], 36600[1], 36640[1], 43752[1], 51040[1], 51102[1], 51700[0], 51701[0], 51702[0], 51703[0], 52000[0], 52001[1], 52005[1], 52204[1], 52214[1], 52224[1], 52234[1], 52235[1], 52240[1], 52270[0], 52275[1], 52276[0], 52281[0], 52283[1], 52287[1], 52305[1], 52310[0], 52315[0], 52400[0], 52441[1], 52450[1], 52500[0], 52601[0], 52630[1], 52640[1], 52647[0], 52648[0], 52700[1], 53000[0], 53010[0], 53020[0], 53025[0], 53600[0], 53601[0], 53605[0], 53620[0], 53621[0], 53660[0], 53661[0], 53665[0], 53855[1], 55000[1], 55200[1], 55250[0], 55700[1], 55705[1], 55706[1], 62320[0], 62321[0], 62322[0], 62323[0], 62324[0], 62325[0], 62326[0], 62327[0], 64400[0], 64405[0], 64408[0], 64415[0], 64416[0], 64417[0], 64418[0], 64420[0], 64421[0], 64425[0], 64430[0], 64435[0], 64445[0], 64446[0], 64447[0], 64448[0], 64449[0], 64450[0], 64451[0], 64454[0], 64461[0], 64462[0], 64463[0], 64479[0], 64480[0], 64483[0], 64484[0], 64486[0], 64487[0], 64488[0], 64489[0], 64490[0], 64491[0], 64492[0], 64493[0], 64494[0], 64495[0], 64505[0], 64510[0], 64517[0], 64520[0], 64530[0], 69990[0], 76000[1], 77001[1], 77002[1], 92012[1], 92014[1], 93000[1], 93005[1], 93010[1], 93040[1], 93041[1], 93042[1], 93318[1], 93355[1], 94002[1], 94200[1], 94680[1], 94681[1], 94690[1], 95812[1], 95813[1], 95816[1], 95819[1], 95822[1], 95829[1], 95955[1], 96360[1], 96361[1], 96365[1], 96366[1], 96367[1], 96368[1], 96372[1], 96374[1], 96375[1], 96376[1], 96377[1], 96523[0], 97597[1], 97598[1], 97602[1], 99155[0], 99156[0], 99157[0], 99211[1], 99212[1], 99213[1], 99214[1], 99215[1], 99217[1], 99218[1], 99219[1], 99220[1], 99221[1], 99222[1], 99223[1], 99231[1], 99232[1], 99233[1], 99234[1], 99235[1], 99236[1], 99238[1], 99239[1], 99241[1], 99242[1], 99243[1], 99244[1], 99245[1], 99251[1], 99252[1], 99253[1], 99254[1], 99255[1], 99291[1], 99292[1], 99304[1], 99305[1], 99306[1], 99307[1], 99308[1], 99309[1], 99310[1], 99315[1], 99316[1], 99334[1], 99335[1], 99336[1], 99337[1], 99347[1], 99348[1], 99349[1], 99350[1], 99374[1], 99375[1], 99377[1], 99378[1], 99446[0], 99447[0], 99448[0], 99449[0], 99451[0], 99452[0], 99495[0], 99496[0], G0463[1], G0471[0], P9612[0]
52700	00910[0], 00914[0], 00916[0], 0213T[0], 0216T[0], 0596T[0], 0597T[0], 0619T[1], 0708T[1], 0709T[1], 12001[1], 12002[1], 12004[1], 12005[1], 12006[1], 12007[1], 12011[1], 12013[1], 12014[1], 12015[1], 12016[1], 12017[1], 12018[1], 12020[1], 12021[1], 12031[1], 12032[1], 12034[1], 12035[1], 12036[1], 12037[1], 12041[1], 12042[1], 12044[1], 12045[1], 12046[1], 12047[1], 12051[1], 12052[1], 12053[1], 12054[1], 12055[1], 12056[1], 12057[1], 13100[1], 13101[1], 13102[1], 13120[1], 13121[1], 13122[1], 13131[1], 13132[1], 13133[1], 13151[1], 13152[1], 13153[1], 36000[1], 36400[1], 36405[1], 36406[1], 36410[1], 36420[1], 36425[1], 36430[1], 36440[1], 36591[0], 36592[0], 36600[1], 36640[1], 43752[1], 51701[0], 51702[0], 51703[0], 52000[0], 52001[1], 52281[0], 52441[1], 53000[0], 53010[0], 53020[0], 53025[0], 53600[0], 53601[0], 53605[0], 53620[0], 53621[0], 53855[1], 62320[0], 62321[0], 62322[0], 62323[0], 62324[0], 62325[0], 62326[0], 62327[0], 64400[0], 64405[0], 64408[0], 64415[0], 64416[0], 64417[0], 64418[0], 64420[0], 64421[0], 64425[0], 64430[0], 64435[0], 64445[0], 64446[0], 64447[0], 64448[0], 64449[0], 64450[0], 64451[0], 64454[0], 64461[0], 64462[0], 64463[0], 64479[0], 64480[0], 64483[0], 64484[0], 64486[0], 64487[0], 64488[0], 64489[0], 64490[0], 64491[0], 64492[0], 64493[0], 64494[0], 64495[0], 64505[0], 64510[0], 64517[0], 64520[0], 64530[0], 69990[0], 76000[1], 77001[1], 77002[1], 92012[1], 92014[1], 93000[1], 93005[1], 93010[1], 93040[1], 93041[1], 93042[1], 93318[1], 93355[1], 94002[1], 94200[1], 94680[1], 94681[1], 94690[1], 95812[1], 95813[1], 95816[1], 95819[1], 95822[1], 95829[1], 95955[1], 96360[1], 96361[1], 96365[1], 96366[1], 96367[1], 96368[1], 96372[1], 96374[1], 96375[1], 96376[1], 96377[1], 96523[0], 99155[0], 99156[0], 99157[0], 99211[1], 99212[1], 99213[1], 99214[1], 99215[1], 99217[1], 99218[1], 99219[1], 99220[1], 99221[1], 99222[1], 99223[1], 99231[1], 99232[1], 99233[1], 99234[1], 99235[1], 99236[1], 99238[1], 99239[1], 99241[1], 99242[1], 99243[1], 99244[1], 99245[1], 99251[1], 99252[1], 99253[1], 99254[1], 99255[1], 99291[1], 99292[1], 99304[1], 99305[1], 99306[1], 99307[1], 99308[1], 99309[1], 99310[1], 99315[1], 99316[1], 99334[1], 99335[1], 99336[1], 99337[1], 99347[1], 99348[1], 99349[1], 99350[1], 99374[1], 99375[1], 99377[1], 99378[1], 99446[0], 99447[0], 99448[0], 99449[0], 99451[0], 99452[0], 99495[0], 99496[0], G0463[1], G0471[0], P9612[0]
53000	0213T[0], 0216T[0], 0708T[1], 0709T[1], 11000[1], 11001[1], 11004[1], 11005[1], 11006[1], 11042[1], 11043[1], 11044[1], 11045[1], 11046[1], 11047[1], 12001[1], 12002[1], 12004[1], 12005[1], 12006[1], 12007[1], 12011[1], 12013[1], 12014[1], 12015[1], 12016[1], 12017[1], 12018[1], 12020[1], 12021[1], 12031[1], 12032[1], 12034[1], 12035[1], 12036[1], 12037[1], 12041[1], 12042[1], 12044[1], 12045[1], 12046[1], 12047[1], 12051[1], 12052[1], 12053[1], 12054[1], 12055[1], 12056[1], 12057[1], 13100[1], 13101[1], 13102[1], 13120[1], 13121[1], 13122[1], 13131[1], 13132[1], 13133[1], 13151[1], 13152[1], 13153[1], 36000[1], 36400[1], 36405[1], 36406[1], 36410[1], 36420[1], 36425[1], 36430[1], 36440[1], 36591[0], 36592[0], 36600[1], 36640[1], 43752[1], 51701[0], 51702[0], 51703[1], 62320[0], 62321[0], 62322[0], 62323[0], 62324[0], 62325[0], 62326[0], 62327[0], 64400[0], 64405[0], 64408[0], 64415[0], 64416[0], 64417[0], 64418[0], 64420[0], 64421[0], 64425[0], 64430[0], 64435[0], 64445[0], 64446[0], 64447[0], 64448[0], 64449[0], 64450[0], 64451[0], 64454[0], 64461[0], 64462[0], 64463[0], 64479[0], 64480[0], 64483[0], 64484[0], 64486[0], 64487[0], 64488[0], 64489[0], 64490[0], 64491[0], 64492[0], 64493[0], 64494[0], 64495[0], 64505[0], 64510[0], 64517[0], 64520[0], 64530[0], 69990[0], 92012[1], 92014[1], 93000[1], 93005[1], 93010[1], 93040[1], 93041[1], 93042[1], 93318[1], 93355[1], 94002[1], 94200[1], 94680[1], 94681[1], 94690[1], 95812[1], 95813[1], 95816[1], 95819[1], 95822[1], 95829[1], 95955[1], 96360[1], 96361[1], 96365[1], 96366[1], 96367[1], 96368[1], 96372[1], 96374[1], 96375[1], 96376[1], 96377[1], 96523[0], 97597[1], 97598[1], 97602[1], 99155[0], 99156[0], 99157[0], 99211[1], 99212[1], 99213[1], 99214[1], 99215[1], 99217[1], 99218[1], 99219[1], 99220[1], 99221[1], 99222[1], 99223[1], 99231[1], 99232[1], 99233[1], 99234[1], 99235[1], 99236[1], 99238[1], 99239[1], 99241[1], 99242[1], 99243[1], 99244[1], 99245[1], 99251[1], 99252[1], 99253[1], 99254[1], 99255[1], 99291[1], 99292[1], 99304[1], 99305[1], 99306[1], 99307[1], 99308[1], 99309[1], 99310[1], 99315[1], 99316[1], 99334[1], 99335[1], 99336[1], 99337[1], 99347[1], 99348[1], 99349[1], 99350[1], 99374[1], 99375[1], 99377[1], 99378[1], 99446[0], 99447[0], 99448[0], 99449[0], 99451[0], 99452[0], 99495[0], 99496[0], G0463[1], G0471[0], J2001[1]
53010	0213T[0], 0216T[0], 0708T[1], 0709T[1], 11000[1], 11001[1], 11004[1], 11005[1], 11006[1], 11042[1], 11043[1], 11044[1], 11045[1], 11046[1], 11047[1], 12001[1], 12002[1], 12004[1], 12005[1], 12006[1], 12007[1], 12011[1], 12013[1], 12014[1], 12015[1], 12016[1], 12017[1], 12018[1], 12020[1], 12021[1], 12031[1], 12032[1], 12034[1], 12035[1], 12036[1], 12037[1], 12041[1], 12042[1], 12044[1], 12045[1], 12046[1], 12047[1], 12051[1], 12052[1], 12053[1], 12054[1], 12055[1], 12056[1], 12057[1], 13100[1], 13101[1], 13102[1], 13120[1], 13121[1], 13122[1], 13131[1], 13132[1], 13133[1], 13151[1], 13152[1], 13153[1], 36000[1], 36400[1], 36405[1], 36406[1], 36410[1], 36420[1], 36425[1], 36430[1], 36440[1], 36591[0], 36592[0], 36600[1], 36640[1], 43752[1], 51701[0], 51702[0], 51703[1], 53000[0], 53020[0], 53025[0], 62320[0], 62321[0], 62322[0], 62323[0], 62324[0], 62325[0], 62326[0], 62327[0], 64400[0], 64405[0], 64408[0], 64415[0], 64416[0], 64417[0], 64418[0], 64420[0], 64421[0], 64425[0], 64430[0], 64435[0], 64445[0], 64446[0], 64447[0], 64448[0], 64449[0], 64450[0], 64451[0], 64454[0], 64461[0], 64462[0], 64463[0], 64479[0], 64480[0], 64483[0], 64484[0], 64486[0], 64487[0], 64488[0], 64489[0], 64490[0], 64491[0], 64492[0], 64493[0], 64494[0], 64495[0], 64505[0], 64510[0], 64517[0], 64520[0], 64530[0], 69990[0], 92012[1], 92014[1], 93000[1], 93005[1], 93010[1], 93040[1], 93041[1], 93042[1], 93318[1], 93355[1], 94002[1], 94200[1], 94680[1], 94681[1], 94690[1], 95812[1], 95813[1], 95816[1], 95819[1], 95822[1], 95829[1], 95955[1], 96360[1], 96361[1], 96365[1], 96366[1], 96367[1], 96368[1], 96372[1], 96374[1], 96375[1], 96376[1], 96377[1], 96523[0], 97597[1], 97598[1], 97602[1], 99155[0], 99156[0], 99157[0], 99211[1], 99212[1], 99213[1], 99214[1], 99215[1], 99217[1], 99218[1], 99219[1], 99220[1], 99221[1], 99222[1], 99223[1], 99231[1], 99232[1], 99233[1], 99234[1], 99235[1], 99236[1], 99238[1], 99239[1], 99241[1], 99242[1], 99243[1], 99244[1], 99245[1], 99251[1], 99252[1], 99253[1], 99254[1], 99255[1], 99291[1], 99292[1], 99304[1], 99305[1], 99306[1], 99307[1], 99308[1], 99309[1], 99310[1], 99315[1], 99316[1], 99334[1], 99335[1], 99336[1], 99337[1], 99347[1], 99348[1], 99349[1], 99350[1], 99374[1], 99375[1], 99377[1], 99378[1], 99446[0], 99447[0], 99448[0], 99449[0], 99451[0], 99452[0], 99495[0], 99496[0], G0463[1], G0471[0]
53020	0213T[0], 0216T[0], 0708T[1], 0709T[1], 11000[1], 11001[1], 11004[1], 11005[1], 11006[1], 11042[1], 11043[1], 11044[1], 11045[1], 11046[1], 11047[1], 12001[1], 12002[1], 12004[1], 12005[1], 12006[1], 12007[1], 12011[1], 12013[1], 12014[1], 12015[1], 12016[1], 12017[1], 12018[1], 12020[1], 12021[1], 12031[1], 12032[1], 12034[1], 12035[1], 12036[1], 12037[1], 12041[1], 12042[1], 12044[1], 12045[1], 12046[1], 12047[1], 12051[1], 12052[1], 12053[1], 12054[1], 12055[1], 12056[1], 12057[1], 13100[1], 13101[1], 13102[1], 13120[1], 13121[1], 13122[1], 13131[1], 13132[1], 13133[1], 13151[1], 13152[1], 13153[1], 36000[1], 36400[1], 36405[1], 36406[1], 36410[1], 36420[1], 36425[1], 36430[1], 36440[1], 36591[0], 36592[0], 36600[1], 36640[1], 43752[1], 51701[0], 51703[1], 53000[0], 62320[0], 62321[0], 62322[0], 62323[0], 62324[0], 62325[0], 62326[0], 62327[0], 64400[0], 64405[0], 64408[0], 64415[0], 64416[0], 64417[0], 64418[0], 64420[0], 64421[0], 64425[0], 64430[0], 64435[0], 64445[0], 64446[0], 64447[0], 64448[0], 64449[0], 64450[0], 64451[0], 64454[0], 64461[0], 64462[0], 64463[0], 64479[0], 64480[0], 64483[0], 64484[0], 64486[0], 64487[0], 64488[0], 64489[0], 64490[0], 64491[0], 64492[0], 64493[0], 64494[0], 64495[0], 64505[0], 64510[0], 64517[0], 64520[0], 64530[0], 69990[0], 92012[1], 92014[1], 93000[1], 93005[1], 93010[1], 93040[1], 93041[1], 93042[1], 93318[1], 93355[1], 94002[1], 94200[1], 94680[1], 94681[1], 94690[1], 95812[1], 95813[1], 95816[1], 95819[1], 95822[1], 95829[1], 95955[1], 96360[1], 96361[1], 96365[1], 96366[1], 96367[1], 96368[1], 96372[1], 96374[1], 96375[1], 96376[1], 96377[1], 96523[0], 97597[1], 97598[1], 97602[1], 99155[0], 99156[0], 99157[0], 99211[1], 99212[1], 99213[1], 99214[1], 99215[1], 99217[1], 99218[1], 99219[1], 99220[1], 99221[1], 99222[1], 99223[1], 99231[1], 99232[1], 99233[1], 99234[1], 99235[1], 99236[1], 99238[1], 99239[1], 99241[1], 99242[1], 99243[1], 99244[1], 99245[1], 99251[1], 99252[1], 99253[1], 99254[1], 99255[1], 99291[1], 99292[1], 99304[1], 99305[1], 99306[1], 99307[1], 99308[1], 99309[1], 99310[1], 99315[1], 99316[1], 99334[1], 99335[1], 99336[1], 99337[1], 99347[1], 99348[1], 99349[1], 99350[1], 99374[1], 99375[1], 99377[1], 99378[1], 99446[0], 99447[0], 99448[0], 99449[0], 99451[0], 99452[0], 99495[1], 99496[1], G0463[1], J0670[1], J2001[1]

0 = Modifier usage not allowed or inappropriate   1 = Modifier usage allowed

Code 1	Code 2
53025	0213T[0], 0216T[0], 0708T[1], 0709T[1], 11000[1], 11001[1], 11004[1], 11005[1], 11006[1], 11042[1], 11043[1], 11044[1], 11045[1], 11046[1], 11047[1], 12001[1], 12002[1], 12004[1], 12005[1], 12006[1], 12007[1], 12011[1], 12013[1], 12014[1], 12015[1], 12016[1], 12017[1], 12018[1], 12020[1], 12021[1], 12031[1], 12032[1], 12034[1], 12035[1], 12036[1], 12037[1], 12041[1], 12042[1], 12044[1], 12045[1], 12046[1], 12047[1], 12051[1], 12052[1], 12053[1], 12054[1], 12055[1], 12056[1], 12057[1], 13100[1], 13101[1], 13102[1], 13120[1], 13121[1], 13122[1], 13131[1], 13132[1], 13133[1], 13151[1], 13152[1], 13153[1], 36000[1], 36400[1], 36405[1], 36406[1], 36410[1], 36420[1], 36425[1], 36430[1], 36440[1], 36591[0], 36592[0], 36600[1], 36640[1], 43752[1], 51701[0], 51703[1], 53000[0], 53020[0], 62320[0], 62321[0], 62322[0], 62323[0], 62324[0], 62325[0], 62326[0], 62327[0], 64400[0], 64405[0], 64408[0], 64415[0], 64416[0], 64417[0], 64418[0], 64420[0], 64421[0], 64425[0], 64430[0], 64435[0], 64445[0], 64446[0], 64447[0], 64448[0], 64449[0], 64450[0], 64451[0], 64454[0], 64461[0], 64462[0], 64463[0], 64479[0], 64480[0], 64483[0], 64484[0], 64486[0], 64487[0], 64488[0], 64489[0], 64490[0], 64491[0], 64492[0], 64493[0], 64494[0], 64495[0], 64505[0], 64510[0], 64517[0], 64520[0], 64530[0], 69990[0], 92012[1], 92014[1], 93000[1], 93005[1], 93010[1], 93040[1], 93041[1], 93042[1], 93318[1], 93355[1], 94002[1], 94200[1], 94680[1], 94681[1], 94690[1], 95812[1], 95813[1], 95816[1], 95819[1], 95822[1], 95829[1], 95955[1], 96360[1], 96361[1], 96365[1], 96366[1], 96367[1], 96368[1], 96372[1], 96374[1], 96375[1], 96376[1], 96377[1], 96523[0], 97597[1], 97598[1], 97602[1], 99155[0], 99156[0], 99157[0], 99211[1], 99212[1], 99213[1], 99214[1], 99215[1], 99217[1], 99218[1], 99219[1], 99220[1], 99221[1], 99222[1], 99223[1], 99231[1], 99232[1], 99233[1], 99234[1], 99235[1], 99236[1], 99238[1], 99239[1], 99241[1], 99242[1], 99243[1], 99244[1], 99245[1], 99251[1], 99252[1], 99253[1], 99254[1], 99255[1], 99291[1], 99292[1], 99304[1], 99305[1], 99306[1], 99307[1], 99308[1], 99309[1], 99310[1], 99315[1], 99316[1], 99334[1], 99335[1], 99336[1], 99337[1], 99347[1], 99348[1], 99349[1], 99350[1], 99374[1], 99375[1], 99377[1], 99378[1], 99446[0], 99447[0], 99448[0], 99449[0], 99451[0], 99452[0], 99495[1], 99496[1], G0463[1], J0670[1], J2001[1]
53040	0213T[0], 0216T[0], 0596T[1], 0597T[1], 0708T[1], 0709T[1], 12001[1], 12002[1], 12004[1], 12005[1], 12006[1], 12007[1], 12011[1], 12013[1], 12014[1], 12015[1], 12016[1], 12017[1], 12018[1], 12020[1], 12021[1], 12031[1], 12032[1], 12034[1], 12035[1], 12036[1], 12037[1], 12041[1], 12042[1], 12044[1], 12045[1], 12046[1], 12047[1], 12051[1], 12052[1], 12053[1], 12054[1], 12055[1], 12056[1], 12057[1], 13100[1], 13101[1], 13102[1], 13120[1], 13121[1], 13122[1], 13131[1], 13132[1], 13133[1], 13151[1], 13152[1], 13153[1], 36000[1], 36400[1], 36405[1], 36406[1], 36410[1], 36420[1], 36425[1], 36430[1], 36440[1], 36591[0], 36592[0], 36600[1], 36640[1], 43752[1], 51701[0], 51702[0], 51703[1], 53000[0], 53010[0], 53020[0], 53025[0], 53060[1], 53080[1], 53265[1], 62320[0], 62321[0], 62322[0], 62323[0], 62324[0], 62325[0], 62326[0], 62327[0], 64400[0], 64405[0], 64408[0], 64415[0], 64416[0], 64417[0], 64418[0], 64420[0], 64421[0], 64425[0], 64430[0], 64435[0], 64445[0], 64446[0], 64447[0], 64448[0], 64449[0], 64450[0], 64451[0], 64454[0], 64461[0], 64462[0], 64463[0], 64479[0], 64480[0], 64483[0], 64484[0], 64486[0], 64487[0], 64488[0], 64489[0], 64490[0], 64491[0], 64492[0], 64493[0], 64494[0], 64495[0], 64505[0], 64510[0], 64517[0], 64520[0], 64530[0], 69990[0], 92012[1], 92014[1], 93000[1], 93005[1], 93010[1], 93040[1], 93041[1], 93042[1], 93318[1], 93355[1], 94002[1], 94200[1], 94680[1], 94681[1], 94690[1], 95812[1], 95813[1], 95816[1], 95819[1], 95822[1], 95829[1], 95955[1], 96360[1], 96361[1], 96365[1], 96366[1], 96367[1], 96368[1], 96372[1], 96374[1], 96375[1], 96376[1], 96377[1], 96523[0], 99155[0], 99156[0], 99157[0], 99211[1], 99212[1], 99213[1], 99214[1], 99215[1], 99217[1], 99218[1], 99219[1], 99220[1], 99221[1], 99222[1], 99223[1], 99231[1], 99232[1], 99233[1], 99234[1], 99235[1], 99236[1], 99238[1], 99239[1], 99241[1], 99242[1], 99243[1], 99244[1], 99245[1], 99251[1], 99252[1], 99253[1], 99254[1], 99255[1], 99291[1], 99292[1], 99304[1], 99305[1], 99306[1], 99307[1], 99308[1], 99309[1], 99310[1], 99315[1], 99316[1], 99334[1], 99335[1], 99336[1], 99337[1], 99347[1], 99348[1], 99349[1], 99350[1], 99374[1], 99375[1], 99377[1], 99378[1], 99446[0], 99447[0], 99448[0], 99449[0], 99451[0], 99452[0], 99495[0], 99496[0], G0463[1], G0471[0], J2001[1]
53060	0213T[0], 0216T[0], 0596T[1], 0597T[1], 0708T[1], 0709T[1], 12001[1], 12002[1], 12004[1], 12005[1], 12006[1], 12007[1], 12011[1], 12013[1], 12014[1], 12015[1], 12016[1], 12017[1], 12018[1], 12020[1], 12021[1], 12031[1], 12032[1], 12034[1], 12035[1], 12036[1], 12037[1], 12041[1], 12042[1], 12044[1], 12045[1], 12046[1], 12047[1], 12051[1], 12052[1], 12053[1], 12054[1], 12055[1], 12056[1], 12057[1], 13100[1], 13101[1], 13102[1], 13120[1], 13121[1], 13122[1], 13131[1], 13132[1], 13133[1], 13151[1], 13152[1], 13153[1], 36000[1], 36400[1], 36405[1], 36406[1], 36410[1], 36420[1], 36425[1], 36430[1], 36440[1], 36591[0], 36592[0], 36600[1], 36640[1], 43752[1], 51701[0], 51702[0], 51703[1], 53000[0], 53010[0], 53020[0], 53025[0], 53080[1], 53270[1], 62320[0], 62321[0], 62322[0], 62323[0], 62324[0], 62325[0], 62326[0], 62327[0], 64400[0], 64405[0], 64408[0], 64415[0], 64416[0], 64417[0], 64418[0], 64420[0], 64421[0], 64425[0], 64430[0], 64435[0], 64445[0], 64446[0], 64447[0], 64448[0], 64449[0], 64450[0], 64451[0], 64454[0], 64461[0], 64462[0], 64463[0], 64479[0], 64480[0], 64483[0], 64484[0], 64486[0], 64487[0], 64488[0], 64489[0], 64490[0], 64491[0], 64492[0], 64493[0], 64494[0], 64495[0], 64505[0], 64510[0], 64517[0], 64520[0], 64530[0], 69990[0], 92012[1], 92014[1], 93000[1], 93005[1], 93010[1], 93040[1], 93041[1], 93042[1], 93318[1], 93355[1], 94002[1], 94200[1], 94680[1], 94681[1], 94690[1], 95812[1], 95813[1], 95816[1], 95819[1], 95822[1], 95829[1], 95955[1], 96360[1], 96361[1], 96365[1], 96366[1], 96367[1], 96368[1], 96372[1], 96374[1], 96375[1], 96376[1], 96377[1], 96523[0], 99155[0], 99156[0], 99157[0], 99211[1], 99212[1], 99213[1], 99214[1], 99215[1], 99217[1], 99218[1], 99219[1], 99220[1], 99221[1], 99222[1], 99223[1], 99231[1], 99232[1], 99233[1], 99234[1], 99235[1], 99236[1], 99238[1], 99239[1], 99241[1], 99242[1], 99243[1], 99244[1], 99245[1], 99251[1], 99252[1], 99253[1], 99254[1], 99255[1], 99291[1], 99292[1], 99304[1], 99305[1], 99306[1], 99307[1], 99308[1], 99309[1], 99310[1], 99315[1], 99316[1], 99334[1], 99335[1], 99336[1], 99337[1], 99347[1], 99348[1], 99349[1], 99350[1], 99374[1], 99375[1], 99377[1], 99378[1], 99446[0], 99447[0], 99448[0], 99449[0], 99451[0], 99452[0], 99495[0], 99496[0], G0463[1], G0471[0], J2001[1]
53080	0213T[0], 0216T[0], 0708T[1], 0709T[1], 12001[1], 12002[1], 12004[1], 12005[1], 12006[1], 12007[1], 12011[1], 12013[1], 12014[1], 12015[1], 12016[1], 12017[1], 12018[1], 12020[1], 12021[1], 12031[1], 12032[1], 12034[1], 12035[1], 12036[1], 12037[1], 12041[1], 12042[1], 12044[1], 12045[1], 12046[1], 12047[1], 12051[1], 12052[1], 12053[1], 12054[1], 12055[1], 12056[1], 12057[1], 13100[1], 13101[1], 13102[1], 13120[1], 13121[1], 13122[1], 13131[1], 13132[1], 13133[1], 13151[1], 13152[1], 13153[1], 36000[1], 36400[1], 36405[1], 36406[1], 36410[1], 36420[1], 36425[1], 36430[1], 36440[1], 36591[0], 36592[0], 36600[1], 36640[1], 43752[1], 51701[1], 51702[1], 53000[0], 53010[0], 53020[0], 53025[0], 62320[0], 62321[0], 62322[0], 62323[0], 62324[0], 62325[0], 62326[0], 62327[0], 64400[0], 64405[0], 64408[0], 64415[0], 64416[0], 64417[0], 64418[0], 64420[0], 64421[0], 64425[0], 64430[0], 64435[0], 64445[0], 64446[0], 64447[0], 64448[0], 64449[0], 64450[0], 64451[0], 64454[0], 64461[0], 64462[0], 64463[0], 64479[0], 64480[0], 64483[0], 64484[0], 64486[0], 64487[0], 64488[0], 64489[0], 64490[0], 64491[0], 64492[0], 64493[0], 64494[0], 64495[0], 64505[0], 64510[0], 64517[0], 64520[0], 64530[0], 69990[0], 92012[1], 92014[1], 93000[1], 93005[1], 93010[1], 93040[1], 93041[1], 93042[1], 93318[1], 93355[1], 94002[1], 94200[1], 94680[1], 94681[1], 94690[1], 95812[1], 95813[1], 95816[1], 95819[1], 95822[1], 95829[1], 95955[1], 96360[1], 96361[1], 96365[1], 96366[1], 96367[1], 96368[1], 96372[1], 96374[1], 96375[1], 96376[1], 96377[1], 96523[0], 99155[0], 99156[0], 99157[0], 99211[1], 99212[1], 99213[1], 99214[1], 99215[1], 99217[1], 99218[1], 99219[1], 99220[1], 99221[1], 99222[1], 99223[1], 99231[1], 99232[1], 99233[1], 99234[1], 99235[1], 99236[1], 99238[1], 99239[1], 99241[1], 99242[1], 99243[1], 99244[1], 99245[1], 99251[1], 99252[1], 99253[1], 99254[1], 99255[1], 99291[1], 99292[1], 99304[1], 99305[1], 99306[1], 99307[1], 99308[1], 99309[1], 99310[1], 99315[1], 99316[1], 99334[1], 99335[1], 99336[1], 99337[1], 99347[1], 99348[1], 99349[1], 99350[1], 99374[1], 99375[1], 99377[1], 99378[1], 99446[0], 99447[0], 99448[0], 99449[0], 99451[0], 99452[0], 99495[0], 99496[0], G0463[1], G0471[1]
53085	0213T[0], 0216T[0], 0596T[1], 0597T[1], 0708T[1], 0709T[1], 12001[1], 12002[1], 12004[1], 12005[1], 12006[1], 12007[1], 12011[1], 12013[1], 12014[1], 12015[1], 12016[1], 12017[1], 12018[1], 12020[1], 12021[1], 12031[1], 12032[1], 12034[1], 12035[1], 12036[1], 12037[1], 12041[1], 12042[1], 12044[1], 12045[1], 12046[1], 12047[1], 12051[1], 12052[1], 12053[1], 12054[1], 12055[1], 12056[1], 12057[1], 13100[1], 13101[1], 13102[1], 13120[1], 13121[1], 13122[1], 13131[1], 13132[1], 13133[1], 13151[1], 13152[1], 13153[1], 36000[1], 36400[1], 36405[1], 36406[1], 36410[1], 36420[1], 36425[1], 36430[1], 36440[1], 36591[0], 36592[0], 36600[1], 36640[1], 43752[1], 51701[0], 51702[0], 51703[1], 53000[0], 53010[0], 53020[0], 53025[0], 53080[0], 62320[0], 62321[0], 62322[0], 62323[0], 62324[0], 62325[0], 62326[0], 62327[0], 64400[0], 64405[0], 64408[0], 64415[0], 64416[0], 64417[0], 64418[0], 64420[0], 64421[0], 64425[0], 64430[0], 64435[0], 64445[0], 64446[0], 64447[0], 64448[0], 64449[0], 64450[0], 64451[0], 64454[0], 64461[0], 64462[0], 64463[0], 64479[0], 64480[0], 64483[0], 64484[0], 64486[0], 64487[0], 64488[0], 64489[0], 64490[0], 64491[0], 64492[0], 64493[0], 64494[0], 64495[0], 64505[0], 64510[0], 64517[0], 64520[0], 64530[0], 69990[0], 92012[1], 92014[1], 93000[1], 93005[1], 93010[1], 93040[1], 93041[1], 93042[1], 93318[1], 93355[1], 94002[1], 94200[1], 94680[1], 94681[1], 94690[1], 95812[1], 95813[1], 95816[1], 95819[1], 95822[1], 95829[1], 95955[1], 96360[1], 96361[1], 96365[1], 96366[1], 96367[1], 96368[1], 96372[1], 96374[1], 96375[1], 96376[1], 96377[1], 96523[0], 99155[0], 99156[0], 99157[0], 99211[1], 99212[1], 99213[1], 99214[1], 99215[1], 99217[1], 99218[1], 99219[1], 99220[1], 99221[1], 99222[1], 99223[1], 99231[1], 99232[1], 99233[1], 99234[1], 99235[1], 99236[1], 99238[1], 99239[1], 99241[1], 99242[1], 99243[1], 99244[1], 99245[1], 99251[1], 99252[1], 99253[1], 99254[1], 99255[1], 99291[1], 99292[1], 99304[1], 99305[1], 99306[1], 99307[1], 99308[1], 99309[1], 99310[1], 99315[1], 99316[1], 99334[1], 99335[1], 99336[1], 99337[1], 99347[1], 99348[1], 99349[1], 99350[1], 99374[1], 99375[1], 99377[1], 99378[1], 99446[0], 99447[0], 99448[0], 99449[0], 99451[0], 99452[0], 99495[0], 99496[0], G0463[1], G0471[0]
53200	0213T[0], 0216T[0], 0596T[1], 0597T[1], 0708T[1], 0709T[1], 10005[1], 10007[1], 10009[1], 10011[1], 10021[1], 12001[1], 12002[1], 12004[1], 12005[1], 12006[1], 12007[1], 12011[1], 12013[1], 12014[1], 12015[1], 12016[1], 12017[1], 12018[1], 12020[1], 12021[1], 12031[1], 12032[1], 12034[1], 12035[1], 12036[1], 12037[1], 12041[1], 12042[1], 12044[1], 12045[1], 12046[1], 12047[1], 12051[1], 12052[1], 12053[1], 12054[1], 12055[1], 12056[1], 12057[1], 13100[1], 13101[1], 13102[1], 13120[1], 13121[1], 13122[1], 13131[1], 13132[1], 13133[1], 13151[1], 13152[1], 13153[1], 36000[1], 36400[1], 36405[1], 36406[1], 36410[1], 36420[1], 36425[1], 36430[1], 36440[1], 36591[0], 36592[0], 36600[1], 36640[1], 43752[1], 51701[0], 51702[0], 51703[1], 52000[0], 53000[0], 53010[0], 53020[0], 53025[0], 62320[0], 62321[0], 62322[0], 62323[0], 62324[0], 62325[0], 62326[0], 62327[0], 64400[0], 64405[0], 64408[0], 64415[0], 64416[0], 64417[0], 64418[0], 64420[0], 64421[0], 64425[0], 64430[0], 64435[0], 64445[0], 64446[0], 64447[0], 64448[0], 64449[0], 64450[0], 64451[0], 64454[0], 64461[0], 64462[0], 64463[0], 64479[0], 64480[0], 64483[0], 64484[0], 64486[0], 64487[0], 64488[0], 64489[0], 64490[0], 64491[0], 64492[0], 64493[0], 64494[0], 64495[0], 64505[0], 64510[0], 64517[0], 64520[0], 64530[0], 69990[0], 92012[1], 92014[1], 93000[1], 93005[1], 93010[1], 93040[1], 93041[1], 93042[1], 93318[1], 93355[1], 94002[1], 94200[1], 94680[1], 94681[1], 94690[1], 95812[1], 95813[1], 95816[1], 95819[1], 95822[1],

0 = Modifier usage not allowed or inappropriate 1 = Modifier usage allowed

Code 1	Code 2
	95829[1], 95955[1], 96360[1], 96361[1], 96365[1], 96366[1], 96367[1], 96368[1], 96372[1], 96374[1], 96375[1], 96376[1], 96377[1], 96523[0], 99155[0], 99156[0], 99157[0], 99211[1], 99212[1], 99213[1], 99214[1], 99215[1], 99217[1], 99218[1], 99219[1], 99220[1], 99221[1], 99222[1], 99223[1], 99231[1], 99232[1], 99233[1], 99234[1], 99235[1], 99236[1], 99238[1], 99239[1], 99241[1], 99242[1], 99243[1], 99244[1], 99245[1], 99251[1], 99252[1], 99253[1], 99254[1], 99255[1], 99291[1], 99292[1], 99304[1], 99305[1], 99306[1], 99307[1], 99308[1], 99309[1], 99310[1], 99315[1], 99316[1], 99334[1], 99335[1], 99336[1], 99337[1], 99347[1], 99348[1], 99349[1], 99350[1], 99374[1], 99375[1], 99377[1], 99378[1], 99446[0], 99447[0], 99448[0], 99449[0], 99451[0], 99452[0], 99495[1], 99496[1], G0463[1], G0471[0], J2001[1]
53210	0213T[0], 0216T[0], 0596T[1], 0597T[1], 0708T[1], 0709T[1], 11000[1], 11001[1], 11004[1], 11005[1], 11006[1], 11042[1], 11043[1], 11044[1], 11045[1], 11046[1], 11047[1], 12001[1], 12002[1], 12004[1], 12005[1], 12006[1], 12007[1], 12011[1], 12013[1], 12014[1], 12015[1], 12016[1], 12017[1], 12018[1], 12020[1], 12021[1], 12031[1], 12032[1], 12034[1], 12035[1], 12036[1], 12037[1], 12041[1], 12042[1], 12044[1], 12045[1], 12046[1], 12047[1], 12051[1], 12052[1], 12053[1], 12054[1], 12055[1], 12056[1], 12057[1], 13100[1], 13101[1], 13102[1], 13120[1], 13121[1], 13122[1], 13131[1], 13132[1], 13133[1], 13151[1], 13152[1], 13153[1], 36000[1], 36400[1], 36405[1], 36406[1], 36410[1], 36420[1], 36425[1], 36430[1], 36440[1], 36591[0], 36592[0], 36600[1], 36640[1], 43752[1], 51701[0], 51702[0], 51703[1], 52000[0], 52301[0], 53000[0], 53010[0], 53020[0], 53025[0], 53080[1], 53200[0], 53220[1], 53250[1], 53260[1], 53265[1], 53270[1], 53275[1], 62320[0], 62321[0], 62322[0], 62323[0], 62324[0], 62325[0], 62326[0], 62327[0], 64400[0], 64405[0], 64408[0], 64415[0], 64416[0], 64417[0], 64418[0], 64420[0], 64421[0], 64425[0], 64430[0], 64435[0], 64445[0], 64446[0], 64447[0], 64448[0], 64449[0], 64450[0], 64451[0], 64454[0], 64461[0], 64462[0], 64463[0], 64479[0], 64480[0], 64483[0], 64484[0], 64486[0], 64487[0], 64488[0], 64489[0], 64490[0], 64491[0], 64492[0], 64493[0], 64494[0], 64495[0], 64505[0], 64510[0], 64517[0], 64520[0], 64530[0], 69990[0], 92012[1], 92014[1], 93000[1], 93005[1], 93010[1], 93040[1], 93041[1], 93042[1], 93318[1], 93355[1], 94002[1], 94200[1], 94680[1], 94681[1], 94690[1], 95812[1], 95813[1], 95816[1], 95819[1], 95822[1], 95829[1], 95955[1], 96360[1], 96361[1], 96365[1], 96366[1], 96367[1], 96368[1], 96372[1], 96374[1], 96375[1], 96376[1], 96377[1], 96523[0], 97597[1], 97598[1], 97602[1], 99155[0], 99156[0], 99157[0], 99211[1], 99212[1], 99213[1], 99214[1], 99215[1], 99217[1], 99218[1], 99219[1], 99220[1], 99221[1], 99222[1], 99223[1], 99231[1], 99232[1], 99233[1], 99234[1], 99235[1], 99236[1], 99238[1], 99239[1], 99241[1], 99242[1], 99243[1], 99244[1], 99245[1], 99251[1], 99252[1], 99253[1], 99254[1], 99255[1], 99291[1], 99292[1], 99304[1], 99305[1], 99306[1], 99307[1], 99308[1], 99309[1], 99310[1], 99315[1], 99316[1], 99334[1], 99335[1], 99336[1], 99337[1], 99347[1], 99348[1], 99349[1], 99350[1], 99374[1], 99375[1], 99377[1], 99378[1], 99446[0], 99447[0], 99448[0], 99449[0], 99451[0], 99452[0], 99495[0], 99496[0], G0463[1], G0471[0]
53215	0213T[0], 0216T[0], 0596T[1], 0597T[1], 0708T[1], 0709T[1], 11000[1], 11001[1], 11004[1], 11005[1], 11006[1], 11042[1], 11043[1], 11044[1], 11045[1], 11046[1], 11047[1], 12001[1], 12002[1], 12004[1], 12005[1], 12006[1], 12007[1], 12011[1], 12013[1], 12014[1], 12015[1], 12016[1], 12017[1], 12018[1], 12020[1], 12021[1], 12031[1], 12032[1], 12034[1], 12035[1], 12036[1], 12037[1], 12041[1], 12042[1], 12044[1], 12045[1], 12046[1], 12047[1], 12051[1], 12052[1], 12053[1], 12054[1], 12055[1], 12056[1], 12057[1], 13100[1], 13101[1], 13102[1], 13120[1], 13121[1], 13122[1], 13131[1], 13132[1], 13133[1], 13151[1], 13152[1], 13153[1], 36000[1], 36400[1], 36405[1], 36406[1], 36410[1], 36420[1], 36425[1], 36430[1], 36440[1], 36591[0], 36592[0], 36600[1], 36640[1], 43752[1], 51701[0], 51702[0], 51703[1], 52000[0], 52301[0], 53000[0], 53010[0], 53020[0], 53025[0], 53080[1], 53200[0], 53210[1], 53220[1], 53235[1], 53250[1], 53260[1], 53265[1], 53270[1], 53275[1], 62320[0], 62321[0], 62322[0], 62323[0], 62324[0], 62325[0], 62326[0], 62327[0], 64400[0], 64405[0], 64408[0], 64415[0], 64416[0], 64417[0], 64418[0], 64420[0], 64421[0], 64425[0], 64430[0], 64435[0], 64445[0], 64446[0], 64447[0], 64448[0], 64449[0], 64450[0], 64451[0], 64454[0], 64461[0], 64462[0], 64463[0], 64479[0], 64480[0], 64483[0], 64484[0], 64486[0], 64487[0], 64488[0], 64489[0], 64490[0], 64491[0], 64492[0], 64493[0], 64494[0], 64495[0], 64505[0], 64510[0], 64517[0], 64520[0], 64530[0], 69990[0], 92012[1], 92014[1], 93000[1], 93005[1], 93010[1], 93040[1], 93041[1], 93042[1], 93318[1], 93355[1], 94002[1], 94200[1], 94680[1], 94681[1], 94690[1], 95812[1], 95813[1], 95816[1], 95819[1], 95822[1], 95829[1], 95955[1], 96360[1], 96361[1], 96365[1], 96366[1], 96367[1], 96368[1], 96372[1], 96374[1], 96375[1], 96376[1], 96377[1], 96523[0], 97597[1], 97598[1], 97602[1], 99155[0], 99156[0], 99157[0], 99211[1], 99212[1], 99213[1], 99214[1], 99215[1], 99217[1], 99218[1], 99219[1], 99220[1], 99221[1], 99222[1], 99223[1], 99231[1], 99232[1], 99233[1], 99234[1], 99235[1], 99236[1], 99238[1], 99239[1], 99241[1], 99242[1], 99243[1], 99244[1], 99245[1], 99251[1], 99252[1], 99253[1], 99254[1], 99255[1], 99291[1], 99292[1], 99304[1], 99305[1], 99306[1], 99307[1], 99308[1], 99309[1], 99310[1], 99315[1], 99316[1], 99334[1], 99335[1], 99336[1], 99337[1], 99347[1], 99348[1], 99349[1], 99350[1], 99374[1], 99375[1], 99377[1], 99378[1], 99446[0], 99447[0], 99448[0], 99449[0], 99451[0], 99452[0], 99495[0], 99496[0], G0463[1], G0471[0]
53220	0213T[0], 0216T[0], 0596T[1], 0597T[1], 0708T[1], 0709T[1], 11000[1], 11001[1], 11004[1], 11005[1], 11006[1], 11042[1], 11043[1], 11044[1], 11045[1], 11046[1], 11047[1], 12001[1], 12002[1], 12004[1], 12005[1], 12006[1], 12007[1], 12011[1], 12013[1], 12014[1], 12015[1], 12016[1], 12017[1], 12018[1], 12020[1], 12021[1], 12031[1], 12032[1], 12034[1], 12035[1], 12036[1], 12037[1], 12041[1], 12042[1], 12044[1], 12045[1], 12046[1], 12047[1], 12051[1], 12052[1], 12053[1], 12054[1], 12055[1], 12056[1], 12057[1], 13100[1], 13101[1], 13102[1], 13120[1], 13121[1], 13122[1], 13131[1], 13132[1], 13133[1], 13151[1], 13152[1], 13153[1], 36000[1], 36400[1], 36405[1], 36406[1], 36410[1], 36420[1], 36425[1], 36430[1], 36440[1], 36591[0], 36592[0], 36600[1], 36640[1], 43752[1], 51701[0], 51702[0], 51703[1], 52000[0], 52301[1], 53000[0], 53010[0], 53020[0], 53025[0], 53080[1], 56740[1], 62320[0], 62321[0], 62322[0], 62323[0], 62324[0], 62325[0], 62326[0], 62327[0], 64400[0], 64405[0], 64408[0], 64415[0], 64416[0], 64417[0], 64418[0], 64420[0], 64421[0], 64425[0], 64430[0], 64435[0], 64445[0], 64446[0], 64447[0], 64448[0], 64449[0], 64450[0], 64451[0], 64454[0], 64461[0], 64462[0], 64463[0], 64479[0], 64480[0], 64483[0], 64484[0], 64486[0], 64487[0], 64488[0], 64489[0], 64490[0], 64491[0], 64492[0], 64493[0], 64494[0], 64495[0], 64505[0], 64510[0], 64517[0], 64520[0], 64530[0], 69990[0], 92012[1], 92014[1], 93000[1], 93005[1], 93010[1], 93040[1], 93041[1], 93042[1], 93318[1], 93355[1], 94002[1], 94200[1], 94680[1], 94681[1], 94690[1], 95812[1], 95813[1], 95816[1], 95819[1], 95822[1], 95829[1], 95955[1], 96360[1], 96361[1], 96365[1], 96366[1], 96367[1], 96368[1], 96372[1], 96374[1], 96375[1], 96376[1], 96377[1], 96523[0], 97597[1], 97598[1], 97602[1], 99155[0], 99156[0], 99157[0], 99211[1], 99212[1], 99213[1], 99214[1], 99215[1], 99217[1], 99218[1], 99219[1], 99220[1], 99221[1], 99222[1], 99223[1], 99231[1], 99232[1], 99233[1], 99234[1], 99235[1], 99236[1], 99238[1], 99239[1], 99241[1], 99242[1], 99243[1], 99244[1], 99245[1], 99251[1], 99252[1], 99253[1], 99254[1], 99255[1], 99291[1], 99292[1], 99304[1], 99305[1], 99306[1], 99307[1], 99308[1], 99309[1], 99310[1], 99315[1], 99316[1], 99334[1], 99335[1], 99336[1], 99337[1], 99347[1], 99348[1], 99349[1], 99350[1], 99374[1], 99375[1], 99377[1], 99378[1], 99446[0], 99447[0], 99448[0], 99449[0], 99451[0], 99452[0], 99495[0], 99496[0], G0463[1], G0471[0]
53230	0213T[0], 0216T[0], 0596T[1], 0597T[1], 0708T[1], 0709T[1], 11000[1], 11001[1], 11004[1], 11005[1], 11006[1], 11042[1], 11043[1], 11044[1], 11045[1], 11046[1], 11047[1], 12001[1], 12002[1], 12004[1], 12005[1], 12006[1], 12007[1], 12011[1], 12013[1], 12014[1], 12015[1], 12016[1], 12017[1], 12018[1], 12020[1], 12021[1], 12031[1], 12032[1], 12034[1], 12035[1], 12036[1], 12037[1], 12041[1], 12042[1], 12044[1], 12045[1], 12046[1], 12047[1], 12051[1], 12052[1], 12053[1], 12054[1], 12055[1], 12056[1], 12057[1], 13100[1], 13101[1], 13102[1], 13120[1], 13121[1], 13122[1], 13131[1], 13132[1], 13133[1], 13151[1], 13152[1], 13153[1], 36000[1], 36400[1], 36405[1], 36406[1], 36410[1], 36420[1], 36425[1], 36430[1], 36440[1], 36591[0], 36592[0], 36600[1], 36640[1], 43752[1], 51701[0], 51702[0], 51703[1], 52000[0], 52301[1], 53000[0], 53010[0], 53020[0], 53025[0], 62320[0], 62321[0], 62322[0], 62323[0], 62324[0], 62325[0], 62326[0], 62327[0], 64400[0], 64405[0], 64408[0], 64415[0], 64416[0], 64417[0], 64418[0], 64420[0], 64421[0], 64425[0], 64430[0], 64435[0], 64445[0], 64446[0], 64447[0], 64448[0], 64449[0], 64450[0], 64451[0], 64454[0], 64461[0], 64462[0], 64463[0], 64479[0], 64480[0], 64483[0], 64484[0], 64486[0], 64487[0], 64488[0], 64489[0], 64490[0], 64491[0], 64492[0], 64493[0], 64494[0], 64495[0], 64505[0], 64510[0], 64517[0], 64520[0], 64530[0], 69990[0], 92012[1], 92014[1], 93000[1], 93005[1], 93010[1], 93040[1], 93041[1], 93042[1], 93318[1], 93355[1], 94002[1], 94200[1], 94680[1], 94681[1], 94690[1], 95812[1], 95813[1], 95816[1], 95819[1], 95822[1], 95829[1], 95955[1], 96360[1], 96361[1], 96365[1], 96366[1], 96367[1], 96368[1], 96372[1], 96374[1], 96375[1], 96376[1], 96377[1], 96523[0], 97597[1], 97598[1], 97602[1], 99155[0], 99156[0], 99157[0], 99211[1], 99212[1], 99213[1], 99214[1], 99215[1], 99217[1], 99218[1], 99219[1], 99220[1], 99221[1], 99222[1], 99223[1], 99231[1], 99232[1], 99233[1], 99234[1], 99235[1], 99236[1], 99238[1], 99239[1], 99241[1], 99242[1], 99243[1], 99244[1], 99245[1], 99251[1], 99252[1], 99253[1], 99254[1], 99255[1], 99291[1], 99292[1], 99304[1], 99305[1], 99306[1], 99307[1], 99308[1], 99309[1], 99310[1], 99315[1], 99316[1], 99334[1], 99335[1], 99336[1], 99337[1], 99347[1], 99348[1], 99349[1], 99350[1], 99374[1], 99375[1], 99377[1], 99378[1], 99446[0], 99447[0], 99448[0], 99449[0], 99451[0], 99452[0], 99495[0], 99496[0], G0463[1], G0471[0]
53235	0213T[0], 0216T[0], 0596T[1], 0597T[1], 0708T[1], 0709T[1], 11000[1], 11001[1], 11004[1], 11005[1], 11006[1], 11042[1], 11043[1], 11044[1], 11045[1], 11046[1], 11047[1], 12001[1], 12002[1], 12004[1], 12005[1], 12006[1], 12007[1], 12011[1], 12013[1], 12014[1], 12015[1], 12016[1], 12017[1], 12018[1], 12020[1], 12021[1], 12031[1], 12032[1], 12034[1], 12035[1], 12036[1], 12037[1], 12041[1], 12042[1], 12044[1], 12045[1], 12046[1], 12047[1], 12051[1], 12052[1], 12053[1], 12054[1], 12055[1], 12056[1], 12057[1], 13100[1], 13101[1], 13102[1], 13120[1], 13121[1], 13122[1], 13131[1], 13132[1], 13133[1], 13151[1], 13152[1], 13153[1], 36000[1], 36400[1], 36405[1], 36406[1], 36410[1], 36420[1], 36425[1], 36430[1], 36440[1], 36591[0], 36592[0], 36600[1], 36640[1], 43752[1], 51701[0], 51702[0], 51703[1], 52000[0], 52301[1], 53000[0], 53010[0], 53020[0], 53025[0], 53080[1], 53230[0], 62320[0], 62321[0], 62322[0], 62323[0], 62324[0], 62325[0], 62326[0], 62327[0], 64400[0], 64405[0], 64408[0], 64415[0], 64416[0], 64417[0], 64418[0], 64420[0], 64421[0], 64425[0], 64430[0], 64435[0], 64445[0], 64446[0], 64447[0], 64448[0], 64449[0], 64450[0], 64451[0], 64454[0], 64461[0], 64462[0], 64463[0], 64479[0], 64480[0], 64483[0], 64484[0], 64486[0], 64487[0], 64488[0], 64489[0], 64490[0], 64491[0], 64492[0], 64493[0], 64494[0], 64495[0], 64505[0], 64510[0], 64517[0], 64520[0], 64530[0], 69990[0], 92012[1], 92014[1], 93000[1], 93005[1], 93010[1], 93040[1], 93041[1], 93042[1], 93318[1], 93355[1], 94002[1], 94200[1], 94680[1], 94681[1], 94690[1], 95812[1], 95813[1], 95816[1], 95819[1], 95822[1], 95829[1], 95955[1], 96360[1], 96361[1], 96365[1], 96366[1], 96367[1], 96368[1], 96372[1], 96374[1], 96375[1], 96376[1], 96377[1], 96523[0], 97597[1], 97598[1], 97602[1], 99155[0], 99156[0], 99157[0], 99211[1], 99212[1], 99213[1], 99214[1], 99215[1], 99217[1], 99218[1], 99219[1], 99220[1], 99221[1], 99222[1], 99223[1], 99231[1], 99232[1], 99233[1], 99234[1], 99235[1], 99236[1], 99238[1], 99239[1], 99241[1], 99242[1], 99243[1], 99244[1], 99245[1], 99251[1], 99252[1], 99253[1], 99254[1], 99255[1], 99291[1], 99292[1], 99304[1], 99305[1], 99306[1], 99307[1], 99308[1], 99309[1], 99310[1], 99315[1], 99316[1], 99334[1], 99335[1], 99336[1], 99337[1], 99347[1], 99348[1], 99349[1], 99350[1], 99374[1], 99375[1],

0 = Modifier usage not allowed or inappropriate   1 = Modifier usage allowed

Code 1	Code 2
	99377[1], 99378[1], 99446[0], 99447[0], 99448[0], 99449[0], 99451[0], 99452[0], 99495[0], 99496[0], G0463[1], G0471[0]
53240	0213T[0], 0216T[0], 0596T[1], 0597T[1], 0708T[1], 0709T[1], 12001[1], 12002[1], 12004[1], 12005[1], 12006[1], 12007[1], 12011[1], 12013[1], 12014[1], 12015[1], 12016[1], 12017[1], 12018[1], 12020[1], 12021[1], 12031[1], 12032[1], 12034[1], 12035[1], 12036[1], 12037[1], 12041[1], 12042[1], 12044[1], 12045[1], 12046[1], 12047[1], 12051[1], 12052[1], 12053[1], 12054[1], 12055[1], 12056[1], 12057[1], 13100[1], 13101[1], 13102[1], 13120[1], 13121[1], 13122[1], 13131[1], 13132[1], 13133[1], 13151[1], 13152[1], 13153[1], 36000[1], 36400[1], 36405[1], 36406[1], 36410[1], 36420[1], 36425[1], 36430[1], 36440[1], 36591[0], 36592[0], 36600[1], 36640[1], 43752[1], 51701[0], 51702[0], 51703[1], 52000[0], 52301[1], 53000[0], 53010[0], 53020[0], 53025[0], 53230[0], 62320[0], 62321[0], 62322[0], 62323[0], 62324[0], 62325[0], 62326[0], 62327[0], 64400[0], 64405[0], 64408[0], 64415[0], 64416[0], 64417[0], 64418[0], 64420[0], 64421[0], 64425[0], 64430[0], 64435[0], 64445[0], 64446[0], 64447[0], 64448[0], 64449[0], 64450[0], 64451[0], 64454[0], 64461[0], 64462[0], 64463[0], 64479[0], 64480[0], 64483[0], 64484[0], 64486[0], 64487[0], 64488[0], 64489[0], 64490[0], 64491[0], 64492[0], 64493[0], 64494[0], 64495[0], 64505[0], 64510[0], 64517[0], 64520[0], 64530[0], 69990[0], 92012[1], 92014[1], 93000[1], 93005[1], 93010[1], 93040[1], 93041[1], 93042[1], 93318[1], 93355[1], 94002[1], 94200[1], 94680[1], 94681[1], 94690[1], 95812[1], 95813[1], 95816[1], 95819[1], 95822[1], 95829[1], 95955[1], 96360[1], 96361[1], 96365[1], 96366[1], 96367[1], 96368[1], 96372[1], 96374[1], 96375[1], 96376[1], 96377[1], 96523[0], 99155[0], 99156[0], 99157[0], 99211[1], 99212[1], 99213[1], 99214[1], 99215[1], 99217[1], 99218[1], 99219[1], 99220[1], 99221[1], 99222[1], 99223[1], 99231[1], 99232[1], 99233[1], 99234[1], 99235[1], 99236[1], 99238[1], 99239[1], 99241[1], 99242[1], 99243[1], 99244[1], 99245[1], 99251[1], 99252[1], 99253[1], 99254[1], 99255[1], 99291[1], 99292[1], 99304[1], 99305[1], 99306[1], 99307[1], 99308[1], 99309[1], 99310[1], 99315[1], 99316[1], 99334[1], 99335[1], 99336[1], 99337[1], 99347[1], 99348[1], 99349[1], 99350[1], 99374[1], 99375[1], 99377[1], 99378[1], 99446[0], 99447[0], 99448[0], 99449[0], 99451[0], 99452[0], 99495[0], 99496[0], G0463[1], G0471[0]
53250	0213T[0], 0216T[0], 0596T[1], 0597T[1], 0708T[1], 0709T[1], 11000[1], 11001[1], 11004[1], 11005[1], 11006[1], 11042[1], 11043[1], 11044[1], 11045[1], 11046[1], 11047[1], 12001[1], 12002[1], 12004[1], 12005[1], 12006[1], 12007[1], 12011[1], 12013[1], 12014[1], 12015[1], 12016[1], 12017[1], 12018[1], 12020[1], 12021[1], 12031[1], 12032[1], 12034[1], 12035[1], 12036[1], 12037[1], 12041[1], 12042[1], 12044[1], 12045[1], 12046[1], 12047[1], 12051[1], 12052[1], 12053[1], 12054[1], 12055[1], 12056[1], 12057[1], 13100[1], 13101[1], 13102[1], 13120[1], 13121[1], 13122[1], 13131[1], 13132[1], 13133[1], 13151[1], 13152[1], 13153[1], 36000[1], 36400[1], 36405[1], 36406[1], 36410[1], 36420[1], 36425[1], 36430[1], 36440[1], 36591[0], 36592[0], 36600[1], 36640[1], 43752[1], 51701[0], 51702[0], 51703[1], 52000[0], 53000[0], 53010[0], 53020[0], 53025[0], 53040[1], 53080[1], 53230[0], 62320[0], 62321[0], 62322[0], 62323[0], 62324[0], 62325[0], 62326[0], 62327[0], 64400[0], 64405[0], 64408[0], 64415[0], 64416[0], 64417[0], 64418[0], 64420[0], 64421[0], 64425[0], 64430[0], 64435[0], 64445[0], 64446[0], 64447[0], 64448[0], 64449[0], 64450[0], 64451[0], 64454[0], 64461[0], 64462[0], 64463[0], 64479[0], 64480[0], 64483[0], 64484[0], 64486[0], 64487[0], 64488[0], 64489[0], 64490[0], 64491[0], 64492[0], 64493[0], 64494[0], 64495[0], 64505[0], 64510[0], 64517[0], 64520[0], 64530[0], 69990[0], 92012[1], 92014[1], 93000[1], 93005[1], 93010[1], 93040[1], 93041[1], 93042[1], 93318[1], 93355[1], 94002[1], 94200[1], 94680[1], 94681[1], 94690[1], 95812[1], 95813[1], 95816[1], 95819[1], 95822[1], 95829[1], 95955[1], 96360[1], 96361[1], 96365[1], 96366[1], 96367[1], 96368[1], 96372[1], 96374[1], 96375[1], 96376[1], 96377[1], 96523[0], 97597[1], 97598[1], 97602[1], 99155[0], 99156[0], 99157[0], 99211[1], 99212[1], 99213[1], 99214[1], 99215[1], 99217[1], 99218[1], 99219[1], 99220[1], 99221[1], 99222[1], 99223[1], 99231[1], 99232[1], 99233[1], 99234[1], 99235[1], 99236[1], 99238[1], 99239[1], 99241[1], 99242[1], 99243[1], 99244[1], 99245[1], 99251[1], 99252[1], 99253[1], 99254[1], 99255[1], 99291[1], 99292[1], 99304[1], 99305[1], 99306[1], 99307[1], 99308[1], 99309[1], 99310[1], 99315[1], 99316[1], 99334[1], 99335[1], 99336[1], 99337[1], 99347[1], 99348[1], 99349[1], 99350[1], 99374[1], 99375[1], 99377[1], 99378[1], 99446[0], 99447[0], 99448[0], 99449[0], 99451[0], 99452[0], 99495[0], 99496[0], G0463[1], G0471[0]
53260	0213T[0], 0216T[0], 0596T[1], 0597T[1], 0708T[1], 0709T[1], 11000[1], 11001[1], 11004[1], 11005[1], 11006[1], 11042[1], 11043[1], 11044[1], 11045[1], 11046[1], 11047[1], 12001[1], 12002[1], 12004[1], 12005[1], 12006[1], 12007[1], 12011[1], 12013[1], 12014[1], 12015[1], 12016[1], 12017[1], 12018[1], 12020[1], 12021[1], 12031[1], 12032[1], 12034[1], 12035[1], 12036[1], 12037[1], 12041[1], 12042[1], 12044[1], 12045[1], 12046[1], 12047[1], 12051[1], 12052[1], 12053[1], 12054[1], 12055[1], 12056[1], 12057[1], 13100[1], 13101[1], 13102[1], 13120[1], 13121[1], 13122[1], 13131[1], 13132[1], 13133[1], 13151[1], 13152[1], 13153[1], 36000[1], 36400[1], 36405[1], 36406[1], 36410[1], 36420[1], 36425[1], 36430[1], 36440[1], 36591[0], 36592[0], 36600[1], 36640[1], 43752[1], 51701[0], 51702[0], 51703[1], 52000[0], 53000[0], 53010[0], 53020[0], 53025[0], 53080[1], 53230[0], 62320[0], 62321[0], 62322[0], 62323[0], 62324[0], 62325[0], 62326[0], 62327[0], 64400[0], 64405[0], 64408[0], 64415[0], 64416[0], 64417[0], 64418[0], 64420[0], 64421[0], 64425[0], 64430[0], 64435[0], 64445[0], 64446[0], 64447[0], 64448[0], 64449[0], 64450[0], 64451[0], 64454[0], 64461[0], 64462[0], 64463[0], 64479[0], 64480[0], 64483[0], 64484[0], 64486[0], 64487[0], 64488[0], 64489[0], 64490[0], 64491[0], 64492[0], 64493[0], 64494[0], 64495[0], 64505[0], 64510[0], 64517[0], 64520[0], 64530[0], 69990[0], 92012[1], 92014[1], 93000[1], 93005[1], 93010[1], 93040[1], 93041[1], 93042[1], 93318[1], 93355[1], 94002[1], 94200[1], 94680[1], 94681[1], 94690[1], 95812[1], 95813[1], 95816[1], 95819[1], 95822[1], 95829[1], 95955[1], 96360[1], 96361[1], 96365[1], 96366[1], 96367[1], 96368[1], 96372[1], 96374[1], 96375[1], 96376[1], 96377[1], 96523[0], 97597[1], 97598[1], 97602[1], 99155[0], 99156[0], 99157[0], 99211[1], 99212[1], 99213[1], 99214[1], 99215[1], 99217[1], 99218[1], 99219[1], 99220[1], 99221[1], 99222[1], 99223[1], 99231[1], 99232[1], 99233[1], 99234[1], 99235[1], 99236[1], 99238[1], 99239[1], 99241[1], 99242[1], 99243[1], 99244[1], 99245[1], 99251[1], 99252[1], 99253[1], 99254[1], 99255[1], 99291[1], 99292[1], 99304[1], 99305[1], 99306[1], 99307[1], 99308[1], 99309[1], 99310[1], 99315[1], 99316[1], 99334[1], 99335[1], 99336[1], 99337[1], 99347[1], 99348[1], 99349[1], 99350[1], 99374[1], 99375[1], 99377[1], 99378[1], 99446[0], 99447[0], 99448[0], 99449[0], 99451[0], 99452[0], 99495[0], 99496[0], G0463[1], G0471[0], J2001[1]
53265	0213T[0], 0216T[0], 0596T[1], 0597T[1], 0708T[1], 0709T[1], 11000[1], 11001[1], 11004[1], 11005[1], 11006[1], 11042[1], 11043[1], 11044[1], 11045[1], 11046[1], 11047[1], 12001[1], 12002[1], 12004[1], 12005[1], 12006[1], 12007[1], 12011[1], 12013[1], 12014[1], 12015[1], 12016[1], 12017[1], 12018[1], 12020[1], 12021[1], 12031[1], 12032[1], 12034[1], 12035[1], 12036[1], 12037[1], 12041[1], 12042[1], 12044[1], 12045[1], 12046[1], 12047[1], 12051[1], 12052[1], 12053[1], 12054[1], 12055[1], 12056[1], 12057[1], 13100[1], 13101[1], 13102[1], 13120[1], 13121[1], 13122[1], 13131[1], 13132[1], 13133[1], 13151[1], 13152[1], 13153[1], 36000[1], 36400[1], 36405[1], 36406[1], 36410[1], 36420[1], 36425[1], 36430[1], 36440[1], 36591[0], 36592[0], 36600[1], 36640[1], 43752[1], 51701[0], 51702[0], 51703[1], 52000[0], 53000[0], 53010[0], 53020[0], 53025[0], 53080[1], 53230[0], 62320[0], 62321[0], 62322[0], 62323[0], 62324[0], 62325[0], 62326[0], 62327[0], 64400[0], 64405[0], 64408[0], 64415[0], 64416[0], 64417[0], 64418[0], 64420[0], 64421[0], 64425[0], 64430[0], 64435[0], 64445[0], 64446[0], 64447[0], 64448[0], 64449[0], 64450[0], 64451[0], 64454[0], 64461[0], 64462[0], 64463[0], 64479[0], 64480[0], 64483[0], 64484[0], 64486[0], 64487[0], 64488[0], 64489[0], 64490[0], 64491[0], 64492[0], 64493[0], 64494[0], 64495[0], 64505[0], 64510[0], 64517[0], 64520[0], 64530[0], 69990[0], 92012[1], 92014[1], 93000[1], 93005[1], 93010[1], 93040[1], 93041[1], 93042[1], 93318[1], 93355[1], 94002[1], 94200[1], 94680[1], 94681[1], 94690[1], 95812[1], 95813[1], 95816[1], 95819[1], 95822[1], 95829[1], 95955[1], 96360[1], 96361[1], 96365[1], 96366[1], 96367[1], 96368[1], 96372[1], 96374[1], 96375[1], 96376[1], 96377[1], 96523[0], 97597[1], 97598[1], 97602[1], 99155[0], 99156[0], 99157[0], 99211[1], 99212[1], 99213[1], 99214[1], 99215[1], 99217[1], 99218[1], 99219[1], 99220[1], 99221[1], 99222[1], 99223[1], 99231[1], 99232[1], 99233[1], 99234[1], 99235[1], 99236[1], 99238[1], 99239[1], 99241[1], 99242[1], 99243[1], 99244[1], 99245[1], 99251[1], 99252[1], 99253[1], 99254[1], 99255[1], 99291[1], 99292[1], 99304[1], 99305[1], 99306[1], 99307[1], 99308[1], 99309[1], 99310[1], 99315[1], 99316[1], 99334[1], 99335[1], 99336[1], 99337[1], 99347[1], 99348[1], 99349[1], 99350[1], 99374[1], 99375[1], 99377[1], 99378[1], 99446[0], 99447[0], 99448[0], 99449[0], 99451[0], 99452[0], 99495[0], 99496[0], G0463[1], G0471[0], J0670[1], J2001[1]
53270	0213T[0], 0216T[0], 0596T[1], 0597T[1], 0708T[1], 0709T[1], 11000[1], 11001[1], 11004[1], 11005[1], 11006[1], 11042[1], 11043[1], 11044[1], 11045[1], 11046[1], 11047[1], 12001[1], 12002[1], 12004[1], 12005[1], 12006[1], 12007[1], 12011[1], 12013[1], 12014[1], 12015[1], 12016[1], 12017[1], 12018[1], 12020[1], 12021[1], 12031[1], 12032[1], 12034[1], 12035[1], 12036[1], 12037[1], 12041[1], 12042[1], 12044[1], 12045[1], 12046[1], 12047[1], 12051[1], 12052[1], 12053[1], 12054[1], 12055[1], 12056[1], 12057[1], 13100[1], 13101[1], 13102[1], 13120[1], 13121[1], 13122[1], 13131[1], 13132[1], 13133[1], 13151[1], 13152[1], 13153[1], 36000[1], 36400[1], 36405[1], 36406[1], 36410[1], 36420[1], 36425[1], 36430[1], 36440[1], 36591[0], 36592[0], 36600[1], 36640[1], 43752[1], 51701[0], 51702[0], 51703[1], 52000[0], 53000[0], 53010[0], 53020[0], 53025[0], 53080[1], 53230[0], 62320[0], 62321[0], 62322[0], 62323[0], 62324[0], 62325[0], 62326[0], 62327[0], 64400[0], 64405[0], 64408[0], 64415[0], 64416[0], 64417[0], 64418[0], 64420[0], 64421[0], 64425[0], 64430[0], 64435[0], 64445[0], 64446[0], 64447[0], 64448[0], 64449[0], 64450[0], 64451[0], 64454[0], 64461[0], 64462[0], 64463[0], 64479[0], 64480[0], 64483[0], 64484[0], 64486[0], 64487[0], 64488[0], 64489[0], 64490[0], 64491[0], 64492[0], 64493[0], 64494[0], 64495[0], 64505[0], 64510[0], 64517[0], 64520[0], 64530[0], 69990[0], 92012[1], 92014[1], 93000[1], 93005[1], 93010[1], 93040[1], 93041[1], 93042[1], 93318[1], 93355[1], 94002[1], 94200[1], 94680[1], 94681[1], 94690[1], 95812[1], 95813[1], 95816[1], 95819[1], 95822[1], 95829[1], 95955[1], 96360[1], 96361[1], 96365[1], 96366[1], 96367[1], 96368[1], 96372[1], 96374[1], 96375[1], 96376[1], 96377[1], 96523[0], 97597[1], 97598[1], 97602[1], 99155[0], 99156[0], 99157[0], 99211[1], 99212[1], 99213[1], 99214[1], 99215[1], 99217[1], 99218[1], 99219[1], 99220[1], 99221[1], 99222[1], 99223[1], 99231[1], 99232[1], 99233[1], 99234[1], 99235[1], 99236[1], 99238[1], 99239[1], 99241[1], 99242[1], 99243[1], 99244[1], 99245[1], 99251[1], 99252[1], 99253[1], 99254[1], 99255[1], 99291[1], 99292[1], 99304[1], 99305[1], 99306[1], 99307[1], 99308[1], 99309[1], 99310[1], 99315[1], 99316[1], 99334[1], 99335[1], 99336[1], 99337[1], 99347[1], 99348[1], 99349[1], 99350[1], 99374[1], 99375[1], 99377[1], 99378[1], 99446[0], 99447[0], 99448[0], 99449[0], 99451[0], 99452[0], 99495[0], 99496[0], G0463[1], G0471[0], J2001[1]
53275	0213T[0], 0216T[0], 0596T[1], 0597T[1], 0708T[1], 0709T[1], 11000[1], 11001[1], 11004[1], 11005[1], 11006[1], 11042[1], 11043[1], 11044[1], 11045[1], 11046[1], 11047[1], 12001[1], 12002[1], 12004[1], 12005[1], 12006[1], 12007[1], 12011[1], 12013[1], 12014[1], 12015[1], 12016[1], 12017[1], 12018[1], 12020[1], 12021[1], 12031[1], 12032[1], 12034[1], 12035[1], 12036[1], 12037[1], 12041[1], 12042[1], 12044[1], 12045[1], 12046[1], 12047[1], 12051[1], 12052[1], 12053[1], 12054[1], 12055[1], 12056[1],

Appendix A: NCCI - CPT Codes

0 = Modifier usage not allowed or inappropriate 1 = Modifier usage allowed

Code 1	Code 2
	12057[1], 13100[1], 13101[1], 13102[1], 13120[1], 13121[1], 13122[1], 13131[1], 13132[1], 13133[1], 13151[1], 13152[1], 13153[1], 36000[1], 36400[1], 36405[1], 36406[1], 36410[1], 36420[1], 36425[1], 36430[1], 36440[1], 36591[0], 36592[0], 36600[1], 36640[1], 43752[1], 51701[0], 51702[0], 51703[1], 52000[0], 53000[0], 53010[0], 53020[0], 53025[0], 53080[1], 53230[0], 62320[0], 62321[0], 62322[0], 62323[0], 62324[0], 62325[0], 62326[0], 62327[0], 64400[0], 64405[0], 64408[0], 64415[0], 64416[0], 64417[0], 64418[0], 64420[0], 64421[0], 64425[0], 64430[0], 64435[0], 64445[0], 64446[0], 64447[0], 64448[0], 64449[0], 64450[0], 64451[0], 64454[0], 64461[0], 64462[0], 64463[0], 64479[0], 64480[0], 64483[0], 64484[0], 64486[0], 64487[0], 64488[0], 64489[0], 64490[0], 64491[0], 64492[0], 64493[0], 64494[0], 64495[0], 64505[0], 64510[0], 64517[0], 64520[0], 64530[0], 69990[0], 92012[1], 92014[1], 93000[1], 93005[1], 93010[1], 93040[1], 93041[1], 93042[1], 93318[1], 93355[1], 94002[1], 94200[1], 94680[1], 94681[1], 94690[1], 95812[1], 95813[1], 95816[1], 95819[1], 95822[1], 95829[1], 95955[1], 96360[1], 96361[1], 96365[1], 96366[1], 96367[1], 96368[1], 96372[1], 96374[1], 96375[1], 96376[1], 96377[1], 96523[0], 97597[1], 97598[1], 97602[1], 99155[0], 99156[0], 99157[0], 99211[1], 99212[1], 99213[1], 99214[1], 99215[1], 99217[1], 99218[1], 99219[1], 99220[1], 99221[1], 99222[1], 99223[1], 99231[1], 99232[1], 99233[1], 99234[1], 99235[1], 99236[1], 99238[1], 99239[1], 99241[1], 99242[1], 99243[1], 99244[1], 99245[1], 99251[1], 99252[1], 99253[1], 99254[1], 99255[1], 99291[1], 99292[1], 99304[1], 99305[1], 99306[1], 99307[1], 99308[1], 99309[1], 99310[1], 99315[1], 99316[1], 99334[1], 99335[1], 99336[1], 99337[1], 99347[1], 99348[1], 99349[1], 99350[1], 99374[1], 99375[1], 99377[1], 99378[1], 99446[0], 99447[0], 99448[0], 99449[0], 99451[0], 99452[0], 99495[0], 99496[0], G0463[1], G0471[0]
53400	0213T[0], 0216T[0], 0596T[1], 0597T[1], 0708T[1], 0709T[1], 11000[1], 11001[1], 11004[1], 11005[1], 11006[1], 11042[1], 11043[1], 11044[1], 11045[1], 11046[1], 11047[1], 12001[1], 12002[1], 12004[1], 12005[1], 12006[1], 12007[1], 12011[1], 12013[1], 12014[1], 12015[1], 12016[1], 12017[1], 12018[1], 12020[1], 12021[1], 12031[1], 12032[1], 12034[1], 12035[1], 12036[1], 12037[1], 12041[1], 12042[1], 12044[1], 12045[1], 12046[1], 12047[1], 12051[1], 12052[1], 12053[1], 12054[1], 12055[1], 12056[1], 12057[1], 13100[1], 13101[1], 13102[1], 13120[1], 13121[1], 13122[1], 13131[1], 13132[1], 13133[1], 13151[1], 13152[1], 13153[1], 36000[1], 36400[1], 36405[1], 36406[1], 36410[1], 36420[1], 36425[1], 36430[1], 36440[1], 36591[0], 36592[0], 36600[1], 36640[1], 43752[1], 51701[0], 51702[0], 51703[1], 52000[1], 52301[1], 53000[0], 53010[0], 53020[0], 53025[0], 53080[1], 53405[1], 53502[1], 53505[1], 53510[1], 53515[1], 53520[1], 62320[0], 62321[0], 62322[0], 62323[0], 62324[0], 62325[0], 62326[0], 62327[0], 64400[0], 64405[0], 64408[0], 64415[0], 64416[0], 64417[0], 64418[0], 64420[0], 64421[0], 64425[0], 64430[0], 64435[0], 64445[0], 64446[0], 64447[0], 64448[0], 64449[0], 64450[0], 64451[0], 64454[0], 64461[0], 64462[0], 64463[0], 64479[0], 64480[0], 64483[0], 64484[0], 64486[0], 64487[0], 64488[0], 64489[0], 64490[0], 64491[0], 64492[0], 64493[0], 64494[0], 64495[0], 64505[0], 64510[0], 64517[0], 64520[0], 64530[0], 69990[0], 92012[1], 92014[1], 93000[1], 93005[1], 93010[1], 93040[1], 93041[1], 93042[1], 93318[1], 93355[1], 94002[1], 94200[1], 94680[1], 94681[1], 94690[1], 95812[1], 95813[1], 95816[1], 95819[1], 95822[1], 95829[1], 95955[1], 96360[1], 96361[1], 96365[1], 96366[1], 96367[1], 96368[1], 96372[1], 96374[1], 96375[1], 96376[1], 96377[1], 96523[0], 97597[1], 97598[1], 97602[1], 99155[0], 99156[0], 99157[0], 99211[1], 99212[1], 99213[1], 99214[1], 99215[1], 99217[1], 99218[1], 99219[1], 99220[1], 99221[1], 99222[1], 99223[1], 99231[1], 99232[1], 99233[1], 99234[1], 99235[1], 99236[1], 99238[1], 99239[1], 99241[1], 99242[1], 99243[1], 99244[1], 99245[1], 99251[1], 99252[1], 99253[1], 99254[1], 99255[1], 99291[1], 99292[1], 99304[1], 99305[1], 99306[1], 99307[1], 99308[1], 99309[1], 99310[1], 99315[1], 99316[1], 99334[1], 99335[1], 99336[1], 99337[1], 99347[1], 99348[1], 99349[1], 99350[1], 99374[1], 99375[1], 99377[1], 99378[1], 99446[0], 99447[0], 99448[0], 99449[0], 99451[0], 99452[0], 99495[0], 99496[0], G0463[1], G0471[0]
53405	0213T[0], 0216T[0], 0596T[1], 0597T[1], 0708T[1], 0709T[1], 11000[1], 11001[1], 11004[1], 11005[1], 11006[1], 11042[1], 11043[1], 11044[1], 11045[1], 11046[1], 11047[1], 12001[1], 12002[1], 12004[1], 12005[1], 12006[1], 12007[1], 12011[1], 12013[1], 12014[1], 12015[1], 12016[1], 12017[1], 12018[1], 12020[1], 12021[1], 12031[1], 12032[1], 12034[1], 12035[1], 12036[1], 12037[1], 12041[1], 12042[1], 12044[1], 12045[1], 12046[1], 12047[1], 12051[1], 12052[1], 12053[1], 12054[1], 12055[1], 12056[1], 12057[1], 13100[1], 13101[1], 13102[1], 13120[1], 13121[1], 13122[1], 13131[1], 13132[1], 13133[1], 13151[1], 13152[1], 13153[1], 36000[1], 36400[1], 36405[1], 36406[1], 36410[1], 36420[1], 36425[1], 36430[1], 36440[1], 36591[0], 36592[0], 36600[1], 36640[1], 43752[1], 51701[0], 51702[0], 51703[1], 52000[1], 52301[1], 53000[0], 53010[0], 53020[0], 53025[0], 53080[1], 53502[1], 53505[1], 53510[1], 53515[1], 53520[1], 62320[0], 62321[0], 62322[0], 62323[0], 62324[0], 62325[0], 62326[0], 62327[0], 64400[0], 64405[0], 64408[0], 64415[0], 64416[0], 64417[0], 64418[0], 64420[0], 64421[0], 64425[0], 64430[0], 64435[0], 64445[0], 64446[0], 64447[0], 64448[0], 64449[0], 64450[0], 64451[0], 64454[0], 64461[0], 64462[0], 64463[0], 64479[0], 64480[0], 64483[0], 64484[0], 64486[0], 64487[0], 64488[0], 64489[0], 64490[0], 64491[0], 64492[0], 64493[0], 64494[0], 64495[0], 64505[0], 64510[0], 64517[0], 64520[0], 64530[0], 69990[0], 92012[1], 92014[1], 93000[1], 93005[1], 93010[1], 93040[1], 93041[1], 93042[1], 93318[1], 93355[1], 94002[1], 94200[1], 94680[1], 94681[1], 94690[1], 95812[1], 95813[1], 95816[1], 95819[1], 95822[1], 95829[1], 95955[1], 96360[1], 96361[1], 96365[1], 96366[1], 96367[1], 96368[1], 96372[1], 96374[1], 96375[1], 96376[1], 96377[1], 96523[0], 97597[1], 97598[1], 97602[1], 99155[0], 99156[0], 99157[0], 99211[1], 99212[1], 99213[1], 99214[1], 99215[1], 99217[1], 99218[1], 99219[1], 99220[1], 99221[1], 99222[1], 99223[1], 99231[1], 99232[1], 99233[1], 99234[1], 99235[1], 99236[1], 99238[1], 99239[1], 99241[1], 99242[1], 99243[1], 99244[1], 99245[1], 99251[1], 99252[1], 99253[1], 99254[1], 99255[1], 99291[1], 99292[1], 99304[1], 99305[1], 99306[1], 99307[1], 99308[1], 99309[1], 99310[1], 99315[1], 99316[1], 99334[1], 99335[1], 99336[1], 99337[1], 99347[1], 99348[1], 99349[1], 99350[1], 99374[1], 99375[1], 99377[1], 99378[1], 99446[0], 99447[0], 99448[0], 99449[0], 99451[0], 99452[0], 99495[0], 99496[0], G0463[1], G0471[0]
53410	0213T[0], 0216T[0], 0596T[1], 0597T[1], 0708T[1], 0709T[1], 11000[1], 11001[1], 11004[1], 11005[1], 11006[1], 11042[1], 11043[1], 11044[1], 11045[1], 11046[1], 11047[1], 12001[1], 12002[1], 12004[1], 12005[1], 12006[1], 12007[1], 12011[1], 12013[1], 12014[1], 12015[1], 12016[1], 12017[1], 12018[1], 12020[1], 12021[1], 12031[1], 12032[1], 12034[1], 12035[1], 12036[1], 12037[1], 12041[1], 12042[1], 12044[1], 12045[1], 12046[1], 12047[1], 12051[1], 12052[1], 12053[1], 12054[1], 12055[1], 12056[1], 12057[1], 13100[1], 13101[1], 13102[1], 13120[1], 13121[1], 13122[1], 13131[1], 13132[1], 13133[1], 13151[1], 13152[1], 13153[1], 36000[1], 36400[1], 36405[1], 36406[1], 36410[1], 36420[1], 36425[1], 36430[1], 36440[1], 36591[0], 36592[0], 36600[1], 36640[1], 43752[1], 51701[0], 51702[0], 51703[1], 51990[1], 51992[1], 52000[0], 52301[1], 53000[0], 53010[0], 53020[0], 53025[0], 53080[1], 53502[1], 53505[1], 53510[1], 53515[1], 53520[1], 62320[0], 62321[0], 62322[0], 62323[0], 62324[0], 62325[0], 62326[0], 62327[0], 64400[0], 64405[0], 64408[0], 64415[0], 64416[0], 64417[0], 64418[0], 64420[0], 64421[0], 64425[0], 64430[0], 64435[0], 64445[0], 64446[0], 64447[0], 64448[0], 64449[0], 64450[0], 64451[0], 64454[0], 64461[0], 64462[0], 64463[0], 64479[0], 64480[0], 64483[0], 64484[0], 64486[0], 64487[0], 64488[0], 64489[0], 64490[0], 64491[0], 64492[0], 64493[0], 64494[0], 64495[0], 64505[0], 64510[0], 64517[0], 64520[0], 64530[0], 69990[0], 92012[1], 92014[1], 93000[1], 93005[1], 93010[1], 93040[1], 93041[1], 93042[1], 93318[1], 93355[1], 94002[1], 94200[1], 94680[1], 94681[1], 94690[1], 95812[1], 95813[1], 95816[1], 95819[1], 95822[1], 95829[1], 95955[1], 96360[1], 96361[1], 96365[1], 96366[1], 96367[1], 96368[1], 96372[1], 96374[1], 96375[1], 96376[1], 96377[1], 96523[0], 97597[1], 97598[1], 97602[1], 99155[0], 99156[0], 99157[0], 99211[1], 99212[1], 99213[1], 99214[1], 99215[1], 99217[1], 99218[1], 99219[1], 99220[1], 99221[1], 99222[1], 99223[1], 99231[1], 99232[1], 99233[1], 99234[1], 99235[1], 99236[1], 99238[1], 99239[1], 99241[1], 99242[1], 99243[1], 99244[1], 99245[1], 99251[1], 99252[1], 99253[1], 99254[1], 99255[1], 99291[1], 99292[1], 99304[1], 99305[1], 99306[1], 99307[1], 99308[1], 99309[1], 99310[1], 99315[1], 99316[1], 99334[1], 99335[1], 99336[1], 99337[1], 99347[1], 99348[1], 99349[1], 99350[1], 99374[1], 99375[1], 99377[1], 99378[1], 99446[0], 99447[0], 99448[0], 99449[0], 99451[0], 99452[0], 99495[0], 99496[0], G0463[1], G0471[0]
53415	0213T[0], 0216T[0], 0596T[1], 0597T[1], 0708T[1], 0709T[1], 11000[1], 11001[1], 11004[1], 11005[1], 11006[1], 11042[1], 11043[1], 11044[1], 11045[1], 11046[1], 11047[1], 12001[1], 12002[1], 12004[1], 12005[1], 12006[1], 12007[1], 12011[1], 12013[1], 12014[1], 12015[1], 12016[1], 12017[1], 12018[1], 12020[1], 12021[1], 12031[1], 12032[1], 12034[1], 12035[1], 12036[1], 12037[1], 12041[1], 12042[1], 12044[1], 12045[1], 12046[1], 12047[1], 12051[1], 12052[1], 12053[1], 12054[1], 12055[1], 12056[1], 12057[1], 13100[1], 13101[1], 13102[1], 13120[1], 13121[1], 13122[1], 13131[1], 13132[1], 13133[1], 13151[1], 13152[1], 13153[1], 36000[1], 36400[1], 36405[1], 36406[1], 36410[1], 36420[1], 36425[1], 36430[1], 36440[1], 36591[0], 36592[0], 36600[1], 36640[1], 43752[1], 51701[0], 51702[0], 51703[1], 51990[1], 51992[1], 52000[1], 52301[1], 52640[1], 53000[0], 53010[0], 53020[0], 53025[0], 53080[1], 53502[1], 53505[1], 53510[1], 53515[1], 53520[1], 62320[0], 62321[0], 62322[0], 62323[0], 62324[0], 62325[0], 62326[0], 62327[0], 64400[0], 64405[0], 64408[0], 64415[0], 64416[0], 64417[0], 64418[0], 64420[0], 64421[0], 64425[0], 64430[0], 64435[0], 64445[0], 64446[0], 64447[0], 64448[0], 64449[0], 64450[0], 64451[0], 64454[0], 64461[0], 64462[0], 64463[0], 64479[0], 64480[0], 64483[0], 64484[0], 64486[0], 64487[0], 64488[0], 64489[0], 64490[0], 64491[0], 64492[0], 64493[0], 64494[0], 64495[0], 64505[0], 64510[0], 64517[0], 64520[0], 64530[0], 69990[0], 92012[1], 92014[1], 93000[1], 93005[1], 93010[1], 93040[1], 93041[1], 93042[1], 93318[1], 93355[1], 94002[1], 94200[1], 94680[1], 94681[1], 94690[1], 95812[1], 95813[1], 95816[1], 95819[1], 95822[1], 95829[1], 95955[1], 96360[1], 96361[1], 96365[1], 96366[1], 96367[1], 96368[1], 96372[1], 96374[1], 96375[1], 96376[1], 96377[1], 96523[0], 97597[1], 97598[1], 97602[1], 99155[0], 99156[0], 99157[0], 99211[1], 99212[1], 99213[1], 99214[1], 99215[1], 99217[1], 99218[1], 99219[1], 99220[1], 99221[1], 99222[1], 99223[1], 99231[1], 99232[1], 99233[1], 99234[1], 99235[1], 99236[1], 99238[1], 99239[1], 99241[1], 99242[1], 99243[1], 99244[1], 99245[1], 99251[1], 99252[1], 99253[1], 99254[1], 99255[1], 99291[1], 99292[1], 99304[1], 99305[1], 99306[1], 99307[1], 99308[1], 99309[1], 99310[1], 99315[1], 99316[1], 99334[1], 99335[1], 99336[1], 99337[1], 99347[1], 99348[1], 99349[1], 99350[1], 99374[1], 99375[1], 99377[1], 99378[1], 99446[0], 99447[0], 99448[0], 99449[0], 99451[0], 99452[0], 99495[0], 99496[0], G0463[1], G0471[0]
53420	0213T[0], 0216T[0], 0596T[1], 0597T[1], 0708T[1], 0709T[1], 11000[1], 11001[1], 11004[1], 11005[1], 11006[1], 11042[1], 11043[1], 11044[1], 11045[1], 11046[1], 11047[1], 12001[1], 12002[1], 12004[1], 12005[1], 12006[1], 12007[1], 12011[1], 12013[1], 12014[1], 12015[1], 12016[1], 12017[1], 12018[1], 12020[1], 12021[1], 12031[1], 12032[1], 12034[1], 12035[1], 12036[1], 12037[1], 12041[1], 12042[1], 12044[1], 12045[1], 12046[1], 12047[1], 12051[1], 12052[1], 12053[1], 12054[1], 12055[1], 12056[1], 12057[1], 13100[1], 13101[1], 13102[1], 13120[1], 13121[1], 13122[1], 13131[1], 13132[1], 13133[1], 13151[1], 13152[1], 13153[1], 36000[1], 36400[1], 36405[1], 36406[1], 36410[1], 36420[1], 36425[1], 36430[1], 36440[1], 36591[0], 36592[0], 36600[1], 36640[1], 43752[1], 51701[0], 51702[0], 51703[1], 51990[1], 51992[1], 52000[1], 52301[1], 52640[1], 53000[0], 53010[0], 53020[0], 53025[0], 53080[1], 53425[1], 53502[1], 53505[1], 53510[1], 53515[1], 53520[1], 62320[0], 62321[0], 62322[0], 62323[0], 62324[0], 62325[0], 62326[0], 62327[0], 64400[0], 64405[0], 64408[0], 64415[0], 64416[0], 64417[0],

0 = Modifier usage not allowed or inappropriate   1 = Modifier usage allowed

Code 1	Code 2
	64418[0], 64420[0], 64421[0], 64425[0], 64430[0], 64435[0], 64445[0], 64446[0], 64447[0], 64448[0], 64449[0], 64450[0], 64451[0], 64454[0], 64461[0], 64462[0], 64463[0], 64479[0], 64480[0], 64483[0], 64484[0], 64486[0], 64487[0], 64488[0], 64489[0], 64490[0], 64491[0], 64492[0], 64493[0], 64494[0], 64495[0], 64505[0], 64510[0], 64517[0], 64520[0], 64530[0], 69990[0], 92012[1], 92014[1], 93000[1], 93005[1], 93010[1], 93040[1], 93041[1], 93042[1], 93318[1], 93355[1], 94002[1], 94200[1], 94680[1], 94681[1], 94690[1], 95812[1], 95813[1], 95816[1], 95819[1], 95822[1], 95829[1], 95955[1], 96360[1], 96361[1], 96365[1], 96366[1], 96367[1], 96368[1], 96372[1], 96374[1], 96375[1], 96376[1], 96377[1], 96523[0], 97597[1], 97598[1], 97602[1], 99155[0], 99156[0], 99157[0], 99211[1], 99212[1], 99213[1], 99214[1], 99215[1], 99217[1], 99218[1], 99219[1], 99220[1], 99221[1], 99222[1], 99223[1], 99231[1], 99232[1], 99233[1], 99234[1], 99235[1], 99236[1], 99238[1], 99239[1], 99241[1], 99242[1], 99243[1], 99244[1], 99245[1], 99251[1], 99252[1], 99253[1], 99254[1], 99255[1], 99291[1], 99292[1], 99304[1], 99305[1], 99306[1], 99307[1], 99308[1], 99309[1], 99310[1], 99315[1], 99316[1], 99334[1], 99335[1], 99336[1], 99337[1], 99347[1], 99348[1], 99349[1], 99350[1], 99374[1], 99375[1], 99377[1], 99378[1], 99446[0], 99447[0], 99448[0], 99449[0], 99451[0], 99452[0], 99495[0], 99496[0], G0463[1], G0471[0]
53425	0213T[0], 0216T[0], 0596T[1], 0597T[1], 0708T[1], 0709T[1], 11000[1], 11001[1], 11004[1], 11005[1], 11006[1], 11042[1], 11043[1], 11044[1], 11045[1], 11046[1], 11047[1], 12001[1], 12002[1], 12004[1], 12005[1], 12006[1], 12007[1], 12011[1], 12013[1], 12014[1], 12015[1], 12016[1], 12017[1], 12018[1], 12020[1], 12021[1], 12031[1], 12032[1], 12034[1], 12035[1], 12036[1], 12037[1], 12041[1], 12042[1], 12044[1], 12045[1], 12046[1], 12047[1], 12051[1], 12052[1], 12053[1], 12054[1], 12055[1], 12056[1], 12057[1], 13100[1], 13101[1], 13102[1], 13120[1], 13121[1], 13122[1], 13131[1], 13132[1], 13133[1], 13151[1], 13152[1], 13153[1], 36000[1], 36400[1], 36405[1], 36406[1], 36410[1], 36420[1], 36425[1], 36430[1], 36440[1], 36591[0], 36592[0], 36600[1], 36640[1], 43752[1], 51701[0], 51702[0], 51703[1], 51990[1], 51992[1], 52000[1], 52301[1], 52640[1], 53000[0], 53010[0], 53020[0], 53025[0], 53080[1], 53502[1], 53505[1], 53510[1], 53515[1], 53520[1], 62320[0], 62321[0], 62322[0], 62323[0], 62324[0], 62325[0], 62326[0], 62327[0], 64400[0], 64405[0], 64408[0], 64415[0], 64416[0], 64417[0], 64418[0], 64420[0], 64421[0], 64425[0], 64430[0], 64435[0], 64445[0], 64446[0], 64447[0], 64448[0], 64449[0], 64450[0], 64451[0], 64454[0], 64461[0], 64462[0], 64463[0], 64479[0], 64480[0], 64483[0], 64484[0], 64486[0], 64487[0], 64488[0], 64489[0], 64490[0], 64491[0], 64492[0], 64493[0], 64494[0], 64495[0], 64505[0], 64510[0], 64517[0], 64520[0], 64530[0], 69990[0], 92012[1], 92014[1], 93000[1], 93005[1], 93010[1], 93040[1], 93041[1], 93042[1], 93318[1], 93355[1], 94002[1], 94200[1], 94680[1], 94681[1], 94690[1], 95812[1], 95813[1], 95816[1], 95819[1], 95822[1], 95829[1], 95955[1], 96360[1], 96361[1], 96365[1], 96366[1], 96367[1], 96368[1], 96372[1], 96374[1], 96375[1], 96376[1], 96377[1], 96523[0], 97597[1], 97598[1], 97602[1], 99155[0], 99156[0], 99157[0], 99211[1], 99212[1], 99213[1], 99214[1], 99215[1], 99217[1], 99218[1], 99219[1], 99220[1], 99221[1], 99222[1], 99223[1], 99231[1], 99232[1], 99233[1], 99234[1], 99235[1], 99236[1], 99238[1], 99239[1], 99241[1], 99242[1], 99243[1], 99244[1], 99245[1], 99251[1], 99252[1], 99253[1], 99254[1], 99255[1], 99291[1], 99292[1], 99304[1], 99305[1], 99306[1], 99307[1], 99308[1], 99309[1], 99310[1], 99315[1], 99316[1], 99334[1], 99335[1], 99336[1], 99337[1], 99347[1], 99348[1], 99349[1], 99350[1], 99374[1], 99375[1], 99377[1], 99378[1], 99446[0], 99447[0], 99448[0], 99449[0], 99451[0], 99452[0], 99495[0], 99496[0], G0463[1], G0471[0]
53430	0213T[0], 0216T[0], 0596T[1], 0597T[1], 0708T[1], 0709T[1], 11000[1], 11001[1], 11004[1], 11005[1], 11006[1], 11042[1], 11043[1], 11044[1], 11045[1], 11046[1], 11047[1], 12001[1], 12002[1], 12004[1], 12005[1], 12006[1], 12007[1], 12011[1], 12013[1], 12014[1], 12015[1], 12016[1], 12017[1], 12018[1], 12020[1], 12021[1], 12031[1], 12032[1], 12034[1], 12035[1], 12036[1], 12037[1], 12041[1], 12042[1], 12044[1], 12045[1], 12046[1], 12047[1], 12051[1], 12052[1], 12053[1], 12054[1], 12055[1], 12056[1], 12057[1], 13100[1], 13101[1], 13102[1], 13120[1], 13121[1], 13122[1], 13131[1], 13132[1], 13133[1], 13151[1], 13152[1], 13153[1], 36000[1], 36400[1], 36405[1], 36406[1], 36410[1], 36420[1], 36425[1], 36430[1], 36440[1], 36591[0], 36592[0], 36600[1], 36640[1], 43752[1], 51701[0], 51702[0], 51703[1], 51990[1], 51992[1], 52000[1], 52301[1], 53000[0], 53010[0], 53020[0], 53025[0], 53080[1], 53502[1], 53505[1], 53510[1], 53515[1], 53520[1], 53860[1], 62320[0], 62321[0], 62322[0], 62323[0], 62324[0], 62325[0], 62326[0], 62327[0], 64400[0], 64405[0], 64408[0], 64415[0], 64416[0], 64417[0], 64418[0], 64420[0], 64421[0], 64425[0], 64430[0], 64435[0], 64445[0], 64446[0], 64447[0], 64448[0], 64449[0], 64450[0], 64451[0], 64454[0], 64461[0], 64462[0], 64463[0], 64479[0], 64480[0], 64483[0], 64484[0], 64486[0], 64487[0], 64488[0], 64489[0], 64490[0], 64491[0], 64492[0], 64493[0], 64494[0], 64495[0], 64505[0], 64510[0], 64517[0], 64520[0], 64530[0], 69990[0], 92012[1], 92014[1], 93000[1], 93005[1], 93010[1], 93040[1], 93041[1], 93042[1], 93318[1], 93355[1], 94002[1], 94200[1], 94680[1], 94681[1], 94690[1], 95812[1], 95813[1], 95816[1], 95819[1], 95822[1], 95829[1], 95955[1], 96360[1], 96361[1], 96365[1], 96366[1], 96367[1], 96368[1], 96372[1], 96374[1], 96375[1], 96376[1], 96377[1], 96523[0], 97597[1], 97598[1], 97602[1], 99155[0], 99156[0], 99157[0], 99211[1], 99212[1], 99213[1], 99214[1], 99215[1], 99217[1], 99218[1], 99219[1], 99220[1], 99221[1], 99222[1], 99223[1], 99231[1], 99232[1], 99233[1], 99234[1], 99235[1], 99236[1], 99238[1], 99239[1], 99241[1], 99242[1], 99243[1], 99244[1], 99245[1], 99251[1], 99252[1], 99253[1], 99254[1], 99255[1], 99291[1], 99292[1], 99304[1], 99305[1], 99306[1], 99307[1], 99308[1], 99309[1], 99310[1], 99315[1], 99316[1], 99334[1], 99335[1], 99336[1], 99337[1], 99347[1], 99348[1], 99349[1], 99350[1], 99374[1], 99375[1], 99377[1], 99378[1], 99446[0], 99447[0], 99448[0], 99449[0], 99451[0], 99452[0], 99495[0], 99496[0], G0463[1], G0471[0]
53431	0213T[0], 0216T[0], 0596T[1], 0597T[1], 0708T[1], 0709T[1], 11000[1], 11001[1], 11004[1], 11005[1], 11006[1], 11042[1], 11043[1], 11044[1], 11045[1], 11046[1], 11047[1], 12001[1], 12002[1], 12004[1], 12005[1], 12006[1], 12007[1], 12011[1], 12013[1], 12014[1], 12015[1], 12016[1], 12017[1], 12018[1], 12020[1], 12021[1], 12031[1], 12032[1], 12034[1], 12035[1], 12036[1], 12037[1], 12041[1], 12042[1], 12044[1], 12045[1], 12046[1], 12047[1], 12051[1], 12052[1], 12053[1], 12054[1], 12055[1], 12056[1], 12057[1], 13100[1], 13101[1], 13102[1], 13120[1], 13121[1], 13122[1], 13131[1], 13132[1], 13133[1], 13151[1], 13152[1], 13153[1], 36000[1], 36400[1], 36405[1], 36406[1], 36410[1], 36420[1], 36425[1], 36430[1], 36440[1], 36591[0], 36592[0], 36600[1], 36640[1], 43752[1], 51701[0], 51702[0], 51703[1], 51990[1], 51992[1], 52000[1], 52301[1], 53000[0], 53010[0], 53020[0], 53025[0], 53080[1], 53502[1], 53505[1], 53510[1], 53515[1], 53520[1], 53860[1], 62320[0], 62321[0], 62322[0], 62323[0], 62324[0], 62325[0], 62326[0], 62327[0], 64400[0], 64405[0], 64408[0], 64415[0], 64416[0], 64417[0], 64418[0], 64420[0], 64421[0], 64425[0], 64430[0], 64435[0], 64445[0], 64446[0], 64447[0], 64448[0], 64449[0], 64450[0], 64451[0], 64454[0], 64461[0], 64462[0], 64463[0], 64479[0], 64480[0], 64483[0], 64484[0], 64486[0], 64487[0], 64488[0], 64489[0], 64490[0], 64491[0], 64492[0], 64493[0], 64494[0], 64495[0], 64505[0], 64510[0], 64517[0], 64520[0], 64530[0], 69990[0], 92012[1], 92014[1], 93000[1], 93005[1], 93010[1], 93040[1], 93041[1], 93042[1], 93318[1], 93355[1], 94002[1], 94200[1], 94680[1], 94681[1], 94690[1], 95812[1], 95813[1], 95816[1], 95819[1], 95822[1], 95829[1], 95955[1], 96360[1], 96361[1], 96365[1], 96366[1], 96367[1], 96368[1], 96372[1], 96374[1], 96375[1], 96376[1], 96377[1], 96523[0], 97597[1], 97598[1], 97602[1], 99155[0], 99156[0], 99157[0], 99211[1], 99212[1], 99213[1], 99214[1], 99215[1], 99217[1], 99218[1], 99219[1], 99220[1], 99221[1], 99222[1], 99223[1], 99231[1], 99232[1], 99233[1], 99234[1], 99235[1], 99236[1], 99238[1], 99239[1], 99241[1], 99242[1], 99243[1], 99244[1], 99245[1], 99251[1], 99252[1], 99253[1], 99254[1], 99255[1], 99291[1], 99292[1], 99304[1], 99305[1], 99306[1], 99307[1], 99308[1], 99309[1], 99310[1], 99315[1], 99316[1], 99334[1], 99335[1], 99336[1], 99337[1], 99347[1], 99348[1], 99349[1], 99350[1], 99374[1], 99375[1], 99377[1], 99378[1], 99446[0], 99447[0], 99448[0], 99449[0], 99451[0], 99452[0], 99495[0], 99496[0], G0463[1], G0471[0]
53440	0213T[0], 0216T[0], 0596T[1], 0597T[1], 0708T[1], 0709T[1], 12001[1], 12002[1], 12004[1], 12005[1], 12006[1], 12007[1], 12011[1], 12013[1], 12014[1], 12015[1], 12016[1], 12017[1], 12018[1], 12020[1], 12021[1], 12031[1], 12032[1], 12034[1], 12035[1], 12036[1], 12037[1], 12041[1], 12042[1], 12044[1], 12045[1], 12046[1], 12047[1], 12051[1], 12052[1], 12053[1], 12054[1], 12055[1], 12056[1], 12057[1], 13100[1], 13101[1], 13102[1], 13120[1], 13121[1], 13122[1], 13131[1], 13132[1], 13133[1], 13151[1], 13152[1], 13153[1], 36000[1], 36400[1], 36405[1], 36406[1], 36410[1], 36420[1], 36425[1], 36430[1], 36440[1], 36591[0], 36592[0], 36600[1], 36640[1], 43752[1], 51701[0], 51702[0], 51703[1], 51990[1], 51992[1], 52000[1], 52301[1], 53000[0], 53010[0], 53020[0], 53025[0], 53080[1], 53444[0], 62320[0], 62321[0], 62322[0], 62323[0], 62324[0], 62325[0], 62326[0], 62327[0], 64400[0], 64405[0], 64408[0], 64415[0], 64416[0], 64417[0], 64418[0], 64420[0], 64421[0], 64425[0], 64430[0], 64435[0], 64445[0], 64446[0], 64447[0], 64448[0], 64449[0], 64450[0], 64451[0], 64454[0], 64461[0], 64462[0], 64463[0], 64479[0], 64480[0], 64483[0], 64484[0], 64486[0], 64487[0], 64488[0], 64489[0], 64490[0], 64491[0], 64492[0], 64493[0], 64494[0], 64495[0], 64505[0], 64510[0], 64517[0], 64520[0], 64530[0], 69990[0], 92012[1], 92014[1], 93000[1], 93005[1], 93010[1], 93040[1], 93041[1], 93042[1], 93318[1], 93355[1], 94002[1], 94200[1], 94680[1], 94681[1], 94690[1], 95812[1], 95813[1], 95816[1], 95819[1], 95822[1], 95829[1], 95955[1], 96360[1], 96361[1], 96365[1], 96366[1], 96367[1], 96368[1], 96372[1], 96374[1], 96375[1], 96376[1], 96377[1], 96523[0], 99155[0], 99156[0], 99157[0], 99211[1], 99212[1], 99213[1], 99214[1], 99215[1], 99217[1], 99218[1], 99219[1], 99220[1], 99221[1], 99222[1], 99223[1], 99231[1], 99232[1], 99233[1], 99234[1], 99235[1], 99236[1], 99238[1], 99239[1], 99241[1], 99242[1], 99243[1], 99244[1], 99245[1], 99251[1], 99252[1], 99253[1], 99254[1], 99255[1], 99291[1], 99292[1], 99304[1], 99305[1], 99306[1], 99307[1], 99308[1], 99309[1], 99310[1], 99315[1], 99316[1], 99334[1], 99335[1], 99336[1], 99337[1], 99347[1], 99348[1], 99349[1], 99350[1], 99374[1], 99375[1], 99377[1], 99378[1], 99446[0], 99447[0], 99448[0], 99449[0], 99451[0], 99452[0], 99495[0], 99496[0], G0463[1], G0471[0]
53442	0213T[0], 0216T[0], 0596T[1], 0597T[1], 0708T[1], 0709T[1], 11000[1], 11001[1], 11004[1], 11005[1], 11006[1], 11042[1], 11043[1], 11044[1], 11045[1], 11046[1], 11047[1], 12001[1], 12002[1], 12004[1], 12005[1], 12006[1], 12007[1], 12011[1], 12013[1], 12014[1], 12015[1], 12016[1], 12017[1], 12018[1], 12020[1], 12021[1], 12031[1], 12032[1], 12034[1], 12035[1], 12036[1], 12037[1], 12041[1], 12042[1], 12044[1], 12045[1], 12046[1], 12047[1], 12051[1], 12052[1], 12053[1], 12054[1], 12055[1], 12056[1], 12057[1], 13100[1], 13101[1], 13102[1], 13120[1], 13121[1], 13122[1], 13131[1], 13132[1], 13133[1], 13151[1], 13152[1], 13153[1], 36000[1], 36400[1], 36405[1], 36406[1], 36410[1], 36420[1], 36425[1], 36430[1], 36440[1], 36591[0], 36592[0], 36600[1], 36640[1], 43752[1], 51701[0], 51702[0], 51703[1], 52000[1], 52301[1], 53000[0], 53010[0], 53020[0], 53025[0], 53440[0], 62320[0], 62321[0], 62322[0], 62323[0], 62324[0], 62325[0], 62326[0], 62327[0], 64400[0], 64405[0], 64408[0], 64415[0], 64416[0], 64417[0], 64418[0], 64420[0], 64421[0], 64425[0], 64430[0], 64435[0], 64445[0], 64446[0], 64447[0], 64448[0], 64449[0], 64450[0], 64451[0], 64454[0], 64461[0], 64462[0], 64463[0], 64479[0], 64480[0], 64483[0], 64484[0], 64486[0], 64487[0], 64488[0], 64489[0], 64490[0], 64491[0], 64492[0], 64493[0], 64494[0], 64495[0], 64505[0], 64510[0], 64517[0], 64520[0], 64530[0], 69990[0], 92012[1], 92014[1], 93000[1], 93005[1], 93010[1], 93040[1], 93041[1], 93042[1], 93318[1], 93355[1], 94002[1], 94200[1], 94680[1], 94681[1], 94690[1], 95812[1], 95813[1], 95816[1], 95819[1], 95822[1], 95829[1], 95955[1], 96360[1], 96361[1], 96365[1], 96366[1], 96367[1], 96368[1], 96372[1], 96374[1], 96375[1], 96376[1], 96377[1], 96523[0], 97597[1], 97598[1], 97602[1], 99155[0], 99156[0], 99157[0], 99211[1], 99212[1],

0 = Modifier usage not allowed or inappropriate 1 = Modifier usage allowed

Code 1	Code 2
	99213[1], 99214[1], 99215[1], 99217[1], 99218[1], 99219[1], 99220[1], 99221[1], 99222[1], 99223[1], 99231[1], 99232[1], 99233[1], 99234[1], 99235[1], 99236[1], 99238[1], 99239[1], 99241[1], 99242[1], 99243[1], 99244[1], 99245[1], 99251[1], 99252[1], 99253[1], 99254[1], 99255[1], 99291[1], 99292[1], 99304[1], 99305[1], 99306[1], 99307[1], 99308[1], 99309[1], 99310[1], 99315[1], 99316[1], 99334[1], 99335[1], 99336[1], 99337[1], 99347[1], 99348[1], 99349[1], 99350[1], 99374[1], 99375[1], 99377[1], 99378[1], 99446[0], 99447[0], 99448[0], 99449[0], 99451[0], 99452[0], 99495[0], 99496[0], G0463[1], G0471[0]
53444	0213T[0], 0216T[0], 0596T[1], 0597T[1], 0708T[1], 0709T[1], 11000[1], 11001[1], 11004[1], 11005[1], 11006[1], 11042[1], 11043[1], 11044[1], 11045[1], 11046[1], 11047[1], 12001[1], 12002[1], 12004[1], 12005[1], 12006[1], 12007[1], 12011[1], 12013[1], 12014[1], 12015[1], 12016[1], 12017[1], 12018[1], 12020[1], 12021[1], 12031[1], 12032[1], 12034[1], 12035[1], 12036[1], 12037[1], 12041[1], 12042[1], 12044[1], 12045[1], 12046[1], 12047[1], 12051[1], 12052[1], 12053[1], 12054[1], 12055[1], 12056[1], 12057[1], 13100[1], 13101[1], 13102[1], 13120[1], 13121[1], 13122[1], 13131[1], 13132[1], 13133[1], 13151[1], 13152[1], 13153[1], 36000[1], 36400[1], 36405[1], 36406[1], 36410[1], 36420[1], 36425[1], 36430[1], 36440[1], 36591[0], 36592[0], 36600[1], 36640[1], 43752[1], 51701[0], 51702[0], 51703[1], 52000[1], 53000[0], 53010[0], 53020[0], 53025[0], 53446[0], 53449[0], 53453[0], 62320[0], 62321[0], 62322[0], 62323[0], 62324[0], 62325[0], 62326[0], 62327[0], 64400[0], 64405[0], 64408[0], 64415[0], 64416[0], 64417[0], 64418[0], 64420[0], 64421[0], 64425[0], 64430[0], 64435[0], 64445[0], 64446[0], 64447[0], 64448[0], 64449[0], 64450[0], 64451[0], 64454[0], 64461[0], 64462[0], 64463[0], 64479[0], 64480[0], 64483[0], 64484[0], 64486[0], 64487[0], 64488[0], 64489[0], 64490[0], 64491[0], 64492[0], 64493[0], 64494[0], 64495[0], 64505[0], 64510[0], 64517[0], 64520[0], 64530[0], 69990[0], 92012[1], 92014[1], 93000[1], 93005[1], 93010[1], 93040[1], 93041[1], 93042[1], 93318[1], 93355[1], 94002[1], 94200[1], 94680[1], 94681[1], 94690[1], 95812[1], 95813[1], 95816[1], 95819[1], 95822[1], 95829[1], 95955[1], 96360[1], 96361[1], 96365[1], 96366[1], 96367[1], 96368[1], 96372[1], 96374[1], 96375[1], 96376[1], 96377[1], 96523[0], 97597[1], 97598[1], 97602[1], 99155[0], 99156[0], 99157[0], 99211[1], 99212[1], 99213[1], 99214[1], 99215[1], 99217[1], 99218[1], 99219[1], 99220[1], 99221[1], 99222[1], 99223[1], 99231[1], 99232[1], 99233[1], 99234[1], 99235[1], 99236[1], 99238[1], 99239[1], 99241[1], 99242[1], 99243[1], 99244[1], 99245[1], 99251[1], 99252[1], 99253[1], 99254[1], 99255[1], 99291[1], 99292[1], 99304[1], 99305[1], 99306[1], 99307[1], 99308[1], 99309[1], 99310[1], 99315[1], 99316[1], 99334[1], 99335[1], 99336[1], 99337[1], 99347[1], 99348[1], 99349[1], 99350[1], 99374[1], 99375[1], 99377[1], 99378[1], 99446[0], 99447[0], 99448[0], 99449[0], 99451[0], 99452[0], 99495[0], 99496[0], G0463[1], G0471[0]
53445	0213T[0], 0216T[0], 0596T[1], 0597T[1], 0708T[1], 0709T[1], 11000[1], 11001[1], 11004[1], 11005[1], 11006[1], 11042[1], 11043[1], 11044[1], 11045[1], 11046[1], 11047[1], 12001[1], 12002[1], 12004[1], 12005[1], 12006[1], 12007[1], 12011[1], 12013[1], 12014[1], 12015[1], 12016[1], 12017[1], 12018[1], 12020[1], 12021[1], 12031[1], 12032[1], 12034[1], 12035[1], 12036[1], 12037[1], 12041[1], 12042[1], 12044[1], 12045[1], 12046[1], 12047[1], 12051[1], 12052[1], 12053[1], 12054[1], 12055[1], 12056[1], 12057[1], 13100[1], 13101[1], 13102[1], 13120[1], 13121[1], 13122[1], 13131[1], 13132[1], 13133[1], 13151[1], 13152[1], 13153[1], 36000[1], 36400[1], 36405[1], 36406[1], 36410[1], 36420[1], 36425[1], 36430[1], 36440[1], 36591[0], 36592[0], 36600[1], 36640[1], 43752[1], 51701[0], 51702[0], 51703[1], 51990[1], 51992[1], 52000[1], 52301[1], 53000[0], 53010[0], 53020[0], 53025[0], 53080[1], 53444[0], 62320[0], 62321[0], 62322[0], 62323[0], 62324[0], 62325[0], 62326[0], 62327[0], 64400[0], 64405[0], 64408[0], 64415[0], 64416[0], 64417[0], 64418[0], 64420[0], 64421[0], 64425[0], 64430[0], 64435[0], 64445[0], 64446[0], 64447[0], 64448[0], 64449[0], 64450[0], 64451[0], 64454[0], 64461[0], 64462[0], 64463[0], 64479[0], 64480[0], 64483[0], 64484[0], 64486[0], 64487[0], 64488[0], 64489[0], 64490[0], 64491[0], 64492[0], 64493[0], 64494[0], 64495[0], 64505[0], 64510[0], 64517[0], 64520[0], 64530[0], 69990[0], 92012[1], 92014[1], 93000[1], 93005[1], 93010[1], 93040[1], 93041[1], 93042[1], 93318[1], 93355[1], 94002[1], 94200[1], 94680[1], 94681[1], 94690[1], 95812[1], 95813[1], 95816[1], 95819[1], 95822[1], 95829[1], 95955[1], 96360[1], 96361[1], 96365[1], 96366[1], 96367[1], 96368[1], 96372[1], 96374[1], 96375[1], 96376[1], 96377[1], 96523[0], 97597[1], 97598[1], 97602[1], 99155[0], 99156[0], 99157[0], 99211[1], 99212[1], 99213[1], 99214[1], 99215[1], 99217[1], 99218[1], 99219[1], 99220[1], 99221[1], 99222[1], 99223[1], 99231[1], 99232[1], 99233[1], 99234[1], 99235[1], 99236[1], 99238[1], 99239[1], 99241[1], 99242[1], 99243[1], 99244[1], 99245[1], 99251[1], 99252[1], 99253[1], 99254[1], 99255[1], 99291[1], 99292[1], 99304[1], 99305[1], 99306[1], 99307[1], 99308[1], 99309[1], 99310[1], 99315[1], 99316[1], 99334[1], 99335[1], 99336[1], 99337[1], 99347[1], 99348[1], 99349[1], 99350[1], 99374[1], 99375[1], 99377[1], 99378[1], 99446[0], 99447[0], 99448[0], 99449[0], 99451[0], 99452[0], 99495[0], 99496[0], G0463[1], G0471[0]
53446	0213T[0], 0216T[0], 0549T[0], 0596T[1], 0597T[1], 0708T[1], 0709T[1], 11000[1], 11001[1], 11004[1], 11005[1], 11006[1], 11042[1], 11043[1], 11044[1], 11045[1], 11046[1], 11047[1], 12001[1], 12002[1], 12004[1], 12005[1], 12006[1], 12007[1], 12011[1], 12013[1], 12014[1], 12015[1], 12016[1], 12017[1], 12018[1], 12020[1], 12021[1], 12031[1], 12032[1], 12034[1], 12035[1], 12036[1], 12037[1], 12041[1], 12042[1], 12044[1], 12045[1], 12046[1], 12047[1], 12051[1], 12052[1], 12053[1], 12054[1], 12055[1], 12056[1], 12057[1], 13100[1], 13101[1], 13102[1], 13120[1], 13121[1], 13122[1], 13131[1], 13132[1], 13133[1], 13151[1], 13152[1], 13153[1], 36000[1], 36400[1], 36405[1], 36406[1], 36410[1], 36420[1], 36425[1], 36430[1], 36440[1], 36591[0], 36592[0], 36600[1], 36640[1], 43752[1], 51701[0], 51702[0], 51703[1], 52000[1], 53000[0], 53010[0], 53020[0], 53025[0], 53080[1], 53445[0], 53451[0], 53452[0], 62320[0], 62321[0], 62322[0], 62323[0], 62324[0], 62325[0], 62326[0], 62327[0], 64400[0], 64405[0], 64408[0], 64415[0], 64416[0], 64417[0], 64418[0], 64420[0], 64421[0], 64425[0], 64430[0], 64435[0], 64445[0], 64446[0], 64447[0], 64448[0], 64449[0], 64450[0], 64451[0], 64454[0], 64461[0], 64462[0], 64463[0], 64479[0], 64480[0], 64483[0], 64484[0], 64486[0], 64487[0], 64488[0], 64489[0], 64490[0], 64491[0], 64492[0], 64493[0], 64494[0], 64495[0], 64505[0], 64510[0], 64517[0], 64520[0], 64530[0], 69990[0], 92012[1], 92014[1], 93000[1], 93005[1], 93010[1], 93040[1], 93041[1], 93042[1], 93318[1], 93355[1], 94002[1], 94200[1], 94680[1], 94681[1], 94690[1], 95812[1], 95813[1], 95816[1], 95819[1], 95822[1], 95829[1], 95955[1], 96360[1], 96361[1], 96365[1], 96366[1], 96367[1], 96368[1], 96372[1], 96374[1], 96375[1], 96376[1], 96377[1], 96523[0], 97597[1], 97598[1], 97602[1], 99155[0], 99156[0], 99157[0], 99211[1], 99212[1], 99213[1], 99214[1], 99215[1], 99217[1], 99218[1], 99219[1], 99220[1], 99221[1], 99222[1], 99223[1], 99231[1], 99232[1], 99233[1], 99234[1], 99235[1], 99236[1], 99238[1], 99239[1], 99241[1], 99242[1], 99243[1], 99244[1], 99245[1], 99251[1], 99252[1], 99253[1], 99254[1], 99255[1], 99291[1], 99292[1], 99304[1], 99305[1], 99306[1], 99307[1], 99308[1], 99309[1], 99310[1], 99315[1], 99316[1], 99334[1], 99335[1], 99336[1], 99337[1], 99347[1], 99348[1], 99349[1], 99350[1], 99374[1], 99375[1], 99377[1], 99378[1], 99446[0], 99447[0], 99448[0], 99449[0], 99451[0], 99452[0], 99495[0], 99496[0], G0463[1], G0471[0]
53447	0213T[0], 0216T[0], 0549T[0], 0596T[1], 0597T[1], 0708T[1], 0709T[1], 11000[1], 11001[1], 11004[1], 11005[1], 11006[1], 11042[1], 11043[1], 11044[1], 11045[1], 11046[1], 11047[1], 12001[1], 12002[1], 12004[1], 12005[1], 12006[1], 12007[1], 12011[1], 12013[1], 12014[1], 12015[1], 12016[1], 12017[1], 12018[1], 12020[1], 12021[1], 12031[1], 12032[1], 12034[1], 12035[1], 12036[1], 12037[1], 12041[1], 12042[1], 12044[1], 12045[1], 12046[1], 12047[1], 12051[1], 12052[1], 12053[1], 12054[1], 12055[1], 12056[1], 12057[1], 13100[1], 13101[1], 13102[1], 13120[1], 13121[1], 13122[1], 13131[1], 13132[1], 13133[1], 13151[1], 13152[1], 13153[1], 36000[1], 36400[1], 36405[1], 36406[1], 36410[1], 36420[1], 36425[1], 36430[1], 36440[1], 36591[0], 36592[0], 36600[1], 36640[1], 43752[1], 51701[0], 51702[0], 51703[1], 52000[1], 52301[1], 53000[0], 53010[0], 53020[0], 53025[0], 53080[0], 53440[0], 53444[0], 53445[0], 53446[0], 53448[0], 53449[0], 53451[0], 53452[0], 53453[0], 62320[0], 62321[0], 62322[0], 62323[0], 62324[0], 62325[0], 62326[0], 62327[0], 64400[0], 64405[0], 64408[0], 64415[0], 64416[0], 64417[0], 64418[0], 64420[0], 64421[0], 64425[0], 64430[0], 64435[0], 64445[0], 64446[0], 64447[0], 64448[0], 64449[0], 64450[0], 64451[0], 64454[0], 64461[0], 64462[0], 64463[0], 64479[0], 64480[0], 64483[0], 64484[0], 64486[0], 64487[0], 64488[0], 64489[0], 64490[0], 64491[0], 64492[0], 64493[0], 64494[0], 64495[0], 64505[0], 64510[0], 64517[0], 64520[0], 64530[0], 69990[0], 92012[1], 92014[1], 93000[1], 93005[1], 93010[1], 93040[1], 93041[1], 93042[1], 93318[1], 93355[1], 94002[1], 94200[1], 94680[1], 94681[1], 94690[1], 95812[1], 95813[1], 95816[1], 95819[1], 95822[1], 95829[1], 95955[1], 96360[1], 96361[1], 96365[1], 96366[1], 96367[1], 96368[1], 96372[1], 96374[1], 96375[1], 96376[1], 96377[1], 96523[0], 97597[1], 97598[1], 97602[1], 99155[0], 99156[0], 99157[0], 99211[1], 99212[1], 99213[1], 99214[1], 99215[1], 99217[1], 99218[1], 99219[1], 99220[1], 99221[1], 99222[1], 99223[1], 99231[1], 99232[1], 99233[1], 99234[1], 99235[1], 99236[1], 99238[1], 99239[1], 99241[1], 99242[1], 99243[1], 99244[1], 99245[1], 99251[1], 99252[1], 99253[1], 99254[1], 99255[1], 99291[1], 99292[1], 99304[1], 99305[1], 99306[1], 99307[1], 99308[1], 99309[1], 99310[1], 99315[1], 99316[1], 99334[1], 99335[1], 99336[1], 99337[1], 99347[1], 99348[1], 99349[1], 99350[1], 99374[1], 99375[1], 99377[1], 99378[1], 99446[0], 99447[0], 99448[0], 99449[0], 99451[0], 99452[0], 99495[0], 99496[0], G0463[1], G0471[0]
53448	0213T[0], 0216T[0], 0549T[0], 0596T[1], 0597T[1], 0708T[1], 0709T[1], 11000[1], 11001[1], 11004[1], 11005[1], 11006[1], 11042[1], 11043[1], 11044[1], 11045[1], 11046[1], 11047[1], 12001[1], 12002[1], 12004[1], 12005[1], 12006[1], 12007[1], 12011[1], 12013[1], 12014[1], 12015[1], 12016[1], 12017[1], 12018[1], 12020[1], 12021[1], 12031[1], 12032[1], 12034[1], 12035[1], 12036[1], 12037[1], 12041[1], 12042[1], 12044[1], 12045[1], 12046[1], 12047[1], 12051[1], 12052[1], 12053[1], 12054[1], 12055[1], 12056[1], 12057[1], 13100[1], 13101[1], 13102[1], 13120[1], 13121[1], 13122[1], 13131[1], 13132[1], 13133[1], 13151[1], 13152[1], 13153[1], 36000[1], 36400[1], 36405[1], 36406[1], 36410[1], 36420[1], 36425[1], 36430[1], 36440[1], 36591[0], 36592[0], 36600[1], 36640[1], 43752[1], 51701[0], 51702[0], 51703[1], 52000[1], 53000[0], 53010[0], 53020[0], 53025[0], 53080[0], 53440[0], 53444[0], 53445[0], 53446[0], 53449[0], 53451[0], 53452[0], 53453[0], 62320[0], 62321[0], 62322[0], 62323[0], 62324[0], 62325[0], 62326[0], 62327[0], 64400[0], 64405[0], 64408[0], 64415[0], 64416[0], 64417[0], 64418[0], 64420[0], 64421[0], 64425[0], 64430[0], 64435[0], 64445[0], 64446[0], 64447[0], 64448[0], 64449[0], 64450[0], 64451[0], 64454[0], 64461[0], 64462[0], 64463[0], 64479[0], 64480[0], 64483[0], 64484[0], 64486[0], 64487[0], 64488[0], 64489[0], 64490[0], 64491[0], 64492[0], 64493[0], 64494[0], 64495[0], 64505[0], 64510[0], 64517[0], 64520[0], 64530[0], 69990[0], 92012[1], 92014[1], 93000[1], 93005[1], 93010[1], 93040[1], 93041[1], 93042[1], 93318[1], 93355[1], 94002[1], 94200[1], 94680[1], 94681[1], 94690[1], 95812[1], 95813[1], 95816[1], 95819[1], 95822[1], 95829[1], 95955[1], 96360[1], 96361[1], 96365[1], 96366[1], 96367[1], 96368[1], 96372[1], 96374[1], 96375[1], 96376[1], 96377[1], 96523[0], 97597[1], 97598[1], 97602[1], 99155[0], 99156[0], 99157[0], 99211[1], 99212[1], 99213[1], 99214[1], 99215[1], 99217[1], 99218[1], 99219[1], 99220[1], 99221[1], 99222[1], 99223[1], 99231[1], 99232[1], 99233[1], 99234[1], 99235[1], 99236[1], 99238[1], 99239[1], 99241[1], 99242[1], 99243[1], 99244[1], 99245[1], 99251[1], 99252[1], 99253[1], 99254[1], 99255[1], 99291[1], 99292[1], 99304[1], 99305[1], 99306[1], 99307[1], 99308[1], 99309[1], 99310[1], 99315[1], 99316[1], 99334[1], 99335[1], 99336[1],

0 = Modifier usage not allowed or inappropriate 1 = Modifier usage allowed

Code 1	Code 2
	99337[1], 99347[1], 99348[1], 99349[1], 99350[1], 99374[1], 99375[1], 99377[1], 99378[1], 99446[0], 99447[0], 99448[0], 99449[0], 99451[0], 99452[0], 99495[0], 99496[0], G0463[1], G0471[0]
53449	0213T[0], 0216T[0], 0596T[1], 0597T[1], 0708T[1], 0709T[1], 12001[1], 12002[1], 12004[1], 12005[1], 12006[1], 12007[1], 12011[1], 12013[1], 12014[1], 12015[1], 12016[1], 12017[1], 12018[1], 12020[1], 12021[1], 12031[1], 12032[1], 12034[1], 12035[1], 12036[1], 12037[1], 12041[1], 12042[1], 12044[1], 12045[1], 12046[1], 12047[1], 12051[1], 12052[1], 12053[1], 12054[1], 12055[1], 12056[1], 12057[1], 13100[1], 13101[1], 13102[1], 13120[1], 13121[1], 13122[1], 13131[1], 13132[1], 13133[1], 13151[1], 13152[1], 13153[1], 36000[1], 36400[1], 36405[1], 36406[1], 36410[1], 36420[1], 36425[1], 36430[1], 36440[1], 36591[0], 36592[0], 36600[1], 36640[1], 43752[1], 51701[0], 51702[0], 51703[1], 52000[1], 52301[1], 53000[0], 53010[0], 53020[0], 53025[0], 53080[0], 62320[0], 62321[0], 62322[0], 62323[0], 62324[0], 62325[0], 62326[0], 62327[0], 64400[0], 64405[0], 64408[0], 64415[0], 64416[0], 64417[0], 64418[0], 64420[0], 64421[0], 64425[0], 64430[0], 64435[0], 64445[0], 64446[0], 64447[0], 64448[0], 64449[0], 64450[0], 64451[0], 64454[0], 64461[0], 64462[0], 64463[0], 64479[0], 64480[0], 64483[0], 64484[0], 64486[0], 64487[0], 64488[0], 64489[0], 64490[0], 64491[0], 64492[0], 64493[0], 64494[0], 64495[0], 64505[0], 64510[0], 64517[0], 64520[0], 64530[0], 69990[0], 92012[1], 92014[1], 93000[1], 93005[1], 93010[1], 93040[1], 93041[1], 93042[1], 93318[1], 93355[1], 94002[1], 94200[1], 94680[1], 94681[1], 94690[1], 95812[1], 95813[1], 95816[1], 95819[1], 95822[1], 95829[1], 95955[1], 96360[1], 96361[1], 96365[1], 96366[1], 96367[1], 96368[1], 96372[1], 96374[1], 96375[1], 96376[1], 96377[1], 96523[0], 99155[0], 99156[0], 99157[0], 99211[1], 99212[1], 99213[1], 99214[1], 99215[1], 99217[1], 99218[1], 99219[1], 99220[1], 99221[1], 99222[1], 99223[1], 99231[1], 99232[1], 99233[1], 99234[1], 99235[1], 99236[1], 99238[1], 99239[1], 99241[1], 99242[1], 99243[1], 99244[1], 99245[1], 99251[1], 99252[1], 99253[1], 99254[1], 99255[1], 99291[1], 99292[1], 99304[1], 99305[1], 99306[1], 99307[1], 99308[1], 99309[1], 99310[1], 99315[1], 99316[1], 99334[1], 99335[1], 99336[1], 99337[1], 99347[1], 99348[1], 99349[1], 99350[1], 99374[1], 99375[1], 99377[1], 99378[1], 99446[0], 99447[0], 99448[0], 99449[0], 99451[0], 99452[0], 99495[0], 99496[0], G0463[1], G0471[0]
53450	0213T[0], 0216T[0], 0596T[1], 0597T[1], 0708T[1], 0709T[1], 11000[1], 11001[1], 11004[1], 11005[1], 11006[1], 11042[1], 11043[1], 11044[1], 11045[1], 11046[1], 11047[1], 12001[1], 12002[1], 12004[1], 12005[1], 12006[1], 12007[1], 12011[1], 12013[1], 12014[1], 12015[1], 12016[1], 12017[1], 12018[1], 12020[1], 12021[1], 12031[1], 12032[1], 12034[1], 12035[1], 12036[1], 12037[1], 12041[1], 12042[1], 12044[1], 12045[1], 12046[1], 12047[1], 12051[1], 12052[1], 12053[1], 12054[1], 12055[1], 12056[1], 12057[1], 13100[1], 13101[1], 13102[1], 13120[1], 13121[1], 13122[1], 13131[1], 13132[1], 13133[1], 13151[1], 13152[1], 13153[1], 36000[1], 36400[1], 36405[1], 36406[1], 36410[1], 36420[1], 36425[1], 36430[1], 36440[1], 36591[0], 36592[0], 36600[1], 36640[1], 43752[1], 51701[0], 51702[0], 51703[1], 52000[0], 52301[1], 53000[0], 53010[0], 53020[0], 53025[0], 53080[0], 53502[1], 53505[1], 53510[1], 53515[1], 53520[1], 62320[0], 62321[0], 62322[0], 62323[0], 62324[0], 62325[0], 62326[0], 62327[0], 64400[0], 64405[0], 64408[0], 64415[0], 64416[0], 64417[0], 64418[0], 64420[0], 64421[0], 64425[0], 64430[0], 64435[0], 64445[0], 64446[0], 64447[0], 64448[0], 64449[0], 64450[0], 64451[0], 64454[0], 64461[0], 64462[0], 64463[0], 64479[0], 64480[0], 64483[0], 64484[0], 64486[0], 64487[0], 64488[0], 64489[0], 64490[0], 64491[0], 64492[0], 64493[0], 64494[0], 64495[0], 64505[0], 64510[0], 64517[0], 64520[0], 64530[0], 69990[0], 92012[1], 92014[1], 93000[1], 93005[1], 93010[1], 93040[1], 93041[1], 93042[1], 93318[1], 93355[1], 94002[1], 94200[1], 94680[1], 94681[1], 94690[1], 95812[1], 95813[1], 95816[1], 95819[1], 95822[1], 95829[1], 95955[1], 96360[1], 96361[1], 96365[1], 96366[1], 96367[1], 96368[1], 96372[1], 96374[1], 96375[1], 96376[1], 96377[1], 96523[0], 97597[1], 97598[1], 97602[1], 99155[0], 99156[0], 99157[0], 99211[1], 99212[1], 99213[1], 99214[1], 99215[1], 99217[1], 99218[1], 99219[1], 99220[1], 99221[1], 99222[1], 99223[1], 99231[1], 99232[1], 99233[1], 99234[1], 99235[1], 99236[1], 99238[1], 99239[1], 99241[1], 99242[1], 99243[1], 99244[1], 99245[1], 99251[1], 99252[1], 99253[1], 99254[1], 99255[1], 99291[1], 99292[1], 99304[1], 99305[1], 99306[1], 99307[1], 99308[1], 99309[1], 99310[1], 99315[1], 99316[1], 99334[1], 99335[1], 99336[1], 99337[1], 99347[1], 99348[1], 99349[1], 99350[1], 99374[1], 99375[1], 99377[1], 99378[1], 99446[0], 99447[0], 99448[0], 99449[0], 99451[0], 99452[0], 99495[0], 99496[0], G0463[1], G0471[0]
53451	0213T[0], 0216T[0], 0549T[0], 11000[1], 11001[1], 11004[1], 11005[1], 11006[1], 11042[1], 11043[1], 11044[1], 11045[1], 11046[1], 11047[1], 12001[1], 12002[1], 12004[1], 12005[1], 12006[1], 12007[1], 12011[1], 12013[1], 12014[1], 12015[1], 12016[1], 12017[1], 12018[1], 12020[1], 12021[1], 12031[1], 12032[1], 12034[1], 12035[1], 12036[1], 12037[1], 12041[1], 12042[1], 12044[1], 12045[1], 12046[1], 12047[1], 12051[1], 12052[1], 12053[1], 12054[1], 12055[1], 12056[1], 12057[1], 13100[1], 13101[1], 13102[1], 13120[1], 13121[1], 13122[1], 13131[1], 13132[1], 13133[1], 13151[1], 13152[1], 13153[1], 36000[1], 36400[1], 36405[1], 36406[1], 36410[1], 36420[1], 36425[1], 36430[1], 36440[1], 36591[0], 36592[0], 36600[1], 36640[1], 43752[1], 51701[1], 51702[1], 51703[1], 51990[1], 51992[1], 52000[0], 52301[1], 53000[0], 53010[0], 53020[0], 53025[0], 53080[1], 53444[0], 53452[0], 53453[0], 53454[0], 62320[0], 62321[0], 62322[0], 62323[0], 62324[0], 62325[0], 62326[0], 62327[0], 64400[0], 64405[0], 64408[0], 64415[0], 64416[0], 64417[0], 64418[0], 64420[0], 64421[0], 64425[0], 64430[0], 64435[0], 64445[0], 64446[0], 64447[0], 64448[0], 64449[0], 64450[0], 64461[0], 64462[0], 64463[0], 64479[0], 64480[0], 64483[0], 64484[0], 64486[0], 64487[0], 64488[0], 64489[0], 64490[0], 64491[0], 64492[0], 64493[0], 64494[0], 64495[0], 64505[0], 64510[0], 64517[0], 64520[0], 64530[0], 69990[0], 76000[1], 76380[1], 76942[1], 76998[1], 77002[1], 77012[1], 77021[1], 92012[1], 92014[1], 93000[1], 93005[1], 93010[1], 93040[1], 93041[1], 93042[1], 93318[1], 93355[1], 94002[1], 94200[1], 94680[1], 94681[1], 94690[1], 95812[1], 95813[1], 95816[1], 95819[1], 95822[1], 95829[1], 95955[1], 96360[1], 96361[1], 96365[1], 96366[1], 96367[1], 96368[1], 96372[1], 96374[1], 96375[1], 96376[1], 96377[1], 96523[0], 97597[1], 97598[1], 97602[1], 99155[0], 99156[0], 99157[0], 99211[1], 99212[1], 99213[1], 99214[1], 99215[1], 99217[1], 99218[1], 99219[1], 99220[1], 99221[1], 99222[1], 99223[1], 99231[1], 99232[1], 99233[1], 99234[1], 99235[1], 99236[1], 99238[1], 99239[1], 99241[1], 99242[1], 99243[1], 99244[1], 99245[1], 99251[1], 99252[1], 99253[1], 99254[1], 99255[1], 99291[1], 99292[1], 99304[1], 99305[1], 99306[1], 99307[1], 99308[1], 99309[1], 99310[1], 99315[1], 99316[1], 99334[1], 99335[1], 99336[1], 99337[1], 99347[1], 99348[1], 99349[1], 99350[1], 99374[1], 99375[1], 99377[1], 99378[1], 99446[0], 99447[0], 99448[0], 99449[0], 99451[0], 99452[0], 99495[0], 99496[0], G0463[1], G0471[0]
53452	0213T[0], 0216T[0], 0596T[1], 0597T[1], 11000[1], 11001[1], 11004[1], 11005[1], 11006[1], 11042[1], 11043[1], 11044[1], 11045[1], 11046[1], 11047[1], 12001[1], 12002[1], 12004[1], 12005[1], 12006[1], 12007[1], 12011[1], 12013[1], 12014[1], 12015[1], 12016[1], 12017[1], 12018[1], 12020[1], 12021[1], 12031[1], 12032[1], 12034[1], 12035[1], 12036[1], 12037[1], 12041[1], 12042[1], 12044[1], 12045[1], 12046[1], 12047[1], 12051[1], 12052[1], 12053[1], 12054[1], 12055[1], 12056[1], 12057[1], 13100[1], 13101[1], 13102[1], 13120[1], 13121[1], 13122[1], 13131[1], 13132[1], 13133[1], 13151[1], 13152[1], 13153[1], 36000[1], 36400[1], 36405[1], 36406[1], 36410[1], 36420[1], 36425[1], 36430[1], 36440[1], 36591[0], 36592[0], 36600[1], 36640[1], 43752[1], 51701[1], 51702[1], 51703[1], 51990[1], 51992[1], 52000[1], 52301[1], 53000[0], 53010[0], 53020[0], 53025[0], 53080[1], 53444[0], 53453[0], 53454[0], 62320[0], 62321[0], 62322[0], 62323[0], 62324[0], 62325[0], 62326[0], 62327[0], 64400[0], 64405[0], 64408[0], 64415[0], 64416[0], 64417[0], 64418[0], 64420[0], 64421[0], 64425[0], 64430[0], 64435[0], 64445[0], 64446[0], 64447[0], 64448[0], 64449[0], 64450[0], 64451[0], 64454[0], 64461[0], 64462[0], 64463[0], 64479[0], 64480[0], 64483[0], 64484[0], 64486[0], 64487[0], 64488[0], 64489[0], 64490[0], 64491[0], 64492[0], 64493[0], 64494[0], 64495[0], 64505[0], 64510[0], 64517[0], 64520[0], 64530[0], 69990[0], 76000[1], 76380[1], 76942[1], 76998[1], 77002[1], 77012[1], 77021[1], 92012[1], 92014[1], 93000[1], 93005[1], 93010[1], 93040[1], 93041[1], 93042[1], 93318[1], 93355[1], 94002[1], 94200[1], 94680[1], 94681[1], 94690[1], 95812[1], 95813[1], 95816[1], 95819[1], 95822[1], 95829[1], 95955[1], 96360[1], 96361[1], 96365[1], 96366[1], 96367[1], 96368[1], 96372[1], 96374[1], 96375[1], 96376[1], 96377[1], 96523[0], 97597[1], 97598[1], 97602[1], 99155[0], 99156[0], 99157[0], 99211[1], 99212[1], 99213[1], 99214[1], 99215[1], 99217[1], 99218[1], 99219[1], 99220[1], 99221[1], 99222[1], 99223[1], 99231[1], 99232[1], 99233[1], 99234[1], 99235[1], 99236[1], 99238[1], 99239[1], 99241[1], 99242[1], 99243[1], 99244[1], 99245[1], 99251[1], 99252[1], 99253[1], 99254[1], 99255[1], 99291[1], 99292[1], 99304[1], 99305[1], 99306[1], 99307[1], 99308[1], 99309[1], 99310[1], 99315[1], 99316[1], 99334[1], 99335[1], 99336[1], 99337[1], 99347[1], 99348[1], 99349[1], 99350[1], 99374[1], 99375[1], 99377[1], 99378[1], 99446[0], 99447[0], 99448[0], 99449[0], 99451[0], 99452[0], 99495[0], 99496[0], G0463[1], G0471[0]
53453	0213T[0], 0216T[0], 0596T[1], 0597T[1], 11000[1], 11001[1], 11004[1], 11005[1], 11006[1], 11042[1], 11043[1], 11044[1], 11045[1], 11046[1], 11047[1], 12001[1], 12002[1], 12004[1], 12005[1], 12006[1], 12007[1], 12011[1], 12013[1], 12014[1], 12015[1], 12016[1], 12017[1], 12018[1], 12020[1], 12021[1], 12031[1], 12032[1], 12034[1], 12035[1], 12036[1], 12037[1], 12041[1], 12042[1], 12044[1], 12045[1], 12046[1], 12047[1], 12051[1], 12052[1], 12053[1], 12054[1], 12055[1], 12056[1], 12057[1], 13100[1], 13101[1], 13102[1], 13120[1], 13121[1], 13122[1], 13131[1], 13132[1], 13133[1], 13151[1], 13152[1], 13153[1], 36000[1], 36400[1], 36405[1], 36406[1], 36410[1], 36420[1], 36425[1], 36430[1], 36440[1], 36591[0], 36592[0], 36600[1], 36640[1], 43752[1], 51701[1], 51702[1], 51703[1], 52000[1], 53000[0], 53010[0], 53020[0], 53025[0], 53080[1], 53445[0], 53454[0], 62320[0], 62321[0], 62322[0], 62323[0], 62324[0], 62325[0], 62326[0], 62327[0], 64400[0], 64405[0], 64408[0], 64415[0], 64416[0], 64417[0], 64418[0], 64420[0], 64421[0], 64425[0], 64430[0], 64435[0], 64445[0], 64446[0], 64447[0], 64448[0], 64449[0], 64450[0], 64461[0], 64462[0], 64463[0], 64479[0], 64480[0], 64483[0], 64484[0], 64486[0], 64487[0], 64488[0], 64489[0], 64490[0], 64491[0], 64492[0], 64493[0], 64494[0], 64495[0], 64505[0], 64510[0], 64517[0], 64520[0], 64530[0], 69990[0], 92012[1], 92014[1], 93000[1], 93005[1], 93010[1], 93040[1], 93041[1], 93042[1], 93318[1], 93355[1], 94002[1], 94200[1], 94680[1], 94681[1], 94690[1], 95812[1], 95813[1], 95816[1], 95819[1], 95822[1], 95829[1], 95955[1], 96360[1], 96361[1], 96365[1], 96366[1], 96367[1], 96368[1], 96372[1], 96374[1], 96375[1], 96376[1], 96377[1], 96523[0], 97597[1], 97598[1], 97602[1], 99155[0], 99156[0], 99157[0], 99211[1], 99212[1], 99213[1], 99214[1], 99215[1], 99217[1], 99218[1], 99219[1], 99220[1], 99221[1], 99222[1], 99223[1], 99231[1], 99232[1], 99233[1], 99234[1], 99235[1], 99236[1], 99238[1], 99239[1], 99241[1], 99242[1], 99243[1], 99244[1], 99245[1], 99251[1], 99252[1], 99253[1], 99254[1], 99255[1], 99291[1], 99292[1], 99304[1], 99305[1], 99306[1], 99307[1], 99308[1], 99309[1], 99310[1], 99315[1], 99316[1], 99334[1], 99335[1], 99336[1], 99337[1], 99347[1], 99348[1], 99349[1], 99350[1], 99374[1], 99375[1], 99377[1], 99378[1], 99446[0], 99447[0], 99448[0], 99449[0], 99451[0], 99452[0], 99495[0], 99496[0], G0463[1], G0471[0]
53454	0213T[0], 0216T[0], 11000[1], 11001[1], 11004[1], 11005[1], 11006[1], 11042[1], 11043[1], 11044[1], 11045[1], 11046[1], 11047[1], 12001[1], 12002[1], 12004[1], 12005[1], 12006[1], 12007[1], 12011[1], 12013[1], 12014[1], 12015[1], 12016[1], 12017[1], 12018[1], 12020[1], 12021[1], 12031[1], 12032[1], 12034[1], 12035[1], 12036[1], 12037[1], 12041[1], 12042[1], 12044[1], 12045[1], 12046[1], 12047[1], 12051[1], 12052[1], 12053[1], 12054[1], 12055[1], 12056[1], 12057[1], 13100[1], 13101[1], 13102[1],

0 = Modifier usage not allowed or inappropriate 1 = Modifier usage allowed

Code 1	Code 2
	13120[1], 13121[1], 13122[1], 13131[1], 13132[1], 13133[1], 13151[1], 13152[1], 13153[1], 36000[1], 36400[1], 36405[1], 36406[1], 36410[1], 36420[1], 36425[1], 36430[1], 36440[1], 36591[0], 36592[0], 36600[1], 36640[1], 43752[1], 51701[1], 51702[1], 51703[1], 62320[0], 62321[0], 62322[0], 62323[0], 62324[0], 62325[0], 62326[0], 62327[0], 64400[0], 64405[0], 64408[0], 64415[0], 64416[0], 64417[0], 64418[0], 64420[0], 64421[0], 64425[0], 64430[0], 64435[0], 64445[0], 64446[0], 64447[0], 64448[0], 64449[0], 64450[0], 64461[0], 64462[0], 64463[0], 64479[0], 64480[0], 64483[0], 64484[0], 64486[0], 64487[0], 64488[0], 64489[0], 64490[0], 64491[0], 64492[0], 64493[0], 64494[0], 64495[0], 64505[0], 64510[0], 64517[0], 64520[0], 64530[0], 69990[0], 92012[1], 92014[1], 93000[1], 93005[1], 93010[1], 93040[1], 93041[1], 93042[1], 93318[1], 94002[1], 94200[1], 94680[1], 94681[1], 94690[1], 95812[1], 95813[1], 95816[1], 95819[1], 95822[1], 95829[1], 95955[1], 96360[1], 96361[1], 96365[1], 96366[1], 96367[1], 96368[1], 96372[1], 96374[1], 96375[1], 96376[1], 96377[1], 96523[0], 97597[1], 97598[1], 97602[1], 99155[0], 99156[0], 99157[0], 99211[1], 99212[1], 99213[1], 99214[1], 99215[1], 99217[1], 99218[1], 99219[1], 99220[1], 99221[1], 99222[1], 99223[1], 99231[1], 99232[1], 99233[1], 99234[1], 99235[1], 99236[1], 99238[1], 99239[1], 99241[1], 99242[1], 99243[1], 99244[1], 99245[1], 99251[1], 99252[1], 99253[1], 99254[1], 99255[1], 99291[1], 99292[1], 99315[1], 99316[1], 99347[1], 99348[1], 99349[1], 99350[1], 99374[1], 99375[1], 99377[1], 99378[1]
53460	0213T[0], 0216T[0], 0596T[1], 0597T[1], 0708T[1], 0709T[1], 11000[1], 11001[1], 11004[1], 11005[1], 11006[1], 11042[1], 11043[1], 11044[1], 11045[1], 11046[1], 11047[1], 12001[1], 12002[1], 12004[1], 12005[1], 12006[1], 12007[1], 12011[1], 12013[1], 12014[1], 12015[1], 12016[1], 12017[1], 12018[1], 12020[1], 12021[1], 12031[1], 12032[1], 12034[1], 12035[1], 12036[1], 12037[1], 12041[1], 12042[1], 12044[1], 12045[1], 12046[1], 12047[1], 12051[1], 12052[1], 12053[1], 12054[1], 12055[1], 12056[1], 12057[1], 13100[1], 13101[1], 13102[1], 13120[1], 13121[1], 13122[1], 13131[1], 13132[1], 13133[1], 13151[1], 13152[1], 13153[1], 36000[1], 36400[1], 36405[1], 36406[1], 36410[1], 36420[1], 36425[1], 36430[1], 36440[1], 36591[0], 36592[0], 36600[1], 36640[1], 43752[1], 51701[0], 51702[0], 51703[1], 52000[0], 52301[1], 53000[0], 53010[0], 53020[0], 53025[0], 53080[1], 53502[1], 53505[1], 53510[1], 53515[1], 53520[1], 62320[0], 62321[0], 62322[0], 62323[0], 62324[0], 62325[0], 62326[0], 62327[0], 64400[0], 64405[0], 64408[0], 64415[0], 64416[0], 64417[0], 64418[0], 64420[0], 64421[0], 64425[0], 64430[0], 64435[0], 64445[0], 64446[0], 64447[0], 64448[0], 64449[0], 64450[0], 64451[0], 64454[0], 64461[0], 64462[0], 64463[0], 64479[0], 64480[0], 64483[0], 64484[0], 64486[0], 64487[0], 64488[0], 64489[0], 64490[0], 64491[0], 64492[0], 64493[0], 64494[0], 64495[0], 64505[0], 64510[0], 64517[0], 64520[0], 64530[0], 69990[0], 92012[1], 92014[1], 93000[1], 93005[1], 93010[1], 93040[1], 93041[1], 93042[1], 93318[1], 93355[1], 94002[1], 94200[1], 94680[1], 94681[1], 94690[1], 95812[1], 95813[1], 95816[1], 95819[1], 95822[1], 95829[1], 95955[1], 96360[1], 96361[1], 96365[1], 96366[1], 96367[1], 96368[1], 96372[1], 96374[1], 96375[1], 96376[1], 96377[1], 96523[0], 97597[1], 97598[1], 97602[1], 99155[0], 99156[0], 99157[0], 99211[1], 99212[1], 99213[1], 99214[1], 99215[1], 99217[1], 99218[1], 99219[1], 99220[1], 99221[1], 99222[1], 99223[1], 99231[1], 99232[1], 99233[1], 99234[1], 99235[1], 99236[1], 99238[1], 99239[1], 99241[1], 99242[1], 99243[1], 99244[1], 99245[1], 99251[1], 99252[1], 99253[1], 99254[1], 99255[1], 99291[1], 99292[1], 99304[1], 99305[1], 99306[1], 99307[1], 99308[1], 99309[1], 99310[1], 99315[1], 99316[1], 99334[1], 99335[1], 99336[1], 99337[1], 99347[1], 99348[1], 99349[1], 99350[1], 99374[1], 99375[1], 99377[1], 99378[1], 99446[0], 99447[0], 99448[0], 99449[0], 99451[0], 99452[0], 99495[0], 99496[0], G0463[1], G0471[0]
53500	00910[0], 0213T[0], 0216T[0], 0596T[1], 0597T[1], 0708T[1], 0709T[1], 12001[1], 12002[1], 12004[1], 12005[1], 12006[1], 12007[1], 12011[1], 12013[1], 12014[1], 12015[1], 12016[1], 12017[1], 12018[1], 12020[1], 12021[1], 12031[1], 12032[1], 12034[1], 12035[1], 12036[1], 12037[1], 12041[1], 12042[1], 12044[1], 12045[1], 12046[1], 12047[1], 12051[1], 12052[1], 12053[1], 12054[1], 12055[1], 12056[1], 12057[1], 13100[1], 13101[1], 13102[1], 13120[1], 13121[1], 13122[1], 13131[1], 13132[1], 13133[1], 13151[1], 13152[1], 13153[1], 36000[1], 36400[1], 36405[1], 36406[1], 36410[1], 36420[1], 36425[1], 36430[1], 36440[1], 36591[0], 36592[0], 36600[1], 36640[1], 43752[1], 51700[1], 51701[1], 51702[1], 51703[1], 52000[0], 52310[0], 52315[0], 53000[0], 53010[0], 53020[0], 53025[0], 53080[1], 53502[0], 53505[1], 53510[1], 53520[1], 53600[1], 53601[1], 53605[1], 53620[1], 53621[1], 53660[1], 53661[1], 53665[1], 62320[0], 62321[0], 62322[0], 62323[0], 62324[0], 62325[0], 62326[0], 62327[0], 64400[0], 64405[0], 64408[0], 64415[0], 64416[0], 64417[0], 64418[0], 64420[0], 64421[0], 64425[0], 64430[0], 64435[0], 64445[0], 64446[0], 64447[0], 64448[0], 64449[0], 64450[0], 64451[0], 64454[0], 64461[0], 64462[0], 64463[0], 64479[0], 64480[0], 64483[0], 64484[0], 64486[0], 64487[0], 64488[0], 64489[0], 64490[0], 64491[0], 64492[0], 64493[0], 64494[0], 64495[0], 64505[0], 64510[0], 64517[0], 64520[0], 64530[0], 69990[0], 92012[1], 92014[1], 93000[1], 93005[1], 93010[1], 93040[1], 93041[1], 93042[1], 93318[1], 93355[1], 94002[1], 94200[1], 94680[1], 94681[1], 94690[1], 95812[1], 95813[1], 95816[1], 95819[1], 95822[1], 95829[1], 95955[1], 96360[1], 96361[1], 96365[1], 96366[1], 96367[1], 96368[1], 96372[1], 96374[1], 96375[1], 96376[1], 96377[1], 96523[0], 99155[0], 99156[0], 99157[0], 99211[1], 99212[1], 99213[1], 99214[1], 99215[1], 99217[1], 99218[1], 99219[1], 99220[1], 99221[1], 99222[1], 99223[1], 99231[1], 99232[1], 99233[1], 99234[1], 99235[1], 99236[1], 99238[1], 99239[1], 99241[1], 99242[1], 99243[1], 99244[1], 99245[1], 99251[1], 99252[1], 99253[1], 99254[1], 99255[1], 99291[1], 99292[1], 99304[1], 99305[1], 99306[1], 99307[1], 99308[1], 99309[1], 99310[1], 99315[1], 99316[1], 99334[1], 99335[1], 99336[1], 99337[1], 99347[1], 99348[1], 99349[1], 99350[1], 99374[1], 99375[1], 99377[1], 99378[1], 99446[0], 99447[0], 99448[0], 99449[0], 99451[0], 99452[0], 99495[0], 99496[0], G0463[1], G0471[1]
53502	0213T[0], 0216T[0], 0596T[1], 0597T[1], 0708T[1], 0709T[1], 12001[1], 12002[1], 12004[1], 12005[1], 12006[1], 12007[1], 12011[1], 12013[1], 12014[1], 12015[1], 12016[1], 12017[1], 12018[1], 12020[1], 12021[1], 12031[1], 12032[1], 12034[1], 12035[1], 12036[1], 12037[1], 12041[1], 12042[1], 12044[1], 12045[1], 12046[1], 12047[1], 12051[1], 12052[1], 12053[1], 12054[1], 12055[1], 12056[1], 12057[1], 13100[1], 13101[1], 13102[1], 13120[1], 13121[1], 13122[1], 13131[1], 13132[1], 13133[1], 13151[1], 13152[1], 13153[1], 36000[1], 36400[1], 36405[1], 36406[1], 36410[1], 36420[1], 36425[1], 36430[1], 36440[1], 36591[0], 36592[0], 36600[1], 36640[1], 43752[1], 51701[0], 51702[0], 51703[1], 52000[1], 52301[1], 53000[0], 53010[0], 53020[0], 53025[0], 53080[1], 62320[0], 62321[0], 62322[0], 62323[0], 62324[0], 62325[0], 62326[0], 62327[0], 64400[0], 64405[0], 64408[0], 64415[0], 64416[0], 64417[0], 64418[0], 64420[0], 64421[0], 64425[0], 64430[0], 64435[0], 64445[0], 64446[0], 64447[0], 64448[0], 64449[0], 64450[0], 64451[0], 64454[0], 64461[0], 64462[0], 64463[0], 64479[0], 64480[0], 64483[0], 64484[0], 64486[0], 64487[0], 64488[0], 64489[0], 64490[0], 64491[0], 64492[0], 64493[0], 64494[0], 64495[0], 64505[0], 64510[0], 64517[0], 64520[0], 64530[0], 69990[0], 92012[1], 92014[1], 93000[1], 93005[1], 93010[1], 93040[1], 93041[1], 93042[1], 93318[1], 93355[1], 94002[1], 94200[1], 94680[1], 94681[1], 94690[1], 95812[1], 95813[1], 95816[1], 95819[1], 95822[1], 95829[1], 95955[1], 96360[1], 96361[1], 96365[1], 96366[1], 96367[1], 96368[1], 96372[1], 96374[1], 96375[1], 96376[1], 96377[1], 96523[0], 99155[0], 99156[0], 99157[0], 99211[1], 99212[1], 99213[1], 99214[1], 99215[1], 99217[1], 99218[1], 99219[1], 99220[1], 99221[1], 99222[1], 99223[1], 99231[1], 99232[1], 99233[1], 99234[1], 99235[1], 99236[1], 99238[1], 99239[1], 99241[1], 99242[1], 99243[1], 99244[1], 99245[1], 99251[1], 99252[1], 99253[1], 99254[1], 99255[1], 99291[1], 99292[1], 99304[1], 99305[1], 99306[1], 99307[1], 99308[1], 99309[1], 99310[1], 99315[1], 99316[1], 99334[1], 99335[1], 99336[1], 99337[1], 99347[1], 99348[1], 99349[1], 99350[1], 99374[1], 99375[1], 99377[1], 99378[1], 99446[0], 99447[0], 99448[0], 99449[0], 99451[0], 99452[0], 99495[0], 99496[0], G0463[1], G0471[0]
53505	0213T[0], 0216T[0], 0596T[1], 0597T[1], 0708T[1], 0709T[1], 12001[1], 12002[1], 12004[1], 12005[1], 12006[1], 12007[1], 12011[1], 12013[1], 12014[1], 12015[1], 12016[1], 12017[1], 12018[1], 12020[1], 12021[1], 12031[1], 12032[1], 12034[1], 12035[1], 12036[1], 12037[1], 12041[1], 12042[1], 12044[1], 12045[1], 12046[1], 12047[1], 12051[1], 12052[1], 12053[1], 12054[1], 12055[1], 12056[1], 12057[1], 13100[1], 13101[1], 13102[1], 13120[1], 13121[1], 13122[1], 13131[1], 13132[1], 13133[1], 13151[1], 13152[1], 13153[1], 36000[1], 36400[1], 36405[1], 36406[1], 36410[1], 36420[1], 36425[1], 36430[1], 36440[1], 36591[0], 36592[0], 36600[1], 36640[1], 43752[1], 51701[0], 51702[0], 51703[1], 52000[1], 52301[1], 53000[0], 53010[0], 53020[0], 53025[0], 53080[0], 53502[1], 62320[0], 62321[0], 62322[0], 62323[0], 62324[0], 62325[0], 62326[0], 62327[0], 64400[0], 64405[0], 64408[0], 64415[0], 64416[0], 64417[0], 64418[0], 64420[0], 64421[0], 64425[0], 64430[0], 64435[0], 64445[0], 64446[0], 64447[0], 64448[0], 64449[0], 64450[0], 64451[0], 64454[0], 64461[0], 64462[0], 64463[0], 64479[0], 64480[0], 64483[0], 64484[0], 64486[0], 64487[0], 64488[0], 64489[0], 64490[0], 64491[0], 64492[0], 64493[0], 64494[0], 64495[0], 64505[0], 64510[0], 64517[0], 64520[0], 64530[0], 69990[0], 92012[1], 92014[1], 93000[1], 93005[1], 93010[1], 93040[1], 93041[1], 93042[1], 93318[1], 93355[1], 94002[1], 94200[1], 94680[1], 94681[1], 94690[1], 95812[1], 95813[1], 95816[1], 95819[1], 95822[1], 95829[1], 95955[1], 96360[1], 96361[1], 96365[1], 96366[1], 96367[1], 96368[1], 96372[1], 96374[1], 96375[1], 96376[1], 96377[1], 96523[0], 99155[0], 99156[0], 99157[0], 99211[1], 99212[1], 99213[1], 99214[1], 99215[1], 99217[1], 99218[1], 99219[1], 99220[1], 99221[1], 99222[1], 99223[1], 99231[1], 99232[1], 99233[1], 99234[1], 99235[1], 99236[1], 99238[1], 99239[1], 99241[1], 99242[1], 99243[1], 99244[1], 99245[1], 99251[1], 99252[1], 99253[1], 99254[1], 99255[1], 99291[1], 99292[1], 99304[1], 99305[1], 99306[1], 99307[1], 99308[1], 99309[1], 99310[1], 99315[1], 99316[1], 99334[1], 99335[1], 99336[1], 99337[1], 99347[1], 99348[1], 99349[1], 99350[1], 99374[1], 99375[1], 99377[1], 99378[1], 99446[0], 99447[0], 99448[0], 99449[0], 99451[0], 99452[0], 99495[0], 99496[0], G0463[1], G0471[0]
53510	0213T[0], 0216T[0], 0596T[1], 0597T[1], 0708T[1], 0709T[1], 12001[1], 12002[1], 12004[1], 12005[1], 12006[1], 12007[1], 12011[1], 12013[1], 12014[1], 12015[1], 12016[1], 12017[1], 12018[1], 12020[1], 12021[1], 12031[1], 12032[1], 12034[1], 12035[1], 12036[1], 12037[1], 12041[1], 12042[1], 12044[1], 12045[1], 12046[1], 12047[1], 12051[1], 12052[1], 12053[1], 12054[1], 12055[1], 12056[1], 12057[1], 13100[1], 13101[1], 13102[1], 13120[1], 13121[1], 13122[1], 13131[1], 13132[1], 13133[1], 13151[1], 13152[1], 13153[1], 36000[1], 36400[1], 36405[1], 36406[1], 36410[1], 36420[1], 36425[1], 36430[1], 36440[1], 36591[0], 36592[0], 36600[1], 36640[1], 43752[1], 51701[0], 51702[0], 51703[1], 52000[1], 52301[1], 53000[0], 53010[0], 53020[0], 53025[0], 53080[0], 62320[0], 62321[0], 62322[0], 62323[0], 62324[0], 62325[0], 62326[0], 62327[0], 64400[0], 64405[0], 64408[0], 64415[0], 64416[0], 64417[0], 64418[0], 64420[0], 64421[0], 64425[0], 64430[0], 64435[0], 64445[0], 64446[0], 64447[0], 64448[0], 64449[0], 64450[0], 64451[0], 64454[0], 64461[0], 64462[0], 64463[0], 64479[0], 64480[0], 64483[0], 64484[0], 64486[0], 64487[0], 64488[0], 64489[0], 64490[0], 64491[0], 64492[0], 64493[0], 64494[0], 64495[0], 64505[0], 64510[0], 64517[0], 64520[0], 64530[0], 69990[0], 92012[1], 92014[1], 93000[1], 93005[1], 93010[1], 93040[1], 93041[1], 93042[1], 93318[1], 93355[1], 94002[1], 94200[1], 94680[1], 94681[1], 94690[1], 95812[1], 95813[1], 95816[1], 95819[1], 95822[1], 95829[1], 95955[1], 96360[1], 96361[1], 96365[1], 96366[1], 96367[1], 96368[1], 96372[1], 96374[1], 96375[1], 96376[1], 96377[1], 96523[0], 99155[0], 99156[0], 99157[0], 99211[1], 99212[1], 99213[1], 99214[1], 99215[1], 99217[1], 99218[1], 99219[1], 99220[1], 99221[1], 99222[1], 99223[1], 99231[1], 99232[1], 99233[1], 99234[1], 99235[1], 99236[1], 99238[1], 99239[1], 99241[1], 99242[1], 99243[1], 99244[1], 99245[1], 99251[1], 99252[1], 99253[1], 99254[1], 99255[1], 99291[1], 99292[1], 99304[1], 99305[1], 99306[1], 99307[1],

0 = Modifier usage not allowed or inappropriate 1 = Modifier usage allowed

Appendix A: NCCI - CPT Codes

Code 1	Code 2
	99308[1], 99309[1], 99310[1], 99315[1], 99316[1], 99334[1], 99335[1], 99336[1], 99337[1], 99347[1], 99348[1], 99349[1], 99350[1], 99374[1], 99375[1], 99377[1], 99378[1], 99446[0], 99447[0], 99448[0], 99449[0], 99451[0], 99452[0], 99495[0], 99496[0], G0463[1], G0471[0]
53515	0213T[0], 0216T[0], 0596T[1], 0597T[1], 0708T[1], 0709T[1], 12001[1], 12002[1], 12004[1], 12005[1], 12006[1], 12007[1], 12011[1], 12013[1], 12014[1], 12015[1], 12016[1], 12017[1], 12018[1], 12020[1], 12021[1], 12031[1], 12032[1], 12034[1], 12035[1], 12036[1], 12037[1], 12041[1], 12042[1], 12044[1], 12045[1], 12046[1], 12047[1], 12051[1], 12052[1], 12053[1], 12054[1], 12055[1], 12056[1], 12057[1], 13100[1], 13101[1], 13102[1], 13120[1], 13121[1], 13122[1], 13131[1], 13132[1], 13133[1], 13151[1], 13152[1], 13153[1], 36000[1], 36400[1], 36405[1], 36406[1], 36410[1], 36420[1], 36425[1], 36430[1], 36440[1], 36591[0], 36592[0], 36600[1], 36640[1], 43752[1], 51701[0], 51702[0], 51703[1], 52000[1], 52301[1], 53000[0], 53010[0], 53020[0], 53025[0], 53080[0], 53500[1], 62320[0], 62321[0], 62322[0], 62323[0], 62324[0], 62325[0], 62326[0], 62327[0], 64400[0], 64405[0], 64408[0], 64415[0], 64416[0], 64417[0], 64418[0], 64420[0], 64421[0], 64425[0], 64430[0], 64435[0], 64445[0], 64446[0], 64447[0], 64448[0], 64449[0], 64450[0], 64451[0], 64454[0], 64461[0], 64462[0], 64463[0], 64479[0], 64480[0], 64483[0], 64484[0], 64486[0], 64487[0], 64488[0], 64489[0], 64490[0], 64491[0], 64492[0], 64493[0], 64494[0], 64495[0], 64505[0], 64510[0], 64517[0], 64520[0], 64530[0], 69990[0], 92012[1], 92014[1], 93000[1], 93005[1], 93010[1], 93040[1], 93041[1], 93042[1], 93318[1], 93355[1], 94002[1], 94200[1], 94680[1], 94681[1], 94690[1], 95812[1], 95813[1], 95816[1], 95819[1], 95822[1], 95829[1], 95955[1], 96360[1], 96361[1], 96365[1], 96366[1], 96367[1], 96368[1], 96372[1], 96374[1], 96375[1], 96376[1], 96377[1], 96523[0], 99155[0], 99156[0], 99157[0], 99211[1], 99212[1], 99213[1], 99214[1], 99215[1], 99217[1], 99218[1], 99219[1], 99220[1], 99221[1], 99222[1], 99223[1], 99231[1], 99232[1], 99233[1], 99234[1], 99235[1], 99236[1], 99238[1], 99239[1], 99241[1], 99242[1], 99243[1], 99244[1], 99245[1], 99251[1], 99252[1], 99253[1], 99254[1], 99255[1], 99291[1], 99292[1], 99304[1], 99305[1], 99306[1], 99307[1], 99308[1], 99309[1], 99310[1], 99315[1], 99316[1], 99334[1], 99335[1], 99336[1], 99337[1], 99347[1], 99348[1], 99349[1], 99350[1], 99374[1], 99375[1], 99377[1], 99378[1], 99446[0], 99447[0], 99448[0], 99449[0], 99451[0], 99452[0], 99495[0], 99496[0], G0463[1], G0471[0]
53520	0213T[0], 0216T[0], 0708T[1], 0709T[1], 11000[1], 11001[1], 11004[1], 11005[1], 11006[1], 11042[1], 11043[1], 11044[1], 11045[1], 11046[1], 11047[1], 12001[1], 12002[1], 12004[1], 12005[1], 12006[1], 12007[1], 12011[1], 12013[1], 12014[1], 12015[1], 12016[1], 12017[1], 12018[1], 12020[1], 12021[1], 12031[1], 12032[1], 12034[1], 12035[1], 12036[1], 12037[1], 12041[1], 12042[1], 12044[1], 12045[1], 12046[1], 12047[1], 12051[1], 12052[1], 12053[1], 12054[1], 12055[1], 12056[1], 12057[1], 13100[1], 13101[1], 13102[1], 13120[1], 13121[1], 13122[1], 13131[1], 13132[1], 13133[1], 13151[1], 13152[1], 13153[1], 36000[1], 36400[1], 36405[1], 36406[1], 36410[1], 36420[1], 36425[1], 36430[1], 36440[1], 36591[0], 36592[0], 36600[1], 36640[1], 43752[1], 51701[0], 51702[0], 51703[1], 52000[1], 52301[1], 53000[0], 53010[0], 53020[0], 53025[0], 53080[0], 62320[0], 62321[0], 62322[0], 62323[0], 62324[0], 62325[0], 62326[0], 62327[0], 64400[0], 64405[0], 64408[0], 64415[0], 64416[0], 64417[0], 64418[0], 64420[0], 64421[0], 64425[0], 64430[0], 64435[0], 64445[0], 64446[0], 64447[0], 64448[0], 64449[0], 64450[0], 64451[0], 64454[0], 64461[0], 64462[0], 64463[0], 64479[0], 64480[0], 64483[0], 64484[0], 64486[0], 64487[0], 64488[0], 64489[0], 64490[0], 64491[0], 64492[0], 64493[0], 64494[0], 64495[0], 64505[0], 64510[0], 64517[0], 64520[0], 64530[0], 69990[0], 92012[1], 92014[1], 93000[1], 93005[1], 93010[1], 93040[1], 93041[1], 93042[1], 93318[1], 93355[1], 94002[1], 94200[1], 94680[1], 94681[1], 94690[1], 95812[1], 95813[1], 95816[1], 95819[1], 95822[1], 95829[1], 95955[1], 96360[1], 96361[1], 96365[1], 96366[1], 96367[1], 96368[1], 96372[1], 96374[1], 96375[1], 96376[1], 96377[1], 96523[0], 97597[1], 97598[1], 97602[1], 99155[0], 99156[0], 99157[0], 99211[1], 99212[1], 99213[1], 99214[1], 99215[1], 99217[1], 99218[1], 99219[1], 99220[1], 99221[1], 99222[1], 99223[1], 99231[1], 99232[1], 99233[1], 99234[1], 99235[1], 99236[1], 99238[1], 99239[1], 99241[1], 99242[1], 99243[1], 99244[1], 99245[1], 99251[1], 99252[1], 99253[1], 99254[1], 99255[1], 99291[1], 99292[1], 99304[1], 99305[1], 99306[1], 99307[1], 99308[1], 99309[1], 99310[1], 99315[1], 99316[1], 99334[1], 99335[1], 99336[1], 99337[1], 99347[1], 99348[1], 99349[1], 99350[1], 99374[1], 99375[1], 99377[1], 99378[1], 99446[0], 99447[0], 99448[0], 99449[0], 99451[0], 99452[0], 99495[0], 99496[0], G0463[1], G0471[0]
53600	0213T[0], 0216T[0], 0708T[1], 0709T[1], 12001[1], 12002[1], 12004[1], 12005[1], 12006[1], 12007[1], 12011[1], 12013[1], 12014[1], 12015[1], 12016[1], 12017[1], 12018[1], 12020[1], 12021[1], 12031[1], 12032[1], 12034[1], 12035[1], 12036[1], 12037[1], 12041[1], 12042[1], 12044[1], 12045[1], 12046[1], 12047[1], 12051[1], 12052[1], 12053[1], 12054[1], 12055[1], 12056[1], 12057[1], 13100[1], 13101[1], 13102[1], 13120[1], 13121[1], 13122[1], 13131[1], 13132[1], 13133[1], 13151[1], 13152[1], 13153[1], 36000[1], 36400[1], 36405[1], 36406[1], 36410[1], 36420[1], 36425[1], 36430[1], 36440[1], 36591[0], 36592[0], 36600[1], 36640[1], 43752[1], 51701[0], 51702[0], 51703[1], 53000[0], 53010[0], 53020[0], 53025[0], 53601[1], 53660[1], 53661[1], 53665[1], 62320[0], 62321[0], 62322[0], 62323[0], 62324[0], 62325[0], 62326[0], 62327[0], 64400[0], 64405[0], 64408[0], 64415[0], 64416[0], 64417[0], 64418[0], 64420[0], 64421[0], 64425[0], 64430[0], 64435[0], 64445[0], 64446[0], 64447[0], 64448[0], 64449[0], 64450[0], 64451[0], 64454[0], 64461[0], 64462[0], 64463[0], 64479[0], 64480[0], 64483[0], 64484[0], 64486[0], 64487[0], 64488[0], 64489[0], 64490[0], 64491[0], 64492[0], 64493[0], 64494[0], 64495[0], 64505[0], 64510[0], 64517[0], 64520[0], 64530[0], 69990[0], 92012[1], 92014[1], 93000[1], 93005[1], 93010[1], 93040[1], 93041[1], 93042[1], 93318[1], 93355[1], 94002[1], 94200[1], 94680[1], 94681[1], 94690[1], 95812[1], 95813[1], 95816[1], 95819[1], 95822[1], 95829[1], 95955[1], 96360[1], 96361[1], 96365[1], 96366[1], 96367[1], 96368[1], 96372[1], 96374[1], 96375[1], 96376[1], 96377[1], 96523[0], 99155[0], 99156[0], 99157[0], 99211[1], 99212[1], 99213[1], 99214[1], 99215[1], 99217[1], 99218[1], 99219[1], 99220[1], 99221[1], 99222[1], 99223[1], 99231[1], 99232[1], 99233[1], 99234[1], 99235[1], 99236[1], 99238[1], 99239[1], 99241[1], 99242[1], 99243[1], 99244[1], 99245[1], 99251[1], 99252[1], 99253[1], 99254[1], 99255[1], 99291[1], 99292[1], 99304[1], 99305[1], 99306[1], 99307[1], 99308[1], 99309[1], 99310[1], 99315[1], 99316[1], 99334[1], 99335[1], 99336[1], 99337[1], 99347[1], 99348[1], 99349[1], 99350[1], 99374[1], 99375[1], 99377[1], 99378[1], 99446[0], 99447[0], 99448[0], 99449[0], 99451[0], 99452[0], 99495[1], 99496[1], G0463[1], G0471[0], J0670[1], J2001[1], P9612[0]
53601	0213T[0], 0216T[0], 0708T[1], 0709T[1], 12001[1], 12002[1], 12004[1], 12005[1], 12006[1], 12007[1], 12011[1], 12013[1], 12014[1], 12015[1], 12016[1], 12017[1], 12018[1], 12020[1], 12021[1], 12031[1], 12032[1], 12034[1], 12035[1], 12036[1], 12037[1], 12041[1], 12042[1], 12044[1], 12045[1], 12046[1], 12047[1], 12051[1], 12052[1], 12053[1], 12054[1], 12055[1], 12056[1], 12057[1], 13100[1], 13101[1], 13102[1], 13120[1], 13121[1], 13122[1], 13131[1], 13132[1], 13133[1], 13151[1], 13152[1], 13153[1], 36000[1], 36400[1], 36405[1], 36406[1], 36410[1], 36420[1], 36425[1], 36430[1], 36440[1], 36591[0], 36592[0], 36600[1], 36640[1], 43752[1], 51701[0], 51702[0], 51703[1], 53000[0], 53010[0], 53020[0], 53025[0], 53660[1], 53661[1], 53665[1], 62320[0], 62321[0], 62322[0], 62323[0], 62324[0], 62325[0], 62326[0], 62327[0], 64400[0], 64405[0], 64408[0], 64415[0], 64416[0], 64417[0], 64418[0], 64420[0], 64421[0], 64425[0], 64430[0], 64435[0], 64445[0], 64446[0], 64447[0], 64448[0], 64449[0], 64450[0], 64451[0], 64454[0], 64461[0], 64462[0], 64463[0], 64479[0], 64480[0], 64483[0], 64484[0], 64486[0], 64487[0], 64488[0], 64489[0], 64490[0], 64491[0], 64492[0], 64493[0], 64494[0], 64495[0], 64505[0], 64510[0], 64517[0], 64520[0], 64530[0], 69990[0], 92012[1], 92014[1], 93000[1], 93005[1], 93010[1], 93040[1], 93041[1], 93042[1], 93318[1], 93355[1], 94002[1], 94200[1], 94680[1], 94681[1], 94690[1], 95812[1], 95813[1], 95816[1], 95819[1], 95822[1], 95829[1], 95955[1], 96360[1], 96361[1], 96365[1], 96366[1], 96367[1], 96368[1], 96372[1], 96374[1], 96375[1], 96376[1], 96377[1], 96523[0], 99155[0], 99156[0], 99157[0], 99211[1], 99212[1], 99213[1], 99214[1], 99215[1], 99217[1], 99218[1], 99219[1], 99220[1], 99221[1], 99222[1], 99223[1], 99231[1], 99232[1], 99233[1], 99234[1], 99235[1], 99236[1], 99238[1], 99239[1], 99241[1], 99242[1], 99243[1], 99244[1], 99245[1], 99251[1], 99252[1], 99253[1], 99254[1], 99255[1], 99291[1], 99292[1], 99304[1], 99305[1], 99306[1], 99307[1], 99308[1], 99309[1], 99310[1], 99315[1], 99316[1], 99334[1], 99335[1], 99336[1], 99337[1], 99347[1], 99348[1], 99349[1], 99350[1], 99374[1], 99375[1], 99377[1], 99378[1], 99446[0], 99447[0], 99448[0], 99449[0], 99451[0], 99452[0], 99495[1], 99496[1], G0463[1], G0471[0], J0670[1], J2001[1], P9612[0]
53605	0213T[0], 0216T[0], 0708T[1], 0709T[1], 12001[1], 12002[1], 12004[1], 12005[1], 12006[1], 12007[1], 12011[1], 12013[1], 12014[1], 12015[1], 12016[1], 12017[1], 12018[1], 12020[1], 12021[1], 12031[1], 12032[1], 12034[1], 12035[1], 12036[1], 12037[1], 12041[1], 12042[1], 12044[1], 12045[1], 12046[1], 12047[1], 12051[1], 12052[1], 12053[1], 12054[1], 12055[1], 12056[1], 12057[1], 13100[1], 13101[1], 13102[1], 13120[1], 13121[1], 13122[1], 13131[1], 13132[1], 13133[1], 13151[1], 13152[1], 13153[1], 36000[1], 36400[1], 36405[1], 36406[1], 36410[1], 36420[1], 36425[1], 36430[1], 36440[1], 36591[0], 36592[0], 36600[1], 36640[1], 43752[1], 51701[0], 51702[0], 51703[1], 53000[0], 53010[0], 53020[0], 53025[0], 53600[0], 53601[1], 53660[1], 53661[1], 53665[1], 62320[0], 62321[0], 62322[0], 62323[0], 62324[0], 62325[0], 62326[0], 62327[0], 64400[0], 64405[0], 64408[0], 64415[0], 64416[0], 64417[0], 64418[0], 64420[0], 64421[0], 64425[0], 64430[0], 64435[0], 64445[0], 64446[0], 64447[0], 64448[0], 64449[0], 64450[0], 64451[0], 64454[0], 64461[0], 64462[0], 64463[0], 64479[0], 64480[0], 64483[0], 64484[0], 64486[0], 64487[0], 64488[0], 64489[0], 64490[0], 64491[0], 64492[0], 64493[0], 64494[0], 64495[0], 64505[0], 64510[0], 64517[0], 64520[0], 64530[0], 69990[0], 92012[1], 92014[1], 93000[1], 93005[1], 93010[1], 93040[1], 93041[1], 93042[1], 93318[1], 93355[1], 94002[1], 94200[1], 94680[1], 94681[1], 94690[1], 95812[1], 95813[1], 95816[1], 95819[1], 95822[1], 95829[1], 95955[1], 96360[1], 96361[1], 96365[1], 96366[1], 96367[1], 96368[1], 96372[1], 96374[1], 96375[1], 96376[1], 96377[1], 96523[0], 99151[0], 99152[0], 99153[0], 99155[0], 99156[0], 99157[0], 99211[1], 99212[1], 99213[1], 99214[1], 99215[1], 99217[1], 99218[1], 99219[1], 99220[1], 99221[1], 99222[1], 99223[1], 99231[1], 99232[1], 99233[1], 99234[1], 99235[1], 99236[1], 99238[1], 99239[1], 99241[1], 99242[1], 99243[1], 99244[1], 99245[1], 99251[1], 99252[1], 99253[1], 99254[1], 99255[1], 99291[1], 99292[1], 99304[1], 99305[1], 99306[1], 99307[1], 99308[1], 99309[1], 99310[1], 99315[1], 99316[1], 99334[1], 99335[1], 99336[1], 99337[1], 99347[1], 99348[1], 99349[1], 99350[1], 99374[1], 99375[1], 99377[1], 99378[1], 99446[0], 99447[0], 99448[0], 99449[0], 99451[0], 99452[0], 99495[1], 99496[1], G0463[1], G0471[0]
53620	0213T[0], 0216T[0], 0708T[1], 0709T[1], 12001[1], 12002[1], 12004[1], 12005[1], 12006[1], 12007[1], 12011[1], 12013[1], 12014[1], 12015[1], 12016[1], 12017[1], 12018[1], 12020[1], 12021[1], 12031[1], 12032[1], 12034[1], 12035[1], 12036[1], 12037[1], 12041[1], 12042[1], 12044[1], 12045[1], 12046[1], 12047[1], 12051[1], 12052[1], 12053[1], 12054[1], 12055[1], 12056[1], 12057[1], 13100[1], 13101[1], 13102[1], 13120[1], 13121[1], 13122[1], 13131[1], 13132[1], 13133[1], 13151[1], 13152[1], 13153[1], 36000[1], 36400[1], 36405[1], 36406[1], 36410[1], 36420[1], 36425[1], 36430[1], 36440[1], 36591[0], 36592[0], 36600[1], 36640[1], 43752[1], 51701[0], 51702[0], 51703[0], 53000[0], 53010[0], 53020[0], 53025[0], 53600[0], 53601[0], 53605[0], 53621[1], 53660[1], 53661[1], 53665[1], 62320[0], 62321[0], 62322[0], 62323[0], 62324[0], 62325[0], 62326[0], 62327[0], 64400[0], 64405[0], 64408[0], 64415[0], 64416[0], 64417[0], 64418[0], 64420[0], 64421[0], 64425[0], 64430[0], 64435[0], 64445[0], 64446[0], 64447[0], 64448[0], 64449[0], 64450[0], 64451[0], 64454[0], 64461[0], 64462[0], 64463[0], 64479[0],

0 = Modifier usage not allowed or inappropriate 1 = Modifier usage allowed

Code 1	Code 2
	64480^0, 64483^0, 64484^0, 64486^0, 64487^0, 64488^0, 64489^0, 64490^0, 64491^0, 64492^0, 64493^0, 64494^0, 64495^0, 64505^0, 64510^0, 64517^0, 64520^0, 64530^0, 69990^0, 92012^1, 92014^1, 93000^1, 93005^1, 93010^1, 93040^1, 93041^1, 93042^1, 93318^1, 93355^1, 94002^1, 94200^1, 94680^1, 94681^1, 94690^1, 95812^1, 95813^1, 95816^1, 95819^1, 95822^1, 95829^1, 95955^1, 96360^1, 96361^1, 96365^1, 96366^1, 96367^1, 96368^1, 96372^1, 96374^1, 96375^1, 96376^1, 96377^1, 96523^0, 99155^0, 99156^0, 99157^0, 99211^1, 99212^1, 99213^1, 99214^1, 99215^1, 99217^1, 99218^1, 99219^1, 99220^1, 99221^1, 99222^1, 99223^1, 99231^1, 99232^1, 99233^1, 99234^1, 99235^1, 99236^1, 99238^1, 99239^1, 99241^1, 99242^1, 99243^1, 99244^1, 99245^1, 99251^1, 99252^1, 99253^1, 99254^1, 99255^1, 99291^1, 99292^1, 99304^1, 99305^1, 99306^1, 99307^1, 99308^1, 99309^1, 99310^1, 99315^1, 99316^1, 99334^1, 99335^1, 99336^1, 99337^1, 99347^1, 99348^1, 99349^1, 99350^1, 99374^1, 99375^1, 99377^1, 99378^1, 99446^0, 99447^0, 99448^0, 99449^0, 99451^0, 99452^0, 99495^1, 99496^1, G0463^1, G0471^0, J0670^1, J2001^1
53621	0213T^0, 0216T^0, 0708T^1, 0709T^1, 12001^1, 12002^1, 12004^1, 12005^1, 12006^1, 12007^1, 12011^1, 12013^1, 12014^1, 12015^1, 12016^1, 12017^1, 12018^1, 12020^1, 12021^1, 12031^1, 12032^1, 12034^1, 12035^1, 12036^1, 12037^1, 12041^1, 12042^1, 12044^1, 12045^1, 12046^1, 12047^1, 12051^1, 12052^1, 12053^1, 12054^1, 12055^1, 12056^1, 12057^1, 13100^1, 13101^1, 13102^1, 13120^1, 13121^1, 13122^1, 13131^1, 13132^1, 13133^1, 13151^1, 13152^1, 13153^1, 36000^1, 36400^1, 36405^1, 36406^1, 36410^1, 36420^1, 36425^1, 36430^1, 36440^1, 36591^0, 36592^0, 36600^1, 36640^1, 43752^1, 51701^0, 51702^0, 51703^1, 53000^0, 53010^0, 53020^0, 53025^0, 53600^0, 53601^0, 53605^0, 62320^0, 62321^0, 62322^0, 62323^0, 62324^0, 62325^0, 62326^0, 62327^0, 64400^0, 64405^0, 64408^0, 64415^0, 64416^0, 64417^0, 64418^0, 64420^0, 64421^0, 64425^0, 64430^0, 64435^0, 64445^0, 64446^0, 64447^0, 64448^0, 64449^0, 64450^0, 64451^0, 64454^0, 64461^0, 64462^0, 64463^0, 64479^0, 64480^0, 64483^0, 64484^0, 64486^0, 64487^0, 64488^0, 64489^0, 64490^0, 64491^0, 64492^0, 64493^0, 64494^0, 64495^0, 64505^0, 64510^0, 64517^0, 64520^0, 64530^0, 69990^0, 92012^1, 92014^1, 93000^1, 93005^1, 93010^1, 93040^1, 93041^1, 93042^1, 93318^1, 93355^1, 94002^1, 94200^1, 94680^1, 94681^1, 94690^1, 95812^1, 95813^1, 95816^1, 95819^1, 95822^1, 95829^1, 95955^1, 96360^1, 96361^1, 96365^1, 96366^1, 96367^1, 96368^1, 96372^1, 96374^1, 96375^1, 96376^1, 96377^1, 96523^0, 99155^0, 99156^0, 99157^0, 99211^1, 99212^1, 99213^1, 99214^1, 99215^1, 99217^1, 99218^1, 99219^1, 99220^1, 99221^1, 99222^1, 99223^1, 99231^1, 99232^1, 99233^1, 99234^1, 99235^1, 99236^1, 99238^1, 99239^1, 99241^1, 99242^1, 99243^1, 99244^1, 99245^1, 99251^1, 99252^1, 99253^1, 99254^1, 99255^1, 99291^1, 99292^1, 99304^1, 99305^1, 99306^1, 99307^1, 99308^1, 99309^1, 99310^1, 99315^1, 99316^1, 99334^1, 99335^1, 99336^1, 99337^1, 99347^1, 99348^1, 99349^1, 99350^1, 99374^1, 99375^1, 99377^1, 99378^1, 99446^0, 99447^0, 99448^0, 99449^0, 99451^0, 99452^0, 99495^1, 99496^1, G0463^1, G0471^0, J0670^1, J2001^1
53660	0213T^0, 0216T^0, 0421T^0, 0708T^1, 0709T^1, 12001^1, 12002^1, 12004^1, 12005^1, 12006^1, 12007^1, 12011^1, 12013^1, 12014^1, 12015^1, 12016^1, 12017^1, 12018^1, 12020^1, 12021^1, 12031^1, 12032^1, 12034^1, 12035^1, 12036^1, 12037^1, 12041^1, 12042^1, 12044^1, 12045^1, 12046^1, 12047^1, 12051^1, 12052^1, 12053^1, 12054^1, 12055^1, 12056^1, 12057^1, 13100^1, 13101^1, 13102^1, 13120^1, 13121^1, 13122^1, 13131^1, 13132^1, 13133^1, 13151^1, 13152^1, 13153^1, 36000^1, 36400^1, 36405^1, 36406^1, 36410^1, 36420^1, 36425^1, 36430^1, 36440^1, 36591^0, 36592^0, 36600^1, 36640^1, 43752^1, 51701^0, 51702^0, 51703^1, 53000^0, 53010^0, 53020^0, 53025^0, 53080^1, 53661^1, 62320^0, 62321^0, 62322^0, 62323^0, 62324^0, 62325^0, 62326^0, 62327^0, 64400^0, 64405^0, 64408^0, 64415^0, 64416^0, 64417^0, 64418^0, 64420^0, 64421^0, 64425^0, 64430^0, 64435^0, 64445^0, 64446^0, 64447^0, 64448^0, 64449^0, 64450^0, 64451^0, 64454^0, 64461^0, 64462^0, 64463^0, 64479^0, 64480^0, 64483^0, 64484^0, 64486^0, 64487^0, 64488^0, 64489^0, 64490^0, 64491^0, 64492^0, 64493^0, 64494^0, 64495^0, 64505^0, 64510^0, 64517^0, 64520^0, 64530^0, 69990^0, 92012^1, 92014^1, 93000^1, 93005^1, 93010^1, 93040^1, 93041^1, 93042^1, 93318^1, 93355^1, 94002^1, 94200^1, 94680^1, 94681^1, 94690^1, 95812^1, 95813^1, 95816^1, 95819^1, 95822^1, 95829^1, 95955^1, 96360^1, 96361^1, 96365^1, 96366^1, 96367^1, 96368^1, 96372^1, 96374^1, 96375^1, 96376^1, 96377^1, 96523^0, 99155^0, 99156^0, 99157^0, 99211^1, 99212^1, 99213^1, 99214^1, 99215^1, 99217^1, 99218^1, 99219^1, 99220^1, 99221^1, 99222^1, 99223^1, 99231^1, 99232^1, 99233^1, 99234^1, 99235^1, 99236^1, 99238^1, 99239^1, 99241^1, 99242^1, 99243^1, 99244^1, 99245^1, 99251^1, 99252^1, 99253^1, 99254^1, 99255^1, 99291^1, 99292^1, 99304^1, 99305^1, 99306^1, 99307^1, 99308^1, 99309^1, 99310^1, 99315^1, 99316^1, 99334^1, 99335^1, 99336^1, 99337^1, 99347^1, 99348^1, 99349^1, 99350^1, 99374^1, 99375^1, 99377^1, 99378^1, 99446^0, 99447^0, 99448^0, 99449^0, 99451^0, 99452^0, 99495^1, 99496^1, G0463^1, G0471^0, J0670^1, J2001^1, P9612^0
53661	0213T^0, 0216T^0, 0421T^0, 0708T^1, 0709T^1, 12001^1, 12002^1, 12004^1, 12005^1, 12006^1, 12007^1, 12011^1, 12013^1, 12014^1, 12015^1, 12016^1, 12017^1, 12018^1, 12020^1, 12021^1, 12031^1, 12032^1, 12034^1, 12035^1, 12036^1, 12037^1, 12041^1, 12042^1, 12044^1, 12045^1, 12046^1, 12047^1, 12051^1, 12052^1, 12053^1, 12054^1, 12055^1, 12056^1, 12057^1, 13100^1, 13101^1, 13102^1, 13120^1, 13121^1, 13122^1, 13131^1, 13132^1, 13133^1, 13151^1, 13152^1, 13153^1, 36000^1, 36400^1, 36405^1, 36406^1, 36410^1, 36420^1, 36425^1, 36430^1, 36440^1, 36591^0, 36592^0, 36600^1, 36640^1, 43752^1, 51700^0, 51701^0, 51702^0, 51703^1, 53000^0, 53010^0, 53020^0, 53025^0, 53080^1, 62320^0, 62321^0, 62322^0, 62323^0, 62324^0, 62325^0, 62326^0, 62327^0, 64400^0, 64405^0, 64408^0, 64415^0, 64416^0, 64417^0, 64418^0, 64420^0, 64421^0, 64425^0, 64430^0, 64435^0, 64445^0, 64446^0, 64447^0, 64448^0, 64449^0, 64450^0, 64451^0, 64454^0, 64461^0, 64462^0, 64463^0, 64479^0, 64480^0, 64483^0, 64484^0, 64486^0, 64487^0, 64488^0, 64489^0, 64490^0, 64491^0, 64492^0, 64493^0, 64494^0, 64495^0, 64505^0, 64510^0, 64517^0, 64520^0, 64530^0, 69990^0, 92012^1, 92014^1, 93000^1, 93005^1, 93010^1, 93040^1, 93041^1, 93042^1, 93318^1, 93355^1, 94002^1, 94200^1, 94680^1, 94681^1, 94690^1, 95812^1, 95813^1, 95816^1, 95819^1, 95822^1, 95829^1, 95955^1, 96360^1, 96361^1, 96365^1, 96366^1, 96367^1, 96368^1, 96372^1, 96374^1, 96375^1, 96376^1, 96377^1, 96523^0, 99155^0, 99156^0, 99157^0, 99211^1, 99212^1, 99213^1, 99214^1, 99215^1, 99217^1, 99218^1, 99219^1, 99220^1, 99221^1, 99222^1, 99223^1, 99231^1, 99232^1, 99233^1, 99234^1, 99235^1, 99236^1, 99238^1, 99239^1, 99241^1, 99242^1, 99243^1, 99244^1, 99245^1, 99251^1, 99252^1, 99253^1, 99254^1, 99255^1, 99291^1, 99292^1, 99304^1, 99305^1, 99306^1, 99307^1, 99308^1, 99309^1, 99310^1, 99315^1, 99316^1, 99334^1, 99335^1, 99336^1, 99337^1, 99347^1, 99348^1, 99349^1, 99350^1, 99374^1, 99375^1, 99377^1, 99378^1, 99446^0, 99447^0, 99448^0, 99449^0, 99451^0, 99452^0, 99495^1, 99496^1, G0463^1, G0471^0, J0670^1, J2001^1, P9612^0
53665	0213T^0, 0216T^0, 0421T^0, 0708T^1, 0709T^1, 12001^1, 12002^1, 12004^1, 12005^1, 12006^1, 12007^1, 12011^1, 12013^1, 12014^1, 12015^1, 12016^1, 12017^1, 12018^1, 12020^1, 12021^1, 12031^1, 12032^1, 12034^1, 12035^1, 12036^1, 12037^1, 12041^1, 12042^1, 12044^1, 12045^1, 12046^1, 12047^1, 12051^1, 12052^1, 12053^1, 12054^1, 12055^1, 12056^1, 12057^1, 13100^1, 13101^1, 13102^1, 13120^1, 13121^1, 13122^1, 13131^1, 13132^1, 13133^1, 13151^1, 13152^1, 13153^1, 36000^1, 36400^1, 36405^1, 36406^1, 36410^1, 36420^1, 36425^1, 36430^1, 36440^1, 36591^0, 36592^0, 36600^1, 36640^1, 43752^1, 51701^0, 51702^0, 51703^1, 53000^0, 53010^0, 53020^0, 53025^0, 53080^1, 53660^0, 53661^1, 62320^0, 62321^0, 62322^0, 62323^0, 62324^0, 62325^0, 62326^0, 62327^0, 64400^0, 64405^0, 64408^0, 64415^0, 64416^0, 64417^0, 64418^0, 64420^0, 64421^0, 64425^0, 64430^0, 64435^0, 64445^0, 64446^0, 64447^0, 64448^0, 64449^0, 64450^0, 64451^0, 64454^0, 64461^0, 64462^0, 64463^0, 64479^0, 64480^0, 64483^0, 64484^0, 64486^0, 64487^0, 64488^0, 64489^0, 64490^0, 64491^0, 64492^0, 64493^0, 64494^0, 64495^0, 64505^0, 64510^0, 64517^0, 64520^0, 64530^0, 69990^0, 92012^1, 92014^1, 93000^1, 93005^1, 93010^1, 93040^1, 93041^1, 93042^1, 93318^1, 93355^1, 94002^1, 94200^1, 94680^1, 94681^1, 94690^1, 95812^1, 95813^1, 95816^1, 95819^1, 95822^1, 95829^1, 95955^1, 96360^1, 96361^1, 96365^1, 96366^1, 96367^1, 96368^1, 96372^1, 96374^1, 96375^1, 96376^1, 96377^1, 96523^0, 99151^0, 99152^0, 99153^0, 99155^0, 99156^0, 99157^0, 99211^1, 99212^1, 99213^1, 99214^1, 99215^1, 99217^1, 99218^1, 99219^1, 99220^1, 99221^1, 99222^1, 99223^1, 99231^1, 99232^1, 99233^1, 99234^1, 99235^1, 99236^1, 99238^1, 99239^1, 99241^1, 99242^1, 99243^1, 99244^1, 99245^1, 99251^1, 99252^1, 99253^1, 99254^1, 99255^1, 99291^1, 99292^1, 99304^1, 99305^1, 99306^1, 99307^1, 99308^1, 99309^1, 99310^1, 99315^1, 99316^1, 99334^1, 99335^1, 99336^1, 99337^1, 99347^1, 99348^1, 99349^1, 99350^1, 99374^1, 99375^1, 99377^1, 99378^1, 99446^0, 99447^0, 99448^0, 99449^0, 99451^0, 99452^0, 99495^1, 99496^1, G0463^1, G0471^0
53850	0213T^0, 0216T^0, 0421T^0, 0596T^0, 0597T^0, 0600T^1, 0601T^1, 0708T^1, 0709T^1, 12001^1, 12002^1, 12004^1, 12005^1, 12006^1, 12007^1, 12011^1, 12013^1, 12014^1, 12015^1, 12016^1, 12017^1, 12018^1, 12020^1, 12021^1, 12031^1, 12032^1, 12034^1, 12035^1, 12036^1, 12037^1, 12041^1, 12042^1, 12044^1, 12045^1, 12046^1, 12047^1, 12051^1, 12052^1, 12053^1, 12054^1, 12055^1, 12056^1, 12057^1, 13100^1, 13101^1, 13102^1, 13120^1, 13121^1, 13122^1, 13131^1, 13132^1, 13133^1, 13151^1, 13152^1, 13153^1, 36000^1, 36400^1, 36405^1, 36406^1, 36410^1, 36420^1, 36425^1, 36430^1, 36440^1, 36591^0, 36592^0, 36600^1, 36640^1, 43752^1, 51700^0, 51701^0, 51702^0, 51703^0, 52000^0, 52001^1, 52005^1, 52276^0, 52281^0, 52441^1, 52630^0, 52640^0, 53000^0, 53010^0, 53020^0, 53025^0, 53600^0, 53601^0, 53605^0, 53620^0, 53621^0, 53855^1, 55700^1, 55706^1, 55873^1, 55880^1, 62320^0, 62321^0, 62322^0, 62323^0, 62324^0, 62325^0, 62326^0, 62327^0, 64400^0, 64405^0, 64408^0, 64415^0, 64416^0, 64417^0, 64418^0, 64420^0, 64421^0, 64425^0, 64430^0, 64435^0, 64445^0, 64446^0, 64447^0, 64448^0, 64449^0, 64450^0, 64451^0, 64454^0, 64461^0, 64462^0, 64463^0, 64479^0, 64480^0, 64483^0, 64484^0, 64486^0, 64487^0, 64488^0, 64489^0, 64490^0, 64491^0, 64492^0, 64493^0, 64494^0, 64495^0, 64505^0, 64510^0, 64517^0, 64520^0, 64530^0, 69990^0, 76872^1, 76873^0, 92012^1, 92014^1, 93000^1, 93005^1, 93010^1, 93040^1, 93041^1, 93042^1, 93318^1, 93355^1, 94002^1, 94200^1, 94680^1, 94681^1, 94690^1, 95812^1, 95813^1, 95816^1, 95819^1, 95822^1, 95829^1, 95955^1, 96360^1, 96361^1, 96365^1, 96366^1, 96367^1, 96368^1, 96372^1, 96374^1, 96375^1, 96376^1, 96377^1, 96523^0, 99155^0, 99156^0, 99157^0, 99211^1, 99212^1, 99213^1, 99214^1, 99215^1, 99217^1, 99218^1, 99219^1, 99220^1, 99221^1, 99222^1, 99223^1, 99231^1, 99232^1, 99233^1, 99234^1, 99235^1, 99236^1, 99238^1, 99239^1, 99241^1, 99242^1, 99243^1, 99244^1, 99245^1, 99251^1, 99252^1, 99253^1, 99254^1, 99255^1, 99291^1, 99292^1, 99304^1, 99305^1, 99306^1, 99307^1, 99308^1, 99309^1, 99310^1, 99315^1, 99316^1, 99334^1, 99335^1, 99336^1, 99337^1, 99347^1, 99348^1, 99349^1, 99350^1, 99374^1, 99375^1, 99377^1, 99378^1, 99446^0, 99447^0, 99448^0, 99449^0, 99451^0, 99452^0, 99495^0, 99496^0, G0463^1, G0471^0, J0670^1, J2001^1, P9612^0

0 = Modifier usage not allowed or inappropriate 1 = Modifier usage allowed

Code 1	Code 2
53852	0213T^0, 0216T^0, 0421T^0, 0596T^0, 0597T^0, 0600T^1, 0601T^1, 0708T^1, 0709T^1, 12001^1, 12002^1, 12004^1, 12005^1, 12006^1, 12007^1, 12011^1, 12013^1, 12014^1, 12015^1, 12016^1, 12017^1, 12018^1, 12020^1, 12021^1, 12031^1, 12032^1, 12034^1, 12035^1, 12036^1, 12037^1, 12041^1, 12042^1, 12044^1, 12045^1, 12046^1, 12047^1, 12051^1, 12052^1, 12053^1, 12054^1, 12055^1, 12056^1, 12057^1, 13100^1, 13101^1, 13102^1, 13120^1, 13121^1, 13122^1, 13131^1, 13132^1, 13133^1, 13151^1, 13152^1, 13153^1, 36000^1, 36400^1, 36405^1, 36406^1, 36410^1, 36420^1, 36425^1, 36430^1, 36440^1, 36591^0, 36592^0, 36600^1, 36640^1, 43752^1, 51102^1, 51700^0, 51701^0, 51702^0, 51703^0, 52000^0, 52001^1, 52281^1, 52441^1, 52500^0, 52630^0, 52640^0, 53000^0, 53010^0, 53020^0, 53025^0, 53600^0, 53601^1, 53605^0, 53620^0, 53621^0, 53850^0, 53855^1, 55700^0, 55706^1, 55873^1, 55880^1, 62320^0, 62321^0, 62322^0, 62323^0, 62324^0, 62325^0, 62326^0, 62327^0, 64400^0, 64405^0, 64408^0, 64415^0, 64416^0, 64417^0, 64418^0, 64420^0, 64421^0, 64425^0, 64430^0, 64435^0, 64445^0, 64446^0, 64447^0, 64448^0, 64449^0, 64450^0, 64451^0, 64454^0, 64461^0, 64462^0, 64463^0, 64479^0, 64480^0, 64483^0, 64484^0, 64486^0, 64487^0, 64488^0, 64489^0, 64490^0, 64491^0, 64492^0, 64493^0, 64494^0, 64495^0, 64505^0, 64510^0, 64517^0, 64520^0, 64530^0, 69990^0, 76872^1, 76873^0, 92012^1, 92014^1, 93000^1, 93005^1, 93010^1, 93040^1, 93041^1, 93042^1, 93318^1, 93355^1, 94002^1, 94200^1, 94680^1, 94681^1, 94690^1, 95812^1, 95813^1, 95816^1, 95819^1, 95822^1, 95829^1, 95955^1, 96360^1, 96361^1, 96365^1, 96366^1, 96367^1, 96368^1, 96372^1, 96374^1, 96375^1, 96376^1, 96377^1, 96523^0, 99155^0, 99156^0, 99157^0, 99211^1, 99212^1, 99213^1, 99214^1, 99215^1, 99217^1, 99218^1, 99219^1, 99220^1, 99221^1, 99222^1, 99223^1, 99231^1, 99232^1, 99233^1, 99234^1, 99235^1, 99236^1, 99238^1, 99239^1, 99241^1, 99242^1, 99243^1, 99244^1, 99245^1, 99251^1, 99252^1, 99253^1, 99254^1, 99255^1, 99291^1, 99292^1, 99304^1, 99305^1, 99306^1, 99307^1, 99308^1, 99309^1, 99310^1, 99315^1, 99316^1, 99334^1, 99335^1, 99336^1, 99337^1, 99347^1, 99348^1, 99349^1, 99350^1, 99374^1, 99375^1, 99377^1, 99378^1, 99446^0, 99447^0, 99448^0, 99449^0, 99451^0, 99452^0, 99495^0, 99496^0, G0463^1, G0471^0, J0670^1, J2001^1, P9612^0
53854	0213T^0, 0216T^0, 0421T^0, 0596T^1, 0597T^1, 0708T^1, 0709T^1, 12001^1, 12002^1, 12004^1, 12005^1, 12006^1, 12007^1, 12011^1, 12013^1, 12014^1, 12015^1, 12016^1, 12017^1, 12018^1, 12020^1, 12021^1, 12031^1, 12032^1, 12034^1, 12035^1, 12036^1, 12037^1, 12041^1, 12042^1, 12044^1, 12045^1, 12046^1, 12047^1, 12051^1, 12052^1, 12053^1, 12054^1, 12055^1, 12056^1, 12057^1, 13100^1, 13101^1, 13102^1, 13120^1, 13121^1, 13122^1, 13131^1, 13132^1, 13133^1, 13151^1, 13152^1, 13153^1, 36000^1, 36400^1, 36405^1, 36406^1, 36410^1, 36420^1, 36425^1, 36430^1, 36440^1, 36591^0, 36592^0, 36600^1, 36640^1, 43752^1, 51102^1, 51700^0, 51701^1, 51702^1, 51703^1, 52000^0, 52001^1, 52281^1, 52441^1, 52500^0, 52640^0, 53000^0, 53010^0, 53020^0, 53025^0, 53600^0, 53601^0, 53605^0, 53620^0, 53621^0, 53850^0, 53852^0, 53855^1, 55700^0, 62320^0, 62321^0, 62322^0, 62323^0, 62324^0, 62325^0, 62326^0, 62327^0, 64400^0, 64405^0, 64408^0, 64415^0, 64416^0, 64417^0, 64418^0, 64420^0, 64421^0, 64425^0, 64430^0, 64435^0, 64445^0, 64446^0, 64447^0, 64448^0, 64449^0, 64450^0, 64451^0, 64454^0, 64461^0, 64462^0, 64463^0, 64479^0, 64480^0, 64483^0, 64484^0, 64486^0, 64487^0, 64488^0, 64489^0, 64490^0, 64491^0, 64492^0, 64493^0, 64494^0, 64495^0, 64505^0, 64510^0, 64517^0, 64520^0, 64530^0, 69990^0, 76872^1, 76873^0, 92012^1, 92014^1, 93000^1, 93005^1, 93010^1, 93040^1, 93041^1, 93042^1, 93318^1, 93355^1, 94002^1, 94200^1, 94680^1, 94681^1, 94690^1, 95812^1, 95813^1, 95816^1, 95819^1, 95822^1, 95829^1, 95955^1, 96360^1, 96361^1, 96365^1, 96366^1, 96367^1, 96368^1, 96372^1, 96374^1, 96375^1, 96376^1, 96377^1, 96523^0, 99155^0, 99156^0, 99157^0, 99211^1, 99212^1, 99213^1, 99214^1, 99215^1, 99217^1, 99218^1, 99219^1, 99220^1, 99221^1, 99222^1, 99223^1, 99231^1, 99232^1, 99233^1, 99234^1, 99235^1, 99236^1, 99238^1, 99239^1, 99241^1, 99242^1, 99243^1, 99244^1, 99245^1, 99251^1, 99252^1, 99253^1, 99254^1, 99255^1, 99291^1, 99292^1, 99304^1, 99305^1, 99306^1, 99307^1, 99308^1, 99309^1, 99310^1, 99315^1, 99316^1, 99334^1, 99335^1, 99336^1, 99337^1, 99347^1, 99348^1, 99349^1, 99350^1, 99374^1, 99375^1, 99377^1, 99378^1, 99446^0, 99447^0, 99448^0, 99449^0, 99495^0, 99496^0, G0463^1, G0471^0, J0670^1, J2001^1, P9612^0
53855	0213T^0, 0216T^0, 0708T^1, 0709T^1, 11000^1, 11001^1, 11004^1, 11005^1, 11006^1, 11042^1, 11043^1, 11044^1, 11045^1, 11046^1, 11047^1, 12001^1, 12002^1, 12004^1, 12005^1, 12006^1, 12007^1, 12011^1, 12013^1, 12014^1, 12015^1, 12016^1, 12017^1, 12018^1, 12020^1, 12021^1, 12031^1, 12032^1, 12034^1, 12035^1, 12036^1, 12037^1, 12041^1, 12042^1, 12044^1, 12045^1, 12046^1, 12047^1, 12051^1, 12052^1, 12053^1, 12054^1, 12055^1, 12056^1, 12057^1, 13100^1, 13101^1, 13102^1, 13120^1, 13121^1, 13122^1, 13131^1, 13132^1, 13133^1, 13151^1, 13152^1, 13153^1, 36000^1, 36400^1, 36405^1, 36406^1, 36410^1, 36420^1, 36425^1, 36430^1, 36440^1, 36591^0, 36592^0, 36600^1, 36640^1, 43752^1, 51701^1, 51702^1, 51703^1, 52000^0, 52442^1, 53000^0, 53010^0, 53020^0, 53025^0, 53080^1, 53520^1, 53600^1, 53601^1, 53605^1, 53620^1, 53621^1, 53660^1, 53661^1, 53665^1, 62320^0, 62321^0, 62322^0, 62323^0, 62324^0, 62325^0, 62326^0, 62327^0, 64400^0, 64405^0, 64408^0, 64415^0, 64416^0, 64417^0, 64418^0, 64420^0, 64421^0, 64425^0, 64430^0, 64435^0, 64445^0, 64446^0, 64447^0, 64448^0, 64449^0, 64450^0, 64451^0, 64454^0, 64461^0, 64462^0, 64463^0, 64479^0, 64480^0, 64483^0, 64484^0, 64486^0, 64487^0, 64488^0, 64489^0, 64490^0, 64491^0, 64492^0, 64493^0, 64494^0, 64495^0, 64505^0, 64510^0, 64517^0, 64520^0, 64530^0, 69990^0, 92012^1, 92014^1, 93000^1, 93005^1, 93010^1, 93040^1, 93041^1, 93042^1, 93318^1, 93355^1, 94002^1, 94200^1, 94680^1, 94681^1, 94690^1, 95812^1, 95813^1, 95816^1, 95819^1, 95822^1, 95829^1, 95955^1, 96360^1, 96361^1, 96365^1, 96366^1, 96367^1, 96368^1, 96372^1, 96374^1, 96375^1, 96376^1, 96377^1, 96523^0, 97597^1, 97598^1, 97602^1, 99155^0, 99156^0, 99157^0, 99211^1, 99212^1, 99213^1, 99214^1, 99215^1, 99217^1, 99218^1, 99219^1, 99220^1, 99221^1, 99222^1, 99223^1, 99231^1, 99232^1, 99233^1, 99234^1, 99235^1, 99236^1, 99238^1, 99239^1, 99241^1, 99242^1, 99243^1, 99244^1, 99245^1, 99251^1, 99252^1, 99253^1, 99254^1, 99255^1, 99291^1, 99292^1, 99304^1, 99305^1, 99306^1, 99307^1, 99308^1, 99309^1, 99310^1, 99315^1, 99316^1, 99334^1, 99335^1, 99336^1, 99337^1, 99347^1, 99348^1, 99349^1, 99350^1, 99374^1, 99375^1, 99377^1, 99378^1, 99446^0, 99447^0, 99448^0, 99449^0, 99451^0, 99452^0, 99495^1, 99496^1, G0463^1, G0471^1, J0670^1, J2001^1
53860	0596T^1, 0597T^1, 0708T^1, 0709T^1, 12001^1, 12002^1, 12004^1, 12005^1, 12006^1, 12007^1, 12011^1, 12013^1, 12014^1, 12015^1, 12016^1, 12017^1, 12018^1, 12020^1, 12021^1, 12031^1, 12032^1, 12034^1, 12035^1, 12036^1, 12037^1, 12041^1, 12042^1, 12044^1, 12045^1, 12046^1, 12047^1, 12051^1, 12052^1, 12053^1, 12054^1, 12055^1, 12056^1, 12057^1, 13100^1, 13101^1, 13102^1, 13120^1, 13121^1, 13122^1, 13131^1, 13132^1, 13133^1, 13151^1, 13152^1, 13153^1, 36000^1, 36400^1, 36405^1, 36406^1, 36410^1, 36420^1, 36425^1, 36430^1, 36440^1, 36591^0, 36592^0, 36600^1, 36640^1, 43752^1, 51102^1, 51700^0, 51701^1, 51702^1, 51703^1, 52000^0, 52001^1, 52281^1, 52285^1, 52310^1, 52315^1, 52500^1, 53000^1, 53010^1, 53020^1, 53025^1, 53080^1, 53660^1, 53661^1, 53665^1, 62320^0, 62321^0, 62322^0, 62323^0, 62324^0, 62325^0, 62326^0, 62327^0, 64400^0, 64405^0, 64408^0, 64415^0, 64416^0, 64417^0, 64418^0, 64420^0, 64421^0, 64425^0, 64430^0, 64435^0, 64445^0, 64446^0, 64447^0, 64448^0, 64449^0, 64450^0, 64451^0, 64454^0, 64461^0, 64462^0, 64463^0, 64479^0, 64480^0, 64483^0, 64484^0, 64486^0, 64487^0, 64488^0, 64489^0, 64490^0, 64491^0, 64492^0, 64493^0, 64494^0, 64495^0, 64505^0, 64510^0, 64517^0, 64520^0, 64530^0, 69990^0, 92012^1, 92014^1, 93000^1, 93005^1, 93010^1, 93040^1, 93041^1, 93042^1, 93318^1, 93355^1, 94002^1, 94200^1, 94680^1, 94681^1, 94690^1, 95812^1, 95813^1, 95816^1, 95819^1, 95822^1, 95829^1, 95955^1, 96360^1, 96361^1, 96365^1, 96366^1, 96367^1, 96368^1, 96372^1, 96374^1, 96375^1, 96376^1, 96377^1, 96523^0, 99155^0, 99156^0, 99157^0, 99211^1, 99212^1, 99213^1, 99214^1, 99215^1, 99217^1, 99218^1, 99219^1, 99220^1, 99221^1, 99222^1, 99223^1, 99231^1, 99232^1, 99233^1, 99234^1, 99235^1, 99236^1, 99238^1, 99239^1, 99241^1, 99242^1, 99243^1, 99244^1, 99245^1, 99251^1, 99252^1, 99253^1, 99254^1, 99255^1, 99291^1, 99292^1, 99304^1, 99305^1, 99306^1, 99307^1, 99308^1, 99309^1, 99310^1, 99315^1, 99316^1, 99334^1, 99335^1, 99336^1, 99337^1, 99347^1, 99348^1, 99349^1, 99350^1, 99374^1, 99375^1, 99377^1, 99378^1, 99446^0, 99447^0, 99448^0, 99449^0, 99451^0, 99452^0, 99495^0, 99496^0, G0463^1, G0471^1, J0670^1, J2001^1, P9612^1
54000	0213T^0, 0216T^0, 0596T^1, 0597T^1, 0708T^1, 0709T^1, 12001^1, 12002^1, 12004^1, 12005^1, 12006^1, 12007^1, 12011^1, 12013^1, 12014^1, 12015^1, 12016^1, 12017^1, 12018^1, 12020^1, 12021^1, 12031^1, 12032^1, 12034^1, 12035^1, 12036^1, 12037^1, 12041^1, 12042^1, 12044^1, 12045^1, 12046^1, 12047^1, 12051^1, 12052^1, 12053^1, 12054^1, 12055^1, 12056^1, 12057^1, 13100^1, 13101^1, 13102^1, 13120^1, 13121^1, 13122^1, 13131^1, 13132^1, 13133^1, 13151^1, 13152^1, 13153^1, 36000^1, 36400^1, 36405^1, 36406^1, 36410^1, 36420^1, 36425^1, 36430^1, 36440^1, 36591^0, 36592^0, 36600^1, 36640^1, 43752^1, 51701^0, 51702^0, 51703^1, 62320^0, 62321^0, 62322^0, 62323^0, 62324^0, 62325^0, 62326^0, 62327^0, 64400^0, 64405^0, 64408^0, 64415^0, 64416^0, 64417^0, 64418^0, 64420^0, 64421^0, 64425^0, 64430^0, 64435^0, 64445^0, 64446^0, 64447^0, 64448^0, 64449^0, 64450^0, 64451^0, 64454^0, 64461^0, 64462^0, 64463^0, 64479^0, 64480^0, 64483^0, 64484^0, 64486^0, 64487^0, 64488^0, 64489^0, 64490^0, 64491^0, 64492^0, 64493^0, 64494^0, 64495^0, 64505^0, 64510^0, 64517^0, 64520^0, 64530^0, 69990^0, 92012^1, 92014^1, 93000^1, 93005^1, 93010^1, 93040^1, 93041^1, 93042^1, 93318^1, 93355^1, 94002^1, 94200^1, 94680^1, 94681^1, 94690^1, 95812^1, 95813^1, 95816^1, 95819^1, 95822^1, 95829^1, 95955^1, 96360^1, 96361^1, 96365^1, 96366^1, 96367^1, 96368^1, 96372^1, 96374^1, 96375^1, 96376^1, 96377^1, 96523^0, 99155^0, 99156^0, 99157^0, 99211^1, 99212^1, 99213^1, 99214^1, 99215^1, 99217^1, 99218^1, 99219^1, 99220^1, 99221^1, 99222^1, 99223^1, 99231^1, 99232^1, 99233^1, 99234^1, 99235^1, 99236^1, 99238^1, 99239^1, 99241^1, 99242^1, 99243^1, 99244^1, 99245^1, 99251^1, 99252^1, 99253^1, 99254^1, 99255^1, 99291^1, 99292^1, 99304^1, 99305^1, 99306^1, 99307^1, 99308^1, 99309^1, 99310^1, 99315^1, 99316^1, 99334^1, 99335^1, 99336^1, 99337^1, 99347^1, 99348^1, 99349^1, 99350^1, 99374^1, 99375^1, 99377^1, 99378^1, 99446^0, 99447^0, 99448^0, 99449^0, 99451^0, 99452^0, 99495^0, 99496^0, G0463^1, G0471^0, J2001^1
54001	0213T^0, 0216T^0, 0596T^1, 0597T^1, 0708T^1, 0709T^1, 12001^1, 12002^1, 12004^1, 12005^1, 12006^1, 12007^1, 12011^1, 12013^1, 12014^1, 12015^1, 12016^1, 12017^1, 12018^1, 12020^1, 12021^1, 12031^1, 12032^1, 12034^1, 12035^1, 12036^1, 12037^1, 12041^1, 12042^1, 12044^1, 12045^1, 12046^1, 12047^1, 12051^1, 12052^1, 12053^1, 12054^1, 12055^1, 12056^1, 12057^1, 13100^1, 13101^1, 13102^1, 13120^1, 13121^1, 13122^1, 13131^1, 13132^1, 13133^1, 13151^1, 13152^1, 13153^1, 36000^1, 36400^1, 36405^1, 36406^1, 36410^1, 36420^1, 36425^1, 36430^1, 36440^1, 36591^0, 36592^0, 36600^1, 36640^1, 43752^1, 51701^0, 51702^0, 51703^1, 62320^0, 62321^0, 62322^0, 62323^0, 62324^0, 62325^0, 62326^0, 62327^0, 64400^0, 64405^0, 64408^0,

0 = Modifier usage not allowed or inappropriate 1 = Modifier usage allowed

Code 1	Code 2
	64415[0], 64416[0], 64417[0], 64418[0], 64420[0], 64421[0], 64425[0], 64430[0], 64435[0], 64445[0], 64446[0], 64447[0], 64448[0], 64449[0], 64450[0], 64451[0], 64454[0], 64461[0], 64462[0], 64463[0], 64479[0], 64480[0], 64483[0], 64484[0], 64486[0], 64487[0], 64488[0], 64489[0], 64490[0], 64491[0], 64492[0], 64493[0], 64494[0], 64495[0], 64505[0], 64510[0], 64517[0], 64520[0], 64530[0], 69990[0], 92012[1], 92014[1], 93000[1], 93005[1], 93010[1], 93040[1], 93041[1], 93042[1], 93318[1], 93355[1], 94002[1], 94200[1], 94680[1], 94681[1], 94690[1], 95812[1], 95813[1], 95816[1], 95819[1], 95822[1], 95829[1], 95955[1], 96360[1], 96361[1], 96365[1], 96366[1], 96367[1], 96368[1], 96372[1], 96374[1], 96375[1], 96376[1], 96377[1], 96523[0], 99155[0], 99156[0], 99157[0], 99211[1], 99212[1], 99213[1], 99214[1], 99215[1], 99217[1], 99218[1], 99219[1], 99220[1], 99221[1], 99222[1], 99223[1], 99231[1], 99232[1], 99233[1], 99234[1], 99235[1], 99236[1], 99238[1], 99239[1], 99241[1], 99242[1], 99243[1], 99244[1], 99245[1], 99251[1], 99252[1], 99253[1], 99254[1], 99255[1], 99291[1], 99292[1], 99304[1], 99305[1], 99306[1], 99307[1], 99308[1], 99309[1], 99310[1], 99315[1], 99316[1], 99334[1], 99335[1], 99336[1], 99337[1], 99347[1], 99348[1], 99349[1], 99350[1], 99374[1], 99375[1], 99377[1], 99378[1], 99446[0], 99447[0], 99448[0], 99449[0], 99451[0], 99452[0], 99495[0], 99496[0], G0463[1], G0471[0], J0670[1], J2001[1]
54015	0213T[0], 0216T[0], 0596T[1], 0597T[1], 0708T[1], 0709T[1], 12001[1], 12002[1], 12004[1], 12005[1], 12006[1], 12007[1], 12011[1], 12013[1], 12014[1], 12015[1], 12016[1], 12017[1], 12018[1], 12020[1], 12021[1], 12031[1], 12032[1], 12034[1], 12035[1], 12036[1], 12037[1], 12041[1], 12042[1], 12044[1], 12045[1], 12046[1], 12047[1], 12051[1], 12052[1], 12053[1], 12054[1], 12055[1], 12056[1], 12057[1], 13100[1], 13101[1], 13102[1], 13120[1], 13121[1], 13122[1], 13131[1], 13132[1], 13133[1], 13151[1], 13152[1], 13153[1], 36000[1], 36400[1], 36405[1], 36406[1], 36410[1], 36420[1], 36425[1], 36430[1], 36440[1], 36591[0], 36592[0], 36600[1], 36640[1], 43752[1], 51701[0], 51702[0], 51703[1], 54001[1], 54450[1], 62320[0], 62321[0], 62322[0], 62323[0], 62324[0], 62325[0], 62326[0], 62327[0], 64400[0], 64405[0], 64408[0], 64415[0], 64416[0], 64417[0], 64418[0], 64420[0], 64421[0], 64425[0], 64430[0], 64435[0], 64445[0], 64446[0], 64447[0], 64448[0], 64449[0], 64450[0], 64451[0], 64454[0], 64461[0], 64462[0], 64463[0], 64479[0], 64480[0], 64483[0], 64484[0], 64486[0], 64487[0], 64488[0], 64489[0], 64490[0], 64491[0], 64492[0], 64493[0], 64494[0], 64495[0], 64505[0], 64510[0], 64517[0], 64520[0], 64530[0], 69990[0], 92012[1], 92014[1], 93000[1], 93005[1], 93010[1], 93040[1], 93041[1], 93042[1], 93318[1], 93355[1], 94002[1], 94200[1], 94680[1], 94681[1], 94690[1], 95812[1], 95813[1], 95816[1], 95819[1], 95822[1], 95829[1], 95955[1], 96360[1], 96361[1], 96365[1], 96366[1], 96367[1], 96368[1], 96372[1], 96374[1], 96375[1], 96376[1], 96377[1], 96523[0], 99155[0], 99156[0], 99157[0], 99211[1], 99212[1], 99213[1], 99214[1], 99215[1], 99217[1], 99218[1], 99219[1], 99220[1], 99221[1], 99222[1], 99223[1], 99231[1], 99232[1], 99233[1], 99234[1], 99235[1], 99236[1], 99238[1], 99239[1], 99241[1], 99242[1], 99243[1], 99244[1], 99245[1], 99251[1], 99252[1], 99253[1], 99254[1], 99255[1], 99291[1], 99292[1], 99304[1], 99305[1], 99306[1], 99307[1], 99308[1], 99309[1], 99310[1], 99315[1], 99316[1], 99334[1], 99335[1], 99336[1], 99337[1], 99347[1], 99348[1], 99349[1], 99350[1], 99374[1], 99375[1], 99377[1], 99378[1], 99446[0], 99447[0], 99448[0], 99449[0], 99451[0], 99452[0], 99495[0], 99496[0], G0463[1], G0471[0], J2001[1]
54050	0213T[0], 0216T[0], 0596T[1], 0597T[1], 0708T[1], 0709T[1], 12001[1], 12002[1], 12004[1], 12005[1], 12006[1], 12007[1], 12011[1], 12013[1], 12014[1], 12015[1], 12016[1], 12017[1], 12018[1], 12020[1], 12021[1], 12031[1], 12032[1], 12034[1], 12035[1], 12036[1], 12037[1], 12041[1], 12042[1], 12044[1], 12045[1], 12046[1], 12047[1], 12051[1], 12052[1], 12053[1], 12054[1], 12055[1], 12056[1], 12057[1], 13100[1], 13101[1], 13102[1], 13120[1], 13121[1], 13122[1], 13131[1], 13132[1], 13133[1], 13151[1], 13152[1], 13153[1], 36000[1], 36400[1], 36405[1], 36406[1], 36410[1], 36420[1], 36425[1], 36430[1], 36440[1], 36591[0], 36592[0], 36600[1], 36640[1], 43752[1], 51701[0], 51702[0], 51703[1], 54060[1], 62320[0], 62321[0], 62322[0], 62323[0], 62324[0], 62325[0], 62326[0], 62327[0], 64400[0], 64405[0], 64408[0], 64415[0], 64416[0], 64417[0], 64418[0], 64420[0], 64421[0], 64425[0], 64430[0], 64435[0], 64445[0], 64446[0], 64447[0], 64448[0], 64449[0], 64450[0], 64451[0], 64454[0], 64461[0], 64462[0], 64463[0], 64479[0], 64480[0], 64483[0], 64484[0], 64486[0], 64487[0], 64488[0], 64489[0], 64490[0], 64491[0], 64492[0], 64493[0], 64494[0], 64495[0], 64505[0], 64510[0], 64517[0], 64520[0], 64530[0], 69990[0], 92012[1], 92014[1], 93000[1], 93005[1], 93010[1], 93040[1], 93041[1], 93042[1], 93318[1], 93355[1], 94002[1], 94200[1], 94680[1], 94681[1], 94690[1], 95812[1], 95813[1], 95816[1], 95819[1], 95822[1], 95829[1], 95955[1], 96360[1], 96361[1], 96365[1], 96366[1], 96367[1], 96368[1], 96372[1], 96374[1], 96375[1], 96376[1], 96377[1], 96523[0], 99155[0], 99156[0], 99157[0], 99211[1], 99212[1], 99213[1], 99214[1], 99215[1], 99217[1], 99218[1], 99219[1], 99220[1], 99221[1], 99222[1], 99223[1], 99231[1], 99232[1], 99233[1], 99234[1], 99235[1], 99236[1], 99238[1], 99239[1], 99241[1], 99242[1], 99243[1], 99244[1], 99245[1], 99251[1], 99252[1], 99253[1], 99254[1], 99255[1], 99291[1], 99292[1], 99304[1], 99305[1], 99306[1], 99307[1], 99308[1], 99309[1], 99310[1], 99315[1], 99316[1], 99334[1], 99335[1], 99336[1], 99337[1], 99347[1], 99348[1], 99349[1], 99350[1], 99374[1], 99375[1], 99377[1], 99378[1], 99446[0], 99447[0], 99448[0], 99449[0], 99451[0], 99452[0], 99495[0], 99496[0], G0463[1], G0471[0]
54055	0213T[0], 0216T[0], 0596T[1], 0597T[1], 0708T[1], 0709T[1], 12001[1], 12002[1], 12004[1], 12005[1], 12006[1], 12007[1], 12011[1], 12013[1], 12014[1], 12015[1], 12016[1], 12017[1], 12018[1], 12020[1], 12021[1], 12031[1], 12032[1], 12034[1], 12035[1], 12036[1], 12037[1], 12041[1], 12042[1], 12044[1], 12045[1], 12046[1], 12047[1], 12051[1], 12052[1], 12053[1], 12054[1], 12055[1], 12056[1], 12057[1], 13100[1], 13101[1], 13102[1], 13120[1], 13121[1], 13122[1], 13131[1], 13132[1], 13133[1], 13151[1], 13152[1], 13153[1], 36000[1], 36400[1], 36405[1], 36406[1], 36410[1], 36420[1], 36425[1], 36430[1], 36440[1], 36591[0], 36592[0], 36600[1], 36640[1], 43752[1], 51701[0], 51702[0], 51703[1], 54060[1], 62320[0], 62321[0], 62322[0], 62323[0], 62324[0], 62325[0], 62326[0], 62327[0], 64400[0], 64405[0], 64408[0], 64415[0], 64416[0], 64417[0], 64418[0], 64420[0], 64421[0], 64425[0], 64430[0], 64435[0], 64445[0], 64446[0], 64447[0], 64448[0], 64449[0], 64450[0], 64451[0], 64454[0], 64461[0], 64462[0], 64463[0], 64479[0], 64480[0], 64483[0], 64484[0], 64486[0], 64487[0], 64488[0], 64489[0], 64490[0], 64491[0], 64492[0], 64493[0], 64494[0], 64495[0], 64505[0], 64510[0], 64517[0], 64520[0], 64530[0], 69990[0], 92012[1], 92014[1], 93000[1], 93005[1], 93010[1], 93040[1], 93041[1], 93042[1], 93318[1], 93355[1], 94002[1], 94200[1], 94680[1], 94681[1], 94690[1], 95812[1], 95813[1], 95816[1], 95819[1], 95822[1], 95829[1], 95955[1], 96360[1], 96361[1], 96365[1], 96366[1], 96367[1], 96368[1], 96372[1], 96374[1], 96375[1], 96376[1], 96377[1], 96523[0], 99155[0], 99156[0], 99157[0], 99211[1], 99212[1], 99213[1], 99214[1], 99215[1], 99217[1], 99218[1], 99219[1], 99220[1], 99221[1], 99222[1], 99223[1], 99231[1], 99232[1], 99233[1], 99234[1], 99235[1], 99236[1], 99238[1], 99239[1], 99241[1], 99242[1], 99243[1], 99244[1], 99245[1], 99251[1], 99252[1], 99253[1], 99254[1], 99255[1], 99291[1], 99292[1], 99304[1], 99305[1], 99306[1], 99307[1], 99308[1], 99309[1], 99310[1], 99315[1], 99316[1], 99334[1], 99335[1], 99336[1], 99337[1], 99347[1], 99348[1], 99349[1], 99350[1], 99374[1], 99375[1], 99377[1], 99378[1], 99446[0], 99447[0], 99448[0], 99449[0], 99451[0], 99452[0], 99495[0], 99496[0], G0463[1], G0471[0]
54056	0213T[0], 0216T[0], 0596T[1], 0597T[1], 0708T[1], 0709T[1], 12001[1], 12002[1], 12004[1], 12005[1], 12006[1], 12007[1], 12011[1], 12013[1], 12014[1], 12015[1], 12016[1], 12017[1], 12018[1], 12020[1], 12021[1], 12031[1], 12032[1], 12034[1], 12035[1], 12036[1], 12037[1], 12041[1], 12042[1], 12044[1], 12045[1], 12046[1], 12047[1], 12051[1], 12052[1], 12053[1], 12054[1], 12055[1], 12056[1], 12057[1], 13100[1], 13101[1], 13102[1], 13120[1], 13121[1], 13122[1], 13131[1], 13132[1], 13133[1], 13151[1], 13152[1], 13153[1], 36000[1], 36400[1], 36405[1], 36406[1], 36410[1], 36420[1], 36425[1], 36430[1], 36440[1], 36591[0], 36592[0], 36600[1], 36640[1], 43752[1], 51701[0], 51702[0], 51703[1], 54050[1], 54055[1], 54060[1], 62320[0], 62321[0], 62322[0], 62323[0], 62324[0], 62325[0], 62326[0], 62327[0], 64400[0], 64405[0], 64408[0], 64415[0], 64416[0], 64417[0], 64418[0], 64420[0], 64421[0], 64425[0], 64430[0], 64435[0], 64445[0], 64446[0], 64447[0], 64448[0], 64449[0], 64450[0], 64451[0], 64454[0], 64461[0], 64462[0], 64463[0], 64479[0], 64480[0], 64483[0], 64484[0], 64486[0], 64487[0], 64488[0], 64489[0], 64490[0], 64491[0], 64492[0], 64493[0], 64494[0], 64495[0], 64505[0], 64510[0], 64517[0], 64520[0], 64530[0], 69990[0], 92012[1], 92014[1], 93000[1], 93005[1], 93010[1], 93040[1], 93041[1], 93042[1], 93318[1], 93355[1], 94002[1], 94200[1], 94680[1], 94681[1], 94690[1], 95812[1], 95813[1], 95816[1], 95819[1], 95822[1], 95829[1], 95955[1], 96360[1], 96361[1], 96365[1], 96366[1], 96367[1], 96368[1], 96372[1], 96374[1], 96375[1], 96376[1], 96377[1], 96523[0], 99155[0], 99156[0], 99157[0], 99211[1], 99212[1], 99213[1], 99214[1], 99215[1], 99217[1], 99218[1], 99219[1], 99220[1], 99221[1], 99222[1], 99223[1], 99231[1], 99232[1], 99233[1], 99234[1], 99235[1], 99236[1], 99238[1], 99239[1], 99241[1], 99242[1], 99243[1], 99244[1], 99245[1], 99251[1], 99252[1], 99253[1], 99254[1], 99255[1], 99291[1], 99292[1], 99304[1], 99305[1], 99306[1], 99307[1], 99308[1], 99309[1], 99310[1], 99315[1], 99316[1], 99334[1], 99335[1], 99336[1], 99337[1], 99347[1], 99348[1], 99349[1], 99350[1], 99374[1], 99375[1], 99377[1], 99378[1], 99446[0], 99447[0], 99448[0], 99449[0], 99451[0], 99452[0], 99495[0], 99496[0], G0463[1], G0471[0], J0670[1], J2001[1]
54057	0213T[0], 0216T[0], 0596T[1], 0597T[1], 0708T[1], 0709T[1], 12001[1], 12002[1], 12004[1], 12005[1], 12006[1], 12007[1], 12011[1], 12013[1], 12014[1], 12015[1], 12016[1], 12017[1], 12018[1], 12020[1], 12021[1], 12031[1], 12032[1], 12034[1], 12035[1], 12036[1], 12037[1], 12041[1], 12042[1], 12044[1], 12045[1], 12046[1], 12047[1], 12051[1], 12052[1], 12053[1], 12054[1], 12055[1], 12056[1], 12057[1], 13100[1], 13101[1], 13102[1], 13120[1], 13121[1], 13122[1], 13131[1], 13132[1], 13133[1], 13151[1], 13152[1], 13153[1], 36000[1], 36400[1], 36405[1], 36406[1], 36410[1], 36420[1], 36425[1], 36430[1], 36440[1], 36591[0], 36592[0], 36600[1], 36640[1], 43752[1], 51701[0], 51702[0], 51703[1], 54050[1], 54055[1], 54056[1], 54060[1], 62320[0], 62321[0], 62322[0], 62323[0], 62324[0], 62325[0], 62326[0], 62327[0], 64400[0], 64405[0], 64408[0], 64415[0], 64416[0], 64417[0], 64418[0], 64420[0], 64421[0], 64425[0], 64430[0], 64435[0], 64445[0], 64446[0], 64447[0], 64448[0], 64449[0], 64450[0], 64451[0], 64454[0], 64461[0], 64462[0], 64463[0], 64479[0], 64480[0], 64483[0], 64484[0], 64486[0], 64487[0], 64488[0], 64489[0], 64490[0], 64491[0], 64492[0], 64493[0], 64494[0], 64495[0], 64505[0], 64510[0], 64517[0], 64520[0], 64530[0], 69990[0], 92012[1], 92014[1], 93000[1], 93005[1], 93010[1], 93040[1], 93041[1], 93042[1], 93318[1], 93355[1], 94002[1], 94200[1], 94680[1], 94681[1], 94690[1], 95812[1], 95813[1], 95816[1], 95819[1], 95822[1], 95829[1], 95955[1], 96360[1], 96361[1], 96365[1], 96366[1], 96367[1], 96368[1], 96372[1], 96374[1], 96375[1], 96376[1], 96377[1], 96523[0], 99155[0], 99156[0], 99157[0], 99211[1], 99212[1], 99213[1], 99214[1], 99215[1], 99217[1], 99218[1], 99219[1], 99220[1], 99221[1], 99222[1], 99223[1], 99231[1], 99232[1], 99233[1], 99234[1], 99235[1], 99236[1], 99238[1], 99239[1], 99241[1], 99242[1], 99243[1], 99244[1], 99245[1], 99251[1], 99252[1], 99253[1], 99254[1], 99255[1], 99291[1], 99292[1], 99304[1], 99305[1], 99306[1], 99307[1], 99308[1], 99309[1], 99310[1], 99315[1], 99316[1], 99334[1], 99335[1], 99336[1], 99337[1], 99347[1], 99348[1], 99349[1], 99350[1], 99374[1], 99375[1], 99377[1], 99378[1], 99446[0], 99447[0], 99448[0], 99449[0], 99451[0], 99452[0], 99495[0], 99496[0], G0463[1], G0471[0], J0670[1], J2001[1]

0 = Modifier usage not allowed or inappropriate 1 = Modifier usage allowed

Code 1	Code 2
54060	0213T^0, 0216T^0, 0596T^1, 0597T^1, 0708T^1, 0709T^1, 11000^1, 11001^1, 11004^1, 11005^1, 11006^1, 11042^1, 11043^1, 11044^1, 11045^1, 11046^1, 11047^1, 12001^1, 12002^1, 12004^1, 12005^1, 12006^1, 12007^1, 12011^1, 12013^1, 12014^1, 12015^1, 12016^1, 12017^1, 12018^1, 12020^1, 12021^1, 12031^1, 12032^1, 12034^1, 12035^1, 12036^1, 12037^1, 12041^1, 12042^1, 12044^1, 12045^1, 12046^1, 12047^1, 12051^1, 12052^1, 12053^1, 12054^1, 12055^1, 12056^1, 12057^1, 13100^1, 13101^1, 13102^1, 13120^1, 13121^1, 13122^1, 13131^1, 13132^1, 13133^1, 13151^1, 13152^1, 13153^1, 36000^1, 36400^1, 36405^1, 36406^1, 36410^1, 36420^1, 36425^1, 36430^1, 36440^1, 36591^0, 36592^0, 36600^1, 36640^1, 43752^1, 51701^0, 51702^0, 51703^1, 62320^0, 62321^0, 62322^0, 62323^0, 62324^0, 62325^0, 62326^0, 62327^0, 64400^0, 64405^0, 64408^0, 64415^0, 64416^0, 64417^0, 64418^0, 64420^0, 64421^0, 64425^0, 64430^0, 64435^0, 64445^0, 64446^0, 64447^0, 64448^0, 64449^0, 64450^0, 64451^0, 64454^0, 64461^0, 64462^0, 64463^0, 64479^0, 64480^0, 64483^0, 64484^0, 64486^0, 64487^0, 64488^0, 64489^0, 64490^0, 64491^0, 64492^0, 64493^0, 64494^0, 64495^0, 64505^0, 64510^0, 64517^0, 64520^0, 64530^0, 69990^0, 92012^1, 92014^1, 93000^1, 93005^1, 93010^1, 93040^1, 93041^1, 93042^1, 93318^1, 93355^1, 94002^1, 94200^1, 94680^1, 94681^1, 94690^1, 95812^1, 95813^1, 95816^1, 95819^1, 95822^1, 95829^1, 95955^1, 96360^1, 96361^1, 96365^1, 96366^1, 96367^1, 96368^1, 96372^1, 96374^1, 96375^1, 96376^1, 96377^1, 96523^0, 97597^1, 97598^1, 97602^1, 99155^0, 99156^0, 99157^0, 99211^1, 99212^1, 99213^1, 99214^1, 99215^1, 99217^1, 99218^1, 99219^1, 99220^1, 99221^1, 99222^1, 99223^1, 99231^1, 99232^1, 99233^1, 99234^1, 99235^1, 99236^1, 99238^1, 99239^1, 99241^1, 99242^1, 99243^1, 99244^1, 99245^1, 99251^1, 99252^1, 99253^1, 99254^1, 99255^1, 99291^1, 99292^1, 99304^1, 99305^1, 99306^1, 99307^1, 99308^1, 99309^1, 99310^1, 99315^1, 99316^1, 99334^1, 99335^1, 99336^1, 99337^1, 99347^1, 99348^1, 99349^1, 99350^1, 99374^1, 99375^1, 99377^1, 99378^1, 99446^0, 99447^0, 99448^0, 99449^0, 99451^0, 99452^0, 99495^0, 99496^0, G0463^1, G0471^0, J0670^1, J2001^1
54065	0213T^0, 0216T^0, 0596T^1, 0597T^1, 0708T^1, 0709T^1, 12001^1, 12002^1, 12004^1, 12005^1, 12006^1, 12007^1, 12011^1, 12013^1, 12014^1, 12015^1, 12016^1, 12017^1, 12018^1, 12020^1, 12021^1, 12031^1, 12032^1, 12034^1, 12035^1, 12036^1, 12037^1, 12041^1, 12042^1, 12044^1, 12045^1, 12046^1, 12047^1, 12051^1, 12052^1, 12053^1, 12054^1, 12055^1, 12056^1, 12057^1, 13100^1, 13101^1, 13102^1, 13120^1, 13121^1, 13122^1, 13131^1, 13132^1, 13133^1, 13151^1, 13152^1, 13153^1, 36000^1, 36400^1, 36405^1, 36406^1, 36410^1, 36420^1, 36425^1, 36430^1, 36440^1, 36591^0, 36592^0, 36600^1, 36640^1, 43752^1, 51701^0, 51702^0, 51703^1, 54050^1, 54055^1, 54056^1, 54057^1, 54060^1, 62320^0, 62321^0, 62322^0, 62323^0, 62324^0, 62325^0, 62326^0, 62327^0, 64400^0, 64405^0, 64408^0, 64415^0, 64416^0, 64417^0, 64418^0, 64420^0, 64421^0, 64425^0, 64430^0, 64435^0, 64445^0, 64446^0, 64447^0, 64448^0, 64449^0, 64450^0, 64451^0, 64454^0, 64461^0, 64462^0, 64463^0, 64479^0, 64480^0, 64483^0, 64484^0, 64486^0, 64487^0, 64488^0, 64489^0, 64490^0, 64491^0, 64492^0, 64493^0, 64494^0, 64495^0, 64505^0, 64510^0, 64517^0, 64520^0, 64530^0, 69990^0, 92012^1, 92014^1, 93000^1, 93005^1, 93010^1, 93040^1, 93041^1, 93042^1, 93318^1, 93355^1, 94002^1, 94200^1, 94680^1, 94681^1, 94690^1, 95812^1, 95813^1, 95816^1, 95819^1, 95822^1, 95829^1, 95955^1, 96360^1, 96361^1, 96365^1, 96366^1, 96367^1, 96368^1, 96372^1, 96374^1, 96375^1, 96376^1, 96377^1, 96523^0, 99155^0, 99156^0, 99157^0, 99211^1, 99212^1, 99213^1, 99214^1, 99215^1, 99217^1, 99218^1, 99219^1, 99220^1, 99221^1, 99222^1, 99223^1, 99231^1, 99232^1, 99233^1, 99234^1, 99235^1, 99236^1, 99238^1, 99239^1, 99241^1, 99242^1, 99243^1, 99244^1, 99245^1, 99251^1, 99252^1, 99253^1, 99254^1, 99255^1, 99291^1, 99292^1, 99304^1, 99305^1, 99306^1, 99307^1, 99308^1, 99309^1, 99310^1, 99315^1, 99316^1, 99334^1, 99335^1, 99336^1, 99337^1, 99347^1, 99348^1, 99349^1, 99350^1, 99374^1, 99375^1, 99377^1, 99378^1, 99446^0, 99447^0, 99448^0, 99449^0, 99451^0, 99452^0, 99495^0, 99496^0, G0463^1, G0471^0, J0670^1, J2001^1
54100	0213T^0, 0216T^0, 0596T^1, 0597T^1, 0708T^1, 0709T^1, 10005^1, 10007^1, 10009^1, 10011^1, 10021^1, 11102^1, 11103^1, 11104^1, 11105^1, 11106^1, 11107^1, 12001^1, 12002^1, 12004^1, 12005^1, 12006^1, 12007^1, 12011^1, 12013^1, 12014^1, 12015^1, 12016^1, 12017^1, 12018^1, 12020^1, 12021^1, 12031^1, 12032^1, 12034^1, 12035^1, 12036^1, 12037^1, 12041^1, 12042^1, 12044^1, 12045^1, 12046^1, 12047^1, 12051^1, 12052^1, 12053^1, 12054^1, 12055^1, 12056^1, 12057^1, 13100^1, 13101^1, 13102^1, 13120^1, 13121^1, 13122^1, 13131^1, 13132^1, 13133^1, 13151^1, 13152^1, 13153^1, 36000^1, 36400^1, 36405^1, 36406^1, 36410^1, 36420^1, 36425^1, 36430^1, 36440^1, 36591^0, 36592^0, 36600^1, 36640^1, 43752^1, 51701^0, 51703^1, 54001^0, 62320^0, 62321^0, 62322^0, 62323^0, 62324^0, 62325^0, 62326^0, 62327^0, 64400^0, 64405^0, 64408^0, 64415^0, 64416^0, 64417^0, 64418^0, 64420^0, 64421^0, 64425^0, 64430^0, 64435^0, 64445^0, 64446^0, 64447^0, 64448^0, 64449^0, 64450^0, 64451^0, 64454^0, 64461^0, 64462^0, 64463^0, 64479^0, 64480^0, 64483^0, 64484^0, 64486^0, 64487^0, 64488^0, 64489^0, 64490^0, 64491^0, 64492^0, 64493^0, 64494^0, 64495^0, 64505^0, 64510^0, 64517^0, 64520^0, 64530^0, 69990^0, 92012^1, 92014^1, 93000^1, 93005^1, 93010^1, 93040^1, 93041^1, 93042^1, 93318^1, 93355^1, 94002^1, 94200^1, 94680^1, 94681^1, 94690^1, 95812^1, 95813^1, 95816^1, 95819^1, 95822^1, 95829^1, 95955^1, 96360^1, 96361^1, 96365^1, 96366^1, 96367^1, 96368^1, 96372^1, 96374^1, 96375^1, 96376^1, 96377^1, 96523^0, 99155^0, 99156^0, 99157^0, 99211^1, 99212^1, 99213^1, 99214^1, 99215^1, 99217^1, 99218^1, 99219^1, 99220^1, 99221^1, 99222^1, 99223^1, 99231^1, 99232^1, 99233^1, 99234^1, 99235^1, 99236^1, 99238^1, 99239^1, 99241^1, 99242^1, 99243^1, 99244^1, 99245^1, 99251^1, 99252^1, 99253^1, 99254^1, 99255^1, 99291^1, 99292^1, 99304^1, 99305^1, 99306^1, 99307^1, 99308^1, 99309^1, 99310^1, 99315^1, 99316^1, 99334^1, 99335^1, 99336^1, 99337^1, 99347^1, 99348^1, 99349^1, 99350^1, 99374^1, 99375^1, 99377^1, 99378^1, 99446^0, 99447^0, 99448^0, 99449^0, 99451^0, 99452^0, 99495^1, 99496^1, G0463^1, J0670^1, J2001^1
54105	0213T^0, 0216T^0, 0596T^1, 0597T^1, 0708T^1, 0709T^1, 10005^1, 10007^1, 10009^1, 10011^1, 10021^1, 12001^1, 12002^1, 12004^1, 12005^1, 12006^1, 12007^1, 12011^1, 12013^1, 12014^1, 12015^1, 12016^1, 12017^1, 12018^1, 12020^1, 12021^1, 12031^1, 12032^1, 12034^1, 12035^1, 12036^1, 12037^1, 12041^1, 12042^1, 12044^1, 12045^1, 12046^1, 12047^1, 12051^1, 12052^1, 12053^1, 12054^1, 12055^1, 12056^1, 12057^1, 13100^1, 13101^1, 13102^1, 13120^1, 13121^1, 13122^1, 13131^1, 13132^1, 13133^1, 13151^1, 13152^1, 13153^1, 36000^1, 36400^1, 36405^1, 36406^1, 36410^1, 36420^1, 36425^1, 36430^1, 36440^1, 36591^0, 36592^0, 36600^1, 36640^1, 43752^1, 51701^0, 51702^0, 51703^1, 54100^1, 62320^0, 62321^0, 62322^0, 62323^0, 62324^0, 62325^0, 62326^0, 62327^0, 64400^0, 64405^0, 64408^0, 64415^0, 64416^0, 64417^0, 64418^0, 64420^0, 64421^0, 64425^0, 64430^0, 64435^0, 64445^0, 64446^0, 64447^0, 64448^0, 64449^0, 64450^0, 64451^0, 64454^0, 64461^0, 64462^0, 64463^0, 64479^0, 64480^0, 64483^0, 64484^0, 64486^0, 64487^0, 64488^0, 64489^0, 64490^0, 64491^0, 64492^0, 64493^0, 64494^0, 64495^0, 64505^0, 64510^0, 64517^0, 64520^0, 64530^0, 69990^0, 92012^1, 92014^1, 93000^1, 93005^1, 93010^1, 93040^1, 93041^1, 93042^1, 93318^1, 93355^1, 94002^1, 94200^1, 94680^1, 94681^1, 94690^1, 95812^1, 95813^1, 95816^1, 95819^1, 95822^1, 95829^1, 95955^1, 96360^1, 96361^1, 96365^1, 96366^1, 96367^1, 96368^1, 96372^1, 96374^1, 96375^1, 96376^1, 96377^1, 96523^0, 99155^0, 99156^0, 99157^0, 99211^1, 99212^1, 99213^1, 99214^1, 99215^1, 99217^1, 99218^1, 99219^1, 99220^1, 99221^1, 99222^1, 99223^1, 99231^1, 99232^1, 99233^1, 99234^1, 99235^1, 99236^1, 99238^1, 99239^1, 99241^1, 99242^1, 99243^1, 99244^1, 99245^1, 99251^1, 99252^1, 99253^1, 99254^1, 99255^1, 99291^1, 99292^1, 99304^1, 99305^1, 99306^1, 99307^1, 99308^1, 99309^1, 99310^1, 99315^1, 99316^1, 99334^1, 99335^1, 99336^1, 99337^1, 99347^1, 99348^1, 99349^1, 99350^1, 99374^1, 99375^1, 99377^1, 99378^1, 99446^0, 99447^0, 99448^0, 99449^0, 99451^0, 99452^0, 99495^0, 99496^0, G0463^1, G0471^0, J0670^1, J2001^1
54110	0213T^0, 0216T^0, 0596T^1, 0597T^1, 0708T^1, 0709T^1, 11000^1, 11001^1, 11004^1, 11005^1, 11006^1, 11042^1, 11043^1, 11044^1, 11045^1, 11046^1, 11047^1, 12001^1, 12002^1, 12004^1, 12005^1, 12006^1, 12007^1, 12011^1, 12013^1, 12014^1, 12015^1, 12016^1, 12017^1, 12018^1, 12020^1, 12021^1, 12031^1, 12032^1, 12034^1, 12035^1, 12036^1, 12037^1, 12041^1, 12042^1, 12044^1, 12045^1, 12046^1, 12047^1, 12051^1, 12052^1, 12053^1, 12054^1, 12055^1, 12056^1, 12057^1, 13100^1, 13101^1, 13102^1, 13120^1, 13121^1, 13122^1, 13131^1, 13132^1, 13133^1, 13151^1, 13152^1, 13153^1, 36000^1, 36400^1, 36405^1, 36406^1, 36410^1, 36420^1, 36425^1, 36430^1, 36440^1, 36591^0, 36592^0, 36600^1, 36640^1, 43752^1, 51701^0, 51702^0, 51703^1, 54100^1, 54105^1, 54200^1, 54205^1, 62320^0, 62321^0, 62322^0, 62323^0, 62324^0, 62325^0, 62326^0, 62327^0, 64400^0, 64405^0, 64408^0, 64415^0, 64416^0, 64417^0, 64418^0, 64420^0, 64421^0, 64425^0, 64430^0, 64435^0, 64445^0, 64446^0, 64447^0, 64448^0, 64449^0, 64450^0, 64451^0, 64454^0, 64461^0, 64462^0, 64463^0, 64479^0, 64480^0, 64483^0, 64484^0, 64486^0, 64487^0, 64488^0, 64489^0, 64490^0, 64491^0, 64492^0, 64493^0, 64494^0, 64495^0, 64505^0, 64510^0, 64517^0, 64520^0, 64530^0, 69990^0, 92012^1, 92014^1, 93000^1, 93005^1, 93010^1, 93040^1, 93041^1, 93042^1, 93318^1, 93355^1, 94002^1, 94200^1, 94680^1, 94681^1, 94690^1, 95812^1, 95813^1, 95816^1, 95819^1, 95822^1, 95829^1, 95955^1, 96360^1, 96361^1, 96365^1, 96366^1, 96367^1, 96368^1, 96372^1, 96374^1, 96375^1, 96376^1, 96377^1, 96523^0, 97597^1, 97598^1, 97602^1, 99155^0, 99156^0, 99157^0, 99211^1, 99212^1, 99213^1, 99214^1, 99215^1, 99217^1, 99218^1, 99219^1, 99220^1, 99221^1, 99222^1, 99223^1, 99231^1, 99232^1, 99233^1, 99234^1, 99235^1, 99236^1, 99238^1, 99239^1, 99241^1, 99242^1, 99243^1, 99244^1, 99245^1, 99251^1, 99252^1, 99253^1, 99254^1, 99255^1, 99291^1, 99292^1, 99304^1, 99305^1, 99306^1, 99307^1, 99308^1, 99309^1, 99310^1, 99315^1, 99316^1, 99334^1, 99335^1, 99336^1, 99337^1, 99347^1, 99348^1, 99349^1, 99350^1, 99374^1, 99375^1, 99377^1, 99378^1, 99446^0, 99447^0, 99448^0, 99449^0, 99451^0, 99452^0, 99495^0, 99496^0, G0463^1, G0471^0
54111	0213T^0, 0216T^0, 0596T^1, 0597T^1, 0708T^1, 0709T^1, 11000^1, 11001^1, 11004^1, 11005^1, 11006^1, 11042^1, 11043^1, 11044^1, 11045^1, 11046^1, 11047^1, 12001^1, 12002^1, 12004^1, 12005^1, 12006^1, 12007^1, 12011^1, 12013^1, 12014^1, 12015^1, 12016^1, 12017^1, 12018^1, 12020^1, 12021^1, 12031^1, 12032^1, 12034^1, 12035^1, 12036^1, 12037^1, 12041^1, 12042^1, 12044^1, 12045^1, 12046^1, 12047^1, 12051^1, 12052^1, 12053^1, 12054^1, 12055^1, 12056^1, 12057^1, 13100^1, 13101^1, 13102^1, 13120^1, 13121^1, 13122^1, 13131^1, 13132^1, 13133^1, 13151^1, 13152^1, 13153^1, 36000^1, 36400^1, 36405^1, 36406^1, 36410^1, 36420^1, 36425^1, 36430^1, 36440^1, 36591^0, 36592^0, 36600^1, 36640^1, 43752^1, 51701^0, 51702^0, 51703^1, 54100^1, 54105^1, 54110^1, 54112^1, 54115^1, 54200^1, 54205^1, 62320^0, 62321^0, 62322^0, 62323^0, 62324^0, 62325^0, 62326^0, 62327^0, 64400^0, 64405^0, 64408^0, 64415^0, 64416^0, 64417^0, 64418^0, 64420^0, 64421^0, 64425^0, 64430^0, 64435^0, 64445^0, 64446^0, 64447^0, 64448^0, 64449^0, 64450^0, 64451^0, 64454^0, 64461^0, 64462^0, 64463^0, 64479^0, 64480^0, 64483^0, 64484^0, 64486^0, 64487^0, 64488^0, 64489^0, 64490^0, 64491^0, 64492^0, 64493^0,

0 = Modifier usage not allowed or inappropriate 1 = Modifier usage allowed

Code 1	Code 2
	64494[0], 64495[0], 64505[0], 64510[0], 64517[0], 64520[0], 64530[0], 69990[0], 92012[1], 92014[1], 93000[1], 93005[1], 93010[1], 93040[1], 93041[1], 93042[1], 93318[1], 93355[1], 94002[1], 94200[1], 94680[1], 94681[1], 94690[1], 95812[1], 95813[1], 95816[1], 95819[1], 95822[1], 95829[1], 95955[1], 96360[1], 96361[1], 96365[1], 96366[1], 96367[1], 96368[1], 96372[1], 96374[1], 96375[1], 96376[1], 96377[1], 96523[0], 97597[1], 97598[1], 97602[1], 99155[0], 99156[0], 99157[0], 99211[1], 99212[1], 99213[1], 99214[1], 99215[1], 99217[1], 99218[1], 99219[1], 99220[1], 99221[1], 99222[1], 99223[1], 99231[1], 99232[1], 99233[1], 99234[1], 99235[1], 99236[1], 99238[1], 99239[1], 99241[1], 99242[1], 99243[1], 99244[1], 99245[1], 99251[1], 99252[1], 99253[1], 99254[1], 99255[1], 99291[1], 99292[1], 99304[1], 99305[1], 99306[1], 99307[1], 99308[1], 99309[1], 99310[1], 99315[1], 99316[1], 99334[1], 99335[1], 99336[1], 99337[1], 99347[1], 99348[1], 99349[1], 99350[1], 99374[1], 99375[1], 99377[1], 99378[1], 99446[0], 99447[0], 99448[0], 99449[0], 99451[0], 99452[0], 99495[0], 99496[0], G0463[1], G0471[0]
54112	0213T[0], 0216T[0], 0596T[1], 0597T[1], 0708T[1], 0709T[1], 11000[1], 11001[1], 11004[1], 11005[1], 11006[1], 11042[1], 11043[1], 11044[1], 11045[1], 11046[1], 11047[1], 12001[1], 12002[1], 12004[1], 12005[1], 12006[1], 12007[1], 12011[1], 12013[1], 12014[1], 12015[1], 12016[1], 12017[1], 12018[1], 12020[1], 12021[1], 12031[1], 12032[1], 12034[1], 12035[1], 12036[1], 12037[1], 12041[1], 12042[1], 12044[1], 12045[1], 12046[1], 12047[1], 12051[1], 12052[1], 12053[1], 12054[1], 12055[1], 12056[1], 12057[1], 13100[1], 13101[1], 13102[1], 13120[1], 13121[1], 13122[1], 13131[1], 13132[1], 13133[1], 13151[1], 13152[1], 13153[1], 36000[1], 36400[1], 36405[1], 36406[1], 36410[1], 36420[1], 36425[1], 36430[1], 36440[1], 36591[0], 36592[0], 36600[1], 36640[1], 43752[1], 51701[0], 51702[0], 51703[1], 54100[1], 54105[1], 54110[1], 54115[1], 54200[1], 54205[1], 62320[0], 62321[0], 62322[0], 62323[0], 62324[0], 62325[0], 62326[0], 62327[0], 64400[0], 64405[0], 64408[0], 64415[0], 64416[0], 64417[0], 64418[0], 64420[0], 64421[0], 64425[0], 64430[0], 64435[0], 64445[0], 64446[0], 64447[0], 64448[0], 64449[0], 64450[0], 64451[0], 64454[0], 64461[0], 64462[0], 64463[0], 64479[0], 64480[0], 64483[0], 64484[0], 64486[0], 64487[0], 64488[0], 64489[0], 64490[0], 64491[0], 64492[0], 64493[0], 64494[0], 64495[0], 64505[0], 64510[0], 64517[0], 64520[0], 64530[0], 69990[0], 92012[1], 92014[1], 93000[1], 93005[1], 93010[1], 93040[1], 93041[1], 93042[1], 93318[1], 93355[1], 94002[1], 94200[1], 94680[1], 94681[1], 94690[1], 95812[1], 95813[1], 95816[1], 95819[1], 95822[1], 95829[1], 95955[1], 96360[1], 96361[1], 96365[1], 96366[1], 96367[1], 96368[1], 96372[1], 96374[1], 96375[1], 96376[1], 96377[1], 96523[0], 97597[1], 97598[1], 97602[1], 99155[0], 99156[0], 99157[0], 99211[1], 99212[1], 99213[1], 99214[1], 99215[1], 99217[1], 99218[1], 99219[1], 99220[1], 99221[1], 99222[1], 99223[1], 99231[1], 99232[1], 99233[1], 99234[1], 99235[1], 99236[1], 99238[1], 99239[1], 99241[1], 99242[1], 99243[1], 99244[1], 99245[1], 99251[1], 99252[1], 99253[1], 99254[1], 99255[1], 99291[1], 99292[1], 99304[1], 99305[1], 99306[1], 99307[1], 99308[1], 99309[1], 99310[1], 99315[1], 99316[1], 99334[1], 99335[1], 99336[1], 99337[1], 99347[1], 99348[1], 99349[1], 99350[1], 99374[1], 99375[1], 99377[1], 99378[1], 99446[0], 99447[0], 99448[0], 99449[0], 99451[0], 99452[0], 99495[0], 99496[0], G0463[1], G0471[0]
54115	0213T[0], 0216T[0], 0596T[1], 0597T[1], 0708T[1], 0709T[1], 11000[1], 11001[1], 11004[1], 11005[1], 11006[1], 11042[1], 11043[1], 11044[1], 11045[1], 11046[1], 11047[1], 12001[1], 12002[1], 12004[1], 12005[1], 12006[1], 12007[1], 12011[1], 12013[1], 12014[1], 12015[1], 12016[1], 12017[1], 12018[1], 12020[1], 12021[1], 12031[1], 12032[1], 12034[1], 12035[1], 12036[1], 12037[1], 12041[1], 12042[1], 12044[1], 12045[1], 12046[1], 12047[1], 12051[1], 12052[1], 12053[1], 12054[1], 12055[1], 12056[1], 12057[1], 13100[1], 13101[1], 13102[1], 13120[1], 13121[1], 13122[1], 13131[1], 13132[1], 13133[1], 13151[1], 13152[1], 13153[1], 36000[1], 36400[1], 36405[1], 36406[1], 36410[1], 36420[1], 36425[1], 36430[1], 36440[1], 36591[0], 36592[0], 36600[1], 36640[1], 43752[1], 51701[0], 51702[0], 51703[1], 54100[1], 54110[0], 62320[0], 62321[0], 62322[0], 62323[0], 62324[0], 62325[0], 62326[0], 62327[0], 64400[0], 64405[0], 64408[0], 64415[0], 64416[0], 64417[0], 64418[0], 64420[0], 64421[0], 64425[0], 64430[0], 64435[0], 64445[0], 64446[0], 64447[0], 64448[0], 64449[0], 64450[0], 64451[0], 64454[0], 64461[0], 64462[0], 64463[0], 64479[0], 64480[0], 64483[0], 64484[0], 64486[0], 64487[0], 64488[0], 64489[0], 64490[0], 64491[0], 64492[0], 64493[0], 64494[0], 64495[0], 64505[0], 64510[0], 64517[0], 64520[0], 64530[0], 69990[0], 92012[1], 92014[1], 93000[1], 93005[1], 93010[1], 93040[1], 93041[1], 93042[1], 93318[1], 93355[1], 94002[1], 94200[1], 94680[1], 94681[1], 94690[1], 95812[1], 95813[1], 95816[1], 95819[1], 95822[1], 95829[1], 95955[1], 96360[1], 96361[1], 96365[1], 96366[1], 96367[1], 96368[1], 96372[1], 96374[1], 96375[1], 96376[1], 96377[1], 96523[0], 97597[1], 97598[1], 97602[1], 99155[0], 99156[0], 99157[0], 99211[1], 99212[1], 99213[1], 99214[1], 99215[1], 99217[1], 99218[1], 99219[1], 99220[1], 99221[1], 99222[1], 99223[1], 99231[1], 99232[1], 99233[1], 99234[1], 99235[1], 99236[1], 99238[1], 99239[1], 99241[1], 99242[1], 99243[1], 99244[1], 99245[1], 99251[1], 99252[1], 99253[1], 99254[1], 99255[1], 99291[1], 99292[1], 99304[1], 99305[1], 99306[1], 99307[1], 99308[1], 99309[1], 99310[1], 99315[1], 99316[1], 99334[1], 99335[1], 99336[1], 99337[1], 99347[1], 99348[1], 99349[1], 99350[1], 99374[1], 99375[1], 99377[1], 99378[1], 99446[0], 99447[0], 99448[0], 99449[0], 99451[0], 99452[0], 99495[0], 99496[0], G0463[1], G0471[0], J0670[1], J2001[1]
54120	0213T[0], 0216T[0], 0596T[1], 0597T[1], 0708T[1], 0709T[1], 12001[1], 12002[1], 12004[1], 12005[1], 12006[1], 12007[1], 12011[1], 12013[1], 12014[1], 12015[1], 12016[1], 12017[1], 12018[1], 12020[1], 12021[1], 12031[1], 12032[1], 12034[1], 12035[1], 12036[1], 12037[1], 12041[1], 12042[1], 12044[1], 12045[1], 12046[1], 12047[1], 12051[1], 12052[1], 12053[1], 12054[1], 12055[1], 12056[1], 12057[1], 13100[1], 13101[1], 13102[1], 13120[1], 13121[1], 13122[1], 13131[1], 13132[1], 13133[1], 13151[1], 13152[1], 13153[1], 36000[1], 36400[1], 36405[1], 36406[1], 36410[1], 36420[1], 36425[1], 36430[1], 36440[1], 36591[0], 36592[0], 36600[1], 36640[1], 43752[1], 51701[0], 51702[0], 51703[1], 54100[1], 54105[1], 54110[1], 54111[1], 54112[1], 54115[1], 62320[0], 62321[0], 62322[0], 62323[0], 62324[0], 62325[0], 62326[0], 62327[0], 64400[0], 64405[0], 64408[0], 64415[0], 64416[0], 64417[0], 64418[0], 64420[0], 64421[0], 64425[0], 64430[0], 64435[0], 64445[0], 64446[0], 64447[0], 64448[0], 64449[0], 64450[0], 64451[0], 64454[0], 64461[0], 64462[0], 64463[0], 64479[0], 64480[0], 64483[0], 64484[0], 64486[0], 64487[0], 64488[0], 64489[0], 64490[0], 64491[0], 64492[0], 64493[0], 64494[0], 64495[0], 64505[0], 64510[0], 64517[0], 64520[0], 64530[0], 69990[0], 92012[1], 92014[1], 93000[1], 93005[1], 93010[1], 93040[1], 93041[1], 93042[1], 93318[1], 93355[1], 94002[1], 94200[1], 94680[1], 94681[1], 94690[1], 95812[1], 95813[1], 95816[1], 95819[1], 95822[1], 95829[1], 95955[1], 96360[1], 96361[1], 96365[1], 96366[1], 96367[1], 96368[1], 96372[1], 96374[1], 96375[1], 96376[1], 96377[1], 96523[0], 99155[0], 99156[0], 99157[0], 99211[1], 99212[1], 99213[1], 99214[1], 99215[1], 99217[1], 99218[1], 99219[1], 99220[1], 99221[1], 99222[1], 99223[1], 99231[1], 99232[1], 99233[1], 99234[1], 99235[1], 99236[1], 99238[1], 99239[1], 99241[1], 99242[1], 99243[1], 99244[1], 99245[1], 99251[1], 99252[1], 99253[1], 99254[1], 99255[1], 99291[1], 99292[1], 99304[1], 99305[1], 99306[1], 99307[1], 99308[1], 99309[1], 99310[1], 99315[1], 99316[1], 99334[1], 99335[1], 99336[1], 99337[1], 99347[1], 99348[1], 99349[1], 99350[1], 99374[1], 99375[1], 99377[1], 99378[1], 99446[0], 99447[0], 99448[0], 99449[0], 99451[0], 99452[0], 99495[0], 99496[0], G0463[1], G0471[0]
54125	0213T[0], 0216T[0], 0596T[1], 0597T[1], 0708T[1], 0709T[1], 12001[1], 12002[1], 12004[1], 12005[1], 12006[1], 12007[1], 12011[1], 12013[1], 12014[1], 12015[1], 12016[1], 12017[1], 12018[1], 12020[1], 12021[1], 12031[1], 12032[1], 12034[1], 12035[1], 12036[1], 12037[1], 12041[1], 12042[1], 12044[1], 12045[1], 12046[1], 12047[1], 12051[1], 12052[1], 12053[1], 12054[1], 12055[1], 12056[1], 12057[1], 13100[1], 13101[1], 13102[1], 13120[1], 13121[1], 13122[1], 13131[1], 13132[1], 13133[1], 13151[1], 13152[1], 13153[1], 36000[1], 36400[1], 36405[1], 36406[1], 36410[1], 36420[1], 36425[1], 36430[1], 36440[1], 36591[0], 36592[0], 36600[1], 36640[1], 43752[1], 51701[0], 51702[0], 51703[1], 54100[0], 54105[0], 54110[1], 54111[1], 54112[1], 54115[1], 54120[1], 62320[0], 62321[0], 62322[0], 62323[0], 62324[0], 62325[0], 62326[0], 62327[0], 64400[0], 64405[0], 64408[0], 64415[0], 64416[0], 64417[0], 64418[0], 64420[0], 64421[0], 64425[0], 64430[0], 64435[0], 64445[0], 64446[0], 64447[0], 64448[0], 64449[0], 64450[0], 64451[0], 64454[0], 64461[0], 64462[0], 64463[0], 64479[0], 64480[0], 64483[0], 64484[0], 64486[0], 64487[0], 64488[0], 64489[0], 64490[0], 64491[0], 64492[0], 64493[0], 64494[0], 64495[0], 64505[0], 64510[0], 64517[0], 64520[0], 64530[0], 69990[0], 92012[1], 92014[1], 93000[1], 93005[1], 93010[1], 93040[1], 93041[1], 93042[1], 93318[1], 93355[1], 94002[1], 94200[1], 94680[1], 94681[1], 94690[1], 95812[1], 95813[1], 95816[1], 95819[1], 95822[1], 95829[1], 95955[1], 96360[1], 96361[1], 96365[1], 96366[1], 96367[1], 96368[1], 96372[1], 96374[1], 96375[1], 96376[1], 96377[1], 96523[0], 99155[0], 99156[0], 99157[0], 99211[1], 99212[1], 99213[1], 99214[1], 99215[1], 99217[1], 99218[1], 99219[1], 99220[1], 99221[1], 99222[1], 99223[1], 99231[1], 99232[1], 99233[1], 99234[1], 99235[1], 99236[1], 99238[1], 99239[1], 99241[1], 99242[1], 99243[1], 99244[1], 99245[1], 99251[1], 99252[1], 99253[1], 99254[1], 99255[1], 99291[1], 99292[1], 99304[1], 99305[1], 99306[1], 99307[1], 99308[1], 99309[1], 99310[1], 99315[1], 99316[1], 99334[1], 99335[1], 99336[1], 99337[1], 99347[1], 99348[1], 99349[1], 99350[1], 99374[1], 99375[1], 99377[1], 99378[1], 99446[0], 99447[0], 99448[0], 99449[0], 99451[0], 99452[0], 99495[0], 99496[0], G0463[1], G0471[0]
54130	0213T[0], 0216T[0], 0596T[1], 0597T[1], 0708T[1], 0709T[1], 11000[1], 11001[1], 11004[1], 11005[1], 11006[1], 11042[1], 11043[1], 11044[1], 11045[1], 11046[1], 11047[1], 12001[1], 12002[1], 12004[1], 12005[1], 12006[1], 12007[1], 12011[1], 12013[1], 12014[1], 12015[1], 12016[1], 12017[1], 12018[1], 12020[1], 12021[1], 12031[1], 12032[1], 12034[1], 12035[1], 12036[1], 12037[1], 12041[1], 12042[1], 12044[1], 12045[1], 12046[1], 12047[1], 12051[1], 12052[1], 12053[1], 12054[1], 12055[1], 12056[1], 12057[1], 13100[1], 13101[1], 13102[1], 13120[1], 13121[1], 13122[1], 13131[1], 13132[1], 13133[1], 13151[1], 13152[1], 13153[1], 36000[1], 36400[1], 36405[1], 36406[1], 36410[1], 36420[1], 36425[1], 36430[1], 36440[1], 36591[0], 36592[0], 36600[1], 36640[1], 38531[0], 38760[1], 43752[1], 51701[0], 51702[0], 51703[1], 54100[0], 54105[0], 62320[0], 62321[0], 62322[0], 62323[0], 62324[0], 62325[0], 62326[0], 62327[0], 64400[0], 64405[0], 64408[0], 64415[0], 64416[0], 64417[0], 64418[0], 64420[0], 64421[0], 64425[0], 64430[0], 64435[0], 64445[0], 64446[0], 64447[0], 64448[0], 64449[0], 64450[0], 64451[0], 64454[0], 64461[0], 64462[0], 64463[0], 64479[0], 64480[0], 64483[0], 64484[0], 64486[0], 64487[0], 64488[0], 64489[0], 64490[0], 64491[0], 64492[0], 64493[0], 64494[0], 64495[0], 64505[0], 64510[0], 64517[0], 64520[0], 64530[0], 69990[0], 92012[1], 92014[1], 93000[1], 93005[1], 93010[1], 93040[1], 93041[1], 93042[1], 93318[1], 93355[1], 94002[1], 94200[1], 94680[1], 94681[1], 94690[1], 95812[1], 95813[1], 95816[1], 95819[1], 95822[1], 95829[1], 95955[1], 96360[1], 96361[1], 96365[1], 96366[1], 96367[1], 96368[1], 96372[1], 96374[1], 96375[1], 96376[1], 96377[1], 96523[0], 97597[1], 97598[1], 97602[1], 99155[0], 99156[0], 99157[0], 99211[1], 99212[1], 99213[1], 99214[1], 99215[1], 99217[1], 99218[1], 99219[1], 99220[1], 99221[1], 99222[1], 99223[1], 99231[1], 99232[1], 99233[1], 99234[1], 99235[1], 99236[1], 99238[1], 99239[1], 99241[1], 99242[1], 99243[1], 99244[1], 99245[1], 99251[1], 99252[1], 99253[1], 99254[1], 99255[1], 99291[1], 99292[1], 99304[1], 99305[1], 99306[1], 99307[1], 99308[1], 99309[1], 99310[1], 99315[1], 99316[1], 99334[1], 99335[1], 99336[1], 99337[1], 99347[1], 99348[1], 99349[1], 99350[1], 99374[1], 99375[1], 99377[1], 99378[1], 99446[0], 99447[0], 99448[0], 99449[0], 99451[0], 99452[0], 99495[0], 99496[0], G0463[1], G0471[0]

0 = Modifier usage not allowed or inappropriate 1 = Modifier usage allowed

Code 1	Code 2
54135	0213T[0], 0216T[0], 0596T[1], 0597T[1], 0708T[1], 0709T[1], 11000[1], 11001[1], 11004[1], 11005[1], 11006[1], 11042[1], 11043[1], 11044[1], 11045[1], 11046[1], 11047[1], 12001[1], 12002[1], 12004[1], 12005[1], 12006[1], 12007[1], 12011[1], 12013[1], 12014[1], 12015[1], 12016[1], 12017[1], 12018[1], 12020[1], 12021[1], 12031[1], 12032[1], 12034[1], 12035[1], 12036[1], 12037[1], 12041[1], 12042[1], 12044[1], 12045[1], 12046[1], 12047[1], 12051[1], 12052[1], 12053[1], 12054[1], 12055[1], 12056[1], 12057[1], 13100[1], 13101[1], 13102[1], 13120[1], 13121[1], 13122[1], 13131[1], 13132[1], 13133[1], 13151[1], 13152[1], 13153[1], 36000[1], 36400[1], 36405[1], 36406[1], 36410[1], 36420[1], 36425[1], 36430[1], 36440[1], 36591[0], 36592[0], 36600[1], 36640[1], 38531[0], 38571[0], 38572[1], 38573[0], 38765[1], 43752[1], 51701[0], 51702[0], 51703[1], 52000[1], 54100[0], 54105[0], 62320[0], 62321[0], 62322[0], 62323[0], 62324[0], 62325[0], 62326[0], 62327[0], 64400[0], 64405[0], 64408[0], 64415[0], 64416[0], 64417[0], 64418[0], 64420[0], 64421[0], 64425[0], 64430[0], 64435[0], 64445[0], 64446[0], 64447[0], 64448[0], 64449[0], 64450[0], 64451[0], 64454[0], 64461[0], 64462[0], 64463[0], 64479[0], 64480[0], 64483[0], 64484[0], 64486[0], 64487[0], 64488[0], 64489[0], 64490[0], 64491[0], 64492[0], 64493[0], 64494[0], 64495[0], 64505[0], 64510[0], 64517[0], 64520[0], 64530[0], 69990[0], 92012[1], 92014[1], 93000[1], 93005[1], 93010[1], 93040[1], 93041[1], 93042[1], 93318[1], 93355[1], 94002[1], 94200[1], 94680[1], 94681[1], 94690[1], 95812[1], 95813[1], 95816[1], 95819[1], 95822[1], 95829[1], 95955[1], 96360[1], 96361[1], 96365[1], 96366[1], 96367[1], 96368[1], 96372[1], 96374[1], 96375[1], 96376[1], 96377[1], 96523[0], 97597[1], 97598[1], 97602[1], 99155[0], 99156[0], 99157[0], 99211[1], 99212[1], 99213[1], 99214[1], 99215[1], 99217[1], 99218[1], 99219[1], 99220[1], 99221[1], 99222[1], 99223[1], 99231[1], 99232[1], 99233[1], 99234[1], 99235[1], 99236[1], 99238[1], 99239[1], 99241[1], 99242[1], 99243[1], 99244[1], 99245[1], 99251[1], 99252[1], 99253[1], 99254[1], 99255[1], 99291[1], 99292[1], 99304[1], 99305[1], 99306[1], 99307[1], 99308[1], 99309[1], 99310[1], 99315[1], 99316[1], 99334[1], 99335[1], 99336[1], 99337[1], 99347[1], 99348[1], 99349[1], 99350[1], 99374[1], 99375[1], 99377[1], 99378[1], 99446[0], 99447[0], 99448[0], 99449[0], 99451[0], 99452[0], 99495[0], 99496[0], G0463[1], G0471[0]
54150	0213T[0], 0216T[0], 0596T[1], 0597T[1], 0708T[1], 0709T[1], 12001[1], 12002[1], 12004[1], 12005[1], 12006[1], 12007[1], 12011[1], 12013[1], 12014[1], 12015[1], 12016[1], 12017[1], 12018[1], 12020[1], 12021[1], 12031[1], 12032[1], 12034[1], 12035[1], 12036[1], 12037[1], 12041[1], 12042[1], 12044[1], 12045[1], 12046[1], 12047[1], 12051[1], 12052[1], 12053[1], 12054[1], 12055[1], 12056[1], 12057[1], 13100[1], 13101[1], 13102[1], 13120[1], 13121[1], 13122[1], 13131[1], 13132[1], 13133[1], 13151[1], 13152[1], 13153[1], 36000[1], 36400[1], 36405[1], 36406[1], 36410[1], 36420[1], 36425[1], 36430[1], 36440[1], 36591[0], 36592[0], 36600[1], 36640[1], 43752[1], 51701[0], 51702[0], 51703[1], 54000[0], 54001[0], 54100[1], 54162[1], 54163[1], 54164[1], 62320[0], 62321[0], 62322[0], 62323[0], 62324[0], 62325[0], 62326[0], 62327[0], 64400[0], 64405[0], 64408[0], 64415[0], 64416[0], 64417[0], 64418[0], 64420[0], 64421[0], 64425[0], 64430[0], 64435[0], 64445[0], 64446[0], 64447[0], 64448[0], 64449[0], 64450[0], 64451[0], 64454[0], 64461[0], 64462[0], 64463[0], 64479[0], 64480[0], 64483[0], 64484[0], 64486[0], 64487[0], 64488[0], 64489[0], 64490[0], 64491[0], 64492[0], 64493[0], 64494[0], 64495[0], 64505[0], 64510[0], 64517[0], 64520[0], 64530[0], 69990[0], 92012[1], 92014[1], 93000[1], 93005[1], 93010[1], 93040[1], 93041[1], 93042[1], 93318[1], 93355[1], 94002[1], 94200[1], 94680[1], 94681[1], 94690[1], 95812[1], 95813[1], 95816[1], 95819[1], 95822[1], 95829[1], 95955[1], 96360[1], 96361[1], 96365[1], 96366[1], 96367[1], 96368[1], 96372[1], 96374[1], 96375[1], 96376[1], 96377[1], 96523[0], 99155[0], 99156[0], 99157[0], 99211[1], 99212[1], 99213[1], 99214[1], 99215[1], 99217[1], 99218[1], 99219[1], 99220[1], 99221[1], 99222[1], 99223[1], 99231[1], 99232[1], 99233[1], 99234[1], 99235[1], 99236[1], 99238[1], 99239[1], 99241[1], 99242[1], 99243[1], 99244[1], 99245[1], 99251[1], 99252[1], 99253[1], 99254[1], 99255[1], 99291[1], 99292[1], 99304[1], 99305[1], 99306[1], 99307[1], 99308[1], 99309[1], 99310[1], 99315[1], 99316[1], 99334[1], 99335[1], 99336[1], 99337[1], 99347[1], 99348[1], 99349[1], 99350[1], 99374[1], 99375[1], 99377[1], 99378[1], 99446[0], 99447[0], 99448[0], 99449[0], 99451[0], 99452[0], 99495[1], 99496[1], G0463[1], G0471[0], J0670[1], J2001[1]
54160	0213T[0], 0216T[0], 0596T[1], 0597T[1], 0708T[1], 0709T[1], 11000[1], 11001[1], 11004[1], 11005[1], 11006[1], 11042[1], 11043[1], 11044[1], 11045[1], 11046[1], 11047[1], 12001[1], 12002[1], 12004[1], 12005[1], 12006[1], 12007[1], 12011[1], 12013[1], 12014[1], 12015[1], 12016[1], 12017[1], 12018[1], 12020[1], 12021[1], 12031[1], 12032[1], 12034[1], 12035[1], 12036[1], 12037[1], 12041[1], 12042[1], 12044[1], 12045[1], 12046[1], 12047[1], 12051[1], 12052[1], 12053[1], 12054[1], 12055[1], 12056[1], 12057[1], 13100[1], 13101[1], 13102[1], 13120[1], 13121[1], 13122[1], 13131[1], 13132[1], 13133[1], 13151[1], 13152[1], 13153[1], 36000[1], 36400[1], 36405[1], 36406[1], 36410[1], 36420[1], 36425[1], 36430[1], 36440[1], 36591[0], 36592[0], 36600[1], 36640[1], 43752[1], 51701[0], 51702[0], 51703[1], 54000[0], 54001[0], 54100[1], 54162[1], 54163[1], 54164[1], 62320[0], 62321[0], 62322[0], 62323[0], 62324[0], 62325[0], 62326[0], 62327[0], 64400[0], 64405[0], 64408[0], 64415[0], 64416[0], 64417[0], 64418[0], 64420[0], 64421[0], 64425[0], 64430[0], 64435[0], 64445[0], 64446[0], 64447[0], 64448[0], 64449[0], 64450[0], 64451[0], 64454[0], 64461[0], 64462[0], 64463[0], 64479[0], 64480[0], 64483[0], 64484[0], 64486[0], 64487[0], 64488[0], 64489[0], 64490[0], 64491[0], 64492[0], 64493[0], 64494[0], 64495[0], 64505[0], 64510[0], 64517[0], 64520[0], 64530[0], 92012[1], 92014[1], 93000[1], 93005[1], 93010[1], 93040[1], 93041[1], 93042[1], 93318[1], 93355[1], 94002[1], 94200[1], 94680[1], 94681[1], 94690[1], 95812[1], 95813[1], 95816[1], 95819[1], 95822[1], 95829[1], 95955[1], 96360[1], 96361[1], 96365[1], 96366[1], 96367[1], 96368[1], 96372[1], 96374[1], 96375[1], 96376[1], 96377[1], 96523[0], 97597[1], 97598[1], 97602[1], 99155[0], 99156[0], 99157[0], 99211[1], 99212[1], 99213[1], 99214[1], 99215[1], 99217[1], 99218[1], 99219[1], 99220[1], 99221[1], 99222[1], 99223[1], 99231[1], 99232[1], 99233[1], 99234[1], 99235[1], 99236[1], 99238[1], 99239[1], 99241[1], 99242[1], 99243[1], 99244[1], 99245[1], 99251[1], 99252[1], 99253[1], 99254[1], 99255[1], 99291[1], 99292[1], 99304[1], 99305[1], 99306[1], 99307[1], 99308[1], 99309[1], 99310[1], 99315[1], 99316[1], 99334[1], 99335[1], 99336[1], 99337[1], 99347[1], 99348[1], 99349[1], 99350[1], 99374[1], 99375[1], 99377[1], 99378[1], 99446[0], 99447[0], 99448[0], 99449[0], 99451[0], 99452[0], 99495[0], 99496[0], G0463[1], G0471[0], J2001[1]
54161	0213T[0], 0216T[0], 0596T[1], 0597T[1], 0708T[1], 0709T[1], 11000[1], 11001[1], 11004[1], 11005[1], 11006[1], 11042[1], 11043[1], 11044[1], 11045[1], 11046[1], 11047[1], 12001[1], 12002[1], 12004[1], 12005[1], 12006[1], 12007[1], 12011[1], 12013[1], 12014[1], 12015[1], 12016[1], 12017[1], 12018[1], 12020[1], 12021[1], 12031[1], 12032[1], 12034[1], 12035[1], 12036[1], 12037[1], 12041[1], 12042[1], 12044[1], 12045[1], 12046[1], 12047[1], 12051[1], 12052[1], 12053[1], 12054[1], 12055[1], 12056[1], 12057[1], 13100[1], 13101[1], 13102[1], 13120[1], 13121[1], 13122[1], 13131[1], 13132[1], 13133[1], 13151[1], 13152[1], 13153[1], 36000[1], 36400[1], 36405[1], 36406[1], 36410[1], 36420[1], 36425[1], 36430[1], 36440[1], 36591[0], 36592[0], 36600[1], 36640[1], 43752[1], 51701[0], 51702[0], 51703[1], 54000[0], 54001[0], 54100[1], 54162[1], 54163[1], 54164[1], 54450[0], 62320[0], 62321[0], 62322[0], 62323[0], 62324[0], 62325[0], 62326[0], 62327[0], 64400[0], 64405[0], 64408[0], 64415[0], 64416[0], 64417[0], 64418[0], 64420[0], 64421[0], 64425[0], 64430[0], 64435[0], 64445[0], 64446[0], 64447[0], 64448[0], 64449[0], 64450[0], 64451[0], 64454[0], 64461[0], 64462[0], 64463[0], 64479[0], 64480[0], 64483[0], 64484[0], 64486[0], 64487[0], 64488[0], 64489[0], 64490[0], 64491[0], 64492[0], 64493[0], 64494[0], 64495[0], 64505[0], 64510[0], 64517[0], 64520[0], 64530[0], 69990[0], 92012[1], 92014[1], 93000[1], 93005[1], 93010[1], 93040[1], 93041[1], 93042[1], 93318[1], 93355[1], 94002[1], 94200[1], 94680[1], 94681[1], 94690[1], 95812[1], 95813[1], 95816[1], 95819[1], 95822[1], 95829[1], 95955[1], 96360[1], 96361[1], 96365[1], 96366[1], 96367[1], 96368[1], 96372[1], 96374[1], 96375[1], 96376[1], 96377[1], 96523[0], 97597[1], 97598[1], 97602[1], 99155[0], 99156[0], 99157[0], 99211[1], 99212[1], 99213[1], 99214[1], 99215[1], 99217[1], 99218[1], 99219[1], 99220[1], 99221[1], 99222[1], 99223[1], 99231[1], 99232[1], 99233[1], 99234[1], 99235[1], 99236[1], 99238[1], 99239[1], 99241[1], 99242[1], 99243[1], 99244[1], 99245[1], 99251[1], 99252[1], 99253[1], 99254[1], 99255[1], 99291[1], 99292[1], 99304[1], 99305[1], 99306[1], 99307[1], 99308[1], 99309[1], 99310[1], 99315[1], 99316[1], 99334[1], 99335[1], 99336[1], 99337[1], 99347[1], 99348[1], 99349[1], 99350[1], 99374[1], 99375[1], 99377[1], 99378[1], 99446[0], 99447[0], 99448[0], 99449[0], 99451[0], 99452[0], 99495[0], 99496[0], G0463[1], G0471[0]
54162	0213T[0], 0216T[0], 0596T[1], 0597T[1], 0708T[1], 0709T[1], 11000[1], 11001[1], 11004[1], 11005[1], 11006[1], 11042[1], 11043[1], 11044[1], 11045[1], 11046[1], 11047[1], 12001[1], 12002[1], 12004[1], 12005[1], 12006[1], 12007[1], 12011[1], 12013[1], 12014[1], 12015[1], 12016[1], 12017[1], 12018[1], 12020[1], 12021[1], 12031[1], 12032[1], 12034[1], 12035[1], 12036[1], 12037[1], 12041[1], 12042[1], 12044[1], 12045[1], 12046[1], 12047[1], 12051[1], 12052[1], 12053[1], 12054[1], 12055[1], 12056[1], 12057[1], 13100[1], 13101[1], 13102[1], 13120[1], 13121[1], 13122[1], 13131[1], 13132[1], 13133[1], 13151[1], 13152[1], 13153[1], 36000[1], 36400[1], 36405[1], 36406[1], 36410[1], 36420[1], 36425[1], 36430[1], 36440[1], 36591[0], 36592[0], 36600[1], 36640[1], 43752[1], 51701[0], 51702[0], 51703[1], 54000[1], 54001[0], 54100[1], 54164[1], 62320[0], 62321[0], 62322[0], 62323[0], 62324[0], 62325[0], 62326[0], 62327[0], 64400[0], 64405[0], 64408[0], 64415[0], 64416[0], 64417[0], 64418[0], 64420[0], 64421[0], 64425[0], 64430[0], 64435[0], 64445[0], 64446[0], 64447[0], 64448[0], 64449[0], 64450[0], 64451[0], 64454[0], 64461[0], 64462[0], 64463[0], 64479[0], 64480[0], 64483[0], 64484[0], 64486[0], 64487[0], 64488[0], 64489[0], 64490[0], 64491[0], 64492[0], 64493[0], 64494[0], 64495[0], 64505[0], 64510[0], 64517[0], 64520[0], 64530[0], 69990[0], 92012[1], 92014[1], 93000[1], 93005[1], 93010[1], 93040[1], 93041[1], 93042[1], 93318[1], 93355[1], 94002[1], 94200[1], 94680[1], 94681[1], 94690[1], 95812[1], 95813[1], 95816[1], 95819[1], 95822[1], 95829[1], 95955[1], 96360[1], 96361[1], 96365[1], 96366[1], 96367[1], 96368[1], 96372[1], 96374[1], 96375[1], 96376[1], 96377[1], 96523[0], 97597[1], 97598[1], 97602[1], 99155[0], 99156[0], 99157[0], 99211[1], 99212[1], 99213[1], 99214[1], 99215[1], 99217[1], 99218[1], 99219[1], 99220[1], 99221[1], 99222[1], 99223[1], 99231[1], 99232[1], 99233[1], 99234[1], 99235[1], 99236[1], 99238[1], 99239[1], 99241[1], 99242[1], 99243[1], 99244[1], 99245[1], 99251[1], 99252[1], 99253[1], 99254[1], 99255[1], 99291[1], 99292[1], 99304[1], 99305[1], 99306[1], 99307[1], 99308[1], 99309[1], 99310[1], 99315[1], 99316[1], 99334[1], 99335[1], 99336[1], 99337[1], 99347[1], 99348[1], 99349[1], 99350[1], 99374[1], 99375[1], 99377[1], 99378[1], 99446[0], 99447[0], 99448[0], 99449[0], 99451[0], 99452[0], 99495[0], 99496[0], G0463[1], G0471[0]
54163	0213T[0], 0216T[0], 0596T[1], 0597T[1], 0708T[1], 0709T[1], 12001[1], 12002[1], 12004[1], 12005[1], 12006[1], 12007[1], 12011[1], 12013[1], 12014[1], 12015[1], 12016[1], 12017[1], 12018[1], 12020[1], 12021[1], 12031[1], 12032[1], 12034[1], 12035[1], 12036[1], 12037[1], 12041[1], 12042[1], 12044[1], 12045[1], 12046[1], 12047[1], 12051[1], 12052[1], 12053[1], 12054[1], 12055[1], 12056[1], 12057[1], 13100[1], 13101[1], 13102[1], 13120[1], 13121[1], 13122[1], 13131[1], 13132[1], 13133[1], 13151[1], 13152[1], 13153[1], 36000[1], 36400[1], 36405[1], 36406[1], 36410[1], 36420[1], 36425[1], 36430[1], 36440[1], 36591[0], 36592[0], 36600[1], 36640[1], 43752[1], 51701[0], 51702[0], 51703[1], 54000[1], 54001[1], 54100[1], 54162[1], 54164[1], 62320[0], 62321[0], 62322[0], 62323[0], 62324[0], 62325[0], 62326[0], 62327[0], 64400[0], 64405[0], 64408[0], 64415[0], 64416[0], 64417[0], 64418[0], 64420[0], 64421[0], 64425[0], 64430[0], 64435[0], 64445[0], 64446[0], 64447[0], 64448[0], 64449[0], 64450[0],

0 = Modifier usage not allowed or inappropriate 1 = Modifier usage allowed

Code 1	Code 2
	64451[0], 64454[0], 64461[0], 64462[0], 64463[0], 64479[0], 64480[0], 64483[0], 64484[0], 64486[0], 64487[0], 64488[0], 64489[0], 64490[0], 64491[0], 64492[0], 64493[0], 64494[0], 64495[0], 64505[0], 64510[0], 64517[0], 64520[0], 64530[0], 69990[0], 92012[1], 92014[1], 93000[1], 93005[1], 93010[1], 93040[1], 93041[1], 93042[1], 93318[1], 93355[1], 94002[1], 94200[1], 94680[1], 94681[1], 94690[1], 95812[1], 95813[1], 95816[1], 95819[1], 95822[1], 95829[1], 95955[1], 96360[1], 96361[1], 96365[1], 96366[1], 96367[1], 96368[1], 96372[1], 96374[1], 96375[1], 96376[1], 96377[1], 96523[0], 99155[0], 99156[0], 99157[0], 99211[1], 99212[1], 99213[1], 99214[1], 99215[1], 99217[1], 99218[1], 99219[1], 99220[1], 99221[1], 99222[1], 99223[1], 99231[1], 99232[1], 99233[1], 99234[1], 99235[1], 99236[1], 99238[1], 99239[1], 99241[1], 99242[1], 99243[1], 99244[1], 99245[1], 99251[1], 99252[1], 99253[1], 99254[1], 99255[1], 99291[1], 99292[1], 99304[1], 99305[1], 99306[1], 99307[1], 99308[1], 99309[1], 99310[1], 99315[1], 99316[1], 99334[1], 99335[1], 99336[1], 99337[1], 99347[1], 99348[1], 99349[1], 99350[1], 99374[1], 99375[1], 99377[1], 99378[1], 99446[0], 99447[0], 99448[0], 99449[0], 99451[0], 99452[0], 99495[0], 99496[0], G0463[1], G0471[0]
54164	0213T[0], 0216T[0], 0596T[1], 0597T[1], 0708T[1], 0709T[1], 11000[1], 11001[1], 11004[1], 11005[1], 11006[1], 11042[1], 11043[1], 11044[1], 11045[1], 11046[1], 11047[1], 12001[1], 12002[1], 12004[1], 12005[1], 12006[1], 12007[1], 12011[1], 12013[1], 12014[1], 12015[1], 12016[1], 12017[1], 12018[1], 12020[1], 12021[1], 12031[1], 12032[1], 12034[1], 12035[1], 12036[1], 12037[1], 12041[1], 12042[1], 12044[1], 12045[1], 12046[1], 12047[1], 12051[1], 12052[1], 12053[1], 12054[1], 12055[1], 12056[1], 12057[1], 13100[1], 13101[1], 13102[1], 13120[1], 13121[1], 13122[1], 13131[1], 13132[1], 13133[1], 13151[1], 13152[1], 13153[1], 36000[1], 36400[1], 36405[1], 36406[1], 36410[1], 36420[1], 36425[1], 36430[1], 36440[1], 36591[0], 36592[0], 36600[1], 36640[1], 43752[1], 51701[0], 51702[0], 51703[1], 54000[1], 54001[1], 54100[1], 62320[0], 62321[0], 62322[0], 62323[0], 62324[0], 62325[0], 62326[0], 62327[0], 64400[0], 64405[0], 64408[0], 64415[0], 64416[0], 64417[0], 64418[0], 64420[0], 64421[0], 64425[0], 64430[0], 64435[0], 64445[0], 64446[0], 64447[0], 64448[0], 64449[0], 64450[0], 64451[0], 64454[0], 64461[0], 64462[0], 64463[0], 64479[0], 64480[0], 64483[0], 64484[0], 64486[0], 64487[0], 64488[0], 64489[0], 64490[0], 64491[0], 64492[0], 64493[0], 64494[0], 64495[0], 64505[0], 64510[0], 64517[0], 64520[0], 64530[0], 69990[0], 92012[1], 92014[1], 93000[1], 93005[1], 93010[1], 93040[1], 93041[1], 93042[1], 93318[1], 93355[1], 94002[1], 94200[1], 94680[1], 94681[1], 94690[1], 95812[1], 95813[1], 95816[1], 95819[1], 95822[1], 95829[1], 95955[1], 96360[1], 96361[1], 96365[1], 96366[1], 96367[1], 96368[1], 96372[1], 96374[1], 96375[1], 96376[1], 96377[1], 96523[0], 97597[1], 97598[1], 97602[1], 99155[0], 99156[0], 99157[0], 99211[1], 99212[1], 99213[1], 99214[1], 99215[1], 99217[1], 99218[1], 99219[1], 99220[1], 99221[1], 99222[1], 99223[1], 99231[1], 99232[1], 99233[1], 99234[1], 99235[1], 99236[1], 99238[1], 99239[1], 99241[1], 99242[1], 99243[1], 99244[1], 99245[1], 99251[1], 99252[1], 99253[1], 99254[1], 99255[1], 99291[1], 99292[1], 99304[1], 99305[1], 99306[1], 99307[1], 99308[1], 99309[1], 99310[1], 99315[1], 99316[1], 99334[1], 99335[1], 99336[1], 99337[1], 99347[1], 99348[1], 99349[1], 99350[1], 99374[1], 99375[1], 99377[1], 99378[1], 99446[0], 99447[0], 99448[0], 99449[0], 99451[0], 99452[0], 99495[0], 99496[0], G0463[1], G0471[0]
54200	0213T[0], 0216T[0], 0596T[1], 0597T[1], 0708T[1], 0709T[1], 12001[1], 12002[1], 12004[1], 12005[1], 12006[1], 12007[1], 12011[1], 12013[1], 12014[1], 12015[1], 12016[1], 12017[1], 12018[1], 12020[1], 12021[1], 12031[1], 12032[1], 12034[1], 12035[1], 12036[1], 12037[1], 12041[1], 12042[1], 12044[1], 12045[1], 12046[1], 12047[1], 12051[1], 12052[1], 12053[1], 12054[1], 12055[1], 12056[1], 12057[1], 13100[1], 13101[1], 13102[1], 13120[1], 13121[1], 13122[1], 13131[1], 13132[1], 13133[1], 13151[1], 13152[1], 13153[1], 36000[1], 36400[1], 36405[1], 36406[1], 36410[1], 36420[1], 36425[1], 36430[1], 36440[1], 36591[0], 36592[0], 36600[1], 36640[1], 43752[1], 51701[0], 51702[0], 51703[1], 62320[0], 62321[0], 62322[0], 62323[0], 62324[0], 62325[0], 62326[0], 62327[0], 64400[0], 64405[0], 64408[0], 64415[0], 64416[0], 64417[0], 64418[0], 64420[0], 64421[0], 64425[0], 64430[0], 64435[0], 64445[0], 64446[0], 64447[0], 64448[0], 64449[0], 64450[0], 64451[0], 64454[0], 64461[0], 64462[0], 64463[0], 64479[0], 64480[0], 64483[0], 64484[0], 64486[0], 64487[0], 64488[0], 64489[0], 64490[0], 64491[0], 64492[0], 64493[0], 64494[0], 64495[0], 64505[0], 64510[0], 64517[0], 64520[0], 64530[0], 69990[0], 92012[1], 92014[1], 93000[1], 93005[1], 93010[1], 93040[1], 93041[1], 93042[1], 93318[1], 93355[1], 94002[1], 94200[1], 94680[1], 94681[1], 94690[1], 95812[1], 95813[1], 95816[1], 95819[1], 95822[1], 95829[1], 95955[1], 96360[1], 96361[1], 96365[1], 96366[1], 96367[1], 96368[1], 96372[1], 96374[1], 96375[1], 96376[1], 96377[1], 96523[0], 99155[0], 99156[0], 99157[0], 99211[1], 99212[1], 99213[1], 99214[1], 99215[1], 99217[1], 99218[1], 99219[1], 99220[1], 99221[1], 99222[1], 99223[1], 99231[1], 99232[1], 99233[1], 99234[1], 99235[1], 99236[1], 99238[1], 99239[1], 99241[1], 99242[1], 99243[1], 99244[1], 99245[1], 99251[1], 99252[1], 99253[1], 99254[1], 99255[1], 99291[1], 99292[1], 99304[1], 99305[1], 99306[1], 99307[1], 99308[1], 99309[1], 99310[1], 99315[1], 99316[1], 99334[1], 99335[1], 99336[1], 99337[1], 99347[1], 99348[1], 99349[1], 99350[1], 99374[1], 99375[1], 99377[1], 99378[1], 99446[0], 99447[0], 99448[0], 99449[0], 99451[0], 99452[0], 99495[0], 99496[0], G0463[1], G0471[0], J0670[1], J2001[1]
54205	0213T[0], 0216T[0], 0596T[1], 0597T[1], 0708T[1], 0709T[1], 12001[1], 12002[1], 12004[1], 12005[1], 12006[1], 12007[1], 12011[1], 12013[1], 12014[1], 12015[1], 12016[1], 12017[1], 12018[1], 12020[1], 12021[1], 12031[1], 12032[1], 12034[1], 12035[1], 12036[1], 12037[1], 12041[1], 12042[1], 12044[1], 12045[1], 12046[1], 12047[1], 12051[1], 12052[1], 12053[1], 12054[1], 12055[1], 12056[1], 12057[1], 13100[1], 13101[1], 13102[1], 13120[1], 13121[1], 13122[1], 13131[1], 13132[1], 13133[1], 13151[1], 13152[1], 13153[1], 36000[1], 36400[1], 36405[1], 36406[1], 36410[1], 36420[1], 36425[1], 36430[1], 36440[1], 36591[0], 36592[0], 36600[1], 36640[1], 43752[1], 51701[0], 51702[0], 51703[1], 54200[1], 62320[0], 62321[0], 62322[0], 62323[0], 62324[0], 62325[0], 62326[0], 62327[0], 64400[0], 64405[0], 64408[0], 64415[0], 64416[0], 64417[0], 64418[0], 64420[0], 64421[0], 64425[0], 64430[0], 64435[0], 64445[0], 64446[0], 64447[0], 64448[0], 64449[0], 64450[0], 64451[0], 64454[0], 64461[0], 64462[0], 64463[0], 64479[0], 64480[0], 64483[0], 64484[0], 64486[0], 64487[0], 64488[0], 64489[0], 64490[0], 64491[0], 64492[0], 64493[0], 64494[0], 64495[0], 64505[0], 64510[0], 64517[0], 64520[0], 64530[0], 69990[0], 92012[1], 92014[1], 93000[1], 93005[1], 93010[1], 93040[1], 93041[1], 93042[1], 93318[1], 93355[1], 94002[1], 94200[1], 94680[1], 94681[1], 94690[1], 95812[1], 95813[1], 95816[1], 95819[1], 95822[1], 95829[1], 95955[1], 96360[1], 96361[1], 96365[1], 96366[1], 96367[1], 96368[1], 96372[1], 96374[1], 96375[1], 96376[1], 96377[1], 96523[0], 99155[0], 99156[0], 99157[0], 99211[1], 99212[1], 99213[1], 99214[1], 99215[1], 99217[1], 99218[1], 99219[1], 99220[1], 99221[1], 99222[1], 99223[1], 99231[1], 99232[1], 99233[1], 99234[1], 99235[1], 99236[1], 99238[1], 99239[1], 99241[1], 99242[1], 99243[1], 99244[1], 99245[1], 99251[1], 99252[1], 99253[1], 99254[1], 99255[1], 99291[1], 99292[1], 99304[1], 99305[1], 99306[1], 99307[1], 99308[1], 99309[1], 99310[1], 99315[1], 99316[1], 99334[1], 99335[1], 99336[1], 99337[1], 99347[1], 99348[1], 99349[1], 99350[1], 99374[1], 99375[1], 99377[1], 99378[1], 99446[0], 99447[0], 99448[0], 99449[0], 99451[0], 99452[0], 99495[0], 99496[0], G0463[1], G0471[0]
54220	0213T[0], 0216T[0], 0596T[1], 0597T[1], 0708T[1], 0709T[1], 12001[1], 12002[1], 12004[1], 12005[1], 12006[1], 12007[1], 12011[1], 12013[1], 12014[1], 12015[1], 12016[1], 12017[1], 12018[1], 12020[1], 12021[1], 12031[1], 12032[1], 12034[1], 12035[1], 12036[1], 12037[1], 12041[1], 12042[1], 12044[1], 12045[1], 12046[1], 12047[1], 12051[1], 12052[1], 12053[1], 12054[1], 12055[1], 12056[1], 12057[1], 13100[1], 13101[1], 13102[1], 13120[1], 13121[1], 13122[1], 13131[1], 13132[1], 13133[1], 13151[1], 13152[1], 13153[1], 36000[1], 36400[1], 36405[1], 36406[1], 36410[1], 36420[1], 36425[1], 36430[1], 36440[1], 36591[0], 36592[0], 36600[1], 36640[1], 43752[1], 51701[0], 51702[0], 51703[1], 62320[0], 62321[0], 62322[0], 62323[0], 62324[0], 62325[0], 62326[0], 62327[0], 64400[0], 64405[0], 64408[0], 64415[0], 64416[0], 64417[0], 64418[0], 64420[0], 64421[0], 64425[0], 64430[0], 64435[0], 64445[0], 64446[0], 64447[0], 64448[0], 64449[0], 64450[0], 64451[0], 64454[0], 64461[0], 64462[0], 64463[0], 64479[0], 64480[0], 64483[0], 64484[0], 64486[0], 64487[0], 64488[0], 64489[0], 64490[0], 64491[0], 64492[0], 64493[0], 64494[0], 64495[0], 64505[0], 64510[0], 64517[0], 64520[0], 64530[0], 69990[0], 92012[1], 92014[1], 93000[1], 93005[1], 93010[1], 93040[1], 93041[1], 93042[1], 93318[1], 93355[1], 94002[1], 94200[1], 94680[1], 94681[1], 94690[1], 95812[1], 95813[1], 95816[1], 95819[1], 95822[1], 95829[1], 95955[1], 96360[1], 96361[1], 96365[1], 96366[1], 96367[1], 96368[1], 96372[1], 96374[1], 96375[1], 96376[1], 96377[1], 96523[0], 99155[0], 99156[0], 99157[0], 99211[1], 99212[1], 99213[1], 99214[1], 99215[1], 99217[1], 99218[1], 99219[1], 99220[1], 99221[1], 99222[1], 99223[1], 99231[1], 99232[1], 99233[1], 99234[1], 99235[1], 99236[1], 99238[1], 99239[1], 99241[1], 99242[1], 99243[1], 99244[1], 99245[1], 99251[1], 99252[1], 99253[1], 99254[1], 99255[1], 99291[1], 99292[1], 99304[1], 99305[1], 99306[1], 99307[1], 99308[1], 99309[1], 99310[1], 99315[1], 99316[1], 99334[1], 99335[1], 99336[1], 99337[1], 99347[1], 99348[1], 99349[1], 99350[1], 99374[1], 99375[1], 99377[1], 99378[1], 99446[0], 99447[0], 99448[0], 99449[0], 99451[0], 99452[0], 99495[1], 99496[1], G0463[1], G0471[0], J0670[1], J2001[1]
54230	0213T[0], 0216T[0], 0596T[1], 0597T[1], 0708T[1], 0709T[1], 12001[1], 12002[1], 12004[1], 12005[1], 12006[1], 12007[1], 12011[1], 12013[1], 12014[1], 12015[1], 12016[1], 12017[1], 12018[1], 12020[1], 12021[1], 12031[1], 12032[1], 12034[1], 12035[1], 12036[1], 12037[1], 12041[1], 12042[1], 12044[1], 12045[1], 12046[1], 12047[1], 12051[1], 12052[1], 12053[1], 12054[1], 12055[1], 12056[1], 12057[1], 13100[1], 13101[1], 13102[1], 13120[1], 13121[1], 13122[1], 13131[1], 13132[1], 13133[1], 13151[1], 13152[1], 13153[1], 36000[1], 36400[1], 36405[1], 36406[1], 36410[1], 36420[1], 36425[1], 36430[1], 36440[1], 36591[0], 36592[0], 36600[1], 36640[1], 43752[1], 51701[0], 51702[0], 51703[1], 62320[0], 62321[0], 62322[0], 62323[0], 62324[0], 62325[0], 62326[0], 62327[0], 64400[0], 64405[0], 64408[0], 64415[0], 64416[0], 64417[0], 64418[0], 64420[0], 64421[0], 64425[0], 64430[0], 64435[0], 64445[0], 64446[0], 64447[0], 64448[0], 64449[0], 64450[0], 64451[0], 64454[0], 64461[0], 64462[0], 64463[0], 64479[0], 64480[0], 64483[0], 64484[0], 64486[0], 64487[0], 64488[0], 64489[0], 64490[0], 64491[0], 64492[0], 64493[0], 64494[0], 64495[0], 64505[0], 64510[0], 64517[0], 64520[0], 64530[0], 69990[0], 76000[1], 77001[1], 77002[1], 92012[1], 92014[1], 93000[1], 93005[1], 93010[1], 93040[1], 93041[1], 93042[1], 93318[1], 93355[1], 94002[1], 94200[1], 94680[1], 94681[1], 94690[1], 95812[1], 95813[1], 95816[1], 95819[1], 95822[1], 95829[1], 95955[1], 96360[1], 96361[1], 96365[1], 96366[1], 96367[1], 96368[1], 96372[1], 96374[1], 96375[1], 96376[1], 96377[1], 96523[0], 99155[0], 99156[0], 99157[0], 99211[1], 99212[1], 99213[1], 99214[1], 99215[1], 99217[1], 99218[1], 99219[1], 99220[1], 99221[1], 99222[1], 99223[1], 99231[1], 99232[1], 99233[1], 99234[1], 99235[1], 99236[1], 99238[1], 99239[1], 99241[1], 99242[1], 99243[1], 99244[1], 99245[1], 99251[1], 99252[1], 99253[1], 99254[1], 99255[1], 99291[1], 99292[1], 99304[1], 99305[1], 99306[1], 99307[1], 99308[1], 99309[1], 99310[1], 99315[1], 99316[1], 99334[1], 99335[1], 99336[1], 99337[1], 99347[1], 99348[1], 99349[1], 99350[1], 99374[1], 99375[1], 99377[1], 99378[1], 99446[0], 99447[0], 99448[0], 99449[0], 99451[0], 99452[0], 99495[1], 99496[1], G0463[1], G0471[0]

0 = Modifier usage not allowed or inappropriate   1 = Modifier usage allowed

Code 1	Code 2
54231	0213T[0], 0216T[0], 0596T[1], 0597T[1], 0708T[1], 0709T[1], 12001[1], 12002[1], 12004[1], 12005[1], 12006[1], 12007[1], 12011[1], 12013[1], 12014[1], 12015[1], 12016[1], 12017[1], 12018[1], 12020[1], 12021[1], 12031[1], 12032[1], 12034[1], 12035[1], 12036[1], 12037[1], 12041[1], 12042[1], 12044[1], 12045[1], 12046[1], 12047[1], 12051[1], 12052[1], 12053[1], 12054[1], 12055[1], 12056[1], 12057[1], 13100[1], 13101[1], 13102[1], 13120[1], 13121[1], 13122[1], 13131[1], 13132[1], 13133[1], 13151[1], 13152[1], 13153[1], 36000[1], 36400[1], 36405[1], 36406[1], 36410[1], 36420[1], 36425[1], 36430[1], 36440[1], 36591[0], 36592[0], 36600[1], 36640[1], 43752[1], 51701[0], 51702[0], 51703[1], 54235[1], 54240[1], 62320[0], 62321[0], 62322[0], 62323[0], 62324[0], 62325[0], 62326[0], 62327[0], 64400[0], 64405[0], 64408[0], 64415[0], 64416[0], 64417[0], 64418[0], 64420[0], 64421[0], 64425[0], 64430[0], 64435[0], 64445[0], 64446[0], 64447[0], 64448[0], 64449[0], 64450[0], 64451[0], 64454[0], 64461[0], 64462[0], 64463[0], 64479[0], 64480[0], 64483[0], 64484[0], 64486[0], 64487[0], 64488[0], 64489[0], 64490[0], 64491[0], 64492[0], 64493[0], 64494[0], 64495[0], 64505[0], 64510[0], 64517[0], 64520[0], 64530[0], 69990[0], 92012[1], 92014[1], 93000[1], 93005[1], 93010[1], 93040[1], 93041[1], 93042[1], 93318[1], 93355[1], 94002[1], 94200[1], 94680[1], 94681[1], 94690[1], 95812[1], 95813[1], 95816[1], 95819[1], 95822[1], 95829[1], 95955[1], 96360[1], 96361[1], 96365[1], 96366[1], 96367[1], 96368[1], 96372[1], 96374[1], 96375[1], 96376[1], 96377[1], 96523[0], 99155[0], 99156[0], 99157[0], 99211[1], 99212[1], 99213[1], 99214[1], 99215[1], 99217[1], 99218[1], 99219[1], 99220[1], 99221[1], 99222[1], 99223[1], 99231[1], 99232[1], 99233[1], 99234[1], 99235[1], 99236[1], 99238[1], 99239[1], 99241[1], 99242[1], 99243[1], 99244[1], 99245[1], 99251[1], 99252[1], 99253[1], 99254[1], 99255[1], 99291[1], 99292[1], 99304[1], 99305[1], 99306[1], 99307[1], 99308[1], 99309[1], 99310[1], 99315[1], 99316[1], 99334[1], 99335[1], 99336[1], 99337[1], 99347[1], 99348[1], 99349[1], 99350[1], 99374[1], 99375[1], 99377[1], 99378[1], 99446[0], 99447[0], 99448[0], 99449[0], 99451[0], 99452[0], 99495[1], 99496[1], G0463[1], G0471[0], J2001[1]
54235	0213T[0], 0216T[0], 0596T[1], 0597T[1], 0708T[1], 0709T[1], 12001[1], 12002[1], 12004[1], 12005[1], 12006[1], 12007[1], 12011[1], 12013[1], 12014[1], 12015[1], 12016[1], 12017[1], 12018[1], 12020[1], 12021[1], 12031[1], 12032[1], 12034[1], 12035[1], 12036[1], 12037[1], 12041[1], 12042[1], 12044[1], 12045[1], 12046[1], 12047[1], 12051[1], 12052[1], 12053[1], 12054[1], 12055[1], 12056[1], 12057[1], 13100[1], 13101[1], 13102[1], 13120[1], 13121[1], 13122[1], 13131[1], 13132[1], 13133[1], 13151[1], 13152[1], 13153[1], 36000[1], 36400[1], 36405[1], 36406[1], 36410[1], 36420[1], 36425[1], 36430[1], 36440[1], 36591[0], 36592[0], 36600[1], 36640[1], 43752[1], 51701[0], 51702[0], 51703[1], 62320[0], 62321[0], 62322[0], 62323[0], 62324[0], 62325[0], 62326[0], 62327[0], 64400[0], 64405[0], 64408[0], 64415[0], 64416[0], 64417[0], 64418[0], 64420[0], 64421[0], 64425[0], 64430[0], 64435[0], 64445[0], 64446[0], 64447[0], 64448[0], 64449[0], 64450[0], 64451[0], 64454[0], 64461[0], 64462[0], 64463[0], 64479[0], 64480[0], 64483[0], 64484[0], 64486[0], 64487[0], 64488[0], 64489[0], 64490[0], 64491[0], 64492[0], 64493[0], 64494[0], 64495[0], 64505[0], 64510[0], 64517[0], 64520[0], 64530[0], 69990[0], 92012[1], 92014[1], 93000[1], 93005[1], 93010[1], 93040[1], 93041[1], 93042[1], 93318[1], 93355[1], 94002[1], 94200[1], 94680[1], 94681[1], 94690[1], 95812[1], 95813[1], 95816[1], 95819[1], 95822[1], 95829[1], 95955[1], 96360[1], 96361[1], 96365[1], 96366[1], 96367[1], 96368[1], 96372[1], 96374[1], 96375[1], 96376[1], 96377[1], 96523[0], 99155[0], 99156[0], 99157[0], 99211[1], 99212[1], 99213[1], 99214[1], 99215[1], 99217[1], 99218[1], 99219[1], 99220[1], 99221[1], 99222[1], 99223[1], 99231[1], 99232[1], 99233[1], 99234[1], 99235[1], 99236[1], 99238[1], 99239[1], 99241[1], 99242[1], 99243[1], 99244[1], 99245[1], 99251[1], 99252[1], 99253[1], 99254[1], 99255[1], 99291[1], 99292[1], 99304[1], 99305[1], 99306[1], 99307[1], 99308[1], 99309[1], 99310[1], 99315[1], 99316[1], 99334[1], 99335[1], 99336[1], 99337[1], 99347[1], 99348[1], 99349[1], 99350[1], 99374[1], 99375[1], 99377[1], 99378[1], 99446[0], 99447[0], 99448[0], 99449[0], 99451[0], 99452[0], 99495[1], 99496[1], G0463[1], G0471[0]
54240	0213T[0], 0216T[0], 0596T[1], 0597T[1], 0708T[1], 0709T[1], 12001[1], 12002[1], 12004[1], 12005[1], 12006[1], 12007[1], 12011[1], 12013[1], 12014[1], 12015[1], 12016[1], 12017[1], 12018[1], 12020[1], 12021[1], 12031[1], 12032[1], 12034[1], 12035[1], 12036[1], 12037[1], 12041[1], 12042[1], 12044[1], 12045[1], 12046[1], 12047[1], 12051[1], 12052[1], 12053[1], 12054[1], 12055[1], 12056[1], 12057[1], 13100[1], 13101[1], 13102[1], 13120[1], 13121[1], 13122[1], 13131[1], 13132[1], 13133[1], 13151[1], 13152[1], 13153[1], 36000[1], 36400[1], 36405[1], 36406[1], 36410[1], 36420[1], 36425[1], 36430[1], 36440[1], 36591[0], 36592[0], 36600[1], 36640[1], 43752[1], 51701[0], 51702[0], 51703[1], 62320[0], 62321[0], 62322[0], 62323[0], 62324[0], 62325[0], 62326[0], 62327[0], 64400[0], 64405[0], 64408[0], 64415[0], 64416[0], 64417[0], 64418[0], 64420[0], 64421[0], 64425[0], 64430[0], 64435[0], 64445[0], 64446[0], 64447[0], 64448[0], 64449[0], 64450[0], 64451[0], 64454[0], 64461[0], 64462[0], 64463[0], 64479[0], 64480[0], 64483[0], 64484[0], 64486[0], 64487[0], 64488[0], 64489[0], 64490[0], 64491[0], 64492[0], 64493[0], 64494[0], 64495[0], 64505[0], 64510[0], 64517[0], 64520[0], 64530[0], 69990[0], 92012[1], 92014[1], 93000[1], 93005[1], 93010[1], 93040[1], 93041[1], 93042[1], 93318[1], 93355[1], 94002[1], 94200[1], 94680[1], 94681[1], 94690[1], 95812[1], 95813[1], 95816[1], 95819[1], 95822[1], 95829[1], 95955[1], 96360[1], 96361[1], 96365[1], 96366[1], 96367[1], 96368[1], 96372[1], 96374[1], 96375[1], 96376[1], 96377[1], 96523[0], 99155[0], 99156[0], 99157[0], 99211[1], 99212[1], 99213[1], 99214[1], 99215[1], 99217[1], 99218[1], 99219[1], 99220[1], 99221[1], 99222[1], 99223[1], 99231[1], 99232[1], 99233[1], 99234[1], 99235[1], 99236[1], 99238[1], 99239[1], 99241[1], 99242[1], 99243[1], 99244[1], 99245[1], 99251[1], 99252[1], 99253[1], 99254[1], 99255[1], 99291[1], 99292[1], 99304[1], 99305[1], 99306[1], 99307[1], 99308[1], 99309[1], 99310[1], 99315[1], 99316[1], 99334[1], 99335[1], 99336[1], 99337[1], 99347[1], 99348[1], 99349[1], 99350[1], 99374[1], 99375[1], 99377[1], 99378[1], 99446[0], 99447[0], 99448[0], 99449[0], 99451[0], 99452[0], 99495[1], 99496[1], G0463[1], G0471[0]
54250	0213T[0], 0216T[0], 0596T[1], 0597T[1], 0708T[1], 0709T[1], 12001[1], 12002[1], 12004[1], 12005[1], 12006[1], 12007[1], 12011[1], 12013[1], 12014[1], 12015[1], 12016[1], 12017[1], 12018[1], 12020[1], 12021[1], 12031[1], 12032[1], 12034[1], 12035[1], 12036[1], 12037[1], 12041[1], 12042[1], 12044[1], 12045[1], 12046[1], 12047[1], 12051[1], 12052[1], 12053[1], 12054[1], 12055[1], 12056[1], 12057[1], 13100[1], 13101[1], 13102[1], 13120[1], 13121[1], 13122[1], 13131[1], 13132[1], 13133[1], 13151[1], 13152[1], 13153[1], 36000[1], 36400[1], 36405[1], 36406[1], 36410[1], 36420[1], 36425[1], 36430[1], 36440[1], 36591[0], 36592[0], 36600[1], 36640[1], 43752[1], 51701[0], 51702[0], 51703[1], 62320[0], 62321[0], 62322[0], 62323[0], 62324[0], 62325[0], 62326[0], 62327[0], 64400[0], 64405[0], 64408[0], 64415[0], 64416[0], 64417[0], 64418[0], 64420[0], 64421[0], 64425[0], 64430[0], 64435[0], 64445[0], 64446[0], 64447[0], 64448[0], 64449[0], 64450[0], 64451[0], 64454[0], 64461[0], 64462[0], 64463[0], 64479[0], 64480[0], 64483[0], 64484[0], 64486[0], 64487[0], 64488[0], 64489[0], 64490[0], 64491[0], 64492[0], 64493[0], 64494[0], 64495[0], 64505[0], 64510[0], 64517[0], 64520[0], 64530[0], 69990[0], 92012[1], 92014[1], 93000[1], 93005[1], 93010[1], 93040[1], 93041[1], 93042[1], 93318[1], 93355[1], 94002[1], 94200[1], 94680[1], 94681[1], 94690[1], 95812[1], 95813[1], 95816[1], 95819[1], 95822[1], 95829[1], 95955[1], 96360[1], 96361[1], 96365[1], 96366[1], 96367[1], 96368[1], 96372[1], 96374[1], 96375[1], 96376[1], 96377[1], 96523[0], 99155[0], 99156[0], 99157[0], 99211[1], 99212[1], 99213[1], 99214[1], 99215[1], 99217[1], 99218[1], 99219[1], 99220[1], 99221[1], 99222[1], 99223[1], 99231[1], 99232[1], 99233[1], 99234[1], 99235[1], 99236[1], 99238[1], 99239[1], 99241[1], 99242[1], 99243[1], 99244[1], 99245[1], 99251[1], 99252[1], 99253[1], 99254[1], 99255[1], 99291[1], 99292[1], 99304[1], 99305[1], 99306[1], 99307[1], 99308[1], 99309[1], 99310[1], 99315[1], 99316[1], 99334[1], 99335[1], 99336[1], 99337[1], 99347[1], 99348[1], 99349[1], 99350[1], 99374[1], 99375[1], 99377[1], 99378[1], 99446[0], 99447[0], 99448[0], 99449[0], 99451[0], 99452[0], 99495[1], 99496[1], G0463[1], G0471[0]
54300	0213T[0], 0216T[0], 0596T[1], 0597T[1], 0708T[1], 0709T[1], 12001[1], 12002[1], 12004[1], 12005[1], 12006[1], 12007[1], 12011[1], 12013[1], 12014[1], 12015[1], 12016[1], 12017[1], 12018[1], 12020[1], 12021[1], 12031[1], 12032[1], 12034[1], 12035[1], 12036[1], 12037[1], 12041[1], 12042[1], 12044[1], 12045[1], 12046[1], 12047[1], 12051[1], 12052[1], 12053[1], 12054[1], 12055[1], 12056[1], 12057[1], 13100[1], 13101[1], 13102[1], 13120[1], 13121[1], 13122[1], 13131[1], 13132[1], 13133[1], 13151[1], 13152[1], 13153[1], 36000[1], 36400[1], 36405[1], 36406[1], 36410[1], 36420[1], 36425[1], 36430[1], 36440[1], 36591[0], 36592[0], 36600[1], 36640[1], 43752[1], 51701[0], 51702[0], 51703[1], 53000[0], 53010[0], 53020[0], 53025[0], 62320[0], 62321[0], 62322[0], 62323[0], 62324[0], 62325[0], 62326[0], 62327[0], 64400[0], 64405[0], 64408[0], 64415[0], 64416[0], 64417[0], 64418[0], 64420[0], 64421[0], 64425[0], 64430[0], 64435[0], 64445[0], 64446[0], 64447[0], 64448[0], 64449[0], 64450[0], 64451[0], 64454[0], 64461[0], 64462[0], 64463[0], 64479[0], 64480[0], 64483[0], 64484[0], 64486[0], 64487[0], 64488[0], 64489[0], 64490[0], 64491[0], 64492[0], 64493[0], 64494[0], 64495[0], 64505[0], 64510[0], 64517[0], 64520[0], 64530[0], 69990[0], 92012[1], 92014[1], 93000[1], 93005[1], 93010[1], 93040[1], 93041[1], 93042[1], 93318[1], 93355[1], 94002[1], 94200[1], 94680[1], 94681[1], 94690[1], 95812[1], 95813[1], 95816[1], 95819[1], 95822[1], 95829[1], 95955[1], 96360[1], 96361[1], 96365[1], 96366[1], 96367[1], 96368[1], 96372[1], 96374[1], 96375[1], 96376[1], 96377[1], 96523[0], 99155[0], 99156[0], 99157[0], 99211[1], 99212[1], 99213[1], 99214[1], 99215[1], 99217[1], 99218[1], 99219[1], 99220[1], 99221[1], 99222[1], 99223[1], 99231[1], 99232[1], 99233[1], 99234[1], 99235[1], 99236[1], 99238[1], 99239[1], 99241[1], 99242[1], 99243[1], 99244[1], 99245[1], 99251[1], 99252[1], 99253[1], 99254[1], 99255[1], 99291[1], 99292[1], 99304[1], 99305[1], 99306[1], 99307[1], 99308[1], 99309[1], 99310[1], 99315[1], 99316[1], 99334[1], 99335[1], 99336[1], 99337[1], 99347[1], 99348[1], 99349[1], 99350[1], 99374[1], 99375[1], 99377[1], 99378[1], 99446[0], 99447[0], 99448[0], 99449[0], 99451[0], 99452[0], 99495[0], 99496[0], G0463[1], G0471[0]
54304	0213T[0], 0216T[0], 0596T[1], 0597T[1], 0708T[1], 0709T[1], 12001[1], 12002[1], 12004[1], 12005[1], 12006[1], 12007[1], 12011[1], 12013[1], 12014[1], 12015[1], 12016[1], 12017[1], 12018[1], 12020[1], 12021[1], 12031[1], 12032[1], 12034[1], 12035[1], 12036[1], 12037[1], 12041[1], 12042[1], 12044[1], 12045[1], 12046[1], 12047[1], 12051[1], 12052[1], 12053[1], 12054[1], 12055[1], 12056[1], 12057[1], 13100[1], 13101[1], 13102[1], 13120[1], 13121[1], 13122[1], 13131[1], 13132[1], 13133[1], 13151[1], 13152[1], 13153[1], 36000[1], 36400[1], 36405[1], 36406[1], 36410[1], 36420[1], 36425[1], 36430[1], 36440[1], 36591[0], 36592[0], 36600[1], 36640[1], 43752[1], 51701[0], 51702[0], 51703[1], 54300[1], 62320[0], 62321[0], 62322[0], 62323[0], 62324[0], 62325[0], 62326[0], 62327[0], 64400[0], 64405[0], 64408[0], 64415[0], 64416[0], 64417[0], 64418[0], 64420[0], 64421[0], 64425[0], 64430[0], 64435[0], 64445[0], 64446[0], 64447[0], 64448[0], 64449[0], 64450[0], 64451[0], 64454[0], 64461[0], 64462[0], 64463[0], 64479[0], 64480[0], 64483[0], 64484[0], 64486[0], 64487[0], 64488[0], 64489[0], 64490[0], 64491[0], 64492[0], 64493[0], 64494[0], 64495[0], 64505[0], 64510[0], 64517[0], 64520[0], 64530[0], 69990[0], 92012[1], 92014[1], 93000[1], 93005[1], 93010[1], 93040[1], 93041[1], 93042[1], 93318[1], 93355[1], 94002[1], 94200[1], 94680[1], 94681[1], 94690[1], 95812[1], 95813[1], 95816[1], 95819[1], 95822[1], 95829[1], 95955[1], 96360[1], 96361[1], 96365[1], 96366[1], 96367[1], 96368[1], 96372[1], 96374[1], 96375[1], 96376[1], 96377[1], 96523[0], 99155[0], 99156[0], 99157[0], 99211[1], 99212[1], 99213[1], 99214[1], 99215[1], 99217[1], 99218[1], 99219[1], 99220[1], 99221[1], 99222[1], 99223[1], 99231[1], 99232[1], 99233[1], 99234[1], 99235[1], 99236[1], 99238[1], 99239[1], 99241[1], 99242[1],

0 = Modifier usage not allowed or inappropriate 1 = Modifier usage allowed

Code 1	Code 2
	99243[1], 99244[1], 99245[1], 99251[1], 99252[1], 99253[1], 99254[1], 99255[1], 99291[1], 99292[1], 99304[1], 99305[1], 99306[1], 99307[1], 99308[1], 99309[1], 99310[1], 99315[1], 99316[1], 99334[1], 99335[1], 99336[1], 99337[1], 99347[1], 99348[1], 99349[1], 99350[1], 99374[1], 99375[1], 99377[1], 99378[1], 99446[0], 99447[0], 99448[0], 99449[0], 99451[0], 99452[0], 99495[0], 99496[0], G0463[1], G0471[0]
54308	0213T[0], 0216T[0], 0596T[1], 0597T[1], 0708T[1], 0709T[1], 11000[1], 11001[1], 11004[1], 11005[1], 11006[1], 11042[1], 11043[1], 11044[1], 11045[1], 11046[1], 11047[1], 12001[1], 12002[1], 12004[1], 12005[1], 12006[1], 12007[1], 12011[1], 12013[1], 12014[1], 12015[1], 12016[1], 12017[1], 12018[1], 12020[1], 12021[1], 12031[1], 12032[1], 12034[1], 12035[1], 12036[1], 12037[1], 12041[1], 12042[1], 12044[1], 12045[1], 12046[1], 12047[1], 12051[1], 12052[1], 12053[1], 12054[1], 12055[1], 12056[1], 12057[1], 13100[1], 13101[1], 13102[1], 13120[1], 13121[1], 13122[1], 13131[1], 13132[1], 13133[1], 13151[1], 13152[1], 13153[1], 36000[1], 36400[1], 36405[1], 36406[1], 36410[1], 36420[1], 36425[1], 36430[1], 36440[1], 36591[0], 36592[0], 36600[1], 36640[1], 43752[1], 51701[0], 51702[0], 51703[1], 52000[0], 53000[0], 53010[0], 53020[0], 53025[0], 54312[1], 62320[0], 62321[0], 62322[0], 62323[0], 62324[0], 62325[0], 62326[0], 62327[0], 64400[0], 64405[0], 64408[0], 64415[0], 64416[0], 64417[0], 64418[0], 64420[0], 64421[0], 64425[0], 64430[0], 64435[0], 64445[0], 64446[0], 64447[0], 64448[0], 64449[0], 64450[0], 64451[0], 64454[0], 64461[0], 64462[0], 64463[0], 64479[0], 64480[0], 64483[0], 64484[0], 64486[0], 64487[0], 64488[0], 64489[0], 64490[0], 64491[0], 64492[0], 64493[0], 64494[0], 64495[0], 64505[0], 64510[0], 64517[0], 64520[0], 64530[0], 69990[0], 92012[1], 92014[1], 93000[1], 93005[1], 93010[1], 93040[1], 93041[1], 93042[1], 93318[1], 93355[1], 94002[1], 94200[1], 94680[1], 94681[1], 94690[1], 95812[1], 95813[1], 95816[1], 95819[1], 95822[1], 95829[1], 95955[1], 96360[1], 96361[1], 96365[1], 96366[1], 96367[1], 96368[1], 96372[1], 96374[1], 96375[1], 96376[1], 96377[1], 96523[0], 97597[1], 97598[1], 97602[1], 99155[0], 99156[0], 99157[0], 99211[1], 99212[1], 99213[1], 99214[1], 99215[1], 99217[1], 99218[1], 99219[1], 99220[1], 99221[1], 99222[1], 99223[1], 99231[1], 99232[1], 99233[1], 99234[1], 99235[1], 99236[1], 99238[1], 99239[1], 99241[1], 99242[1], 99243[1], 99244[1], 99245[1], 99251[1], 99252[1], 99253[1], 99254[1], 99255[1], 99291[1], 99292[1], 99304[1], 99305[1], 99306[1], 99307[1], 99308[1], 99309[1], 99310[1], 99315[1], 99316[1], 99334[1], 99335[1], 99336[1], 99337[1], 99347[1], 99348[1], 99349[1], 99350[1], 99374[1], 99375[1], 99377[1], 99378[1], 99446[0], 99447[0], 99448[0], 99449[0], 99451[0], 99452[0], 99495[0], 99496[0], G0463[1], G0471[0]
54312	0213T[0], 0216T[0], 0596T[1], 0597T[1], 0708T[1], 0709T[1], 11000[1], 11001[1], 11004[1], 11005[1], 11006[1], 11042[1], 11043[1], 11044[1], 11045[1], 11046[1], 11047[1], 12001[1], 12002[1], 12004[1], 12005[1], 12006[1], 12007[1], 12011[1], 12013[1], 12014[1], 12015[1], 12016[1], 12017[1], 12018[1], 12020[1], 12021[1], 12031[1], 12032[1], 12034[1], 12035[1], 12036[1], 12037[1], 12041[1], 12042[1], 12044[1], 12045[1], 12046[1], 12047[1], 12051[1], 12052[1], 12053[1], 12054[1], 12055[1], 12056[1], 12057[1], 13100[1], 13101[1], 13102[1], 13120[1], 13121[1], 13122[1], 13131[1], 13132[1], 13133[1], 13151[1], 13152[1], 13153[1], 36000[1], 36400[1], 36405[1], 36406[1], 36410[1], 36420[1], 36425[1], 36430[1], 36440[1], 36591[0], 36592[0], 36600[1], 36640[1], 43752[1], 51701[0], 51702[0], 51703[1], 52000[0], 53000[0], 53010[0], 53020[0], 53025[0], 62320[0], 62321[0], 62322[0], 62323[0], 62324[0], 62325[0], 62326[0], 62327[0], 64400[0], 64405[0], 64408[0], 64415[0], 64416[0], 64417[0], 64418[0], 64420[0], 64421[0], 64425[0], 64430[0], 64435[0], 64445[0], 64446[0], 64447[0], 64448[0], 64449[0], 64450[0], 64451[0], 64454[0], 64461[0], 64462[0], 64463[0], 64479[0], 64480[0], 64483[0], 64484[0], 64486[0], 64487[0], 64488[0], 64489[0], 64490[0], 64491[0], 64492[0], 64493[0], 64494[0], 64495[0], 64505[0], 64510[0], 64517[0], 64520[0], 64530[0], 69990[0], 92012[1], 92014[1], 93000[1], 93005[1], 93010[1], 93040[1], 93041[1], 93042[1], 93318[1], 93355[1], 94002[1], 94200[1], 94680[1], 94681[1], 94690[1], 95812[1], 95813[1], 95816[1], 95819[1], 95822[1], 95829[1], 95955[1], 96360[1], 96361[1], 96365[1], 96366[1], 96367[1], 96368[1], 96372[1], 96374[1], 96375[1], 96376[1], 96377[1], 96523[0], 97597[1], 97598[1], 97602[1], 99155[0], 99156[0], 99157[0], 99211[1], 99212[1], 99213[1], 99214[1], 99215[1], 99217[1], 99218[1], 99219[1], 99220[1], 99221[1], 99222[1], 99223[1], 99231[1], 99232[1], 99233[1], 99234[1], 99235[1], 99236[1], 99238[1], 99239[1], 99241[1], 99242[1], 99243[1], 99244[1], 99245[1], 99251[1], 99252[1], 99253[1], 99254[1], 99255[1], 99291[1], 99292[1], 99304[1], 99305[1], 99306[1], 99307[1], 99308[1], 99309[1], 99310[1], 99315[1], 99316[1], 99334[1], 99335[1], 99336[1], 99337[1], 99347[1], 99348[1], 99349[1], 99350[1], 99374[1], 99375[1], 99377[1], 99378[1], 99446[0], 99447[0], 99448[0], 99449[0], 99451[0], 99452[0], 99495[0], 99496[0], G0463[1], G0471[0]
54316	0213T[0], 0216T[0], 0596T[1], 0597T[1], 0708T[1], 0709T[1], 11000[1], 11001[1], 11004[1], 11005[1], 11006[1], 11042[1], 11043[1], 11044[1], 11045[1], 11046[1], 11047[1], 12001[1], 12002[1], 12004[1], 12005[1], 12006[1], 12007[1], 12011[1], 12013[1], 12014[1], 12015[1], 12016[1], 12017[1], 12018[1], 12020[1], 12021[1], 12031[1], 12032[1], 12034[1], 12035[1], 12036[1], 12037[1], 12041[1], 12042[1], 12044[1], 12045[1], 12046[1], 12047[1], 12051[1], 12052[1], 12053[1], 12054[1], 12055[1], 12056[1], 12057[1], 13100[1], 13101[1], 13102[1], 13120[1], 13121[1], 13122[1], 13131[1], 13132[1], 13133[1], 13151[1], 13152[1], 13153[1], 36000[1], 36400[1], 36405[1], 36406[1], 36410[1], 36420[1], 36425[1], 36430[1], 36440[1], 36591[0], 36592[0], 36600[1], 36640[1], 43752[1], 51701[0], 51702[0], 51703[1], 52000[0], 53000[0], 53010[0], 53020[0], 53025[0], 62320[0], 62321[0], 62322[0], 62323[0], 62324[0], 62325[0], 62326[0], 62327[0], 64400[0], 64405[0], 64408[0], 64415[0], 64416[0], 64417[0], 64418[0], 64420[0], 64421[0], 64425[0], 64430[0], 64435[0], 64445[0], 64446[0], 64447[0], 64448[0], 64449[0], 64450[0], 64451[0], 64454[0], 64461[0], 64462[0], 64463[0], 64479[0], 64480[0], 64483[0], 64484[0], 64486[0], 64487[0], 64488[0], 64489[0], 64490[0], 64491[0], 64492[0], 64493[0], 64494[0], 64495[0], 64505[0], 64510[0], 64517[0], 64520[0], 64530[0], 69990[0], 92012[1], 92014[1], 93000[1], 93005[1], 93010[1], 93040[1], 93041[1], 93042[1], 93318[1], 93355[1], 94002[1], 94200[1], 94680[1], 94681[1], 94690[1], 95812[1], 95813[1], 95816[1], 95819[1], 95822[1], 95829[1], 95955[1], 96360[1], 96361[1], 96365[1], 96366[1], 96367[1], 96368[1], 96372[1], 96374[1], 96375[1], 96376[1], 96377[1], 96523[0], 97597[1], 97598[1], 97602[1], 99155[0], 99156[0], 99157[0], 99211[1], 99212[1], 99213[1], 99214[1], 99215[1], 99217[1], 99218[1], 99219[1], 99220[1], 99221[1], 99222[1], 99223[1], 99231[1], 99232[1], 99233[1], 99234[1], 99235[1], 99236[1], 99238[1], 99239[1], 99241[1], 99242[1], 99243[1], 99244[1], 99245[1], 99251[1], 99252[1], 99253[1], 99254[1], 99255[1], 99291[1], 99292[1], 99304[1], 99305[1], 99306[1], 99307[1], 99308[1], 99309[1], 99310[1], 99315[1], 99316[1], 99334[1], 99335[1], 99336[1], 99337[1], 99347[1], 99348[1], 99349[1], 99350[1], 99374[1], 99375[1], 99377[1], 99378[1], 99446[0], 99447[0], 99448[0], 99449[0], 99451[0], 99452[0], 99495[0], 99496[0], G0463[1], G0471[0]
54318	0213T[0], 0216T[0], 0596T[1], 0597T[1], 0708T[1], 0709T[1], 11000[1], 11001[1], 11004[1], 11005[1], 11006[1], 11042[1], 11043[1], 11044[1], 11045[1], 11046[1], 11047[1], 12001[1], 12002[1], 12004[1], 12005[1], 12006[1], 12007[1], 12011[1], 12013[1], 12014[1], 12015[1], 12016[1], 12017[1], 12018[1], 12020[1], 12021[1], 12031[1], 12032[1], 12034[1], 12035[1], 12036[1], 12037[1], 12041[1], 12042[1], 12044[1], 12045[1], 12046[1], 12047[1], 12051[1], 12052[1], 12053[1], 12054[1], 12055[1], 12056[1], 12057[1], 13100[1], 13101[1], 13102[1], 13120[1], 13121[1], 13122[1], 13131[1], 13132[1], 13133[1], 13151[1], 13152[1], 13153[1], 36000[1], 36400[1], 36405[1], 36406[1], 36410[1], 36420[1], 36425[1], 36430[1], 36440[1], 36591[0], 36592[0], 36600[1], 36640[1], 43752[1], 51701[0], 51702[0], 51703[1], 52000[0], 53000[0], 53010[0], 53020[0], 53025[0], 62320[0], 62321[0], 62322[0], 62323[0], 62324[0], 62325[0], 62326[0], 62327[0], 64400[0], 64405[0], 64408[0], 64415[0], 64416[0], 64417[0], 64418[0], 64420[0], 64421[0], 64425[0], 64430[0], 64435[0], 64445[0], 64446[0], 64447[0], 64448[0], 64449[0], 64450[0], 64451[0], 64454[0], 64461[0], 64462[0], 64463[0], 64479[0], 64480[0], 64483[0], 64484[0], 64486[0], 64487[0], 64488[0], 64489[0], 64490[0], 64491[0], 64492[0], 64493[0], 64494[0], 64495[0], 64505[0], 64510[0], 64517[0], 64520[0], 64530[0], 69990[0], 92012[1], 92014[1], 93000[1], 93005[1], 93010[1], 93040[1], 93041[1], 93042[1], 93318[1], 93355[1], 94002[1], 94200[1], 94680[1], 94681[1], 94690[1], 95812[1], 95813[1], 95816[1], 95819[1], 95822[1], 95829[1], 95955[1], 96360[1], 96361[1], 96365[1], 96366[1], 96367[1], 96368[1], 96372[1], 96374[1], 96375[1], 96376[1], 96377[1], 96523[0], 97597[1], 97598[1], 97602[1], 99155[0], 99156[0], 99157[0], 99211[1], 99212[1], 99213[1], 99214[1], 99215[1], 99217[1], 99218[1], 99219[1], 99220[1], 99221[1], 99222[1], 99223[1], 99231[1], 99232[1], 99233[1], 99234[1], 99235[1], 99236[1], 99238[1], 99239[1], 99241[1], 99242[1], 99243[1], 99244[1], 99245[1], 99251[1], 99252[1], 99253[1], 99254[1], 99255[1], 99291[1], 99292[1], 99304[1], 99305[1], 99306[1], 99307[1], 99308[1], 99309[1], 99310[1], 99315[1], 99316[1], 99334[1], 99335[1], 99336[1], 99337[1], 99347[1], 99348[1], 99349[1], 99350[1], 99374[1], 99375[1], 99377[1], 99378[1], 99446[0], 99447[0], 99448[0], 99449[0], 99451[0], 99452[0], 99495[0], 99496[0], G0463[1], G0471[0]
54322	0213T[0], 0216T[0], 0596T[1], 0597T[1], 0708T[1], 0709T[1], 12001[1], 12002[1], 12004[1], 12005[1], 12006[1], 12007[1], 12011[1], 12013[1], 12014[1], 12015[1], 12016[1], 12017[1], 12018[1], 12020[1], 12021[1], 12031[1], 12032[1], 12034[1], 12035[1], 12036[1], 12037[1], 12041[1], 12042[1], 12044[1], 12045[1], 12046[1], 12047[1], 12051[1], 12052[1], 12053[1], 12054[1], 12055[1], 12056[1], 12057[1], 13100[1], 13101[1], 13102[1], 13120[1], 13121[1], 13122[1], 13131[1], 13132[1], 13133[1], 13151[1], 13152[1], 13153[1], 36000[1], 36400[1], 36405[1], 36406[1], 36410[1], 36420[1], 36425[1], 36430[1], 36440[1], 36591[0], 36592[0], 36600[1], 36640[1], 43752[1], 51701[0], 51702[0], 51703[1], 53000[0], 53010[0], 53020[0], 53025[0], 62320[0], 62321[0], 62322[0], 62323[0], 62324[0], 62325[0], 62326[0], 62327[0], 64400[0], 64405[0], 64408[0], 64415[0], 64416[0], 64417[0], 64418[0], 64420[0], 64421[0], 64425[0], 64430[0], 64435[0], 64445[0], 64446[0], 64447[0], 64448[0], 64449[0], 64450[0], 64451[0], 64454[0], 64461[0], 64462[0], 64463[0], 64479[0], 64480[0], 64483[0], 64484[0], 64486[0], 64487[0], 64488[0], 64489[0], 64490[0], 64491[0], 64492[0], 64493[0], 64494[0], 64495[0], 64505[0], 64510[0], 64517[0], 64520[0], 64530[0], 69990[0], 92012[1], 92014[1], 93000[1], 93005[1], 93010[1], 93040[1], 93041[1], 93042[1], 93318[1], 93355[1], 94002[1], 94200[1], 94680[1], 94681[1], 94690[1], 95812[1], 95813[1], 95816[1], 95819[1], 95822[1], 95829[1], 95955[1], 96360[1], 96361[1], 96365[1], 96366[1], 96367[1], 96368[1], 96372[1], 96374[1], 96375[1], 96376[1], 96377[1], 96523[0], 99155[0], 99156[0], 99157[0], 99211[1], 99212[1], 99213[1], 99214[1], 99215[1], 99217[1], 99218[1], 99219[1], 99220[1], 99221[1], 99222[1], 99223[1], 99231[1], 99232[1], 99233[1], 99234[1], 99235[1], 99236[1], 99238[1], 99239[1], 99241[1], 99242[1], 99243[1], 99244[1], 99245[1], 99251[1], 99252[1], 99253[1], 99254[1], 99255[1], 99291[1], 99292[1], 99304[1], 99305[1], 99306[1], 99307[1], 99308[1], 99309[1], 99310[1], 99315[1], 99316[1], 99334[1], 99335[1], 99336[1], 99337[1], 99347[1], 99348[1], 99349[1], 99350[1], 99374[1], 99375[1], 99377[1], 99378[1], 99446[0], 99447[0], 99448[0], 99449[0], 99451[0], 99452[0], 99495[0], 99496[0], G0463[1], G0471[0]
54324	0213T[0], 0216T[0], 0596T[1], 0597T[1], 0708T[1], 0709T[1], 11000[1], 11001[1], 11004[1], 11005[1], 11006[1], 11042[1], 11043[1], 11044[1], 11045[1], 11046[1], 11047[1], 12001[1], 12002[1], 12004[1], 12005[1], 12006[1], 12007[1], 12011[1], 12013[1], 12014[1], 12015[1], 12016[1], 12017[1], 12018[1], 12020[1], 12021[1], 12031[1], 12032[1], 12034[1], 12035[1], 12036[1], 12037[1], 12041[1], 12042[1], 12044[1], 12045[1], 12046[1], 12047[1], 12051[1], 12052[1], 12053[1], 12054[1], 12055[1], 12056[1], 12057[1], 13100[1], 13101[1], 13102[1], 13120[1], 13121[1], 13122[1], 13131[1], 13132[1], 13133[1],

0 = Modifier usage not allowed or inappropriate 1 = Modifier usage allowed

Code 1	Code 2
	13151[1], 13152[1], 13153[1], 36000[1], 36400[1], 36405[1], 36406[1], 36410[1], 36420[1], 36425[1], 36430[1], 36440[1], 36591[0], 36592[0], 36600[1], 36640[1], 43752[1], 51701[0], 51702[0], 51703[1], 52000[0], 53000[0], 53010[0], 53020[0], 53025[0], 62320[0], 62321[0], 62322[0], 62323[0], 62324[0], 62325[0], 62326[0], 62327[0], 64400[0], 64405[0], 64408[0], 64415[0], 64416[0], 64417[0], 64418[0], 64420[0], 64421[0], 64425[0], 64430[0], 64435[0], 64445[0], 64446[0], 64447[0], 64448[0], 64449[0], 64450[0], 64451[0], 64454[0], 64461[0], 64462[0], 64463[0], 64479[0], 64480[0], 64483[0], 64484[0], 64486[0], 64487[0], 64488[0], 64489[0], 64490[0], 64491[0], 64492[0], 64493[0], 64494[0], 64495[0], 64505[0], 64510[0], 64517[0], 64520[0], 64530[0], 69990[0], 92012[1], 92014[1], 93000[1], 93005[1], 93010[1], 93040[1], 93041[1], 93042[1], 93318[1], 93355[1], 94002[1], 94200[1], 94680[1], 94681[1], 94690[1], 95812[1], 95813[1], 95816[1], 95819[1], 95822[1], 95829[1], 95955[1], 96360[1], 96361[1], 96365[1], 96366[1], 96367[1], 96368[1], 96372[1], 96374[1], 96375[1], 96376[1], 96377[1], 96523[0], 97597[1], 97598[1], 97602[1], 99155[0], 99156[0], 99157[0], 99211[1], 99212[1], 99213[1], 99214[1], 99215[1], 99217[1], 99218[1], 99219[1], 99220[1], 99221[1], 99222[1], 99223[1], 99231[1], 99232[1], 99233[1], 99234[1], 99235[1], 99236[1], 99238[1], 99239[1], 99241[1], 99242[1], 99243[1], 99244[1], 99245[1], 99251[1], 99252[1], 99253[1], 99254[1], 99255[1], 99291[1], 99292[1], 99304[1], 99305[1], 99306[1], 99307[1], 99308[1], 99309[1], 99310[1], 99315[1], 99316[1], 99334[1], 99335[1], 99336[1], 99337[1], 99347[1], 99348[1], 99349[1], 99350[1], 99374[1], 99375[1], 99377[1], 99378[1], 99446[0], 99447[0], 99448[0], 99449[0], 99451[0], 99452[0], 99495[0], 99496[0], G0463[1], G0471[0]
54326	0213T[0], 0216T[0], 0596T[1], 0597T[1], 0708T[1], 0709T[1], 11000[1], 11001[1], 11004[1], 11005[1], 11006[1], 11042[1], 11043[1], 11044[1], 11045[1], 11046[1], 11047[1], 12001[1], 12002[1], 12004[1], 12005[1], 12006[1], 12007[1], 12011[1], 12013[1], 12014[1], 12015[1], 12016[1], 12017[1], 12018[1], 12020[1], 12021[1], 12031[1], 12032[1], 12034[1], 12035[1], 12036[1], 12037[1], 12041[1], 12042[1], 12044[1], 12045[1], 12046[1], 12047[1], 12051[1], 12052[1], 12053[1], 12054[1], 12055[1], 12056[1], 12057[1], 13100[1], 13101[1], 13102[1], 13120[1], 13121[1], 13122[1], 13131[1], 13132[1], 13133[1], 13151[1], 13152[1], 13153[1], 36000[1], 36400[1], 36405[1], 36406[1], 36410[1], 36420[1], 36425[1], 36430[1], 36440[1], 36591[0], 36592[0], 36600[1], 36640[1], 43752[1], 51701[0], 51702[0], 51703[1], 52000[0], 53000[0], 53010[0], 53020[0], 53025[0], 54324[1], 62320[0], 62321[0], 62322[0], 62323[0], 62324[0], 62325[0], 62326[0], 62327[0], 64400[0], 64405[0], 64408[0], 64415[0], 64416[0], 64417[0], 64418[0], 64420[0], 64421[0], 64425[0], 64430[0], 64435[0], 64445[0], 64446[0], 64447[0], 64448[0], 64449[0], 64450[0], 64451[0], 64454[0], 64461[0], 64462[0], 64463[0], 64479[0], 64480[0], 64483[0], 64484[0], 64486[0], 64487[0], 64488[0], 64489[0], 64490[0], 64491[0], 64492[0], 64493[0], 64494[0], 64495[0], 64505[0], 64510[0], 64517[0], 64520[0], 64530[0], 69990[0], 92012[1], 92014[1], 93000[1], 93005[1], 93010[1], 93040[1], 93041[1], 93042[1], 93318[1], 93355[1], 94002[1], 94200[1], 94680[1], 94681[1], 94690[1], 95812[1], 95813[1], 95816[1], 95819[1], 95822[1], 95829[1], 95955[1], 96360[1], 96361[1], 96365[1], 96366[1], 96367[1], 96368[1], 96372[1], 96374[1], 96375[1], 96376[1], 96377[1], 96523[0], 97597[1], 97598[1], 97602[1], 99155[0], 99156[0], 99157[0], 99211[1], 99212[1], 99213[1], 99214[1], 99215[1], 99217[1], 99218[1], 99219[1], 99220[1], 99221[1], 99222[1], 99223[1], 99231[1], 99232[1], 99233[1], 99234[1], 99235[1], 99236[1], 99238[1], 99239[1], 99241[1], 99242[1], 99243[1], 99244[1], 99245[1], 99251[1], 99252[1], 99253[1], 99254[1], 99255[1], 99291[1], 99292[1], 99304[1], 99305[1], 99306[1], 99307[1], 99308[1], 99309[1], 99310[1], 99315[1], 99316[1], 99334[1], 99335[1], 99336[1], 99337[1], 99347[1], 99348[1], 99349[1], 99350[1], 99374[1], 99375[1], 99377[1], 99378[1], 99446[0], 99447[0], 99448[0], 99449[0], 99451[0], 99452[0], 99495[0], 99496[0], G0463[1], G0471[0]
54328	0213T[0], 0216T[0], 0596T[1], 0597T[1], 0708T[1], 0709T[1], 11000[1], 11001[1], 11004[1], 11005[1], 11006[1], 11042[1], 11043[1], 11044[1], 11045[1], 11046[1], 11047[1], 12001[1], 12002[1], 12004[1], 12005[1], 12006[1], 12007[1], 12011[1], 12013[1], 12014[1], 12015[1], 12016[1], 12017[1], 12018[1], 12020[1], 12021[1], 12031[1], 12032[1], 12034[1], 12035[1], 12036[1], 12037[1], 12041[1], 12042[1], 12044[1], 12045[1], 12046[1], 12047[1], 12051[1], 12052[1], 12053[1], 12054[1], 12055[1], 12056[1], 12057[1], 13100[1], 13101[1], 13102[1], 13120[1], 13121[1], 13122[1], 13131[1], 13132[1], 13133[1], 13151[1], 13152[1], 13153[1], 36000[1], 36400[1], 36405[1], 36406[1], 36410[1], 36420[1], 36425[1], 36430[1], 36440[1], 36591[0], 36592[0], 36600[1], 36640[1], 43752[1], 51701[0], 51702[0], 51703[1], 52000[0], 53000[0], 53010[0], 53020[0], 53025[0], 54326[1], 62320[0], 62321[0], 62322[0], 62323[0], 62324[0], 62325[0], 62326[0], 62327[0], 64400[0], 64405[0], 64408[0], 64415[0], 64416[0], 64417[0], 64418[0], 64420[0], 64421[0], 64425[0], 64430[0], 64435[0], 64445[0], 64446[0], 64447[0], 64448[0], 64449[0], 64450[0], 64451[0], 64454[0], 64461[0], 64462[0], 64463[0], 64479[0], 64480[0], 64483[0], 64484[0], 64486[0], 64487[0], 64488[0], 64489[0], 64490[0], 64491[0], 64492[0], 64493[0], 64494[0], 64495[0], 64505[0], 64510[0], 64517[0], 64520[0], 64530[0], 69990[0], 92012[1], 92014[1], 93000[1], 93005[1], 93010[1], 93040[1], 93041[1], 93042[1], 93318[1], 93355[1], 94002[1], 94200[1], 94680[1], 94681[1], 94690[1], 95812[1], 95813[1], 95816[1], 95819[1], 95822[1], 95829[1], 95955[1], 96360[1], 96361[1], 96365[1], 96366[1], 96367[1], 96368[1], 96372[1], 96374[1], 96375[1], 96376[1], 96377[1], 96523[0], 97597[1], 97598[1], 97602[1], 99155[0], 99156[0], 99157[0], 99211[1], 99212[1], 99213[1], 99214[1], 99215[1], 99217[1], 99218[1], 99219[1], 99220[1], 99221[1], 99222[1], 99223[1], 99231[1], 99232[1], 99233[1], 99234[1], 99235[1], 99236[1], 99238[1], 99239[1], 99241[1], 99242[1], 99243[1], 99244[1], 99245[1], 99251[1], 99252[1], 99253[1], 99254[1], 99255[1], 99291[1], 99292[1], 99304[1], 99305[1], 99306[1], 99307[1], 99308[1], 99309[1], 99310[1], 99315[1], 99316[1], 99334[1], 99335[1], 99336[1], 99337[1], 99347[1], 99348[1], 99349[1], 99350[1], 99374[1], 99375[1], 99377[1], 99378[1], 99446[0], 99447[0], 99448[0], 99449[0], 99451[0], 99452[0], 99495[0], 99496[0], G0463[1], G0471[0]
54332	0213T[0], 0216T[0], 0596T[1], 0597T[1], 0708T[1], 0709T[1], 11000[1], 11001[1], 11004[1], 11005[1], 11006[1], 11042[1], 11043[1], 11044[1], 11045[1], 11046[1], 11047[1], 12001[1], 12002[1], 12004[1], 12005[1], 12006[1], 12007[1], 12011[1], 12013[1], 12014[1], 12015[1], 12016[1], 12017[1], 12018[1], 12020[1], 12021[1], 12031[1], 12032[1], 12034[1], 12035[1], 12036[1], 12037[1], 12041[1], 12042[1], 12044[1], 12045[1], 12046[1], 12047[1], 12051[1], 12052[1], 12053[1], 12054[1], 12055[1], 12056[1], 12057[1], 13100[1], 13101[1], 13102[1], 13120[1], 13121[1], 13122[1], 13131[1], 13132[1], 13133[1], 13151[1], 13152[1], 13153[1], 36000[1], 36400[1], 36405[1], 36406[1], 36410[1], 36420[1], 36425[1], 36430[1], 36440[1], 36591[0], 36592[0], 36600[1], 36640[1], 43752[1], 51701[0], 51702[0], 51703[1], 52000[0], 53000[0], 53010[0], 53020[0], 53025[0], 53452[1], 54352[1], 62320[0], 62321[0], 62322[0], 62323[0], 62324[0], 62325[0], 62326[0], 62327[0], 64400[0], 64405[0], 64408[0], 64415[0], 64416[0], 64417[0], 64418[0], 64420[0], 64421[0], 64425[0], 64430[0], 64435[0], 64445[0], 64446[0], 64447[0], 64448[0], 64449[0], 64450[0], 64451[0], 64454[0], 64461[0], 64462[0], 64463[0], 64479[0], 64480[0], 64483[0], 64484[0], 64486[0], 64487[0], 64488[0], 64489[0], 64490[0], 64491[0], 64492[0], 64493[0], 64494[0], 64495[0], 64505[0], 64510[0], 64517[0], 64520[0], 64530[0], 69990[0], 92012[1], 92014[1], 93000[1], 93005[1], 93010[1], 93040[1], 93041[1], 93042[1], 93318[1], 93355[1], 94002[1], 94200[1], 94680[1], 94681[1], 94690[1], 95812[1], 95813[1], 95816[1], 95819[1], 95822[1], 95829[1], 95955[1], 96360[1], 96361[1], 96365[1], 96366[1], 96367[1], 96368[1], 96372[1], 96374[1], 96375[1], 96376[1], 96377[1], 96523[0], 97597[1], 97598[1], 97602[1], 99155[0], 99156[0], 99157[0], 99211[1], 99212[1], 99213[1], 99214[1], 99215[1], 99217[1], 99218[1], 99219[1], 99220[1], 99221[1], 99222[1], 99223[1], 99231[1], 99232[1], 99233[1], 99234[1], 99235[1], 99236[1], 99238[1], 99239[1], 99241[1], 99242[1], 99243[1], 99244[1], 99245[1], 99251[1], 99252[1], 99253[1], 99254[1], 99255[1], 99291[1], 99292[1], 99304[1], 99305[1], 99306[1], 99307[1], 99308[1], 99309[1], 99310[1], 99315[1], 99316[1], 99334[1], 99335[1], 99336[1], 99337[1], 99347[1], 99348[1], 99349[1], 99350[1], 99374[1], 99375[1], 99377[1], 99378[1], 99446[0], 99447[0], 99448[0], 99449[0], 99451[0], 99452[0], 99495[0], 99496[0], G0463[1], G0471[0]
54336	0213T[0], 0216T[0], 0596T[1], 0597T[1], 0708T[1], 0709T[1], 11000[1], 11001[1], 11004[1], 11005[1], 11006[1], 11042[1], 11043[1], 11044[1], 11045[1], 11046[1], 11047[1], 12001[1], 12002[1], 12004[1], 12005[1], 12006[1], 12007[1], 12011[1], 12013[1], 12014[1], 12015[1], 12016[1], 12017[1], 12018[1], 12020[1], 12021[1], 12031[1], 12032[1], 12034[1], 12035[1], 12036[1], 12037[1], 12041[1], 12042[1], 12044[1], 12045[1], 12046[1], 12047[1], 12051[1], 12052[1], 12053[1], 12054[1], 12055[1], 12056[1], 12057[1], 13100[1], 13101[1], 13102[1], 13120[1], 13121[1], 13122[1], 13131[1], 13132[1], 13133[1], 13151[1], 13152[1], 13153[1], 36000[1], 36400[1], 36405[1], 36406[1], 36410[1], 36420[1], 36425[1], 36430[1], 36440[1], 36591[0], 36592[0], 36600[1], 36640[1], 43752[1], 51701[0], 51702[0], 51703[1], 52000[0], 53000[0], 53010[0], 53020[0], 53025[0], 62320[0], 62321[0], 62322[0], 62323[0], 62324[0], 62325[0], 62326[0], 62327[0], 64400[0], 64405[0], 64408[0], 64415[0], 64416[0], 64417[0], 64418[0], 64420[0], 64421[0], 64425[0], 64430[0], 64435[0], 64445[0], 64446[0], 64447[0], 64448[0], 64449[0], 64450[0], 64451[0], 64454[0], 64461[0], 64462[0], 64463[0], 64479[0], 64480[0], 64483[0], 64484[0], 64486[0], 64487[0], 64488[0], 64489[0], 64490[0], 64491[0], 64492[0], 64493[0], 64494[0], 64495[0], 64505[0], 64510[0], 64517[0], 64520[0], 64530[0], 69990[0], 92012[1], 92014[1], 93000[1], 93005[1], 93010[1], 93040[1], 93041[1], 93042[1], 93318[1], 93355[1], 94002[1], 94200[1], 94680[1], 94681[1], 94690[1], 95812[1], 95813[1], 95816[1], 95819[1], 95822[1], 95829[1], 95955[1], 96360[1], 96361[1], 96365[1], 96366[1], 96367[1], 96368[1], 96372[1], 96374[1], 96375[1], 96376[1], 96377[1], 96523[0], 97597[1], 97598[1], 97602[1], 99155[0], 99156[0], 99157[0], 99211[1], 99212[1], 99213[1], 99214[1], 99215[1], 99217[1], 99218[1], 99219[1], 99220[1], 99221[1], 99222[1], 99223[1], 99231[1], 99232[1], 99233[1], 99234[1], 99235[1], 99236[1], 99238[1], 99239[1], 99241[1], 99242[1], 99243[1], 99244[1], 99245[1], 99251[1], 99252[1], 99253[1], 99254[1], 99255[1], 99291[1], 99292[1], 99304[1], 99305[1], 99306[1], 99307[1], 99308[1], 99309[1], 99310[1], 99315[1], 99316[1], 99334[1], 99335[1], 99336[1], 99337[1], 99347[1], 99348[1], 99349[1], 99350[1], 99374[1], 99375[1], 99377[1], 99378[1], 99446[0], 99447[0], 99448[0], 99449[0], 99451[0], 99452[0], 99495[0], 99496[0], G0463[1], G0471[0]
54340	0213T[0], 0216T[0], 0596T[1], 0597T[1], 0708T[1], 0709T[1], 11000[1], 11001[1], 11004[1], 11005[1], 11006[1], 11042[1], 11043[1], 11044[1], 11045[1], 11046[1], 11047[1], 12001[1], 12002[1], 12004[1], 12005[1], 12006[1], 12007[1], 12011[1], 12013[1], 12014[1], 12015[1], 12016[1], 12017[1], 12018[1], 12020[1], 12021[1], 12031[1], 12032[1], 12034[1], 12035[1], 12036[1], 12037[1], 12041[1], 12042[1], 12044[1], 12045[1], 12046[1], 12047[1], 12051[1], 12052[1], 12053[1], 12054[1], 12055[1], 12056[1], 12057[1], 13100[1], 13101[1], 13102[1], 13120[1], 13121[1], 13122[1], 13131[1], 13132[1], 13133[1], 13151[1], 13152[1], 13153[1], 36000[1], 36400[1], 36405[1], 36406[1], 36410[1], 36420[1], 36425[1], 36430[1], 36440[1], 36591[0], 36592[0], 36600[1], 36640[1], 43752[1], 51701[0], 51702[0], 51703[1], 53000[0], 53010[0], 53020[0], 53025[0], 62320[0], 62321[0], 62322[0], 62323[0], 62324[0], 62325[0], 62326[0], 62327[0], 64400[0], 64405[0], 64408[0], 64415[0], 64416[0], 64417[0], 64418[0], 64420[0], 64421[0], 64425[0], 64430[0], 64435[0], 64445[0], 64446[0], 64447[0], 64448[0], 64449[0], 64450[0], 64451[0], 64454[0], 64461[0], 64462[0], 64463[0], 64479[0], 64480[0], 64483[0], 64484[0], 64486[0], 64487[0], 64488[0], 64489[0], 64490[0], 64491[0], 64492[0], 64493[0], 64494[0], 64495[0], 64505[0], 64510[0], 64517[0], 64520[0], 64530[0], 69990[0], 92012[1], 92014[1], 93000[1], 93005[1], 93010[1], 93040[1], 93041[1], 93042[1], 93318[1], 93355[1], 94002[1], 94200[1], 94680[1], 94681[1], 94690[1], 95812[1], 95813[1], 95816[1], 95819[1], 95822[1], 95829[1], 95955[1], 96360[1], 96361[1], 96365[1], 96366[1], 96367[1], 96368[1], 96372[1], 96374[1], 96375[1], 96376[1], 96377[1], 96523[0], 97597[1],

0 = Modifier usage not allowed or inappropriate 1 = Modifier usage allowed

Code 1	Code 2
	97598[1], 97602[1], 99155[0], 99156[0], 99157[0], 99211[1], 99212[1], 99213[1], 99214[1], 99215[1], 99217[1], 99218[1], 99219[1], 99220[1], 99221[1], 99222[1], 99223[1], 99231[1], 99232[1], 99233[1], 99234[1], 99235[1], 99236[1], 99238[1], 99239[1], 99241[1], 99242[1], 99243[1], 99244[1], 99245[1], 99251[1], 99252[1], 99253[1], 99254[1], 99255[1], 99291[1], 99292[1], 99304[1], 99305[1], 99306[1], 99307[1], 99308[1], 99309[1], 99310[1], 99315[1], 99316[1], 99334[1], 99335[1], 99336[1], 99337[1], 99347[1], 99348[1], 99349[1], 99350[1], 99374[1], 99375[1], 99377[1], 99378[1], 99446[0], 99447[0], 99448[0], 99449[0], 99451[0], 99452[0], 99495[0], 99496[0], G0463[1], G0471[0]
54344	0213T[0], 0216T[0], 0596T[1], 0597T[1], 0708T[1], 0709T[1], 11000[1], 11001[1], 11004[1], 11005[1], 11006[1], 11042[1], 11043[1], 11044[1], 11045[1], 11046[1], 11047[1], 12001[1], 12002[1], 12004[1], 12005[1], 12006[1], 12007[1], 12011[1], 12013[1], 12014[1], 12015[1], 12016[1], 12017[1], 12018[1], 12020[1], 12021[1], 12031[1], 12032[1], 12034[1], 12035[1], 12036[1], 12037[1], 12041[1], 12042[1], 12044[1], 12045[1], 12046[1], 12047[1], 12051[1], 12052[1], 12053[1], 12054[1], 12055[1], 12056[1], 12057[1], 13100[1], 13101[1], 13102[1], 13120[1], 13121[1], 13122[1], 13131[1], 13132[1], 13133[1], 13151[1], 13152[1], 13153[1], 36000[1], 36400[1], 36405[1], 36406[1], 36410[1], 36420[1], 36425[1], 36430[1], 36440[1], 36591[0], 36592[0], 36600[1], 36640[1], 43752[1], 51701[0], 51702[0], 51703[1], 52000[0], 53000[0], 53010[0], 53020[0], 53025[0], 62320[0], 62321[0], 62322[0], 62323[0], 62324[0], 62325[0], 62326[0], 62327[0], 64400[0], 64405[0], 64408[0], 64415[0], 64416[0], 64417[0], 64418[0], 64420[0], 64421[0], 64425[0], 64430[0], 64435[0], 64445[0], 64446[0], 64447[0], 64448[0], 64449[0], 64450[0], 64451[0], 64454[0], 64461[0], 64462[0], 64463[0], 64479[0], 64480[0], 64483[0], 64484[0], 64486[0], 64487[0], 64488[0], 64489[0], 64490[0], 64491[0], 64492[0], 64493[0], 64494[0], 64495[0], 64505[0], 64510[0], 64517[0], 64520[0], 64530[0], 69990[0], 92012[1], 92014[1], 93000[1], 93005[1], 93010[1], 93040[1], 93041[1], 93042[1], 93318[1], 93355[1], 94002[1], 94200[1], 94680[1], 94681[1], 94690[1], 95812[1], 95813[1], 95816[1], 95819[1], 95822[1], 95829[1], 95955[1], 96360[1], 96361[1], 96365[1], 96366[1], 96367[1], 96368[1], 96372[1], 96374[1], 96375[1], 96376[1], 96377[1], 96523[0], 97597[1], 97598[1], 97602[1], 99155[0], 99156[0], 99157[0], 99211[1], 99212[1], 99213[1], 99214[1], 99215[1], 99217[1], 99218[1], 99219[1], 99220[1], 99221[1], 99222[1], 99223[1], 99231[1], 99232[1], 99233[1], 99234[1], 99235[1], 99236[1], 99238[1], 99239[1], 99241[1], 99242[1], 99243[1], 99244[1], 99245[1], 99251[1], 99252[1], 99253[1], 99254[1], 99255[1], 99291[1], 99292[1], 99304[1], 99305[1], 99306[1], 99307[1], 99308[1], 99309[1], 99310[1], 99315[1], 99316[1], 99334[1], 99335[1], 99336[1], 99337[1], 99347[1], 99348[1], 99349[1], 99350[1], 99374[1], 99375[1], 99377[1], 99378[1], 99446[0], 99447[0], 99448[0], 99449[0], 99451[0], 99452[0], 99495[0], 99496[0], G0463[1], G0471[0]
54348	0213T[0], 0216T[0], 0596T[1], 0597T[1], 0708T[1], 0709T[1], 11000[1], 11001[1], 11004[1], 11005[1], 11006[1], 11042[1], 11043[1], 11044[1], 11045[1], 11046[1], 11047[1], 12001[1], 12002[1], 12004[1], 12005[1], 12006[1], 12007[1], 12011[1], 12013[1], 12014[1], 12015[1], 12016[1], 12017[1], 12018[1], 12020[1], 12021[1], 12031[1], 12032[1], 12034[1], 12035[1], 12036[1], 12037[1], 12041[1], 12042[1], 12044[1], 12045[1], 12046[1], 12047[1], 12051[1], 12052[1], 12053[1], 12054[1], 12055[1], 12056[1], 12057[1], 13100[1], 13101[1], 13102[1], 13120[1], 13121[1], 13122[1], 13131[1], 13132[1], 13133[1], 13151[1], 13152[1], 13153[1], 36000[1], 36400[1], 36405[1], 36406[1], 36410[1], 36420[1], 36425[1], 36430[1], 36440[1], 36591[0], 36592[0], 36600[1], 36640[1], 43752[1], 51701[0], 51702[0], 51703[1], 52000[0], 53000[0], 53010[0], 53020[0], 53025[0], 62320[0], 62321[0], 62322[0], 62323[0], 62324[0], 62325[0], 62326[0], 62327[0], 64400[0], 64405[0], 64408[0], 64415[0], 64416[0], 64417[0], 64418[0], 64420[0], 64421[0], 64425[0], 64430[0], 64435[0], 64445[0], 64446[0], 64447[0], 64448[0], 64449[0], 64450[0], 64451[0], 64454[0], 64461[0], 64462[0], 64463[0], 64479[0], 64480[0], 64483[0], 64484[0], 64486[0], 64487[0], 64488[0], 64489[0], 64490[0], 64491[0], 64492[0], 64493[0], 64494[0], 64495[0], 64505[0], 64510[0], 64517[0], 64520[0], 64530[0], 69990[0], 92012[1], 92014[1], 93000[1], 93005[1], 93010[1], 93040[1], 93041[1], 93042[1], 93318[1], 93355[1], 94002[1], 94200[1], 94680[1], 94681[1], 94690[1], 95812[1], 95813[1], 95816[1], 95819[1], 95822[1], 95829[1], 95955[1], 96360[1], 96361[1], 96365[1], 96366[1], 96367[1], 96368[1], 96372[1], 96374[1], 96375[1], 96376[1], 96377[1], 96523[0], 97597[1], 97598[1], 97602[1], 99155[0], 99156[0], 99157[0], 99211[1], 99212[1], 99213[1], 99214[1], 99215[1], 99217[1], 99218[1], 99219[1], 99220[1], 99221[1], 99222[1], 99223[1], 99231[1], 99232[1], 99233[1], 99234[1], 99235[1], 99236[1], 99238[1], 99239[1], 99241[1], 99242[1], 99243[1], 99244[1], 99245[1], 99251[1], 99252[1], 99253[1], 99254[1], 99255[1], 99291[1], 99292[1], 99304[1], 99305[1], 99306[1], 99307[1], 99308[1], 99309[1], 99310[1], 99315[1], 99316[1], 99334[1], 99335[1], 99336[1], 99337[1], 99347[1], 99348[1], 99349[1], 99350[1], 99374[1], 99375[1], 99377[1], 99378[1], 99446[0], 99447[0], 99448[0], 99449[0], 99451[0], 99452[0], 99495[0], 99496[0], G0463[1], G0471[0]
54352	0213T[0], 0216T[0], 0596T[1], 0597T[1], 0708T[1], 0709T[1], 11000[1], 11001[1], 11004[1], 11005[1], 11006[1], 11042[1], 11043[1], 11044[1], 11045[1], 11046[1], 11047[1], 12001[1], 12002[1], 12004[1], 12005[1], 12006[1], 12007[1], 12011[1], 12013[1], 12014[1], 12015[1], 12016[1], 12017[1], 12018[1], 12020[1], 12021[1], 12031[1], 12032[1], 12034[1], 12035[1], 12036[1], 12037[1], 12041[1], 12042[1], 12044[1], 12045[1], 12046[1], 12047[1], 12051[1], 12052[1], 12053[1], 12054[1], 12055[1], 12056[1], 12057[1], 13100[1], 13101[1], 13102[1], 13120[1], 13121[1], 13122[1], 13131[1], 13132[1], 13133[1], 13151[1], 13152[1], 13153[1], 15276[1], 15277[1], 15278[1], 36000[1], 36400[1], 36405[1], 36406[1], 36410[1], 36420[1], 36425[1], 36430[1], 36440[1], 36591[0], 36592[0], 36600[1], 36640[1], 43752[1], 51701[0], 51702[0], 51703[1], 52000[0], 53000[0], 53010[0], 53020[0], 53025[0], 54304[0], 54308[0], 54312[0], 54316[0], 54318[0], 54322[0], 54324[0], 54326[0], 54328[0], 62320[0], 62321[0], 62322[0], 62323[0], 62324[0], 62325[0], 62326[0], 62327[0], 64400[0], 64405[0], 64408[0], 64415[0], 64416[0], 64417[0], 64418[0], 64420[0], 64421[0], 64425[0], 64430[0], 64435[0], 64445[0], 64446[0], 64447[0], 64448[0], 64449[0], 64450[0], 64451[0], 64454[0], 64461[0], 64462[0], 64463[0], 64479[0], 64480[0], 64483[0], 64484[0], 64486[0], 64487[0], 64488[0], 64489[0], 64490[0], 64491[0], 64492[0], 64493[0], 64494[0], 64495[0], 64505[0], 64510[0], 64517[0], 64520[0], 64530[0], 69990[0], 92012[1], 92014[1], 93000[1], 93005[1], 93010[1], 93040[1], 93041[1], 93042[1], 93318[1], 93355[1], 94002[1], 94200[1], 94680[1], 94681[1], 94690[1], 95812[1], 95813[1], 95816[1], 95819[1], 95822[1], 95829[1], 95955[1], 96360[1], 96361[1], 96365[1], 96366[1], 96367[1], 96368[1], 96372[1], 96374[1], 96375[1], 96376[1], 96377[1], 96523[0], 97597[1], 97598[1], 97602[1], 99155[0], 99156[0], 99157[0], 99211[1], 99212[1], 99213[1], 99214[1], 99215[1], 99217[1], 99218[1], 99219[1], 99220[1], 99221[1], 99222[1], 99223[1], 99231[1], 99232[1], 99233[1], 99234[1], 99235[1], 99236[1], 99238[1], 99239[1], 99241[1], 99242[1], 99243[1], 99244[1], 99245[1], 99251[1], 99252[1], 99253[1], 99254[1], 99255[1], 99291[1], 99292[1], 99304[1], 99305[1], 99306[1], 99307[1], 99308[1], 99309[1], 99310[1], 99315[1], 99316[1], 99334[1], 99335[1], 99336[1], 99337[1], 99347[1], 99348[1], 99349[1], 99350[1], 99374[1], 99375[1], 99377[1], 99378[1], 99446[0], 99447[0], 99448[0], 99449[0], 99451[0], 99452[0], 99495[0], 99496[0], G0463[1], G0471[0]
54360	0213T[0], 0216T[0], 0596T[1], 0597T[1], 0708T[1], 0709T[1], 12001[1], 12002[1], 12004[1], 12005[1], 12006[1], 12007[1], 12011[1], 12013[1], 12014[1], 12015[1], 12016[1], 12017[1], 12018[1], 12020[1], 12021[1], 12031[1], 12032[1], 12034[1], 12035[1], 12036[1], 12037[1], 12041[1], 12042[1], 12044[1], 12045[1], 12046[1], 12047[1], 12051[1], 12052[1], 12053[1], 12054[1], 12055[1], 12056[1], 12057[1], 13100[1], 13101[1], 13102[1], 13120[1], 13121[1], 13122[1], 13131[1], 13132[1], 13133[1], 13151[1], 13152[1], 13153[1], 36000[1], 36400[1], 36405[1], 36406[1], 36410[1], 36420[1], 36425[1], 36430[1], 36440[1], 36591[0], 36592[0], 36600[1], 36640[1], 43752[1], 51701[0], 51702[0], 51703[1], 54437[0], 54440[1], 62320[0], 62321[0], 62322[0], 62323[0], 62324[0], 62325[0], 62326[0], 62327[0], 64400[0], 64405[0], 64408[0], 64415[0], 64416[0], 64417[0], 64418[0], 64420[0], 64421[0], 64425[0], 64430[0], 64435[0], 64445[0], 64446[0], 64447[0], 64448[0], 64449[0], 64450[0], 64451[0], 64454[0], 64461[0], 64462[0], 64463[0], 64479[0], 64480[0], 64483[0], 64484[0], 64486[0], 64487[0], 64488[0], 64489[0], 64490[0], 64491[0], 64492[0], 64493[0], 64494[0], 64495[0], 64505[0], 64510[0], 64517[0], 64520[0], 64530[0], 69990[0], 92012[1], 92014[1], 93000[1], 93005[1], 93010[1], 93040[1], 93041[1], 93042[1], 93318[1], 93355[1], 94002[1], 94200[1], 94680[1], 94681[1], 94690[1], 95812[1], 95813[1], 95816[1], 95819[1], 95822[1], 95829[1], 95955[1], 96360[1], 96361[1], 96365[1], 96366[1], 96367[1], 96368[1], 96372[1], 96374[1], 96375[1], 96376[1], 96377[1], 96523[0], 99155[0], 99156[0], 99157[0], 99211[1], 99212[1], 99213[1], 99214[1], 99215[1], 99217[1], 99218[1], 99219[1], 99220[1], 99221[1], 99222[1], 99223[1], 99231[1], 99232[1], 99233[1], 99234[1], 99235[1], 99236[1], 99238[1], 99239[1], 99241[1], 99242[1], 99243[1], 99244[1], 99245[1], 99251[1], 99252[1], 99253[1], 99254[1], 99255[1], 99291[1], 99292[1], 99304[1], 99305[1], 99306[1], 99307[1], 99308[1], 99309[1], 99310[1], 99315[1], 99316[1], 99334[1], 99335[1], 99336[1], 99337[1], 99347[1], 99348[1], 99349[1], 99350[1], 99374[1], 99375[1], 99377[1], 99378[1], 99446[0], 99447[0], 99448[0], 99449[0], 99451[0], 99452[0], 99495[0], 99496[0], G0463[1], G0471[0]
54380	0213T[0], 0216T[0], 0596T[1], 0597T[1], 0708T[1], 0709T[1], 12001[1], 12002[1], 12004[1], 12005[1], 12006[1], 12007[1], 12011[1], 12013[1], 12014[1], 12015[1], 12016[1], 12017[1], 12018[1], 12020[1], 12021[1], 12031[1], 12032[1], 12034[1], 12035[1], 12036[1], 12037[1], 12041[1], 12042[1], 12044[1], 12045[1], 12046[1], 12047[1], 12051[1], 12052[1], 12053[1], 12054[1], 12055[1], 12056[1], 12057[1], 13100[1], 13101[1], 13102[1], 13120[1], 13121[1], 13122[1], 13131[1], 13132[1], 13133[1], 13151[1], 13152[1], 13153[1], 36000[1], 36400[1], 36405[1], 36406[1], 36410[1], 36420[1], 36425[1], 36430[1], 36440[1], 36591[0], 36592[0], 36600[1], 36640[1], 43752[1], 51701[0], 51702[0], 51703[1], 53000[0], 53010[0], 53020[0], 53025[0], 54110[1], 54111[1], 54112[1], 54200[1], 54205[1], 62320[0], 62321[0], 62322[0], 62323[0], 62324[0], 62325[0], 62326[0], 62327[0], 64400[0], 64405[0], 64408[0], 64415[0], 64416[0], 64417[0], 64418[0], 64420[0], 64421[0], 64425[0], 64430[0], 64435[0], 64445[0], 64446[0], 64447[0], 64448[0], 64449[0], 64450[0], 64451[0], 64454[0], 64461[0], 64462[0], 64463[0], 64479[0], 64480[0], 64483[0], 64484[0], 64486[0], 64487[0], 64488[0], 64489[0], 64490[0], 64491[0], 64492[0], 64493[0], 64494[0], 64495[0], 64505[0], 64510[0], 64517[0], 64520[0], 64530[0], 69990[0], 92012[1], 92014[1], 93000[1], 93005[1], 93010[1], 93040[1], 93041[1], 93042[1], 93318[1], 93355[1], 94002[1], 94200[1], 94680[1], 94681[1], 94690[1], 95812[1], 95813[1], 95816[1], 95819[1], 95822[1], 95829[1], 95955[1], 96360[1], 96361[1], 96365[1], 96366[1], 96367[1], 96368[1], 96372[1], 96374[1], 96375[1], 96376[1], 96377[1], 96523[0], 99155[0], 99156[0], 99157[0], 99211[1], 99212[1], 99213[1], 99214[1], 99215[1], 99217[1], 99218[1], 99219[1], 99220[1], 99221[1], 99222[1], 99223[1], 99231[1], 99232[1], 99233[1], 99234[1], 99235[1], 99236[1], 99238[1], 99239[1], 99241[1], 99242[1], 99243[1], 99244[1], 99245[1], 99251[1], 99252[1], 99253[1], 99254[1], 99255[1], 99291[1], 99292[1], 99304[1], 99305[1], 99306[1], 99307[1], 99308[1], 99309[1], 99310[1], 99315[1], 99316[1], 99334[1], 99335[1], 99336[1], 99337[1], 99347[1], 99348[1], 99349[1], 99350[1], 99374[1], 99375[1], 99377[1], 99378[1], 99446[0], 99447[0], 99448[0], 99449[0], 99451[0], 99452[0], 99495[0], 99496[0], G0463[1], G0471[0]
54385	0213T[0], 0216T[0], 0596T[1], 0597T[1], 0708T[1], 0709T[1], 12001[1], 12002[1], 12004[1], 12005[1], 12006[1], 12007[1], 12011[1], 12013[1], 12014[1], 12015[1], 12016[1], 12017[1], 12018[1], 12020[1], 12021[1], 12031[1], 12032[1], 12034[1], 12035[1], 12036[1], 12037[1], 12041[1], 12042[1], 12044[1],

0 = Modifier usage not allowed or inappropriate 1 = Modifier usage allowed

Code 1	Code 2
	12045[1], 12046[1], 12047[1], 12051[1], 12052[1], 12053[1], 12054[1], 12055[1], 12056[1], 12057[1], 13100[1], 13101[1], 13102[1], 13120[1], 13121[1], 13122[1], 13131[1], 13132[1], 13133[1], 13151[1], 13152[1], 13153[1], 36000[1], 36400[1], 36405[1], 36406[1], 36410[1], 36420[1], 36425[1], 36430[1], 36440[1], 36591[0], 36592[0], 36600[1], 36640[1], 43752[1], 51701[0], 51702[0], 51703[1], 53000[0], 53010[0], 53020[0], 53025[0], 54380[1], 62320[0], 62321[0], 62322[0], 62323[0], 62324[0], 62325[0], 62326[0], 62327[0], 64400[0], 64405[0], 64408[0], 64415[0], 64416[0], 64417[0], 64418[0], 64420[0], 64421[0], 64425[0], 64430[0], 64435[0], 64445[0], 64446[0], 64447[0], 64448[0], 64449[0], 64450[0], 64451[0], 64454[0], 64461[0], 64462[0], 64463[0], 64479[0], 64480[0], 64483[0], 64484[0], 64486[0], 64487[0], 64488[0], 64489[0], 64490[0], 64491[0], 64492[0], 64493[0], 64494[0], 64495[0], 64505[0], 64510[0], 64517[0], 64520[0], 64530[0], 69990[0], 92012[1], 92014[1], 93000[1], 93005[1], 93010[1], 93040[1], 93041[1], 93042[1], 93318[1], 93355[1], 94002[1], 94200[1], 94680[1], 94681[1], 94690[1], 95812[1], 95813[1], 95816[1], 95819[1], 95822[1], 95829[1], 95955[1], 96360[1], 96361[1], 96365[1], 96366[1], 96367[1], 96368[1], 96372[1], 96374[1], 96375[1], 96376[1], 96377[1], 96523[0], 99155[0], 99156[0], 99157[0], 99211[1], 99212[1], 99213[1], 99214[1], 99215[1], 99217[1], 99218[1], 99219[1], 99220[1], 99221[1], 99222[1], 99223[1], 99231[1], 99232[1], 99233[1], 99234[1], 99235[1], 99236[1], 99238[1], 99239[1], 99241[1], 99242[1], 99243[1], 99244[1], 99245[1], 99251[1], 99252[1], 99253[1], 99254[1], 99255[1], 99291[1], 99292[1], 99304[1], 99305[1], 99306[1], 99307[1], 99308[1], 99309[1], 99310[1], 99315[1], 99316[1], 99334[1], 99335[1], 99336[1], 99337[1], 99347[1], 99348[1], 99349[1], 99350[1], 99374[1], 99375[1], 99377[1], 99378[1], 99446[0], 99447[0], 99448[0], 99449[0], 99451[0], 99452[0], 99495[0], 99496[0], G0463[1], G0471[0]
54390	0213T[0], 0216T[0], 0596T[1], 0597T[1], 0708T[1], 0709T[1], 12001[1], 12002[1], 12004[1], 12005[1], 12006[1], 12007[1], 12011[1], 12013[1], 12014[1], 12015[1], 12016[1], 12017[1], 12018[1], 12020[1], 12021[1], 12031[1], 12032[1], 12034[1], 12035[1], 12036[1], 12037[1], 12041[1], 12042[1], 12044[1], 12045[1], 12046[1], 12047[1], 12051[1], 12052[1], 12053[1], 12054[1], 12055[1], 12056[1], 12057[1], 13100[1], 13101[1], 13102[1], 13120[1], 13121[1], 13122[1], 13131[1], 13132[1], 13133[1], 13151[1], 13152[1], 13153[1], 36000[1], 36400[1], 36405[1], 36406[1], 36410[1], 36420[1], 36425[1], 36430[1], 36440[1], 36591[0], 36592[0], 36600[1], 36640[1], 43752[1], 51701[0], 51702[0], 51703[1], 51940[1], 52000[0], 53000[0], 53010[0], 53020[0], 53025[0], 54380[1], 62320[0], 62321[0], 62322[0], 62323[0], 62324[0], 62325[0], 62326[0], 62327[0], 64400[0], 64405[0], 64408[0], 64415[0], 64416[0], 64417[0], 64418[0], 64420[0], 64421[0], 64425[0], 64430[0], 64435[0], 64445[0], 64446[0], 64447[0], 64448[0], 64449[0], 64450[0], 64451[0], 64454[0], 64461[0], 64462[0], 64463[0], 64479[0], 64480[0], 64483[0], 64484[0], 64486[0], 64487[0], 64488[0], 64489[0], 64490[0], 64491[0], 64492[0], 64493[0], 64494[0], 64495[0], 64505[0], 64510[0], 64517[0], 64520[0], 64530[0], 69990[0], 92012[1], 92014[1], 93000[1], 93005[1], 93010[1], 93040[1], 93041[1], 93042[1], 93318[1], 93355[1], 94002[1], 94200[1], 94680[1], 94681[1], 94690[1], 95812[1], 95813[1], 95816[1], 95819[1], 95822[1], 95829[1], 95955[1], 96360[1], 96361[1], 96365[1], 96366[1], 96367[1], 96368[1], 96372[1], 96374[1], 96375[1], 96376[1], 96377[1], 96523[0], 99155[0], 99156[0], 99157[0], 99211[1], 99212[1], 99213[1], 99214[1], 99215[1], 99217[1], 99218[1], 99219[1], 99220[1], 99221[1], 99222[1], 99223[1], 99231[1], 99232[1], 99233[1], 99234[1], 99235[1], 99236[1], 99238[1], 99239[1], 99241[1], 99242[1], 99243[1], 99244[1], 99245[1], 99251[1], 99252[1], 99253[1], 99254[1], 99255[1], 99291[1], 99292[1], 99304[1], 99305[1], 99306[1], 99307[1], 99308[1], 99309[1], 99310[1], 99315[1], 99316[1], 99334[1], 99335[1], 99336[1], 99337[1], 99347[1], 99348[1], 99349[1], 99350[1], 99374[1], 99375[1], 99377[1], 99378[1], 99446[0], 99447[0], 99448[0], 99449[0], 99451[0], 99452[0], 99495[0], 99496[0], G0463[1], G0471[0]
54400	0213T[0], 0216T[0], 0596T[1], 0597T[1], 0708T[1], 0709T[1], 12001[1], 12002[1], 12004[1], 12005[1], 12006[1], 12007[1], 12011[1], 12013[1], 12014[1], 12015[1], 12016[1], 12017[1], 12018[1], 12020[1], 12021[1], 12031[1], 12032[1], 12034[1], 12035[1], 12036[1], 12037[1], 12041[1], 12042[1], 12044[1], 12045[1], 12046[1], 12047[1], 12051[1], 12052[1], 12053[1], 12054[1], 12055[1], 12056[1], 12057[1], 13100[1], 13101[1], 13102[1], 13120[1], 13121[1], 13122[1], 13131[1], 13132[1], 13133[1], 13151[1], 13152[1], 13153[1], 36000[1], 36400[1], 36405[1], 36406[1], 36410[1], 36420[1], 36425[1], 36430[1], 36440[1], 36591[0], 36592[0], 36600[1], 36640[1], 43752[1], 51701[0], 51702[0], 51703[1], 54161[1], 54401[1], 54405[1], 62320[0], 62321[0], 62322[0], 62323[0], 62324[0], 62325[0], 62326[0], 62327[0], 64400[0], 64405[0], 64408[0], 64415[0], 64416[0], 64417[0], 64418[0], 64420[0], 64421[0], 64425[0], 64430[0], 64435[0], 64445[0], 64446[0], 64447[0], 64448[0], 64449[0], 64450[0], 64451[0], 64454[0], 64461[0], 64462[0], 64463[0], 64479[0], 64480[0], 64483[0], 64484[0], 64486[0], 64487[0], 64488[0], 64489[0], 64490[0], 64491[0], 64492[0], 64493[0], 64494[0], 64495[0], 64505[0], 64510[0], 64517[0], 64520[0], 64530[0], 69990[0], 92012[1], 92014[1], 93000[1], 93005[1], 93010[1], 93040[1], 93041[1], 93042[1], 93318[1], 93355[1], 94002[1], 94200[1], 94680[1], 94681[1], 94690[1], 95812[1], 95813[1], 95816[1], 95819[1], 95822[1], 95829[1], 95955[1], 96360[1], 96361[1], 96365[1], 96366[1], 96367[1], 96368[1], 96372[1], 96374[1], 96375[1], 96376[1], 96377[1], 96523[0], 99155[0], 99156[0], 99157[0], 99211[1], 99212[1], 99213[1], 99214[1], 99215[1], 99217[1], 99218[1], 99219[1], 99220[1], 99221[1], 99222[1], 99223[1], 99231[1], 99232[1], 99233[1], 99234[1], 99235[1], 99236[1], 99238[1], 99239[1], 99241[1], 99242[1], 99243[1], 99244[1], 99245[1], 99251[1], 99252[1], 99253[1], 99254[1], 99255[1], 99291[1], 99292[1], 99304[1], 99305[1], 99306[1], 99307[1], 99308[1], 99309[1], 99310[1], 99315[1], 99316[1], 99334[1], 99335[1], 99336[1], 99337[1], 99347[1], 99348[1], 99349[1], 99350[1], 99374[1], 99375[1], 99377[1], 99378[1], 99446[0], 99447[0], 99448[0], 99449[0], 99451[0], 99452[0], 99495[0], 99496[0], G0463[1], G0471[0]
54401	0213T[0], 0216T[0], 0596T[1], 0597T[1], 0708T[1], 0709T[1], 12001[1], 12002[1], 12004[1], 12005[1], 12006[1], 12007[1], 12011[1], 12013[1], 12014[1], 12015[1], 12016[1], 12017[1], 12018[1], 12020[1], 12021[1], 12031[1], 12032[1], 12034[1], 12035[1], 12036[1], 12037[1], 12041[1], 12042[1], 12044[1], 12045[1], 12046[1], 12047[1], 12051[1], 12052[1], 12053[1], 12054[1], 12055[1], 12056[1], 12057[1], 13100[1], 13101[1], 13102[1], 13120[1], 13121[1], 13122[1], 13131[1], 13132[1], 13133[1], 13151[1], 13152[1], 13153[1], 36000[1], 36400[1], 36405[1], 36406[1], 36410[1], 36420[1], 36425[1], 36430[1], 36440[1], 36591[0], 36592[0], 36600[1], 36640[1], 43752[1], 51701[0], 51702[0], 51703[1], 54405[1], 62320[0], 62321[0], 62322[0], 62323[0], 62324[0], 62325[0], 62326[0], 62327[0], 64400[0], 64405[0], 64408[0], 64415[0], 64416[0], 64417[0], 64418[0], 64420[0], 64421[0], 64425[0], 64430[0], 64435[0], 64445[0], 64446[0], 64447[0], 64448[0], 64449[0], 64450[0], 64451[0], 64454[0], 64461[0], 64462[0], 64463[0], 64479[0], 64480[0], 64483[0], 64484[0], 64486[0], 64487[0], 64488[0], 64489[0], 64490[0], 64491[0], 64492[0], 64493[0], 64494[0], 64495[0], 64505[0], 64510[0], 64517[0], 64520[0], 64530[0], 69990[0], 92012[1], 92014[1], 93000[1], 93005[1], 93010[1], 93040[1], 93041[1], 93042[1], 93318[1], 93355[1], 94002[1], 94200[1], 94680[1], 94681[1], 94690[1], 95812[1], 95813[1], 95816[1], 95819[1], 95822[1], 95829[1], 95955[1], 96360[1], 96361[1], 96365[1], 96366[1], 96367[1], 96368[1], 96372[1], 96374[1], 96375[1], 96376[1], 96377[1], 96523[0], 99155[0], 99156[0], 99157[0], 99211[1], 99212[1], 99213[1], 99214[1], 99215[1], 99217[1], 99218[1], 99219[1], 99220[1], 99221[1], 99222[1], 99223[1], 99231[1], 99232[1], 99233[1], 99234[1], 99235[1], 99236[1], 99238[1], 99239[1], 99241[1], 99242[1], 99243[1], 99244[1], 99245[1], 99251[1], 99252[1], 99253[1], 99254[1], 99255[1], 99291[1], 99292[1], 99304[1], 99305[1], 99306[1], 99307[1], 99308[1], 99309[1], 99310[1], 99315[1], 99316[1], 99334[1], 99335[1], 99336[1], 99337[1], 99347[1], 99348[1], 99349[1], 99350[1], 99374[1], 99375[1], 99377[1], 99378[1], 99446[0], 99447[0], 99448[0], 99449[0], 99451[0], 99452[0], 99495[0], 99496[0], G0463[1], G0471[0]
54405	0213T[0], 0216T[0], 0596T[1], 0597T[1], 0708T[1], 0709T[1], 12001[1], 12002[1], 12004[1], 12005[1], 12006[1], 12007[1], 12011[1], 12013[1], 12014[1], 12015[1], 12016[1], 12017[1], 12018[1], 12020[1], 12021[1], 12031[1], 12032[1], 12034[1], 12035[1], 12036[1], 12037[1], 12041[1], 12042[1], 12044[1], 12045[1], 12046[1], 12047[1], 12051[1], 12052[1], 12053[1], 12054[1], 12055[1], 12056[1], 12057[1], 13100[1], 13101[1], 13102[1], 13120[1], 13121[1], 13122[1], 13131[1], 13132[1], 13133[1], 13151[1], 13152[1], 13153[1], 36000[1], 36400[1], 36405[1], 36406[1], 36410[1], 36420[1], 36425[1], 36430[1], 36440[1], 36591[0], 36592[0], 36600[1], 36640[1], 43752[1], 49000[1], 49002[1], 49010[0], 51701[0], 51702[0], 51703[1], 54110[1], 54161[1], 54408[0], 62270[1], 62320[0], 62321[0], 62322[0], 62323[0], 62324[0], 62325[0], 62326[0], 62327[0], 62328[1], 64400[0], 64405[0], 64408[0], 64415[0], 64416[0], 64417[0], 64418[0], 64420[0], 64421[0], 64425[0], 64430[0], 64435[0], 64445[0], 64446[0], 64447[0], 64448[0], 64449[0], 64450[0], 64451[0], 64454[0], 64461[0], 64462[0], 64463[0], 64479[0], 64480[0], 64483[0], 64484[0], 64486[0], 64487[0], 64488[0], 64489[0], 64490[0], 64491[0], 64492[0], 64493[0], 64494[0], 64495[0], 64505[0], 64510[0], 64517[0], 64520[0], 64530[0], 69990[0], 92012[1], 92014[1], 93000[1], 93005[1], 93010[1], 93040[1], 93041[1], 93042[1], 93318[1], 93355[1], 94002[1], 94200[1], 94680[1], 94681[1], 94690[1], 95812[1], 95813[1], 95816[1], 95819[1], 95822[1], 95829[1], 95955[1], 96360[1], 96361[1], 96365[1], 96366[1], 96367[1], 96368[1], 96372[1], 96374[1], 96375[1], 96376[1], 96377[1], 96523[0], 99155[0], 99156[0], 99157[0], 99211[1], 99212[1], 99213[1], 99214[1], 99215[1], 99217[1], 99218[1], 99219[1], 99220[1], 99221[1], 99222[1], 99223[1], 99231[1], 99232[1], 99233[1], 99234[1], 99235[1], 99236[1], 99238[1], 99239[1], 99241[1], 99242[1], 99243[1], 99244[1], 99245[1], 99251[1], 99252[1], 99253[1], 99254[1], 99255[1], 99291[1], 99292[1], 99304[1], 99305[1], 99306[1], 99307[1], 99308[1], 99309[1], 99310[1], 99315[1], 99316[1], 99334[1], 99335[1], 99336[1], 99337[1], 99347[1], 99348[1], 99349[1], 99350[1], 99374[1], 99375[1], 99377[1], 99378[1], 99446[0], 99447[0], 99448[0], 99449[0], 99451[0], 99452[0], 99495[0], 99496[0], G0463[1], G0471[0], P9612[0]
54406	0213T[0], 0216T[0], 0596T[1], 0597T[1], 0708T[1], 0709T[1], 12001[1], 12002[1], 12004[1], 12005[1], 12006[1], 12007[1], 12011[1], 12013[1], 12014[1], 12015[1], 12016[1], 12017[1], 12018[1], 12020[1], 12021[1], 12031[1], 12032[1], 12034[1], 12035[1], 12036[1], 12037[1], 12041[1], 12042[1], 12044[1], 12045[1], 12046[1], 12047[1], 12051[1], 12052[1], 12053[1], 12054[1], 12055[1], 12056[1], 12057[1], 13100[1], 13101[1], 13102[1], 13120[1], 13121[1], 13122[1], 13131[1], 13132[1], 13133[1], 13151[1], 13152[1], 13153[1], 36000[1], 36400[1], 36405[1], 36406[1], 36410[1], 36420[1], 36425[1], 36430[1], 36440[1], 36591[0], 36592[0], 36600[1], 36640[1], 43752[1], 51701[0], 51702[0], 51703[1], 54405[0], 54416[0], 62320[0], 62321[0], 62322[0], 62323[0], 62324[0], 62325[0], 62326[0], 62327[0], 64400[0], 64405[0], 64408[0], 64415[0], 64416[0], 64417[0], 64418[0], 64420[0], 64421[0], 64425[0], 64430[0], 64435[0], 64445[0], 64446[0], 64447[0], 64448[0], 64449[0], 64450[0], 64451[0], 64454[0], 64461[0], 64462[0], 64463[0], 64479[0], 64480[0], 64483[0], 64484[0], 64486[0], 64487[0], 64488[0], 64489[0], 64490[0], 64491[0], 64492[0], 64493[0], 64494[0], 64495[0], 64505[0], 64510[0], 64517[0], 64520[0], 64530[0], 69990[0], 92012[1], 92014[1], 93000[1], 93005[1], 93010[1], 93040[1], 93041[1], 93042[1], 93318[1], 93355[1], 94002[1], 94200[1], 94680[1], 94681[1], 94690[1], 95812[1], 95813[1], 95816[1], 95819[1], 95822[1], 95829[1], 95955[1], 96360[1], 96361[1], 96365[1], 96366[1], 96367[1], 96368[1], 96372[1], 96374[1], 96375[1], 96376[1], 96377[1], 96523[0], 99155[0], 99156[0], 99157[0], 99211[1], 99212[1], 99213[1], 99214[1], 99215[1], 99217[1], 99218[1], 99219[1], 99220[1], 99221[1], 99222[1], 99223[1], 99231[1], 99232[1], 99233[1], 99234[1], 99235[1], 99236[1], 99238[1], 99239[1], 99241[1], 99242[1], 99243[1], 99244[1], 99245[1], 99251[1], 99252[1], 99253[1], 99254[1], 99255[1], 99291[1], 99292[1], 99304[1], 99305[1], 99306[1], 99307[1], 99308[1], 99309[1], 99310[1], 99315[1], 99316[1],

0 = Modifier usage not allowed or inappropriate 1 = Modifier usage allowed

Code 1	Code 2
	99334[1], 99335[1], 99336[1], 99337[1], 99347[1], 99348[1], 99349[1], 99350[1], 99374[1], 99375[1], 99377[1], 99378[1], 99446[0], 99447[0], 99448[0], 99449[0], 99451[0], 99452[0], 99495[0], 99496[0], G0463[1], G0471[0]
54408	0213T[0], 0216T[0], 0596T[1], 0597T[1], 0708T[1], 0709T[1], 12001[1], 12002[1], 12004[1], 12005[1], 12006[1], 12007[1], 12011[1], 12013[1], 12014[1], 12015[1], 12016[1], 12017[1], 12018[1], 12020[1], 12021[1], 12031[1], 12032[1], 12034[1], 12035[1], 12036[1], 12037[1], 12041[1], 12042[1], 12044[1], 12045[1], 12046[1], 12047[1], 12051[1], 12052[1], 12053[1], 12054[1], 12055[1], 12056[1], 12057[1], 13100[1], 13101[1], 13102[1], 13120[1], 13121[1], 13122[1], 13131[1], 13132[1], 13133[1], 13151[1], 13152[1], 13153[1], 36000[1], 36400[1], 36405[1], 36406[1], 36410[1], 36420[1], 36425[1], 36430[1], 36440[1], 36591[0], 36592[0], 36600[1], 36640[1], 43752[1], 51701[0], 51702[0], 51703[1], 54400[0], 54401[0], 54406[0], 54416[0], 62320[0], 62321[0], 62322[0], 62323[0], 62324[0], 62325[0], 62326[0], 62327[0], 64400[0], 64405[0], 64408[0], 64415[0], 64416[0], 64417[0], 64418[0], 64420[0], 64421[0], 64425[0], 64430[0], 64435[0], 64445[0], 64446[0], 64447[0], 64448[0], 64449[0], 64450[0], 64451[0], 64454[0], 64461[0], 64462[0], 64463[0], 64479[0], 64480[0], 64483[0], 64484[0], 64486[0], 64487[0], 64488[0], 64489[0], 64490[0], 64491[0], 64492[0], 64493[0], 64494[0], 64495[0], 64505[0], 64510[0], 64517[0], 64520[0], 64530[0], 69990[0], 92012[1], 92014[1], 93000[1], 93005[1], 93010[1], 93040[1], 93041[1], 93042[1], 93318[1], 93355[1], 94002[1], 94200[1], 94680[1], 94681[1], 94690[1], 95812[1], 95813[1], 95816[1], 95819[1], 95822[1], 95829[1], 95955[1], 96360[1], 96361[1], 96365[1], 96366[1], 96367[1], 96368[1], 96372[1], 96374[1], 96375[1], 96376[1], 96377[1], 96523[0], 99155[0], 99156[0], 99157[0], 99211[1], 99212[1], 99213[1], 99214[1], 99215[1], 99217[1], 99218[1], 99219[1], 99220[1], 99221[1], 99222[1], 99223[1], 99231[1], 99232[1], 99233[1], 99234[1], 99235[1], 99236[1], 99238[1], 99239[1], 99241[1], 99242[1], 99243[1], 99244[1], 99245[1], 99251[1], 99252[1], 99253[1], 99254[1], 99255[1], 99291[1], 99292[1], 99304[1], 99305[1], 99306[1], 99307[1], 99308[1], 99309[1], 99310[1], 99315[1], 99316[1], 99334[1], 99335[1], 99336[1], 99337[1], 99347[1], 99348[1], 99349[1], 99350[1], 99374[1], 99375[1], 99377[1], 99378[1], 99446[0], 99447[0], 99448[0], 99449[0], 99451[0], 99452[0], 99495[0], 99496[0], G0463[1], G0471[0]
54410	0213T[0], 0216T[0], 0596T[1], 0597T[1], 0708T[1], 0709T[1], 12001[1], 12002[1], 12004[1], 12005[1], 12006[1], 12007[1], 12011[1], 12013[1], 12014[1], 12015[1], 12016[1], 12017[1], 12018[1], 12020[1], 12021[1], 12031[1], 12032[1], 12034[1], 12035[1], 12036[1], 12037[1], 12041[1], 12042[1], 12044[1], 12045[1], 12046[1], 12047[1], 12051[1], 12052[1], 12053[1], 12054[1], 12055[1], 12056[1], 12057[1], 13100[1], 13101[1], 13102[1], 13120[1], 13121[1], 13122[1], 13131[1], 13132[1], 13133[1], 13151[1], 13152[1], 13153[1], 36000[1], 36400[1], 36405[1], 36406[1], 36410[1], 36420[1], 36425[1], 36430[1], 36440[1], 36591[0], 36592[0], 36600[1], 36640[1], 43752[1], 51701[0], 51702[0], 51703[1], 54400[0], 54401[0], 54405[0], 54406[0], 54408[0], 54411[0], 54415[0], 54416[0], 54417[0], 62320[0], 62321[0], 62322[0], 62323[0], 62324[0], 62325[0], 62326[0], 62327[0], 64400[0], 64405[0], 64408[0], 64415[0], 64416[0], 64417[0], 64418[0], 64420[0], 64421[0], 64425[0], 64430[0], 64435[0], 64445[0], 64446[0], 64447[0], 64448[0], 64449[0], 64450[0], 64451[0], 64454[0], 64461[0], 64462[0], 64463[0], 64479[0], 64480[0], 64483[0], 64484[0], 64486[0], 64487[0], 64488[0], 64489[0], 64490[0], 64491[0], 64492[0], 64493[0], 64494[0], 64495[0], 64505[0], 64510[0], 64517[0], 64520[0], 64530[0], 69990[0], 92012[1], 92014[1], 93000[1], 93005[1], 93010[1], 93040[1], 93041[1], 93042[1], 93318[1], 93355[1], 94002[1], 94200[1], 94680[1], 94681[1], 94690[1], 95812[1], 95813[1], 95816[1], 95819[1], 95822[1], 95829[1], 95955[1], 96360[1], 96361[1], 96365[1], 96366[1], 96367[1], 96368[1], 96372[1], 96374[1], 96375[1], 96376[1], 96377[1], 96523[0], 99155[0], 99156[0], 99157[0], 99211[1], 99212[1], 99213[1], 99214[1], 99215[1], 99217[1], 99218[1], 99219[1], 99220[1], 99221[1], 99222[1], 99223[1], 99231[1], 99232[1], 99233[1], 99234[1], 99235[1], 99236[1], 99238[1], 99239[1], 99241[1], 99242[1], 99243[1], 99244[1], 99245[1], 99251[1], 99252[1], 99253[1], 99254[1], 99255[1], 99291[1], 99292[1], 99304[1], 99305[1], 99306[1], 99307[1], 99308[1], 99309[1], 99310[1], 99315[1], 99316[1], 99334[1], 99335[1], 99336[1], 99337[1], 99347[1], 99348[1], 99349[1], 99350[1], 99374[1], 99375[1], 99377[1], 99378[1], 99446[0], 99447[0], 99448[0], 99449[0], 99451[0], 99452[0], 99495[0], 99496[0], G0463[1], G0471[0]
54411	0213T[0], 0216T[0], 0596T[1], 0597T[1], 0708T[1], 0709T[1], 11000[1], 11001[1], 11004[1], 11005[1], 11006[1], 11042[1], 11043[1], 11044[1], 11045[1], 11046[1], 11047[1], 12001[1], 12002[1], 12004[1], 12005[1], 12006[1], 12007[1], 12011[1], 12013[1], 12014[1], 12015[1], 12016[1], 12017[1], 12018[1], 12020[1], 12021[1], 12031[1], 12032[1], 12034[1], 12035[1], 12036[1], 12037[1], 12041[1], 12042[1], 12044[1], 12045[1], 12046[1], 12047[1], 12051[1], 12052[1], 12053[1], 12054[1], 12055[1], 12056[1], 12057[1], 13100[1], 13101[1], 13102[1], 13120[1], 13121[1], 13122[1], 13131[1], 13132[1], 13133[1], 13151[1], 13152[1], 13153[1], 36000[1], 36400[1], 36405[1], 36406[1], 36410[1], 36420[1], 36425[1], 36430[1], 36440[1], 36591[0], 36592[0], 36600[1], 36640[1], 43752[1], 51701[0], 51702[0], 51703[1], 54400[0], 54401[0], 54405[0], 54406[0], 54408[0], 54415[0], 54416[0], 54417[0], 62320[0], 62321[0], 62322[0], 62323[0], 62324[0], 62325[0], 62326[0], 62327[0], 64400[0], 64405[0], 64408[0], 64415[0], 64416[0], 64417[0], 64418[0], 64420[0], 64421[0], 64425[0], 64430[0], 64435[0], 64445[0], 64446[0], 64447[0], 64448[0], 64449[0], 64450[0], 64451[0], 64454[0], 64461[0], 64462[0], 64463[0], 64479[0], 64480[0], 64483[0], 64484[0], 64486[0], 64487[0], 64488[0], 64489[0], 64490[0], 64491[0], 64492[0], 64493[0], 64494[0], 64495[0], 64505[0], 64510[0], 64517[0], 64520[0], 64530[0], 69990[0], 92012[1], 92014[1], 93000[1], 93005[1], 93010[1], 93040[1], 93041[1], 93042[1], 93318[1], 93355[1], 94002[1], 94200[1], 94680[1], 94681[1], 94690[1], 95812[1], 95813[1], 95816[1], 95819[1], 95822[1], 95829[1], 95955[1], 96360[1], 96361[1], 96365[1], 96366[1], 96367[1], 96368[1], 96372[1], 96374[1], 96375[1], 96376[1], 96377[1], 96523[0], 97597[1], 97598[1], 97602[1], 99155[0], 99156[0], 99157[0], 99211[1], 99212[1], 99213[1], 99214[1], 99215[1], 99217[1], 99218[1], 99219[1], 99220[1], 99221[1], 99222[1], 99223[1], 99231[1], 99232[1], 99233[1], 99234[1], 99235[1], 99236[1], 99238[1], 99239[1], 99241[1], 99242[1], 99243[1], 99244[1], 99245[1], 99251[1], 99252[1], 99253[1], 99254[1], 99255[1], 99291[1], 99292[1], 99304[1], 99305[1], 99306[1], 99307[1], 99308[1], 99309[1], 99310[1], 99315[1], 99316[1], 99334[1], 99335[1], 99336[1], 99337[1], 99347[1], 99348[1], 99349[1], 99350[1], 99374[1], 99375[1], 99377[1], 99378[1], 99446[0], 99447[0], 99448[0], 99449[0], 99451[0], 99452[0], 99495[0], 99496[0], G0463[1], G0471[0]
54415	0213T[0], 0216T[0], 0596T[1], 0597T[1], 0708T[1], 0709T[1], 12001[1], 12002[1], 12004[1], 12005[1], 12006[1], 12007[1], 12011[1], 12013[1], 12014[1], 12015[1], 12016[1], 12017[1], 12018[1], 12020[1], 12021[1], 12031[1], 12032[1], 12034[1], 12035[1], 12036[1], 12037[1], 12041[1], 12042[1], 12044[1], 12045[1], 12046[1], 12047[1], 12051[1], 12052[1], 12053[1], 12054[1], 12055[1], 12056[1], 12057[1], 13100[1], 13101[1], 13102[1], 13120[1], 13121[1], 13122[1], 13131[1], 13132[1], 13133[1], 13151[1], 13152[1], 13153[1], 36000[1], 36400[1], 36405[1], 36406[1], 36410[1], 36420[1], 36425[1], 36430[1], 36440[1], 36591[0], 36592[0], 36600[1], 36640[1], 43752[1], 51701[0], 51702[0], 51703[1], 54400[0], 54401[0], 62320[0], 62321[0], 62322[0], 62323[0], 62324[0], 62325[0], 62326[0], 62327[0], 64400[0], 64405[0], 64408[0], 64415[0], 64416[0], 64417[0], 64418[0], 64420[0], 64421[0], 64425[0], 64430[0], 64435[0], 64445[0], 64446[0], 64447[0], 64448[0], 64449[0], 64450[0], 64451[0], 64454[0], 64461[0], 64462[0], 64463[0], 64479[0], 64480[0], 64483[0], 64484[0], 64486[0], 64487[0], 64488[0], 64489[0], 64490[0], 64491[0], 64492[0], 64493[0], 64494[0], 64495[0], 64505[0], 64510[0], 64517[0], 64520[0], 64530[0], 69990[0], 92012[1], 92014[1], 93000[1], 93005[1], 93010[1], 93040[1], 93041[1], 93042[1], 93318[1], 93355[1], 94002[1], 94200[1], 94680[1], 94681[1], 94690[1], 95812[1], 95813[1], 95816[1], 95819[1], 95822[1], 95829[1], 95955[1], 96360[1], 96361[1], 96365[1], 96366[1], 96367[1], 96368[1], 96372[1], 96374[1], 96375[1], 96376[1], 96377[1], 96523[0], 99155[0], 99156[0], 99157[0], 99211[1], 99212[1], 99213[1], 99214[1], 99215[1], 99217[1], 99218[1], 99219[1], 99220[1], 99221[1], 99222[1], 99223[1], 99231[1], 99232[1], 99233[1], 99234[1], 99235[1], 99236[1], 99238[1], 99239[1], 99241[1], 99242[1], 99243[1], 99244[1], 99245[1], 99251[1], 99252[1], 99253[1], 99254[1], 99255[1], 99291[1], 99292[1], 99304[1], 99305[1], 99306[1], 99307[1], 99308[1], 99309[1], 99310[1], 99315[1], 99316[1], 99334[1], 99335[1], 99336[1], 99337[1], 99347[1], 99348[1], 99349[1], 99350[1], 99374[1], 99375[1], 99377[1], 99378[1], 99446[0], 99447[0], 99448[0], 99449[0], 99451[0], 99452[0], 99495[0], 99496[0], G0463[1], G0471[0]
54416	0213T[0], 0216T[0], 0596T[1], 0597T[1], 0708T[1], 0709T[1], 12001[1], 12002[1], 12004[1], 12005[1], 12006[1], 12007[1], 12011[1], 12013[1], 12014[1], 12015[1], 12016[1], 12017[1], 12018[1], 12020[1], 12021[1], 12031[1], 12032[1], 12034[1], 12035[1], 12036[1], 12037[1], 12041[1], 12042[1], 12044[1], 12045[1], 12046[1], 12047[1], 12051[1], 12052[1], 12053[1], 12054[1], 12055[1], 12056[1], 12057[1], 13100[1], 13101[1], 13102[1], 13120[1], 13121[1], 13122[1], 13131[1], 13132[1], 13133[1], 13151[1], 13152[1], 13153[1], 36000[1], 36400[1], 36405[1], 36406[1], 36410[1], 36420[1], 36425[1], 36430[1], 36440[1], 36591[0], 36592[0], 36600[1], 36640[1], 43752[1], 51701[0], 51702[0], 51703[1], 54400[0], 54401[0], 54405[0], 54415[0], 54417[0], 62320[0], 62321[0], 62322[0], 62323[0], 62324[0], 62325[0], 62326[0], 62327[0], 64400[0], 64405[0], 64408[0], 64415[0], 64416[0], 64417[0], 64418[0], 64420[0], 64421[0], 64425[0], 64430[0], 64435[0], 64445[0], 64446[0], 64447[0], 64448[0], 64449[0], 64450[0], 64451[0], 64454[0], 64461[0], 64462[0], 64463[0], 64479[0], 64480[0], 64483[0], 64484[0], 64486[0], 64487[0], 64488[0], 64489[0], 64490[0], 64491[0], 64492[0], 64493[0], 64494[0], 64495[0], 64505[0], 64510[0], 64517[0], 64520[0], 64530[0], 69990[0], 92012[1], 92014[1], 93000[1], 93005[1], 93010[1], 93040[1], 93041[1], 93042[1], 93318[1], 93355[1], 94002[1], 94200[1], 94680[1], 94681[1], 94690[1], 95812[1], 95813[1], 95816[1], 95819[1], 95822[1], 95829[1], 95955[1], 96360[1], 96361[1], 96365[1], 96366[1], 96367[1], 96368[1], 96372[1], 96374[1], 96375[1], 96376[1], 96377[1], 96523[0], 99155[0], 99156[0], 99157[0], 99211[1], 99212[1], 99213[1], 99214[1], 99215[1], 99217[1], 99218[1], 99219[1], 99220[1], 99221[1], 99222[1], 99223[1], 99231[1], 99232[1], 99233[1], 99234[1], 99235[1], 99236[1], 99238[1], 99239[1], 99241[1], 99242[1], 99243[1], 99244[1], 99245[1], 99251[1], 99252[1], 99253[1], 99254[1], 99255[1], 99291[1], 99292[1], 99304[1], 99305[1], 99306[1], 99307[1], 99308[1], 99309[1], 99310[1], 99315[1], 99316[1], 99334[1], 99335[1], 99336[1], 99337[1], 99347[1], 99348[1], 99349[1], 99350[1], 99374[1], 99375[1], 99377[1], 99378[1], 99446[0], 99447[0], 99448[0], 99449[0], 99451[0], 99452[0], 99495[0], 99496[0], G0463[1], G0471[0]
54417	0213T[0], 0216T[0], 0596T[1], 0597T[1], 0708T[1], 0709T[1], 11000[1], 11001[1], 11004[1], 11005[1], 11006[1], 11042[1], 11043[1], 11044[1], 11045[1], 11046[1], 11047[1], 12001[1], 12002[1], 12004[1], 12005[1], 12006[1], 12007[1], 12011[1], 12013[1], 12014[1], 12015[1], 12016[1], 12017[1], 12018[1], 12020[1], 12021[1], 12031[1], 12032[1], 12034[1], 12035[1], 12036[1], 12037[1], 12041[1], 12042[1], 12044[1], 12045[1], 12046[1], 12047[1], 12051[1], 12052[1], 12053[1], 12054[1], 12055[1], 12056[1], 12057[1], 13100[1], 13101[1], 13102[1], 13120[1], 13121[1], 13122[1], 13131[1], 13132[1], 13133[1], 13151[1], 13152[1], 13153[1], 36000[1], 36400[1], 36405[1], 36406[1], 36410[1], 36420[1], 36425[1], 36430[1], 36440[1], 36591[0], 36592[0], 36600[1], 36640[1], 43752[1], 51701[0], 51702[0], 51703[1], 54400[0], 54401[0], 54405[0], 54406[0], 54408[0], 54415[0], 62320[0], 62321[0], 62322[0], 62323[0], 62324[0], 62325[0], 62326[0], 62327[0], 64400[0], 64405[0], 64408[0], 64415[0], 64416[0], 64417[0],

0 = Modifier usage not allowed or inappropriate　　1 = Modifier usage allowed

Code 1	Code 2
	64418[0], 64420[0], 64421[0], 64425[0], 64430[0], 64435[0], 64445[0], 64446[0], 64447[0], 64448[0], 64449[0], 64450[0], 64451[0], 64454[0], 64461[0], 64462[0], 64463[0], 64479[0], 64480[0], 64483[0], 64484[0], 64486[0], 64487[0], 64488[0], 64489[0], 64490[0], 64491[0], 64492[0], 64493[0], 64494[0], 64495[0], 64505[0], 64510[0], 64517[0], 64520[0], 64530[0], 69990[0], 92012[1], 92014[1], 93000[1], 93005[1], 93010[1], 93040[1], 93041[1], 93042[1], 93318[1], 93355[1], 94002[1], 94200[1], 94680[1], 94681[1], 94690[1], 95812[1], 95813[1], 95816[1], 95819[1], 95822[1], 95829[1], 95955[1], 96360[1], 96361[1], 96365[1], 96366[1], 96367[1], 96368[1], 96372[1], 96374[1], 96375[1], 96376[1], 96377[1], 96523[0], 97597[1], 97598[1], 97602[1], 99155[0], 99156[0], 99157[0], 99211[1], 99212[1], 99213[1], 99214[1], 99215[1], 99217[1], 99218[1], 99219[1], 99220[1], 99221[1], 99222[1], 99223[1], 99231[1], 99232[1], 99233[1], 99234[1], 99235[1], 99236[1], 99238[1], 99239[1], 99241[1], 99242[1], 99243[1], 99244[1], 99245[1], 99251[1], 99252[1], 99253[1], 99254[1], 99255[1], 99291[1], 99292[1], 99304[1], 99305[1], 99306[1], 99307[1], 99308[1], 99309[1], 99310[1], 99315[1], 99316[1], 99334[1], 99335[1], 99336[1], 99337[1], 99347[1], 99348[1], 99349[1], 99350[1], 99374[1], 99375[1], 99377[1], 99378[1], 99446[0], 99447[0], 99448[0], 99449[0], 99451[0], 99452[0], 99495[0], 99496[0], G0463[1], G0471[0]
54420	0213T[0], 0216T[0], 0596T[1], 0597T[1], 0708T[1], 0709T[1], 12001[1], 12002[1], 12004[1], 12005[1], 12006[1], 12007[1], 12011[1], 12013[1], 12014[1], 12015[1], 12016[1], 12017[1], 12018[1], 12020[1], 12021[1], 12031[1], 12032[1], 12034[1], 12035[1], 12036[1], 12037[1], 12041[1], 12042[1], 12044[1], 12045[1], 12046[1], 12047[1], 12051[1], 12052[1], 12053[1], 12054[1], 12055[1], 12056[1], 12057[1], 13100[1], 13101[1], 13102[1], 13120[1], 13121[1], 13122[1], 13131[1], 13132[1], 13133[1], 13151[1], 13152[1], 13153[1], 36000[1], 36400[1], 36405[1], 36406[1], 36410[1], 36420[1], 36425[1], 36430[1], 36440[1], 36591[0], 36592[0], 36600[1], 36640[1], 43752[1], 51701[0], 51702[0], 51703[1], 54430[0], 54435[0], 62320[0], 62321[0], 62322[0], 62323[0], 62324[0], 62325[0], 62326[0], 62327[0], 64400[0], 64405[0], 64408[0], 64415[0], 64416[0], 64417[0], 64418[0], 64420[0], 64421[0], 64425[0], 64430[0], 64435[0], 64445[0], 64446[0], 64447[0], 64448[0], 64449[0], 64450[0], 64451[0], 64454[0], 64461[0], 64462[0], 64463[0], 64479[0], 64480[0], 64483[0], 64484[0], 64486[0], 64487[0], 64488[0], 64489[0], 64490[0], 64491[0], 64492[0], 64493[0], 64494[0], 64495[0], 64505[0], 64510[0], 64517[0], 64520[0], 64530[0], 69990[0], 92012[1], 92014[1], 93000[1], 93005[1], 93010[1], 93040[1], 93041[1], 93042[1], 93318[1], 93355[1], 94002[1], 94200[1], 94680[1], 94681[1], 94690[1], 95812[1], 95813[1], 95816[1], 95819[1], 95822[1], 95829[1], 95955[1], 96360[1], 96361[1], 96365[1], 96366[1], 96367[1], 96368[1], 96372[1], 96374[1], 96375[1], 96376[1], 96377[1], 96523[0], 99155[0], 99156[0], 99157[0], 99211[1], 99212[1], 99213[1], 99214[1], 99215[1], 99217[1], 99218[1], 99219[1], 99220[1], 99221[1], 99222[1], 99223[1], 99231[1], 99232[1], 99233[1], 99234[1], 99235[1], 99236[1], 99238[1], 99239[1], 99241[1], 99242[1], 99243[1], 99244[1], 99245[1], 99251[1], 99252[1], 99253[1], 99254[1], 99255[1], 99291[1], 99292[1], 99304[1], 99305[1], 99306[1], 99307[1], 99308[1], 99309[1], 99310[1], 99315[1], 99316[1], 99334[1], 99335[1], 99336[1], 99337[1], 99347[1], 99348[1], 99349[1], 99350[1], 99374[1], 99375[1], 99377[1], 99378[1], 99446[0], 99447[0], 99448[0], 99449[0], 99451[0], 99452[0], 99495[0], 99496[0], G0463[1], G0471[0]
54430	0213T[0], 0216T[0], 0596T[1], 0597T[1], 0708T[1], 0709T[1], 12001[1], 12002[1], 12004[1], 12005[1], 12006[1], 12007[1], 12011[1], 12013[1], 12014[1], 12015[1], 12016[1], 12017[1], 12018[1], 12020[1], 12021[1], 12031[1], 12032[1], 12034[1], 12035[1], 12036[1], 12037[1], 12041[1], 12042[1], 12044[1], 12045[1], 12046[1], 12047[1], 12051[1], 12052[1], 12053[1], 12054[1], 12055[1], 12056[1], 12057[1], 13100[1], 13101[1], 13102[1], 13120[1], 13121[1], 13122[1], 13131[1], 13132[1], 13133[1], 13151[1], 13152[1], 13153[1], 36000[1], 36400[1], 36405[1], 36406[1], 36410[1], 36420[1], 36425[1], 36430[1], 36440[1], 36591[0], 36592[0], 36600[1], 36640[1], 43752[1], 51701[0], 51702[0], 51703[1], 62320[0], 62321[0], 62322[0], 62323[0], 62324[0], 62325[0], 62326[0], 62327[0], 64400[0], 64405[0], 64408[0], 64415[0], 64416[0], 64417[0], 64418[0], 64420[0], 64421[0], 64425[0], 64430[0], 64435[0], 64445[0], 64446[0], 64447[0], 64448[0], 64449[0], 64450[0], 64451[0], 64454[0], 64461[0], 64462[0], 64463[0], 64479[0], 64480[0], 64483[0], 64484[0], 64486[0], 64487[0], 64488[0], 64489[0], 64490[0], 64491[0], 64492[0], 64493[0], 64494[0], 64495[0], 64505[0], 64510[0], 64517[0], 64520[0], 64530[0], 69990[0], 92012[1], 92014[1], 93000[1], 93005[1], 93010[1], 93040[1], 93041[1], 93042[1], 93318[1], 93355[1], 94002[1], 94200[1], 94680[1], 94681[1], 94690[1], 95812[1], 95813[1], 95816[1], 95819[1], 95822[1], 95829[1], 95955[1], 96360[1], 96361[1], 96365[1], 96366[1], 96367[1], 96368[1], 96372[1], 96374[1], 96375[1], 96376[1], 96377[1], 96523[0], 99155[0], 99156[0], 99157[0], 99211[1], 99212[1], 99213[1], 99214[1], 99215[1], 99217[1], 99218[1], 99219[1], 99220[1], 99221[1], 99222[1], 99223[1], 99231[1], 99232[1], 99233[1], 99234[1], 99235[1], 99236[1], 99238[1], 99239[1], 99241[1], 99242[1], 99243[1], 99244[1], 99245[1], 99251[1], 99252[1], 99253[1], 99254[1], 99255[1], 99291[1], 99292[1], 99304[1], 99305[1], 99306[1], 99307[1], 99308[1], 99309[1], 99310[1], 99315[1], 99316[1], 99334[1], 99335[1], 99336[1], 99337[1], 99347[1], 99348[1], 99349[1], 99350[1], 99374[1], 99375[1], 99377[1], 99378[1], 99446[0], 99447[0], 99448[0], 99449[0], 99451[0], 99452[0], 99495[0], 99496[0], G0463[1], G0471[0]
54435	0213T[0], 0216T[0], 0596T[1], 0597T[1], 0708T[1], 0709T[1], 10005[1], 10007[1], 10009[1], 10011[1], 10021[1], 12001[1], 12002[1], 12004[1], 12005[1], 12006[1], 12007[1], 12011[1], 12013[1], 12014[1], 12015[1], 12016[1], 12017[1], 12018[1], 12020[1], 12021[1], 12031[1], 12032[1], 12034[1], 12035[1], 12036[1], 12037[1], 12041[1], 12042[1], 12044[1], 12045[1], 12046[1], 12047[1], 12051[1], 12052[1], 12053[1], 12054[1], 12055[1], 12056[1], 12057[1], 13100[1], 13101[1], 13102[1], 13120[1], 13121[1], 13122[1], 13131[1], 13132[1], 13133[1], 13151[1], 13152[1], 13153[1], 36000[1], 36400[1], 36405[1], 36406[1], 36410[1], 36420[1], 36425[1], 36430[1], 36440[1], 36591[0], 36592[0], 36600[1], 36640[1], 43752[1], 51701[0], 51702[0], 51703[1], 54430[1], 62320[0], 62321[0], 62322[0], 62323[0], 62324[0], 62325[0], 62326[0], 62327[0], 64400[0], 64405[0], 64408[0], 64415[0], 64416[0], 64417[0], 64418[0], 64420[0], 64421[0], 64425[0], 64430[0], 64435[0], 64445[0], 64446[0], 64447[0], 64448[0], 64449[0], 64450[0], 64451[0], 64454[0], 64461[0], 64462[0], 64463[0], 64479[0], 64480[0], 64483[0], 64484[0], 64486[0], 64487[0], 64488[0], 64489[0], 64490[0], 64491[0], 64492[0], 64493[0], 64494[0], 64495[0], 64505[0], 64510[0], 64517[0], 64520[0], 64530[0], 69990[0], 92012[1], 92014[1], 93000[1], 93005[1], 93010[1], 93040[1], 93041[1], 93042[1], 93318[1], 93355[1], 94002[1], 94200[1], 94680[1], 94681[1], 94690[1], 95812[1], 95813[1], 95816[1], 95819[1], 95822[1], 95829[1], 95955[1], 96360[1], 96361[1], 96365[1], 96366[1], 96367[1], 96368[1], 96372[1], 96374[1], 96375[1], 96376[1], 96377[1], 96523[0], 99155[0], 99156[0], 99157[0], 99211[1], 99212[1], 99213[1], 99214[1], 99215[1], 99217[1], 99218[1], 99219[1], 99220[1], 99221[1], 99222[1], 99223[1], 99231[1], 99232[1], 99233[1], 99234[1], 99235[1], 99236[1], 99238[1], 99239[1], 99241[1], 99242[1], 99243[1], 99244[1], 99245[1], 99251[1], 99252[1], 99253[1], 99254[1], 99255[1], 99291[1], 99292[1], 99304[1], 99305[1], 99306[1], 99307[1], 99308[1], 99309[1], 99310[1], 99315[1], 99316[1], 99334[1], 99335[1], 99336[1], 99337[1], 99347[1], 99348[1], 99349[1], 99350[1], 99374[1], 99375[1], 99377[1], 99378[1], 99446[0], 99447[0], 99448[0], 99449[0], 99451[0], 99452[0], 99495[0], 99496[0], G0463[1], G0471[0]
54437	0213T[0], 0216T[0], 0596T[1], 0597T[1], 0708T[1], 0709T[1], 12001[1], 12002[1], 12004[1], 12005[1], 12006[1], 12007[1], 12011[1], 12013[1], 12014[1], 12015[1], 12016[1], 12017[1], 12018[1], 12020[1], 12021[1], 12031[1], 12032[1], 12034[1], 12035[1], 12036[1], 12037[1], 12041[1], 12042[1], 12044[1], 12045[1], 12046[1], 12047[1], 12051[1], 12052[1], 12053[1], 12054[1], 12055[1], 12056[1], 12057[1], 13100[1], 13101[1], 13102[1], 13120[1], 13121[1], 13122[1], 13131[1], 13132[1], 13133[1], 13151[1], 13152[1], 13153[1], 36000[1], 36400[1], 36405[1], 36406[1], 36410[1], 36420[1], 36425[1], 36430[1], 36440[1], 36591[0], 36592[0], 36600[1], 36640[1], 43752[1], 51701[0], 51702[0], 51703[1], 54440[0], 62320[0], 62321[0], 62322[0], 62323[0], 62324[0], 62325[0], 62326[0], 62327[0], 64400[0], 64405[0], 64408[0], 64415[0], 64416[0], 64417[0], 64418[0], 64420[0], 64421[0], 64425[0], 64430[0], 64435[0], 64445[0], 64446[0], 64447[0], 64448[0], 64449[0], 64450[0], 64451[0], 64454[0], 64461[0], 64462[0], 64463[0], 64479[0], 64480[0], 64483[0], 64484[0], 64486[0], 64487[0], 64488[0], 64489[0], 64490[0], 64491[0], 64492[0], 64493[0], 64494[0], 64495[0], 64505[0], 64510[0], 64517[0], 64520[0], 64530[0], 69990[0], 92012[1], 92014[1], 93000[1], 93005[1], 93010[1], 93040[1], 93041[1], 93042[1], 93318[1], 93355[1], 94002[1], 94200[1], 94680[1], 94681[1], 94690[1], 95812[1], 95813[1], 95816[1], 95819[1], 95822[1], 95829[1], 95955[1], 96360[1], 96361[1], 96365[1], 96366[1], 96367[1], 96368[1], 96372[1], 96374[1], 96375[1], 96376[1], 96377[1], 96523[0], 99155[0], 99156[0], 99157[0], 99211[1], 99212[1], 99213[1], 99214[1], 99215[1], 99217[1], 99218[1], 99219[1], 99220[1], 99221[1], 99222[1], 99223[1], 99231[1], 99232[1], 99233[1], 99234[1], 99235[1], 99236[1], 99238[1], 99239[1], 99241[1], 99242[1], 99243[1], 99244[1], 99245[1], 99251[1], 99252[1], 99253[1], 99254[1], 99255[1], 99291[1], 99292[1], 99304[1], 99305[1], 99306[1], 99307[1], 99308[1], 99309[1], 99310[1], 99315[1], 99316[1], 99334[1], 99335[1], 99336[1], 99337[1], 99347[1], 99348[1], 99349[1], 99350[1], 99374[1], 99375[1], 99377[1], 99378[1], 99446[0], 99447[0], 99448[0], 99449[0], 99451[0], 99452[0], 99495[0], 99496[0], G0463[1], G0471[0]
54438	0213T[0], 0216T[0], 0596T[1], 0597T[1], 0708T[1], 0709T[1], 12001[1], 12002[1], 12004[1], 12005[1], 12006[1], 12007[1], 12011[1], 12013[1], 12014[1], 12015[1], 12016[1], 12017[1], 12018[1], 12020[1], 12021[1], 12031[1], 12032[1], 12034[1], 12035[1], 12036[1], 12037[1], 12041[1], 12042[1], 12044[1], 12045[1], 12046[1], 12047[1], 12051[1], 12052[1], 12053[1], 12054[1], 12055[1], 12056[1], 12057[1], 13100[1], 13101[1], 13102[1], 13120[1], 13121[1], 13122[1], 13131[1], 13132[1], 13133[1], 13151[1], 13152[1], 13153[1], 36000[1], 36400[1], 36405[1], 36406[1], 36410[1], 36420[1], 36425[1], 36430[1], 36440[1], 36591[0], 36592[0], 36600[1], 36640[1], 43752[1], 51701[0], 51702[0], 51703[1], 53410[0], 53415[0], 54360[0], 54437[0], 54440[0], 62320[0], 62321[0], 62322[0], 62323[0], 62324[0], 62325[0], 62326[0], 62327[0], 64400[0], 64405[0], 64408[0], 64415[0], 64416[0], 64417[0], 64418[0], 64420[0], 64421[0], 64425[0], 64430[0], 64435[0], 64445[0], 64446[0], 64447[0], 64448[0], 64449[0], 64450[0], 64451[0], 64454[0], 64461[0], 64462[0], 64463[0], 64479[0], 64480[0], 64483[0], 64484[0], 64486[0], 64487[0], 64488[0], 64489[0], 64490[0], 64491[0], 64492[0], 64493[0], 64494[0], 64495[0], 64505[0], 64510[0], 64517[0], 64520[0], 64530[0], 69990[0], 92012[1], 92014[1], 93000[1], 93005[1], 93010[1], 93040[1], 93041[1], 93042[1], 93318[1], 93355[1], 94002[1], 94200[1], 94680[1], 94681[1], 94690[1], 95812[1], 95813[1], 95816[1], 95819[1], 95822[1], 95829[1], 95955[1], 96360[1], 96361[1], 96365[1], 96366[1], 96367[1], 96368[1], 96372[1], 96374[1], 96375[1], 96376[1], 96377[1], 96523[0], 99155[0], 99156[0], 99157[0], 99211[1], 99212[1], 99213[1], 99214[1], 99215[1], 99217[1], 99218[1], 99219[1], 99220[1], 99221[1], 99222[1], 99223[1], 99231[1], 99232[1], 99233[1], 99234[1], 99235[1], 99236[1], 99238[1], 99239[1], 99241[1], 99242[1], 99243[1], 99244[1], 99245[1], 99251[1], 99252[1], 99253[1], 99254[1], 99255[1], 99291[1], 99292[1], 99304[1], 99305[1], 99306[1], 99307[1], 99308[1], 99309[1], 99310[1], 99315[1], 99316[1], 99334[1], 99335[1], 99336[1], 99337[1], 99347[1], 99348[1], 99349[1], 99350[1], 99374[1], 99375[1], 99377[1], 99378[1], 99446[0], 99447[0], 99448[0], 99449[0], 99451[0], 99452[0], 99495[0], 99496[0], G0463[1], G0471[0]
54440	0213T[0], 0216T[0], 0596T[1], 0597T[1], 0708T[1], 0709T[1], 12001[1], 12002[1], 12004[1], 12005[1], 12006[1], 12007[1], 12011[1], 12013[1], 12014[1], 12015[1], 12016[1], 12017[1], 12018[1], 12020[1],

0 = Modifier usage not allowed or inappropriate 1 = Modifier usage allowed

Code 1	Code 2
	12021[1], 12031[1], 12032[1], 12034[1], 12035[1], 12036[1], 12037[1], 12041[1], 12042[1], 12044[1], 12045[1], 12046[1], 12047[1], 12051[1], 12052[1], 12053[1], 12054[1], 12055[1], 12056[1], 12057[1], 13100[1], 13101[1], 13102[1], 13120[1], 13121[1], 13122[1], 13131[1], 13132[1], 13133[1], 13151[1], 13152[1], 13153[1], 36000[1], 36400[1], 36405[1], 36406[1], 36410[1], 36420[1], 36425[1], 36430[1], 36440[1], 36591[0], 36592[0], 36600[1], 36640[1], 43752[1], 51701[0], 51702[0], 51703[1], 62320[0], 62321[0], 62322[0], 62323[0], 62324[0], 62325[0], 62326[0], 62327[0], 64400[0], 64405[0], 64408[0], 64415[0], 64416[0], 64417[0], 64418[0], 64420[0], 64421[0], 64425[0], 64430[0], 64435[0], 64445[0], 64446[0], 64447[0], 64448[0], 64449[0], 64450[0], 64451[0], 64454[0], 64461[0], 64462[0], 64463[0], 64479[0], 64480[0], 64483[0], 64484[0], 64486[0], 64487[0], 64488[0], 64489[0], 64490[0], 64491[0], 64492[0], 64493[0], 64494[0], 64495[0], 64505[0], 64510[0], 64517[0], 64520[0], 64530[0], 69990[0], 92012[1], 92014[1], 93000[1], 93005[1], 93010[1], 93040[1], 93041[1], 93042[1], 93318[1], 93355[1], 94002[1], 94200[1], 94680[1], 94681[1], 94690[1], 95812[1], 95813[1], 95816[1], 95819[1], 95822[1], 95829[1], 95955[1], 96360[1], 96361[1], 96365[1], 96366[1], 96367[1], 96368[1], 96372[1], 96374[1], 96375[1], 96376[1], 96377[1], 96523[0], 99155[0], 99156[0], 99157[0], 99211[1], 99212[1], 99213[1], 99214[1], 99215[1], 99217[1], 99218[1], 99219[1], 99220[1], 99221[1], 99222[1], 99223[1], 99231[1], 99232[1], 99233[1], 99234[1], 99235[1], 99236[1], 99238[1], 99239[1], 99241[1], 99242[1], 99243[1], 99244[1], 99245[1], 99251[1], 99252[1], 99253[1], 99254[1], 99255[1], 99291[1], 99292[1], 99304[1], 99305[1], 99306[1], 99307[1], 99308[1], 99309[1], 99310[1], 99315[1], 99316[1], 99334[1], 99335[1], 99336[1], 99337[1], 99347[1], 99348[1], 99349[1], 99350[1], 99374[1], 99375[1], 99377[1], 99378[1], 99446[0], 99447[0], 99448[0], 99449[0], 99451[0], 99452[0], 99495[0], 99496[0], G0463[1], G0471[0]
54450	0213T[0], 0216T[0], 0596T[1], 0597T[1], 0708T[1], 0709T[1], 12001[1], 12002[1], 12004[1], 12005[1], 12006[1], 12007[1], 12011[1], 12013[1], 12014[1], 12015[1], 12016[1], 12017[1], 12018[1], 12020[1], 12021[1], 12031[1], 12032[1], 12034[1], 12035[1], 12036[1], 12037[1], 12041[1], 12042[1], 12044[1], 12045[1], 12046[1], 12047[1], 12051[1], 12052[1], 12053[1], 12054[1], 12055[1], 12056[1], 12057[1], 13100[1], 13101[1], 13102[1], 13120[1], 13121[1], 13122[1], 13131[1], 13132[1], 13133[1], 13151[1], 13152[1], 13153[1], 36000[1], 36400[1], 36405[1], 36406[1], 36410[1], 36420[1], 36425[1], 36430[1], 36440[1], 36591[0], 36592[0], 36600[1], 36640[1], 43752[1], 51701[1], 51702[1], 51703[1], 54000[0], 54001[0], 62320[0], 62321[0], 62322[0], 62323[0], 62324[0], 62325[0], 62326[0], 62327[0], 64400[0], 64405[0], 64408[0], 64415[0], 64416[0], 64417[0], 64418[0], 64420[0], 64421[0], 64425[0], 64430[0], 64435[0], 64445[0], 64446[0], 64447[0], 64448[0], 64449[0], 64450[0], 64451[0], 64454[0], 64461[0], 64462[0], 64463[0], 64479[0], 64480[0], 64483[0], 64484[0], 64486[0], 64487[0], 64488[0], 64489[0], 64490[0], 64491[0], 64492[0], 64493[0], 64494[0], 64495[0], 64505[0], 64510[0], 64517[0], 64520[0], 64530[0], 69990[0], 92012[1], 92014[1], 93000[1], 93005[1], 93010[1], 93040[1], 93041[1], 93042[1], 93318[1], 93355[1], 94002[1], 94200[1], 94680[1], 94681[1], 94690[1], 95812[1], 95813[1], 95816[1], 95819[1], 95822[1], 95829[1], 95955[1], 96360[1], 96361[1], 96365[1], 96366[1], 96367[1], 96368[1], 96372[1], 96374[1], 96375[1], 96376[1], 96377[1], 96523[0], 99155[0], 99156[0], 99157[0], 99211[1], 99212[1], 99213[1], 99214[1], 99215[1], 99217[1], 99218[1], 99219[1], 99220[1], 99221[1], 99222[1], 99223[1], 99231[1], 99232[1], 99233[1], 99234[1], 99235[1], 99236[1], 99238[1], 99239[1], 99241[1], 99242[1], 99243[1], 99244[1], 99245[1], 99251[1], 99252[1], 99253[1], 99254[1], 99255[1], 99291[1], 99292[1], 99304[1], 99305[1], 99306[1], 99307[1], 99308[1], 99309[1], 99310[1], 99315[1], 99316[1], 99334[1], 99335[1], 99336[1], 99337[1], 99347[1], 99348[1], 99349[1], 99350[1], 99374[1], 99375[1], 99377[1], 99378[1], 99446[0], 99447[0], 99448[0], 99449[0], 99451[0], 99452[0], 99495[1], 99496[1], G0463[1], G0471[1]
54500	0213T[0], 0216T[0], 0596T[1], 0597T[1], 0708T[1], 0709T[1], 10005[1], 10007[1], 10009[1], 10011[1], 10021[1], 12001[1], 12002[1], 12004[1], 12005[1], 12006[1], 12007[1], 12011[1], 12013[1], 12014[1], 12015[1], 12016[1], 12017[1], 12018[1], 12020[1], 12021[1], 12031[1], 12032[1], 12034[1], 12035[1], 12036[1], 12037[1], 12041[1], 12042[1], 12044[1], 12045[1], 12046[1], 12047[1], 12051[1], 12052[1], 12053[1], 12054[1], 12055[1], 12056[1], 12057[1], 13100[1], 13101[1], 13102[1], 13120[1], 13121[1], 13122[1], 13131[1], 13132[1], 13133[1], 13151[1], 13152[1], 13153[1], 36000[1], 36400[1], 36405[1], 36406[1], 36410[1], 36420[1], 36425[1], 36430[1], 36440[1], 36591[0], 36592[0], 36600[1], 36640[1], 43752[1], 51701[1], 51702[1], 51703[1], 54660[1], 62320[0], 62321[0], 62322[0], 62323[0], 62324[0], 62325[0], 62326[0], 62327[0], 64400[0], 64405[0], 64408[0], 64415[0], 64416[0], 64417[0], 64418[0], 64420[0], 64421[0], 64425[0], 64430[0], 64435[0], 64445[0], 64446[0], 64447[0], 64448[0], 64449[0], 64450[0], 64451[0], 64454[0], 64461[0], 64462[0], 64463[0], 64479[0], 64480[0], 64483[0], 64484[0], 64486[0], 64487[0], 64488[0], 64489[0], 64490[0], 64491[0], 64492[0], 64493[0], 64494[0], 64495[0], 64505[0], 64510[0], 64517[0], 64520[0], 64530[0], 69990[0], 92012[1], 92014[1], 93000[1], 93005[1], 93010[1], 93040[1], 93041[1], 93042[1], 93318[1], 93355[1], 94002[1], 94200[1], 94680[1], 94681[1], 94690[1], 95812[1], 95813[1], 95816[1], 95819[1], 95822[1], 95829[1], 95955[1], 96360[1], 96361[1], 96365[1], 96366[1], 96367[1], 96368[1], 96372[1], 96374[1], 96375[1], 96376[1], 96377[1], 96523[0], 99155[0], 99156[0], 99157[0], 99211[1], 99212[1], 99213[1], 99214[1], 99215[1], 99217[1], 99218[1], 99219[1], 99220[1], 99221[1], 99222[1], 99223[1], 99231[1], 99232[1], 99233[1], 99234[1], 99235[1], 99236[1], 99238[1], 99239[1], 99241[1], 99242[1], 99243[1], 99244[1], 99245[1], 99251[1], 99252[1], 99253[1], 99254[1], 99255[1], 99291[1], 99292[1], 99304[1], 99305[1], 99306[1], 99307[1], 99308[1], 99309[1], 99310[1], 99315[1], 99316[1], 99334[1], 99335[1], 99336[1], 99337[1], 99347[1], 99348[1], 99349[1], 99350[1], 99374[1], 99375[1], 99377[1], 99378[1], 99446[0], 99447[0], 99448[0], 99449[0], 99451[0], 99452[0], 99495[1], 99496[1], G0463[1], G0471[1]
54505	0213T[0], 0216T[0], 0596T[1], 0597T[1], 0708T[1], 0709T[1], 10005[1], 10007[1], 10009[1], 10011[1], 10021[1], 12001[1], 12002[1], 12004[1], 12005[1], 12006[1], 12007[1], 12011[1], 12013[1], 12014[1], 12015[1], 12016[1], 12017[1], 12018[1], 12020[1], 12021[1], 12031[1], 12032[1], 12034[1], 12035[1], 12036[1], 12037[1], 12041[1], 12042[1], 12044[1], 12045[1], 12046[1], 12047[1], 12051[1], 12052[1], 12053[1], 12054[1], 12055[1], 12056[1], 12057[1], 13100[1], 13101[1], 13102[1], 13120[1], 13121[1], 13122[1], 13131[1], 13132[1], 13133[1], 13151[1], 13152[1], 13153[1], 36000[1], 36400[1], 36405[1], 36406[1], 36410[1], 36420[1], 36425[1], 36430[1], 36440[1], 36591[0], 36592[0], 36600[1], 36640[1], 43752[1], 51701[1], 51702[1], 51703[1], 62320[0], 62321[0], 62322[0], 62323[0], 62324[0], 62325[0], 62326[0], 62327[0], 64400[0], 64405[0], 64408[0], 64415[0], 64416[0], 64417[0], 64418[0], 64420[0], 64421[0], 64425[0], 64430[0], 64435[0], 64445[0], 64446[0], 64447[0], 64448[0], 64449[0], 64450[0], 64451[0], 64454[0], 64461[0], 64462[0], 64463[0], 64479[0], 64480[0], 64483[0], 64484[0], 64486[0], 64487[0], 64488[0], 64489[0], 64490[0], 64491[0], 64492[0], 64493[0], 64494[0], 64495[0], 64505[0], 64510[0], 64517[0], 64520[0], 64530[0], 69990[0], 92012[1], 92014[1], 93000[1], 93005[1], 93010[1], 93040[1], 93041[1], 93042[1], 93318[1], 93355[1], 94002[1], 94200[1], 94680[1], 94681[1], 94690[1], 95812[1], 95813[1], 95816[1], 95819[1], 95822[1], 95829[1], 95955[1], 96360[1], 96361[1], 96365[1], 96366[1], 96367[1], 96368[1], 96372[1], 96374[1], 96375[1], 96376[1], 96377[1], 96523[0], 99155[0], 99156[0], 99157[0], 99211[1], 99212[1], 99213[1], 99214[1], 99215[1], 99217[1], 99218[1], 99219[1], 99220[1], 99221[1], 99222[1], 99223[1], 99231[1], 99232[1], 99233[1], 99234[1], 99235[1], 99236[1], 99238[1], 99239[1], 99241[1], 99242[1], 99243[1], 99244[1], 99245[1], 99251[1], 99252[1], 99253[1], 99254[1], 99255[1], 99291[1], 99292[1], 99304[1], 99305[1], 99306[1], 99307[1], 99308[1], 99309[1], 99310[1], 99315[1], 99316[1], 99334[1], 99335[1], 99336[1], 99337[1], 99347[1], 99348[1], 99349[1], 99350[1], 99374[1], 99375[1], 99377[1], 99378[1], 99446[0], 99447[0], 99448[0], 99449[0], 99451[0], 99452[0], 99495[0], 99496[0], G0463[1], G0471[1]
54512	0213T[0], 0216T[0], 0596T[1], 0597T[1], 0708T[1], 0709T[1], 12001[1], 12002[1], 12004[1], 12005[1], 12006[1], 12007[1], 12011[1], 12013[1], 12014[1], 12015[1], 12016[1], 12017[1], 12018[1], 12020[1], 12021[1], 12031[1], 12032[1], 12034[1], 12035[1], 12036[1], 12037[1], 12041[1], 12042[1], 12044[1], 12045[1], 12046[1], 12047[1], 12051[1], 12052[1], 12053[1], 12054[1], 12055[1], 12056[1], 12057[1], 13100[1], 13101[1], 13102[1], 13120[1], 13121[1], 13122[1], 13131[1], 13132[1], 13133[1], 13151[1], 13152[1], 13153[1], 36000[1], 36400[1], 36405[1], 36406[1], 36410[1], 36420[1], 36425[1], 36430[1], 36440[1], 36591[0], 36592[0], 36600[1], 36640[1], 43752[1], 51701[1], 51702[1], 51703[1], 54500[1], 54505[1], 54620[1], 54660[1], 54700[1], 55110[0], 62320[0], 62321[0], 62322[0], 62323[0], 62324[0], 62325[0], 62326[0], 62327[0], 64400[0], 64405[0], 64408[0], 64415[0], 64416[0], 64417[0], 64418[0], 64420[0], 64421[0], 64425[0], 64430[0], 64435[0], 64445[0], 64446[0], 64447[0], 64448[0], 64449[0], 64450[0], 64451[0], 64454[0], 64461[0], 64462[0], 64463[0], 64479[0], 64480[0], 64483[0], 64484[0], 64486[0], 64487[0], 64488[0], 64489[0], 64490[0], 64491[0], 64492[0], 64493[0], 64494[0], 64495[0], 64505[0], 64510[0], 64517[0], 64520[0], 64530[0], 69990[0], 92012[1], 92014[1], 93000[1], 93005[1], 93010[1], 93040[1], 93041[1], 93042[1], 93318[1], 93355[1], 94002[1], 94200[1], 94680[1], 94681[1], 94690[1], 95812[1], 95813[1], 95816[1], 95819[1], 95822[1], 95829[1], 95955[1], 96360[1], 96361[1], 96365[1], 96366[1], 96367[1], 96368[1], 96372[1], 96374[1], 96375[1], 96376[1], 96377[1], 96523[0], 99155[0], 99156[0], 99157[0], 99211[1], 99212[1], 99213[1], 99214[1], 99215[1], 99217[1], 99218[1], 99219[1], 99220[1], 99221[1], 99222[1], 99223[1], 99231[1], 99232[1], 99233[1], 99234[1], 99235[1], 99236[1], 99238[1], 99239[1], 99241[1], 99242[1], 99243[1], 99244[1], 99245[1], 99251[1], 99252[1], 99253[1], 99254[1], 99255[1], 99291[1], 99292[1], 99304[1], 99305[1], 99306[1], 99307[1], 99308[1], 99309[1], 99310[1], 99315[1], 99316[1], 99334[1], 99335[1], 99336[1], 99337[1], 99347[1], 99348[1], 99349[1], 99350[1], 99374[1], 99375[1], 99377[1], 99378[1], 99446[0], 99447[0], 99448[0], 99449[0], 99451[0], 99452[0], 99495[0], 99496[0], G0463[1], G0471[1]
54520	0213T[0], 0216T[0], 0596T[1], 0597T[1], 0708T[1], 0709T[1], 12001[1], 12002[1], 12004[1], 12005[1], 12006[1], 12007[1], 12011[1], 12013[1], 12014[1], 12015[1], 12016[1], 12017[1], 12018[1], 12020[1], 12021[1], 12031[1], 12032[1], 12034[1], 12035[1], 12036[1], 12037[1], 12041[1], 12042[1], 12044[1], 12045[1], 12046[1], 12047[1], 12051[1], 12052[1], 12053[1], 12054[1], 12055[1], 12056[1], 12057[1], 13100[1], 13101[1], 13102[1], 13120[1], 13121[1], 13122[1], 13131[1], 13132[1], 13133[1], 13151[1], 13152[1], 13153[1], 36000[1], 36400[1], 36405[1], 36406[1], 36410[1], 36420[1], 36425[1], 36430[1], 36440[1], 36591[0], 36592[0], 36600[1], 36640[1], 43752[1], 49000[1], 49002[1], 49010[0], 51701[1], 51702[1], 51703[1], 54500[1], 54505[1], 54512[1], 54522[0], 54660[1], 54690[1], 55040[1], 55041[1], 55110[0], 62320[0], 62321[0], 62322[0], 62323[0], 62324[0], 62325[0], 62326[0], 62327[0], 64400[0], 64405[0], 64408[0], 64415[0], 64416[0], 64417[0], 64418[0], 64420[0], 64421[0], 64425[0], 64430[0], 64435[0], 64445[0], 64446[0], 64447[0], 64448[0], 64449[0], 64450[0], 64451[0], 64454[0], 64461[0], 64462[0], 64463[0], 64479[0], 64480[0], 64483[0], 64484[0], 64486[0], 64487[0], 64488[0], 64489[0], 64490[0], 64491[0], 64492[0], 64493[0], 64494[0], 64495[0], 64505[0], 64510[0], 64517[0], 64520[0], 64530[0], 69990[0], 92012[1], 92014[1], 93000[1], 93005[1], 93010[1], 93040[1], 93041[1], 93042[1], 93318[1], 93355[1], 94002[1], 94200[1], 94680[1], 94681[1], 94690[1], 95812[1], 95813[1], 95816[1], 95819[1], 95822[1], 95829[1], 95955[1], 96360[1], 96361[1], 96365[1], 96366[1], 96367[1], 96368[1], 96372[1], 96374[1], 96375[1], 96376[1], 96377[1], 96523[0], 99155[0], 99156[0], 99157[0], 99211[1], 99212[1], 99213[1], 99214[1], 99215[1], 99217[1], 99218[1], 99219[1], 99220[1], 99221[1], 99222[1], 99223[1], 99231[1], 99232[1], 99233[1], 99234[1], 99235[1], 99236[1], 99238[1], 99239[1], 99241[1], 99242[1], 99243[1], 99244[1], 99245[1], 99251[1], 99252[1], 99253[1], 99254[1], 99255[1], 99291[1],

0 = Modifier usage not allowed or inappropriate 1 = Modifier usage allowed

Code 1	Code 2
	99292[1], 99304[1], 99305[1], 99306[1], 99307[1], 99308[1], 99309[1], 99310[1], 99315[1], 99316[1], 99334[1], 99335[1], 99336[1], 99337[1], 99347[1], 99348[1], 99349[1], 99350[1], 99374[1], 99375[1], 99377[1], 99378[1], 99446[0], 99447[0], 99448[0], 99449[0], 99451[0], 99452[0], 99495[0], 99496[0], G0463[1], G0471[1]
54522	0213T[0], 0216T[0], 0596T[1], 0597T[1], 0708T[1], 0709T[1], 11000[1], 11001[1], 11004[1], 11005[1], 11006[1], 11042[1], 11043[1], 11044[1], 11045[1], 11046[1], 11047[1], 12001[1], 12002[1], 12004[1], 12005[1], 12006[1], 12007[1], 12011[1], 12013[1], 12014[1], 12015[1], 12016[1], 12017[1], 12018[1], 12020[1], 12021[1], 12031[1], 12032[1], 12034[1], 12035[1], 12036[1], 12037[1], 12041[1], 12042[1], 12044[1], 12045[1], 12046[1], 12047[1], 12051[1], 12052[1], 12053[1], 12054[1], 12055[1], 12056[1], 12057[1], 13100[1], 13101[1], 13102[1], 13120[1], 13121[1], 13122[1], 13131[1], 13132[1], 13133[1], 13151[1], 13152[1], 13153[1], 36000[1], 36400[1], 36405[1], 36406[1], 36410[1], 36420[1], 36425[1], 36430[1], 36440[1], 36591[0], 36592[0], 36600[1], 36640[1], 43752[1], 51701[1], 51702[1], 51703[1], 54500[1], 54505[1], 54512[1], 54620[1], 54660[1], 55110[0], 62320[0], 62321[0], 62322[0], 62323[0], 62324[0], 62325[0], 62326[0], 62327[0], 64400[0], 64405[0], 64408[0], 64415[0], 64416[0], 64417[0], 64418[0], 64420[0], 64421[0], 64425[0], 64430[0], 64435[0], 64445[0], 64446[0], 64447[0], 64448[0], 64449[0], 64450[0], 64451[0], 64454[0], 64461[0], 64462[0], 64463[0], 64479[0], 64480[0], 64483[0], 64484[0], 64486[0], 64487[0], 64488[0], 64489[0], 64490[0], 64491[0], 64492[0], 64493[0], 64494[0], 64495[0], 64505[0], 64510[0], 64517[0], 64520[0], 64530[0], 69990[0], 92012[1], 92014[1], 93000[1], 93005[1], 93010[1], 93040[1], 93041[1], 93042[1], 93318[1], 93355[1], 94002[1], 94200[1], 94680[1], 94681[1], 94690[1], 95812[1], 95813[1], 95816[1], 95819[1], 95822[1], 95829[1], 95955[1], 96360[1], 96361[1], 96365[1], 96366[1], 96367[1], 96368[1], 96372[1], 96374[1], 96375[1], 96376[1], 96377[1], 96523[0], 97597[1], 97598[1], 97602[1], 99155[0], 99156[0], 99157[0], 99211[1], 99212[1], 99213[1], 99214[1], 99215[1], 99217[1], 99218[1], 99219[1], 99220[1], 99221[1], 99222[1], 99223[1], 99231[1], 99232[1], 99233[1], 99234[1], 99235[1], 99236[1], 99238[1], 99239[1], 99241[1], 99242[1], 99243[1], 99244[1], 99245[1], 99251[1], 99252[1], 99253[1], 99254[1], 99255[1], 99291[1], 99292[1], 99304[1], 99305[1], 99306[1], 99307[1], 99308[1], 99309[1], 99310[1], 99315[1], 99316[1], 99334[1], 99335[1], 99336[1], 99337[1], 99347[1], 99348[1], 99349[1], 99350[1], 99374[1], 99375[1], 99377[1], 99378[1], 99446[0], 99447[0], 99448[0], 99449[0], 99451[0], 99452[0], 99495[0], 99496[0], G0463[1], G0471[1]
54530	0213T[0], 0216T[0], 0596T[1], 0597T[1], 0708T[1], 0709T[1], 11000[1], 11001[1], 11004[1], 11005[1], 11006[1], 11042[1], 11043[1], 11044[1], 11045[1], 11046[1], 11047[1], 12001[1], 12002[1], 12004[1], 12005[1], 12006[1], 12007[1], 12011[1], 12013[1], 12014[1], 12015[1], 12016[1], 12017[1], 12018[1], 12020[1], 12021[1], 12031[1], 12032[1], 12034[1], 12035[1], 12036[1], 12037[1], 12041[1], 12042[1], 12044[1], 12045[1], 12046[1], 12047[1], 12051[1], 12052[1], 12053[1], 12054[1], 12055[1], 12056[1], 12057[1], 13100[1], 13101[1], 13102[1], 13120[1], 13121[1], 13122[1], 13131[1], 13132[1], 13133[1], 13151[1], 13152[1], 13153[1], 36000[1], 36400[1], 36405[1], 36406[1], 36410[1], 36420[1], 36425[1], 36430[1], 36440[1], 36591[0], 36592[0], 36600[1], 36640[1], 43752[1], 51701[1], 51702[1], 51703[1], 54505[1], 54512[1], 54520[1], 54522[1], 54535[1], 54620[0], 54660[0], 54690[1], 55110[0], 62320[0], 62321[0], 62322[0], 62323[0], 62324[0], 62325[0], 62326[0], 62327[0], 64400[0], 64405[0], 64408[0], 64415[0], 64416[0], 64417[0], 64418[0], 64420[0], 64421[0], 64425[0], 64430[0], 64435[0], 64445[0], 64446[0], 64447[0], 64448[0], 64449[0], 64450[0], 64451[0], 64454[0], 64461[0], 64462[0], 64463[0], 64479[0], 64480[0], 64483[0], 64484[0], 64486[0], 64487[0], 64488[0], 64489[0], 64490[0], 64491[0], 64492[0], 64493[0], 64494[0], 64495[0], 64505[0], 64510[0], 64517[0], 64520[0], 64530[0], 69990[0], 92012[1], 92014[1], 93000[1], 93005[1], 93010[1], 93040[1], 93041[1], 93042[1], 93318[1], 93355[1], 94002[1], 94200[1], 94680[1], 94681[1], 94690[1], 95812[1], 95813[1], 95816[1], 95819[1], 95822[1], 95829[1], 95955[1], 96360[1], 96361[1], 96365[1], 96366[1], 96367[1], 96368[1], 96372[1], 96374[1], 96375[1], 96376[1], 96377[1], 96523[0], 97597[1], 97598[1], 97602[1], 99155[0], 99156[0], 99157[0], 99211[1], 99212[1], 99213[1], 99214[1], 99215[1], 99217[1], 99218[1], 99219[1], 99220[1], 99221[1], 99222[1], 99223[1], 99231[1], 99232[1], 99233[1], 99234[1], 99235[1], 99236[1], 99238[1], 99239[1], 99241[1], 99242[1], 99243[1], 99244[1], 99245[1], 99251[1], 99252[1], 99253[1], 99254[1], 99255[1], 99291[1], 99292[1], 99304[1], 99305[1], 99306[1], 99307[1], 99308[1], 99309[1], 99310[1], 99315[1], 99316[1], 99334[1], 99335[1], 99336[1], 99337[1], 99347[1], 99348[1], 99349[1], 99350[1], 99374[1], 99375[1], 99377[1], 99378[1], 99446[0], 99447[0], 99448[0], 99449[0], 99451[0], 99452[0], 99495[0], 99496[0], G0463[1], G0471[1]
54535	0213T[0], 0216T[0], 0596T[1], 0597T[1], 0708T[1], 0709T[1], 11000[1], 11001[1], 11004[1], 11005[1], 11006[1], 11042[1], 11043[1], 11044[1], 11045[1], 11046[1], 11047[1], 12001[1], 12002[1], 12004[1], 12005[1], 12006[1], 12007[1], 12011[1], 12013[1], 12014[1], 12015[1], 12016[1], 12017[1], 12018[1], 12020[1], 12021[1], 12031[1], 12032[1], 12034[1], 12035[1], 12036[1], 12037[1], 12041[1], 12042[1], 12044[1], 12045[1], 12046[1], 12047[1], 12051[1], 12052[1], 12053[1], 12054[1], 12055[1], 12056[1], 12057[1], 13100[1], 13101[1], 13102[1], 13120[1], 13121[1], 13122[1], 13131[1], 13132[1], 13133[1], 13151[1], 13152[1], 13153[1], 36000[1], 36400[1], 36405[1], 36406[1], 36410[1], 36420[1], 36425[1], 36430[1], 36440[1], 36591[0], 36592[0], 36600[1], 36640[1], 43752[1], 44005[0], 44180[0], 44820[0], 44850[0], 44950[0], 44970[0], 49000[0], 49002[1], 49010[0], 49255[0], 49320[1], 49321[1], 51701[1], 51702[1], 51703[1], 54500[1], 54505[1], 54512[1], 54522[1], 54620[0], 54660[0], 54690[1], 55110[0], 62320[0], 62321[0], 62322[0], 62323[0], 62324[0], 62325[0], 62326[0], 62327[0], 64400[0], 64405[0], 64408[0], 64415[0], 64416[0], 64417[0], 64418[0], 64420[0], 64421[0], 64425[0], 64430[0], 64435[0], 64445[0], 64446[0], 64447[0], 64448[0], 64449[0], 64450[0], 64451[0], 64454[0], 64461[0], 64462[0], 64463[0], 64479[0], 64480[0], 64483[0], 64484[0], 64486[0], 64487[0], 64488[0], 64489[0], 64490[0], 64491[0], 64492[0], 64493[0], 64494[0], 64495[0], 64505[0], 64510[0], 64517[0], 64520[0], 64530[0], 69990[0], 92012[1], 92014[1], 93000[1], 93005[1], 93010[1], 93040[1], 93041[1], 93042[1], 93318[1], 93355[1], 94002[1], 94200[1], 94680[1], 94681[1], 94690[1], 95812[1], 95813[1], 95816[1], 95819[1], 95822[1], 95829[1], 95955[1], 96360[1], 96361[1], 96365[1], 96366[1], 96367[1], 96368[1], 96372[1], 96374[1], 96375[1], 96376[1], 96377[1], 96523[0], 97597[1], 97598[1], 97602[1], 99155[0], 99156[0], 99157[0], 99211[1], 99212[1], 99213[1], 99214[1], 99215[1], 99217[1], 99218[1], 99219[1], 99220[1], 99221[1], 99222[1], 99223[1], 99231[1], 99232[1], 99233[1], 99234[1], 99235[1], 99236[1], 99238[1], 99239[1], 99241[1], 99242[1], 99243[1], 99244[1], 99245[1], 99251[1], 99252[1], 99253[1], 99254[1], 99255[1], 99291[1], 99292[1], 99304[1], 99305[1], 99306[1], 99307[1], 99308[1], 99309[1], 99310[1], 99315[1], 99316[1], 99334[1], 99335[1], 99336[1], 99337[1], 99347[1], 99348[1], 99349[1], 99350[1], 99374[1], 99375[1], 99377[1], 99378[1], 99446[0], 99447[0], 99448[0], 99449[0], 99451[0], 99452[0], 99495[0], 99496[0], G0463[1], G0471[1]
54550	0213T[0], 0216T[0], 0596T[1], 0597T[1], 0708T[1], 0709T[1], 12001[1], 12002[1], 12004[1], 12005[1], 12006[1], 12007[1], 12011[1], 12013[1], 12014[1], 12015[1], 12016[1], 12017[1], 12018[1], 12020[1], 12021[1], 12031[1], 12032[1], 12034[1], 12035[1], 12036[1], 12037[1], 12041[1], 12042[1], 12044[1], 12045[1], 12046[1], 12047[1], 12051[1], 12052[1], 12053[1], 12054[1], 12055[1], 12056[1], 12057[1], 13100[1], 13101[1], 13102[1], 13120[1], 13121[1], 13122[1], 13131[1], 13132[1], 13133[1], 13151[1], 13152[1], 13153[1], 36000[1], 36400[1], 36405[1], 36406[1], 36410[1], 36420[1], 36425[1], 36430[1], 36440[1], 36591[0], 36592[0], 36600[1], 36640[1], 43752[1], 51701[1], 51702[1], 51703[1], 54500[1], 54505[1], 54560[1], 54660[1], 55110[0], 62320[0], 62321[0], 62322[0], 62323[0], 62324[0], 62325[0], 62326[0], 62327[0], 64400[0], 64405[0], 64408[0], 64415[0], 64416[0], 64417[0], 64418[0], 64420[0], 64421[0], 64425[0], 64430[0], 64435[0], 64445[0], 64446[0], 64447[0], 64448[0], 64449[0], 64450[0], 64451[0], 64454[0], 64461[0], 64462[0], 64463[0], 64479[0], 64480[0], 64483[0], 64484[0], 64486[0], 64487[0], 64488[0], 64489[0], 64490[0], 64491[0], 64492[0], 64493[0], 64494[0], 64495[0], 64505[0], 64510[0], 64517[0], 64520[0], 64530[0], 69990[0], 92012[1], 92014[1], 93000[1], 93005[1], 93010[1], 93040[1], 93041[1], 93042[1], 93318[1], 93355[1], 94002[1], 94200[1], 94680[1], 94681[1], 94690[1], 95812[1], 95813[1], 95816[1], 95819[1], 95822[1], 95829[1], 95955[1], 96360[1], 96361[1], 96365[1], 96366[1], 96367[1], 96368[1], 96372[1], 96374[1], 96375[1], 96376[1], 96377[1], 96523[0], 99155[0], 99156[0], 99157[0], 99211[1], 99212[1], 99213[1], 99214[1], 99215[1], 99217[1], 99218[1], 99219[1], 99220[1], 99221[1], 99222[1], 99223[1], 99231[1], 99232[1], 99233[1], 99234[1], 99235[1], 99236[1], 99238[1], 99239[1], 99241[1], 99242[1], 99243[1], 99244[1], 99245[1], 99251[1], 99252[1], 99253[1], 99254[1], 99255[1], 99291[1], 99292[1], 99304[1], 99305[1], 99306[1], 99307[1], 99308[1], 99309[1], 99310[1], 99315[1], 99316[1], 99334[1], 99335[1], 99336[1], 99337[1], 99347[1], 99348[1], 99349[1], 99350[1], 99374[1], 99375[1], 99377[1], 99378[1], 99446[0], 99447[0], 99448[0], 99449[0], 99451[0], 99452[0], 99495[0], 99496[0], G0463[1], G0471[1]
54560	0213T[0], 0216T[0], 0596T[1], 0597T[1], 0708T[1], 0709T[1], 12001[1], 12002[1], 12004[1], 12005[1], 12006[1], 12007[1], 12011[1], 12013[1], 12014[1], 12015[1], 12016[1], 12017[1], 12018[1], 12020[1], 12021[1], 12031[1], 12032[1], 12034[1], 12035[1], 12036[1], 12037[1], 12041[1], 12042[1], 12044[1], 12045[1], 12046[1], 12047[1], 12051[1], 12052[1], 12053[1], 12054[1], 12055[1], 12056[1], 12057[1], 13100[1], 13101[1], 13102[1], 13120[1], 13121[1], 13122[1], 13131[1], 13132[1], 13133[1], 13151[1], 13152[1], 13153[1], 36000[1], 36400[1], 36405[1], 36406[1], 36410[1], 36420[1], 36425[1], 36430[1], 36440[1], 36591[0], 36592[0], 36600[1], 36640[1], 43752[1], 44005[0], 44180[0], 44602[1], 44603[1], 44604[1], 44605[1], 44820[0], 44850[0], 44950[0], 44970[0], 49000[0], 49002[1], 49010[0], 49255[0], 49320[1], 51701[1], 51702[1], 51703[1], 54500[1], 54505[1], 54620[0], 62320[0], 62321[0], 62322[0], 62323[0], 62324[0], 62325[0], 62326[0], 62327[0], 64400[0], 64405[0], 64408[0], 64415[0], 64416[0], 64417[0], 64418[0], 64420[0], 64421[0], 64425[0], 64430[0], 64435[0], 64445[0], 64446[0], 64447[0], 64448[0], 64449[0], 64450[0], 64451[0], 64454[0], 64461[0], 64462[0], 64463[0], 64479[0], 64480[0], 64483[0], 64484[0], 64486[0], 64487[0], 64488[0], 64489[0], 64490[0], 64491[0], 64492[0], 64493[0], 64494[0], 64495[0], 64505[0], 64510[0], 64517[0], 64520[0], 64530[0], 69990[0], 92012[1], 92014[1], 93000[1], 93005[1], 93010[1], 93040[1], 93041[1], 93042[1], 93318[1], 93355[1], 94002[1], 94200[1], 94680[1], 94681[1], 94690[1], 95812[1], 95813[1], 95816[1], 95819[1], 95822[1], 95829[1], 95955[1], 96360[1], 96361[1], 96365[1], 96366[1], 96367[1], 96368[1], 96372[1], 96374[1], 96375[1], 96376[1], 96377[1], 96523[0], 99155[0], 99156[0], 99157[0], 99211[1], 99212[1], 99213[1], 99214[1], 99215[1], 99217[1], 99218[1], 99219[1], 99220[1], 99221[1], 99222[1], 99223[1], 99231[1], 99232[1], 99233[1], 99234[1], 99235[1], 99236[1], 99238[1], 99239[1], 99241[1], 99242[1], 99243[1], 99244[1], 99245[1], 99251[1], 99252[1], 99253[1], 99254[1], 99255[1], 99291[1], 99292[1], 99304[1], 99305[1], 99306[1], 99307[1], 99308[1], 99309[1], 99310[1], 99315[1], 99316[1], 99334[1], 99335[1], 99336[1], 99337[1], 99347[1], 99348[1], 99349[1], 99350[1], 99374[1], 99375[1], 99377[1], 99378[1], 99446[0], 99447[0], 99448[0], 99449[0], 99451[0], 99452[0], 99495[0], 99496[0], G0463[1], G0471[1]
54600	0213T[0], 0216T[0], 0596T[1], 0597T[1], 0708T[1], 0709T[1], 12001[1], 12002[1], 12004[1], 12005[1], 12006[1], 12007[1], 12011[1], 12013[1], 12014[1], 12015[1], 12016[1], 12017[1], 12018[1], 12020[1], 12021[1], 12031[1], 12032[1], 12034[1], 12035[1], 12036[1], 12037[1], 12041[1], 12042[1], 12044[1], 12045[1], 12046[1], 12047[1], 12051[1], 12052[1], 12053[1], 12054[1], 12055[1], 12056[1], 12057[1],

Appendix A: NCCI - CPT Codes

0 = Modifier usage not allowed or inappropriate 1 = Modifier usage allowed

Code 1	Code 2
	13100[1], 13101[1], 13102[1], 13120[1], 13121[1], 13122[1], 13131[1], 13132[1], 13133[1], 13151[1], 13152[1], 13153[1], 36000[1], 36400[1], 36405[1], 36406[1], 36410[1], 36420[1], 36425[1], 36430[1], 36440[1], 36591[0], 36592[0], 36600[1], 36640[1], 43752[1], 51701[1], 51702[1], 51703[1], 54500[1], 54505[1], 54620[0], 55110[0], 62320[0], 62321[0], 62322[0], 62323[0], 62324[0], 62325[0], 62326[0], 62327[0], 64400[0], 64405[0], 64408[0], 64415[0], 64416[0], 64417[0], 64418[0], 64420[0], 64421[0], 64425[0], 64430[0], 64435[0], 64445[0], 64446[0], 64447[0], 64448[0], 64449[0], 64450[0], 64451[0], 64454[0], 64461[0], 64462[0], 64463[0], 64479[0], 64480[0], 64483[0], 64484[0], 64486[0], 64487[0], 64488[0], 64489[0], 64490[0], 64491[0], 64492[0], 64493[0], 64494[0], 64495[0], 64505[0], 64510[0], 64517[0], 64520[0], 64530[0], 69990[0], 92012[1], 92014[1], 93000[1], 93005[1], 93010[1], 93040[1], 93041[1], 93042[1], 93318[1], 93355[1], 94002[1], 94200[1], 94680[1], 94681[1], 94690[1], 95812[1], 95813[1], 95816[1], 95819[1], 95822[1], 95829[1], 95955[1], 96360[1], 96361[1], 96365[1], 96366[1], 96367[1], 96368[1], 96372[1], 96374[1], 96375[1], 96376[1], 96377[1], 96523[0], 99155[0], 99156[0], 99157[0], 99211[1], 99212[1], 99213[1], 99214[1], 99215[1], 99217[1], 99218[1], 99219[1], 99220[1], 99221[1], 99222[1], 99223[1], 99231[1], 99232[1], 99233[1], 99234[1], 99235[1], 99236[1], 99238[1], 99239[1], 99241[1], 99242[1], 99243[1], 99244[1], 99245[1], 99251[1], 99252[1], 99253[1], 99254[1], 99255[1], 99291[1], 99292[1], 99304[1], 99305[1], 99306[1], 99307[1], 99308[1], 99309[1], 99310[1], 99315[1], 99316[1], 99334[1], 99335[1], 99336[1], 99337[1], 99347[1], 99348[1], 99349[1], 99350[1], 99374[1], 99375[1], 99377[1], 99378[1], 99446[0], 99447[0], 99448[0], 99449[0], 99451[0], 99452[0], 99495[0], 99496[0], G0463[1], G0471[1]
54620	0213T[0], 0216T[0], 0596T[1], 0597T[1], 0708T[1], 0709T[1], 12001[1], 12002[1], 12004[1], 12005[1], 12006[1], 12007[1], 12011[1], 12013[1], 12014[1], 12015[1], 12016[1], 12017[1], 12018[1], 12020[1], 12021[1], 12031[1], 12032[1], 12034[1], 12035[1], 12036[1], 12037[1], 12041[1], 12042[1], 12044[1], 12045[1], 12046[1], 12047[1], 12051[1], 12052[1], 12053[1], 12054[1], 12055[1], 12056[1], 12057[1], 13100[1], 13101[1], 13102[1], 13120[1], 13121[1], 13122[1], 13131[1], 13132[1], 13133[1], 13151[1], 13152[1], 13153[1], 36000[1], 36400[1], 36405[1], 36406[1], 36410[1], 36420[1], 36425[1], 36430[1], 36440[1], 36591[0], 36592[0], 36600[1], 36640[1], 43752[1], 51701[1], 51702[1], 51703[1], 54505[0], 55110[0], 62320[0], 62321[0], 62322[0], 62323[0], 62324[0], 62325[0], 62326[0], 62327[0], 64400[0], 64405[0], 64408[0], 64415[0], 64416[0], 64417[0], 64418[0], 64420[0], 64421[0], 64425[0], 64430[0], 64435[0], 64445[0], 64446[0], 64447[0], 64448[0], 64449[0], 64450[0], 64451[0], 64454[0], 64461[0], 64462[0], 64463[0], 64479[0], 64480[0], 64483[0], 64484[0], 64486[0], 64487[0], 64488[0], 64489[0], 64490[0], 64491[0], 64492[0], 64493[0], 64494[0], 64495[0], 64505[0], 64510[0], 64517[0], 64520[0], 64530[0], 69990[0], 92012[1], 92014[1], 93000[1], 93005[1], 93010[1], 93040[1], 93041[1], 93042[1], 93318[1], 93355[1], 94002[1], 94200[1], 94680[1], 94681[1], 94690[1], 95812[1], 95813[1], 95816[1], 95819[1], 95822[1], 95829[1], 95955[1], 96360[1], 96361[1], 96365[1], 96366[1], 96367[1], 96368[1], 96372[1], 96374[1], 96375[1], 96376[1], 96377[1], 96523[0], 99155[0], 99156[0], 99157[0], 99211[1], 99212[1], 99213[1], 99214[1], 99215[1], 99217[1], 99218[1], 99219[1], 99220[1], 99221[1], 99222[1], 99223[1], 99231[1], 99232[1], 99233[1], 99234[1], 99235[1], 99236[1], 99238[1], 99239[1], 99241[1], 99242[1], 99243[1], 99244[1], 99245[1], 99251[1], 99252[1], 99253[1], 99254[1], 99255[1], 99291[1], 99292[1], 99304[1], 99305[1], 99306[1], 99307[1], 99308[1], 99309[1], 99310[1], 99315[1], 99316[1], 99334[1], 99335[1], 99336[1], 99337[1], 99347[1], 99348[1], 99349[1], 99350[1], 99374[1], 99375[1], 99377[1], 99378[1], 99446[0], 99447[0], 99448[0], 99449[0], 99451[0], 99452[0], 99495[0], 99496[0], G0463[1], G0471[1]
54640	0213T[0], 0216T[0], 0437T[1], 0596T[1], 0597T[1], 0708T[1], 0709T[1], 12001[1], 12002[1], 12004[1], 12005[1], 12006[1], 12007[1], 12011[1], 12013[1], 12014[1], 12015[1], 12016[1], 12017[1], 12018[1], 12020[1], 12021[1], 12031[1], 12032[1], 12034[1], 12035[1], 12036[1], 12037[1], 12041[1], 12042[1], 12044[1], 12045[1], 12046[1], 12047[1], 12051[1], 12052[1], 12053[1], 12054[1], 12055[1], 12056[1], 12057[1], 13100[1], 13101[1], 13102[1], 13120[1], 13121[1], 13122[1], 13131[1], 13132[1], 13133[1], 13151[1], 13152[1], 13153[1], 15777[1], 36000[1], 36400[1], 36405[1], 36406[1], 36410[1], 36420[1], 36425[1], 36430[1], 36440[1], 36591[0], 36592[0], 36600[1], 36640[1], 43752[1], 49568[1], 51701[1], 51702[1], 51703[1], 54500[1], 54505[1], 54512[1], 54550[1], 54650[1], 54692[1], 55110[0], 57267[1], 62320[0], 62321[0], 62322[0], 62323[0], 62324[0], 62325[0], 62326[0], 62327[0], 64400[0], 64405[0], 64408[0], 64415[0], 64416[0], 64417[0], 64418[0], 64420[0], 64421[0], 64425[0], 64430[0], 64435[0], 64445[0], 64446[0], 64447[0], 64448[0], 64449[0], 64450[0], 64451[0], 64454[0], 64461[0], 64462[0], 64463[0], 64479[0], 64480[0], 64483[0], 64484[0], 64486[0], 64487[0], 64488[0], 64489[0], 64490[0], 64491[0], 64492[0], 64493[0], 64494[0], 64495[0], 64505[0], 64510[0], 64517[0], 64520[0], 64530[0], 69990[0], 92012[1], 92014[1], 93000[1], 93005[1], 93010[1], 93040[1], 93041[1], 93042[1], 93318[1], 93355[1], 94002[1], 94200[1], 94680[1], 94681[1], 94690[1], 95812[1], 95813[1], 95816[1], 95819[1], 95822[1], 95829[1], 95955[1], 96360[1], 96361[1], 96365[1], 96366[1], 96367[1], 96368[1], 96372[1], 96374[1], 96375[1], 96376[1], 96377[1], 96523[0], 99155[0], 99156[0], 99157[0], 99211[1], 99212[1], 99213[1], 99214[1], 99215[1], 99217[1], 99218[1], 99219[1], 99220[1], 99221[1], 99222[1], 99223[1], 99231[1], 99232[1], 99233[1], 99234[1], 99235[1], 99236[1], 99238[1], 99239[1], 99241[1], 99242[1], 99243[1], 99244[1], 99245[1], 99251[1], 99252[1], 99253[1], 99254[1], 99255[1], 99291[1], 99292[1], 99304[1], 99305[1], 99306[1], 99307[1], 99308[1], 99309[1], 99310[1], 99315[1], 99316[1], 99334[1], 99335[1], 99336[1], 99337[1], 99347[1], 99348[1], 99349[1], 99350[1], 99374[1], 99375[1], 99377[1], 99378[1], 99446[0], 99447[0], 99448[0], 99449[0], 99451[0], 99452[0], 99495[0], 99496[0], G0463[1], G0471[1]
54650	0213T[0], 0216T[0], 0596T[1], 0597T[1], 0708T[1], 0709T[1], 12001[1], 12002[1], 12004[1], 12005[1], 12006[1], 12007[1], 12011[1], 12013[1], 12014[1], 12015[1], 12016[1], 12017[1], 12018[1], 12020[1], 12021[1], 12031[1], 12032[1], 12034[1], 12035[1], 12036[1], 12037[1], 12041[1], 12042[1], 12044[1], 12045[1], 12046[1], 12047[1], 12051[1], 12052[1], 12053[1], 12054[1], 12055[1], 12056[1], 12057[1], 13100[1], 13101[1], 13102[1], 13120[1], 13121[1], 13122[1], 13131[1], 13132[1], 13133[1], 13151[1], 13152[1], 13153[1], 36000[1], 36400[1], 36405[1], 36406[1], 36410[1], 36420[1], 36425[1], 36430[1], 36440[1], 36591[0], 36592[0], 36600[1], 36640[1], 43752[1], 44005[0], 44180[0], 44602[1], 44603[1], 44604[1], 44605[1], 44820[0], 44850[0], 44950[0], 44970[0], 49000[0], 49002[1], 49010[0], 49255[0], 49320[1], 51701[1], 51702[1], 51703[1], 54500[1], 54505[1], 54512[1], 54560[1], 54692[1], 55110[0], 62320[0], 62321[0], 62322[0], 62323[0], 62324[0], 62325[0], 62326[0], 62327[0], 64400[0], 64405[0], 64408[0], 64415[0], 64416[0], 64417[0], 64418[0], 64420[0], 64421[0], 64425[0], 64430[0], 64435[0], 64445[0], 64446[0], 64447[0], 64448[0], 64449[0], 64450[0], 64451[0], 64454[0], 64461[0], 64462[0], 64463[0], 64479[0], 64480[0], 64483[0], 64484[0], 64486[0], 64487[0], 64488[0], 64489[0], 64490[0], 64491[0], 64492[0], 64493[0], 64494[0], 64495[0], 64505[0], 64510[0], 64517[0], 64520[0], 64530[0], 69990[0], 92012[1], 92014[1], 93000[1], 93005[1], 93010[1], 93040[1], 93041[1], 93042[1], 93318[1], 93355[1], 94002[1], 94200[1], 94680[1], 94681[1], 94690[1], 95812[1], 95813[1], 95816[1], 95819[1], 95822[1], 95829[1], 95955[1], 96360[1], 96361[1], 96365[1], 96366[1], 96367[1], 96368[1], 96372[1], 96374[1], 96375[1], 96376[1], 96377[1], 96523[0], 99155[0], 99156[0], 99157[0], 99211[1], 99212[1], 99213[1], 99214[1], 99215[1], 99217[1], 99218[1], 99219[1], 99220[1], 99221[1], 99222[1], 99223[1], 99231[1], 99232[1], 99233[1], 99234[1], 99235[1], 99236[1], 99238[1], 99239[1], 99241[1], 99242[1], 99243[1], 99244[1], 99245[1], 99251[1], 99252[1], 99253[1], 99254[1], 99255[1], 99291[1], 99292[1], 99304[1], 99305[1], 99306[1], 99307[1], 99308[1], 99309[1], 99310[1], 99315[1], 99316[1], 99334[1], 99335[1], 99336[1], 99337[1], 99347[1], 99348[1], 99349[1], 99350[1], 99374[1], 99375[1], 99377[1], 99378[1], 99446[0], 99447[0], 99448[0], 99449[0], 99451[0], 99452[0], 99495[0], 99496[0], G0463[1], G0471[1]
54660	0213T[0], 0216T[0], 0596T[1], 0597T[1], 0708T[1], 0709T[1], 12001[1], 12002[1], 12004[1], 12005[1], 12006[1], 12007[1], 12011[1], 12013[1], 12014[1], 12015[1], 12016[1], 12017[1], 12018[1], 12020[1], 12021[1], 12031[1], 12032[1], 12034[1], 12035[1], 12036[1], 12037[1], 12041[1], 12042[1], 12044[1], 12045[1], 12046[1], 12047[1], 12051[1], 12052[1], 12053[1], 12054[1], 12055[1], 12056[1], 12057[1], 13100[1], 13101[1], 13102[1], 13120[1], 13121[1], 13122[1], 13131[1], 13132[1], 13133[1], 13151[1], 13152[1], 13153[1], 36000[1], 36400[1], 36405[1], 36406[1], 36410[1], 36420[1], 36425[1], 36430[1], 36440[1], 36591[0], 36592[0], 36600[1], 36640[1], 43752[1], 51701[1], 51702[1], 51703[1], 54505[1], 55110[0], 62320[0], 62321[0], 62322[0], 62323[0], 62324[0], 62325[0], 62326[0], 62327[0], 64400[0], 64405[0], 64408[0], 64415[0], 64416[0], 64417[0], 64418[0], 64420[0], 64421[0], 64425[0], 64430[0], 64435[0], 64445[0], 64446[0], 64447[0], 64448[0], 64449[0], 64450[0], 64451[0], 64454[0], 64461[0], 64462[0], 64463[0], 64479[0], 64480[0], 64483[0], 64484[0], 64486[0], 64487[0], 64488[0], 64489[0], 64490[0], 64491[0], 64492[0], 64493[0], 64494[0], 64495[0], 64505[0], 64510[0], 64517[0], 64520[0], 64530[0], 69990[0], 92012[1], 92014[1], 93000[1], 93005[1], 93010[1], 93040[1], 93041[1], 93042[1], 93318[1], 93355[1], 94002[1], 94200[1], 94680[1], 94681[1], 94690[1], 95812[1], 95813[1], 95816[1], 95819[1], 95822[1], 95829[1], 95955[1], 96360[1], 96361[1], 96365[1], 96366[1], 96367[1], 96368[1], 96372[1], 96374[1], 96375[1], 96376[1], 96377[1], 96523[0], 99155[0], 99156[0], 99157[0], 99211[1], 99212[1], 99213[1], 99214[1], 99215[1], 99217[1], 99218[1], 99219[1], 99220[1], 99221[1], 99222[1], 99223[1], 99231[1], 99232[1], 99233[1], 99234[1], 99235[1], 99236[1], 99238[1], 99239[1], 99241[1], 99242[1], 99243[1], 99244[1], 99245[1], 99251[1], 99252[1], 99253[1], 99254[1], 99255[1], 99291[1], 99292[1], 99304[1], 99305[1], 99306[1], 99307[1], 99308[1], 99309[1], 99310[1], 99315[1], 99316[1], 99334[1], 99335[1], 99336[1], 99337[1], 99347[1], 99348[1], 99349[1], 99350[1], 99374[1], 99375[1], 99377[1], 99378[1], 99446[0], 99447[0], 99448[0], 99449[0], 99451[0], 99452[0], 99495[0], 99496[0], G0463[1], G0471[1]
54670	0213T[0], 0216T[0], 0596T[1], 0597T[1], 0708T[1], 0709T[1], 12001[1], 12002[1], 12004[1], 12005[1], 12006[1], 12007[1], 12011[1], 12013[1], 12014[1], 12015[1], 12016[1], 12017[1], 12018[1], 12020[1], 12021[1], 12031[1], 12032[1], 12034[1], 12035[1], 12036[1], 12037[1], 12041[1], 12042[1], 12044[1], 12045[1], 12046[1], 12047[1], 12051[1], 12052[1], 12053[1], 12054[1], 12055[1], 12056[1], 12057[1], 13100[1], 13101[1], 13102[1], 13120[1], 13121[1], 13122[1], 13131[1], 13132[1], 13133[1], 13151[1], 13152[1], 13153[1], 36000[1], 36400[1], 36405[1], 36406[1], 36410[1], 36420[1], 36425[1], 36430[1], 36440[1], 36591[0], 36592[0], 36600[1], 36640[1], 43752[1], 51701[1], 51702[1], 51703[1], 54500[1], 54505[1], 54620[0], 55110[0], 62320[0], 62321[0], 62322[0], 62323[0], 62324[0], 62325[0], 62326[0], 62327[0], 64400[0], 64405[0], 64408[0], 64415[0], 64416[0], 64417[0], 64418[0], 64420[0], 64421[0], 64425[0], 64430[0], 64435[0], 64445[0], 64446[0], 64447[0], 64448[0], 64449[0], 64450[0], 64451[0], 64454[0], 64461[0], 64462[0], 64463[0], 64479[0], 64480[0], 64483[0], 64484[0], 64486[0], 64487[0], 64488[0], 64489[0], 64490[0], 64491[0], 64492[0], 64493[0], 64494[0], 64495[0], 64505[0], 64510[0], 64517[0], 64520[0], 64530[0], 69990[0], 92012[1], 92014[1], 93000[1], 93005[1], 93010[1], 93040[1], 93041[1], 93042[1], 93318[1], 93355[1], 94002[1], 94200[1], 94680[1], 94681[1], 94690[1], 95812[1], 95813[1], 95816[1], 95819[1], 95822[1], 95829[1], 95955[1], 96360[1], 96361[1], 96365[1], 96366[1], 96367[1], 96368[1], 96372[1], 96374[1], 96375[1], 96376[1], 96377[1], 96523[0], 99155[0], 99156[0], 99157[0], 99211[1], 99212[1], 99213[1], 99214[1], 99215[1], 99217[1], 99218[1], 99219[1], 99220[1], 99221[1], 99222[1], 99223[1], 99231[1], 99232[1], 99233[1], 99234[1], 99235[1], 99236[1], 99238[1],

0 = Modifier usage not allowed or inappropriate 1 = Modifier usage allowed

Code 1	Code 2
	99239[1], 99241[1], 99242[1], 99243[1], 99244[1], 99245[1], 99251[1], 99252[1], 99253[1], 99254[1], 99255[1], 99291[1], 99292[1], 99304[1], 99305[1], 99306[1], 99307[1], 99308[1], 99309[1], 99310[1], 99315[1], 99316[1], 99334[1], 99335[1], 99336[1], 99337[1], 99347[1], 99348[1], 99349[1], 99350[1], 99374[1], 99375[1], 99377[1], 99378[1], 99446[0], 99447[0], 99448[0], 99449[0], 99451[0], 99452[0], 99495[0], 99496[0], G0463[1], G0471[1]
54680	0213T[0], 0216T[0], 0596T[1], 0597T[1], 0708T[1], 0709T[1], 12001[1], 12002[1], 12004[1], 12005[1], 12006[1], 12007[1], 12011[1], 12013[1], 12014[1], 12015[1], 12016[1], 12017[1], 12018[1], 12020[1], 12021[1], 12031[1], 12032[1], 12034[1], 12035[1], 12036[1], 12037[1], 12041[1], 12042[1], 12044[1], 12045[1], 12046[1], 12047[1], 12051[1], 12052[1], 12053[1], 12054[1], 12055[1], 12056[1], 12057[1], 13100[1], 13101[1], 13102[1], 13120[1], 13121[1], 13122[1], 13131[1], 13132[1], 13133[1], 13151[1], 13152[1], 13153[1], 36000[1], 36400[1], 36405[1], 36406[1], 36410[1], 36420[1], 36425[1], 36430[1], 36440[1], 36591[0], 36592[0], 36600[1], 36640[1], 43752[1], 51701[1], 51702[1], 51703[1], 54500[0], 54505[0], 54620[0], 54670[1], 55110[0], 62320[0], 62321[0], 62322[0], 62323[0], 62324[0], 62325[0], 62326[0], 62327[0], 64400[0], 64405[0], 64408[0], 64415[0], 64416[0], 64417[0], 64418[0], 64420[0], 64421[0], 64425[0], 64430[0], 64435[0], 64445[0], 64446[0], 64447[0], 64448[0], 64449[0], 64450[0], 64451[0], 64454[0], 64461[0], 64462[0], 64463[0], 64479[0], 64480[0], 64483[0], 64484[0], 64486[0], 64487[0], 64488[0], 64489[0], 64490[0], 64491[0], 64492[0], 64493[0], 64494[0], 64495[0], 64505[0], 64510[0], 64517[0], 64520[0], 64530[0], 69990[0], 92012[1], 92014[1], 93000[1], 93005[1], 93010[1], 93040[1], 93041[1], 93042[1], 93318[1], 93355[1], 94002[1], 94200[1], 94680[1], 94681[1], 94690[1], 95812[1], 95813[1], 95816[1], 95819[1], 95822[1], 95829[1], 95955[1], 96360[1], 96361[1], 96365[1], 96366[1], 96367[1], 96368[1], 96372[1], 96374[1], 96375[1], 96376[1], 96377[1], 96523[0], 99155[0], 99156[0], 99157[0], 99211[1], 99212[1], 99213[1], 99214[1], 99215[1], 99217[1], 99218[1], 99219[1], 99220[1], 99221[1], 99222[1], 99223[1], 99231[1], 99232[1], 99233[1], 99234[1], 99235[1], 99236[1], 99238[1], 99239[1], 99241[1], 99242[1], 99243[1], 99244[1], 99245[1], 99251[1], 99252[1], 99253[1], 99254[1], 99255[1], 99291[1], 99292[1], 99304[1], 99305[1], 99306[1], 99307[1], 99308[1], 99309[1], 99310[1], 99315[1], 99316[1], 99334[1], 99335[1], 99336[1], 99337[1], 99347[1], 99348[1], 99349[1], 99350[1], 99374[1], 99375[1], 99377[1], 99378[1], 99446[0], 99447[0], 99448[0], 99449[0], 99451[0], 99452[0], 99495[0], 99496[0], G0463[1], G0471[1]
54690	0213T[0], 0216T[0], 0596T[1], 0597T[1], 0708T[1], 0709T[1], 11000[1], 11001[1], 11004[1], 11005[1], 11006[1], 11042[1], 11043[1], 11044[1], 11045[1], 11046[1], 11047[1], 12001[1], 12002[1], 12004[1], 12005[1], 12006[1], 12007[1], 12011[1], 12013[1], 12014[1], 12015[1], 12016[1], 12017[1], 12018[1], 12020[1], 12021[1], 12031[1], 12032[1], 12034[1], 12035[1], 12036[1], 12037[1], 12041[1], 12042[1], 12044[1], 12045[1], 12046[1], 12047[1], 12051[1], 12052[1], 12053[1], 12054[1], 12055[1], 12056[1], 12057[1], 13100[1], 13101[1], 13102[1], 13120[1], 13121[1], 13122[1], 13131[1], 13132[1], 13133[1], 13151[1], 13152[1], 13153[1], 36000[1], 36400[1], 36405[1], 36406[1], 36410[1], 36420[1], 36425[1], 36430[1], 36440[1], 36591[0], 36592[0], 36600[1], 36640[1], 43653[0], 43752[1], 44005[0], 44180[0], 44602[1], 44603[1], 44604[1], 44605[1], 44950[0], 44970[1], 49082[1], 49083[1], 49084[1], 49320[0], 49321[1], 49400[0], 50715[1], 51701[1], 51702[1], 51703[1], 54512[1], 54522[1], 55110[0], 62320[0], 62321[0], 62322[0], 62323[0], 62324[0], 62325[0], 62326[0], 62327[0], 64400[0], 64405[0], 64408[0], 64415[0], 64416[0], 64417[0], 64418[0], 64420[0], 64421[0], 64425[0], 64430[0], 64435[0], 64445[0], 64446[0], 64447[0], 64448[0], 64449[0], 64450[0], 64451[0], 64454[0], 64461[0], 64462[0], 64463[0], 64479[0], 64480[0], 64483[0], 64484[0], 64486[0], 64487[0], 64488[0], 64489[0], 64490[0], 64491[0], 64492[0], 64493[0], 64494[0], 64495[0], 64505[0], 64510[0], 64517[0], 64520[0], 64530[0], 69990[0], 76000[1], 77001[1], 77002[1], 92012[1], 92014[1], 93000[1], 93005[1], 93010[1], 93040[1], 93041[1], 93042[1], 93318[1], 93355[1], 94002[1], 94200[1], 94680[1], 94681[1], 94690[1], 95812[1], 95813[1], 95816[1], 95819[1], 95822[1], 95829[1], 95955[1], 96360[1], 96361[1], 96365[1], 96366[1], 96367[1], 96368[1], 96372[1], 96374[1], 96375[1], 96376[1], 96377[1], 96523[0], 97597[1], 97598[1], 97602[1], 99155[0], 99156[0], 99157[0], 99211[1], 99212[1], 99213[1], 99214[1], 99215[1], 99217[1], 99218[1], 99219[1], 99220[1], 99221[1], 99222[1], 99223[1], 99231[1], 99232[1], 99233[1], 99234[1], 99235[1], 99236[1], 99238[1], 99239[1], 99241[1], 99242[1], 99243[1], 99244[1], 99245[1], 99251[1], 99252[1], 99253[1], 99254[1], 99255[1], 99291[1], 99292[1], 99304[1], 99305[1], 99306[1], 99307[1], 99308[1], 99309[1], 99310[1], 99315[1], 99316[1], 99334[1], 99335[1], 99336[1], 99337[1], 99347[1], 99348[1], 99349[1], 99350[1], 99374[1], 99375[1], 99377[1], 99378[1], 99446[0], 99447[0], 99448[0], 99449[0], 99451[0], 99452[0], 99495[0], 99496[0], G0463[1], G0471[1]
54692	0213T[0], 0216T[0], 0596T[1], 0597T[1], 0708T[1], 0709T[1], 12001[1], 12002[1], 12004[1], 12005[1], 12006[1], 12007[1], 12011[1], 12013[1], 12014[1], 12015[1], 12016[1], 12017[1], 12018[1], 12020[1], 12021[1], 12031[1], 12032[1], 12034[1], 12035[1], 12036[1], 12037[1], 12041[1], 12042[1], 12044[1], 12045[1], 12046[1], 12047[1], 12051[1], 12052[1], 12053[1], 12054[1], 12055[1], 12056[1], 12057[1], 13100[1], 13101[1], 13102[1], 13120[1], 13121[1], 13122[1], 13131[1], 13132[1], 13133[1], 13151[1], 13152[1], 13153[1], 36000[1], 36400[1], 36405[1], 36406[1], 36410[1], 36420[1], 36425[1], 36430[1], 36440[1], 36591[0], 36592[0], 36600[1], 36640[1], 43653[0], 43752[1], 44005[0], 44180[0], 44602[1], 44603[1], 44604[1], 44605[1], 44950[0], 44970[1], 49082[1], 49083[1], 49084[1], 49320[0], 49400[0], 50715[1], 51701[1], 51702[1], 51703[1], 55110[0], 58660[0], 62320[0], 62321[0], 62322[0], 62323[0], 62324[0], 62325[0], 62326[0], 62327[0], 64400[0], 64405[0], 64408[0], 64415[0], 64416[0], 64417[0], 64418[0], 64420[0], 64421[0], 64425[0], 64430[0], 64435[0], 64445[0], 64446[0], 64447[0], 64448[0], 64449[0], 64450[0], 64451[0], 64454[0], 64461[0], 64462[0], 64463[0], 64479[0], 64480[0], 64483[0], 64484[0], 64486[0], 64487[0], 64488[0], 64489[0], 64490[0], 64491[0], 64492[0], 64493[0], 64494[0], 64495[0], 64505[0], 64510[0], 64517[0], 64520[0], 64530[0], 69990[0], 76000[1], 77001[1], 77002[1], 92012[1], 92014[1], 93000[1], 93005[1], 93010[1], 93040[1], 93041[1], 93042[1], 93318[1], 93355[1], 94002[1], 94200[1], 94680[1], 94681[1], 94690[1], 95812[1], 95813[1], 95816[1], 95819[1], 95822[1], 95829[1], 95955[1], 96360[1], 96361[1], 96365[1], 96366[1], 96367[1], 96368[1], 96372[1], 96374[1], 96375[1], 96376[1], 96377[1], 96523[0], 99155[0], 99156[0], 99157[0], 99211[1], 99212[1], 99213[1], 99214[1], 99215[1], 99217[1], 99218[1], 99219[1], 99220[1], 99221[1], 99222[1], 99223[1], 99231[1], 99232[1], 99233[1], 99234[1], 99235[1], 99236[1], 99238[1], 99239[1], 99241[1], 99242[1], 99243[1], 99244[1], 99245[1], 99251[1], 99252[1], 99253[1], 99254[1], 99255[1], 99291[1], 99292[1], 99304[1], 99305[1], 99306[1], 99307[1], 99308[1], 99309[1], 99310[1], 99315[1], 99316[1], 99334[1], 99335[1], 99336[1], 99337[1], 99347[1], 99348[1], 99349[1], 99350[1], 99374[1], 99375[1], 99377[1], 99378[1], 99446[0], 99447[0], 99448[0], 99449[0], 99451[0], 99452[0], 99495[0], 99496[0], G0463[1], G0471[1]
54700	0213T[0], 0216T[0], 0596T[1], 0597T[1], 0708T[1], 0709T[1], 12001[1], 12002[1], 12004[1], 12005[1], 12006[1], 12007[1], 12011[1], 12013[1], 12014[1], 12015[1], 12016[1], 12017[1], 12018[1], 12020[1], 12021[1], 12031[1], 12032[1], 12034[1], 12035[1], 12036[1], 12037[1], 12041[1], 12042[1], 12044[1], 12045[1], 12046[1], 12047[1], 12051[1], 12052[1], 12053[1], 12054[1], 12055[1], 12056[1], 12057[1], 13100[1], 13101[1], 13102[1], 13120[1], 13121[1], 13122[1], 13131[1], 13132[1], 13133[1], 13151[1], 13152[1], 13153[1], 36000[1], 36400[1], 36405[1], 36406[1], 36410[1], 36420[1], 36425[1], 36430[1], 36440[1], 36591[0], 36592[0], 36600[1], 36640[1], 43752[1], 51701[1], 51702[1], 51703[1], 54500[1], 54505[1], 55100[1], 55110[0], 62320[0], 62321[0], 62322[0], 62323[0], 62324[0], 62325[0], 62326[0], 62327[0], 64400[0], 64405[0], 64408[0], 64415[0], 64416[0], 64417[0], 64418[0], 64420[0], 64421[0], 64425[0], 64430[0], 64435[0], 64445[0], 64446[0], 64447[0], 64448[0], 64449[0], 64450[0], 64451[0], 64454[0], 64461[0], 64462[0], 64463[0], 64479[0], 64480[0], 64483[0], 64484[0], 64486[0], 64487[0], 64488[0], 64489[0], 64490[0], 64491[0], 64492[0], 64493[0], 64494[0], 64495[0], 64505[0], 64510[0], 64517[0], 64520[0], 64530[0], 69990[0], 92012[1], 92014[1], 93000[1], 93005[1], 93010[1], 93040[1], 93041[1], 93042[1], 93318[1], 93355[1], 94002[1], 94200[1], 94680[1], 94681[1], 94690[1], 95812[1], 95813[1], 95816[1], 95819[1], 95822[1], 95829[1], 95955[1], 96360[1], 96361[1], 96365[1], 96366[1], 96367[1], 96368[1], 96372[1], 96374[1], 96375[1], 96376[1], 96377[1], 96523[0], 99155[0], 99156[0], 99157[0], 99211[1], 99212[1], 99213[1], 99214[1], 99215[1], 99217[1], 99218[1], 99219[1], 99220[1], 99221[1], 99222[1], 99223[1], 99231[1], 99232[1], 99233[1], 99234[1], 99235[1], 99236[1], 99238[1], 99239[1], 99241[1], 99242[1], 99243[1], 99244[1], 99245[1], 99251[1], 99252[1], 99253[1], 99254[1], 99255[1], 99291[1], 99292[1], 99304[1], 99305[1], 99306[1], 99307[1], 99308[1], 99309[1], 99310[1], 99315[1], 99316[1], 99334[1], 99335[1], 99336[1], 99337[1], 99347[1], 99348[1], 99349[1], 99350[1], 99374[1], 99375[1], 99377[1], 99378[1], 99446[0], 99447[0], 99448[0], 99449[0], 99451[0], 99452[0], 99495[0], 99496[0], G0463[1], G0471[1], J2001[1]
54800	0213T[0], 0216T[0], 0596T[1], 0597T[1], 0708T[1], 0709T[1], 10005[1], 10007[1], 10009[1], 10011[1], 10021[1], 12001[1], 12002[1], 12004[1], 12005[1], 12006[1], 12007[1], 12011[1], 12013[1], 12014[1], 12015[1], 12016[1], 12017[1], 12018[1], 12020[1], 12021[1], 12031[1], 12032[1], 12034[1], 12035[1], 12036[1], 12037[1], 12041[1], 12042[1], 12044[1], 12045[1], 12046[1], 12047[1], 12051[1], 12052[1], 12053[1], 12054[1], 12055[1], 12056[1], 12057[1], 13100[1], 13101[1], 13102[1], 13120[1], 13121[1], 13122[1], 13131[1], 13132[1], 13133[1], 13151[1], 13152[1], 13153[1], 36000[1], 36400[1], 36405[1], 36406[1], 36410[1], 36420[1], 36425[1], 36430[1], 36440[1], 36591[0], 36592[0], 36600[1], 36640[1], 43752[1], 51701[1], 51702[1], 51703[1], 54500[1], 54505[1], 62320[0], 62321[0], 62322[0], 62323[0], 62324[0], 62325[0], 62326[0], 62327[0], 64400[0], 64405[0], 64408[0], 64415[0], 64416[0], 64417[0], 64418[0], 64420[0], 64421[0], 64425[0], 64430[0], 64435[0], 64445[0], 64446[0], 64447[0], 64448[0], 64449[0], 64450[0], 64451[0], 64454[0], 64461[0], 64462[0], 64463[0], 64479[0], 64480[0], 64483[0], 64484[0], 64486[0], 64487[0], 64488[0], 64489[0], 64490[0], 64491[0], 64492[0], 64493[0], 64494[0], 64495[0], 64505[0], 64510[0], 64517[0], 64520[0], 64530[0], 69990[0], 92012[1], 92014[1], 93000[1], 93005[1], 93010[1], 93040[1], 93041[1], 93042[1], 93318[1], 93355[1], 94002[1], 94200[1], 94680[1], 94681[1], 94690[1], 95812[1], 95813[1], 95816[1], 95819[1], 95822[1], 95829[1], 95955[1], 96360[1], 96361[1], 96365[1], 96366[1], 96367[1], 96368[1], 96372[1], 96374[1], 96375[1], 96376[1], 96377[1], 96523[0], 99155[0], 99156[0], 99157[0], 99211[1], 99212[1], 99213[1], 99214[1], 99215[1], 99217[1], 99218[1], 99219[1], 99220[1], 99221[1], 99222[1], 99223[1], 99231[1], 99232[1], 99233[1], 99234[1], 99235[1], 99236[1], 99238[1], 99239[1], 99241[1], 99242[1], 99243[1], 99244[1], 99245[1], 99251[1], 99252[1], 99253[1], 99254[1], 99255[1], 99291[1], 99292[1], 99304[1], 99305[1], 99306[1], 99307[1], 99308[1], 99309[1], 99310[1], 99315[1], 99316[1], 99334[1], 99335[1], 99336[1], 99337[1], 99347[1], 99348[1], 99349[1], 99350[1], 99374[1], 99375[1], 99377[1], 99378[1], 99446[0], 99447[0], 99448[0], 99449[0], 99451[0], 99452[0], 99495[1], 99496[1], G0463[1], G0471[1]
54830	0213T[0], 0216T[0], 0596T[1], 0597T[1], 0708T[1], 0709T[1], 11000[1], 11001[1], 11004[1], 11005[1], 11006[1], 11042[1], 11043[1], 11044[1], 11045[1], 11046[1], 11047[1], 12001[1], 12002[1], 12004[1], 12005[1], 12006[1], 12007[1], 12011[1], 12013[1], 12014[1], 12015[1], 12016[1], 12017[1], 12018[1], 12020[1], 12021[1], 12031[1], 12032[1], 12034[1], 12035[1], 12036[1], 12037[1], 12041[1], 12042[1], 12044[1], 12045[1], 12046[1], 12047[1], 12051[1], 12052[1], 12053[1], 12054[1], 12055[1], 12056[1], 12057[1], 13100[1], 13101[1], 13102[1], 13120[1], 13121[1], 13122[1], 13131[1], 13132[1], 13133[1],

0 = Modifier usage not allowed or inappropriate 1 = Modifier usage allowed

Code 1	Code 2
	13151[1], 13152[1], 13153[1], 36000[1], 36400[1], 36405[1], 36406[1], 36410[1], 36420[1], 36425[1], 36430[1], 36440[1], 36591[0], 36592[0], 36600[1], 36640[1], 43752[1], 51701[1], 51702[1], 51703[1], 54500[1], 54505[1], 55110[0], 62320[0], 62321[0], 62322[0], 62323[0], 62324[0], 62325[0], 62326[0], 62327[0], 64400[0], 64405[0], 64408[0], 64415[0], 64416[0], 64417[0], 64418[0], 64420[0], 64421[0], 64425[0], 64430[0], 64435[0], 64445[0], 64446[0], 64447[0], 64448[0], 64449[0], 64450[0], 64451[0], 64454[0], 64461[0], 64462[0], 64463[0], 64479[0], 64480[0], 64483[0], 64484[0], 64486[0], 64487[0], 64488[0], 64489[0], 64490[0], 64491[0], 64492[0], 64493[0], 64494[0], 64495[0], 64505[0], 64510[0], 64517[0], 64520[0], 64530[0], 69990[0], 92012[1], 92014[1], 93000[1], 93005[1], 93010[1], 93040[1], 93041[1], 93042[1], 93318[1], 93355[1], 94002[1], 94200[1], 94680[1], 94681[1], 94690[1], 95812[1], 95813[1], 95816[1], 95819[1], 95822[1], 95829[1], 95955[1], 96360[1], 96361[1], 96365[1], 96366[1], 96367[1], 96368[1], 96372[1], 96374[1], 96375[1], 96376[1], 96377[1], 96523[0], 97597[1], 97598[1], 97602[1], 99155[0], 99156[0], 99157[0], 99211[1], 99212[1], 99213[1], 99214[1], 99215[1], 99217[1], 99218[1], 99219[1], 99220[1], 99221[1], 99222[1], 99223[1], 99231[1], 99232[1], 99233[1], 99234[1], 99235[1], 99236[1], 99238[1], 99239[1], 99241[1], 99242[1], 99243[1], 99244[1], 99245[1], 99251[1], 99252[1], 99253[1], 99254[1], 99255[1], 99291[1], 99292[1], 99304[1], 99305[1], 99306[1], 99307[1], 99308[1], 99309[1], 99310[1], 99315[1], 99316[1], 99334[1], 99335[1], 99336[1], 99337[1], 99347[1], 99348[1], 99349[1], 99350[1], 99374[1], 99375[1], 99377[1], 99378[1], 99446[0], 99447[0], 99448[0], 99449[0], 99451[0], 99452[0], 99495[0], 99496[0], G0463[1], G0471[1]
54840	0213T[0], 0216T[0], 0596T[1], 0597T[1], 0708T[1], 0709T[1], 11000[1], 11001[1], 11004[1], 11005[1], 11006[1], 11042[1], 11043[1], 11044[1], 11045[1], 11046[1], 11047[1], 12001[1], 12002[1], 12004[1], 12005[1], 12006[1], 12007[1], 12011[1], 12013[1], 12014[1], 12015[1], 12016[1], 12017[1], 12018[1], 12020[1], 12021[1], 12031[1], 12032[1], 12034[1], 12035[1], 12036[1], 12037[1], 12041[1], 12042[1], 12044[1], 12045[1], 12046[1], 12047[1], 12051[1], 12052[1], 12053[1], 12054[1], 12055[1], 12056[1], 12057[1], 13100[1], 13101[1], 13102[1], 13120[1], 13121[1], 13122[1], 13131[1], 13132[1], 13133[1], 13151[1], 13152[1], 13153[1], 36000[1], 36400[1], 36405[1], 36406[1], 36410[1], 36420[1], 36425[1], 36430[1], 36440[1], 36591[0], 36592[0], 36600[1], 36640[1], 43752[1], 51701[1], 51702[1], 51703[1], 54500[1], 54505[1], 55110[0], 62320[0], 62321[0], 62322[0], 62323[0], 62324[0], 62325[0], 62326[0], 62327[0], 64400[0], 64405[0], 64408[0], 64415[0], 64416[0], 64417[0], 64418[0], 64420[0], 64421[0], 64425[0], 64430[0], 64435[0], 64445[0], 64446[0], 64447[0], 64448[0], 64449[0], 64450[0], 64451[0], 64454[0], 64461[0], 64462[0], 64463[0], 64479[0], 64480[0], 64483[0], 64484[0], 64486[0], 64487[0], 64488[0], 64489[0], 64490[0], 64491[0], 64492[0], 64493[0], 64494[0], 64495[0], 64505[0], 64510[0], 64517[0], 64520[0], 64530[0], 69990[0], 92012[1], 92014[1], 93000[1], 93005[1], 93010[1], 93040[1], 93041[1], 93042[1], 93318[1], 93355[1], 94002[1], 94200[1], 94680[1], 94681[1], 94690[1], 95812[1], 95813[1], 95816[1], 95819[1], 95822[1], 95829[1], 95955[1], 96360[1], 96361[1], 96365[1], 96366[1], 96367[1], 96368[1], 96372[1], 96374[1], 96375[1], 96376[1], 96377[1], 96523[0], 97597[1], 97598[1], 97602[1], 99155[0], 99156[0], 99157[0], 99211[1], 99212[1], 99213[1], 99214[1], 99215[1], 99217[1], 99218[1], 99219[1], 99220[1], 99221[1], 99222[1], 99223[1], 99231[1], 99232[1], 99233[1], 99234[1], 99235[1], 99236[1], 99238[1], 99239[1], 99241[1], 99242[1], 99243[1], 99244[1], 99245[1], 99251[1], 99252[1], 99253[1], 99254[1], 99255[1], 99291[1], 99292[1], 99304[1], 99305[1], 99306[1], 99307[1], 99308[1], 99309[1], 99310[1], 99315[1], 99316[1], 99334[1], 99335[1], 99336[1], 99337[1], 99347[1], 99348[1], 99349[1], 99350[1], 99374[1], 99375[1], 99377[1], 99378[1], 99446[0], 99447[0], 99448[0], 99449[0], 99451[0], 99452[0], 99495[0], 99496[0], G0463[1], G0471[1]
54860	0213T[0], 0216T[0], 0596T[1], 0597T[1], 0708T[1], 0709T[1], 11000[1], 11001[1], 11004[1], 11005[1], 11006[1], 11042[1], 11043[1], 11044[1], 11045[1], 11046[1], 11047[1], 12001[1], 12002[1], 12004[1], 12005[1], 12006[1], 12007[1], 12011[1], 12013[1], 12014[1], 12015[1], 12016[1], 12017[1], 12018[1], 12020[1], 12021[1], 12031[1], 12032[1], 12034[1], 12035[1], 12036[1], 12037[1], 12041[1], 12042[1], 12044[1], 12045[1], 12046[1], 12047[1], 12051[1], 12052[1], 12053[1], 12054[1], 12055[1], 12056[1], 12057[1], 13100[1], 13101[1], 13102[1], 13120[1], 13121[1], 13122[1], 13131[1], 13132[1], 13133[1], 13151[1], 13152[1], 13153[1], 36000[1], 36400[1], 36405[1], 36406[1], 36410[1], 36420[1], 36425[1], 36430[1], 36440[1], 36591[0], 36592[0], 36600[1], 36640[1], 43752[1], 51701[1], 51702[1], 51703[1], 54500[1], 54505[1], 55110[0], 62320[0], 62321[0], 62322[0], 62323[0], 62324[0], 62325[0], 62326[0], 62327[0], 64400[0], 64405[0], 64408[0], 64415[0], 64416[0], 64417[0], 64418[0], 64420[0], 64421[0], 64425[0], 64430[0], 64435[0], 64445[0], 64446[0], 64447[0], 64448[0], 64449[0], 64450[0], 64451[0], 64454[0], 64461[0], 64462[0], 64463[0], 64479[0], 64480[0], 64483[0], 64484[0], 64486[0], 64487[0], 64488[0], 64489[0], 64490[0], 64491[0], 64492[0], 64493[0], 64494[0], 64495[0], 64505[0], 64510[0], 64517[0], 64520[0], 64530[0], 69990[0], 92012[1], 92014[1], 93000[1], 93005[1], 93010[1], 93040[1], 93041[1], 93042[1], 93318[1], 93355[1], 94002[1], 94200[1], 94680[1], 94681[1], 94690[1], 95812[1], 95813[1], 95816[1], 95819[1], 95822[1], 95829[1], 95955[1], 96360[1], 96361[1], 96365[1], 96366[1], 96367[1], 96368[1], 96372[1], 96374[1], 96375[1], 96376[1], 96377[1], 96523[0], 97597[1], 97598[1], 97602[1], 99155[0], 99156[0], 99157[0], 99211[1], 99212[1], 99213[1], 99214[1], 99215[1], 99217[1], 99218[1], 99219[1], 99220[1], 99221[1], 99222[1], 99223[1], 99231[1], 99232[1], 99233[1], 99234[1], 99235[1], 99236[1], 99238[1], 99239[1], 99241[1], 99242[1], 99243[1], 99244[1], 99245[1], 99251[1], 99252[1], 99253[1], 99254[1], 99255[1], 99291[1], 99292[1], 99304[1], 99305[1], 99306[1], 99307[1], 99308[1], 99309[1], 99310[1], 99315[1], 99316[1], 99334[1], 99335[1], 99336[1], 99337[1], 99347[1], 99348[1], 99349[1], 99350[1], 99374[1], 99375[1], 99377[1], 99378[1], 99446[0], 99447[0], 99448[0], 99449[0], 99451[0], 99452[0], 99495[0], 99496[0], G0463[1], G0471[1]
54861	0213T[0], 0216T[0], 0596T[1], 0597T[1], 0708T[1], 0709T[1], 11000[1], 11001[1], 11004[1], 11005[1], 11006[1], 11042[1], 11043[1], 11044[1], 11045[1], 11046[1], 11047[1], 12001[1], 12002[1], 12004[1], 12005[1], 12006[1], 12007[1], 12011[1], 12013[1], 12014[1], 12015[1], 12016[1], 12017[1], 12018[1], 12020[1], 12021[1], 12031[1], 12032[1], 12034[1], 12035[1], 12036[1], 12037[1], 12041[1], 12042[1], 12044[1], 12045[1], 12046[1], 12047[1], 12051[1], 12052[1], 12053[1], 12054[1], 12055[1], 12056[1], 12057[1], 13100[1], 13101[1], 13102[1], 13120[1], 13121[1], 13122[1], 13131[1], 13132[1], 13133[1], 13151[1], 13152[1], 13153[1], 36000[1], 36400[1], 36405[1], 36406[1], 36410[1], 36420[1], 36425[1], 36430[1], 36440[1], 36591[0], 36592[0], 36600[1], 36640[1], 43752[1], 51701[1], 51702[1], 51703[1], 54500[0], 54505[0], 54860[1], 55110[0], 62320[0], 62321[0], 62322[0], 62323[0], 62324[0], 62325[0], 62326[0], 62327[0], 64400[0], 64405[0], 64408[0], 64415[0], 64416[0], 64417[0], 64418[0], 64420[0], 64421[0], 64425[0], 64430[0], 64435[0], 64445[0], 64446[0], 64447[0], 64448[0], 64449[0], 64450[0], 64451[0], 64454[0], 64461[0], 64462[0], 64463[0], 64479[0], 64480[0], 64483[0], 64484[0], 64486[0], 64487[0], 64488[0], 64489[0], 64490[0], 64491[0], 64492[0], 64493[0], 64494[0], 64495[0], 64505[0], 64510[0], 64517[0], 64520[0], 64530[0], 69990[0], 92012[1], 92014[1], 93000[1], 93005[1], 93010[1], 93040[1], 93041[1], 93042[1], 93318[1], 93355[1], 94002[1], 94200[1], 94680[1], 94681[1], 94690[1], 95812[1], 95813[1], 95816[1], 95819[1], 95822[1], 95829[1], 95955[1], 96360[1], 96361[1], 96365[1], 96366[1], 96367[1], 96368[1], 96372[1], 96374[1], 96375[1], 96376[1], 96377[1], 96523[0], 97597[1], 97598[1], 97602[1], 99155[0], 99156[0], 99157[0], 99211[1], 99212[1], 99213[1], 99214[1], 99215[1], 99217[1], 99218[1], 99219[1], 99220[1], 99221[1], 99222[1], 99223[1], 99231[1], 99232[1], 99233[1], 99234[1], 99235[1], 99236[1], 99238[1], 99239[1], 99241[1], 99242[1], 99243[1], 99244[1], 99245[1], 99251[1], 99252[1], 99253[1], 99254[1], 99255[1], 99291[1], 99292[1], 99304[1], 99305[1], 99306[1], 99307[1], 99308[1], 99309[1], 99310[1], 99315[1], 99316[1], 99334[1], 99335[1], 99336[1], 99337[1], 99347[1], 99348[1], 99349[1], 99350[1], 99374[1], 99375[1], 99377[1], 99378[1], 99446[0], 99447[0], 99448[0], 99449[0], 99451[0], 99452[0], 99495[0], 99496[0], G0463[1], G0471[1]
54865	0213T[0], 0216T[0], 0596T[1], 0597T[1], 0708T[1], 0709T[1], 10005[1], 10007[1], 10009[1], 10011[1], 10021[1], 12001[1], 12002[1], 12004[1], 12005[1], 12006[1], 12007[1], 12011[1], 12013[1], 12014[1], 12015[1], 12016[1], 12017[1], 12018[1], 12020[1], 12021[1], 12031[1], 12032[1], 12034[1], 12035[1], 12036[1], 12037[1], 12041[1], 12042[1], 12044[1], 12045[1], 12046[1], 12047[1], 12051[1], 12052[1], 12053[1], 12054[1], 12055[1], 12056[1], 12057[1], 13100[1], 13101[1], 13102[1], 13120[1], 13121[1], 13122[1], 13131[1], 13132[1], 13133[1], 13151[1], 13152[1], 13153[1], 36000[1], 36400[1], 36405[1], 36406[1], 36410[1], 36420[1], 36425[1], 36430[1], 36440[1], 36591[0], 36592[0], 36600[1], 36640[1], 43752[1], 51701[1], 51702[1], 51703[1], 54500[1], 54505[1], 55110[0], 62320[0], 62321[0], 62322[0], 62323[0], 62324[0], 62325[0], 62326[0], 62327[0], 64400[0], 64405[0], 64408[0], 64415[0], 64416[0], 64417[0], 64418[0], 64420[0], 64421[0], 64425[0], 64430[0], 64435[0], 64445[0], 64446[0], 64447[0], 64448[0], 64449[0], 64450[0], 64451[0], 64454[0], 64461[0], 64462[0], 64463[0], 64479[0], 64480[0], 64483[0], 64484[0], 64486[0], 64487[0], 64488[0], 64489[0], 64490[0], 64491[0], 64492[0], 64493[0], 64494[0], 64495[0], 64505[0], 64510[0], 64517[0], 64520[0], 64530[0], 69990[0], 92012[1], 92014[1], 93000[1], 93005[1], 93010[1], 93040[1], 93041[1], 93042[1], 93318[1], 93355[1], 94002[1], 94200[1], 94680[1], 94681[1], 94690[1], 95812[1], 95813[1], 95816[1], 95819[1], 95822[1], 95829[1], 95955[1], 96360[1], 96361[1], 96365[1], 96366[1], 96367[1], 96368[1], 96372[1], 96374[1], 96375[1], 96376[1], 96377[1], 96523[0], 99155[0], 99156[0], 99157[0], 99211[1], 99212[1], 99213[1], 99214[1], 99215[1], 99217[1], 99218[1], 99219[1], 99220[1], 99221[1], 99222[1], 99223[1], 99231[1], 99232[1], 99233[1], 99234[1], 99235[1], 99236[1], 99238[1], 99239[1], 99241[1], 99242[1], 99243[1], 99244[1], 99245[1], 99251[1], 99252[1], 99253[1], 99254[1], 99255[1], 99291[1], 99292[1], 99304[1], 99305[1], 99306[1], 99307[1], 99308[1], 99309[1], 99310[1], 99315[1], 99316[1], 99334[1], 99335[1], 99336[1], 99337[1], 99347[1], 99348[1], 99349[1], 99350[1], 99374[1], 99375[1], 99377[1], 99378[1], 99446[0], 99447[0], 99448[0], 99449[0], 99451[0], 99452[0], 99495[0], 99496[0], G0463[1], G0471[1]
54900	0213T[0], 0216T[0], 0596T[1], 0597T[1], 0708T[1], 0709T[1], 12001[1], 12002[1], 12004[1], 12005[1], 12006[1], 12007[1], 12011[1], 12013[1], 12014[1], 12015[1], 12016[1], 12017[1], 12018[1], 12020[1], 12021[1], 12031[1], 12032[1], 12034[1], 12035[1], 12036[1], 12037[1], 12041[1], 12042[1], 12044[1], 12045[1], 12046[1], 12047[1], 12051[1], 12052[1], 12053[1], 12054[1], 12055[1], 12056[1], 12057[1], 13100[1], 13101[1], 13102[1], 13120[1], 13121[1], 13122[1], 13131[1], 13132[1], 13133[1], 13151[1], 13152[1], 13153[1], 36000[1], 36400[1], 36405[1], 36406[1], 36410[1], 36420[1], 36425[1], 36430[1], 36440[1], 36591[0], 36592[0], 36600[1], 36640[1], 43752[1], 51701[1], 51702[1], 51703[1], 54500[1], 54505[1], 55110[0], 62320[0], 62321[0], 62322[0], 62323[0], 62324[0], 62325[0], 62326[0], 62327[0], 64400[0], 64405[0], 64408[0], 64415[0], 64416[0], 64417[0], 64418[0], 64420[0], 64421[0], 64425[0], 64430[0], 64435[0], 64445[0], 64446[0], 64447[0], 64448[0], 64449[0], 64450[0], 64451[0], 64454[0], 64461[0], 64462[0], 64463[0], 64479[0], 64480[0], 64483[0], 64484[0], 64486[0], 64487[0], 64488[0], 64489[0], 64490[0], 64491[0], 64492[0], 64493[0], 64494[0], 64495[0], 64505[0], 64510[0], 64517[0], 64520[0], 64530[0], 69990[0], 92012[1], 92014[1], 93000[1], 93005[1], 93010[1], 93040[1], 93041[1], 93042[1], 93318[1], 93355[1], 94002[1], 94200[1], 94680[1], 94681[1], 94690[1], 95812[1], 95813[1], 95816[1], 95819[1], 95822[1], 95829[1], 95955[1], 96360[1], 96361[1], 96365[1], 96366[1], 96367[1], 96368[1], 96372[1], 96374[1], 96375[1], 96376[1], 96377[1], 96523[0], 99155[0], 99156[0], 99157[0], 99211[1], 99212[1], 99213[1], 99214[1], 99215[1], 99217[1], 99218[1], 99219[1], 99220[1], 99221[1], 99222[1], 99223[1], 99231[1], 99232[1], 99233[1], 99234[1], 99235[1], 99236[1], 99238[1], 99239[1], 99241[1], 99242[1], 99243[1], 99244[1], 99245[1], 99251[1], 99252[1], 99253[1], 99254[1], 99255[1],

0 = Modifier usage not allowed or inappropriate   1 = Modifier usage allowed

Code 1	Code 2
	99291[1], 99292[1], 99304[1], 99305[1], 99306[1], 99307[1], 99308[1], 99309[1], 99310[1], 99315[1], 99316[1], 99334[1], 99335[1], 99336[1], 99337[1], 99347[1], 99348[1], 99349[1], 99350[1], 99374[1], 99375[1], 99377[1], 99378[1], 99446[0], 99447[0], 99448[0], 99449[0], 99451[0], 99452[0], 99495[0], 99496[0], G0463[1], G0471[1]
54901	0213T[0], 0216T[0], 0596T[1], 0597T[1], 0708T[1], 0709T[1], 12001[1], 12002[1], 12004[1], 12005[1], 12006[1], 12007[1], 12011[1], 12013[1], 12014[1], 12015[1], 12016[1], 12017[1], 12018[1], 12020[1], 12021[1], 12031[1], 12032[1], 12034[1], 12035[1], 12036[1], 12037[1], 12041[1], 12042[1], 12044[1], 12045[1], 12046[1], 12047[1], 12051[1], 12052[1], 12053[1], 12054[1], 12055[1], 12056[1], 12057[1], 13100[1], 13101[1], 13102[1], 13120[1], 13121[1], 13122[1], 13131[1], 13132[1], 13133[1], 13151[1], 13152[1], 13153[1], 36000[1], 36400[1], 36405[1], 36406[1], 36410[1], 36420[1], 36425[1], 36430[1], 36440[1], 36591[0], 36592[0], 36600[1], 36640[1], 43752[1], 51701[1], 51702[1], 51703[1], 54500[0], 54505[0], 54900[1], 55110[0], 62320[0], 62321[0], 62322[0], 62323[0], 62324[0], 62325[0], 62326[0], 62327[0], 64400[0], 64405[0], 64408[0], 64415[0], 64416[0], 64417[0], 64418[0], 64420[0], 64421[0], 64425[0], 64430[0], 64435[0], 64445[0], 64446[0], 64447[0], 64448[0], 64449[0], 64450[0], 64451[0], 64454[0], 64461[0], 64462[0], 64463[0], 64479[0], 64480[0], 64483[0], 64484[0], 64486[0], 64487[0], 64488[0], 64489[0], 64490[0], 64491[0], 64492[0], 64493[0], 64494[0], 64495[0], 64505[0], 64510[0], 64517[0], 64520[0], 64530[0], 69990[0], 92012[1], 92014[1], 93000[1], 93005[1], 93010[1], 93040[1], 93041[1], 93042[1], 93318[1], 93355[1], 94002[1], 94200[1], 94680[1], 94681[1], 94690[1], 95812[1], 95813[1], 95816[1], 95819[1], 95822[1], 95829[1], 95955[1], 96360[1], 96361[1], 96365[1], 96366[1], 96367[1], 96368[1], 96372[1], 96374[1], 96375[1], 96376[1], 96377[1], 96523[0], 99155[0], 99156[0], 99157[0], 99211[1], 99212[1], 99213[1], 99214[1], 99215[1], 99217[1], 99218[1], 99219[1], 99220[1], 99221[1], 99222[1], 99223[1], 99231[1], 99232[1], 99233[1], 99234[1], 99235[1], 99236[1], 99238[1], 99239[1], 99241[1], 99242[1], 99243[1], 99244[1], 99245[1], 99251[1], 99252[1], 99253[1], 99254[1], 99255[1], 99291[1], 99292[1], 99304[1], 99305[1], 99306[1], 99307[1], 99308[1], 99309[1], 99310[1], 99315[1], 99316[1], 99334[1], 99335[1], 99336[1], 99337[1], 99347[1], 99348[1], 99349[1], 99350[1], 99374[1], 99375[1], 99377[1], 99378[1], 99446[0], 99447[0], 99448[0], 99449[0], 99451[0], 99452[0], 99495[0], 99496[0], G0463[1], G0471[1]
55000	0213T[0], 0216T[0], 0596T[1], 0597T[1], 0708T[1], 0709T[1], 12001[1], 12002[1], 12004[1], 12005[1], 12006[1], 12007[1], 12011[1], 12013[1], 12014[1], 12015[1], 12016[1], 12017[1], 12018[1], 12020[1], 12021[1], 12031[1], 12032[1], 12034[1], 12035[1], 12036[1], 12037[1], 12041[1], 12042[1], 12044[1], 12045[1], 12046[1], 12047[1], 12051[1], 12052[1], 12053[1], 12054[1], 12055[1], 12056[1], 12057[1], 13100[1], 13101[1], 13102[1], 13120[1], 13121[1], 13122[1], 13131[1], 13132[1], 13133[1], 13151[1], 13152[1], 13153[1], 36000[1], 36400[1], 36405[1], 36406[1], 36410[1], 36420[1], 36425[1], 36430[1], 36440[1], 36591[0], 36592[0], 36600[1], 36640[1], 43752[1], 51701[1], 51702[1], 51703[1], 54500[1], 54505[1], 55110[0], 62320[0], 62321[0], 62322[0], 62323[0], 62324[0], 62325[0], 62326[0], 62327[0], 64400[0], 64405[0], 64408[0], 64415[0], 64416[0], 64417[0], 64418[0], 64420[0], 64421[0], 64425[0], 64430[0], 64435[0], 64445[0], 64446[0], 64447[0], 64448[0], 64449[0], 64450[0], 64451[0], 64454[0], 64461[0], 64462[0], 64463[0], 64479[0], 64480[0], 64483[0], 64484[0], 64486[0], 64487[0], 64488[0], 64489[0], 64490[0], 64491[0], 64492[0], 64493[0], 64494[0], 64495[0], 64505[0], 64510[0], 64517[0], 64520[0], 64530[0], 69990[0], 92012[1], 92014[1], 93000[1], 93005[1], 93010[1], 93040[1], 93041[1], 93042[1], 93318[1], 93355[1], 94002[1], 94200[1], 94680[1], 94681[1], 94690[1], 95812[1], 95813[1], 95816[1], 95819[1], 95822[1], 95829[1], 95955[1], 96360[1], 96361[1], 96365[1], 96366[1], 96367[1], 96368[1], 96372[1], 96374[1], 96375[1], 96376[1], 96377[1], 96523[0], 99155[0], 99156[0], 99157[0], 99211[1], 99212[1], 99213[1], 99214[1], 99215[1], 99217[1], 99218[1], 99219[1], 99220[1], 99221[1], 99222[1], 99223[1], 99231[1], 99232[1], 99233[1], 99234[1], 99235[1], 99236[1], 99238[1], 99239[1], 99241[1], 99242[1], 99243[1], 99244[1], 99245[1], 99251[1], 99252[1], 99253[1], 99254[1], 99255[1], 99291[1], 99292[1], 99304[1], 99305[1], 99306[1], 99307[1], 99308[1], 99309[1], 99310[1], 99315[1], 99316[1], 99334[1], 99335[1], 99336[1], 99337[1], 99347[1], 99348[1], 99349[1], 99350[1], 99374[1], 99375[1], 99377[1], 99378[1], 99446[0], 99447[0], 99448[0], 99449[0], 99451[0], 99452[0], 99495[1], 99496[1], G0463[1], G0471[1], J0670[1], J2001[1]
55040	0213T[0], 0216T[0], 0596T[1], 0597T[1], 0708T[1], 0709T[1], 11000[1], 11001[1], 11004[1], 11005[1], 11006[1], 11042[1], 11043[1], 11044[1], 11045[1], 11046[1], 11047[1], 12001[1], 12002[1], 12004[1], 12005[1], 12006[1], 12007[1], 12011[1], 12013[1], 12014[1], 12015[1], 12016[1], 12017[1], 12018[1], 12020[1], 12021[1], 12031[1], 12032[1], 12034[1], 12035[1], 12036[1], 12037[1], 12041[1], 12042[1], 12044[1], 12045[1], 12046[1], 12047[1], 12051[1], 12052[1], 12053[1], 12054[1], 12055[1], 12056[1], 12057[1], 13100[1], 13101[1], 13102[1], 13120[1], 13121[1], 13122[1], 13131[1], 13132[1], 13133[1], 13151[1], 13152[1], 13153[1], 36000[1], 36400[1], 36405[1], 36406[1], 36410[1], 36420[1], 36425[1], 36430[1], 36440[1], 36591[0], 36592[0], 36600[1], 36640[1], 43752[1], 51701[1], 51702[1], 51703[1], 54500[1], 54505[1], 54840[1], 55110[0], 62320[0], 62321[0], 62322[0], 62323[0], 62324[0], 62325[0], 62326[0], 62327[0], 64400[0], 64405[0], 64408[0], 64415[0], 64416[0], 64417[0], 64418[0], 64420[0], 64421[0], 64425[0], 64430[0], 64435[0], 64445[0], 64446[0], 64447[0], 64448[0], 64449[0], 64450[0], 64451[0], 64454[0], 64461[0], 64462[0], 64463[0], 64479[0], 64480[0], 64483[0], 64484[0], 64486[0], 64487[0], 64488[0], 64489[0], 64490[0], 64491[0], 64492[0], 64493[0], 64494[0], 64495[0], 64505[0], 64510[0], 64517[0], 64520[0], 64530[0], 69990[0], 92012[1], 92014[1], 93000[1], 93005[1], 93010[1], 93040[1], 93041[1], 93042[1], 93318[1], 93355[1], 94002[1], 94200[1], 94680[1], 94681[1], 94690[1], 95812[1], 95813[1], 95816[1], 95819[1], 95822[1], 95829[1], 95955[1], 96360[1], 96361[1], 96365[1], 96366[1], 96367[1], 96368[1], 96372[1], 96374[1], 96375[1], 96376[1], 96377[1], 96523[0], 97597[1], 97598[1], 97602[1], 99155[0], 99156[0], 99157[0], 99211[1], 99212[1], 99213[1], 99214[1], 99215[1], 99217[1], 99218[1], 99219[1], 99220[1], 99221[1], 99222[1], 99223[1], 99231[1], 99232[1], 99233[1], 99234[1], 99235[1], 99236[1], 99238[1], 99239[1], 99241[1], 99242[1], 99243[1], 99244[1], 99245[1], 99251[1], 99252[1], 99253[1], 99254[1], 99255[1], 99291[1], 99292[1], 99304[1], 99305[1], 99306[1], 99307[1], 99308[1], 99309[1], 99310[1], 99315[1], 99316[1], 99334[1], 99335[1], 99336[1], 99337[1], 99347[1], 99348[1], 99349[1], 99350[1], 99374[1], 99375[1], 99377[1], 99378[1], 99446[0], 99447[0], 99448[0], 99449[0], 99451[0], 99452[0], 99495[0], 99496[0], G0463[1], G0471[1]
55041	0213T[0], 0216T[0], 0596T[1], 0597T[1], 0708T[1], 0709T[1], 11000[1], 11001[1], 11004[1], 11005[1], 11006[1], 11042[1], 11043[1], 11044[1], 11045[1], 11046[1], 11047[1], 12001[1], 12002[1], 12004[1], 12005[1], 12006[1], 12007[1], 12011[1], 12013[1], 12014[1], 12015[1], 12016[1], 12017[1], 12018[1], 12020[1], 12021[1], 12031[1], 12032[1], 12034[1], 12035[1], 12036[1], 12037[1], 12041[1], 12042[1], 12044[1], 12045[1], 12046[1], 12047[1], 12051[1], 12052[1], 12053[1], 12054[1], 12055[1], 12056[1], 12057[1], 13100[1], 13101[1], 13102[1], 13120[1], 13121[1], 13122[1], 13131[1], 13132[1], 13133[1], 13151[1], 13152[1], 13153[1], 36000[1], 36400[1], 36405[1], 36406[1], 36410[1], 36420[1], 36425[1], 36430[1], 36440[1], 36591[0], 36592[0], 36600[1], 36640[1], 43752[1], 51701[1], 51702[1], 51703[1], 54500[0], 54505[0], 55040[1], 55110[0], 62320[0], 62321[0], 62322[0], 62323[0], 62324[0], 62325[0], 62326[0], 62327[0], 64400[0], 64405[0], 64408[0], 64415[0], 64416[0], 64417[0], 64418[0], 64420[0], 64421[0], 64425[0], 64430[0], 64435[0], 64445[0], 64446[0], 64447[0], 64448[0], 64449[0], 64450[0], 64451[0], 64454[0], 64461[0], 64462[0], 64463[0], 64479[0], 64480[0], 64483[0], 64484[0], 64486[0], 64487[0], 64488[0], 64489[0], 64490[0], 64491[0], 64492[0], 64493[0], 64494[0], 64495[0], 64505[0], 64510[0], 64517[0], 64520[0], 64530[0], 69990[0], 92012[1], 92014[1], 93000[1], 93005[1], 93010[1], 93040[1], 93041[1], 93042[1], 93318[1], 93355[1], 94002[1], 94200[1], 94680[1], 94681[1], 94690[1], 95812[1], 95813[1], 95816[1], 95819[1], 95822[1], 95829[1], 95955[1], 96360[1], 96361[1], 96365[1], 96366[1], 96367[1], 96368[1], 96372[1], 96374[1], 96375[1], 96376[1], 96377[1], 96523[0], 97597[1], 97598[1], 97602[1], 99155[0], 99156[0], 99157[0], 99211[1], 99212[1], 99213[1], 99214[1], 99215[1], 99217[1], 99218[1], 99219[1], 99220[1], 99221[1], 99222[1], 99223[1], 99231[1], 99232[1], 99233[1], 99234[1], 99235[1], 99236[1], 99238[1], 99239[1], 99241[1], 99242[1], 99243[1], 99244[1], 99245[1], 99251[1], 99252[1], 99253[1], 99254[1], 99255[1], 99291[1], 99292[1], 99304[1], 99305[1], 99306[1], 99307[1], 99308[1], 99309[1], 99310[1], 99315[1], 99316[1], 99334[1], 99335[1], 99336[1], 99337[1], 99347[1], 99348[1], 99349[1], 99350[1], 99374[1], 99375[1], 99377[1], 99378[1], 99446[0], 99447[0], 99448[0], 99449[0], 99451[0], 99452[0], 99495[0], 99496[0], G0463[1], G0471[1]
55060	0213T[0], 0216T[0], 0596T[1], 0597T[1], 0708T[1], 0709T[1], 12001[1], 12002[1], 12004[1], 12005[1], 12006[1], 12007[1], 12011[1], 12013[1], 12014[1], 12015[1], 12016[1], 12017[1], 12018[1], 12020[1], 12021[1], 12031[1], 12032[1], 12034[1], 12035[1], 12036[1], 12037[1], 12041[1], 12042[1], 12044[1], 12045[1], 12046[1], 12047[1], 12051[1], 12052[1], 12053[1], 12054[1], 12055[1], 12056[1], 12057[1], 13100[1], 13101[1], 13102[1], 13120[1], 13121[1], 13122[1], 13131[1], 13132[1], 13133[1], 13151[1], 13152[1], 13153[1], 36000[1], 36400[1], 36405[1], 36406[1], 36410[1], 36420[1], 36425[1], 36430[1], 36440[1], 36591[0], 36592[0], 36600[1], 36640[1], 43752[1], 49010[0], 51701[1], 51702[1], 51703[1], 55110[0], 62320[0], 62321[0], 62322[0], 62323[0], 62324[0], 62325[0], 62326[0], 62327[0], 64400[0], 64405[0], 64408[0], 64415[0], 64416[0], 64417[0], 64418[0], 64420[0], 64421[0], 64425[0], 64430[0], 64435[0], 64445[0], 64446[0], 64447[0], 64448[0], 64449[0], 64450[0], 64451[0], 64454[0], 64461[0], 64462[0], 64463[0], 64479[0], 64480[0], 64483[0], 64484[0], 64486[0], 64487[0], 64488[0], 64489[0], 64490[0], 64491[0], 64492[0], 64493[0], 64494[0], 64495[0], 64505[0], 64510[0], 64517[0], 64520[0], 64530[0], 69990[0], 92012[1], 92014[1], 93000[1], 93005[1], 93010[1], 93040[1], 93041[1], 93042[1], 93318[1], 93355[1], 94002[1], 94200[1], 94680[1], 94681[1], 94690[1], 95812[1], 95813[1], 95816[1], 95819[1], 95822[1], 95829[1], 95955[1], 96360[1], 96361[1], 96365[1], 96366[1], 96367[1], 96368[1], 96372[1], 96374[1], 96375[1], 96376[1], 96377[1], 96523[0], 99155[0], 99156[0], 99157[0], 99211[1], 99212[1], 99213[1], 99214[1], 99215[1], 99217[1], 99218[1], 99219[1], 99220[1], 99221[1], 99222[1], 99223[1], 99231[1], 99232[1], 99233[1], 99234[1], 99235[1], 99236[1], 99238[1], 99239[1], 99241[1], 99242[1], 99243[1], 99244[1], 99245[1], 99251[1], 99252[1], 99253[1], 99254[1], 99255[1], 99291[1], 99292[1], 99304[1], 99305[1], 99306[1], 99307[1], 99308[1], 99309[1], 99310[1], 99315[1], 99316[1], 99334[1], 99335[1], 99336[1], 99337[1], 99347[1], 99348[1], 99349[1], 99350[1], 99374[1], 99375[1], 99377[1], 99378[1], 99446[0], 99447[0], 99448[0], 99449[0], 99451[0], 99452[0], 99495[0], 99496[0], G0463[1], G0471[1]
55100	0213T[0], 0216T[0], 0596T[1], 0597T[1], 0708T[1], 0709T[1], 12001[1], 12002[1], 12004[1], 12005[1], 12006[1], 12007[1], 12011[1], 12013[1], 12014[1], 12015[1], 12016[1], 12017[1], 12018[1], 12020[1], 12021[1], 12031[1], 12032[1], 12034[1], 12035[1], 12036[1], 12037[1], 12041[1], 12042[1], 12044[1], 12045[1], 12046[1], 12047[1], 12051[1], 12052[1], 12053[1], 12054[1], 12055[1], 12056[1], 12057[1], 13100[1], 13101[1], 13102[1], 13120[1], 13121[1], 13122[1], 13131[1], 13132[1], 13133[1], 13151[1], 13152[1], 13153[1], 36000[1], 36400[1], 36405[1], 36406[1], 36410[1], 36420[1], 36425[1], 36430[1], 36440[1], 36591[0], 36592[0], 36600[1], 36640[1], 43752[1], 51701[1], 51702[1], 51703[1], 54500[0], 54505[0], 55110[0], 62320[0], 62321[0], 62322[0], 62323[0], 62324[0], 62325[0], 62326[0], 62327[0], 64400[0], 64405[0], 64408[0], 64415[0], 64416[0], 64417[0], 64418[0], 64420[0], 64421[0], 64425[0],

0 = Modifier usage not allowed or inappropriate 1 = Modifier usage allowed

Code 1	Code 2
	64430[0], 64435[0], 64445[0], 64446[0], 64447[0], 64448[0], 64449[0], 64450[0], 64451[0], 64454[0], 64461[0], 64462[0], 64463[0], 64479[0], 64480[0], 64483[0], 64484[0], 64486[0], 64487[0], 64488[0], 64489[0], 64490[0], 64491[0], 64492[0], 64493[0], 64494[0], 64495[0], 64505[0], 64510[0], 64517[0], 64520[0], 64530[0], 69990[0], 92012[1], 92014[1], 93000[1], 93005[1], 93010[1], 93040[1], 93041[1], 93042[1], 93318[1], 93355[1], 94002[1], 94200[1], 94680[1], 94681[1], 94690[1], 95812[1], 95813[1], 95816[1], 95819[1], 95822[1], 95829[1], 95955[1], 96360[1], 96361[1], 96365[1], 96366[1], 96367[1], 96368[1], 96372[1], 96374[1], 96375[1], 96376[1], 96377[1], 96523[0], 99155[0], 99156[0], 99157[0], 99211[1], 99212[1], 99213[1], 99214[1], 99215[1], 99217[1], 99218[1], 99219[1], 99220[1], 99221[1], 99222[1], 99223[1], 99231[1], 99232[1], 99233[1], 99234[1], 99235[1], 99236[1], 99238[1], 99239[1], 99241[1], 99242[1], 99243[1], 99244[1], 99245[1], 99251[1], 99252[1], 99253[1], 99254[1], 99255[1], 99291[1], 99292[1], 99304[1], 99305[1], 99306[1], 99307[1], 99308[1], 99309[1], 99310[1], 99315[1], 99316[1], 99334[1], 99335[1], 99336[1], 99337[1], 99347[1], 99348[1], 99349[1], 99350[1], 99374[1], 99375[1], 99377[1], 99378[1], 99446[0], 99447[0], 99448[0], 99449[0], 99451[0], 99452[0], 99495[0], 99496[0], G0463[1], G0471[1], J0670[1], J2001[1]
55110	0213T[0], 0216T[0], 0596T[1], 0597T[1], 0708T[1], 0709T[1], 12001[1], 12002[1], 12004[1], 12005[1], 12006[1], 12007[1], 12011[1], 12013[1], 12014[1], 12015[1], 12016[1], 12017[1], 12018[1], 12020[1], 12021[1], 12031[1], 12032[1], 12034[1], 12035[1], 12036[1], 12037[1], 12041[1], 12042[1], 12044[1], 12045[1], 12046[1], 12047[1], 12051[1], 12052[1], 12053[1], 12054[1], 12055[1], 12056[1], 12057[1], 13100[1], 13101[1], 13102[1], 13120[1], 13121[1], 13122[1], 13131[1], 13132[1], 13133[1], 13151[1], 13152[1], 13153[1], 36000[1], 36400[1], 36405[1], 36406[1], 36410[1], 36420[1], 36425[1], 36430[1], 36440[1], 36591[0], 36592[0], 36600[1], 36640[1], 43752[1], 51701[1], 51702[1], 51703[1], 54500[0], 54505[0], 62320[0], 62321[0], 62322[0], 62323[0], 62324[0], 62325[0], 62326[0], 62327[0], 64400[0], 64405[0], 64408[0], 64415[0], 64416[0], 64417[0], 64418[0], 64420[0], 64421[0], 64425[0], 64430[0], 64435[0], 64445[0], 64446[0], 64447[0], 64448[0], 64449[0], 64450[0], 64451[0], 64454[0], 64461[0], 64462[0], 64463[0], 64479[0], 64480[0], 64483[0], 64484[0], 64486[0], 64487[0], 64488[0], 64489[0], 64490[0], 64491[0], 64492[0], 64493[0], 64494[0], 64495[0], 64505[0], 64510[0], 64517[0], 64520[0], 64530[0], 69990[0], 92012[1], 92014[1], 93000[1], 93005[1], 93010[1], 93040[1], 93041[1], 93042[1], 93318[1], 93355[1], 94002[1], 94200[1], 94680[1], 94681[1], 94690[1], 95812[1], 95813[1], 95816[1], 95819[1], 95822[1], 95829[1], 95955[1], 96360[1], 96361[1], 96365[1], 96366[1], 96367[1], 96368[1], 96372[1], 96374[1], 96375[1], 96376[1], 96377[1], 96523[0], 99155[0], 99156[0], 99157[0], 99211[1], 99212[1], 99213[1], 99214[1], 99215[1], 99217[1], 99218[1], 99219[1], 99220[1], 99221[1], 99222[1], 99223[1], 99231[1], 99232[1], 99233[1], 99234[1], 99235[1], 99236[1], 99238[1], 99239[1], 99241[1], 99242[1], 99243[1], 99244[1], 99245[1], 99251[1], 99252[1], 99253[1], 99254[1], 99255[1], 99291[1], 99292[1], 99304[1], 99305[1], 99306[1], 99307[1], 99308[1], 99309[1], 99310[1], 99315[1], 99316[1], 99334[1], 99335[1], 99336[1], 99337[1], 99347[1], 99348[1], 99349[1], 99350[1], 99374[1], 99375[1], 99377[1], 99378[1], 99446[0], 99447[0], 99448[0], 99449[0], 99451[0], 99452[0], 99495[0], 99496[0], G0463[1], G0471[1]
55120	0213T[0], 0216T[0], 0596T[1], 0597T[1], 0708T[1], 0709T[1], 11000[1], 11001[1], 11004[1], 11005[1], 11006[1], 11042[1], 11043[1], 11044[1], 11045[1], 11046[1], 11047[1], 12001[1], 12002[1], 12004[1], 12005[1], 12006[1], 12007[1], 12011[1], 12013[1], 12014[1], 12015[1], 12016[1], 12017[1], 12018[1], 12020[1], 12021[1], 12031[1], 12032[1], 12034[1], 12035[1], 12036[1], 12037[1], 12041[1], 12042[1], 12044[1], 12045[1], 12046[1], 12047[1], 12051[1], 12052[1], 12053[1], 12054[1], 12055[1], 12056[1], 12057[1], 13100[1], 13101[1], 13102[1], 13120[1], 13121[1], 13122[1], 13131[1], 13132[1], 13133[1], 13151[1], 13152[1], 13153[1], 36000[1], 36400[1], 36405[1], 36406[1], 36410[1], 36420[1], 36425[1], 36430[1], 36440[1], 36591[0], 36592[0], 36600[1], 36640[1], 43752[1], 51701[1], 51702[1], 51703[1], 54500[0], 54505[0], 55100[1], 55110[1], 62320[0], 62321[0], 62322[0], 62323[0], 62324[0], 62325[0], 62326[0], 62327[0], 64400[0], 64405[0], 64408[0], 64415[0], 64416[0], 64417[0], 64418[0], 64420[0], 64421[0], 64425[0], 64430[0], 64435[0], 64445[0], 64446[0], 64447[0], 64448[0], 64449[0], 64450[0], 64451[0], 64454[0], 64461[0], 64462[0], 64463[0], 64479[0], 64480[0], 64483[0], 64484[0], 64486[0], 64487[0], 64488[0], 64489[0], 64490[0], 64491[0], 64492[0], 64493[0], 64494[0], 64495[0], 64505[0], 64510[0], 64517[0], 64520[0], 64530[0], 69990[0], 92012[1], 92014[1], 93000[1], 93005[1], 93010[1], 93040[1], 93041[1], 93042[1], 93318[1], 93355[1], 94002[1], 94200[1], 94680[1], 94681[1], 94690[1], 95812[1], 95813[1], 95816[1], 95819[1], 95822[1], 95829[1], 95955[1], 96360[1], 96361[1], 96365[1], 96366[1], 96367[1], 96368[1], 96372[1], 96374[1], 96375[1], 96376[1], 96377[1], 96523[0], 97597[1], 97598[1], 97602[1], 99155[0], 99156[0], 99157[0], 99211[1], 99212[1], 99213[1], 99214[1], 99215[1], 99217[1], 99218[1], 99219[1], 99220[1], 99221[1], 99222[1], 99223[1], 99231[1], 99232[1], 99233[1], 99234[1], 99235[1], 99236[1], 99238[1], 99239[1], 99241[1], 99242[1], 99243[1], 99244[1], 99245[1], 99251[1], 99252[1], 99253[1], 99254[1], 99255[1], 99291[1], 99292[1], 99304[1], 99305[1], 99306[1], 99307[1], 99308[1], 99309[1], 99310[1], 99315[1], 99316[1], 99334[1], 99335[1], 99336[1], 99337[1], 99347[1], 99348[1], 99349[1], 99350[1], 99374[1], 99375[1], 99377[1], 99378[1], 99446[0], 99447[0], 99448[0], 99449[0], 99451[0], 99452[0], 99495[0], 99496[0], G0463[1], G0471[1], J2001[1]
55150	0213T[0], 0216T[0], 0596T[1], 0597T[1], 0708T[1], 0709T[1], 11000[1], 11001[1], 11004[1], 11005[1], 11006[1], 11042[1], 11043[1], 11044[1], 11045[1], 11046[1], 11047[1], 12001[1], 12002[1], 12004[1], 12005[1], 12006[1], 12007[1], 12011[1], 12013[1], 12014[1], 12015[1], 12016[1], 12017[1], 12018[1], 12020[1], 12021[1], 12031[1], 12032[1], 12034[1], 12035[1], 12036[1], 12037[1], 12041[1], 12042[1], 12044[1], 12045[1], 12046[1], 12047[1], 12051[1], 12052[1], 12053[1], 12054[1], 12055[1], 12056[1], 12057[1], 13100[1], 13101[1], 13102[1], 13120[1], 13121[1], 13122[1], 13131[1], 13132[1], 13133[1], 13151[1], 13152[1], 13153[1], 36000[1], 36400[1], 36405[1], 36406[1], 36410[1], 36420[1], 36425[1], 36430[1], 36440[1], 36591[0], 36592[0], 36600[1], 36640[1], 43752[1], 51701[1], 51702[1], 51703[1], 54500[0], 54505[0], 55110[0], 55180[1], 62320[0], 62321[0], 62322[0], 62323[0], 62324[0], 62325[0], 62326[0], 62327[0], 64400[0], 64405[0], 64408[0], 64415[0], 64416[0], 64417[0], 64418[0], 64420[0], 64421[0], 64425[0], 64430[0], 64435[0], 64445[0], 64446[0], 64447[0], 64448[0], 64449[0], 64450[0], 64451[0], 64454[0], 64461[0], 64462[0], 64463[0], 64479[0], 64480[0], 64483[0], 64484[0], 64486[0], 64487[0], 64488[0], 64489[0], 64490[0], 64491[0], 64492[0], 64493[0], 64494[0], 64495[0], 64505[0], 64510[0], 64517[0], 64520[0], 64530[0], 69990[0], 92012[1], 92014[1], 93000[1], 93005[1], 93010[1], 93040[1], 93041[1], 93042[1], 93318[1], 93355[1], 94002[1], 94200[1], 94680[1], 94681[1], 94690[1], 95812[1], 95813[1], 95816[1], 95819[1], 95822[1], 95829[1], 95955[1], 96360[1], 96361[1], 96365[1], 96366[1], 96367[1], 96368[1], 96372[1], 96374[1], 96375[1], 96376[1], 96377[1], 96523[0], 97597[1], 97598[1], 97602[1], 99155[0], 99156[0], 99157[0], 99211[1], 99212[1], 99213[1], 99214[1], 99215[1], 99217[1], 99218[1], 99219[1], 99220[1], 99221[1], 99222[1], 99223[1], 99231[1], 99232[1], 99233[1], 99234[1], 99235[1], 99236[1], 99238[1], 99239[1], 99241[1], 99242[1], 99243[1], 99244[1], 99245[1], 99251[1], 99252[1], 99253[1], 99254[1], 99255[1], 99291[1], 99292[1], 99304[1], 99305[1], 99306[1], 99307[1], 99308[1], 99309[1], 99310[1], 99315[1], 99316[1], 99334[1], 99335[1], 99336[1], 99337[1], 99347[1], 99348[1], 99349[1], 99350[1], 99374[1], 99375[1], 99377[1], 99378[1], 99446[0], 99447[0], 99448[0], 99449[0], 99451[0], 99452[0], 99495[0], 99496[0], G0463[1], G0471[1]
55175	0213T[0], 0216T[0], 0596T[1], 0597T[1], 0708T[1], 0709T[1], 11000[1], 11001[1], 11004[1], 11005[1], 11006[1], 11042[1], 11043[1], 11044[1], 11045[1], 11046[1], 11047[1], 12001[1], 12002[1], 12004[1], 12005[1], 12006[1], 12007[1], 12011[1], 12013[1], 12014[1], 12015[1], 12016[1], 12017[1], 12018[1], 12020[1], 12021[1], 12031[1], 12032[1], 12034[1], 12035[1], 12036[1], 12037[1], 12041[1], 12042[1], 12044[1], 12045[1], 12046[1], 12047[1], 12051[1], 12052[1], 12053[1], 12054[1], 12055[1], 12056[1], 12057[1], 13100[1], 13101[1], 13102[1], 13120[1], 13121[1], 13122[1], 13131[1], 13132[1], 13133[1], 13151[1], 13152[1], 13153[1], 36000[1], 36400[1], 36405[1], 36406[1], 36410[1], 36420[1], 36425[1], 36430[1], 36440[1], 36591[0], 36592[0], 36600[1], 36640[1], 43752[1], 51701[1], 51702[1], 51703[1], 55110[0], 55150[1], 62320[0], 62321[0], 62322[0], 62323[0], 62324[0], 62325[0], 62326[0], 62327[0], 64400[0], 64405[0], 64408[0], 64415[0], 64416[0], 64417[0], 64418[0], 64420[0], 64421[0], 64425[0], 64430[0], 64435[0], 64445[0], 64446[0], 64447[0], 64448[0], 64449[0], 64450[0], 64451[0], 64454[0], 64461[0], 64462[0], 64463[0], 64479[0], 64480[0], 64483[0], 64484[0], 64486[0], 64487[0], 64488[0], 64489[0], 64490[0], 64491[0], 64492[0], 64493[0], 64494[0], 64495[0], 64505[0], 64510[0], 64517[0], 64520[0], 64530[0], 69990[0], 92012[1], 92014[1], 93000[1], 93005[1], 93010[1], 93040[1], 93041[1], 93042[1], 93318[1], 93355[1], 94002[1], 94200[1], 94680[1], 94681[1], 94690[1], 95812[1], 95813[1], 95816[1], 95819[1], 95822[1], 95829[1], 95955[1], 96360[1], 96361[1], 96365[1], 96366[1], 96367[1], 96368[1], 96372[1], 96374[1], 96375[1], 96376[1], 96377[1], 96523[0], 97597[1], 97598[1], 97602[1], 99155[0], 99156[0], 99157[0], 99211[1], 99212[1], 99213[1], 99214[1], 99215[1], 99217[1], 99218[1], 99219[1], 99220[1], 99221[1], 99222[1], 99223[1], 99231[1], 99232[1], 99233[1], 99234[1], 99235[1], 99236[1], 99238[1], 99239[1], 99241[1], 99242[1], 99243[1], 99244[1], 99245[1], 99251[1], 99252[1], 99253[1], 99254[1], 99255[1], 99291[1], 99292[1], 99304[1], 99305[1], 99306[1], 99307[1], 99308[1], 99309[1], 99310[1], 99315[1], 99316[1], 99334[1], 99335[1], 99336[1], 99337[1], 99347[1], 99348[1], 99349[1], 99350[1], 99374[1], 99375[1], 99377[1], 99378[1], 99446[0], 99447[0], 99448[0], 99449[0], 99451[0], 99452[0], 99495[0], 99496[0], G0463[1], G0471[1]
55180	0213T[0], 0216T[0], 0596T[1], 0597T[1], 0708T[1], 0709T[1], 11000[1], 11001[1], 11004[1], 11005[1], 11006[1], 11042[1], 11043[1], 11044[1], 11045[1], 11046[1], 11047[1], 12001[1], 12002[1], 12004[1], 12005[1], 12006[1], 12007[1], 12011[1], 12013[1], 12014[1], 12015[1], 12016[1], 12017[1], 12018[1], 12020[1], 12021[1], 12031[1], 12032[1], 12034[1], 12035[1], 12036[1], 12037[1], 12041[1], 12042[1], 12044[1], 12045[1], 12046[1], 12047[1], 12051[1], 12052[1], 12053[1], 12054[1], 12055[1], 12056[1], 12057[1], 13100[1], 13101[1], 13102[1], 13120[1], 13121[1], 13122[1], 13131[1], 13132[1], 13133[1], 13151[1], 13152[1], 13153[1], 36000[1], 36400[1], 36405[1], 36406[1], 36410[1], 36420[1], 36425[1], 36430[1], 36440[1], 36591[0], 36592[0], 36600[1], 36640[1], 43752[1], 51701[1], 51702[1], 51703[1], 55110[0], 55175[1], 62320[0], 62321[0], 62322[0], 62323[0], 62324[0], 62325[0], 62326[0], 62327[0], 64400[0], 64405[0], 64408[0], 64415[0], 64416[0], 64417[0], 64418[0], 64420[0], 64421[0], 64425[0], 64430[0], 64435[0], 64445[0], 64446[0], 64447[0], 64448[0], 64449[0], 64450[0], 64451[0], 64454[0], 64461[0], 64462[0], 64463[0], 64479[0], 64480[0], 64483[0], 64484[0], 64486[0], 64487[0], 64488[0], 64489[0], 64490[0], 64491[0], 64492[0], 64493[0], 64494[0], 64495[0], 64505[0], 64510[0], 64517[0], 64520[0], 64530[0], 69990[0], 92012[1], 92014[1], 93000[1], 93005[1], 93010[1], 93040[1], 93041[1], 93042[1], 93318[1], 93355[1], 94002[1], 94200[1], 94680[1], 94681[1], 94690[1], 95812[1], 95813[1], 95816[1], 95819[1], 95822[1], 95829[1], 95955[1], 96360[1], 96361[1], 96365[1], 96366[1], 96367[1], 96368[1], 96372[1], 96374[1], 96375[1], 96376[1], 96377[1], 96523[0], 97597[1], 97598[1], 97602[1], 99155[0], 99156[0], 99157[0], 99211[1], 99212[1], 99213[1], 99214[1], 99215[1], 99217[1], 99218[1], 99219[1], 99220[1], 99221[1], 99222[1], 99223[1], 99231[1], 99232[1], 99233[1], 99234[1], 99235[1], 99236[1], 99238[1], 99239[1], 99241[1], 99242[1], 99243[1], 99244[1], 99245[1], 99251[1], 99252[1], 99253[1], 99254[1], 99255[1], 99291[1], 99292[1], 99304[1], 99305[1], 99306[1], 99307[1], 99308[1], 99309[1], 99310[1], 99315[1], 99316[1], 99334[1], 99335[1], 99336[1], 99337[1], 99347[1], 99348[1],

0 = Modifier usage not allowed or inappropriate 1 = Modifier usage allowed

Appendix A: NCCI - CPT Codes

Code 1	Code 2
	99349[1], 99350[1], 99374[1], 99375[1], 99377[1], 99378[1], 99446[0], 99447[0], 99448[0], 99449[0], 99451[0], 99452[0], 99495[0], 99496[0], G0463[1], G0471[1]
55200	00921[0], 0213T[0], 0216T[0], 0596T[1], 0597T[1], 0708T[1], 0709T[1], 11000[1], 11001[1], 11004[1], 11005[1], 11006[1], 11042[1], 11043[1], 11044[1], 11045[1], 11046[1], 11047[1], 12001[1], 12002[1], 12004[1], 12005[1], 12006[1], 12007[1], 12011[1], 12013[1], 12014[1], 12015[1], 12016[1], 12017[1], 12018[1], 12020[1], 12021[1], 12031[1], 12032[1], 12034[1], 12035[1], 12036[1], 12037[1], 12041[1], 12042[1], 12044[1], 12045[1], 12046[1], 12047[1], 12051[1], 12052[1], 12053[1], 12054[1], 12055[1], 12056[1], 12057[1], 13100[1], 13101[1], 13102[1], 13120[1], 13121[1], 13122[1], 13131[1], 13132[1], 13133[1], 13151[1], 13152[1], 13153[1], 36000[1], 36400[1], 36405[1], 36406[1], 36410[1], 36420[1], 36425[1], 36430[1], 36440[1], 36591[0], 36592[0], 36600[1], 36640[1], 43752[1], 51701[1], 51702[1], 51703[1], 62320[0], 62321[0], 62322[0], 62323[0], 62324[0], 62325[0], 62326[0], 62327[0], 64400[0], 64405[0], 64408[0], 64415[0], 64416[0], 64417[0], 64418[0], 64420[0], 64421[0], 64425[0], 64430[0], 64435[0], 64445[0], 64446[0], 64447[0], 64448[0], 64449[0], 64450[0], 64451[0], 64454[0], 64461[0], 64462[0], 64463[0], 64479[0], 64480[0], 64483[0], 64484[0], 64486[0], 64487[0], 64488[0], 64489[0], 64490[0], 64491[0], 64492[0], 64493[0], 64494[0], 64495[0], 64505[0], 64510[0], 64517[0], 64520[0], 64530[0], 69990[0], 92012[1], 92014[1], 93000[1], 93005[1], 93010[1], 93040[1], 93041[1], 93042[1], 93318[1], 93355[1], 94002[1], 94200[1], 94680[1], 94681[1], 94690[1], 95812[1], 95813[1], 95816[1], 95819[1], 95822[1], 95829[1], 95955[1], 96360[1], 96361[1], 96365[1], 96366[1], 96367[1], 96368[1], 96372[1], 96374[1], 96375[1], 96376[1], 96377[1], 96523[0], 97597[1], 97598[1], 97602[1], 99155[0], 99156[0], 99157[0], 99211[1], 99212[1], 99213[1], 99214[1], 99215[1], 99217[1], 99218[1], 99219[1], 99220[1], 99221[1], 99222[1], 99223[1], 99231[1], 99232[1], 99233[1], 99234[1], 99235[1], 99236[1], 99238[1], 99239[1], 99241[1], 99242[1], 99243[1], 99244[1], 99245[1], 99251[1], 99252[1], 99253[1], 99254[1], 99255[1], 99291[1], 99292[1], 99304[1], 99305[1], 99306[1], 99307[1], 99308[1], 99309[1], 99310[1], 99315[1], 99316[1], 99334[1], 99335[1], 99336[1], 99337[1], 99347[1], 99348[1], 99349[1], 99350[1], 99374[1], 99375[1], 99377[1], 99378[1], 99446[0], 99447[0], 99448[0], 99449[0], 99451[0], 99452[0], 99495[0], 99496[0], G0463[1], G0471[1], J0670[1], J2001[1]
55250	00921[0], 0213T[0], 0216T[0], 0596T[1], 0597T[1], 0708T[1], 0709T[1], 11000[1], 11001[1], 11004[1], 11005[1], 11006[1], 11042[1], 11043[1], 11044[1], 11045[1], 11046[1], 11047[1], 12001[1], 12002[1], 12004[1], 12005[1], 12006[1], 12007[1], 12011[1], 12013[1], 12014[1], 12015[1], 12016[1], 12017[1], 12018[1], 12020[1], 12021[1], 12031[1], 12032[1], 12034[1], 12035[1], 12036[1], 12037[1], 12041[1], 12042[1], 12044[1], 12045[1], 12046[1], 12047[1], 12051[1], 12052[1], 12053[1], 12054[1], 12055[1], 12056[1], 12057[1], 13100[1], 13101[1], 13102[1], 13120[1], 13121[1], 13122[1], 13131[1], 13132[1], 13133[1], 13151[1], 13152[1], 13153[1], 36000[1], 36400[1], 36405[1], 36406[1], 36410[1], 36420[1], 36425[1], 36430[1], 36440[1], 36591[0], 36592[0], 36600[1], 36640[1], 43752[1], 51701[1], 51702[1], 51703[1], 54500[0], 54505[0], 55200[1], 62320[0], 62321[0], 62322[0], 62323[0], 62324[0], 62325[0], 62326[0], 62327[0], 64400[0], 64405[0], 64408[0], 64415[0], 64416[0], 64417[0], 64418[0], 64420[0], 64421[0], 64425[0], 64430[0], 64435[0], 64445[0], 64446[0], 64447[0], 64448[0], 64449[0], 64450[0], 64451[0], 64454[0], 64461[0], 64462[0], 64463[0], 64479[0], 64480[0], 64483[0], 64484[0], 64486[0], 64487[0], 64488[0], 64489[0], 64490[0], 64491[0], 64492[0], 64493[0], 64494[0], 64495[0], 64505[0], 64510[0], 64517[0], 64520[0], 64530[0], 69990[0], 92012[1], 92014[1], 93000[1], 93005[1], 93010[1], 93040[1], 93041[1], 93042[1], 93318[1], 93355[1], 94002[1], 94200[1], 94680[1], 94681[1], 94690[1], 95812[1], 95813[1], 95816[1], 95819[1], 95822[1], 95829[1], 95955[1], 96360[1], 96361[1], 96365[1], 96366[1], 96367[1], 96368[1], 96372[1], 96374[1], 96375[1], 96376[1], 96377[1], 96523[0], 97597[1], 97598[1], 97602[1], 99155[0], 99156[0], 99157[0], 99211[1], 99212[1], 99213[1], 99214[1], 99215[1], 99217[1], 99218[1], 99219[1], 99220[1], 99221[1], 99222[1], 99223[1], 99231[1], 99232[1], 99233[1], 99234[1], 99235[1], 99236[1], 99238[1], 99239[1], 99241[1], 99242[1], 99243[1], 99244[1], 99245[1], 99251[1], 99252[1], 99253[1], 99254[1], 99255[1], 99291[1], 99292[1], 99304[1], 99305[1], 99306[1], 99307[1], 99308[1], 99309[1], 99310[1], 99315[1], 99316[1], 99334[1], 99335[1], 99336[1], 99337[1], 99347[1], 99348[1], 99349[1], 99350[1], 99374[1], 99375[1], 99377[1], 99378[1], 99446[0], 99447[0], 99448[0], 99449[0], 99451[0], 99452[0], 99495[0], 99496[0], G0463[1], G0471[1], J0670[1], J2001[1]
55300	0213T[0], 0216T[0], 0596T[1], 0597T[1], 0708T[1], 0709T[1], 11000[1], 11001[1], 11004[1], 11005[1], 11006[1], 11042[1], 11043[1], 11044[1], 11045[1], 11046[1], 11047[1], 12001[1], 12002[1], 12004[1], 12005[1], 12006[1], 12007[1], 12011[1], 12013[1], 12014[1], 12015[1], 12016[1], 12017[1], 12018[1], 12020[1], 12021[1], 12031[1], 12032[1], 12034[1], 12035[1], 12036[1], 12037[1], 12041[1], 12042[1], 12044[1], 12045[1], 12046[1], 12047[1], 12051[1], 12052[1], 12053[1], 12054[1], 12055[1], 12056[1], 12057[1], 13100[1], 13101[1], 13102[1], 13120[1], 13121[1], 13122[1], 13131[1], 13132[1], 13133[1], 13151[1], 13152[1], 13153[1], 36000[1], 36400[1], 36405[1], 36406[1], 36410[1], 36420[1], 36425[1], 36430[1], 36440[1], 36591[0], 36592[0], 36600[1], 36640[1], 43752[1], 51701[1], 51702[1], 51703[1], 55200[0], 55250[1], 62320[0], 62321[0], 62322[0], 62323[0], 62324[0], 62325[0], 62326[0], 62327[0], 64400[0], 64405[0], 64408[0], 64415[0], 64416[0], 64417[0], 64418[0], 64420[0], 64421[0], 64425[0], 64430[0], 64435[0], 64445[0], 64446[0], 64447[0], 64448[0], 64449[0], 64450[0], 64451[0], 64454[0], 64461[0], 64462[0], 64463[0], 64479[0], 64480[0], 64483[0], 64484[0], 64486[0], 64487[0], 64488[0], 64489[0], 64490[0], 64491[0], 64492[0], 64493[0], 64494[0], 64495[0], 64505[0], 64510[0], 64517[0], 64520[0], 64530[0], 69990[0], 76000[1], 76942[1], 76998[1], 77001[1], 77002[1], 92012[1], 92014[1], 93000[1], 93005[1], 93010[1], 93040[1], 93041[1], 93042[1], 93318[1], 93355[1], 94002[1], 94200[1], 94680[1], 94681[1], 94690[1], 95812[1], 95813[1], 95816[1], 95819[1], 95822[1], 95829[1], 95955[1], 96360[1], 96361[1], 96365[1], 96366[1], 96367[1], 96368[1], 96372[1], 96374[1], 96375[1], 96376[1], 96377[1], 96523[0], 97597[1], 97598[1], 97602[1], 99155[0], 99156[0], 99157[0], 99211[1], 99212[1], 99213[1], 99214[1], 99215[1], 99217[1], 99218[1], 99219[1], 99220[1], 99221[1], 99222[1], 99223[1], 99231[1], 99232[1], 99233[1], 99234[1], 99235[1], 99236[1], 99238[1], 99239[1], 99241[1], 99242[1], 99243[1], 99244[1], 99245[1], 99251[1], 99252[1], 99253[1], 99254[1], 99255[1], 99291[1], 99292[1], 99304[1], 99305[1], 99306[1], 99307[1], 99308[1], 99309[1], 99310[1], 99315[1], 99316[1], 99334[1], 99335[1], 99336[1], 99337[1], 99347[1], 99348[1], 99349[1], 99350[1], 99374[1], 99375[1], 99377[1], 99378[1], 99446[0], 99447[0], 99448[0], 99449[0], 99451[0], 99452[0], 99495[1], 99496[1], G0463[1], G0471[1]
55400	0213T[0], 0216T[0], 0596T[1], 0597T[1], 0708T[1], 0709T[1], 12001[1], 12002[1], 12004[1], 12005[1], 12006[1], 12007[1], 12011[1], 12013[1], 12014[1], 12015[1], 12016[1], 12017[1], 12018[1], 12020[1], 12021[1], 12031[1], 12032[1], 12034[1], 12035[1], 12036[1], 12037[1], 12041[1], 12042[1], 12044[1], 12045[1], 12046[1], 12047[1], 12051[1], 12052[1], 12053[1], 12054[1], 12055[1], 12056[1], 12057[1], 13100[1], 13101[1], 13102[1], 13120[1], 13121[1], 13122[1], 13131[1], 13132[1], 13133[1], 13151[1], 13152[1], 13153[1], 36000[1], 36400[1], 36405[1], 36406[1], 36410[1], 36420[1], 36425[1], 36430[1], 36440[1], 36591[0], 36592[0], 36600[1], 36640[1], 43752[1], 51701[1], 51702[1], 51703[1], 55200[1], 55250[1], 62320[0], 62321[0], 62322[0], 62323[0], 62324[0], 62325[0], 62326[0], 62327[0], 64400[0], 64405[0], 64408[0], 64415[0], 64416[0], 64417[0], 64418[0], 64420[0], 64421[0], 64425[0], 64430[0], 64435[0], 64445[0], 64446[0], 64447[0], 64448[0], 64449[0], 64450[0], 64451[0], 64454[0], 64461[0], 64462[0], 64463[0], 64479[0], 64480[0], 64483[0], 64484[0], 64486[0], 64487[0], 64488[0], 64489[0], 64490[0], 64491[0], 64492[0], 64493[0], 64494[0], 64495[0], 64505[0], 64510[0], 64517[0], 64520[0], 64530[0], 69990[0], 92012[1], 92014[1], 93000[1], 93005[1], 93010[1], 93040[1], 93041[1], 93042[1], 93318[1], 93355[1], 94002[1], 94200[1], 94680[1], 94681[1], 94690[1], 95812[1], 95813[1], 95816[1], 95819[1], 95822[1], 95829[1], 95955[1], 96360[1], 96361[1], 96365[1], 96366[1], 96367[1], 96368[1], 96372[1], 96374[1], 96375[1], 96376[1], 96377[1], 96523[0], 99155[0], 99156[0], 99157[0], 99211[1], 99212[1], 99213[1], 99214[1], 99215[1], 99217[1], 99218[1], 99219[1], 99220[1], 99221[1], 99222[1], 99223[1], 99231[1], 99232[1], 99233[1], 99234[1], 99235[1], 99236[1], 99238[1], 99239[1], 99241[1], 99242[1], 99243[1], 99244[1], 99245[1], 99251[1], 99252[1], 99253[1], 99254[1], 99255[1], 99291[1], 99292[1], 99304[1], 99305[1], 99306[1], 99307[1], 99308[1], 99309[1], 99310[1], 99315[1], 99316[1], 99334[1], 99335[1], 99336[1], 99337[1], 99347[1], 99348[1], 99349[1], 99350[1], 99374[1], 99375[1], 99377[1], 99378[1], 99446[0], 99447[0], 99448[0], 99449[0], 99451[0], 99452[0], 99495[0], 99496[0], G0463[1], G0471[1]
55500	0213T[0], 0216T[0], 0596T[1], 0597T[1], 0708T[1], 0709T[1], 11000[1], 11001[1], 11004[1], 11005[1], 11006[1], 11042[1], 11043[1], 11044[1], 11045[1], 11046[1], 11047[1], 12001[1], 12002[1], 12004[1], 12005[1], 12006[1], 12007[1], 12011[1], 12013[1], 12014[1], 12015[1], 12016[1], 12017[1], 12018[1], 12020[1], 12021[1], 12031[1], 12032[1], 12034[1], 12035[1], 12036[1], 12037[1], 12041[1], 12042[1], 12044[1], 12045[1], 12046[1], 12047[1], 12051[1], 12052[1], 12053[1], 12054[1], 12055[1], 12056[1], 12057[1], 13100[1], 13101[1], 13102[1], 13120[1], 13121[1], 13122[1], 13131[1], 13132[1], 13133[1], 13151[1], 13152[1], 13153[1], 36000[1], 36400[1], 36405[1], 36406[1], 36410[1], 36420[1], 36425[1], 36430[1], 36440[1], 36591[0], 36592[0], 36600[1], 36640[1], 43752[1], 51701[1], 51702[1], 51703[1], 62320[0], 62321[0], 62322[0], 62323[0], 62324[0], 62325[0], 62326[0], 62327[0], 64400[0], 64405[0], 64408[0], 64415[0], 64416[0], 64417[0], 64418[0], 64420[0], 64421[0], 64425[0], 64430[0], 64435[0], 64445[0], 64446[0], 64447[0], 64448[0], 64449[0], 64450[0], 64451[0], 64454[0], 64461[0], 64462[0], 64463[0], 64479[0], 64480[0], 64483[0], 64484[0], 64486[0], 64487[0], 64488[0], 64489[0], 64490[0], 64491[0], 64492[0], 64493[0], 64494[0], 64495[0], 64505[0], 64510[0], 64517[0], 64520[0], 64530[0], 69990[0], 92012[1], 92014[1], 93000[1], 93005[1], 93010[1], 93040[1], 93041[1], 93042[1], 93318[1], 93355[1], 94002[1], 94200[1], 94680[1], 94681[1], 94690[1], 95812[1], 95813[1], 95816[1], 95819[1], 95822[1], 95829[1], 95955[1], 96360[1], 96361[1], 96365[1], 96366[1], 96367[1], 96368[1], 96372[1], 96374[1], 96375[1], 96376[1], 96377[1], 96523[0], 97597[1], 97598[1], 97602[1], 99155[0], 99156[0], 99157[0], 99211[1], 99212[1], 99213[1], 99214[1], 99215[1], 99217[1], 99218[1], 99219[1], 99220[1], 99221[1], 99222[1], 99223[1], 99231[1], 99232[1], 99233[1], 99234[1], 99235[1], 99236[1], 99238[1], 99239[1], 99241[1], 99242[1], 99243[1], 99244[1], 99245[1], 99251[1], 99252[1], 99253[1], 99254[1], 99255[1], 99291[1], 99292[1], 99304[1], 99305[1], 99306[1], 99307[1], 99308[1], 99309[1], 99310[1], 99315[1], 99316[1], 99334[1], 99335[1], 99336[1], 99337[1], 99347[1], 99348[1], 99349[1], 99350[1], 99374[1], 99375[1], 99377[1], 99378[1], 99446[0], 99447[0], 99448[0], 99449[0], 99451[0], 99452[0], 99495[0], 99496[0], G0463[1], G0471[1]
55520	0213T[0], 0216T[0], 0596T[1], 0597T[1], 0708T[1], 0709T[1], 11000[1], 11001[1], 11004[1], 11005[1], 11006[1], 11042[1], 11043[1], 11044[1], 11045[1], 11046[1], 11047[1], 12001[1], 12002[1], 12004[1], 12005[1], 12006[1], 12007[1], 12011[1], 12013[1], 12014[1], 12015[1], 12016[1], 12017[1], 12018[1], 12020[1], 12021[1], 12031[1], 12032[1], 12034[1], 12035[1], 12036[1], 12037[1], 12041[1], 12042[1], 12044[1], 12045[1], 12046[1], 12047[1], 12051[1], 12052[1], 12053[1], 12054[1], 12055[1], 12056[1], 12057[1], 13100[1], 13101[1], 13102[1], 13120[1], 13121[1], 13122[1], 13131[1], 13132[1], 13133[1], 13151[1], 13152[1], 13153[1], 36000[1], 36400[1], 36405[1], 36406[1], 36410[1], 36420[1], 36425[1], 36430[1], 36440[1], 36591[0], 36592[0], 36600[1], 36640[1], 43752[1], 49000[0], 49002[1], 51701[1],

Appendix A: NCCI - CPT Codes

0 = Modifier usage not allowed or inappropriate 1 = Modifier usage allowed

Code 1	Code 2
	51702[1], 51703[1], 55500[1], 62320[0], 62321[0], 62322[0], 62323[0], 62324[0], 62325[0], 62326[0], 62327[0], 64400[0], 64405[0], 64408[0], 64415[0], 64416[0], 64417[0], 64418[0], 64420[0], 64421[0], 64425[0], 64430[0], 64435[0], 64445[0], 64446[0], 64447[0], 64448[0], 64449[0], 64450[0], 64451[0], 64454[0], 64461[0], 64462[0], 64463[0], 64479[0], 64480[0], 64483[0], 64484[0], 64486[0], 64487[0], 64488[0], 64489[0], 64490[0], 64491[0], 64492[0], 64493[0], 64494[0], 64495[0], 64505[0], 64510[0], 64517[0], 64520[0], 64530[0], 69990[0], 92012[1], 92014[1], 93000[1], 93005[1], 93010[1], 93040[1], 93041[1], 93042[1], 93318[1], 93355[1], 94002[1], 94200[1], 94680[1], 94681[1], 94690[1], 95812[1], 95813[1], 95816[1], 95819[1], 95822[1], 95829[1], 95955[1], 96360[1], 96361[1], 96365[1], 96366[1], 96367[1], 96368[1], 96372[1], 96374[1], 96375[1], 96376[1], 96377[1], 96523[0], 97597[1], 97598[1], 97602[1], 99155[0], 99156[0], 99157[0], 99211[1], 99212[1], 99213[1], 99214[1], 99215[1], 99217[1], 99218[1], 99219[1], 99220[1], 99221[1], 99222[1], 99223[1], 99231[1], 99232[1], 99233[1], 99234[1], 99235[1], 99236[1], 99238[1], 99239[1], 99241[1], 99242[1], 99243[1], 99244[1], 99245[1], 99251[1], 99252[1], 99253[1], 99254[1], 99255[1], 99291[1], 99292[1], 99304[1], 99305[1], 99306[1], 99307[1], 99308[1], 99309[1], 99310[1], 99315[1], 99316[1], 99334[1], 99335[1], 99336[1], 99337[1], 99347[1], 99348[1], 99349[1], 99350[1], 99374[1], 99375[1], 99377[1], 99378[1], 99446[0], 99447[0], 99448[0], 99449[0], 99451[0], 99452[0], 99495[0], 99496[0], G0463[1], G0471[1]
55530	0213T[0], 0216T[0], 0596T[1], 0597T[1], 0708T[1], 0709T[1], 11000[1], 11001[1], 11004[1], 11005[1], 11006[1], 11042[1], 11043[1], 11044[1], 11045[1], 11046[1], 11047[1], 12001[1], 12002[1], 12004[1], 12005[1], 12006[1], 12007[1], 12011[1], 12013[1], 12014[1], 12015[1], 12016[1], 12017[1], 12018[1], 12020[1], 12021[1], 12031[1], 12032[1], 12034[1], 12035[1], 12036[1], 12037[1], 12041[1], 12042[1], 12044[1], 12045[1], 12046[1], 12047[1], 12051[1], 12052[1], 12053[1], 12054[1], 12055[1], 12056[1], 12057[1], 13100[1], 13101[1], 13102[1], 13120[1], 13121[1], 13122[1], 13131[1], 13132[1], 13133[1], 13151[1], 13152[1], 13153[1], 36000[1], 36400[1], 36405[1], 36406[1], 36410[1], 36420[1], 36425[1], 36430[1], 36440[1], 36591[0], 36592[0], 36600[1], 36640[1], 43752[1], 51701[1], 51702[1], 51703[1], 55500[1], 55520[1], 55550[1], 62320[0], 62321[0], 62322[0], 62323[0], 62324[0], 62325[0], 62326[0], 62327[0], 64400[0], 64405[0], 64408[0], 64415[0], 64416[0], 64417[0], 64418[0], 64420[0], 64421[0], 64425[0], 64430[0], 64435[0], 64445[0], 64446[0], 64447[0], 64448[0], 64449[0], 64450[0], 64451[0], 64454[0], 64461[0], 64462[0], 64463[0], 64479[0], 64480[0], 64483[0], 64484[0], 64486[0], 64487[0], 64488[0], 64489[0], 64490[0], 64491[0], 64492[0], 64493[0], 64494[0], 64495[0], 64505[0], 64510[0], 64517[0], 64520[0], 64530[0], 69990[0], 92012[1], 92014[1], 93000[1], 93005[1], 93010[1], 93040[1], 93041[1], 93042[1], 93318[1], 93355[1], 94002[1], 94200[1], 94680[1], 94681[1], 94690[1], 95812[1], 95813[1], 95816[1], 95819[1], 95822[1], 95829[1], 95955[1], 96360[1], 96361[1], 96365[1], 96366[1], 96367[1], 96368[1], 96372[1], 96374[1], 96375[1], 96376[1], 96377[1], 96523[0], 97597[1], 97598[1], 97602[1], 99155[0], 99156[0], 99157[0], 99211[1], 99212[1], 99213[1], 99214[1], 99215[1], 99217[1], 99218[1], 99219[1], 99220[1], 99221[1], 99222[1], 99223[1], 99231[1], 99232[1], 99233[1], 99234[1], 99235[1], 99236[1], 99238[1], 99239[1], 99241[1], 99242[1], 99243[1], 99244[1], 99245[1], 99251[1], 99252[1], 99253[1], 99254[1], 99255[1], 99291[1], 99292[1], 99304[1], 99305[1], 99306[1], 99307[1], 99308[1], 99309[1], 99310[1], 99315[1], 99316[1], 99334[1], 99335[1], 99336[1], 99337[1], 99347[1], 99348[1], 99349[1], 99350[1], 99374[1], 99375[1], 99377[1], 99378[1], 99446[0], 99447[0], 99448[0], 99449[0], 99451[0], 99452[0], 99495[0], 99496[0], G0463[1], G0471[1]
55535	0213T[0], 0216T[0], 0596T[1], 0597T[1], 0708T[1], 0709T[1], 11000[1], 11001[1], 11004[1], 11005[1], 11006[1], 11042[1], 11043[1], 11044[1], 11045[1], 11046[1], 11047[1], 12001[1], 12002[1], 12004[1], 12005[1], 12006[1], 12007[1], 12011[1], 12013[1], 12014[1], 12015[1], 12016[1], 12017[1], 12018[1], 12020[1], 12021[1], 12031[1], 12032[1], 12034[1], 12035[1], 12036[1], 12037[1], 12041[1], 12042[1], 12044[1], 12045[1], 12046[1], 12047[1], 12051[1], 12052[1], 12053[1], 12054[1], 12055[1], 12056[1], 12057[1], 13100[1], 13101[1], 13102[1], 13120[1], 13121[1], 13122[1], 13131[1], 13132[1], 13133[1], 13151[1], 13152[1], 13153[1], 36000[1], 36400[1], 36405[1], 36406[1], 36410[1], 36420[1], 36425[1], 36430[1], 36440[1], 36591[0], 36592[0], 36600[1], 36640[1], 43752[1], 44602[1], 44603[1], 44604[1], 44605[1], 44950[0], 44970[0], 49000[0], 49002[1], 49320[1], 51701[1], 51702[1], 51703[1], 55500[1], 55550[1], 62320[0], 62321[0], 62322[0], 62323[0], 62324[0], 62325[0], 62326[0], 62327[0], 64400[0], 64405[0], 64408[0], 64415[0], 64416[0], 64417[0], 64418[0], 64420[0], 64421[0], 64425[0], 64430[0], 64435[0], 64445[0], 64446[0], 64447[0], 64448[0], 64449[0], 64450[0], 64451[0], 64454[0], 64461[0], 64462[0], 64463[0], 64479[0], 64480[0], 64483[0], 64484[0], 64486[0], 64487[0], 64488[0], 64489[0], 64490[0], 64491[0], 64492[0], 64493[0], 64494[0], 64495[0], 64505[0], 64510[0], 64517[0], 64520[0], 64530[0], 69990[0], 92012[1], 92014[1], 93000[1], 93005[1], 93010[1], 93040[1], 93041[1], 93042[1], 93318[1], 93355[1], 94002[1], 94200[1], 94680[1], 94681[1], 94690[1], 95812[1], 95813[1], 95816[1], 95819[1], 95822[1], 95829[1], 95955[1], 96360[1], 96361[1], 96365[1], 96366[1], 96367[1], 96368[1], 96372[1], 96374[1], 96375[1], 96376[1], 96377[1], 96523[0], 97597[1], 97598[1], 97602[1], 99155[0], 99156[0], 99157[0], 99211[1], 99212[1], 99213[1], 99214[1], 99215[1], 99217[1], 99218[1], 99219[1], 99220[1], 99221[1], 99222[1], 99223[1], 99231[1], 99232[1], 99233[1], 99234[1], 99235[1], 99236[1], 99238[1], 99239[1], 99241[1], 99242[1], 99243[1], 99244[1], 99245[1], 99251[1], 99252[1], 99253[1], 99254[1], 99255[1], 99291[1], 99292[1], 99304[1], 99305[1], 99306[1], 99307[1], 99308[1], 99309[1], 99310[1], 99315[1], 99316[1], 99334[1], 99335[1], 99336[1], 99337[1], 99347[1], 99348[1], 99349[1], 99350[1], 99374[1], 99375[1], 99377[1], 99378[1], 99446[0], 99447[0], 99448[0], 99449[0], 99451[0], 99452[0], 99495[0], 99496[0], G0463[1], G0471[1]
55540	0213T[0], 0216T[0], 0437T[1], 0596T[1], 0597T[1], 0708T[1], 0709T[1], 11000[1], 11001[1], 11004[1], 11005[1], 11006[1], 11042[1], 11043[1], 11044[1], 11045[1], 11046[1], 11047[1], 12001[1], 12002[1], 12004[1], 12005[1], 12006[1], 12007[1], 12011[1], 12013[1], 12014[1], 12015[1], 12016[1], 12017[1], 12018[1], 12020[1], 12021[1], 12031[1], 12032[1], 12034[1], 12035[1], 12036[1], 12037[1], 12041[1], 12042[1], 12044[1], 12045[1], 12046[1], 12047[1], 12051[1], 12052[1], 12053[1], 12054[1], 12055[1], 12056[1], 12057[1], 13100[1], 13101[1], 13102[1], 13120[1], 13121[1], 13122[1], 13131[1], 13132[1], 13133[1], 13151[1], 13152[1], 13153[1], 15777[1], 36000[1], 36400[1], 36405[1], 36406[1], 36410[1], 36420[1], 36425[1], 36430[1], 36440[1], 36591[0], 36592[0], 36600[1], 36640[1], 43752[1], 49491[1], 49492[1], 49495[1], 49500[1], 49501[1], 49505[1], 49507[1], 49520[1], 49521[1], 49525[1], 49568[1], 49650[1], 49651[1], 51701[1], 51702[1], 51703[1], 55500[1], 55520[1], 55530[1], 55550[1], 57267[1], 62320[0], 62321[0], 62322[0], 62323[0], 62324[0], 62325[0], 62326[0], 62327[0], 64400[0], 64405[0], 64408[0], 64415[0], 64416[0], 64417[0], 64418[0], 64420[0], 64421[0], 64425[0], 64430[0], 64435[0], 64445[0], 64446[0], 64447[0], 64448[0], 64449[0], 64450[0], 64451[0], 64454[0], 64461[0], 64462[0], 64463[0], 64479[0], 64480[0], 64483[0], 64484[0], 64486[0], 64487[0], 64488[0], 64489[0], 64490[0], 64491[0], 64492[0], 64493[0], 64494[0], 64495[0], 64505[0], 64510[0], 64517[0], 64520[0], 64530[0], 69990[0], 92012[1], 92014[1], 93000[1], 93005[1], 93010[1], 93040[1], 93041[1], 93042[1], 93318[1], 93355[1], 94002[1], 94200[1], 94680[1], 94681[1], 94690[1], 95812[1], 95813[1], 95816[1], 95819[1], 95822[1], 95829[1], 95955[1], 96360[1], 96361[1], 96365[1], 96366[1], 96367[1], 96368[1], 96372[1], 96374[1], 96375[1], 96376[1], 96377[1], 96523[0], 97597[1], 97598[1], 97602[1], 99155[0], 99156[0], 99157[0], 99211[1], 99212[1], 99213[1], 99214[1], 99215[1], 99217[1], 99218[1], 99219[1], 99220[1], 99221[1], 99222[1], 99223[1], 99231[1], 99232[1], 99233[1], 99234[1], 99235[1], 99236[1], 99238[1], 99239[1], 99241[1], 99242[1], 99243[1], 99244[1], 99245[1], 99251[1], 99252[1], 99253[1], 99254[1], 99255[1], 99291[1], 99292[1], 99304[1], 99305[1], 99306[1], 99307[1], 99308[1], 99309[1], 99310[1], 99315[1], 99316[1], 99334[1], 99335[1], 99336[1], 99337[1], 99347[1], 99348[1], 99349[1], 99350[1], 99374[1], 99375[1], 99377[1], 99378[1], 99446[0], 99447[0], 99448[0], 99449[0], 99451[0], 99452[0], 99495[0], 99496[0], G0463[1], G0471[1]
55550	0213T[0], 0216T[0], 0596T[1], 0597T[1], 0708T[1], 0709T[1], 12001[1], 12002[1], 12004[1], 12005[1], 12006[1], 12007[1], 12011[1], 12013[1], 12014[1], 12015[1], 12016[1], 12017[1], 12018[1], 12020[1], 12021[1], 12031[1], 12032[1], 12034[1], 12035[1], 12036[1], 12037[1], 12041[1], 12042[1], 12044[1], 12045[1], 12046[1], 12047[1], 12051[1], 12052[1], 12053[1], 12054[1], 12055[1], 12056[1], 12057[1], 13100[1], 13101[1], 13102[1], 13120[1], 13121[1], 13122[1], 13131[1], 13132[1], 13133[1], 13151[1], 13152[1], 13153[1], 36000[1], 36400[1], 36405[1], 36406[1], 36410[1], 36420[1], 36425[1], 36430[1], 36440[1], 36591[0], 36592[0], 36600[1], 36640[1], 43653[0], 43752[1], 44005[0], 44180[0], 44602[1], 44603[1], 44604[1], 44605[1], 44950[0], 44970[0], 49082[1], 49083[1], 49084[1], 49320[0], 49400[0], 50715[1], 51701[1], 51702[1], 51703[1], 62320[0], 62321[0], 62322[0], 62323[0], 62324[0], 62325[0], 62326[0], 62327[0], 64400[0], 64405[0], 64408[0], 64415[0], 64416[0], 64417[0], 64418[0], 64420[0], 64421[0], 64425[0], 64430[0], 64435[0], 64445[0], 64446[0], 64447[0], 64448[0], 64449[0], 64450[0], 64451[0], 64454[0], 64461[0], 64462[0], 64463[0], 64479[0], 64480[0], 64483[0], 64484[0], 64486[0], 64487[0], 64488[0], 64489[0], 64490[0], 64491[0], 64492[0], 64493[0], 64494[0], 64495[0], 64505[0], 64510[0], 64517[0], 64520[0], 64530[0], 69990[0], 76000[1], 77001[1], 77002[1], 92012[1], 92014[1], 93000[1], 93005[1], 93010[1], 93040[1], 93041[1], 93042[1], 93318[1], 93355[1], 94002[1], 94200[1], 94680[1], 94681[1], 94690[1], 95812[1], 95813[1], 95816[1], 95819[1], 95822[1], 95829[1], 95955[1], 96360[1], 96361[1], 96365[1], 96366[1], 96367[1], 96368[1], 96372[1], 96374[1], 96375[1], 96376[1], 96377[1], 96523[0], 99155[0], 99156[0], 99157[0], 99211[1], 99212[1], 99213[1], 99214[1], 99215[1], 99217[1], 99218[1], 99219[1], 99220[1], 99221[1], 99222[1], 99223[1], 99231[1], 99232[1], 99233[1], 99234[1], 99235[1], 99236[1], 99238[1], 99239[1], 99241[1], 99242[1], 99243[1], 99244[1], 99245[1], 99251[1], 99252[1], 99253[1], 99254[1], 99255[1], 99291[1], 99292[1], 99304[1], 99305[1], 99306[1], 99307[1], 99308[1], 99309[1], 99310[1], 99315[1], 99316[1], 99334[1], 99335[1], 99336[1], 99337[1], 99347[1], 99348[1], 99349[1], 99350[1], 99374[1], 99375[1], 99377[1], 99378[1], 99446[0], 99447[0], 99448[0], 99449[0], 99451[0], 99452[0], 99495[0], 99496[0], G0463[1], G0471[1]
55600	0213T[0], 0216T[0], 0596T[1], 0597T[1], 0708T[1], 0709T[1], 11000[1], 11001[1], 11004[1], 11005[1], 11006[1], 11042[1], 11043[1], 11044[1], 11045[1], 11046[1], 11047[1], 12001[1], 12002[1], 12004[1], 12005[1], 12006[1], 12007[1], 12011[1], 12013[1], 12014[1], 12015[1], 12016[1], 12017[1], 12018[1], 12020[1], 12021[1], 12031[1], 12032[1], 12034[1], 12035[1], 12036[1], 12037[1], 12041[1], 12042[1], 12044[1], 12045[1], 12046[1], 12047[1], 12051[1], 12052[1], 12053[1], 12054[1], 12055[1], 12056[1], 12057[1], 13100[1], 13101[1], 13102[1], 13120[1], 13121[1], 13122[1], 13131[1], 13132[1], 13133[1], 13151[1], 13152[1], 13153[1], 36000[1], 36400[1], 36405[1], 36406[1], 36410[1], 36420[1], 36425[1], 36430[1], 36440[1], 36591[0], 36592[0], 36600[1], 36640[1], 43752[1], 44602[1], 44603[1], 44604[1], 44605[1], 44950[0], 44970[0], 49000[0], 49002[1], 49320[1], 51701[1], 51702[1], 51703[1], 62320[0], 62321[0], 62322[0], 62323[0], 62324[0], 62325[0], 62326[0], 62327[0], 64400[0], 64405[0], 64408[0], 64415[0], 64416[0], 64417[0], 64418[0], 64420[0], 64421[0], 64425[0], 64430[0], 64435[0], 64445[0], 64446[0], 64447[0], 64448[0], 64449[0], 64450[0], 64451[0], 64454[0], 64461[0], 64462[0], 64463[0], 64479[0], 64480[0], 64483[0], 64484[0], 64486[0], 64487[0], 64488[0], 64489[0], 64490[0], 64491[0], 64492[0], 64493[0], 64494[0], 64495[0], 64505[0], 64510[0], 64517[0], 64520[0], 64530[0], 69990[0], 92012[1], 92014[1], 93000[1], 93005[1], 93010[1], 93040[1], 93041[1], 93042[1], 93318[1], 93355[1], 94002[1], 94200[1], 94680[1], 94681[1], 94690[1], 95812[1], 95813[1], 95816[1], 95819[1], 95822[1],

0 = Modifier usage not allowed or inappropriate 1 = Modifier usage allowed

Code 1	Code 2
	95829[1], 95955[1], 96360[1], 96361[1], 96365[1], 96366[1], 96367[1], 96368[1], 96372[1], 96374[1], 96375[1], 96376[1], 96377[1], 96523[0], 97597[1], 97598[1], 97602[1], 99155[0], 99156[0], 99157[0], 99211[1], 99212[1], 99213[1], 99214[1], 99215[1], 99217[1], 99218[1], 99219[1], 99220[1], 99221[1], 99222[1], 99223[1], 99231[1], 99232[1], 99233[1], 99234[1], 99235[1], 99236[1], 99238[1], 99239[1], 99241[1], 99242[1], 99243[1], 99244[1], 99245[1], 99251[1], 99252[1], 99253[1], 99254[1], 99255[1], 99291[1], 99292[1], 99304[1], 99305[1], 99306[1], 99307[1], 99308[1], 99309[1], 99310[1], 99315[1], 99316[1], 99334[1], 99335[1], 99336[1], 99337[1], 99347[1], 99348[1], 99349[1], 99350[1], 99374[1], 99375[1], 99377[1], 99378[1], 99446[0], 99447[0], 99448[0], 99449[0], 99451[0], 99452[0], 99495[0], 99496[0], G0463[1], G0471[1]
55605	0213T[0], 0216T[0], 0596T[1], 0597T[1], 0708T[1], 0709T[1], 11000[1], 11001[1], 11004[1], 11005[1], 11006[1], 11042[1], 11043[1], 11044[1], 11045[1], 11046[1], 11047[1], 12001[1], 12002[1], 12004[1], 12005[1], 12006[1], 12007[1], 12011[1], 12013[1], 12014[1], 12015[1], 12016[1], 12017[1], 12018[1], 12020[1], 12021[1], 12031[1], 12032[1], 12034[1], 12035[1], 12036[1], 12037[1], 12041[1], 12042[1], 12044[1], 12045[1], 12046[1], 12047[1], 12051[1], 12052[1], 12053[1], 12054[1], 12055[1], 12056[1], 12057[1], 13100[1], 13101[1], 13102[1], 13120[1], 13121[1], 13122[1], 13131[1], 13132[1], 13133[1], 13151[1], 13152[1], 13153[1], 36000[1], 36400[1], 36405[1], 36406[1], 36410[1], 36420[1], 36425[1], 36430[1], 36440[1], 36591[0], 36592[0], 36600[1], 36640[1], 43752[1], 44602[1], 44603[1], 44604[1], 44605[1], 44950[0], 44970[0], 49000[0], 49002[1], 49320[1], 51701[1], 51702[1], 51703[1], 55600[1], 62320[0], 62321[0], 62322[0], 62323[0], 62324[0], 62325[0], 62326[0], 62327[0], 64400[0], 64405[0], 64408[0], 64415[0], 64416[0], 64417[0], 64418[0], 64420[0], 64421[0], 64425[0], 64430[0], 64435[0], 64445[0], 64446[0], 64447[0], 64448[0], 64449[0], 64450[0], 64451[0], 64454[0], 64461[0], 64462[0], 64463[0], 64479[0], 64480[0], 64483[0], 64484[0], 64486[0], 64487[0], 64488[0], 64489[0], 64490[0], 64491[0], 64492[0], 64493[0], 64494[0], 64495[0], 64505[0], 64510[0], 64517[0], 64520[0], 64530[0], 69990[0], 92012[1], 92014[1], 93000[1], 93005[1], 93010[1], 93040[1], 93041[1], 93042[1], 93318[1], 93355[1], 94002[1], 94200[1], 94680[1], 94681[1], 94690[1], 95812[1], 95813[1], 95816[1], 95819[1], 95822[1], 95829[1], 95955[1], 96360[1], 96361[1], 96365[1], 96366[1], 96367[1], 96368[1], 96372[1], 96374[1], 96375[1], 96376[1], 96377[1], 96523[0], 97597[1], 97598[1], 97602[1], 99155[0], 99156[0], 99157[0], 99211[1], 99212[1], 99213[1], 99214[1], 99215[1], 99217[1], 99218[1], 99219[1], 99220[1], 99221[1], 99222[1], 99223[1], 99231[1], 99232[1], 99233[1], 99234[1], 99235[1], 99236[1], 99238[1], 99239[1], 99241[1], 99242[1], 99243[1], 99244[1], 99245[1], 99251[1], 99252[1], 99253[1], 99254[1], 99255[1], 99291[1], 99292[1], 99304[1], 99305[1], 99306[1], 99307[1], 99308[1], 99309[1], 99310[1], 99315[1], 99316[1], 99334[1], 99335[1], 99336[1], 99337[1], 99347[1], 99348[1], 99349[1], 99350[1], 99374[1], 99375[1], 99377[1], 99378[1], 99446[0], 99447[0], 99448[0], 99449[0], 99451[0], 99452[0], 99495[0], 99496[0], G0463[1], G0471[1]
55650	0213T[0], 0216T[0], 0596T[1], 0597T[1], 0708T[1], 0709T[1], 11000[1], 11001[1], 11004[1], 11005[1], 11006[1], 11042[1], 11043[1], 11044[1], 11045[1], 11046[1], 11047[1], 12001[1], 12002[1], 12004[1], 12005[1], 12006[1], 12007[1], 12011[1], 12013[1], 12014[1], 12015[1], 12016[1], 12017[1], 12018[1], 12020[1], 12021[1], 12031[1], 12032[1], 12034[1], 12035[1], 12036[1], 12037[1], 12041[1], 12042[1], 12044[1], 12045[1], 12046[1], 12047[1], 12051[1], 12052[1], 12053[1], 12054[1], 12055[1], 12056[1], 12057[1], 13100[1], 13101[1], 13102[1], 13120[1], 13121[1], 13122[1], 13131[1], 13132[1], 13133[1], 13151[1], 13152[1], 13153[1], 36000[1], 36400[1], 36405[1], 36406[1], 36410[1], 36420[1], 36425[1], 36430[1], 36440[1], 36591[0], 36592[0], 36600[1], 36640[1], 43752[1], 44602[1], 44603[1], 44604[1], 44605[1], 44950[0], 44970[0], 49000[0], 49002[1], 49320[1], 51701[1], 51702[1], 51703[1], 55600[1], 55605[1], 62320[0], 62321[0], 62322[0], 62323[0], 62324[0], 62325[0], 62326[0], 62327[0], 64400[0], 64405[0], 64408[0], 64415[0], 64416[0], 64417[0], 64418[0], 64420[0], 64421[0], 64425[0], 64430[0], 64435[0], 64445[0], 64446[0], 64447[0], 64448[0], 64449[0], 64450[0], 64451[0], 64454[0], 64461[0], 64462[0], 64463[0], 64479[0], 64480[0], 64483[0], 64484[0], 64486[0], 64487[0], 64488[0], 64489[0], 64490[0], 64491[0], 64492[0], 64493[0], 64494[0], 64495[0], 64505[0], 64510[0], 64517[0], 64520[0], 64530[0], 69990[0], 92012[1], 92014[1], 93000[1], 93005[1], 93010[1], 93040[1], 93041[1], 93042[1], 93318[1], 93355[1], 94002[1], 94200[1], 94680[1], 94681[1], 94690[1], 95812[1], 95813[1], 95816[1], 95819[1], 95822[1], 95829[1], 95955[1], 96360[1], 96361[1], 96365[1], 96366[1], 96367[1], 96368[1], 96372[1], 96374[1], 96375[1], 96376[1], 96377[1], 96523[0], 97597[1], 97598[1], 97602[1], 99155[0], 99156[0], 99157[0], 99211[1], 99212[1], 99213[1], 99214[1], 99215[1], 99217[1], 99218[1], 99219[1], 99220[1], 99221[1], 99222[1], 99223[1], 99231[1], 99232[1], 99233[1], 99234[1], 99235[1], 99236[1], 99238[1], 99239[1], 99241[1], 99242[1], 99243[1], 99244[1], 99245[1], 99251[1], 99252[1], 99253[1], 99254[1], 99255[1], 99291[1], 99292[1], 99304[1], 99305[1], 99306[1], 99307[1], 99308[1], 99309[1], 99310[1], 99315[1], 99316[1], 99334[1], 99335[1], 99336[1], 99337[1], 99347[1], 99348[1], 99349[1], 99350[1], 99374[1], 99375[1], 99377[1], 99378[1], 99446[0], 99447[0], 99448[0], 99449[0], 99451[0], 99452[0], 99495[0], 99496[0], G0463[1], G0471[1]
55680	0213T[0], 0216T[0], 0596T[1], 0597T[1], 0708T[1], 0709T[1], 11000[1], 11001[1], 11004[1], 11005[1], 11006[1], 11042[1], 11043[1], 11044[1], 11045[1], 11046[1], 11047[1], 12001[1], 12002[1], 12004[1], 12005[1], 12006[1], 12007[1], 12011[1], 12013[1], 12014[1], 12015[1], 12016[1], 12017[1], 12018[1], 12020[1], 12021[1], 12031[1], 12032[1], 12034[1], 12035[1], 12036[1], 12037[1], 12041[1], 12042[1], 12044[1], 12045[1], 12046[1], 12047[1], 12051[1], 12052[1], 12053[1], 12054[1], 12055[1], 12056[1], 12057[1], 13100[1], 13101[1], 13102[1], 13120[1], 13121[1], 13122[1], 13131[1], 13132[1], 13133[1], 13151[1], 13152[1], 13153[1], 36000[1], 36400[1], 36405[1], 36406[1], 36410[1], 36420[1], 36425[1], 36430[1], 36440[1], 36591[0], 36592[0], 36600[1], 36640[1], 43752[1], 44602[1], 44603[1], 44604[1], 44605[1], 44950[0], 44970[0], 49000[0], 49002[1], 49320[1], 51701[1], 51702[1], 51703[1], 62320[0], 62321[0], 62322[0], 62323[0], 62324[0], 62325[0], 62326[0], 62327[0], 64400[0], 64405[0], 64408[0], 64415[0], 64416[0], 64417[0], 64418[0], 64420[0], 64421[0], 64425[0], 64430[0], 64435[0], 64445[0], 64446[0], 64447[0], 64448[0], 64449[0], 64450[0], 64451[0], 64454[0], 64461[0], 64462[0], 64463[0], 64479[0], 64480[0], 64483[0], 64484[0], 64486[0], 64487[0], 64488[0], 64489[0], 64490[0], 64491[0], 64492[0], 64493[0], 64494[0], 64495[0], 64505[0], 64510[0], 64517[0], 64520[0], 64530[0], 69990[0], 92012[1], 92014[1], 93000[1], 93005[1], 93010[1], 93040[1], 93041[1], 93042[1], 93318[1], 93355[1], 94002[1], 94200[1], 94680[1], 94681[1], 94690[1], 95812[1], 95813[1], 95816[1], 95819[1], 95822[1], 95829[1], 95955[1], 96360[1], 96361[1], 96365[1], 96366[1], 96367[1], 96368[1], 96372[1], 96374[1], 96375[1], 96376[1], 96377[1], 96523[0], 97597[1], 97598[1], 97602[1], 99155[0], 99156[0], 99157[0], 99211[1], 99212[1], 99213[1], 99214[1], 99215[1], 99217[1], 99218[1], 99219[1], 99220[1], 99221[1], 99222[1], 99223[1], 99231[1], 99232[1], 99233[1], 99234[1], 99235[1], 99236[1], 99238[1], 99239[1], 99241[1], 99242[1], 99243[1], 99244[1], 99245[1], 99251[1], 99252[1], 99253[1], 99254[1], 99255[1], 99291[1], 99292[1], 99304[1], 99305[1], 99306[1], 99307[1], 99308[1], 99309[1], 99310[1], 99315[1], 99316[1], 99334[1], 99335[1], 99336[1], 99337[1], 99347[1], 99348[1], 99349[1], 99350[1], 99374[1], 99375[1], 99377[1], 99378[1], 99446[0], 99447[0], 99448[0], 99449[0], 99451[0], 99452[0], 99495[0], 99496[0], G0463[1], G0471[1]
55700	0213T[0], 0216T[0], 0596T[1], 0597T[1], 0600T[1], 0601T[1], 0708T[1], 0709T[1], 10005[1], 10007[1], 10009[1], 10011[1], 10021[1], 12001[1], 12002[1], 12004[1], 12005[1], 12006[1], 12007[1], 12011[1], 12013[1], 12014[1], 12015[1], 12016[1], 12017[1], 12018[1], 12020[1], 12021[1], 12031[1], 12032[1], 12034[1], 12035[1], 12036[1], 12037[1], 12041[1], 12042[1], 12044[1], 12045[1], 12046[1], 12047[1], 12051[1], 12052[1], 12053[1], 12054[1], 12055[1], 12056[1], 12057[1], 13100[1], 13101[1], 13102[1], 13120[1], 13121[1], 13122[1], 13131[1], 13132[1], 13133[1], 13151[1], 13152[1], 13153[1], 36000[1], 36400[1], 36405[1], 36406[1], 36410[1], 36420[1], 36425[1], 36430[1], 36440[1], 36591[0], 36592[0], 36600[1], 36640[1], 43752[1], 44950[0], 44970[0], 51701[0], 51703[1], 55873[1], 55880[1], 62320[0], 62321[0], 62322[0], 62323[0], 62324[0], 62325[0], 62326[0], 62327[0], 64400[0], 64405[0], 64408[0], 64415[0], 64416[0], 64417[0], 64418[0], 64420[0], 64421[0], 64425[0], 64430[0], 64435[0], 64445[0], 64446[0], 64447[0], 64448[0], 64449[0], 64450[0], 64451[0], 64454[0], 64461[0], 64462[0], 64463[0], 64479[0], 64480[0], 64483[0], 64484[0], 64486[0], 64487[0], 64488[0], 64489[0], 64490[0], 64491[0], 64492[0], 64493[0], 64494[0], 64495[0], 64505[0], 64510[0], 64517[0], 64520[0], 64530[0], 69990[0], 76000[1], 77001[1], 92012[1], 92014[1], 93000[1], 93005[1], 93010[1], 93040[1], 93041[1], 93042[1], 93318[1], 93355[1], 94002[1], 94200[1], 94680[1], 94681[1], 94690[1], 95812[1], 95813[1], 95816[1], 95819[1], 95822[1], 95829[1], 95955[1], 96360[1], 96361[1], 96365[1], 96366[1], 96367[1], 96368[1], 96372[1], 96374[1], 96375[1], 96376[1], 96377[1], 96523[0], 99155[0], 99156[0], 99157[0], 99211[1], 99212[1], 99213[1], 99214[1], 99215[1], 99217[1], 99218[1], 99219[1], 99220[1], 99221[1], 99222[1], 99223[1], 99231[1], 99232[1], 99233[1], 99234[1], 99235[1], 99236[1], 99238[1], 99239[1], 99241[1], 99242[1], 99243[1], 99244[1], 99245[1], 99251[1], 99252[1], 99253[1], 99254[1], 99255[1], 99291[1], 99292[1], 99304[1], 99305[1], 99306[1], 99307[1], 99308[1], 99309[1], 99310[1], 99315[1], 99316[1], 99334[1], 99335[1], 99336[1], 99337[1], 99347[1], 99348[1], 99349[1], 99350[1], 99374[1], 99375[1], 99377[1], 99378[1], 99446[0], 99447[0], 99448[0], 99449[0], 99451[0], 99452[0], 99495[1], 99496[1], G0463[1], J0670[1], J2001[1]
55705	0213T[0], 0216T[0], 0596T[1], 0597T[1], 0600T[1], 0601T[1], 0708T[1], 0709T[1], 10005[1], 10007[1], 10009[1], 10011[1], 10021[1], 12001[1], 12002[1], 12004[1], 12005[1], 12006[1], 12007[1], 12011[1], 12013[1], 12014[1], 12015[1], 12016[1], 12017[1], 12018[1], 12020[1], 12021[1], 12031[1], 12032[1], 12034[1], 12035[1], 12036[1], 12037[1], 12041[1], 12042[1], 12044[1], 12045[1], 12046[1], 12047[1], 12051[1], 12052[1], 12053[1], 12054[1], 12055[1], 12056[1], 12057[1], 13100[1], 13101[1], 13102[1], 13120[1], 13121[1], 13122[1], 13131[1], 13132[1], 13133[1], 13151[1], 13152[1], 13153[1], 36000[1], 36400[1], 36405[1], 36406[1], 36410[1], 36420[1], 36425[1], 36430[1], 36440[1], 36591[0], 36592[0], 36600[1], 36640[1], 43752[1], 44950[0], 44970[0], 51701[0], 51702[0], 51703[1], 55700[1], 55873[1], 55880[1], 62320[0], 62321[0], 62322[0], 62323[0], 62324[0], 62325[0], 62326[0], 62327[0], 64400[0], 64405[0], 64408[0], 64415[0], 64416[0], 64417[0], 64418[0], 64420[0], 64421[0], 64425[0], 64430[0], 64435[0], 64445[0], 64446[0], 64447[0], 64448[0], 64449[0], 64450[0], 64451[0], 64454[0], 64461[0], 64462[0], 64463[0], 64479[0], 64480[0], 64483[0], 64484[0], 64486[0], 64487[0], 64488[0], 64489[0], 64490[0], 64491[0], 64492[0], 64493[0], 64494[0], 64495[0], 64505[0], 64510[0], 64517[0], 64520[0], 64530[0], 69990[0], 92012[1], 92014[1], 93000[1], 93005[1], 93010[1], 93040[1], 93041[1], 93042[1], 93318[1], 93355[1], 94002[1], 94200[1], 94680[1], 94681[1], 94690[1], 95812[1], 95813[1], 95816[1], 95819[1], 95822[1], 95829[1], 95955[1], 96360[1], 96361[1], 96365[1], 96366[1], 96367[1], 96368[1], 96372[1], 96374[1], 96375[1], 96376[1], 96377[1], 96523[0], 99155[0], 99156[0], 99157[0], 99211[1], 99212[1], 99213[1], 99214[1], 99215[1], 99217[1], 99218[1], 99219[1], 99220[1], 99221[1], 99222[1], 99223[1], 99231[1], 99232[1], 99233[1], 99234[1], 99235[1], 99236[1], 99238[1], 99239[1], 99241[1], 99242[1], 99243[1], 99244[1], 99245[1], 99251[1], 99252[1], 99253[1], 99254[1], 99255[1], 99291[1], 99292[1], 99304[1], 99305[1], 99306[1], 99307[1], 99308[1], 99309[1], 99310[1], 99315[1], 99316[1], 99334[1], 99335[1], 99336[1], 99337[1], 99347[1], 99348[1], 99349[1], 99350[1], 99374[1], 99375[1],

Appendix A: NCCI - CPT Codes

0 = Modifier usage not allowed or inappropriate 1 = Modifier usage allowed

Code 1	Code 2
	99377[1], 99378[1], 99446[0], 99447[0], 99448[0], 99449[0], 99451[0], 99452[0], 99495[0], 99496[0], G0463[1], G0471[0]
55706	0213T[1], 0216T[1], 0421T[1], 0582T[1], 0596T[1], 0597T[1], 0655T[1], 0708T[1], 0709T[1], 10005[1], 10007[1], 10009[1], 10011[1], 10021[1], 12001[1], 12002[1], 12004[1], 12005[1], 12006[1], 12007[1], 12011[1], 12013[1], 12014[1], 12015[1], 12016[1], 12017[1], 12018[1], 12020[1], 12021[1], 12031[1], 12032[1], 12034[1], 12035[1], 12036[1], 12037[1], 12041[1], 12042[1], 12044[1], 12045[1], 12046[1], 12047[1], 12051[1], 12052[1], 12053[1], 12054[1], 12055[1], 12056[1], 12057[1], 13100[1], 13101[1], 13102[1], 13120[1], 13121[1], 13122[1], 13131[1], 13132[1], 13133[1], 13151[1], 13152[1], 13153[1], 36000[1], 36400[1], 36405[1], 36406[1], 36410[1], 36420[1], 36425[1], 36430[1], 36440[1], 36591[0], 36592[0], 36600[1], 36640[1], 43752[1], 51701[1], 51702[1], 51703[1], 53854[1], 55700[1], 55705[1], 62320[0], 62321[0], 62322[0], 62323[0], 62324[0], 62325[0], 62326[0], 62327[0], 64400[0], 64405[0], 64408[0], 64415[1], 64416[1], 64417[1], 64418[0], 64420[0], 64421[0], 64425[0], 64430[0], 64435[0], 64445[0], 64446[0], 64447[0], 64448[0], 64449[0], 64450[1], 64451[0], 64454[1], 64461[0], 64462[0], 64463[0], 64479[0], 64480[0], 64483[0], 64484[0], 64486[0], 64487[0], 64488[0], 64489[0], 64490[1], 64491[0], 64492[0], 64493[1], 64494[0], 64495[0], 64505[0], 64510[0], 64517[0], 64520[0], 64530[0], 69990[0], 76000[1], 76942[1], 76998[1], 77001[1], 77002[1], 92012[1], 92014[1], 93000[1], 93005[1], 93010[1], 93040[1], 93041[1], 93042[1], 93318[1], 93355[1], 94002[1], 94200[1], 94680[1], 94681[1], 94690[1], 95812[1], 95813[1], 95816[1], 95819[1], 95822[1], 95829[1], 95955[1], 96360[1], 96361[1], 96365[1], 96366[1], 96367[1], 96368[1], 96372[1], 96374[1], 96375[1], 96376[1], 96377[1], 96523[0], 99155[0], 99156[0], 99157[0], 99211[1], 99212[1], 99213[1], 99214[1], 99215[1], 99217[1], 99218[1], 99219[1], 99220[1], 99221[1], 99222[1], 99223[1], 99231[1], 99232[1], 99233[1], 99234[1], 99235[1], 99236[1], 99238[1], 99239[1], 99241[1], 99242[1], 99243[1], 99244[1], 99245[1], 99251[1], 99252[1], 99253[1], 99254[1], 99255[1], 99291[1], 99292[1], 99304[1], 99305[1], 99306[1], 99307[1], 99308[1], 99309[1], 99310[1], 99315[1], 99316[1], 99334[1], 99335[1], 99336[1], 99337[1], 99347[1], 99348[1], 99349[1], 99350[1], 99374[1], 99375[1], 99377[1], 99378[1], 99446[0], 99447[0], 99448[0], 99449[0], 99451[0], 99452[0], 99495[0], 99496[0], G0463[1], G0471[1]
55720	0213T[0], 0216T[0], 0596T[1], 0597T[1], 0708T[1], 0709T[1], 11000[1], 11001[1], 11004[1], 11005[1], 11006[1], 11042[1], 11043[1], 11044[1], 11045[1], 11046[1], 11047[1], 12001[1], 12002[1], 12004[1], 12005[1], 12006[1], 12007[1], 12011[1], 12013[1], 12014[1], 12015[1], 12016[1], 12017[1], 12018[1], 12020[1], 12021[1], 12031[1], 12032[1], 12034[1], 12035[1], 12036[1], 12037[1], 12041[1], 12042[1], 12044[1], 12045[1], 12046[1], 12047[1], 12051[1], 12052[1], 12053[1], 12054[1], 12055[1], 12056[1], 12057[1], 13100[1], 13101[1], 13102[1], 13120[1], 13121[1], 13122[1], 13131[1], 13132[1], 13133[1], 13151[1], 13152[1], 13153[1], 36000[1], 36400[1], 36405[1], 36406[1], 36410[1], 36420[1], 36425[1], 36430[1], 36440[1], 36591[0], 36592[0], 36600[1], 36640[1], 43752[1], 44005[1], 44180[0], 44820[0], 44850[0], 44950[0], 44970[0], 49000[0], 49002[1], 49010[0], 49255[1], 51701[0], 51702[0], 51703[1], 52000[1], 62320[0], 62321[0], 62322[0], 62323[0], 62324[0], 62325[0], 62326[0], 62327[0], 64400[0], 64405[0], 64408[0], 64415[0], 64416[0], 64417[0], 64418[0], 64420[0], 64421[0], 64425[0], 64430[0], 64435[0], 64445[0], 64446[0], 64447[0], 64448[0], 64449[0], 64450[0], 64451[0], 64454[0], 64461[0], 64462[0], 64463[0], 64479[0], 64480[0], 64483[0], 64484[0], 64486[0], 64487[0], 64488[0], 64489[0], 64490[0], 64491[0], 64492[0], 64493[0], 64494[0], 64495[0], 64505[0], 64510[0], 64517[0], 64520[0], 64530[0], 69990[0], 92012[1], 92014[1], 93000[1], 93005[1], 93010[1], 93040[1], 93041[1], 93042[1], 93318[1], 93355[1], 94002[1], 94200[1], 94680[1], 94681[1], 94690[1], 95812[1], 95813[1], 95816[1], 95819[1], 95822[1], 95829[1], 95955[1], 96360[1], 96361[1], 96365[1], 96366[1], 96367[1], 96368[1], 96372[1], 96374[1], 96375[1], 96376[1], 96377[1], 96523[0], 97597[1], 97598[1], 97602[1], 99155[0], 99156[0], 99157[0], 99211[1], 99212[1], 99213[1], 99214[1], 99215[1], 99217[1], 99218[1], 99219[1], 99220[1], 99221[1], 99222[1], 99223[1], 99231[1], 99232[1], 99233[1], 99234[1], 99235[1], 99236[1], 99238[1], 99239[1], 99241[1], 99242[1], 99243[1], 99244[1], 99245[1], 99251[1], 99252[1], 99253[1], 99254[1], 99255[1], 99291[1], 99292[1], 99304[1], 99305[1], 99306[1], 99307[1], 99308[1], 99309[1], 99310[1], 99315[1], 99316[1], 99334[1], 99335[1], 99336[1], 99337[1], 99347[1], 99348[1], 99349[1], 99350[1], 99374[1], 99375[1], 99377[1], 99378[1], 99446[0], 99447[0], 99448[0], 99449[0], 99451[0], 99452[0], 99495[0], 99496[0], G0463[1], G0471[0]
55725	0213T[0], 0216T[0], 0596T[1], 0597T[1], 0708T[1], 0709T[1], 11000[1], 11001[1], 11004[1], 11005[1], 11006[1], 11042[1], 11043[1], 11044[1], 11045[1], 11046[1], 11047[1], 12001[1], 12002[1], 12004[1], 12005[1], 12006[1], 12007[1], 12011[1], 12013[1], 12014[1], 12015[1], 12016[1], 12017[1], 12018[1], 12020[1], 12021[1], 12031[1], 12032[1], 12034[1], 12035[1], 12036[1], 12037[1], 12041[1], 12042[1], 12044[1], 12045[1], 12046[1], 12047[1], 12051[1], 12052[1], 12053[1], 12054[1], 12055[1], 12056[1], 12057[1], 13100[1], 13101[1], 13102[1], 13120[1], 13121[1], 13122[1], 13131[1], 13132[1], 13133[1], 13151[1], 13152[1], 13153[1], 36000[1], 36400[1], 36405[1], 36406[1], 36410[1], 36420[1], 36425[1], 36430[1], 36440[1], 36591[0], 36592[0], 36600[1], 36640[1], 43752[1], 44005[1], 44180[0], 44820[0], 44850[0], 44950[0], 44970[0], 49000[0], 49002[1], 49010[0], 49255[1], 51701[0], 51702[0], 51703[1], 52000[1], 55720[1], 62320[0], 62321[0], 62322[0], 62323[0], 62324[0], 62325[0], 62326[0], 62327[0], 64400[0], 64405[0], 64408[0], 64415[0], 64416[0], 64417[0], 64418[0], 64420[0], 64421[0], 64425[0], 64430[0], 64435[0], 64445[0], 64446[0], 64447[0], 64448[0], 64449[0], 64450[0], 64451[0], 64454[0], 64461[0], 64462[0], 64463[0], 64479[0], 64480[0], 64483[0], 64484[0], 64486[0], 64487[0], 64488[0], 64489[0], 64490[0], 64491[0], 64492[0], 64493[0], 64494[0], 64495[0], 64505[0], 64510[0], 64517[0], 64520[0], 64530[0], 69990[0], 92012[1], 92014[1], 93000[1], 93005[1], 93010[1], 93040[1], 93041[1], 93042[1], 93318[1], 93355[1], 94002[1], 94200[1], 94680[1], 94681[1], 94690[1], 95812[1], 95813[1], 95816[1], 95819[1], 95822[1], 95829[1], 95955[1], 96360[1], 96361[1], 96365[1], 96366[1], 96367[1], 96368[1], 96372[1], 96374[1], 96375[1], 96376[1], 96377[1], 96523[0], 97597[1], 97598[1], 97602[1], 99155[0], 99156[0], 99157[0], 99211[1], 99212[1], 99213[1], 99214[1], 99215[1], 99217[1], 99218[1], 99219[1], 99220[1], 99221[1], 99222[1], 99223[1], 99231[1], 99232[1], 99233[1], 99234[1], 99235[1], 99236[1], 99238[1], 99239[1], 99241[1], 99242[1], 99243[1], 99244[1], 99245[1], 99251[1], 99252[1], 99253[1], 99254[1], 99255[1], 99291[1], 99292[1], 99304[1], 99305[1], 99306[1], 99307[1], 99308[1], 99309[1], 99310[1], 99315[1], 99316[1], 99334[1], 99335[1], 99336[1], 99337[1], 99347[1], 99348[1], 99349[1], 99350[1], 99374[1], 99375[1], 99377[1], 99378[1], 99446[0], 99447[0], 99448[0], 99449[0], 99451[0], 99452[0], 99495[0], 99496[0], G0463[1], G0471[0]
55801	0213T[0], 0216T[0], 0421T[0], 0582T[0], 0596T[1], 0597T[1], 0655T[0], 0708T[1], 0709T[1], 11000[1], 11001[1], 11004[1], 11005[1], 11006[1], 11042[1], 11043[1], 11044[1], 11045[1], 11046[1], 11047[1], 12001[1], 12002[1], 12004[1], 12005[1], 12006[1], 12007[1], 12011[1], 12013[1], 12014[1], 12015[1], 12016[1], 12017[1], 12018[1], 12020[1], 12021[1], 12031[1], 12032[1], 12034[1], 12035[1], 12036[1], 12037[1], 12041[1], 12042[1], 12044[1], 12045[1], 12046[1], 12047[1], 12051[1], 12052[1], 12053[1], 12054[1], 12055[1], 12056[1], 12057[1], 13100[1], 13101[1], 13102[1], 13120[1], 13121[1], 13122[1], 13131[1], 13132[1], 13133[1], 13151[1], 13152[1], 13153[1], 36000[1], 36400[1], 36405[1], 36406[1], 36410[1], 36420[1], 36425[1], 36430[1], 36440[1], 36591[0], 36592[0], 36600[1], 36640[1], 43752[1], 44950[0], 44970[0], 51701[0], 51702[0], 51703[1], 51800[0], 52000[1], 52601[0], 52630[0], 52640[0], 52647[0], 52648[0], 53020[0], 53850[0], 53852[0], 53854[0], 55250[0], 55650[1], 55706[1], 55821[0], 55831[0], 55875[1], 55876[1], 62320[0], 62321[0], 62322[0], 62323[0], 62324[0], 62325[0], 62326[0], 62327[0], 64400[0], 64405[0], 64408[0], 64415[0], 64416[0], 64417[0], 64418[0], 64420[0], 64421[0], 64425[0], 64430[0], 64435[0], 64445[0], 64446[0], 64447[0], 64448[0], 64449[0], 64450[0], 64451[0], 64454[0], 64461[0], 64462[0], 64463[0], 64479[0], 64480[0], 64483[0], 64484[0], 64486[0], 64487[0], 64488[0], 64489[0], 64490[0], 64491[0], 64492[0], 64493[0], 64494[0], 64495[0], 64505[0], 64510[0], 64517[0], 64520[0], 64530[0], 69990[0], 92012[1], 92014[1], 93000[1], 93005[1], 93010[1], 93040[1], 93041[1], 93042[1], 93318[1], 93355[1], 94002[1], 94200[1], 94680[1], 94681[1], 94690[1], 95812[1], 95813[1], 95816[1], 95819[1], 95822[1], 95829[1], 95955[1], 96360[1], 96361[1], 96365[1], 96366[1], 96367[1], 96368[1], 96372[1], 96374[1], 96375[1], 96376[1], 96377[1], 96523[0], 97597[1], 97598[1], 97602[1], 99155[0], 99156[0], 99157[0], 99211[1], 99212[1], 99213[1], 99214[1], 99215[1], 99217[1], 99218[1], 99219[1], 99220[1], 99221[1], 99222[1], 99223[1], 99231[1], 99232[1], 99233[1], 99234[1], 99235[1], 99236[1], 99238[1], 99239[1], 99241[1], 99242[1], 99243[1], 99244[1], 99245[1], 99251[1], 99252[1], 99253[1], 99254[1], 99255[1], 99291[1], 99292[1], 99304[1], 99305[1], 99306[1], 99307[1], 99308[1], 99309[1], 99310[1], 99315[1], 99316[1], 99334[1], 99335[1], 99336[1], 99337[1], 99347[1], 99348[1], 99349[1], 99350[1], 99374[1], 99375[1], 99377[1], 99378[1], 99446[0], 99447[0], 99448[0], 99449[0], 99451[0], 99452[0], 99495[0], 99496[0], G0463[1], G0471[0]
55810	0213T[0], 0216T[0], 0421T[0], 0582T[0], 0596T[1], 0597T[1], 0655T[0], 0708T[1], 0709T[1], 11000[1], 11001[1], 11004[1], 11005[1], 11006[1], 11042[1], 11043[1], 11044[1], 11045[1], 11046[1], 11047[1], 12001[1], 12002[1], 12004[1], 12005[1], 12006[1], 12007[1], 12011[1], 12013[1], 12014[1], 12015[1], 12016[1], 12017[1], 12018[1], 12020[1], 12021[1], 12031[1], 12032[1], 12034[1], 12035[1], 12036[1], 12037[1], 12041[1], 12042[1], 12044[1], 12045[1], 12046[1], 12047[1], 12051[1], 12052[1], 12053[1], 12054[1], 12055[1], 12056[1], 12057[1], 13100[1], 13101[1], 13102[1], 13120[1], 13121[1], 13122[1], 13131[1], 13132[1], 13133[1], 13151[1], 13152[1], 13153[1], 36000[1], 36400[1], 36405[1], 36406[1], 36410[1], 36420[1], 36425[1], 36430[1], 36440[1], 36591[0], 36592[0], 36600[1], 36640[1], 38573[0], 43752[1], 44950[0], 44970[0], 51701[0], 51702[0], 51703[1], 51800[0], 52000[1], 52601[0], 52630[0], 52640[0], 52647[0], 52648[0], 53850[0], 53852[0], 53854[0], 55650[1], 55706[1], 55801[0], 55821[0], 55831[0], 55875[1], 55876[1], 62320[0], 62321[0], 62322[0], 62323[0], 62324[0], 62325[0], 62326[0], 62327[0], 64400[0], 64405[0], 64408[0], 64415[0], 64416[0], 64417[0], 64418[0], 64420[0], 64421[0], 64425[0], 64430[0], 64435[0], 64445[0], 64446[0], 64447[0], 64448[0], 64449[0], 64450[0], 64451[0], 64454[0], 64461[0], 64462[0], 64463[0], 64479[0], 64480[0], 64483[0], 64484[0], 64486[0], 64487[0], 64488[0], 64489[0], 64490[0], 64491[0], 64492[0], 64493[0], 64494[0], 64495[0], 64505[0], 64510[0], 64517[0], 64520[0], 64530[0], 69990[0], 92012[1], 92014[1], 93000[1], 93005[1], 93010[1], 93040[1], 93041[1], 93042[1], 93318[1], 93355[1], 94002[1], 94200[1], 94680[1], 94681[1], 94690[1], 95812[1], 95813[1], 95816[1], 95819[1], 95822[1], 95829[1], 95955[1], 96360[1], 96361[1], 96365[1], 96366[1], 96367[1], 96368[1], 96372[1], 96374[1], 96375[1], 96376[1], 96377[1], 96523[0], 97597[1], 97598[1], 97602[1], 99155[0], 99156[0], 99157[0], 99211[1], 99212[1], 99213[1], 99214[1], 99215[1], 99217[1], 99218[1], 99219[1], 99220[1], 99221[1], 99222[1], 99223[1], 99231[1], 99232[1], 99233[1], 99234[1], 99235[1], 99236[1], 99238[1], 99239[1], 99241[1], 99242[1], 99243[1], 99244[1], 99245[1], 99251[1], 99252[1], 99253[1], 99254[1], 99255[1], 99291[1], 99292[1], 99304[1], 99305[1], 99306[1], 99307[1], 99308[1], 99309[1], 99310[1], 99315[1], 99316[1], 99334[1], 99335[1], 99336[1], 99337[1], 99347[1], 99348[1], 99349[1], 99350[1], 99374[1], 99375[1], 99377[1], 99378[1], 99446[0], 99447[0], 99448[0], 99449[0], 99451[0], 99452[0], 99495[0], 99496[0], G0463[1], G0471[0]
55812	0213T[0], 0216T[0], 0421T[0], 0582T[0], 0596T[1], 0597T[1], 0600T[1], 0601T[1], 0655T[0], 0708T[1], 0709T[1], 10005[1], 10007[1], 10009[1], 10011[1], 10021[1], 11000[1], 11001[1], 11004[1], 11005[1],

0 = Modifier usage not allowed or inappropriate   1 = Modifier usage allowed

Appendix A: NCCI - CPT Codes

Code 1	Code 2
	11006[1], 11042[1], 11043[1], 11044[1], 11045[1], 11046[1], 11047[1], 12001[1], 12002[1], 12004[1], 12005[1], 12006[1], 12007[1], 12011[1], 12013[1], 12014[1], 12015[1], 12016[1], 12017[1], 12018[1], 12020[1], 12021[1], 12031[1], 12032[1], 12034[1], 12035[1], 12036[1], 12037[1], 12041[1], 12042[1], 12044[1], 12045[1], 12046[1], 12047[1], 12051[1], 12052[1], 12053[1], 12054[1], 12055[1], 12056[1], 12057[1], 13100[1], 13101[1], 13102[1], 13120[1], 13121[1], 13122[1], 13131[1], 13132[1], 13133[1], 13151[1], 13152[1], 13153[1], 36000[1], 36400[1], 36405[1], 36406[1], 36410[1], 36420[1], 36425[1], 36430[1], 36440[1], 36591[0], 36592[0], 36600[1], 36640[1], 38562[0], 38573[0], 43752[1], 44950[0], 44970[0], 49000[0], 49002[1], 51701[0], 51702[0], 51703[1], 51800[0], 52000[1], 52601[0], 52630[0], 52640[0], 52647[0], 52648[0], 53850[0], 53852[0], 53854[0], 55650[1], 55706[1], 55801[0], 55810[0], 55821[0], 55831[0], 55840[0], 55842[0], 55873[1], 55875[1], 55876[1], 55880[1], 62320[0], 62321[0], 62322[0], 62323[0], 62324[0], 62325[0], 62326[0], 62327[0], 64400[0], 64405[0], 64408[0], 64415[0], 64416[0], 64417[0], 64418[0], 64420[0], 64421[0], 64425[0], 64430[0], 64435[0], 64445[0], 64446[0], 64447[0], 64448[0], 64449[0], 64450[0], 64451[0], 64454[0], 64461[0], 64462[0], 64463[0], 64479[0], 64480[0], 64483[0], 64484[0], 64486[0], 64487[0], 64488[0], 64489[0], 64490[0], 64491[0], 64492[0], 64493[0], 64494[0], 64495[0], 64505[0], 64510[0], 64517[0], 64520[0], 64530[0], 69990[0], 92012[1], 92014[1], 93000[1], 93005[1], 93010[1], 93040[1], 93041[1], 93042[1], 93318[1], 93355[1], 94002[1], 94200[1], 94680[1], 94681[1], 94690[1], 95812[1], 95813[1], 95816[1], 95819[1], 95822[1], 95829[1], 95955[1], 96360[1], 96361[1], 96365[1], 96366[1], 96367[1], 96368[1], 96372[1], 96374[1], 96375[1], 96376[1], 96377[1], 96523[0], 97597[1], 97598[1], 97602[1], 99155[0], 99156[0], 99157[0], 99211[1], 99212[1], 99213[1], 99214[1], 99215[1], 99217[1], 99218[1], 99219[1], 99220[1], 99221[1], 99222[1], 99223[1], 99231[1], 99232[1], 99233[1], 99234[1], 99235[1], 99236[1], 99238[1], 99239[1], 99241[1], 99242[1], 99243[1], 99244[1], 99245[1], 99251[1], 99252[1], 99253[1], 99254[1], 99255[1], 99291[1], 99292[1], 99304[1], 99305[1], 99306[1], 99307[1], 99308[1], 99309[1], 99310[1], 99315[1], 99316[1], 99334[1], 99335[1], 99336[1], 99337[1], 99347[1], 99348[1], 99349[1], 99350[1], 99374[1], 99375[1], 99377[1], 99378[1], 99446[0], 99447[0], 99448[0], 99449[0], 99451[0], 99452[0], 99495[0], 99496[0], G0463[1], G0471[0]
55815	0213T[0], 0216T[0], 0421T[0], 0582T[0], 0596T[1], 0597T[1], 0600T[1], 0601T[1], 0655T[0], 0708T[1], 0709T[1], 11000[1], 11001[1], 11004[1], 11005[1], 11006[1], 11042[1], 11043[1], 11044[1], 11045[1], 11046[1], 11047[1], 12001[1], 12002[1], 12004[1], 12005[1], 12006[1], 12007[1], 12011[1], 12013[1], 12014[1], 12015[1], 12016[1], 12017[1], 12018[1], 12020[1], 12021[1], 12031[1], 12032[1], 12034[1], 12035[1], 12036[1], 12037[1], 12041[1], 12042[1], 12044[1], 12045[1], 12046[1], 12047[1], 12051[1], 12052[1], 12053[1], 12054[1], 12055[1], 12056[1], 12057[1], 13100[1], 13101[1], 13102[1], 13120[1], 13121[1], 13122[1], 13131[1], 13132[1], 13133[1], 13151[1], 13152[1], 13153[1], 36000[1], 36400[1], 36405[1], 36406[1], 36410[1], 36420[1], 36425[1], 36430[1], 36440[1], 36591[0], 36592[0], 36600[1], 36640[1], 38562[0], 38571[1], 38572[1], 38573[0], 38770[0], 38780[1], 43752[1], 44005[0], 44180[0], 44602[1], 44603[1], 44604[1], 44605[1], 44820[0], 44850[0], 44950[0], 44970[0], 49000[0], 49002[1], 49010[0], 49255[0], 49320[1], 49321[1], 51701[0], 51702[0], 51703[1], 51800[0], 52000[1], 52601[0], 52630[0], 52640[0], 52647[0], 52648[0], 53850[0], 53852[0], 53854[0], 55650[1], 55706[1], 55801[0], 55810[0], 55812[0], 55821[0], 55831[0], 55840[0], 55842[0], 55845[0], 55866[0], 55873[1], 55875[1], 55876[1], 55880[1], 62320[0], 62321[0], 62322[0], 62323[0], 62324[0], 62325[0], 62326[0], 62327[0], 64400[0], 64405[0], 64408[0], 64415[0], 64416[0], 64417[0], 64418[0], 64420[0], 64421[0], 64425[0], 64430[0], 64435[0], 64445[0], 64446[0], 64447[0], 64448[0], 64449[0], 64450[0], 64451[0], 64454[0], 64461[0], 64462[0], 64463[0], 64479[0], 64480[0], 64483[0], 64484[0], 64486[0], 64487[0], 64488[0], 64489[0], 64490[0], 64491[0], 64492[0], 64493[0], 64494[0], 64495[0], 64505[0], 64510[0], 64517[0], 64520[0], 64530[0], 69990[0], 92012[1], 92014[1], 93000[1], 93005[1], 93010[1], 93040[1], 93041[1], 93042[1], 93318[1], 93355[1], 94002[1], 94200[1], 94680[1], 94681[1], 94690[1], 95812[1], 95813[1], 95816[1], 95819[1], 95822[1], 95829[1], 95955[1], 96360[1], 96361[1], 96365[1], 96366[1], 96367[1], 96368[1], 96372[1], 96374[1], 96375[1], 96376[1], 96377[1], 96523[0], 97597[1], 97598[1], 97602[1], 99155[0], 99156[0], 99157[0], 99211[1], 99212[1], 99213[1], 99214[1], 99215[1], 99217[1], 99218[1], 99219[1], 99220[1], 99221[1], 99222[1], 99223[1], 99231[1], 99232[1], 99233[1], 99234[1], 99235[1], 99236[1], 99238[1], 99239[1], 99241[1], 99242[1], 99243[1], 99244[1], 99245[1], 99251[1], 99252[1], 99253[1], 99254[1], 99255[1], 99291[1], 99292[1], 99304[1], 99305[1], 99306[1], 99307[1], 99308[1], 99309[1], 99310[1], 99315[1], 99316[1], 99334[1], 99335[1], 99336[1], 99337[1], 99347[1], 99348[1], 99349[1], 99350[1], 99374[1], 99375[1], 99377[1], 99378[1], 99446[0], 99447[0], 99448[0], 99449[0], 99451[0], 99452[0], 99495[0], 99496[0], G0463[1], G0471[0]
55821	0213T[0], 0216T[0], 0421T[0], 0582T[0], 0596T[1], 0597T[1], 0600T[1], 0601T[1], 0655T[0], 0708T[1], 0709T[1], 11000[1], 11001[1], 11004[1], 11005[1], 11006[1], 11042[1], 11043[1], 11044[1], 11045[1], 11046[1], 11047[1], 12001[1], 12002[1], 12004[1], 12005[1], 12006[1], 12007[1], 12011[1], 12013[1], 12014[1], 12015[1], 12016[1], 12017[1], 12018[1], 12020[1], 12021[1], 12031[1], 12032[1], 12034[1], 12035[1], 12036[1], 12037[1], 12041[1], 12042[1], 12044[1], 12045[1], 12046[1], 12047[1], 12051[1], 12052[1], 12053[1], 12054[1], 12055[1], 12056[1], 12057[1], 13100[1], 13101[1], 13102[1], 13120[1], 13121[1], 13122[1], 13131[1], 13132[1], 13133[1], 13151[1], 13152[1], 13153[1], 35840[1], 36000[1], 36400[1], 36405[1], 36406[1], 36410[1], 36420[1], 36425[1], 36430[1], 36440[1], 36591[0], 36592[0], 36600[1], 36640[1], 43752[1], 44005[0], 44180[0], 44602[1], 44603[1], 44604[1], 44605[1], 44820[0], 44850[0], 44950[0], 44970[0], 49000[0], 49002[1], 49010[0], 49255[0], 49320[1], 49321[1], 51040[1], 51050[1], 51102[1], 51700[0], 51701[0], 51702[0], 51703[1], 51800[0], 52000[1], 52281[1], 52601[0], 52630[0], 52640[0], 52647[0], 52648[0], 53020[1], 53600[1], 53850[0], 53852[0], 53854[0], 55250[1], 55650[1], 55706[1], 55873[1], 55875[1], 55876[1], 55880[1], 62320[0], 62321[0], 62322[0], 62323[0], 62324[0], 62325[0], 62326[0], 62327[0], 64400[0], 64405[0], 64408[0], 64415[0], 64416[0], 64417[0], 64418[0], 64420[0], 64421[0], 64425[0], 64430[0], 64435[0], 64445[0], 64446[0], 64447[0], 64448[0], 64449[0], 64450[0], 64451[0], 64454[0], 64461[0], 64462[0], 64463[0], 64479[0], 64480[0], 64483[0], 64484[0], 64486[0], 64487[0], 64488[0], 64489[0], 64490[0], 64491[0], 64492[0], 64493[0], 64494[0], 64495[0], 64505[0], 64510[0], 64517[0], 64520[0], 64530[0], 69990[0], 92012[1], 92014[1], 93000[1], 93005[1], 93010[1], 93040[1], 93041[1], 93042[1], 93318[1], 93355[1], 94002[1], 94200[1], 94680[1], 94681[1], 94690[1], 95812[1], 95813[1], 95816[1], 95819[1], 95822[1], 95829[1], 95955[1], 96360[1], 96361[1], 96365[1], 96366[1], 96367[1], 96368[1], 96372[1], 96374[1], 96375[1], 96376[1], 96377[1], 96523[0], 97597[1], 97598[1], 97602[1], 99155[0], 99156[0], 99157[0], 99211[1], 99212[1], 99213[1], 99214[1], 99215[1], 99217[1], 99218[1], 99219[1], 99220[1], 99221[1], 99222[1], 99223[1], 99231[1], 99232[1], 99233[1], 99234[1], 99235[1], 99236[1], 99238[1], 99239[1], 99241[1], 99242[1], 99243[1], 99244[1], 99245[1], 99251[1], 99252[1], 99253[1], 99254[1], 99255[1], 99291[1], 99292[1], 99304[1], 99305[1], 99306[1], 99307[1], 99308[1], 99309[1], 99310[1], 99315[1], 99316[1], 99334[1], 99335[1], 99336[1], 99337[1], 99347[1], 99348[1], 99349[1], 99350[1], 99374[1], 99375[1], 99377[1], 99378[1], 99446[0], 99447[0], 99448[0], 99449[0], 99451[0], 99452[0], 99495[0], 99496[0], G0463[1], G0471[0]
55831	0213T[0], 0216T[0], 0421T[0], 0582T[0], 0596T[1], 0597T[1], 0600T[1], 0601T[1], 0655T[0], 0708T[1], 0709T[1], 11000[1], 11001[1], 11004[1], 11005[1], 11006[1], 11042[1], 11043[1], 11044[1], 11045[1], 11046[1], 11047[1], 12001[1], 12002[1], 12004[1], 12005[1], 12006[1], 12007[1], 12011[1], 12013[1], 12014[1], 12015[1], 12016[1], 12017[1], 12018[1], 12020[1], 12021[1], 12031[1], 12032[1], 12034[1], 12035[1], 12036[1], 12037[1], 12041[1], 12042[1], 12044[1], 12045[1], 12046[1], 12047[1], 12051[1], 12052[1], 12053[1], 12054[1], 12055[1], 12056[1], 12057[1], 13100[1], 13101[1], 13102[1], 13120[1], 13121[1], 13122[1], 13131[1], 13132[1], 13133[1], 13151[1], 13152[1], 13153[1], 36000[1], 36400[1], 36405[1], 36406[1], 36410[1], 36420[1], 36425[1], 36430[1], 36440[1], 36591[0], 36592[0], 36600[1], 36640[1], 43752[1], 44005[0], 44180[0], 44602[1], 44603[1], 44604[1], 44605[1], 44820[0], 44850[0], 44950[0], 44970[0], 49000[0], 49002[1], 49010[0], 49255[0], 49320[1], 49321[1], 51040[1], 51050[1], 51102[1], 51700[0], 51701[0], 51702[0], 51703[1], 51800[0], 52000[1], 52281[1], 52601[0], 52630[0], 52640[0], 52647[0], 52648[0], 53020[1], 53600[1], 53850[0], 53852[0], 53854[0], 55250[1], 55650[1], 55706[1], 55821[0], 55873[1], 55875[1], 55876[1], 55880[1], 62320[0], 62321[0], 62322[0], 62323[0], 62324[0], 62325[0], 62326[0], 62327[0], 64400[0], 64405[0], 64408[0], 64415[0], 64416[0], 64417[0], 64418[0], 64420[0], 64421[0], 64425[0], 64430[0], 64435[0], 64445[0], 64446[0], 64447[0], 64448[0], 64449[0], 64450[0], 64451[0], 64454[0], 64461[0], 64462[0], 64463[0], 64479[0], 64480[0], 64483[0], 64484[0], 64486[0], 64487[0], 64488[0], 64489[0], 64490[0], 64491[0], 64492[0], 64493[0], 64494[0], 64495[0], 64505[0], 64510[0], 64517[0], 64520[0], 64530[0], 69990[0], 92012[1], 92014[1], 93000[1], 93005[1], 93010[1], 93040[1], 93041[1], 93042[1], 93318[1], 93355[1], 94002[1], 94200[1], 94680[1], 94681[1], 94690[1], 95812[1], 95813[1], 95816[1], 95819[1], 95822[1], 95829[1], 95955[1], 96360[1], 96361[1], 96365[1], 96366[1], 96367[1], 96368[1], 96372[1], 96374[1], 96375[1], 96376[1], 96377[1], 96523[0], 97597[1], 97598[1], 97602[1], 99155[0], 99156[0], 99157[0], 99211[1], 99212[1], 99213[1], 99214[1], 99215[1], 99217[1], 99218[1], 99219[1], 99220[1], 99221[1], 99222[1], 99223[1], 99231[1], 99232[1], 99233[1], 99234[1], 99235[1], 99236[1], 99238[1], 99239[1], 99241[1], 99242[1], 99243[1], 99244[1], 99245[1], 99251[1], 99252[1], 99253[1], 99254[1], 99255[1], 99291[1], 99292[1], 99304[1], 99305[1], 99306[1], 99307[1], 99308[1], 99309[1], 99310[1], 99315[1], 99316[1], 99334[1], 99335[1], 99336[1], 99337[1], 99347[1], 99348[1], 99349[1], 99350[1], 99374[1], 99375[1], 99377[1], 99378[1], 99446[0], 99447[0], 99448[0], 99449[0], 99451[0], 99452[0], 99495[0], 99496[0], G0463[1], G0471[0]
55840	0213T[0], 0216T[0], 0421T[0], 0582T[0], 0596T[1], 0597T[1], 0655T[0], 0708T[1], 0709T[1], 11000[1], 11001[1], 11004[1], 11005[1], 11006[1], 11042[1], 11043[1], 11044[1], 11045[1], 11046[1], 11047[1], 12001[1], 12002[1], 12004[1], 12005[1], 12006[1], 12007[1], 12011[1], 12013[1], 12014[1], 12015[1], 12016[1], 12017[1], 12018[1], 12020[1], 12021[1], 12031[1], 12032[1], 12034[1], 12035[1], 12036[1], 12037[1], 12041[1], 12042[1], 12044[1], 12045[1], 12046[1], 12047[1], 12051[1], 12052[1], 12053[1], 12054[1], 12055[1], 12056[1], 12057[1], 13100[1], 13101[1], 13102[1], 13120[1], 13121[1], 13122[1], 13131[1], 13132[1], 13133[1], 13151[1], 13152[1], 13153[1], 36000[1], 36400[1], 36405[1], 36406[1], 36410[1], 36420[1], 36425[1], 36430[1], 36440[1], 36591[0], 36592[0], 36600[1], 36640[1], 38573[0], 43752[1], 44005[0], 44180[0], 44602[1], 44603[1], 44604[1], 44605[1], 44820[0], 44850[0], 44950[0], 44970[0], 49000[0], 49002[1], 49010[0], 49255[0], 51701[0], 51702[0], 51703[1], 51800[0], 52000[1], 52601[0], 52630[0], 52640[0], 52647[0], 52648[0], 53850[0], 53852[0], 53854[0], 55650[1], 55706[1], 55801[0], 55810[0], 55821[0], 55831[0], 55875[1], 55876[1], 62320[0], 62321[0], 62322[0], 62323[0], 62324[0], 62325[0], 62326[0], 62327[0], 64400[0], 64405[0], 64408[0], 64415[0], 64416[0], 64417[0], 64418[0], 64420[0], 64421[0], 64425[0], 64430[0], 64435[0], 64445[0], 64446[0], 64447[0], 64448[0], 64449[0], 64450[0], 64451[0], 64454[0], 64461[0], 64462[0], 64463[0], 64479[0], 64480[0], 64483[0], 64484[0], 64486[0], 64487[0], 64488[0], 64489[0], 64490[0], 64491[0], 64492[0], 64493[0], 64494[0], 64495[0], 64505[0], 64510[0], 64517[0], 64520[0], 64530[0], 69990[0], 92012[1], 92014[1], 93000[1], 93005[1], 93010[1], 93040[1], 93041[1], 93042[1], 93318[1], 93355[1], 94002[1], 94200[1], 94680[1], 94681[1], 94690[1], 95812[1], 95813[1], 95816[1], 95819[1], 95822[1], 95829[1], 95955[1], 96360[1], 96361[1], 96365[1], 96366[1], 96367[1], 96368[1], 96372[1], 96374[1], 96375[1], 96376[1], 96377[1], 96523[0], 97597[1], 97598[1], 97602[1], 99155[0], 99156[0], 99157[0], 99211[1], 99212[1], 99213[1],

0 = Modifier usage not allowed or inappropriate 1 = Modifier usage allowed

Code 1	Code 2
	99214[1], 99215[1], 99217[1], 99218[1], 99219[1], 99220[1], 99221[1], 99222[1], 99223[1], 99231[1], 99232[1], 99233[1], 99234[1], 99235[1], 99236[1], 99238[1], 99239[1], 99241[1], 99242[1], 99243[1], 99244[1], 99245[1], 99251[1], 99252[1], 99253[1], 99254[1], 99255[1], 99291[1], 99292[1], 99304[1], 99305[1], 99306[1], 99307[1], 99308[1], 99309[1], 99310[1], 99315[1], 99316[1], 99334[1], 99335[1], 99336[1], 99337[1], 99347[1], 99348[1], 99349[1], 99350[1], 99374[1], 99375[1], 99377[1], 99378[1], 99446[0], 99447[0], 99448[0], 99449[0], 99451[0], 99452[0], 99495[0], 99496[0], G0463[1], G0471[0]
55842	0213T[0], 0216T[0], 0421T[0], 0582T[0], 0596T[1], 0597T[1], 0600T[1], 0601T[1], 0655T[0], 0708T[1], 0709T[1], 10005[1], 10007[1], 10009[1], 10011[1], 10021[1], 11000[1], 11001[1], 11004[1], 11005[1], 11006[1], 11042[1], 11043[1], 11044[1], 11045[1], 11046[1], 11047[1], 12001[1], 12002[1], 12004[1], 12005[1], 12006[1], 12007[1], 12011[1], 12013[1], 12014[1], 12015[1], 12016[1], 12017[1], 12018[1], 12020[1], 12021[1], 12031[1], 12032[1], 12034[1], 12035[1], 12036[1], 12037[1], 12041[1], 12042[1], 12044[1], 12045[1], 12046[1], 12047[1], 12051[1], 12052[1], 12053[1], 12054[1], 12055[1], 12056[1], 12057[1], 13100[1], 13101[1], 13102[1], 13120[1], 13121[1], 13122[1], 13131[1], 13132[1], 13133[1], 13151[1], 13152[1], 13153[1], 36000[1], 36400[1], 36405[1], 36406[1], 36410[1], 36420[1], 36425[1], 36430[1], 36440[1], 36591[0], 36592[0], 36600[1], 36640[1], 38562[0], 38573[0], 43752[1], 44005[0], 44180[0], 44602[1], 44603[1], 44604[1], 44605[1], 44820[0], 44850[0], 44950[0], 44970[0], 49000[0], 49002[1], 49010[0], 49255[0], 49320[1], 51701[0], 51702[0], 51703[1], 51800[0], 52000[1], 52601[0], 52630[0], 52640[0], 52647[0], 52648[0], 53850[0], 53852[0], 53854[0], 55650[1], 55706[1], 55801[0], 55810[0], 55821[0], 55831[0], 55840[0], 55873[1], 55875[1], 55876[1], 55880[1], 62320[0], 62321[0], 62322[0], 62323[0], 62324[0], 62325[0], 62326[0], 62327[0], 64400[0], 64405[0], 64408[0], 64415[0], 64416[0], 64417[0], 64418[0], 64420[0], 64421[0], 64425[0], 64430[0], 64435[0], 64445[0], 64446[0], 64447[0], 64448[0], 64449[0], 64450[0], 64451[0], 64454[0], 64461[0], 64462[0], 64463[0], 64479[0], 64480[0], 64483[0], 64484[0], 64486[0], 64487[0], 64488[0], 64489[0], 64490[0], 64491[0], 64492[0], 64493[0], 64494[0], 64495[0], 64505[0], 64510[0], 64517[0], 64520[0], 64530[0], 69990[0], 92012[1], 92014[1], 93000[1], 93005[1], 93010[1], 93040[1], 93041[1], 93042[1], 93318[1], 93355[1], 94002[1], 94200[1], 94680[1], 94681[1], 94690[1], 95812[1], 95813[1], 95816[1], 95819[1], 95822[1], 95829[1], 95955[1], 96360[1], 96361[1], 96365[1], 96366[1], 96367[1], 96368[1], 96372[1], 96374[1], 96375[1], 96376[1], 96377[1], 96523[0], 97597[1], 97598[1], 97602[1], 99155[0], 99156[0], 99157[0], 99211[1], 99212[1], 99213[1], 99214[1], 99215[1], 99217[1], 99218[1], 99219[1], 99220[1], 99221[1], 99222[1], 99223[1], 99231[1], 99232[1], 99233[1], 99234[1], 99235[1], 99236[1], 99238[1], 99239[1], 99241[1], 99242[1], 99243[1], 99244[1], 99245[1], 99251[1], 99252[1], 99253[1], 99254[1], 99255[1], 99291[1], 99292[1], 99304[1], 99305[1], 99306[1], 99307[1], 99308[1], 99309[1], 99310[1], 99315[1], 99316[1], 99334[1], 99335[1], 99336[1], 99337[1], 99347[1], 99348[1], 99349[1], 99350[1], 99374[1], 99375[1], 99377[1], 99378[1], 99446[0], 99447[0], 99448[0], 99449[0], 99451[0], 99452[0], 99495[0], 99496[0], G0463[1], G0471[0]
55845	0213T[0], 0216T[0], 0421T[0], 0582T[0], 0596T[1], 0597T[1], 0600T[1], 0601T[1], 0655T[0], 0708T[1], 0709T[1], 11000[1], 11001[1], 11004[1], 11005[1], 11006[1], 11042[1], 11043[1], 11044[1], 11045[1], 11046[1], 11047[1], 12001[1], 12002[1], 12004[1], 12005[1], 12006[1], 12007[1], 12011[1], 12013[1], 12014[1], 12015[1], 12016[1], 12017[1], 12018[1], 12020[1], 12021[1], 12031[1], 12032[1], 12034[1], 12035[1], 12036[1], 12037[1], 12041[1], 12042[1], 12044[1], 12045[1], 12046[1], 12047[1], 12051[1], 12052[1], 12053[1], 12054[1], 12055[1], 12056[1], 12057[1], 13100[1], 13101[1], 13102[1], 13120[1], 13121[1], 13122[1], 13131[1], 13132[1], 13133[1], 13151[1], 13152[1], 13153[1], 27070[1], 36000[1], 36400[1], 36405[1], 36406[1], 36410[1], 36420[1], 36425[1], 36430[1], 36440[1], 36591[0], 36592[0], 36600[1], 36640[1], 38562[0], 38571[0], 38572[0], 38573[0], 38770[0], 38780[1], 43752[1], 44005[0], 44180[0], 44602[1], 44603[1], 44604[1], 44605[1], 44820[0], 44850[0], 44950[0], 44970[0], 49000[0], 49002[1], 49010[0], 49255[0], 49320[1], 49321[1], 51040[1], 51050[1], 51102[1], 51550[1], 51700[0], 51701[0], 51702[0], 51703[1], 51800[0], 52000[0], 52601[0], 52630[0], 52640[0], 52647[0], 52648[0], 53020[1], 53620[1], 53850[0], 53852[0], 53854[0], 55250[1], 55650[0], 55706[1], 55801[0], 55810[0], 55812[0], 55821[0], 55831[0], 55840[0], 55842[0], 55866[0], 55873[1], 55875[1], 55876[0], 55880[1], 62320[0], 62321[0], 62322[0], 62323[0], 62324[0], 62325[0], 62326[0], 62327[0], 64400[0], 64405[0], 64408[0], 64415[0], 64416[0], 64417[0], 64418[0], 64420[0], 64421[0], 64425[0], 64430[0], 64435[0], 64445[0], 64446[0], 64447[0], 64448[0], 64449[0], 64450[0], 64451[0], 64454[0], 64461[0], 64462[0], 64463[0], 64479[0], 64480[0], 64483[0], 64484[0], 64486[0], 64487[0], 64488[0], 64489[0], 64490[0], 64491[0], 64492[0], 64493[0], 64494[0], 64495[0], 64505[0], 64510[0], 64517[0], 64520[0], 64530[0], 69990[0], 92012[1], 92014[1], 93000[1], 93005[1], 93010[1], 93040[1], 93041[1], 93042[1], 93318[1], 93355[1], 94002[1], 94200[1], 94680[1], 94681[1], 94690[1], 95812[1], 95813[1], 95816[1], 95819[1], 95822[1], 95829[1], 95955[1], 96360[1], 96361[1], 96365[1], 96366[1], 96367[1], 96368[1], 96372[1], 96374[1], 96375[1], 96376[1], 96377[1], 96523[0], 97597[1], 97598[1], 97602[1], 99155[0], 99156[0], 99157[0], 99211[1], 99212[1], 99213[1], 99214[1], 99215[1], 99217[1], 99218[1], 99219[1], 99220[1], 99221[1], 99222[1], 99223[1], 99231[1], 99232[1], 99233[1], 99234[1], 99235[1], 99236[1], 99238[1], 99239[1], 99241[1], 99242[1], 99243[1], 99244[1], 99245[1], 99251[1], 99252[1], 99253[1], 99254[1], 99255[1], 99291[1], 99292[1], 99304[1], 99305[1], 99306[1], 99307[1], 99308[1], 99309[1], 99310[1], 99315[1], 99316[1], 99334[1], 99335[1], 99336[1], 99337[1], 99347[1], 99348[1], 99349[1], 99350[1], 99374[1], 99375[1], 99377[1], 99378[1], 99446[0], 99447[0], 99448[0], 99449[0], 99451[0], 99452[0], 99495[0], 99496[0], G0463[1], G0471[0]
55860	0213T[0], 0216T[0], 0596T[1], 0597T[1], 0600T[1], 0601T[1], 0708T[1], 0709T[1], 11000[1], 11001[1], 11004[1], 11005[1], 11006[1], 11042[1], 11043[1], 11044[1], 11045[1], 11046[1], 11047[1], 12001[1], 12002[1], 12004[1], 12005[1], 12006[1], 12007[1], 12011[1], 12013[1], 12014[1], 12015[1], 12016[1], 12017[1], 12018[1], 12020[1], 12021[1], 12031[1], 12032[1], 12034[1], 12035[1], 12036[1], 12037[1], 12041[1], 12042[1], 12044[1], 12045[1], 12046[1], 12047[1], 12051[1], 12052[1], 12053[1], 12054[1], 12055[1], 12056[1], 12057[1], 13100[1], 13101[1], 13102[1], 13120[1], 13121[1], 13122[1], 13131[1], 13132[1], 13133[1], 13151[1], 13152[1], 13153[1], 36000[1], 36400[1], 36405[1], 36406[1], 36410[1], 36420[1], 36425[1], 36430[1], 36440[1], 36591[0], 36592[0], 36600[1], 36640[1], 43752[1], 44602[1], 44603[1], 44604[1], 44605[1], 44950[0], 44970[0], 49000[0], 49002[1], 49320[1], 51701[0], 51702[0], 51703[1], 55873[1], 55875[1], 55880[1], 62320[0], 62321[0], 62322[0], 62323[0], 62324[0], 62325[0], 62326[0], 62327[0], 64400[0], 64405[0], 64408[0], 64415[0], 64416[0], 64417[0], 64418[0], 64420[0], 64421[0], 64425[0], 64430[0], 64435[0], 64445[0], 64446[0], 64447[0], 64448[0], 64449[0], 64450[0], 64451[0], 64454[0], 64461[0], 64462[0], 64463[0], 64479[0], 64480[0], 64483[0], 64484[0], 64486[0], 64487[0], 64488[0], 64489[0], 64490[0], 64491[0], 64492[0], 64493[0], 64494[0], 64495[0], 64505[0], 64510[0], 64517[0], 64520[0], 64530[0], 69990[0], 92012[1], 92014[1], 93000[1], 93005[1], 93010[1], 93040[1], 93041[1], 93042[1], 93318[1], 93355[1], 94002[1], 94200[1], 94680[1], 94681[1], 94690[1], 95812[1], 95813[1], 95816[1], 95819[1], 95822[1], 95829[1], 95955[1], 96360[1], 96361[1], 96365[1], 96366[1], 96367[1], 96368[1], 96372[1], 96374[1], 96375[1], 96376[1], 96377[1], 96523[0], 97597[1], 97598[1], 97602[1], 99155[0], 99156[0], 99157[0], 99211[1], 99212[1], 99213[1], 99214[1], 99215[1], 99217[1], 99218[1], 99219[1], 99220[1], 99221[1], 99222[1], 99223[1], 99231[1], 99232[1], 99233[1], 99234[1], 99235[1], 99236[1], 99238[1], 99239[1], 99241[1], 99242[1], 99243[1], 99244[1], 99245[1], 99251[1], 99252[1], 99253[1], 99254[1], 99255[1], 99291[1], 99292[1], 99304[1], 99305[1], 99306[1], 99307[1], 99308[1], 99309[1], 99310[1], 99315[1], 99316[1], 99334[1], 99335[1], 99336[1], 99337[1], 99347[1], 99348[1], 99349[1], 99350[1], 99374[1], 99375[1], 99377[1], 99378[1], 99446[0], 99447[0], 99448[0], 99449[0], 99451[0], 99452[0], 99495[0], 99496[0], G0463[1], G0471[0]
55862	0213T[0], 0216T[0], 0596T[1], 0597T[1], 0708T[1], 0709T[1], 10005[1], 10007[1], 10009[1], 10011[1], 10021[1], 11000[1], 11001[1], 11004[1], 11005[1], 11006[1], 11042[1], 11043[1], 11044[1], 11045[1], 11046[1], 11047[1], 12001[1], 12002[1], 12004[1], 12005[1], 12006[1], 12007[1], 12011[1], 12013[1], 12014[1], 12015[1], 12016[1], 12017[1], 12018[1], 12020[1], 12021[1], 12031[1], 12032[1], 12034[1], 12035[1], 12036[1], 12037[1], 12041[1], 12042[1], 12044[1], 12045[1], 12046[1], 12047[1], 12051[1], 12052[1], 12053[1], 12054[1], 12055[1], 12056[1], 12057[1], 13100[1], 13101[1], 13102[1], 13120[1], 13121[1], 13122[1], 13131[1], 13132[1], 13133[1], 13151[1], 13152[1], 13153[1], 36000[1], 36400[1], 36405[1], 36406[1], 36410[1], 36420[1], 36425[1], 36430[1], 36440[1], 36591[0], 36592[0], 36600[1], 36640[1], 38562[0], 43752[1], 44602[1], 44603[1], 44604[1], 44605[1], 44950[0], 44970[0], 49000[0], 49002[1], 49320[1], 49321[1], 51701[0], 51702[0], 51703[1], 55860[1], 55875[1], 62320[0], 62321[0], 62322[0], 62323[0], 62324[0], 62325[0], 62326[0], 62327[0], 64400[0], 64405[0], 64408[0], 64415[0], 64416[0], 64417[0], 64418[0], 64420[0], 64421[0], 64425[0], 64430[0], 64435[0], 64445[0], 64446[0], 64447[0], 64448[0], 64449[0], 64450[0], 64451[0], 64454[0], 64461[0], 64462[0], 64463[0], 64479[0], 64480[0], 64483[0], 64484[0], 64486[0], 64487[0], 64488[0], 64489[0], 64490[0], 64491[0], 64492[0], 64493[0], 64494[0], 64495[0], 64505[0], 64510[0], 64517[0], 64520[0], 64530[0], 69990[0], 92012[1], 92014[1], 93000[1], 93005[1], 93010[1], 93040[1], 93041[1], 93042[1], 93318[1], 93355[1], 94002[1], 94200[1], 94680[1], 94681[1], 94690[1], 95812[1], 95813[1], 95816[1], 95819[1], 95822[1], 95829[1], 95955[1], 96360[1], 96361[1], 96365[1], 96366[1], 96367[1], 96368[1], 96372[1], 96374[1], 96375[1], 96376[1], 96377[1], 96523[0], 97597[1], 97598[1], 97602[1], 99155[0], 99156[0], 99157[0], 99211[1], 99212[1], 99213[1], 99214[1], 99215[1], 99217[1], 99218[1], 99219[1], 99220[1], 99221[1], 99222[1], 99223[1], 99231[1], 99232[1], 99233[1], 99234[1], 99235[1], 99236[1], 99238[1], 99239[1], 99241[1], 99242[1], 99243[1], 99244[1], 99245[1], 99251[1], 99252[1], 99253[1], 99254[1], 99255[1], 99291[1], 99292[1], 99304[1], 99305[1], 99306[1], 99307[1], 99308[1], 99309[1], 99310[1], 99315[1], 99316[1], 99334[1], 99335[1], 99336[1], 99337[1], 99347[1], 99348[1], 99349[1], 99350[1], 99374[1], 99375[1], 99377[1], 99378[1], 99446[0], 99447[0], 99448[0], 99449[0], 99451[0], 99452[0], 99495[0], 99496[0], G0463[1], G0471[0]
55865	0213T[0], 0216T[0], 0596T[1], 0597T[1], 0600T[1], 0601T[1], 0708T[1], 0709T[1], 11000[1], 11001[1], 11004[1], 11005[1], 11006[1], 11042[1], 11043[1], 11044[1], 11045[1], 11046[1], 11047[1], 12001[1], 12002[1], 12004[1], 12005[1], 12006[1], 12007[1], 12011[1], 12013[1], 12014[1], 12015[1], 12016[1], 12017[1], 12018[1], 12020[1], 12021[1], 12031[1], 12032[1], 12034[1], 12035[1], 12036[1], 12037[1], 12041[1], 12042[1], 12044[1], 12045[1], 12046[1], 12047[1], 12051[1], 12052[1], 12053[1], 12054[1], 12055[1], 12056[1], 12057[1], 13100[1], 13101[1], 13102[1], 13120[1], 13121[1], 13122[1], 13131[1], 13132[1], 13133[1], 13151[1], 13152[1], 13153[1], 36000[1], 36400[1], 36405[1], 36406[1], 36410[1], 36420[1], 36425[1], 36430[1], 36440[1], 36591[0], 36592[0], 36600[1], 36640[1], 38562[0], 38571[1], 38572[1], 38573[0], 38770[0], 38780[1], 43752[1], 44005[0], 44180[0], 44602[1], 44603[1], 44604[1], 44605[1], 44820[0], 44850[0], 44950[0], 44970[0], 49000[0], 49002[1], 49010[0], 49255[0], 49320[1], 49321[1], 51701[0], 51702[0], 51703[1], 52000[1], 55860[1], 55862[1], 55873[1], 55880[1], 62320[0], 62321[0], 62322[0], 62323[0], 62324[0], 62325[0], 62326[0], 62327[0], 64400[0], 64405[0], 64408[0], 64415[0], 64416[0], 64417[0], 64418[0], 64420[0], 64421[0], 64425[0], 64430[0], 64435[0], 64445[0], 64446[0], 64447[0], 64448[0], 64449[0], 64450[0], 64451[0], 64454[0], 64461[0], 64462[0], 64463[0], 64479[0], 64480[0], 64483[0], 64484[0], 64486[0], 64487[0], 64488[0], 64489[0], 64490[0], 64491[0],

0 = Modifier usage not allowed or inappropriate 1 = Modifier usage allowed

Code 1	Code 2
	64492[0], 64493[0], 64494[0], 64495[0], 64505[0], 64510[0], 64517[0], 64520[0], 64530[0], 69990[0], 92012[1], 92014[1], 93000[1], 93005[1], 93010[1], 93040[1], 93041[1], 93042[1], 93318[1], 93355[1], 94002[1], 94200[1], 94680[1], 94681[1], 94690[1], 95812[1], 95813[1], 95816[1], 95819[1], 95822[1], 95829[1], 95955[1], 96360[1], 96361[1], 96365[1], 96366[1], 96367[1], 96368[1], 96372[1], 96374[1], 96375[1], 96376[1], 96377[1], 96523[0], 97597[1], 97598[1], 97602[1], 99155[0], 99156[0], 99157[0], 99211[1], 99212[1], 99213[1], 99214[1], 99215[1], 99217[1], 99218[1], 99219[1], 99220[1], 99221[1], 99222[1], 99223[1], 99231[1], 99232[1], 99233[1], 99234[1], 99235[1], 99236[1], 99238[1], 99239[1], 99241[1], 99242[1], 99243[1], 99244[1], 99245[1], 99251[1], 99252[1], 99253[1], 99254[1], 99255[1], 99291[1], 99292[1], 99304[1], 99305[1], 99306[1], 99307[1], 99308[1], 99309[1], 99310[1], 99315[1], 99316[1], 99334[1], 99335[1], 99336[1], 99337[1], 99347[1], 99348[1], 99349[1], 99350[1], 99374[1], 99375[1], 99377[1], 99378[1], 99446[0], 99447[0], 99448[0], 99449[0], 99451[0], 99452[0], 99495[0], 99496[0], G0463[1], G0471[0]
55866	0213T[0], 0216T[0], 0421T[1], 0596T[1], 0597T[1], 0600T[1], 0601T[1], 0708T[1], 0709T[1], 11000[1], 11001[1], 11004[1], 11005[1], 11006[1], 11042[1], 11043[1], 11044[1], 11045[1], 11046[1], 11047[1], 12001[1], 12002[1], 12004[1], 12005[1], 12006[1], 12007[1], 12011[1], 12013[1], 12014[1], 12015[1], 12016[1], 12017[1], 12018[1], 12020[1], 12021[1], 12031[1], 12032[1], 12034[1], 12035[1], 12036[1], 12037[1], 12041[1], 12042[1], 12044[1], 12045[1], 12046[1], 12047[1], 12051[1], 12052[1], 12053[1], 12054[1], 12055[1], 12056[1], 12057[1], 13100[1], 13101[1], 13102[1], 13120[1], 13121[1], 13122[1], 13131[1], 13132[1], 13133[1], 13151[1], 13152[1], 13153[1], 35840[1], 36000[1], 36400[1], 36405[1], 36406[1], 36410[1], 36420[1], 36425[1], 36430[1], 36440[1], 36591[0], 36592[0], 36600[1], 36640[1], 43653[0], 43752[1], 44005[0], 44180[0], 44602[1], 44603[1], 44604[1], 44605[1], 44950[0], 44970[1], 49082[1], 49083[1], 49084[1], 49320[0], 49321[1], 49400[0], 50715[1], 51701[0], 51702[0], 51703[1], 51800[0], 52000[1], 52601[0], 52630[1], 52640[1], 52647[1], 52648[1], 52649[1], 55700[1], 55705[1], 55706[1], 55801[0], 55810[0], 55812[0], 55821[0], 55831[0], 55840[0], 55842[0], 55860[1], 55862[1], 55865[1], 55873[1], 55875[1], 55876[1], 55880[1], 58660[0], 62320[0], 62321[0], 62322[0], 62323[0], 62324[0], 62325[0], 62326[0], 62327[0], 64400[0], 64405[0], 64408[0], 64415[0], 64416[0], 64417[0], 64418[0], 64420[0], 64421[0], 64425[0], 64430[0], 64435[0], 64445[0], 64446[0], 64447[0], 64448[0], 64449[0], 64450[0], 64451[0], 64454[0], 64461[0], 64462[0], 64463[0], 64479[0], 64480[0], 64483[0], 64484[0], 64486[0], 64487[0], 64488[0], 64489[0], 64490[0], 64491[0], 64492[0], 64493[0], 64494[0], 64495[0], 64505[0], 64510[0], 64517[0], 64520[0], 64530[0], 69990[0], 76000[1], 77001[1], 77002[1], 92012[1], 92014[1], 93000[1], 93005[1], 93010[1], 93040[1], 93041[1], 93042[1], 93318[1], 93355[1], 94002[1], 94200[1], 94680[1], 94681[1], 94690[1], 95812[1], 95813[1], 95816[1], 95819[1], 95822[1], 95829[1], 95955[1], 96360[1], 96361[1], 96365[1], 96366[1], 96367[1], 96368[1], 96372[1], 96374[1], 96375[1], 96376[1], 96377[1], 96523[0], 97597[1], 97598[1], 97602[1], 99155[0], 99156[0], 99157[0], 99211[1], 99212[1], 99213[1], 99214[1], 99215[1], 99217[1], 99218[1], 99219[1], 99220[1], 99221[1], 99222[1], 99223[1], 99231[1], 99232[1], 99233[1], 99234[1], 99235[1], 99236[1], 99238[1], 99239[1], 99241[1], 99242[1], 99243[1], 99244[1], 99245[1], 99251[1], 99252[1], 99253[1], 99254[1], 99255[1], 99291[1], 99292[1], 99304[1], 99305[1], 99306[1], 99307[1], 99308[1], 99309[1], 99310[1], 99315[1], 99316[1], 99334[1], 99335[1], 99336[1], 99337[1], 99347[1], 99348[1], 99349[1], 99350[1], 99374[1], 99375[1], 99377[1], 99378[1], 99446[0], 99447[0], 99448[0], 99449[0], 99451[0], 99452[0], 99495[0], 99496[0], G0463[1], G0471[0]
55870	0213T[0], 0216T[0], 0596T[1], 0597T[1], 0708T[1], 0709T[1], 12001[1], 12002[1], 12004[1], 12005[1], 12006[1], 12007[1], 12011[1], 12013[1], 12014[1], 12015[1], 12016[1], 12017[1], 12018[1], 12020[1], 12021[1], 12031[1], 12032[1], 12034[1], 12035[1], 12036[1], 12037[1], 12041[1], 12042[1], 12044[1], 12045[1], 12046[1], 12047[1], 12051[1], 12052[1], 12053[1], 12054[1], 12055[1], 12056[1], 12057[1], 13100[1], 13101[1], 13102[1], 13120[1], 13121[1], 13122[1], 13131[1], 13132[1], 13133[1], 13151[1], 13152[1], 13153[1], 36000[1], 36400[1], 36405[1], 36406[1], 36410[1], 36420[1], 36425[1], 36430[1], 36440[1], 36591[0], 36592[0], 36600[1], 36640[1], 43752[1], 51701[0], 51703[1], 62320[0], 62321[0], 62322[0], 62323[0], 62324[0], 62325[0], 62326[0], 62327[0], 64400[0], 64405[0], 64408[0], 64415[0], 64416[0], 64417[0], 64418[0], 64420[0], 64421[0], 64425[0], 64430[0], 64435[0], 64445[0], 64446[0], 64447[0], 64448[0], 64449[0], 64450[0], 64451[0], 64454[0], 64461[0], 64462[0], 64463[0], 64479[0], 64480[0], 64483[0], 64484[0], 64486[0], 64487[0], 64488[0], 64489[0], 64490[0], 64491[0], 64492[0], 64493[0], 64494[0], 64495[0], 64505[0], 64510[0], 64517[0], 64520[0], 64530[0], 69990[0], 92012[1], 92014[1], 93000[1], 93005[1], 93010[1], 93040[1], 93041[1], 93042[1], 93318[1], 93355[1], 94002[1], 94200[1], 94680[1], 94681[1], 94690[1], 95812[1], 95813[1], 95816[1], 95819[1], 95822[1], 95829[1], 95955[1], 96360[1], 96361[1], 96365[1], 96366[1], 96367[1], 96368[1], 96372[1], 96374[1], 96375[1], 96376[1], 96377[1], 96523[0], 99155[0], 99156[0], 99157[0], 99211[1], 99212[1], 99213[1], 99214[1], 99215[1], 99217[1], 99218[1], 99219[1], 99220[1], 99221[1], 99222[1], 99223[1], 99231[1], 99232[1], 99233[1], 99234[1], 99235[1], 99236[1], 99238[1], 99239[1], 99241[1], 99242[1], 99243[1], 99244[1], 99245[1], 99251[1], 99252[1], 99253[1], 99254[1], 99255[1], 99291[1], 99292[1], 99304[1], 99305[1], 99306[1], 99307[1], 99308[1], 99309[1], 99310[1], 99315[1], 99316[1], 99334[1], 99335[1], 99336[1], 99337[1], 99347[1], 99348[1], 99349[1], 99350[1], 99374[1], 99375[1], 99377[1], 99378[1], 99446[0], 99447[0], 99448[0], 99449[0], 99451[0], 99452[0], 99495[1], 99496[1], G0463[1]
55873	0213T[0], 0216T[0], 0421T[1], 0582T[1], 0596T[1], 0597T[1], 0619T[1], 0655T[1], 0708T[1], 0709T[1], 12001[1], 12002[1], 12004[1], 12005[1], 12006[1], 12007[1], 12011[1], 12013[1], 12014[1], 12015[1], 12016[1], 12017[1], 12018[1], 12020[1], 12021[1], 12031[1], 12032[1], 12034[1], 12035[1], 12036[1], 12037[1], 12041[1], 12042[1], 12044[1], 12045[1], 12046[1], 12047[1], 12051[1], 12052[1], 12053[1], 12054[1], 12055[1], 12056[1], 12057[1], 13100[1], 13101[1], 13102[1], 13120[1], 13121[1], 13122[1], 13131[1], 13132[1], 13133[1], 13151[1], 13152[1], 13153[1], 35840[1], 36000[1], 36400[1], 36405[1], 36406[1], 36410[1], 36420[1], 36425[1], 36430[1], 36440[1], 36591[0], 36592[0], 36600[1], 36640[1], 43752[1], 44005[1], 44820[1], 44850[1], 49000[0], 49010[0], 49255[1], 51040[1], 51050[1], 51102[1], 51700[1], 51701[1], 51702[1], 51703[1], 52000[0], 52270[1], 52275[1], 52281[1], 52450[1], 52500[1], 52649[1], 52700[1], 53020[1], 53080[1], 53600[1], 53601[1], 53605[1], 53620[1], 53621[1], 53660[1], 53661[1], 53665[1], 53854[1], 55250[1], 55706[1], 55801[1], 55810[1], 55840[1], 55862[1], 55875[1], 55876[1], 62320[0], 62321[0], 62322[0], 62323[0], 62324[0], 62325[0], 62326[0], 62327[0], 64400[0], 64405[0], 64408[0], 64415[0], 64416[0], 64417[0], 64418[0], 64420[0], 64421[0], 64425[0], 64430[0], 64435[0], 64445[0], 64446[0], 64447[0], 64448[0], 64449[0], 64450[0], 64451[0], 64454[0], 64461[0], 64462[0], 64463[0], 64479[0], 64480[0], 64483[0], 64484[0], 64486[0], 64487[0], 64488[0], 64489[0], 64490[0], 64491[0], 64492[0], 64493[0], 64494[0], 64495[0], 64505[0], 64510[0], 64517[0], 64520[0], 64530[0], 69990[0], 76380[1], 76872[1], 76940[0], 76942[0], 76998[1], 77013[0], 77022[0], 92012[1], 92014[1], 93000[1], 93005[1], 93010[1], 93040[1], 93041[1], 93042[1], 93318[1], 93355[1], 94002[1], 94200[1], 94680[1], 94681[1], 94690[1], 95812[1], 95813[1], 95816[1], 95819[1], 95822[1], 95829[1], 95955[1], 96360[1], 96361[1], 96365[1], 96366[1], 96367[1], 96368[1], 96372[1], 96374[1], 96375[1], 96376[1], 96377[1], 96523[0], 99155[0], 99156[0], 99157[0], 99211[1], 99212[1], 99213[1], 99214[1], 99215[1], 99217[1], 99218[1], 99219[1], 99220[1], 99221[1], 99222[1], 99223[1], 99231[1], 99232[1], 99233[1], 99234[1], 99235[1], 99236[1], 99238[1], 99239[1], 99241[1], 99242[1], 99243[1], 99244[1], 99245[1], 99251[1], 99252[1], 99253[1], 99254[1], 99255[1], 99291[1], 99292[1], 99304[1], 99305[1], 99306[1], 99307[1], 99308[1], 99309[1], 99310[1], 99315[1], 99316[1], 99334[1], 99335[1], 99336[1], 99337[1], 99347[1], 99348[1], 99349[1], 99350[1], 99374[1], 99375[1], 99377[1], 99378[1], 99446[0], 99447[0], 99448[0], 99449[0], 99451[0], 99452[0], 99495[0], 99496[0], G0463[1], G0471[1], J0670[1], J2001[1]
55874	0213T[0], 0216T[0], 0596T[1], 0597T[1], 0708T[1], 0709T[1], 12001[1], 12002[1], 12004[1], 12005[1], 12006[1], 12007[1], 12011[1], 12013[1], 12014[1], 12015[1], 12016[1], 12017[1], 12018[1], 12020[1], 12021[1], 12031[1], 12032[1], 12034[1], 12035[1], 12036[1], 12037[1], 12041[1], 12042[1], 12044[1], 12045[1], 12046[1], 12047[1], 12051[1], 12052[1], 12053[1], 12054[1], 12055[1], 12056[1], 12057[1], 13100[1], 13101[1], 13102[1], 13120[1], 13121[1], 13122[1], 13131[1], 13132[1], 13133[1], 13151[1], 13152[1], 13153[1], 36000[1], 36400[1], 36405[1], 36406[1], 36410[1], 36420[1], 36425[1], 36430[1], 36440[1], 36591[0], 36592[0], 36600[1], 36640[1], 43752[1], 51701[1], 51702[1], 51703[1], 62320[0], 62321[0], 62322[0], 62323[0], 62324[0], 62325[0], 62326[0], 62327[0], 64400[0], 64405[0], 64408[0], 64415[0], 64416[0], 64417[0], 64418[0], 64420[0], 64421[0], 64425[0], 64430[0], 64435[0], 64445[0], 64446[0], 64447[0], 64448[0], 64449[0], 64450[0], 64451[0], 64454[0], 64461[0], 64462[0], 64463[0], 64479[0], 64480[0], 64483[0], 64484[0], 64486[0], 64487[0], 64488[0], 64489[0], 64490[0], 64491[0], 64492[0], 64493[0], 64494[0], 64495[0], 64505[0], 64510[0], 64517[0], 64520[0], 64530[0], 69990[0], 76000[1], 76942[1], 76998[1], 77002[1], 77003[1], 77012[1], 77021[1], 92012[1], 92014[1], 93000[1], 93005[1], 93010[1], 93040[1], 93041[1], 93042[1], 93318[1], 94002[1], 94200[1], 94680[1], 94681[1], 94690[1], 95812[1], 95813[1], 95816[1], 95819[1], 95822[1], 95829[1], 95955[1], 96360[1], 96361[1], 96365[1], 96366[1], 96367[1], 96368[1], 96372[1], 96374[1], 96375[1], 96376[1], 96377[1], 96523[0], 99155[0], 99156[0], 99157[0], 99211[1], 99212[1], 99213[1], 99214[1], 99215[1], 99217[1], 99218[1], 99219[1], 99220[1], 99221[1], 99222[1], 99223[1], 99231[1], 99232[1], 99233[1], 99234[1], 99235[1], 99236[1], 99238[1], 99239[1], 99241[1], 99242[1], 99243[1], 99244[1], 99245[1], 99251[1], 99252[1], 99253[1], 99254[1], 99255[1], 99291[1], 99292[1], 99304[1], 99305[1], 99306[1], 99307[1], 99308[1], 99309[1], 99310[1], 99315[1], 99316[1], 99334[1], 99335[1], 99336[1], 99337[1], 99347[1], 99348[1], 99349[1], 99350[1], 99374[1], 99375[1], 99377[1], 99378[1]
55875	00860[0], 0213T[0], 0216T[0], 0596T[0], 0597T[0], 0708T[1], 0709T[1], 10035[1], 10036[1], 12001[1], 12002[1], 12004[1], 12005[1], 12006[1], 12007[1], 12011[1], 12013[1], 12014[1], 12015[1], 12016[1], 12017[1], 12018[1], 12020[1], 12021[1], 12031[1], 12032[1], 12034[1], 12035[1], 12036[1], 12037[1], 12041[1], 12042[1], 12044[1], 12045[1], 12046[1], 12047[1], 12051[1], 12052[1], 12053[1], 12054[1], 12055[1], 12056[1], 12057[1], 13100[1], 13101[1], 13102[1], 13120[1], 13121[1], 13122[1], 13131[1], 13132[1], 13133[1], 13151[1], 13152[1], 13153[1], 36000[1], 36400[1], 36405[1], 36406[1], 36410[1], 36420[1], 36425[1], 36430[1], 36440[1], 36591[0], 36592[0], 36600[1], 36640[1], 43752[1], 51701[0], 51702[0], 51703[0], 52000[0], 52250[0], 55920[1], 62320[0], 62321[0], 62322[0], 62323[0], 62324[0], 62325[0], 62326[0], 62327[0], 64400[0], 64405[0], 64408[0], 64415[0], 64416[0], 64417[0], 64418[0], 64420[0], 64421[0], 64425[0], 64430[0], 64435[0], 64445[0], 64446[0], 64447[0], 64448[0], 64449[0], 64450[0], 64451[0], 64454[0], 64461[0], 64462[0], 64463[0], 64479[0], 64480[0], 64483[0], 64484[0], 64486[0], 64487[0], 64488[0], 64489[0], 64490[0], 64491[0], 64492[0], 64493[0], 64494[0], 64495[0], 64505[0], 64510[0], 64517[0], 64520[0], 64530[0], 69990[0], 76942[1], 76998[1], 92012[1], 92014[1], 93000[1], 93005[1], 93010[1], 93040[1], 93041[1], 93042[1], 93318[1], 93355[1], 94002[1], 94200[1], 94680[1], 94681[1], 94690[1], 95812[1], 95813[1], 95816[1], 95819[1], 95822[1], 95829[1], 95955[1], 96360[1], 96361[1], 96365[1], 96366[1], 96367[1], 96368[1], 96372[1], 96374[1], 96375[1], 96376[1], 96377[1], 96523[0], 99155[0], 99156[0], 99157[0], 99211[1], 99212[1], 99213[1], 99214[1], 99215[1], 99217[1], 99218[1], 99219[1], 99220[1], 99221[1], 99222[1], 99223[1], 99231[1], 99232[1], 99233[1],

0 = Modifier usage not allowed or inappropriate   1 = Modifier usage allowed

Code 1	Code 2
	99234[1], 99235[1], 99236[1], 99238[1], 99239[1], 99241[1], 99242[1], 99243[1], 99244[1], 99245[1], 99251[1], 99252[1], 99253[1], 99254[1], 99255[1], 99291[1], 99292[1], 99304[1], 99305[1], 99306[1], 99307[1], 99308[1], 99309[1], 99310[1], 99315[1], 99316[1], 99334[1], 99335[1], 99336[1], 99337[1], 99347[1], 99348[1], 99349[1], 99350[1], 99374[1], 99375[1], 99377[1], 99378[1], 99446[0], 99447[0], 99448[0], 99449[0], 99451[0], 99452[0], 99495[0], 99496[0], G0463[1], G0471[0], P9612[0]
55876	00860[0], 0213T[0], 0216T[0], 0596T[1], 0597T[1], 0708T[1], 0709T[1], 10035[1], 10036[1], 12001[1], 12002[1], 12004[1], 12005[1], 12006[1], 12007[1], 12011[1], 12013[1], 12014[1], 12015[1], 12016[1], 12017[1], 12018[1], 12020[1], 12021[1], 12031[1], 12032[1], 12034[1], 12035[1], 12036[1], 12037[1], 12041[1], 12042[1], 12044[1], 12045[1], 12046[1], 12047[1], 12051[1], 12052[1], 12053[1], 12054[1], 12055[1], 12056[1], 12057[1], 13100[1], 13101[1], 13102[1], 13120[1], 13121[1], 13122[1], 13131[1], 13132[1], 13133[1], 13151[1], 13152[1], 13153[1], 36000[1], 36400[1], 36405[1], 36406[1], 36410[1], 36420[1], 36425[1], 36430[1], 36440[1], 36591[0], 36592[0], 36600[1], 36640[1], 43752[1], 49327[0], 49411[0], 49412[0], 51701[1], 51702[1], 51703[1], 62320[0], 62321[0], 62322[0], 62323[0], 62324[0], 62325[0], 62326[0], 62327[0], 64400[0], 64405[0], 64408[0], 64415[0], 64416[0], 64417[0], 64418[0], 64420[0], 64421[0], 64425[0], 64430[0], 64435[0], 64445[0], 64446[0], 64447[0], 64448[0], 64449[0], 64450[0], 64451[0], 64454[0], 64461[0], 64462[0], 64463[0], 64479[0], 64480[0], 64483[0], 64484[0], 64486[0], 64487[0], 64488[0], 64489[0], 64490[0], 64491[0], 64492[0], 64493[0], 64494[0], 64495[0], 64505[0], 64510[0], 64517[0], 64520[0], 64530[0], 69990[0], 76000[1], 76998[1], 92012[1], 92014[1], 93000[1], 93005[1], 93010[1], 93040[1], 93041[1], 93042[1], 93318[1], 93355[1], 94002[1], 94200[1], 94680[1], 94681[1], 94690[1], 95812[1], 95813[1], 95816[1], 95819[1], 95822[1], 95829[1], 95955[1], 96360[1], 96361[1], 96365[1], 96366[1], 96367[1], 96368[1], 96372[1], 96374[1], 96375[1], 96376[1], 96377[1], 96523[0], 99155[0], 99156[0], 99157[0], 99211[1], 99212[1], 99213[1], 99214[1], 99215[1], 99217[1], 99218[1], 99219[1], 99220[1], 99221[1], 99222[1], 99223[1], 99231[1], 99232[1], 99233[1], 99234[1], 99235[1], 99236[1], 99238[1], 99239[1], 99241[1], 99242[1], 99243[1], 99244[1], 99245[1], 99251[1], 99252[1], 99253[1], 99254[1], 99255[1], 99291[1], 99292[1], 99304[1], 99305[1], 99306[1], 99307[1], 99308[1], 99309[1], 99310[1], 99315[1], 99316[1], 99334[1], 99335[1], 99336[1], 99337[1], 99347[1], 99348[1], 99349[1], 99350[1], 99374[1], 99375[1], 99377[1], 99378[1], 99446[0], 99447[0], 99448[0], 99449[0], 99451[0], 99452[0], 99495[1], 99496[1], G0463[1], G0471[1], J0670[1], J2001[1]
55880	0213T[0], 0216T[0], 0421T[1], 0582T[1], 0655T[1], 0708T[1], 0709T[1], 12001[1], 12002[1], 12004[1], 12005[1], 12006[1], 12007[1], 12011[1], 12013[1], 12014[1], 12015[1], 12016[1], 12017[1], 12018[1], 12020[1], 12021[1], 12031[1], 12032[1], 12034[1], 12035[1], 12036[1], 12037[1], 12041[1], 12042[1], 12044[1], 12045[1], 12046[1], 12047[1], 12051[1], 12052[1], 12053[1], 12054[1], 12055[1], 12056[1], 12057[1], 13100[1], 13101[1], 13102[1], 13120[1], 13121[1], 13122[1], 13131[1], 13132[1], 13133[1], 13151[1], 13152[1], 13153[1], 35840[1], 36000[1], 36400[1], 36405[1], 36406[1], 36410[1], 36420[1], 36425[1], 36430[1], 36440[1], 36591[0], 36592[0], 36600[1], 36640[1], 43752[1], 44005[1], 44820[1], 44850[1], 49000[0], 49010[0], 49255[1], 51040[1], 51050[1], 51102[1], 51700[1], 51701[1], 51702[1], 51703[1], 52000[0], 52270[1], 52275[1], 52281[1], 52450[1], 52500[1], 52649[1], 52700[1], 53020[1], 53080[1], 53600[1], 53601[1], 53605[1], 53620[1], 53621[1], 53660[1], 53661[1], 53665[1], 53854[1], 55250[1], 55706[1], 55801[1], 55810[1], 55840[1], 55862[1], 55875[1], 55876[1], 62320[0], 62321[0], 62322[0], 62323[0], 62324[0], 62325[0], 62326[0], 62327[0], 64400[0], 64405[0], 64408[0], 64415[0], 64416[0], 64417[0], 64418[0], 64420[0], 64421[0], 64425[0], 64430[0], 64435[0], 64445[0], 64446[0], 64447[0], 64448[0], 64449[0], 64450[0], 64451[0], 64454[0], 64461[0], 64462[0], 64463[0], 64479[0], 64480[0], 64483[0], 64484[0], 64486[0], 64487[0], 64488[0], 64489[0], 64490[0], 64491[0], 64492[0], 64493[0], 64494[0], 64495[0], 64505[0], 64510[0], 64517[0], 64520[0], 64530[0], 69990[0], 76380[1], 76872[1], 76940[0], 76942[1], 76998[1], 77013[0], 77022[0], 92012[1], 92014[1], 93000[1], 93005[1], 93010[1], 93040[1], 93041[1], 93042[1], 93318[1], 93355[1], 94002[1], 94200[1], 94680[1], 94681[1], 94690[1], 95812[1], 95813[1], 95816[1], 95819[1], 95822[1], 95829[1], 95955[1], 96360[1], 96361[1], 96365[1], 96366[1], 96367[1], 96368[1], 96372[1], 96374[1], 96375[1], 96376[1], 96377[1], 96523[0], 99155[0], 99156[0], 99157[0], 99211[1], 99212[1], 99213[1], 99214[1], 99215[1], 99217[1], 99218[1], 99219[1], 99220[1], 99221[1], 99222[1], 99223[1], 99231[1], 99232[1], 99233[1], 99234[1], 99235[1], 99236[1], 99238[1], 99239[1], 99241[1], 99242[1], 99243[1], 99244[1], 99245[1], 99251[1], 99252[1], 99253[1], 99254[1], 99255[1], 99291[1], 99292[1], 99304[1], 99305[1], 99306[1], 99307[1], 99308[1], 99309[1], 99310[1], 99315[1], 99316[1], 99334[1], 99335[1], 99336[1], 99337[1], 99347[1], 99348[1], 99349[1], 99350[1], 99374[1], 99375[1], 99377[1], 99378[1], 99446[0], 99447[0], 99448[0], 99449[0], 99451[0], 99452[0], 99495[0], 99496[0], G0463[1], G0471[1], J0670[1], J2001[1]
55920	0213T[0], 0216T[0], 0347T[1], 0708T[1], 0709T[1], 10035[1], 10036[1], 12001[1], 12002[1], 12004[1], 12005[1], 12006[1], 12007[1], 12011[1], 12013[1], 12014[1], 12015[1], 12016[1], 12017[1], 12018[1], 12020[1], 12021[1], 12031[1], 12032[1], 12034[1], 12035[1], 12036[1], 12037[1], 12041[1], 12042[1], 12044[1], 12045[1], 12046[1], 12047[1], 12051[1], 12052[1], 12053[1], 12054[1], 12055[1], 12056[1], 12057[1], 13100[1], 13101[1], 13102[1], 13120[1], 13121[1], 13122[1], 13131[1], 13132[1], 13133[1], 13151[1], 13152[1], 13153[1], 20555[1], 36000[1], 36400[1], 36405[1], 36406[1], 36410[1], 36420[1], 36425[1], 36430[1], 36440[1], 36591[0], 36592[0], 36600[1], 36640[1], 43752[1], 57155[1], 57156[0], 58346[1], 62320[0], 62321[0], 62322[0], 62323[0], 62324[0], 62325[0], 62326[0], 62327[0], 64400[0], 64405[0], 64408[0], 64415[0], 64416[0], 64417[0], 64418[0], 64420[0], 64421[0], 64425[0], 64430[0], 64435[0], 64445[0], 64446[0], 64447[0], 64448[0], 64449[0], 64450[0], 64451[0], 64454[0], 64461[0], 64462[0], 64463[0], 64479[0], 64480[0], 64483[0], 64484[0], 64486[0], 64487[0], 64488[0], 64489[0], 64490[0], 64491[0], 64492[0], 64493[0], 64494[0], 64495[0], 64505[0], 64510[0], 64517[0], 64520[0], 64530[0], 69990[0], 92012[1], 92014[1], 93000[1], 93005[1], 93010[1], 93040[1], 93041[1], 93042[1], 93318[1], 93355[1], 94002[1], 94200[1], 94680[1], 94681[1], 94690[1], 95812[1], 95813[1], 95816[1], 95819[1], 95822[1], 95829[1], 95955[1], 96360[1], 96361[1], 96365[1], 96366[1], 96367[1], 96368[1], 96372[1], 96374[1], 96375[1], 96376[1], 96377[1], 96523[0], 99155[0], 99156[0], 99157[0], 99211[1], 99212[1], 99213[1], 99214[1], 99215[1], 99217[1], 99218[1], 99219[1], 99220[1], 99221[1], 99222[1], 99223[1], 99231[1], 99232[1], 99233[1], 99234[1], 99235[1], 99236[1], 99238[1], 99239[1], 99241[1], 99242[1], 99243[1], 99244[1], 99245[1], 99251[1], 99252[1], 99253[1], 99254[1], 99255[1], 99291[1], 99292[1], 99304[1], 99305[1], 99306[1], 99307[1], 99308[1], 99309[1], 99310[1], 99315[1], 99316[1], 99334[1], 99335[1], 99336[1], 99337[1], 99347[1], 99348[1], 99349[1], 99350[1], 99374[1], 99375[1], 99377[1], 99378[1], 99446[0], 99447[0], 99448[0], 99449[0], 99451[0], 99452[0], 99495[1], 99496[1], G0463[1]
57220	00940[0], 0213T[0], 0216T[0], 0596T[0], 0597T[0], 0708T[1], 0709T[1], 12001[1], 12002[1], 12004[1], 12005[1], 12006[1], 12007[1], 12011[1], 12013[1], 12014[1], 12015[1], 12016[1], 12017[1], 12018[1], 12020[1], 12021[1], 12031[1], 12032[1], 12034[1], 12035[1], 12036[1], 12037[1], 12041[1], 12042[1], 12044[1], 12045[1], 12046[1], 12047[1], 12051[1], 12052[1], 12053[1], 12054[1], 12055[1], 12056[1], 12057[1], 13100[1], 13101[1], 13102[1], 13120[1], 13121[1], 13122[1], 13131[1], 13132[1], 13133[1], 13151[1], 13152[1], 13153[1], 36000[1], 36400[1], 36405[1], 36406[1], 36410[1], 36420[1], 36425[1], 36430[1], 36440[1], 36591[0], 36592[0], 36600[1], 36640[1], 43752[1], 44950[0], 44970[0], 45560[1], 50715[1], 51701[0], 51702[0], 51703[0], 52000[1], 53000[0], 53010[0], 53020[0], 53025[0], 53200[1], 56810[0], 57000[1], 57061[1], 57065[1], 57100[0], 57105[1], 57150[0], 57180[0], 57210[1], 57268[0], 57410[0], 57420[0], 57452[0], 57500[1], 57800[1], 58100[0], 62320[0], 62321[0], 62322[0], 62323[0], 62324[0], 62325[0], 62326[0], 62327[0], 64400[0], 64405[0], 64408[0], 64415[0], 64416[0], 64417[0], 64418[0], 64420[0], 64421[0], 64425[0], 64430[0], 64435[0], 64445[0], 64446[0], 64447[0], 64448[0], 64449[0], 64450[0], 64451[0], 64454[0], 64461[0], 64462[0], 64463[0], 64479[0], 64480[0], 64483[0], 64484[0], 64486[0], 64487[0], 64488[0], 64489[0], 64490[0], 64491[0], 64492[0], 64493[0], 64494[0], 64495[0], 64505[0], 64510[0], 64517[0], 64520[0], 64530[0], 69990[0], 92012[1], 92014[1], 93000[1], 93005[1], 93010[1], 93040[1], 93041[1], 93042[1], 93318[1], 93355[1], 94002[1], 94200[1], 94680[1], 94681[1], 94690[1], 95812[1], 95813[1], 95816[1], 95819[1], 95822[1], 95829[1], 95955[1], 96360[1], 96361[1], 96365[1], 96366[1], 96367[1], 96368[1], 96372[1], 96374[1], 96375[1], 96376[1], 96377[1], 96523[0], 99155[0], 99156[0], 99157[0], 99211[1], 99212[1], 99213[1], 99214[1], 99215[1], 99217[1], 99218[1], 99219[1], 99220[1], 99221[1], 99222[1], 99223[1], 99231[1], 99232[1], 99233[1], 99234[1], 99235[1], 99236[1], 99238[1], 99239[1], 99241[1], 99242[1], 99243[1], 99244[1], 99245[1], 99251[1], 99252[1], 99253[1], 99254[1], 99255[1], 99291[1], 99292[1], 99304[1], 99305[1], 99306[1], 99307[1], 99308[1], 99309[1], 99310[1], 99315[1], 99316[1], 99334[1], 99335[1], 99336[1], 99337[1], 99347[1], 99348[1], 99349[1], 99350[1], 99374[1], 99375[1], 99377[1], 99378[1], 99446[0], 99447[0], 99448[0], 99449[0], 99451[0], 99452[0], 99495[0], 99496[0], G0463[1], G0471[0], P9612[0]
57230	00940[0], 0213T[0], 0216T[0], 0596T[0], 0597T[0], 0708T[1], 0709T[1], 12001[1], 12002[1], 12004[1], 12005[1], 12006[1], 12007[1], 12011[1], 12013[1], 12014[1], 12015[1], 12016[1], 12017[1], 12018[1], 12020[1], 12021[1], 12031[1], 12032[1], 12034[1], 12035[1], 12036[1], 12037[1], 12041[1], 12042[1], 12044[1], 12045[1], 12046[1], 12047[1], 12051[1], 12052[1], 12053[1], 12054[1], 12055[1], 12056[1], 12057[1], 13100[1], 13101[1], 13102[1], 13120[1], 13121[1], 13122[1], 13131[1], 13132[1], 13133[1], 13151[1], 13152[1], 13153[1], 36000[1], 36400[1], 36405[1], 36406[1], 36410[1], 36420[1], 36425[1], 36430[1], 36440[1], 36591[0], 36592[0], 36600[1], 36640[1], 43752[1], 44950[0], 44970[0], 45560[1], 50715[1], 51701[0], 51702[0], 51703[0], 52000[1], 53000[0], 53010[0], 53020[0], 53025[0], 53200[1], 53275[1], 53450[1], 53460[1], 56810[0], 57100[0], 57105[1], 57150[0], 57180[0], 57220[1], 57268[0], 57410[0], 57420[0], 57452[0], 57500[1], 57800[1], 58100[0], 62320[0], 62321[0], 62322[0], 62323[0], 62324[0], 62325[0], 62326[0], 62327[0], 64400[0], 64405[0], 64408[0], 64415[0], 64416[0], 64417[0], 64418[0], 64420[0], 64421[0], 64425[0], 64430[0], 64435[0], 64445[0], 64446[0], 64447[0], 64448[0], 64449[0], 64450[0], 64451[0], 64454[0], 64461[0], 64462[0], 64463[0], 64479[0], 64480[0], 64483[0], 64484[0], 64486[0], 64487[0], 64488[0], 64489[0], 64490[0], 64491[0], 64492[0], 64493[0], 64494[0], 64495[0], 64505[0], 64510[0], 64517[0], 64520[0], 64530[0], 69990[0], 92012[1], 92014[1], 93000[1], 93005[1], 93010[1], 93040[1], 93041[1], 93042[1], 93318[1], 93355[1], 94002[1], 94200[1], 94680[1], 94681[1], 94690[1], 95812[1], 95813[1], 95816[1], 95819[1], 95822[1], 95829[1], 95955[1], 96360[1], 96361[1], 96365[1], 96366[1], 96367[1], 96368[1], 96372[1], 96374[1], 96375[1], 96376[1], 96377[1], 96523[0], 99155[0], 99156[0], 99157[0], 99211[1], 99212[1], 99213[1], 99214[1], 99215[1], 99217[1], 99218[1], 99219[1], 99220[1], 99221[1], 99222[1], 99223[1], 99231[1], 99232[1], 99233[1], 99234[1], 99235[1], 99236[1], 99238[1], 99239[1], 99241[1], 99242[1], 99243[1], 99244[1], 99245[1], 99251[1], 99252[1], 99253[1], 99254[1], 99255[1], 99291[1], 99292[1], 99304[1], 99305[1], 99306[1], 99307[1], 99308[1], 99309[1], 99310[1], 99315[1], 99316[1], 99334[1], 99335[1], 99336[1], 99337[1], 99347[1], 99348[1], 99349[1], 99350[1], 99374[1], 99375[1], 99377[1], 99378[1], 99446[0], 99447[0], 99448[0], 99449[0], 99451[0], 99452[0], 99495[0], 99496[0], G0463[1], G0471[0], P9612[0]
57240	00940[0], 0213T[0], 0216T[0], 0437T[1], 0596T[0], 0597T[0], 0708T[1], 0709T[1], 12001[1], 12002[1], 12004[1], 12005[1], 12006[1], 12007[1], 12011[1], 12013[1], 12014[1], 12015[1], 12016[1], 12017[1],

0 = Modifier usage not allowed or inappropriate   1 = Modifier usage allowed

Code 1	Code 2
	12018[1], 12020[1], 12021[1], 12031[1], 12032[1], 12034[1], 12035[1], 12036[1], 12037[1], 12041[1], 12042[1], 12044[1], 12045[1], 12046[1], 12047[1], 12051[1], 12052[1], 12053[1], 12054[1], 12055[1], 12056[1], 12057[1], 13100[1], 13101[1], 13102[1], 13120[1], 13121[1], 13122[1], 13131[1], 13132[1], 13133[1], 13151[1], 13152[1], 13153[1], 15777[1], 36000[1], 36400[1], 36405[1], 36406[1], 36410[1], 36420[1], 36425[1], 36430[1], 36440[1], 36591[0], 36592[0], 36600[1], 36640[1], 43752[1], 44950[0], 44970[0], 49568[1], 50715[1], 51701[0], 51702[0], 51703[0], 52000[0], 53000[0], 53010[0], 53020[0], 53025[0], 56810[0], 57000[0], 57065[1], 57100[0], 57105[1], 57106[1], 57150[0], 57180[0], 57200[0], 57220[1], 57230[1], 57250[0], 57285[0], 57410[0], 57420[0], 57452[0], 57500[1], 57800[1], 58100[0], 62320[0], 62321[0], 62322[0], 62323[0], 62324[0], 62325[0], 62326[0], 62327[0], 64400[0], 64405[0], 64408[0], 64415[0], 64416[0], 64417[0], 64418[0], 64420[0], 64421[0], 64425[0], 64430[0], 64435[0], 64445[0], 64446[0], 64447[0], 64448[0], 64449[0], 64450[0], 64451[0], 64454[0], 64461[0], 64462[0], 64463[0], 64479[0], 64480[0], 64483[0], 64484[0], 64486[0], 64487[0], 64488[0], 64489[0], 64490[0], 64491[0], 64492[0], 64493[0], 64494[0], 64495[0], 64505[0], 64510[0], 64517[0], 64520[0], 64530[0], 69990[0], 92012[1], 92014[1], 93000[1], 93005[1], 93010[1], 93040[1], 93041[1], 93042[1], 93318[1], 93355[1], 94002[1], 94200[1], 94680[1], 94681[1], 94690[1], 95812[1], 95813[1], 95816[1], 95819[1], 95822[1], 95829[1], 95955[1], 96360[1], 96361[1], 96365[1], 96366[1], 96367[1], 96368[1], 96372[1], 96374[1], 96375[1], 96376[1], 96377[1], 96523[0], 99155[0], 99156[0], 99157[0], 99211[1], 99212[1], 99213[1], 99214[1], 99215[1], 99217[1], 99218[1], 99219[1], 99220[1], 99221[1], 99222[1], 99223[1], 99231[1], 99232[1], 99233[1], 99234[1], 99235[1], 99236[1], 99238[1], 99239[1], 99241[1], 99242[1], 99243[1], 99244[1], 99245[1], 99251[1], 99252[1], 99253[1], 99254[1], 99255[1], 99291[1], 99292[1], 99304[1], 99305[1], 99306[1], 99307[1], 99308[1], 99309[1], 99310[1], 99315[1], 99316[1], 99334[1], 99335[1], 99336[1], 99337[1], 99347[1], 99348[1], 99349[1], 99350[1], 99374[1], 99375[1], 99377[1], 99378[1], 99446[0], 99447[0], 99448[0], 99449[0], 99451[0], 99452[0], 99495[0], 99496[0], G0463[1], G0471[0], P9612[0]
57284	00940[0], 0213T[0], 0216T[0], 0596T[0], 0597T[0], 0708T[1], 0709T[1], 12001[1], 12002[1], 12004[1], 12005[1], 12006[1], 12007[1], 12011[1], 12013[1], 12014[1], 12015[1], 12016[1], 12017[1], 12018[1], 12020[1], 12021[1], 12031[1], 12032[1], 12034[1], 12035[1], 12036[1], 12037[1], 12041[1], 12042[1], 12044[1], 12045[1], 12046[1], 12047[1], 12051[1], 12052[1], 12053[1], 12054[1], 12055[1], 12056[1], 12057[1], 13100[1], 13101[1], 13102[1], 13120[1], 13121[1], 13122[1], 13131[1], 13132[1], 13133[1], 13151[1], 13152[1], 13153[1], 36000[1], 36400[1], 36405[1], 36406[1], 36410[1], 36420[1], 36425[1], 36430[1], 36440[1], 36591[0], 36592[0], 36600[1], 36640[1], 43653[0], 43752[1], 44005[0], 44180[0], 44602[1], 44603[1], 44604[1], 44605[1], 44820[1], 44850[1], 44950[0], 44970[0], 49000[0], 49002[1], 49010[0], 49255[0], 49320[0], 49570[1], 50715[1], 51701[0], 51702[0], 51703[0], 51715[1], 51840[0], 51841[0], 51990[0], 52000[0], 57100[0], 57240[0], 57260[0], 57268[0], 57270[0], 57285[0], 57410[0], 57420[0], 57423[0], 57452[0], 57500[1], 57800[1], 58100[0], 58660[0], 62320[0], 62321[0], 62322[0], 62323[0], 62324[0], 62325[0], 62326[0], 62327[0], 64400[0], 64405[0], 64408[0], 64415[0], 64416[0], 64417[0], 64418[0], 64420[0], 64421[0], 64425[0], 64430[0], 64435[0], 64445[0], 64446[0], 64447[0], 64448[0], 64449[0], 64450[0], 64451[0], 64454[0], 64461[0], 64462[0], 64463[0], 64479[0], 64480[0], 64483[0], 64484[0], 64486[0], 64487[0], 64488[0], 64489[0], 64490[0], 64491[0], 64492[0], 64493[0], 64494[0], 64495[0], 64505[0], 64510[0], 64517[0], 64520[0], 64530[0], 69990[0], 92012[1], 92014[1], 93000[1], 93005[1], 93010[1], 93040[1], 93041[1], 93042[1], 93318[1], 93355[1], 94002[1], 94200[1], 94680[1], 94681[1], 94690[1], 95812[1], 95813[1], 95816[1], 95819[1], 95822[1], 95829[1], 95955[1], 96360[1], 96361[1], 96365[1], 96366[1], 96367[1], 96368[1], 96372[1], 96374[1], 96375[1], 96376[1], 96377[1], 96523[0], 99155[0], 99156[0], 99157[0], 99211[1], 99212[1], 99213[1], 99214[1], 99215[1], 99217[1], 99218[1], 99219[1], 99220[1], 99221[1], 99222[1], 99223[1], 99231[1], 99232[1], 99233[1], 99234[1], 99235[1], 99236[1], 99238[1], 99239[1], 99241[1], 99242[1], 99243[1], 99244[1], 99245[1], 99251[1], 99252[1], 99253[1], 99254[1], 99255[1], 99291[1], 99292[1], 99304[1], 99305[1], 99306[1], 99307[1], 99308[1], 99309[1], 99310[1], 99315[1], 99316[1], 99334[1], 99335[1], 99336[1], 99337[1], 99347[1], 99348[1], 99349[1], 99350[1], 99374[1], 99375[1], 99377[1], 99378[1], 99446[0], 99447[0], 99448[0], 99449[0], 99451[0], 99452[0], 99495[0], 99496[0], G0463[1], G0471[0], P9612[0]
57285	00940[1], 0213T[0], 0216T[0], 0437T[1], 0596T[1], 0597T[1], 0708T[1], 0709T[1], 12001[1], 12002[1], 12004[1], 12005[1], 12006[1], 12007[1], 12011[1], 12013[1], 12014[1], 12015[1], 12016[1], 12017[1], 12018[1], 12020[1], 12021[1], 12031[1], 12032[1], 12034[1], 12035[1], 12036[1], 12037[1], 12041[1], 12042[1], 12044[1], 12045[1], 12046[1], 12047[1], 12051[1], 12052[1], 12053[1], 12054[1], 12055[1], 12056[1], 12057[1], 13100[1], 13101[1], 13102[1], 13120[1], 13121[1], 13122[1], 13131[1], 13132[1], 13133[1], 13151[1], 13152[1], 13153[1], 15777[1], 36000[1], 36400[1], 36405[1], 36406[1], 36410[1], 36420[1], 36425[1], 36430[1], 36440[1], 36591[0], 36592[0], 36600[1], 36640[1], 43752[1], 49568[1], 51701[1], 51702[1], 51703[1], 51840[0], 52000[0], 56810[0], 57020[1], 57100[0], 57150[0], 57180[0], 57268[0], 57400[1], 57410[1], 57415[0], 57420[1], 57423[1], 57452[1], 57500[1], 57530[1], 57800[1], 58100[1], 62320[0], 62321[0], 62322[0], 62323[0], 62324[0], 62325[0], 62326[0], 62327[0], 64400[0], 64405[0], 64408[0], 64415[0], 64416[0], 64417[0], 64418[0], 64420[0], 64421[0], 64425[0], 64430[0], 64435[0], 64445[0], 64446[0], 64447[0], 64448[0], 64449[0], 64450[0], 64451[0], 64454[0], 64461[0], 64462[0], 64463[0], 64479[0], 64480[0], 64483[0], 64484[0], 64486[0], 64487[0], 64488[0], 64489[0], 64490[0], 64491[0], 64492[0], 64493[0], 64494[0], 64495[0], 64505[0], 64510[0], 64517[0], 64520[0], 64530[0], 69990[0], 92012[1], 92014[1], 93000[1], 93005[1], 93010[1], 93040[1], 93041[1], 93042[1], 93318[1], 93355[1], 94002[1], 94200[1], 94680[1], 94681[1], 94690[1], 95812[1], 95813[1], 95816[1], 95819[1], 95822[1], 95829[1], 95955[1], 96360[1], 96361[1], 96365[1], 96366[1], 96367[1], 96368[1], 96372[1], 96374[1], 96375[1], 96376[1], 96377[1], 96523[0], 99155[0], 99156[0], 99157[0], 99211[1], 99212[1], 99213[1], 99214[1], 99215[1], 99217[1], 99218[1], 99219[1], 99220[1], 99221[1], 99222[1], 99223[1], 99231[1], 99232[1], 99233[1], 99234[1], 99235[1], 99236[1], 99238[1], 99239[1], 99241[1], 99242[1], 99243[1], 99244[1], 99245[1], 99251[1], 99252[1], 99253[1], 99254[1], 99255[1], 99291[1], 99292[1], 99304[1], 99305[1], 99306[1], 99307[1], 99308[1], 99309[1], 99310[1], 99315[1], 99316[1], 99334[1], 99335[1], 99336[1], 99337[1], 99347[1], 99348[1], 99349[1], 99350[1], 99374[1], 99375[1], 99377[1], 99378[1], 99446[0], 99447[0], 99448[0], 99449[0], 99451[0], 99452[0], 99495[0], 99496[0], G0463[1], G0471[1], P9612[1]
57287	00940[0], 0213T[0], 0216T[0], 0596T[1], 0597T[1], 0708T[1], 0709T[1], 11000[1], 11001[1], 11004[1], 11005[1], 11006[1], 11042[1], 11043[1], 11044[1], 11045[1], 11046[1], 11047[1], 12001[1], 12002[1], 12004[1], 12005[1], 12006[1], 12007[1], 12011[1], 12013[1], 12014[1], 12015[1], 12016[1], 12017[1], 12018[1], 12020[1], 12021[1], 12031[1], 12032[1], 12034[1], 12035[1], 12036[1], 12037[1], 12041[1], 12042[1], 12044[1], 12045[1], 12046[1], 12047[1], 12051[1], 12052[1], 12053[1], 12054[1], 12055[1], 12056[1], 12057[1], 13100[1], 13101[1], 13102[1], 13120[1], 13121[1], 13122[1], 13131[1], 13132[1], 13133[1], 13151[1], 13152[1], 13153[1], 36000[1], 36400[1], 36405[1], 36406[1], 36410[1], 36420[1], 36425[1], 36430[1], 36440[1], 36591[0], 36592[0], 36600[1], 36640[1], 43752[1], 44950[0], 44970[0], 50715[1], 51701[1], 51702[1], 51703[1], 51992[0], 52000[1], 53000[0], 53010[0], 53020[0], 53025[0], 57000[0], 57020[1], 57100[0], 57150[0], 57180[0], 57220[1], 57268[1], 57288[0], 57289[1], 57410[0], 57420[0], 57452[0], 57500[1], 57800[1], 58100[1], 58267[1], 62320[0], 62321[0], 62322[0], 62323[0], 62324[0], 62325[0], 62326[0], 62327[0], 64400[0], 64405[0], 64408[0], 64415[0], 64416[0], 64417[0], 64418[0], 64420[0], 64421[0], 64425[0], 64430[0], 64435[0], 64445[0], 64446[0], 64447[0], 64448[0], 64449[0], 64450[0], 64451[0], 64454[0], 64461[0], 64462[0], 64463[0], 64479[0], 64480[0], 64483[0], 64484[0], 64486[0], 64487[0], 64488[0], 64489[0], 64490[0], 64491[0], 64492[0], 64493[0], 64494[0], 64495[0], 64505[0], 64510[0], 64517[0], 64520[0], 64530[0], 69990[0], 92012[1], 92014[1], 93000[1], 93005[1], 93010[1], 93040[1], 93041[1], 93042[1], 93318[1], 93355[1], 94002[1], 94200[1], 94680[1], 94681[1], 94690[1], 95812[1], 95813[1], 95816[1], 95819[1], 95822[1], 95829[1], 95955[1], 96360[1], 96361[1], 96365[1], 96366[1], 96367[1], 96368[1], 96372[1], 96374[1], 96375[1], 96376[1], 96377[1], 96523[0], 97597[1], 97598[1], 97602[1], 99155[0], 99156[0], 99157[0], 99211[1], 99212[1], 99213[1], 99214[1], 99215[1], 99217[1], 99218[1], 99219[1], 99220[1], 99221[1], 99222[1], 99223[1], 99231[1], 99232[1], 99233[1], 99234[1], 99235[1], 99236[1], 99238[1], 99239[1], 99241[1], 99242[1], 99243[1], 99244[1], 99245[1], 99251[1], 99252[1], 99253[1], 99254[1], 99255[1], 99291[1], 99292[1], 99304[1], 99305[1], 99306[1], 99307[1], 99308[1], 99309[1], 99310[1], 99315[1], 99316[1], 99334[1], 99335[1], 99336[1], 99337[1], 99347[1], 99348[1], 99349[1], 99350[1], 99374[1], 99375[1], 99377[1], 99378[1], 99446[0], 99447[0], 99448[0], 99449[0], 99451[0], 99452[0], 99495[0], 99496[0], G0463[1], G0471[1], P9612[1]
57288	00940[0], 0213T[0], 0216T[0], 0596T[0], 0597T[0], 0708T[1], 0709T[1], 12001[1], 12002[1], 12004[1], 12005[1], 12006[1], 12007[1], 12011[1], 12013[1], 12014[1], 12015[1], 12016[1], 12017[1], 12018[1], 12020[1], 12021[1], 12031[1], 12032[1], 12034[1], 12035[1], 12036[1], 12037[1], 12041[1], 12042[1], 12044[1], 12045[1], 12046[1], 12047[1], 12051[1], 12052[1], 12053[1], 12054[1], 12055[1], 12056[1], 12057[1], 13100[1], 13101[1], 13102[1], 13120[1], 13121[1], 13122[1], 13131[1], 13132[1], 13133[1], 13151[1], 13152[1], 13153[1], 36000[1], 36400[1], 36405[1], 36406[1], 36410[1], 36420[1], 36425[1], 36430[1], 36440[1], 36591[0], 36592[0], 36600[1], 36640[1], 43752[1], 44950[0], 44970[0], 50715[1], 51701[0], 51702[0], 51703[0], 51992[0], 52000[0], 53000[0], 53010[0], 53020[0], 53025[0], 56810[0], 57000[0], 57100[0], 57150[0], 57180[0], 57220[1], 57267[1], 57268[0], 57289[1], 57410[0], 57420[0], 57452[0], 57500[1], 57800[1], 58100[0], 58267[1], 62320[0], 62321[0], 62322[0], 62323[0], 62324[0], 62325[0], 62326[0], 62327[0], 64400[0], 64405[0], 64408[0], 64415[0], 64416[0], 64417[0], 64418[0], 64420[0], 64421[0], 64425[0], 64430[0], 64435[0], 64445[0], 64446[0], 64447[0], 64448[0], 64449[0], 64450[0], 64451[0], 64454[0], 64461[0], 64462[0], 64463[0], 64479[0], 64480[0], 64483[0], 64484[0], 64486[0], 64487[0], 64488[0], 64489[0], 64490[0], 64491[0], 64492[0], 64493[0], 64494[0], 64495[0], 64505[0], 64510[0], 64517[0], 64520[0], 64530[0], 92012[1], 92014[1], 93000[1], 93005[1], 93010[1], 93040[1], 93041[1], 93042[1], 93318[1], 93355[1], 94002[1], 94200[1], 94680[1], 94681[1], 94690[1], 95812[1], 95813[1], 95816[1], 95819[1], 95822[1], 95829[1], 95955[1], 96360[1], 96361[1], 96365[1], 96366[1], 96367[1], 96368[1], 96372[1], 96374[1], 96375[1], 96376[1], 96377[1], 96523[0], 99155[0], 99156[0], 99157[0], 99211[1], 99212[1], 99213[1], 99214[1], 99215[1], 99217[1], 99218[1], 99219[1], 99220[1], 99221[1], 99222[1], 99223[1], 99231[1], 99232[1], 99233[1], 99234[1], 99235[1], 99236[1], 99238[1], 99239[1], 99241[1], 99242[1], 99243[1], 99244[1], 99245[1], 99251[1], 99252[1], 99253[1], 99254[1], 99255[1], 99291[1], 99292[1], 99304[1], 99305[1], 99306[1], 99307[1], 99308[1], 99309[1], 99310[1], 99315[1], 99316[1], 99334[1], 99335[1], 99336[1], 99337[1], 99347[1], 99348[1], 99349[1], 99350[1], 99374[1], 99375[1], 99377[1], 99378[1], 99446[0], 99447[0], 99448[0], 99449[0], 99451[0], 99452[0], 99495[0], 99496[0], G0463[1], G0471[0], P9612[0]
57289	00940[0], 0213T[0], 0216T[0], 0596T[0], 0597T[0], 0708T[1], 0709T[1], 12001[1], 12002[1], 12004[1], 12005[1], 12006[1], 12007[1], 12011[1], 12013[1], 12014[1], 12015[1], 12016[1], 12017[1], 12018[1], 12020[1], 12021[1], 12031[1], 12032[1], 12034[1], 12035[1], 12036[1], 12037[1], 12041[1], 12042[1], 12044[1], 12045[1], 12046[1], 12047[1], 12051[1], 12052[1], 12053[1], 12054[1], 12055[1], 12056[1],

Appendix A: NCCI - CPT Codes

0 = Modifier usage not allowed or inappropriate 1 = Modifier usage allowed

Code 1	Code 2
	12057[1], 13100[1], 13101[1], 13102[1], 13120[1], 13121[1], 13122[1], 13131[1], 13132[1], 13133[1], 13151[1], 13152[1], 13153[1], 36000[1], 36400[1], 36405[1], 36406[1], 36410[1], 36420[1], 36425[1], 36430[1], 36440[1], 36591[0], 36592[0], 36600[1], 36640[1], 43752[1], 44950[0], 44970[0], 50715[1], 51701[0], 51702[0], 51703[0], 51840[1], 52000[1], 56810[0], 57000[0], 57100[0], 57150[0], 57180[0], 57200[1], 57230[1], 57240[1], 57260[0], 57268[0], 57410[0], 57420[0], 57452[0], 57500[1], 57800[1], 58100[0], 62320[0], 62321[0], 62322[0], 62323[0], 62324[0], 62325[0], 62326[0], 62327[0], 64400[0], 64405[0], 64408[0], 64415[0], 64416[0], 64417[0], 64418[0], 64420[0], 64421[0], 64425[0], 64430[0], 64435[0], 64445[0], 64446[0], 64447[0], 64448[0], 64449[0], 64450[0], 64451[0], 64454[0], 64461[0], 64462[0], 64463[0], 64479[0], 64480[0], 64483[0], 64484[0], 64486[0], 64487[0], 64488[0], 64489[0], 64490[0], 64491[0], 64492[0], 64493[0], 64494[0], 64495[0], 64505[0], 64510[0], 64517[0], 64520[0], 64530[0], 69990[0], 92012[1], 92014[1], 93000[1], 93005[1], 93010[1], 93040[1], 93041[1], 93042[1], 93318[1], 93355[1], 94002[1], 94200[1], 94680[1], 94681[1], 94690[1], 95812[1], 95813[1], 95816[1], 95819[1], 95822[1], 95829[1], 95955[1], 96360[1], 96361[1], 96365[1], 96366[1], 96367[1], 96368[1], 96372[1], 96374[1], 96375[1], 96376[1], 96377[1], 96523[0], 99155[0], 99156[0], 99157[0], 99211[1], 99212[1], 99213[1], 99214[1], 99215[1], 99217[1], 99218[1], 99219[1], 99220[1], 99221[1], 99222[1], 99223[1], 99231[1], 99232[1], 99233[1], 99234[1], 99235[1], 99236[1], 99238[1], 99239[1], 99241[1], 99242[1], 99243[1], 99244[1], 99245[1], 99251[1], 99252[1], 99253[1], 99254[1], 99255[1], 99291[1], 99292[1], 99304[1], 99305[1], 99306[1], 99307[1], 99308[1], 99309[1], 99310[1], 99315[1], 99316[1], 99334[1], 99335[1], 99336[1], 99337[1], 99347[1], 99348[1], 99349[1], 99350[1], 99374[1], 99375[1], 99377[1], 99378[1], 99446[0], 99447[0], 99448[0], 99449[0], 99451[0], 99452[0], 99495[0], 99496[0], G0463[1], G0471[0], P9612[0]
57423	0213T[0], 0216T[0], 0596T[1], 0597T[1], 0708T[1], 0709T[1], 12001[1], 12002[1], 12004[1], 12005[1], 12006[1], 12007[1], 12011[1], 12013[1], 12014[1], 12015[1], 12016[1], 12017[1], 12018[1], 12020[1], 12021[1], 12031[1], 12032[1], 12034[1], 12035[1], 12036[1], 12037[1], 12041[1], 12042[1], 12044[1], 12045[1], 12046[1], 12047[1], 12051[1], 12052[1], 12053[1], 12054[1], 12055[1], 12056[1], 12057[1], 13100[1], 13101[1], 13102[1], 13120[1], 13121[1], 13122[1], 13131[1], 13132[1], 13133[1], 13151[1], 13152[1], 13153[1], 36000[1], 36400[1], 36405[1], 36406[1], 36410[1], 36420[1], 36425[1], 36430[1], 36440[1], 36591[0], 36592[0], 36600[1], 36640[1], 43752[1], 44180[0], 44602[1], 44603[1], 44604[1], 44605[1], 49082[1], 49083[1], 49084[1], 49320[0], 49400[0], 51701[1], 51702[1], 51703[1], 51840[1], 51841[1], 51990[1], 52000[0], 57180[0], 57240[1], 57260[1], 57265[0], 57410[1], 58660[0], 62320[0], 62321[0], 62322[0], 62323[0], 62324[0], 62325[0], 62326[0], 62327[0], 64400[0], 64405[0], 64408[0], 64415[0], 64416[0], 64417[0], 64418[0], 64420[0], 64421[0], 64425[0], 64430[0], 64435[0], 64445[0], 64446[0], 64447[0], 64448[0], 64449[0], 64450[0], 64451[0], 64454[0], 64461[0], 64462[0], 64463[0], 64479[0], 64480[0], 64483[0], 64484[0], 64486[0], 64487[0], 64488[0], 64489[0], 64490[0], 64491[0], 64492[0], 64493[0], 64494[0], 64495[0], 64505[0], 64510[0], 64517[0], 64520[0], 64530[0], 69990[0], 76000[1], 77001[1], 77002[1], 92012[1], 92014[1], 93000[1], 93005[1], 93010[1], 93040[1], 93041[1], 93042[1], 93318[1], 93355[1], 94002[1], 94200[1], 94680[1], 94681[1], 94690[1], 95812[1], 95813[1], 95816[1], 95819[1], 95822[1], 95829[1], 95955[1], 96360[1], 96361[1], 96365[1], 96366[1], 96367[1], 96368[1], 96372[1], 96374[1], 96375[1], 96376[1], 96377[1], 96523[0], 99155[0], 99156[0], 99157[0], 99211[1], 99212[1], 99213[1], 99214[1], 99215[1], 99217[1], 99218[1], 99219[1], 99220[1], 99221[1], 99222[1], 99223[1], 99231[1], 99232[1], 99233[1], 99234[1], 99235[1], 99236[1], 99238[1], 99239[1], 99241[1], 99242[1], 99243[1], 99244[1], 99245[1], 99251[1], 99252[1], 99253[1], 99254[1], 99255[1], 99291[1], 99292[1], 99304[1], 99305[1], 99306[1], 99307[1], 99308[1], 99309[1], 99310[1], 99315[1], 99316[1], 99334[1], 99335[1], 99336[1], 99337[1], 99347[1], 99348[1], 99349[1], 99350[1], 99374[1], 99375[1], 99377[1], 99378[1], 99446[0], 99447[0], 99448[0], 99449[0], 99451[0], 99452[0], 99495[0], 99496[0], G0463[1], G0471[1]
60540	0213T[0], 0216T[0], 0596T[1], 0597T[1], 0708T[1], 0709T[1], 10005[1], 10007[1], 10009[1], 10011[1], 10021[1], 11000[1], 11001[1], 11004[1], 11005[1], 11006[1], 11042[1], 11043[1], 11044[1], 11045[1], 11046[1], 11047[1], 12001[1], 12002[1], 12004[1], 12005[1], 12006[1], 12007[1], 12011[1], 12013[1], 12014[1], 12015[1], 12016[1], 12017[1], 12018[1], 12020[1], 12021[1], 12031[1], 12032[1], 12034[1], 12035[1], 12036[1], 12037[1], 12041[1], 12042[1], 12044[1], 12045[1], 12046[1], 12047[1], 12051[1], 12052[1], 12053[1], 12054[1], 12055[1], 12056[1], 12057[1], 13100[1], 13101[1], 13102[1], 13120[1], 13121[1], 13122[1], 13131[1], 13132[1], 13133[1], 13151[1], 13152[1], 13153[1], 36000[1], 36400[1], 36405[1], 36406[1], 36410[1], 36420[1], 36425[1], 36430[1], 36440[1], 36591[0], 36592[0], 36600[1], 36640[1], 43752[1], 44602[1], 44603[1], 44604[1], 44605[1], 49000[0], 49002[1], 49010[0], 51701[1], 51702[1], 51703[1], 60545[1], 60650[1], 62320[0], 62321[0], 62322[0], 62323[0], 62324[0], 62325[0], 62326[0], 62327[0], 64400[0], 64405[0], 64408[0], 64415[0], 64416[0], 64417[0], 64418[0], 64420[0], 64421[0], 64425[0], 64430[0], 64435[0], 64445[0], 64446[0], 64447[0], 64448[0], 64449[0], 64450[0], 64451[0], 64454[0], 64461[0], 64462[0], 64463[0], 64479[0], 64480[0], 64483[0], 64484[0], 64486[0], 64487[0], 64488[0], 64489[0], 64490[0], 64491[0], 64492[0], 64493[0], 64494[0], 64495[0], 64505[0], 64510[0], 64517[0], 64520[0], 64530[0], 69990[0], 92012[1], 92014[1], 93000[1], 93005[1], 93010[1], 93040[1], 93041[1], 93042[1], 93318[1], 93355[1], 94002[1], 94200[1], 94680[1], 94681[1], 94690[1], 95812[1], 95813[1], 95816[1], 95819[1], 95822[1], 95829[1], 95955[1], 96360[1], 96361[1], 96365[1], 96366[1], 96367[1], 96368[1], 96372[1], 96374[1], 96375[1], 96376[1], 96377[1], 96523[0], 97597[1], 97598[1], 97602[1], 99155[0], 99156[0], 99157[0], 99211[1], 99212[1], 99213[1], 99214[1], 99215[1], 99217[1], 99218[1], 99219[1], 99220[1], 99221[1], 99222[1], 99223[1], 99231[1], 99232[1], 99233[1], 99234[1], 99235[1], 99236[1], 99238[1], 99239[1], 99241[1], 99242[1], 99243[1], 99244[1], 99245[1], 99251[1], 99252[1], 99253[1], 99254[1], 99255[1], 99291[1], 99292[1], 99304[1], 99305[1], 99306[1], 99307[1], 99308[1], 99309[1], 99310[1], 99315[1], 99316[1], 99334[1], 99335[1], 99336[1], 99337[1], 99347[1], 99348[1], 99349[1], 99350[1], 99374[1], 99375[1], 99377[1], 99378[1], 99446[0], 99447[0], 99448[0], 99449[0], 99451[0], 99452[0], 99495[0], 99496[0], G0463[1], G0471[1]
60545	0213T[0], 0216T[0], 0596T[1], 0597T[1], 0708T[1], 0709T[1], 10005[1], 10007[1], 10009[1], 10011[1], 10021[1], 11000[1], 11001[1], 11004[1], 11005[1], 11006[1], 11042[1], 11043[1], 11044[1], 11045[1], 11046[1], 11047[1], 12001[1], 12002[1], 12004[1], 12005[1], 12006[1], 12007[1], 12011[1], 12013[1], 12014[1], 12015[1], 12016[1], 12017[1], 12018[1], 12020[1], 12021[1], 12031[1], 12032[1], 12034[1], 12035[1], 12036[1], 12037[1], 12041[1], 12042[1], 12044[1], 12045[1], 12046[1], 12047[1], 12051[1], 12052[1], 12053[1], 12054[1], 12055[1], 12056[1], 12057[1], 13100[1], 13101[1], 13102[1], 13120[1], 13121[1], 13122[1], 13131[1], 13132[1], 13133[1], 13151[1], 13152[1], 13153[1], 36000[1], 36400[1], 36405[1], 36406[1], 36410[1], 36420[1], 36425[1], 36430[1], 36440[1], 36591[0], 36592[0], 36600[1], 36640[1], 43752[1], 44602[1], 44603[1], 44604[1], 44605[1], 49000[0], 49002[1], 49010[0], 51701[1], 51702[1], 51703[1], 60650[1], 62320[0], 62321[0], 62322[0], 62323[0], 62324[0], 62325[0], 62326[0], 62327[0], 64400[0], 64405[0], 64408[0], 64415[0], 64416[0], 64417[0], 64418[0], 64420[0], 64421[0], 64425[0], 64430[0], 64435[0], 64445[0], 64446[0], 64447[0], 64448[0], 64449[0], 64450[0], 64451[0], 64454[0], 64461[0], 64462[0], 64463[0], 64479[0], 64480[0], 64483[0], 64484[0], 64486[0], 64487[0], 64488[0], 64489[0], 64490[0], 64491[0], 64492[0], 64493[0], 64494[0], 64495[0], 64505[0], 64510[0], 64517[0], 64520[0], 64530[0], 69990[0], 92012[1], 92014[1], 93000[1], 93005[1], 93010[1], 93040[1], 93041[1], 93042[1], 93318[1], 93355[1], 94002[1], 94200[1], 94680[1], 94681[1], 94690[1], 95812[1], 95813[1], 95816[1], 95819[1], 95822[1], 95829[1], 95955[1], 96360[1], 96361[1], 96365[1], 96366[1], 96367[1], 96368[1], 96372[1], 96374[1], 96375[1], 96376[1], 96377[1], 96523[0], 97597[1], 97598[1], 97602[1], 99155[0], 99156[0], 99157[0], 99211[1], 99212[1], 99213[1], 99214[1], 99215[1], 99217[1], 99218[1], 99219[1], 99220[1], 99221[1], 99222[1], 99223[1], 99231[1], 99232[1], 99233[1], 99234[1], 99235[1], 99236[1], 99238[1], 99239[1], 99241[1], 99242[1], 99243[1], 99244[1], 99245[1], 99251[1], 99252[1], 99253[1], 99254[1], 99255[1], 99291[1], 99292[1], 99304[1], 99305[1], 99306[1], 99307[1], 99308[1], 99309[1], 99310[1], 99315[1], 99316[1], 99334[1], 99335[1], 99336[1], 99337[1], 99347[1], 99348[1], 99349[1], 99350[1], 99374[1], 99375[1], 99377[1], 99378[1], 99446[0], 99447[0], 99448[0], 99449[0], 99451[0], 99452[0], 99495[0], 99496[0], G0463[1], G0471[1]
60650	0213T[0], 0216T[0], 0596T[1], 0597T[1], 0708T[1], 0709T[1], 10005[1], 10007[1], 10009[1], 10011[1], 10021[1], 11000[1], 11001[1], 11004[1], 11005[1], 11006[1], 11042[1], 11043[1], 11044[1], 11045[1], 11046[1], 11047[1], 12001[1], 12002[1], 12004[1], 12005[1], 12006[1], 12007[1], 12011[1], 12013[1], 12014[1], 12015[1], 12016[1], 12017[1], 12018[1], 12020[1], 12021[1], 12031[1], 12032[1], 12034[1], 12035[1], 12036[1], 12037[1], 12041[1], 12042[1], 12044[1], 12045[1], 12046[1], 12047[1], 12051[1], 12052[1], 12053[1], 12054[1], 12055[1], 12056[1], 12057[1], 13100[1], 13101[1], 13102[1], 13120[1], 13121[1], 13122[1], 13131[1], 13132[1], 13133[1], 13151[1], 13152[1], 13153[1], 35840[1], 36000[1], 36400[1], 36405[1], 36406[1], 36410[1], 36420[1], 36425[1], 36430[1], 36440[1], 36591[0], 36592[0], 36600[1], 36640[1], 43653[0], 43752[1], 44180[0], 44602[1], 44603[1], 44604[1], 44605[1], 44950[0], 44970[1], 49082[1], 49083[1], 49084[1], 49320[0], 49321[1], 49400[0], 50715[1], 51701[1], 51702[1], 51703[1], 58660[0], 62320[0], 62321[0], 62322[0], 62323[0], 62324[0], 62325[0], 62326[0], 62327[0], 64400[0], 64405[0], 64408[0], 64415[0], 64416[0], 64417[0], 64418[0], 64420[0], 64421[0], 64425[0], 64430[0], 64435[0], 64445[0], 64446[0], 64447[0], 64448[0], 64449[0], 64450[0], 64451[0], 64454[0], 64461[0], 64462[0], 64463[0], 64479[0], 64480[0], 64483[0], 64484[0], 64486[0], 64487[0], 64488[0], 64489[0], 64490[0], 64491[0], 64492[0], 64493[0], 64494[0], 64495[0], 64505[0], 64510[0], 64517[0], 64520[0], 64530[0], 69990[0], 76000[1], 77001[1], 77002[1], 92012[1], 92014[1], 93000[1], 93005[1], 93010[1], 93040[1], 93041[1], 93042[1], 93318[1], 93355[1], 94002[1], 94200[1], 94680[1], 94681[1], 94690[1], 95812[1], 95813[1], 95816[1], 95819[1], 95822[1], 95829[1], 95955[1], 96360[1], 96361[1], 96365[1], 96366[1], 96367[1], 96368[1], 96372[1], 96374[1], 96375[1], 96376[1], 96377[1], 96523[0], 97597[1], 97598[1], 97602[1], 99155[0], 99156[0], 99157[0], 99211[1], 99212[1], 99213[1], 99214[1], 99215[1], 99217[1], 99218[1], 99219[1], 99220[1], 99221[1], 99222[1], 99223[1], 99231[1], 99232[1], 99233[1], 99234[1], 99235[1], 99236[1], 99238[1], 99239[1], 99241[1], 99242[1], 99243[1], 99244[1], 99245[1], 99251[1], 99252[1], 99253[1], 99254[1], 99255[1], 99291[1], 99292[1], 99304[1], 99305[1], 99306[1], 99307[1], 99308[1], 99309[1], 99310[1], 99315[1], 99316[1], 99334[1], 99335[1], 99336[1], 99337[1], 99347[1], 99348[1], 99349[1], 99350[1], 99374[1], 99375[1], 99377[1], 99378[1], 99446[0], 99447[0], 99448[0], 99449[0], 99451[0], 99452[0], 99495[0], 99496[0], G0463[1], G0471[1]
64566	0333T[0], 0464T[0], 0588T[1], 0589T[0], 0590T[0], 0596T[1], 0597T[1], 0708T[1], 0709T[1], 12001[1], 12002[1], 12004[1], 12005[1], 12006[1], 12007[1], 12011[1], 12013[1], 12014[1], 12015[1], 12016[1], 12017[1], 12018[1], 12020[1], 12021[1], 12031[1], 12032[1], 12034[1], 12035[1], 12036[1], 12037[1], 12041[1], 12042[1], 12044[1], 12045[1], 12046[1], 12047[1], 12051[1], 12052[1], 12053[1], 12054[1], 12055[1], 12056[1], 12057[1], 13100[1], 13101[1], 13102[1], 13120[1], 13121[1], 13122[1], 13131[1], 13132[1], 13133[1], 13151[1], 13152[1], 13153[1], 36000[1], 36400[1], 36405[1], 36406[1], 36410[1], 36420[1], 36425[1], 36430[1], 36440[1], 36591[0], 36592[0], 36600[1], 36640[1], 43752[1], 51701[1], 51702[1], 51703[1], 62320[0], 62321[0], 62322[0], 62323[0], 62324[0], 62325[0], 62326[0], 62327[0], 64400[0], 64405[0], 64408[0], 64415[0], 64416[0], 64417[0], 64418[0], 64420[0], 64421[0], 64425[0],

0 = Modifier usage not allowed or inappropriate 1 = Modifier usage allowed

Code 1	Code 2
	64430[0], 64435[0], 64445[0], 64446[0], 64447[0], 64448[0], 64449[0], 64450[0], 64451[0], 64454[0], 64461[0], 64462[0], 64463[0], 64479[0], 64480[0], 64483[0], 64484[0], 64486[0], 64487[0], 64488[0], 64489[0], 64490[0], 64491[0], 64492[0], 64493[0], 64494[0], 64495[0], 64505[0], 64510[0], 64517[0], 64520[0], 64530[0], 64585[1], 69990[0], 76000[1], 76942[1], 76998[1], 77002[1], 92012[1], 92014[1], 92652[0], 92653[0], 93000[1], 93005[1], 93010[1], 93040[1], 93041[1], 93042[1], 93318[1], 93355[1], 94002[1], 94200[1], 94680[1], 94681[1], 94690[1], 95812[1], 95813[1], 95816[1], 95819[1], 95822[0], 95829[1], 95860[0], 95861[0], 95863[0], 95864[0], 95865[0], 95866[0], 95867[0], 95868[0], 95869[0], 95870[0], 95907[0], 95908[0], 95909[0], 95910[0], 95911[0], 95912[0], 95913[0], 95925[0], 95926[0], 95927[0], 95928[0], 95929[0], 95930[0], 95933[0], 95937[0], 95938[0], 95939[0], 95940[0], 95955[1], 95970[1], 95971[1], 95972[1], 96360[1], 96361[1], 96365[1], 96366[1], 96367[1], 96368[1], 96372[1], 96374[1], 96375[1], 96376[1], 96377[1], 96523[0], 99155[0], 99156[0], 99157[0], 99211[1], 99212[1], 99213[1], 99214[1], 99215[1], 99217[1], 99218[1], 99219[1], 99220[1], 99221[1], 99222[1], 99223[1], 99231[1], 99232[1], 99233[1], 99234[1], 99235[1], 99236[1], 99238[1], 99239[1], 99241[1], 99242[1], 99243[1], 99244[1], 99245[1], 99251[1], 99252[1], 99253[1], 99254[1], 99255[1], 99291[1], 99292[1], 99304[1], 99305[1], 99306[1], 99307[1], 99308[1], 99309[1], 99310[1], 99315[1], 99316[1], 99334[1], 99335[1], 99336[1], 99337[1], 99347[1], 99348[1], 99349[1], 99350[1], 99374[1], 99375[1], 99377[1], 99378[1], 99446[0], 99447[0], 99448[0], 99449[0], 99451[0], 99452[0], 99495[1], 99496[1], G0453[0], G0463[1], G0471[1], J0670[1], J2001[1]
64581	0213T[0], 0216T[0], 0333T[0], 0464T[0], 0589T[0], 0590T[0], 0596T[1], 0597T[1], 0708T[1], 0709T[1], 12001[1], 12002[1], 12004[1], 12005[1], 12006[1], 12007[1], 12011[1], 12013[1], 12014[1], 12015[1], 12016[1], 12017[1], 12018[1], 12020[1], 12021[1], 12031[1], 12032[1], 12034[1], 12035[1], 12036[1], 12037[1], 12041[1], 12042[1], 12044[1], 12045[1], 12046[1], 12047[1], 12051[1], 12052[1], 12053[1], 12054[1], 12055[1], 12056[1], 12057[1], 13100[1], 13101[1], 13102[1], 13120[1], 13121[1], 13122[1], 13131[1], 13132[1], 13133[1], 13151[1], 13152[1], 13153[1], 36000[1], 36400[1], 36405[1], 36406[1], 36410[1], 36420[1], 36425[1], 36430[1], 36440[1], 36591[0], 36592[0], 36600[1], 36640[1], 43752[1], 51701[1], 51702[1], 51703[1], 62320[0], 62321[0], 62322[0], 62323[0], 62324[0], 62325[0], 62326[0], 62327[0], 64400[0], 64405[0], 64408[0], 64415[0], 64416[0], 64417[0], 64418[0], 64420[0], 64421[0], 64425[0], 64430[0], 64435[0], 64445[0], 64446[0], 64447[0], 64448[0], 64449[0], 64450[0], 64451[0], 64454[0], 64461[0], 64462[0], 64463[0], 64479[0], 64480[0], 64483[0], 64484[0], 64486[0], 64487[0], 64488[0], 64489[0], 64490[0], 64491[0], 64492[0], 64493[0], 64494[0], 64495[0], 64505[0], 64510[0], 64517[0], 64520[0], 64530[0], 69990[0], 92012[1], 92014[1], 92652[0], 92653[0], 93000[1], 93005[1], 93010[1], 93040[1], 93041[1], 93042[1], 93318[1], 93355[1], 94002[1], 94200[1], 94680[1], 94681[1], 94690[1], 95812[1], 95813[1], 95816[1], 95819[1], 95822[0], 95829[1], 95860[0], 95861[0], 95863[0], 95864[0], 95865[0], 95866[0], 95867[0], 95868[0], 95869[0], 95870[0], 95907[0], 95908[0], 95909[0], 95910[0], 95911[0], 95912[0], 95913[0], 95925[0], 95926[0], 95927[0], 95928[0], 95929[0], 95930[0], 95933[0], 95937[0], 95938[0], 95939[0], 95940[0], 95955[1], 95970[1], 96360[1], 96361[1], 96365[1], 96366[1], 96367[1], 96368[1], 96372[1], 96374[1], 96375[1], 96376[1], 96377[1], 96523[0], 99155[0], 99156[0], 99157[0], 99211[1], 99212[1], 99213[1], 99214[1], 99215[1], 99217[1], 99218[1], 99219[1], 99220[1], 99221[1], 99222[1], 99223[1], 99231[1], 99232[1], 99233[1], 99234[1], 99235[1], 99236[1], 99238[1], 99239[1], 99241[1], 99242[1], 99243[1], 99244[1], 99245[1], 99251[1], 99252[1], 99253[1], 99254[1], 99255[1], 99291[1], 99292[1], 99304[1], 99305[1], 99306[1], 99307[1], 99308[1], 99309[1], 99310[1], 99315[1], 99316[1], 99334[1], 99335[1], 99336[1], 99337[1], 99347[1], 99348[1], 99349[1], 99350[1], 99374[1], 99375[1], 99377[1], 99378[1], 99446[0], 99447[0], 99448[0], 99449[0], 99451[0], 99452[0], 99495[0], 99496[0], G0453[0], G0463[1], G0471[1]

Appendix A: NCCI - CPT Codes

0 = Modifier usage not allowed or inappropriate 1 = Modifier usage allowed

Code 1	Code 2
G0102	36591[0], 36592[0], 96523[0], 99446[0], 99447[0], 99448[0], 99449[0], 99451[0], 99452[0], 99463[0]
G0103	84153[0], 84154[1]
G0491	0596T[1], 0597T[1], 0708T[1], 0709T[1], 12001[1], 12002[1], 12004[1], 12005[1], 12006[1], 12007[1], 12011[1], 12013[1], 12014[1], 12015[1], 12016[1], 12017[1], 12018[1], 12020[1], 12021[1], 12031[1], 12032[1], 12034[1], 12035[1], 12036[1], 12037[1], 12041[1], 12042[1], 12044[1], 12045[1], 12046[1], 12047[1], 12051[1], 12052[1], 12053[1], 12054[1], 12055[1], 12056[1], 12057[1], 13100[1], 13101[1], 13102[1], 13120[1], 13121[1], 13122[1], 13131[1], 13132[1], 13133[1], 13151[1], 13152[1], 13153[1], 36000[1], 36400[1], 36405[1], 36406[1], 36410[1], 36420[1], 36425[1], 36430[1], 36440[1], 36591[0], 36592[0], 36600[1], 36901[1], 36902[1], 36903[1], 36904[1], 36905[1], 36906[1], 36907[1], 36908[1], 36909[1], 43752[1], 51701[1], 51702[1], 51703[1], 62320[0], 62321[0], 62322[0], 62323[0], 62324[0], 62325[0], 62326[0], 62327[0], 64400[0], 64405[0], 64408[0], 64415[0], 64416[0], 64417[0], 64418[0], 64420[0], 64421[0], 64425[0], 64430[0], 64435[0], 64445[0], 64446[0], 64447[0], 64448[0], 64449[0], 64450[0], 64451[0], 64454[0], 64461[0], 64462[0], 64463[0], 64479[0], 64480[0], 64483[0], 64484[0], 64486[0], 64487[0], 64488[0], 64489[0], 64490[0], 64491[0], 64492[0], 64493[0], 64494[0], 64495[0], 64505[0], 64510[0], 64517[0], 64520[0], 64530[0], 90997[1], 92012[1], 92014[1], 93000[1], 93005[1], 93010[1], 93040[1], 93041[1], 93042[1], 93318[1], 93355[1], 94002[1], 94200[1], 94680[1], 94681[1], 94690[1], 95812[1], 95813[1], 95816[1], 95819[1], 95822[1], 95829[1], 95955[1], 96360[1], 96361[1], 96365[1], 96366[1], 96367[1], 96368[1], 96372[1], 96374[1], 96375[1], 96376[1], 96377[1], 96523[0], 97802[0], 97803[0], 97804[0], 99155[0], 99156[0], 99157[0], 99202[1], 99203[1], 99204[1], 99205[1], 99211[1], 99212[1], 99213[1], 99214[1], 99215[1], 99217[0], 99218[0], 99219[0], 99220[0], 99221[1], 99222[1], 99223[1], 99224[0], 99225[0], 99226[0], 99231[0], 99232[0], 99233[0], 99234[0], 99235[0], 99236[0], 99238[1], 99239[1], 99241[1], 99242[1], 99243[1], 99244[1], 99245[1], 99251[1], 99252[1], 99253[1], 99254[1], 99255[1], 99281[0], 99282[0], 99283[0], 99284[0], 99285[0], 99291[1], 99292[1], 99304[0], 99305[0], 99306[0], 99307[0], 99308[0], 99309[0], 99310[0], 99315[0], 99316[0], 99318[0], 99324[0], 99325[0], 99326[0], 99327[0], 99328[0], 99334[0], 99335[0], 99336[0], 99337[0], 99341[0], 99342[0], 99343[0], 99344[0], 99345[0], 99347[0], 99348[0], 99349[0], 99350[0], 99354[0], 99355[0], 99356[0], 99357[0], 99358[0], 99359[0], 99360[0], 99374[1], 99375[1], 99377[1], 99378[1], 99415[0], 99416[0], 99446[0], 99447[0], 99448[0], 99449[0], 99451[0], 99452[0], 99455[0], 99456[0], 99460[0], 99461[0], 99462[0], 99463[0], 99464[0], 99465[0], 99466[0], 99467[0], 99468[0], 99469[0], 99471[0], 99472[0], 99475[0], 99476[0], 99477[0], 99478[0], 99479[0], 99480[0], 99483[1], 99485[0], 99495[1], 99496[1], 99497[1], G0270[0], G0271[0], G0380[1], G0381[1], G0382[1], G0383[1], G0384[1], G0406[1], G0407[1], G0408[1], G0425[1], G0426[1], G0427[1], G0463[1], G0471[1], G0508[1], G0509[1]
G0492	0596T[1], 0597T[1], 0708T[1], 0709T[1], 12001[1], 12002[1], 12004[1], 12005[1], 12006[1], 12007[1], 12011[1], 12013[1], 12014[1], 12015[1], 12016[1], 12017[1], 12018[1], 12020[1], 12021[1], 12031[1], 12032[1], 12034[1], 12035[1], 12036[1], 12037[1], 12041[1], 12042[1], 12044[1], 12045[1], 12046[1], 12047[1], 12051[1], 12052[1], 12053[1], 12054[1], 12055[1], 12056[1], 12057[1], 13100[1], 13101[1], 13102[1], 13120[1], 13121[1], 13122[1], 13131[1], 13132[1], 13133[1], 13151[1], 13152[1], 13153[1], 36000[1], 36400[1], 36405[1], 36406[1], 36410[1], 36420[1], 36425[1], 36430[1], 36440[1], 36591[0], 36592[0], 36600[1], 36901[1], 36902[1], 36903[1], 36904[1], 36905[1], 36906[1], 36907[1], 36908[1], 36909[1], 43752[1], 51701[1], 51702[1], 51703[1], 62320[0], 62321[0], 62322[0], 62323[0], 62324[0], 62325[0], 62326[0], 62327[0], 64400[0], 64405[0], 64408[0], 64415[0], 64416[0], 64417[0], 64418[0], 64420[0], 64421[0], 64425[0], 64430[0], 64435[0], 64445[0], 64446[0], 64447[0], 64448[0], 64449[0], 64450[0], 64451[0], 64454[0], 64461[0], 64462[0], 64463[0], 64479[0], 64480[0], 64483[0], 64484[0], 64486[0], 64487[0], 64488[0], 64489[0], 64490[0], 64491[0], 64492[0], 64493[0], 64494[0], 64495[0], 64505[0], 64510[0], 64517[0], 64520[0], 64530[0], 90997[1], 92012[1], 92014[1], 93000[1], 93005[1], 93010[1], 93040[1], 93041[1], 93042[1], 93318[1], 93355[1], 94002[1], 94200[1], 94680[1], 94681[1], 94690[1], 95812[1], 95813[1], 95816[1], 95819[1], 95822[1], 95829[1], 95955[1], 96360[1], 96361[1], 96365[1], 96366[1], 96367[1], 96368[1], 96372[1], 96374[1], 96375[1], 96376[1], 96377[1], 96523[0], 97802[0], 97803[0], 97804[0], 99155[0], 99156[0], 99157[0], 99202[1], 99203[1], 99204[1], 99205[1], 99211[1], 99212[1], 99213[1], 99214[1], 99215[1], 99217[0], 99218[0], 99219[0], 99220[0], 99221[1], 99222[1], 99223[1], 99224[0], 99225[0], 99226[0], 99231[0], 99232[0], 99233[0], 99234[0], 99235[0], 99236[0], 99238[1], 99239[1], 99241[1], 99242[1], 99243[1], 99244[1], 99245[1], 99251[1], 99252[1], 99253[1], 99254[1], 99255[1], 99281[0], 99282[0], 99283[0], 99284[0], 99285[0], 99291[1], 99292[1], 99304[0], 99305[0], 99306[0], 99307[0], 99308[0], 99309[0], 99310[0], 99315[0], 99316[0], 99318[0], 99324[0], 99325[0], 99326[0], 99327[0], 99328[0], 99334[0], 99335[0], 99336[0], 99337[0], 99341[0], 99342[0], 99343[0], 99344[0], 99345[0], 99347[0], 99348[0], 99349[0], 99350[0], 99354[0], 99355[0], 99356[0], 99357[0], 99358[0], 99359[0], 99360[0], 99374[1], 99375[1], 99377[1], 99378[1], 99415[0], 99416[0], 99446[0], 99447[0], 99448[0], 99449[0], 99451[0], 99452[0], 99455[0], 99456[0], 99460[0], 99461[0], 99462[0], 99463[0], 99464[0], 99465[0], 99466[0], 99467[0], 99468[0], 99469[0], 99471[0], 99472[0], 99475[0], 99476[0], 99477[0], 99478[0], 99479[0], 99480[0], 99483[1], 99485[0], 99495[1], 99496[1], 99497[1], G0270[0], G0271[0], G0380[1], G0381[1], G0382[1], G0383[1], G0384[1], G0406[1], G0407[1], G0408[1], G0425[1], G0426[1], G0427[1], G0463[1], G0471[1], G0508[1], G0509[1]

0 = Modifier usage not allowed or inappropriate 1 = Modifier usage allowed

APPENDIX B

Clinical Documentation Checklists

Introduction

Appendix B provides checklists for common diagnoses and other conditions which are designed to be used for review of current records to help identify any documentation deficiencies. The checklists begin with the applicable ICD-10-CM categories, subcategories, and/or codes being covered. Definitions and other information pertinent to coding the condition are then provided. This is followed by a checklist that identifies each element needed for assignment of the most specific code. If one or more of the required elements are not documented, this information should be shared with the physician and a corrective action plan initiated to ensure that the necessary information is captured in the future.

Similar documentation and coding checklists for conditions not addressed in this book can be created using the checklists provided as a template. There are a few different formats and styles of checklists so users can determine which style works best for their practice and then create additional checklists using that format and style.

Undescended/Retractile Testes

ICD-10-CM Categories/Codes

Q53	Undescended and ectopic testicle
Q55.22	Retractile testis

ICD-10-CM Definitions

Abdominal testis – An undescended testis that does not descend into the scrotum before birth, remaining instead in the retroperitoneum or abdomen which is where the testes originate during fetal development.

Cryptorchidism (undescended testis) – Congenital anomaly in which one or both testes do not descend into the normal position in the scrotum before birth.

Ectopic testis – Variant of undescended testis in which the testis lies outside the usual pathway of descent.

Perineal ectopic testis – An ectopic testis that has descended into an abnormal position between the penoscrotal raphe and the genitofemoral fold.

Retractile testis – The tendency of a descended testis to ascend to the upper part of the scrotum or into the inguinal canal.

Checklist

1. Identify condition:
   - ☐ Abdominal testis
     - ☐ inguinal
     - ☐ intraabdominal
   - ☐ Ectopic perineal testis
   - ☐ Ectopic testis
   - ☐ High scrotal
   - ☐ Retractile testis
   - ☐ Unspecified undescended testicle
2. Specify laterality:
   - ☐ Bilateral
   - ☐ Unilateral
   - ☐ Unspecified

Note: Laterality is not required for retractile testis.

Documentation Guidelines for Evaluation and Management (E/M) Services

I. Introduction

What is documentation and why is it important?

Medical record documentation is required to record pertinent facts, findings, and observations about an individual's health history including past and present illnesses, examinations, tests, treatments, and outcomes. The medical record chronologically documents the care of the patient and is an important element contributing to high-quality care. The medical record facilitates:

- the ability of the physician and other health care professionals to evaluate and plan the patient's immediate treatment, and to monitor his/her health care over time;
- communication and continuity of care among physicians and other health care professionals involved in the patient's care;
- accurate and timely claims review and payment;
- appropriate utilization review and quality of care evaluations; and
- collection of data that may be useful for research and education.

An appropriately documented medical record can reduce many of the "hassles" associated with claims processing and may serve as a legal document to verify the care provided, if necessary.

What do payers want and why?

Because payers have a contractual obligation to enrollees, they may require reasonable documentation that services are consistent with the insurance coverage provided. They may request information to validate:

- the site of service;
- the medical necessity and appropriateness of the diagnostic and/or therapeutic services provided; and/or
- that services provided have been accurately reported.

II. General Principles of Medical Record Documentation

The principles of documentation listed below are applicable to all types of medical and surgical services in all settings. For Evaluation and Management (E/M) services, the nature and amount of physician work and documentation varies by type of service, place of service and the patient's status. The general principles listed below may be modified to account for these variable circumstances in providing E/M services.

1. The medical record should be complete and legible.
2. The documentation of each patient encounter should include:
    - reason for the encounter and relevant history, physical examination findings and prior diagnostic test results;
    - assessment, clinical impression or diagnosis;
    - plan for care; and
    - date and legible identity of the observer.
3. If not documented, the rationale for ordering diagnostic and other ancillary services should be easily inferred.
4. Past and present diagnoses should be accessible to the treating and/or consulting physician.
5. Appropriate health risk factors should be identified.
6. The patient's progress, response to and changes in treatment, and revision of diagnosis should be documented.
7. The CPT® and ICD-10-CM codes reported on the health insurance claim form or billing statement should be supported by the documentation in the medical record.

III. Documentation of E/M Services

This publication provides definitions and documentation guidelines for the three *key* components of E/M services and for visits which consist predominately of counseling or coordination of care. The three key components — history, examination, and medical decision-making — appear in the descriptors for many outpatient services, hospital observation services, hospital inpatient services, consultations, emergency department services, nursing facility services, domiciliary care services and home services. Note: Starting Jan. 1, 2021, the guidelines for E/M office visit codes 99202-99215 will be based on medical decision-making or time. The guidelines in this Appendix pertain to the remainder of the E/M code set, excluding 99202-99215. While some of the text of CPT® has been repeated in this publication, the reader should refer to CPT® for the complete descriptors for E/M services and instructions for selecting a level of service.

Documentation Guidelines are identified by the symbol • *DG*.

The descriptors for the levels of E/M services recognize seven components which are used in defining the levels of E/M services. These components are:

- history;
- examination;
- medical decision-making;
- counseling;
- coordination of care;
- nature of presenting problem; and
- time.

The first three of these components (i.e., history, examination and medical decision-making) are the key components in selecting the level of E/M services. In the case of visits which consist predominantly of counseling or coordination of care, time is the key or controlling factor to qualify for a particular level of E/M service.

Because the level of E/M service is dependent on two or three *key* components, performance and documentation of one component (e.g., examination) at the highest level does not necessarily mean that the encounter in its entirety qualifies for the highest level of E/M service.

These documentation guidelines for E/M services reflect the needs of the typical adult population. For certain groups of patients, the recorded information may vary slightly from that described here. Specifically, the medical records of infants, children, adolescents and pregnant women may have additional or modified information recorded in each history and examination area.

As an example, newborn records may include under history of the present illness (HPI) the details of mother's pregnancy and the infant's status at birth; social history will focus on family structure; family history will focus on congenital anomalies and hereditary disorders in the family. In addition, the content of a pediatric examination will vary with the age and development of the child. Although not specifically defined in these documentation guidelines, these patient group variations on history and examination are appropriate.

A. Documentation of History

The levels of E/M services are based on four types of history (Problem Focused, Expanded Problem Focused, Detailed and Comprehensive). Each type of history includes some or all of the following elements:

- Chief complaint (CC);
- History of present illness (HPI);
- Review of systems (ROS); and
- Past, family and/or social history (PFSH).

The extent of history of present illness, review of systems and past, family and/or social history that is obtained and documented is dependent upon clinical judgment and the nature of the presenting problem(s).

The chart below shows the progression of the elements required for each type of history. To qualify for a given type of history all three elements in the table must be met. (A chief complaint is indicated at all levels.)

History of Present Illness (HPI)	Review of Systems (ROS)	Past, Family, and/or Social History (PFSH)	Type of History
Brief	N/A	N/A	Problem Focused
Brief	Problem Pertinent	Problem Pertinent	Expanded Problem Focused
Extended	Extended	Pertinent	Detailed
Extended	Complete	Complete	Comprehensive

• *DG: The CC, ROS and PFSH may be listed as separate elements of history, or they may be included in the description of the history of the present illness.*

• *DG: A ROS and/or a PFSH obtained during an earlier encounter does not need to be re-recorded if there is evidence that the physician reviewed and updated the previous information. This may occur when a physician updates his or her own record or in an institutional setting or group practice where many physicians use a common record. The review and update may be documented by:*

- *describing any new ROS and/or PFSH information or noting there has been no change in the information; and*
- *noting the date and location of the earlier ROS and/or PFSH.*

• *DG: The ROS and/or PFSH may be recorded by ancillary staff or on a form completed by the patient. To document that the physician reviewed the information, there must be a notation supplementing or confirming the information recorded by others.*

• *DG: If the physician is unable to obtain a history from the patient or other source, the record should describe the patient's condition or other circumstance which precludes obtaining a history.*

Definitions and specific documentation guidelines for each of the elements of history are listed below.

Chief Complaint (CC)

The CC is a concise statement describing the symptom, problem, condition, diagnosis, physician recommended return, or other factor that is the reason for the encounter, usually stated in the patient's words.

• *DG: The medical record should clearly reflect the chief complaint.*

History of Present Illness (HPI)

The HPI is a chronological description of the development of the patient's present illness from the first sign and/or symptom or from the previous encounter to the present. It includes the following elements:

- location,
- quality,
- severity,
- duration,
- timing,
- context,
- modifying factors, and
- associated signs and symptoms.

Brief and ***extended*** HPIs are distinguished by the amount of detail needed to accurately characterize the clinical problem(s).

A brief HPI consists of one to three elements of the HPI.

• *DG: The medical record should describe one to three elements of the present illness (HPI).*

An ***extended*** HPI consists of at least four elements of the HPI or the status of at least three chronic or inactive conditions.

• *DG: The medical record should describe at least four elements of the present illness (HPI), or the status of at least three chronic or inactive conditions.*

Review of Systems (ROS)

A ROS is an inventory of body systems obtained through a series of questions seeking to identify signs and/or symptoms which the patient may be experiencing or has experienced.

For purposes of ROS, the following systems are recognized:

- Constitutional symptoms (e.g., fever, weight loss)
- Eyes
- Ears, Nose, Mouth, Throat
- Cardiovascular
- Respiratory
- Gastrointestinal
- Genitourinary
- Musculoskeletal
- Integumentary (skin and/or breast)
- Neurological
- Psychiatric
- Endocrine
- Hematologic/Lymphatic
- Allergic/Immunologic

A ***problem*** pertinent ROS inquires about the system directly related to the problem(s) identified in the HPI.

• *DG: The patient's positive responses and pertinent negatives for the system related to the problem should be documented.*

An ***extended*** ROS inquires about the system directly related to the problem(s) identified in the HPI and a

limited number of additional systems.

• *DG: The patient's positive responses and pertinent negatives for two to nine systems should be documented.*

A ***complete*** ROS inquires about the system(s) directly related to the problem(s) identified in the HPI plus all additional body systems.

• *DG: At least 10 organ systems must be reviewed. Those systems with positive or pertinent negative responses must be individually documented. For the remaining systems, a notation indicating all other systems are negative is permissible. In the absence of such a notation, at least 10 systems must be individually documented.*

Past, Family and/or Social History (PFSH)

The PFSH consists of a review of three areas: past history (the patient's past experiences with illnesses, operations, injuries and treatments); family history (a review of medical events in the patient's family, including diseases which may be hereditary or place the patient at risk); and social history (an age-appropriate review of past and current activities).

For certain categories of E/M services that include only an interval history, it is not necessary to record information about the PFSH. Those categories are subsequent hospital care, follow-up inpatient consultations and subsequent nursing facility care.

A ***pertinent*** PFSH is a review of the history area(s) directly related to the problem(s) identified in the HPI.

• *DG: At least one specific item from any of the three history areas must be documented for a pertinent PFSH.*

A ***complete*** PFSH is of a review of two or all three of the PFSH history areas, depending on the category of the E/M service. A review of all three history areas is required for services that by their nature include a comprehensive assessment or reassessment of the patient. A review of two of the three history areas is sufficient for other services.

• *DG: At least one specific item from two of the three history areas must be documented for a complete PFSH for the following categories of E/M services: office or other outpatient services, established patient; emergency department; domiciliary care, established patient; and home care, established patient.*

• *DG: At least one specific item from each of the three history areas must be documented for a complete PFSH for the following categories of E/M services: office or other outpatient services, new patient; hospital observation services; hospital inpatient services, initial care; consultations; comprehensive nursing facility assessments; domiciliary care, new patient; and home care, new patient.*

B. Documentation of Examination

The levels of E/M services are based on four types of examination:

- ***Problem Focused*** — a limited examination of the affected body area or organ system.
- ***Expanded Problem Focused*** — a limited examination of the affected body area or organ system and any other symptomatic or related body area(s) or organ system(s).

- *Detailed* — an extended examination of the affected body area(s) or organ system(s) and any other symptomatic or related body area(s) or organ system(s).
- *Comprehensive* — a general multi-system examination, or complete examination of a single organ system and other symptomatic or related body area(s) or organ system(s).

These types of examinations have been defined for general multi-system and the following single organ systems:

- Cardiovascular
- Ears, Nose, Mouth and Throat
- Eyes
- Genitourinary (Female)
- Genitourinary (Male)
- Hematologic/Lymphatic/Immunologic
- Musculoskeletal
- Neurological
- Psychiatric
- Respiratory
- Skin

A general multi-system examination or a single organ system examination may be performed by any physician regardless of specialty. The type (general multi-system or single organ system) and content of examination are selected by the examining physician and are based upon clinical judgment, the patient's history, and the nature of the presenting problem(s).

The content and documentation requirements for each type and level of examination are summarized below and described in detail in tables. In the tables, organ systems and body areas recognized by CPT® for purposes of describing examinations are shown in the left column. The content, or individual elements, of the examination pertaining to that body area or organ system are identified by bullets (•) in the right column.

Parenthetical examples, "(e.g., ...)", have been used for clarification and to provide guidance regarding documentation. Documentation for each element must satisfy any numeric requirements (such as "Measurement of any three of the following seven ... ") included in the description of the element. Elements with multiple components but with no specific numeric requirement (such as "Examination of liver and spleen") require documentation of at least one component. It is possible for a given examination to be expanded beyond what is defined here. When that occurs, findings related to the additional systems and/or areas should be documented.

• *DG: Specific abnormal and relevant negative findings of the examination of the affected or symptomatic body area(s) or organ system(s) should be documented. A notation of "abnormal" without elaboration is insufficient.*

• *DG: Abnormal or unexpected findings of the examination of any asymptomatic body area(s) or organ system(s) should be described.*

• *DG: A brief statement or notation indicating "negative" or "normal" is sufficient to document normal findings related to unaffected area(s) or asymptomatic organ system(s).*

General Multi-System Examinations

General multi-system examinations are described in detail below. To qualify for a given level of multi-system examination, the following content and documentation requirements should be met:

- *Problem Focused Examination* — should include performance and documentation of one to five elements identified by a bullet (•) in one or more organ system(s) or body area(s).
- *Expanded Problem Focused Examination* — should include performance and documentation of at least six elements identified by a bullet (•) in one or more organ system(s) or body area(s).
- *Detailed Examination* — should include at least six organ systems or body areas. For each system/area selected, performance and documentation of at least two elements identified by a bullet (•) is expected. Alternatively, a detailed examination may include performance and documentation of at least 12 elements identified by a bullet (•) in two or more organ systems or body areas.
- *Comprehensive Examination* — should include at least nine organ systems or body areas. For each system/area selected, all elements of the examination identified by a bullet (•) should be performed, unless specific directions limit the content of the examination. For each area/system, documentation of at least two elements identified by a bullet is expected.

Single Organ System Examinations

The single organ system examinations recognized by CPT® are described in detail previously. Variations among these examinations in the organ systems and body areas identified in the left columns and in the elements of the examinations described in the right columns reflect differing emphases among specialties. To qualify for a given level of single organ system examination, the following content and documentation requirements should be met:

- *Problem Focused Examination* — should include performance and documentation of one to five elements identified by a bullet (•), whether in a box with a shaded or unshaded border.
- *Expanded Problem Focused Examination* — should include performance and documentation of at least six elements identified by a bullet (•), whether in a box with a shaded or unshaded border.
- *Detailed Examination* — examinations other than the eye and psychiatric examinations should include performance and documentation of at least 12 elements identified by a bullet (•), whether in box with a shaded or unshaded border.

Eye and psychiatric examinations should include the performance and documentation of at least nine elements identified by a bullet (•), whether in a box with a shaded or unshaded border.

- *Comprehensive Examination* — should include performance of all elements identified by a bullet (•), whether in a shaded or unshaded box. Documentation of every element in each box with a shaded border and at least one element in each box with an unshaded border is expected.

General Multi-System Examination

System/Body Area	Elements of Examination
Constitutional	Measurement of **any three of the following seven** vital signs: 1) sitting or standing blood pressure, 2) supine blood pressure, 3) pulse rate and regularity, 4) respiration, 5) temperature, 6) height, 7) weight (May be measured and recorded by ancillary staff) General appearance of patient (e.g., development, nutrition, body habitus, deformities, attention to grooming)
Eyes	Inspection of conjunctivae and lids Examination of pupils and irises (e.g., reaction to light and accommodation, size and symmetry) Ophthalmoscopic examination of optic discs (e.g., size, C/D ratio, appearance) and posterior segments (e.g., vessel changes, exudates, hemorrhages)
Ears, Nose, Mouth, and Throat	External inspection of ears and nose (e.g., overall appearance, scars, lesions, masses) Otoscopic examination of external auditory canals and tympanic membranes Assessment of hearing (e.g., whispered voice, finger rub, tuning fork) Inspection of nasal mucosa, septum and turbinates Inspection of lips, teeth and gums Examination of oropharynx: oral mucosa, salivary glands, hard and soft palates, tongue, tonsils and posterior pharynx
Neck	Examination of neck (e.g., masses, overall appearance, symmetry, tracheal position, crepitus Examination of thyroid (e.g., enlargement, tenderness, mass)
Respiratory	Assessment of respiratory effort (e.g., intercostal retractions, use of accessory muscles, diaphragmatic movement) Percussion of chest (e.g., dullness, flatness, hyperresonance) Palpation of chest (e.g., tactile fremitus) Auscultation of lungs (e.g., breath sounds, adventitious sounds, rubs)
Cardiovascular	Palpation of heart (e.g., location, size, thrills) Auscultation of heart with notation of abnormal sounds and murmurs Examination of: Carotid arteries (e.g., pulse amplitude, bruits) Abdominal aorta (e.g., size, bruits) Femoral arteries (e.g., pulse amplitude, bruits) Pedal pulses (e.g., pulse amplitude) Extremities for edema and/or varicosities
Chest (Breasts)	Inspection of breasts (e.g., symmetry, nipple discharge) Palpation of breasts and axillae (e.g., masses or lumps, tenderness)
Gastrointestinal (Abdomen)	Examination of abdomen with notation of presence of masses or tenderness Examination of liver and spleen Examination for presence or absence of hernia Examination (when indicated) of anus, perineum and rectum, including sphincter tone, presence of hemorrhoids, rectal masses Obtain stool sample for occult blood test when indicated
Genitourinary	Male: Examination of the scrotal contents (e.g., hydrocele, spermatocele, tenderness of cord, testicular mass) Examination of the penis Digital rectal examination of prostate gland (e.g., size, symmetry, nodularity, tenderness) Female: Pelvic examination (with or without specimen collection for smears and cultures), including: Examination of external genitalia (e.g., general appearance, hair distribution, lesions) and vagina (e.g., general appearance, estrogen effect, discharge, lesions, pelvic support, cystocele, rectocele) Examination of urethra (e.g., masses, tenderness, scarring) Examination of bladder (e.g., fullness, masses, tenderness) Cervix (e.g., general appearance, lesions, discharge) Uterus (e.g., size, contour, position, mobility, tenderness, consistency, descent or support) Adnexa/parametria (e.g., masses, tenderness, organomegaly, nodularity)
Lymphatic	Palpation of lymph nodes in **two or more** areas: Neck Axillae Groin Other

System/Body Area	Elements of Examination
Musculoskeletal	Examination of gait and station Inspection and/or palpation of digits and nails (e.g., clubbing, cyanosis, inflammatory conditions, petechiae, ischemia, infections, nodes) Examination of joints, bones and muscles of **one or more of the following six** areas: 1) head and neck; 2) spine, ribs and pelvis; 3) right upper extremity; 4) left upper extremity; 5) right lower extremity; and 6) left lower extremity. The examination of a given area includes: Inspection and/or palpation with notation of presence of any misalignment, asymmetry, crepitation, defects, tenderness, masses, effusions Assessment of range of motion with notation of any pain, crepitation or contracture Assessment of stability with notation of any dislocation (luxation), subluxation or laxity Assessment of muscle strength and tone (e.g., flaccid, cog wheel, spastic) with notation of any atrophy or abnormal movements
Skin	Inspection of skin and subcutaneous tissue (e.g., rashes, lesions, ulcers) Palpation of skin and subcutaneous tissue (e.g., induration, subcutaneous nodules, tightening)
Neurologic	Test cranial nerves with notation of any deficits Examination of deep tendon reflexes with notation of pathological reflexes (e.g., Babinski) Examination of sensation (e.g., by touch, pin, vibration, proprioception)
Psychiatric	Description of patient's judgment and insight Brief assessment of mental status including: Orientation to time, place and person Recent and remote memory Mood and affect (e.g., depression, anxiety, agitation)

General Multi-System Examination Content and Documentation Requirements

Level of Exam	Perform and Document
Problem Focused	**One to five** elements identified by a bullet
Expanded Problem Focused	**At least six** elements identified by a bullet
Detailed	**At least two** elements identified by a bullet **from each of six areas/systems** OR **at least 12** elements identified by a bullet **in two or more areas/systems.**
Comprehensive	Perform **all elements** identified by a bullet in **at least nine** organ systems or body areas and document **at least two** elements identified by a bullet **from each of nine areas/systems.**

Cardiovascular Examination

System/Body Area	Elements of Examination
Constitutional	Measurement of **any three of the following seven** vital signs: 1) sitting or standing blood pressure, 2) supine blood pressure, 3) pulse rate and regularity, 4) respiration, 5) temperature, 6) height, 7) weight (May be measured and recorded by ancillary staff) General appearance of patient (e.g., development, nutrition, body habitus, deformities, attention to grooming)
Eyes	Inspection of conjunctivae and lids (e.g., xanthelasma)
Ears, Nose, Mouth, and Throat	Inspection of teeth, gums and palate Inspection of oral mucosa with notation of presence of pallor or cyanosis
Neck	Examination of jugular veins (e.g., distension; a, v or cannon a waves) Examination of thyroid (e.g., enlargement, tenderness, mass)
Respiratory	Assessment of respiratory effort (e.g., intercostal retractions, use of accessory muscles, diaphragmatic movement) Auscultation of lungs (e.g., breath sounds, adventitious sounds, rubs)
Cardiovascular	Palpation of heart (e.g., location, size and forcefulness of the point of maximal impact; thrills; lifts; palpable S3 or S4) Auscultation of heart including sounds, abnormal sounds and murmurs Measurement of blood pressure in two or more extremities when indicated (e.g., aortic dissection, coarctation) Examination of: Carotid arteries (e.g., waveform, pulse amplitude, bruits, apical-carotid delay) Abdominal aorta (e.g., size, bruits) Femoral arteries (e.g., pulse amplitude, bruits) Pedal pulses (e.g., pulse amplitude) Extremities for peripheral edema and/or varicosities
Gastrointestinal (Abdomen)	Examination of abdomen with notation of presence of masses or tenderness Examination of liver and spleen Obtain stool sample for occult blood from patients who are being considered for thrombolytic or anticoagulant therapy
Musculoskeletal	Examination of the back with notation of kyphosis or scoliosis Examination of gait with notation of ability to undergo exercise testing and/or participation in exercise programs Assessment of muscle strength and tone (e.g., flaccid, cog wheel, spastic) with notation of any atrophy and abnormal movements
Extremities	Inspection and palpation of digits and nails (e.g., clubbing, cyanosis, inflammation, petechiae, ischemia, infections, Osler's nodes)

System/Body Area	Elements of Examination
Skin	Inspection and/or palpation of skin and subcutaneous tissue (e.g., stasis dermatitis, ulcers, scars, xanthomas)
Neurological/ Psychiatric	Brief assessment of mental status including: Orientation to time, place and person, Mood and affect (e.g., depression, anxiety, agitation)

Cardiovascular Examination Content and Documentation Requirements

Level of Exam	Perform and Document
Problem Focused	**One to five** elements identified by a bullet
Expanded Problem Focused	**At least six** elements identified by a bullet
Detailed	**At least 12** elements identified by a bullet
Comprehensive	Perform all elements identified by a bullet; document every element in each box with a shaded border and at least one element in each box with an unshaded border.

C. Documentation of the Complexity of Medical Decision-Making

The levels of E/M services recognize four types of medical decision-making (Straightforward, Low Complexity, Moderate Complexity and High Complexity). Medical decision-making refers to the complexity of establishing a diagnosis and/or selecting a management option as measured by:

- the number of possible diagnoses and/or the number of management options that must be considered;
- the amount and/or complexity of medical records, diagnostic tests, and/or other information that must be obtained, reviewed and analyzed; and
- the risk of significant complications, morbidity and/or mortality, as well as comorbidities associated with the patient's presenting problem(s), the diagnostic procedure(s) and/or the possible management options.

The chart below shows the progression of the elements required for each level of medical decision-making. To qualify for a given type of decision-making, two of the three elements in the table must be either met or exceeded.

Number of diagnoses or management options	Amount and/or complexity of data	Risk of complications and/or morbidity or mortality	Type of decision-making
Minimal	Minimal or None	Minimal	**Straightforward**
Limited	Limited	Low	**Low Complexity**
Multiple	Moderate	Moderate	**Moderate Complexity**
Extensive	Extensive	High	**High Complexity**

The following is a description of elements of medical decision-making.

Number of Diagnoses of Management Options

The number of possible diagnoses and/or the number of management options that must be considered is based on the number and types of problems addressed during the encounter, the complexity of establishing a diagnosis and the management decisions that are made by the physician.

Generally, decision-making with respect to a diagnosed problem is easier than that for an identified but undiagnosed problem. The number and type of diagnostic tests employed may be an indicator of the number of possible diagnoses. Problems which are improving or resolving are less complex than those which are worsening or failing to change as expected. The need to seek advice from others is another indicator of complexity of diagnostic or management problems.

• *DG: For each encounter, an assessment, clinical impression, or diagnosis should be documented. It may be explicitly stated or implied in documented decisions regarding management plans and/or further evaluation.*

- For a presenting problem with an established diagnosis the record should reflect whether the problem is: a) improved, well controlled, resolving or resolved; or, b) inadequately controlled, worsening, or failing to change as expected.
- For a presenting problem without an established diagnosis, the assessment or clinical impression may be stated in the form of differential diagnoses or as a "possible," "probable," or "rule out" (R/O) diagnosis.

• *DG: The initiation of, or changes in, treatment should be documented. Treatment includes a wide range of management options including patient instructions, nursing instructions, therapies, and medications.*

• *DG: If referrals are made, consultations requested or advice sought, the record should indicate to whom or where the referral or consultation is made or from whom the advice is requested.*

Amount and/or Complexity of Data to be Reviewed

The amount and complexity of data to be reviewed is based on the types of diagnostic testing ordered or reviewed. A decision to obtain and review old medical records and/or obtain history from sources other than the patient increases the amount and complexity of data to be reviewed.

Discussion of contradictory or unexpected test results with the physician who performed or interpreted the test is an indication of the complexity of data being reviewed. On occasion the physician who ordered a test may personally review the image, tracing or specimen to supplement information from the physician who prepared the test report or interpretation; this is another indication of the complexity of data being reviewed.

A clinician who ordered a diagnostic test, performed the interpretation and billed for the test may not count it toward the MDM data amount/complexity of the E/M service.

Tests that do not require clinician interpretation (such as clinical lab tests, which are results only), may be counted toward tests ordered or reviewed during an E/M service.

• *DG: If a diagnostic service (test or procedure) is ordered, planned, scheduled, or performed at the time of the E/M encounter, the type of service, e.g., lab or X-ray, should be documented.*

• *DG: The review of lab, radiology and/or other diagnostic tests should be documented. A simple notation such as "WB elevated" or "chest X-ray unremarkable" is acceptable. Alternatively, the review may be documented by initialing and dating the report containing the test results.*

• *DG: A decision to obtain old records or decision to obtain additional history from the family, caretaker or other source to supplement that obtained from the patient should be documented.*

• *DG: Relevant findings from the review of old records, and/or the receipt of additional history from the family, caretaker or other source to supplement that obtained from the patient should be documented. If there is no relevant information beyond that already obtained, that fact should be documented. A notation of "old records reviewed" or "additional history obtained from family" without elaboration is insufficient.*

• *DG: The results of discussion of laboratory, radiology or other diagnostic tests with the physician who performed or interpreted the study should be documented.*

• *DG: The direct visualization and independent interpretation of an image, tracing or specimen previously or subsequently interpreted by another physician should be documented.*

Risk of Significant Complications, Morbidity and/or Mortality

The risk of significant complications, morbidity and/or mortality is based on the risks associated with the presenting problem(s), the diagnostic procedure(s) and the possible management options.

• *DG: Comorbidities/underlying diseases or other factors that increase the complexity of medical decision-making by increasing the risk of complications, morbidity, and/or mortality should be documented.*

• *DG: If a surgical or invasive diagnostic procedure is ordered, planned or scheduled at the time of the E/M encounter, the type of procedure, e.g., laparoscopy, should be documented.*

• *DG: If a surgical or invasive diagnostic procedure is performed at the time of the E/M encounter, the specific procedure should be documented.*

• *DG: The referral for or decision to perform a surgical or invasive diagnostic procedure on an urgent basis should be documented or implied.*

The following table may be used to help determine whether the risk of significant complications, morbidity and/or mortality is minimal, low, moderate or high. Because the determination of risk is complex and not readily quantifiable, the table includes common clinical examples rather than absolute measures of risk. The assessment of risk of the presenting problem(s) is based on the risk related to the disease process anticipated between the present encounter and the next one. The assessment of risk of selecting diagnostic procedures and management options is based on the risk during and immediately following any procedures or treatment. **The highest level of risk in any one category (presenting problem(s), diagnostic procedure(s) or management options) determines the overall risk.**

D. Documentation of an Encounter Dominated by Counseling or Coordination of Care

In the case where counseling and/or coordination of care dominates (more than 50%) of the physician/patient and/or family encounter (face-to-face time in the office or other or outpatient setting, floor/unit time in the hospital or nursing facility), time is considered the key or controlling factor to qualify for a particular level of E/M services.

• *DG: If the physician elects to report the level of service based on counseling and/or coordination of care, the total length of time of the encounter (face-to-face or floor time, as appropriate) should be documented and the record should describe the counseling and/or activities to coordinate care.*

Table of Risk

Level of Risk	Presenting Problem(s)	Diagnostic Procedure(s) Ordered	Management Options Selected
Minimal	One self-limited or minor problem, e.g., cold, insect bite, tinea corporis	Laboratory tests requiring venipuncture Chest X-rays EKG/EEG Urinalysis Ultrasound, e.g., echocardiography KOH prep	Rest Gargles Elastic bandages Superficial dressings
Low	Two or more self-limited or minor problems One stable chronic illness, e.g., well controlled hypertension, non-insulin dependent diabetes, cataract, BPH Acute uncomplicated illness or injury, e.g., cystitis, allergic rhinitis, simple sprain	Physiologic tests not under stress, e.g., pulmonary function test Non-cardiovascular imaging studies with contrast, e.g., barium enema Superficial needle biopsies Clinical laboratory tests requiring arterial puncture Skin biopsies	Over-the-counter drugs Minor surgery with no identified risk factors Physical therapy Occupational therapy IV fluids without additives
Moderate	One or more chronic illnesses with mild exacerbation, progression, or side effects of treatment Two or more stable chronic illnesses Undiagnosed new problem with uncertain prognosis, e.g., lump in breast Acute illness with systemic symptoms, e.g., pyelonephritis, pneumonitis, colitis Acute complicated injury, e.g., head injury with brief loss of consciousness	Physiologic tests under stress, e.g., cardio stress test, fetal contraction stress test Diagnostic endoscopies with no identified risk factors Deep needle or incisional biopsy Cardiovascular imaging studies with contrast and no identified risk factors, e.g., arteriogram, cardiac catheterization Obtain fluid from body cavity, e.g. lumbar puncture, thoracentesis, culdocentesis	Minor surgery with identified risk factors Elective major surgery (open, percutaneous or endoscopic) with no identified risk factors Prescription drug management Therapeutic nuclear medicine IV fluids with additives Closed treatment of fracture or dislocation without manipulation
High	One or more chronic illnesses with severe exacerbation, progression, or side effects of treatment Acute or chronic illnesses or injuries that pose a threat to life or bodily function, e.g., multiple trauma, acute MI, pulmonary embolus, severe respiratory distress, progressive severe rheumatoid arthritis, psychiatric illness with potential threat to self or others, peritonitis, acute renal failure An abrupt change in neurologic status, e.g., seizure, TIA, weakness, sensory loss	Cardiovascular imaging studies with contrast with identified risk factors Cardiac electrophysiological tests Diagnostic endoscopies with identified risk factors Discography	Elective major surgery (open, percutaneous or endoscopic) with identified risk factors Emergency major surgery (open, percutaneous or endoscopic) Parenteral controlled substances Drug therapy requiring intensive monitoring for toxicity Decision not to resuscitate or to deescalate care because of poor prognosis